OTHER PMIC TITLES OF INTEREST

CODING AND REIMBURSEMENT TITLES

Collections Made Easy!
CPT Coders Choice®, Thumb Indexed
CPT & HCPCS Coding Made Easy!
CPT Easy Links
CPT Plus!
DRG Plus!
E/M Coding Made Easy!
Getting Paid for What You Do
HCPCS Coders Choice®, Color Coded, Thumb Indexed
Health Insurance Carrier Directory
HIPAA Compliance Manual
ICD-9-CM, Coders Choice®, Thumb Indexed
ICD-9-CM Coding for Physicians' Offices
ICD-9-CM Coding Made Easy!
ICD-9-CM, Home Health Edition
Medical Fees in the United States
Medicare Compliance Manual
Medicare Rules & Regulations
Physicians Fee Guide
Reimbursement Manual for the Medical Office

PRACTICE MANAGEMENT TITLES

Accounts Receivable Management for the Medical Practice
Achieving Profitability With a Medical Office System
Encyclopedia of Practice and Financial Management
Managed Care Organizations
Managing Medical Office Personnel
Marketing Strategies for Physicians
Medical Marketing Handbook
Medical Office Policy Manual
Medical Practice Forms
Medical Practice Handbook
Medical Staff Privileges
Negotiating Managed Care Contracts
Patient Satisfaction
Performance Standards for the Laboratory
Professional and Practice Development
Promoting Your Medical Practice
Starting in Medical Practice
Working With Insurance and Managed Care Plans

**AVAILABLE FROM YOUR LOCAL MEDICAL
BOOK STORE OR CALL 1-800-MED-SHOP**

OTHER PMIC TITLES OF INTEREST

RISK MANAGEMENT TITLES
Malpractice Depositions
Medical Risk Management
Preparing for Your Deposition
Preventing Emergency Malpractice
Testifying in Court

FINANCIAL MANAGEMENT TITLES
A Physician's Guide to Financial Independence
Business Ventures for Physicians
Financial Valuation of Your Practice
Personal Money Management for Physicians
Personal Pension Plan Strategies for Physicians
Securing Your Assets

DICTIONARIES AND OTHER REFERENCE TITLES
Drugs of Abuse
Health and Medicine on the Internet
Medical Acronyms and Abbreviations
Medical Phrase Index
Medical Word Building
Medico Mnemonica
Medico-Legal Glossary
Spanish/English Handbook for Medical Professionals

MEDICAL REFERENCE AND CLINICAL TITLES
Advance Medical Directives
Clinical Research Opportunities
Gastroenterology: Problems in Primary Care
Manual of IV Therapy
Medical Care of the Adolescent Athlete
Medical Procedures for Referral
Neurology: Problems in Primary Care
Orthopaedics: Problems in Primary Care
Patient Care Emergency Handbook
Patient Care Flowchart Manual
Patient Care Procedures for Your Practice
Physician's Office Laboratory
Pulmonary Medicine: Problems in Primary Care
Questions and Answers on AIDS

**AVAILABLE FROM YOUR LOCAL MEDICAL
BOOK STORE OR CALL 1-800-MED-SHOP**

ICD·9·CM

International Classification of Diseases
9th Revision

Clinical Modification
Sixth Edition

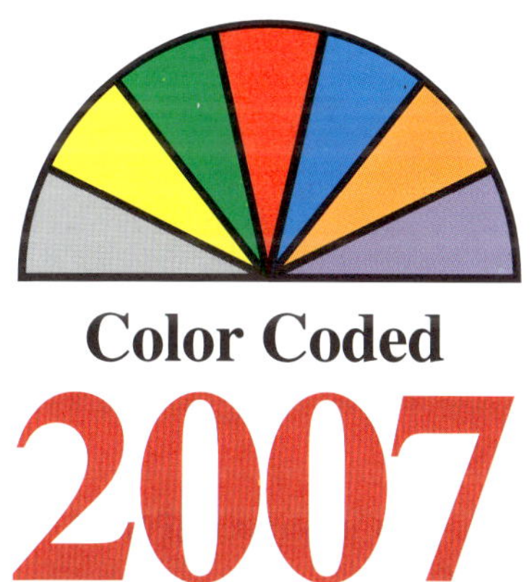

Color Coded
2007

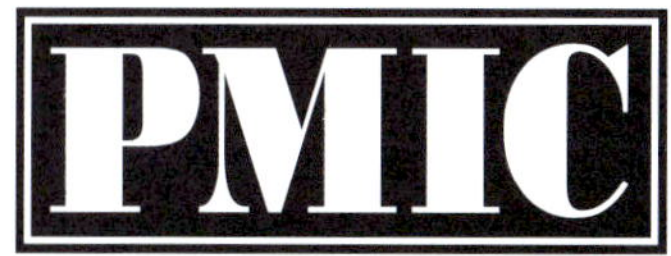

Volumes 1 & 2

ISBN 1-57066-408-0 (Soft cover)
ISBN 1-57066-410-2 (Spiral)

Volumes 1, 2, & 3

ISBN 1-57066-411-0 (Soft cover)
ISBN 1-57066-413-7 (Spiral)
ISBN 1-57066-421-8 (Home Health Edition)

Non-indexed versions

ISBN 1-57066-409-9 (Volumes 1 & 2)
ISBN 1-57066-412-9 (Volumes 1, 2, & 3)

Practice Management Information Corporation [PMIC]
4727 Wilshire Boulevard, Suite 300
Los Angeles, California 90010
1-800-MED-SHOP
http://www.pmiconline.com

Printed in China

Preface

Health care professionals have long used coding systems to describe procedures, services, and supplies. However, most described the reason for the procedure, service or supply with a diagnostic statement. Of those health care professionals who do code the diagnosis, either due to a requirement for a computer billing system and/or electronic claims filing, many do not code completely or accurately. With the passage of the Medicare Catastrophic Coverage Act of 1988, diagnostic coding using *ICD-9-CM* became mandatory for Medicare claims. In the area of health care reimbursement rules and regulations, the typical progression is that changes required for Medicare are followed shortly by similar changes for Medicaid and private insurance carriers.

To some professionals, the requirement to use diagnostic coding may have seemed like a burden or simply another excuse for Medicare intermediaries to delay or deny payment. However, it is important to understand that the proper use of coding systems for both procedures and diagnoses gives the professional absolute control over his or her billing and reimbursement. Accurate diagnosis coding is not easy. It requires a good working knowledge of medical terminology and a fundamental understanding of *ICD-9-CM*. In addition, the coder must know the rules and regulations required to comply with Medicare requirements for coding.

This edition of the *International Classification of Diseases, 9th Revision, Clinical Modification (ICD-9-CM)* is published by Practice Management Information Corporation in recognition of its responsibility to promulgate this classification throughout the United States for morbidity coding and billing purposes. *The International Classification of Diseases, 9th Revision*, originally published by the World Health Organization (WHO) is the foundation of the *ICD-9-CM* and continues to be the classification employed in cause-of-death coding in the United States.

The *ICD-9-CM* is recommended for use in all clinical settings, but is required for reporting diagnoses and diseases to all U.S. Public Health Service and Department of Health and Human Services programs, such as Medicare and Medicaid. This version faithfully follows and contains the same information found in the official U.S. government version of the *ICD-9-CM*.

All official authorized addenda effective October 1, 2006, have been included in this edition. A new revision will be available approximately September 15th of each year. Revised editions may be purchased from:

Practice Management Information Corporation
4727 Wilshire Boulevard, Suite 300
Los Angeles, California 90010
1-800-MED-SHOP

Or by contacting our web site at http://www.pmiconline.com.

Disclaimer

This publication includes all official ICD-9-CM codes, descriptions, annotations and guidelines as maintained by the U.S. Department of Health and Human Services with the exception that this publication includes special symbols to indicate additions and revisions from the previous edition and special symbols to facilitate identification of diagnostic codes that require 4th or 5th digit specificity, the use of color coding to alert the user to special coding considerations, and thumb indexing to make locating codes easier. This publication is revised annually so that we may present the most current information possible. Though all of the information is carefully researched and checked for accuracy and completeness, the publisher accepts no responsibility with regard to errors, omissions, misuse or misinterpretation.

Table of Contents

ICD-9-CM CODING FUNDAMENTALS 21

[1] These listings appear only in the three volume edition

Introduction to ICD-9-CM

ICD-9-CM is an acronym for *International Classification of Diseases, 9th Revision, Clinical Modification*, published under different names since 1900. *ICD-9-CM* is a statistical classification system that arranges diseases and injuries into groups according to established criteria. Most *ICD-9-CM* codes are numeric and consist of three, four or five numbers and a description. The codes are revised approximately every 10 years by the World Health Organization and annual updates are published by Center for Medicare and Medicaid Services (CMS).

HISTORICAL PERSPECTIVE

The *International Classification of Diseases, 9th Revision, Clinical Modification (ICD-9-CM)* is based on the official version of the *World Health Organization's (WHO) 9th Revision, International Classification of Diseases (ICD-9)*. *ICD-9* is designed for the classification of morbidity and mortality information for statistical purposes, and for the indexing of medical records by disease and operations, and for data storage and retrieval. *ICD-9-CM* replaced the Eighth Revision International Classification of Diseases, Adapted for Use in the United States commonly referred to as *ICDA*.

The concept of extending the International Classification of Diseases for use in hospital indexing was originally developed in response to a need for a more efficient basis for storage and retrieval of diagnostic data. In 1950, the U.S. Public Health Service and the Veterans Administration began independent tests of the International Classification of Diseases for hospital indexing purposes. In the following year, the Columbia Presbyterian Medical Center in New York City adopted the International Classification of Diseases, 6th Revision for use in its medical record department. A few years later, the Commission on Professional and Hospital Activities adopted the International Classification of Diseases for use in hospitals participating in the Professional Activity Study (PAS).

In view of the growing interest in the use of the International Classification of Diseases for hospital indexing, a study was undertaken in 1956 by the American Medical Association and the American Medical Record Association of the relative efficiencies of coding systems for diagnostic indexing. Following this study, the major uses of the International Classification of Diseases for hospital indexing purposes consolidated their experiences and an adaptation was published in December 1959. A revision containing the first "Classification of Operations and Treatments" was published in 1962.

In 1968, following a study by the American Hospital Association, the United States Public Health Service published the Eighth Revision International Classification of Diseases, Adapted for Use in the United States. This publication became commonly known as ICDA, and served as the basis for coding diagnostic data for official morbidity and mortality statistics in the United States.

ICD-9-CM Background

In February 1977, a committee was convened by the National Center for Health Statistics to provide advice and counsel for the development of clinical modification of the ICD-9. The organizations represented on the committee included:

> American Association of Health Data Systems
> American Hospital Association
> American Medical Record Association
> Association for Health Records
> Commission on Professional and Hospital Activities
> Council on Clinical Classifications, sponsored by:
>
> > American Academy of Pediatrics
> > American College of Obstetricians and Gynecologists
> > American College of Physicians
> > American College of Surgeons
> > American Psychiatric Association
>
> > Health Care Financing Administration
> > WHO Center for Classification of Diseases

The resulting *ICD-9-CM* is a clinical modification of the *World Health Organization's International Classification of Diseases, 9th Revision (ICD-9)*. The term "clinical" is used to emphasize the modifications intent; namely, to serve as a useful tool in the area of classification of morbidity data for indexing of medical records, medical care review, ambulatory and other medical care programs, as well as for basic health statistics.

In use since January 1979, *ICD-9-CM* provides a diagnostic coding system that is more precise than those needed only for statistical groupings and trend analysis. Official addenda (updates) to *ICD-9-CM* are issued in October each year by the National Center for Health Statistics (NCHS), part of the Centers for Disease Control (CDC).

Use of ICD-9-CM Codes for Professional Billing

Until passage of the Medicare Catastrophic Coverage Act of 1988, health care professionals were not required to report *ICD-9-CM* codes when billing government or private insurance carriers for reimbursement. The exception to this requirement was for those health care professionals who filed insurance claims electronically and those who used "code driven" computer billing services or computer systems.

Most health care professionals simply included the text or description of the injury, illness, sign or symptom that was the reason for the encounter. Insurance carriers who used *ICD-9-CM* coding had to code the diagnostic statements prior to input into their computer systems for reimbursement processing.

A specific requirement of the Medicare Catastrophic Coverage Act of 1988 required health care professionals to include *ICD-9-CM* codes on their Medicare claim forms effective April 1, 1989. A two-month grace period, to June 1, 1989, was allowed at the request of the American Medical Association, to allow health care professionals additional time to develop the knowledge and systems necessary to implement the requirement.

TERMINOLOGY

There are terms used throughout this publication that are important for a proper understanding of *ICD-9-CM*. The following terms are defined specifically as they are used for *ICD-9-CM* with the knowledge that some terms may have other definitions and meanings.

acute	refers to the condition that is the primary reason for the current encounter.
addenda	official updates to ICD-9-CM published continuously since 1986, that become effective on October 1st of each year.
adverse	any response to a drug that is noxious and unintended and occurs with proper dosage.
aftercare	an encounter for something planned in advance, for example, cast removal.
AHFS	American Hospital Formulary Service.
alphabetic index	the portion of ICD-9-CM that lists definitions and codes in alphabetic order. Also called Volume 2.
category	refers to diagnoses codes listed within a specific three-digit category, for example category 250, Diabetes Mellitus.
cause	that which brings about any condition or produces any effect.
chronic	continuing over a long period of time or recurring frequently.
coding	the process of transferring written or verbal descriptions of diseases, injuries and procedures into numerical designations.
combination	a code that combines a diagnosis with an associated secondary process or complication.
complication	the occurrence of two or more diseases in the same patient at the same time.
concurrent	when a patient is being treated by more than one provider for different care conditions at the same time.
conventions	refers to the use of certain abbreviations, punctuation, symbols, type faces, and other instructions that must be clearly understood in order to use ICD-9-CM.
CPT	Current Procedural Terminology. Listing of codes and descriptions for procedures, services and supplies published by the American Medical Association. Used to bill insurance carriers.
diagnosis	a written description of the reason(s) for the procedure, service, supply or encounter.
down coding	the process where insurance carriers reduce the value of a procedure, and the resulting reimbursement, due to either 1) a mismatch of CPT code and description or 2) ICD-9-CM code does not justify the procedure or level of service.
E codes	specific ICD-9-CM codes used to identify the cause of injury, poisoning and other adverse effects.
eponyms	medical procedures or conditions named after a person or a place.
etiology	the cause(s) or origin of a disease.

HCFA1500 — Uniform health insurance claim form used for billing services to Medicare and other insurance carriers.

hierarchy — a system that ranks items one above another.

ICD-9-CM — International Classification of Diseases, 9th Revision, Clinical Modification.

ICD-10 — International Classification of Diseases, 10th Revision

late effect — a residual effect (condition produced) after the acute phase of an illness or injury has ended.

main term — refers to listings in the Alphabetic Index appearing **BOLDFACE** type.

manifestation — characteristic signs or symptoms of an illness.

multiple — refers to the need to use more than one ICD-9-CM code to fully identify coding a condition.

primary code — the ICD-9-CM code that defines the main reason for the current encounter.

residual — the long-term condition(s) resulting from a previous acute illness or injury.

rule out — refers to a method used to indicate that a condition is probable, suspected, or questionable but unconfirmed. ICD-9-CM has no provisions for the use of this term.

secondary — code(s) listed after the primary code that further indicate the cause(s) code for the current encounter or define the need for higher levels of care.

sections — refers to portions of the Tabular List that are organized in groups of three-digit code numbers. For example, Malignant Neoplasm of Lip, Oral Cavity and Pharynx (140-149).

sequencing — the process of listing ICD-9-CM codes in the proper order.

specificity — refers to the requirement to code to the highest number of digits possible, 3, 4 or 5, when choosing an ICD-9-CM code.

sub term — refers to listings appearing in the Alphabetic Index under MAIN TERMS and always indented two spaces to the right.

subcategories — refers to groupings of four-digit codes listed under three-digit categories.

Tabular List — the portion of ICD-9-CM that lists codes and definitions in numeric order. Also referred to as Volume 1.

V codes — specific ICD-9-CM codes used to identify encounters for reasons other than illness or injury, for example, immunization.

Volume 1 — see TABULAR LIST

Volume 2 — see ALPHABETIC INDEX

Volume 3 — procedure codes used only for hospital coding. Volume 3 contains both a numeric listing and an alphabetic index.

FORMAT OF ICD-9-CM

The *International Classification of Diseases, 9th Revision, Clinical Modification* was originally published as a three volume set (2nd edition). Newer versions of *ICD-9-CM* are available as two separate books containing Volume 1 and Volume 2 in one book and Volumes 1, 2 and 3 in the other. It is also now available on CD-ROM from the U.S. Government.

This edition of *ICD-9-CM* includes all official addenda from October 1986 through October 2006.

The Tabular List (Volume 1)

The Tabular List (Volume 1) is a *numeric* listing of diagnosis codes and descriptions consisting of 17 chapters that classify diseases and injuries, two sections containing supplementary codes (V codes and E codes) and six appendices.

Classification of Diseases and Injuries

The Classification of Diseases and Injuries includes the following 17 chapters:

Chapter 1	Infectious and Parasitic Diseases (001-139)
Chapter 2	Neoplasms (140-239)
Chapter 3	Endocrine, Nutritional and Metabolic Diseases, and Immunity Disorders (240-279)
Chapter 4	Diseases of the Blood and Blood-Forming Organs (280-289)
Chapter 5	Mental Disorders (290-319)
Chapter 6	Diseases of the Nervous System and Sense Organs (320-389)
Chapter 7	Diseases of the Circulatory System (390-459)
Chapter 8	Diseases of the Respiratory System (460-519)
Chapter 9	Diseases of the Digestive System (520-579)
Chapter 10	Diseases of the Genitourinary System (580-629)
Chapter 11	Complications of Pregnancy, Childbirth, and the Puerperium (630-677)
Chapter 12	Diseases of the Skin and Subcutaneous Tissue (680-709)
Chapter 13	Diseases of the Musculoskeletal System and Connective Tissue (710-739)
Chapter 14	Congenital Anomalies (740-759)
Chapter 15	Certain Conditions Originating in the Perinatal Period (760-779)
Chapter 16	Symptoms, Signs and Ill-defined Conditions (780-799)
Chapter 17	Injury and Poisoning (800-999)

Each chapter of the Tabular List (Volume 1) is structured into four components, namely:

    Sections: groups of three-digit code numbers

    Categories: three-digit code numbers

    Subcategories: four-digit code numbers

    Fifth-Digit Subclassifications: five-digit code numbers

Supplementary Classifications

There are two supplementary classifications included in the Tabular List (Volume 1). These are:

V Codes   Supplementary Classification of Factors Influencing Health Status and Contact with Health Services (V01-V85)

E Codes   Supplementary Classification of External Causes of Injury and Poisoning (E800-E999)

Appendices

The Tabular List (Volume 1) includes four appendices. These are:

Appendix A   Morphology of Neoplasms

Appendix C   Classification of Drugs by American Hospital Formulary Service List Number and Their ICD-9-CM Equivalents

Appendix D   Classification of Industrial Accidents According to Agency

Appendix E   List of Three-Digit Categories

Specifications for the Tabular List

1.   Three-digit rubrics and their contents are unchanged from *ICD-9*.

2.   The sequence of three-digit rubrics is unchanged from *ICD-9*.

3.   Three-digit rubrics are not added to the main body of the classification.

4.   Unsubdivided three-digit rubrics are subdivided where necessary to:

    a) Add clinical detail

    b) Isolate terms for clinical accuracy

5.   The modification in *ICD-9-CM* is accomplished by the addition of a fifth digit to existing *ICD-9* rubrics, except as noted under number 7 below.

6.   Four-digit rubrics are added to subdivided three-digit codes only when there is no other means of achieving desired detail. These codes, unique to *ICD-9-CM* (28 three-digit categories) are marked with the symbol in the Tabular List.

7.   The optional dual classification in *ICD-9* is modified.

    a) Duplicate rubrics are deleted:

        1) Four-digit manifestation categories duplicating etiology entries.

        2) Manifestation inclusion terms duplicating etiology entries.

    b) Manifestations of diseases are identified, to the extent possible, by creating five digit codes in the etiology rubrics.

    c) When the manifestation of a disease cannot be included in the etiology rubrics, provision for its identification is made by retaining the *ICD-9* rubrics used for classifying manifestations of disease.

8.   The format of *ICD-9-CM* is revised from that used in *ICD-9*.

    a) American spelling of medical terms is used.

    b) Inclusion terms are indented beneath the titles of codes.

    c) Codes not to be used for primary tabulation of disease are printed in italics with the notation, "code also underlying disease."

The Alphabetic Index (Volume 2)

The Alphabetic Index (Volume 2) of *ICD-9-CM* consists of an alphabetic list of terms and codes, two supplementary Sections following the alphabetic listing, plus two special tables found within the alphabetic listing. The Alphabetic Index (Volume 2) is structured as follows:

MAIN TERMS: appear in **BOLDFACE** type

SUBHERBS: are always indented two spaces to the right under main terms

CARRY-OVER LINES: are always indented more than two spaces from the level of the preceding line

Supplementary Sections

The supplementary sections following the Alphabetic Index are:

TABLE OF DRUGS AND CHEMICALS

> This table contains a classification of drugs and other chemical substances to identify poisoning states and external causes of adverse effects.

INDEX TO EXTERNAL CAUSES OF INJURIES & POISONINGS (E-CODES)

> This section contains the index to the codes that classify environmental events, circumstances, and other conditions as the cause of injury and other adverse effects.

Special Tables

The two special tables, located within the Alphabetic Index, and found under the main terms as underlined below, are:

HYPERTENSION TABLE

NEOPLASM TABLE

Specifications for the Alphabetic Index

1. Format of the Alphabetic Index follows the format of the ICD-9.

2. Main terms in the Alphabetic Index are printed in bold face type.

3. When two codes are required to indicate etiology and manifestation, the optional manifestation code appears in brackets, e.g., diabetic cataract 250.5 *[366.41]*.

Procedures: Tabular List and Alphabetic Index (Volume 3)

Volume 3 consists of two sections, a Tabular List of codes and an alphabetic index. These codes define procedures instead of diagnoses. Frequently used incorrectly by health care professionals, codes from Volume 3 are intended only for use by hospitals. The Fourth Edition of ICD-9-CM printed by the U.S. Government Printing Office did not include Volume 3. The Fifth and subsequent Editions of ICD-9-CM issued by the U.S. Government included Volume 3 on a CD-ROM.

The ICD-9-CM Procedure Classification is a modification of WHO's *Fascicle V, Surgical Procedures*, and is published as Volume 3 of ICD-9-CM. It contains both a Tabular List and an Alphabetic Index. Greater detail has been added to the ICD-9-CM Procedure Classification necessitating expansion of the codes from three to four digits. Approximately 90% of the rubrics refer to surgical procedures with the remaining 10% accounting for other investigative and therapeutic procedures.

Tabular List of Procedures

The Tabular List includes 16 chapters containing codes and descriptions for surgical procedures and miscellaneous diagnostic and therapeutic procedures.

Alphabetic Index to Procedures

The Alphabetic Index provides an alphabetic index to the Tabular List of Volume 3

Specifications for the Procedure Classification

1.   The ICD-9-CM Procedure Classification is published in its own volume containing both a Tabular List and an Alphabetic Index.

2.   The classification is a modification of *Fascicle V Surgical Procedures* of the ICD-9 Classification of Procedures in Medicine, working from the draft dated Geneva, 30 September-6 October 1975, and labeled WHO/ICD-9/Rev. Conf. 75.4.

3.   All three-digit rubrics in the range 01-86 are maintained as they appear in *Fascicle V*, whenever feasible.

4.   Nonsurgical procedures are segregated from the surgical procedures and confined to the rubrics 87-99, whenever feasible.

5.   Selected detail contained in the remaining fascicles of the *ICD-9 Classification of Procedures in Medicine* is accommodated where possible.

6.   The structure of the classification is based on anatomy rather than surgical specialty.

7.   The *ICD-9-CM* Procedure Classification is numeric only, i.e., no alphabetic characters are used.

8.   The classification is based on a two-digit structure with two decimal digits where necessary.

9.   Compatibility with the *ICD-9 Classification of Procedures in Medicine* was not maintained when a different axis was deemed more clinically appropriate.

CONVENTIONS USED IN THE TABULAR LIST

The *ICD-9-CM* Tabular List (Volume 1) makes use of certain abbreviations, punctuation, symbols, and other conventions that must be clearly understood. The purpose of these conventions is to first, provide special coding instructions, and second, to conserve space.

Abbreviations

NOS   Not Otherwise Specified. Equivalent to Unspecified. This abbreviation refers to a lack of sufficient detail in the statement of diagnosis to be able to assign it to a more specific sub division within the classification.

NEC   Not Elsewhere Classified. Used with ill-defined terms to alert the coder that a specified form of the condition is classified differently. The category number for the term including NEC is to be used only when the coder lacks the information necessary to code the term to a more specific category.

Punctuation

( )   PARENTHESES are used to enclose supplementary words that may be present or absent in a statement of disease without affecting the code assignment.

[ ]   SQUARE BRACKETS are used to enclose synonyms, alternate wordings or explanatory phrases.

:   COLONS are used after an incomplete phrase or term that requires one or more of the modifiers indented under it to make it assignable to a given category. EXCEPTION to this rule pertains to the abbreviation NOS.

Symbols

●   A filled BLACK CIRCLE preceding a code indicates that the code is new to this revision of ICD-9-CM. A symbol key appears on all left-hand pages of the Tabular List, Volume 1 and Volume 3.

▲   A filled BLACK TRIANGLE preceding a code indicates that there is a revision to the text of an existing code. A symbol key appears on all left-hand pages of the Tabular List, Volume 1 and Volume 3.

④ ⑤   A circle containing the number 4 or the number 5 preceding a code indicates that a fourth or fifth digit is required for coding to the highest level of specificity. Valid digits are in [brackets] under each code if the fourth- and fifth-digit codes themselves are not listed. Definitions of valid fifth digits are found under the major category.

Other conventions

Type Face:

BOLD: Bold type face is used for all codes and titles in the Tabular List.

Italics: Italicized type face is used for all exclusion notes and to identify those rubrics that are not to be used for primary tabulations of disease.

Format: ICD-9-CM uses an indented format for ease in reference.

Instructional Notations

Instructional terms define what is, or what is not, included in a given subdivision. This is accomplished by using both inclusion and exclusion terms.

INCLUDES: Indicates separate terms, such as, modifying adjectives, sites and conditions, entered under a subdivision, such as a category, to further define or give examples of, the content of the category.

Excludes: Exclusion terms are enclosed in a box and are printed in italics to draw attention to their presence. The importance of this instructional term is its use as a guideline to direct the coder to the proper code assignment. In other words, all terms following the word EXCLUDES: are to be coded elsewhere as indicated in each instance.

NOTES These are used to define terms and give coding instructions. Often used to list the fifth-digit subclassifications for certain categories.

SEE The "see" instruction following a main term in the index indicates that another term should be referenced. It is necessary to go to the main term referenced with the "see" note to locate the correct code.

SEE CATEGORY A variation of the instructional term SEE. This refers the coder to a specific category. You must *always* follow this instructional term.

SEE ALSO A "see also" instruction following a main term in the index instructs that there is another main term that may also be referenced that may provide additional index entries that may be useful. It is not necessary to follow the "see also" note when the original main term provides the necessary code.

CODE FIRST This instructional note is used for those codes not intended to be used as a principal diagnosis, or not to be sequenced before the underlying disease. The note requires that the underlying disease (etiology) be coded first with the code the note is applied to being coded second. This note appears only in the Tabular List (Vol. 1).

USE ADDITIONAL CODE This instruction is placed in the Tabular List in those categories where the coder may wish to add further information, by using an additional code, to give a more complete picture of the diagnosis or procedure.

Related terms

AND The word "and" should be interpreted to mean either "and" or "or" when it appears in a title.

WITH The word "with" in the alphabetic index is sequenced immediately following the main term, not in alphabetical order.

COLOR CODING

A PMIC versions of ICD-9-CM include color-coding to alert the user to special coding situations or conditions that require additional attention. The use of color-coding is found in the Tabular List of Volume 1 and the Tabular List of Volume 3. The color is applied as solid rectangular bars over the codes only so that the descriptions remain clear and legible. The color codes and definitions are printed at the bottom of all right-sided pages of Volume 1 and Volume 3.

Volume 1

Three digit codes. Coding to fourth or fifth digit specificity is required.

Unspecified code. Descriptions include the term "unspecified." Use only if a more specific diagnosis is not known or available.

Nonspecific code. Descriptions include the term "nonspecific, unspecified, other specified or other." A report *may* be required by insurance carriers.

Manifestation codes. Used only to code the manifestation of an underlying disease. Code the underlying disease first.

Medicare secondary payer (MSP) alert. Diagnoses that may trigger a post-payment review by Medicare. Medicare is usually the secondary payer for these diagnoses.

Secondary diagnosis only. V codes that may only be used as additional codes, not as first-listed codes.

Primary diagnosis only. V codes which are only acceptable as first listed codes.

Volume 3 [*]

Noncovered operating room procedure. An operating room procedure that is not covered by Medicare.

Non-operating room procedure. A procedure that is not performed in the operating room that affects DRG assignment.

Bilateral procedure.

Valid operating room procedure. Prompts a change in DRG assignment.

Nonspecific operating room procedure. Choose a more precise code if possible.

---

*These colors appear only in the three-volume edition

MEDICARE REQUIREMENTS FOR ICD-9-CM CODING

The Medicare Catastrophic Coverage Act of 1988 (PL 100-330) requires that health care professionals submit an appropriate diagnosis code, using the *International Classification of Diseases, 9th Revision, Clinical Modification (ICD-9-CM)* for each procedure, service, or supply billed under Medicare Part B.

To comply with the regulations, health care professionals must convert the reason(s) for the procedures, services or supplies, performed or issued, from written diagnostic statements that may include specific diagnoses, signs, symptoms and/or complaints, into ICD-9-CM diagnosis codes. The Health Care Financing Administration (now CMS) originally set the implementation date for this requirement as April 1, 1989, however, it was subsequently delayed until June 1, 1989, at the request of the American Medical Association, to give health care providers additional time to prepare for the change.

CMS Guidelines for Using ICD-9-CM Codes

The Center for Medicare and Medicaid Services (CMS, formerly HCFA) has prepared guidelines for using ICD-9-CM codes and instructions on how to report them on claim forms. In addition, CMS has directed your medicare intermediary to provide you with a written copy of these instructions. The basic CMS guidelines are summarized below, however, it is very important that you obtain a copy of the guidelines from your Medicare intermediary as implementation of CMS requirements varies from one intermediary to another.

These guidelines are a set of rules that have been developed to accompany and complement the official conventions and instructions provided within the ICD-9-CM itself. These guidelines are based on the coding and sequencing instructions in Volumes 1, 2 and 3 of ICD-9-CM, but provide additional instruction. Adherence to these guidelines when assigning ICD-9-CM diagnosis and procedure codes is required under the Health Insurance Portability and Accountability Act (HIPAA). The diagnosis codes (Volumes 1-2) have been adopted under HIPAA for all healthcare settings. Volume 3 procedure codes have been adopted for inpatient procedures reported by hospitals.

A joint effort between the healthcare provider and the coder is essential to achieve complete and accurate documentation, code assignment, and reporting of diagnoses and procedures. These guidelines have been developed to assist both the healthcare provider and the coder in identifying those diagnoses and procedures that are to be reported. The importance of consistent, complete documentation in the medical record cannot be overemphasized. Without such documentation, accurate coding cannot be achieved.

The entire record should be reviewed to determine the specific reason for the encounter and the conditions treated.

The term encounter is used for all settings, including hospital admissions. In the context of these guidelines, the term provider is used throughout the guidelines to mean physician or any qualified health care practitioner who is legally accountable for establishing the patient's diagnosis. Only this set of guidelines, approved by the Cooperating Parties, is official.

1. Indicate on the claim form or itemized statement the appropriate code(s) from the ICD-9-CM code range 001.0 through V84.8 to identify diagnoses, symptoms, conditions, problems, complaints or other reason(s) for the procedure, service or supply provided.

    A. In choosing codes to describe the reason for the encounter, the health care professional will frequently be using codes within the range from 001.0 through 999.9, the section of ICD-9-CM for the classification of diseases and injuries (e.g. infectious and parasitic diseases; neoplasms; signs, symptoms and ill-defined conditions). Codes that describe symptoms as opposed to diagnoses are acceptable if this is the highest level of certainty documented by the physician.

    B. ICD-9-CM also provides codes to deal with visits for circumstances other than a disease or injury, such as an encounter for a laboratory test only. These codes are found in the V-code section and range from V01.0 through V84.8.

2. The ICD-9-CM code for the diagnosis, condition, problem, or other reason for the encounter documented in the medical record as the main reason for the procedure, service or supply provided should be listed first. Additional ICD-9-CM codes that describe any current coexisting conditions are then listed. Do not include codes for conditions that were previously treated and no longer exist.

3. ICD-9-CM codes should be used at their highest level of specificity.

    A. Assign three digit codes only if there are no four digit codes within the coding category.

    B. Assign four digit codes only if there is no fifth digit subclassification for that category.

    C. Assign the fifth digit subclassification code for those categories where it exists.

    Claims submitted with three or four digit codes where four and five digit codes are available may be returned to you by the Medicare intermediary for proper coding. It is recognized that a very specific diagnosis may not be known at the time of the initial encounter. However, that is not an acceptable reason to submit a three digit code when four or five digits are available.

    For example, if the patient has chronic bronchitis, ICD-9-CM code 491, and the physician has not yet documented whether the bronchitis is simple, mucopurulent, or obstructive, the code for unspecified chronic bronchitis, ICD-9-CM code 491.9, should be listed.

4. Diagnoses documented as "probable," "suspected," "questionable," or "rule out" should not be coded as if the diagnosis is confirmed. The condition(s) should be coded to the highest degree of certainty for the encounter, such as describing symptoms, signs, abnormal test results, or other reasons for the encounter.

5. Chronic disease(s) treated on an ongoing basis may be coded and reported as many times as the patient receives treatment and care for the condition(s).

6. When patients receive ancillary diagnostic services only during an encounter, the appropriate "V code" for the service should be listed first, and the diagnosis or problem for which the diagnostic procedures are being performed should be listed second.

    A. V codes will be used frequently by radiologists who perform radiological examinations on referrals. For example, ICD-9-CM code V72.5, Radiological examination, not elsewhere classified, describes the reason for the encounter and should be listed first on the claim form or statement. If the reason for the referral is known, a second ICD-9-CM code that describes the signs or symptoms for which the examination was ordered should be listed.

    B. Failure to list a second ICD-9-CM code in addition to the V code may result in claim delays or denials. The ICD-9-CM code V72.5, Radiological examination, not elsewhere classified, includes referrals for routine chest x-rays that are not covered by the Medicare program. Medicare intermediaries may establish screening programs to verify that the referrals were not for routine chest x-rays. By supplying a second ICD-9-CM code to describe the reason for the referral, these claims can be clearly identified by the Medicare intermediary as referrals to evaluate symptoms, signs or diagnoses. The mission of a second ICD-9-CM code may lead to requests for additional information from Medicare intermediaries prior to processing the claim.

7. For patients receiving only ancillary therapeutic services during an encounter, list the appropriate V code first, followed by the ICD-9-CM code for the diagnosis or problem for which the services are being performed. For example, a patient with multiple sclerosis presenting for rehabilitation services would be coded using either V57.1 Other physical therapy, or V57.89 Other care involving use of rehabilitation procedures, followed by code 340 Multiple sclerosis.

8. For surgical procedures, use the ICD-9-CM code for the diagnosis for which the surgery was performed. If the postoperative diagnosis is known to be different at the time the claim is filed, use the ICD-9-CM code for the post-operative diagnosis.

9. Code all documented conditions that coexist at the time of the visit that require or affect patient care, treatment or management. Do not code conditions that were previously treated and no longer exist.

Completing the CMS1500 Claim Form

Health care professionals using the Uniform Health Insurance Claim Form, CMS1500, to file claims for services provided to Medicare beneficiaries must list a minimum of one ICD-9-CM code and may list up to four total ICD-9-CM codes on the claim form.

The ICD-9-CM code for the diagnosis, condition, problem or other reason for the encounter is listed first, followed by up to three additional codes that describe any coexisting conditions. At times, there may be several conditions that equally resulted in the encounter. In these cases, the health care professional is free to select the one that will be listed first.

The ICD-9-CM codes are listed in Box 23 of the "old" HCFA1500 (10/84) claim form and Box 21 of the "new" CMS1500 (12/90) claim form (see example). In addition, in Box 24 D of both versions of the form, you must indicate by a number from 1 to 4, or combination of numbers, which diagnoses from Box 23 support the procedure, service or supply listed in Box 24 C.

Due to space limitations on the claim form you may use only up to four ICD-9-CM codes for diagnoses, conditions, or signs and symptoms. Frequently the patient may have more than four conditions present at the time of the encounter, however, you must choose only four codes to be listed on the claim form.

If you strongly believe that additional diagnostic information is needed by the Medicare intermediary for proper claim processing you may attach additional supporting documentation to your manual claim. Keep in mind that in most cases the additional documentation will be ignored by the claims examiners, and, in other cases will result in reimbursement delay while someone reviews your documentation.

Medicare Penalties for Non-compliance

The Medicare Catastrophic Coverage Act of 1988 mandates submission of an appropriate ICD-9-CM diagnosis code or codes for each procedure, service, or supply furnished by the health care professional to Medicare Part B beneficiaries. The Act further specifies that compliance is mandatory and that penalties may be assessed for noncompliance.

The penalties for noncompliance differ depending upon whether or not the health care professional has agreed to accept assignment or not.

1.   For health care professionals who accept assignment on a Medicare claim and who fail to include ICD-9-CM codes as required will have their claim(s) returned for proper coding and may be subject to post-payment review by the Medicare intermediary, as well as payment denials.

2.   For health care professionals who do not accept assignment, the penalties are more severe.

    A.   If the original claim form does not include ICD-9-CM codes as required, and the health care professional refuses to provide the codes promptly on request to the Medicare intermediary, the professional may be subject to a civil monetary penalty in an amount not to exceed $2,000, per claim.

    B.   If the health care professional continuously fails to provide ICD-9-CM codes as requested, the professional may be subject to the sanction process described in section 1842 (j) (2) (A), that mandates that the professional may be barred from participation in the Medicare program for a period not to exceed five years.

CODING AND BILLING ISSUES

Diagnosis Codes Must Support Procedure Codes

Each service or procedure performed for a patient should be represented by a diagnosis that would substantiate those particular services or procedures as necessary in the investigation or treatment of their condition based on currently accepted standards of practice by the medical profession.

Place (Location) of Service

The actual setting that the services are rendered in for particular diagnoses plays an important part in reimbursement. Many people became accustomed to using emergency rooms for any type of illness or injury. By utilizing highly specialized places of service for conditions that were not true emergencies, third party payer were being billed with CPT codes indicating emergency services were rendered. Since the cost of services rendered on an emergency basis is considerably more expensive than those services in an non-emergency situation, third party payers began watching for those claims with diagnoses that did not indicate that a true emergency existed. Payment then was based on what the cost would have been had the patient been treated in the proper setting.

Level of Service Provided

The patient's condition and the treatment of that condition must be billed according to the criteria, as published by the AMA, for each level of service (i.e., minimal, brief, limited, intermediate, extended, comprehensive). Many practices bill the office visit level that they know will pay better rather than to consider the criteria that must be met to use a particular level of service. Again, the patient's diagnosis enters into this concept as well as it is often the diagnosis that indicates the complexity of the level of service to be used.

Frequency of Services

Many times claims are submitted for a patient with the same diagnosis and the same procedure(s) time after time. When the diagnosis indicates a chronic condition and the claims do not indicate any change in the patient's treatment or, give any indication that the patient's condition has been altered (i.e., exacerbated, other symptomology) the third party payer may deny payment based on the frequency of services for the reported condition.

Concurrent Care

Reimbursement problems often arise when a patient is being treated by different professionals, within the same billing entity (medical group or clinic), for different problems at the same time. This is known as concurrent care. For example, a patient may be hospitalized by a clinic's general surgeon for an operation and may also be seen while hospitalized by the group's cardiologist for an unrelated cardiac condition.

ICD-9-CM Coding Fundamentals

Learning and following the basic steps of coding will increase your chances of better and faster reimbursement from third party payers, as well as establish meaningful profiles for future reimbursement rates. To become a proficient coder, two basic principles always must be considered.

First, it is imperative that you use both the Alphabetic Index (Volume 2) and the Tabular List (Volume 1) when locating and assigning codes. Coding only from the Alphabetic Index will cause you to miss any additional information provided only in the Tabular List, such as exclusions, instructions to use additional codes or the need for a fifth-digit.

Second, the level of specificity is important in all coding situations. A three-digit code that has subdivisions indicates you must use the appropriate subdivision code. Also, any time a fifth-digit subclassification is provided, you must use the fifth-digit code.

NINE STEPS FOR ACCURATE ICD-9-CM CODING

1.   Locate the main term within the diagnostic statement.

2.   Locate that main term in the Alphabetic Index (Volume 2). Keep in mind that the primary arrangement for main terms is by condition in the Alphabetic Index (Volume 2); main terms can be referred to in outmoded, ill-defined and lay terms as well as proper medical terms; main terms can be expressed in broad or specific terms, as nouns, adjectives or eponyms and can be with or without modifiers. Certain conditions may be listed under more than one main term.

3.   Remember to refer to all notes under the main term. Be guided by the instructions in any notes appearing in a box immediately after the main term.

4.   Examine any modifiers appearing in parentheses next to the main term. See if any of these modifiers apply to any of the qualifying terms used in the diagnostic statement.

5.   Take note of the subterms indented beneath the main term. Subterms differ from main terms in that they provide greater specificity, becoming more specific the further they are indented to the right of the main term in 2-space increments; also, they provide the anatomical sites affected by the disease or injury.

6.   Be sure to follow any cross reference instructions. These instructional terms ("see" or "see also") must be followed to locate the correct code.

7.   Confirm the code selection in the Tabular List (Volume 1). Make certain you have selected the appropriate classification in accordance with the diagnosis.

8.   Follow instructional terms in the Tabular List (Volume 1). Watch for exclusion terms, notes and fifth-digit instructions that apply to the code number you are verifying. It is necessary to search not only the selected code number for instructions but also the category, section and chapter in which the code number is collapsible. Many times the instructional information is located one or more pages preceding the actual page you find the code number on.

9.   Finally, assign the code number you have determined to be correct.

ITALICIZED ENTRIES

During the process of designating a code to identify a principal diagnosis it is important to remember that italicized entries or codes in slanted brackets cannot be used. In these instances, it is required that the etiology code be sequenced first and the manifestation code be listed second even if the physician recorded them in the opposite order.

OTHER AND UNSPECIFIED CODES

Subcategories for diagnoses listed as "Other" and "Unspecified" are referred to as residual subcategories. Remember, the subdivisions are arranged in a hierarchy starting with the more specific and ending with the least specific. In the Tabular List (Volume 1), in most instances, the four-digit subcategory ".8" has been reserved for "Other" specified conditions not classifiable elsewhere and the four-digit subcategory ".9" has been reserved for "Unspecified" conditions. Following is an example demonstrating this principle.

005   Other food poisoning (bacterial)

| *Excludes:* |

Excludes: salmonella infections (003.0-003.9)
toxic effect of:
   food contaminants (989.7)
   noxious foodstuffs (988-0-988.9)

005.0   Staphylococcal food poisoning
Staphylococcal toxemia specified as due to food

005.1   Botulism
Food poisoning due to Clostridium botulinum

005.2   Food poisoning due to Clostridium perfringens [C. welchii]
Enteritis necroticans

005.3   Food poisoning due to other Clostridia

005.4   Food poisoning due to Vibrio parahaemolyticus

005.8   Other bacterial food poisoning
Excludes: salmonella food poisoning (003.0-003.9)

005.81   Food poisoning due to Vibrio vulnificus

005.89   Other bacterial food poisoning
Food poisoning due to Bacillus cereus

005.9   Food poisoning, unspecified

As you look at Category 005, note that codes 005.0-005.4 indicate that the food poisoning is related to specific types of organisms. Therefore, subcategories 005.0-005.4 are regarded as more specific than subcategory 005.9. Fifth-digit subclassification 005.89 *Other bacterial food poisoning* would include other specific types of bacterial food poisoning not classified elsewhere, as well as bacterial food poisoning NOS. Whereas subcategory 005.9 *Food poisoning unspecified* would be used for a diagnostic statement of "Food poisoning NOS" where the causative organism is not mentioned.

The hierarchy from more specific to less specific is not consistently maintained at the fifth-digit level. The level of specificity at the fifth-digit level is usually (not always) indicated by the use of 0 and 9. The digit 9 identifies the entry for "Other specified" while the digit 0 identifies the "Unspecified" entry. Below is an example.

279   Disorders involving the immune mechanism

    279.0   Deficiency of humoral immunity

        279.00   Hypogammaglobulinemia, unspecified
            Agammaglobulinemia NOS

        279.01   Selective IgA immunodeficiency

        279.02   Selective IgM immunodeficiency

        279.03   Other selective immunoglobulin deficiencies
            Selective deficiency of IgG

        279.04   Congenital hypogammaglobulinemia
            Agammaglobulinemia:
                Bruton's type
                X-linked

        279.05   Immunodeficiency with increased IgM
            Immunodeficiency with hyper-IgM:
                autosomal recessive
                X-linked

        279.06   Common variable immunodeficiency
            Dysgammaglobulinemia (acquired)
                (congenital) (primary)
            Hypogammaglobulinemia:
                acquired primary
                congenital non-sex-linked
                sporadic

        279.09   Other
            Transient hypogammaglobulinemia of infancy

Notice that the fifth-digit 0 identifies "Unspecified" and the fifth-digit 9 identifies "Other specified."

ACUTE AND CHRONIC CODING

Whenever a particular condition is described as both acute and chronic, code according to the subentries in the Alphabetic Index (Volume 2) for the stated condition. The following directions should be considered:

1. If there are separate subentries listed for acute, subacute and chronic, then use both codes, sequencing the code for the acute condition first.

2. If there are no subentries to identify acute, subacute or chronic, ignore these adjectives when selecting the code for the particular condition.

3. If a certain condition is described as a subacute condition and the index does not provide a subentry designating subacute, then code the condition as if it were acute.

CODING SUSPECTED CONDITIONS

Whenever the diagnosis is stated as "questionable," "probable," "likely," or "rule out," it is advisable to code documented symptoms or complaints by the patient. The reason for this is that you do not want an insurance carrier to include a disease code in the patient's history if in fact the "suspected" condition is never proven.

Keep in mind that there are no "rule out" codes per se in the ICD-9-CM coding system. If your diagnostic statement is "Rule out Breast Carcinoma" and you use code 174.9 *Malignant neoplasm of female breast, unspecified*, the code definition does not state "rule out." Therefore, the insurance carrier processes the code 174.9 as is, which results in the patient having an insurance history of breast cancer.

To avoid what could become a problem for you and your patient (including the potential of litigation), you should use codes for signs and symptoms in these cases. For example, use code 611.72 *Lump or mass in breast*, or 611.71 *Mastodynia (breast pain)* if these symptoms exist and this is the highest degree of certainty you can code to.

If the patient is asymptomatic but there is a family history of breast cancer then you should consider using a V-code, such as V16.3 *Family history of malignant neoplasm, breast* as your diagnosis code. There are also V-codes to indicate screening for a particular illness or disease. In the above example, code V76.1 *Special screening for malignant neoplasm, breast* could also have been used.

It is important to note that when you use a screening code from the V-code section you should also code signs or symptoms. The reason for doing so is because most health insurance carriers do not provide coverage for routine screening procedures or preventive medicine.

COMBINATION CODES

A combination code is used to fully identify an instance where two diagnoses or a diagnosis with an associated secondary process (manifestation) or complication is included in the description of a single code number. These combination codes are identified by referring to the subterms in the Alphabetic Index (Volume 2) and the inclusion and exclusion terms in the Tabular List (Volume 1).

Examples of commonly used combination codes include 034.0 *Streptococcal sore throat* and 404 *Hypertensive heart and renal disease.* Code 034.0 exists because the throat is often infected with Streptococcus and code 404 must be used whenever a patient has both heart and renal disease instead of assigning codes from categories 402 and 403.

Two main terms may be joined together by combination terms listed in the Alphabetic Index (Volume 2) as subterms such as:

associated with   *in*
complicated (by) *secondary to*
due to   *with*
during   *without*
following

The listing for the above terms advises the coder to use one or two codes depending on the condition.

MULTIPLE CODING

There are single conditions that require more than one code. "Use additional code" notes are found in the Tabular List at codes that are not part of an etiology/ manifestation pair where a secondary code is useful to fully describe a condition. The sequencing rule is the same: "use additional code" indicates that a secondary code should be added.

For example, for infections that are not included in Chapter 1, a secondary code from category 041, *Bacterial infection in conditions classified elsewhere and of unspecified site,* may be required to identify the bacterial organism causing the infection. A "use additional code" note will normally be found at the infection code and indicates a need for the organism code to be added as the secondary code.

There are also "code first" notes under certain codes that are not specifically manifestation codes but may be due to an underlying cause. When a "code first" note is present and an underlying condition is present, the underlying condition should be sequenced first.

"Code, if applicable, any causal condition first" notes indicate that this code may be assigned as a principal diagnosis when the causal condition is unknown or not applicable. If a causal condition is known, then the code for that condition should be sequenced as the principal or first-listed diagnosis.

Multiple codes may be needed for late effects, complication codes and obstetric codes to more fully describe a condition. See the specific guidelines for these sections for further instruction.

When is multiple coding mandatory? Only if the instructional term "code also" appears in italics under an italicized subdivision in the Tabular List (Volume 1). In this instance, you should interpret mandatory as: "requires the use of both codes, and these codes must be sequenced with the code for the etiology being listed first and the code identifying the manifestation listed second." You will recognize mandatory multiple coding situations by instructional terms used in the Tabular List (Volume 1). Terms to watch for are: "Code also....," "Use additional code...," and "Note:...."

If you turn to Category 330 in the Tabular List (Volume 1), you will notice the instructional term cited: "Use additional code to identify associated mental retardation." The phrase "...identify associated mental retardation" should be interpreted as "...identify associated mental retardation, if stated to be present in the diagnostic statement." With this understood, these diagnostic statements would be coded as below.

Coding Examples

Cerebral degeneration in childhood with mental retardation

    330.9   Unspecified cerebral degeneration in childhood

    319   Unspecified mental retardation

Cerebral degeneration in childhood

    330.9   Unspecified cerebral degeneration in childhood

In the Alphabetic Index (Volume 2), if two codes are listed, the first should be sequenced first with the code in italicized brackets listed second to indicate the additional code. However, the fact that two codes appear after a subterm in the Alphabetic Index does not automatically indicate mandatory multiple coding. It is necessary to verify both code numbers in the Tabular List. If, in the Tabular List, the code number is also in italics as in the Alphabetical Index and, the instructional term "Code also" appears in italics, then both criteria have been met for mandatory multiple coding.

Coding Example

Diabetic neuropathy

    250.60 Diabetes with neurological manifestations

    357.2   Polyneuropathy in diabetes

In the Alphabetic Index (Volume 2) under "Diabetes," you will find "Neuropathy" listed followed by the codes 250.6 and *[357.2]* in brackets.

It should also be noted at this point, that even though mandatory multiple coding is always indicated by the presence of the instructional term "Code first" in italics beneath the italicized code number and title for the manifestation, this does not always hold true under the code number for the etiology. Multiple coding is not to be used in those instances when a combination code accurately identifies all of the elements within the diagnostic statement.

CODING LATE EFFECTS

A late effect is the residual effect (condition produced) after the acute phase of an illness or injury has terminated. There is no time limit on when a late effect code can be used. The residual may be apparent early, such as in cerebrovascular accident cases, or it may occur months or years later, such as that due to a previous injury. Coding of late effects generally requires two codes sequenced in the following order: The condition or nature of the late effect first; the late effect code second.

An exception to the above guideline is when the code for late effect is followed by a manifestation code identified in the Tabular List and title, or when the late effect code has been expanded (at the fourth and fifth-digit levels) to include the manifestation(s). The code for the acute phase of an illness or injury that led to the late effect is never used with a code for the late effect.

Coding Example

Hemiplegia due to previous cerebral vascular accident

    342.90 Hemiplegia, unspecified, affecting unspecified side

    438.20 Late effects of cerebrovascular disease, Hemiplegia affecting unspecified side

The *residual* for this statement is "Hemiplegia" as it is the long term condition that resulted from a previous acute illness. The *cause* for this statement is "Cerebral vascular accident" as it is the original illness no longer in its acute phase but which did cause the long term residual condition now present.

How do you recognize when to use late effects coding and when not to? Often, the diagnostic statement will contain key words to help identify a late effects situation. Key words used in defining late effects include:

> *late*
> *due to an old injury*
> *due to a previous illness/injury*
> *due to an illness/injury occurring one year or more ago*

In cases where these key words (phrases) are not included within the diagnostic statement, an effect is considered to be late if sufficient time has elapsed between the occurrence of the acute illness/injury and the development of the residual effect.

Coding Example

Excessive scar tissue due to third degree burn, right leg

    709.2 Scar conditions and fibrosis of skin

    906.7 Late effect of burn of other extremities

The previous diagnostic statement does not indicate the time element with any modifying terms as "old" or "previous." The fact that enough time has elapsed for the development of scar tissue indicates that the acute phase of the injury has subsided and the scarring should be coded as a late effect.

If a diagnostic statement only specifies the cause of the late effect and does not indicate the residual, then use the code number for the cause.

Coding Example

Residuals of tuberculosis

    137 Late effects of tuberculosis

The above statement does not identify the actual residuals, so you would use the code for the cause.

To find the code for such a statement in the Alphabetic Index (Volume 2), refer to the main term "LATE" and the subterm "EFFECTS OF." The only codes available for causes of late effects are:

137	**Late effects of tuberculosis**
138	**Late effects of acute poliomyelitis**
139	**Late effects of other infectious and parasitic diseases**
268.1	**Rickets, late effect**
326	**Late effects of intracranial abscess or pyogenic infection**
438	**Late effects of cerebrovascular disease**
677	**Late effect of complication of pregnancy, childbirth and the puerperium**
905	**Late effects of musculoskeletal and connective tissue injuries**
906	**Late effects of injuries to skin and subcutaneous tissues**
907	**Late effects of injuries to the nervous system**
908	**Late effects of other and unspecified injuries**
909	**Late effects of other and unspecified external causes**

Be sure to distinguish between a late effect and a historical statement in a diagnosis. Whenever the statement uses the terms "effects of old...," "sequela of...," or "residuals of...," then code as late effects. If the diagnosis is expressed in terms as "history of...," these are coded to personal history of the illness or injury and are coded to the V-Codes (V-10 to V-15).

CODING IMPENDING OR THREATENED CONDITIONS

Code any condition described at the time of discharge as impending or threatened as follows:

1.   If it did occur, code as confirmed diagnosis.

2.   If it did not occur, reference the Alphabetic Index to determine if the condition has a subentry term for impending or threatened and also reference main term entries for Impending and for Threatened.

3.   If the subterms are listed, assign the given code.

4.   If the subterms are not listed, code the existing underlying condition(s) and not the condition described as impending or threatened.

CODING INJURIES

Injuries comprise a major section of ICD-9-CM. Categories 800-959 include fractures, dislocations, sprains and various other types of injuries. Injuries are classified first according to the general type of injury and within each type there is a further breakdown by anatomical site.

When coding injuries, assign separate codes for each injury unless a combination code is provided, in which case the combination code is assigned. Multiple injury codes are provided in ICD-9-CM, but should not be assigned unless information for a more specific code is not available. These codes are not to be used for normal, healing surgical wounds or to identify complications of surgical wounds.

The code for the most serious injury, as determined by the physician, is sequenced first.

1.	Superficial injuries such as abrasions or contusions are not coded when associated with more severe injuries of the same site.

2.	When a primary injury results in minor damage to peripheral nerves or blood vessels, the primary injury is sequenced first with additional code(s) from categories 950-957, *Injury to nerves and spinal cord*, and/ or 900-904, *Injury to blood vessels*. When the primary injury is to the blood vessels or nerves, that injury should be sequenced first.

In cases where a patient has multiple injuries, the most severe injury is the principal diagnosis. Where multiple sites of injury are specified in the diagnosis, you should interpret the term "with" as indicating involvement of both sites, and interpret the term "and" as indicating involvement of either or both sites. You will also note that fifth-digits are commonly used when coding injuries to provide information regarding level of consciousness, specific anatomical sites and severity of injuries.

Coding Fractures

The principles of multiple coding of injuries should be followed in coding fractures. Fractures of specified sites are coded individually by site in accordance with both the provisions within categories 800-829 and the level of detail furnished by medical record content. Combination categories for multiple fractures are provided for use when there is insufficient detail in the medical record (such as trauma cases transferred to another hospital), when the reporting form limits the number of codes that can be used in reporting pertinent clinical data, or when there is insufficient specificity at the fourth-digit or fifth-digit level. More specific guidelines are as follows:

1.	Multiple fractures of same limb classifiable to the same three-digit or four-digit category are coded to that category.

2.	Multiple unilateral or bilateral fractures of same bone(s) but classified to different fourth-digit subdivisions (bone part) within the same three-digit category are coded individually by site.

3.	Multiple fracture categories 819 and 828 classify bilateral fractures of both upper limbs (819) and both lower limbs (828), but without any detail at the fourth-digit level other than open and closed type of fractures.

4.   Multiple fractures are sequenced in accordance with the severity of the fracture and the physician should be asked to list the fracture diagnoses in the order of severity.

Some general rules to apply when coding fractures follow. Fractures can either be "open" or "closed." An "open" fracture is when the skin has been broken and there is communication with the bone and the outside of the body. Whereas, with a "closed" fracture the bone does not have contact with the outside of the body.

Note the following descriptions as set forth in the ICD-9-CM at the four-digit subdivision level to help distinguish between an "open" and "closed" fracture.

Closed Fractures

comminuted	*simple*
linear	*greenstick*
fissured	*depressed*
spiral	*march*
impacted	*fractured NOS*
elevated	*slipped epiphysis*

Open Fractures

compound	*with foreign body*
missile	*infected*
puncture	

Anytime that it is not indicated whether a fracture is open or closed, code it as if it were closed. Fracture-dislocations are classified as fractures. Pathological fractures are classified to the condition causing the fracture (i.e. osteoporosis) with the use of an additional code to identify the *Pathologic fracture* (733.1).

Coding Burns

Current burns (940-949) are classified by depth, extent and by agent (E code). Burns are classified by depth as first degree (erythema), second degree (blistering), and third degree (full-thickness involvement).

1.   Sequence first the code that reflects the highest degree of burn when more than one burn is present.

    A. When the reason for the admission or encounter is for treatment of external multiple burns, sequence first the code that reflects the burn of the highest degree.

    B. When a patient has both internal and external burns, the circumstances of admission govern the selection of the principal diagnosis or first-listed diagnosis.

    C. When a patient is admitted for burn injuries and other related conditions such as smoke inhalation and/or respiratory failure, the circumstances of admission govern the selection of the principal or first-listed diagnosis.

2.   Classify burns of the same local site (three-digit category level, 940-947) but of different degrees to the subcategory identifying the highest degree recorded in the diagnosis.

3.   Non-healing burns are coded as acute burns. Necrosis of burned skin should be coded as a non-healed burn.

4.   Assign code 958.3, *Posttraumatic wound infection, not elsewhere classified*, as an additional code for any documented infected burn site.

5.   When coding burns, assign separate codes for each burn site. Category 946 *Burns of Multiple specified sites,* should only be used if the location of the burns are not documented. Category 949, *Burn, unspecified*, is extremely vague and should rarely be used.

6.   Assign codes from category 948, *Burns classified according to extent of body surface involved*, when the site of the burn is not specified or when there is a need for additional data. It is advisable to use category 948 as additional coding when needed to provide data for evaluating burn mortality, such as that needed by burn units. It is also advisable to use category 948 as an additional code for reporting purposes when there is mention of a third-degree burn involving 20 percent or more of the body surface.

     In assigning a code from category 948:

     A.   Fourth-digit codes are used to identify the percentage of total body surface involved in a burn (all degree).

     B.   Fifth-digits are assigned to identify the percentage of body surface involved in third-degree burn.

     C.   Fifth-digit zero (0) is assigned when less than 10 percent or when no body surface is involved in a third-degree burn.

     Category 948 is based on the classic rule of nines in estimating body surface involved: head and neck are assigned nine percent, each arm nine percent, each leg 18 percent, the anterior trunk 18 percent, posterior trunk 18 percent, and genitalia one percent. Physicians may change these percentage assignments where necessary to accommodate infants and children who have proportionately larger heads than adults and patients who have large buttocks, thighs, or abdomen that involve burns.

7.   Encounters for the treatment of the late effects of burns (i.e., scars or joint contractures) should be coded to the residual condition (sequelae) followed by the appropriate late effect code (906.5-906.9). A late effect E code may also be used, if desired.

8.   When appropriate, both a sequelae with a late effect code, and a current burn code may be assigned on the same record.

9.   Excisional debridement involves an excisional debridement (surgical removal or cutting away), as opposed to a mechanical (brushing, scrubbing, washing) debridement. For coding purposes, excisional debridement is assigned to code 86.22.

     Nonexcisional debridement is assigned to code 86.28.

Remember when coding burns, code only the most severe degree of burns when the burns are of the same site but of different degrees. In cases of burns where it is noted that there is an infection, assign the code for the burn and also the code for the infection (958.3 *Posttraumatic wound infection NEC*).

POISONING AND ADVERSE EFFECTS OF DRUGS

There are two different sets of code numbers to use to differentiate between poisoning and adverse reactions to the correct substances properly administered. First, you must make the distinction between poisoning and adverse reaction. Poisoning by drugs includes:

Poisoning

Accidental

1.   Given in error during diagnostic or therapeutic procedures.

2.   Given in error by one person to another (for example, mother to child).

3.   Taken in error by self.

Purposeful

1.   Suicide attempt.

2.   Homicide attempt.

Adverse Reaction in Spite of Proper Administration of Correct Substance

1.   In therapeutic of diagnostic procedure.

2.   Taken by self or given to another as prescribed.

3.   Accumulative effect (intoxication due to....).

4.   Interaction of prescribed drugs.

5.   Synergistic reaction (enhancing the effect of another drug).

6.   Allergic reaction.

7.   Hypersensitivity.

To code poisoning by drugs, use the Alphabetic Index (Volume 2) which contains the Table of Drugs and Chemicals. This table includes one column to identify the poisoning code (960-989) and four columns of External Cause Codes to classify whether the poisoning was an accident, suicide, assault or undetermined.

The column labeled "Therapeutic Use" is not used for poisonings but in coding adverse reactions to correct substances properly administered. The External Cause Codes are optional but may be used if a facility's coding policy requires their use.

Note that in the Alphabetic Index (Volume 2) that the subterm entry "Drug" under the main term of "Poisoning" refers the coder to the Table of Drugs and Chemicals for the code assignment. Because the Table of Drugs and Chemicals is so extensive, it is acceptable to code directly from the Table without verifying the code obtained in Volume 1.

What if the drug which caused the poisoning is not listed in the Table of Drugs and Chemicals?

1.   Refer to Appendix C in Volume 1 (American Hospital Formulary Service) and locate the name of the drug.

2.   Note the AHFS category number listed.

3.   Turn to the Table of Drugs and Chemicals in the Alphabetic Index (Volume 2) of ICD-9-CM.

4.   Locate the term "Drug."

5.   Refer to the subterm "AHFS List."

6.   Look through the list until you find the AHFS Category Number determined in step 2 above. The AHFS Category Numbers are listed in numeric order.

7.   Assign the code.

How Do You Identify Poisoning by Drugs?

The statement of diagnosis will usually have descriptive terms that would indicate poisoning. Look for terms such as:

Intoxication	*Toxic effect*
Overdose	*Wrong drug given/taken in error*
Poisoning	*Wrong dosage given/taken in error*

Adverse effects of a medicine taken in combination with alcohol or from taking a prescribed drug in combination with a drug the patient took on his/her own initiative (for example antihistamines) are coded as poisonings. If you wish to code a manifestation of the poisoning as well, this code is always listed second, after listing the code identifying the poison first.

Adverse Effects of Drugs

The World Health Organization (WHO) defines adverse drug reaction as any response to a drug "which is noxious and unintended and which occurs at doses used in man for prophylaxis, diagnosis or therapy." Notice that this definition does not include the terms "overdose" or "poisoning."

Why does ICD-9-CM differentiate between poisoning and adverse drug reaction? Tabulation of statistical data indicates how often a drug reaction occurred because of the drug itself versus how often the drug was either not given or taken properly. Two codes are required when coding adverse drug reactions to the correct substance properly administered. One code is used to identify the manifestation or the nature of the adverse reaction such as urticaria, vertigo, gastritis, etc. This code is assigned from Categories 001-799 in Volume 1.

Refer to the main term identifying the manifestation in the Alphabetic Index (Volume 2). But remember that the Table of Drugs and Chemicals is not used to locate the code for the manifestation, and the code used to identify the manifestation does not identify the drug responsible for the adverse reaction.

A second code is required to identify the drug causing the adverse reaction. In ICD-9-CM, the only codes provided to identify the drug causing an adverse reaction to a substance properly administered are E930 through E949. Anytime a code is selected from the E930-E949 range, it can never be sequenced first or be a solo code.

When the drug was correctly prescribed and properly administered, code the reaction plus the appropriate code from the E930-E949 series. Codes from the E930-E949 series must be used to identify the causative substance for an adverse effect of drug, medicinal and biological substances, correctly prescribed and properly administered. The effect, such as tachycardia, delirium, gastrointestinal hemorrhaging, vomiting, hypokalemia, hepatitis, renal failure, or respiratory failure, is coded and followed by the appropriate code from the E930-E949 series.

Adverse effects of therapeutic substances correctly prescribed and properly administered (toxicity, synergistic reaction, side effect, and idiosyncratic reaction) may be due to (1) differences among patients, such as age, sex, disease, and genetic factors, and (2) drug-related factors, such as type of drug, route of administration, duration of therapy, dosage, and bioavailability.

Poisoning

1. Errors made in drug prescription or in the administration of the drug by provider, nurse, patient, or other person, use the appropriate poisoning code from the 960-979 series.

2. If an overdose of a drug was intentionally taken or administered and resulted in drug toxicity, it would be coded as a poisoning (960-979 series).

3. If a nonprescribed drug or medicinal agent was taken in combination with a correctly prescribed and properly administered drug, any drug toxicity or other reaction resulting from the interaction of the two drugs would be classified as a poisoning.

4. When coding a poisoning or reaction to the improper use of a medication (e.g., wrong dose, wrong substance, wrong route of administration), the poisoning code is sequenced first, followed by a code for the manifestation. If there is also a diagnosis of drug abuse or dependence to the substance, the abuse or dependence is coded as an additional code.

Toxic Effects

1. When a harmful substance is ingested or comes in contact with a person, this is classified as a toxic effect. The toxic effect codes are in categories 980-989.

2. A toxic effect code should be sequenced first, followed by the code(s) that identify the result of the toxic effect.

3. An external cause code from categories E860-E869 for accidental exposure, codes E950.6 or E950.7 for intentional self-harm, category E962 for assault, or categories E980-E982 (undetermined), should also be assigned to indicate intent.

Locating the Proper E Code

How do you locate the proper E code to identify the drug which was responsible for causing an adverse reaction to a correct substance properly administered? Turn to the Table of Drugs and Chemicals in the Alphabetic Index (Volume 2). Earlier we noted that the column labeled "Therapeutic Use" was not used for coding instances involving poisoning. However, for adverse drug reactions to a correct substance properly administered, the "Therapeutic Use" column is used to find the proper code within the range E930 through E949 to identify the drug.

Drug Interactions Between Two or More Drugs

Drug interactions between two or more prescribed drugs are classified as adverse drug reactions to a correct substance properly administered. This holds true regardless of whether the drugs were prescribed by the same physician or different physicians.

Two types of drug interactions should be noted:

1. Synergistic interaction. One drug enhances the action of another drug so that the combined effect is greater than the sum of the effects of each used alone.

2. Antagonistic interaction. One drug represses the action of another drug.

To properly code drug interactions, first code the manifestation. Then code each drug involved in the interaction using the E codes from the column labeled "Therapeutic Use" from the Table of Drugs and Chemicals.

Coding Example

Gastritis due to interaction between Motrin and Procainamide

535.50 Unspecified gastritis and gastroduodenitis

List the manifestation first

E935.8 Other specified analgesics and antipyretics

E942.0 Cardiac rhythm regulators

Coding Example

When a diagnostic statement does not state specifically the manifestation or nature of the adverse reaction, you should use the code provided to identify an adverse drug reaction of unspecified nature, 995.2 *Unspecified adverse effect of drug, medicinal and biological substance.* For example:

Allergic reaction to Motrin, proper dose

995.2 Unspecified adverse effect of drug, medicinal and biological substance

E935.8 Other specified analgesics and antipyretics

Note in the above example that the code indicating the manifestation, although unspecified as to the nature, is listed first followed by the E code to identify the drug. When the drug causing an adverse effect is unknown or unspecified, use code E947.9 *Unspecified drug or medicinal substance.*

It is very important to remember that codes in the range 960 through 979 are never used in combination with codes in the range E930 through E949 because codes in the range 960-979 identify poisonings and codes in the range E930-E949 identify the external cause of adverse reactions to the correct substance properly administered.

CODING COMPLICATIONS OF MEDICAL AND SURGICAL CARE

A complication is when you have the occurrence of two or more diseases in the same patient. Recent studies have revealed serious deficiencies in properly coding complications for insurance claims processing. Often the complication is never mentioned. Complications are responsible for many of the procedures that are ordered for patients, therefore the complication should be coded and submitted on your insurance claims.

Postoperative complications that affect a specific anatomical site or body system are classified to the appropriate Chapter 1 through 16 of the Tabular Index (Volume 1). Postoperative complications affecting more than one anatomical site or body system are classified in the chapter on injury and poisoning (Chapter 17, Categories 996-999). If the Alphabetic Index (Volume 2) does not provide a specific main term and subterm to identify a postoperative complication, classify the complication to categories 996-999.

Coding Example

Postcholecystectomy syndrome

576.0   Postcholecystectomy syndrome

The Alphabetic Index (Volume 2) specifically classifies the postoperative condition to one of the categories from 001 through 799. See main term "Complication," subterms "surgical procedure" and "postcholecystectomy syndrome."

Coding Examples

Postoperative wound infection

998.5   Postoperative infection

The Alphabetic Index (Volume 2) has a main term "Infection" and subterms "wound, postoperative" for this condition. Note that this code appears in Chapter 17 within categories 996-999.

Postoperative atelectasis

997.3   Respiratory complications

Refer to the main term "Atelectasis" in the Alphabetic Index (Volume 2). Note there is no subterm for postoperative beneath this main term. Therefore, you must presume this complication is classified to one of the categories in the range 969-999. You may also code 518.0 *Pulmonary collapse*, to identify the nature of the respiratory complication for statistical purposes; however, the code for the complication must be listed first.

Complications From Mechanical Devices

Subcategories in the range 996.0 through 996.5 are used to identify mechanical complications of devices. Mechanical complications are the result of a malfunction on the part of the internal prosthetic implant or device. What indicates a mechanical complication? Breakdown or obstruction, displacement, leakage, perforation or protrusion of the devices are all forms of mechanical complications.

Coding Examples

Displacement of cardiac pacemaker electrode

> **996.01 Mechanical complication of cardiac device, implant, and graft due to cardiac pacemaker (electrode)**

Protrusion of nail into acetabulum

> **996.4 Mechanical complication of internal orthopedic device, implant, and graft**

Other complications of devices, such as infection or hemorrhage, are due to an abnormal reaction of the body to an otherwise properly functioning device. All complications involving infection are coded to category 996.7 *Other complications of internal prosthetic device, implant and graft.*

Coding Examples

Infected arteriovenous shunt

> **996.6 Infection and inflammatory reaction due to internal prosthetic device, implant, and graft**

Anterior chamber hemorrhage due to displaced prosthetic lens

> **996.7 Other complications of internal (biological) (synthetic) prosthetic device, implant, and graft**

Cardiac Complications

In the case of cardiac complications, ICD-9-CM defines the "immediate postoperative period" as "the period between surgery and the time of discharge from the hospital." This definition is the basis of whether to code cardiac complications under subcategory 997.1 *Cardiac complications affecting specified body systems, not elsewhere classified*, or under subcategory 429.4 *Functional disturbances following cardiac surgery.*

Use 997.1 for a cardiac complication that occurs anytime between surgery and hospital discharge from any type of procedure performed. Use subcategory 429.4 to code long-term cardiac complications resulting from cardiac surgery.

It is important to distinguish between complications and aftercare. Aftercare is usually an encounter for something planned in advance (example, removal of Kirshner wire). Aftercare is classified using codes in the range of V51-V58. An encounter for a complication occurs from unforeseen circumstances, such as wound infection, resulting in complication of the patient's condition.

Transplant Complications

1. **Transplant complications other than kidney:** Codes under subcategory 996.8, *Complications of transplanted organ,* are for use for both complications and rejection of transplanted organs. A transplant complication code is only assigned if the complication affects the function of the transplanted organ. Two codes are required to fully describe a transplant complication, the appropriate code from subcategory 996.8 and a secondary code that identifies the complication.

    Pre-existing conditions or conditions that develop after the transplant are not coded as complications unless they affect the function of the transplanted organs.

    Post-transplants surgical complications that do not relate to the function of the transplanted organ are classified to the specific complication. For example, a surgical wound dehiscence would be coded to the wound dehiscence, not as a transplant complication.

    Post-transplant patients who are seen for treatment unrelated to the transplanted organ should be assigned a code from category V42, *Organ or tissue replaced by transplant,* to identify the transplant status of the patient. A code from category V42 should never be used with a code from subcategory 996.8.

2. **Kidney transplant and chronic kidney disease:** Patients with chronic kidney disease (CKD) following a transplant should not be assumed to have transplant failure or rejection unless it is documented by the provider. If documentation supports the presence of failure or rejection, then it is appropriate to assign code 996.81, *Complications of tranplanted organs, kidney,* followed by the appropriate CKD code.

SPECIAL CODING SITUATIONS

As you become an experienced coder you will encounter situations where the standard rules do not seem to apply, or which require a special understanding in order to code properly. These situations include coding of circulatory diseases, diabetes, mental disorders, infectious diseases, manifestations, neoplasms, and pregnancy and childbirth. The following sections address these specific special coding situations.

CODING DISEASES OF BLOOD AND BLOOD FORMING ORGANS

Subcategory 285.2, *Anemia in chronic illness,* has codes for anemia in chronic kidney disease, code 285.21; anemia in neoplastic disease, code 285.22; and anemia in other chronic illness, code 285.29. These codes can be used as the principal/first listed code if the reason for the encounter is to treat the anemia. They may also be used as secondary codes if treatment of the anemia is a component of an encounter, but not the primary reason for the encounter. When using a code from subcategory 285, it is also necessary to use the code for the chronic condition causing the anemia.

1. When assigning code 285.21, *Anemia in chronic kidney disease,* it is also necessary to assign a code from category 585, *Chronic kidney disease,* to indicate the stage of chronic kidney disease.

2.   When assigning code 285.22, *Anemia in neoplastic disease*, it is also necessary to assign the neoplasm code that is responsible for the anemia. Code 285.22 is for use for anemia that is due to the malignancy, not for anemia due to antineoplastic chemotherapy drugs, which is an adverse effect.

CODING CIRCULATORY DISEASES

Because of the variety of terms and phrases used by physicians to identify diseases of the circulatory system, you will often experience difficulty in coding. To accurately code disorders of the circulatory system, it is imperative that the coder carefully read all inclusion, exclusion and "use additional code" notations contained in the Tabular List (Volume 1).

Fifth digit subclassifications are also frequently used to code combination disorders or to provide further specificity in this section. Even those in specialties other than cardiology will frequently find themselves coding circulatory system diagnoses due to the prevalence of circulatory disorders in this country.

Chapter 7 of the Tabular List (Volume 1), titled Diseases of the Circulatory System, contains the following major sections:

Acute Rheumatic Fever (390-392)

Chronic Rheumatic Heart Disease (393-398)

Hypertensive Disease (401-405)

Ischemic Heart Disease (410-414)

Diseases of Pulmonary Circulation (415-417)

Other Forms of Heart Disease (420-429)

Cerebrovascular Disease (430-438)

Diseases of Arteries, Arterioles, and Capillaries (440-448)

Diseases of Veins, Lymphatics, and Other Diseases of the Circulatory System (451-459)

Diseases of Mitral and Aortic Valves

Certain diseases of the mitral valve of unspecified etiology are presumed to be of rheumatic origin and others are not. None of the disorders of the aortic valve of unspecified etiology are presumed to be of rheumatic origin. When you have disorders involving both the mitral and aortic valves of unspecified etiology, then they are presumed to be of rheumatic origin.

Coding Examples

Mitral valve insufficiency

    424.0   Mitral valve disorders

Refer to the main term "Insufficiency" in the Alphabetic Index (Volume 2). Note the subterm "mitral (valve)."

Mitral valve stenosis

394.0   Mitral stenosis

Refer to the main term "Stenosis" and the sub-term "mitral (valve)" in the Alphabetic Index (Volume 2).

Aortic valve insufficiency

424.1   Aortic valve disorders

Aortic valve stenosis

424.1   Aortic valve disorders

Look up the main term "Stenosis" and the subterm "aortic" in the Alphabetic Index (Volume 2). Remember that aortic valve disorders of unspecified etiology are not considered rheumatic in nature or origin.

Insufficiency of mitral and aortic valves

396.3   Mitral valve insufficiency and aortic valve insufficiency

Under the main term "Insufficiency" in the Alphabetic Index (Volume 2) you will find the subterm "aortic." Further review will locate "with," "mitral valve disease," "insufficiency, incompetence or regurgitation" which directs you to code 396.3.

Ischemic Heart Disease

In ischemic heart disease, the manifestations are due to a lack of blood flow to the heart rather than to the anatomical lesion of the coronary arteries. The most common cause of coronary heart disease is coronary atherosclerosis. However, ischemic heart disease can be due to non-coronary disease, such as aortic valvular stenosis, as well. There are many synonyms used to indicate ischemic heart disease such as: coronary artery heart disease, ASHD, and coronary ischemia. Categories in the range 410-414, Ischemic Heart Disease, includes that with mention of hypertension. Use an additional code to identify the presence of hypertension.

Coding Examples

Angina pectoris

413.9   Other and unspecified angina pectoris

As no mention of hypertension is made in the diagnostic statement, a single code is all that is required.

Angina pectoris with essential hypertension

413.9   Other and unspecified angina pectoris

401.9   Essential hypertension, unspecified

In this example, the mention of hypertension in the diagnostic statement requires the use of a second code.

Myocardial Infarction

A myocardial infarction is classified as acute if it is either specified as "acute" in the diagnostic statement or with a stated duration of eight weeks or less. When a myocardial infarction is specified as "chronic" or with symptoms after eight weeks from the date of the onset, it should be coded to subcategory 414.8 *Other specified forms of chronic ischemic heart disease.* If a myocardial infarction is specified as old or healed or has been diagnosed by special investigation (EKG) but is currently not presenting any symptoms, code using category 412 *Old myocardial infarction.*

1. The ICD-9-CM codes for acute myocardial infarction (AMI) identify the site, such as anterolateral wall or true posterior wall. Subcategories 410.0-410.6 and 410.8 are used for ST elevation myocardial infarction (STEMI). Subcategory 410.7, *Subendocardial infarction,* is used for non-ST elevation myocardial infarction (NSTEMI) and nontransmural MIs.

2. Subcategory 410.9 is the default for the unspecified term acute myocardial infarction. If only STEMI or transmural MI without the site is documented, query the provider as to the site, or assign a code from subcategory 410.9.

3. If an AMI is documented as nontransmural or subendocardial, but the site is provided, it is still coded as a subendocardial AMI. If NSTEMI evolves to STEMI, assign the STEMI code. If STEMI converts to NSTEMI due to thrombolytic therapy, it is still coded as STEMI.

Coding Examples

Myocardial infarction three weeks ago

410.92   Acute myocardial infarction, unspecified site

Chronic myocardial infarction with angina

414.8   Other specified forms of chronic ischemic heart disease

413.9   Other and unspecified angina pectoris

Myocardial infarction diagnoses by EKG, symptomatic

412   Old myocardial infarction

Arteriosclerotic Cardiovascular Disease (ASCVD)

Arteriosclerotic cardiovascular disease (ASCVD) is classified to subcategory 429.2 *Cardiovascular disease, unspecified.* You should use an additional code to identify the presence of arteriosclerosis when coding ASCVD. For example, the diagnostic statement "generalized arteriosclerotic cardiovascular disease" should be coded using 429.2 followed by 440.9 *Generalized and unspecified atherosclerosis.*

"Other forms of heart disease," categories 420-429, are used for multiple coding purposes to fully identify a stated diagnosis. The exception to this rule is if the Alphabetic Index (Volume 2) or Tabular List (Volume 1) specifically instructs you otherwise.

Coding Examples

Arteriosclerotic heart disease with acute pulmonary edema

> **428.1   Left heart failure**

> **414.00   Coronary atherosclerosis, of unspecified type of vessel, native or graft**

Note that the code for ASHD (414.00) is listed second as a possible underlying cause of the acute situation.

Arteriosclerotic heart disease with congestive heart failure

> **428.0   Congestive heart failure, unspecified**

> **414.00   Coronary atherosclerosis, of unspecified type of vessel, native or graft**

Cerebrovascular Disease

When coding cerebrovascular disease (codes 430-438), you should code the component parts of the diagnostic statement identifying the cerebrovascular disease, unless specifically instructed to do otherwise in the Alphabetic Index (Volume 2) or Tabular List (Volume 1).

Coding Examples

Cerebrovascular arteriosclerosis with subarachnoid hemorrhage

> **430   Subarachnoid hemorrhage**

> **437.0   Cerebral atherosclerosis**

Cerebrovascular accident secondary to thrombosis

> **434.00   Cerebral thrombosis, without mention of cerebral infarction**

In this example, you use only one code because of the instructions in the Alphabetic Index (Volume 2). When you look up the main term "Accident" with subterm "cerebrovascular," you are instructed to "(see also Disease, cerebrovascular, acute) 436." When you locate the main term "Disease" and subterms "cerebrovascular," "acute" and "thrombotic," you are further instructed to "see Thrombosis, brain." This is where you finally locate the single code for this diagnosis, 434.0. When you look up the code in the Tabular List (Volume 1), you are instructed to add a fifth digit "0" if it is without mention of cerebral infarction, and "1" if it is with cerebral infarction.

Whenever there are conditions resulting from the acute cerebrovascular disease, code them if they are stated to be residual(s). If the resulting condition is stated to be transient, do not code them.

Coding Examples

Cerebrovascular accident with residual aphasia

436   Acute, but ill-defined, cerebrovascular disease

784.3   Aphasia

Cerebrovascular accident with transient hemiparesis

436   Acute, but ill-defined, cerebrovascular disease

Cerebral Infarction/Stroke/Cerebrovascular Accident (CVA)

The terms stroke and CVA are often used interchangeably to refer to a cerebral infarction. The terms stroke, CVA, and cerebral infarction NOS are all indexed to the default code 434.91, *Cerebral artery occlusion, unspecified, with infarction.* Code 436, *Acute, but ill-defined, cerebrovascular disease,* should not be used when the documentation states stroke or CVA.

A cerebrovascular hemorrhage or infarction that occurs as a result of medical intervention is coded to 997.02, *Iatrogenic cerebrovascular infarction or hemorrhage.* Medical record documentation should clearly specify the cause-and-effect relationship between the medical intervention and the cerebrovascular accident in order to assign this code. A secondary code from the code range 430-432 or from a code from subcategories 433 or 434 with a fifth digit of "1" should also be used to identify the type of hemorrhage or infarct.

This guideline conforms to the use additional code note instruction at category 997. Code 436, *Acute, but ill-defined, cerebrovascular disease,* should not be used as a secondary code with code 997.02.

Late Effects of Cerebrovascular Disease

Category 438 is used to indicate conditions classifiable to categories 430-437 as the causes of late effects (neurologic deficits), themselves classified elsewhere. These late effects include neurologic deficits that persist after initial onset of conditions classifiable to 430-437. The neurologic deficits caused by cerebrovascular disease may be present from the onset or may arise at any time after the onset of the condition classifiable to 430-437.

Codes from category 438 may be assigned on a health care record with codes from 430-437, if the patient has a current cerebrovascular accident (CVA) and deficits from an old CVA. Assign code V12.59 (and not a code from category 438) as an additional code for history of cerebrovascular disease when no neurologic deficits are present.

Hypertensive Disease

As demonstrated earlier with ischemic heart disease, conditions that are classified to cerebrovascular disease (codes 430-438) include that with mention of hypertension, but you must identify the hypertension with another code (401-405) and list it second.

Hypertension is frequently the cause of various forms of heart and vascular disease. However, the mention of hypertension with some heart conditions should not be interpreted as a combination resulting in hypertensive heart disease. The combination is only to be made if there is a cause-and-effect relationship between hypertension and a heart condition classified to subcategories 425.8, 428.0-428.9, 429.0-429.3 and 429.8-429.9.

Hypertensive disease is classified to the categories 401-405. The Table of Hypertension is located in the Alphabetic Index (Volume 2) under the main term "Hypertension." This Table contains subterms to identify types of hypertension and complications. It contains a complete listing of all conditions due to or associated with hypertension and classifies them according to malignant, benign, and unspecified.

1. Hypertension, Essential or NOS

    Assign hypertension (arterial) (essential) (primary) (systemic) (NOS) to category code 401 with the appropriate fourth digit to indicate malignant (.0), benign (.1), or unspecified (.9). Do not use either .0 malignant or .1 benign unless medical record documentation supports such a designation.

2. Hypertension with Heart Disease

    Heart conditions (425.8, 429.0-429.3, 429.8, 429.9) are assigned to a code from category 402 when a causal relationship is stated (due to hypertension) or implied (hypertensive). Use an additional code from category 428 to identify the type of heart failure in those patients with heart failure. More than one code from category 428 may be assigned if the patient has systolic or diastolic failure and congestive heart failure.

    The same heart conditions (425.8, 429.0-429.3, 429.8, 429.9) with hypertension, but without a stated causal relationship, are coded separately. Sequence according to the circumstances of the admission/encounter.

3. Hypertensive Kidney Disease

    Assign codes from category 403, *Hypertensive kidney disease*, when conditions classified to categories 585-587 are present. Unlike hypertension with heart disease, ICD-9-CM presumes a cause-and-effect relationship and classifies renal failure with hypertension as hypertensive kidney disease.

4. Hypertensive Heart and Kidney Disease

    Assign codes from combination category 404, *Hypertensive heart and kidney disease*, when both hypertensive kidney disease and hypertensive heart disease are stated in the diagnosis. Assume a relationship between the hypertension and the kidney disease, whether or not the condition is so designated. Assign an additional code from category 428, to identify the type of heart failure. More than one code from category 428 may be assigned if the patient has systolic or diastolic failure and congestive heart failure.

5. Hypertensive Cerebrovascular Disease

    First assign codes from 430-438, *Cerebrovascular disease*, then the appropriate hypertension code from categories 401-405.

6.   Hypertensive Retinopathy

Two codes are necessary to identify the condition. First assign the code from subcategory 362.11, *Hypertensive retinopathy*, then the appropriate code from categories 401-405 to indicate the type of hypertension.

7.   Hypertension, Secondary

Two codes are required: one to identify the underlying etiology and one from category 405 to identify the hypertension. Sequencing of codes is determined by the reason for admission/encounter.

8.   Hypertension, Transient

Assign code 796.2, *Elevated blood pressure reading without diagnosis of hypertension*, unless patient has an established diagnosis of hypertension. Assign code 642.3x for transient hypertension of pregnancy.

9.   Hypertension, Controlled

Assign appropriate code from categories 401-405. This diagnostic statement usually refers to an existing state of hypertension under control by therapy.

10.   Hypertension, Uncontrolled

Uncontrolled hypertension may refer to untreated hypertension or hypertension not responding to current therapeutic regimen. In either case, assign the appropriate code from categories 401-405 to designate the stage and type of hypertension. Code to the type of hypertension.

11.   Elevated Blood Pressure

For a statement of elevated blood pressure without further specificity, assign code 796.2, *Elevated blood pressure reading without diagnosis of hypertension*, rather than a code from category 401.

First you need to be able to make a distinction between conditions specified as "due to" or "with" hypertension. Keep in mind that the phrase "due to hypertension" and the word "hypertensive" are considered synonymous.

Coding Examples

Hypertensive heart disease

402.90   Hypertensive heart disease, unspecified, without heart failure

Heart disease due to hypertension

402.90   Hypertensive heart disease, unspecified, without heart failure

Each of the above diagnostic statements indicate clearly a cause-and-effect relationship between hypertension and the condition by specifying that the condition is "due to." Therefore, both statements are coded using 402.90.

If the phrase "with hypertension" is stated or, the diagnostic statement mentions the conditions separately, then you code the conditions separately.

Coding Example

Myocarditis with hypertension

> **429.0   Myocarditis, unspecified**
>
> **401.9   Essential hypertension, unspecified**

As a cause-and-effect relationship is not indicated in the diagnostic statement, the conditions are coded separately.

High Blood Pressure Versus Elevated Blood Pressure

With the ICD-9-CM coding system there is a differentiation made between high blood pressure (hypertension) and elevated blood pressure without a diagnosis of hypertension. If the diagnostic statement indicates elevated blood pressure without the diagnosis of hypertension, it is coded to subcategory 796.2 *Elevated blood pressure reading without diagnosis of hypertension.* If the diagnostic statement indicates high blood pressure or hypertension, it is coded to category 401 *Essential hypertension.*

DISEASES OF THE RESPIRATORY SYSTEM

Chronic Obstructive Pulmonary Disease [COPD] and Asthma

1. Conditions that comprise COPD and asthma

    The conditions that comprise COPD are obstructive chronic bronchitis, subcategory 491.2, and emphysema, category 492. All asthma codes are under category 493, *Asthma.* Code 496, *Chronic airway obstruction, not elsewhere classified,* is a nonspecific code that should be used only when the documentation in a medical record does not specify the type of COPD being treated.

2. Acute exacerbation of chronic obstructive bronchitis and asthma

    The codes for chronic obstructive bronchitis and asthma distinguish between uncomplicated cases and those in acute exacerbation. An acute exacerbation is a worsening or a decompensation of a chronic condition. An acute exacerbation is not equivalent to an infection superimposed on a chronic condition, though an exacerbation may be triggered by an infection.

3. Overlapping nature of the conditions that comprise COPD and asthma

    Due to the overlapping nature of the conditions that make up COPD and asthma, there are many variations in the way these conditions are documented. Code selection must be based on the terms as documented. When selecting the correct code for the documented type of COPD and asthma, it is essential to first review the index and then verify the code in the tabular list. There are many instructional notes under the different COPD subcategories and codes. It is important that all such notes be reviewed to assure correct code assignment.

4.   Acute exacerbation of asthma and status asthmaticus

An acute exacerbation of asthma is an increased severity of the asthma symptoms, such as wheezing and shortness of breath. Status asthmaticus refers to a patient's failure to respond to therapy administered during an asthmatic episode and is a life-threatening complication that requires emergency care. If status asthmaticus is documented by the provider with any type of COPD or with acute bronchitis, the status asthmaticus should be sequenced first. It supersedes any type of COPD including that with acute exacerbation or acute bronchitis. It is inappropriate to assign an asthma code with fifth-digit 2, with acute exacerbation, together with an asthma code with fifth-digit 1, with status asthmatics. Only the fifth-digit 1 should be assigned.

Chronic Obstructive Pulmonary Disease [COPD] and Bronchitis

Acute bronchitis, code 466.0, is due to an infectious organism. When acute bronchitis is documented with COPD, code 491.22, *Obstructive chronic bronchitis with acute bronchitis,* should be assigned. It is not necessary to also assign code 466.0. If a medical record documents acute bronchitis with COPD with acute exacerbation, only code 491.22 should be assigned. The acute bronchitis included in code 491.22 supersedes the acute exacerbation. If a medical record documents COPD with acute exacerbation without mention of acute bronchitis, only code 491.21 should be assigned.

DIABETES MELLITUS CODING (250)

Diabetes mellitus codes under category 250, *Diabetes mellitus,* identify complications/manifestations associated with diabetes mellitus. A fifth digit is required for all category 250 codes to identify the type of diabetes mellitus and whether the diabetes is controlled or uncontrolled.

1.   The following are the fifth digits for the codes under category 250:

0   type II or unspecified type, not stated as uncontrolled

1   type I, [juvenile type], not stated as uncontrolled

2   type II or unspecified type, uncontrolled

3   type I, [juvenile type], uncontrolled

The age of a patient is not the sole determining factor, though most type I diabetics develop the condition before reaching puberty. For this reason type I diabetes mellitus is also referred to as juvenile diabetes.

2.   If the type of diabetes mellitus is not documented in the medical record, the default is type II.

3.   All type I diabetics must use insulin to replace what their bodies do not produce. However, the use of insulin does not mean that a patient is a type I diabetic. Some patients with type II diabetes mellitus are unable to control their blood sugar through diet and oral medication alone and do require insulin. If the documentation in a medical record does not indicate the type of diabetes but does indicate that the patient uses insulin, the appropriate fifth digit for type II must be used. For type II patients who routinely use insulin, code V58.67, *Long-term (current) use of insulin*, should also be assigned to

indicate that the patient uses insulin. Code V58.67 should not be assigned if insulin is given temporarily to bring a type II patient's blood sugar under control during an encounter.

4.　　When assigning codes for diabetes and its associated conditions, the code(s) from category 250 must be sequenced before the codes for the associated conditions. The diabetes codes and the secondary codes that correspond to them are paired codes that follow the etiology/manifestation convention of the classification (see Section I.A.6., Etiology/manifestation convention). Assign as many codes from category 250 as needed to identify all of the associated conditions that the patient has. The corresponding secondary codes are listed under each of the diabetes codes.

A.　Diabetic retinopathy/diabetic macular edema

Diabetic macular edema, code 362.07, is only present with diabetic retinopathy. Another code from subcategory 362.0, *Diabetic retinopathy*, must be used with code 362.07. Codes under subcategory 362.0 are diabetes manifestation codes, so they must be used following the appropriate diabetes codes.

5.　　Insulin pump malfunction is handled as follows:

A.　Underdose of insulin due to insulin pump failure

An underdose of insulin due to an insulin pump failure should be assigned 996.57, *Mechanical complication due to insulin pump*, as the principal or first listed code, followed by the appropriate diabetes mellitus code based on documentation.

B.　Overdose of insulin due to insulin pump failure

The principal or first listed code for an encounter due to an insulin pump malfunction resulting in an overdose of insulin should also be 996.57, *Mechanical complication due to insulin pump*, followed by code 962.3, *Poisoning by insulins and antidiabetic agents*, and the appropriate diabetes mellitus code based on documentation.

Do not assume a patient has insulin-dependent diabetes simply because the patient is receiving insulin, as some non-dependent diabetics may require temporary use when they encounter stressful situations such as surgery or physical or mental illness.

Anytime diabetes is described as "brittle" or "uncontrolled" you should interpret it as diabetes mellitus complicated and assign code 250.9 with the appropriate fifth-digit, 0, 1, 2 or 3. However, if there is also a specific complication present, then assign the code identifying that specific complication, for example, Diabetes mellitus, brittle, with ketoacidosis would be 250.13.

CODING MENTAL DISORDERS

You should be aware of the existence of the glossary of mental disorders in Appendix B of the Tabular List (Volume 1). This glossary is not used for coding purposes but rather as a guide to provide a common frame of reference for statistical comparisons. It is simply an alphabetized listing of mental disorders with definitions.

The coder should choose code assignments based on the terminology used by the physician or psychiatrist and not by the coder's impression of the content of the categories and subcategories. The chapter on mental disorders has many fifth digit subclassifications to watch for when selecting your code.

INFECTIOUS AND PARASITIC DISEASES

There are two categories for identifying the organism causing diseases classified elsewhere. These codes may be used as either additional codes, or as solo codes depending on the diagnostic statement.

041   **Bacterial infection in conditions classified elsewhere and of unspecified site**

079   **Viral and chlamydial infection in conditions classified elsewhere and of unspecified site**

Coding Examples

Acute UTI due to Escherichia coli

599.0   **Urinary tract infection, site not specified**

041.4   **Escherichia coli [E. coli]**

Staphylococcus infection

041.11 **Staphylococcus aureus**

Bacterial infection

041.9   **Bacterial infection, unspecified**

The basic coding principles regarding combination codes (one code accurately identifies the components of the condition) applies throughout the chapter on Infectious and Parasitic Diseases.

In the Alphabetic Index (Volume 2), a subterm that identifies an infectious organism takes precedence in code assignment over a subterm at the same indentation level that identifies a site or other descriptive term.

Coding Example

Chronic syphilitic cystitis

095.8   **Other specified forms of late symptomatic syphilis**

Using the Alphabetic Index (Volume 2) to look up the main term "Cystitis (bacillary)," you will note the subterms "chronic 595.2" and "syphilitic 095.8" at the same indentation level under the main term. Therefore, code 095.8 is assigned to this diagnostic statement, as the organism has precedence over other descriptive terms or anatomical sites.

Human Immunodeficiency Virus (HIV) Disease

1. Code only confirmed cases of HIV infection/illness. This is an exception to the hospital inpatient guideline Section II, H.

    In this context, confirmation does not require documentation of positive serology or culture for HIV; the physician's diagnostic statement that the patient is HIV positive, or has an HIV-related illness is sufficient.

2. Selection and sequencing

    A. If a patient is admitted for an HIV-related condition, the principal diagnosis should be 042, followed by additional diagnosis codes for all reported HIV-related conditions.

    B. If a patient with HIV disease is admitted for an unrelated condition (such as a traumatic injury), the code for the unrelated condition (e.g., the nature of injury code) should be the principal diagnosis. Other diagnoses would be 042 followed by additional diagnosis codes for all reported HIV-related conditions.

    C. Whether the patient is newly diagnosed or has had previous admissions/ encounters for HIV conditions is irrelevant to the sequencing decision.

    D. V08 *Asymptomatic human immunodeficiency virus [HIV] infection status*, is to be applied when the patient without any documentation of symptoms is listed as being HIV positive, known HIV, HIV test positive, or similar terminology. Do not use this code if the term AIDS is used or if the patient is treated for any HIV-related illness or is described as having any condition(s) resulting from his/her HIV positive status; use 042 instead.

    E. Patients with inconclusive HIV serology, but no definitive diagnosis or manifestations of the illness, may be assigned code 795.71, *Nonspecific serologic evidence of human immunodeficiency virus [HIV]*.

    F. Previously diagnosed HIV-related illness: Patients with any known prior diagnosis of an HIV-related illness should be coded to 042. Once a patient had developed an HIV-related illness, the patient should always be assigned code 042 on every subsequent admission/encounter. Patients previously diagnosed with any HIV illness (042) should never be assigned to 795.71 or V08.

    G. HIV Infection in Pregnancy, Childbirth and the Puerperium: During pregnancy, childbirth or the puerperium, a patient admitted (or presenting for a health care encounter) because of an HIV-related illness should receive a principal diagnosis of 647.6X, *Other viral diseases in the mother classifiable elsewhere, but complicating the pregnancy, childbirth or the puerperium*, followed by 042 and the code(s) for the HIV-related illness(es). Codes from Chapter 11 *Pregnancy, Childbirth and the Puerperium* always take sequencing priority.

        Patients with asymptomatic HIV infection status admitted (or presenting for a health care encounter) during pregnancy, childbirth, or the puerperium should receive codes of 647.6X and V08.

H. Encounters for Testing for HIV: If a patient is being seen to determine his/her HIV status, use code V73.89, *Screening for other specified viral disease*. Use code V69.8, *Other problems related to lifestyle*, as a secondary code if an asymptomatic patient is in a known high risk group for HIV. Should a patient with signs or symptoms or illness, or a confirmed HIV related diagnosis be tested for HIV, code the signs and symptoms or the diagnosis. An additional code V65.44 *HIV counseling* may be used if counseling is provided during the encounter for the test.

When a patient returns to be informed of his/her HIV test results use code V65.44, *HIV counseling*, if the results of the test are negative.

If the results are positive but the patient is asymptomatic use code V08, *Asymptomatic HIV infection*. If the results are positive and the patient is symptomatic use code 042, *HIV disease*, with codes for the HIV related symptoms or diagnosis. The HIV counseling code may also be used if counseling is provided for patients with positive test results.

Septicemia, Systemic Inflammatory Response Syndrome (SIRS), Sepsis, Severe Sepsis and Septic Shock

1. Sepsis may be coded as a principal diagnosis or secondary diagnosis.

    A. If sepsis is present on admission, and meets the definition of principal diagnosis, the underlying systemic infection code (e.g., 038.xx, 112.5, etc.) should be assigned as the principal diagnosis, followed by code 995.91, Systemic inflammatory response syndrome due to infectious process without organ dysfunction, as required by the sequencing rules in the Tabular List. Codes from subcategory 995.9 can never be assigned as a principal diagnosis.

    B. When sepsis develops during the encounter (it was not present on admission), the sepsis codes may be assigned as secondary diagnoses, following the sequencing rules provided in the Tabular List.

    C. If the documentation is not clear whether the sepsis was present on admission, the provider should be queried. After provider query, if sepsis is determined at that point to have met the definition of principal diagnosis, the underlying systemic infection (038.xx, 112.5, etc.) may be used as principal diagnosis along with code 995.91, *Systemic inflammatory response syndrome due to infectious process without organ dysfunction*.

2. In most cases, it will be a code from category 038 *Septicemia* that will be used in conjunction with a code from subcategory 995.9.

    A. If the documentation in the record states streptococcal sepsis, codes 038.0 and code 995.91 should be used, in that sequence.

    B. If the documentation states streptococcal septicemia, only code 038.0 should be assigned, however, the physician should be queried whether the patient has sepsis, and infection with SIRS.

    C. Either the term sepsis or SIRS must be documented to assign a code from subcategory 995.9.

3. If the terms sepsis, severe sepsis, or SIRS are used with an underlying infection other than septicemia, such as pneumonia, cellulitis or a nonspecified urinary tract infection, code 038.9 should be assigned first, then code 995.91, followed by the code for the initial infection. The use of the terms sepsis or SIRS indicates that the patient's infection has advanced to the point of a systemic infection so the systemic infection should be sequenced before the localized infection. The instructional note under subcategory 995.9 instructs to assign the underlying condition first.

    Note: The term urosepsis is a nonspecific term. If that is the only term documented then only code 599.0 should be assigned based on the default for the term in the ICD-9-CM index, in addition to the code for the causal organism if known.

4. For patients with severe sepsis, the code for the systemic infection (038.x) or trauma should be sequenced first, followed by either code 995.92 *Systemic inflammatory response syndrome due to infectious process with organ dysfunction*, or code 995.94 *Systemic inflammatory response syndrome due to noninfectious process with organ dysfunction*. Codes for the specific organ dysfunction should also be assigned.

5. Documentation of septic shock is handled as follows:

    A. Septic shock is a form of organ dysfunction associated with severe sepsis. A code for the initiating underlying systemic infection followed by a code for SIRS (code 995.92) must be assigned before the code for septic shock. As noted in the sequencing instructions in the Tabular List, the code for septic shock cannot be assigned as a principal diagnosis.

    B. Septic shock cannot occur in the absence of severe sepsis. A code from subcategory 995.9 must be sequenced before the code for septic shock. The use additional code notes and the code first note provide sequencing instructions.

6. Sepsis and septic shock associated with abortion, ectopic pregnancy, and molar pregnancy are classified to category codes in Chapter 11 (630-639).

7. Negative or inconclusive blood cultures do not preclude a diagnosis of septicemia or sepsis in patients with clinical evidence of the condition, however, the physician should be queried.

8. Sepsis resulting from a postprocedural infection is a complication of care. For such cases code 998.59, *Other postoperative infections*, should be coded first followed by the appropriate codes for the sepsis. The other guidelines for coding sepsis should then be followed for the assignment of additional codes.

9. An external cause code is not needed with codes 995.91, *Systemic inflammatory response syndrome due to infectious process without organ dysfunction*, or code 995.92, *Systemic inflammatory response syndrome due to infectious process with organ dysfunction*.

MANIFESTATIONS

Manifestations are characteristic signs or symptoms of an illness. Signs and symptoms that point rather definitely to a given diagnosis are assigned to the appropriate chapter of ICD-9-CM. For example, hematuria is assigned to the Genitourinary System chapter. However, Chapter 16 *Symptoms, Signs and*

Ill-Defined Conditions (780-799), includes ill-defined conditions and symptoms that may suggest two or more diseases or may point to two or more systems of the body, and are used in cases lacking the necessary study to make a final diagnosis. Conditions allocated to Chapter 16 include:

1. Cases for which no more specific diagnosis can be made even after all facts bearing on the case have been investigated; for example code 784.0 *Headache.*

2. Signs or symptoms existing at the time of initial encounter that proved to be transient and whose cause could not be determined; for example code 780.2 *Syncope and collapse.*

3. Provisional diagnoses in a patient who failed to return for further investigation or care; for example code 782.4 *Jaundice, unspecified, not of newborn.*

4. Cases referred elsewhere for investigation or treatment before the diagnosis was made; for example code 782.5 *Cyanosis.*

5. Cases in which a more precise diagnosis was not available for any other reason; for example code 780.4 *Dizziness and giddiness.*

6. Certain symptoms which represent important problems in medical care and which it might be desired to classify in addition to a known cause; for example, code 780.01 *Coma.*

In the last case, if the cause of a symptom or sign is stated in the diagnosis, assign the code identifying the cause. An additional code may be assigned to further identify this symptom or sign if there is a need to further identify the symptom or sign. In such cases, the code identifying the cause will ordinarily be listed as the principal diagnosis.

Etiology/Manifestation Convention

Certain conditions have both an underlying etiology and multiple body system manifestations. For such conditions, the ICD-9-CM has a coding convention that requires the underlying condition be sequenced first followed by the manifestation. Wherever such a combination exists there is a "Use additional code" note at the etiology code, and a "Code first" note at the manifestation code. These instructional notes indicate the proper sequencing order of the codes, etiology followed by manifestation.

In most cases, the manifestation codes will have "in diseases classified elsewhere" in the code title. Such codes are a component of the etiology/manifestation convention. The code title indicates that it is a manifestation code. The "diseases classified elsewhere" codes are never permitted to be used as first listed or principal diagnosis codes. They must be used in conjunction with an underlying condition code and they must be listed following the underlying condition.

There are manifestation codes that do not have "in diseases classified elsewhere" in their title. For such codes a "Use additional code" note will still be present and the rules for sequencing apply. In addition to the notes in the Tabular Listing, these conditions also have a specific index entry structure. In the alphabetical index, both conditions are listed together with the etiology code first followed by the manifestation codes in [brackets]. The code in brackets is always to be sequenced second.

The most commonly used etiology/manifestation combinations are the codes for *Diabetes mellitus,* category 250. For each code under category 250 there is a "Use additional code" note for the manifestation that is specific for that particular diabetic manifestation. Should a patient have more than one manifestation of diabetes, more than one code from category 250 may be used with as many manifestation codes as are needed to fully describe the patient's complete diabetic condition. The diabetes category 250 codes should be sequenced first, followed by the manifestation codes.

"Code first" and "Use additional code" notes are also used as sequencing rules in the classification for certain codes that are not part of an etiology/manifestation combination.

CODING OF NEOPLASMS

General Guidelines

Chapter 2 of the ICD-9-CM contains the codes for most benign and all malignant neoplasms. Certain benign neoplasms, such as prostatic adenomas, may be found in the specific body system chapters. To properly code a neoplasm it is necessary to determine from the record if the neoplasm is benign, in-situ, malignant, or of uncertain histologic behavior. If malignant, any secondary (metastatic) sites should also be determined.

The Neoplasm Table in the Alphabetic Index should be referenced first. However, if the histological term is documented, that term should be referenced first, rather than going immediately to the Neoplasm Table, in order to determine which column in the Neoplasm Table is appropriate. For example, if the documentation indicates "adenoma," refer to the term in the Alphabetic Index to review the entries under this term and the instructional note to "see also neoplasm, by site, benign." The table provides the proper code based on the type of neoplasm and the site. It is important to select the proper column in the table that corresponds to the type of neoplasm. The tabular should then be referenced to verify that the correct code has been selected from the table and that a more specific site code does not exist.

1.   If the treatment is directed at the malignancy, designate the malignancy as the principal diagnosis.

2.   When a patient is admitted because of a primary neoplasm with metastasis and treatment is directed toward the secondary site only, the secondary neoplasm is designated as the principal diagnosis even though the primary malignancy is still present.

3.   Coding and sequencing of complications associated with the malignancies or with the therapy thereof are subject to the following guidelines:

     A. When admission/encounter is for management of an anemia associated with the malignancy, and the treatment is only for anemia, the appropriate anemia code (such as code 285.22, *Anemia in neoplastic disease*) is designated at the principal diagnosis and is followed by the appropriate code(s) for the malignancy.

     Code 285.22 may also be used as a secondary code if the patient suffers from anemia and is being treated for the malignancy.

B. When the admission/encounter is for management of an anemia associated with chemotherapy, immunotherapy or radiotherapy and the only treatment is for the anemia, the anemia is sequenced first followed by code E933.1. The appropriate neoplasm code should be assigned as an additional code.

C. When the admission/encounter is for management of dehydration due to the malignancy or the therapy, or a combination of both, and only the dehydration is being treated (intravenous rehydration), the dehydration is sequenced first, followed by the code(s) for the malignancy.

D. When the admission/encounter is for treatment of a complication resulting from a surgical procedure, designate the complication as the principal or first-listed diagnosis if treatment is directed at resolving the complication.

4. When a primary malignancy has been previously excised or eradicated from its site and there is no further treatment directed to that site and there is no evidence of any existing primary malignancy, a code from category V10, *Personal history of malignant neoplasm*, should be used to indicate the former site of the malignancy. Any mention of extension, invasion, or metastasis to another site is coded as a secondary malignant neoplasm to that site. The secondary site may be the principal or first-listed with the V10 code used as a secondary code.

5. Admissions/encounters involving chemotherapy, immunotherapy and radiation therapy are handled as follows:

A. When an episode of care involves the surgical removal of a neoplasm, primary or secondary site, followed by adjunct chemotherapy or radiation treatment during the same episode of care, the neoplasm code should be assigned as principal or first-listed diagnosis, using codes in the 140-198 series or where appropriate in the 200-203 series.

B. If a patient admission/encounter is solely for the administration of chemotherapy, immunotherapy or radiation therapy, assign code V58.0, *Encounter for radiation therapy*, or V58.11, *Encounter for antineoplastic chemotherapy*, or V58.12, *Encounter for antineoplastic immunotherapy*, as the first-listed or principal diagnosis. If a patient receives more than one of these therapies during the same admission, more than one of these codes may be assigned, in any sequence.

C. When a patient is admitted for the purpose of radiotherapy, immunotherapy or chemotherapy and develops complications such as uncontrolled nausea and vomiting or dehydration, the principal or first-listed diagnosis is V58.0, *Encounter for radiotherapy*, or V58.11, *Encounter for antineoplastic chemotherapy*, or V58.12, *Encounter for antineoplastic immunotherapy*, followed by any codes for the complications.

6. When the reason for admission/encounter is to determine the extent of the malignancy, or for a procedure such as paracentesis or thoracentesis, the primary malignancy or appropriate metastatic site is designated as the principal or first-listed diagnosis, even though chemotherapy or radiotherapy is administered.

7. Symptoms, signs, and ill-defined conditions listed in Chapter 16 characteristic of, or associated with, an existing primary or secondary site malignancy cannot be used to replace the malignancy as principal or first-listed diagnosis, regardless of the number of admissions or encounters for treatment and care of the neoplasm.

8.   For encounters specifically for prophylactic removal of breasts, ovaries, or another organ due to a genetic susceptibility to cancer or a family history of cancer, the principal or first-listed code should be a code from subcategory V50.4, *Prophylactic organ removal,* followed by the appropriate genetic susceptibility code and the appropriate family history code.

   If the patient has a malignancy of one site and is having prophylactic removal of another site to prevent either a new primary malignancy or metastatic disease, a code for the malignancy should also be assigned in addition to a code from subcategory V50.4. A V50.4 code should not be assigned if the patient is having organ removal for treatment of a malignancy, such as the removal of the testes for the treatment of prostate cancer.

The coding of neoplasms requires a good understanding of medical terminology. All neoplasms are classified in the Tabular List (Volume 1) in Chapter 2 *Neoplasms* 140-239 which contains the following broad groups:

140-195   Malignant neoplasms, stated or presumed to be primary, of specified sites, except of lymphatic and hematopoietic tissue

196-198   Malignant neoplasms, stated or presumed to be secondary, of specified sites

199   Malignant neoplasms, without specification of site

200-208   Malignant neoplasms, stated or presumed to be primary of lymphatic and hematopoietic tissue

210-229   Benign neoplasms

230-234   Carcinoma in situ

235-238   Neoplasms of uncertain behavior

239   Neoplasms of unspecified nature

Table of Neoplasms

The Table of Neoplasms appears in the Alphabetic Index (Volume 2) under the main term "Neoplasms." This table gives the code numbers for neoplasms of anatomical site. For each anatomical site there are six possible code numbers according to whether the neoplasm in questions is either:

   Malignant:
      Primary
      Secondary
      Ca in situ
   Benign
   Of uncertain behavior
   Of unspecified nature

Definitions of Site and Behaviors of Neoplasms

Primary

Identifies the stated or presumed site of origin.

Secondary

Identifies site(s) to which the primary site has spread (direct extension) or metastasized by lymphatic spread, invading local blood vessels, or by implantation as tumor cells shed into body cavities.

In-situ

Tumor cells that are undergoing malignant changes but are still confined to the point of origin without invasion of surrounding normal tissue (non-infiltrating, non-invasive or pre-invasive carcinoma).

Benign

Tumor does not invade adjacent structures or spread to distant sites but may displace or exert pressure on adjacent structures.

Of Uncertain Behavior

The pathologist is not able to determine whether the tumor is benign or malignant because some features of each are present.

Of Unspecified Nature

Neither the behavior nor the histological type of tumors are specified in the diagnostic statement. This type of diagnosis may be encountered when the patient has been treated elsewhere and comes in terminally ill without accompanying information, is referred elsewhere for work-up, or no work-up is performed because of advanced age or poor condition of the patient.

Steps to Coding Neoplasms

1. ICD-9-CM disregards classification of neoplasms by histological type (according to tissue origin) with the exception of lymphatic and hematopoietic neoplasms, malignant melanoma of skin, lipoma, and a few common tumors of bone, uterus, ovary, etc. All other tumors are classified by system, organ or site. The existence of these exceptions makes it necessary to first consult the Alphabetic Index (Volume 2) to determine whether a specific code has been assigned to a specified histological type. For example, *Malignant melanoma of skin of scalp* is coded 172.4 although the code specified in the "Malignant: Primary Column" of the Neoplasm Table for skin of scalp is 173.4.

2. The General Alphabetical Index (Volume 2) also provides guidance to the appropriate column for neoplasms which are not assigned a specific code by histological type. For example, if you look up *Lipomyoma, specified site* in the Alphabetic Index (Volume 2), you will find "see Neoplasm, connective tissue, benign."

   The guidance in the Alphabetic Index (Volume 2) can be over-ridden if a descriptor is present. For example, *Malignant adenoma of colon* is coded as 153.9 and not as 211.3 because the adjective "malignant" overrides the entry "adenoma — *see also* Neoplasm, benign."

3. The Neoplasm Table may be consulted directly if a specific neoplasm diagnosis indicates which column of the table is appropriate but does not delineate a specific type of tumor.

4. Sites marked with an asterisk (*), such as buttock NEC* or calf*, should be classified to malignant neoplasm of skin of these sites if the variety of neoplasm is a squamous cell carcinoma or an epidermoid carcinoma and to benign neoplasm of skin of these sites if the variety of neoplasm is a papilloma (of any type).

5. Primary malignant neoplasms are classified to the site of origin of the neoplasm. In some cases, it may not be possible to identify the site of origin, such as malignant neoplasms originating from contiguous sites.

    Neoplasms with overlapping site boundaries are classified to the fourth-digit subcategory .8 "other." For example, code 151.8 *Malignant neoplasm of contiguous or overlapping sites of stomach* whose point of origin cannot be determined.

6. Neoplasms which demonstrate functional activity require an additional code to identify the functional activity.

Coding Example

Cushing's syndrome due to malignant pheochromocytoma

    194.0   **Malignant neoplasm of adrenal gland**

    255.0   **Disorders of adrenal glands; Cushing's syndrome**

Code sequencing depends on the circumstances of the encounter.

7. Two categories in the malignant neoplasm section represent departures from the usual principles of classification in that the fourth-digit subdivisions in each case are not mutually exclusive. These categories are 150 *Malignant neoplasm of esophagus* and 201 *Hodgkin's disease*. The dual axis is provided to account for differing terminology, for there is no uniform international agreement on the use of these terms.

Coding Example

Malignant neoplasm of the esophagus

    150.0   **Cervical esophagus**

    150.1   **Thoracic esophagus**

    150.2   **Abdominal esophagus**

or using alternate coding

    150.3   **Upper third of esophagus**

    150.4   **Middle third of esophagus**

    150.5   **Lower third of esophagus**

8. When the treatment is directed at the primary site of the malignancy, designate the primary site as the principal diagnosis, except when the encounter or hospital admission is solely for *Radiotherapy* (V58.0) or, for *Chemotherapy* (V58.1).

9. When surgical intervention for removal of a primary site or secondary site malignancy is followed by adjunct chemotherapy or radiotherapy, code the malignancy using codes in the 140-198 series, or, where appropriate, in the 200-203 series as long as chemotherapy or radiotherapy is being actively administered. If the admission is for chemotherapy or radiotherapy, the malignancy code is listed second.

10. When the primary malignancy has been previously excised or eradicated from its site and there is no adjunct treatment directed to that site, and there is no evidence of any remaining malignancy at the primary site, use the appropriate code from the V10 series to indicate the site of the primary malignancy. Any mention of extension, invasion or metastasis to a nearby structure or organ, or to a distant site, is coded as a secondary malignant neoplasm to that site and may be the principal diagnosis in the absence of the primary site.

11. If the patient has no secondary malignancy and if the reason for admission or for the visit is follow-up of the malignancy, two codes are used and sequenced.

Coding Example

Follow-up of breast cancer treated with chemotherapy. No evidence of recurrence.

V67.2 Follow-up examination following chemotherapy

V10.3 Personal history of carcinoma of breast

12. Malignancies of hematopoietic and lymphatic tissue are always coded to the 200.0-208.9 series unless specified as "in remission." If they are in remission, they are coded as V10.60-V10.79.

13. If the primary malignant neoplasm previously excised or eradicated has recurred, code it as primary malignancy of the stated site unless the Alphabetic Index (Volume 2) directs you to do otherwise.

Coding Examples

Recurrence of prostate carcinoma

185 Malignant neoplasm of prostate

Recurrence of breast carcinoma in mastectomy site

198.2 Secondary malignant neoplasm of other specified sites, skin of breast

Make sure to code any mention of secondary site(s).

14. Terminology referring to metastatic cancer is often ambiguous, so when there is doubt as to the meaning intended, the following rules should be used:

A. Cancer described as metastatic "from" a site should be interpreted as primary of that site.

B. Cancer described as metastatic "to" a site should be interpreted as secondary of that site.

Coding Examples

Carcinoma in axillary lymph nodes and lungs metastatic from breast

> **174.9**   **Malignant neoplasm of breast (female), unspecified**
>
> **196.3**   **Secondary and unspecified malignant neoplasm of lymph nodes of axilla and upper limb**
>
> **197.0**   **Secondary malignant neoplasm of lung**

Adenocarcinoma of colon with extension to peritoneum

> **153.9**   **Malignant neoplasm of colon, unspecified**
>
> **197.6**   **Secondary malignant neoplasm of retroperitoneum and peritoneum**

15. Diagnostic statements when only one site is identified as metastatic:

    A. Code to the category for "primary of unspecified site" for the morphological type concerned UNLESS the code thus obtained is either 199.0 or 199.1.

    B. If the code obtained in the above step is 199.0 or 199.1, then code the site qualified as "metastatic" as for a primary malignant neoplasm of the stated site EXCEPT for the sites listed below, which should always be coded as secondary neoplasm of the state site:

Bone	*Mediastinum*
Brain	*Meninges*
Diaphragm	*Peritoneum*
Heart	*Pleura*
Liver	*Retroperitoneum*
Lymph nodes	*Spinal cord*

    Sites classifiable to 195

    C. Also assign the appropriate code for primary or secondary malignant neoplasm of specified or unspecified site, depending on the diagnostic statement you are coding.

Coding Examples

Metastatic renal cell carcinoma of lung

> **189.0**   **Malignant neoplasm of kidney, except pelvis**
>
> **197.0**   **Secondary malignant neoplasm of lung**

Metastatic carcinoma of lung

> **162.9**   **Malignant neoplasm of bronchus and lung, unspecified**
>
> **199.1**   **Malignant neoplasm without specification of site, other**

This code is assigned to identify "secondary neoplasm of unspecified site" per the instructions in step C above.

Metastatic carcinoma of brain

> **198.3**   **Secondary malignant neoplasm of other specified sites, brain and spinal cord**
>
> **199.1**   **Malignant neoplasm without specification of site, other**

In this case, the brain is one of the sites listed in Step B as an exception. So for this diagnostic statement, the code assignment is for secondary neoplasm of the brain and primary malignant neoplasm of unspecified site.

16. When two or more sites are stated in the diagnostic statement and all are qualified to be "metastatic," you should code as for "primary site unknown" and code the stated sites as secondary neoplasms of those sites.

Coding Example

Metastatic melanoma of lung and liver

> **172.9**   **Malignant melanoma of skin, site unspecified**
>
> **197.0**   **Secondary malignant neoplasm of lung**
>
> **197.7**   **Secondary malignant neoplasm of liver, specified as secondary**

17. When there is no site specified in the diagnostic statement, but the morphological type is qualified as "metastatic," code as for "primary site unknown." Then assign the code for secondary neoplasms of unspecified site.

Coding Example

Metastatic apocrine adenocarcinoma

> **173.9**   **Other malignant neoplasms of skin, site unspecified**
>
> **199.1**   **Malignant neoplasm without specification of site, other**

18. When two or more sites are stated in the diagnosis and only some are qualified as "metastatic" while others are not, code as for "primary site unknown." However, you should interpret the following sites as secondary neoplasms:

> *Bone*   *Meninges*
> *Brain*   *Peritoneum*
> *Diaphragm*   *Pleura*
> *Heart*   *Retroperitoneum*
> *Liver*   *Spinal Cord*
>
> *Sites classifiable to category 195*

Coding Example

Carcinoma of lung, metastatic, and brain

198.3 **Secondary malignant neoplasm of brain and spinal cord**

197.0 **Secondary malignant neoplasm of lung**

199.1 **Malignant neoplasm without specification of site, other**

CHRONIC KIDNEY DISEASE

Stages of Chronic Kidney Disease (CKD)

The ICD-9-CM classifies CKD based on severity. The severity of CKD is designated by stages I-V. Stage II, code 585.2, equates to mild CKD; stage III, code 585.3, equates to moderate CKD; and stage IV, code 585.4, equates to severe CKD. Code 585.6, *End stage renal disease (ESRD),* is assigned when the provider has documented end-stage renal disease (ESRD).

If both a stage of CKD and ESRD are documented, assign code 585.6 only.

Chronic Kidney Disease and Kidney Transplant Status

Patients who have undergone kidney transplant may still have some form of CKD because the kidney transplant may not fully restore kidney function. Code V42.0 may be assigned with the appropriate CKD code for patients who are status post-kidney transplant, based on the patient's post-transplant stage. The *use additional code* note under category 585 provides this instruction.

Use of a 585 code with V42.0 does not necessarily indicate transplant rejection or failure. Patients with mild or moderate CKD following a transplant should not be coded as having transplant failure, unless it is documented in the medical record. For patients with severe CKD or ESRD it is appropriate to assign code 996.81, *Complications of transplanted organ, kidney transplant,* when kidney transplant failure is documented. If a post kidney transplant patient has CKD and it is unclear from the documentation whether there is transplant failure or rejection, it is necessary to query the provider.

Chronic Kidney Disease With Other Conditions

Patients with CKD may also suffer from other serious conditions, most commonly diabetes mellitus and hypertension. The sequencing of the CKD code in relationship to codes for other contributing conditions is based on the conventions in the tabular list.

PREGNANCY, CHILDBIRTH, AND THE PUERPERIUM

Chapter 11 of the Tabular List (Volume 1) uses fifth-digit subclassifications extensively. In general, the fifth digit is not given in the Alphabetic Index (Volume 2), so each code must be verified in the Tabular List (Volume 1).

General Rules for Obstetrics Cases

1. Obstetric cases require codes from Chapter 11, codes in the range 630-677, *Complications of Pregnancy, Childbirth, and the Puerperium.* Should the physician document that the pregnancy is incidental to the encounter, then code V22.2 should be used in place of any Chapter 11 codes. It is the physician's responsibility to state that the condition being treated is not affecting the pregnancy.

2. Chapter 11 codes have sequencing priority over codes from other chapters. Additional codes from other chapters may be used in conjunction with Chapter 11 codes to further specify conditions. For example, sepsis and septic shock associated with abortion, ectopic pregnancy, and molar pregnancy are classified to category codes in Chapter 11 (630-639).

3. Chapter 11 codes are to be used only on the maternal record, never on the record of the newborn.

4. Categories 640-648 and 651-676 have required fifth-digits, which indicate whether the encounter is antepartum or postpartum, and whether a delivery has also occurred.

5. The fifth-digits that are appropriate for each code number, are listed in brackets under each code. The fifth-digits on each code should all be consistent with each other. That is, should a delivery occur, all of the fifth-digits should indicate that the delivery occurred.

Selection of OB Principal or First-Listed Diagnosis

1. For routine outpatient prenatal visits when no complications are present, codes V22.0, *Supervision of normal first pregnancy*, and V22.1, *Supervision of other normal pregnancy,* should be used as the first-listed diagnoses. These codes should not be used in conjunction with Chapter 11 codes.

2. For prenatal outpatient visits for patients with high-risk pregnancies, a code from category V23, *Supervision of high-risk pregnancy*, should be used as the principal or first-listed diagnosis. Secondary Chapter 11 codes may be used in conjunction with these codes if appropriate.

3. In episodes when no delivery occurs, the principal diagnosis should correspond to the principal complication of the pregnancy that necessitated the encounter. Should more than one complication exist, all of which are treated or monitored, any of the complications codes may be sequenced first.

4. When a delivery occurs, the principal diagnosis should correspond to the main circumstances or complication of the delivery. In cases of cesarean delivery, the selection of the principal diagnosis should correspond to the reason the cesarean delivery was performed unless the reason for admission/encounter was unrelated to the condition resulting in the cesarean delivery.

5. An outcome of delivery code, V27.0-V27.9, should be included on every maternal record when a delivery has occurred. These codes are not to be used on subsequent records or on the newborn record.

Fetal Conditions Affecting the Management of the Mother

Codes from category 655, *Known or suspected fetal abnormality affecting management of the mother,* and category 656, *Other fetal and placental problems affecting the management of the mother,* are assigned only when the fetal condition is actually responsible for modifying the management of the mother, i.e., by requiring diagnostic studies, additional observation, special care, or termination of pregnancy. The fact that the fetal condition exists does not justify assigning a code from this series to the mother's record.

In cases when surgery is performed on the fetus, a diagnosis code from category 655, *Known or suspected fetal abnormalities affecting management of the mother,* should be assigned identifying the fetal condition. Procedure code 75.36, *Correction of fetal defect,* should be assigned on the hospital inpatient record.

No code from Chapter 15, the perinatal codes, should be used on the mother's record to identify fetal conditions. Surgery performed in utero on a fetus is still to be coded as an obstetric encounter.

HIV Infection in Pregnancy, Childbirth and the Puerperium

During pregnancy, childbirth or the puerperium, a patient admitted because of an HIV-related illness should receive a principal diagnosis of 647.6x, *Other viral diseases in the mother classifiable elsewhere, but complicating the pregnancy, childbirth or the puerperium,* followed by 042 *HIV disease,* and the code(s) for the HIV-related illness(es). This is an exception to the sequencing rule found in above.

Patients with asymptomatic HIV infection status admitted during pregnancy, childbirth, or the puerperium should receive codes of 647.6x and V08.

Current Conditions Complicating Pregnancy

Assign a code from subcategory 648.x for patients that have current conditions when the condition affects the management of the pregnancy, childbirth, or the puerperium. Use additional secondary codes from other chapters to identify the conditions, as appropriate.

Diabetes Mellitus in Pregnancy

Diabetes mellitus is a significant complicating factor in pregnancy. Pregnant women who are diabetic should be assigned code 648.0x, *Diabetes mellitus complicating pregnancy,* and a secondary code from category 250, *Diabetes mellitus,* to identify the type of diabetes. Code V58.67, *Long-term (current) use of insulin,* should also be assigned if the diabetes mellitus is being treated with insulin.

Gestational Diabetes

Gestational diabetes can occur during the second and third trimester of pregnancy in women who were not diabetic prior to pregnancy. Gestational diabetes can cause complications in the pregnancy similar to those of pre-existing diabetes mellitus. It also puts the woman at greater risk of developing diabetes after the pregnancy. Gestational diabetes is coded to 648.8x, *Abnormal glucose tolerance.* Codes 648.0x and 648.8x should never be used together on the same record.

Code V58.67, *Long-term (current) use of insulin*, should also be assigned if the gestational diabetes is being treated with insulin.

Normal Delivery

1. Code 650, *Normal delivery*, is for use in cases when a woman is admitted for a full-term normal delivery and delivers a single, healthy infant without any complications antepartum, during the delivery, or postpartum during the delivery episode. Code 650 is always a principal diagnosis. It is not to be used if any other code from Chapter 11 is needed to describe a current complication of the antenatal, delivery, or perinatal period. Additional codes from other chapters may be used with code 650 if they are not related to or are in any way complicating the pregnancy.

2. Code 650 may be used if the patient had a complication at some point during her pregnancy but the complication is not present at the time of the admission for delivery.

3. Code 650 is always a principal diagnosis. It is not to be used if any other code from Chapter 11 is needed to describe a current complication of the antenatal, delivery, or perinatal period. Additional codes from other chapters may be used with code 650 if they are not related to or are in any way complicating the pregnancy.

4. V27.0, *Single liveborn*, is the only outcome of delivery code appropriate for use with 650.

The Postpartum Period

1. The postpartum period begins immediately after delivery and continues for six weeks following delivery.

2. A postpartum complication is any complication occurring within the six-week period.

3. Chapter 11 codes may also be used to describe pregnancy-related complications after the six-week period should the physician document that a condition is pregnancy related.

4. Postpartum complications that occur during the same admission as the delivery are identified with a fifth-digit of subsequent admissions/encounters for postpartum complications, should identified with a fifth-digit of "4.".

5. When the mother delivers outside the hospital prior to admission and is admitted for routine postpartum care and no complications are noted, code V24.0, *Postpartum care and examination immediately after delivery,* should be assigned as the principal diagnosis.

6. A delivery diagnosis code should not be used for a woman who has delivered prior to admission to the hospital. Any postpartum procedures should be coded.

Late Effect of Complication of Pregnancy, Childbirth, and the Puerperium

1. Code 677, *Late effect of complication of pregnancy, childbirth, and the puerperium* is for use in those cases when an initial complication of a pregnancy develops a sequelae requiring care or treatment at a future date.

2. This code may be used at any time after the initial postpartum period.

3. This code, like all late effect codes, is to be sequenced following the code describing the sequelae of the complication.

Abortions

1. Fifth-digits are required for abortion categories 634-637. Fifth-digit 1, *Incomplete*, indicates that all of the products of conception have not been expelled from the uterus. Fifth-digit 2, *Complete*, indicates that all products of conception have been expelled from the uterus prior to the episode of care.

2. A code from categories 640-648 and 651-657 may be used as additional codes with an abortion code to indicate the complication leading to the abortion.

   Fifth-digit 3 is assigned with codes from these categories when used with an abortion code because the other fifth-digits will not apply. Codes from the 660-669 series are not to be used for complications of abortion.

3. Code 639, *Complications following abortion and ectopic and molar pregnancies*, is to be used for all complications following abortion. Code 639 cannot be assigned with codes from categories 634-638.

4. When an attempted termination of pregnancy results in a liveborn fetus, assign code 644.21, *Early onset of delivery*, with an appropriate code from category V27, *Outcome of delivery.* The procedure code for the attempted termination of pregnancy should also be assigned.

5. Subsequent admissions for retained products of conception following a spontaneous or legally induced abortion are assigned the appropriate code from category 634, *Abortion*, or 635, *Legally induced abortion*, with a fifth digit of 1, *Incomplete.* This advice is appropriate even when the patient was discharged previously with a discharge diagnosis of "complete abortion."

Pregnancy Coding Examples

Pregnancy, 3 months gestation complicated by benign essential hypertension

642.03 Benign essential hypertension complicating pregnancy, childbirth, and the puerperium, antepartum condition or complication

Categories 647 and 648 are used for conditions that are usually classified elsewhere, but which have been classified here because they are complications of pregnancy. The interaction of certain conditions with the pregnant state complicates the pregnancy and/or aggravates the non-obstetrical condition (i.e., diabetes mellitus, drug dependence, thyroid dysfunction) and are the main reasons for the obstetrical care provided.

Coding Example

Rubella in woman, 7 months gestation

647.53 Infectious and parasitic conditions in the mother classifiable elsewhere, but complicating pregnancy, childbirth or the puerperium, rubella, antepartum condition or complication

Pregnancy with diabetes mellitus

648.03 Other current conditions in the mother classifiable elsewhere, but complicating pregnancy, childbirth or the puerperium, diabetes mellitus, antepartum condition or complication

If greater detail is needed for the complication, use an additional code to identify the complication more completely.

Coding Example

Pregnancy with pernicious anemia

648.23 Other current conditions in the mother classifiable elsewhere, but complicating pregnancy, childbirth or the puerperium, anemia, antepartum condition or complication

281.0   Pernicious anemia

NEWBORN (PERINATAL) GUIDELINES

For coding and reporting purposes, the perinatal period is defined as birth through the 28th day following birth. The following guidelines are provided for reporting purposes. Hospitals may record other diagnoses as needed for internal data use.

General Perinatal Rules

1. Chapter 15 codes are *never* for use on the maternal record. Codes from Chapter 11, the obstetric chapter, are never permitted on the newborn record. Chapter 15 code may be used throughout the life of the patient if the condition is still present.

2. Generally, codes from Chapter 15 should be sequenced as the principal/first-listed diagnosis on the newborn record, with the exception of the appropriate V30 code for the birth episode, followed by codes from any other chapter that provide additional detail. The "use additional code" note at the beginning of the chapter supports this guideline. If the index does not provide a specific code for a perinatal condition, assign code 779.89, *Other specified conditions originating in the perinatal period*, followed by the code from another chapter that specifies the condition. Codes for signs and symptoms may be assigned when a definitive diagnosis has not been established.

3. If a newborn has a condition that may be either due to the birth process or community-acquired and the documentation does not indicate which it is, the default is due to the birth process and the code from Chapter 15 should be used. If the condition is community-acquired, a code from Chapter 15 should not be assigned.

4.   All clinically significant conditions noted on routine newborn examination should be coded. A condition is clinically significant if it requires:

   - clinical evaluation; or
   - therapeutic treatment; or
   - diagnostic procedures; or
   - extended length of hospital stay; or
   - increased nursing care and/or monitoring; or
   - has implications for future health care needs

Note: The perinatal guidelines listed above are the same as the general coding guidelines for "additional diagnoses," except for the final point regarding implications for future health care needs. Codes should be assigned for conditions that have been specified by the provider as having implications for future health care needs. Codes from the perinatal chapter should not be assigned unless the provider has established a definitive diagnosis.

Use of Codes V30-V39

When coding the birth of an infant, assign a code from categories V30-V39, according to the type of birth. A code from this series is assigned as a principal diagnosis and assigned only once to a newborn at the time of birth.

Newborn Transfers

If the newborn is transferred to another institution, the V30 series is not used at the receiving hospital.

Use of Category V29

1.   Assign a code from category V29, *Observation and evaluation of newborns and infants for suspected conditions not found*, to identify those instances when a healthy newborn is evaluated for a suspected condition that is determined after study not to be present. Do not use a code from category V29 when the patient has identified signs or symptoms of a suspected problem; in such cases, code the sign or symptom.

   A code from category V29 may also be assigned as a principal code for readmissions or encounters when the V30 code no longer applies. Codes from category V29 are for use only for healthy newborns and infants for which no condition after study is found to be present.

2.   A V29 code is to be used as a secondary code after the V30, *Outcome of delivery*, code.

Use of Other V Codes on Perinatal Records

V codes other than V30 and V29 may be assigned on a perinatal or newborn record code. The codes may be used as a principal or first-listed diagnosis for specific types of encounters or for readmissions or encounters when the V30 code no longer applies.

Maternal Causes of Perinatal Morbidity

Codes from categories 760-763, *Maternal causes of perinatal morbidity and mortality,* are assigned only when the maternal condition has actually affected the fetus or newborn. The fact that the mother has an associated medical condition or experiences some complication of pregnancy, labor or delivery does not justify the routine assignment of codes from these categories to the newborn record.

Congenital Anomalies

For the birth admission, the appropriate code from category V30, *Liveborn infants according to type of birth,* should be sequenced as the principal diagnosis, followed by any congenital anomaly codes, categories 740-759. Use additional secondary codes from other chapters to specify conditions associated with the anomaly, if applicable. Assign an appropriate code(s) from categories 740-759, *Congenital Anomalies,* when an anomaly is documented.

When a congenital anomaly does not have a unique code assignment, assign additional code(s) for any manifestations that may be present. When the code assignment specifically identifies the congenital anomaly, manifestations that are an inherent component of the anomaly should not be coded separately. Additional codes should be assigned for manifestations that are not an inherent component.

A congenital anomaly may be the principal/first-listed diagnosis on a record or a secondary diagnosis. Use additional secondary codes from other chapters to specify conditions associated with the anomaly, if applicable. Codes from Chapter 14 may be used throughout the life of the patient. If a congenital anomaly has been corrected, a personal history code should be used to identify the history of the anomaly. Although present at birth, a congenital anomaly may not be identified until later in life. Whenever the condition is diagnosed by the physician, it is appropriate to assign a code from codes 740-759.

Coding of Additional Perinatal Diagnoses

1. Assign codes for conditions that require treatment or further investigation, prolong the length of stay, or require resource utilization.

2. Assign codes for conditions that have been specified by the physician as having implications for future health care needs.

    Note: This guideline should not be used for adult patients.

3. Assign a code for *Newborn conditions originating in the perinatal period* (categories 760-779), as well as complications arising during the current episode of care classified in other chapters, only if the diagnoses have been documented by the responsible physician at the time of transfer or discharge as having affected the fetus or newborn.

Prematurity and Fetal Growth Retardation

Codes from category 764, *Slow fetal growth and fetal malnutrition,* and subcategories 765.0, *Extreme immaturity,* and 765.1, *Other preterm infant,* should not be assigned based solely on recorded birthweight or estimated gestational age, but on the attending physician's clinical assessment of maturity of the infant. Note: since physicians may utilize different criteria in determining prematurity, do not code the diagnosis of prematurity unless the physician documents this condition.

A code from subcategory 765.2x, *Weeks of gestation,* should be assigned as an additional code with category 764 and codes 765.0 and 765.1 in order to specify weeks of gestation as documented by the physician.

Newborn Sepsis

Code 771.81, *Septicemia [sepsis] of newborn,* should be assigned with a secondary code from category 041, *Bacterial infections in conditions classified elsewhere and of unspecified site,* to identify the organism. It is not necessary to use a code from subcategory 995.9, *Systemic inflammatory response syndrome (SIRS),* on a newborn record. A code from category 038, *Septicemia,* should not be used on a newborn record. Code 771.81 describes the sepsis.

V CODES: CLASSIFICATION OF FACTORS INFLUENCING HEALTH STATUS AND CONTACT WITH HEALTH SERVICE

ICD-9-CM provides codes to deal with encounters for circumstances other than a disease or injury. *The Supplementary Classification of Factors Influencing Health Status and Contact with Health Services* (V01.0-V84.8) is provided to deal with occasions when circumstances other than a disease or injury (codes 001-999) are recorded as a diagnosis or problem.

V codes are used for four primary circumstances:

1. When a person who is not currently sick encounters the health services for some specific reason, such as to act as an organ donor, to receive prophylactic care such as inoculations or health screenings, or to receive counseling on health related issue.

2. When a person with a resolving disease or injury, or a chronic, long-term condition requiring continuous care, encounters the health care system for specific aftercare of that disease or injury (e.g., dialysis for renal disease, chemotherapy for malignancy, or a cast change). Note: A diagnosis/symptom code should be used whenever a current/acute diagnosis is being treated or a sign or symptom is being studied.

3. When circumstances or problems influence a person's health status but are not in themselves a current illness or injury.

4. For newborns, to indicate birth status.

V codes are for use in both the inpatient and outpatient setting but are generally more applicable to the outpatient setting. V codes may be used as either a first listed (principal diagnosis code in the inpatient setting) or secondary code depending on the circumstances of the encounter. Certain V codes may only be used as first listed, and others only as secondary codes.

V codes indicate a reason for an encounter. They are not procedure codes. A corresponding procedure code must accompany a V code to describe the procedure performed. Key words found in diagnostic statements which may result in selection of a V code include:

Admission for	*Health or healthy*
Aftercare	*History (of)*
Attention to	*Maintenance*
Care (of)	*Maladjustment*
Carrier	*Observation*
Checking/checkup	*Problem (with)*
Contact	*Prophylactic*
Contraception	*Replacement (by)(of)*
Counseling	*Screening*
Dialysis	*Status*
Donor	*Supervision (of)*
Examination	*Test*
Fitting of	*Transplant*
Follow up	*Vaccination*

Categories of V Codes

Contact/Exposure

Category V01 indicates *Contact with or exposure to communicable diseases*. These codes are for patients who do not show any sign or symptom of a disease but have been exposed to it by close personal contact with an infected individual or are in an area where a disease is epidemic. These codes may be used as a first-listed code to explain an encounter for testing, or, more commonly, as a secondary code to identify a potential risk.

Inoculations and Vaccinations

Categories V03-V06 are used for encounters for inoculations and vaccinations. These codes indicate that a patient is being seen to receive a prophylactic inoculation against a disease. The injection itself must be represented by the appropriate procedure code. A code from V03-V06 may be used as a secondary code if the inoculation is given as a routine part of preventive health care, such as well-baby visit.

Status

Status codes indicate that a patient is either a carrier of a disease or has the sequelae or residual of a past disease or condition. This includes such things as the presence of prosthetic or mechanical devices resulting from past treatment. A status code is informative because the status may affect the current course of treatment and its outcome. A status code is distinct from a history code. The history code indicates that the patient no longer has the condition.

Status V codes/categories

V02   *Carrier or suspected carrier of infectious diseases*

    Carrier status indicates that a person harbors the specific organisms of a disease without manifest symptoms and is capable of transmitting the infection.

V08   *Asymptomatic HIV infection status*

    This code indicates that a patient has tested positive for HIV but has manifested no signs or symptoms of the disease.

V09   *Infection with drug-resistant microorganisms*

> This category indicates that a patient has an infection which is resistant to drug treatment. Sequence the infection code first.

V21   *Constitutional states in development*

V22.2 *Pregnant state, incidental*

> This code is a secondary code only for use when the pregnancy is in no way complicating the reason for visit. Otherwise, a code from the obstetric chapter is required.

V26.5X *Sterilization status*

V42   *Organ or tissue replaced by transplant*

V43   *Organ or tissue replaced by other means*

V44   *Artificial opening status*

V45   *Other postprocedural states*

V46   *Other dependence on machines*

V49.6 *Upper limb amputation status*

V49.7 *Lower limb amputation status*

V49.8 *Other specific conditions influencing health status*

> Categories V42-V46, and subcategories V49.6, V49.7 and V49.8 are for use only if there are no complications or malfunctions of the organ or tissue replaced, the amputation site or the equipment on which the patient is dependent. These are always secondary codes.

V49.83 *Awaiting organ transplant status*

V58.6 *Long-term (current) drug use*

> This subcategory indicates a patient's continuous use of a prescribed drug (including such things as aspirin therapy) for the long-term treatment of a condition or for prophylactic use. It is not for use for patients who have addictions to drugs.
>
> Assign a code from subcategory V58.6, *Long-term (current) drug use,* if the patient is receiving a medication for an extended period as a prophylactic measure (such as for the prevention of deep vein thrombosis) or as treatment of a chronic condition (such as arthritis) or a disease requiring a lengthy course of treatment (such as cancer). Do not assign a code from subcategory V58.6 for medication being administered for a brief period of time to treat an acute illness or injury (such as a course of antibiotics to treat acute bronchitis).

V83   *Genetic carrier status*

Genetic carrier status indicates that a person carries a gene, associated with a particular disease, which may be passed to offspring who may develop that disease. The person does not have the disease and is not at risk of developing the disease.

V84   *Genetic susceptibility status*

Genetic susceptibility indicates that a person has a gene that increases the risk of that person developing the disease.

Codes from category V84, *Genetic susceptibility to disease*, should not be used as principal or first-listed codes. If the patient has the condition to which he/she is susceptible, and that condition is the reason for the encounter, the code for the current condition should be sequenced first. If the patient is being seen for follow-up after completed treatment for this condition, and the condition no longer exists, a follow-up code should be sequenced first, followed by the appropriate personal history and genetic susceptibility codes. If the purpose of the encounter is genetic counseling associated with procreative management, a code from subcategory V26.3, *Genetic counseling and testing*, should be assigned as the first-listed code, followed by a code from category V84. Additional codes should be assigned for any applicable family or personal history.

Note: Categories V42-V46 and subcategories V49.6, V49.7 are for use only if there are no complications or malfunctions of the organ or tissue replaced, the amputation site or the equipment on which the patient is dependent.

History (of)

There are two types of history V codes: personal and family. Personal history codes explain a patient's past medical condition that no longer exists and is not receiving any treatment, but that has the potential for recurrence and, therefore, may require continued monitoring. The exceptions to this general rule are category V14, *Personal history of allergy to medicinal agents* and subcategory V15.0, *Allergy, other than to medicinal agents*. A person who has had an allergic episode to a substance or food in the past should always be considered allergic to the substance.

Family history codes are used when a patient has a family member(s) who has had a particular disease that causes the patient to be at higher risk of also contracting the disease.

Personal history codes may be used in conjunction with follow-up codes and family history codes may be used in conjunction with screening codes to explain the need for a test or procedure. History codes are also acceptable on any medical record regardless of the reason for visit. A history of an illness, even if no longer present, is important information that may alter the type of treatment ordered.

History V codes/categories:

V10   *Personal history of malignant neoplasm*

V12   *Personal history of certain other diseases*

V13	*Personal history of other diseases*

> Except: V13.4, *Personal history of arthritis*, and V13.6, *Personal history of congenital malformations.* These are lifelong conditions so are not true history codes.

V14	*Personal history of allergy to medicinal agents*
V15	*Other personal history presenting hazards to health*

> Except: V15.7, *Personal history of contraception.*

V16	*Family history of malignant neoplasm*
V17	*Family history of certain chronic disabling diseases*
V18	*Family history of certain other specific conditions*
V19	*Family history of other conditions*

Screening

Screening is the testing for disease or disease precursors in seemingly well individuals so that early detection and treatment can be provided for those who test positive for the disease. Screenings that are recommended for many subgroups in a population include: routine mammograms for women over 40 or a fecal occult blood test for everyone over 50, because the incidence of breast cancer and colon cancer in these subgroups is higher than in the general population; or an amniocentesis to rule out a fetal anomaly for pregnant women over 35, because the incidence of Down's syndrome is higher in older mothers.

The testing of a person to rule out or confirm a suspected diagnosis because the patient has some sign or symptom is a diagnostic examination, not a screening. In these cases, the sign or symptom is used to explain the reason for the test.

A screening code may be a first-listed code if the reason for the visit is specifically the screening exam. It may also be used as an additional code if the screening is done during an office visit for other health problems. A screening code is not necessary if the screening is inherent to a routine examination, such as a pap smear done during a routine pelvic examination.

Should a condition be discovered during the screening then the code for the condition may be assigned as an additional diagnosis.

The V code indicates that a screening exam is planned. A procedure code is required to confirm that the screening was performed.

Screening V codes/categories:

V28	*Antenatal screening*
V73-V82	*Special screening examinations*

Observation

There are two observation V code categories. They are for use in very limited circumstances when a person is being observed for a suspected condition that is ruled out. The observation codes are not for use if an injury or illness or any signs or symptoms related to the suspected condition are present. In such cases the diagnosis/ symptom code is used with the corresponding E code to identify any external cause.

The observation codes are to be used as principal diagnosis only. The only exception to this is when the principal diagnosis is required to be a code from category V30, *Live born infant*. Then the V29 observation code is sequenced after the V30 code. Additional codes may be used in addition to the observation code but only if they are unrelated to the suspected condition being observed.

Observation V codes/categories:

V29　　　　　*Observation and evaluation of newborns for suspected condition not found*

　　　　　　　　　For the birth encounter, a code from category V30 should be sequenced before the V29 code.

V71　　　　　*Observation and evaluation for suspected conditions not found*

Aftercare

Aftercare visit codes cover situations when the initial treatment of a disease or injury has been performed and the patient requires continued care during the healing or recovery phase, or for the long-term consequences of the disease. The aftercare V code should not be used if treatment is directed at a current, acute disease or injury. The diagnosis code is to be used in these cases. Exceptions to this rule are codes V58.0, *Radiotherapy,* and codes from subcategory V58.1, *Encounter for chemotherapy and immunotherapy for neoplastic conditions.* These codes are to be first listed, followed by the diagnosis code when a patient's encounter is solely to receive radiation therapy or chemotherapy for the treatment of a neoplasm. Should a patient receive both chemotherapy and radiation therapy during the same encounter, codes V58.0 and V58.1 may be used together with either one being sequenced first.

The aftercare codes are generally first listed to explain the specific reason for the encounter. An aftercare code may be used as an additional code when some type of aftercare is provided in addition to the reason for admission and no diagnosis code is applicable. An example of this would be the closure of a colostomy during an encounter for treatment of another condition.

Certain aftercare V code categories need a secondary diagnosis code to describe the resolving condition or sequelae. For others, the condition is inherent in the code title. Additional V code aftercare category terms include, "fitting and adjustment," and "attention to artificial openings."

Status V codes may be used with aftercare V codes to indicate the nature of the aftercare. For example, code V45.81, *Aortocoronary bypass status*, may be used with code V58.73, *Aftercare following surgery of the circulatory system, NEC*, to indicate the surgery for which the aftercare is being performed. Also, a transplant status code may be used following code V58.44, *Aftercare following organ transplant*, to identify the organ transplanted. A status code should not be used when the aftercare code indicates the type of status, such as using V55.0, *Attention to tracheostomy* with V44.0, *Tracheostomy status*.

Aftercare V codes/categories:

V52	*Fitting and adjustment of prosthetic device and implant*
V53	*Fitting and adjustment of other device*
V54	*Other orthopedic aftercare*
V55	*Attention to artificial openings*
V56	*Encounter for dialysis and dialysis catheter care*
V57	*Care involving the use of rehabilitation procedures*
V58.0	*Radiotherapy*
V58.11	*Encounter for antineoplastic chemotherapy*
V58.12	*Encounter for antineoplastic immunotherapy*
V58.3	*Attention to surgical dressings and sutures*
V58.41	*Encounter for planned post-operative wound closure*
V58.42	*Aftercare following surgery for neoplasm*
V58.43	*Aftercare following surgery for injury and trauma*
V58.44	*Aftercare following organ transplant*
V58.49	*Other specified aftercare following surgery*
V58.71- V58.78	*Aftercare following surgery to specified body systems NEC*
V58.81	*Fitting and adjustment of vascular catheter*
V58.82	*Fitting and adjustment of non-vascular catheter NEC*
V58.83	*Encounter for therapeutic drug monitoring*
V58.89	*Other specified aftercare*

Follow-Up

The follow-up codes are for use to explain continuing surveillance following completed treatment of a disease, condition, or injury. They infer that the condition has been fully treated and no longer exists. They should not be confused with aftercare codes which explain current treatment for a healing condition or its sequelae.

Follow-up codes may be used in conjunction with history codes to provide the full picture of the healed condition and its treatment. The follow-up code is sequenced first, followed by the history code.

A follow-up code may be used to explain repeated visits. Should a condition be found to have recurred on the follow-up visit, then the diagnosis code should be used in place of the follow-up code.

Follow-up V codes/categories:

V24   *Postpartum care and evaluation*

V67   *Follow-up examination*

Donor

Category V59 is the donor codes. They are for use for living individuals who are donating blood or other body tissue. These codes are only for individuals donating for others, not for self donations. They are not to identify cadaveric donations.

Counseling

Counseling V codes are for use for when a patient or family member receives assistance in the aftermath of an illness or injury, or when support is required in coping with family or social problems. They are not necessary for use in conjunction with a diagnosis code when the counseling component of care is considered integral to standard treatment.

Counseling V codes/categories:

V25.0   *General counseling and advice for contraceptive management*

V26.3   *Genetic counseling and testing*

V26.4   *General counseling and advice for procreative management*

V61   *Other family circumstances*

V65.1   *Person consulting on behalf of another person*

V65.3   *Dietary surveillance and counseling*

V65.4   *Other counseling, not elsewhere classified*

Obstetrics and Related Conditions

See the Obstetrics guidelines for further instruction on the use of these codes. V codes for pregnancy are for use in those circumstances when none of the problems or complications included in the codes from the Obstetrics chapter exist, such as a routine prenatal visit or postpartum care. V22.0, *Supervision of normal first pregnancy,* and V22.1, *Supervision of other normal pregnancy,* are always first listed and are not to be used with any other code from the Obstetrics chapter.

Category V27, *Outcome of delivery,* should be included on all maternal delivery records. It is always a secondary code. V codes for family planning (contraceptive) or procreative management and counseling should be included on an obstetric record either during the pregnancy or the postpartum stage, if applicable.

Obstetrics and related conditions V codes/categories:

V22   *Normal pregnancy*

V23	*Supervision of high-risk pregnancy*

Except: V23.2, *Pregnancy with history of abortion.* Code 646.3, *Habitual aborter,* from the OB chapter is required to indicate a history of abortion during a pregnancy.

V24	*Postpartum care and evaluation*

V25	*Encounter for contraceptive management*

Except: V25.0X (See counseling above)

V26	*Procreative management*

Except: V26.5x, *Sterilization status*, V26.3 and V26.4 (*Counseling*)

V27	*Outcome of delivery*

V28	*Antenatal screening*

Newborn, Infant and Child

See the Newborn Guidelines for further instruction on the use of these codes.

Newborn V codes/categories:

V20	*Health supervision of infant or child*

V29	*Observation and evaluation of newborns for suspected condition not found*

V30-V39	*Liveborn infant according to type of birth*

Routine and Administrative Examinations

The V codes allow for the description of encounters for routine examinations, such as a general check-up, or examinations for administrative purposes, such as a pre-employment physical. The codes are for use as first-listed codes only and are not to be used if the examination is for diagnosis of a suspected condition or for treatment purposes. In such cases the diagnosis code is used. During a routine exam, should a diagnosis or condition be discovered, it should be coded as an additional code. Pre-existing and chronic conditions, and history codes may also be included as additional codes as long as the examination is for administrative purposes and not focused on any particular condition.

Pre-operative examination V codes are for use only in those situations when a patient is being cleared for surgery and no treatment is given.

Routine and administrative examinations V codes/categories:

V20.2	*Routine infant or child health check*

Any injections given should have a corresponding procedure code.

V70	*General medical examination*

V72	*Special investigations and examinations* Except V72.5 and V72.6

Miscellaneous V Codes

The miscellaneous V codes capture a number of other health care encounters that do not fall into one of the other categories. Certain of these codes identify the reason for the encounter, others are for use as additional codes which provide useful information on circumstances which may affect a patient's care and treatment.

For encounters specifically for prophylactic removal of breasts, ovaries, or another organ due to a genetic susceptibility to cancer or a family history of cancer, the principal or first listed code should be a code from subcategory V50.4, *Prophylactic organ removal*, followed by the appropriate genetic susceptibility code and the appropriate family history code.

If the patient has a malignancy of one site and is having prophylactic removal at another site to prevent either a new primary malignancy or metastatic disease, a code for the malignancy should also be assigned in addition to a code from subcategory V50.4. A V50.4 code should not be assigned if the patient is having organ removal for treatment of a malignancy, such as the removal of the testes for the treatment of prostate cancer.

Miscellaneous V codes/categories:

V07	*Need for isolation and other prophylactic measures*
V50	*Elective surgery for purposes other than remedying health states*
V58.5	*Orthodontics*
V60	*Housing, household, and economic circumstances*
V62	*Other psychosocial circumstances*
V63	*Unavailability of other medical facilities for care*
V64	*Persons encountering health services for specific procedures, not carried out*
V66	*Convalescence and palliative care*
V68	*Encounters for administrative purposes*
V69	*Problems related to lifestyle*

Nonspecific V Codes

Certain V codes are so non-specific, or potentially redundant with other codes in the classification, that there can be little justification for their use in the inpatient setting. Their use in the outpatient setting should be limited to those instances when there is no further documentation to permit more precise coding. Otherwise, any sign or symptom, or any other reason for the visit which is captured in another code, should be used instead.

Nonspecific V codes/categories:

V11	*Personal history of mental disorder*

> A code from the mental disorders chapter, with an in remission fifth-digit, should be used.

V13.4   *Personal history of arthritis*

V13.69   *Personal history of congenital malformations*

V15.7   *Personal history of contraception*

V40   *Mental and behavioral problems*

V41   *Problems with special senses and other special functions*

V47   *Other problems with internal organs*

V48   *Problems with head, neck, and trunk*

V49.0   Deficiencies of limbs

V49.1   *Mechanical problems with limbs*

V49.2   *Motor problems with limbs*

V49.3   *Sensory problems with limbs*

V49.4   *Disfigurements in limbs*

V49.5   *Other problems with limbs*

V49.9   *Unspecified condition influencing health status*

V51   *Aftercare involving the use of plastic surgery*

V58.2   *Blood transfusion, without reported diagnosis*

V58.5   *Orthodontics*

V58.9   *Unspecified aftercare*

V72.5   *Radiological examination, NEC*

V72.6   *Laboratory examination*

> Codes V72.5 and V72.6 are not to be used if any sign or symptoms, or reason for a test is documented.

V Code Coding Example

Colostomy status with colostomy malfunction

569.60 Colostomy and enterostomy complications, unspecified

The code V44.3 *Artificial opening status, colostomy* would not be used in this case because of the complication.

V CODE TABLE

First Listed Only

V Codes/Categories/Subcategories That Are Only Acceptable as Principal/First Listed

Codes:

V22.0   *Supervision of normal first pregnancy*

V22.1   *Supervision of other normal pregnancy*

V46.12   *Encounter for respirator dependence during power failure*

V46.13   *Encounter for weaning from respirator [ventilator]*

V56.0   *Extracorporeal dialysis*

V58.0   *Radiotherapy*

> V58.0 and V58.11 may be used together on a record with either one being sequenced first, when a patient receives both chemotherapy and radiation therapy during the same encounter.

V58.11   *Encounter for antineoplastic chemotherapy*

> V58.0 and V58.11 may be used together on a record with either one being sequenced first, when a patient receives both chemotherapy and radiation therapy during the same encounter.

V58.12   *Encounter for antineoplastic immunotherapy*

Categories/Subcategories:

V20   *Health supervision of infant or child*

V24   *Postpartum care and examination*

V29   *Observation and evaluation of newborns for suspected condition not found*

> Exception: A code from V30-V39 may be sequenced before V29 if it is the newborn record.

V30-V39   *Liveborn infants according to type of birth*

V57   *Care involving use of rehabilitation procedures*

V59   *Donors*

V66   *Convalescence and palliative care*

> Exception: V66.7 *Palliative care*

V68   *Encounters for administrative purposes*

V70	*General medical examination*

        Exception: V70.7 *Examination of participant in clinical trial*

V71	*Observation and evaluation for suspected conditions not found*
V72	*Special investigations and examinations*

        Exceptions:
V72.4 *Pregnancy examination or test*
V72.5 *Radiological examination, NEC*
V72.6 *Laboratory examination*
V72.86 *Encounter for blood typing*

First or Additional

V Codes/Categories/Subcategories That May Be Either Principal/First-Listed or Additional Codes

Codes:

V15.88	*History of fall*
V43.22	*Fully implantable artificial heart status*
V46.14	*Mechanical complication of respiratory [ventilator]*
V49.81	*Asymptomatic postmenopausal status (age-related) (natural)*
V49.84	*Bed confinement status*
V49.89	*Other specified conditions influencing health status*
V70.7	*Examination of participant in clinical trial*
V72.5	*Radiological examination, NEC*
V72.6	*Laboratory examination*
V72.86	*Encounter for blood typing*

Categories/Subcategories:

V01	*Contact with or exposure to communicable diseases*
V02	*Carrier or suspected carrier of infectious diseases*
V03-V06	*Need for prophylactic vaccination and inoculations*
V07	*Need for isolation and other prophylactic measures*
V08	*Asymptomatic HIV infection status*
V10	*Personal history of malignant neoplasm*
V12	*Personal history of certain other diseases*

V13	*Personal history of other diseases*

        Exceptions:
        V13.4 *Personal history of arthritis*
        V13.69 *Personal history of other congenital malformations*

V16-V19	*Family history of disease*
V23	*Supervision of high-risk pregnancy*
V25	*Encounter for contraceptive management*
V26	*Procreative management*

        Exception: V26.5 *Sterilization status*

V28	*Antenatal screening*
V45.7	*Acquired absence of organ*
V49.6x	*Upper limb amputation status*
V49.7x	*Lower limb amputation status*
V50	*Elective surgery for purposes other than remedying health states*
V52	*Fitting and adjustment of prosthetic device and implant*
V53	*Fitting and adjustment of other device*
V54	*Other orthopedic aftercare*
V55	*Attention to artificial openings*
V56	*Encounter for dialysis and dialysis catheter care*

        Exception: V56.0 *Extracorporeal dialysis*

V58.3	*Attention to surgical dressings and sutures*
V58.4	*Other aftercare following surgery*
V58.7	*Aftercare following surgery to specified body systems, not elsewhere classified*
V58.8	*Other specified procedures and aftercare*
V61	*Other family circumstances*
V63	*Unavailability of other medical facilities for care*
V65	*Other persons seeking consultation without complaint or sickness*
V67	*Follow-up examination*
V69	*Problems related to lifestyle*

V72.4	*Pregnancy examination or test*
V73-V82	*Special screening examinations*
V83	*Genetic carrier status*

Additional Only

V Codes/Categories/Subcategories That May Only Be Used As Additional Codes, Not As Principal/First Listed

Codes:

V13.61	*Personal history of hypospadias*
V22.2	*Pregnancy state, incidental*
V46.11	*Dependence on respirator, status*
V49.82	*Dental sealant status*
V49.83	*Awaiting organ transplant status*
V66.7	*Palliative care*

Categories/Subcategories:

V09	*Infection with drug-resistant microorganisms*
V14	*Personal history of allergy to medicinal agents*
V15	*Other personal history presenting hazards to health*

Exception:
V15.7 *Personal history of contraception*
V15.88 *History of fall*

V21	*Constitutional states in development*
V26.5	*Sterilization status*
V27	*Outcome of delivery*
V42	*Organ or tissue replaced by transplant*
V43	*Organ or tissue replaced by other means*

Exception: V43.22 *Fully implantable artificial heart status*

V44	*Artificial opening status*
V45	*Other postsurgical states*

Exception: Subcategory V45.7 *Acquired absence of organ*

V46	*Other dependence on machines*

> Exceptions:
> V46.12 *Encounter for respirator dependence during power failure*
> V46.13 *Encounter for weaning from respirator [ventilator]*

V58.6	*Long-term (current) drug use*
V60	*Housing, household, and economic circumstances*
V62	*Other psychosocial circumstances*
V64	*Persons encountering health services for specified procedure, not carried out*
V84	*Genetic susceptibility to disease*
V85	*Body mass index*

E CODES: SUPPLEMENTAL CLASSIFICATION OF EXTERNAL CAUSES OF INJURY AND POISONING

E-codes permit the classification of environmental events, circumstances and conditions as the cause of injury, poisoning and other adverse effects. The use of E-codes, together with the code identifying the injury or condition, provides additional information of particular concern to industrial medicine, insurance carriers, national safety programs and public health agencies. External causes of injury and poisoning codes (E codes) are intended to provide data for injury research and evaluation of injury prevention strategies. E codes capture how the injury or poisoning happened (cause), the intent (unintentional or accidental; or intentional, such as suicide or assault), and the place where the event occurred.

The following guidelines are provided for those who are currently collecting E codes in order that there will be standardization in the process. If your institution plans to begin collecting E codes, these guidelines are to be applied. The use of E codes is supplemental to the application of ICD-9-CM diagnosis codes. E codes are <u>never</u> to be recorded as a principal diagnosis (first-listed in non-inpatient setting) and are not required for reporting to CMS.

These guidelines apply for the coding and collection of E codes from records in hospitals, outpatient clinics, emergency departments, other ambulatory care settings and physician offices, and nonacute care settings, except when other specific guidelines apply.

Some major categories of E codes include:

- transport accidents;
- poisoning and adverse effects of drugs, medicinal substances and biologicals;
- accidental falls;
- accidents caused by fire and flames;
- accidents due to natural and environmental factors;
- late effects of accidents, assaults or self injury;
- assaults or purposely inflicted injury;
- suicide or self inflicted injury.

General E Code Coding Guidelines

1.   An E code may be used with any code in the range of 001-V83.89, which indicates an injury, poisoning, or adverse effect due to an external cause.

2.   Assign the appropriate E code for all initial treatments of an injury, poisoning, or adverse effect of drugs, not for subsequent treatment.

3.   Use the full range of E codes to completely describe the cause, the intent and the place of occurrence, if applicable, for all injuries, poisonings and adverse effects of drugs.

4.   Assign as many E codes as necessary to fully explain each cause. If only one E code can be recorded, assign the E code most related to the principal diagnosis.

5.   The selection of the appropriate E code is guided by the Index to External Causes, which is located after the alphabetical index to diseases, and by "Inclusion" and "Exclusion" notes in the Tabular List.

6.   An E code can never be a principal (first-listed) diagnosis.

7.   An external cause code(s) may be used with codes 995.93, Systemic inflammatory response syndrome due to noninfectious process without organ dysfunction, and 995.94, Systemic inflammatory response syndrome due to noninfectious process with organ dysfunction, if trauma was the initiating insult that precipitated the SIRS. The external cause(s) code should correspond to the most serious injury resulting from the trauma. The external cause code(s) should be assigned only if the trauma necessitated the admission in which the patient also developed SIRS. If a patient is admitted with SIRS but the trauma has been treated previously, the external cause codes should not be used.

Place of Occurrence Guideline

Use an additional code from category E849 to indicate the *Place of Occurrence* for injuries and poisonings. This describes the place where the event occurred and not the patient's activity at the time of the event.

Note: Do not use E849.9 if the place of occurrence is not stated.

Adverse Effects of Drugs, Medicinal and Biological Substances Guidelines

1.   Do not code directly from the Table of Drugs and Chemicals. Always refer back to the Tabular List.

2.   Use as many codes as necessary to describe completely all drugs, medicinal or biological substances.

3.   If the same E code would describe the causative agent for more than one adverse reaction, assign the code only once.

4.   If two or more drugs, medicinal or biological substances are reported, code each individually unless the combination code is listed in the Table of Drugs and Chemicals. In that case, assign the E code for the combination.

5.   When a reaction results from the interaction of a drug(s) and alcohol, use poisoning codes and E codes for both.

6.   If the reporting format limits the number of E codes that can be used in reporting clinical data, code the one most related to the principal diagnosis. Include at least one from each category (cause, intent, place) if possible.

      If there are different fourth-digit codes in the same three-digit category, use the code for *Other specified* of that category. If there is no *Other specified* code in that category, use the appropriate *Unspecified* code in that category.

      If the codes are in different three-digit categories, assign the appropriate E code for other multiple drugs and medicinal substances.

7.   Codes from the E930-E949 series must be used to identify the causative substance for an adverse effect of drug, medicinal and biological substances, correctly prescribed and properly administered. The effect, such as tachycardia, delirium, gastrointestinal hemorrhaging, vomiting, hypokalemia, hepatitis, renal failure, or respiratory failure, etc., is coded and followed by the appropriate code from the E930-E949 series.

Multiple Cause Coding Guidelines

If two or more events cause separate injuries, an E code should be assigned for each cause. The first-listed E code will be selected in the following order:

1.   E codes for child and adult abuse take priority over all other E codes—see Child and Adult Abuse Guidelines below.

2.   E codes for terrorism events take priority over all other E codes except child and adult abuse.

3.   E codes for cataclysmic events take priority over all other E codes except child and adult abuse, and terrorism.

4.   E codes for transport accidents take priority over all other E codes except cataclysmic events, and child and adult abuse, and terrorism.

5.   The first-listed E code should correspond to the cause of the most serious diagnosis due to an assault, accident or self-harm, following the order of hierarchy listed above.

Child and Adult Abuse Guidelines

1.   When the cause of an injury or neglect is intentional child or adult abuse, the first-listed E code should be assigned from categories E960-E969, *Homicide and injury purposely inflicted by other persons*, (except category E967). An E code from category E967, *Perpetrator of child and adult abuse*, should be added as an additional code to identify the perpetrator, if known.

2.   In cases of neglect when the intent is determined to be accidental, E code E904.0, *Abandonment or neglect of infants and helpless persons*, should be the first listed E code.

Unknown or Suspected Intent Guidelines

1. If the intent (accident, self-harm, assault) of the cause of an injury or poisoning is unknown or unspecified, code the intent as undetermined E980-E989.

2. If the intent (accident, self-harm, assault) of the cause of an injury or poisoning is questionable, probable or suspected, code the intent as undetermined E980-E989.

Undetermined Cause Guidelines

When the intent of an injury or poisoning is known, but the cause is unknown, use codes: E928.9, *Unspecified accident*; E958.9, *Suicide and self-inflicted injury by unspecified means*; or E968.9, *Assault by unspecified means*.

These E codes should rarely be used, since the documentation in the medical record, in inpatient, outpatient and other setting, should normally provide sufficient detail to determine the cause of the injury.

Late Effects of External Cause Guidelines

1. Late effect E codes exist for injuries and poisonings but not for adverse effects of drugs, misadventures and surgical complications.

2. A late effect E code (E929, E959, E969, E977, E989, or E999.1) should be used with any report of a late effect or sequela resulting from a previous injury or poisoning (905-909).

3. A late effect E code should never be used with a related current "nature of injury" code.

4. Use a late effect E code for subsequent visits when a late effect of the initial injury or poisoning is being treated. There is no late effect E code for adverse effects of drugs. Do not use a late effect E code for subsequent visits for follow-up care (e.g., to assess healing, to receive rehabilitative therapy) of the injury or poisoning when no late effect of the injury has been documented.

Misadventures and Complications of Care Guidelines

1. Assign a code in the range of E870-E876 if misadventures are stated by the physician.

2. Assign a code in the range of E878-E879 if the physician attributes an abnormal reaction or later complication to a surgical or medical procedure, but does not mention misadventure at the time of the procedure as the cause of the reaction.

Terrorism Guidelines

1. When the cause of an injury is identified by the Federal Government (FBI) as terrorism, the first-listed E code should be from category E979, *Terrorism*. The definition of terrorism employed by the FBI is found at the inclusion note at E979. The terrorism E code is the only E code that should be assigned. Additional E codes from the assault categories should not be assigned.

2. When the cause of an injury is only *suspected* to be the result of terrorism, a code from category E979 should *not* be assigned. Assign an E code based on circumstances in the documentation of intent and mechanism.

3. Assign code E979.9, *Terrorism, secondary effects*, for conditions occurring subsequent to the terrorist event. This code should not be assigned for conditions that are due to the initial terrorist act.

4. For statistical purposes, these codes will be tabulated within the category for assault, expanding the current category from E960-E969 to include E979 and E999.1.

Examples Using E Codes

When using E-codes, search the Alphabetic Index (Volume 2) for the main term identifying the cause such as "accident," "fire," "shooting," "fall," or "collision." To find the E-code for an adverse reaction to surgical or medical treatment, use the main term "reaction."

Coding Example

Burns to right arm, occurred while burning trash

943.00 Burn of upper limb, except wrist and hand, unspecified degree

E897   Accident caused by controlled fire not in building or structure

E-codes are important for providing the details of an accident to an insurance carrier to enable them to issue faster and more accurate reimbursement. Most insurance carriers want to be sure they reimburse only for services covered under their policy and not for services covered under worker's compensation, automobile or homeowner's insurance. A clear understanding of the circumstances will eliminate questions from the insurance carrier which cause delays in reimbursements.

Coding Example

Fractured ribs due to fall from ladder at home

807.00 Fracture of ribs, closed, unspecified

E881.0 Fall from ladder

E849.0 Place of occurrence, home

Using the above E-codes to provide important information regarding the circumstances of the injury to the insurance carrier eliminates any doubt about the insurer's responsibility for coverage. When using E-codes always list the E-codes as secondary or supplemental to the code(s) describing the injury.

PRINCIPAL AND ADDITIONAL DIAGNOSIS(ES): GUIDELINES FOR INPATIENT, SHORT-TERM, ACUTE CARE HOSPITAL RECORDS

Selecting Principal Diagnoses

The circumstances of inpatient admission always govern the selection of principal diagnosis. The principal diagnosis is defined in the Uniform Hospital Discharge Data Set (UHDDS) as that condition established after study to be chiefly responsible for occasioning the admission of the patient to the hospital for care.

The UHDDS definitions are used by all non-outpatient settings including acute care, short term, long term care and psychiatric hospitals; home health agencies; rehab facilities; and nursing homes. In determining principal diagnosis, the coding conventions in the ICD-9-CM, Volumes I and II take precedence over these official coding guidelines. (See Section IA).

The importance of consistent, complete documentation in the medical record cannot be overemphasized. Without such documentation the application of all coding guidelines is a difficult, if not impossible, task.

1. Codes for symptoms, signs, and ill-defined conditions.

   Codes for symptoms, signs, and ill-defined conditions from Chapter 16 are not to be used as principal diagnosis when a related definitive diagnosis has been established.

2. Two or more interrelated conditions, each potentially meeting the definition for principal diagnosis.

   When there are two or more interrelated conditions (such as diseases in the same ICD-9-CM chapter or manifestations characteristically associated with a certain disease) potentially meeting the definition of principal diagnosis, either condition may be sequenced first, unless the circumstances of the admission, the therapy provided, the Tabular List, or the Alphabetic Index indicate otherwise.

3. Two or more diagnoses that equally meet the definition for principal diagnosis.

   In the unusual instance when two or more diagnoses equally meet the criteria for principal diagnosis as determined by the circumstances of admission, diagnostic workup and/or therapy provided, and the Alphabetic Index, Tabular List, or other coding guideline does not provide sequencing direction, any one of the diagnoses may be sequenced first.

4. Two or more comparative or contrasting conditions.

   In those rare instances when two or more contrasting or comparative diagnoses are documented as either/or (or similar terminology), they are coded as if the diagnoses were confirmed. The diagnoses are sequenced according to the circumstances of the admission. If no further determination can be made as to which diagnosis should be principal, either diagnosis may be sequenced first.

5. Symptom(s) followed by contrasting/comparative diagnoses.

    When a symptom(s) is followed by contrasting/comparative diagnoses, the symptom code is sequenced first. All the contrasting/comparative diagnoses should be coded as additional diagnoses.

6. Original treatment plan not carried out.

    Sequence as the principal diagnosis the condition, which after study occasioned the admission to the hospital, even though treatment may not have been carried out due to unforeseen circumstances.

7. Complications of surgery and other medical care.

    When the admission is for treatment of a complication resulting from surgery or other medical care, the complication code is sequenced as the principal diagnosis. If the complication is classified to the 996-999 series and the code lacks the necessary specificity in describing the complication, an additional code for the specific complication may be assigned.

8. Uncertain Diagnosis.

    If the diagnosis documented at the time of discharge is qualified as "probable," "possible," "suspected," "likely," "questionable," or "still to be ruled out," code the condition as if it existed or was established. The basis for these guidelines are the diagnostic workup, arrangements for further workup or observation, and initial therapeutic approach that correspond the closest to the established diagnosis. Note: This guideline is applicable only to short-term, acute, long-term care and psychiatric hospitals.

9. Admission from Observation Unit

    A. Admission Following Medical Observation

       When a patient is admitted to an observation unit for a medical condition, which either worsens or does not improve, and is subsequently admitted as an inpatient of the same hospital for this same medical condition, the principal diagnosis would be the medical condition which led to the hospital admission.

    B. Admission Following Post-Operative Observation

       When a patient is admitted to an observation unit to monitor a condition (or complication) that develops following outpatient surgery, and then is subsequently admitted as an inpatient of the same hospital, hospitals should apply the Uniform Hospital Discharge Data Set (UHDDS) definition of principal diagnosis as "that condition established after study to be chiefly responsible for occasioning the admission of the patient to the hospital for care."

10. Admission from Outpatient Surgery

    When a patient receives surgery in the hospital's outpatient surgery department and is subsequently admitted for continuing inpatient care at the same hospital, the following guidelines should be followed in selecting the principal diagnosis for the inpatient admission:

- If the reason for the inpatient admission is a complication, assign the complication as the principal diagnosis.

- If no complication or other condition is documented as the reason for the inpatient admission, assign the reason for the outpatient surgery as the principal diagnosis.

- If the reason for the inpatient admission is another condition unrelated to the surgery, assign the unrelated condition as the principal diagnosis.

Rules For Reporting Additional Diagnoses

For reporting purposes, the definition for "other diagnoses" is interpreted as additional conditions that affect patient care in terms of requiring: clinical evaluation; or therapeutic treatment; or diagnostic procedures; or extended length of hospital stay; or increased nursing care and/or monitoring.

The UHDDS item #11-b defines *Other Diagnoses* as "all conditions that coexist at the time of admission, that develop subsequently, or that affect the treatment received and/or the length of stay. Diagnoses that relate to an earlier episode which have no bearing on the current hospital stay are to be excluded."

UHDDS definitions apply to all non-outpatient settings including: acute care, short term, long term care and psychiatric hospitals; home health agencies; rehab facilities; and nursing homes. The UHDDS definitions are used by acute care short-term and long-term care hospitals to report inpatient data elements in a standardized manner.

The following guidelines are to be applied in designating other diagnoses when neither the Alphabetic Index nor the Tabular List in ICD-9-CM provide direction. The listing of the diagnoses in the patient record is the responsibility of the attending physician.

1. Previous conditions

   If the physician has included a diagnosis in the final diagnostic statement, such as the discharge summary or the face sheet, it should ordinarily be coded. Some physicians include in the diagnostic statement: resolved conditions or diagnoses and status-post procedures from previous admission that have no bearing on the current stay. Such conditions are not to be reported and are coded only if required by hospital policy.

   However, history codes (V10-V19) may be used as secondary codes if the historical condition or family history has an impact on current care or if it influences treatment.

2. Abnormal findings

   Abnormal findings (laboratory, x-ray, pathologic, and other diagnostic results) are not coded and reported unless the physician indicates their clinical significance. If the findings are outside the normal range and the attending physician has ordered other tests to evaluate the condition or prescribed treatment, it is appropriate to ask the physician whether the abnormal finding should be added.

   Note: This differs from the coding practices in the outpatient setting for coding encounters for diagnostic tests that have been interpreted by a physician.

3.   Uncertain Diagnosis

If the diagnosis documented at the time of discharge is qualified as probable, possible, suspected, likely, questionable, or still to be ruled out, code the condition as if it existed or was established. The basis for these guidelines are the diagnostic workup, arrangements for further workup or observation, and initial therapeutic approach that correspond most closely with the established diagnosis.

DIAGNOSTIC CODING AND REPORTING GUIDELINES FOR OUTPATIENT SERVICES

These coding guidelines for outpatient diagnoses have been approved for use by hospitals/physicians in coding and reporting hospital-based outpatient services and physician office visits.

Information about the use of certain abbreviations, punctuation, symbols, and other conventions used in the ICD-9-CM Tabular List (code numbers and titles), can be found under Conventions Used in the Tabular List. Information about the correct sequence to use in finding a code is also described previously in Section I.

The terms "encounter" and "visit" are often used interchangeably in describing outpatient service contacts and, therefore, appear together in these guidelines without distinguishing one from the other.

Though the conventions and general guidelines apply to all settings, coding guidelines for outpatient and physician reporting of diagnoses will vary in a number of instances from those for inpatient/hospital diagnoses, recognizing that:

The Uniform Hospital Discharge Data Set (UHDDS) definition of "principal diagnosis" applies only to inpatients in acute, short-term, general and long-term care and psychiatric hospitals.

Coding guidelines for inconclusive diagnoses (probable, suspected, rule out, etc.) were developed for inpatient reporting and do not apply to outpatients.

1.   Selection of first-listed condition

In the outpatient setting, the term "first-listed diagnosis" is used in lieu of "principal diagnosis."

In determining the first-listed diagnosis, the coding conventions of ICD-9-CM —as well as the general and disease-specific guidelines—take precedence over the outpatient guidelines.

Diagnoses often are not established at the time of the initial encounter/visit. It may take two or more visits before the diagnosis is confirmed.

The most critical rule involves beginning the search for the correct code assignment through the Alphabetic Index. Never begin searching initially in the Tabular List as this will lead to coding errors.

2.   The appropriate code or codes from 001.0 through V84.8 must be used to identify diagnoses, symptoms, conditions, problems, complaints, or other reason(s) for the encounter/visit.

3.   For accurate reporting of ICD-9-CM diagnosis codes, the documentation should describe the patient's condition using terminology which includes specific diagnoses as well as symptoms, problems, or reasons for the encounter. There are ICD-9-CM codes to describe all of these.

4.   The selection of codes 001.0 through 999.9 will frequently be used to describe the reason for the encounter. These codes are from the section of ICD-9-CM for the classification of diseases and injuries (e.g. infectious and parasitic diseases; neoplasms; symptoms, signs, and ill-defined conditions, etc.).

5.   Codes that describe symptoms and signs, as opposed to diagnoses, are acceptable for reporting purposes when a diagnosis has not been established (confirmed) by the physician. Chapter 16 of ICD-9-CM, *Symptoms, Signs, and Ill-defined Conditions* (codes 780.0 to 799.9) contain many, but not all codes for symptoms.

6.   ICD-9-CM provides codes to deal with encounters for circumstances other than a disease or injury. *The Supplementary Classification of Factors Influencing Health Status and Contact with Health Services* (V01.0-V83.89) is provided to deal with occasions when circumstances other than a disease or injury are recorded as diagnosis or problems.

7.   Level of Detail in Coding

   a.   ICD-9-CM is composed of codes with either 3, 4, or 5 digits. Codes with three digits are included in ICD-9-CM as the heading of a category of codes that may be further subdivided by the use of fourth and/or fifth digits, which provide greater specificity.

   b.   A three-digit code is to be used only if it is not further subdivided. Where fourth-digit subcategories and/or fifth-digit subclassifications are provided, they must be assigned. A code is invalid if it has not been coded to the full number of digits required for that code.

8.   List first the ICD-9-CM code for the diagnosis, condition, problem, or other reason for encounter/visit shown in the medical record to be chiefly responsible for the services provided. List additional codes that describe any coexisting conditions. In some cases the first-listed diagnosis may be a symptom when a diagnosis has not been established (confirmed) by the physician.

9.   Do not code diagnoses documented as probable, suspected, questionable, rule out, or working diagnosis. Rather, code the condition(s) to the highest degree of certainty for that encounter/visit, such as symptoms, signs, abnormal test results, or other reason for the visit.

   Note: This differs from the coding practices used by hospital medical record departments for coding the diagnosis of acute care, short-term hospital inpatients.

10.   Chronic diseases treated on an ongoing basis may be coded and reported as many times as the patient receives treatment and care for the condition(s).

11.   Code all documented conditions that coexist at the time of the encounter/visit, and require or affect patient care treatment or management. Do not code conditions that were previously treated and no longer exist. However, history codes (V10-V19) may be used as secondary codes if the historical condition or family history has an impact on current care or influences treatment.

12. For patients receiving *diagnostic* services only during an encounter/visit, sequence first the diagnosis, condition, problem, or other reason for encounter/ visit shown in the medical record to be chiefly responsible for the outpatient services provided during the encounter/visit. Codes for other diagnoses (e.g., chronic conditions) may be sequenced as additional diagnoses. For outpatient encounters for diagnostic tests that have been interpreted by a physician, and the final report is available at the time of coding, code any confirmed or definitive diagnosis(es) documented in the interpretation. Do not code related signs and symptoms as additional diagnoses.

Note: This differs from the coding practice in the hospital inpatient setting regarding abnormal findings on test results.

13. For patients receiving *therapeutic* services only during an encounter/visit, sequence first the diagnosis, condition, problem, or other reason for encounter/ visit shown in the medical record to be chiefly responsible for the outpatient services provided during the encounter/visit. Codes for other diagnoses (e.g., chronic conditions) may be sequenced as additional diagnoses.

The only exception to this rule is that when the primary reason for the admission/encounter is chemotherapy, radiation therapy, or rehabilitation, the appropriate V code for the service is listed first, and the diagnosis or problem for which the service is being performed listed second.

14. For patient's receiving preoperative evaluations only, sequence a code from category V72.8, *Other specified examinations*, to describe the pre-op consultations. Assign a code for the condition to describe the reason for the surgery as an additional diagnosis. Code also any findings related to the pre-op evaluation.

15. For ambulatory surgery, code the diagnosis for which the surgery was performed. If the postoperative diagnosis is known to be different from the preoperative diagnosis at the time the diagnosis is confirmed, select the postoperative diagnosis for coding, since it is the most definitive.

16. For routine outpatient prenatal visits when no complications are present, codes V22.0, *Supervision of normal first pregnancy*, and V22.1, *Supervision of other normal pregnancy*, should be used as principal diagnoses. These codes should not be used in conjunction with Chapter 11 *Pregnancy, Childbirth and the Puerperium* codes.

Anatomical Illustrations

A fundamental knowledge and understanding of basic human anatomy and physiology is a prerequisite for accurate diagnosis coding. While a comprehensive treatment of anatomy and physiology is beyond the scope of this text, the large scale, full color anatomical illustrations on the following pages are designed to facilitate the diagnosis coding process for both beginning and experienced coders.

The illustrations provide an anatomical perspective of diagnosis coding by providing a side-by-side view of the major systems of the human body and a corresponding list of the most common diagnoses categories used to support medical, surgical and diagnostic services performed on the illustrated system.

The diagnostic categories listed on the left facing page of each anatomical illustration are three-digit categories and may not be used for coding. These categories are provided as "pointers" to the appropriate section of the ICD-9-CM Volume 1 where the complete listings, including 4th and 5th digits if appropriate, may be found.

PLATE 1. SKIN AND SUBCUTANEOUS TISSUE — MALE

Viral diseases accompanied by exanthem	050-057

Neoplasms

Malignant melanoma of skin	172
Other malignant neoplasm of skin	173
Malignant neoplasm of male breast	175
Kaposi's sarcoma	176
Benign neoplasm of skin	216
Carcinoma in situ of skin	232

Infections of skin and subcutaneous tissue

Carbuncle and furuncle	680
Cellulitis and abscess of finger and toe	681
Other cellulitis and abscess	682
Acute lymphadenitis	683
Impetigo	684
Pilonidal cyst	685
Other local infections of skin and subcutaneous tissue	686

Other inflammatory conditions of skin and subcutaneous tissue

Erythematosquamous dermatosis	690
Atopic dermatitis and related conditions	691
Contact dermatitis and other eczema	692
Dermatitis due to substances taken internally	693
Bullous dermatoses	694
Erythematous conditions	695
Psoriasis and similar disorders	696
Lichen	697
Pruritus and related conditions	698

Other diseases of skin and subcutaneous tissue

Corns and callosities	700
Other hypertrophic and atrophic conditions of skin	701
Diseases of nail	703
Diseases of hair and hair follicles	704
Disorders of sweat glands	705
Diseases of sebaceous glands	706
Chronic ulcer of skin	707
Urticaria	708
Other disorders of skin and subcutaneous tissue	709
Symptoms involving skin and other integumentary tissue	782

Symptoms, signs and ill-defined conditions	780-799

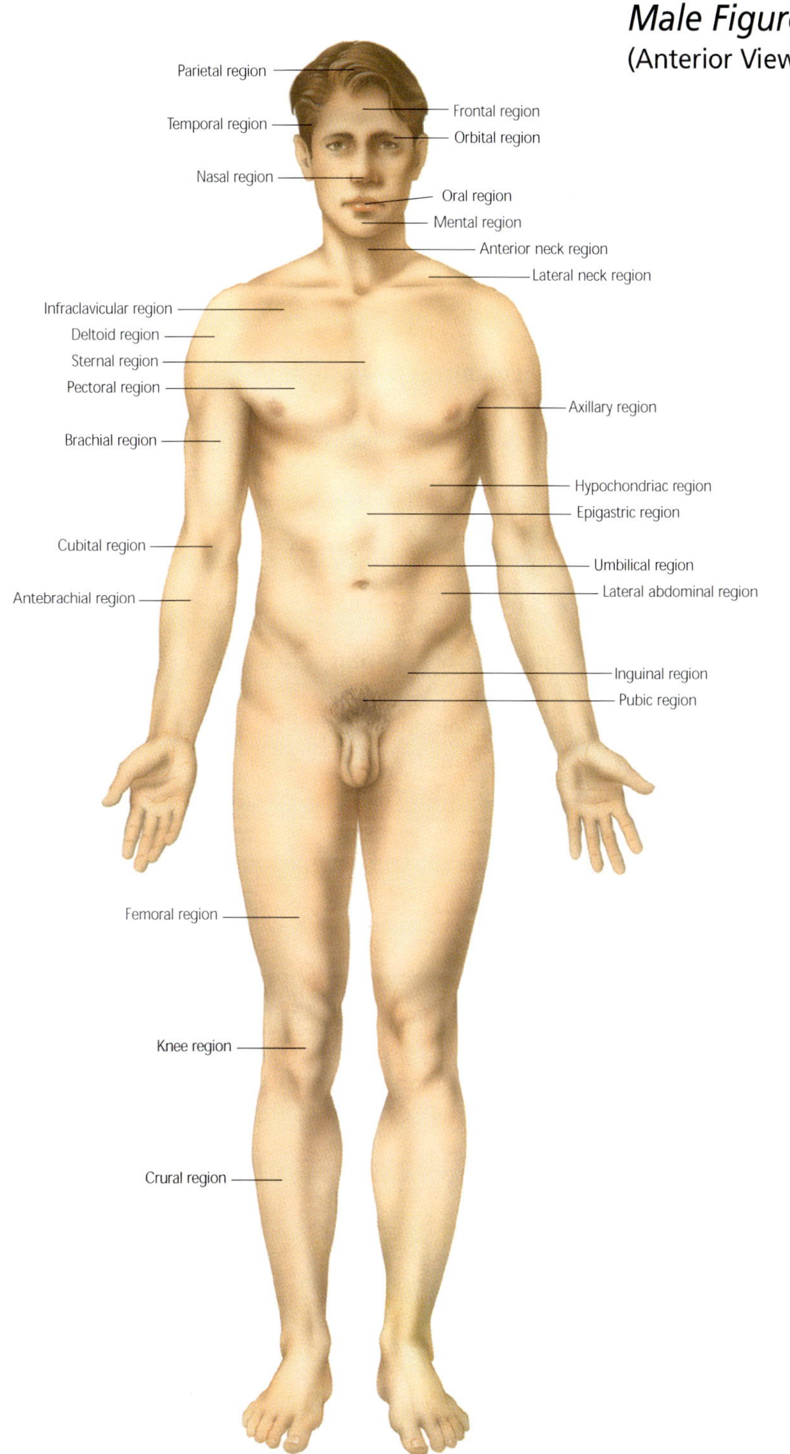

©Practice Management Information Corp., Los Angeles, CA

PLATE 2. SKIN AND SUBCUTANEOUS TISSUE — FEMALE

Female Figure
(Anterior View)

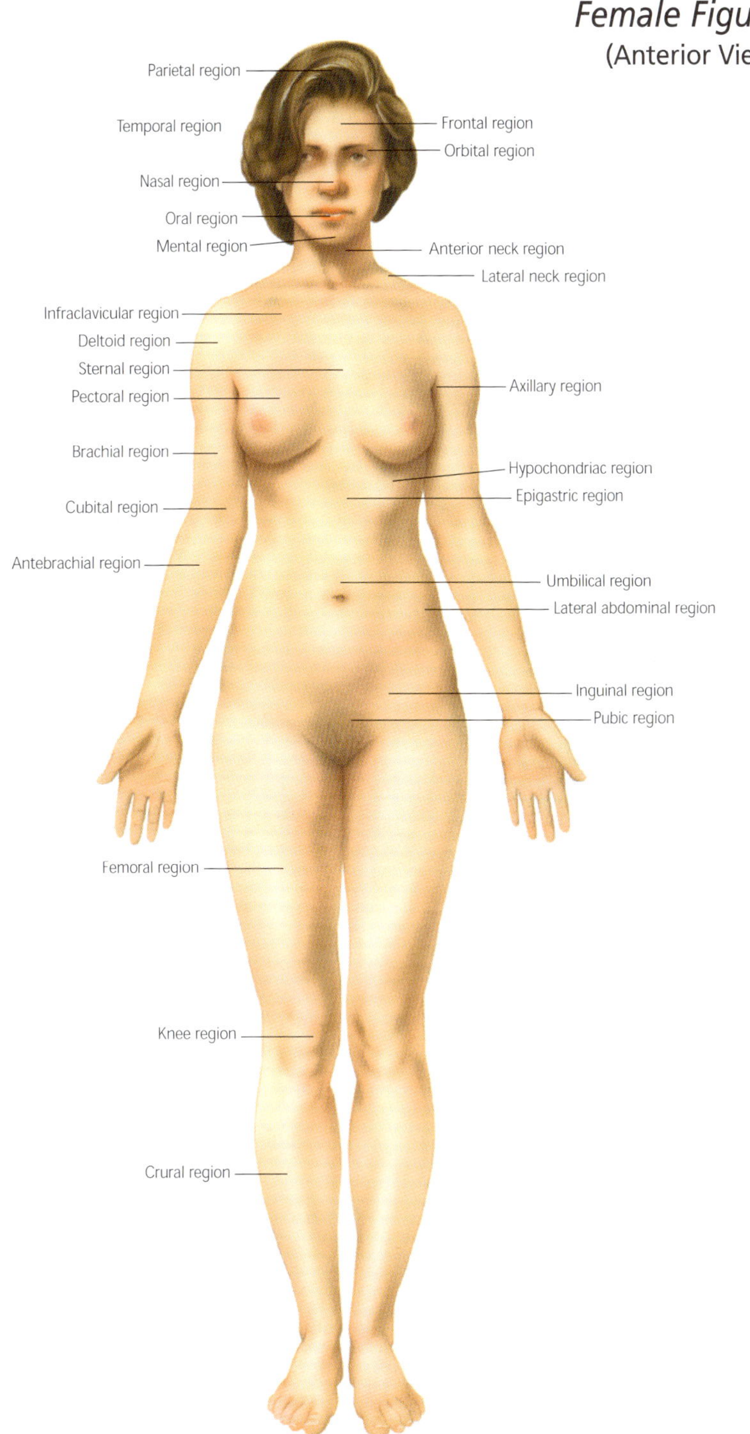

©Practice Management Information Corp., Los Angeles, CA

PLATE 3. FEMALE BREAST

Female Breast

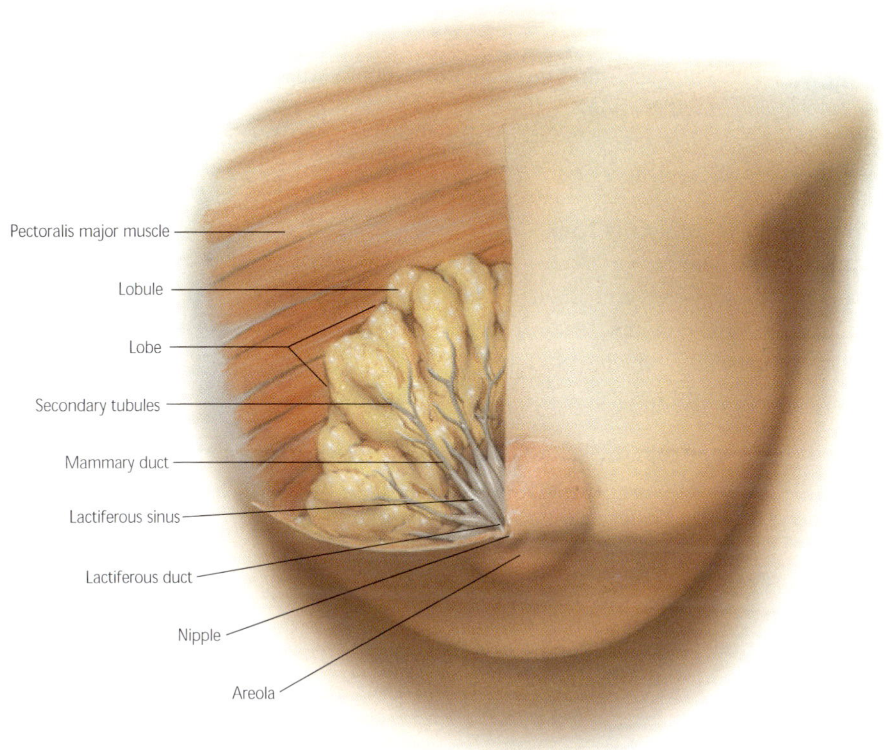

PLATE 4. MUSCULAR SYSTEM AND CONNECTIVE TISSUE — ANTERIOR VIEW

Muscular System
(Anterior View)

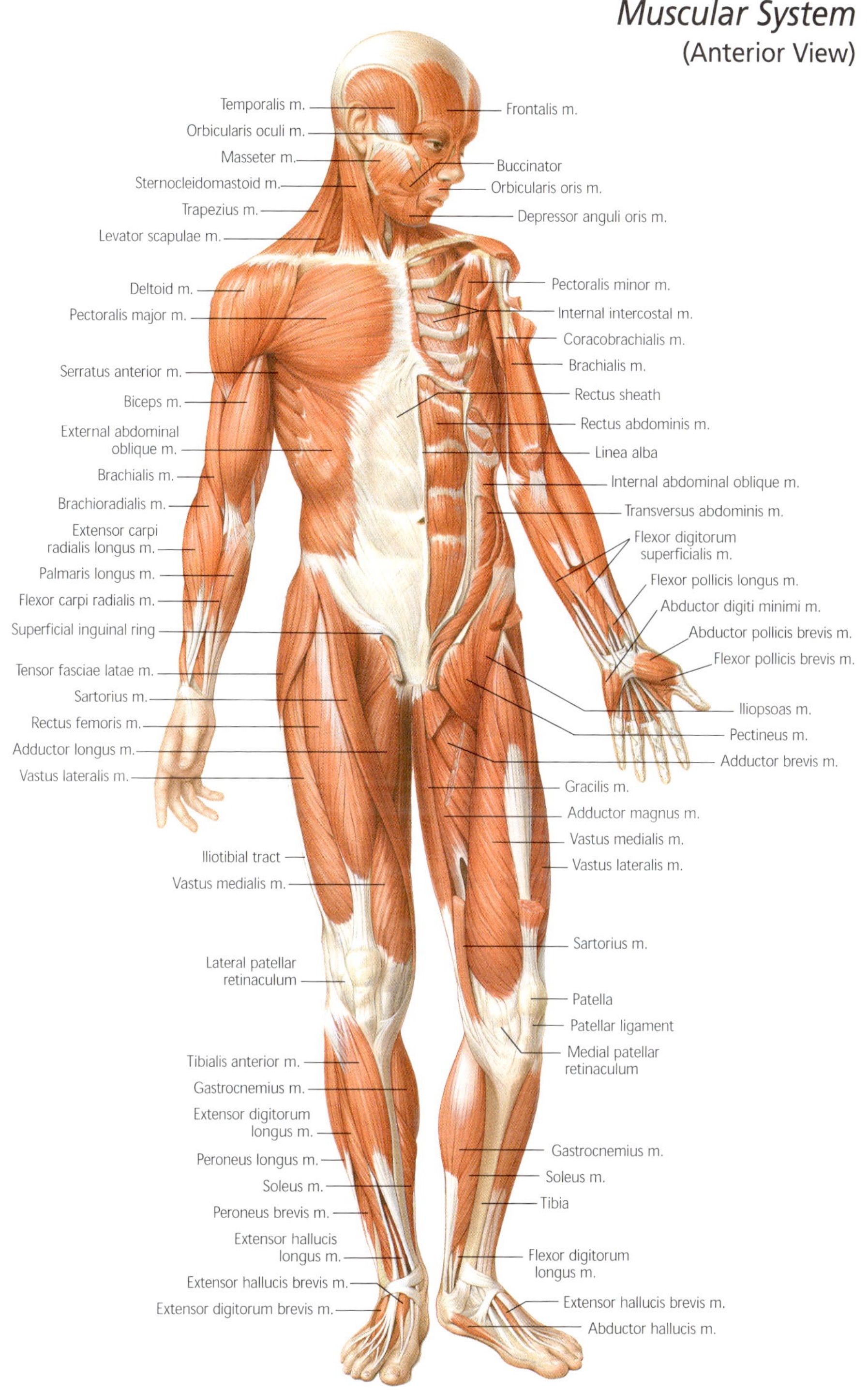

PLATE 5. MUSCULAR SYSTEM AND CONNECTIVE TISSUE — POSTERIOR VIEW

Muscular System
(Posterior View)

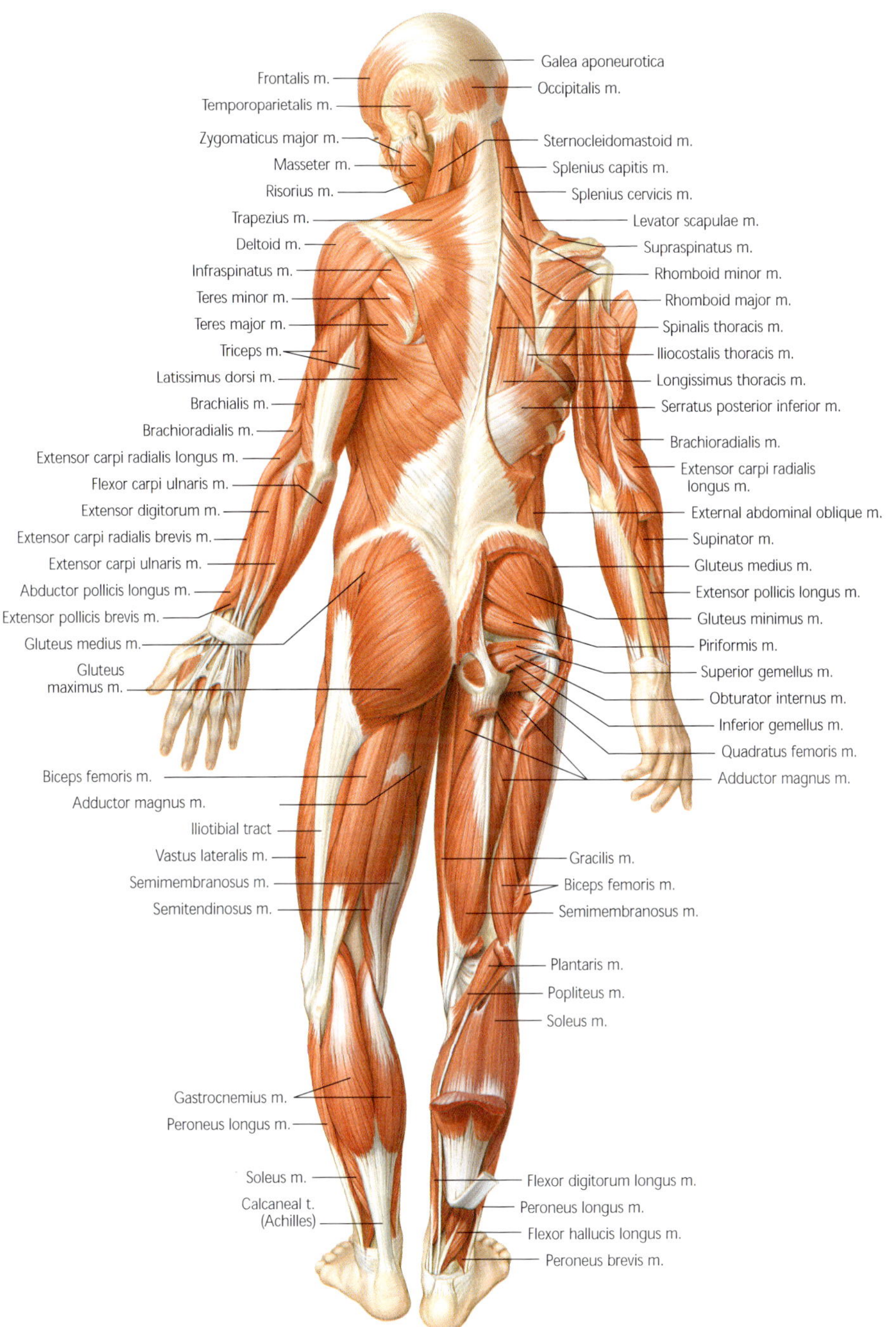

PLATE 6. MUSCULAR SYSTEM — SHOULDER AND ELBOW

Shoulder and Elbow
(Anterior View)

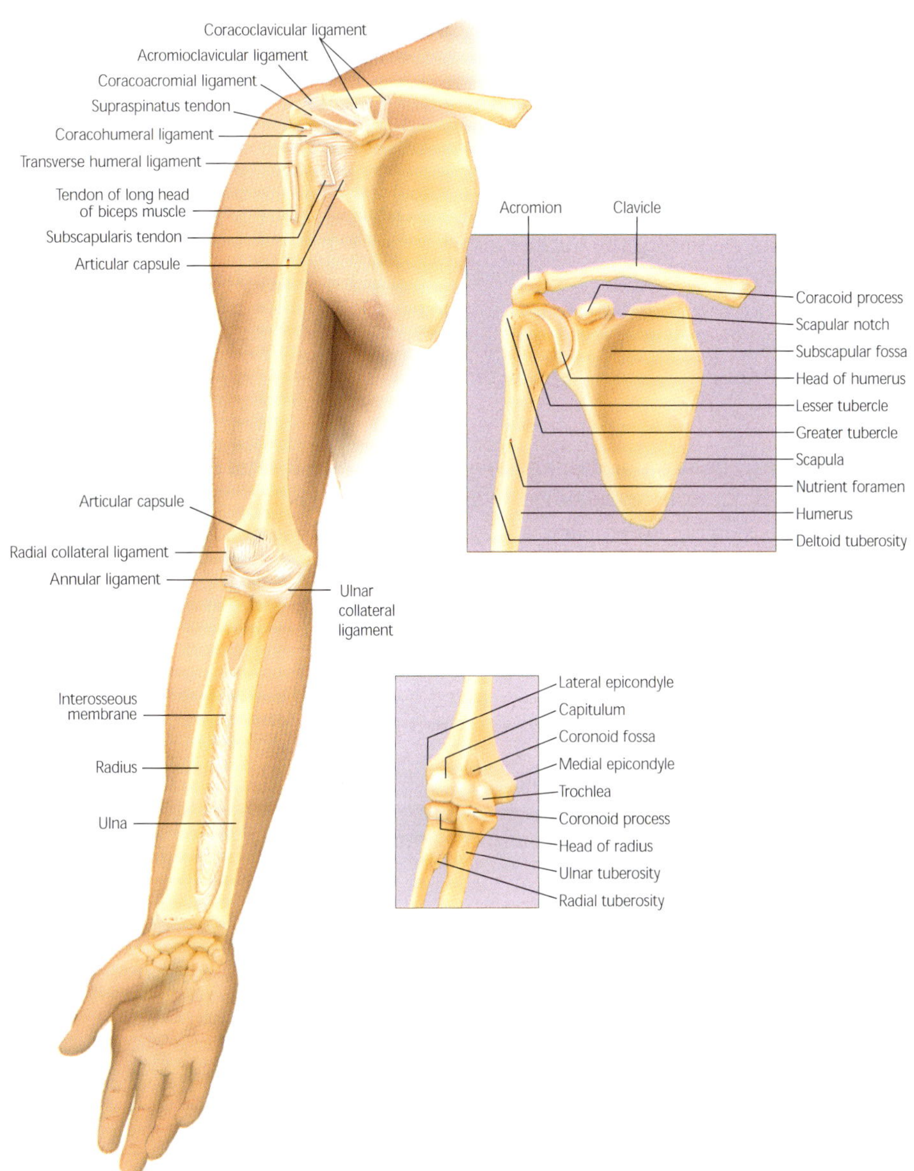

PLATE 7. MUSCULAR SYSTEM — HAND AND WRIST

Hand and Wrist

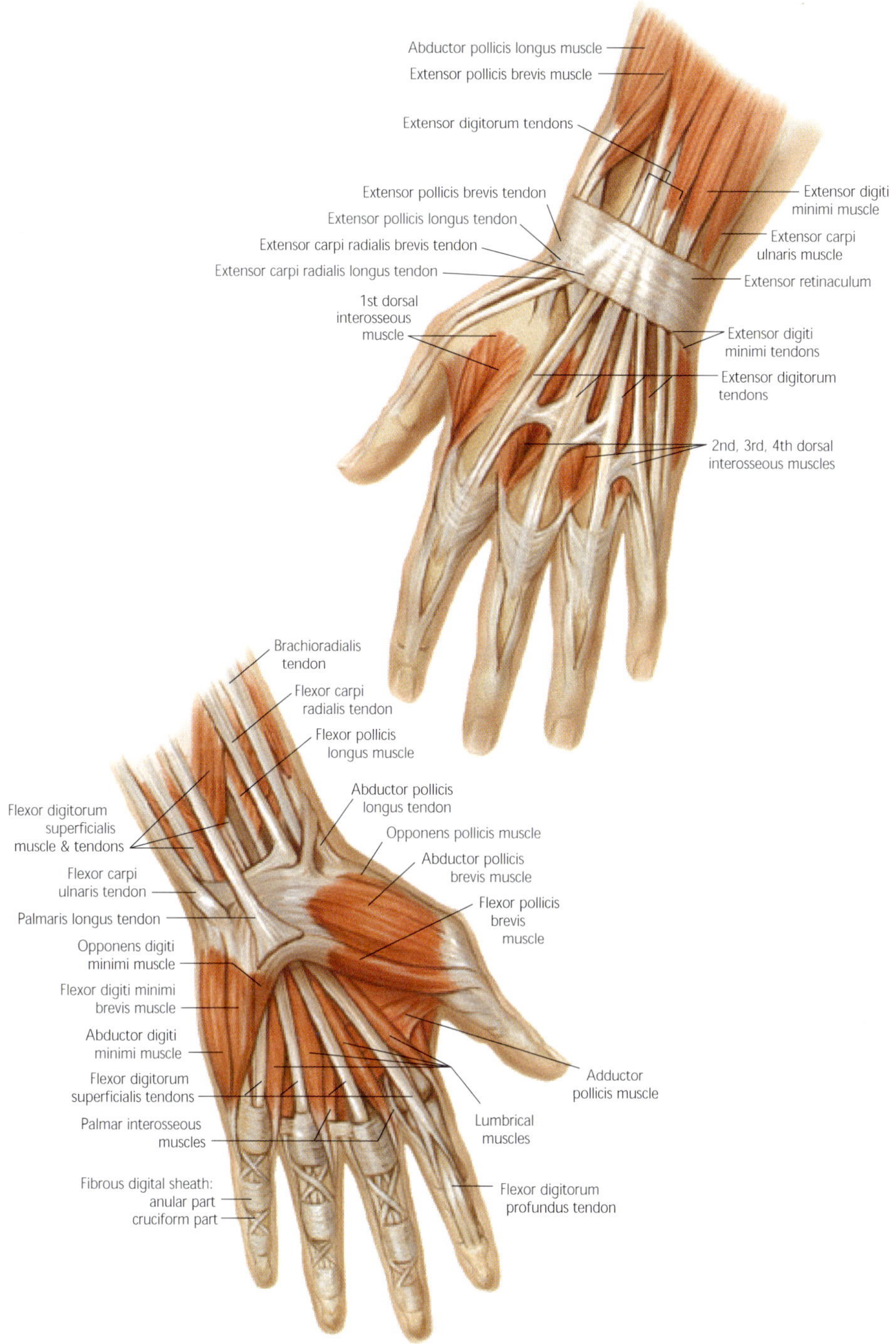

PLATE 8. MUSCULOSKELETAL SYSTEM — HIP AND KNEE

Hip and Knee
(Anterior View)

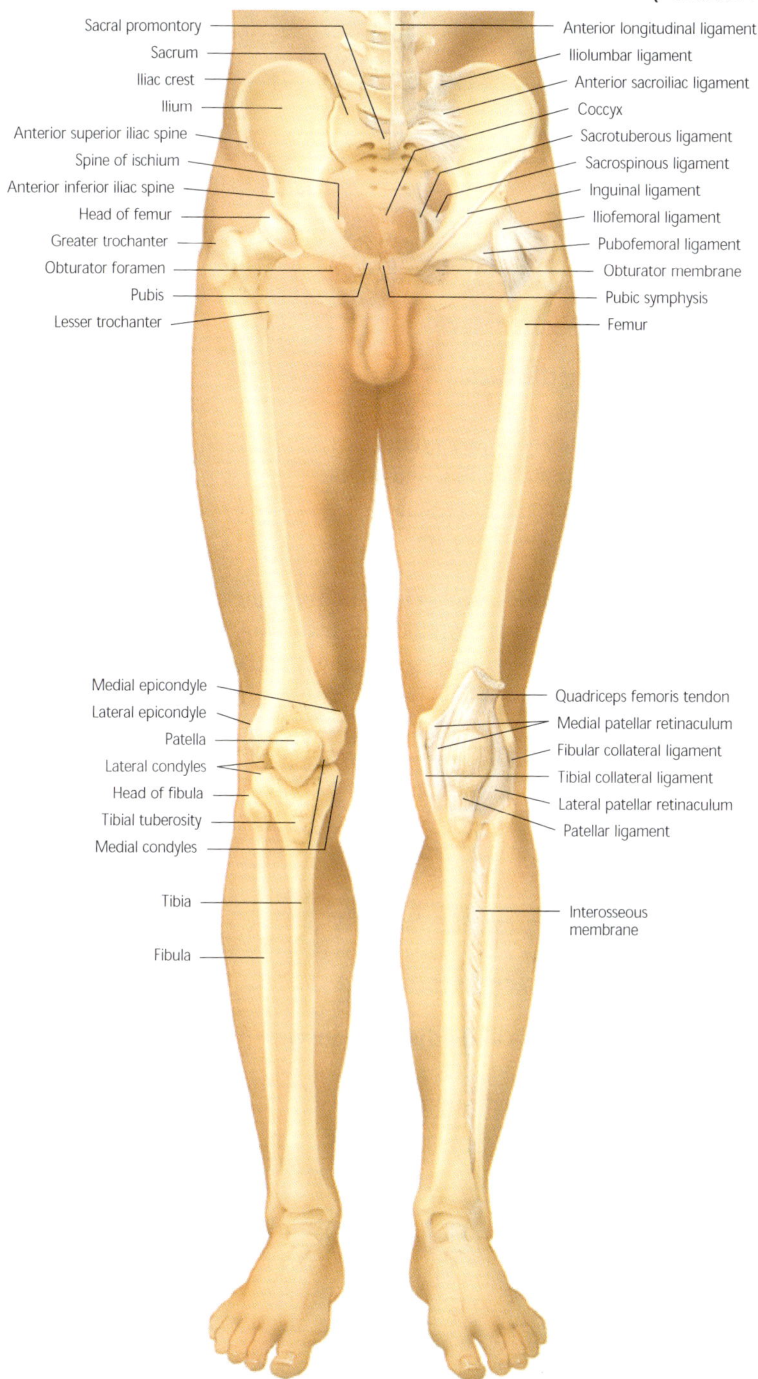

PLATE 9. MUSCULOSKELETAL SYSTEM — FOOT AND ANKLE

Foot and Ankle

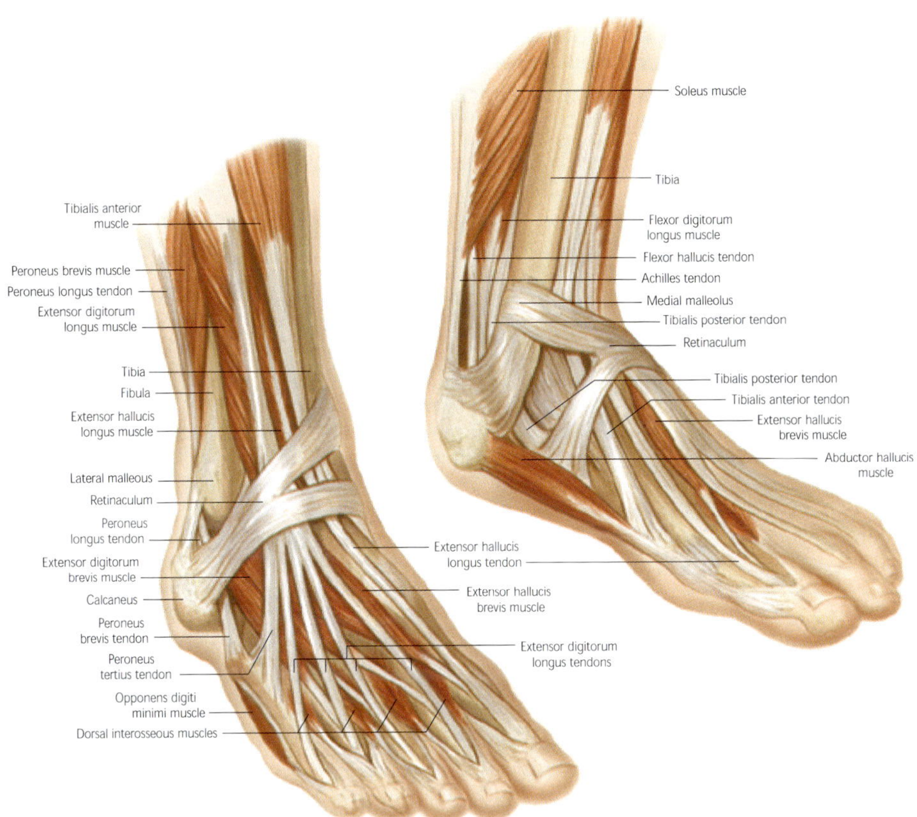

PLATE 10. SKELETAL SYSTEM — ANTERIOR VIEW

Skeletal System
(Anterior View)

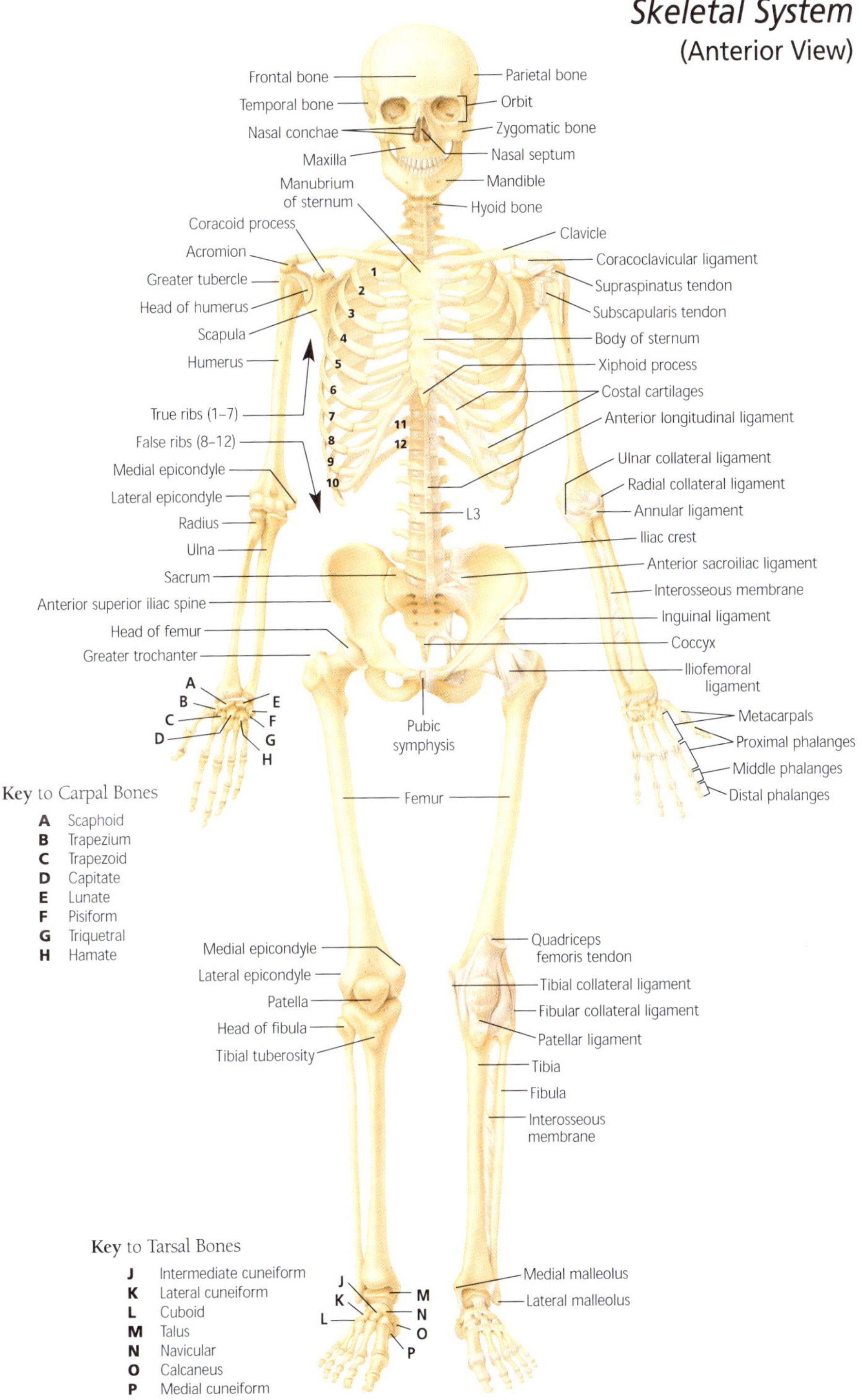

PLATE 11. SKELETAL SYSTEM — POSTERIOR VIEW

Symptoms, signs and ill-defined conditions   780-799

Fracture of skull

Fracture of vault of skull	800
Fracture of base of skull	801
Fracture of face bones	802
Multiple fractures involving skull or face with other bones	804

Fracture of neck and trunk

Fracture of vertebral column without mention of spinal cord injury	805
Fracture of vertebral column with spinal cord injury	806
Fracture of rib(s), sternum, larynx and trachea	807
Fracture of pelvis	808

Fracture of upper limb

Fracture of clavicle	810
Fracture of scapula	811
Fracture of humerus	812
Fracture of radius and ulna	813
Fracture of carpal bone(s)	814
Fracture of metacarpal bone(s)	815
Fracture of one or more phalanges of hand	816
Multiple fractures of hand bones	817

Fracture of lower limb

Fracture of neck of femur	820
Fracture of other and unspecified parts of femur	821
Fracture of patella	822
Fracture of tibia and fibula	823
Fracture of ankle	824
Fracture of one or more tarsal and metatarsal bones	825
Fracture of one or more phalanges of foot	826

Dislocation

Dislocation of jaw	830
Dislocation of shoulder	831
Dislocation of elbow	832
Dislocation of wrist	833
Dislocation of finger	834
Dislocation of hip	835
Dislocation of knee	836
Dislocation of ankle	837
Dislocation of foot	838

Skeletal System
(Posterior View)

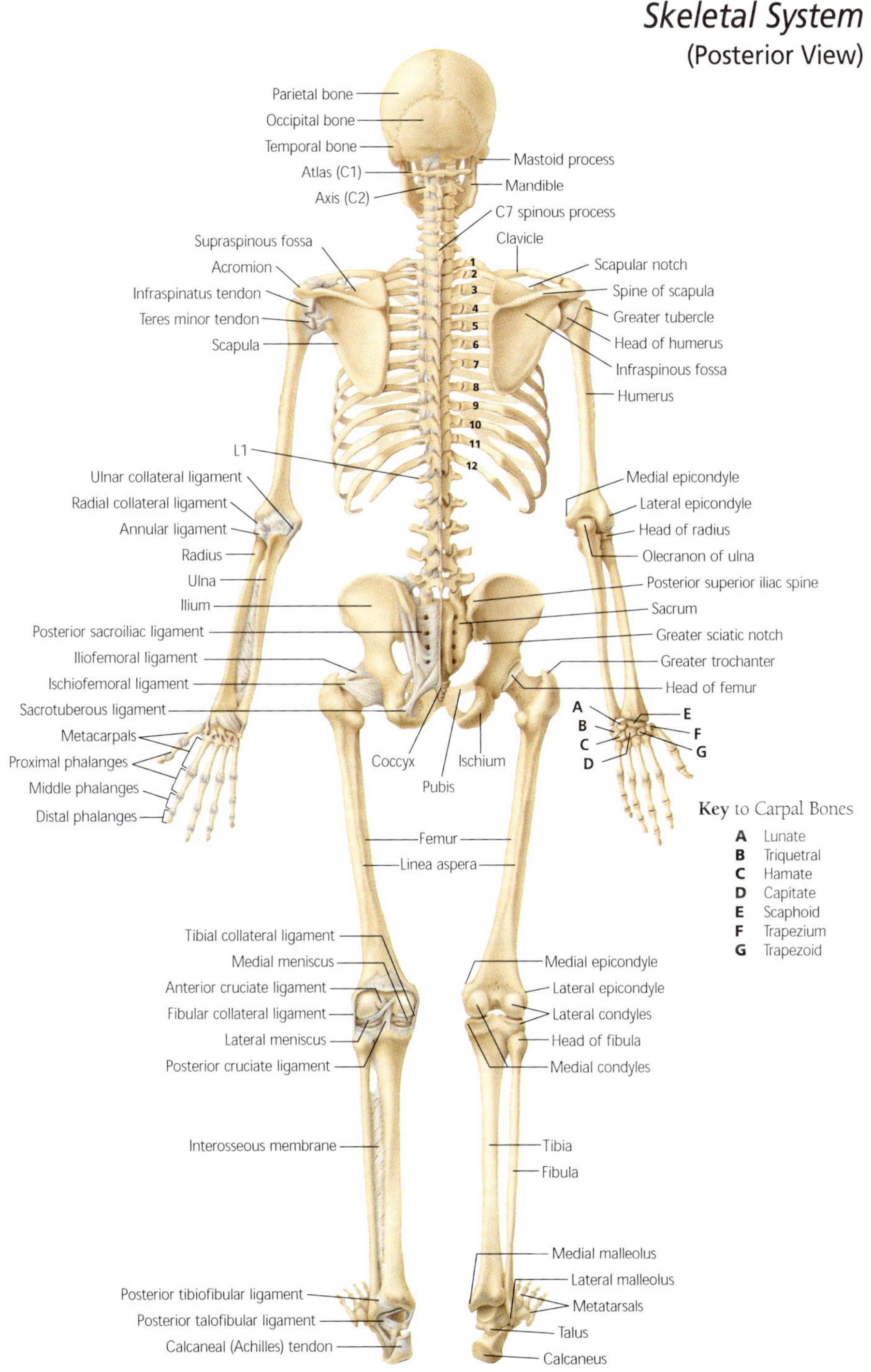

PLATE 12. SKELETAL SYSTEM — VERTEBRAL COLUMN

Vertebral Column
(Lateral View)

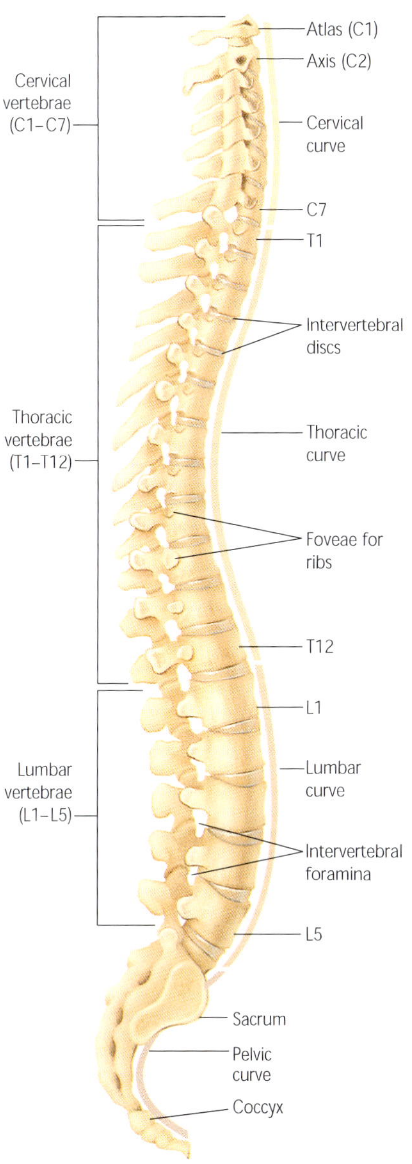

PLATE 13. RESPIRATORY SYSTEM

Respiratory System

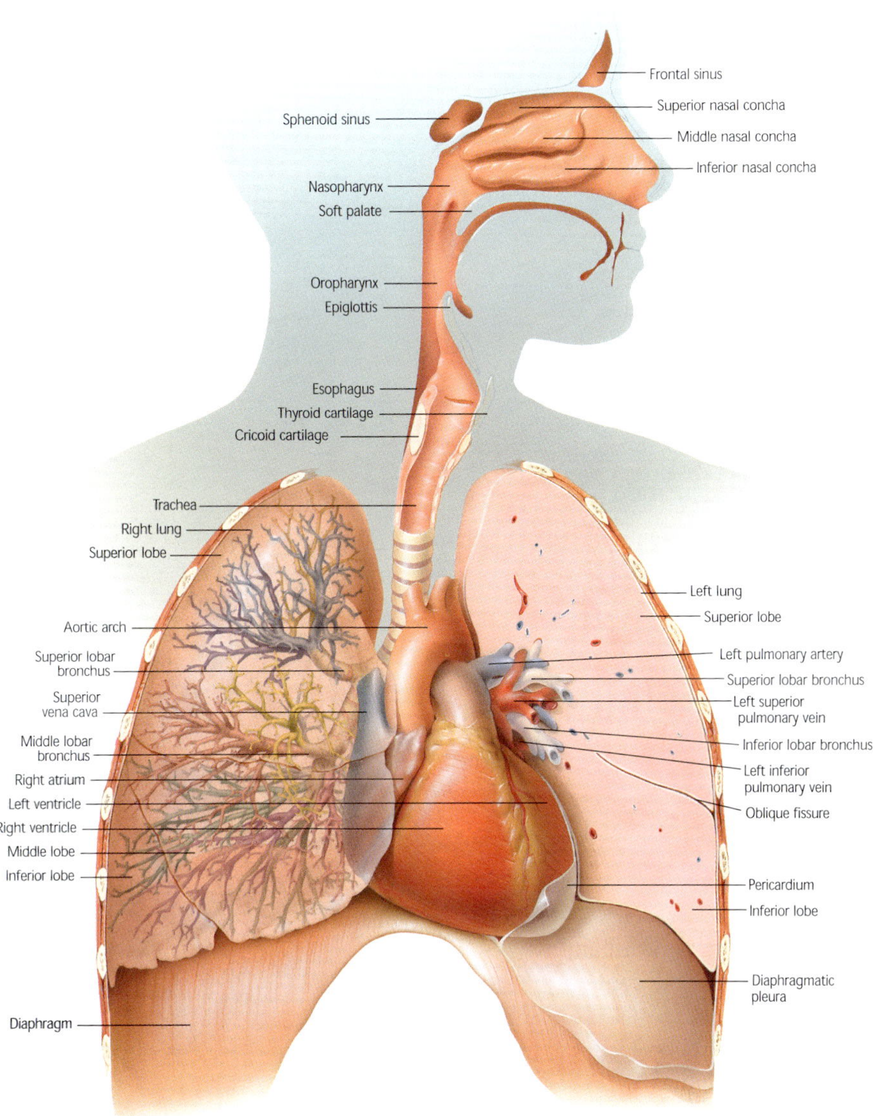

PLATE 14. HEART AND PERICARDIUM

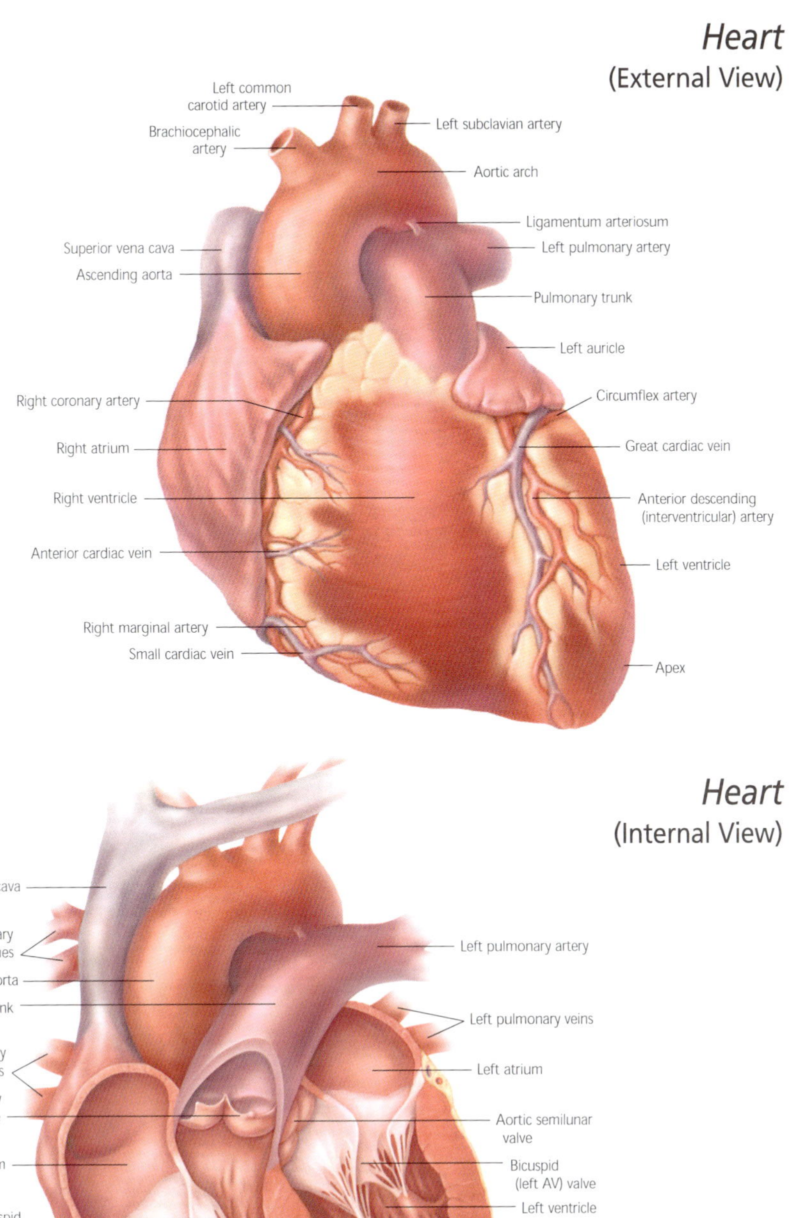
Heart
(External View)
Left common carotid artery
Brachiocephalic artery
Left subclavian artery
Aortic arch
Ligamentum arteriosum
Left pulmonary artery
Superior vena cava
Ascending aorta
Pulmonary trunk
Left auricle
Right coronary artery
Circumflex artery
Great cardiac vein
Right atrium
Right ventricle
Anterior descending (interventricular) artery
Anterior cardiac vein
Left ventricle
Right marginal artery
Small cardiac vein
Apex
Heart
(Internal View)
Superior vena cava
Right pulmonary artery branches
Left pulmonary artery
Aorta
Pulmonary trunk
Left pulmonary veins
Right pulmonary veins
Left atrium
Pulmonary semilunar valve
Aortic semilunar valve
Right atrium
Bicuspid (left AV) valve
Left ventricle
Tricuspid (right AV) valve
Papillary muscle
Interventricular septum
Chordae tendineae
Inferior vena cava
Myocardium
Right ventricle
Trabeculae carneae

PLATE 15. CIRCULATORY SYSTEM

Vascular System

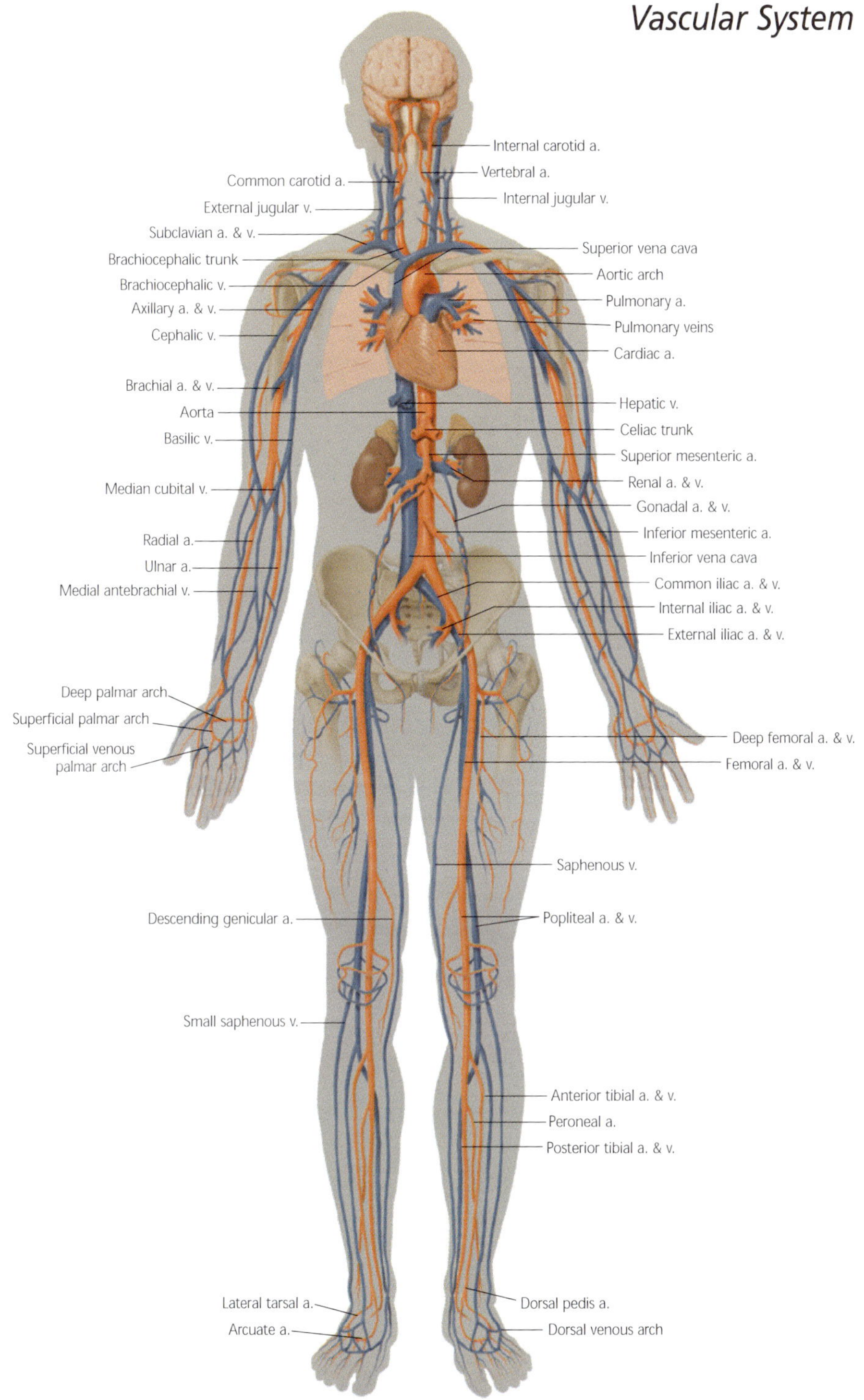

PLATE 16. DIGESTIVE SYSTEM

Digestive System

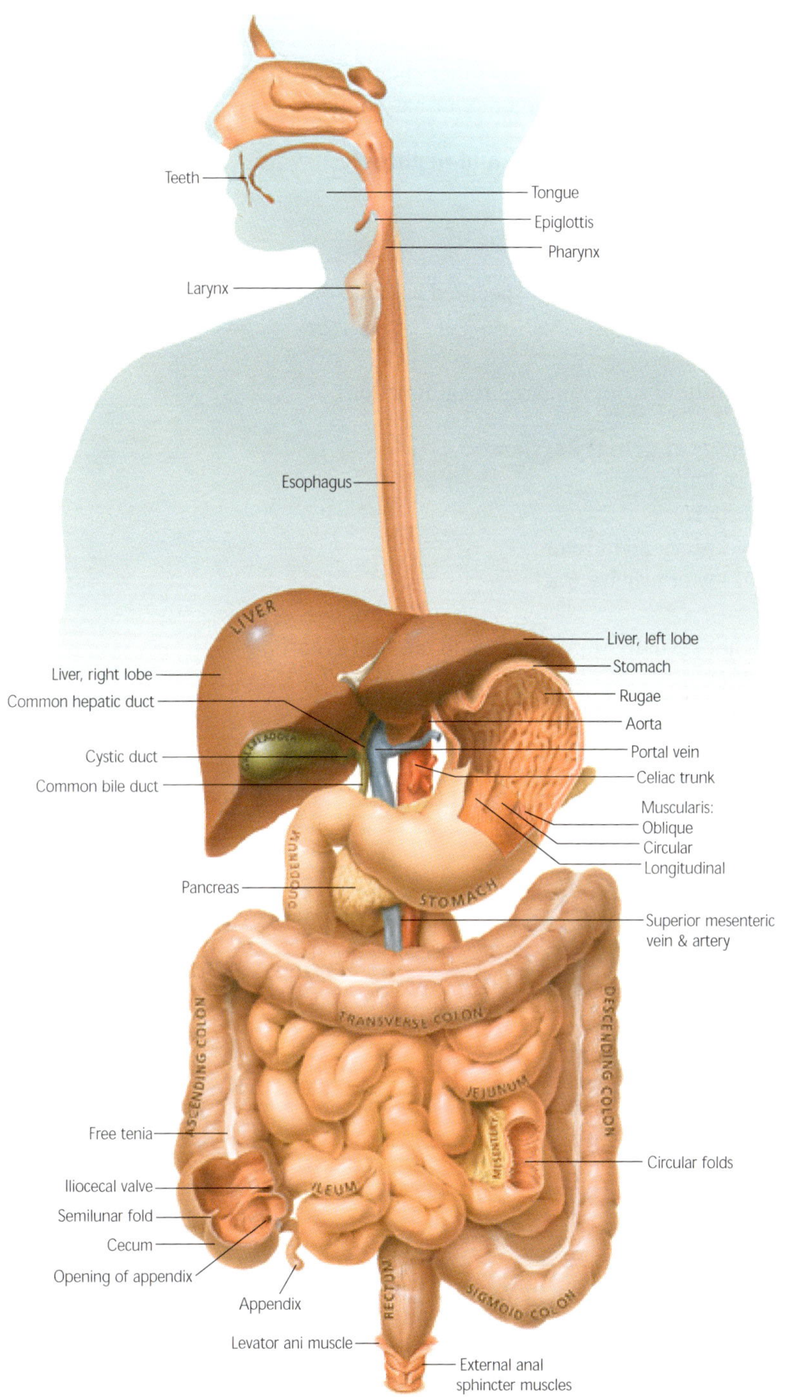

PLATE 17. GENITOURINARY SYSTEM

Urinary System

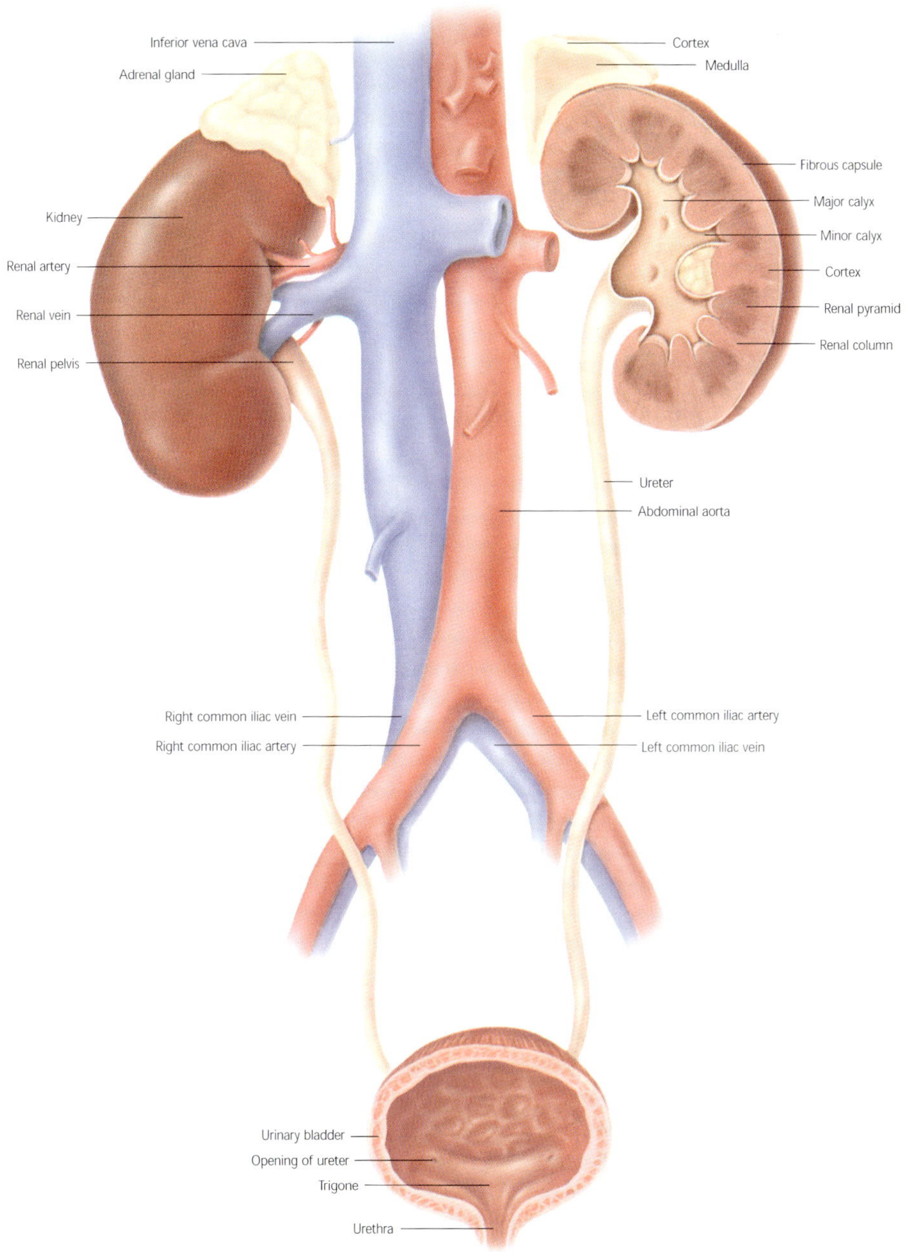

PLATE 18. MALE REPRODUCTIVE SYSTEM

Neoplasms

Diseases of male genital organs

Male Reproductive System

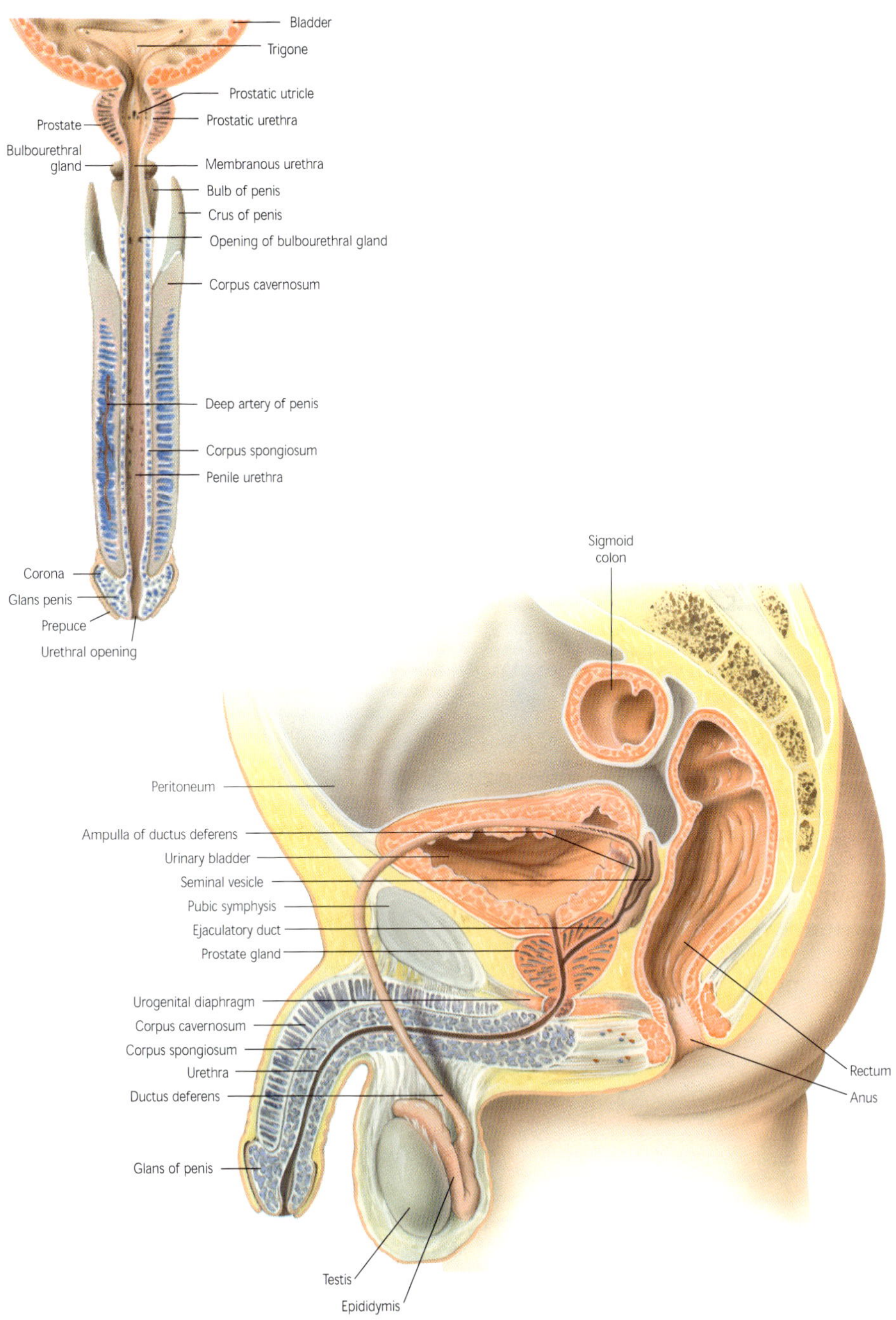

PLATE 19. FEMALE REPRODUCTIVE SYSTEM

Female Reproductive System

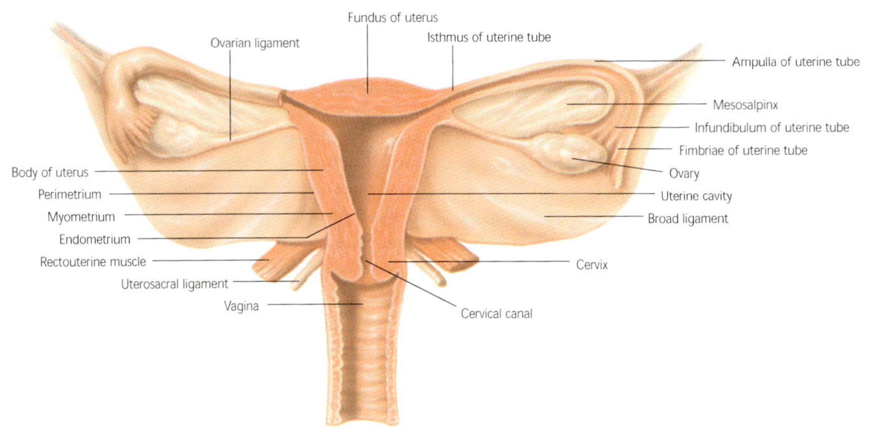

PLATE 20. PREGNANCY, CHILDBIRTH AND THE PUERPERIUM

Female Reproductive System: Pregnancy
(Lateral View)

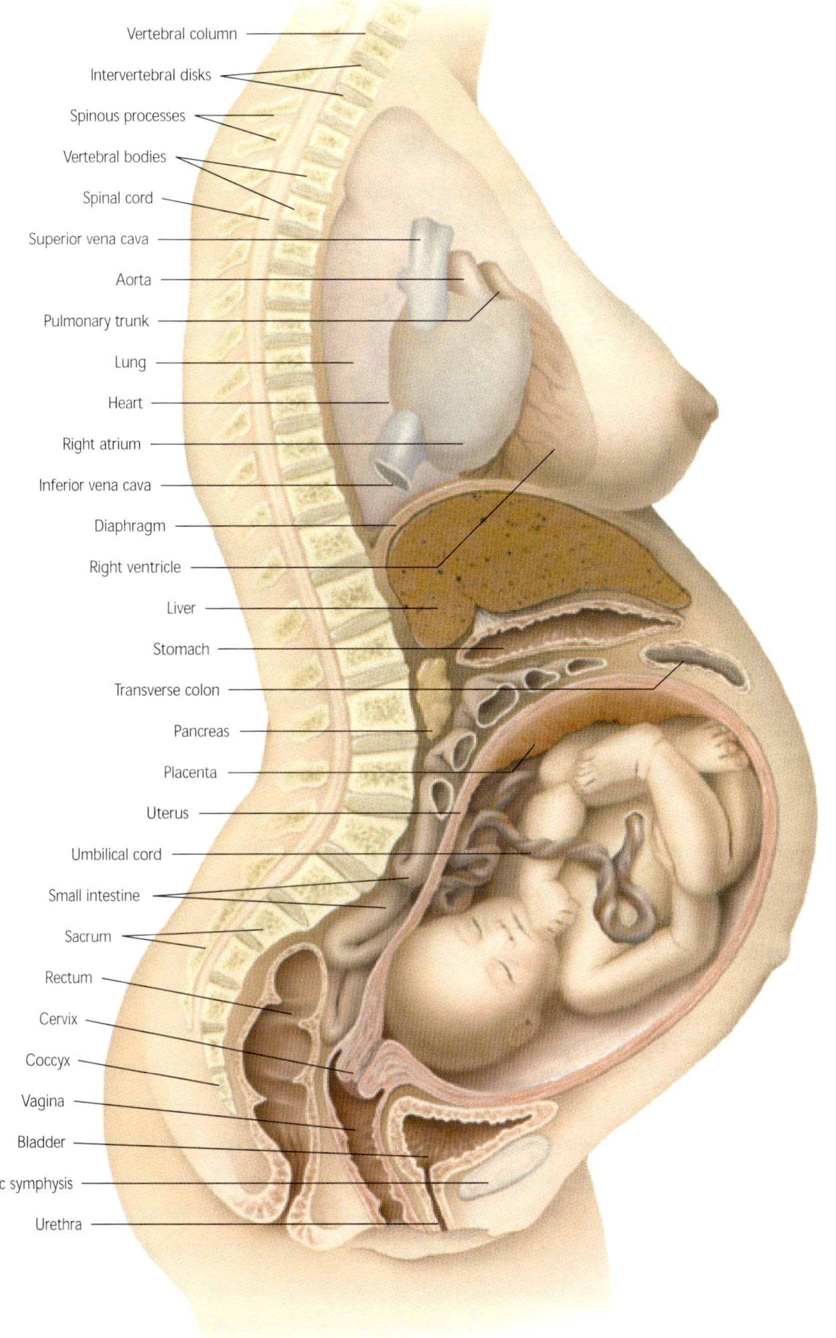

©Practice Management Information Corp., Los Angeles, CA

PLATE 21. NERVOUS SYSTEM — BRAIN

Brain
(Base View)

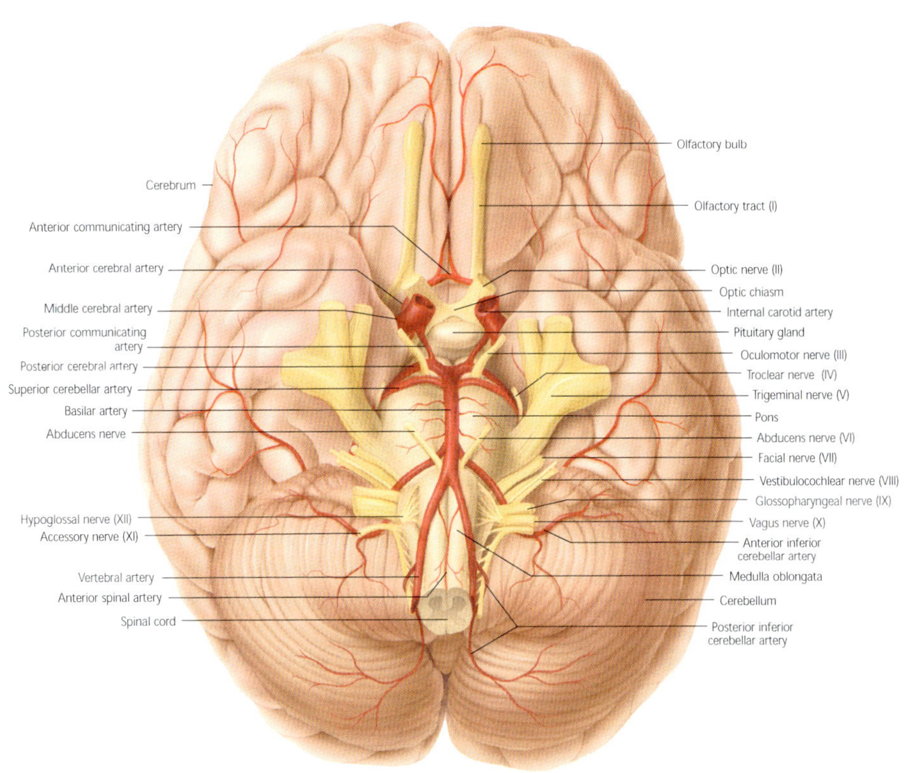

PLATE 22. NERVOUS SYSTEM

Nervous System

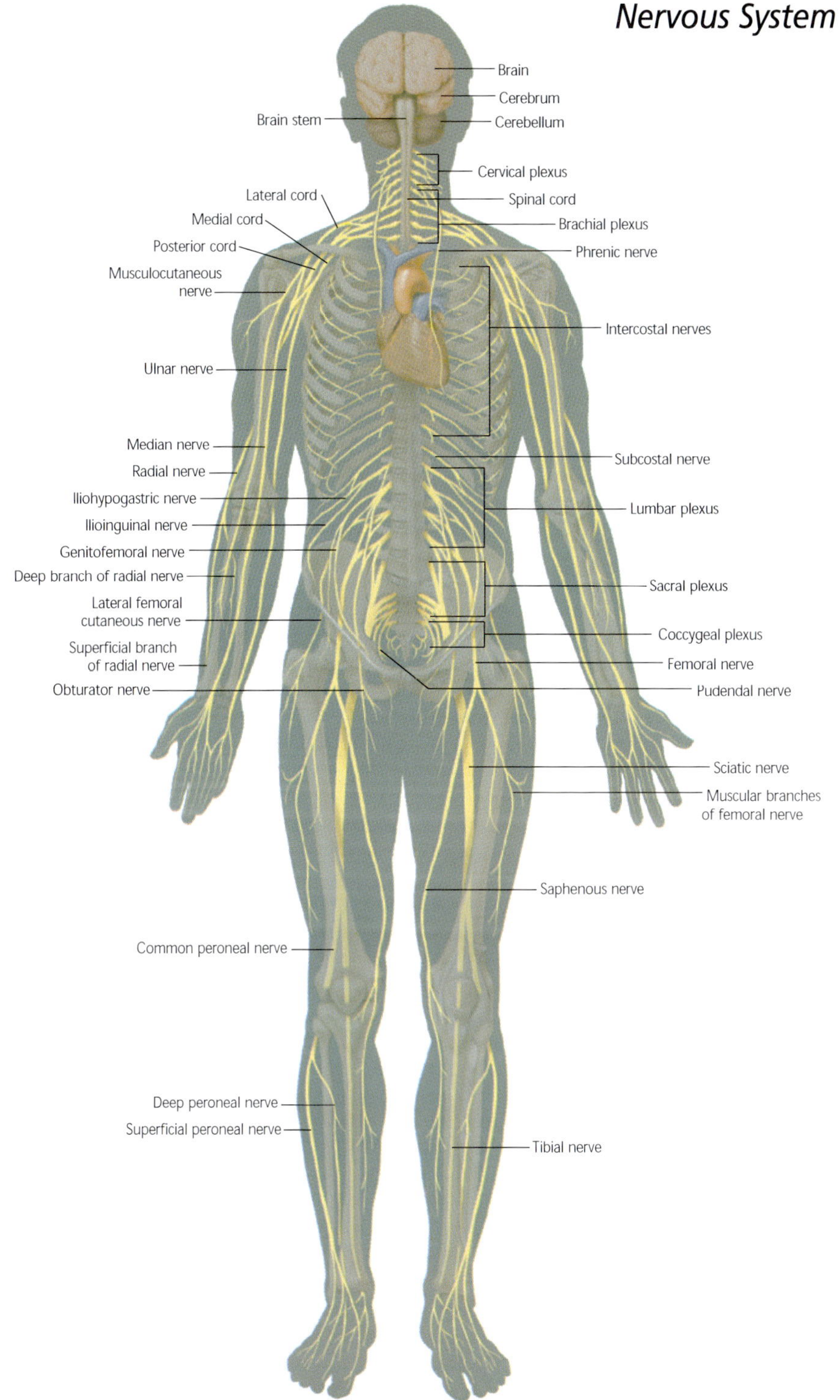

PLATE 23. EYE AND OCULAR ADNEXA

Right Eye
(Horizontal Section)

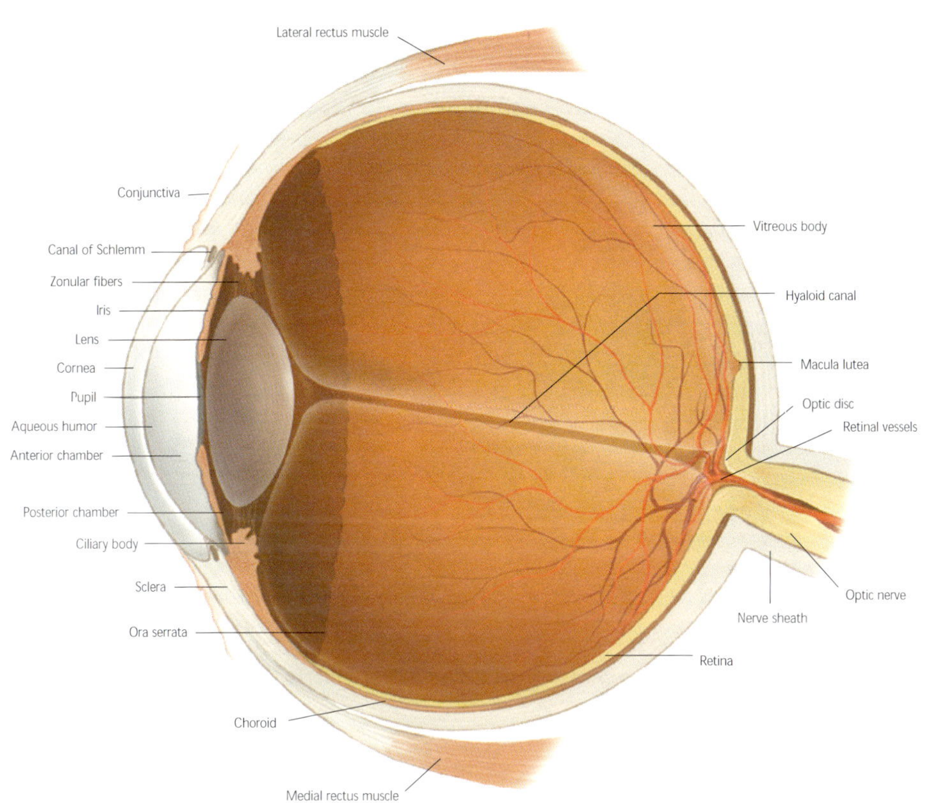

PLATE 24. AUDITORY SYSTEM

The Ear

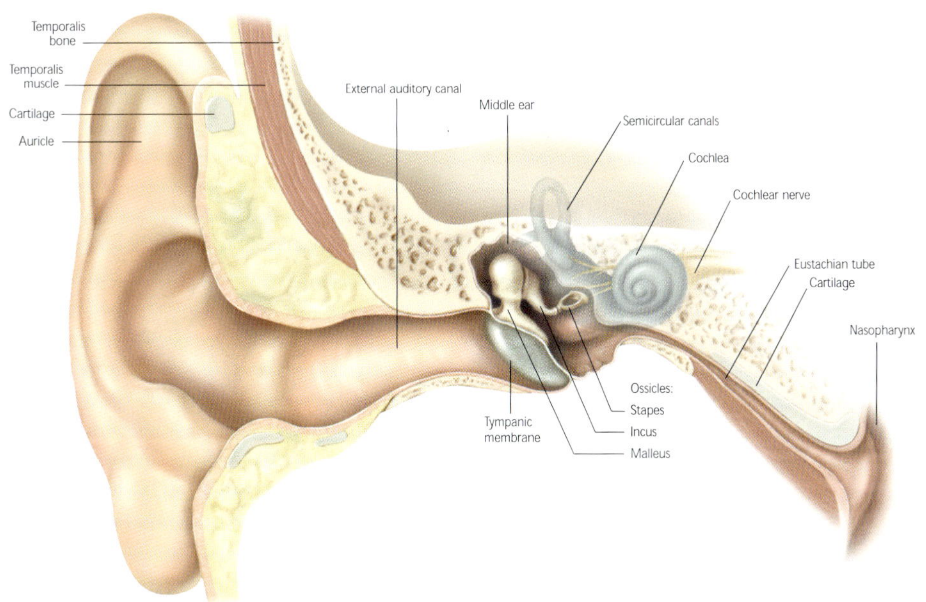

Temporalis bone
Temporalis muscle
Cartilage
Auricle
External auditory canal
Middle ear
Semicircular canals
Cochlea
Cochlear nerve
Eustachian tube
Cartilage
Nasopharynx
Ossicles:
Stapes
Incus
Malleus
Tympanic membrane

DISEASES: TABULAR LIST

VOLUME 1

1. INFECTIOUS AND PARASITIC DISEASES (001-139)

Note: Categories for "late effects" of infectious and parasitic diseases are to be found at 137-139.

Includes: diseases generally recognized as communicable or transmissible as well as a few diseases of unknown but possibly infectious origin

Excludes: *acute respiratory infections (460-466)*

carrier or suspected carrier of infectious organism (V02.0-V02.9)
certain localized infections
influenza (487.0-487.8)

INTESTINAL INFECTIOUS DISEASES (001-009)

Excludes: *helminthiases (120.0-129)*

001 Cholera

    001.0 Due to Vibrio cholerae

    001.1 Due to Vibrio cholerae el tor

    001.9 Cholera, unspecified

002 Typhoid and paratyphoid fevers

    002.0 Typhoid fever
        Typhoid (fever) (infection) [any site]

    002.1 Paratyphoid fever A

    002.2 Paratyphoid fever B

    002.3 Paratyphoid fever C

    002.9 Paratyphoid fever, unspecified

003 Other salmonella infections
    Includes: infection or food poisoning by Salmonella [any serotype]

    003.0 Salmonella gastroenteritis
        Salmonellosis

    003.1 Salmonella septicemia

    ⑤ **003.2 Localized salmonella infections**

        003.20 Localized salmonella infection, unspecified

        003.21 Salmonella meningitis

        003.22 Salmonella pneumonia

        003.23 Salmonella arthritis

        003.24 Salmonella osteomyelitis

        003.29 Other

    003.8 Other specified salmonella infections

    003.9 Salmonella infection, unspecified

004 Shigellosis
    Includes: bacillary dysentery

    004.0 Shigella dysenteriae
        Infection by group A Shigella (Schmitz) (Shiga)

    004.1 Shigella flexneri
        Infection by group B Shigella

    004.2 Shigella boydii
        Infection by group C Shigella

    004.3 Shigella sonnei
        Infection by group D Shigella

    004.8 Other specified shigella infections

    004.9 Shigellosis, unspecified

005 Other food poisoning (bacterial)

    Excludes: *salmonella infections (003.0-003.9)*

        toxic effect of:
          food contaminants (989.7)
          noxious foodstuffs (988.0-988.9)

    005.0 Staphylococcal food poisoning
        Staphylococcal toxemia specified as due to food

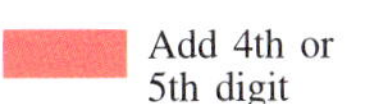

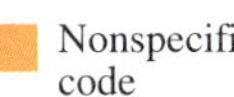

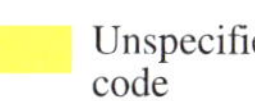

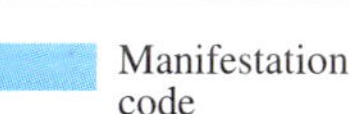

005.1 Botulism
Food poisoning due to Clostridium botulinum

005.2 Food poisoning due to Clostridium perfringens [C. welchii]
Enteritis necroticans

005.3 Food poisoning due to other Clostridia

005.4 Food poisoning due to Vibrio parahaemolyticus

⑤ **005.8 Other bacterial food poisoning**
Excludes: salmonella food poisoning (003.0-003.9)

　　005.81 Food poisoning due to Vibrio vulnificus

　　005.89 Other bacterial food poisoning
　　Food poisoning due to Bacillus cereus

005.9 Food poisoning, unspecified

006 Amebiasis
Includes: infection due to Entamoeba histolytica
Excludes: amebiasis due to organisms other than Entamoeba histolytica (007.8)

006.0 Acute amebic dysentery without mention of abscess
Acute amebiasis

006.1 Chronic intestinal amebiasis without mention of abscess
Chronic:
　amebiasis
　amebic dysentery

006.2 Amebic nondysenteric colitis

006.3 Amebic liver abscess
Hepatic amebiasis

006.4 Amebic lung abscess
Amebic abscess of lung (and liver)

006.5 Amebic brain abscess
Amebic abscess of brain (and liver) (and lung)

006.6 Amebic skin ulceration
Cutaneous amebiasis

006.8 Amebic infection of other sites
Amebic:　　　　　　　　　Ameboma
　appendicitis
　balanitis

Excludes: specific infections by free-living amebae (136.2)

006.9 Amebiasis, unspecified
Amebiasis NOS

007 Other protozoal intestinal diseases
Includes: protozoal:
　　　colitis
　　　diarrhea
　　　dysentery

007.0 Balantidiasis
Infection by Balantidium coli

007.1 Giardiasis
Infection by Giardia lamblia
Lambliasis

007.2 Coccidiosis
Infection by Isospora belli and Isospora hominis
Isosporiasis

007.3 Intestinal trichomoniasis

007.4 Cryptosporidiosis

007.5 Cyclosporiasis

007.8 Other specified protozoal intestinal diseases
Amebiasis due to organisms other than Entamoeba histolytica

007.9 Unspecified protozoal intestinal disease
Flagellate diarrhea　　　　　　Protozoal dysentery NOS

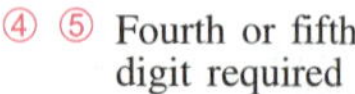

008 **Intestinal infections due to other organisms**
Includes: any condition classifiable to 009.0-009.3 with mention of the responsible organisms

Excludes: *food poisoning by these organisms (005.0-005.9)*

⑤ **008.0** **Escherichia coli [E. coli]**

008.00 **E. coli, unspecified**
E. coli enteritis NOS

008.01 **Enteropathogenic E. coli**

008.02 **Enterotoxigenic E. coli**

008.03 **Enteroinvasive E. coli**

008.04 **Enterohemorrhagic E. coli**

008.09 **Other intestinal E. coli infections**

008.1 **Arizona group of paracolon bacilli**

008.2 **Aerobacter aerogenes**
Enterobacter aerogenes

008.3 **Proteus (mirabilis) (morganii)**

⑤ **008.4** **Other specified bacteria**

008.41 **Staphylococcus**
Staphylococcal enterocolitis

008.42 **Pseudomonas**

008.43 **Campylobacter**

008.44 **Yersinia enterocolitica**

008.45 **Clostridium difficile**
Pseudomembranous colitis

008.46 **Other anaerobes**
Anaerobic enteritis NOS
Bacteroides (fragilis)
Gram-negative anaerobes

008.47 **Other Gram-negative bacteria**
Gram-negative enteritis NOS

Excludes: *Gram-negative anaerobes (008.46)*

008.49 **Other**

008.5 **Bacterial enteritis, unspecified**

⑤ **008.6** **Enteritis due to specified virus**

008.61 **Rotavirus**

008.62 **Adenovirus**

008.63 **Norwalk virus**
Norwalk-like agent

008.64 **Other small round viruses [SRV's]**
Small round virus NOS

008.65 **Calcivirus**

008.66 **Astrovirus**

008.67 **Enterovirus NEC**
Coxsackie virus
Echovirus

Excludes: *poliovirus (045.0-045.9)*

008.69 **Other viral enteritis**
Torovirus

008.8 **Other organism, not elsewhere classified**
Viral:
enteritis NOS
gastroenteritis

Excludes: *influenza with involvement of gastrointestinal tract (487.8)*

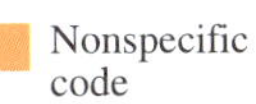

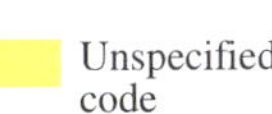

009 Ill-defined intestinal infections

> *Excludes:* *diarrheal disease or intestinal infection due to specified organism (001.0-008.8)*
> *diarrhea following gastrointestinal surgery (564.4)*
> *intestinal malabsorption (579.0-579.9)*
> *ischemic enteritis (557.0-557.9)*
> *other noninfectious gastroenteritis and colitis (558.1-558.9)*
> *regional enteritis (555.0-555.9)*
> *ulcerative colitis (556)*

009.0 Infectious colitis, enteritis, and gastroenteritis

Colitis, septic	Dysentery:
Enteritis, septic	NOS
Gastroenteritis, septic	catarrhal
	hemorrhagic

009.1 Colitis, enteritis, and gastroenteritis of presumed infectious origin

> *Excludes:* *colitis NOS (558.9)*
> *enteritis NOS (558.9)*
> *gastroenteritis NOS (558.9)*

009.2 Infectious diarrhea

Diarrhea: Infectious diarrheal disease NOS
  dysenteric
  epidemic

009.3 Diarrhea of presumed infectious origin

> *Excludes:* *diarrhea NOS (787.91)*

TUBERCULOSIS (010-018)

Includes: infection by Mycobacterium tuberculosis (human) (bovine)

> *Excludes:* *congenital tuberculosis (771.2)*
> *late effects of tuberculosis (137.0-137.4)*

The following fifth-digit subclassification is for use with categories 010-018:

0 unspecified

1 bacteriological or histological examination not done

2 bacteriological or histological examination unknown (at present)

3 tubercle bacilli found (in sputum) by microscopy

4 tubercle bacilli not found (in sputum) by microscopy, but found by bacterial culture

5 tubercle bacilli not found by bacteriological examination, but tuberculosis confirmed histologically

6 tubercle bacilli not found by bacteriological or histological examination but tuberculosis confirmed by other methods [inoculation of animals]

⑤ **010 Primary tuberculous infection**

> *Excludes:* *nonspecific reaction to tuberculin skin test without active tuberculosis (795.5)*
> *positive PPD (795.5)*
> *positive tuberculin skin test without active tuberculosis (795.5)*

⑤ **010.0 Primary tuberculous complex**

⑤ **010.1 Tuberculous pleurisy in primary progressive tuberculosis**

⑤ **010.8 Other primary progressive tuberculosis**

> *Excludes:* *tuberculous erythema nodosum (017.1)*

⑤ **010.9 Primary tuberculous infection, unspecified**

⑤ **011 Pulmonary tuberculosis**

Use additional code, if desired, to identify any associated silicosis (502)

⑤ **011.0 Tuberculosis of lung, infiltrative**

⑤ **011.1 Tuberculosis of lung, nodular**

⑤ **011.2 Tuberculosis of lung with cavitation**

⑤ **011.3 Tuberculosis of bronchus**

> *Excludes:* *isolated bronchial tuberculosis (012.2)*

⑤ **011.4 Tuberculous fibrosis of lung**

⑤ **011.5 Tuberculous bronchiectasis**

● Code new   ▲ Revision of   ④ ⑤ Fourth or fifth
  to this edition   existing code   digit required

⑤ **011.6 Tuberculous pneumonia [any form]**

⑤ **011.7 Tuberculous pneumothorax**

⑤ **011.8 Other specified pulmonary tuberculosis**

⑤ **011.9 Pulmonary tuberculosis, unspecified**
Respiratory tuberculosis NOS
Tuberculosis of lung NOS

⑤ **012 Other respiratory tuberculosis**

> *Excludes:* *respiratory tuberculosis, unspecified (011.9)*

⑤ **012.0 Tuberculous pleurisy**
Tuberculosis of pleura   Tuberculous hydrothorax
Tuberculous empyema

> *Excludes:* *pleurisy with effusion without mention of cause (511.9)*
> *tuberculous pleurisy in primary progressive tuberculosis (010.1)*

⑤ **012.1 Tuberculosis of intrathoracic lymph nodes**
Tuberculosis of lymph nodes:
hilar
mediastinal
tracheobronchial
Tuberculous tracheobronchial adenopathy

> *Excludes:* *that specified as primary (010.0-010.9)*

⑤ **012.2 Isolated tracheal or bronchial tuberculosis**

⑤ **012.3 Tuberculous laryngitis**
Tuberculosis of glottis

⑤ **012.8 Other specified respiratory tuberculosis**
Tuberculosis of: Tuberculosis of:
mediastinum   nose (septum)
nasopharynx   sinus [any nasal]

⑤ **013 Tuberculosis of meninges and central nervous system**

⑤ **013.0 Tuberculous meningitis**
Tuberculosis of meninges   Tuberculous:
(cerebral) (spinal)   leptomeningitis
meningoencephalitis

> *Excludes:* *tuberculoma of meninges (013.1)*

⑤ **013.1 Tuberculoma of meninges**

⑤ **013.2 Tuberculoma of brain**
Tuberculosis of brain (current disease)

⑤ **013.3 Tuberculous abscess of brain**

⑤ **013.4 Tuberculoma of spinal cord**

⑤ **013.5 Tuberculous abscess of spinal cord**

⑤ **013.6 Tuberculous encephalitis or myelitis**

⑤ **013.8 Other specified tuberculosis of central nervous system**

⑤ **013.9 Unspecified tuberculosis of central nervous system**
Tuberculosis of central nervous system NOS

⑤ **014 Tuberculosis of intestines, peritoneum, and mesenteric glands**

⑤ **014.0 Tuberculous peritonitis**
Tuberculous ascites

⑤ **014.8 Other**
Tuberculosis (of):   Tuberculous enteritis
anus
intestine (large) (small)
mesenteric glands
rectum
retroperitoneal (lymph nodes)

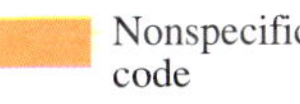

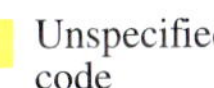

⑤ **015 Tuberculosis of bones and joints**
Use additional code, if desired, to identify manifestation, as:
    tuberculous:
        arthropathy (711.4)
        necrosis of bone (730.8)
        osteitis (730.8)
        osteomyelitis (730.8)
        synovitis (727.01)
        tenosynovitis (727.01)

⑤ **015.0 Vertebral column**
        Pott's disease
Use additional code, if desired, to identify manifestation, as:
            curvature of spine [Pott's] (737.4)
            kyphosis (737.4)
            spondylitis (720.81)

⑤ **015.1 Hip**

⑤ **015.2 Knee**

⑤ **015.5 Limb bones**
        Tuberculous dactylitis

⑤ **015.6 Mastoid**
        Tuberculous mastoiditis

⑤ **015.7 Other specified bone**

⑤ **015.8 Other specified joint**

⑤ **015.9 Tuberculosis of unspecified bones and joints**

⑤ **016 Tuberculosis of genitourinary system**

⑤ **016.0 Kidney**
        Renal tuberculosis
Use additional code, if desired, to identify manifestation, as:
            tuberculous:
                nephropathy (583.81)
                pyelitis (590.81)
                pyelonephritis (590.81)

⑤ **016.1 Bladder**

⑤ **016.2 Ureter**

⑤ **016.3 Other urinary organs**

⑤ **016.4 Epididymis**

⑤ **016.5 Other male genital organs**
Use additional code, if desired, to identify manifestation, as:
            tuberculosis of:
                prostate (601.4)
                seminal vesicle (608.81)
                testis (608.81)

⑤ **016.6 Tuberculous oophoritis and salpingitis**

⑤ **016.7 Other female genital organs**
        Tuberculous:
            cervicitis
            endometritis

⑤ **016.9 Genitourinary tuberculosis, unspecified**

⑤ **017 Tuberculosis of other organs**

⑤ **017.0 Skin and subcutaneous cellular tissue**

Lupus:	Tuberculosis:
exedens	colliquativa
vulgaris	cutis
Scrofuloderma	lichenoides
	papulonecrotica
	verrucosa cutis

Excludes: *lupus erythematosus (695.4)*
            disseminated (710.0)
            lupus NOS (710.0)
            nonspecific reaction to tuberculin skin test without active tuberculosis (795.5)
            positive PPD (795.5)
            positive tuberculin skin test without active tuberculosis (795.5)

    ● Code new   ▲ Revision of   ④ ⑤ Fourth or fifth
        to this edition   existing code   digit required

⑤ **017.1 Erythema nodosum with hypersensitivity reaction in tuberculosis**
  Bazin's disease   Tuberculosis indurativa
  Erythema:
   induratum
   nodosum, tuberculous

  Excludes: *erythema nodosum NOS (695.2)*

⑤ **017.2 Peripheral lymph nodes**
  Scrofula   Tuberculous adenitis
  Scrofulous abscess

  Excludes: *tuberculosis of lymph nodes:*
     bronchial and mediastinal (012.1)
     mesenteric and retroperitoneal (014.8)
     tuberculous tracheobronchial adenopathy (012.1)

⑤ **017.3 Eye**
Use additional code, if desired, to identify manifestation, as:
   tuberculous:
    chorioretinitis, disseminated (363.13)
    episcleritis (379.09)
    interstitial keratitis (370.59)
    iridocyclitis, chronic (364.11)
    keratoconjunctivitis (phlyctenular) (370.31)

⑤ **017.4 Ear**
  Tuberculosis of ear
  Tuberculous otitis media

  Excludes: *tuberculous mastoiditis (015.6)*

⑤ **017.5 Thyroid gland**

⑤ **017.6 Adrenal glands**
  Addison's disease, tuberculous

⑤ **017.7 Spleen**

⑤ **017.8 Esophagus**

⑤ **017.9 Other specified organs**
Use additional code, if desired, to identify manifestation, as:
   tuberculosis of:
    endocardium [any valve] (424.91)
    myocardium (422.0)
    pericardium (420.0)

⑤ **018 Miliary tuberculosis**
  Includes: tuberculosis:
     disseminated
     generalized
     miliary, whether of a single specified site, multiple sites, or unspecified site
     polyserositis

⑤ **018.0 Acute miliary tuberculosis**

⑤ **018.8 Other specified miliary tuberculosis**

⑤ **018.9 Miliary tuberculosis, unspecified**

ZOONOTIC BACTERIAL DISEASES (020-027)

020 Plague
  Includes: infection by Yersinia [Pasteurella] pestis

 020.0 Bubonic

 020.1 Cellulocutaneous

 020.2 Septicemic

 020.3 Primary pneumonic

 020.4 Secondary pneumonic

 020.5 Pneumonic, unspecified

 020.8 Other specified types of plague
  Abortive plague   Pestis minor
  Ambulatory plague

 020.9 Plague, unspecified

	Add 4th or 5th digit		Nonspecific code		Unspecified code		Manifestation code

021 Tularemia
Includes: deerfly fever
infection by Francisella [Pasteurella] tularensis
rabbit fever

021.0 Ulceroglandular tularemia

021.1 Enteric tularemia
Tularemia:
cryptogenic
intestinal
typhoidal

021.2 Pulmonary tularemia
Bronchopneumonic tularemia

021.3 Oculoglandular tularemia

021.8 Other specified tularemia
Tularemia:
generalized or disseminated
glandular

021.9 Unspecified tularemia

022 Anthrax

022.0 Cutaneous anthrax
Malignant pustule

022.1 Pulmonary anthrax
Respiratory anthrax
Wool-sorters' disease

022.2 Gastrointestinal anthrax

022.3 Anthrax septicemia

022.8 Other specified manifestations of anthrax

022.9 Anthrax, unspecified

023 Brucellosis
Includes: fever:
Malta
Mediterranean
undulant

023.0 Brucella melitensis

023.1 Brucella abortus

023.2 Brucella suis

023.3 Brucella canis

023.8 Other brucellosis
Infection by more than one organism

023.9 Brucellosis, unspecified

024 Glanders
Infection by: Farcy
Actinobacillus mallei   Malleus
Malleomyces mallei
Pseudomonas mallei

025 Melioidosis
Infection by:
Malleomyces pseudomallei
Pseudomonas pseudomallei
Whitmore's bacillus
Pseudoglanders

026 Rat-bite fever

026.0 Spirillary fever
Rat-bite fever due to Spirillum minor [S. minus]
Sodoku

026.1 Streptobacillary fever
Epidemic arthritic erythema
Haverhill fever
Rat-bite fever due to Streptobacillus moniliformis

026.9 Unspecified rat-bite fever

● Code new
to this edition

▲ Revision of
existing code

④ ⑤ Fourth or fifth
digit required

027 Other zoonotic bacterial diseases

027.0 Listeriosis
Infection by Listeria monocytogenes
Septicemia by Listeria monocytogenes

Use additional code to identify manifestations, as meningitis (320.7)

> *Excludes:* *congenital listeriosis (771.2)*

027.1 Erysipelothrix infection
Erysipeloid (of Rosenbach)
Infection by Erysipelothrix insidiosa [E. rhusiopathiae]
Septicemia by Erysipelothrix insidiosa [E. rhusiopathiae]

027.2 Pasteurellosis
Pasteurella pseudotuberculosis infection
Mesenteric adenitis by Pasteurella multocida [P. septica]
Septic infection (cat bite) (dog bite) by Pasteurella multocida [P. septica]

> *Excludes:* *infection by:*
> *Francisella [Pasteurella] tularensis (021.0-021.9)*
> *Yersinia [Pasteurella] pestis (020.0-020.9)*

027.8 Other specified zoonotic bacterial diseases

027.9 Unspecified zoonotic bacterial disease

OTHER BACTERIAL DISEASES (030-041)

> *Excludes:* *bacterial venereal diseases (098.0-099.9)*
> *bartonellosis (088.0)*

030 Leprosy
Includes: Hansen's disease
infection by Mycobacterium leprae

030.0 Lepromatous [type L]
Lepromatous leprosy (macular) (diffuse) (infiltrated) (nodular) (neuritic)

030.1 Tuberculoid [type T]
Tuberculoid leprosy (macular) (maculoanesthetic) (major) (minor) (neuritic)

030.2 Indeterminate [group I]
Indeterminate [uncharacteristic] leprosy (macular) (neuritic)

030.3 Borderline [group B]
Borderline or dimorphous leprosy (infiltrated) (neuritic)

030.8 Other specified leprosy

030.9 Leprosy, unspecified

031 Diseases due to other mycobacteria

031.0 Pulmonary
Infection by Mycobacterium:
avium
intracellulare [Battey bacillus]
kansasii
Battey disease

031.1 Cutaneous
Buruli ulcer
Infection by Mycobacterium:
marinum [M. balnei]
ulcerans

031.2 Disseminated
Disseminated mycobacterium avium-intracellulare complex (DMAC)
Mycobacterium avium-intracellulare complex (MAC) bacteremia

031.8 Other specified mycobacterial diseases

031.9 Unspecified diseases due to mycobacteria
Atypical mycobacterium infection NOS

032 Diphtheria
Includes: infection by Corynebacterium diphtheriae

032.0 Faucial diphtheria
Membranous angina, diphtheritic

032.1 Nasopharyngeal diphtheria

032.2 Anterior nasal diphtheria

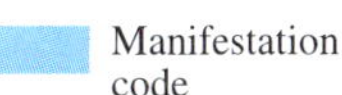

| Add 4th or 5th digit | Nonspecific code | Unspecified code | Manifestation code |

032.3 Laryngeal diphtheria
Laryngotracheitis, diphtheritic

⑤ **032.8 Other specified diphtheria**

032.81 Conjunctival diphtheria
Pseudomembranous diphtheritic conjunctivitis

032.82 Diphtheritic myocarditis

032.83 Diphtheritic peritonitis

032.84 Diphtheritic cystitis

032.85 Cutaneous diphtheria

032.89 Other

032.9 Diphtheria, unspecified

033 Whooping cough
Includes: pertussis

Use additional code, if desired, to identify any associated pneumonia (484.3)

033.0 Bordetella pertussis [B. pertussis]

033.1 Bordetella parapertussis [B. parapertussis]

033.8 Whooping cough due to other specified organism
Bordetella bronchiseptica [B. bronchiseptica]

033.9 Whooping cough, unspecified organism

034 Streptococcal sore throat and scarlet fever

034.0 Streptococcal sore throat

Septic:
  angina
   sore throat

Streptococcal:
  angina
  laryngitis
  pharyngitis
  tonsillitis

034.1 Scarlet fever
Scarlatina

Excludes: parascarlatina (057.8)

035 Erysipelas

Excludes: postpartum or puerperal erysipelas (670)

036 Meningococcal infection

036.0 Meningococcal meningitis

Cerebrospinal fever
  (meningococcal)

Meningitis:
  cerebrospinal
  epidemic

036.1 Meningococcal encephalitis

036.2 Meningococcemia
Meningococcal septicemia

036.3 Waterhouse-Friderichsen syndrome, meningococcal
Meningococcal hemorrhagic adrenalitis
Meningococcic adrenal syndrome
Waterhouse-Friderichsen syndrome NOS

⑤ **036.4 Meningococcal carditis**

036.40 Meningococcal carditis, unspecified

036.41 Meningococcal pericarditis

036.42 Meningococcal endocarditis

036.43 Meningococcal myocarditis

⑤ **036.8 Other specified meningococcal infections**

036.81 Meningococcal optic neuritis

036.82 Meningococcal arthropathy

036.89 Other

036.9 Meningococcal infection, unspecified
Meningococcal infection NOS

   ● Code new
to this edition   ▲ Revision of
existing code   ④ ⑤ Fourth or fifth
digit required

037 Tetanus

Excludes: *tetanus:*

  complicating:
   abortion (634-638 with .0, 639.0)
   ectopic or molar pregnancy (639.0)
  neonatorum (771.3)
  puerperal (670)

038 Septicemia

Excludes: *bacteremia (790.7)*

  during labor (659.3)
  following ectopic or molar pregnancy (639.0)
  following infusion, injection, transfusion, or vaccination (999.3)
  postpartum, puerperal (670)
  septicemia (sepsis) of newborn (771.81)
  that complicating abortion (634-638 with .0, 639.0)

Use additional code for systemic inflammatory response syndrome (SIRS) (995.91-995.92)

038.0 Streptococcal septicemia

038.1 Staphylococcal septicemia

 038.10 Staphylococcal septicemia, unspecified

 038.11 Staphylococcus aureus septicemia

 038.19 Other staphylococcal septicemia

038.2 Pneumococcal septicemia

038.3 Septicemia due to anaerobes
 Septicemia due to bacteroides

 Excludes: *gas gangrene (040.0)*

  that due to anaerobic streptococci (038.0)

038.4 Septicemia due to other gram-negative organisms

 038.40 Gram-negative organism, unspecified
  Gram-negative septicemia NOS

 038.41 Hemophilus influenzae [H. influenzae]

 038.42 Escherichia coli [E. coli]

 038.43 Pseudomonas

 038.44 Serratia

 038.49 Other

038.8 Other specified septicemias

 Excludes: *septicemia (due to):*

  anthrax (022.3)
  gonococcal (098.89)
  herpetic (054.5)
  meningococcal (036.2)
 septicemic plague (020.2)

038.9 Unspecified septicemia
 Septicemia NOS

 Excludes: *bacteremia NOS (790.7)*

039 Actinomycotic infections
 Includes: actinomycotic mycetoma
   infection by Actinomycetales, such as species of Actinomyces, Actinomadura,
    Nocardia, Streptomyces
   maduromycosis (actinomycotic)
   schizomycetoma (actinomycotic)

039.0 Cutaneous
 Erythrasma   Trichomycosis axillaris

039.1 Pulmonary
 Thoracic actinomycosis

039.2 Abdominal

039.3 Cervicofacial

039.4 Madura foot

 Excludes: *madura foot due to mycotic infection (117.4)*

039.8 Of other specified sites

Add 4th or 5th digit Nonspecific code Unspecified code Manifestation code

039.9 Of unspecified site
Actinomycosis NOS
Maduromycosis NOS   Nocardiosis NOS

040 Other bacterial diseases
Excludes: bacteremia NOS (790.7)
              bacterial infection NOS (041.9)

040.0 Gas gangrene
Gas bacillus infection   Malignant edema
   or gangrene   Myonecrosis, clostridial
Infection by Clostridium: Myositis, clostridial
   histolyticum
   oedematiens
   perfringens [welchii]
   septicum
   sordellii

040.1 Rhinoscleroma

040.2 Whipple's disease
Intestinal lipodystrophy

040.3 Necrobacillosis

⑤ **040.8 Other specified bacterial diseases**

    040.81 Tropical pyomyositis

    040.82 Toxic shock syndrome
Use additional code to identify the organism

    040.89 Other

041 Bacterial infection in conditions classified elsewhere and of unspecified site
Note: This category is provided to be used as an additional code where it is desired to identify
      the bacterial agent in diseases classified elsewhere. This category will also be used to
      classify bacterial infections of unspecified nature or site.
Excludes: bacteremia NOS (790.7)
              septicemia (038.0-038.9)

⑤ **041.0 Streptococcus**

    041.00 Streptococcus, unspecified

    041.01 Group A

    041.02 Group B

    041.03 Group C

    041.04 Group D [Enterococcus]

    041.05 Group G

    041.09 Other Streptococcus

⑤ **041.1 Staphylococcus**

    041.10 Staphylococcus, unspecified

    041.11 Staphylococcus aureus

    041.19 Other Staphylococcus

041.2 Pneumococcus

041.3 Friedländer's bacillus
Infection by Klebsiella pneumoniae

041.4 Escherichia coli [E. coli]

041.5 Hemophilus influenzae [H. influenzae]

041.6 Proteus (mirabilis) (morganii)

041.7 Pseudomonas

⑤ **041.8 Other specified bacterial infections**

    041.81 Mycoplasma
Eaton's agent
Pleuropneumonia-like organisms [PPLO]

    041.82 Bacteroides fragilis

    041.83 Clostridium perfringens

● Code new   ▲ Revision of   ④ ⑤ Fourth or fifth
   to this edition   existing code   digit required

041.84 Other anaerobes
Gram-negative anaerobes

Excludes: *Helicobacter pylori (041.86)*

041.85 Other Gram-negative organisms
Aerobacter aerogenes
Gram-negative bacteria NOS
Mima polymorpha
Serratia

Excludes: *Gram-negative anaerobes (041.84)*

041.86 Helicobacter pylori (H. pylori)

041.89 Other specified bacteria

041.9 Bacterial infection, unspecified

HUMAN IMMUNODEFICIENCY VIRUS (HIV) INFECTION (042)

042 Human immunodeficiency virus [HIV] disease
Acquired immune deficiency syndrome
Acquired immunodeficiency syndrome
AIDS
AIDS-like syndrome
AIDS-related complex
ARC
HIV infection, symptomatic

Use additional code(s) to identify all manifestations of HIV

Use additional code, if desired, to identify HIV-2 infection (079.53)

Excludes: *asymptomatic HIV infection status (V08)*
exposure to HIV virus (V01.79)
nonspecific serologic evidence of HIV (795.71)

POLIOMYELITIS AND OTHER NON-ARTHROPOD-BORNE VIRAL DISEASES OF CENTRAL NERVOUS SYSTEM (045-049)

⑤ **045 Acute poliomyelitis**

Excludes: *late effects of acute poliomyelitis (138)*

The following fifth-digit subclassification is for use with category 045:

0 poliovirus, unspecified type

1 poliovirus type I

2 poliovirus type II

3 poliovirus type III

⑤ **045.0 Acute paralytic poliomyelitis specified as bulbar**
Infantile paralysis (acute) specified as bulbar
Poliomyelitis (acute) (anterior) specified as bulbar
Polioencephalitis (acute) (bulbar)
Polioencephalomyelitis (acute) (anterior) (bulbar)

⑤ **045.1 Acute poliomyelitis with other paralysis**
Paralysis:
acute atrophic, spinal
infantile, paralytic
Poliomyelitis (acute):
anterior, with paralysis except bulbar
epidemic, with paralysis except bulbar

⑤ **045.2 Acute nonparalytic poliomyelitis**
Poliomyelitis (acute):
anterior, specified as nonparalytic
epidemic, specified as nonparalytic

⑤ **045.9 Acute poliomyelitis, unspecified**
Infantile paralysis, unspecified whether paralytic or nonparalytic
Poliomyelitis (acute):
anterior, unspecified whether paralytic or nonparalytic
epidemic, unspecified whether paralytic or nonparalytic

046 Slow virus infection of central nervous system

046.0 Kuru

046.1 Jakob-Creutzfeldt disease
Subacute spongiform encephalopathy

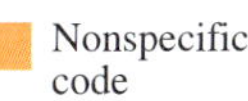

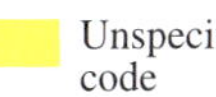

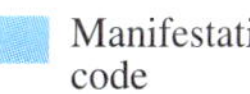

Manifestation
code

046.2 Subacute sclerosing panencephalitis
Dawson's inclusion body encephalitis
Van Bogaert's sclerosing leukoencephalitis

046.3 Progressive multifocal leukoencephalopathy
Multifocal leukoencephalopathy NOS

046.8 Other specified slow virus infection of central nervous system

046.9 Unspecified slow virus infection of central nervous system

047 Meningitis due to enterovirus
Includes: meningitis:
abacterial
aseptic
viral

Excludes: *meningitis due to:*
adenovirus (049.1)
arthropod-borne virus (060.0-066.9)
leptospira (100.81)
virus of:
herpes simplex (054.72)
herpes zoster (053.0)
lymphocytic choriomeningitis (049.0)
mumps (072.1)
poliomyelitis (045.0-045.9)
any other infection specifically classified elsewhere

047.0 Coxsackie virus

047.1 ECHO virus
Meningo-eruptive syndrome

047.8 Other specified viral meningitis

047.9 Unspecified viral meningitis
Viral meningitis NOS

048 Other enterovirus diseases of central nervous system
Boston exanthem

049 Other non-arthropod-borne viral diseases of central nervous system

Excludes: *late effects of viral encephalitis (139.0)*

049.0 Lymphocytic choriomeningitis
Lymphocytic:
meningitis (serous) (benign)
meningoencephalitis (serous) (benign)

049.1 Meningitis due to adenovirus

049.8 Other specified non-arthropod-borne viral diseases of central nervous system

Encephalitis:	Encephalitis:
acute:	lethargica
inclusion body	Rio Bravo
necrotizing	von Economo's disease
epidemic	

049.9 Unspecified non-arthropod-borne viral diseases of central nervous system
Viral encephalitis NOS

VIRAL DISEASES ACCOMPANIED BY EXANTHEM (050-057)

Excludes: *arthropod-borne viral diseases (060.0-066.9)*
Boston exanthem (048)

050 Smallpox

050.0 Variola major

Hemorrhagic (pustular)	Malignant smallpox
smallpox	Purpura variolosa

050.1 Alastrim
Variola minor

050.2 Modified smallpox
Varioloid

050.9 Smallpox, unspecified

● Code new
to this edition   ▲ Revision of
existing code   ④ ⑤ Fourth or fifth
digit required

051 Cowpox and paravaccinia

051.0 Cowpox
Vaccinia not from vaccination

Excludes: vaccinia (generalized) (from vaccination) (999.0)

051.1 Pseudocowpox
Milkers' node

051.2 Contagious pustular dermatitis
Ecthyma contagiosum Orf

051.9 Paravaccinia, unspecified

052 Chickenpox

052.0 Postvaricella encephalitis
Postchickenpox encephalitis

052.1 Varicella (hemorrhagic) pneumonitis

● **052.2 Postvaricella myelitis**
Postchickenpox myelitis

052.7 With other specified complications

052.8 With unspecified complication

052.9 Varicella without mention of complication
Chickenpox NOS
Varicella NOS

053 Herpes zoster
Includes: shingles
zona

053.0 With meningitis

⑤ **053.1 With other nervous system complications**

053.10 With unspecified nervous system complication

053.11 Geniculate herpes zoster
Herpetic geniculate ganglionitis

053.12 Postherpetic trigeminal neuralgia

053.13 Postherpetic polyneuropathy

● **053.14 Herpes zoster myelitis**

053.19 Other

⑤ **053.2 With ophthalmic complications**

053.20 Herpes zoster dermatitis of eyelid
Herpes zoster ophthalmicus

053.21 Herpes zoster keratoconjunctivitis

053.22 Herpes zoster iridocyclitis

053.29 Other

⑤ **053.7 With other specified complications**

053.71 Otitis externa due to herpes zoster

053.79 Other

053.8 With unspecified complication

053.9 Herpes zoster without mention of complication
Herpes zoster NOS

054 Herpes simplex

Excludes: congenital herpes simplex (771.2)

054.0 Eczema herpeticum
Kaposi's varicelliform eruption

⑤ **054.1 Genital herpes**

054.10 Genital herpes, unspecified
Herpes progenitalis

054.11 Herpetic vulvovaginitis

054.12 Herpetic ulceration of vulva

054.13 Herpetic infection of penis

054.19 Other

054.2 Herpetic gingivostomatitis

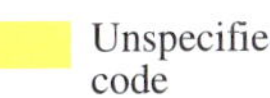

054.3 Herpetic meningoencephalitis
　　　Herpes encephalitis
　　　Simian B disease

⑤ **054.4 With ophthalmic complications**

　　　054.40 With unspecified ophthalmic complication

　　　054.41 Herpes simplex dermatitis of eyelid

　　　054.42 Dendritic keratitis

　　　054.43 Herpes simplex disciform keratitis

　　　054.44 Herpes simplex iridocyclitis

　　　054.49 Other

054.5 Herpetic septicemia

054.6 Herpetic whitlow
　　　Herpetic felon

⑤ **054.7 With other specified complications**

　　　054.71 Visceral herpes simplex

　　　054.72 Herpes simplex meningitis

　　　054.73 Herpes simplex otitis externa

　● **054.74 Herpes simplex myelitis**

　　　054.79 Other

054.8 With unspecified complication

054.9 Herpes simplex without mention of complication

055 Measles
　　　Includes: morbilli
　　　　　　　　rubeola

055.0 Postmeasles encephalitis

055.1 Postmeasles pneumonia

055.2 Postmeasles otitis media

⑤ **055.7 With other specified complications**

　　　055.71 Measles keratoconjunctivitis
　　　　　　Measles keratitis

　　　055.79 Other

055.8 With unspecified complication

055.9 Measles without mention of complication

056 Rubella
　　　Includes: German measles

　　　Excludes: *congenital rubella (771.0)*

⑤ **056.0 With neurological complications**

　　　056.00 With unspecified neurological complication

　　　056.01 Encephalomyelitis due to rubella
　　　　　　Encephalitis due to rubella
　　　　　　Meningoencephalitis due to rubella

　　　056.09 Other

⑤ **056.7 With other specified complications**

　　　056.71 Arthritis due to rubella

　　　056.79 Other

056.8 With unspecified complications

056.9 Rubella without mention of complication

057 Other viral exanthemata

057.0 Erythema infectiosum [fifth disease]

057.8 Other specified viral exanthemata
　　　Dukes (-Filatow) disease　　　Parascarlatina
　　　Exanthema subitum　　　　　Pseudoscarlatina
　　　　[sixth disease]　　　　　Roseola infantum
　　　Fourth disease

057.9 Viral exanthem, unspecified

● Code new
to this edition

▲ Revision of
existing code

④ ⑤ Fourth or fifth
digit required

ARTHROPOD-BORNE VIRAL DISEASES (060-066)

Use additional code, if desired, to identify any associated meningitis (321.2)

> *Excludes:* *late effects of viral encephalitis (139.0)*

060 Yellow fever

060.0 Sylvatic
Yellow fever:
jungle
sylvan

060.1 Urban

060.9 Yellow fever, unspecified

061 Dengue
Breakbone fever

> *Excludes:* *hemorrhagic fever caused by dengue virus (065.4)*

062 Mosquito-borne viral encephalitis

062.0 Japanese encephalitis
Japanese B encephalitis

062.1 Western equine encephalitis

062.2 Eastern equine encephalitis

> *Excludes:* *Venezuelan equine encephalitis (066.2)*

062.3 St. Louis encephalitis

062.4 Australian encephalitis
Australian arboencephalitis
Australian X disease
Murray Valley encephalitis

062.5 California virus encephalitis
Encephalitis: Tahyna fever
California
La Crosse

062.8 Other specified mosquito-borne viral encephalitis
Encephalitis by Ilheus virus

> *Excludes:* *West Nile virus (066.40-066.49)*

062.9 Mosquito-borne viral encephalitis, unspecified

063 Tick-borne viral encephalitis
Includes: diphasic meningoencephalitis

063.0 Russian spring-summer [taiga] encephalitis

063.1 Louping ill

063.2 Central European encephalitis

063.8 Other specified tick-borne viral encephalitis
Langat encephalitis
Powassan encephalitis

063.9 Tick-borne viral encephalitis, unspecified

064 Viral encephalitis transmitted by other and unspecified arthropods
Arthropod-borne viral encephalitis, vector unknown
Negishi virus encephalitis

> *Excludes:* *viral encephalitis NOS (049.9)*

065 Arthropod-borne hemorrhagic fever

065.0 Crimean hemorrhagic fever [CHF Congo virus]
Central Asian hemorrhagic fever

065.1 Omsk hemorrhagic fever

065.2 Kyasanur Forest disease

065.3 Other tick-borne hemorrhagic fever

065.4 Mosquito-borne hemorrhagic fever
Chikungunya hemorrhagic fever
Dengue hemorrhagic fever

> *Excludes:* *Chikungunya fever (066.3)*
> *dengue (061)*
> *yellow fever (060.0-060.9)*

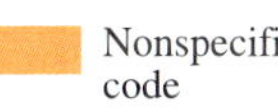

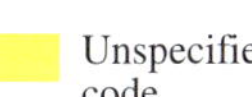

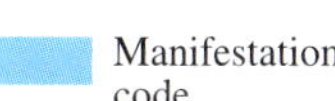

065.8 Other specified arthropod-borne hemorrhagic fever
Mite-borne hemorrhagic fever

065.9 Arthropod-borne hemorrhagic fever, unspecified
Arbovirus hemorrhagic fever NOS

066 Other arthropod-borne viral diseases

066.0 Phlebotomus fever
Changuinola fever
Sandfly fever

066.1 Tick-borne fever
Nairobi sheep disease
Tick fever:
  American mountain
  Colorado
Tick fever:
  Kemerovo
  Quaranfil

066.2 Venezuelan equine fever
Venezuelan equine encephalitis

066.3 Other mosquito-borne fever
Fever (viral):
  Bunyamwera
  Bwamba
  Chikungunya
  GuamaR Mayaro
  Mucambo
  O'nyong-nyong
Fever (viral):
  Oropouche
  Pixuna
  Rift valley
  Ross river
  Wesselsbron
  Zika

Excludes: *dengue (061)*
yellow fever (060.0-060.9)

⑤ **066.4 West Nile fever**

066.40 West Nile fever, unspecified
West Nile fever NOS
West Nile fever without complications
West Nile virus NOS

066.41 West Nile fever with encephalitis
West Nile encephalitis
West Nile encephalomyelitis

066.42 West Nile fever with other neurologic manifestation
Use additional code to specify the neurologic manifestation

066.49 West Nile fever with other complications
Use additional code to specify the other conditions

066.8 Other specified arthropod-borne viral diseases
Chandipura fever
Piry fever

066.9 Arthropod-borne viral disease, unspecified
Arbovirus infection NOS

OTHER DISEASES DUE TO VIRUSES AND CHLAMYDIAE (070-079)

070 Viral hepatitis
Includes: viral hepatitis (acute) (chronic)

Excludes: *cytomegalic inclusion virus hepatitis (078.5)*
The following fifth-digit subclassification is for use with categories 070.2 and 070.3:

0 acute or unspecified, without mention of hepatitis delta

1 acute or unspecified, with hepatitis delta

2 chronic, without mention of hepatitis delta

3 chronic, with hepatitis delta

070.0 Viral hepatitis A with hepatic coma

070.1 Viral hepatitis A without mention of hepatic coma
Infectious hepatitis

⑤ **070.2 Viral hepatitis B with hepatic coma**

⑤ **070.3 Viral hepatitis B without mention of hepatic coma**
Serum hepatitis

⑤ **070.4 Other specified viral hepatitis with hepatic coma**

070.41 Acute hepatitis C with hepatic coma

     ● Code new   ▲ Revision of   ④ ⑤ Fourth or fifth
    to this edition   existing code   digit required

070.42 Hepatitis delta without mention of active hepatitis B disease with hepatic coma
Hepatitis delta with hepatitis B carrier state

070.43 Hepatitis E with hepatic coma

070.44 Chronic hepatitis C with hepatic coma

070.49 Other specified viral hepatitis with hepatic coma

⑤ **070.5 Other specified viral hepatitis without mention of hepatic coma**

070.51 Acute hepatitis C without mention of hepatic coma

070.52 Hepatitis delta without mention of active hepatitis B disease or hepatic coma

070.53 Hepatitis E without mention of hepatic coma

070.54 Chronic hepatitis C without mention of hepatic coma

070.59 Other specified viral hepatitis without mention of hepatic coma

070.6 Unspecified viral hepatitis with hepatic coma

Excludes: *unspecified viral hepatitis C with hepatic coma (070.71)*

⑤ **070.7 Unspecified viral hepatitis C**

070.70 Unspecified viral hepatitis C without hepatic coma
Unspecified viral hepatitis C NOS

070.71 Unspecified viral hepatitis C with hepatic coma

070.9 Unspecified viral hepatitis without mention of hepatic coma
Viral hepatitis NOS

Excludes: *unspecified viral hepatitis C without hepatic coma (070.70)*

071 Rabies
Hydrophobia   Lyssa

072 Mumps

072.0 Mumps orchitis

072.1 Mumps meningitis

072.2 Mumps encephalitis
Mumps meningoencephalitis

072.3 Mumps pancreatitis

⑤ **072.7 Mumps with other specified complications**

072.71 Mumps hepatitis

072.72 Mumps polyneuropathy

072.79 Other

072.8 Mumps with unspecified complication

072.9 Mumps without mention of complication
Epidemic parotitis
Infectious parotitis

073 Ornithosis
Includes: parrot fever
psittacosis

073.0 With pneumonia
Lobular pneumonitis due to ornithosis

073.7 With other specified complications

073.8 With unspecified complication

073.9 Ornithosis, unspecified

074 Specific diseases due to Coxsackie virus

Excludes: *Coxsackie virus:*
infection NOS (079.2)
meningitis (047.0)

074.0 Herpangina
Vesicular pharyngitis

074.1 Epidemic pleurodynia
Bornholm disease   Epidemic:
Devil's grip   myalgia
myositis

⑤ **074.2 Coxsackie carditis**

Add 4th or 5th digit	Nonspecific code	Unspecified code	Manifestation code

074.20 **Coxsackie carditis, unspecified**

074.21 **Coxsackie pericarditis**

074.22 **Coxsackie endocarditis**

074.23 **Coxsackie myocarditis**
Aseptic myocarditis of newborn

074.3 **Hand, foot, and mouth disease**
Vesicular stomatitis and exanthem

074.8 **Other specified diseases due to Coxsackie virus**
Acute lymphonodular pharyngitis

075 Infectious mononucleosis
Glandular fever   Pfeiffer's disease
Monocytic angina

076 Trachoma
Excludes: *late effect of trachoma (139.1)*

076.0 **Initial stage**
Trachoma dubium

076.1 **Active stage**
Granular conjunctivitis (trachomatous)
Trachomatous:
    follicular conjunctivitis
    pannus

076.9 **Trachoma, unspecified**
Trachoma NOS

077 Other diseases of conjunctiva due to viruses and Chlamydiae
Excludes: *ophthalmic complications of viral diseases classified elsewhere*

077.0 **Inclusion conjunctivitis**
Paratrachoma
Swimming pool conjunctivitis

Excludes: *inclusion blennorrhea (neonatal) (771.6)*

077.1 **Epidemic keratoconjunctivitis**
Shipyard eye

077.2 **Pharyngoconjunctival fever**
Viral pharyngoconjunctivitis

077.3 **Other adenoviral conjunctivitis**
Acute adenoviral follicular conjunctivitis

077.4 **Epidemic hemorrhagic conjunctivitis**
Apollo:
    conjunctivitis
    disease
Conjunctivitis due to enterovirus type 70
Hemorrhagic conjunctivitis (acute) (epidemic)

077.8 **Other viral conjunctivitis**
Newcastle conjunctivitis

⑤ **077.9** **Unspecified diseases of conjunctiva due to viruses and Chlamydiae**

077.98 **Due to Chlamydiae**

077.99 **Due to viruses**
Viral conjunctivitis NOS

078 Other diseases due to viruses and Chlamydiae
Excludes: *viral infection NOS (079.0-079.9)*
        viremia NOS (790.8)

078.0 **Molluscum contagiosum**

⑤ **078.1** **Viral warts**
Viral warts due to Human papillomavirus

078.10 **Viral warts, unspecified**
Condyloma NOS
Verruca:
    NOS
    vulgaris
Warts (infectious)

078.11 **Condyloma acuminatum**

● Code new   ▲ Revision of   ④ ⑤ Fourth or fifth
  to this edition   existing code   digit required

078.19 **Other specified viral warts**
Genital warts NOS
Verruca:
plana
plantaris

078.2 **Sweating fever**
Miliary fever
Sweating disease

078.3 **Cat-scratch disease**
Benign lymphoreticulosis (of inoculation)
Cat-scratch fever

078.4 **Foot and mouth disease**
Aphthous fever
Epizootic:
aphthae
stomatitis

078.5 **Cytomegaloviral disease**
Cytomegalic inclusion disease
Salivary gland virus disease
Use additional code, if desired, to identify manifestation, as:
cytomegalic inclusion virus:
hepatitis (573.1)
pneumonia (484.1)
Excludes: *congenital cytomegalovirus infection (771.1)*

078.6 **Hemorrhagic nephrosonephritis**
Hemorrhagic fever:
epidemic
Korean

Hemorrhagic fever:
Russian
with renal syndrome

078.7 **Arenaviral hemorrhagic fever**
Hemorrhagic fever:
Argentine
Bolivian

Hemorrhagic fever:
Junin virus
Machupo virus

⑤ **078.8** **Other specified diseases due to viruses and Chlamydiae**
Excludes: *epidemic diarrhea (009.2)*

lymphogranuloma venereum (099.1)

078.81 **Epidemic vertigo**

078.82 **Epidemic vomiting syndrome**
Winter vomiting disease

078.88 **Other specified diseases due to Chlamydiae**

078.89 **Other specified diseases due to viruses**
Epidemic cervical myalgia
Marburg disease
Tanapox

079 **Viral and Chlamydial infection in conditions classified elsewhere and of unspecified site**
Note: This category is provided to be used as an additional code where it is desired to identify
the viral agent in diseases classifiable elsewhere. This category will also be used to
classify virus infection of unspecified nature or site.

079.0 **Adenovirus**

079.1 **ECHO virus**

079.2 **Coxsackievirus**

079.3 **Rhinovirus**

079.4 **Human papillomavirus**

⑤ **079.5** **Retrovirus**
Excludes: *human immunodeficiency virus, type 1 [HIV-1] (042)*

human T-cell lymphotrophic virus, type III [HTLV-III] (042)
lymphadenopathy-associated virus [LAV] (042)

079.50 **Retrovirus, unspecified**

079.51 **Human T-cell lymphotrophic virus, type I [HTLV-I]**

079.52 **Human T-cell lymphotrophic virus, type II [HTLV-II]**

079.53 **Human immunodeficiency virus, type 2 [HIV-2]**

079.59 **Other specified retrovirus**

	Add 4th or 5th digit		Nonspecific code		Unspecified code		Manifestation code

079.6 Respiratory syncytial virus (RSV)

⑤ **079.8 Other specified viral and chlamydial infections**

    079.81 Hantavirus

    079.82 SARS-associated coronavirus

    079.88 Other specified chlamydial infection

    079.89 Other specified viral infection

⑤ **079.9 Unspecified viral and chlamydial infections**

    Excludes: *viremia NOS (790.8)*

    079.98 Unspecified chlamydial infection
      Chlamydial infection NOS

    079.99 Unspecified viral infection
      Viral infection NOS

RICKETTSIOSES AND OTHER ARTHROPOD-BORNE DISEASES (080-088)

Excludes: *arthropod-borne viral diseases (060.0-066.9)*

080 Louse-borne [epidemic] typhus
Typhus (fever):   Typhus (fever):
  classical   exanthematic NOS
  epidemic   louse-borne

081 Other typhus

    081.0 Murine [endemic] typhus
      Typhus (fever):
        endemic
        flea-borne

    081.1 Brill's disease
      Brill-Zinsser disease
      Recrudescent typhus (fever)

    081.2 Scrub typhus
      Japanese river fever   Mite-borne typhus
      Kedani fever   Tsutsugamushi

    081.9 Typhus, unspecified
      Typhus (fever) NOS

082 Tick-borne rickettsioses

    082.0 Spotted fevers
      Rocky mountain spotted fever
      São Paulo fever

    082.1 Boutonneuse fever
      African tick typhus   Marseilles fever
      India tick typhus   Mediterranean tick fever
      Kenya tick typhus

    082.2 North Asian tick fever
      Siberian tick typhus

    082.3 Queensland tick typhus

⑤   **082.4 Ehrlichiosis**

      082.40 Ehrlichiosis, unspecified

      082.41 Ehrlichiosis chafeensis (E. chafeensis)

      082.49 Other ehrlichiosis

    082.8 Other specified tick-borne rickettsioses
      Lone star fever

    082.9 Tick-borne rickettsiosis, unspecified
      Tick-borne typhus NOS

083 Other rickettsioses

    083.0 Q fever

    083.1 Trench fever
      Quintan fever
      Wolhynian fever

    083.2 Rickettsialpox
      Vesicular rickettsiosis

    083.8 Other specified rickettsioses

● Code new to this edition   ▲ Revision of existing code   ④ ⑤ Fourth or fifth digit required

083.9 Rickettsiosis, unspecified

084 Malaria

Note: Subcategories 084.0-084.6 exclude the listed conditions with mention of pernicious complications (084.8-084.9).

> | Excludes: | congenital malaria (771.2)

084.0 Falciparum malaria [malignant tertian]
Malaria (fever):
  by Plasmodium falciparum
  subtertian

084.1 Vivax malaria [benign tertian]
Malaria (fever) by Plasmodium vivax

084.2 Quartan malaria
Malaria (fever) by Plasmodium malariae
Malariae malaria

084.3 Ovale malaria
Malaria (fever) by Plasmodium ovale

084.4 Other malaria
Monkey malaria

084.5 Mixed malaria
Malaria (fever) by more than one parasite

084.6 Malaria, unspecified
Malaria (fever) NOS

084.7 Induced malaria
Therapeutically induced malaria

> | Excludes: | accidental infection from syringe, blood transfusion, etc. (084.0-084.6, above, according to parasite species)
> transmission from mother to child during delivery (771.2)

084.8 Blackwater fever
Hemoglobinuric: Malarial hemoglobinuria
  fever (bilious)
  malaria

084.9 Other pernicious complications of malaria
Algid malaria
Cerebral malaria
Use additional code, if desired, to identify complication, as:
  malarial:
    hepatitis (573.2)
    nephrosis (581.81)

085 Leishmaniasis

085.0 Visceral [kala-azar]
Dumdum fever   Leishmaniasis:
Infection by Leishmania: dermal, post-kala-azar
  donovani   Mediterranean
  infantum   visceral (Indian)

085.1 Cutaneous, urban
Aleppo boil   Leishmaniasis, cutaneous:
Baghdad boil   dry form
Delhi boil   late
Infection by Leishmania   recurrent
  tropica (minor)   ulcerating
                              Oriental sore

085.2 Cutaneous, Asian desert
Infection by Leishmania tropica major
Leishmaniasis, cutaneous:
  acute necrotizing
  rural
  wet form
  zoonotic form

085.3 Cutaneous, Ethiopian
Infection by Leishmania ethiopica
Leishmaniasis, cutaneous:
  diffuse
  lepromatous

Add 4th or 5th digit   Nonspecific code   Unspecified code   Manifestation code

085.4 Cutaneous, American
    Chiclero ulcer
    Infection by Leishmania mexicana
    Leishmaniasis tegumentaria diffusa

085.5 Mucocutaneous (American)
    Espundia
    Infection by Leishmania braziliensis
    Uta

085.9 Leishmaniasis, unspecified

086 Trypanosomiasis

Use additional code, if desired, to identify manifestations, as:
  trypanosomiasis:
    encephalitis (323.2)
    meningitis (321.3)

086.0 Chagas' disease with heart involvement
    American trypanosomiasis with heart involvement
    Infection by Trypanosoma cruzi with heart involvement
    Any condition classifiable to 086.2 with heart involvement

086.1 Chagas' disease with other organ involvement
    American trypanosomiasis with involvement of organ other than heart
    Infection by Trypanosoma cruzi with involvement of organ other than heart
    Any condition classifiable to 086.2 with involvement of organ other than heart

086.2 Chagas' disease without mention of organ involvement
    American trypanosomiasis
    Infection by Trypanosoma cruzi

086.3 Gambian trypanosomiasis
    Gambian sleeping sickness
    Infection by Trypanosoma gambiense

086.4 Rhodesian trypanosomiasis
    Infection by Trypanosoma rhodesiense
    Rhodesian sleeping sickness

086.5 African trypanosomiasis, unspecified
    Sleeping sickness NOS

086.9 Trypanosomiasis, unspecified

087 Relapsing fever
    Includes: recurrent fever

087.0 Louse-borne

087.1 Tick-borne

087.9 Relapsing fever, unspecified

088 Other arthropod-borne diseases

088.0 Bartonellosis
    Carrión's disease   Verruga peruana
    Oroya fever

⑤ **088.8 Other specified arthropod-borne diseases**

    088.81 Lyme Disease
        Erythema chronicum migrans

    088.82 Babesiosis
        Babesiasis

    088.89 Other

088.9 Arthropod-borne disease, unspecified

● Code new
   to this edition
▲ Revision of
   existing code
④ ⑤ Fourth or fifth
     digit required

SYPHILIS AND OTHER VENEREAL DISEASES (090-099)

Excludes: nonvenereal endemic syphilis (104.0)
urogenital trichomoniasis (131.0)

090 Congenital syphilis

090.0 Early congenital syphilis, symptomatic

Congenital syphilitic:
choroiditis
coryza (chronic)
hepatomegaly
mucous patches
periostitis
splenomegaly

Syphilitic (congenital):
epiphysitis
osteochondritis
pemphigus
Any congenital syphilitic condition specified as early or manifest less than two years after birth

090.1 Early congenital syphilis, latent

Congenital syphilis without clinical manifestations, with positive serological reaction and negative spinal fluid test, less than two years after birth

090.2 Early congenital syphilis, unspecified

Congenital syphilis NOS, less than two years after birth

090.3 Syphilitic interstitial keratitis

Syphilitic keratitis:
parenchymatous
punctata profunda

Excludes: interstitial keratitis NOS (370.50)

⑤ 090.4 Juvenile neurosyphilis

Use additional code, if desired, to identify any associated mental disorder

090.40 Juvenile neurosyphilis, unspecified

Congenital neurosyphilis
Dementia paralytica juvenilis
Juvenile:
general paresis
tabes
taboparesis

090.41 Congenital syphilitic encephalitis

090.42 Congenital syphilitic meningitis

090.49 Other

090.5 Other late congenital syphilis, symptomatic

Gumma due to congenital syphilis
Hutchinson's teeth
Syphilitic saddle nose
Any congenital syphilitic condition specified as late or manifest two years or more after birth

090.6 Late congenital syphilis, latent

Congenital syphilis without clinical manifestations, with positive serological reaction and negative spinal fluid test, two years or more after birth

090.7 Late congenital syphilis, unspecified

Congenital syphilis NOS, two years or more after birth

090.9 Congenital syphilis, unspecified

091 Early syphilis, symptomatic

Excludes: early cardiovascular syphilis (093.0-093.9)
early neurosyphilis (094.0-094.9)

091.0 Genital syphilis (primary)

Genital chancre

091.1 Primary anal syphilis

091.2 Other primary syphilis

Primary syphilis of:
breast
fingers

Primary syphilis of:
lip
tonsils

091.3 Secondary syphilis of skin or mucous membranes

Condyloma latum
Secondary syphilis of:
anus
mouth
pharynx

Secondary syphilis of:
skin
tonsils
vulva

	Add 4th or 5th digit		Nonspecific code		Unspecified code		Manifestation code

091.4 Adenopathy due to secondary syphilis
Syphilitic adenopathy (secondary)
Syphilitic lymphadenitis (secondary)

⑤ **091.5 Uveitis due to secondary syphilis**

091.50 Syphilitic uveitis, unspecified

091.51 Syphilitic chorioretinitis (secondary)

091.52 Syphilitic iridocyclitis (secondary)

⑤ **091.6 Secondary syphilis of viscera and bone**

091.61 Secondary syphilitic periostitis

091.62 Secondary syphilitic hepatitis
Secondary syphilis of liver

091.69 Other viscera

091.7 Secondary syphilis, relapse
Secondary syphilis, relapse (treated) (untreated)

⑤ **091.8 Other forms of secondary syphilis**

091.81 Acute syphilitic meningitis (secondary)

091.82 Syphilitic alopecia

091.89 Other

091.9 Unspecified secondary syphilis

092 Early syphilis, latent
Includes: syphilis (acquired) without clinical manifestations, with positive serological
reaction and negative spinal fluid test, less than two years after infection

092.0 Early syphilis, latent, serological relapse after treatment

092.9 Early syphilis, latent, unspecified

093 Cardiovascular syphilis

093.0 Aneurysm of aorta, specified as syphilitic
Dilatation of aorta, specified as syphilitic

093.1 Syphilitic aortitis

⑤ **093.2 Syphilitic endocarditis**

093.20 Valve, unspecified
Syphilitic ostial coronary disease

093.21 Mitral valve

093.22 Aortic valve
Syphilitic aortic incompetence or stenosis

093.23 Tricuspid valve

093.24 Pulmonary valve

⑤ **093.8 Other specified cardiovascular syphilis**

093.81 Syphilitic pericarditis

093.82 Syphilitic myocarditis

093.89 Other

093.9 Cardiovascular syphilis, unspecified

094 Neurosyphilis
Use additional code, if desired, to identify any associated mental disorder

094.0 Tabes dorsalis
Locomotor ataxia (progressive)
Posterior spinal sclerosis (syphilitic)
Tabetic neurosyphilis
Use additional code, if desired, to identify manifestation, as:
neurogenic arthropathy [Charcot's joint disease] (713.5)

094.1 General paresis
Dementia paralytica   Paretic neurosyphilis
General paralysis (of the   Taboparesis
insane) (progressive)

094.2 Syphilitic meningitis
Meningovascular syphilis

Excludes: *acute syphilitic meningitis (secondary) (091.81)*

094.3 Asymptomatic neurosyphilis

   ● Code new   ▲ Revision of   ④ ⑤ Fourth or fifth
     to this edition   existing code   digit required

⑤ **094.8 Other specified neurosyphilis**

  094.81 Syphilitic encephalitis

  094.82 Syphilitic Parkinsonism

  094.83 Syphilitic disseminated retinochoroiditis

  094.84 Syphilitic optic atrophy

  094.85 Syphilitic retrobulbar neuritis

  094.86 Syphilitic acoustic neuritis

  094.87 Syphilitic ruptured cerebral aneurysm

  094.89 Other

094.9 Neurosyphilis, unspecified
  Gumma (syphilitic) of central nervous system NOS
  Syphilis (early) (late) of central nervous system NOS
  Syphiloma of central nervous system NOS

095 Other forms of late syphilis, with symptoms
  Includes: gumma (syphilitic)
        syphilis, late, tertiary, or unspecified stage

095.0 Syphilitic episcleritis

095.1 Syphilis of lung

095.2 Syphilitic peritonitis

095.3 Syphilis of liver

095.4 Syphilis of kidney

095.5 Syphilis of bone

095.6 Syphilis of muscle
  Syphilitic myositis

095.7 Syphilis of synovium, tendon, and bursa
  Syphilitic:
   bursitis
   synovitis

095.8 Other specified forms of late symptomatic syphilis

  Excludes: cardiovascular syphilis (093.0-093.9)
        neurosyphilis (094.0-094.9)

095.9 Late symptomatic syphilis, unspecified

096 Late syphilis, latent
  Syphilis (acquired) without clinical manifestations, with positive serological reaction and
    negative spinal fluid test, two years or more after infection

097 Other and unspecified syphilis

  097.0 Late syphilis, unspecified

  097.1 Latent syphilis, unspecified
    Positive serological reaction for syphilis

  097.9 Syphilis, unspecified
    Syphilis (acquired) NOS

  Excludes: syphilis NOS causing death under two years of age (090.9)

098 Gonococcal infections

  098.0 Acute, of lower genitourinary tract
    Gonococcal: Gonorrhea (acute):
     Bartholinitis (acute)   NOS
     urethritis (acute)   genitourinary (tract) NOS
     vulvovaginitis (acute)

⑤ **098.1 Acute, of upper genitourinary tract**

  098.10 Gonococcal infection (acute) of upper genitourinary tract, site unspecified

  098.11 Gonococcal cystitis (acute)
    Gonorrhea (acute) of bladder

  098.12 Gonococcal prostatitis (acute)

  098.13 Gonococcal epididymo-orchitis (acute)
    Gonococcal orchitis (acute)

  098.14 Gonococcal seminal vesiculitis (acute)
    Gonorrhea (acute) of seminal vesicle

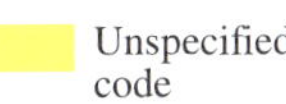

098.15 Gonococcal cervicitis (acute)
Gonorrhea (acute) of cervix

098.16 Gonococcal endometritis (acute)
Gonorrhea (acute) of uterus

098.17 Gonococcal salpingitis, specified as acute

098.19 Other

098.2 Chronic, of lower genitourinary tract
Gonococcal:
Bartholinitis specified as chronic or with duration of two months or more
urethritis specified as chronic or with duration of two months or more
vulvovaginitis specified as chronic or with duration of two months or more
Gonorrhea:
NOS specified as chronic or with duration of two months or more
genitourinary (tract) specified as chronic or with duration of two months or more
Any condition classifiable to 098.0 specified as chronic or with duration of two months
or more

⑤ **098.3 Chronic, of upper genitourinary tract**
Includes: any condition classifiable to 098.1 stated as chronic or with a duration of two
months or more

098.30 Chronic gonococcal infection of upper genitourinary tract, site unspecified

098.31 Gonococcal cystitis, chronic
Any condition classifiable to 098.11, specified as chronic
Gonorrhea of bladder, chronic

098.32 Gonococcal prostatitis, chronic
Any condition classifiable to 098.12, specified as chronic

098.33 Gonococcal epididymo-orchitis, chronic
Any condition classifiable to 098.13, specified as chronic
Chronic gonococcal orchitis

098.34 Gonococcal seminal vesiculitis, chronic
Any condition classifiable to 098.14, specified as chronic
Gonorrhea of seminal vesicle, chronic

098.35 Gonococcal cervicitis, chronic
Any condition classifiable to 098.15, specified as chronic
Gonorrhea of cervix, chronic

098.36 Gonococcal endometritis, chronic
Any condition classifiable to 098.16, specified as chronic

098.37 Gonococcal salpingitis (chronic)

098.39 Other

⑤ **098.4 Gonococcal infection of eye**

098.40 Gonococcal conjunctivitis (neonatorum)
Gonococcal ophthalmia (neonatorum)

098.41 Gonococcal iridocyclitis

098.42 Gonococcal endophthalmia

098.43 Gonococcal keratitis

098.49 Other

⑤ **098.5 Gonococcal infection of joint**

098.50 Gonococcal arthritis
Gonococcal infection of joint NOS

098.51 Gonococcal synovitis and tenosynovitis

098.52 Gonococcal bursitis

098.53 Gonococcal spondylitis

098.59 Other
Gonococcal rheumatism

098.6 Gonococcal infection of pharynx

098.7 Gonococcal infection of anus and rectum
Gonococcal proctitis

⑤ **098.8 Gonococcal infection of other specified sites**

098.81 Gonococcal keratosis (blennorrhagica)

098.82 Gonococcal meningitis

098.83 Gonococcal pericarditis

 ● Code new   ▲ Revision of   ④ ⑤ Fourth or fifth
to this edition   existing code   digit required

098.84 Gonococcal endocarditis

098.85 Other gonococcal heart disease

098.86 Gonococcal peritonitis

098.89 Other
Gonococcemia

099 Other venereal diseases

099.0 Chancroid
Bubo (inguinal):   Chancre:
 chancroidal   Ducrey's
 due to Hemophilus ducreyi simple
           soft
          Ulcus molle (cutis) (skin)

099.1 Lymphogranuloma venereum
Climatic or tropical bubo Esthiomene
(Durand-) Nicolas- Favre Lymphogranuloma inguinale
 disease

099.2 Granuloma inguinale
Donovanosis   Granuloma venereum
Granuloma pudendi   Pudendal ulcer
 (ulcerating)

099.3 Reiter's disease
Reiter's syndrome
Use additional code for associated:
 arthropathy (711.1)
 conjunctivitis (372.33)

⑤ **099.4 Other nongonococcal urethritis [NGU]**

 099.40 Unspecified
  Nonspecific urethritis

 099.41 Chlamydia trachomatis

 099.49 Other specified organism

⑤ **099.5 Other venereal diseases due to Chlamydia trachomatis**
Excludes: *Chlamydia trachomatis infection of conjunctiva (076.0-076.9, 077.0, 077.9)*
     Lymphogranuloma venereum (099.1)

 099.50 Unspecified site

 099.51 Pharynx

 099.52 Anus and rectum

 099.53 Lower genitourinary sites
Excludes: *urethra (099.41)*
Use additional code, if desired, to specify site of infection, such as:
   bladder (595.4)
   cervix (616.0)
   vagina and vulva (616.11)

 099.54 Other genitourinary sites
Use additional code, if desired, to specify site of infection, such as:
   pelvic inflammatory disease NOS (614.9)
   testis and epididymis (604.91)

 099.55 Unspecified genitourinary site

 099.56 Peritoneum
  Perihepatitis

 099.59 Other specified site

099.8 Other specified venereal diseases

099.9 Venereal disease, unspecified

OTHER SPIROCHETAL DISEASES (100-104)

100 Leptospirosis

100.0 Leptospirosis icterohemorrhagica
Leptospiral or spirochetal jaundice (hemorrhagic)
Weil's disease

⑤ **100.8 Other specified leptospiral infections**

 100.81 Leptospiral meningitis (aseptic)

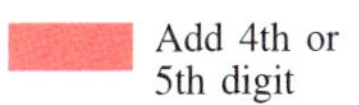

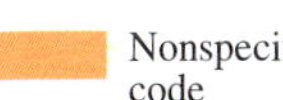

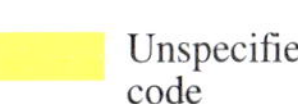

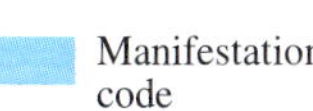

100.89 Other

Fever:

Fort Bragg

pretibial

swamp

Infection by Leptospira:

australis

bataviae

pyrogenes

100.9 Leptospirosis, unspecified

101 Vincent's angina

Acute necrotizing ulcerative:

gingivitis

stomatitis

Fusospirochetal pharyngitis

Spirochetal stomatitis

Trench mouth

Vincent's:

gingivitis

infection [any site]

102 Yaws

Includes: frambesia

pian

102.0 Initial lesions

Chancre of yaws

Frambesia, initial or primary

Initial frambesial ulcer

Mother yaw

102.1 Multiple papillomata and wet crab yaws

Butter yaws

Frambesioma

Pianoma

Planter or palmer papilloma of yaws

102.2 Other early skin lesions

Early yaws (cutaneous) (macular) (papular) (maculopapular) (micropapular)

Frambeside of early yaws

Cutaneous yaws, less than five years after infection

102.3 Hyperkeratosis

Ghoul hand

Hyperkeratosis, palmer or plantar (early) (late) due to yaws

Worm-eaten soles

102.4 Gummata and ulcers

Nodular late yaws (ulcerated)

Gummatous frambeside

102.5 Gangosa

Rhinopharyngitis mutilans

102.6 Bone and joint lesions

Goundou, of yaws (late)

Gumma, bone, of yaws (late)

Gummatous osteitis or periostitis, of yaws (late)

Hydrarthrosis, of yaws (early) (late)

Osteitis, of yaws (early) (late)

Periostitis (hypertrophic), of yaws (early) (late)

102.7 Other manifestations

Juxta-articular nodules of yaws

Mucosal yaws

102.8 Latent yaws

Yaws without clinical manifestations, with positive serology

102.9 Yaws, unspecified

103 Pinta

103.0 Primary lesions

Chancre (primary) of pinta [carate]

Papule (primary) of pinta [carate]

Pintid of pinta [carate]

103.1 Intermediate lesions

Erythematous plaques of pinta [carate]

Hyperchromic lesions of pinta [carate]

Hyperkeratosis of pinta [carate]

103.2 Late lesions

Cardiovascular lesions, of pinta [carate]

Skin lesions:

achromic of pinta [carate]

cicatricial of pinta [carate]

dyschromic of pinta [carate]

Vitiligo of pinta [carate]

● Code new
to this edition

▲ Revision of
existing code

④ ⑤ Fourth or fifth
digit required

103.3 Mixed lesions
Achromic and hyperchromic skin lesions of pinta [carate]

103.9 Pinta, unspecified

104 Other spirochetal infection

104.0 Nonvenereal endemic syphilis
Bejel   Njovera

104.8 Other specified spirochetal infections
Excludes: relapsing fever (087.0-087.9)
syphilis (090.0-097.9)

104.9 Spirochetal infection, unspecified

MYCOSES (110-118)

Use additional code, if desired, to identify manifestation, as:
arthropathy (711.6)
meningitis (321.0-321.1)
otitis externa (380.15)

Excludes: infection by Actinomycetales, such as species of Actinomyces, Actinomadura,
Nocardia, Streptomyces (039.0-039.9)

110 Dermatophytosis
Includes: infection by species of Epidermophyton, Microsporum, and Trichophyton
tinea, any type except those in 111

110.0 Of scalp and beard
Kerion
Sycosis, mycotic
Trichophytic tinea [black dot tinea], scalp

110.1 Of nail
Dermatophytic onychia   Tinea unguium
Onychomycosis

110.2 Of hand
Tinea manuum

110.3 Of groin and perianal area
Dhobie itch   Tinea cruris
Eczema marginatum

110.4 Of foot
Athlete's foot   Tinea pedis

110.5 Of the body
Herpes circinatus
Tinea imbricata [Tokelau]

110.6 Deep seated dermatophytosis
Granuloma trichophyticum
Majocchi's granuloma

110.8 Of other specified sites

110.9 Of unspecified site
Favus NOS   Ringworm NOS
Microsporic tinea NOS

111 Dermatomycosis, other and unspecified

111.0 Pityriasis versicolor
Infection by Malassezia [Pityrosporum] furfur
Tinea flava
Tinea versicolor

111.1 Tinea nigra
Infection by   Microsporosis nigra
Cladosporium species   Pityriasis nigra
Keratomycosis nigricans   Tinea palmaris nigra

111.2 Tinea blanca
Infection by Trichosporon (beigelii) cutaneum
White piedra

111.3 Black piedra
Infection by Piedraia hortai

111.8 Other specified dermatomycoses

111.9 Dermatomycosis, unspecified

Add 4th or   Nonspecific   Unspecified   Manifestation
5th digit   code   code   code

112 Candidiasis
Includes: infection by Candida species
moniliasis

Excludes: neonatal monilial infection (771.7)

112.0 Of mouth
Thrush (oral)

112.1 Of vulva and vagina
Candidal vulvovaginitis   Monilial vulvovaginitis

112.2 Of other urogenital sites
Candidal balanitis

112.3 Of skin and nails
Candidal intertrigo   Candidal perionyxis [paronychia]
Candidal onychia

112.4 Of lung
Candidal pneumonia

112.5 Disseminated
Systemic candidiasis

⑤ **112.8 Of other specified sites**

112.81 Candidal endocarditis

112.82 Candidal otitis externa
Otomycosis in moniliasis

112.83 Candidal meningitis

112.84 Candidal esophagitis

112.85 Candidal enteritis

112.89 Other

112.9 Of unspecified site

114 Coccidioidomycosis
Includes: infection by Coccidioides (immitis)
Posada-Wernicke disease

114.0 Primary coccidioidomycosis (pulmonary)
Acute pulmonary coccidioidomycosis
Coccidioidomycotic pneumonitis
Desert rheumatism
Pulmonary coccidioidomycosis
San Joaquin Valley fever

114.1 Primary extrapulmonary coccidioidomycosis
Chancriform syndrome
Primary cutaneous coccidioidomycosis

114.2 Coccidioidal meningitis

114.3 Other forms of progressive coccidioidomycosis
Coccidioidal granuloma
Disseminated coccidioidomycosis

114.4 Chronic pulmonary coccidioidomycosis

114.5 Pulmonary coccidioidomycosis, unspecified

114.9 Coccidioidomycosis, unspecified

⑤ **115 Histoplasmosis**
The following fifth-digit subclassification is for use with category 115:

0 without mention of manifestation

1 meningitis

2 retinitis

3 pericarditis

4 endocarditis

5 pneumonia

9 other

⑤ **115.0 Infection by Histoplasma capsulatum**
American histoplasmosis
Darling's disease
Reticuloendothelial cytomycosis
Small form histoplasmosis

● Code new
to this edition   ▲ Revision of
existing code   ④ ⑤ Fourth or fifth
digit required

⑤ **115.1 Infection by Histoplasma duboisii**
African histoplasmosis
Large form histoplasmosis

⑤ **115.9 Histoplasmosis, unspecified**
Histoplasmosis NOS

116 Blastomycotic infection

116.0 Blastomycosis
Blastomycotic dermatitis
Chicago disease
Cutaneous blastomycosis
Disseminated blastomycosis
Gilchrist's disease
Infection by Blastomyces [Ajellomyces] dermatitidis
North American blastomycosis
Primary pulmonary blastomycosis

116.1 Paracoccidioidomycosis
Brazilian blastomycosis
Infection by Paracoccidioides [Blastomyces] brasiliensis
Lutz-Splendore-Almeida disease
Mucocutaneous-lymphangitic paracoccidioidomycosis
Pulmonary paracoccidioidomycosis
South American blastomycosis
Visceral paracoccidioidomycosis

116.2 Lobomycosis
Infections by Loboa [Blastomyces] loboi
Keloidal blastomycosis
Lobo's disease

117 Other mycoses

117.0 Rhinosporidiosis
Infection by Rhinosporidium seeberi

117.1 Sporotrichosis
Cutaneous sporotrichosis
Disseminated sporotrichosis
Infection by Sporothrix [Sporotrichum] schenckii
Lymphocutaneous sporotrichosis
Pulmonary sporotrichosis
Sporotrichosis of the bones

117.2 Chromoblastomycosis
Chromomycosis
Infection by Cladosporidium carrionii, Fonsecaea compactum, Fonsecaea pedrosoi,
Phialophora verrucosa

117.3 Aspergillosis
Infection by Aspergillus species, mainly A. fumigatus, A. flavus group, A. terreus group

117.4 Mycotic mycetomas
Infection by various genera and species of Ascomycetes and Deuteromycetes, such as
Acremonium [Cephalosporium] falciforme, Neotestudina rosatii, Madurella grisea,
Madurella mycetomii, Pyrenochaeta romeroi, Zopfia [Leptosphaeria] senegalensis
Madura foot, mycotic
Maduromycosis, mycotic

| Excludes: | actinomycotic mycetomas (039.0-039.9) |

117.5 Cryptococcosis

Busse-Buschke's disease	Pulmonary cryptococcosis
European cryptococcosis	Systemic cryptococcosis
Infection by Cryptococcus neoformans	Torula

117.6 Allescheriosis [Petriellidosis]
Infections by Allescheria [Petriellidium] boydii [Monosporium apiospermum]

| Excludes: | mycotic mycetoma (117.4) |

117.7 Zygomycosis [Phycomycosis or Mucormycosis]
Infection by species of Absidia, Basidiobolus, Conidiobolus, Cunninghamella,
Entomophthora, Mucor, Rhizopus, Saksenaea

117.8 Infection by dematiacious fungi, [Phaehyphomycosis]
Infection by dematiacious fungi, such as Cladosporium trichoides [bantianum],
Dreschlera hawaiiensis, Phialophora gougerotii, Phialophora jeanselmi

117.9 Other and unspecified mycoses

Add 4th or 5th digit   Nonspecific code   Unspecified code   Manifestation code

118 Opportunistic mycoses
Infection of skin, subcutaneous tissues, and/or organs by a wide variety of fungi generally considered to be pathogenic to compromised hosts only (e.g., infection by species of Alternaria, Dreschlera, Fusarium)

HELMINTHIASES (120-129)

120 Schistosomiasis [bilharziasis]

120.0 Schistosoma haematobium
Vesical schistosomiasis NOS

120.1 Schistosoma mansoni
Intestinal schistosomiasis NOS

120.2 Schistosoma japonicum
Asiatic schistosomiasis NOS
Katayama disease or fever

120.3 Cutaneous
Cercarial dermatitis   Schistosome dermatitis
Infection by cercariae   Swimmers' itch
  of Schistosoma

120.8 Other specified schistosomiasis
Infection by Schistosoma: Infection by Schistosoma spindale
  bovis   Schistosomiasis chestermani
  intercalatum
  mattheii

120.9 Schistosomiasis, unspecified
Blood flukes NOS   Hemic distomiasis

121 Other trematode infections

121.0 Opisthorchiasis
Infection by:
  cat liver fluke
  Opisthorchis (felineus) (tenuicollis) (viverrini)

121.1 Clonorchiasis
Biliary cirrhosis due to clonorchiasis
Chinese liver fluke disease
Hepatic distomiasis due to Clonorchis sinensis
Oriental liver fluke disease

121.2 Paragonimiasis
Infection by Paragonimus   Pulmonary distomiasis
Lung fluke disease (oriental)

121.3 Fascioliasis
Infection by Fasciola: Liver flukes NOS
  gigantica   Sheep liver fluke infection
  hepatica

121.4 Fasciolopsiasis
Infection by Fasciolopsis [buski]
Intestinal distomiasis

121.5 Metagonimiasis
Infection by Metagonimus yokogawai

121.6 Heterophyiasis
Infection by:
  Heterophyes heterophyes
  Stellantchasmus falcatus

121.8 Other specified trematode infections
Infection by:
  Dicrocoelium dendriticum
  Echinostoma ilocanum
  Gastrodiscoides hominis

121.9 Trematode infection, unspecified
Distomiasis NOS   Fluke disease NOS

122 Echinococcosis
Includes: echinococciasis
           hydatid disease
           hydatidosis

122.0 Echinococcus granulosus infection of liver

122.1 Echinococcus granulosus infection of lung

● Code new   ▲ Revision of   ④ ⑤ Fourth or fifth
  to this edition   existing code   digit required

122.2 Echinococcus granulosus infection of thyroid

122.3 Echinococcus granulosus infection, other

122.4 Echinococcus granulosus infection, unspecified

122.5 Echinococcus multilocularis infection of liver

122.6 Echinococcus multilocularis infection, other

122.7 Echinococcus multilocularis infection, unspecified

122.8 Echinococcosis, unspecified, of liver

122.9 Echinococcosis, other and unspecified

123 **Other cestode infection**

123.0 **Taenia solium infection, intestinal form**
Pork tapeworm (adult) (infection)

123.1 **Cysticercosis**
Cysticerciasis
Infection by Cysticercus cellulosae [larval form of Taenia solium]

123.2 **Taenia saginata infection**
Beef tapeworm (infection)
Infection by Taeniarhynchus saginatus

123.3 **Taeniasis, unspecified**

123.4 **Diphyllobothriasis, intestinal**
Diphyllobothrium (adult) (latum) (pacificum) infection
Fish tapeworm (infection)

123.5 **Sparganosis [larval diphyllobothriasis]**
Infection by:
Diphyllobothrium larvae
Sparganum (mansoni) (proliferum)
Spirometra larvae

123.6 **Hymenolepiasis**
Dwarf tapeworm (infection)
Hymenolepis (diminuta) (nana) infection
Rat tapeworm (infection)

123.8 **Other specified cestode infection**
Diplogonoporus (grandis) infection
Dipylidium (caninum) infection
Dog tapeworm (infection) infection

123.9 **Cestode infection, unspecified**
Tapeworm (infection) NOS

124 **Trichinosis**
Trichinella spiralis infection
Trichinellosis
Trichiniasis

125 **Filarial infection and dracontiasis**

125.0 **Bancroftian filariasis**
Chyluria due to Wuchereria bancrofti
Elephantiasis due to Wuchereria bancrofti
Infection due to Wuchereria bancrofti
Lymphadenitis due to Wuchereria bancrofti
Lymphangitis due to Wuchereria bancrofti
Wuchereriasis

125.1 **Malayan filariasis**
Brugia filariasis due to Brugia [Wuchereria] malayi
Chyluria due to Brugia [Wuchereria] malayi
Elephantiasis due to Brugia [Wuchereria] malayi
Infection due to Brugia [Wuchereria] malayi
Lymphadenitis due to Brugia [Wuchereria] malayi
Lymphangitis due to Brugia [Wuchereria] malayi

125.2 **Loiasis**
Eyeworm disease of Africa
Loa loa infection

125.3 **Onchocerciasis**
Onchocerca volvulus infection
Onchocercosis

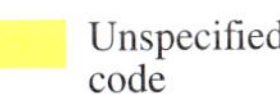

	Add 4th or 5th digit		Nonspecific code		Unspecified code		Manifestation code

125.4 Dipetalonemiasis
Infection by:
Acanthocheilonema perstans
Dipetalonema perstans

125.5 Mansonella ozzardi infection
Filariasis ozzardi

125.6 Other specified filariasis
Dirofilaria infection
Infection by:
Acanthocheilonema streptocerca
Dipetalonema streptocerca

125.7 Dracontiasis
Guinea-worm infection
Infection by Dracunculus medinensis

125.9 Unspecified filariasis

126 Ancylostomiasis and necatoriasis
Includes: cutaneous larva migrans due to Ancylostoma
hookworm (disease) (infection)
uncinariasis

126.0 Ancylostoma duodenale

126.1 Necator americanus

126.2 Ancylostoma braziliense

126.3 Ancylostoma ceylanicum

126.8 Other specified Ancylostoma

126.9 Ancylostomiasis and necatoriasis, unspecified
Creeping eruption NOS
Cutaneous larva migrans NOS

127 Other intestinal helminthiases

127.0 Ascariasis
Ascaridiasis
Infection by Ascaris lumbricoides
Roundworm infection

127.1 Anisakiasis
Infection by Anisakis larva

127.2 Strongyloidiasis
Infection by Strongyloides stercoralis
> *Excludes:* *trichostrongyliasis (127.6)*

127.3 Trichuriasis
Infection by Trichuris trichiuria
Trichocephaliasis
Whipworm (disease) (infection)

127.4 Enterobiasis
Infection by Enterobius vermicularis
Oxyuriasis
Oxyuris vermicularis infection
Pinworn (disease) (infection)
Threadworm infection

127.5 Capillariasis
Infection by Capillaria philippinensis
> *Excludes:* *infection by Capillaria hepatica (128.8)*

127.6 Trichostrongyliasis
Infection by Trichostrongylus species

127.7 Other specified intestinal helminthiasis
Infection by:
Oesophagostomum apiostomum and related species
Ternidens diminutus
other specified intestinal helminth
Physalopteriasis

127.8 Mixed intestinal helminthiasis
Infection by intestinal helminths classified to more than one of the categories
120.0-127.7
Mixed helminthiasis NOS

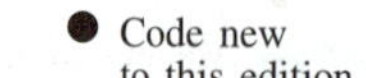

● Code new   ▲ Revision of   ④ ⑤ Fourth or fifth
to this edition   existing code   digit required

127.9 Intestinal helminthiasis, unspecified

128 Other and unspecified helminthiases

128.0 Toxocariasis
Larva migrans visceralis
Toxocara (canis) (cati) infection
Visceral larva migrans syndrome

128.1 Gnathostomiasis
Infection by Gnathostoma spinigerum and related species

128.8 Other specified helminthiasis
Infection by:
Angiostrongylus cantonensis
Capillaria hepatica
other specified helminth

128.9 Helminth infection, unspecified
Helminthiasis NOS
Worms NOS

129 Intestinal parasitism, unspecified

OTHER INFECTIOUS AND PARASITIC DISEASES (130-136)

130 Toxoplasmosis
Includes: infection by toxoplasma gondii
toxoplasmosis (acquired)

Excludes: *congenital toxoplasmosis (771.2)*

130.0 Meningoencephalitis due to toxoplasmosis
Encephalitis due to acquired toxoplasmosis

130.1 Conjunctivitis due to toxoplasmosis

130.2 Chorioretinitis due to toxoplasmosis
Focal retinochoroiditis due to acquired toxoplasmosis

130.3 Myocarditis due to toxoplasmosis

130.4 Pneumonitis due to toxoplasmosis

130.5 Hepatitis due to toxoplasmosis

130.7 Toxoplasmosis of other specified sites

130.8 Multisystemic disseminated toxoplasmosis
Toxoplasmosis of multiple sites

130.9 Toxoplasmosis, unspecified

131 Trichomoniasis
Includes: infection due to Trichomonas (vaginalis)

⑤ **131.0** Urogenital trichomoniasis

131.00 Urogenital trichomoniasis, unspecified
Fluor (vaginalis) trichomonal or due to Trichomonas (vaginalis)
Leukorrhea (vaginalis) trichomonal or due to Trichomonas (vaginalis)

131.01 Trichomonal vulvovaginitis
Vaginitis, trichomonal or due to Trichomonas (vaginalis)

131.02 Trichomonal urethritis

131.03 Trichomonal prostatitis

131.09 Other

131.8 Other specified sites

Excludes: *intestinal (007.3)*

131.9 Trichomoniasis, unspecified

132 Pediculosis and phthirus infestation

132.0 Pediculus capitis [head louse]

132.1 Pediculus corporis [body louse]

132.2 Phthirus pubis [pubic louse]
Pediculus pubis

132.3 Mixed infestation
Infestation classifiable to more than one of the categories 132.0-132.2

132.9 Pediculosis, unspecified

133 Acariasis

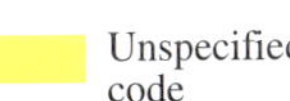

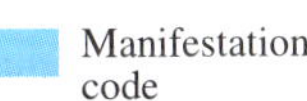

133.0 Scabies
Infestation by Sarcoptes scabiei
Norwegian scabies
Sarcoptic itch

133.8 Other acariasis
Chiggers
Infestation by:
Demodex folliculorum
Trombicula

133.9 Acariasis, unspecified
Infestation by mites NOS

134 Other infestation

134.0 Myiasis
Infestation by:
Dermatobia (hominis)
fly larvae
Gasterophilus (intestinalis)
Infestation by:
maggots
Oestrus ovis

134.1 Other arthropod infestation
Infestation by:
chigoe
sand flea
Tunga penetrans
Jigger disease
Scarabiasis
Tungiasis

134.2 Hirudiniasis
Hirudiniasis (external) (internal)
Leeches (aquatic) (land)

134.8 Other specified infestations

134.9 Infestation, unspecified
Infestation (skin) NOS
Skin parasites NOS

135 Sarcoidosis
Besnier-Boeck- Schaumann disease
Lupoid (miliary) of Boeck
Lupus pernio (Besnier)
Lymphogranulomatosis, benign
(Schaumann's)
Sarcoid (any site):
NOS
Boeck
Darier-Roussy
Uveoparotid fever

136 Other and unspecified infectious and parasitic diseases

136.0 Ainhum
Dactylolysis spontanea

136.1 Behçet's syndrome

136.2 Specific infections by free-living amebae
Meningoencephalitis due to Naegleria

136.3 Pneumocystosis
Pneumonia due to Pneumocystis carinii
Pneumonia due to Pneumocystis jiroveci

136.4 Psorospermiasis

136.5 Sarcosporidiosis
Infection by Sarcocystis lindemanni

136.8 Other specified infectious and parasitic diseases
Candiru infestation

136.9 Unspecified infectious and parasitic diseases
Infectious disease NOS
Parasitic disease NOS

LATE EFFECTS OF INFECTIOUS AND PARASITIC DISEASES (137-139)

137 Late effects of tuberculosis
Note: This category is to be used to indicate conditions classifiable to 010-018 as the cause of
late effects, which are themselves classified elsewhere. The "late effects" include those
specified as such, as sequelae, or as due to old or inactive tuberculosis, without evidence
of active disease.

137.0 Late effects of respiratory or unspecified tuberculosis

137.1 Late effects of central nervous system tuberculosis

137.2 Late effects of genitourinary tuberculosis

137.3 Late effects of tuberculosis of bones and joints

● Code new
to this edition
▲ Revision of
existing code
④ ⑤ Fourth or fifth
digit required

137.4 Late effects of tuberculosis of other specified organs

138 Late effects of acute poliomyelitis
> Note: This category is to be used to indicate conditions classifiable to 045 as the cause of late effects, which are themselves classified elsewhere. The "late effects" include conditions specified as such, or as sequelae, or as due to old or inactive poliomyelitis, without evidence of active disease.

139 Late effects of other infectious and parasitic diseases
> Note: This category is to be used to indicate conditions classifiable to categories 001-009, 020-041, 046-136 as the cause of late effects, which are themselves classified elsewhere. The "late effects" include conditions specified as such; they also include sequela of diseases classifiable to the above categories if there is evidence that the disease itself is no longer present.

139.0 Late effects of viral encephalitis
> Late effects of conditions classifiable to 049.8-049.9, 062-064

139.1 Late effects of trachoma
> Late effects of conditions classifiable to 076

139.8 Late effects of other and unspecified infectious and parasitic diseases

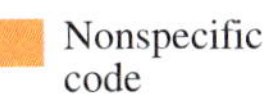

● Code new
to this edition

▲ Revision of
existing code

④ ⑤ Fourth or fifth
digit required

2. NEOPLASMS (140-239)

Notes:

1. Content

This chapter contains the following broad groups:

140-195   **Malignant neoplasms, stated or presumed to be primary, of specified sites, except of lymphatic and hematopoietic tissue**

196-198   **Malignant neoplasms, stated or presumed to be secondary, of specified sites**

199   **Malignant neoplasms, without specification of site**

200-208   **Malignant neoplasms, stated or presumed to be primary, of lymphatic and hematopoietic tissue**

210-229   **Benign neoplasms**

230-234   **Carcinoma in situ**

235-238   **Neoplasms of uncertain behavior**

239   **Neoplasms of unspecified nature**

2. Functional activity

All neoplasms are classified in this chapter, whether or not functionally active. An additional code from Chapter 3 may be used, if desired, to identify such functional activity associated with any neoplasm, e.g.:

catecholamine-producing malignant pheochromocytoma of adrenal:
code 194.0, additional code 255.6

basophil adenoma of pituitary with Cushing's syndrome:
code 227.3, additional code 255.0

3. Morphology [Histology]

For those wishing to identify the histological type of neoplasms, a comprehensive coded nomenclature, which comprises the morphology rubrics of the ICD-Oncology, is given in Appendix A.

4. Malignant neoplasms overlapping site boundaries

Categories 140-195 are for the classification of primary malignant neoplasms according to their point of origin. A malignant neoplasm that overlaps two or more subcategories within a three-digit rubric and whose point of origin cannot be determined should be classified to the subcategory .8 "Other." For example, "carcinoma involving tip and ventral surface of tongue" should be assigned to 141.8. On the other hand, "carcinoma of tip of tongue, extending to involve the ventral surface" should be coded to 141.2, as the point of origin, the tip, is known. Three subcategories (149.8, 159.8, 165.8) have been provided for malignant neoplasms that overlap the boundaries of three-digit rubrics within certain systems. Overlapping malignant neoplasms that cannot be classified as indicated above should be assigned to the appropriate subdivision of category 195 (Malignant neoplasm of other and ill-defined sites).

MALIGNANT NEOPLASM OF LIP, ORAL CAVITY, AND PHARYNX (140-149)

Excludes: carcinoma in situ (230.0)

140 Malignant neoplasm of lip

Excludes: skin of lip (173.0)

140.0 Upper lip, vermilion border
Upper lip:
NOS
external
lipstick area

140.1 Lower lip, vermilion border
Lower lip:
NOS
external
lipstick area

140.3 Upper lip, inner aspect

Upper lip
  buccal aspect
  frenulum

Upper lip:
  mucosa
  oral aspect

140.4 Lower lip, inner aspect

Lower lip:
  buccal aspect
  frenulum

Lower lip:
  mucosa
  oral aspect

140.5 Lip, unspecified, inner aspect
Lip, not specified whether upper or lower:
  buccal aspect   frenulum
  mucosa   oral aspect

140.6 Commissure of lip
Labial commissure

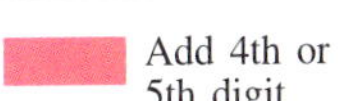 Add 4th or 5th digit
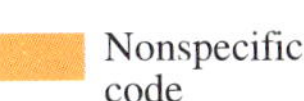 Nonspecific code
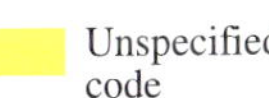 Unspecified code
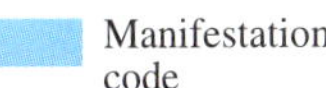 Manifestation code

140.8 Other sites of lip
Malignant neoplasm of contiguous or overlapping sites of lip whose point of origin cannot be determined

140.9 Lip, unspecified, vermilion border
Lip, not specified as upper or lower:
NOS
external
lipstick area

141 Malignant neoplasm of tongue

141.0 Base of tongue
Dorsal surface of base of tongue
Fixed part of tongue NOS

141.1 Dorsal surface of tongue
Anterior two-thirds of tongue, dorsal surface
Dorsal tongue NOS
Midline of tongue

> Excludes: *dorsal surface of base of tongue (141.0)*

141.2 Tip and lateral border of tongue

141.3 Ventral surface of tongue
Anterior two-thirds of tongue, ventral surface
Frenulum linguae

141.4 Anterior two-thirds of tongue, part unspecified
Mobile part of tongue NOS

141.5 Junctional zone
Border of tongue at junction of fixed and mobile parts at insertion of anterior tonsillar pillar

141.6 Lingual tonsil

141.8 Other sites of tongue
Malignant neoplasm of contiguous or overlapping sites of tongue whose point of origin cannot be determined

141.9 Tongue, unspecified
Tongue NOS

142 Malignant neoplasm of major salivary glands
Includes: salivary ducts

> Excludes: *malignant neoplasm of minor salivary glands:*
> *NOS (145.9)*
> *buccal mucosa (145.0)*
> *soft palate (145.3)*
> *tongue (141.0-141.9)*
> *tonsil, palatine (146.0)*

142.0 Parotid gland

142.1 Submandibular gland
Submaxillary gland

142.2 Sublingual gland

142.8 Other major salivary glands
Malignant neoplasm of contiguous or overlapping sites of salivary glands and ducts whose point of origin cannot be determined

142.9 Salivary gland, unspecified
Salivary gland (major) NOS

143 Malignant neoplasm of gum
Includes: alveolar (ridge) mucosa
gingiva (alveolar) (marginal)
interdental papillae

> Excludes: *malignant odontogenic neoplasms (170.0-170.1)*

143.0 Upper gum

143.1 Lower gum

143.8 Other sites of gum
Malignant neoplasm of contiguous or overlapping sites of gum whose point of origin cannot be determined

143.9 Gum, unspecified

144 Malignant neoplasm of floor of mouth

● Code new to this edition   ▲ Revision of existing code   ④ ⑤ Fourth or fifth digit required

144.0 Anterior portion
Anterior to the premolar-canine junction

144.1 Lateral portion

144.8 Other sites of floor of mouth
Malignant neoplasm of contiguous or overlapping sites of floor of mouth whose point of origin cannot be determined

144.9 Floor of mouth, part unspecified

145 Malignant neoplasm of other and unspecified parts of mouth
Excludes: *mucosa of lips (140.0-140.9)*

145.0 Cheek mucosa
Buccal mucosa   Cheek, inner aspect

145.1 Vestibule of mouth
Buccal sulcus (upper) (lower)
Labial sulcus (upper) (lower)

145.2 Hard palate

145.3 Soft palate
Excludes: *nasopharyngeal [posterior] [superior] surface of soft palate (147.3)*

145.4 Uvula

145.5 Palate, unspecified
Junction of hard and soft palate
Roof of mouth

145.6 Retromolar area

145.8 Other specified parts of mouth
Malignant neoplasm of contiguous or overlapping sites of mouth whose point of origin cannot be determined

145.9 Mouth, unspecified
Buccal cavity NOS
Minor salivary gland, unspecified site
Oral cavity NOS

146 Malignant neoplasm of oropharynx

146.0 Tonsil
Tonsil:
  NOS
  faucial
  palatine
Excludes: *lingual tonsil (141.6)*
         pharyngeal tonsil (147.1)

146.1 Tonsillar fossa

146.2 Tonsillar pillars (anterior) (posterior)
Faucial pillar   Palatoglossal arch
Glossopalatine fold   Palatopharyngeal arch

146.3 Vallecula
Anterior and medial surface of the pharyngoepiglottic fold

146.4 Anterior aspect of epiglottis
Epiglottis, free border [margin]
Glossoepiglottic fold(s)
Excludes: *epiglottis:*
         NOS (161.1)
         suprahyoid portion (161.1)

146.5 Junctional region
Junction of the free margin of the epiglottis, the aryepiglottic fold, and the pharyngoepiglottic fold

146.6 Lateral wall of oropharynx

146.7 Posterior wall of oropharynx

146.8 Other specified sites of oropharynx
Branchial cleft
Malignant neoplasm of contiguous or overlapping sites of oropharynx whose point of origin cannot be determined

146.9 Oropharynx, unspecified

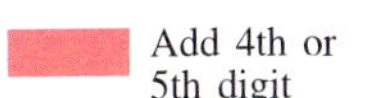

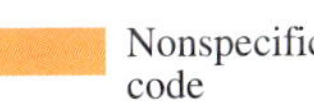

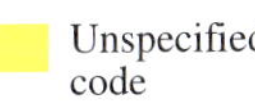

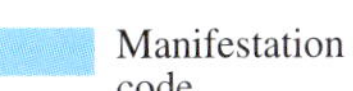

147 **Malignant neoplasm of nasopharynx**

147.0 **Superior wall**
Roof of nasopharynx

147.1 **Posterior wall**
Adenoid   Pharyngeal tonsil

147.2 **Lateral wall**
Fossa of Rosenmüller   Pharyngeal recess
Opening of auditory tube

147.3 **Anterior wall**
Floor of nasopharynx
Nasopharyngeal [posterior] [superior] surface of soft palate
Posterior margin of nasal septum and choanae

147.8 **Other specified sites of nasopharynx**
Malignant neoplasm of contiguous or overlapping sites of nasopharynx whose point of
origin cannot be determined

147.9 **Nasopharynx, unspecified**
Nasopharyngeal wall NOS

148 **Malignant neoplasm of hypopharynx**

148.0 **Postcricoid region**

148.1 **Pyriform sinus**
Pyriform fossa

148.2 **Aryepiglottic fold, hypopharyngeal aspect**
Aryepiglottic fold or interarytenoid fold:
NOS
marginal zone

| Excludes: | aryepiglottic fold or interarytenoid fold, laryngeal aspect (161.1) |

148.3 **Posterior hypopharyngeal wall**

148.8 **Other specified sites of hypopharynx**
Malignant neoplasm of contiguous or overlapping sites of hypopharynx whose point of
origin cannot be determined

148.9 **Hypopharynx, unspecified**
Hypopharyngeal wall NOS   Hypopharynx NOS

149 **Malignant neoplasm of other and ill-defined sites within the lip, oral cavity, and pharynx**

149.0 **Pharynx, unspecified**

149.1 **Waldeyer's ring**

149.8 **Other**
Malignant neoplasms of lip, oral cavity, and pharynx whose point of origin cannot be
assigned to any one of the categories 140-148

| Excludes: | "book leaf" neoplasm [ventral surface of tongue and floor of mouth] (145.8) |

149.9 **Ill-defined**

MALIGNANT NEOPLASM OF DIGESTIVE ORGANS AND PERITONEUM (150-159)

| Excludes: | carcinoma in situ (230.1-230.9) |

150 **Malignant neoplasm of esophagus**

150.0 **Cervical esophagus**

150.1 **Thoracic esophagus**

150.2 **Abdominal esophagus**

| Excludes: | adenocarcinoma (151.0) |
| | cardio-esophageal junction (151.0) |

150.3 **Upper third of esophagus**
Proximal third of esophagus

150.4 **Middle third of esophagus**

150.5 **Lower third of esophagus**
Distal third of esophagus

| Excludes: | adenocarcinoma (151.0) |
| | cardio-esophageal junction (151.0) |

150.8 **Other specified part**
Malignant neoplasm of contiguous or overlapping sites of esophagus whose point of
origin cannot be determined

● Code new
to this edition   ▲ Revision of
existing code   ④ ⑤ Fourth or fifth
digit required

150.9 Esophagus, unspecified

151 Malignant neoplasm of stomach
> *Excludes:* malignant stromal tumor of stomach (171.5)

151.0 Cardia
Cardiac orifice   Cardio-esophageal junction
> *Excludes:* squamous cell carcinoma (150.2, 150.5)

151.1 Pylorus
Prepylorus   Pyloric canal

151.2 Pyloric antrum
Antrum of stomach NOS

151.3 Fundus of stomach

151.4 Body of stomach

151.5 Lesser curvature, unspecified
Lesser curvature, not classifiable to 151.1-151.4

151.6 Greater curvature, unspecified
Greater curvature, not classifiable to 151.0-151.4

151.8 Other specified sites of stomach
Anterior wall, not classifiable to 151.0-151.4
Posterior wall, not classifiable to 151.0-151.4
Malignant neoplasm of contiguous or overlapping sites of stomach whose point of
origin cannot be determined

151.9 Stomach, unspecified
Carcinoma ventriculi   Gastric cancer

152 Malignant neoplasm of small intestine, including duodenum
> *Excludes:* malignant stromal tumor of small intestine (171.5)

152.0 Duodenum

152.1 Jejunum

152.2 Ileum
> *Excludes:* ileocecal valve (153.4)

152.3 Meckel's diverticulum

152.8 Other specified sites of small intestine
Duodenojejunal junction
Malignant neoplasm of contiguous or overlapping sites of small intestine whose point of
origin cannot be determined

152.9 Small intestine, unspecified

153 Malignant neoplasm of colon

153.0 Hepatic flexure

153.1 Transverse colon

153.2 Descending colon
Left colon

153.3 Sigmoid colon
Sigmoid (flexure)
> *Excludes:* rectosigmoid junction (154.0)

153.4 Cecum
Ileocecal valve

153.5 Appendix

153.6 Ascending colon
Right colon

153.7 Splenic flexure

153.8 Other specified sites of large intestine
Malignant neoplasm of contiguous or overlapping sites of colon whose point of origin
cannot be determined
> *Excludes:* ileocecal valve (153.4)
> rectosigmoid junction (154.0)

153.9 Colon, unspecified
Large intestine NOS

154 Malignant neoplasm of rectum, rectosigmoid junction, and anus

	Add 4th or 5th digit		Nonspecific code		Unspecified code		Manifestation code

154.0 Rectosigmoid junction
  Colon with rectum   Rectosigmoid (colon)

154.1 Rectum
  Rectal ampulla

154.2 Anal canal
  Anal sphincter
  | Excludes: | *skin of anus (172.5, 173.5)*

154.3 Anus, unspecified
  | Excludes: | *anus:*
        margin (172.5, 173.5)
        skin (172.5, 173.5)
        perianal skin (172.5, 173.5)

154.8 Other
  Anorectum
  Cloacogenic zone
  Malignant neoplasm of contiguous or overlapping sites of rectum, rectosigmoid junction,
      and anus whose point of origin cannot be determined

155 Malignant neoplasm of liver and intrahepatic bile ducts

155.0 Liver, primary
  Carcinoma:
      liver, specified as primary
      hepatocellular
      liver cell
  Hepatoblastoma

155.1 Intrahepatic bile ducts
  Canaliculi biliferi   Intrahepatic:
  Interlobular: biliary passages
      bile ducts   canaliculi
      biliary canals   gall duct
  | Excludes: | *hepatic duct (156.1)*

155.2 Liver, not specified as primary or secondary

156 Malignant neoplasm of gallbladder and extrahepatic bile ducts

156.0 Gallbladder

156.1 Extrahepatic bile ducts
  Biliary duct or passage NOS   Cystic duct
  Common bile duct   Hepatic duct
                                 Sphincter of Oddi

156.2 Ampulla of Vater

156.8 Other specified sites of gallbladder and extrahepatic bile ducts
  Malignant neoplasm of contiguous or overlapping sites of gallbladder and extrahepatic
      bile ducts whose point of origin cannot be determined

156.9 Biliary tract, part unspecified
  Malignant neoplasm involving both intrahepatic and extrahepatic bile ducts

157 Malignant neoplasm of pancreas

157.0 Head of pancreas

157.1 Body of pancreas

157.2 Tail of pancreas

157.3 Pancreatic duct
  Duct of:
      Santorini
      Wirsung

157.4 Islets of Langerhans
  Islets of Langerhans, any part of pancreas
Use additional code, if desired, to identify any functional activity

157.8 Other specified sites of pancreas
  Ectopic pancreatic tissue
  Malignant neoplasm of contiguous or overlapping sites of pancreas whose point of
      origin cannot be determined

157.9 Pancreas, part unspecified

158 Malignant neoplasm of retroperitoneum and peritoneum

   ● Code new   ▲ Revision of   ④ ⑤ Fourth or fifth
       to this edition   existing code   digit required

158.0 Retroperitoneum
Periadrenal tissue
Perinephric tissue
Perirenal tissue
Retrocecal tissue

158.8 Specified parts of peritoneum
Cul-de-sac (of Douglas)
Mesentery
Mesocolon
Omentum
Peritoneum:
  parietal
  pelvic
Rectouterine pouch
Malignant neoplasm of contiguous or overlapping sites of retroperitoneum and peritoneum whose point of origin cannot be determined

158.9 Peritoneum, unspecified

159 Malignant neoplasm of other and ill-defined sites within the digestive organs and peritoneum

159.0 Intestinal tract, part unspecified
Intestine NOS

159.1 Spleen, not elsewhere classified
Angiosarcoma of spleen
Fibrosarcoma of spleen

Excludes: *Hodgkin's disease (201.0-201.9)*
lymphosarcoma (200.1)
reticulosarcoma (200.0)

159.8 Other sites of digestive system and intra-abdominal organs
Malignant neoplasm of digestive organs and peritoneum whose point of origin cannot be assigned to any one of the categories 150-158

Excludes: *anus and rectum (154.8)*
cardio-esophageal junction (151.0)
colon and rectum ORANGE (154.0)

159.9 Ill-defined
Alimentary canal or tract NOS
Gastrointestinal tract NOS

Excludes: *abdominal NOS (195.2)*
intra-abdominal NOS (195.2)

MALIGNANT NEOPLASM OF RESPIRATORY AND INTRATHORACIC ORGANS (160-165)

Excludes: *carcinoma in situ (231.0-231.9)*

160 Malignant neoplasm of nasal cavities, middle ear, and accessory sinuses

160.0 Nasal cavities
Cartilage of nose
Conchae, nasal
Internal nose
Septum of nose
Vestibule of nose

Excludes: *nasal bone (170.0)*
nose NOS (195.0)
olfactory bulb (192.0)
posterior margin of septum and choanae (147.3)
skin of nose (172.3, 173.3)
turbinates (170.0)

160.1 Auditory tube, middle ear, and mastoid air cells
Antrum tympanicum
Eustachian tube
Tympanic cavity

Excludes: *auditory canal (external) (172.2, 173.2)*
bone of ear (meatus) (170.0)
cartilage of ear (171.0)
ear (external) (skin) (172.2, 173.2)

160.2 Maxillary sinus
Antrum (Highmore) (maxillary)

160.3 Ethmoidal sinus

160.4 Frontal sinus

160.5 Sphenoidal sinus

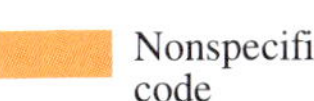
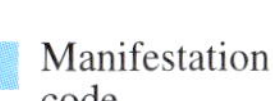

Add 4th or 5th digit   Nonspecific code   Unspecified code   Manifestation code

160.8 Other
Malignant neoplasm of contiguous or overlapping sites of nasal cavities, middle ear, and accessory sinuses whose point of origin cannot be determined

160.9 Accessory sinus, unspecified

161 Malignant neoplasm of larynx

161.0 Glottis
Intrinsic larynx
Laryngeal commissure
  (anterior) (posterior)
True vocal cord
Vocal cord NOS

161.1 Supraglottis
Aryepiglottic fold or interarytenoid fold, laryngeal aspect
Epiglottis (suprahyoid portion) NOS
Extrinsic larynx
False vocal cords
Posterior (laryngeal) surface of epiglottis
Ventricular bands

Excludes: *anterior aspect of epiglottis (146.4)*
      aryepiglottic fold or interarytenoid fold:
        NOS (148.2)
        hypopharyngeal aspect (148.2)
        marginal zone (148.2)

161.2 Subglottis

161.3 Laryngeal cartilages
Cartilage:
  arytenoid
  cricoid
Cartilage:
  cuneiform
  thyroid

161.8 Other specified sites of larynx
Malignant neoplasm of contiguous or overlapping sites of larynx whose point of origin cannot be determined

161.9 Larynx, unspecified

162 Malignant neoplasm of trachea, bronchus, and lung

162.0 Trachea
Cartilage of trachea
Mucosa of trachea

162.2 Main bronchus
Carina
Hilus of lung

162.3 Upper lobe, bronchus or lung

162.4 Middle lobe, bronchus or lung

162.5 Lower lobe, bronchus or lung

162.8 Other parts of bronchus or lung
Malignant neoplasm of contiguous or overlapping sites of bronchus or lung whose point of origin cannot be determined

162.9 Bronchus and lung, unspecified

163 Malignant neoplasm of pleura

163.0 Parietal pleura

163.1 Visceral pleura

163.8 Other specified sites of pleura
Malignant neoplasm of contiguous or overlapping sites of pleura whose point of origin cannot be determined

163.9 Pleura, unspecified

164 Malignant neoplasm of thymus, heart, and mediastinum

164.0 Thymus

164.1 Heart
Endocardium
Epicardium
Myocardium
Pericardium

Excludes: *great vessels (171.4)*

164.2 Anterior mediastinum

164.3 Posterior mediastinum

● Code new
  to this edition
▲ Revision of
  existing code
④ ⑤ Fourth or fifth
    digit required

164.8 Other
Malignant neoplasm of contiguous or overlapping sites of thymus, heart, and mediastinum whose point of origin cannot be determined

164.9 Mediastinum, part unspecified

165 Malignant neoplasm of other and ill-defined sites within the respiratory system and intrathoracic organs

165.0 Upper respiratory trace, part unspecified

165.8 Other
Malignant neoplasm of respiratory and intrathoracic organs whose point of origin cannot be assigned to any one of the categories 160-164

165.9 Ill-defined sites within the respiratory system
Respiratory tract NOS

Excludes: *intrathoracic NOS (195.1)*
thoracic NOS (195.1)

MALIGNANT NEOPLASM OF BONE, CONNECTIVE TISSUE, SKIN, AND BREAST (170-176)

Excludes: *carcinoma in situ:*
breast (233.0)
skin (232.0-232.9)

170 Malignant neoplasm of bone and articular cartilage
Includes: cartilage (articular) (joint)
periosteum

Excludes: *bone marrow NOS (202.9)*

cartilage:
ear (171.0)
eyelid (171.0)
larynx (161.3)
nose (160.0)
synovia (171.0-171.9)

170.0 Bones of skull and face, except mandible

Bone:	Bone:
ethmoid	sphenoid
frontal	temporal
malar	zygomatic
nasal	Maxilla (superior)
occipital	Turbinate
orbital	Upper jaw bone
parietal	Vomer

Excludes: *carcinoma, any type except intraosseous or odontogenic:*
maxilla, maxillary (sinus) (160.2)
upper jaw bone (143.0)
jaw bone (lower) (170.1)

170.1 Mandible

Inferior maxilla	Lower jaw bone
Jaw bone NOS	

Excludes: *carcinoma, any type except intraosseous or odontogenic:*
jaw bone NOS (143.9)
lower (143.1)
upper jaw bone (170.0)

170.2 Vertebral column, excluding sacrum and coccyx

Spinal column	Vertebra
Spine	

Excludes: *sacrum and coccyx (170.6)*

170.3 Ribs, sternum, and clavicle

Costal cartilage	Xiphoid process
Costovertebral joint	

170.4 Scapula and long bones of upper limb

Acromion	Radius
Bones NOS of upper limb	Ulna
Humerus	

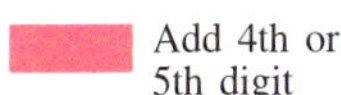

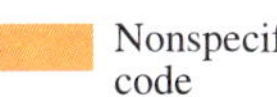

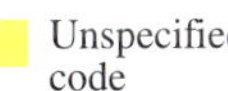

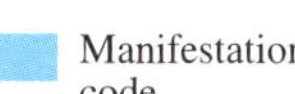

170.5 Short bones of upper limb

Carpal	Scaphoid (of hand)
Cuneiform, wrist	Semilunar or lunate
Metacarpal	Trapezium
Navicular, of hand	Trapezoid
Phalanges of hand	Unciform
Pisiform	

170.6 Pelvic bones, sacrum, and coccyx

Coccygeal vertebra	Pubic bone
Ilium	Sacral vertebra
Ischium	

170.7 Long bones of lower limb

Bones NOS of lower limb	Fibula
Femur	Tibia

170.8 Short bones of lower limb

Astragalus [talus]	Navicular (of ankle)
Calcaneus	Patella
Cuboid	Phalanges of foot
Cuneiform, ankle	Tarsal
Metatarsal	

170.9 Bone and articular cartilage, site unspecified

171 Malignant neoplasm of connective and other soft tissue

Includes: blood vessel
bursa
fascia
fat
ligament, except uterine
malignant stromal tumors
muscle
peripheral, sympathetic, and parasympathetic nerves and ganglia
synovia
tendon (sheath)

Excludes: *cartilage (of):*
articular (170.0-170.9)
larynx (161.3)
nose (160.0)
connective tissue:
breast (174.0-175.9)
internal organs (except stromal tumors)—code to malignant neoplasm of the site
[e.g., leiomyosarcoma of stomach, 151.9]
heart (164.1)
uterine ligament (183.4)

171.0 Head, face, and neck

Cartilage of:
ear
eyelid

171.2 Upper limb, including shoulder

Arm	Forearm
Finger	Hand

171.3 Lower limb, including hip

Foot	Thigh
Leg	Toe
Popliteal space	

171.4 Thorax

Axilla	Great vessels
Diaphragm	

Excludes: *heart (164.1)*
mediastinum (164.2-164.9)
thymus (164.0)

171.5 Abdomen

Abdominal wall
Hypochondrium

Excludes: *peritoneum (158.8)*
retroperitoneum (158.0)

● Code new
to this edition

▲ Revision of
existing code

④ ⑤ Fourth or fifth
digit required

171.6 Pelvis

Buttock

Groin

Inguinal region

Perineum

Excludes: *pelvic peritoneum (158.8)*

retroperitoneum (158.0)

uterine ligament, any (183.3-183.5)

171.7 Trunk, unspecified

Back NOS

Flank NOS

171.8 Other specified sites of connective and other soft tissue

Malignant neoplasm of contiguous or overlapping sites of connective tissue whose point of origin cannot be determined

171.9 Connective and other soft tissue, site unspecified

172 Malignant melanoma of skin

Includes: melanocarcinoma

melanoma (skin) NOS

Excludes: *skin of genital organs (184.0-184.9, 187.1-187.9)*

sites other than skin—code to malignant neoplasm of the site

172.0 Lip

Excludes: *vermilion border of lip (140.0-140.1, 140.9)*

172.1 Eyelid, including canthus

172.2 Ear and external auditory canal

Auricle (ear)

Auricular canal, external

External [acoustic] meatus

Pinna

172.3 Other and unspecified parts of face

Cheek (external)

Chin

Eyebrow

Forehead

Nose, external

Temple

172.4 Scalp and neck

172.5 Trunk, except scrotum

Axilla

Breast

Buttock

Groin

Perianal skin

Perineum

Umbilicus

Excludes: *anal canal (154.2)*

anus NOS (154.3)

scrotum (187.7)

172.6 Upper limb, including shoulder

Arm

Finger

Forearm

Hand

172.7 Lower limb, including hip

Ankle

Foot

Heel

Knee

Leg

Popliteal area

Thigh

Toe

172.8 Other specified sites of skin

Malignant melanoma of contiguous or overlapping sites of skin whose point of origin cannot be determined

172.9 Melanoma of skin, site unspecified

173 Other malignant neoplasm of skin

Includes: malignant neoplasm of:

sebaceous glands

sudoriferous, sudoriparous glands

sweat glands

Excludes: *Kaposi's sarcoma (176.0-176.9)*

malignant melanoma of skin (172.0-172.9)

skin of genital organs (184.0-184.9, 187.1-187.9)

173.0 Skin of lip

Excludes: *vermilion border of lip (140.0-140.1, 140.9)*

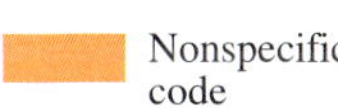

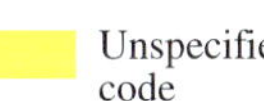

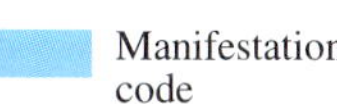

Manifestation
code

173.1 Eyelid, including canthus

> *Excludes:* *cartilage of eyelid (171.0)*

173.2 Skin of ear and external auditory canal

Auricle (ear)
Auricular canal, external
External meatus
Pinna

> *Excludes:* *cartilage of ear (171.0)*

173.3 Skin of other and unspecified parts of face

Cheek, external
Chin
Eyebrow
Forehead
Nose, external
Temple

173.4 Scalp and skin of neck

173.5 Skin of trunk, except scrotum

Axillary fold
Perianal skin
Skin of:
  abdominal wall
  anus
  back
  breast
Skin of:
  buttock
  chest wall
  groin
  perineum
Umbilicus

> *Excludes:* *anal canal (154.2)*
> *anus NOS (154.3)*
> *skin of scrotum (187.7)*

173.6 Skin of upper limb, including shoulder

Arm
Finger
Forearm
Hand

173.7 Skin of lower limb, including hip

Ankle
Foot
Heel
Knee
Leg
Popliteal area
Thigh
Toe

173.8 Other specified sites of skin

Malignant neoplasm of contiguous or overlapping sites of skin whose point of origin cannot be determined

173.9 Skin, site unspecified

174 Malignant neoplasm of female breast

Use additional code to identify estrogen receptor status (V86.0,V86.1)

Includes: breast (female)
    connective tissue
    soft parts
    Paget's disease of:
      breast
      nipple

> *Excludes:* *skin of breast (172.5, 173.5)*

174.0 Nipple and areola

174.1 Central portion

174.2 Upper-inner quadrant

174.3 Lower-inner quadrant

174.4 Upper-outer quadrant

174.5 Lower-outer quadrant

174.6 Axillary tail

174.8 Other specified sites of female breast

Ectopic sites
Inner breast
Lower breast
Midline of breast
Outer breast
Upper breast
Malignant neoplasm of contiguous or overlapping sites of breast whose point of origin cannot be determined

174.9 Breast (female), unspecified

● Code new to this edition   ▲ Revision of existing code   ④ ⑤ Fourth or fifth digit required

175 **Malignant neoplasm of male breast**
Use additional code to identify estrogen receptor status (V86.0,V86.1)

Excludes: *skin of breast (172.5, 173.5)*

175.0 **Nipple and areola**

175.9 **Other and unspecified sites of male breast**
Ectopic breast tissue, male

176 **Kaposi's sarcoma**

176.0 **Skin**

176.1 **Soft tissue**
Includes: Blood vessel
Connective tissue
Fascia
Ligament
Lymphatic(s) NEC
Muscle

Excludes: *lymph glands and nodes (176.5)*

176.2 **Palate**

176.3 **Gastrointestinal sites**

176.4 **Lung**

176.5 **Lymph nodes**

176.8 **Other specified sites**
Includes: Oral cavity NEC

176.9 **Unspecified**
Viscera NOS

MALIGNANT NEOPLASM OF GENITOURINARY ORGANS (179-189)

Excludes: *carcinoma in situ (233.1-233.9)*

179 **Malignant neoplasm of uterus, part unspecified**

180 **Malignant neoplasm of cervix uteri**
Includes: invasive malignancy [carcinoma]

Excludes: *carcinoma in situ (233.1)*

180.0 **Endocervix**
Cervical canal NOS   Endocervical gland
Endocervical canal

180.1 **Exocervix**

180.8 **Other specified sites of cervix**
Cervical stump
Squamocolumnar junction of cervix
Malignant neoplasm of contiguous or overlapping sites of cervix uteri whose point of
origin cannot be determined

180.9 **Cervix uteri, unspecified**

181 **Malignant neoplasm of placenta**
Choriocarcinoma NOS
Chorioepithelioma NOS

Excludes: *chorioadenoma (destruens) (236.1)*
hydatidiform mole (630)
malignant (236.1)
invasive mole (236.1)
male choriocarcinoma NOS (186.0-186.9)

182 **Malignant neoplasm of body of uterus**

Excludes: *carcinoma in situ (233.2)*

182.0 **Corpus uteri, except isthmus**
Cornu   Fundus
Endometrium   Myometrium

182.1 **Isthmus**
Lower uterine segment

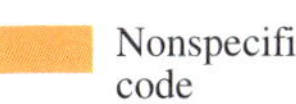

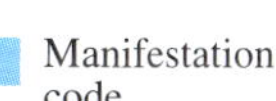

182.8 Other specified sites of body of uterus
Malignant neoplasm of contiguous or overlapping sites of body of uterus whose point of origin cannot be determined
Excludes: uterus NOS (179)

183 Malignant neoplasm of ovary and other uterine adnexa
Excludes: Douglas' cul-de-sac (158.8)

183.0 Ovary
Use additional code, if desired, to identify any functional activity

183.2 Fallopian tube
Oviduct
Uterine tube

183.3 Broad ligament
Mesovarium
Parovarian region

183.4 Parametrium
Uterine ligament NOS
Uterosacral ligament

183.5 Round ligament

183.8 Other specified sites of uterine adnexa
Tubo-ovarian
Utero-ovarian
Malignant neoplasm of contiguous or overlapping sites of ovary and other uterine adnexa whose point of origin cannot be determined

183.9 Uterine adnexa, unspecified

184 Malignant neoplasm of other and unspecified female genital organs
Excludes: carcinoma in situ (233.3)

184.0 Vagina
Gartner's duct
Vaginal vault

184.1 Labia majora
Greater vestibular [Bartholin's] gland

184.2 Labia minora

184.3 Clitoris

184.4 Vulva, unspecified
External female genitalia NOS
Pudendum

184.8 Other specified sites of female genital organs
Malignant neoplasm of contiguous or overlapping sites of female genital organs whose point of origin cannot be determined

184.9 Female genital organ, site unspecified
Female genitourinary tract NOS

185 Malignant neoplasm of prostate
Excludes: seminal vesicles (187.8)

186 Malignant neoplasm of testis
Use additional code, if desired, to identify any functional activity

186.0 Undescended testis
Ectopic testis
Retained testis

186.9 Other and unspecified testis
Testis:
NOS
descended
scrotal

187 Malignant neoplasm of penis and other male genital organs

187.1 Prepuce
Foreskin

187.2 Glans penis

187.3 Body of penis
Corpus cavernosum

● Code new to this edition   ▲ Revision of existing code   ④ ⑤ Fourth or fifth digit required

187.4 **Penis, part unspecified**
Skin of penis NOS

187.5 **Epididymis**

187.6 **Spermatic cord**
Vas deferens

187.7 **Scrotum**
Skin of scrotum

187.8 **Other specified sites of male genital organs**
Seminal vesicle
Tunica vaginalis
Malignant neoplasm of contiguous or overlapping sites of penis and other male genital organs whose point of origin cannot be determined

187.9 **Male genital organ, site unspecified**
Male genital organ or tract NOS

188 **Malignant neoplasm of bladder**

Excludes: *carcinoma in situ (233.7)*

188.0 **Trigone of urinary bladder**

188.1 **Dome of urinary bladder**

188.2 **Lateral wall of urinary bladder**

188.3 **Anterior wall of urinary bladder**

188.4 **Posterior wall of urinary bladder**

188.5 **Bladder neck**
Internal urethral orifice

188.6 **Ureteric orifice**

188.7 **Urachus**

188.8 **Other specified sites of bladder**
Malignant neoplasm of contiguous or overlapping sites of bladder whose point of origin cannot be determined

188.9 **Bladder, part unspecified**
Bladder wall NOS

189 **Malignant neoplasm of kidney and other and unspecified urinary organs**

189.0 **Kidney, except pelvis**
Kidney NOS
Kidney parenchyma

189.1 **Renal pelvis**
Renal calyces
Ureteropelvic junction

189.2 **Ureter**

Excludes: *ureteric orifice of bladder (188.6)*

189.3 **Urethra**

Excludes: *urethral orifice of bladder (188.5)*

189.4 **Paraurethral glands**

189.8 **Other specified sites of urinary organs**
Malignant neoplasm of contiguous or overlapping sites of kidney and other urinary organs whose point of origin cannot be determined

189.9 **Urinary organ, site unspecified**
Urinary system NOS

MALIGNANT NEOPLASM OF OTHER AND UNSPECIFIED SITES (190-199)

Excludes: *carcinoma in situ (234.0-234.9)*

190 **Malignant neoplasm of eye**

Excludes: *carcinoma in situ (234.0)*
eyelid (skin) (172.1, 173.1)
cartilage (171.0)
optic nerve (192.0)
orbital bone (170.0)

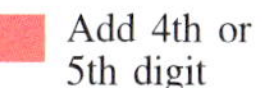

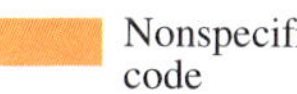

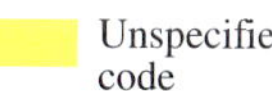

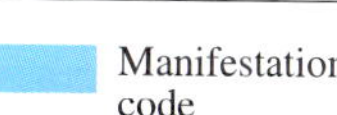

190.0 Eyeball, except conjunctiva, cornea, retina, and choroid
Ciliary body   Sclera
Crystalline lens   Uveal tract
Iris

190.1 Orbit
Connective tissue of orbit
Extraocular muscle
Retrobulbar

Excludes: bone of orbit (170.0)

190.2 Lacrimal gland

190.3 Conjunctiva

190.4 Cornea

190.5 Retina

190.6 Choroid

190.7 Lacrimal duct
Lacrimal sac
Nasolacrimal duct

190.8 Other specified sites of eye
Malignant neoplasm of contiguous or overlapping sites of eye whose point of origin cannot be determined

190.9 Eye, part unspecified

191 Malignant neoplasm of brain

Excludes: cranial nerves (192.0)
retrobulbar area (190.1)

191.0 Cerebrum, except lobes and ventricles
Basal ganglia   Globus pallidus
Cerebral cortex   Hypothalamus
Corpus striatum   Thalamus

191.1 Frontal lobe

191.2 Temporal lobe
Hippocampus
Uncus

191.3 Parietal lobe

191.4 Occipital lobe

191.5 Ventricles
Choroid plexus
Floor of ventricle

191.6 Cerebellum NOS
Cerebellopontine angle

191.7 Brain stem
Cerebral peduncle   Midbrain
Medulla oblongata   Pons

191.8 Other parts of brain
Corpus callosum
Tapetum
Malignant neoplasm of contiguous or overlapping sites of brain whose point of origin cannot be determined

191.9 Brain, unspecified
Cranial fossa NOS

192 Malignant neoplasm of other and unspecified parts of nervous system

Excludes: peripheral, sympathetic, and parasympathetic nerves and ganglia (171.0-171.9)

192.0 Cranial nerves
Olfactory bulb

192.1 Cerebral meninges
Dura (mater)   Meninges NOS
Falx (cerebelli) (cerebri)   Tentorium

192.2 Spinal cord
Cauda equina

192.3 Spinal meninges

    ● Code new
to this edition   ▲ Revision of
existing code   ④ ⑤ Fourth or fifth
digit required

192.8 Other specified sites of nervous system
Malignant neoplasm of contiguous or overlapping sites of other parts of nervous system whose point of origin cannot be determined

192.9 Nervous system, part unspecified
Nervous system (central) NOS

> Excludes: meninges NOS (192.1)

193 Malignant neoplasm of thyroid gland
Sipple's syndrome
Thyroglossal duct

Use additional code, if desired, to identify any functional activity

194 Malignant neoplasm of other endocrine glands and related structures
Use additional code, if desired, to identify any functional activity

> Excludes: islets of Langerhans (157.4)
> ovary (183.0)
> testis (186.0-186.9)
> thymus (164.0)

194.0 Adrenal gland
Adrenal cortex   Suprarenal gland
Adrenal medulla

194.1 Parathyroid gland

194.3 Pituitary gland and craniopharyngeal duct
Craniobuccal pouch   Rathke's pouch
Hypophysis   Sella turcica

194.4 Pineal gland

194.5 Carotid body

194.6 Aortic body and other paraganglia
Coccygeal body   Para-aortic body
Glomus jugulare

194.8 Other
Pluriglandular involvement NOS

Note: If the sites of multiple involvements are known, they should be coded separately.

194.9 Endocrine gland, site unspecified

195 Malignant neoplasm of other and ill-defined sites
Includes: malignant neoplasms of contiguous sites, not elsewhere classified, whose point of origin cannot be determined

> Excludes: malignant neoplasm:
> lymphatic and hematopoietic tissue (200.0-208.9)
> secondary sites (196.0-198.8)
> unspecified site (199.0-199.1)

195.0 Head, face, and neck
Cheek NOS   Nose NOS
Jaw NOS   Supraclavicular region NOS

195.1 Thorax
Axilla   Intrathoracic NOS
Chest (wall) NOS

195.2 Abdomen
Intra-abdominal NOS

195.3 Pelvis
Groin
Inguinal region NOS
Presacral region
Sacrococcygeal region
Sites overlapping systems within pelvis, as:
rectovaginal (septum)
rectovesical (septum)

195.4 Upper limb

195.5 Lower limb

195.8 Other specified sites
Back NOS   Trunk NOS
Flank NOS

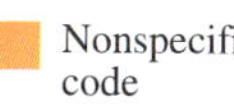

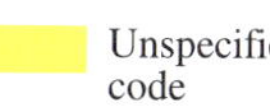

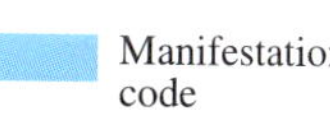

Manifestation
code

196 Secondary and unspecified malignant neoplasm of lymph nodes

Excludes: *any malignant neoplasm of lymph nodes, specified as primary (200.0-202.9)*
Hodgkin's disease (201.0-201.9)
lymphosarcoma (200.1)
reticulosarcoma (200.0)
other forms of lymphoma (202.0-202.9)

196.0 Lymph nodes of head, face, and neck
Cervical
Cervicofacial
Scalene
Supraclavicular

196.1 Intrathoracic lymph nodes
Bronchopulmonary
Intercostal
Mediastinal
Tracheobronchial

196.2 Intra-abdominal lymph nodes
Intestinal
Mesenteric
Retroperitoneal

196.3 Lymph nodes of axilla and upper limb
Brachial
Epitrochlear
Infraclavicular
Pectoral

196.5 Lymph nodes of inguinal region and lower limb
Femoral
Groin
Popliteal
Tibial

196.6 Intrapelvic lymph nodes
Hypogastric
Iliac
Obturator
Parametrial

196.8 Lymph nodes of multiple sites

196.9 Site unspecified
Lymph nodes NOS

197 Secondary malignant neoplasm of respiratory and digestive systems

Excludes: *lymph node metastasis (196.0-196.9)*

197.0 Lung
Bronchus

197.1 Mediastinum

197.2 Pleura

197.3 Other respiratory organs
Trachea

197.4 Small intestine, including duodenum

197.5 Large intestine and rectum

197.6 Retroperitoneum and peritoneum

197.7 Liver, specified as secondary

197.8 Other digestive organs and spleen

198 Secondary malignant neoplasm of other specified sites

Excludes: *lymph node metastasis (196.0-196.9)*

198.0 Kidney

198.1 Other urinary organs

198.2 Skin
Skin of breast

198.3 Brain and spinal cord

198.4 Other parts of nervous system
Meninges (cerebral) (spinal)

198.5 Bone and bone marrow

198.6 Ovary

198.7 Adrenal gland
Suprarenal gland

⑤ **198.8 Other specified sites**

198.81 Breast

Excludes: *skin of breast (198.2)*

198.82 Genital organs

  ● Code new
to this edition   ▲ Revision of
existing code   ④ ⑤ Fourth or fifth
digit required

198.89 Other

Excludes: retroperitoneal lymph nodes (196.2)

199 **Malignant neoplasm without specification of site**

199.0 **Disseminated**
Carcinomatosis unspecified site (primary) (secondary)
Generalized:
  cancer unspecified site (primary) (secondary)
  malignancy unspecified site (primary) (secondary)
Multiple cancer unspecified site (primary) (secondary)

199.1 **Other**
Cancer unspecified site (primary) (secondary)
Carcinoma unspecified site (primary) (secondary)
Malignancy unspecified site (primary) (secondary)

MALIGNANT NEOPLASM OF LYMPHATIC AND HEMATOPOIETIC TISSUE (200-208)

Excludes: secondary neoplasm of:
  bone marrow (198.5)
  spleen (197.8)
  secondary and unspecified neoplasm of lymph nodes (196.0-196.9)

The following fifth-digit subclassification is for use with categories 200-202:

0 unspecified site, extranodal and solid organ sites

1 lymph nodes of head, face, and neck

2 intrathoracic lymph nodes

3 intra-abdominal lymph nodes

4 lymph nodes of axilla and upper limb

5 lymph nodes of inguinal region and lower limb

6 intrapelvic lymph nodes

7 spleen

8 lymph nodes of multiple sites

⑤ **200** **Lymphosarcoma and reticulosarcoma**

⑤ **200.0** **Reticulosarcoma**
Lymphoma (malignant):
  histiocytic (diffuse):
    nodular
      pleomorphic cell type
    reticulum cell type
  Reticulum cell sarcoma:
    NOS
    pleomorphic cell type

⑤ **200.1** **Lymphosarcoma**

Lymphoblastoma (diffuse)
Lymphoma (malignant):
  lymphoblastic (diffuse)
  lymphocytic (cell type)
    (diffuse)
  lymphosarcoma type

Lymphosarcoma:
  NOS
  diffuse NOS
  lymphoblastic (diffuse)
  lymphocytic (diffuse)
  prolymphocytic

Excludes: lymphosarcoma:
  follicular or nodular (202.0)
  mixed cell type (200.8)
  lymphosarcoma cell leukemia (207.8)

⑤ **200.2** **Burkitt's tumor or lymphoma**
Malignant lymphoma, Burkitt's type

⑤ **200.8** **Other named variants**
Lymphoma (malignant):
  lymphoplasmacytoid type
  mixed lymphocytic-histiocytic (diffuse)
Lymphosarcoma, mixed cell type (diffuse)
Reticulolymphosarcoma (diffuse)

⑤ **201** **Hodgkin's disease**

⑤ **201.0** **Hodgkin's paragranuloma**

⑤ **201.1** **Hodgkin's granuloma**

⑤ **201.2** **Hodgkin's sarcoma**

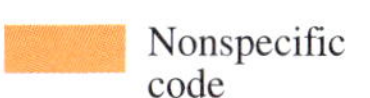

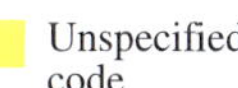

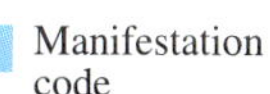

Manifestation
code

⑤ **201.4 Lymphocytic-histiocytic predominance**

⑤ **201.5 Nodular sclerosis**
Hodgkin's disease, nodular sclerosis:
NOS
cellular phase

⑤ **201.6 Mixed cellularity**

⑤ **201.7 Lymphocytic depletion**
Hodgkin's disease, lymphocytic depletion:
NOS
diffuse fibrosis
reticular type

⑤ **201.9 Hodgkin's disease, unspecified**
Hodgkin's: Malignant:
disease NOS   lymphogranuloma
lymphoma NOS   lymphogranulomatosis

⑤ **202 Other malignant neoplasms of lymphoid and histiocytic tissue**

⑤ **202.0 Nodular lymphoma**
Brill-Symmers disease   Lymphosarcoma:
Lymphoma: follicular (giant)
follicular (giant)   nodular
lymphocytic, nodular

⑤ **202.1 Mycosis fungoides**

⑤ **202.2 Sézary's disease**

⑤ **202.3 Malignant histiocytosis**
Histiocytic medullary reticulosis
Malignant:
reticuloendotheliosis
reticulosis

⑤ **202.4 Leukemic reticuloendotheliosis**
Hairy-cell leukemia

⑤ **202.5 Letterer-Siwe disease**
Acute:
differentiated progressive histiocytosis
histiocytosis X (progressive)
infantile reticuloendotheliosis
reticulosis of infancy

Excludes: *Hand-Schüller-Christian disease (277.89)*
histiocytosis (acute) (chronic) (277.89)
histiocytosis X (chronic) (277.89)

⑤ **202.6 Malignant mast cell tumors**
Malignant: Mast cell sarcoma
mastocytoma   Systemic tissue mast cell disease
mastocytosis

Excludes: *mast cell leukemia (207.8)*

⑤ **202.8 Other lymphomas**
Lymphoma (malignant):
NOS
diffuse

Excludes: *benign lymphoma (229.0)*

⑤ **202.9 Other and unspecified malignant neoplasms of lymphoid and histiocytic tissue**
Follicular dendritic cell sarcoma
Interdigitating dendritic cell sarcoma
Langerhans cell sarcoma
Malignant neoplasm of bone marrow NOS

⑤ **203 Multiple myeloma and immunoproliferative neoplasms**
The following fifth-digit subclassification is for use with category 203

0   without mention of remission

1   in remission

⑤ **203.0 Multiple myeloma**
Kahler's disease
Myelomatosis

Excludes: *solitary myeloma (238.6)*

● Code new   ▲ Revision of   ④ ⑤ Fourth or fifth
to this edition   existing code   digit required

⑤ **203.1 Plasma cell leukemia**
Plasmacytic leukemia

⑤ **203.8 Other immunoproliferative neoplasms**

⑤ **204 Lymphoid leukemia**
Includes: leukemia:
lymphatic
lymphoblastic
lymphocytic
lymphogenous

The following fifth-digit subclassification is for use with category 204

0 without mention of remission

1 in remission

⑤ **204.0 Acute**
Excludes: acute exacerbation of chronic lymphoid leukemia (204.1)

⑤ **204.1 Chronic**

⑤ **204.2 Subacute**

⑤ **204.8 Other lymphoid leukemia**
Aleukemic leukemia:
lymphatic
lymphocytic
lymphoid

⑤ **204.9 Unspecified lymphoid leukemia**

⑤ **205 Myeloid leukemia**
Includes: leukemia:
granulocytic   myelomonocytic
myeloblastic   myelosclerotic
myelocytic   myelosis
myelogenous

The following fifth-digit subclassification is for use with category 205

0 without mention of remission

1 in remission

⑤ **205.0 Acute**
Acute promyelocytic leukemia
Excludes: acute exacerbation of chronic myeloid leukemia (205.1)

⑤ **205.1 Chronic**
Eosinophilic leukemia   Neutrophilic leukemia

⑤ **205.2 Subacute**

⑤ **205.3 Myeloid sarcoma**
Chloroma
Granulocytic sarcoma

⑤ **205.8 Other myeloid leukemia**
Aleukemic leukemia:
granulocytic
myelogenous
myeloid
Aleukemic myelosis

⑤ **205.9 Unspecified myeloid leukemia**

⑤ **206 Monocytic leukemia**
Includes: leukemia:
histiocytic
monoblastic
monocytoid

The following fifth-digit subclassification is for use with category 206

0 without mention of remission

1 in remission

⑤ **206.0 Acute**
Excludes: acute exacerbation of chronic monocytic leukemia (206.1)

⑤ **206.1 Chronic**

⑤ **206.2 Subacute**

⑤ **206.8 Other monocytic leukemia**
Aleukemic:
monocytic leukemia
monocytoid leukemia

⑤ **206.9 Unspecified monocytic leukemia**

⑤ **207 Other specified leukemia**
Excludes: leukemic reticuloendotheliosis (202.4)
plasma cell leukemia (203.1)

The following fifth-digit subclassification is for use with category 207

0 without mention of remission

1 in remission

⑤ **207.0 Acute erythremia and erythroleukemia**
Acute erythremic myelosis
Di Guglielmo's disease
Erythremic myelosis

⑤ **207.1 Chronic erythremia**
Heilmeyer-Schöner disease

⑤ **207.2 Megakaryocytic leukemia**
Megakaryocytic myelosis
Thrombocytic leukemia

⑤ **207.8 Other specified leukemia**
Lymphosarcoma cell leukemia

⑤ **208 Leukemia of unspecified cell type**
The following fifth-digit subclassification is for use with category 208

0 without mention of remission

1 in remission

⑤ **208.0 Acute**
Acute leukemia NOS
Blast cell leukemia
Stem cell leukemia
Excludes: acute exacerbation of chronic unspecified leukemia (208.1)

⑤ **208.1 Chronic**
Chronic leukemia NOS

⑤ **208.2 Subacute**
Subacute leukemia NOS

⑤ **208.8 Other leukemia of unspecified cell type**

⑤ **208.9 Unspecified leukemia**
Leukemia NOS

BENIGN NEOPLASMS (210-229)

210 Benign neoplasm of lip, oral cavity, and pharynx
Excludes: cyst (of):
jaw (526.0-526.2, 526.89)
oral soft tissue (528.4)
radicular (522.8)

210.0 Lip
Frenulum labii
Lip (inner aspect) (mucosa) (vermilion border)
Excludes: labial commissure (210.4)
skin of lip (216.0)

210.1 Tongue
Lingual tonsil

● Code new
to this edition
▲ Revision of
existing code
④ ⑤ Fourth or fifth
digit required

210.2 Major salivary glands
Gland:
  parotid
  sublingual
  submandibular

Excludes: benign neoplasms of minor salivary glands:
    NOS (210.4)
    buccal mucosa (210.4)
    lips (210.0)
    palate (hard) (soft) (210.4)
    tongue (210.1)
    tonsil, palatine (210.5)

210.3 Floor of mouth

210.4 Other and unspecified parts of mouth
Gingiva   Oral mucosa
Gum (upper) (lower)   Palate (hard) (soft)
Labial commissure   Uvula
Oral cavity NOS

Excludes: benign odontogenic neoplasms of bone (213.0-213.1)
    developmental odontogenic cysts (526.0)
    mucosa of lips (210.0)
    nasopharyngeal [posterior] [superior] surface of soft palate (210.7)

210.5 Tonsil
Tonsil (faucial) (palatine)

Excludes: lingual tonsil (210.1)
    pharyngeal tonsil (210.7)
    tonsillar:
      fossa (210.6)
      pillars (210.6)

210.6 Other parts of oropharynx
Branchial cleft or vestiges
Epiglottis, anterior aspect
Fauces NOS
Mesopharynx NOS
Tonsillar:
  fossa
  pillars
Vallecula

Excludes: epiglottis:
    NOS (212.1)
    suprahyoid portion (212.1)

210.7 Nasopharynx
Adenoid tissue   Pharyngeal tonsil
Lymphadenoid tissue   Posterior nasal septum

210.8 Hypopharynx
Arytenoid fold   Postcricoid region
Laryngopharynx   Pyriform fossa

210.9 Pharynx, unspecified
Throat NOS

211 Benign neoplasm of other parts of digestive system

Excludes: benign stromal tumors of digestive system (215.5)

211.0 Esophagus

211.1 Stomach
Body of stomach
Cardia of stomach
Fundus of stomach
Cardiac orifice
Pylorus

211.2 Duodenum, jejunum, and ileum
Small intestine NOS

Excludes: ampulla of Vater (211.5)
    ileocecal valve (211.3)

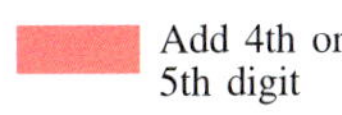
Add 4th or
5th digit

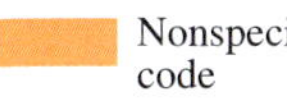
Nonspecific
code

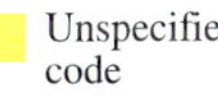
Unspecified
code

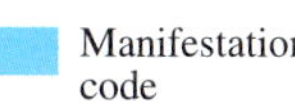
Manifestation
code

211.3 Colon

Appendix
Cecum

Ileocecal valve
Large intestine NOS

Excludes: *rectosigmoid junction (211.4)*

211.4 Rectum and anal canal

Anal canal or sphincter
Anus NOS

Rectosigmoid junction

Excludes: *anus:*

margin (216.5)
skin (216.5)
perianal skin (216.5)

211.5 Liver and biliary passages

Ampulla of Vater
Common bile duct
Cystic duct

Gallbladder
Hepatic duct
Sphincter of Oddi

211.6 Pancreas, except islets of Langerhans

211.7 Islets of Langerhans

Islet cell tumor

Use additional code, if desired, to identify any functional activity

211.8 Retroperitoneum and peritoneum

Mesentery
Mesocolon

Omentum
Retroperitoneal tissue

211.9 Other and unspecified site

Alimentary tract NOS
Digestive system NOS
Gastrointestinal tract NOS

Intestinal tract NOS
Intestine NOS
Spleen, not elsewhere classified

212 Benign neoplasm of respiratory and intrathoracic organs

212.0 Nasal cavities, middle ear, and accessory sinuses

Cartilage of nose
Eustachian tube
Nares
Septum of nose

Sinus:
ethmoidal
frontal
maxillary
sphenoidal

Excludes: *auditory canal (external) (216.2)*

bone of:
ear (213.0)
nose [turbinates] (213.0)
cartilage of ear (215.0)
ear (external) (skin) (216.2)
nose NOS (229.8)
skin (216.3)
olfactory bulb (225.1)
polyp of:
accessory sinus (471.8)
ear (385.30-385.35)
nasal cavity (471.0)
posterior margin of septum and choanae (210.7)

212.1 Larynx

Cartilage:
arytenoid
cricoid
cuneiform
thyroid

Epiglottis (suprahyoid portion) NOS
Glottis
Vocal cords (false) (true)

Excludes: *epiglottis, anterior aspect (210.6)*

polyp of vocal cord or larynx (478.4)

212.2 Trachea

212.3 Bronchus and lung

Carina

Hilus of lung

212.4 Pleura

212.5 Mediastinum

212.6 Thymus

212.7 Heart

Excludes: *great vessels (215.4)*

● Code new
  to this edition

▲ Revision of
  existing code

④ ⑤ Fourth or fifth
  digit required

212.8 Other specified sites

212.9 Site unspecified
        Respiratory organ NOS
        Upper respiratory tract NOS

    Excludes: *intrathoracic NOS (229.8)*
           thoracic NOS (229.8)

213 Benign neoplasm of bone and articular cartilage
    Includes: cartilage (articular) (joint)
              periosteum

    Excludes: *cartilage of:*
            ear (215.0)
            eyelid (215.0)
            larynx (212.1)
            nose (212.0)
        exostosis NOS (726.91)
        synovia (215.0-215.9)

213.0 Bones of skull and face
    Excludes: *lower jaw bone (213.1)*

213.1 Lower jaw bone

213.2 Vertebral column, excluding sacrum and coccyx

213.3 Ribs, sternum, and clavicle

213.4 Scapula and long bones of upper limb

213.5 Short bones of upper limb

213.6 Pelvic bones, sacrum, and coccyx

213.7 Long bones of lower limb

213.8 Short bones of lower limb

213.9 Bone and articular cartilage, site unspecified

214 Lipoma
    Includes: angiolipoma
              fibrolipoma
              hibernoma
              lipoma (fetal) (infiltrating) (intramuscular)
              myelolipoma
              myxolipoma

214.0 Skin and subcutaneous tissue of face

214.1 Other skin and subcutaneous tissue

214.2 Intrathoracic organs

214.3 Intra-abdominal organs

214.4 Spermatic cord

214.8 Other specified sites

214.9 Lipoma, unspecified site

215 Other benign neoplasm of connective and other soft tissue
    Includes: blood vessel
              bursa
              fascia
              ligament
              muscle
              peripheral, sympathetic, and parasympathetic nerves and ganglia
              synovia
              tendon (sheath)

    Excludes: *cartilage:*
            articular (213.0-213.9)
            larynx (212.1)
             nose (212.0)
        connective tissue of:
            breast (217)
            internal organ, except lipoma and hemangioma — code to benign neoplasm of
              the site
        lipoma (214.0-214.9)

215.0 Head, face, and neck

215.2 Upper limb, including shoulder

215.3 Lower limb, including hip

215.4 Thorax
> *Excludes:* *heart (212.7)*
> *mediastinum (212.5)*
> *thymus (212.6)*

215.5 Abdomen
Abdominal wall
Benign stromal tumors of abdomen
Hypochondrium

215.6 Pelvis

Buttock	Inguinal region
Groin	Perineum

> *Excludes:* *uterine:*
> *leiomyoma (218.0-218.9)*
> *ligament, any (221.0)*

215.7 Trunk, unspecified
Back NOS
Flank NOS

215.8 Other specified sites

215.9 Site unspecified

216 Benign neoplasm of skin
Includes: blue nevus
dermatofibroma
hydrocystoma
pigmented nevus
syringoadenoma
syringoma

> *Excludes:* *skin of genital organs (221.0-222.9)*

216.0 Skin of lip
> *Excludes:* *vermilion border of lip (210.0)*

216.1 Eyelid, including canthus
> *Excludes:* *cartilage of eyelid (215.0)*

216.2 Ear and external auditory canal

Auricle (ear)	External meatus
Auricular canal, external	Pinna

> *Excludes:* *cartilage of ear (215.0)*

216.3 Skin of other and unspecified parts of face

Cheek, external	Nose, external
Eyebrow	Temple

216.4 Scalp and skin of neck

216.5 Skin of trunk, except scrotum

Axillary fold	Skin of:
Perianal skin	buttock
Skin of:	chest wall
abdominal wall	groin
anus	perineum
back	Umbilicus
breast	

> *Excludes:* *anal canal (211.4)*
> *anus NOS (211.4)*
> *skin of scrotum (222.4)*

216.6 Skin of upper limb, including shoulder

216.7 Skin of lower limb, including hip

216.8 Other specified sites of skin

216.9 Skin, site unspecified

● Code new to this edition	▲ Revision of existing code	④ ⑤ Fourth or fifth digit required

217 Benign neoplasm of breast
Breast (male) (female)
  connective tissue
  glandular tissue
  soft parts

> *Excludes:* *adenofibrosis (610.2)*
> *benign cyst of breast (610.0)*
> *fibrocystic disease (610.1)*
> *skin of breast (216.5)*

218 Uterine leiomyoma
Includes: fibroid (bleeding) (uterine)
  uterine:
    fibromyoma
    myoma

218.0 Submucous leiomyoma of uterus

218.1 Intramural leiomyoma of uterus
Interstitial leiomyoma of uterus

218.2 Subserous leiomyoma of uterus
Subperitoneal leiomyoma of uterus

218.9 Leiomyoma of uterus, unspecified

219 Other benign neoplasm of uterus

219.0 Cervix uteri

219.1 Corpus uteri
Endometrium   Myometrium
Fundus

219.8 Other specified parts of uterus

219.9 Uterus, part unspecified

220 Benign neoplasm of ovary
Use additional code, if desired, to identify any functional activity (256.0-256.1)

> *Excludes:* *cyst:*
> *corpus albicans (620.2)*
> *corpus luteum (620.1)*
> *endometrial (617.1)*
> *follicular (atretic) (620.0)*
> *graafian follicle (620.0)*
> *ovarian NOS (620.2)*
> *retention (620.2)*

221 Benign neoplasm of other female genital organs
Includes: adenomatous polyp
  benign teratoma

> *Excludes:* *cyst:*
> *epoophoron (752.11)*
> *fimbrial (752.11)*
> *Gartner's duct (752.11)*
> *parovarian (752.11)*

221.0 Fallopian tube and uterine ligaments
Oviduct   Uterine ligament (broad) (round) (uterosacral)
Parametrium   Uterine tube

221.1 Vagina

221.2 Vulva
Clitoris
External female genitalia NOS
Greater vestibular [Bartholin's] gland
Labia (majora) (minora)
Pudendum

> *Excludes:* *Bartholin's (duct) (gland) cyst (616.2)*

221.8 Other specified sites of female genital organs

221.9 Female genital organ, site unspecified
Female genitourinary tract NOS

222 Benign neoplasm of male genital organs

222.0 Testis
Use additional code, if desired, to identify any functional activity

	Add 4th or 5th digit		Nonspecific code		Unspecified code		Manifestation code

222.1 Penis
    Corpus cavernosum   Prepuce
    Glans penis

222.2 Prostate
    Excludes: adenomatous hyperplasia of prostate (600.20-600.21)
        prostatic:
           adenoma (600.20-600.21)
           enlargement (600.00-600.01)
           hypertrophy (600.00-600.01)

222.3 Epididymis

222.4 Scrotum
    Skin of scrotum

222.8 Other specified sites of male genital organs
    Seminal vesicle
    Spermatic cord

222.9 Male genital organ, site unspecified
    Male genitourinary tract NOS

223 Benign neoplasm of kidney and other urinary organs

223.0 Kidney, except pelvis
    Kidney NOS
    Excludes: renal:
        calyces (223.1)
        pelvis (223.1)

223.1 Renal pelvis

223.2 Ureter
    Excludes: ureteric orifice of bladder (223.3)

223.3 Bladder

⑤ 223.8 Other specified sites of urinary organs

    223.81 Urethra
    Excludes: urethral orifice of bladder (223.3)

    223.89 Other
        Paraurethral glands

223.9 Urinary organ, site unspecified
    Urinary system NOS

224 Benign neoplasm of eye
    Excludes: cartilage of eyelid (215.0)
        eyelid (skin) (216.1)
        optic nerve (225.1)
        orbital bone (213.0)

224.0 Eyeball, except conjunctiva, cornea, retina, and choroid
    Ciliary body   Sclera
    Iris   Uveal tract

224.1 Orbit
    Excludes: bone of orbit (213.0)

224.2 Lacrimal gland

224.3 Conjunctiva

224.4 Cornea

224.5 Retina
    Excludes: hemangioma of retina (228.03)

224.6 Choroid

224.7 Lacrimal duct
    Lacrimal sac
    Nasolacrimal duct

224.8 Other specified parts of eye

224.9 Eye, part unspecified

● Code new to this edition   ▲ Revision of existing code   ④ ⑤ Fourth or fifth digit required

225 Benign neoplasm of brain and other parts of nervous system
> *Excludes:* *hemangioma (228.02)*
> *neurofibromatosis (237.7)*
> *peripheral, sympathetic, and parasympathetic nerves and ganglia (215.0-215.9)*
> *retrobulbar (224.1)*

225.0 Brain

225.1 Cranial nerves

225.2 Cerebral meninges
Meninges NOS
Meningioma (cerebral)

225.3 Spinal cord
Cauda equina

225.4 Spinal meninges
Spinal meningioma

225.8 Other specified sites of nervous system

225.9 Nervous system, part unspecified
Nervous system (central) NOS
> *Excludes:* *meninges NOS (225.2)*

226 Benign neoplasm of thyroid glands
Use additional code, if desired, to identify any functional activity

227 Benign neoplasm of other endocrine glands and related structures
Use additional code, if desired, to identify any functional activity
> *Excludes:* *ovary (220)*
> *pancreas (211.6)*
> *testis (222.0)*

227.0 Adrenal gland
Suprarenal gland

227.1 Parathyroid gland

227.3 Pituitary gland and craniopharyngeal duct (pouch)
Craniobuccal pouch   Rathke's pouch
Hypophysis   Sella turcica

227.4 Pineal gland
Pineal body

227.5 Carotid body

227.6 Aortic body and other paraganglia
Coccygeal body   Para-aortic body
Glomus jugulare

227.8 Other

227.9 Endocrine gland, site unspecified

228 Hemangioma and lymphangioma, any site
Includes: angioma (benign) (cavernous) (congenital) NOS
cavernous nevus
glomus tumor
hemangioma (benign) (congenital)
> *Excludes:* *benign neoplasm of spleen, except hemangioma and lymphangioma (211.9)*
> *glomus jugulare (227.6)*
> *nevus:*
> *NOS (216.0-216.9)*
> *blue or pigmented (216.0-216.9)*
> *vascular (757.32)*

⑤ **228.0 Hemangioma, any site**

228.00 Of unspecified site

228.01 Of skin and subcutaneous tissue

228.02 Of intracranial structures

228.03 Of retina

228.04 Of intra-abdominal structures
Peritoneum
Retroperitoneal tissue

228.09 Of other sites
Systemic angiomatosis

Add 4th or 5th digit	Nonspecific code	Unspecified code	Manifestation code

228.1 Lymphangioma, any site
　　　Congenital lymphangioma
　　　Lymphatic nevus

229 Benign neoplasm of other and unspecified sites

229.0 Lymph nodes
　　　Excludes: *lymphangioma (228.1)*

229.8 Other specified sites
　　　Intrathoracic NOS
　　　Thoracic NOS

229.9 Site unspecified

CARCINOMA IN SITU (230-234)

　　Includes:　Bowen's disease
　　　　　　erythroplasia
　　　　　　Queyrat's erythroplasia
　　Excludes: *leukoplakia—see Alphabetic Index*

230 Carcinoma in situ of digestive organs

230.0 Lip, oral cavity, and pharynx

Gingiva	Oropharynx
Hypopharynx	Salivary gland or duct
Mouth [any part]	Tongue
Nasopharynx	

　　Excludes: *aryepiglottic fold or interarytenoid fold, laryngeal aspect (231.0)*
　　　　　epiglottis:
　　　　　　NOS (231.0)
　　　　　　suprahyoid portion (231.0)
　　　　skin of lip (232.0)

230.1 Esophagus

230.2 Stomach

Body of stomach	Cardiac orifice
Cardia of stomach	Pylorus
Fundus of stomach	

230.3 Colon

Appendix	Ileocecal valve
Cecum	Large intestine NOS

　　Excludes: *rectosigmoid junction (230.4)*

230.4 Rectum
　　　Rectosigmoid junction

230.5 Anal canal
　　　Anal sphincter

230.6 Anus, unspecified
　　Excludes: *anus:*
　　　　　margin (232.5)
　　　　　skin (232.5)
　　　　perianal skin (232.5)

230.7 Other and unspecified parts of intestine

Duodenum	Jejunum
Ileum	Small intestine NOS

　　Excludes: *ampulla of Vater (230.8)*

230.8 Liver and biliary system

Ampulla of Vater	Gallbladder
Common bile duct	Hepatic duct
Cystic duct	Sphincter of Oddi

230.9 Other and unspecified digestive organs

Digestive organ NOS	Pancreas
Gastrointestinal tract NOS	Spleen

231 Carcinoma in situ of respiratory system

● Code new
　to this edition
　　　▲ Revision of
　　　　existing code
　　　　　　④ ⑤ Fourth or fifth
　　　　　　　　digit required

231.0 Larynx
    Cartilage: Epiglottis:
      arytenoid   NOS
      cricoid   posterior surface
      cuneiform   suprahyoid portion
      thyroid   Vocal cords (false) (true)

> *Excludes:* *aryepiglottic fold or interarytenoid fold:*
>   *NOS (230.0)*
>   *hypopharyngeal aspect (230.0)*
>   *marginal zone (230.0)*

231.1 Trachea

231.2 Bronchus and lung
    Carina
    Hilus of lung

231.8 Other specified parts of respiratory system
    Accessory sinuses   Nasal cavities
    Middle ear   Pleura

> *Excludes:* *ear (external) (skin) (232.2)*
>   *nose NOS (234.8)*
>   *skin (232.3)*

231.9 Respiratory system, part unspecified
    Respiratory organ NOS

232 Carcinoma in situ of skin
    Includes: pigment cells

232.0 Skin of lip

> *Excludes:* *vermilion border of lip (230.0)*

232.1 Eyelid, including canthus

232.2 Ear and external auditory canal

232.3 Skin of other and unspecified parts of face

232.4 Scalp and skin of neck

232.5 Skin of trunk, except scrotum
    Anus, margin   Skin of:
    Axillary fold   breast
    Perianal skin   buttock
    Skin of: chest wall
     abdominal wall   groin
     anus   perineum
     back   Umbilicus

> *Excludes:* *anal canal (230.5)*
>   *anus NOS (230.6)*
>   *skin of genital organs (233.3, 233.5-233.6)*

232.6 Skin of upper limb, including shoulder

232.7 Skin of lower limb, including hip

232.8 Other specified sites of skin

232.9 Skin, site unspecified

233 Carcinoma in situ of breast and genitourinary system

233.0 Breast

> *Excludes:* *Paget's disease (174.0-174.9)*
>   *skin of breast (232.5)*

233.1 Cervix uteri
    Cervical intraepithelial glandular neoplasia
    Cervical intraepithelial neoplasia III [CIN III]
    Severe dysplasia of cervix

> *Excludes:* *cervical intraepithelial neoplasia II [CIN II] (622.12)*
>   *cytologic evidence of malignancy without histologic confirmation (795.06)*
>   *high grade squamous intraepithelial lesion (HGSIL) (795.04)*
>   *moderate dysplasia of cervix (622.12)*

233.2 Other and unspecified parts of uterus

233.3 Other and unspecified female genital organs

233.4 Prostate

233.5 Penis

233.6 Other and unspecified male genital organs

233.7 Bladder

233.9 Other and unspecified urinary organs

234 Carcinoma in situ of other and unspecified sites

234.0 Eye

> *Excludes:* *cartilage of eyelid (234.8)*
> *eyelid (skin) (232.1)*
> *optic nerve (234.8)*
> *orbital bone (234.8)*

234.8 Other specified sites
Endocrine gland [any]

234.9 Site unspecified
Carcinoma in situ NOS

NEOPLASMS OF UNCERTAIN BEHAVIOR (235-238)

Note: Categories 235-238 classify by site certain histo-morphologically well-defined neoplasms, the subsequent behavior of which cannot be predicted from the present appearance.

235 Neoplasm of uncertain behavior of digestive and respiratory systems

> *Excludes:* *stromal tumors of uncertain behavior of digestive system (238.1)*

235.0 Major salivary glands
Gland:
   parotid
   sublingual
   submandibular

> *Excludes:* *minor salivary glands (235.1)*

235.1 Lip, oral cavity, and pharynx

Gingiva	Nasopharynx
Hypopharynx	Oropharynx
Minor salivary glands	Tongue
Mouth	

> *Excludes:* *aryepiglottic fold or interarytenoid fold, laryngeal aspect (235.6)*
> *epiglottis:*
>   *NOS (235.6)*
>   *suprahyoid portion (235.6)*
> *skin of lip (238.2)*

235.2 Stomach, intestines, and rectum

235.3 Liver and biliary passages

Ampulla of Vater	Gallbladder
Bile ducts [any]	Liver

235.4 Retroperitoneum and peritoneum

235.5 Other and unspecified digestive organs

Anal:	Esophagus
canal	Pancreas
sphincter	Spleen
Anus NOS	

> *Excludes:* *anus:*
>   *margin (238.2)*
>   *skin (238.2)*
> *perianal skin (238.2)*

235.6 Larynx

> *Excludes:* *aryepiglottic fold or interarytenoid fold:*
>   *NOS (235.1)*
>   *hypopharyngeal aspect (235.1)*
>   *marginal zone (235.1)*

235.7 Trachea, bronchus, and lung

235.8 Pleura, thymus, and mediastinum

● Code new
to this edition

▲ Revision of
existing code

④ ⑤ Fourth or fifth
digit required

235.9 Other and unspecified respiratory organs
Accessory sinuses
Middle ear
Nasal cavities
Respiratory organ NOS

Excludes: *ear (external) (skin) (238.2)*
nose (238.8)
skin (238.2)

236 Neoplasm of uncertain behavior of genitourinary organs

236.0 Uterus

236.1 Placenta
Chorioadenoma (destruens)
Invasive mole
Malignant hydatid(iform) mole

236.2 Ovary
Use additional code, if desired, to identify any functional activity

236.3 Other and unspecified female genital organs

236.4 Testis
Use additional code, if desired, to identify any functional activity

236.5 Prostate

236.6 Other and unspecified male genital organs

236.7 Bladder

⑤ **236.9 Other and unspecified urinary organs**

236.90 Urinary organ, unspecified

236.91 Kidney and ureter

236.99 Other

237 Neoplasm of uncertain behavior of endocrine glands and nervous system

237.0 Pituitary gland and craniopharyngeal duct
Use additional code, if desired, to identify any functional activity

237.1 Pineal gland

237.2 Adrenal gland
Suprarenal gland
Use additional code, if desired, to identify any functional activity

237.3 Paraganglia
Aortic body
Carotid body
Coccygeal body
Glomus jugulare

237.4 Other and unspecified endocrine glands
Parathyroid gland
Thyroid gland

237.5 Brain and spinal cord

237.6 Meninges
Meninges:
NOS
cerebral
spinal

⑤ **237.7 Neurofibromatosis**
von Recklinghausen's disease

237.70 Neurofibromatosis, unspecified

237.71 Neurofibromatosis, Type I [von Recklinghausen's disease]

237.72 Neurofibromatosis, Type II [acoustic neurofibromatosis]

237.9 Other and unspecified parts of nervous system
Cranial nerves

Excludes: *peripheral, sympathetic, and parasympathetic nerves and ganglia (238.1)*

238 Neoplasm of uncertain behavior of other and unspecified sites and tissues

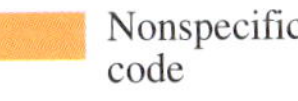
Add 4th or 5th digit

Nonspecific code

Unspecified code

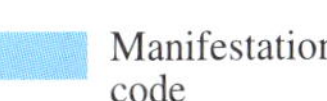
Manifestation code

238.0 Bone and articular cartilage

> *Excludes:* *cartilage:*
>> *ear (238.1)*
>> *eyelid (238.1)*
>> *larynx (235.6)*
>> *nose (235.9)*
>> *synovia (238.1)*

238.1 Connective and other soft tissue
Peripheral, sympathetic, and parasympathetic nerves and ganglia
Stromal tumors of digestive system

> *Excludes:* *cartilage (of):*
>> *articular (238.0)*
>> *larynx (235.6)*
>> *nose (235.9)*
>> *connective tissue of breast (238.3)*

238.2 Skin

> *Excludes:* *anus NOS (235.5)*
>> *skin of genital organs (236.3, 236.6)*
>> *vermilion border of lip (235.1)*

238.3 Breast

> *Excludes:* *skin of breast (238.2)*

238.4 Polycythemia vera

238.5 Histiocytic and mast cells
Mast cell tumor NOS
Mastocytoma NOS

238.6 Plasma cells
Plasmacytoma NOS
Solitary myeloma

⑤ **238.7 Other lymphatic and hematopoietic tissues**

> *Excludes:* *acute myelogenous leukemia (205.0)*
>> *chronic myelomonocytic leukemia (205.1)*
>> *myelofibrosis (289.83)*
>> *myelosclerosis NOS (289.89)*
>> *myelosis:*
>>> *NOS (205.9)*
>>> *megakaryocytic (207.2)*

● **238.71 Essential thrombocythemia**
Essential hemorrhagic thrombocythemia
Essential thrombocytosis
Idiopathic (hemorrhagic) thrombocythemia
Primary thrombocytosis

● **238.72 Low grade myelodysplastic syndrome lesions**
Refractory anemia (RA)
Refractory anemia with ringed sideroblasts (RARS)
Refractory cytopenia with multilineage dysplasia (RCMD)
Refractory cytopenia with multilineage dysplasia and ringed sideroblasts (RCMD-RS)

● **238.73 High grade myelodysplastic syndrome lesions**
Refractory anemia with excess blasts-1 (RAEB-1)
Refractory anemia with excess blasts-2 (RAEB-2)

● **238.74 Myelodysplastic syndrome with 5q deletion**
5q minus syndrome NOS

> *Excludes:* *constitutional 5q deletion (758.39)*
>> *high grade myelodysplastic syndrome with 5q deletion (238.73)*

● **238.75 Myelodysplastic syndrome, unspecified**

● Code new
to this edition

▲ Revision of
existing code

④ ⑤ Fourth or fifth
digit required

● **238.76 Myelofibrosis with myeloid metaplasia**
Agnogenic myeloid metaplasia
Idiopathic myelofibrosis (chronic)
Myelosclerosis with myeloid metaplasia
Primary myelofibrosis

Excludes: *myelofibrosis NOS (289.83)*
myelophthisic anemia (284.2)
myelophthisis (284.2)
secondary myelofibrosis (289.83)

● **238.79 Other lymphatic and hematopoietic tissues**
Lymphoproliferative disease (chronic) NOS
Megakaryocytic myelosclerosis
Myeloproliferative disease (chronic) NOS
Panmyelosis (acute)

238.8 Other specified sites
Eye
Heart

Excludes: *eyelid (skin) (238.2)*
cartilage (238.1)

238.9 Site unspecified

NEOPLASMS OF UNSPECIFIED NATURE (239)

239 Neoplasms of unspecified nature
Note: Category 239 classifies by site neoplasms of unspecified morphology and behavior. The term "mass," unless otherwise stated, is not to be regarded as a neoplastic growth.
Includes: "growth" NOS
neoplasm NOS
new growth NOS
tumor NOS

239.0 Digestive system

Excludes: *anus:*
margin (239.2)
skin (239.2)
perianal skin (239.2)

239.1 Respiratory system

239.2 Bone, soft tissue, and skin

Excludes: *anal canal (239.0)*
anus NOS (239.0)
bone marrow (202.9)
cartilage:
larynx (239.1)
nose (239.1)
connective tissue of breast (239.3)
skin of genital organs (239.5)
vermilion border of lip (239.0)

239.3 Breast

Excludes: *skin of breast (239.2)*

239.4 Bladder

239.5 Other genitourinary organs

239.6 Brain

Excludes: *cerebral meninges (239.7)*
cranial nerves (239.7)

239.7 Endocrine glands and other parts of nervous system

Excludes: *peripheral, sympathetic, and parasympathetic nerves and ganglia (239.2)*

239.8 Other specified sites

Excludes: *eyelids (skin) (239.2)*
cartilage (239.2)
great vessels (239.2)
optic nerve (239.7)

239.9 Site unspecified

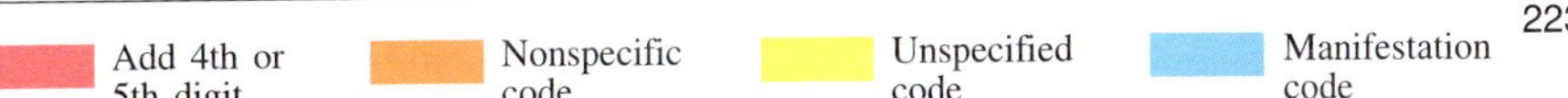

● Code new to this edition   ▲ Revision of existing code   ④ ⑤ Fourth or fifth digit required

3. ENDOCRINE, NUTRITIONAL AND METABOLIC DISEASES, AND IMMUNITY DISORDERS (240-279)

> Excludes: *endocrine and metabolic disturbances specific to the fetus and newborn (775.0-775.9)*

Note: All neoplasms, whether functionally active or not, are classified in Chapter 2. Codes in Chapter 3 (i.e., 242.8, 246.0, 251-253, 255-259) may be used, if desired, to identify such functional activity associated with any neoplasm, or by ectopic endocrine tissue.

DISORDERS OF THYROID GLAND (240-246)

240 Simple and unspecified goiter

240.0 Goiter, specified as simple
Any condition classifiable to 240.9, specified as simple

240.9 Goiter, unspecified
Enlargement of thyroid
Goiter or struma:
  NOS
  diffuse colloid
  endemic
Goiter or struma:
  hyperplastic
  nontoxic (diffuse)
  parenchymatous
  sporadic

> Excludes: *congenital (dyshormonogenic) goiter (246.1)*

241 Nontoxic nodular goiter

> Excludes: *adenoma of thyroid (226)*
> *cystadenoma of thyroid (226)*

241.0 Nontoxic uninodular goiter
Thyroid nodule
Uninodular goiter (nontoxic)

241.1 Nontoxic multinodular goiter
Multinodular goiter (nontoxic)

241.9 Unspecified nontoxic nodular goiter
Adenomatous goiter
Nodular goiter (nontoxic) NOS
Struma nodosa (simplex)

242 Thyrotoxicosis with or without goiter

> Excludes: *neonatal thyrotoxicosis (775.3)*

The following fifth-digit subclassification is for use with category 242:

  0 without mention of thyrotoxic crisis or storm

  1 with mention of thyrotoxic crisis or storm

242.0 Toxic diffuse goiter
Basedow's disease
Exophthalmic or toxic goiter NOS
Graves' disease
Primary thyroid hyperplasia

242.1 Toxic uninodular goiter
Thyroid nodule, toxic or with hyperthyroidism
Uninodular goiter, toxic or with hyperthyroidism

242.2 Toxic multinodular goiter
Secondary thyroid hyperplasia

242.3 Toxic nodular goiter, unspecified
Adenomatous goiter, toxic or with hyperthyroidism
Nodular goiter, toxic or with hyperthyroidism
Struma nodosa, toxic or with hyperthyroidism
Any condition classifiable to 241.9 specified as toxic or with hyperthyroidism

242.4 Thyrotoxicosis from ectopic thyroid nodule

242.8 Thyrotoxicosis of other specified origin
Overproduction of thyroid-stimulating hormone [TSH]
Thyrotoxicosis:
  factitia
  from ingestion of excessive thyroid material

Use additional E code to identify cause, if drug-induced

242.9 Thyrotoxicosis without mention of goiter or other cause
Hyperthyroidism NOS
Thyrotoxicosis NOS

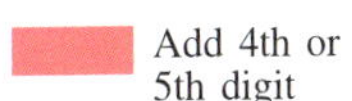

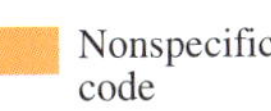

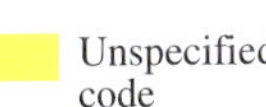

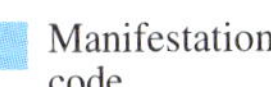

243 Congenital hypothyroidism
Congenital thyroid insufficiency
Cretinism (athyrotic) (endemic)

Use additional code to identify associated mental retardation

Excludes: *congenital (dyshormonogenic) goiter (246.1)*

244 Acquired hypothyroidism
Includes: athyroidism (acquired)
hypothyroidism (acquired)
myxedema (adult) (juvenile)
thyroid (gland) insufficiency (acquired)

244.0 Postsurgical hypothyroidism

244.1 Other postablative hypothyroidism
Hypothyroidism following therapy, such as irradiation

244.2 Iodine hypothyroidism
Hypothyroidism resulting from administration or ingestion of iodide

Use additional E code to identify drug

244.3 Other iatrogenic hypothyroidism
Hypothyroidism resulting from:
P-aminosalicylic acid [PAS]
Phenylbutazone
Resorcinol
Iatrogenic hypothyroidism NOS

Use additional E code to identify drug

244.8 Other specified acquired hypothyroidism
Secondary hypothyroidism NEC

244.9 Unspecified hypothyroidism
Hypothyroidism, primary or NOS
Myxedema, primary or NOS

245 Thyroiditis

245.0 Acute thyroiditis
Abscess of thyroid
Thyroiditis:
nonsuppurative, acute
pyogenic
suppurative

Use additional code to identify organism

245.1 Subacute thyroiditis
Thyroiditis:
de Quervain's
giant cell

Thyroiditis:
granulomatous
viral

245.2 Chronic lymphocytic thyroiditis
Hashimoto's disease
Struma lymphomatosa

Thyroiditis:
autoimmune
lymphocytic (chronic)

245.3 Chronic fibrous thyroiditis
Struma fibrosa
Thyroiditis:
invasive (fibrous)
ligneous
Riedel's

245.4 Iatrogenic thyroiditis
Use additional code to identify cause

245.8 Other and unspecified chronic thyroiditis
Chronic thyroiditis:
NOS
nonspecific

245.9 Thyroiditis, unspecified
Thyroiditis NOS

246 Other disorders of thyroid

246.0 Disorders of thyrocalcitonin secretion
Hypersecretion of calcitonin or thyrocalcitonin

● Code new
to this edition

▲ Revision of
existing code

④ ⑤ Fourth or fifth
digit required

246.1 Dyshormonogenic goiter
Congenital (dyshormonogenic) goiter
Goiter due to enzyme defect in synthesis of thyroid hormone
Goitrous cretinism (sporadic)

246.2 Cyst of thyroid
Excludes: *cystadenoma of thyroid (226)*

246.3 Hemorrhage and infarction of thyroid

246.8 Other specified disorders of thyroid
Abnormality of   Hyper-TBG-nemia
thyroid-binding globulin   Hypo-TBG-nemia
Atrophy of thyroid

246.9 Unspecified disorder of thyroid

DISEASES OF OTHER ENDOCRINE GLANDS (250-259)

⑤ **250 Diabetes mellitus**
Excludes: *gestational diabetes (648.8)*
hyperglycemia NOS (790.6)
neonatal diabetes mellitus (775.1)
nonclinical diabetes (790.29)

The following fifth-digit subclassification is for use with category 250:

0 type II or unspecified type, not stated as uncontrolled

Fifth-digit 0 is for use with type II patients, even if the patient requires insulin
Use additional code, if applicable, for associated long-term (current) insulin use V58.67

1 type I [juvenile type], not stated as uncontrolled

2 type II or unspecified type, uncontrolled

Fifth-digit 2 is for use with type II patients, even if the patient requires insulin
Use additional code, if applicable, for associated long-term (current) insulin use V58.67

3 type I [juvenile type], uncontrolled

⑤ **250.0 Diabetes mellitus without mention of complication**
Diabetes mellitus without mention of complication or manifestation classifiable to
250.1-250.9
Diabetes (mellitus) NOS

⑤ **250.1 Diabetes with ketoacidosis**
Diabetic:
acidosis without mention of coma
ketosis without mention of coma

⑤ **250.2 Diabetes with hyperosmolarity**
Hyperosmolar (nonketotic) coma

⑤ **250.3 Diabetes with other coma**
Diabetic coma (with ketoacidosis)
Diabetic hypoglycemic coma
Insulin coma NOS

Excludes: *diabetes with hyperosmolar coma (250.2)*

⑤ **250.4 Diabetes with renal manifestations**
Use additional code to identify manifestation, as:
chronic kidney disease (585.1-585.9)
diabetic:
nephropathy NOS (583.81)
nephrosis (581.81)
intercapillary glomerulosclerosis (581.81)
Kimmelstiel-Wilson syndrome (581.81)

⑤ **250.5 Diabetes with ophthalmic manifestations**
Use additional code to identify manifestation, as:
diabetic:
blindness (369.00-369.9)
cataract (366.41)
glaucoma (365.44)
macular edema (362.07)
retinal edema (362.07)
retinopathy (362.01-362.07)

⑤ **250.6 Diabetes with neurological manifestations**
Use additional code to identify manifestation, as:
    diabetic:
      amyotrophy (358.1)
      gastroparalysis (536.3)
      gastroparesis (536.3)
      mononeuropathy (354.0-355.9)
      neurogenic arthropathy (713.5)
      peripheral autonomic neuropathy (337.1)
      polyneuropathy (357.2)

⑤ **250.7 Diabetes with peripheral circulatory disorders**
Use additional code to identify manifestation, as:
    diabetic:
      gangrene (785.4)
      peripheral angiopathy (443.81)

⑤ **250.8 Diabetes with other specified manifestations**
    Diabetic hypoglycemia
    Hypoglycemic shock

Use additional code to identify manifestation, as:
    any associated ulceration (707.10-707.9)
    diabetic bone changes (731.8)

Use additional E code to identify cause, if drug-induced

⑤ **250.9 Diabetes with unspecified complication**

251 Other disorders of pancreatic internal secretion

251.0 Hypoglycemic coma
    Iatrogenic hyperinsulinism
    Non-diabetic insulin coma

Use additional E code to identify cause, if drug-induced

    Excludes: *hypoglycemic coma in diabetes mellitus (250.3)*

251.1 Other specified hypoglycemia
    Hyperinsulinism:
      NOS
      ectopic
      functional
    Hyperplasia of pancreatic islet beta cells NOS

    Excludes: *hypoglycemia in diabetes mellitus (250.8)*
        hypoglycemia in infant of diabetic mother (775.0)
        hypoglycemic coma (251.0)
        neonatal hypoglycemia (775.6)

Use additional E code to identify cause, if drug-induced

251.2 Hypoglycemia, unspecified
    Hypoglycemia:
      NOS
      reactive
      spontaneous

    Excludes: *hypoglycemia:*
        with coma (251.0)
        in diabetes mellitus (250.8)
      leucine-induced (270.3)

251.3 Postsurgical hypoinsulinemia
    Hypoinsulinemia following complete or partial pancreatectomy
    Postpancreatectomy hyperglycemia

251.4 Abnormality of secretion of glucagon
    Hyperplasia of pancreatic islet alpha cells with glucagon excess

251.5 Abnormality of secretion of gastrin
    Hyperplasia of pancreatic alpha cells with gastrin excess
    Zollinger-Ellison syndrome

251.8 Other specified disorders of pancreatic internal secretion

251.9 Unspecified disorder of pancreatic internal secretion
    Islet cell hyperplasia NOS

● Code new
to this edition
    ▲ Revision of
existing code
    ④ ⑤ Fourth or fifth
digit required

252 Disorders of parathyroid gland

⑤ **252.0 Hyperparathyroidism**

Excludes: ectopic hyperparathyroidism (259.3)

252.00 Hyperparathyroidism, unspecified

252.01 Primary hyperparathyroidism
Hyperplasia of parathyroid

252.02 Secondary hyperparathyroidism, non-renal

Excludes: secondary hyperparathyroidism (of renal origin) (588.81)

252.08 Other hyperparathyroidism
Tertiary hyperparathyroidism

252.1 Hypoparathyroidism
Parathyroiditis (autoimmune)
Tetany:
   parathyroid
   parathyroprival

Excludes: pseudohypoparathyroidism (275.4)
   pseudo-pseudohypoparathyroidism (275.4)
   tetany NOS (781.7)
   transitory neonatal hypoparathyroidism (775.4)

252.8 Other specified disorders of parathyroid gland
Cyst of parathyroid gland
Hemorrhage of parathyroid gland

252.9 Unspecified disorder of parathyroid gland

253 Disorders of the pituitary gland and its hypothalamic control
Includes: the listed conditions whether the disorder is in the pituitary or the hypothalamus

Excludes: Cushing's syndrome (255.0)

253.0 Acromegaly and gigantism
Overproduction of growth hormone

253.1 Other and unspecified anterior pituitary hyperfunction
Forbes-Albright syndrome

Excludes: overproduction of:
   ACTH (255.3)
   thyroid-stimulating hormone [TSH] (242.8)

253.2 Panhypopituitarism
Cachexia, pituitary   Sheehan's syndrome
Necrosis of pituitary   Simmonds' disease
   (postpartum)
Pituitary insufficiency NOS

Excludes: iatrogenic hypopituitarism (253.7)

253.3 Pituitary dwarfism
Isolated deficiency of (human) growth hormone [HGH]
Lorain-Levi dwarfism

253.4 Other anterior pituitary disorders
Isolated or partial deficiency of an anterior pituitary hormone, other than growth
   hormone
Prolactin deficiency

253.5 Diabetes insipidus
Vasopressin deficiency

Excludes: nephrogenic diabetes insipidus (588.1)

253.6 Other disorders of neurohypophysis
Syndrome of inappropriate secretion of antidiuretic hormone [ADH]

Excludes: ectopic antidiuretic hormone secretion (259.3)

253.7 Iatrogenic pituitary disorders
Hypopituitarism:
   hormone-induced
   hypophysectomy-induced
   postablative
   radiotherapy-induced
Use additional E code to identify cause

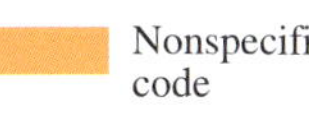

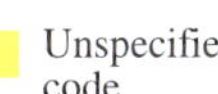

Unspecified
code

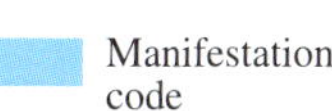

253.8 **Other disorders of the pituitary and other syndromes of diencephalohypophyseal origin**
Abscess of pituitary   Cyst of Rathke's pouch
Adiposogenital dystrophy   Fröhlich's syndrome

Excludes: *craniopharyngioma (237.0)*

253.9 **Unspecified**
Dyspituitarism

254 **Diseases of thymus gland**

Excludes: *aplasia or dysplasia with immunodeficiency (279.2)*
hypoplasia with immunodeficiency (279.2)
myasthenia gravis (358.00-358.01)

254.0 **Persistent hyperplasia of thymus**
Hypertrophy of thymus

254.1 **Abscess of thymus**

254.8 **Other specified diseases of thymus gland**
Atrophy of thymus
Cyst of thymus

Excludes *thymoma (212.6)*

254.9 **Unspecified disease of thymus gland**

255 **Disorders of adrenal glands**
Includes: the listed conditions whether the basic disorder is in the adrenals or is pituitary-induced

255.0 **Cushing's syndrome**
Adrenal hyperplasia due to   Ectopic ACTH syndrome
   excess ACTH   Iatrogenic syndrome of excess cortisol
Cushing's syndrome: Overproduction of cortisol
   NOS
   iatrogenic
   idiopathic
   pituitary-dependent

Excludes: *congenital adrenal hyperplasia (255.2)*
Use additional E code to identify cause, if drug-induced

⑤ **255.1** **Hyperaldosteronism**

▲ **255.10** **Hyperaldosteronism, unspecified**
Aldosteronism NOS
Primary aldosteronism, unspecified

Excludes: *Conn's syndrome (255.12)*

255.11 **Glucocorticoid-remediable aldosteronism**
Familial aldosteronism type I

Excludes: *Conn's syndrome (255.12)*

255.12 **Conn's syndrome**

255.13 **Bartter's syndrome**

255.14 **Other secondary aldosteronism**

255.2 **Adrenogenital disorders**
Adrenogenital syndromes, virilizing or feminizing, whether acquired or associated with congenital adrenal hyperplasia consequent on inborn enzyme defects in hormone synthesis
Achard-Thiers syndrome
Congenital adrenal hyperplasia
Female adrenal pseudohermaphroditism
Male:
   macrogenitosomia praecox
   sexual precocity with adrenal hyperplasia
Virilization (female) (suprarenal)

Excludes: *adrenal hyperplasia due to excess ACTH (255.0)*
isosexual virilization (256.4)

255.3 **Other corticoadrenal overactivity**
Acquired benign adrenal androgenic overactivity
Overproduction of ACTH

● Code new
  to this edition
▲ Revision of
  existing code
④ ⑤ Fourth or fifth
  digit required

255.4 Corticoadrenal insufficiency
Addisonian crisis
Addison's disease NOS
Adrenal:
 atrophy (autoimmune)
 calcification
Adrenal:
 crisis
 hemorrhage
 infarction
 insufficiency NOS

Excludes: *tuberculous Addison's disease (017.6)*

255.5 Other adrenal hypofunction
Adrenal medullary insufficiency

Excludes: *Waterhouse-Friderichsen syndrome (meningococcal) (036.3)*

255.6 Medulloadrenal hyperfunction
Catecholamine secretion by pheochromocytoma

255.8 Other specified disorders of adrenal glands
Abnormality of cortisol-binding globulin

255.9 Unspecified disorder of adrenal glands

256 Ovarian dysfunction

256.0 Hyperestrogenism

256.1 Other ovarian hyperfunction
Hypersecretion of ovarian androgens

256.2 Postablative ovarian failure
Use additional code for states associated with artifical menopause (627.4)
Ovarian failure:
 iatrogenic
 postirradiation
 postsurgical

Excludes: *asymptomatic age-related (natural) postmenopausal status (V49.81)*
 acquired absence of ovary (V45.77)

⑤ **256.3 Other ovarian failure**
Use additional code for states associated with natural menopause (627.2)

Excludes: *asymptomatic age-related (natural) postmenopausal status (V49.81)*

256.31 Premature menopause

256.39 Other ovarian failure
Delayed menarche
Ovarian hypofunction
Primary ovarian failure NOS

256.4 Polycystic ovaries
Isosexual virilization
Stein-Leventhal syndrome

256.8 Other ovarian dysfunction

256.9 Unspecified ovarian dysfunction

257 Testicular dysfunction

257.0 Testicular hyperfunction
Hypersecretion of testicular hormones

257.1 Postablative testicular hypofunction
Testicular hypofunction:
 iatrogenic
 postirradiation
 postsurgical

257.2 Other testicular hypofunction
Defective biosynthesis of testicular androgen
Eunuchoidism:
 NOS
 hypogonadotropic
Failure:
 Leydig's cell, adult
 seminiferous tubule, adult
Testicular hypogonadism

Excludes: *azoospermia (606.0)*

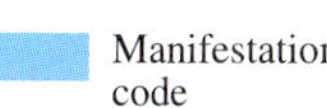

257.8 Other testicular dysfunction
> *Excludes:* androgen insensitivity syndrome (259.5)

257.9 Unspecified testicular dysfunction

258 Polyglandular dysfunction and related disorders

258.0 Polyglandular activity in multiple endocrine adenomatosis
Wermer's syndrome

258.1 Other combinations of endocrine dysfunction
Lloyd's syndrome   Schmidt's syndrome

258.8 Other specified polyglandular dysfunction

258.9 Polyglandular dysfunction, unspecified

259 Other endocrine disorders

259.0 Delay in sexual development and puberty, not elsewhere classified
Delayed puberty

259.1 Precocious sexual development and puberty, not elsewhere classified
Sexual precocity:
NOS
constitutional
cryptogenic
idiopathic

259.2 Carcinoid syndrome
Hormone secretion by carcinoid tumors

259.3 Ectopic hormone secretion, not elsewhere classified
Ectopic:
antidiuretic hormone secretion [ADH]
hyperparathyroidism
> *Excludes:* ectopic ACTH syndrome (255.0)

259.4 Dwarfism, not elsewhere classified
Dwarfism:
NOS
constitutional
> *Excludes:* dwarfism:
>> achondroplastic (756.4)
>> intrauterine (759.7)
>> nutritional (263.2)
>> pituitary (253.3)
>> renal (588.0)
> progeria (259.8)

259.5 Androgen insensitivity syndrome
Partial androgen insensitivity
Reifenstein syndrome

259.8 Other specified endocrine disorders
Pineal gland dysfunction   Werner's syndrome
Progeria

259.9 Unspecified endocrine disorder
Disturbance: Infantilism NOS
endocrine NOS
hormone NOS

NUTRITIONAL DEFICIENCIES (260-269)

> *Excludes:* deficiency anemias (280.0-281.9)

260 Kwashiorkor
Nutritional edema with dyspigmentation of skin and hair

261 Nutritional marasmus
Nutritional atrophy   Severe malnutrition NOS
Severe calorie deficiency

262 Other severe protein-calorie malnutrition
Nutritional edema without mention of dyspigmentation of skin and hair

263 Other and unspecified protein-calorie malnutrition

263.0 Malnutrition of moderate degree

263.1 Malnutrition of mild degree

● Code new   ▲ Revision of   ④ ⑤ Fourth or fifth
   to this edition   existing code   digit required

263.2 Arrested development following protein-calorie malnutrition
Nutritional dwarfism
Physical retardation due to malnutrition

263.8 Other protein-calorie malnutrition

263.9 Unspecified protein-calorie malnutrition
Dystrophy due to malnutrition
Malnutrition (calorie) NOS

> *Excludes:* *nutritional deficiency NOS (269.9)*

264 Vitamin A deficiency

264.0 With conjunctival xerosis

264.1 With conjunctival xerosis and Bitot's spot
Bitot's spot in the young child

264.2 With corneal xerosis

264.3 With corneal ulceration and xerosis

264.4 With keratomalacia

264.5 With night blindness

264.6 With xerophthalmic scars of cornea

264.7 Other ocular manifestations of vitamin A deficiency
Xerophthalmia due to vitamin A deficiency

264.8 Other manifestations of vitamin A deficiency
Follicular keratosis due to vitamin A deficiency
Xeroderma due to vitamin A deficiency

264.9 Unspecified vitamin A deficiency
Hypovitaminosis A NOS

265 Thiamine and niacin deficiency states

265.0 Beriberi

265.1 Other and unspecified manifestations of thiamine deficiency
Other vitamin B_1 deficiency states

265.2 Pellagra
Deficiency:
    niacin (-tryptophan)
    nicotinamide
    nicotinic acid
    vitamin PP
Pellagra (alcoholic)

266 Deficiency of B-complex components

266.0 Ariboflavinosis
Riboflavin [vitamin B_2] deficiency

266.1 Vitamin B_6 deficiency
Deficiency: Vitamin B_6 deficiency syndrome
    pyridoxal
    pyridoxamine
    pyridoxine

> *Excludes:* *vitamin B_6-responsive sideroblastic anemia (285.0)*

266.2 Other B-complex deficiencies
Deficiency:
    cyanocobalamin
    folic acid
    vitamin B_{12}

> *Excludes:* *combined system disease with anemia (281.0-281.1)*
>   *deficiency anemias (281.0-281.9)*
>   *subacute degeneration of spinal cord with anemia (281.0-281.1)*

266.9 Unspecified vitamin B deficiency

267 Ascorbic acid deficiency
Deficiency of vitamin C
Scurvy

> *Excludes:* *scorbutic anemia (281.8)*

Add 4th or 5th digit   Nonspecific code   Unspecified code   Manifestation code

268 Vitamin D deficiency

> *Excludes:* *vitamin D-resistant:*
>> *osteomalacia (275.3)*
>> *rickets (275.3)*

268.0 Rickets, active

> *Excludes:* *celiac rickets (579.0)*
>> *renal rickets (588.0)*

268.1 Rickets, late effect

Any condition specified as due to rickets and stated to be a late effect or sequela of rickets

Use additional code to identify the nature of late effect

268.2 Osteomalacia, unspecified

268.9 Unspecified vitamin D deficiency

Avitaminosis D

269 Other nutritional deficiencies

269.0 Deficiency of vitamin K

> *Excludes:* *deficiency of coagulation factor due to vitamin K deficiency (286.7)*
>> *vitamin K deficiency of newborn (776.0)*

269.1 Deficiency of other vitamins

Deficiency:
> vitamin E
> vitamin P

269.2 Unspecified vitamin deficiency

Multiple vitamin deficiency NOS

269.3 Mineral deficiency, not elsewhere classified

Deficiency:
> calcium, dietary
> iodine

> *Excludes:* *deficiency:*
>> *calcium NOS (275.4)*
>> *potassium (276.8)*
>> *sodium (276.1)*

269.8 Other nutritional deficiency

> *Excludes:* *adult failure to thrive (783.7)*
>> *failure to thrive in childhood (783.41)*
>> *feeding problems (783.3)*
>>> *newborn (779.3)*

269.9 Unspecified nutritional deficiency

OTHER METABOLIC AND IMMUNITY DISORDERS (270-279)

Use additional code to identify any associated mental retardation

270 Disorders of amino-acid transport and metabolism

> *Excludes:* *abnormal findings without manifest disease (790.0-796.9)*
>> *disorders of purine and pyrimidine metabolism (277.1-277.2)*
>> *gout (274.0-274.9)*

270.0 Disturbances of amino-acid transport

Cystinosis
Cystinuria
Fanconi (-de Toni) (-Debré) syndrome
Glycinuria (renal)
Hartnup disease

270.1 Phenylketonuria [PKU]

Hyperphenylalaninemia

● Code new
to this edition

▲ Revision of
existing code

④ ⑤ Fourth or fifth
digit required

270.2 Other disturbances of aromatic amino-acid metabolism

Albinism
Alkaptonuria
Alkaptonuric ochronosis
Disturbances of metabolism
  of tyrosine and
  tryptophan
Homogentisic acid defects
Hydroxykynureninuria

Hypertyrosinemia
Indicanuria
Kynureninase defects
Oasthouse urine disease
Ochronosis
Tyrosinosis
Tyrosinuria
Waardenburg syndrome

Excludes: *vitamin B₆-deficiency syndrome (266.1)*

270.3 Disturbances of branched-chain amino-acid metabolism

Disturbances of metabolism of leucine, isoleucine, and valine
Hypervalinemia
Intermittent branched-chain ketonuria
Leucine-induced hypoglycemia
Leucinosis
Maple syrup urine disease

270.4 Disturbances of sulphur-bearing amino-acid metabolism

Cystathioninemia
Cystathioninuria
Disturbances of metabolism of methionine, homocystine, and cystathionine
Homocystinuria
Hypermethioninemia
Methioninemia

270.5 Disturbances of histidine metabolism

Carnosinemia
Histidinemia
Hyperhistidinemia
Imidazole aminoaciduria

270.6 Disorders of urea cycle metabolism

Argininosuccinic aciduria
Citrullinemia
Disorders of metabolism of ornithine, citrulline, argininosuccinic acid, arginine, and
  ammonia
Hyperammonemia
Hyperornithinemia

270.7 Other disturbances of straight-chain amino-acid metabolism

Glucoglycinuria
Glycinemia (with methyl-
  malonic acidemia)
Hyperglycinemia
Hyperlysinemia
Pipecolic acidemia

Saccharopinuria
Other disturbances of metabolism of glycine, threonine,
  serine, glutamine, and lysine

270.8 Other specified disorders of amino-acid metabolism

Alaninemia
Ethanolaminuria
Glycoprolinuria
Hydroxyprolinemia
Hyperprolinemia

Iminoacidopathy
Prolinemia
Prolinuria
Sarcosinemia

270.9 Unspecified disorder of amino-acid metabolism

271 Disorders of carbohydrate transport and metabolism

Excludes: *abnormality of secretion of glucagon (251.4)*
  diabetes mellitus (250.0-250.9)
  hypoglycemia NOS (251.2)
  mucopolysaccharidosis (277.5)

271.0 Glycogenosis

Amylopectinosis
Glucose-6-phosphatase
  deficiency
Glycogen storage disease

McArdle's disease
Pompe's disease
von Gierke's disease

271.1 Galactosemia

Galactose-1-phosphate uridyl transferase deficiency
Galactosuria

271.2 Hereditary fructose intolerance

Essential benign fructosuria
Fructosemia

271.3 Intestinal disaccharidase deficiencies and disaccharide malabsorption
Intolerance or malabsorption (congenital) (of):
glucose-galactose
lactose
sucrose-isomaltose

271.4 Renal glycosuria
Renal diabetes

271.8 Other specified disorders of carbohydrate transport and metabolism
Essential benign pentosuria   Mannosidosis
Fucosidosis   Oxalosis
Glycolic aciduria   Xylosuria
Hyperoxaluria (primary)   Xylulosuria

271.9 Unspecified disorder of carbohydrate transport and metabolism

272 Disorders of lipoid metabolism
Excludes: localized cerebral lipidoses (330.1)

272.0 Pure hypercholesterolemia
Familial hypercholesterolemia
Fredrickson Type IIa hyperlipoproteinemia
Hyperbetalipoproteinemia
Hyperlipidemia, Group A
Low-density-lipoid-type [LDL] hyperlipoproteinemia

272.1 Pure hyperglyceridemia
Endogenous hyperglyceridemia
Frederickson Type IV hyperlipoproteinemia
Hyperlipidemia, Group B
Hyperprebetalipoproteinemia
Hypertriglyceridemia, essential
Very-low-density-lipoid-type [VLDL] hyperlipoproteinemia

272.2 Mixed hyperlipidemia
Broad- or floating-betalipoproteinemia
Fredrickson Type IIb or III hyperlipoproteinemia
Hypercholesterolemia with endogenous hyperglyceridemia
Hyperbetalipoproteinemia with prebetalipoproteinemia
Tubo-eruptive xanthoma
Xanthoma tuberosum

272.3 Hyperchylomicronemia
Bürger-Grütz syndrome
Fredrickson type I or V hyperlipoproteinemia
Hyperlipidemia, Group D
Mixed hyperglyceridemia

272.4 Other and unspecified hyperlipidemia
Alpha-lipoproteinemia
Combined hyperlipidemia
Hyperlipidemia NOS
Hyperlipoproteinemia NOS

272.5 Lipoprotein deficiencies
Abetalipoproteinemia
Bassen-Kornzweig syndrome
High-density lipoid deficiency
Hypoalphalipoproteinemia
Hypobetalipoproteinemia (familial)

272.6 Lipodystrophy
Barraquer-Simons disease
Progressive lipodystrophy
Use additional E code to identify cause, if iatrogenic
Excludes: intestinal lipodystrophy (040.2)

● Code new
to this edition   ▲ Revision of
existing code   ④ ⑤ Fourth or fifth
digit required

272.7 Lipidoses
Chemically-induced lipidosis
Disease:
 Anderson's
 Fabry's
 Gaucher's
 I cell [mucolipidosis I]
 lipoid storage NOS
 Neimann-Pick
 pseudo-Hurler's or
 mucolipidosis III
Disease:
 triglyceride storage, Type I or II
 Wolman's or triglyceride storage, Type III
Mucolipidosis II
Primary familial xanthomatosis

> **Excludes:** *cerebral lipidoses (330.1)*
> *Tay-Sachs disease (330.1)*

272.8 Other disorders of lipoid metabolism
Hoffa's disease or liposynovitis prepatellaris
Launois-Bensaude's lipomatosis
Lipoid dermatoarthritis

272.9 Unspecified disorder of lipoid metabolism

273 Disorders of plasma protein metabolism

> **Excludes:** *agammaglobulinemia and hypogammaglobulinemia (279.0 -279.2)*
> *coagulation defects (286.0-286.9)*
> *hereditary hemolytic anemias (282.0-282.9)*

273.0 Polyclonal hypergammaglobulinemia
Hypergammaglobulinemic purpura:
 benign primary
 Waldenström's

273.1 Monoclonal paraproteinemia
Benign monoclonal hypergammaglobulinemia [BMH]
Monoclonal gammopathy:
 NOS
 associated with lymphoplasmacytic dyscrasias
 benign
Paraproteinemia:
 benign (familial)
 secondary to malignant or inflammatory disease

273.2 Other paraproteinemias
Cryoglobulinemic:
 purpura
 vasculitis
Mixed cryoglobulinemia

273.3 Macroglobulinemia
Macroglobulinemia (idiopathic) (primary)
Waldenström's macroglobulinemia

273.4 Alpha-1-antitrypsin deficiency
AAT deficiency

273.8 Other disorders of plasma protein metabolism
Abnormality of transport protein
Bisalbuminemia

273.9 Unspecified disorder of plasma protein metabolism

274 Gout

> **Excludes:** *lead gout (984.0-984.9)*

274.0 Gouty arthropathy

⑤ **274.1 Gouty nephropathy**

    274.10 Gouty nephropathy, unspecified

    274.11 Uric acid nephrolithiasis

    274.19 Other

⑤ **274.8 Gout with other specified manifestations**

    274.81 Gouty tophi of ear

    274.82 Gouty tophi of other sites
      Gouty tophi of heart

274.89 Other
Use additional code to identify manifestations, as:
　　　gouty:
　　　　iritis (364.11)
　　　　neuritis (357.4)

274.9 Gout, unspecified

275 Disorders of mineral metabolism
　Excludes: *abnormal findings without manifest disease (790.0-796.9)*

275.0 Disorders of iron metabolism
　　Bronzed diabetes　　　　　Pigmentary cirrhosis (of liver)
　　Hemochromatosis
　Excludes: *anemia:*
　　　　iron deficiency (280.0-280.9)
　　　　sideroblastic (285.0)

275.1 Disorders of copper metabolism
　　Hepatolenticular degeneration
　　Wilson's disease

275.2 Disorders of magnesium metabolism
　　Hypermagnesemia
　　Hypomagnesemia

275.3 Disorders of phosphorus metabolism
　　Familial hypophosphatemia
　　Hypophosphatasia
　　Vitamin D-resistant:
　　　osteomalacia
　　　rickets

⑤ **275.4 Disorders of calcium metabolism**
　Excludes: *parathyroid disorders (252.00-252.9)*
　　　　vitamin D deficiency (268.0-268.9)

　　275.40 Unspecified disorder of calcium metabolism

　　275.41 Hypocalcemia

　　275.42 Hypercalcemia

　　275.49 Other disorders of calcium metabolism
　　　　Nephrocalcinosis
　　　　Pseudohypoparathyroidism
　　　　Pseudopseudohypoparathyroidism

275.8 Other specified disorders of mineral metabolism

275.9 Unspecified disorder of mineral metabolism

276 Disorders of fluid, electrolyte, and acid-base balance
　Excludes: *diabetes insipidus (253.5)*
　　　　familial periodic paralysis (359.3)

276.0 Hyperosmolality and/or hypernatremia
　　Sodium [Na] excess
　　Sodium [Na] overload

276.1 Hyposmolality and/or hyponatremia
　　Sodium [Na] deficiency

276.2 Acidosis
　　Acidosis:
　　　NOS
　　　lactic
　　　metabolic
　　　respiratory
　Excludes: *diabetic acidosis (250.1)*

276.3 Alkalosis
　　Alkalosis:
　　　NOS
　　　metabolic
　　　respiratory

276.4 Mixed acid-base balance disorder
　　Hypercapnia with mixed acid-base disorder

276.5 Volume depletion

● Code new　　　　▲ Revision of　　　　④ ⑤ Fourth or fifth
　to this edition　　　existing code　　　　　digit required

276.50 Volume depletion, unspecified

276.51 Dehydration

276.52 Hypovolemia
Depletion of volume of plasma

276.6 Fluid overload
Fluid retention

| *Excludes:* | *ascites (789.5)* |
| | *localized edema (782.3)* |

276.7 Hyperpotassemia
Hyperkalemia
Potassium [K]:
  excess
  intoxication
  overload

276.8 Hypopotassemia
Hypokalemia
Potassium [K] deficiency

276.9 Electrolyte and fluid disorders not elsewhere classified
Electrolyte imbalance
Hyperchloremia
Hypochloremia

Excludes:	*electrolyte imbalance:*
	associated with hyperemesis gravidarum (643.1)
	complicating labor and delivery (669.0)
	following abortion and ectopic or molar pregnancy (634-638 with .4, 639.4)

277 Other and unspecified disorders of metabolism

277.0 Cystic fibrosis
Fibrocystic disease of the pancreas
Mucoviscidosis

  277.00 Without mention of meconium ileus
  Cystic fibrosis NOS

  277.01 With meconium ileus
  Meconium:
    ileus (of newborn)
    obstruction of intestine in mucoviscidosis

  277.02 With pulmonary manifestations
  Cystic fibrosis with pulmonary exacerbation
Use additional code to identify any infectious organism present, such as:
    pseudomonas (041.7)

  277.03 With gastrointestinal manifestations

| *Excludes:* | *with meconium ileus (277.01)* |

  277.09 With other manifestations

277.1 Disorders of porphyrin metabolism
Hematoporphyria
Hematoporphyrinuria
Hereditary coproporphyria
Porphyria
Porphyrinuria
Protocoproporphyria
Protoporphyria
Pyrroloporphyria

277.2 Other disorders of purine and pyrimidine metabolism
Hypoxanthine-guanine-phosphoribosyltransferase deficiency [HG-PRT deficiency]
Lesch-Nyhan syndrome
Xanthinuria

| *Excludes:* | *gout (274.0-274.9)* |
| | *orotic aciduric anemia (281.4)* |

277.3 Amyloidosis

  ● **277.30 Amyloidosis, unspecified**
  Amyloidosis NOS

  ● **277.31 Familial Mediterranean fever**
  Benign paroxysmal peritonitis
  Hereditary amyloid nephropathy
  Periodic familial polyserositis
  Recurrent polyserositis

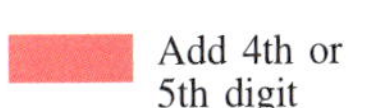

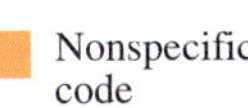

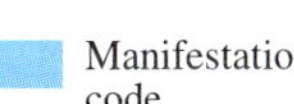

● **277.39** **Other amyloidosis**
Hereditary cardiac amyloidosis
Inherited systemic amyloidosis
Neuropathic (Portuguese) (Swiss) amyloidosis
Secondary amyloidosis

277.4 **Disorders of bilirubin excretion**
Hyperbilirubinemia:
  congenital
  constitutional
Syndrome:
  Crigler-Najjar
  Dubin-Johnson
  Gilbert's
  Rotor's

| Excludes: | *hyperbilirubinemias specific to the perinatal period (774.0-774.7)* |

277.5 **Mucopolysaccharidosis**
Gargoylism
Hunter's syndrome
Hurler's syndrome
Lipochondrodystrophy
Maroteaux-Lamy syndrome
Morquio-Brailsford disease
Osteochondrodystrophy
Sanfilippo's syndrome
Scheie's syndrome

277.6 **Other deficiencies of circulating enzymes**
Hereditary angioedema

277.7 **Dysmetabolic syndrome X**
Use additional code for associated manifestation, such as:
  cardiovascular disease (414.00-414.07)
  obesity (278.00-278.01)

⑤ **277.8** **Other specified disorders of metabolism**

277.81 **Primary carnitine deficiency**

277.82 **Carnitine deficiency due to inborn errors of metabolism**

277.83 **Iatrogenic carnitine deficiency**
Carnitine deficiency due to:
  hemodialysis
  valproic acid therapy

277.84 **Other secondary carnitine deficiency**

277.85 **Disorders of fatty acid oxidation**
Carnitine palmitoyltransferase deficiencies (CPT1, CPT2)
Glutaric aciduria type II (type IIA, IIB, IIC)
Long chain 3-hydroxyacyl CoA dehydrogenase deficiency (LCHAD)
Long chain/very long chain acyl CoA dehydrogenase deficiency (LCAD, VLCAD)
Medium chain acyl CoA dehydrogenase deficiency (MCAD)
Short chain acyl CoA dehydrogenase deficiency (SCAD)

| Excludes: | *primary carnitine deficiency (277.81)* |

277.86 **Peroxisomal disorders**
Adrenomyeloneuropathy
Neonatal adrenoleukodystrophy
Rhizomelic chrondrodysplasia punctata
X-linked adrenoleukodystrophy
Zellweger syndrome

| Excludes: | *infantile Refsum disease (356.3)* |

277.87 **Disorders of mitochondrial metabolism**
Kearns-Sayre syndrome
Mitochondrial Encephalopathy, Lactic Acidosis and Stroke-like episodes (MELAS syndrome)
Mitochondrial Neurogastrointestinal Encephalopathy syndrome (MNGIE)
Myoclonus with Epilepsy and with Ragged Red Fibers (MERRF syndrome)
Neuropathy, Ataxia and Retinitis Pigmentosa (NARP syndrome)
Use additional code for associated conditions

Excludes:	*disorders of pyruvate metabolism (271.8)*
	Leber's optic atrophy (377.16)
	Leigh's subacute necrotizing encephalopathy (330.8)
	Reye's syndrome (331.81)

● Code new
to this edition

▲ Revision of
existing code

④ ⑤ Fourth or fifth
digit required

277.89 **Other specified disorders of metabolism**
Hand-Schuller-Christian disease
Histiocytosis (acute) (chronic)
Histiocytosis X (chronic)

Excludes: *histiocytosis:*
acute differentiatied progressive (202.5)
X, acute (progressive) (202.5)

277.9 **Unspecified disorder of metabolism**
Enzymopathy NOS

278 **Overweight, obesity and other hyperalimentation**

Excludes: *hyperalimentation NOS (783.6)*
poisoning by vitamins NOS (963.5)
polyphagia (783.6)

Use additional code to identify Body Mass Index (BMI), if known (V85.21-V85.25, V85.30-V85.39, V85.4, V85.53, V85.54)

⑤ **278.0** **Overweight and obesity**
Use additional code to identify Body Mass Index (BMI), if known (V85.0-V85.54)

Excludes: *adiposogenital dystrophy (253.8)*
obesity of endocrine origin NOS (259.9)

278.00 **Obesity, unspecified**
Obesity NOS

278.01 **Morbid obesity**
Severe obesity

278.02 **Overweight**

278.1 **Localized adiposity**
Fat pad

278.2 **Hypervitaminosis A**

278.3 **Hypercarotinemia**

278.4 **Hypervitaminosis D**

278.8 **Other hyperalimentation**

279 **Disorders involving the immune mechanism**

⑤ **279.0** **Deficiency of humoral immunity**

279.00 **Hypogammaglobulinemia, unspecified**
Agammaglobulinemia NOS

279.01 **Selective IgA immunodeficiency**

279.02 **Selective IgM immunodeficiency**

279.03 **Other selective immunoglobulin deficiencies**
Selective deficiency of IgG

279.04 **Congenital hypogammaglobulinemia**
Agammaglobulinemia:
Bruton's type
X-linked

279.05 **Immunodeficiency with increased IgM**
Immunodeficiency with hyper-IgM:
autosomal recessive
X-linked

279.06 **Common variable immunodeficiency**
Dysgammaglobulinemia (acquired) (congenital) (primary)
Hypogammaglobulinemia:
acquired primary
congenital non-sex-linked
sporadic

279.09 **Other**
Transient hypogammaglobulinemia of infancy

⑤ **279.1** **Deficiency of cell-mediated immunity**

279.10 **Immunodeficiency with predominant T-cell defect, unspecified**

279.11 **DiGeorge's syndrome**
Pharyngeal pouch syndrome
Thymic hypoplasia

279.12 **Wiskott-Aldrich syndrome**

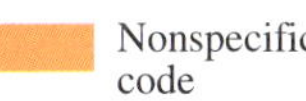

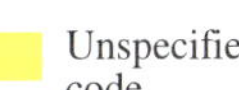

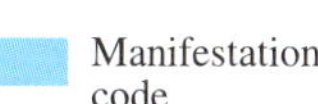

279.13 Nezelof's syndrome
Cellular immunodeficiency with abnormal immunoglobulin deficiency

279.19 Other

Excludes: *ataxia-telangiectasia (334.8)*

279.2 Combined immunity deficiency
Agammaglobulinemia:
autosomal recessive
Swiss-type
x-linked recessive
Severe combined immunodeficiency [SCID]
Thymic:
alymphoplasia
aplasia or dysplasia with immunodeficiency

Excludes: *thymic hypoplasia (279.11)*

279.3 Unspecified immunity deficiency

279.4 Autoimmune disease, not elsewhere classified
Autoimmune disease NOS

Excludes: *transplant failure or rejection (996.80-996.89)*

279.8 Other specified disorders involving the immune mechanism
Single complement [C_1-C_9] deficiency or dysfunction

279.9 Unspecified disorder of immune mechanism

● Code new
to this edition

▲ Revision of
existing code

④ ⑤ Fourth or fifth
digit required

4. DISEASES OF THE BLOOD AND BLOOD-FORMING ORGANS (280-289)

> Excludes: *anemia complicating pregnancy or the puerperium (648.2)*

280 Iron deficiency anemias
Includes: anemia:
      asiderotic
      hypochromic-microcytic
      sideropenic

> Excludes: *familial microcytic anemia (282.49)*

280.0 Secondary to blood loss (chronic)
    Normocytic anemia due to blood loss

> Excludes: *acute posthemorrhagic anemia (285.1)*

280.1 Secondary to inadequate dietary iron intake

280.8 Other specified iron deficiency anemias
    Paterson-Kelly syndrome
    Plummer-Vinson syndrome
    Sideropenic dysphagia

280.9 Iron deficiency anemia, unspecified
    Anemia:
      achlorhydric
      chlorotic
      idiopathic hypochromic
      iron [Fe] deficiency NOS

281 Other deficiency anemias

281.0 Pernicious anemia
    Anemia: Congenital intrinsic factor [Castle's] deficiency
      Addison's
      Biermer's
      congenital pernicious

> Excludes: *combined system disease without mention of anemia (266.2)*
> *subacute degeneration of spinal cord without mention of anemia (266.2)*

281.1 Other vitamin B$_{12}$ deficiency anemia
    Anemia:
      vegan's
      vitamin B$_{12}$ deficiency (dietary)
      due to selective vitamin B$_{12}$ malabsorption with proteinuria
    Syndrome:
      Imerslund's
      Imerslund-Gräsbeck

> Excludes: *combined system disease without mention of anemia (266.2)*
> *subacute degeneration of spinal cord without mention of anemia (266.2)*

281.2 Folate-deficiency anemia
    Congenital folate malabsorption
    Folate or folic acid deficiency anemia:
      NOS
      dietary
      drug-induced
    Goat's milk anemia
    Nutritional megaloblastic anemia (of infancy)
Use additional E code, if desired, to identify drug

281.3 Other specified megaloblastic anemias not elsewhere classified
    Combined B$_{12}$ and folate-deficiency anemia
    Refractory megaloblastic anemia

281.4 Protein-deficiency anemia
    Amino-acid-deficiency anemia

281.8 Anemia associated with other specified nutritional deficiency
    Scorbutic anemia

281.9 Unspecified deficiency anemia
    Anemia: Anemia:
      dimorphic   nutritional NOS
      macrocytic   simple chronic
      megaloblastic NOS

	Add 4th or 5th digit		Nonspecific code		Unspecified code		Manifestation code

282 Hereditary hemolytic anemias

282.0 Hereditary spherocytosis
Acholuric (familial) jaundice
Congenital hemolytic anemia (spherocytic)
Congenital spherocytosis
Minkowski-Chauffard syndrome
Spherocytosis (familial)

Excludes: hemolytic anemia of newborn (773.0-773.5)

282.1 Hereditary elliptocytosis
Elliptocytosis (congenital)
Ovalocytosis (congenital) (hereditary)

282.2 Anemias due to disorders of glutathione metabolism
Anemia:
6-phosphogluconic dehydrogenase deficiency
enzyme deficiency, drug-induced
erythrocytic glutathione deficiency
glucose-6-phosphate dehydrogenase [G-6-PD] deficiency
glutathione-reductase deficiency
hemolytic nonspherocytic (hereditary), type I
Disorder of pentose phosphate pathway
Favism

282.3 Other hemolytic anemias due to enzyme deficiency
Anemia:
hemolytic nonspherocytic (hereditary), type II
hexokinase deficiency
pyruvate kinase [PK] deficiency
triosephosphate isomerase deficiency

⑤ **282.4 Thalassemias**

Excludes: sickle-cell:
disease (282.60-282.69)
trait (282.5)

282.41 Sickle-cell thalassemia without crisis
Sickle-cell thalassemia NOS
Thalassemia Hb-S disease without crisis

282.42 Sickle-cell thalassemia with crisis
Sickle-cell thalassemia with vaso-occlusive pain
Thalassemia Hb-S disease with crisis

Use additional code for types of crisis, such as:
acute chest syndrome (517.3)
splenic sequestration (289.52)

282.49 Other thalassemia
Cooley's anemia
Hb-Bart's disease
Hereditary leptocytosis
Mediterranean anemia (with other hemoglobinopathy)
Microdrepanocytosis
Thalassemia (alpha) (beta) (intermedia) (major) (minima) (minor) (mixed)
(trait) (with other hemoglobinopathy)
Thalassemia NOS

282.5 Sickle-cell trait
Hb-AS genotype   Heterozygous:
Hemoglobin S [Hb-S] trait   hemoglobin S
                                           Hb-S

Excludes: that with other hemoglobinopathy (282.60-282.69)
that with thalassemia (282.49)

⑤ **282.6 Sickle-cell disease**
Sickle-cell anemia

Excludes: sickle-cell thalassemia (282.41-282.42)
sickle-cell trait (282.5)

282.60 Sickle-cell disease, unspecified
Sickle-cell anemia NOS

282.61 Hb-SS disease without crisis

● Code new
to this edition

▲ Revision of
existing code

④ ⑤ Fourth or fifth
digit required

282.62 Hb-SS disease with crisis
Hb-SS disease with vaso-occlusive pain
Sickle-cell crisis NOS

Use additional code for type of crisis, such as:
acute chest syndrome (517.3)
splenic sequestration (289.52)

282.63 Sickle-cell/Hb-C disease without crisis
Hb-S/Hb-C disease without crisis

282.64 Sickle-cell/Hb-C disease with crisis
Hb-S/Hb-C disease with crisis
Sickle-cell/Hb-C disease with vaso-occlusive pain

Use additional code for type of crisis, such as:
acute chest syndrome (517.3)
splenic sequestration (289.52)

282.68 Other sickle-cell disease without crisis
Hb-S/Hb-D disease without crisis
Hb-S/Hb-E disease without crisis
Sickle-cell/Hb-D disease without crisis
Sickle-cell/Hb-E disease without crisis

282.69 Other sickle-cell disease with crisis
Hb-S/Hb-D disease with crisis
Hb-S/Hb-E disease with crisis
Other sickle-cell disease with vaso-occlusive pain
Sickle-cell/Hb-D disease with crisis
Sickle-cell/Hb-E disease with crisis

Use additional code for type of crisis, such as:
acute chest syndrome (517.3)
splenic sequestration (289.52)

282.7 Other hemoglobinopathies
Abnormal hemoglobin NOS
Congenital Heinz-body anemia
Disease:
hemoglobin C [Hb-C]
hemoglobin D [Hb-D]
hemoglobin E [Hb-E]
hemoglobin Zurich [Hb-Zurich]
Hemoglobinopathy NOS
Hereditary persistence of fetal hemoglobin [HPFH]
Unstable hemoglobin hemolytic disease

Excludes:	*familial polycythemia (289.6)*
	hemoglobin M [Hb-M] disease (289.7)
	high-oxygen-affinity hemoglobin (289.0)

282.8 Other specified hereditary hemolytic anemias
Stomatocytosis

282.9 Hereditary hemolytic anemia, unspecified
Hereditary hemolytic anemia NOS

283 Acquired hemolytic anemias

283.0 Autoimmune hemolytic anemias
Autoimmune hemolytic anemias (cold type) (warm type)
Chronic cold hemagglutinin disease
Cold agglutinin disease or hemoglobinuria
Hemolytic anemia:
cold type (secondary) (symptomatic)
drug-induced
warm type (secondary) (symptomatic)

Use additional E code, if desired, to identify cause, if drug-induced

Excludes:	*Evans' syndrome (287.32)*
	hemolytic disease of newborn (773.0-773.5)

⑤ **283.1 Non-autoimmune hemolytic anemias**

283.10 Non-autoimmune hemolytic anemia, unspecified

283.11 Hemolytic-uremic syndrome

Add 4th or 5th digit	Nonspecific code	Unspecified code	Manifestation code

283.19 Other non-autoimmune hemolytic anemias
Hemolytic anemia:
  mechanical
  microangiopathic
  toxic

Use additional E code, if desired, to identify cause

283.2 Hemoglobinuria due to hemolysis from external causes
Acute intravascular hemolysis
Hemoglobinuria:
  from exertion
  march
  paroxysmal (cold) (nocturnal)
  due to other hemolysis
Marchiafava-Micheli syndrome

Use additional E code, if desired, to identify cause

283.9 Acquired hemolytic anemia, unspecified
Acquired hemolytic anemia NOS
Chronic idiopathic hemolytic anemia

▲ **284 Aplastic anemia and other bone marrow failure syndromes**

⑤ **284.0 Constitutional aplastic anemia**

● **284.01 Constitutional red blood cell aplasia**
Aplasia, (pure) red cell:
  congenital
  of infants
  primary
Blackfan-Diamond syndrome
Familial hypoplastic anemia

● **284.09 Other constitutional aplastic anemia**
Fanconi's anemia
Pancytopenia with malformations

● **284.1 Pancytopenia**
Excludes: *pancytopenia (due to) (with):*

aplastic anemia NOS (284.9)
bone marrow infiltration (284.2)
constitutional red blood cell aplasia (284.01)
drug induced (284.8)
hairy cell leukemia (202.4)
human immunodeficiency virus disease (042)
leukoerythroblastic anemia (284.2)
malformations (284.09)
myelodysplastic syndromes (238.72-238.75)
myeloproliferative disease (238.79)
other constitutional aplastic anemia (284.09)

● **284.2 Myelophthisis**
Leukoerythroblastic anemia
Myelophthisic anemia

Code first the underlying disorder, such as:
  malignant neoplasm of breast (174.0-174.9, 175.0-175.9)
  tuberculosis (015.0-015.9)

Excludes: *idiopathic myelofibrosis (238.76)*

myelofibrosis NOS (289.83)
myelofibrosis with myeloid metaplasia (238.76)
primary myelofibrosis (238.76)
secondary myelofibrosis (289.83)

284.8 Other specified aplastic anemias

Aplastic anemia (due to):	toxic (paralytic)
chronic systemic disease	Red cell aplasia (acquired) (adult) (pure) (with
drugs	thymoma)
infection	
radiation	

Use additional E code, if desired, to identify cause

● Code new
to this edition

▲ Revision of
existing code

④ ⑤ Fourth or fifth
digit required

284.9   Aplastic anemia, unspecified
  Anemia: Anemia:
   aplastic (idiopathic) NOS nonregenerative
   aregenerative   Medullary hypoplasia
   hypoplastic NOS

  Excludes: *refractory anemia (238.72)*

285   Other and unspecified anemias

285.0   Sideroblastic anemia
  Anemia:
   hypochromic with iron loading
   sideroachrestic
   sideroblastic:
    acquired
    congenital
    hereditary
    primary
    secondary (drug-induced) (due to disease)
    sex-linked hypochromic
    vitamin B_6-responsive
  Pyridoxine-responsive (hypochromic) anemia
Use additional E code, if desired, to identify cause, if drug induced

  Excludes: *refractory sideroblastic anemia (238.72)*

285.1   Acute posthemorrhagic anemia
  Anemia due to acute blood loss

  Excludes: *anemia due to chronic blood loss (280.0)*
     blood loss anemia NOS (280.0)

▲ **285.2   Anemia of chronic disease**
  Anemia in chronic illness

  285.21   Anemia in chronic kidney disease
    Anemia in end stage renal disease
    Erythropoietin-resistant anemia (EPO resistant anemia)

  285.22   Anemia in neoplastic disease

  ▲ **285.29   Anemia of other chronic disease**
    Anemia in other chronic illness

285.8   Other specified anemias
  Anemia:
   dyserythropoietic (congenital)
   dyshematopoietic (congenital)
   von Jaksch's
  Infantile pseudoleukemia

285.9   Anemia, unspecified
  Anemia: Anemia:
   NOS   profound
   essential   progressive
   normocytic, not due to blood secondary
    loss   Oligocythemia

  Excludes: *anemia (due to):*
    blood loss:
     acute (285.1)
     chronic or unspecified (280.0)
    iron deficiency (280.0-280.9)

286   Coagulation defects

286.0   Congenital factor VIII disorder
  Antihemophilic globulin [AHG] deficiency
  Factor VIII (functional) deficiency
  Hemophilia:
   NOS
   A
   classical
   familial
   hereditary
  Subhemophilia

  Excludes: *factor VIII deficiency with vascular defect (286.4)*

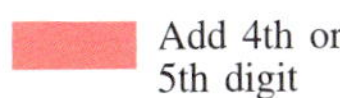

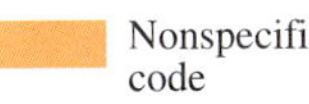

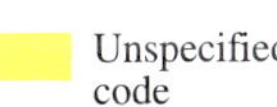

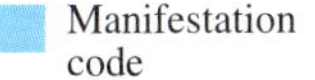

286.1 Congenital factor IX disorder
Christmas disease
Deficiency:
  factor IX (functional)
  plasma thromboplastin component [PTC]
Hemophilia B

286.2 Congenital factor XI deficiency
Hemophilia C
Plasma thromboplastin antecedent [PTA] deficiency
Rosenthal's disease

286.3 Congenital deficiency of other clotting factors
Congenital afibrinogenemia
Deficiency:
  AC globulin factor:
    I [fibrinogen]
    II [prothrombin]
    V [labile]
    VII [stable]
    X [Stuart-Prower]
    XII [Hageman]
    XIII [fibrin stabilizing]
Deficiency:
  Laki-Lorand factor
  proaccelerin
Disease:
  Owren's
  Stuart-Prower
Dysfibrinogenemia (congenital)
Dysprothrombinemia (constitutional)
Hypoproconvertinemia
Hypoprothrombinemia (hereditary)
Parahemophilia

286.4 von Willebrand's disease
Angiohemophilia (A) (B)
Constitutional thrombopathy
Factor VIII deficiency with vascular defect
Pseudohemophilia type B
Vascular hemophilia
von Willebrand's (-Jürgens') disease

Excludes: *factor VIII deficiency:*
NOS (286.0)
with functional defect (286.0)
hereditary capillary fragility (287.8)

286.5 Hemorrhagic disorder due to intrinsic circulating anticoagulants
Antithrombinemia
Antithromboplastinemia
Antithromboplastinogenemia
Hyperheparinemia
Increase in:
  anti-VIIIa
  anti-IXa
Increase in:
  anti-Xa
  anti-XIa
  antithrombin
Secondary hemophilia

Systemic lupus erythematosus [SLE] inhibitor

286.6 Defibrination syndrome
Afibrinogenemia, acquired
Consumption coagulopathy
Diffuse or disseminated intravascular coagulation [DIC syndrome]
Fibrinolytic hemorrhage, acquired
Hemorrhagic fibrinogenolysis
Pathologic fibrinolysis
Purpura:
  fibrinolytic
  fulminans

Excludes: *that complicating:*
abortion (634-638 with .1, 639.1)
pregnancy or the puerperium (641.3, 666.3)
disseminated intravascular coagulation in newborn (776.2)

286.7 Acquired coagulation factor deficiency
Deficiency of coagulation factor due to:
  liver disease
  vitamin K deficiency
Hypoprothrombinemia, acquired

Excludes: *vitamin K deficiency of newborn (776.0)*
Use additional E-code, if desired, to identify cause, if drug induced

● Code new
  to this edition

▲ Revision of
  existing code

④ ⑤ Fourth or fifth
  digit required

286.9 Other and unspecified coagulation defects
Defective coagulation NOS
Deficiency, coagulation factor NOS
Delay, coagulation
Disorder:
    coagulation
    hemostasis

Excludes: *abnormal coagulation profile (790.92)*
    hemorrhagic disease of newborn (776.0)
    that complicating:
        abortion (634-638 with .1, 639.1)
        pregnancy or the puerperium (641.3, 666.3)

287 Purpura and other hemorrhagic conditions

Excludes: *hemorrhagic thrombocythemia (238.79)*
    purpura fulminans (286.6)

287.0 Allergic purpura
Peliosis rheumatica
Purpura:
    anaphylactoid
    autoimmune
    Henoch's
Purpura:
    nonthrombocytopenic:
        hemorrhagic
        idiopathic
    rheumatica
    Schönlein-Henoch
    vascular
Vasculitis, allergic

Excludes: *hemorrhagic purpura (287.39)*
    purpura annularis telangiectodes (709.1)

287.1 Qualitative platelet defects
Thrombasthenia (hemorrhagic) (hereditary)
Thrombocytasthenia
Thrombocytopathy (dystrophic)
Thrombopathy (Bernard-Soulier)

Excludes: *von Willebrand's disease (286.4)*

287.2 Other nonthrombocytopenic purpuras
Purpura:
    NOS
    senile
    simplex

⑤ **287.3 Primary thrombocytopenia**

287.30 Primary thrombocytopenia, unspecified
Megakaryocytic hypoplasia

287.31 Immune thrombocytopenic purpura
Idiopathic thrombocytopenic purpura
Tidal platelet dysgenesis

287.32 Evans' syndrome

287.33 Congenital and hereditary thrombocytopenic purpura
Congenital and hereditary thrombocytopenia
Thrombocytopenia with absent radii (TAR) syndrome

Excludes: *Wiskott-Aldrich syndrome (279.12)*

287.39 Other primary thrombocytopenia

287.4 Secondary thrombocytopenia
Posttransfusion purpura
Thrombocytopenia (due to):
    dilutional
    drugs
    extracorporeal circulation of blood
    massive blood transfusion
    platelet alloimmunization
Use additional E code, if desired, to identify cause

Excludes: *transient thrombocytopenia of newborn (776.1)*

287.5 Thrombocytopenia, unspecified

287.8 Other specified hemorrhagic conditions
Capillary fragility (hereditary)
Vascular pseudohemophilia

Add 4th or 5th digit	Nonspecific code	Unspecified code	Manifestation code

287.9 **Unspecified hemorrhagic conditions**
Hemorrhagic diathesis (familial)

288 **Diseases of white blood cells**
Excludes: *leukemia (204.0-208.9)*

▲ **288.0** **Neutropenia**
Decreased Absolute Neutrophil Count (ANC)
Use additional code for any associated fever (780.6)
Excludes: *neutropenic splenomegaly (289.53)*
transitory neonatal neutropenia (776.7)

● **288.00** **Neutropenia, unspecified**

● **288.01** **Congenital neutropenia**
Congenital agranulocytosis
Infantile genetic agranulocytosis
Kostmann's syndrome

● **288.02** **Cyclic neutropenia**
Cyclic hematopoiesis
Periodic neutropenia

● **288.03** **Drug induced neutropenia**
Use additional E code to identify drug

● **288.04** **Neutropenia due to infection**

● **288.09** **Other neutropenia**
Agranulocytosis
Neutropenia:
immune
toxic

288.1 **Functional disorders of polymorphonuclear neutrophils**
Chronic (childhood) granulomatous disease
Congenital dysphagocytosis
Job's syndrome
Lipochrome histiocytosis (familial)
Progressive septic granulomatosis

288.2 **Genetic anomalies of leukocytes**
Anomaly (granulation) (granulocyte) or syndrome:
Alder's (-Reilly)
Chédiak-Steinbrinck (-Higashi)
Jordan's
May-Hegglin
Pelger-Huet
Hereditary:
hypersegmentation
hyposegmentation
leukomelanopathy

288.3 **Eosinophilia**
Eosinophilia
allergic
hereditary
idiopathic
secondary
Eosinophilic leukocytosis
Excludes: *Löffler's syndrome (518.3)*
pulmonary eosinophilia (518.3)

● **288.4** **Hemophagocytic syndromes**
Familial hemophagocytic lymphohistiocytosis
Familial hemophagocytic reticulosis
Hemophagocytic syndrome, infection-associated
Histiocytic syndromes
Macrophage activation syndrome

● **288.5** **Decreased white blood cell count**
Excludes: *neutropenia (288.01-288.09)*

● **288.50** **Leukocytopenia, unspecified**
Decreased leukocytes, unspecified
Decreased white blood cell count, unspecified
Leukopenia NOS

● Code new
to this edition

▲ Revision of
existing code

④ ⑤ Fourth or fifth
digit required

5. MENTAL DISORDERS (290-319)

PSYCHOSES (290-299)

> *Excludes:* *mental retardation (317-319)*

ORGANIC PSYCHOTIC CONDITIONS (290-294)

Includes: psychotic organic brain syndrome

> *Excludes:* *nonpsychotic syndromes of organic etiology (310.0-310.9)*
>
> *psychoses classifiable to 295-298 and without impairment of orientation, comprehension, calculation, learning capacity, and judgement, but associated with physical disease, injury, or condition affecting the brain [e.g., following childbirth] (295.0-298.8)*

290 Dementias

Code first the associated neurological condition

> *Excludes:* *dementia due to alcohol (291.0-291.2)*
>
> *dementia due to drugs (292.82)*
>
> *dementia not classified as senile, presenile, or arteriosclerotic (294.10-294.11)*
>
> *psychoses classifiable to 295-298 occurring in the senium without dementia or delirium (295.0-298.8)*
>
> *senility with mental changes of nonpsychotic severity (310.1)*
>
> *transient organic psychotic conditions (293.0-293.9)*

290.0 Senile dementia, uncomplicated

Senile dementia:
  NOS
  simple type

> *Excludes:* *mild memory disturbances, not amounting to dementia, associated with senile brain disease (310.1)*
>
> *senile dementia with:*
>   *delirium or confusion (290.3)*
>   *delusional [paranoid] features (290.20)*
>   *depressive features (290.21)*

290.1 Presenile dementia

Brain syndrome with presenile brain disease

> *Excludes:* *arteriosclerotic dementia (290.40-290.43)*
>
> *dementia associated with other cerebral conditions (294.10-294.11)*

290.10 Presenile dementia, uncomplicated

Presenile dementia:
  NOS
  simple type

290.11 Presenile dementia with delirium

Presenile dementia with acute confusional state

290.12 Presenile dementia with delusional features

Presenile dementia, paranoid type

290.13 Presenile dementia with depressive features

Presenile dementia, depressed type

290.2 Senile dementia with delusional or depressive features

> *Excludes:* *senile dementia:*
>   *NOS (290.0)*
>   *with delirium and/or confusion (290.3)*

290.20 Senile dementia with delusional features

Senile dementia, paranoid type
Senile psychosis NOS

290.21 Senile dementia with depressive features

290.3 Senile dementia with delirium

Senile dementia with acute confusional state

> *Excludes:* *senile:*
>   *dementia NOS (290.0)*
>   *psychosis NOS (290.20)*

290.4 Vascular dementia

Multi-infarct dementia or psychosis

Use additional code to identify cerebral atherosclerosis (437.0)

> *Excludes:* *suspected cases with no clear evidence of arteriosclerosis (290.9)*

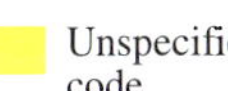
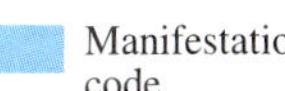

Add 4th or 5th digit   Nonspecific code   Unspecified code   Manifestation code

290.40 Vascular dementia, uncomplicated
Arteriosclerotic dementia:
  NOS
  simple type

290.41 Vascular dementia with delirium
Arteriosclerotic dementia with acute confusional state

290.42 Vascular dementia with delusions
Arteriosclerotic dementia, paranoid type

290.43 Vascular dementia with depressed mood
Arteriosclerotic dementia, depressed type

290.8 Other specified senile psychotic conditions
Presbyophrenic psychosis

290.9 Unspecified senile psychotic condition

291 Alcohol-induced mental disorders
Excludes: *alcoholism without psychosis (303.0-303.9)*

291.0 Alcohol withdrawal delirium
Alcoholic delirium
Delirium tremens
Excludes: *alcohol withdrawal (291.81)*

291.1 Alcohol-induced persisting amnestic disorder
Alcoholic polyneuritic psychosis
Korsakoff's psychosis, alcoholic
Wernicke-Korsakoff syndrome (alcoholic)

291.2 Alcohol-induced persisting dementia
Alcoholic dementia NOS
Alcoholism associated with dementia NOS
Chronic alcoholic brain syndrome

291.3 Alcohol-induced psychotic disorder with hallucinations
Alcoholic:
  hallucinosis (acute)
  psychosis with hallucinosis
Excludes: *alcohol withdrawal with delirium (291.0)*
      schizophrenia (295.0-295.9) and paranoid states (297.0-297.9) taking the form of chronic hallucinosis with clear consciousness in an alcoholic

291.4 Idiosyncratic alcohol intoxication
Pathologic:
  alcohol intoxication
  drunkenness
Excludes: *acute alcohol intoxication (305.0)*
      in alcoholism (303.0)
      simple drunkenness (305.0)

291.5 Alcohol-induced psychotic disorder with delusions
Alcoholic:
  paranoia
  psychosis, paranoid type
Excludes: *nonalcoholic paranoid states (297.0-297.9)*
      schizophrenia, paranoid type (295.3)

⑤ **291.8 Other specified alcohol induced mental disorders**

291.81 Alcohol withdrawal
Alcohol:
  withdrawal syndrome or symptoms
  abstinence syndrome or symptoms
Excludes: *alcohol withdrawal:*
      delirium (291.0)
      hallucinosis (291.3)
      delirium tremens (291.0)

291.82 Alcohol induced sleep disorders
Alcohol induced circadian rhythm sleep disorders
Alcohol induced hypersomnia
Alcohol induced insomnia
Alcohol induced parasomnia

● Code new to this edition   ▲ Revision of existing code   ④ ⑤ Fourth or fifth digit required

291.89 **Other**
Alcohol induced anxiety disorder
Alcohol induced mood disorder
Alcohol induced sexual dysfunction

291.9 **Unspecified alcohol-induced mental disorders**
Alcohol-related disorder NOS
Alcoholic:
mania NOS
psychosis NOS
Alcoholism (chronic) with psychosis

292 **Drug induced mental disorders**
Includes: organic brain syndrome associated with consumption of drugs

Use additional code for any associated drug dependence (304.0-304.9)

Use additional E code, if desired, to identify drug

292.0 **Drug withdrawal**
Drug:
abstinence syndrome or symptoms
withdrawal syndrome or symptoms

⑤ **292.1** **Drug-induced psychotic disorders**

292.11 **Drug-induced psychotic disorder with delusions**
Paranoid state induced by drugs

292.12 **Drug-induced psychotic disorder with hallucinations**
Hallucinatory state induced by drugs

Excludes: *states following LSD or other hallucinogens, lasting only a few days or less ["bad trips"] (305.3)*

292.2 **Pathological drug intoxication**
Drug reaction:
NOS resulting in brief psychotic states
idiosyncratic resulting in brief psychotic states
pathologic resulting in brief psychotic states

Excludes: *expected brief psychotic reactions to hallucinogens ["bad trips"] (305.3)*
physiological side-effects of drugs (e.g., dystonias)

⑤ **292.8** **Other specified drug induced mental disorders**

292.81 **Drug induced delirium**

292.82 **Drug induced persisting dementia**

292.83 **Drug induced persisting amnestic disorder**

292.84 **Drug induced mood disorder**
Depressive state induced by drugs

292.85 **Drug induced sleep disorders**
Drug induced circadian rhythm sleep disorder
Drug induced hypersomnia
Drug induced insomnia
Drug induced parasomnia

292.89 **Other**
Drug induced anxiety disorder
Drug induced organic personality syndrome
Drug induced sexual dysfunction
Drug intoxication

292.9 **Unspecified drug-induced mental disorder**
Drug-related disorder NOS
Organic psychosis NOS due to or associated with drugs

293 **Transient mental disorders due to conditions classified elsewhere**
Includes: transient organic mental disorders not associated with alcohol or drugs
Code first the associated physical or neurological condition

Excludes: *confusional state or delirium superimposed on senile dementia (290.3)*
dementia due to:
alcohol (291.0-291.9)
arteriosclerosis (290.40-290.43)
drugs (292.82)
senility (290.0)

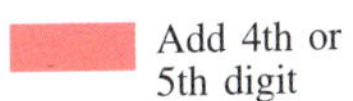

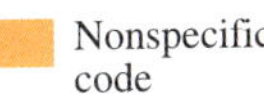

Unspecified
code

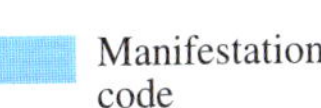

293.0 ***Delirium due to conditions classified elsewhere***
Acute:
  confusional state
  infective psychosis
  organic reaction
  posttraumatic organic psychosis
  psycho-organic syndrome
Acute psychosis associated with endocrine, metabolic, or cerebrovascular disorder
Epileptic:
  confusional state
  twilight state

293.1 ***Subacute delirium***
Subacute:
  confusional state
  infective psychosis
  organic reaction
  posttraumatic organic psychosis
  psycho-organic syndrome
  psychosis associated with endocrine or metabolic disorder

⑤ **293.8** ***Other specified transient mental disorders due to conditions classified elsewhere***

293.81 ***Psychotic disorder with delusions in conditions classified elsewhere***
Transient organic psychotic condition, paranoid type

293.82 ***Psychotic disorder with hallucinations in conditions classified elsewhere***
Transient organic psychotic condition, hallucinatory type

293.83 ***Mood disorder in conditions classified elsewhere***
Transient organic psychotic condition, depressive type

293.84 ***Anxiety disorder in conditions classified elsewhere***

293.89 ***Other***
Catatonic disorder in conditions classified elsewhere

293.9 ***Unspecified transient mental disorder in conditions classified elsewhere***
Organic psychosis:
  infective NOS
  posttraumatic NOS
  transient NOS
Psycho-organic syndrome

294 **Persistent mental disorders due to conditions classified elsewhere**
Includes: organic psychotic brain syndromes (chronic), not elsewhere classified

294.0 ***Amnestic disorder in conditions classified elsewhere***
Code first underlying condition
Korsakoff's psychosis or syndrome (nonalcoholic)

Excludes:	*alcoholic:*

  amnestic syndrome (291.1)
  Korsakoff's psychosis (291.1)

⑤ **294.1** ***Dementia in conditions classified elsewhere***
Dementia of the Alzheimer's type
Code first any underlying physical condition, as:
dementia in:
  Alzheimer's disease (331.0)
  cerebral lipidoses (330.1)
  dementia with Lewy bodies (331.82)
  dementia with Parkinsonism (331.82)
  epilepsy (345.0-345.9)
  frontal dementia (331.19)
  frontotemporal dementia (331.19)
  general paresis [syphilis] (094.1)
  hepatolenticular degeneration (275.1)
  Huntington's chorea (333.4)
  Jakob-Creutzfeldt disease (046.1)
  multiple sclerosis (340)
  Pick's disease of the brain (331.11)
  polyarteritis nodosa (446.0)
  syphilis (094.1)

Excludes:	*dementia:*

  arteriosclerotic (290.40-290.43)
  presenile (290.10-290.13)
  senile (290.0)
  epileptic psychosis NOS (294.8)

● Code new
to this edition

▲ Revision of
existing code

④ ⑤ Fourth or fifth
digit required

294.10 *Dementia in conditions classified elsewhere without behavioral disturbance*
Dementia in conditions classified elsewhere NOS

294.11 *Dementia in conditions classified elsewhere with behavioral disturbance*
Aggressive behavior
Combative behavior
Violent behavior
Wandering off

294.8 *Other persistent mental disorders due to conditions classified elsewhere*
Amnestic disorder NOS
Dementia NOS
Epileptic psychosis NOS
Mixed paranoid and affective organic psychotic states

Use additional code for associated epilepsy (345.0-345.9)

Excludes: *mild memory disturbances, not amounting to dementia (310.1)*

294.9 *Unspecified persistent mental disorders due to conditions classified elsewhere*
Cognitive disorder NOS
Organic psychosis (chronic)

OTHER PSYCHOSES (295-299)

Use additional code to identify any associated physical disease, injury, or condition affecting the brain with psychoses classifiable to 295-298

295 **Schizophrenic disorders**
Includes: schizophrenia of the types described in 295.0-295.9 occurring in children

Excludes: *childhood type schizophrenia (299.9)*

infantile autism (299.0)

The following fifth-digit subclassification is for use with category 295:

0 **unspecified**

1 **subchronic**

2 **chronic**

3 **subchronic with acute exacerbation**

4 **chronic with acute exacerbation**

5 **in remission**

295.0 **Simple type**
Schizophrenia simplex

Excludes: *latent schizophrenia (295.5)*

295.1 **Disorganized type**
Hebephrenia
Hebephrenic type schizophrenia

295.2 **Catatonic type**
Catatonic (schizophrenia):
  agitation
  excitation
  excited type
  stupor
  withdrawn type
Schizophrenic:
  catalepsy
  catatonia
  flexibilitas cerea

295.3 **Paranoid type**
Paraphrenic schizophrenia

Excludes: *involutional paranoid state (297.2)*

paranoia (297.1)
paraphrenia (297.2)

295.4 **Schizophreniform disorder**
Oneirophrenia
Schizophreniform:
  attack
  psychosis, confusional type

Excludes: *acute forms of schizophrenia of:*

catatonic type (295.2)
hebephrenic type (295.1)
paranoid type (295.3)
simple type (295.0)
undifferentiated type (295.8)

⑤ **295.5 Latent schizophrenia**
Latent schizophrenic reaction
Schizophrenia:
  borderline
  incipient
Schizophrenia:
  prepsychotic
  prodromal
  pseudoneurotic
  pseudopsychopathic

Excludes: *schizoid personality (301.20-301.22)*

⑤ **295.6 Residual type**
Chronic undifferentiated schizophrenia
Restzustand (schizophrenic)
Schizophrenic residual state

⑤ **295.7 Schizoaffective disorder**
Cyclic schizophrenia
Mixed schizophrenic and affective psychosis
Schizoaffective psychosis
Schizophreniform psychosis, affective type

⑤ **295.8 Other specified types of schizophrenia**
Acute (undifferentiated) schizophrenia
Atypical schizophrenia
Cenesthopathic schizophrenia

Excludes: *infantile autism (299.0)*

⑤ **295.9 Unspecified schizophrenia**
Schizophrenia:
  NOS
  mixed NOS
  undifferentiated NOS
  undifferentiated type
Schizophrenic reaction NOS
Schizophreniform psychosis NOS

296 Episodic mood disorders
Includes: episodic affective disorders

Excludes: *neurotic depression (300.4)*
     reactive depressive psychosis (298.0)
     reactive excitation (298.1)

The following fifth-digit subclassification is for use with categories 296.0-296.6:

  0 unspecified

  1 mild

  2 moderate

  3 severe, without mention of psychotic behavior

  4 severe, specified as with psychotic behavior

  5 in partial or unspecified remission

  6 in full remission

⑤ **296.0 Bipolar I disorder, single manic episode**
Hypomania (mild) NOS, single episode or unspecified
Hypomanic psychosis, single episode or unspecified
Mania (monopolar) NOS, single episode or unspecified
Manic-depressive psychosis or reaction:
  hypomanic, single episode or unspecified
  manic, single episode or unspecified

Excludes: *circular type, if there was a previous attack of depression (296.4)*

⑤ **296.1 Manic disorder, recurrent episode**
Any condition classifiable to 296.0, stated to be recurrent

Excludes: *circular type, if there was a previous attack of depression (296.4)*

  ● Code new
    to this edition
  ▲ Revision of
    existing code
  ④ ⑤ Fourth or fifth
      digit required

⑤ **296.2 Major depressive disorder, single episode**
 Depressive psychosis, single episode or unspecified
 Endogenous depression, single episode or unspecified
 Involutional melancholia, single episode or unspecified
 Manic-depressive psychosis or reaction, depressed type, single episode or unspecified
 Monopolar depression, single episode or unspecified
 Psychotic depression, single episode or unspecified

 Excludes: *circular type, if previous attack was of manic type (296.5)*
  depression NOS (311)
  reactive depression (neurotic) (300.4)
   psychotic (298.0)

⑤ **296.3 Major depressive disorder, recurrent episode**
 Any condition classifiable to 296.2, stated to be recurrent

 Excludes: *circular type, if previous attack was of manic type (296.5)*
  depression NOS (311)
  reactive depression (neurotic) (300.4)
   psychotic (298.0)

⑤ **296.4 Bipolar I disorder, most recent episode (or current) manic**
 Bipolar disorder, now manic
 Manic-depressive psychosis, circular type but currently manic

 Excludes: *brief compensatory or rebound mood swings (296.99)*

⑤ **296.5 Bipolar I disorder, most recent episode (or current) depressed**
 Bipolar disorder, now depressed
 Manic-depressive psychosis, circular type but currently depressed

 Excludes: *brief compensatory or rebound mood swings (296.99)*

⑤ **296.6 Bipolar I disorder, most recent episode (or current) mixed**
 Manic-depressive psychosis, circular type, mixed

296.7 Bipolar I disorder, most recent episode (or current) unspecified
 Atypical bipolar affective disorder NOS
 Manic-depressive psychosis, circular type, current condition not specified as either
  manic or depressive

⑤ **296.8 Other and unspecified bipolar disorders**

 296.80 Bipolar disorder, unspecified
  Bipolar disorder NOS
  Manic-depressive:
   reaction NOS
   syndrome NOS

 296.81 Atypical manic disorder

 296.82 Atypical depressive disorder

 296.89 Other
  Bipolar II disorder
  Manic-depressive psychosis, mixed type

⑤ **296.9 Other and unspecified episodic mood disorder**

 Excludes: *psychogenic affective psychoses (298.0-298.8)*

 296.90 Unspecified episodic mood disorder
  Affective psychosis NOS
  Melancholia NOS
  Mood disorder NOS

 296.99 Other specified episodic mood disorder
  Mood swings:
   brief compensatory
   rebound

297 Delusional disorders
 Includes: paranoid disorders

 Excludes: *acute paranoid reaction (298.3)*
  alcoholic jealousy or paranoid state (291.5)
  paranoid schizophrenia (295.3)

297.0 Paranoid state, simple

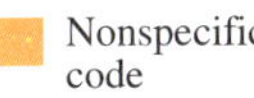

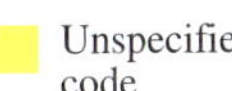

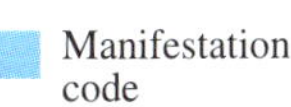

Manifestation
code

297.1 Delusional disorder
Chronic paranoid psychosis
Sander's disease
Systematized delusions

Excludes: paranoid personality disorder (301.0)

297.2 Paraphrenia
Involutional paranoid state
Late paraphrenia
Paraphrenia (involutional)

297.3 Shared psychotic disorder
Folie à deux
Induced psychosis or paranoid disorder

297.8 Other specified paranoid states
Paranoia querulans
Sensitiver Beziehungswahn

Excludes: acute paranoid reaction or state (298.3)
senile paranoid state (290.20)

297.9 Unspecified paranoid state

Paranoid: Paranoid:
  disorder NOS   reaction NOS
  psychosis   state NOS

298 Other nonorganic psychoses
Includes: psychotic conditions due to or provoked by:
emotional stress
environmental factors as major part of etiology

298.0 Depressive type psychosis
Psychogenic depressive psychosis
Psychotic reactive depression
Reactive depressive psychosis

Excludes: manic-depressive psychosis, depressed type (296.2-296.3)
neurotic depression (300.4)
reactive depression NOS (300.4)

298.1 Excitative type psychosis
Acute hysterical psychosis   Reactive excitation
Psychogenic excitation

Excludes: manic-depressive psychosis, manic type (296.0-296.1)

298.2 Reactive confusion
Psychogenic confusion
Psychogenic twilight state

Excludes: acute confusional state (293.0)

298.3 Acute paranoid reaction
Acute psychogenic paranoid psychosis
Bouffée délirante

Excludes: paranoid states (297.0-297.9)

298.4 Psychogenic paranoid psychosis
Protracted reactive paranoid psychosis

298.8 Other and unspecified reactive psychosis
Brief psychotic disorder
Brief reactive psychosis NOS
Hysterical psychosis
Psychogenic psychosis NOS
Psychogenic stupor

Excludes: acute hysterical psychosis (298.1)

298.9 Unspecified psychosis
Atypical psychosis
Psychosis NOS
Psychotic disorder NOS

● Code new to this edition   ▲ Revision of existing code   ④ ⑤ Fourth or fifth digit required

⑤ **299** **Pervasive developmental disorders**

> *Excludes:* *adult type psychoses occurring in childhood, as:*
> *affective disorders (296.0-296.9)*
> *manic-depressive disorders (296.0-296.9)*
> *schizophrenia (295.0-295.9)*

The following fifth-digit subclassification is for use with category 299:

0 **current or active state**

1 **residual state**

⑤ **299.0** **Autistic disorder**
Childhood autism   Kanner's syndrome
Infantile psychosis

> *Excludes:* *disintegrative psychosis (299.1)*
> *Heller's syndrome (299.1)*
> *schizophrenic syndrome of childhood (299.9)*

⑤ **299.1** **Childhood disintegrative disorder**
Heller's syndrome

Use additional code to identify any associated neurological disorder

> *Excludes:* *infantile autism (299.0)*
> *schizophrenic syndrome of childhood (299.9)*

⑤ **299.8** **Other specified pervasive developmental disorders**
Asperger's disorder
Atypical childhood psychosis
Borderline psychosis of childhood

> *Excludes:* *simple stereotypies without psychotic disturbance (307.3)*

⑤ **299.9** **Unspecified pervasive developmental disorder**
Child psychosis NOS
Pervasive developmental disorder NOS
Schizophrenia, childhood type NOS
Schizophrenic syndrome of childhood NOS

> *Excludes:* *schizophrenia of adult type occurring in childhood (295.0-295.9)*

NEUROTIC DISORDERS, PERSONALITY DISORDERS, AND OTHER NONPSYCHOTIC MENTAL DISORDERS (300-316)

300 **Anxiety, dissociative and somatoform disorders**

⑤ **300.0** **Anxiety states**

> *Excludes:* *anxiety in:*
> *acute stress reaction (308.0)*
> *transient adjustment reaction (309.24)*
> *neurasthenia (300.5)*
> *psychophysiological disorders (306.0-306.9)*
> *separation anxiety (309.21)*

300.00 **Anxiety state, unspecified**
Anxiety:
neurosis
reaction
state (neurotic)
Atypical anxiety disorder

300.01 **Panic disorder without agoraphobia**
Panic:
attack
state

> *Excludes:* *panic disorder with agoraphobia (300.21)*

300.02 **Generalized anxiety disorder**

300.09 **Other**

⑤ **300.1** **Dissociative, conversion and factitious disorders**

> *Excludes:* *adjustment reaction (309.0-309.9)*
> *anorexia nervosa (307.1)*
> *gross stress reaction (308.0-308.9)*
> *hysterical personality (301.50-301.59)*
> *psychophysiologic disorders (306.0-306.9)*

300.10 **Hysteria, unspecified**

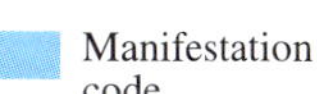

300.11 Conversion disorder
   Astasia-abasia, hysterical
   Conversion hysteria or reaction
   Hysterical:
     blindness
     deafness
     paralysis

300.12 Dissociative amnesia
   Hysterical amnesia

300.13 Dissociative fugue
   Hysterical fugue

300.14 Dissociative identity disorder

300.15 Dissociative disorder or reaction, unspecified

300.16 Factitious disorder with predominantly psychological signs and symptoms
   Compensation neurosis
   Ganser's syndrome, hysterical

300.19 Other and unspecified factitious illness
   Factitious disorder (with combined psychological and physical signs and
     symptoms) (with predominantly physical signs and symptoms) NOS

| Excludes: | *multiple operations or hospital addiction syndrome (301.51)* |

⑤ **300.2 Phobic disorders**

| Excludes: | *anxiety state not associated with a specific situation or object (300.0-300.09)* |
| | *obsessional phobias (300.3)* |

300.20 Phobia, unspecified
   Anxiety-hysteria NOS
   Phobia NOS

300.21 Agoraphobia with panic disorder
   Fear of:
       open spaces with panic attacks
       streets with panic attacks
       travel with panic attacks
   Panic disorder with agoraphobia

| Excludes: | *agoraphobia without panic disorder (300.22)* |
| | *panic disorder without agoraphobia (300.01)* |

300.22 Agoraphobia without mention of panic attacks
   Any condition classifiable to 300.21 without mention of panic attacks

300.23 Social phobia
   Fear of:
       eating in public
       public speaking
       washing in public

300.29 Other isolated or specific phobias
   Acrophobia   Claustrophobia
   Animal phobias   Fear of crowds

300.3 Obsessive-compulsive disorders
   Anancastic neurosis   Obsessional phobia [any]
   Compulsive neurosis

Excludes:	*obsessive-compulsive symptoms occurring in:*
	endogenous depression (296.2-296.3)
	organic states (e.g., encephalitis)
	schizophrenia (295.0-295.9)

300.4 Dysthymic disorder
   Anxiety depression   Neurotic depressive state
   Depression with anxiety   Reactive depression
   Depressive reaction

Excludes:	*adjustment reaction with depressive symptoms (309.0-309.1)*
	depression NOS (311)
	manic-depressive psychosis, depressed type (296.2-296.3)
	reactive depressive psychosis (298.0)

● Code new   ▲ Revision of   ④ ⑤ Fourth or fifth
   to this edition   existing code   digit required

300.5 Neurasthenia
Fatigue neurosis
Nervous debility
Psychogenic:
  asthenia
  general fatigue
Use additional code to identify any associated physical disorder

Excludes: *anxiety state (300.00-300.09)*

neurotic depression (300.4)
psychophysiological disorders (306.0-306.9)
specific nonpsychotic mental disorders following organic brain damage
  (310.0-310.9)

300.6 Depersonalization disorder
Derealization (neurotic)
Neurotic state with depersonalization episode

Excludes: *depersonalization associated with:*

anxiety (300.00-300.09)
depression (300.4)
manic-depressive disorder or psychosis (296.0-296.9)
schizophrenia (295.0-295.9)

300.7 Hypochondriasis
Body dysmorphic disorder

Excludes: *hypochondriasis in:*

hysteria (300.10-300.19)
manic-depressive psychosis, depressed type (296.2-296.3)
neurasthenia (300.5)
obsessional disorder (300.3)
schizophrenia (295.0-295.9)

⑤ **300.8 Somatoform disorders**

300.81 Somatization disorder
Briquet's disorder
Severe somatoform disorder

300.82 Undifferentiated somatoform disorder
Atypical somatoform disorder
Somatoform disorder NOS

300.89 Other somatoform disorders
Occupational neurosis, including writers' cramp
Psychasthenia
Psychasthenic neurosis

300.9 Unspecified nonpsychotic mental disorder
Psychoneurosis NOS

301 Personality disorders
Includes: character neurosis
Use additional code to identify any associated neurosis or psychosis, or physical condition

Excludes: *nonpsychotic personality disorder associated with organic brain syndromes*
  (310.0-310.9)

301.0 Paranoid personality disorder
Fanatic personality
Paranoid personality (disorder)
Paranoid traits

Excludes: *acute paranoid reaction (298.3)*

alcoholic paranoia (291.5)
paranoid schizophrenia (295.3)
paranoid states (297.0-297.9)

⑤ **301.1 Affective personality disorder**

Excludes: *affective psychotic disorders (296.0-296.9)*

neurasthenia (300.5)
neurotic depression (300.4)

301.10 Affective personality disorder, unspecified

301.11 Chronic hypomanic personality disorder
Chronic hypomanic disorder
Hypomanic personality

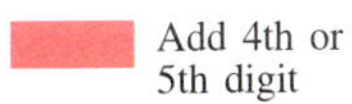

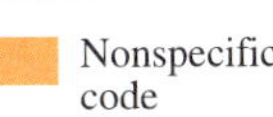

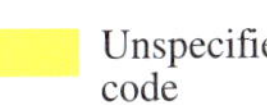

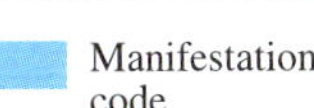

301.12 **Chronic depressive personality disorder**
Chronic depressive disorder
Depressive character or personality

301.13 **Cyclothymic disorder**
Cycloid personality
Cyclothymia
Cyclothymic personality

⑤ **301.2** **Schizoid personality disorder**
Excludes: *schizophrenia (295.0-295.9)*

301.20 **Schizoid personality disorder, unspecified**

301.21 **Introverted personality**

301.22 **Schizotypal personality disorder**

301.3 **Explosive personality disorder**

Aggressive: Emotional instability (excessive)
  personality   Pathological emotionality
  reaction   Quarrelsomeness
Aggressiveness

Excludes: *dyssocial personality (301.7)*
hysterical neurosis (300.10-300.19)

301.4 **Obsessive-compulsive personality disorder**
Anancastic personality
Obsessional personality

Excludes: *obsessive-compulsive disorder (300.3)*
phobic state (300.20-300.29)

⑤ **301.5** **Histrionic personality disorder**
Excludes: *hysterical neurosis (300.10-300.19)*

301.50 **Histrionic personality disorder, unspecified**
Hysterical personality NOS

301.51 **Chronic factitious illness with physical symptoms**
Hospital addiction syndrome
Multiple operations syndrome
Munchausen syndrome

301.59 **Other histrionic personality disorder**
Personality:
  emotionally unstable
  labile
  psychoinfantile

301.6 **Dependent personality disorder**
Asthenic personality   Passive personality
Inadequate personality

Excludes: *neurasthenia (300.5)*
passive-aggressive personality (301.84)

301.7 **Antisocial personality disorder**
Amoral personality
Asocial personality
Dyssocial personality
Personality disorder with predominantly sociopathic or asocial manifestation

Excludes: *disturbance of conduct without specifiable personality disorder (312.0-312.9)*
explosive personality (301.3)

⑤ **301.8** **Other personality disorders**

301.81 **Narcissistic personality disorder**

301.82 **Avoidant personality disorder**

301.83 **Borderline personality disorder**

301.84 **Passive-aggressive personality**

301.89 **Other**
Personality: Personality:
  eccentric   masochistic
  "haltlose" type   psychoneurotic
  immature

Excludes: *psychoinfantile personality (301.59)*

● Code new
  to this edition
    ▲ Revision of
     existing code
    ④ ⑤ Fourth or fifth
     digit required

301.9 Unspecified personality disorder
Pathological personality NOS
Personality disorder NOS
Psychopathic:
constitutional state
personality (disorder)

302 Sexual and gender identity disorders

Excludes: *sexual disorder manifest in:*
organic brain syndrome (290.0-294.9, 310.0-310.9)
psychosis (295.0-298.9)

302.0 Ego-dystonic sexual orientation
Ego-dystonic lesbianism
Sexual orientation conflict disorder

Excludes: *homosexual pedophilia (302.2)*

302.1 Zoophilia
Bestiality

302.2 Pedophilia

302.3 Transvestic fetishism

Excludes: *trans-sexualism (302.5)*

302.4 Exhibitionism

302.5 Trans-sexualism

Excludes: *transvestism (302.3)*

    302.50 With unspecified sexual history

    302.51 With asexual history

    302.52 With homosexual history

    302.53 With heterosexual history

302.6 Gender identity disorder in children
Feminism in boys
Gender identity disorder NOS

Excludes: *gender identity disorder in adult (302.85)*
trans-sexualism (302.50-302.53)
transvestism (302.3)

302.7 Psychosexual dysfunction

Excludes: *impotence of organic origin (607.84)*
normal transient symptoms from ruptured hymen
transient or occasional failures of erection due to fatigue, anxiety, alcohol, or drugs

    302.70 Psychosexual dysfunction, unspecified
Sexual dysfunction NOS

    302.71 Hypoactive sexual desire disorder

Excludes: *decreased sexual desire NOS (799.81)*

    302.72 With inhibited sexual excitement
Female sexual arousal disorder
Frigidity
Impotence
Male erectile disorder

    302.73 Female orgasmic disorder

    302.74 Male orgasmic disorder

    302.75 Premature ejaculation

    302.76 Dyspareunia, psychogenic

    302.79 With other specified psychosexual dysfunctions
Sexual aversion disorder

302.8 Other specified psychosexual disorders

    302.81 Fetishism

    302.82 Voyeurism

    302.83 Sexual masochism

    302.84 Sexual sadism

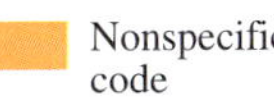

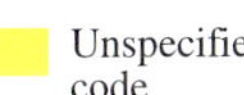

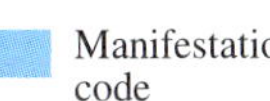

302.85 Gender identity disorder in adolescents or adults
Excludes: *gender identity disorder NOS (302.6)*
gender identity disorder in children (302.6)

302.89 Other
Frotteurism
Nymphomania
Satyriasis

302.9 Unspecified psychosexual disorder
Paraphilia NOS
Pathologic sexuality NOS
Sexual deviation NOS
Sexual disorder NOS

⑤ **303 Alcohol dependence syndrome**
Use additional code to identify any associated condition, as:
alcoholic psychoses (291.0-291.9)
drug dependence (304.0-304.9)
physical complications of alcohol, such as:
cerebral degeneration (331.7)
cirrhosis of liver (571.2)
epilepsy (345.0-345.9)
gastritis (535.3)
hepatitis (571.1)
liver damage NOS (571.3)

Excludes: *drunkenness NOS (305.0)*

The following fifth-digit subclassification is for use with category 303:

0 unspecified

1 continuous

2 episodic

3 in remission

⑤ **303.0 Acute alcoholic intoxication**
Acute drunkenness in alcoholism

⑤ **303.9 Other and unspecified alcohol dependence**
Chronic alcoholism
Dipsomania

⑤ **304 Drug dependence**
Excludes: *nondependent abuse of drugs (305.1-305.9)*

The following fifth-digit subclassification is for use with category 304:

0 unspecified

1 continuous

2 episodic

3 in remission

⑤ **304.0 Opioid type dependence**
Heroin   Opium alkaloids and their derivatives
Meperidine   Synthetics with morphine-like effects
Methadone
Morphine
Opium

⑤ **304.1 Sedative, hypnotic or anxiolytic dependence**
Barbiturates
Nonbarbiturate sedatives and tranquilizers with a similar effect:
chlordiazepoxide
diazepam
glutethimide
meprobamate
methaqualone

⑤ **304.2 Cocaine dependence**
Coca leaves and derivatives

● Code new   ▲ Revision of   ④ ⑤ Fourth or fifth
to this edition   existing code   digit required

⑤ **304.3 Cannabis dependence**
  Hashish
  Hemp
  Marihuana

⑤ **304.4 Amphetamine and other psychostimulant dependence**
  Methylphenidate
  Phenmetrazine

⑤ **304.5 Hallucinogen dependence**
  Dimethyltryptamine [DMT]
  Lysergic acid diethylamide [LSD] and derivatives
  Mescaline
  Psilocybin

⑤ **304.6 Other specified drug dependence**
  Absinthe addiction
  Glue sniffing
  Inhalant dependence
  Phencyclidine dependence

  Excludes: tobacco dependence (305.1)

⑤ **304.7 Combinations of opioid type drug with any other**
⑤ **304.8 Combinations of drug dependence excluding opioid type drug**
⑤ **304.9 Unspecified drug dependence**
  Drug addiction NOS
  Drug dependence NOS

305 Nondependent abuse of drugs
  Note: Includes cases where a person, for whom no other diagnosis is possible, has come under
  medical care because of the maladaptive effect of a drug on which he is not dependent
  and that he has taken on his own initiative to the detriment of his health or social
  functioning.

  Excludes: alcohol dependence syndrome (303.0-303.9)
  drug dependence (304.0-304.9)
  drug withdrawal syndrome (292.0)
  poisoning by drugs or medicinal substances (960.0-979.9)

The following fifth-digit subclassification is for use with codes 305.0, 305.2-305.9:

  0 unspecified

  1 continuous

  2 episodic

  3 in remission

⑤ **305.0 Alcohol abuse**
  Drunkenness NOS   "Hangover" (alcohol)
  Excessive drinking of alcohol NOS   Inebriety NOS

  Excludes: acute alcohol intoxication in alcoholism (303.0)
  alcoholic psychoses (291.0-291.9)

  305.1 Tobacco use disorder
  Tobacco dependence

  Excludes: history of tobacco use (V15.82)
  smoking complicating pregnancy (649.0)
  tobacco use disorder complicating pregnancy (649.0)

⑤ **305.2 Cannabis abuse**
⑤ **305.3 Hallucinogen abuse**
  Acute intoxication from hallucinogens ["bad trips"]
  LSD reaction

⑤ **305.4 Sedative, hypnotic or anxiolytic abuse**
⑤ **305.5 Opioid abuse**
⑤ **305.6 Cocaine abuse**
⑤ **305.7 Amphetamine or related acting sympathomimetic abuse**
⑤ **305.8 Antidepressant type abuse**

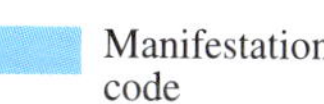

	Add 4th or 5th digit		Nonspecific code		Unspecified code		Manifestation code

⑤ **305.9** **Other, mixed, or unspecified drug abuse**
Caffeine intoxication
Inhalant abuse
"Laxative habit"
Misuse of drugs NOS
Nonprescribed use of drugs or patent medicinals
Phencyclidine abuse

306 **Physiological malfunction arising from mental factors**
Includes: psychogenic:
physical symptoms not involving tissue damage
physiological manifestation not involving tissue damage

Excludes: *hysteria (300.11-300.19)*

physical symptoms secondary to a psychiatric disorder classified elsewhere
psychic factors associated with physical conditions involving tissue damage
classified elsewhere (316)
specific nonpsychotic mental disorders following organic brain damage
(310.0-310.9)

306.0 Musculoskeletal
Psychogenic paralysis
Psychogenic torticollis

Excludes: *Gilles de la Tourette's syndrome (307.23)*

paralysis as hysterical or conversion reaction (300.11)
tics (307.20-307.22)

306.1 Respiratory
Psychogenic:
air hunger
cough
hiccough

Psychogenic:
hyperventilation
yawning

Excludes: *psychogenic asthma (316 and 493.9)*

306.2 Cardiovascular
Cardiac neurosis
Cardiovascular neurosis
Neurocirculatory asthenia
Psychogenic cardiovascular disorder

Excludes: *psychogenic paroxysmal tachycardia (316 and 427.2)*

306.3 Skin
Psychogenic pruritus

Excludes: *psychogenic:*

alopecia (316 and 704.00)
dermatitis (316 and 692.9)
eczema (316 and 691.8 or 692.9)
urticaria (316 and 708.0-708.9)

306.4 Gastrointestinal
Aerophagy
Cyclical vomiting,
psychogenic

Diarrhea, psychogenic
Nervous gastritis
Psychogenic dyspepsia

Excludes: *cyclical vomiting NOS (536.2)*

globus hystericus (300.11)
mucous colitis (316 and 564.9)
psychogenic:
cardiospasm (316 and 530.0)
duodenal ulcer (316 and 532.0-532.9)
gastric ulcer (316 and 531.0-531.9)
peptic ulcer NOS (316 and 533.0-533.9)
vomiting NOS (307.54)

⑤ **306.5 Genitourinary**

Excludes: *enuresis, psychogenic (307.6)*

frigidity (302.72)
impotence (302.72)
psychogenic dyspareunia (302.76)

306.50 **Psychogenic genitourinary malfunction, unspecified**

306.51 **Psychogenic vaginismus**
Functional vaginismus

306.52 **Psychogenic dysmenorrhea**

   ● Code new
to this edition

▲ Revision of
existing code

④ ⑤ Fourth or fifth
digit required

306.53 **Psychogenic dysuria**

306.59 **Other**

306.6 **Endocrine**

306.7 **Organs of special sense**

Excludes: *hysterical blindness or deafness (300.11)*

psychophysical visual disturbances (368.16)

306.8 **Other specified psychophysiological malfunction**
Bruxism
Teeth grinding

306.9 **Unspecified psychophysiological malfunction**
Psychophysiologic disorder NOS
Psychosomatic disorder NOS

307 **Special symptoms or syndromes, not elsewhere classified**
Note: This category is intended for use if the psychopathology is manifested by a single specific
symptom or group of symptoms which is not part of an organic illness or other mental
disorder classifiable elsewhere.

Excludes: *those due to mental disorders classified elsewhere*

those of organic origin

307.0 **Stuttering**

Excludes: *dysphasia (784.5)*

lisping or lalling (307.9)
retarded development of speech (315.31-315.39)

307.1 **Anorexia nervosa**

Excludes: *eating disturbance NOS (307.50)*

feeding problem (783.3)
of nonorganic origin (307.59)
loss of appetite (783.0)
of nonorganic origin (307.59)

⑤ **307.2** **Tics**

Excludes: *nail-biting or thumb-sucking (307.9)*

stereotypies occurring in isolation (307.3)
tics of organic origin (333.3)

307.20 **Tic disorder, unspecified**
Tic disorder NOS

307.21 **Transient tic disorder**

307.22 **Chronic motor or vocal tic disorder**

307.23 **Tourette's disorder**
Motor-verbal tic disorder

307.3 **Stereotypic movement disorder**
Body-rocking   Spasmus nutans
Head banging   Stereotypies NOS

Excludes: *tics (307.20-307.23)*

of organic origin (333.3)

⑤ **307.4** **Specific disorders of sleep of nonorganic origin**

Excludes: *narcolepsy (347.00-347.11)*

organic hypersomnia (327.10-327.19)
organic insomnia (327.00-327.09)
those of unspecified cause (780.50-780.59)

307.40 **Nonorganic sleep disorder, unspecified**

307.41 **Transient disorder of initiating or maintaining sleep**
Adjustment insomnia
Hyposomnia associated with acute or intermittent emotional reactions or
conflicts
Insomnia associated with acute or intermittent emotional reactions or conflicts
Sleeplessness associated with acute or intermittent emotional reactions or
conflicts

307.42   Persistent disorder of initiating or maintaining sleep
Hyposomnia, insomnia, or sleeplessness associated with:
   anxiety
   conditioned arousal
   depression (major) (minor)
   psychosis
Idiopathic insomnia
Paradoxical insomnia
Primary insomnia
Psychophysiological insomnia

307.43   Transient disorder of initiating or maintaining wakefulness
Hypersomnia associated with acute or intermittent emotional reactions or conflicts

307.44   Persistent disorder of initiating or maintaining wakefulness
Hypersomnia associated with depression (major) (minor)
Insufficient sleep syndrome
Primary hypersomnia

Excludes: *sleep deprivation (V69.4)*

307.45   Circadian rhythm sleep disorder of nonorganic origin

307.46   Sleep arousal disorder
Night terror disorder
Night terrors
Sleep terror disorder
Sleepwalking
Somnambulism

307.47   Other dysfunctions of sleep stages or arousal from sleep
Dyssomnia NOS
Nightmare disorder
Nightmares:
   NOS
   REM-sleep type
Parasomnia NOS
Sleep drunkenness

307.48   Repetitive intrusions of sleep
Repetitive intrusion of sleep with:
   atypical polysomnographic features
   environmental disturbances
   repeated REM-sleep interruptions

307.49   Other
"Short-sleeper"
Subjective insomnia complaint

⑤ **307.5   Other and unspecified disorders of eating**

Excludes: *anorexia:*
   nervosa (307.1)
   of unspecified cause (783.0)
overeating, of unspecified cause (783.6)
vomiting:
   NOS (787.0)
   cyclical (536.2)
   psychogenic (306.4)

307.50   Eating disorder, unspecified
Eating disorder NOS

307.51   Bulimia nervosa
Overeating of nonorganic origin

307.52   Pica
Perverted appetite of nonorganic origin

307.53   Rumination disorder
Regurgitation, of nonorganic origin, of food with reswallowing

Excludes: *obsessional rumination (300.3)*

307.54   Psychogenic vomiting

307.59   Other
Feeding disorder of infancy or early childhood of nonorganic origin
Infantile feeding disturbances of nonorganic origin
Loss of appetite of nonorganic origin

   ● Code new   ▲ Revision of   ④ ⑤ Fourth or fifth
   to this edition   existing code   digit required

307.6 Enuresis
Enuresis (primary) (secondary) of nonorganic origin

Excludes: *enuresis of unspecified cause (788.3)*

307.7 Encopresis
Encopresis (continuous) (discontinuous) of nonorganic origin

Excludes: *encopresis of unspecified cause (787.6)*

⑤ **307.8 Pain disorders related to psychological factors**

307.80 Psychogenic pain, site unspecified

307.81 Tension headache

Excludes: *headache:*
NOS (784.0)
migraine (346.0-346.9)

307.89 Other
Code first to type or site of pain

Excludes: *pain disorder exclusively attributed to psychological factors (307.80)*
psychogenic pain (307.80)

307.9 Other and unspecified special symptoms or syndromes, not elsewhere classified
Communication disorder NOS
Hair plucking
Lalling
Lisping
Masturbation
Nail-biting
Thumb-sucking

308 Acute reaction to stress
Includes: catastrophic stress
combat fatigue
gross stress reaction (acute)
transient disorders in response to exceptional physical or mental stress which
usually subside within hours or days

Excludes: *adjustment reaction or disorder (309.0-309.9)*
chronic stress reaction (309.1-309.9)

308.0 Predominant disturbance of emotions
Anxiety as acute reaction to exceptional [gross] stress
Emotional crisis as acute reaction to exceptional [gross] stress
Panic state as acute reaction to exceptional [gross] stress

308.1 Predominant disturbance of consciousness
Fugues as acute reaction to exceptional [gross] stress

308.2 Predominant psychomotor disturbance
Agitation states as acute reaction to exceptional [gross] stress
Stupor as acute reaction to exceptional [gross] stress

308.3 Other acute reactions to stress
Acute situational disturbance
Acute stress disorder

Excludes: *prolonged posttraumatic emotional disturbance (309.81)*

308.4 Mixed disorders as reaction to stress

308.9 Unspecified acute reaction to stress

309 Adjustment reaction
Includes: adjustment disorders
reaction (adjustment) to chronic stress

Excludes: *acute reaction to major stress (308.0-308.9)*
neurotic disorders (300.0-300.9)

309.0 Adjustment disorder with depressed mood
Grief reaction

Excludes: *affective psychoses (296.0-296.9)*
neurotic depression (300.4)
prolonged depressive reaction (309.1)
psychogenic depressive psychosis (298.0)

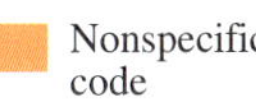

Nonspecific
code

Unspecified
code

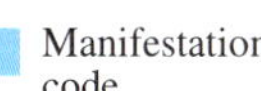

309.1 Prolonged depressive reaction

> *Excludes:* *affective psychoses (296.0-296.9)*
> *brief depressive reaction (309.0)*
> *neurotic depression (300.4)*
> *psychogenic depressive psychosis (298.0)*

⑤ **309.2 With predominant disturbance of other emotions**

309.21 Separation anxiety disorder

309.22 Emancipation disorder of adolescence and early adult life

309.23 Specific academic or work inhibition

309.24 Adjustment disorder with anxiety

309.28 Adjustment disorder with mixed anxiety and depressed mood
Adjustment reaction with anxiety and depression

309.29 Other
Culture shock

309.3 Adjustment disorder with disturbance of conduct
Conduct disturbance as adjustment reaction
Destructiveness as adjustment reaction

> *Excludes:* *destructiveness in child (312.9)*
> *disturbance of conduct NOS (312.9)*
> *dyssocial behavior without manifest psychiatric disorder (V71.01-V71.02)*
> *personality disorder with predominantly sociopathic or asocial manifestations (301.7)*

309.4 Adjustment disorder with mixed disturbance of emotions and conduct

⑤ **309.8 Other specified adjustment reactions**

309.81 Posttraumatic stress disorder
Chronic posttraumatic stress disorder
Concentration camp syndrome
Posttraumatic stress disorder NOS
Post-Traumatic Stress Disorder (PTSD)

> *Excludes:* *acute stress disorder (308.3)*
> *posttraumatic brain syndrome:*
> *nonpsychotic (310.2)*
> *psychotic (293.0-293.9)*

309.82 Adjustment reaction with physical symptoms

309.83 Adjustment reaction with withdrawal
Elective mutism as adjustment reaction
Hospitalism (in children) NOS

309.89 Other

309.9 Unspecified adjustment reaction
Adaptation reaction NOS
Adjustment reaction NOS

310 Specific nonpsychotic mental disorders due to brain damage

> *Excludes:* *neuroses, personality disorders, or other nonpsychotic conditions occurring in a form similar to that seen with functional disorders but in association with a physical condition (300.0-300.9, 301.0-301.9)*

310.0 Frontal lobe syndrome
Lobotomy syndrome
Postleucotomy syndrome [state]

> *Excludes:* *postcontusion syndrome (310.2)*

310.1 Personality change due to conditions classified elsewhere
Cognitive or personality change of other type, of nonpsychotic severity
Organic psychosyndrome of nonpsychotic severity
Presbyophrenia NOS
Senility with mental changes of nonpsychotic severity

> *Excludes:* *memory loss of unknown cause (780.93)*

● Code new to this edition   ▲ Revision of existing code   ④ ⑤ Fourth or fifth digit required

310.2 Postconcussion syndrome
      Postcontusion syndrome or encephalopathy
      Posttraumatic brain syndrome, nonpsychotic
      Status postcommotio cerebri

> *Excludes:* *frontal lobe syndrome (310.0)*
>   *postencephalitic syndrome (310.8)*
>   *any organic psychotic conditions following head injury (293.0—294.0)*

310.8 Other specified nonpsychotic mental disorders following organic brain damage
      Mild memory disturbance
      Postencephalitic syndrome
      Other focal (partial) organic psychosyndromes

310.9 Unspecified nonpsychotic mental disorder following organic brain damage

311 Depressive disorder, not elsewhere classified
    Depressive disorder NOS
    Depressive state NOS
    Depression NOS

> *Excludes:* *acute reaction to major stress with depressive symptoms (308.0)*
>   *affective personality disorder (301.10-301.13)*
>   *affective psychoses (296.0-296.9)*
>   *brief depressive reaction (309.0)*
>   *depressive states associated with stressful events (309.0-309.1)*
>   *disturbance of emotions specific to childhood and adolescence, with misery and*
>   *unhappiness (313.1)*
>   *mixed adjustment reaction with depressive symptoms (309.4)*
>   *neurotic depression (300.4)*
>   *prolonged depressive adjustment reaction (309.1)*
>   *psychogenic depressive psychosis (298.0)*

312 Disturbance of conduct, not elsewhere classified

> *Excludes:* *adjustment reaction with disturbance of conduct (309.3)*
>   *drug dependence (304.0-304.9)*
>   *dyssocial behavior without manifest psychiatric disorder (V71.01-V71.02)*
>   *personality disorder with predominantly sociopathic or asocial manifestations*
>   *(301.7)*
>   *sexual deviations (302.0-302.9)*

The following fifth-digit subclassification is for use with categories 312.0-312.2:

    0 unspecified

    1 mild

    2 moderate

    3 severe

⑤ **312.0 Undersocialized conduct disorder, aggressive type**
      Aggressive outburst   Unsocialized aggressive disorder
      Anger reaction

⑤ **312.1 Undersocialized conduct disorder, unaggressive type**
      Childhood truancy,   Solitary stealing
        unsocialized   Tantrums

⑤ **312.2 Socialized conduct disorder**
      Childhood truancy, socialized
      Group delinquency

> *Excludes:* *gang activity without manifest psychiatric disorder (V71.01)*

⑤ **312.3 Disorders of impulse control, not elsewhere classified**

    312.30 Impulse control disorder, unspecified

    312.31 Pathological gambling

    312.32 Kleptomania

    312.33 Pyromania

    312.34 Intermittent explosive disorder

    312.35 Isolated explosive disorder

    312.39 Other
        Trichotillomania

312.4 Mixed disturbance of conduct and emotions
      Neurotic delinquency

> *Excludes:* *compulsive conduct disorder (312.3)*

Add 4th or 5th digit	Nonspecific code	Unspecified code	Manifestation code

⑤ **312.8** **Other specified disturbances of conduct, not elsewhere classified**

    312.81 **Conduct disorder, childhood onset type**

    312.82 **Conduct disorder, adolescent onset type**

    312.89 **Other conduct disorder**
        Conduct disorder of unspecified onset

312.9 **Unspecified disturbance of conduct**
    Delinquency (juvenile)
    Disruptive behavior disorder NOS

313 **Disturbance of emotions specific to childhood and adolescence**

    Excludes: *adjustment reaction (309.0-309.9)*

        emotional disorder of neurotic type (300.0-300.9)
        masturbation, nail-biting, thumb-sucking, and other isolated symptoms
          (307.0-307.9)

313.0 **Overanxious disorder**
    Anxiety and fearfulness of childhood and adolescence
    Overanxious disorder of childhood and adolescence

    Excludes: *abnormal separation anxiety (309.21)*

        anxiety states (300.00-300.09)
        hospitalism in children (309.83)
        phobic state (300.20-300.29)

313.1 **Misery and unhappiness disorder**
    Excludes: *depressive neurosis (300.4)*

⑤ **313.2** **Sensitivity, shyness, and social withdrawal disorder**
    Excludes: *infantile autism (299.0)*

        schizoid personality (301.20-301.22)
        schizophrenia (295.0-295.9)

    313.21 **Shyness disorder of childhood**
        Sensitivity reaction of childhood or adolescence

    313.22 **Introverted disorder of childhood**
        Social withdrawal of childhood and adolescence
        Withdrawal reaction of childhood and adolescence

    313.23 **Selective mutism**
    Excludes: *elective mutism as adjustment reaction (309.83)*

313.3 **Relationship problems**
    Sibling jealousy

    Excludes: *relationship problems associated with aggression, destruction, or other forms of*
        conduct disturbance (312.0-312.9)

⑤ **313.8** **Other or mixed emotional disturbances of childhood or adolescence**

    313.81 **Oppositional defiant disorder**

    313.82 **Identity disorder**
        Identity problem

    313.83 **Academic underachievement disorder**

    313.89 **Other**
        Reactive attachment disorder of infancy or early childhood

313.9 **Unspecified emotional disturbance of childhood or adolescence**
    Mental disorder of infancy, childhood or adolescence NOS

314 **Hyperkinetic syndrome of childhood**

    Excludes: *hyperkinesis as symptom of underlying disorder—code the underlying disorder*

⑤ **314.0** **Attention deficit disorder**
    Adult
    Child

    314.00 **Without mention of hyperactivity**
        Predominantly inattentive type

    314.01 **With hyperactivity**
        Combined type
        Overactivity NOS
        Predominantly hyperactive/impulsive type
        Simple disturbance of attention with overactivity

  ● Code new
    to this edition
    ▲ Revision of
      existing code
    ④ ⑤ Fourth or fifth
        digit required

314.1 Hyperkinesis with developmental delay
Developmental disorder of hyperkinesis

Use additional code to identify any associated neurological disorder

314.2 Hyperkinetic conduct disorder
Hyperkinetic conduct disorder without developmental delay

Excludes: *hyperkinesis with significant delays in specific skills (314.1)*

314.8 Other specified manifestations of hyperkinetic syndrome

314.9 Unspecified hyperkinetic syndrome
Hyperkinetic reaction of childhood or adolescence NOS
Hyperkinetic syndrome NOS

315 Specific delays in development
Excludes: *that due to a neurological disorder (320.0-389.9)*

⑤ **315.0 Specific reading disorder**

315.00 Reading disorder, unspecified

315.01 Alexia

315.02 Developmental dyslexia

315.09 Other
Specific spelling difficulty

315.1 Mathematics disorder
Dyscalculia

315.2 Other specific learning difficulties
Disorder of written expression

Excludes: *specific arithmetical disorder (315.1)*
specific reading disorder (315.00-315.09)

⑤ **315.3 Developmental speech or language disorder**

315.31 Expressive language disorder
Developmental aphasia
Word deafness

Excludes: *acquired aphasia (784.3)*
elective mutism (309.83, 313.0, 313.23)

315.32 Mixed receptive-expressive language disorder

315.39 Other
Developmental articulation disorder
Dyslalia
Phonological disorder

Excludes: *lisping and lalling (307.9)*
stammering and stuttering (307.0)

315.4 Developmental coordination disorder
Clumsiness syndrome
Dyspraxia syndrome
Specific motor development disorder

315.5 Mixed development disorder

315.8 Other specified delays in development

315.9 Unspecified delay in development
Developmental disorder NOS
Learning disorder NOS

Add 4th or 5th digit	Nonspecific code	Unspecified code	Manifestation code

316 Psychic factors associated with diseases classified elsewhere
Psychologic factors in physical conditions classified elsewhere

Use additional code to identify the associated physical condition, as:
    psychogenic:
        asthma (493.9)
        dermatitis (692.9)
        duodenal ulcer (532.0-532.9)
        eczema (691.8, 692.9)
        gastric ulcer (531.0-531.9)
        mucous colitis (564.9)
        paroxysmal tachycardia (427.2)
        ulcerative colitis (556)
        urticaria (708.0-708.9)
    psychosocial dwarfism (259.4)

> *Excludes:* *physical symptoms and physiological malfunctions, not involving tissue damage, of mental origin (306.0-306.9)*

MENTAL RETARDATION (317-319)

Use additional code(s) to identify any associated psychiatric or physical condition(s)

317 Mild mental retardation
    High-grade defect   Mild mental subnormality
    IQ 50-70

318 Other specified mental retardation

    318.0 Moderate mental retardation
        IQ 35-49
        Moderate mental subnormality

    318.1 Severe mental retardation
        IQ 20-34
        Severe mental subnormality

    318.2 Profound mental retardation
        IQ under 20
        Profound mental subnormality

319 Unspecified mental retardation
    Mental deficiency NOS
    Mental subnormality NOS

● Code new to this edition   ▲ Revision of existing code   ④ ⑤ Fourth or fifth digit required

6. DISEASES OF THE NERVOUS SYSTEM AND SENSE ORGANS (320-389)

INFLAMMATORY DISEASES OF THE CENTRAL NERVOUS SYSTEM (320-326)

320 Bacterial meningitis

Includes: arachnoiditis, bacterial
leptomeningitis, bacterial
meningitis, bacterial
meningoencephalitis, bacterial
meningomyelitis, bacterial
pachymeningitis, bacterial

320.0 Hemophilus meningitis
Meningitis due to Hemophilus influenzae [H. influenzae]

320.1 Pneumococcal meningitis

320.2 Streptococcal meningitis

320.3 Staphylococcal meningitis

320.7 *Meningitis in other bacterial diseases classified elsewhere*
Code first underlying disease, as:
actinomycosis (039.8)
listeriosis (027.0)
typhoid fever (002.0)
whooping cough (033.0-033.9)

Excludes: *meningitis (in):*

epidemic (036.0)
gonococcal (098.82)
meningococcal (036.0)
salmonellosis (003.21)
syphilis:
  NOS (094.2)
  congenital (090.42)
  meningovascular (094.2)
  secondary (091.81)
tuberculous (013.0)

⑤ **320.8 Meningitis due to other specified bacteria**

320.81 Anaerobic meningitis
Bacteroides (fragilis)
Gram-negative anaerobes

320.82 Meningitis due to Gram-negative bacteria, not elsewhere classified
Aerobacter aerogenes
Escherichia coli [E. coli]
Friedlander bacillus
Klebsiella pneumoniae
Proteus morganii
Pseudomonas

Excludes: *Gram-negative anaerobes (320.81)*

320.89 Meningitis due to other specified bacteria
Bacillus pyocyaneus

320.9 Meningitis due to unspecified bacterium

Meningitis:
  bacterial NOS
  purulent NOS

Meningitis:
  pyogenic NOS
  suppurative NOS

321 Meningitis due to other organisms
Includes: arachnoiditis due to organisms other than bacteria
leptomeningitis due to organisms other than bacteria
meningitis due to organisms other than bacteria
pachymeningitis due to organisms other than bacteria

321.0 *Cryptococcal meningitis*
Code first underlying disease (117.5)

321.1 *Meningitis in other fungal diseases*
Code first underlying disease (110.0-118)

Excludes: *meningitis in:*

candidiasis (112.83)
coccidioidomycosis (114.2)
histoplasmosis (115.01, 115.11, 115.91)

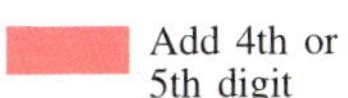

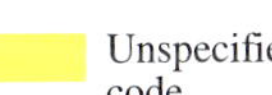

Manifestation
code

321.2 Meningitis due to viruses not elsewhere classified
    Code first underlying disease, as:
      meningitis due to arbovirus (060.0-066.9)

      Excludes: *meningitis (due to):*
          abacterial (047.0-047.9)
          adenovirus (049.1)
          aseptic NOS (047.9)
          Coxsackie (virus) (047.0)
          ECHO virus (047.1)
          enterovirus (047.0-047.9)
          herpes simplex virus (054.72)
          herpes zoster virus (053.0)
          lymphocytic choriomeningitis virus (049.0)
          mumps (072.1)
          viral NOS (047.9)
          meningo-eruptive syndrome (047.1)

321.3 Meningitis due to trypanosomiasis
    Code first underlying disease (086.0-086.9)

321.4 Meningitis in sarcoidosis
    Code first underlying disease (135)

321.8 Meningitis due to other nonbacterial organisms classified elsewhere
    Code first underlying disease

      Excludes: *leptospiral meningitis (100.81)*

322 Meningitis of unspecified cause
    Includes: arachnoiditis with no organism specified as cause
              leptomeningitis with no organism specified as cause
              meningitis with no organism specified as cause
              pachymeningitis with no organism specified as cause

322.0 Nonpyogenic meningitis
    Meningitis with clear cerebrospinal fluid

322.1 Eosinophilic meningitis

322.2 Chronic meningitis

322.9 Meningitis, unspecified

323 Encephalitis, myelitis, and encephalomyelitis
    Includes: acute disseminated encephalomyelitis
              meningoencephalitis, except bacterial
              meningomyelitis, except bacterial
              myelitis:
                  ascending
                  transverse

      Excludes: *acute transverse myelitis NOS (341.20)*

          acute transverse myelitis in conditions classified elsewhere (341.21)
          bacterial:
              meningoencephalitis (320.0-320.9)
              meningomyelitis (320.0-320.9)
              idiopathic transverse myelitis (341.22)
          idiopathic transverse myelitis (341.22)

▲ **323.0 Encephalitis, myelitis, and encephalomyelitis in viral diseases classified elsewhere**
    Code first underlying disease, as:
      cat-scratch disease (078.3)
      infectious mononucleosis (075)
      ornithosis (073.7)

    ● **323.01 Encephalitis and encephalomyelitis in viral diseases classified elsewhere**
      Excludes: *encephalitis (in):*

          arthropod-borne viral (062.0-064)
          herpes simplex (054.3)
          mumps (072.2)
          other viral diseases of central nervous system (049.8-049.9)
          poliomyelitis (045.0-045.9)
          rubella (056.01)
          slow virus infections of central nervous system (046.0-046.9)
          viral NOS (049.9)
          West Nile (066.41)

  ● Code new   ▲ Revision of   ④ ⑤ Fourth or fifth
     to this edition   existing code   digit required

● **323.02 Myelitis in viral diseases classified elsewhere**

Excludes: myelitis (in):
> herpes simplex (054.74)
> herpes zoster (053.14)
> poliomyelitis (045.0-045.9)
> rubella (056.01)
> other viral diseases of central nervous system (049.8-049.9)

▲ **323.1 Encephalitis, myelitis, and encephalomyelitis in rickettsial diseases classified elsewhere**
> Code first underlying disease (080-083.9)

▲ **323.2 Encephalitis, myelitis, and encephalomyelitis in protozoal diseases classified elsewhere**
> Code first underlying disease, as:
> malaria (084.0-084.9)
> trypanosomiasis (086.0-086.9)

▲ **323.4 Other encephalitis, myelitis, and encephalomyelitis due to infection classified elsewhere**
> Code first underlying disease

● **323.41 Other encephalitis and encephalomyelitis due to infection classified elsewhere**

Excludes: encephalitis (in):
> meningococcal (036.1)
> syphilis:
>> NOS (094.81)
>> congenital (090.41)
> toxoplasmosis (130.0)
> tuberculosis (013.6)
> meningoencephalitis due to free-living ameba [Naegleria] ((136.2)

● **323.42 Other myelitis due to infection classified elsewhere**

Excludes: myelitis (in):
> syphilis (094.89)
> tuberculosis (013.6)

▲ **323.5 Encephalitis, myelitis, and encephalomyelitis following immunization procedures**
Use additional E code, if desired, to identify vaccine

● **323.51 Encephalitis and encephalomyelitis following immunization procedures**
> Encephalitis postimmunization or postvaccinal
> Encephalomyelitis postimmunization or postvaccinal

● **323.52 Myelitis following immunization procedures**
> Myelitis postimmunization or postvaccinal

▲ **323.6 Postinfectious encephalitis, myelitis, and encephalomyelitis**
> Code first underlying disease

● **323.61 Infectious acute disseminated encephalomyelitis (ADEM)**
> Acute necrotizing hemorrhagic encephalopathy

Excludes: noninfectious acute disseminated encephalomyelitis (ADEM) (323.81)

● **323.62 Other postinfectious encephalitis and encephalomyelitis**

Excludes: encephalitis:
> postchickenpox (052.0)
> postmeasles (055.0)

● **323.63 Postinfectious myelitis**

Excludes: postchickenpox myelitis (052.2)
> herpes simplex myelitis (054.74)
> herpes zoster myelitis (053.14)

▲ **323.7 Toxic encephalitis, myelitis, and encephalomyelitis**
> Code first underlying cause, as:
> carbon tetrachloride (982.1)
> hydroxyquinoline derivatives (961.3)
> lead (984.0-984.9)
> mercury (985.0)
> thallium (985.8)

● **323.71 Toxic encephalitis and encephalomyelitis**

● **323.72 Toxic myelitis**

▲ **323.8 Other causes of encephalitis, myelitis, and encephalomyelitis**

● **323.81 Other causes of encephalitis and encephalomyelitis**
> Noninfectious acute disseminated encephalomyelitis (ADEM)

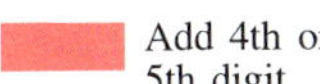

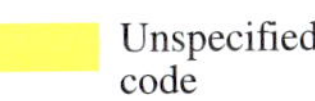

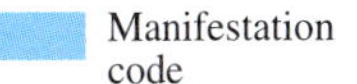

● **323.82** **Other causes of myelitis**
Transverse myelitis NOS

▲ **323.9** **Unspecified causes of encephalitis, myelitis, and encephalomyelitis**

324 **Intracranial and intraspinal abscess**

324.0 **Intracranial abscess**

Abscess (embolic):
cerebellar
cerebral

Abscess (embolic) of brain [any part]:
epidural
extradural
otogenic
subdural

Excludes: *tuberculous (013.3)*

324.1 **Intraspinal abscess**
Abscess (embolic) of spinal cord [any part]:
epidural
extradural
subdural

Excludes: *tuberculous (013.5)*

324.9 **Of unspecified site**
Extradural or subdural abscess NOS

325 **Phlebitis and thrombophlebitis of intracranial venous sinuses**
Embolism, of cavernous, lateral, or other intracranial or unspecified intracranial venous sinus
Endophlebitis, of cavernous, lateral, or other intracranial or unspecified intracranial venous sinus
Phlebitis, septic or suppurative, of cavernous, lateral, or other intracranial or unspecified intracranial venous sinus
Thrombophlebitis of cavernous, lateral, or other intracranial or unspecified intracranial venous sinus
Thrombosis of cavernous, lateral, or other intracranial or unspecified intracranial venous sinus

Excludes: *that specified as:*

complicating pregnancy, childbirth, or the puerperium (671.5)
of nonpyogenic origin (437.6)

326 **Late effects of intracranial abscess or pyogenic infection**
Note: This category is to be used to indicate conditions whose primary classification is to 320-325 [excluding 320.7, 321.0-321.8, 323.01-323.42, 323.61-323.72] as the cause of late effects, themselves classifiable elsewhere. The "late effects" include conditions specified as such, or as sequelae, which may occur at any time after the resolution of the causal condition.

Use additional code, if desired, to identify condition, as:
hydrocephalus (331.4)
paralysis (342.0-342.9, 344.0-344.9)

ORGANIC SLEEP DISORDERS (327)

327 **Organic sleep disorders**

⑤ **327.0** **Organic disorders of initiating and maintaining sleep [Organic insomnia]**
Excludes: *insomnia NOS (780.52)*

insomnia not due to a substance or known physiological condition (307.41-307.42)
insomnia with sleep apnea NOS (780.51)

327.00 **Organic insomnia, unspecified**

327.01 **Insomnia due to medical condition classified elsewhere**
Code first underlying condition

Excludes: *insomnia due to mental disorder (327.02)*

327.02 **Insomnia due to mental disorder**
Code first mental disorder

Excludes: *alcohol induced insomnia (291.82)*

drug induced insomnia (292.85)

327.09 **Other organic insomnia**

⑤ **327.1** **Organic disorder of excessive somnolence [Organic hypersomnia]**
Excludes: *hypersomnia NOS (780.54)*

hypersomnia not due to a substance or known physiological condition (307.43-307.44)
hypersomnia with sleep apnea NOS (780.53)

327.10 **Organic hypersomnia, unspecified**

● Code new
to this edition

▲ Revision of
existing code

④ ⑤ Fourth or fifth
digit required

327.11 **Idiopathic hypersomnia with long sleep time**

327.12 **Idiopathic hypersomnia without long sleep time**

327.13 **Recurrent hypersomnia**
Kleine-Levin syndrome
Menstrual related hypersomnia

327.14 **Hypersomnia due to medical condition classified elsewhere**
Code first underlying condition

Excludes: hypersomnia due to mental disorder (327.15)

327.15 **Hypersomnia due to mental disorder**
Code first mental disorder

Excludes: alcohol induced hypersomnia (291.82)
drug induced hypersomnia (292.85)

327.19 **Other organic hypersomnia**

⑤ **327.2 Organic sleep apnea**

Excludes: Cheyne-Stokes breathing (786.04)
hypersomnia with sleep apnea NOS (780.53)
insomnia with sleep apnea NOS (780.51)
sleep apnea in newborn (770.81-770.82)
sleep apnea NOS (780.57)

327.20 **Organic sleep apnea, unspecified**

327.21 **Primary central sleep apnea**

327.22 **High altitude periodic breathing**

327.23 **Obstructive sleep apnea (adult) (pediatric)**

327.24 **Idiopathic sleep related nonobstructive alveolar hypoventilation**
Sleep related hypoxia

327.25 **Congenital central alveolar hypoventilation syndrome**

327.26 **Sleep related hypoventilation/hypoxemia in conditions classifiable elsewhere**
Code first underlying condition

327.27 **Central sleep apnea in conditions classified elsewhere**
Code first underlying condition

327.29 **Other organic sleep apnea**

⑤ **327.3 Circadian rhythm sleep disorder**
Organic disorder of sleep wake cycle
Organic disorder of sleep wake schedule

Excludes: alcohol induced circadian rhythm sleep disorder (291.82)
circadian rhythm sleep disorder of nonorganic origin (307.45)
disruption of 24 hour sleep wake cycle NOS (780.55)
drug induced circadian rhythm sleep disorder (292.85)

327.30 **Circadian rhythm sleep disorder, unspecified**

327.31 **Circadian rhythm sleep disorder, delayed sleep phase type**

327.32 **Circadian rhythm sleep disorder, advanced sleep phase type**

327.33 **Circadian rhythm sleep disorder, irregular sleep-wake type**

327.34 **Circadian rhythm sleep disorder, free-running type**

327.35 **Circadian rhythm sleep disorder, jet lag type**

327.36 **Circadian rhythm sleep disorder, shift work type**

327.37 **Circadian rhythm sleep disorder in conditions classified elsewhere**
Code first underlying condition

327.39 **Other circadian rhythm sleep disorder**

⑤ **327.4 Organic parasomnia**

Excludes: alcohol induced parasomnia (291.82)
drug induced parasomnia (292.85)
parasomnia not due to a known physiological condition (307.47)

327.40 **Organic parasomnia, unspecified**

327.41 **Confusional arousals**

327.42 **REM sleep behavior disorder**

327.43 **Recurrent isolated sleep paralysis**

327.44 **Parasomnia in conditions classified elsewhere**
Code first underlying condition

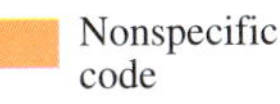

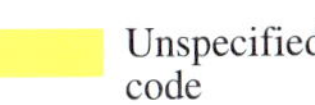

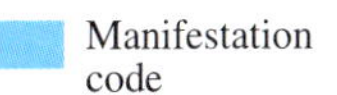

Manifestation
code

327.49 Other organic parasomnia

⑤ **327.5 Organic sleep related movement disorders**

> *Excludes:* *restless legs syndrome (333.94)*
> *sleep related movement disorder NOS (780.58)*

327.51 Periodic limb movement disorder
Periodic limb movement sleep disorder

327.52 Sleep related leg cramps

327.53 Sleep related bruxism

327.59 Other organic sleep related movement disorders

327.8 Other organic sleep disorders

HEREDITARY AND DEGENERATIVE DISEASES OF THE CENTRAL NERVOUS SYSTEM (330-337)

> *Excludes:* *hepatolenticular degeneration (275.1)*
> *multiple sclerosis (340)*
> *other demyelinating diseases of central nervous system (341.0-341.9)*

330 Cerebral degenerations usually manifest in childhood
Use additional code, if desired, to identify associated mental retardation

330.0 Leukodystrophy
Krabbe's disease
Leukodystrophy:
  NOS
  globoid cell
Leukodystrophy:
  metachromatic
  sudanophilic
Pelizaeus-Merzbacher disease
Sulfatide lipidosis

330.1 Cerebral lipidoses
Amaurotic (familial) idiocy
Disease:
  Batten
  Jansky-Bielschowsky
Disease:
  Kufs'
  Spielmeyer-Vogt
  Tay-Sachs
Gangliosidosis

330.2 *Cerebral degeneration in generalized lipidoses*
Code first underlying disease, as:
Fabry's disease (272.7)
Gaucher's disease (272.7)
Neimann-Pick disease (272.7)
sphingolipidosis (272.7)

330.3 *Cerebral degeneration of childhood in other diseases classified elsewhere*
Code first underlying disease, as:
Hunter's disease (277.5)
mucopolysaccharidosis (277.5)

330.8 Other specified cerebral degenerations in childhood
Alpers' disease or gray-matter degeneration
Infantile necrotizing encephalomyelopathy
Leigh's disease
Subacute necrotizing encephalopathy or encephalomyelopathy

330.9 Unspecified cerebral degeneration in childhood

331 Other cerebral degenerations

331.0 Alzheimer's disease

⑤ **331.1 Frontotemporal dementia**
Use additional code for associated behavioral disturbance (294.10-294.11)

331.11 Pick's disease

331.19 Other frontotemporal dementia
Frontal dementia

331.2 Senile degeneration of brain

> *Excludes:* *senility NOS (797)*

331.3 Communicating hydrocephalus

> *Excludes:* *congenital hydrocephalus (741.0, 742.3)*

331.4 Obstructive hydrocephalus
Acquired hydrocephalus NOS

> *Excludes:* *congenital hydrocephalus (741.0, 742.3)*

● Code new
to this edition

▲ Revision of
existing code

④ ⑤ Fourth or fifth
digit required

331.7 *Cerebral degeneration in diseases classified elsewhere*
Code first underlying disease, as:
alcoholism (303.0-303.9)
beriberi (265.0)
cerebrovascular disease (430-438)
congenital hydrocephalus (741.0, 742.3)
neoplastic disease (140.0-239.9)
myxedema (244.0-244.9)
vitamin B_{12} deficiency (266.2)

Excludes: *cerebral degeneration in:*
Jakob-Creutzfeldt disease (046.1)
progressive multifocal leukoencephalopathy (046.3)
subacute spongiform encephalopathy (046.1)

⑤ **331.8 Other cerebral degeneration**

331.81 Reye's syndrome

331.82 Dementia with Lewy bodies
Dementia with Parkinsonism
Lewy body dementia
Lewy body disease

Use additional code for associated behavioral disturbance (294.10-294.11)

● **331.83 Mild cognitive impairment, so stated**

Excludes: *altered mental status (780.97)*
cerebral degeneration (331.0-331.9)
change in mental status (780.97)
cognitive deficits following (late effects of) cerebral hemorrhage or infarction (438.0)
cognitive impairment due to intracranial or head injury (850-854, 959.01)
cognitive impairment due to late effect of intracranial injury (907.0)
dementia (290.0-290.43, 294.8)
mild memory disturbance (310.8)
neurologic neglect syndrome (781.8)
personality change, nonpsychotic (310.1)

331.89 Other
Cerebral ataxia

331.9 Cerebral degeneration, unspecified

332 Parkinson's disease

Excludes: *dementia with Parkinsonism (331.82)*

332.0 Paralysis agitans
Parkinsonism or Parkinson's disease:
NOS
idiopathic
primary

332.1 Secondary Parkinsonism
Neuroleptic-induced Parkinsonism
Parkinsonism due to drugs

Use additional E code, if desired, to identify drug, if drug-induced

Excludes: *Parkinsonism (in):*
Huntington's disease (333.4)
progressive supranuclear palsy (333.0)
Shy-Drager syndrome (333.0)
syphilitic (094.82)

333 Other extrapyramidal disease and abnormal movement disorders
Includes: other forms of extrapyramidal, basal ganglia, or striatopallidal disease

Excludes: *abnormal movements of head NOS (781.0)*
sleep related movement disorders (327.51-327.59)

333.0 Other degenerative diseases of the basal ganglia
Atrophy or degeneration:
olivopontocerebellar [Déjérine-Thomas syndrome]
pigmentary pallidal [Hallervorden-Spatz disease]
striatonigral
Parkinsonian syndrome associated with:
idiopathic orthostatic hypotension
symptomatic orthostatic hypotension
Progressive supranuclear ophthalmoplegia
Shy-Drager syndrome

Add 4th or 5th digit | Nonspecific code | Unspecified code | Manifestation code

333.1 Essential and other specified forms of tremor
Benign essential tremor
Familial tremor
Medication-induced postural tremor
Use additional E code, if desired, to identify drug, if drug-induced
> *Excludes:* *tremor NOS (781.0)*

333.2 Myoclonus
Familial essential myoclonus
Progressive myoclonic epilepsy
Unverricht-Lundborg disease
Use additional E code, if desired, to identify drug, if drug-induced

333.3 Tics of organic origin
> *Excludes:* *Gilles de la Tourette's syndrome (307.23)*
> *habit spasm (307.22)*
> *tic NOS (307.20)*
Use additional E code, if desired, to identify drug, if drug-induced

333.4 Huntington's chorea

333.5 Other choreas
Hemiballism(us)
Paroxysmal choreo-athetosis
> *Excludes:* *Sydenham's or rheumatic chorea (392.0-392.9)*
Use additional E code, if desired, to identify drug, if drug-induced

▲ **333.6 Genetic torsion dystonia**
Dystonia:
deformans progressiva
musculorum deformans
(Schwalbe-) Ziehen-Oppenheim disease

▲ **333.7 Acquired torsion dystonia**

● **333.71 Athetoid cerebral palsy**
Double athetosis (syndrome)
Vogt's disease
> *Excludes:* *infantile cerebral palsy (343.0-343.9)*

● **333.72 Acute dystonia due to drugs**
Acute dystonic reaction due to drugs
Neuroleptic induced acute dystonia
Use additional E code to identify drug
> *Excludes:* *blepharospasm due to drugs (333.85)*
> *orofacial dyskinesia due to drugs (333.85)*
> *secondary Parkinsonism (332.1)*
> *subacute dyskinesia due to drugs (333.85)*
> *tardive dyskinesia (333.85)*

● **333.79 Other acquired torsion dystonia**

⑤ **333.8 Fragments of torsion dystonia**
Use additional E code, if desired, to identify drug, if drug-induced

333.81 Blepharospasm
> *Excludes:* *blepharospasm due to drugs (333.85)*

333.82 Orofacial dyskinesia
> *Excludes:* *orofacial dyskinesia due to drugs (333.85)*

333.83 Spasmodic torticollis
> *Excludes:* *torticollis:*
> *NOS (723.5)*
> *hysterical (300.11)*
> *psychogenic (306.0)*

333.84 Organic writers' cramp
> *Excludes:* *psychogenic (300.89)*

● Code new
to this edition
▲ Revision of
existing code
④ ⑤ Fourth or fifth
digit required

● **333.85 Subacute dyskinesia due to drugs**
Blepharospasm due to drugs
Orofacial dyskinesia due to drugs
Tardive dyskinesia

Use additional E code to identify drug

Excludes: *acute dystonia due to drugs (333.72)*
acute dystonic reaction due to drugs (333.72)
secondary Parkinsonism (332.1)

333.89 Other

⑤ **333.9 Other and unspecified extrapyramidal diseases and abnormal movement disorders**

333.90 Unspecified extrapyramidal disease and abnormal movement disorder
Medication-induced movement disorders NOS
Use additional E code to identify drug, if drug-induced

333.91 Stiff-man syndrome

333.92 Neuroleptic malignant syndrome
Use additional E code to identify drug

Excludes: *neuroleptic induced Parkinsonism (332.1)*

333.93 Benign shuddering attacks

● **333.94 Restless legs syndrome (RLS)**

333.99 Other
Neuroleptic-induced acute akathisia
Use additional E code to identify drug, if drug-induced

334 Spinocerebellar disease

Excludes: *olivopontocerebellar degeneration (333.0)*
peroneal muscular atrophy (356.1)

334.0 Friedreich's ataxia

334.1 Hereditary spastic paraplegia

334.2 Primary cerebellar degeneration
Cerebellar ataxia:
  Marie's
  Sanger-Brown
Dyssynergia cerebellaris myoclonica
Primary cerebellar degeneration:
  NOS
  hereditary
  sporadic

334.3 Other cerebellar ataxia
Cerebellar ataxia NOS

Use additional E code, if desired, to identify drug, if drug-induced

334.4 *Cerebellar ataxia in diseases classified elsewhere*
Code first underlying disease, as:
  alcoholism (303.0-303.9)
  myxedema (244.0-244.9)
  neoplastic disease (140.0-239.9)

334.8 Other spinocerebellar diseases
Ataxia-telangiectasia [Louis-Bar syndrome]
Corticostriatal-spinal degeneration

334.9 Spinocerebellar disease, unspecified

335 Anterior horn cell disease

335.0 Werdnig-Hoffmann disease
Infantile spinal muscular atrophy
Progressive muscular atrophy of infancy

⑤ **335.1 Spinal muscular atrophy**

335.10 Spinal muscular atrophy, unspecified

335.11 Kugelberg-Welander disease
Spinal muscular atrophy:
  familial
  juvenile

335.19 Other
Adult spinal muscular atrophy

⑤ **335.2 Motor neuron disease**

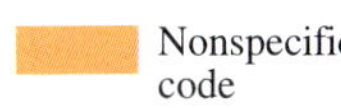

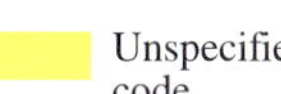

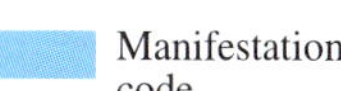

Manifestation
code

335.20 **Amyotrophic lateral sclerosis**
Motor neuron disease (bulbar) (mixed type)

335.21 **Progressive muscular atrophy**
Duchenne-Aran muscular atrophy
Progressive muscular atrophy (pure)

335.22 **Progressive bulbar palsy**

335.23 **Pseudobulbar palsy**

335.24 **Primary lateral sclerosis**

335.29 **Other**

335.8 **Other anterior horn cell diseases**

335.9 **Anterior horn cell disease, unspecified**

336 **Other diseases of spinal cord**

336.0 **Syringomyelia and syringobulbia**

336.1 **Vascular myelopathies**
Acute infarction of spinal cord (embolic) (nonembolic)
Arterial thrombosis of spinal cord
Edema of spinal cord
Hematomyelia
Subacute necrotic myelopathy

336.2 *Subacute combined degeneration of spinal cord in diseases classified elsewhere*
Code first underlying disease, as:
pernicious anemia (281.0)
other vitamin B_{12} deficiency anemia (281.1)
vitamin B_{12} deficiency (266.2)

336.3 *Myelopathy in other diseases classified elsewhere*
Code first underlying disease, as:
myelopathy in neoplastic disease (140.0-239.9)

Excludes: *myelopathy in:*
intervertebral disc disorder (722.70-722.73)
spondylosis (721.1, 721.41-721.42, 721.91)

336.8 **Other myelopathy**
Myelopathy:
drug-induced
radiation-induced

Use additional E code, if desired, to identify cause

336.9 **Unspecified disease of spinal cord**
Cord compression NOS   Myelopathy NOS

Excludes: *myelitis (323.02, 323.1, 323.2, 323.42, 323.52, 323.63, 323.72, 323.82, 323.9)*
spinal (canal) stenosis (723.0, 724.00-724.09)

337 **Disorders of the autonomic nervous system**
Includes: disorders of peripheral autonomic, sympathetic, parasympathetic, or vegetative
system

Excludes: *familial dysautonomia [Riley-Day syndrome] (742.8)*

337.0 **Idiopathic peripheral autonomic neuropathy**
Carotid sinus syncope or syndrome
Cervical sympathetic dystrophy or paralysis

337.1 *Peripheral autonomic neuropathy in disorders classified elsewhere*
Code first underlying disease, as:
amyloidosis (277.30-277.39)
diabetes (250.6)

⑤ **337.2** **Reflex sympathetic dystrophy**

337.20 **Reflex sympathetic dystrophy, unspecified**

337.21 **Reflex sympathetic dystrophy of the upper limb**

337.22 **Reflex sympathetic dystrophy of the lower limb**

337.29 **Reflex sympathetic dystrophy of other specified site**

337.3 **Autonomic dysreflexia**
Use additional code to identify the cause, such as:
decubitus ulcer (707.00-707.09)
fecal impaction (560.39)
urinary tract infection (599.0)

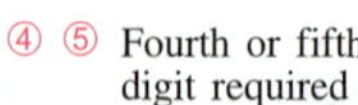

337.9 Unspecified disorder of autonomic nervous system

PAIN (338)

● **338** **Pain, not elsewhere classified**
Use additional code to identify:
pain associated with psychological factors (307.89)
Excludes: *generalized pain (780.96)*
localized pain, unspecified type – code to pain by site
pain disorder exclusively attributed to psychological factors (307.80)

● **338.0** **Central pain syndrome**
Déjérine-Roussy syndrome
Myelopathic pain syndrome
Thalamic pain syndrome (hyperesthetic)

● **338.1** **Acute pain**

● **338.11** **Acute pain due to trauma**

● **338.12** **Acute post-thoracotomy pain**
Post-thoracotomy pain NOS

● **338.18** **Other acute postoperative pain**
Postoperative pain NOS

● **338.19** **Other acute pain**
Excludes: *neoplasm related acute pain (338.3)*

● **338.2** **Chronic pain**
Excludes: *causalgia (355.9)*
lower limb (355.71)
upper limb (354.4)
chronic pain syndrome (338.4)
myofascial pain syndrome (729.1)
neoplasm related chronic pain (338.3)
reflex sympathetic dystrophy (337.20-337.29)

● **338.21** **Chronic pain due to trauma**

● **338.22** **Chronic post-thoracotomy pain**

● **338.28** **Other chronic postoperative pain**

● **338.29** **Other chronic pain**

● **338.3** **Neoplasm related pain (acute) (chronic)**
Cancer associated pain
Pain due to malignancy (primary) (secondary)
Tumor associated pain

● **338.4** **Chronic pain syndrome**
Chronic pain associated with significant psychosocial dysfunction

OTHER DISORDERS OF THE CENTRAL NERVOUS SYSTEM (340-349)

340 **Multiple sclerosis**
Disseminated or multiple sclerosis:
NOS
brain stem
cord
generalized

341 **Other demyelinating diseases of central nervous system**

341.0 **Neuromyelitis optica**

341.1 **Schilder's disease**
Baló's concentric sclerosis
Encephalitis periaxialis:
concentrica [Baló's]
diffusa [Schilder's]

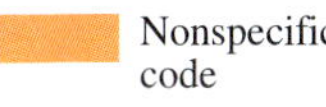

● **341.2** **Acute (transverse) myelitis**

Excludes: *acute (transverse)myelitis (in) (due to):*

    following immunization procedures (323.52)
    infection classified elsewhere (323.42)
    postinfectious (323.63)
    protozoal diseases classified elsewhere (323.2)
    rickettsial diseases classified elsewhere (323.1)
    toxic (323.72)
    viral diseases classified elsewhere (323.02)
  transverse myelitis NOS (323.82)

  ● **341.20** **Acute (transverse) myelitis NOS**

  ● **341.21** **Acute (transverse) myelitis in conditions classified elsewhere**
    Code first underlying condition

  ● **341.22** **Idiopathic transverse myelitis**

341.8 **Other demyelinating diseases of central nervous system**
  Central demyelination of corpus callosum
  Central pontine myelinosis
  Marchiafava (-Bignami) disease

341.9 **Demyelinating disease of central nervous system, unspecified**

342 **Hemiplegia and hemiparesis**

Excludes: *congenital (343.1)*

  hemiplegia due to late effect of cerebrovascular accident (438.20-438.22)
  infantile NOS (343.4)

Note: This category is to be used when hemiplegia (complete) (incomplete) is reported without further specification, or is stated to be old or long-standing but of unspecified cause. The category is also for use in multiple coding to identify these types of hemiplegia resulting from any cause.

The following fifth-digits are for use with codes 342.0-342.9

  0 **affecting unspecified site**

  1 **affecting dominant site**

  2 **affecting nondominant site**

⑤ **342.0** **Flaccid hemiplegia**

⑤ **342.1** **Spastic hemiplegia**

⑤ **342.8** **Other specified hemiplegia**

⑤ **342.9** **Hemiplegia, unspecified**

343 **Infantile cerebral palsy**
  Includes: cerebral:
    palsy NOS
    spastic infantile paralysis
    congenital spastic paralysis (cerebral)
    Little's disease
    paralysis (spastic) due to birth injury:
      intracranial
      spinal

Excludes: *athetoid cerebral palsy (333.71)*

  hereditary cerebral paralysis, such as:
    hereditary spastic paraplegia (334.1)
    Vogt's disease (333.71)
  spastic paralysis specified as noncongenital or noninfantile (344.0-344.9)

343.0 **Diplegic**
  Congenital diplegia   Congenital paraplegia

343.1 **Hemiplegic**
  Congenital hemiplegia

Excludes: *infantile hemiplegia NOS (343.4)*

343.2 **Quadriplegic**
  Tetraplegic

343.3 **Monoplegic**

343.4 **Infantile hemiplegia**
  Infantile hemiplegia (postnatal) NOS

343.8 **Other specified infantile cerebral palsy**

● Code new to this edition   ▲ Revision of existing code   ④ ⑤ Fourth or fifth digit required

343.9 Infantile cerebral palsy, unspecified
> Cerebral palsy NOS

344 Other paralytic syndromes

Note: This category is to be used when the listed conditions are reported without further specification or are stated to be old or long-standing but of unspecified cause. The category is also for use in multiple coding to identify these conditions resulting from any cause.

Includes: paralysis (complete) (incomplete), except as classifiable to 342 and 343

Excludes: *congenital or infantile cerebral palsy (343.0-343.9)*
> *hemiplegia (342.0-342.9)*
> > *congenital or infantile (343.1, 343.4)*

⑤ **344.0 Quadriplegia and quadriparesis**

344.00 Quadriplegia, unspecified

344.01 C1-C4, complete

344.02 C1-C4, incomplete

344.03 C5-C7, complete

344.04 C5-C7, incomplete

344.09 Other

344.1 Paraplegia
> Paralysis of both lower limbs
> Paraplegia (lower)

344.2 Diplegia of upper limbs
> Diplegia (upper)
> Paralysis of both upper limbs

⑤ **344.3 Monoplegia of lower limb**
> Paralysis of lower limb

Excludes: *monoplegia of lower limb due to late effect of cerebrovascular accident (438.40-438.42)*

344.30 affecting unspecified side

344.31 affecting dominant side

344.32 affecting nondominant side

⑤ **344.4 Monoplegia of upper limb**
> Paralysis of upper limb

Excludes: *monoplegia of upper limb due to late effect of cerebrovascular accident (438.30-438.32)*

344.40 affecting unspecified side

344.41 affecting dominant side

344.42 affecting nondominant side

344.5 Unspecified monoplegia

⑤ **344.6 Cauda equina syndrome**

344.60 Without mention of neurogenic bladder

344.61 With neurogenic bladder
> Acontractile bladder
> Autonomic hyperreflexia of bladder
> Cord bladder
> Detrusor hyperreflexia

⑤ **344.8 Other specified paralytic syndromes**

344.81 Locked-in state

344.89 Other specified paralytic syndrome

344.9 Paralysis, unspecified

▲ **345 Epilepsy and recurrent seizures**

The following fifth-digit subclassification is for use with categories 345.0, 345.1, 345.4-345.9:

0 without mention of intractable epilepsy

1 with intractable epilepsy

Excludes: *progressive myoclonic epilepsy (333.2)*

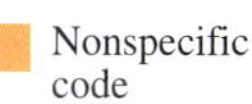

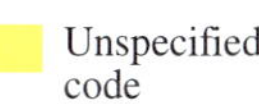

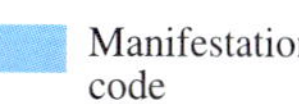

Manifestation
code

⑤ **345.0 Generalized nonconvulsive epilepsy**
Absences: Pykno-epilepsy
  atonic   Seizures:
  typical   akinetic
Minor epilepsy   atonic
Petit mal

⑤ **345.1 Generalized convulsive epilepsy**
Epileptic seizures: Grand mal
  clonic   Major epilepsy
  myoclonic
  tonic
  tonic-clonic

> *Excludes:* *convulsions:*
> > *NOS (780.39)*
> > *infantile (780.39)*
> > *newborn (779.0)*
> > *infantile spasms (345.6)*

345.2 Petit mal status
Epileptic absence status

345.3 Grand mal status
Status epilepticus NOS

> *Excludes:* *epilepsia partialis continua (345.7)*
> > *status:*
> > > *psychomotor (345.7)*
> > > *temporal lobe (345.7)*

▲ **345.4 Localization-related (focal) (partial) epilepsy and epileptic syndromes with complex partial seizures**
Epilepsy:
  limbic system
  partial:
    secondarily generalized
    with impairment of consciousness
    with memory and ideational disturbances
  psychomotor
  psychosensory
  temporal lobe
Epileptic automatism

⑤ **345.5 Localization-related (focal) (partial) epilepsy and epileptic syndromes with simple partial seizures**
Epilepsy: Epilepsy:
  Bravais-Jacksonian NOS   sensory-induced
  focal (motor) NOS   somatomotor
  Jacksonian NOS   somatosensory
  motor partial   visceral
  partial NOS: visual
    without impairment of consciousness

⑤ **345.6 Infantile spasms**
Hypsarrhythmia   Salaam attacks
Lightning spasms

> *Excludes:* *salaam tic (781.0)*

⑤ **345.7 Epilepsia partialis continua**
Kojevnikov's epilepsy

▲ **345.8 Other forms of epilepsy and recurrent seizures**
Epilepsy:
  cursive [running]
  gelastic

⑤ **345.9 Epilepsy, unspecified**
Epileptic convulsions, fits, or seizures NOS
Recurrent seizures NOS
Seizure disorder NOS

> *Excludes:* *convulsion (convulsive) disorder (780.39)*
> > *convulsive seizure or fit NOS (780.39)*
> > *recurrent convulsions (780.39)*

● Code new to this edition   ▲ Revision of existing code   ④ ⑤ Fourth or fifth digit required

⑤ **346 Migraine**

The following fifth-digit subclassification is for use with category 346:

0   without mention of intractable migraine

1   with intractable migraine, so stated

⑤ **346.0 Classical migraine**
Migraine preceded or accompanied by transient focal neurological phenomena
Migraine with aura

⑤ **346.1 Common migraine**
Atypical migraine
Sick headache

⑤ **346.2 Variants of migraine**

Cluster headache
Histamine cephalgia
Horton's neuralgia
Migraine:
 abdominal
 basilar

Migraine:
 lower half
 retinal
Neuralgia:
 ciliary
 migrainous

⑤ **346.8 Other forms of migraine**
Migraine:
 hemiplegic
 ophthalmoplegic

⑤ **346.9 Migraine, unspecified**

347 Cataplexy and narcolepsy

⑤ **347.0 Narcolepsy**

347.00   Without cataplexy
Narcolepsy NOS

347.01   With cataplexy

⑤ **347.1 Narcolepsy in conditions classified elsewhere**
Code first underlying condition

347.10   Without cataplexy

347.11   With cataplexy

348 Other conditions of brain

348.0 Cerebral cysts

Arachnoid cyst
Porencephalic cyst

Porencephaly, acquired
Pseudoporencephaly

Excludes: *porencephaly (congenital) (742.4)*

348.1 Anoxic brain damage

Excludes: *that occurring in:*
abortion (634-638 with .7, 639.8)
ectopic or molar pregnancy (639.8)
labor or delivery (668.2, 669.4)
that of newborn (767.0, 768.0-768.9, 772.1-772.2)

Use additional E code, if desired, to identify cause

348.2 Benign intracranial hypertension
Pseudotumor cerebri

Excludes: *hypertensive encephalopathy (437.2)*

⑤ **348.3 Encephalopathy, not elsewhere classified**

348.30   Encephalopathy, unspecified

348.31   Metabolic encephalopathy
Septic encephalopathy

Excludes: *toxic metabolic encephalopathy (349.82)*

348.39   Other encephalopathy

Excludes: *encephalopathy:*
alcoholic (291.2)
hepatic (572.2)
hypertensive (437.2)
toxic (349.82)

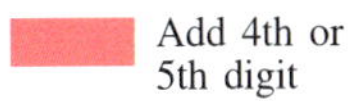
Add 4th or
5th digit

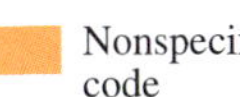
Nonspecific
code

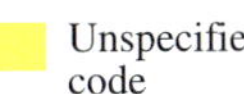
Unspecified
code

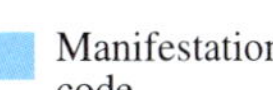
Manifestation
code

348.4 Compression of brain
Compression, brain (stem)
Herniation, brain (stem)
Posterior fossa compression syndrome

348.5 Cerebral edema

348.8 Other conditions of brain
Cerebral:
calcification
fungus

348.9 Unspecified condition of brain

349 Other and unspecified disorders of the nervous system

349.0 Reaction to spinal or lumbar puncture
Headache following lumbar puncture

349.1 Nervous system complications from surgically implanted device

349.2 Disorders of meninges, not elsewhere classified
| Excludes: | *immediate postoperative complications (997.00-997.09)* |

mechanical complications of nervous system device (996.2)
Adhesions, meningeal (cerebral) (spinal)
Cyst, spinal meninges
Meningocele, acquired
Pseudomeningocele, acquired

⑤ **349.8 Other specified disorders of nervous system**

349.81 Cerebrospinal fluid rhinorrhea
| Excludes: | *cerebrospinal fluid otorrhea (388.61)* |

349.82 Toxic encephalopathy
Toxic metabolic encephalopathy
Use additional E code, if desired, to identify cause

349.89 Other

349.9 Unspecified disorders of nervous system
Disorder of nervous system (central) NOS

DISORDERS OF THE PERIPHERAL NERVOUS SYSTEM (350-359)

| Excludes: | *diseases of:* |

acoustic [8th] nerve (388.5)
oculomotor [3rd, 4th, 6th] nerves (378.0-378.9)
optic [2nd] nerve (377.0-377.9)
peripheral autonomic nerves (337.0-337.9)
neuralgia NOS or "rheumatic" (729.2)
neuritis NOS or "rheumatic" (729.2)
radiculitis NOS or "rheumatic" (729.2)
peripheral neuritis in pregnancy (646.4)

350 Trigeminal nerve disorders
Includes: disorders of 5th cranial nerve

350.1 Trigeminal neuralgia
Tic douloureux   Trigeminal neuralgia NOS
Trifacial neuralgia

| Excludes: | *postherpetic (053.12)* |

350.2 Atypical face pain

350.8 Other specified trigeminal nerve disorders

350.9 Trigeminal nerve disorder, unspecified

351 Facial nerve disorders
Includes: disorders of 7th cranial nerve
| Excludes: | *that in newborn (767.5)* |

351.0 Bell's palsy
Facial palsy

351.1 Geniculate ganglionitis
Geniculate ganglionitis NOS
| Excludes: | *herpetic (053.11)* |

● Code new
to this edition

▲ Revision of
existing code

④ ⑤ Fourth or fifth
digit required

351.8 Other facial nerve disorders
Facial myokymia
Melkersson's syndrome

351.9 Facial nerve disorder, unspecified

352 Disorders of other cranial nerves

352.0 Disorders of olfactory [1st] nerve

352.1 Glossopharyngeal neuralgia

352.2 Other disorders of glossopharyngeal [9th] nerve

352.3 Disorders of pneumogastric [10th] nerve
Disorders of vagal nerve
Excludes: *paralysis of vocal cords or larynx (478.30-478.34)*

352.4 Disorders of accessory [11th] nerve

352.5 Disorders of hypoglossal [12th] nerve

352.6 Multiple cranial nerve palsies
Collet-Sicard syndrome
Polyneuritis cranialis

352.9 Unspecified disorder of cranial nerves

353 Nerve root and plexus disorders
Excludes: *conditions due to:*
intervertebral disc disorders (722.0-722.9)
spondylosis (720.0-721.9)
vertebrogenic disorders (723.0-724.9)

353.0 Brachial plexus lesions
Cervical rib syndrome   Scalenus anticus syndrome
Costoclavicular syndrome   Thoracic outlet syndrome
Excludes: *brachial neuritis or radiculitis NOS (723.4)*
that in newborn (767.6)

353.1 Lumbosacral plexus lesions

353.2 Cervical root lesions, not elsewhere classified

353.3 Thoracic root lesions, not elsewhere classified

353.4 Lumbosacral root lesions, not elsewhere classified

353.5 Neuralgic amyotrophy
Parsonage-Aldren-Turner syndrome

353.6 Phantom limb (syndrome)

353.8 Other nerve root and plexus disorders

353.9 Unspecified nerve root and plexus disorder

354 Mononeuritis of upper limb and mononeuritis multiplex

354.0 Carpal tunnel syndrome
Median nerve entrapment
Partial thenar atrophy

354.1 Other lesion of median nerve
Median nerve neuritis

354.2 Lesion of ulnar nerve
Cubital tunnel syndrome
Tardy ulnar nerve palsy

354.3 Lesion of radial nerve
Acute radial nerve palsy

354.4 Causalgia of upper limb
Excludes: *causalgia:*
NOS (355.9)
lower limb (355.71)

354.5 Mononeuritis multiplex
Combinations of single conditions classifiable to 354 or 355

354.8 Other mononeuritis of upper limb

354.9 Mononeuritis of upper limb, unspecified

355 Mononeuritis of lower limb and unspecified site

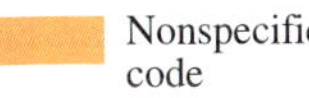

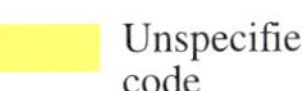

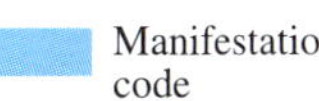

355.0 Lesion of sciatic nerve
Excludes: sciatica NOS (724.3)

355.1 Meralgia paresthetica
Lateral cutaneous femoral nerve of thigh compression or syndrome

355.2 Other lesion of femoral nerve

355.3 Lesion of lateral popliteal nerve
Lesion of common peroneal nerve

355.4 Lesion of medial popliteal nerve

355.5 Tarsal tunnel syndrome

355.6 Lesion of plantar nerve
Morton's metatarsalgia, neuralgia, or neuroma

⑤ **355.7 Other mononeuritis of lower limb**

    355.71 Causalgia of lower limb
Excludes: causalgia:
    NOS (355.9)
    upper limb (354.4)

    355.79 Other mononeuritis of lower limb

355.8 Mononeuritis of lower limb, unspecified

355.9 Mononeuritis of unspecified site
Causalgia NOS
Excludes: causalgia:
    lower limb (355.71)
    upper limb (354.4)

356 Hereditary and idiopathic peripheral neuropathy

356.0 Hereditary peripheral neuropathy
Déjérine-Sottas disease

356.1 Peroneal muscular atrophy
Charcot-Marie-Tooth disease
Neuropathic muscular atrophy

356.2 Hereditary sensory neuropathy

356.3 Refsum's disease
Heredopathia atactica polyneuritiformis

356.4 Idiopathic progressive polyneuropathy

356.8 Other specified idiopathic peripheral neuropathy
Supranuclear paralysis

356.9 Unspecified

357 Inflammatory and toxic neuropathy

357.0 Acute infective polyneuritis
Guillain-Barré syndrome
Postinfectious polyneuritis

357.1 *Polyneuropathy in collagen vascular disease*
Code first underlying disease, as:
disseminated lupus erythematosus (710.0)
polyarteritis nodosa (446.0)
rheumatoid arthritis (714.0)

357.2 *Polyneuropathy in diabetes*
Code first underlying disease (250.6)

357.3 *Polyneuropathy in malignant disease*
Code first underlying disease (140.0-208.9)

● Code new to this edition ▲ Revision of existing code ④ ⑤ Fourth or fifth digit required

357.4 *Polyneuropathy in other diseases classified elsewhere*
Code first underlying disease, as:
amyloidosis (277.30-277.39)
beriberi (265.0)
chronic uremia (585.9)
deficiency of B vitamins (266.0-266.9)
diphtheria (032.0-032.9)
hypoglycemia (251.2)
pellagra (265.2)
porphyria (277.1)
sarcoidosis (135)
uremia NOS (586)

Excludes: *polyneuropathy in:*
herpes zoster (053.13)
mumps (072.72)

357.5 Alcoholic polyneuropathy

357.6 Polyneuropathy due to drugs
Use additional E code, if desired, to identify drug

357.7 Polyneuropathy due to other toxic agents
Use additional E code, if desired, to identify toxic agent

⑤ **357.8 Other**

    357.81 Chronic inflammatory demyelinating polyneuritis

    357.82 Critical illness polyneuropathy
    Acute motor neuropathy

    357.89 Other inflammatory and toxic neuropathy

357.9 Unspecified

358 Myoneural disorders

⑤ **358.0 Myasthenia gravis**

    358.00 Myasthenia gravis without (acute) exacerbation
    Myasthenia gravis NOS

    358.01 Myasthenia gravis with (acute) exacerbation
    Myasthenia gravis in crisis

358.1 *Myasthenic syndromes in diseases classified elsewhere*
Amyotrophy from stated cause classified elsewhere
Eaton-Lambert syndrome from stated cause classified elsewhere
Code first underlying disease, as:
botulism (005.1)
diabetes mellitus (250.6)
hypothyroidism (244.0-244.9)
malignant neoplasm (140.0-208.9)
pernicious anemia (281.0)
thyrotoxicosis (242.0-242.9)

358.2 Toxic myoneural disorders
Use additional E code, if desired, to identify toxic agent

358.8 Other specified myoneural disorders

358.9 Myoneural disorders, unspecified

359 Muscular dystrophies and other myopathies
Excludes: *idiopathic polymyositis (710.4)*

359.0 Congenital hereditary muscular dystrophy
Benign congenital myopathy
Central core disease
Centronuclear myopathy
Myotubular myopathy
Nemaline body disease

Excludes: *arthrogryposis multiplex congenita (754.89)*

359.1 Hereditary progressive muscular dystrophy

Muscular dystrophy:	Muscular dystrophy:
NOS	Gower's
distal	Landouzy-Déjérine
Duchenne	limb-girdle
Erb's	ocular
fascioscapulohumeral	oculopharyngeal

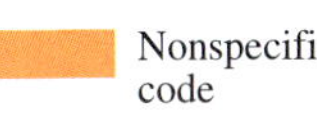

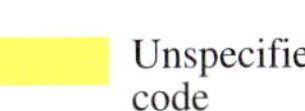

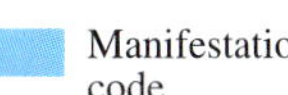

359.2 Myotonic disorders
Dystrophia myotonica
Eulenburg's disease
Myotonia congenita
Paramyotonia congenita
Steinert's disease
Thomsen's disease

359.3 Familial periodic paralysis
Hypokalemic familial periodic paralysis

359.4 Toxic myopathy
Use additional E code, if desired, to identify toxic agent

359.5 *Myopathy in endocrine diseases classified elsewhere*
Code first underlying disease, as:
Addison's disease (255.4)
Cushing's syndrome (255.0)
hypopituitarism (253.2)
myxedema (244.0-244.9)
thyrotoxicosis (242.0-242.9)

359.6 *Symptomatic inflammatory myopathy in diseases classified elsewhere*
Code first underlying disease, as:
amyloidosis (277.30-277.39)
disseminated lupus erythematosus (710.0)
malignant neoplasm (140.0-208.9)
polyarteritis nodosa (446.0)
rheumatoid arthritis (714.0)
sarcoidosis (135)
scleroderma (710.1)
Sjögren's disease (710.2)

⑤ **359.8 Other myopathies**

359.81 Critical illness myopathy
Acute necrotizing myopathy
Acute quadriplegic myopathy
Intensive care (ICU) myopathy
Myopathy of critical illness

359.89 Other myopathies

359.9 Myopathy, unspecified

DISORDERS OF THE EYE AND ADNEXA (360-379)

360 Disorders of the globe
Includes: disorders affecting multiple structures of eye

⑤ **360.0 Purulent endophthalmitis**
Excludes: *bleb associated endophthalmitis (379.63)*

360.00 Purulent endophthalmitis, unspecified

360.01 Acute endophthalmitis

360.02 Panophthalmitis

360.03 Chronic endophthalmitis

360.04 Vitreous abscess

⑤ **360.1 Other endophthalmitis**
Excludes: *bleb associated endophthalmitis (379.63)*

360.11 Sympathetic uveitis

360.12 Panuveitis

360.13 Parasitic endophthalmitis NOS

360.14 Ophthalmia nodosa

360.19 Other
Phacoanaphylactic endophthalmitis

⑤ **360.2 Degenerative disorders of globe**

360.20 Degenerative disorder of globe, unspecified

360.21 Progressive high (degenerative) myopia
Malignant myopia

360.23 Siderosis

360.24 Other metallosis
Chalcosis

● Code new
to this edition

▲ Revision of
existing code

④ ⑤ Fourth or fifth
digit required

      360.29   **Other**

      Excludes: xerophthalmia (264.7)

⑤ **360.3** **Hypotony of eye**

      360.30   **Hypotony, unspecified**

      360.31   **Primary hypotony**

      360.32   **Ocular fistula causing hypotony**

      360.33   **Hypotony associated with other ocular disorders**

      360.34   **Flat anterior chamber**

⑤ **360.4** **Degenerated conditions of globe**

      360.40   **Degenerated globe or eye, unspecified**

      360.41   **Blind hypotensive eye**
            Atrophy of globe
            Phthisis bulbi

      360.42   **Blind hypertensive eye**
            Absolute glaucoma

      360.43   **Hemophthalmos, except current injury**

      Excludes: traumatic (871.0-871.9, 921.0-921.9)

      360.44   **Leucocoria**

⑤ **360.5** **Retained (old) intraocular foreign body, magnetic**

      Excludes: current penetrating injury with magnetic foreign body (871.5)
                 retained (old) foreign body of orbit (376.6)

      360.50   **Foreign body, magnetic, intraocular, unspecified**

      360.51   **Foreign body, magnetic, in anterior chamber**

      360.52   **Foreign body, magnetic, in iris or ciliary body**

      360.53   **Foreign body, magnetic, in lens**

      360.54   **Foreign body, magnetic, in vitreous**

      360.55   **Foreign body, magnetic, in posterior wall**

      360.59   **Foreign body, magnetic, in other or multiple sites**

⑤ **360.6** **Retained (old) intraocular foreign body, nonmagnetic**
      Retained (old) foreign body:
        NOS
      nonmagnetic

      Excludes: current penetrating injury with (nonmagnetic) foreign body (871.6)
                 retained (old) foreign body in orbit (376.6)

      360.60   **Foreign body, intraocular, unspecified**

      360.61   **Foreign body in anterior chamber**

      360.62   **Foreign body in iris or ciliary body**

      360.63   **Foreign body in lens**

      360.64   **Foreign body in vitreous**

      360.65   **Foreign body in posterior wall**

      360.69   **Foreign body in other or multiple sites**

⑤ **360.8** **Other disorders of globe**

      360.81   **Luxation of globe**

      360.89   **Other**

360.9 **Unspecified disorder of globe**

361 **Retinal detachments and defects**

⑤ **361.0** **Retinal detachment with retinal defect**
      Rhegmatogenous retinal detachment

      Excludes: detachment of retinal pigment epithelium (362.42-362.43)
                 retinal detachment (serous) (without defect) (361.2)

      361.00   **Retinal detachment with retinal defect, unspecified**

      361.01   **Recent detachment, partial, with single defect**

      361.02   **Recent detachment, partial, with multiple defects**

      361.03   **Recent detachment, partial, with giant tear**

Add 4th or 5th digit	Nonspecific code	Unspecified code	Manifestation code

361.04 Recent detachment, partial, with retinal dialysis
Dialysis (juvenile) of retina (with detachment)

361.05 Recent detachment, total or subtotal

361.06 Old detachment, partial
Delimited old retinal detachment

361.07 Old detachment, total or subtotal

⑤ **361.1 Retinoschisis and retinal cysts**

Excludes: *juvenile retinoschisis (362.73)*

microcystoid degeneration of retina (362.62)
parasitic cyst of retina (360.13)

361.10 Retinoschisis, unspecified

361.11 Flat retinoschisis

361.12 Bullous retinoschisis

361.13 Primary retinal cysts

361.14 Secondary retinal cysts

361.19 Other
Pseudocyst of retina

361.2 Serous retinal detachment
Retinal detachment without retinal defect

Excludes: *central serous retinopathy (362.41)*

retinal pigment epithelium detachment (362.42-362.43)

⑤ **361.3 Retinal defects without detachment**

Excludes: *chorioretinal scars after surgery for detachment (363.30-363.35)*

peripheral retinal degeneration without defect (362.60-362.66)

361.30 Retinal defect, unspecified
Retinal break(s) NOS

361.31 Round hole of retina without detachment

361.32 Horseshoe tear of retina without detachment
Operculum of retina without mention of detachment

361.33 Multiple defects of retina without detachment

⑤ **361.8 Other forms of retinal detachment**

361.81 Traction detachment of retina
Traction detachment with vitreoretinal organization

361.89 Other

361.9 Unspecified retinal detachment

362 Other retinal disorders

Excludes: *chorioretinal scars (363.30-363.35)*

chorioretinitis (363.0-363.2)

⑤ *362.0 Diabetic retinopathy*
Code first diabetes (250.5)

362.01 *Background diabetic retinopathy*
Diabetic retinal microaneurysms
Diabetic retinopathy NOS

362.02 *Proliferative diabetic retinopathy*

362.03 Nonproliferative diabetic retinopathy NOS

362.04 Mild nonproliferative diabetic retinopathy

362.05 Moderate nonproliferative diabetic retinopathy

362.06 Severe nonproliferative diabetic retinopathy

362.07 Diabetic macular edema
Diabetic retinal edema
Note: Code 362.07 must be used with a code for diabetic retinopathy (362.01-362.06)

⑤ **362.1 Other background retinopathy and retinal vascular changes**

362.10 Background retinopathy, unspecified

362.11 Hypertensive retinopathy

362.12 Exudative retinopathy
Coats' syndrome

● Code new
to this edition   ▲ Revision of
existing code   ④ ⑤ Fourth or fifth
digit required

362.13 Changes in vascular appearance
Vascular sheathing of retina

Use additional code for any associated atherosclerosis (440.8)

362.14 Retinal microaneurysms NOS

362.15 Retinal telangiectasia

362.16 Retinal neovascularization NOS
Neovascularization:
 choroidal
 subretinal

362.17 Other intraretinal microvascular abnormalities
Retinal varices

362.18 Retinal vasculitis
Eales' disease   Retinal:
Retinal: perivasculitis
 arteritis   phlebitis
 endarteritis

⑤ **362.2 Other proliferative retinopathy**

362.21 Retrolental fibroplasia

362.29 Other nondiabetic proliferative retinopathy

⑤ **362.3 Retinal vascular occlusion**

362.30 Retinal vascular occlusion, unspecified

362.31 Central retinal artery occlusion

362.32 Arterial branch occlusion

362.33 Partial arterial occlusion
Hollenhorst plaque
Retinal microembolism

362.34 Transient arterial occlusion
Amaurosis fugax

362.35 Central retinal vein occlusion

362.36 Venous tributary (branch) occlusion

362.37 Venous engorgement
Occlusion:
 incipient of retinal vein
 partial of retinal vein

⑤ **362.4 Separation of retinal layers**

Excludes: *retinal detachment (serous) (361.2)*
rhegmatogenous (361.00-361.07)

362.40 Retinal layer separation, unspecified

362.41 Central serous retinopathy

362.42 Serous detachment of retinal pigment epithelium
Exudative detachment of retinal pigment epithelium

362.43 Hemorrhagic detachment of retinal pigment epithelium

⑤ **362.5 Degeneration of macula and posterior pole**

Excludes: *degeneration of optic disc (377.21-377.24)*
hereditary retinal degeneration [dystrophy] (362.70-362.77)

362.50 Macular degeneration (senile), unspecified

362.51 Nonexudative senile macular degeneration
Senile macular degeneration:
 atrophic
 dry

362.52 Exudative senile macular degeneration
Kuhnt-Junius degeneration
Senile macular degeneration:
 disciform
 wet

362.53 Cystoid macular degeneration
Cystoid macular edema

362.54 Macular cyst, hole, or pseudohole

362.55 Toxic maculopathy

Use additional E code, if desired, to identify drug, if drug induced

---

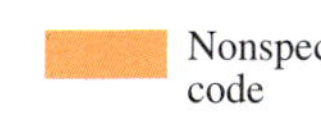

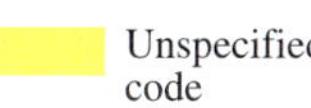

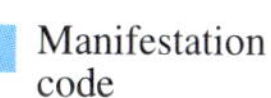

362.56 Macular puckering
Preretinal fibrosis

362.57 Drusen (degenerative)

⑤ **362.6 Peripheral retinal degenerations**
Excludes: *hereditary retinal degeneration [dystrophy] (362.70-362.77)*
retinal degeneration with retinal defect (361.00-361.07)

362.60 Peripheral retinal degeneration, unspecified

362.61 Paving stone degeneration

362.62 Microcystoid degeneration
Blessig's cysts   Iwanoff's cysts

362.63 Lattice degeneration
Palisade degeneration of retina

362.64 Senile reticular degeneration

362.65 Secondary pigmentary degeneration
Pseudoretinitis pigmentosa

362.66 Secondary vitreoretinal degenerations

⑤ **362.7 Hereditary retinal dystrophies**

362.70 Hereditary retinal dystrophy, unspecified

362.71 *Retinal dystrophy in systemic or cerebroretinal lipidoses*
Code first underlying disease, as:
cerebroretinal lipidoses (330.1)
systemic lipidoses (272.7)

362.72 *Retinal dystrophy in other systemic disorders and syndromes*
Code first underlying disease, as:
Bassen-Kornzweig syndrome (272.5)
Refsum's disease (356.3)

362.73 Vitreoretinal dystrophies
Juvenile retinoschisis

362.74 Pigmentary retinal dystrophy
Retinal dystrophy, albipunctate
Retinitis pigmentosa

362.75 Other dystrophies primarily involving the sensory retina
Progressive cone (-rod) dystrophy
Stargardt's disease

362.76 Dystrophies primarily involving the retinal pigment epithelium
Fundus flavimaculatus
Vitelliform dystrophy

362.77 Dystrophies primarily involving Bruch's membrane
Dystrophy:
hyaline
pseudoinflammatory foveal
Hereditary drusen

⑤ **362.8 Other retinal disorders**
Excludes: *chorioretinal inflammations (363.0-363.2)*
chorioretinal scars (363.30-363.35)

362.81 Retinal hemorrhage
Hemorrhage:
preretinal
retinal (deep) (superficial)
subretinal

362.82 Retinal exudates and deposits

362.83 Retinal edema
Retinal:
cotton wool spots
edema (localized) (macular) (peripheral)

362.84 Retinal ischemia

362.85 Retinal nerve fiber bundle defects

362.89 Other retinal disorders

362.9 Unspecified retinal disorder

363 Chorioretinal inflammations, scars, and other disorders of choroid

● Code new
to this edition

▲ Revision of
existing code

④ ⑤ Fourth or fifth
digit required

⑤ **363.0 Focal chorioretinitis and focal retinochoroiditis**

Excludes: *focal chorioretinitis or retinochoroiditis in:*
  histoplasmosis (115.02, 115.12, 115.92)
  toxoplasmosis (130.2)
    congenital infection (771.2)

363.00 Focal chorioretinitis, unspecified
  Focal:
    choroiditis or chorioretinitis NOS
    retinitis or retinochoroiditis NOS

363.01 Focal choroiditis and chorioretinitis, juxtapapillary

363.03 Focal choroiditis and chorioretinitis of other posterior pole

363.04 Focal choroiditis and chorioretinitis, peripheral

363.05 Focal retinitis and retinochoroiditis, juxtapapillary
  Neuroretinitis

363.06 Focal retinitis and retinochoroiditis, macular or paramacular

363.07 Focal retinitis and retinochoroiditis of other posterior pole

363.08 Focal retinitis and retinochoroiditis, peripheral

⑤ **363.1 Disseminated chorioretinitis and disseminated retinochoroiditis**

Excludes: *disseminated choroiditis or chorioretinitis in secondary syphilis (091.51)*
  neurosyphilitic disseminated retinitis or retinochoroiditis (094.83)
  retinal (peri)vasculitis (362.18)

363.10 Disseminated chorioretinitis, unspecified
  Disseminated:
    choroiditis or chorioretinitis NOS
    retinitis or retinochoroiditis NOS

363.11 Disseminated choroiditis and chorioretinitis, posterior pole

363.12 Disseminated choroiditis and chorioretinitis, peripheral

363.13 Disseminated choroiditis and chorioretinitis, generalized
  Code first any underlying disease, as:
    tuberculosis (017.3)

363.14 Disseminated retinitis and retinochoroiditis, metastatic

363.15 Disseminated retinitis and retinochoroiditis, pigment epitheliopathy
  Acute posterior multifocal placoid pigment epitheliopathy

⑤ **363.2 Other and unspecified forms of chorioretinitis and retinochoroiditis**

Excludes: *panophthalmitis (360.02)*
  sympathetic uveitis (360.11)
  uveitis NOS (364.3)

363.20 Chorioretinitis, unspecified
  Choroiditis NOS
  Retinitis NOS
  Uveitis, posterior NOS

363.21 Pars planitis
  Posterior cyclitis

363.22 Harada's disease

⑤ **363.3 Chorioretinal scars**
  Scar (postinflammatory) (postsurgical) (posttraumatic):
    choroid
    retina

363.30 Chorioretinal scar, unspecified

363.31 Solar retinopathy

363.32 Other macular scars

363.33 Other scars of posterior pole

363.34 Peripheral scars

363.35 Disseminated scars

⑤ **363.4 Choroidal degenerations**

363.40 Choroidal degeneration, unspecified
  Choroidal sclerosis NOS

363.41 Senile atrophy of choroid

363.42 Diffuse secondary atrophy of choroid

Add 4th or 5th digit   Nonspecific code   Unspecified code   Manifestation code

363.43   **Angioid streaks of choroid**

⑤ **363.5**   **Hereditary choroidal dystrophies**
Hereditary choroidal atrophy:
  partial [choriocapillaris]
  total [all vessels]

363.50   **Hereditary choroidal dystrophy or atrophy, unspecified**

363.51   **Circumpapillary dystrophy of choroid, partial**

363.52   **Circumpapillary dystrophy of choroid, total**
Helicoid dystrophy of choroid

363.53   **Central dystrophy of choroid, partial**
Dystrophy, choroidal:
  central areolar
  circinate

363.54   **Central choroidal atrophy, total**
Dystrophy, choroidal:
  central gyrate
  serpiginous

363.55   **Choroideremia**

363.56   **Other diffuse or generalized dystrophy, partial**
Diffuse choroidal sclerosis

363.57   **Other diffuse or generalized dystrophy, total**
Generalized gyrate atrophy, choroid

⑤ **363.6**   **Choroidal hemorrhage and rupture**

363.61   **Choroidal hemorrhage, unspecified**

363.62   **Expulsive choroidal hemorrhage**

363.63   **Choroidal rupture**

⑤ **363.7**   **Choroidal detachment**

363.70   **Choroidal detachment, unspecified**

363.71   **Serous choroidal detachment**

363.72   **Hemorrhagic choroidal detachment**

363.8   **Other disorders of choroid**

363.9   **Unspecified disorder of choroid**

364   **Disorders of iris and ciliary body**

⑤ **364.0**   **Acute and subacute iridocyclitis**
Anterior uveitis, acute, subacute
Cyclitis, acute, subacute
Iridocyclitis, acute, subacute
Iritis, acute, subacute

Excludes: *gonococcal (098.41)*
    herpes simplex (054.44)
    herpes zoster (053.22)

364.00   **Acute and subacute iridocyclitis, unspecified**

364.01   **Primary iridocyclitis**

364.02   **Recurrent iridocyclitis**

364.03   **Secondary iridocyclitis, infectious**

364.04   **Secondary iridocyclitis, noninfectious**
Aqueous:
  cells
  fibrin
  flare

364.05   **Hypopyon**

⑤ **364.1**   **Chronic iridocyclitis**

Excludes: *posterior cyclitis (363.21)*

364.10   **Chronic iridocyclitis, unspecified**

364.11   ***Chronic iridocyclitis in diseases classified elsewhere***
Code first underlying disease, as:
  sarcoidosis (135)
  tuberculosis (017.3)

Excludes: *syphilitic iridocyclitis (091.52)*

   ● Code new   ▲ Revision of   ④ ⑤ Fourth or fifth
      to this edition   existing code   digit required

⑤ **364.2   Certain types of iridocyclitis**

> *Excludes:* *posterior cyclitis (363.21)*
> *sympathetic uveitis (360.11)*

364.21   Fuchs' heterochromic cyclitis

364.22   Glaucomatocyclitic crises

364.23   Lens-induced iridocyclitis

364.24   Vogt-Koyanagi syndrome

364.3   Unspecified iridocyclitis
Uveitis NOS

⑤ **364.4   Vascular disorders of iris and ciliary body**

364.41   Hyphema
Hemorrhage of iris or ciliary body

364.42   Rubeosis iridis
Neovascularization of iris or ciliary body

⑤ **364.5   Degenerations of iris and ciliary body**

364.51   Essential or progressive iris atrophy

364.52   Iridoschisis

364.53   Pigmentary iris degeneration
Acquired heterochromia of iris
Pigment dispersion syndrome of iris
Translucency of iris

364.54   Degeneration of pupillary margin
Atrophy of sphincter of iris
Ectropion of pigment epithelium of iris

364.55   Miotic cysts of pupillary margin

364.56   Degenerative changes of chamber angle

364.57   Degenerative changes of ciliary body

364.59   Other iris atrophy
Iris atrophy (generalized) (sector shaped)

⑤ **364.6   Cysts of iris, ciliary body, and anterior chamber**

> *Excludes:* *miotic pupillary cyst (364.55)*
> *parasitic cyst (360.13)*

364.60   Idiopathic cysts

364.61   Implantation cysts
Epithelial down-growth, anterior chamber
Implantation cysts (surgical) (traumatic)

364.62   Exudative cysts of iris or anterior chamber

364.63   Primary cyst of pars plana

364.64   Exudative cyst of pars plana

⑤ **364.7   Adhesions and disruptions of iris and ciliary body**

> *Excludes:* *flat anterior chamber (360.34)*

364.70   Adhesions of iris, unspecified
Synechiae (iris) NOS

364.71   Posterior synechiae

364.72   Anterior synechiae

364.73   Goniosynechiae
Peripheral anterior synechiae

364.74   Pupillary membranes
Iris bombé
Pupillary:
  occlusion
  seclusion

364.75   Pupillary abnormalities
Deformed pupil   Rupture of sphincter, pupil
Ectopic pupil

364.76   Iridodialysis

364.77   Recession of chamber angle

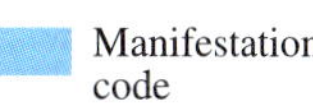

Add 4th or 5th digit	Nonspecific code	Unspecified code	Manifestation code

364.8 **Other disorders of iris and ciliary body**
Prolapse of iris NOS

Excludes: prolapse of iris in recent wound (871.1)

364.9 **Unspecified disorder of iris and ciliary body**

365 **Glaucoma**

Excludes: blind hypertensive eye [absolute glaucoma] (360.42)
congenital glaucoma (743.20-743.22)

⑤ **365.0** **Borderline glaucoma [glaucoma suspect]**

365.00 **Preglaucoma, unspecified**

365.01 **Open angle with borderline findings**
Open angle with:
borderline intraocular pressure
cupping of optic discs

365.02 **Anatomical narrow angle**

365.03 **Steroid responders**

365.04 **Ocular hypertension**

⑤ **365.1** **Open-angle glaucoma**

365.10 **Open-angle glaucoma, unspecified**
Wide-angle glaucoma NOS

365.11 **Primary open angle glaucoma**
Chronic simple glaucoma

365.12 **Low tension glaucoma**

365.13 **Pigmentary glaucoma**

365.14 **Glaucoma of childhood**
Infantile or juvenile glaucoma

365.15 **Residual stage of open angle glaucoma**

⑤ **365.2** **Primary angle-closure glaucoma**

365.20 **Primary angle-closure glaucoma, unspecified**

365.21 **Intermittent angle-closure glaucoma**
Angle-closure glaucoma:
interval
subacute

365.22 **Acute angle-closure glaucoma**

365.23 **Chronic angle-closure glaucoma**

365.24 **Residual stage of angle-closure glaucoma**

⑤ **365.3** **Corticosteroid-induced glaucoma**

365.31 **Glaucomatous stage**

365.32 **Residual stage**

⑤ **365.4** **Glaucoma associated with congenital anomalies, dystrophies, and systemic syndromes**

365.41 *Glaucoma associated with chamber angle anomalies*
Code first associated disorder, as:
Axenfeld's anomaly (743.44)
Rieger's anomaly or syndrome (743.44)

365.42 *Glaucoma associated with anomalies of iris*
Code first associated disorder, as:
aniridia (743.45)
essential iris atrophy (364.51)

365.43 *Glaucoma associated with other anterior segment anomalies*
Code first associated disorder, as:
microcornea (743.41)

365.44 *Glaucoma associated with systemic syndromes*
Code first associated disease, as:
neurofibromatosis (237.7)
Sturge-Weber (-Dimitri) syndrome (759.6)

⑤ **365.5** **Glaucoma associated with disorders of the lens**

365.51 **Phacolytic glaucoma**
Use additional code for associated hypermature cataract (366.18)

365.52 **Pseudoexfoliation glaucoma**
Use additional code for associated pseudoexfoliation of capsule (366.11)

● Code new
to this edition

▲ Revision of
existing code

④ ⑤ Fourth or fifth
digit required

365.59   Glaucoma associated with other lens disorders
Use additional code for associated disorder, as:
    dislocation of lens (379.33-379.34)
    spherophakia (743.36)

⑤ **365.6   Glaucoma associated with other ocular disorders**

365.60   Glaucoma associated with unspecified ocular disorder

365.61   Glaucoma associated with pupillary block
Use additional code for associated disorder, as:
    seclusion of pupil [iris bombé] (364.74)

365.62   Glaucoma associated with ocular inflammations
Use additional code for associated disorder, as:
    glaucomatocyclitic crises (364.22)
    iridocyclitis (364.0-364.3)

365.63   Glaucoma associated with vascular disorders
Use additional code for associated disorder, as:
    central retinal vein occlusion (362.35)
    hyphema (364.41)

365.64   Glaucoma associated with tumors or cysts
Use additional code for associated disorder, as:
    benign neoplasm (224.0-224.9)
    epithelial down-growth (364.61)
    malignant neoplasm (190.0-190.9)

365.65   Glaucoma associated with ocular trauma
Use additional code for associated condition, as:
    contusion of globe (921.3)
    recession of chamber angle (364.77)

⑤ **365.8   Other specified forms of glaucoma**

365.81   Hypersecretion glaucoma

365.82   Glaucoma with increased episcleral venous pressure

365.83   Aqueous misdirection
    Malignant glaucoma

365.89   Other specified glaucoma

365.9   Unspecified glaucoma

366   Cataract
    Excludes: congenital cataract (743.30-743.34)

⑤ **366.0   Infantile, juvenile, and presenile cataract**

366.00   Nonsenile cataract, unspecified

366.01   Anterior subcapsular polar cataract

366.02   Posterior subcapsular polar cataract

366.03   Cortical, lamellar, or zonular cataract

366.04   Nuclear cataract

366.09   Other and combined forms of nonsenile cataract

⑤ **366.1   Senile cataract**

366.10   Senile cataract, unspecified

366.11   Pseudoexfoliation of lens capsule

366.12   Incipient cataract
    Cataract: Water clefts
      coronary
      immature NOS
      punctate

366.13   Anterior subcapsular polar senile cataract

366.14   Posterior subcapsular polar senile cataract

366.15   Cortical senile cataract

366.16   Nuclear sclerosis
    Cataracta brunescens
    Nuclear cataract

366.17   Total or mature cataract

366.18   Hypermature cataract
    Morgagni cataract

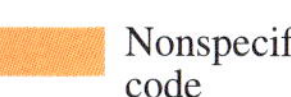

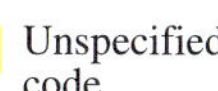

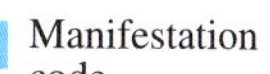

Manifestation
code

366.19   **Other and combined forms of senile cataract**

⑤ **366.2**   **Traumatic cataract**

    366.20   **Traumatic cataract, unspecified**

    366.21   **Localized traumatic opacities**
        Vossius' ring

    366.22   **Total traumatic cataract**

    366.23   **Partially resolved traumatic cataract**

⑤ **366.3**   **Cataract secondary to ocular disorders**

    366.30   **Cataracts complicata, unspecified**

    366.31   *Glaucomatous flecks (subcapsular)*
        Code first underlying glaucoma (365.0-365.9)

    366.32   *Cataract in inflammatory disorders*
        Code first underlying condition, as:
          chronic choroiditis (363.0-363.2)

    366.33   *Cataract with neovascularization*
        Code first underlying condition, as:
          chronic iridocyclitis (364.10)

    366.34   *Cataract in degenerative disorders*
        Sunflower cataract
        Code first underlying condition, as:
          chalcosis (360.24)
          degenerative myopia (360.21)
          pigmentary retinal dystrophy (362.74)

⑤ **366.4**   **Cataract associated with other disorders**

    366.41   *Diabetic cataract*
        Code first diabetes (250.5)

    366.42   *Tetanic cataract*
        Code first underlying disease, as:
          calcinosis (275.4)
          hypoparathyroidism (252.1)

    366.43   *Myotonic cataract*
        Code first underlying disorder (359.2)

    366.44   *Cataract associated with other syndromes*
        Code first underlying condition, as:
          craniofacial dysostosis (756.0)
          galactosemia (271.1)

    366.45   **Toxic cataract**
        Drug-induced cataract
    Use additional E code, if desired, to identify drug or other toxic substance

    366.46   **Cataract associated with radiation and other physical influences**
    Use additional E code, if desired, to identify cause

⑤ **366.5**   **After-cataract**

    366.50   **After-cataract, unspecified**
        Secondary cataract NOS

    366.51   **Soemmering's ring**

    366.52   **Other after-cataract, not obscuring vision**

    366.53   **After-cataract, obscuring vision**

366.8   **Other cataract**
    Calcification of lens

366.9   **Unspecified cataract**

367   **Disorders of refraction and accommodation**

  367.0   **Hypermetropia**
    Far-sightedness
    Hyperopia

  367.1   **Myopia**
    Near-sightedness

⑤ 367.2   **Astigmatism**

    367.20   **Astigmatism, unspecified**

    367.21   **Regular astigmatism**

    367.22   **Irregular astigmatism**

● Code new to this edition   ▲ Revision of existing code   ④ ⑤ Fourth or fifth digit required

⑤ **367.3 Anisometropia and aniseikonia**

    367.31 Anisometropia

    367.32 Aniseikonia

367.4 Presbyopia

⑤ **367.5 Disorders of accommodation**

    367.51 Paresis of accommodation
        Cycloplegia

    367.52 Total or complete internal ophthalmoplegia

    367.53 Spasm of accommodation

⑤ **367.8 Other disorders of refraction and accommodation**

    367.81 Transient refractive change

    367.89 Other
        Drug-induced disorders of refraction and accommodation
        Toxic disorders of refraction and accommodation

367.9 Unspecified disorder of refraction and accommodation

368 Visual disturbances

    Excludes: *electrophysiological disturbances (794.11-794.14)*

⑤ **368.0 Amblyopia ex anopsia**

    368.00 Amblyopia, unspecified

    368.01 Strabismic amblyopia
        Suppression amblyopia

    368.02 Deprivation amblyopia

    368.03 Refractive amblyopia

⑤ **368.1 Subjective visual disturbances**

    368.10 Subjective visual disturbance, unspecified

    368.11 Sudden visual loss

    368.12 Transient visual loss
        Concentric fading
        Scintillating scotoma

    368.13 Visual discomfort
        Asthenopia   Photophobia
        Eye strain

    368.14 Visual distortions of shape and size
        Macropsia   Micropsia
        Metamorphopsia

    368.15 Other visual distortions and entoptic phenomena
        Photopsia   Visual halos
        Refractive:
          diplopia
          polyopia

    368.16 Psychophysical visual disturbances
        Visual:
          agnosia
          disorientation syndrome
          hallucinations

368.2 Diplopia
    Double vision

⑤ **368.3 Other disorders of binocular vision**

    368.30 Binocular vision disorder, unspecified

    368.31 Suppression of binocular vision

    368.32 Simultaneous visual perception without fusion

    368.33 Fusion with defective stereopsis

    368.34 Abnormal retinal correspondence

⑤ **368.4 Visual field defects**

    368.40 Visual field defect, unspecified

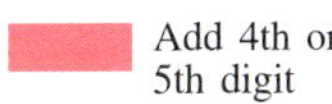

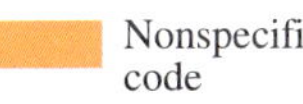

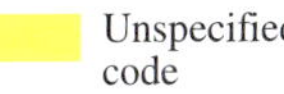

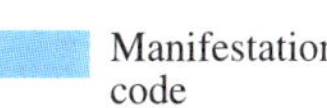

368.41 Scotoma involving central area
Scotoma:
central
centrocecal
paracentral

368.42 Scotoma of blind spot area
Enlarged: Paracecal scotoma
angioscotoma
blind spot

368.43 Sector or arcuate defects
Scotoma:
arcuate
Bjerrum
Seidel

368.44 Other localized visual field defect
Scotoma: Visual field defect:
NOS   nasal step
ring   peripheral

368.45 Generalized contraction or constriction

368.46 Homonymous bilateral field defects
Hemianopsia (altitudinal) (homonymous)
Quadrant anopia

368.47 Heteronymous bilateral field defects
Hemianopsia:
binasal
bitemporal

⑤ **368.5 Color vision deficiencies**
Color blindness

368.51 Protan defect
Protanomaly
Protanopia

368.52 Deutan defect
Deuteranomaly
Deuteranopia

368.53 Tritan defect
Tritanomaly
Tritanopia

368.54 Achromatopsia
Monochromatism (cone) (rod)

368.55 Acquired color vision deficiencies

368.59 Other color vision deficiencies

⑤ **368.6 Night blindness**
Nyctalopia

368.60 Night blindness, unspecified

368.61 Congenital night blindness
Hereditary night blindness
Oguchi's disease

368.62 Acquired night blindness

Excludes: that due to vitamin A deficiency (264.5)

368.63 Abnormal dark adaptation curve
Abnormal threshold of cones or rods
Delayed adaptation of cones or rods

368.69 Other night blindness

368.8 Other specified visual disturbances
Blurred vision NOS

368.9 Unspecified visual disturbance

     ● Code new   ▲ Revision of   ④ ⑤ Fourth or fifth
        to this edition   existing code   digit required

369 Blindness and low vision

Note: Visual impairment refers to a functional limitation of the eye (e.g., limited visual acuity or visual field). It should be distinguished from visual disability, indicating a limitation of the abilities of the individual (e.g., limited reading skills, vocational skills), and from visual handicap, indicating a limitation of personal and socioeconomic independence (e.g., limited mobility, limited employability.)

The levels of impairment defined in the table in this section are based on the recommendations of the WHO Study Group on Prevention of Blindness (Geneva, November 6-10, 1972; WHO Technical Report Series 518), and of the International Council of Ophthalmology (1976).

Note that definitions of blindness vary in different settings.

For international reporting WHO defines blindness as profound impairment. This definition can be applied to blindness of one eye (369.1, 369.6) and to blindness of the individual (369.0).

For determination of benefits in the U.S.A., the definition of legal blindness as severe impairment is often used. This definition applies to blindness of the individual only.

| Excludes: | *correctable impaired vision due to refractive errors (367.0-367.9)* |

⑤ **369.0 Profound impairment, both eyes**

369.00 Impairment level not further specified
Blindness:
  NOS according to WHO definition
  both eyes

369.01 Better eye: total impairment;
  lesser eye: total impairment

369.02 Better eye: near-total impairment;
  lesser eye: not further specified

369.03 Better eye: near-total impairment;
  lesser eye: total impairment

369.04 Better eye: near-total impairment;
  lesser eye: near-total impairment

369.05 Better eye: profound impairment;
  lesser eye: not further specified

369.06 Better eye: profound impairment;
  lesser eye: total impairment

369.07 Better eye: profound impairment;
  lesser eye: near-total impairment

369.08 Better eye: profound impairment;
  lesser eye: profound impairment

⑤ **369.1 Moderate or severe impairment, better eye, profound impairment lesser eye**

369.10 Impairment level not further specified
Blindness, one eye, low vision other eye

369.11 Better eye: severe impairment;
  lesser eye: blind, not further specified

369.12 Better eye: severe impairment;
  lesser eye: total impairment

369.13 Better eye: severe impairment;
  lesser eye: near-total impairment

369.14 Better eye: severe impairment;
  lesser eye: profound impairment

369.15 Better eye: moderate impairment;
  lesser eye: blind, not further specified

369.16 Better eye: moderate impairment;
  lesser eye: total impairment

369.17 Better eye: moderate impairment;
  lesser eye: near-total impairment

369.18 Better eye: moderate impairment;
  lesser eye: profound impairment

⑤ **369.2 Moderate or severe impairment, both eyes**

369.20 Impairment level not further specified
Low vision, both eyes NOS

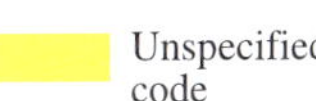

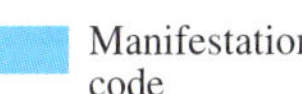

Add 4th or
5th digit

Manifestation
code

369.21 **Better eye: severe impairment;**
    lesser eye: not further specified

369.22 **Better eye: severe impairment;**
    lesser eye: severe impairment

369.23 **Better eye: moderate impairment;**
    lesser eye: not further specified

369.24 **Better eye: moderate impairment;**
    lesser eye: severe impairment

369.25 **Better eye: moderate impairment;**
    lesser eye: moderate impairment

369.3 Unqualified visual loss, both eyes

> Excludes: *blindness NOS:*
>   *legal [U.S.A. definition] (369.4)*
>   *WHO definition (369.00)*

369.4 Legal blindness, as defined in U.S.A.
Blindness NOS according to U.S.A. definition

> Excludes: *legal blindness with specification of impairment level (369.01-369.08,*
>   *369.11-369.14, 369.21-369.22)*

⑤ **369.6 Profound impairment, one eye**

369.60 **Impairment level not further specified**
Blindness, one eye

369.61 **One eye: total impairment; other eye: not specified**

369.62 **One eye: total impairment; other eye: near-normal vision**

369.63 **One eye: total impairment; other eye: normal vision**

369.64 **One eye: near-total impairment; other eye: not specified**

369.65 **One eye: near-total impairment; other eye: near-normal vision**

369.66 **One eye: near-total impairment; other eye: normal vision**

369.67 **One eye: profound impairment; other eye: not specified**

369.68 **One eye: profound impairment; other eye: near-normal vision**

369.69 **One eye: profound impairment; other eye: normal vision**

⑤ **369.7 Moderate or severe impairment, one eye**

369.70 **Impairment level not further specified**
Low vision, one eye

369.71 **One eye: severe impairment; other eye: not specified**

369.72 **One eye: severe impairment; other eye: near-normal vision**

369.73 **One eye: severe impairment; other eye: normal vision**

369.74 **One eye: moderate impairment; other eye: not specified**

369.75 **One eye: moderate impairment; other eye: near-normal vision**

369.76 **One eye: moderate impairment; other eye: normal vision**

369.8 Unqualified visual loss, one eye

369.9 Unspecified visual loss

● Code new to this edition   ▲ Revision of existing code   ④ ⑤ Fourth or fifth digit required

Classification		LEVELS OF VISUAL IMPAIRMENT					Additional Descriptors which may be encountered
"legal"	WHO	Visual Acuity and/or Visual Field Limitation (whichever is worse)					
LEGAL BLINDNESS (USA) both eyes	(NEAR-) NORMAL VISION	**RANGE OF NORMAL VISION** 20/10 — 0.7	20/13 — 0.6	20/16 — 0.5	20/20 — 0.4	20/25 — 0.8	
		NEAR-NORMAL VISION 0.7	20/30 — 0.6	20/40 — 0.5	20/50 — 0.4	20/60 — 0.4	
	LOW VISION	**MODERATE VISUAL IMPAIRMENT** 20/70	20/80 — 0.25	20/100 — 0.20	20/125 — 0.16	20/160 — 0.12	Moderate low vision
		SEVERE VISUAL IMPAIRMENT 20/200 — 0.10	20/250 — 0.08	20/320 — 0.06	20/400 — 0.05		Severe low vision, "legal blindness"
		Visual Field: 20 degrees or less					
	BLINDNESS (WHO) one or both eyes	**PROFOUND VISUAL IMPAIRMENT** 20/500 — 0.04	20/630 — 0.03	20/800 — 0.025	20/1000 — 0.02		Profound low vision, moderate blindness
		Count Fingers at: less than 3 m (10ft) Visual Field: 10 degrees or less					
		NEAR-TOTAL VISUAL IMPAIRMENT Visual Acuity: less than 0.02 (20/1000) Count Fingers at: 1 m (3 ft) or less Hand Movements: 5m (15ft) or less Light projection, light perception Visual Field: 5 degrees or less					Severe blindness Near-Total blindness
		TOTAL VISUAL IMPAIRMENT No light perception (NLP)					Total blindness

Visual acuity refers to best achievable acuity with correction

Non-listed Snellen fractions may be classified by converting to the nearest decimal equivalent, e.g., 10/200=0.05, 6/30=0.20

CF (count fingers) without designation of distance, may be classified to profound impairment

HM (hand motion) without designation of distance, may be classified to near-total impairment.

Visual field measurements refer to the largest field diameter for a 1/100 white test object.

370 Keratitis

⑤ **370.0 Corneal ulcer**

> *Excludes:* that due to vitamin A deficiency (264.3)

370.00 Corneal ulcer, unspecified

370.01 Marginal corneal ulcer

370.02 Ring corneal ulcer

370.03 Central corneal ulcer

370.04 Hypopyon ulcer
Serpiginous ulcer

370.05 Mycotic corneal ulcer

370.06 Perforated corneal ulcer

370.07 Mooren's ulcer

⑤ **370.2 Superficial keratitis without conjunctivitis**

> *Excludes:* dendritic [herpes simplex] keratitis (054.42)

370.20 Superficial keratitis, unspecified

370.21 Punctate keratitis
Thygeson's superficial punctate keratitis

370.22 Macular keratitis
Keratitis: Keratitis:
  areolar stellate
  nummular striate

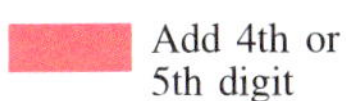

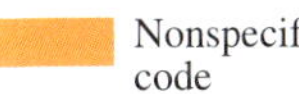

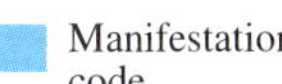

370.23 Filamentary keratitis

370.24 Photokeratitis
Snow blindness
Welders' keratitis

⑤ **370.3 Certain types of keratoconjunctivitis**

370.31 Phlyctenular keratoconjunctivitis
Phlyctenulosis

Use additional code for any associated tuberculosis (017.3)

370.32 Limbar and corneal involvement in vernal conjunctivitis
Use additional code for vernal conjunctivitis (372.13)

370.33 Keratoconjunctivitis sicca, not specified as Sjögren's
Excludes: *Sjögren's syndrome (710.2)*

370.34 Exposure keratoconjunctivitis

370.35 Neurotrophic keratoconjunctivitis

⑤ **370.4 Other and unspecified keratoconjunctivitis**

370.40 Keratoconjunctivitis, unspecified
Superficial keratitis with conjunctivitis NOS

370.44 *Keratitis or keratoconjunctivitis in exanthema*
Code first underlying condition (050.0-052.9)
Excludes: *herpes simplex (054.43)*
herpes zoster (053.21)
measles (055.71)

370.49 Other
Excludes: *epidemic keratoconjunctivitis (077.1)*

⑤ **370.5 Interstitial and deep keratitis**

370.50 Interstitial keratitis, unspecified

370.52 Diffuse interstitial keratitis
Cogan's syndrome

370.54 Sclerosing keratitis

370.55 Corneal abscess

370.59 Other
Excludes: *disciform herpes simplex keratitis (054.43)*
syphilitic keratitis (090.3)

⑤ **370.6 Corneal neovascularization**

370.60 Corneal neovascularization, unspecified

370.61 Localized vascularization of cornea

370.62 Pannus (corneal)

370.63 Deep vascularization of cornea

370.64 Ghost vessels (corneal)

370.8 Other forms of keratitis

370.9 Unspecified keratitis

371 Corneal opacity and other disorders of cornea

⑤ **371.0 Corneal scars and opacities**
Excludes: *that due to vitamin A deficiency (264.6)*

371.00 Corneal opacity, unspecified
Corneal scar NOS

371.01 Minor opacity of cornea
Corneal nebula

371.02 Peripheral opacity of cornea
Corneal macula not interfering with central vision

371.03 Central opacity of cornea
Corneal:
leucoma interfering with central vision
macula interfering with central vision

371.04 Adherent leucoma

371.05 *Phthisical cornea*
Code first underlying tuberculosis (017.3)

● Code new to this edition   ▲ Revision of existing code   ④ ⑤ Fourth or fifth digit required

⑤ **371.1   Corneal pigmentations and deposits**

    371.10   Corneal deposit, unspecified

    371.11   Anterior pigmentations
        Stähli's lines

    371.12   Stromal pigmentations
        Hematocornea

    371.13   Posterior pigmentations
        Krukenberg spindle

    371.14   Kayser-Fleischer ring

    371.15   Other deposits associated with metabolic disorders

    371.16   Argentous deposits

⑤ **371.2   Corneal edema**

    371.20   Corneal edema, unspecified

    371.21   Idiopathic corneal edema

    371.22   Secondary corneal edema

    371.23   Bullous keratopathy

    371.24   Corneal edema due to wearing of contact lenses

⑤ **371.3   Changes of corneal membranes**

    371.30   Corneal membrane change, unspecified

    371.31   Folds and rupture of Bowman's membrane

    371.32   Folds in Descemet's membrane

    371.33   Rupture in Descemet's membrane

⑤ **371.4   Corneal degenerations**

    371.40   Corneal degeneration, unspecified

    371.41   Senile corneal changes
        Arcus senilis
        Hassall-Henle bodies

    371.42   Recurrent erosion of cornea

Excludes:	Mooren's ulcer (370.07)

    371.43   Band-shaped keratopathy

    371.44   Other calcerous degenerations of cornea

    371.45   Keratomalacia NOS

Excludes:	that due to vitamin A deficiency (264.4)

    371.46   Nodular degeneration of cornea
        Salzmann's nodular dystrophy

    371.48   Peripheral degenerations of cornea
        Marginal degeneration of cornea [Terrien's]

    371.49   Other
        Discrete colliquative keratopathy

⑤ **371.5   Hereditary corneal dystrophies**

    371.50   Corneal dystrophy, unspecified

    371.51   Juvenile epithelial corneal dystrophy

    371.52   Other anterior corneal dystrophies
        Corneal dystrophy:
          microscopic cystic
          ring-like

    371.53   Granular corneal dystrophy

    371.54   Lattice corneal dystrophy

    371.55   Macular corneal dystrophy

    371.56   Other stromal corneal dystrophies
        Crystalline corneal dystrophy

    371.57   Endothelial corneal dystrophy
        Combined corneal dystrophy
        Cornea guttata
        Fuchs' endothelial dystrophy

    371.58   Other posterior corneal dystrophies
        Polymorphous corneal dystrophy

	Add 4th or 5th digit		Nonspecific code		Unspecified code		Manifestation code

⑤ **371.6 Keratoconus**

      371.60 Keratoconus, unspecified

      371.61 **Keratoconus, stable condition**

      371.62 **Keratoconus, acute hydrops**

⑤ **371.7 Other corneal deformities**

      371.70 Corneal deformity, unspecified

      371.71 **Corneal ectasia**

      371.72 **Descemetocele**

      371.73 **Corneal staphyloma**

⑤ **371.8 Other corneal disorders**

      371.81 **Corneal anesthesia and hypoesthesia**

      371.82 **Corneal disorder due to contact lens**

      Excludes: *corneal edema due to contact lens (371.24)*

      371.89 Other

371.9 Unspecified corneal disorder

372 Disorders of conjunctiva

      Excludes: *keratoconjunctivitis (370.3-370.4)*

⑤ **372.0 Acute conjunctivitis**

      372.00 Acute conjunctivitis, unspecified

      372.01 **Serous conjunctivitis, except viral**

      Excludes: *viral conjunctivitis NOS (077.9)*

      372.02 **Acute follicular conjunctivitis**
          Conjunctival folliculosis NOS

      Excludes: *conjunctivitis:*
            adenoviral (acute follicular) (077.3)
            epidemic hemorrhagic (077.4)
            inclusion (077.0)
            Newcastle (077.8)
        epidemic keratoconjunctivitis (077.1)
        pharyngoconjunctival fever (077.2)

      372.03 Other mucopurulent conjunctivitis
          Catarrhal conjunctivitis

      Excludes: *blennorrhea neonatorum (gonococcal) (098.40)*
         neonatal conjunctivitis (771.6)
         ophthalmia neonatorum NOS (771.6)

      372.04 **Pseudomembranous conjunctivitis**
          Membranous conjunctivitis

      Excludes: *diphtheritic conjunctivitis (032.81)*

      372.05 **Acute atopic conjunctivitis**

⑤ **372.1 Chronic conjunctivitis**

      372.10 Chronic conjunctivitis, unspecified

      372.11 **Simple chronic conjunctivitis**

      372.12 **Chronic follicular conjunctivitis**

      372.13 **Vernal conjunctivitis**

      372.14 Other chronic allergic conjunctivitis

      372.15 *Parasitic conjunctivitis*
          Code first underlying disease, as:
            filariasis (125.0-125.9)
            mucocutaneous leishmaniasis (085.5)

⑤ **372.2 Blepharoconjunctivitis**

      372.20 Blepharoconjunctivitis, unspecified

      372.21 **Angular blepharoconjunctivitis**

      372.22 **Contact blepharoconjunctivitis**

⑤ **372.3 Other and unspecified conjunctivitis**

      372.30 Conjunctivitis, unspecified

● Code new
to this edition   ▲ Revision of
existing code   ④ ⑤ Fourth or fifth
digit required

372.31 *Rosacea conjunctivitis*
Code first underlying rosacea dermatitis (695.3)

372.33 *Conjunctivitis in mucocutaneous disease*
Code first underlying disease, as:
erythema multiforme (695.1)
Reiter's disease (099.3)

Excludes: *ocular pemphigoid (694.61)*

372.39 **Other**

⑤ **372.4 Pterygium**

Excludes: *pseudopterygium (372.52)*

372.40 **Pterygium, unspecified**

372.41 **Peripheral pterygium, stationary**

372.42 **Peripheral pterygium, progressive**

372.43 **Central pterygium**

372.44 **Double pterygium**

372.45 **Recurrent pterygium**

⑤ **372.5 Conjunctival degenerations and deposits**

372.50 **Conjunctival degeneration, unspecified**

372.51 **Pinguecula**

372.52 **Pseudopterygium**

372.53 **Conjunctival xerosis**

Excludes: *conjunctival xerosis due to vitamin A deficiency (264.0, 264.1, 264.7)*

372.54 **Conjunctival concretions**

372.55 **Conjunctival pigmentations**
Conjunctival argyrosis

372.56 **Conjunctival deposits**

⑤ **372.6 Conjunctival scars**

372.61 **Granuloma of conjunctiva**

372.62 **Localized adhesions and strands of conjunctiva**

372.63 **Symblepharon**
Extensive adhesions of conjunctiva

372.64 **Scarring of conjunctiva**
Contraction of eye socket (after enucleation)

⑤ **372.7 Conjunctival vascular disorders and cysts**

372.71 **Hyperemia of conjunctiva**

372.72 **Conjunctival hemorrhage**
Hyposphagma
Subconjunctival hemorrhage

372.73 **Conjunctival edema**
Chemosis of conjunctiva
Subconjunctival edema

372.74 **Vascular abnormalities of conjunctiva**
Aneurysm(ata) of conjunctiva

372.75 **Conjunctival cysts**

⑤ **372.8 Other disorders of conjunctiva**

372.81 **Conjunctivochalasis**

372.89 **Other disorders of conjunctiva**

372.9 **Unspecified disorder of conjunctiva**

373 **Inflammation of eyelids**

⑤ **373.0 Blepharitis**

Excludes: *blepharoconjunctivitis (372.20-372.22)*

373.00 **Blepharitis, unspecified**

373.01 **Ulcerative blepharitis**

373.02 **Squamous blepharitis**

⑤ **373.1 Hordeolum and other deep inflammation of eyelid**

373.11 Hordeolum externum
Hordeolum NOS
Stye

373.12 Hordeolum internum
Infection of meibomian gland

373.13 Abscess of eyelid
Furuncle of eyelid

373.2 Chalazion
Meibomian (gland) cyst

Excludes: *infected meibomian gland (373.12)*

⑤ **373.3 Noninfectious dermatoses of eyelid**

373.31 Eczematous dermatitis of eyelid

373.32 Contact and allergic dermatitis of eyelid

373.33 Xeroderma of eyelid

373.34 Discoid lupus erythematosus of eyelid

373.4 *Infective dermatitis of eyelid of types resulting in deformity*
Code first underlying disease, as:
leprosy (030.0-030.9)
lupus vulgaris (tuberculous) (017.0)
yaws (102.0-102.9)

373.5 *Other infective dermatitis of eyelid*
Code first underlying disease, as:
actinomycosis (039.3)
impetigo (684)
mycotic dermatitis (110.0-111.9)
vaccinia (051.0)
postvaccination (999.0)

Excludes: *herpes:*
simplex (054.41)
zoster (053.20)

373.6 *Parasitic infestation of eyelid*
Code first underlying disease, as:
leishmaniasis (085.0-085.9)
loiasis (125.2)
onchocerciasis (125.3)
pediculosis (132.0)

373.8 Other inflammations of eyelids

373.9 Unspecified inflammation of eyelid

374 Other disorders of eyelids

⑤ **374.0 Entropion and trichiasis of eyelid**

374.00 Entropion, unspecified

374.01 Senile entropion

374.02 Mechanical entropion

374.03 Spastic entropion

374.04 Cicatricial entropion

374.05 Trichiasis without entropion

⑤ **374.1 Ectropion**

374.10 Ectropion, unspecified

374.11 Senile ectropion

374.12 Mechanical ectropion

374.13 Spastic ectropion

374.14 Cicatricial ectropion

⑤ **374.2 Lagophthalmos**

374.20 Lagophthalmos, unspecified

374.21 Paralytic lagophthalmos

374.22 Mechanical lagophthalmos

374.23 Cicatricial lagophthalmos

⑤ **374.3 Ptosis of eyelid**

● Code new
to this edition

▲ Revision of
existing code

④ ⑤ Fourth or fifth
digit required

374.30 **Ptosis of eyelid, unspecified**

374.31 **Paralytic ptosis**

374.32 **Myogenic ptosis**

374.33 **Mechanical ptosis**

374.34 **Blepharochalasis**
Pseudoptosis

⑤ 374.4 **Other disorders affecting eyelid function**
Excludes: blepharoclonus (333.81)
blepharospasm (333.81)
facial nerve palsy (351.0)
third nerve palsy or paralysis (378.51-378.52)
tic (psychogenic) (307.20-307.23)
organic (333.3)

374.41 **Lid retraction or lag**

374.43 **Abnormal innervation syndrome**
Jaw-blinking
Paradoxical facial movements

374.44 **Sensory disorders**

374.45 **Other sensorimotor disorders**
Deficient blink reflex

374.46 **Blepharophimosis**
Ankyloblepharon

⑤ 374.5 **Degenerative disorders of eyelid and periocular area**

374.50 **Degenerative disorder of eyelid, unspecified**

374.51 *Xanthelasma*
Xanthoma (planum) (tuberosum) of eyelid
Code first underlying condition (272.0-272.9)

374.52 **Hyperpigmentation of eyelid**
Chloasma
Dyspigmentation

374.53 **Hypopigmentation of eyelid**
Vitiligo of eyelid

374.54 **Hypertrichosis of eyelid**

374.55 **Hypotrichosis of eyelid**
Madarosis of eyelid

374.56 **Other degenerative disorders of skin affecting eyelid**

⑤ 374.8 **Other disorders of eyelid**

374.81 **Hemorrhage of eyelid**
Excludes: black eye (921.0)

374.82 **Edema of eyelid**
Hyperemia of eyelid

374.83 **Elephantiasis of eyelid**

374.84 **Cysts of eyelids**
Sebaceous cyst of eyelid

374.85 **Vascular anomalies of eyelid**

374.86 **Retained foreign body of eyelid**

374.87 **Dermatochalasis**

374.89 **Other disorders of eyelid**

374.9 **Unspecified disorder of eyelid**

375 **Disorders of lacrimal system**

⑤ 375.0 **Dacryoadenitis**

375.00 **Dacryoadenitis, unspecified**

375.01 **Acute dacryoadenitis**

375.02 **Chronic dacryoadenitis**

375.03 **Chronic enlargement of lacrimal gland**

⑤ 375.1 **Other disorders of lacrimal gland**

375.11 **Dacryops**

Add 4th or 5th digit	Nonspecific code	Unspecified code	Manifestation code

375.12   **Other lacrimal cysts and cystic degeneration**

375.13   **Primary lacrimal atrophy**

375.14   **Secondary lacrimal atrophy**

375.15   **Tear film insufficiency, unspecified**
    Dry eye syndrome

375.16   **Dislocation of lacrimal gland**

⑤ **375.2**   **Epiphora**

375.20   **Epiphora, unspecified as to cause**

375.21   **Epiphora due to excess lacrimation**

375.22   **Epiphora due to insufficient drainage**

⑤ **375.3**   **Acute and unspecified inflammation of lacrimal passages**
    Excludes: neonatal dacryocystitis (771.6)

375.30   **Dacryocystitis, unspecified**

375.31   **Acute canaliculitis, lacrimal**

375.32   **Acute dacryocystitis**
    Acute peridacryocystitis

375.33   **Phlegmonous dacryocystitis**

⑤ **375.4**   **Chronic inflammation of lacrimal passages**

375.41   **Chronic canaliculitis**

375.42   **Chronic dacryocystitis**

375.43   **Lacrimal mucocele**

⑤ **375.5**   **Stenosis and insufficiency of lacrimal passages**

375.51   **Eversion of lacrimal punctum**

375.52   **Stenosis of lacrimal punctum**

375.53   **Stenosis of lacrimal canaliculi**

375.54   **Stenosis of lacrimal sac**

375.55   **Obstruction of nasolacrimal duct, neonatal**
    Excludes: congenital anomaly of nasolacrimal duct (743.65)

375.56   **Stenosis of nasolacrimal duct, acquired**

375.57   **Dacryolith**

⑤ **375.6**   **Other changes of lacrimal passages**

375.61   **Lacrimal fistula**

375.69   **Other**

⑤ **375.8**   **Other disorders of lacrimal system**

375.81   **Granuloma of lacrimal passages**

375.89   **Other**

375.9   **Unspecified disorder of lacrimal system**

376   **Disorders of the orbit**

⑤ **376.0**   **Acute inflammation of orbit**

376.00   **Acute inflammation of orbit, unspecified**

376.01   **Orbital cellulitis**
    Abscess of orbit

376.02   **Orbital periostitis**

376.03   **Orbital osteomyelitis**

376.04   **Tenonitis**

⑤ **376.1**   **Chronic inflammatory disorders of orbit**

376.10   **Chronic inflammation of orbit, unspecified**

376.11   **Orbital granuloma**
    Pseudotumor (inflammatory) of orbit

376.12   **Orbital myositis**

376.13   *Parasitic infestation of orbit*
    Code first underlying disease, as:
      hydatid infestation of orbit (122.3, 122.6, 122.9)
      myiasis of orbit (134.0)

● Code new
to this edition   ▲ Revision of
existing code   ④ ⑤ Fourth or fifth
digit required

⑤ **376.2** *Endocrine exophthalmos*
Code first underlying thyroid disorder (242.0-242.9)

376.21 *Thyrotoxic exophthalmos*

376.22 *Exophthalmic ophthalmoplegia*

⑤ **376.3 Other exophthalmic conditions**

376.30 Exophthalmos, unspecified

376.31 Constant exophthalmos

376.32 Orbital hemorrhage

376.33 Orbital edema or congestion

376.34 Intermittent exophthalmos

376.35 Pulsating exophthalmos

376.36 Lateral displacement of globe

⑤ **376.4 Deformity of orbit**

376.40 Deformity of orbit, unspecified

376.41 Hypertelorism of orbit

376.42 Exostosis of orbit

376.43 Local deformities due to bone disease

376.44 Orbital deformities associated with craniofacial deformities

376.45 Atrophy of orbit

376.46 Enlargement of orbit

376.47 Deformity due to trauma or surgery

⑤ **376.5 Enophthalmos**

376.50 Enophthalmos, unspecified as to cause

376.51 Enophthalmos due to atrophy of orbital tissue

376.52 Enophthalmos due to trauma or surgery

376.6 Retained (old) foreign body following penetrating wound of orbit
Retrobulbar foreign body

⑤ **376.8 Other orbital disorders**

376.81 Orbital cysts
Encephalocele of orbit

376.82 Myopathy of extraocular muscles

376.89 Other

376.9 Unspecified disorder of orbit

377 Disorders of optic nerve and visual pathways

⑤ **377.0 Papilledema**

377.00 Papilledema, unspecified

377.01 Papilledema associated with increased intracranial pressure

377.02 Papilledema associated with decreased ocular pressure

377.03 Papilledema associated with retinal disorder

377.04 Foster-Kennedy syndrome

⑤ **377.1 Optic atrophy**

377.10 Optic atrophy, unspecified

377.11 Primary optic atrophy

Excludes: *neurosyphilitic optic atrophy (094.84)*

377.12 Postinflammatory optic atrophy

377.13 Optic atrophy associated with retinal dystrophies

377.14 Glaucomatous atrophy [cupping] of optic disc

377.15 Partial optic atrophy
Temporal pallor of optic disc

377.16 Hereditary optic atrophy
Optic atrophy:
dominant hereditary
Leber's

⑤ **377.2 Other disorders of optic disc**

	Add 4th or 5th digit		Nonspecific code		Unspecified code		Manifestation code

377.21   **Drusen of optic disc**

377.22   **Crater-like holes of optic disc**

377.23   **Coloboma of optic disc**

377.24   **Pseudopapilledema**

⑤ **377.3 Optic neuritis**

Excludes: meningococcal optic neuritis (036.81)

377.30   **Optic neuritis, unspecified**

377.31   **Optic papillitis**

377.32   **Retrobulbar neuritis (acute)**

Excludes: syphilitic retrobulbar neuritis (094.85)

377.33   **Nutritional optic neuropathy**

377.34   **Toxic optic neuropathy**
Toxic amblyopia

377.39   **Other**

Excludes: ischemic optic neuropathy (377.41)

⑤ **377.4 Other disorders of optic nerve**

377.41   **Ischemic optic neuropathy**

377.42   **Hemorrhage in optic nerve sheaths**

● 377.43   **Optic nerve hypoplasia**

377.49   **Other**
Compression of optic nerve

⑤ **377.5 Disorders of optic chiasm**

377.51   **Associated with pituitary neoplasms and disorders**

377.52   **Associated with other neoplasms**

377.53   **Associated with vascular disorders**

377.54   **Associated with inflammatory disorders**

⑤ **377.6 Disorders of other visual pathways**

377.61   **Associated with neoplasms**

377.62   **Associated with vascular disorders**

377.63   **Associated with inflammatory disorders**

⑤ **377.7 Disorders of visual cortex**

Excludes: visual:

agnosia (368.16)
hallucinations (368.16)
halos (368.15)

377.71   **Associated with neoplasms**

377.72   **Associated with vascular disorders**

377.73   **Associated with inflammatory disorders**

377.75   **Cortical blindness**

377.9 **Unspecified disorder of optic nerve and visual pathways**

378 **Strabismus and other disorders of binocular eye movements**

Excludes: nystagmus and other irregular eye movements (379.50-379.59)

⑤ **378.0 Esotropia**
Convergent concomitant strabismus

Excludes: intermittent esotropia (378.20-378.22)

378.00   **Esotropia, unspecified**

378.01   **Monocular esotropia**

378.02   **Monocular esotropia with A pattern**

378.03   **Monocular esotropia with V pattern**

378.04   **Monocular esotropia with other noncomitancies**
Monocular esotropia with X or Y pattern

378.05   **Alternating esotropia**

378.06   **Alternating esotropia with A pattern**

● Code new
to this edition

▲ Revision of
existing code

④ ⑤ Fourth or fifth
digit required

378.07 **Alternating esotropia with V pattern**

378.08 **Alternating esotropia with other noncomitancies**
Alternating esotropia with X or Y pattern

⑤ **378.1 Exotropia**
Divergent concomitant strabismus
Excludes: *intermittent exotropia (378.20, 378.23-378.24)*

378.10 **Exotropia, unspecified**

378.11 **Monocular exotropia**

378.12 **Monocular exotropia with A pattern**

378.13 **Monocular exotropia with V pattern**

378.14 **Monocular exotropia with other noncomitancies**
Monocular exotropia with X or Y pattern

378.15 **Alternating exotropia**

378.16 **Alternating exotropia with A pattern**

378.17 **Alternating exotropia with V pattern**

378.18 **Alternating exotropia with other noncomitancies**
Alternating exotropia with X or Y pattern

⑤ **378.2 Intermittent heterotropia**
Excludes: *vertical heterotropia (intermittent) (378.31)*

378.20 **Intermittent heterotropia, unspecified**
Intermittent:
esotropia NOS
exotropia NOS

378.21 **Intermittent esotropia, monocular**

378.22 **Intermittent esotropia, alternating**

378.23 **Intermittent exotropia, monocular**

378.24 **Intermittent exotropia, alternating**

⑤ **378.3 Other and unspecified heterotropia**

378.30 **Heterotropia, unspecified**

378.31 **Hypertropia**
Vertical heterotropia (constant) (intermittent)

378.32 **Hypotropia**

378.33 **Cyclotropia**

378.34 **Monofixation syndrome**
Microtropia

378.35 **Accommodative component in esotropia**

⑤ **378.4 Heterophoria**

378.40 **Heterophoria, unspecified**

378.41 **Esophoria**

378.42 **Exophoria**

378.43 **Vertical heterophoria**

378.44 **Cyclophoria**

378.45 **Alternating hyperphoria**

⑤ **378.5 Paralytic strabismus**

378.50 **Paralytic strabismus, unspecified**

378.51 **Third or oculomotor nerve palsy, partial**

378.52 **Third or oculomotor nerve palsy, total**

378.53 **Fourth or trochlear nerve palsy**

378.54 **Sixth or abducens nerve palsy**

378.55 **External ophthalmoplegia**

378.56 **Total ophthalmoplegia**

⑤ **378.6 Mechanical strabismus**

378.60 **Mechanical strabismus, unspecified**

378.61 **Brown's (tendon) sheath syndrome**

378.62 **Mechanical strabismus from other musculofascial disorders**

Add 4th or 5th digit | Nonspecific code | Unspecified code | Manifestation code

378.63 Limited duction associated with other conditions

⑤ **378.7** Other specified strabismus

378.71 Duane's syndrome

378.72 Progressive external ophthalmoplegia

378.73 Strabismus in other neuromuscular disorders

⑤ **378.8** Other disorders of binocular eye movements

Excludes: nystagmus (379.50-379.56)

378.81 Palsy of conjugate gaze

378.82 Spasm of conjugate gaze

378.83 Convergence insufficiency or palsy

378.84 Convergence excess or spasm

378.85 Anomalies of divergence

378.86 Internuclear ophthalmoplegia

378.87 Other dissociated deviation of eye movements
Skew deviation

378.9 Unspecified disorder of eye movements
Ophthalmoplegia NOS
Strabismus NOS

379 Other disorders of eye

⑤ **379.0** Scleritis and episcleritis

Excludes: syphilitic episcleritis (095.0)

379.00 Scleritis, unspecified
Episcleritis NOS

379.01 Episcleritis periodica fugax

379.02 Nodular episcleritis

379.03 Anterior scleritis

379.04 Scleromalacia perforans

379.05 Scleritis with corneal involvement
Scleroperikeratitis

379.06 Brawny scleritis

379.07 Posterior scleritis
Sclerotenonitis

379.09 Other
Scleral abscess

⑤ **379.1** Other disorders of sclera

Excludes: blue sclera (743.47)

379.11 Scleral ectasia
Scleral staphyloma NOS

379.12 Staphyloma posticum

379.13 Equatorial staphyloma

379.14 Anterior staphyloma, localized

379.15 Ring staphyloma

379.16 Other degenerative disorders of sclera

379.19 Other

⑤ **379.2** Disorders of vitreous body

379.21 Vitreous degeneration
Vitreous:
cavitation
detachment
liquefaction

379.22 Crystalline deposits in vitreous
Asteroid hyalitis
Synchysis scintillans

379.23 Vitreous hemorrhage

379.24 Other vitreous opacities
Vitreous floaters

● Code new
to this edition

▲ Revision of
existing code

④ ⑤ Fourth or fifth
digit required

379.25   **Vitreous membranes and strands**

379.26   **Vitreous prolapse**

379.29   **Other disorders of vitreous**
Excludes: *vitreous abscess (360.04)*

⑤ **379.3   Aphakia and other disorders of lens**
Excludes: *after-cataract (366.50-366.53)*

   379.31   **Aphakia**
Excludes: *cataract extraction status (V45.61)*

379.32   **Subluxation of lens**

379.33   **Anterior dislocation of lens**

379.34   **Posterior dislocation of lens**

379.39   **Other disorders of lens**

⑤ **379.4   Anomalies of pupillary function**

379.40   **Abnormal pupillary function, unspecified**

379.41   **Anisocoria**

379.42   **Miosis (persistent), not due to miotics**

379.43   **Mydriasis (persistent) not due to mydriatics**

379.45   **Argyll Robertson pupil, atypical**
Argyll Robertson phenomenon or pupil, nonsyphilitic

Excludes: *Argyll Robertson pupil (syphilitic) (094.89)*

379.46   **Tonic pupillary reaction**
Adie's pupil or syndrome

379.49   **Other**
Hippus
Pupillary paralysis

⑤ **379.5   Nystagmus and other irregular eye movements**

379.50   **Nystagmus, unspecified**

379.51   **Congenital nystagmus**

379.52   **Latent nystagmus**

379.53   **Visual deprivation nystagmus**

379.54   **Nystagmus associated with disorders of the vestibular system**

379.55   **Dissociated nystagmus**

379.56   **Other forms of nystagmus**

379.57   **Deficiencies of saccadic eye movements**
Abnormal optokinetic response

379.58   **Deficiencies of smooth pursuit movements**

379.59   **Other irregularities of eye movements**
Opsoclonus

● **379.6   Inflammation (infection) of postprocedural bleb**
Postprocedural blebitis

  ● **379.60**   **Inflammation (infection) of postprocedural bleb, unspecified**

  ● **379.61**   **Inflammation (infection) of postprocedural bleb, stage 1**

  ● **379.62**   **Inflammation (infection) of postprocedural bleb, stage 2**

  ● **379.63**   **Inflammation (infection) of postprocedural bleb, stage 3**
Bleb associated endophthalmitis

379.8   Other specified disorders of eye and adnexa

⑤ **379.9   Unspecified disorder of eye and adnexa**

379.90   **Disorder of eye, unspecified**

379.91   **Pain in or around eye**

379.92   **Swelling or mass of eye**

379.93   **Redness or discharge of eye**

379.99   **Other ill-defined disorders of eye**

Excludes: *blurred vision NOS (368.8)*

DISEASES OF THE EAR AND MASTOID PROCESS (380-389)

380 Disorders of external ear

⑤ **380.0 Perichondritis and chondritis of pinna**
Chondritis of auricle
Perichondritis of auricle

380.00 Perichondritis of pinna, unspecified

380.01 Acute perichondritis of pinna

380.02 Chronic perichondritis of pinna

380.03 Chondritis of pinna

⑤ **380.1 Infective otitis externa**

380.10 Infective otitis externa, unspecified
Otitis externa (acute):
NOS
circumscribed
diffuse
hemorrhagica
infective NOS

380.11 Acute infection of pinna
Excludes: furuncular otitis externa (680.0)

380.12 Acute swimmers' ear
Beach ear
Tank ear

380.13 *Other acute infections of external ear*
Code first underlying disease, as:
erysipelas (035)
impetigo (684)
seborrheic dermatitis (690.10-690.18)
Excludes: herpes simplex (054.73)
herpes zoster (053.71)

380.14 Malignant otitis externa

380.15 *Chronic mycotic otitis externa*
Code first underlying disease, as:
aspergillosis (117.3)
otomycosis NOS (111.9)
Excludes: candidal otitis externa (112.82)

380.16 Other chronic infective otitis externa
Chronic infective otitis externa NOS

⑤ **380.2 Other otitis externa**

380.21 Cholesteatoma of external ear
Keratosis obturans of external ear (canal)
Excludes: cholesteatoma NOS (385.30-385.35)
postmastoidectomy (383.32)

380.22 Other acute otitis externa
Acute otitis externa:
actinic
chemical
contact
eczematoid
reactive

380.23 Other chronic otitis externa
Chronic otitis externa NOS

⑤ **380.3 Noninfectious disorders of pinna**

380.30 Disorder of pinna, unspecified

380.31 Hematoma of auricle or pinna

380.32 Acquired deformities of auricle or pinna
Excludes: cauliflower ear (738.7)

380.39 Other
Excludes: gouty tophi of ear (274.81)

380.4 Impacted cerumen
Wax in ear

● Code new to this edition   ▲ Revision of existing code   ④ ⑤ Fourth or fifth digit required

⑤ **380.5 Acquired stenosis of external ear canal**
Collapse of external ear canal

380.50 **Acquired stenosis of external ear canal, unspecified as to cause**

380.51 Secondary to trauma

380.52 Secondary to surgery

380.53 Secondary to inflammation

⑤ **380.8 Other disorders of external ear**

380.81 Exostosis of external ear canal

380.89 Other

380.9 Unspecified disorder of external ear

381 Nonsuppurative otitis media and Eustachian tube disorders

⑤ **381.0 Acute nonsuppurative otitis media**
Acute tubotympanic catarrh
Otitis media, acute or subacute:
   catarrhal
   exudative
   transudative
   with effusion

Excludes: otitic barotrauma (993.0)

381.00 **Acute nonsuppurative otitis media, unspecified**

381.01 Acute serous otitis media
Acute or subacute secretory otitis media

381.02 Acute mucoid otitis media
Acute or subacute seromucinous otitis media
Blue drum syndrome

381.03 Acute sanguinous otitis media

381.04 Acute allergic serous otitis media

381.05 Acute allergic mucoid otitis media

381.06 Acute allergic sanguinous otitis media

⑤ **381.1 Chronic serous otitis media**
Chronic tubotympanic catarrh

381.10 Chronic serous otitis media, simple or unspecified

381.19 Other
Serosanguinous chronic otitis media

⑤ **381.2 Chronic mucoid otitis media**
Glue ear

Excludes: adhesive middle ear disease (385.10-385.19)

381.20 Chronic mucoid otitis media, simple or unspecified

381.29 Other
Mucosanguinous chronic otitis media

381.3 Other and unspecified chronic nonsuppurative otitis media
Otitis media, chronic: Otitis media, chronic:
   allergic   seromucinous
   exudative   transudative
   secretory   with effusion

381.4 Nonsuppurative otitis media, not specified as acute or chronic
Otitis media: Otitis media:
   allergic   secretory
   catarrhal   seromucinous
   exudative   serous
   mucoid   transudative
                  with effusion

⑤ **381.5 Eustachian salpingitis**

381.50 **Eustachian salpingitis, unspecified**

381.51 Acute Eustachian salpingitis

381.52 Chronic Eustachian salpingitis

⑤ **381.6 Obstruction of Eustachian tube**
Stenosis of Eustachian tube
Stricture of Eustachian tube

Add 4th or 5th digit	Nonspecific code	Unspecified code	Manifestation code

381.60 **Obstruction of Eustachian tube, unspecified**

381.61 **Osseous obstruction of Eustachian tube**
Obstruction of Eustachian tube from cholesteatoma, polyp, or other osseous lesion

381.62 **Intrinsic cartilagenous obstruction of Eustachian tube**

381.63 **Extrinsic cartilagenous obstruction of Eustachian tube**
Compression of Eustachian tube

381.7 **Patulous Eustachian tube**

⑤ **381.8** **Other disorders of Eustachian tube**

381.81 **Dysfunction of Eustachian tube**

381.89 **Other**

381.9 **Unspecified Eustachian tube disorder**

382 **Suppurative and unspecified otitis media**

⑤ **382.0** **Acute suppurative otitis media**
Otitis media, acute:
necrotizing NOS
purulent

382.00 **Acute suppurative otitis media without spontaneous rupture of ear drum**

382.01 **Acute suppurative otitis media with spontaneous rupture of ear drum**

382.02 **Acute suppurative otitis media in diseases classified elsewhere**
Code first underlying disease, as:
influenza (487.8)
scarlet fever (034.1)

Excludes: *postmeasles otitis (055.2)*

382.1 **Chronic tubotympanic suppurative otitis media**
Benign chronic suppurative otitis media (with anterior perforation of ear drum)
Chronic tubotympanic disease (with anterior perforation of ear drum)

382.2 **Chronic atticoantral suppurative otitis media**
Chronic atticoantral disease (with posterior or superior marginal perforation of ear drum)
Persistent mucosal disease (with posterior or superior marginal perforation of ear drum)

382.3 **Unspecified chronic suppurative otitis media**
Chronic purulent otitis media

Excludes: *tuberculous otitis media (017.4)*

382.4 **Unspecified suppurative otitis media**
Purulent otitis media NOS

382.9 **Unspecified otitis media**
Otitis media:
NOS
acute NOS
chronic NOS

383 **Mastoiditis and related conditions**

⑤ **383.0** **Acute mastoiditis**
Abscess of mastoid
Empyema of mastoid

383.00 **Acute mastoiditis without complications**

383.01 **Subperiosteal abscess of mastoid**

383.02 **Acute mastoiditis with other complications**
Gradenigo's syndrome

383.1 **Chronic mastoiditis**
Caries of mastoid
Fistula of mastoid

Excludes: *tuberculous mastoiditis (015.6)*

⑤ **383.2** **Petrositis**
Coalescing osteitis of petrous bone
Inflammation of petrous bone
Osteomyelitis of petrous bone

383.20 **Petrositis, unspecified**

383.21 **Acute petrositis**

383.22 **Chronic petrositis**

● Code new to this edition   ▲ Revision of existing code   ④ ⑤ Fourth or fifth digit required

⑤ **383.3 Complications following mastoidectomy**

    383.30 Postmastoidectomy complication, unspecified

    383.31 Mucosal cyst of postmastoidectomy cavity

    383.32 Recurrent cholesteatoma of postmastoidectomy cavity

    383.33 Granulations of postmastoidectomy cavity
        Chronic inflammation of postmastoidectomy cavity

⑤ **383.8 Other disorders of mastoid**

    383.81 Postauricular fistula

    383.89 Other

383.9 Unspecified mastoiditis

384 Other disorders of tympanic membrane

⑤ **384.0 Acute myringitis without mention of otitis media**

    384.00 Acute myringitis, unspecified
        Acute tympanitis NOS

    384.01 Bullous myringitis
        Myringitis bullosa hemorrhagica

    384.09 Other

384.1 Chronic myringitis without mention of otitis media
    Chronic tympanitis

⑤ **384.2 Perforation of tympanic membrane**
    Perforation of ear drum:
      NOS
      persistent posttraumatic
      postinflammatory

    Excludes: *otitis media with perforation of tympanic membrane (382.00-382.9)*
        traumatic perforation [current injury] (872.61)

    384.20 Perforation of tympanic membrane, unspecified

    384.21 Central perforation of tympanic membrane

    384.22 Attic perforation of tympanic membrane
        Pars flaccida

    384.23 Other marginal perforation of tympanic membrane

    384.24 Multiple perforations of tympanic membrane

    384.25 Total perforation of tympanic membrane

⑤ **384.8 Other specified disorders of tympanic membrane**

    384.81 Atrophic flaccid tympanic membrane
        Healed perforation of ear drum

    384.82 Atrophic nonflaccid tympanic membrane

384.9 Unspecified disorder of tympanic membrane

385 Other disorders of middle ear and mastoid

    Excludes: *mastoiditis (383.0-383.9)*

⑤ **385.0 Tympanosclerosis**

    385.00 Tympanosclerosis, unspecified as to involvement

    385.01 Tympanosclerosis involving tympanic membrane only

    385.02 Tympanosclerosis involving tympanic membrane and ear ossicles

    385.03 Tympanosclerosis involving tympanic membrane, ear ossicles, and middle ear

    385.09 Tympanosclerosis involving other combination of structures

⑤ **385.1 Adhesive middle ear disease**
    Adhesive otitis
    Otitis media:
      chronic adhesive
      fibrotic

    Excludes: *glue ear (381.20-381.29)*

    385.10 Adhesive middle ear disease, unspecified as to involvement

    385.11 Adhesions of drum head to incus

    385.12 Adhesions of drum head to stapes

Add 4th or 5th digit	Nonspecific code	Unspecified code	Manifestation code

385.13 **Adhesions of drum head to promontorium**

385.19 **Other adhesions and combinations**

⑤ **385.2** **Other acquired abnormality of ear ossicles**

385.21 **Impaired mobility of malleus**
Ankylosis of malleus

385.22 **Impaired mobility of other ear ossicles**
Ankylosis of ear ossicles, except malleus

385.23 **Discontinuity or dislocation of ear ossicles**

385.24 **Partial loss or necrosis of ear ossicles**

⑤ **385.3** **Cholesteatoma of middle ear and mastoid**
Cholesterosis of (middle) ear
Epidermosis of (middle) ear
Keratosis of (middle) ear
Polyp of (middle) ear

Excludes: *cholesteatoma:*

external ear canal (380.21)
recurrent of postmastoidectomy cavity (383.32)

385.30 **Cholesteatoma, unspecified**

385.31 **Cholesteatoma of attic**

385.32 **Cholesteatoma of middle ear**

385.33 **Cholesteatoma of middle ear and mastoid**

385.35 **Diffuse cholesteatosis**

⑤ **385.8** **Other disorders of middle ear and mastoid**

385.82 **Cholesterin granuloma**

385.83 **Retained foreign body of middle ear**

385.89 **Other**

385.9 **Unspecified disorder of middle ear and mastoid**

386 **Vertiginous syndromes and other disorders of vestibular system**

Excludes: *vertigo NOS (780.4)*

⑤ **386.0** **Ménière's disease**
Endolymphatic hydrops   Ménière's syndrome or vertigo
Lermoyez's syndrome

386.00 **Ménière's disease, unspecified**
Ménière's disease (active)

386.01 **Active Ménière's disease, cochleovestibular**

386.02 **Active Ménière's disease, cochlear**

386.03 **Active Ménière's disease, vestibular**

386.04 **Inactive Ménière's disease**
Ménière's disease in remission

⑤ **386.1** **Other and unspecified peripheral vertigo**

Excludes: *epidemic vertigo (078.81)*

386.10 **Peripheral vertigo, unspecified**

386.11 **Benign paroxysmal positional vertigo**
Benign paroxysmal positional nystagmus

386.12 **Vestibular neuronitis**
Acute (and recurrent) peripheral vestibulopathy

386.19 **Other**
Aural vertigo
Otogenic vertigo

386.2 **Vertigo of central origin**
Central positional nystagmus
Malignant positional vertigo

⑤ **386.3** **Labyrinthitis**

386.30 **Labyrinthitis, unspecified**

386.31 **Serous labyrinthitis**
Diffuse labyrinthitis

386.32 **Circumscribed labyrinthitis**
Focal labyrinthitis

     ● Code new   ▲ Revision of   ④ ⑤ Fourth or fifth
   to this edition   existing code   digit required

386.33 **Suppurative labyrinthitis**
Purulent labyrinthitis

386.34 **Toxic labyrinthitis**

386.35 **Viral labyrinthitis**

⑤ 386.4 **Labyrinthine fistula**

386.40 **Labyrinthine fistula, unspecified**

386.41 **Round window fistula**

386.42 **Oval window fistula**

386.43 **Semicircular canal fistula**

386.48 **Labyrinthine fistula of combined sites**

⑤ 386.5 **Labyrinthine dysfunction**

386.50 **Labyrinthine dysfunction, unspecified**

386.51 **Hyperactive labyrinth, unilateral**

386.52 **Hyperactive labyrinth, bilateral**

386.53 **Hypoactive labyrinth, unilateral**

386.54 **Hypoactive labyrinth, bilateral**

386.55 **Loss of labyrinthine reactivity, unilateral**

386.56 **Loss of labyrinthine reactivity, bilateral**

386.58 **Other forms and combinations**

386.8 **Other disorders of labyrinth**

386.9 **Unspecified vertiginous syndromes and labyrinthine disorders**

387 **Otosclerosis**
Includes: otospongiosis

387.0 **Otosclerosis involving oval window, nonobliterative**

387.1 **Otosclerosis involving oval window, obliterative**

387.2 **Cochlear otosclerosis**
Otosclerosis involving:
otic capsule
round window

387.8 **Other otosclerosis**

387.9 **Otosclerosis, unspecified**

388 **Other disorders of ear**

⑤ 388.0 **Degenerative and vascular disorders of ear**

388.00 **Degenerative and vascular disorders, unspecified**

388.01 **Presbyacusis**

388.02 **Transient ischemic deafness**

⑤ 388.1 **Noise effects on inner ear**

388.10 **Noise effects on inner ear, unspecified**

388.11 **Acoustic trauma (explosive) to ear**
Otitic blast injury

388.12 **Noise-induced hearing loss**

388.2 **Sudden hearing loss, unspecified**

⑤ 388.3 **Tinnitus**

388.30 **Tinnitus, unspecified**

388.31 **Subjective tinnitus**

388.32 **Objective tinnitus**

⑤ 388.4 **Other abnormal auditory perception**

388.40 **Abnormal auditory perception, unspecified**

388.41 **Diplacusis**

388.42 **Hyperacusis**

388.43 **Impairment of auditory discrimination**

388.44 **Recruitment**

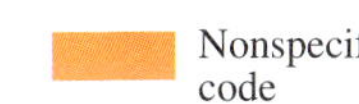

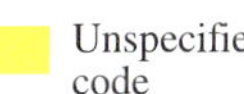

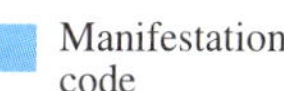

Manifestation
code

388.5 Disorders of acoustic nerve
Acoustic neuritis
Degeneration of acoustic or eighth nerve
Disorder of acoustic or eighth nerve
Excludes: acoustic neuroma (225.1)
syphilitic acoustic neuritis (094.86)

⑤ **388.6 Otorrhea**

388.60 Otorrhea, unspecified
Discharging ear NOS

388.61 Cerebrospinal fluid otorrhea
Excludes: cerebrospinal fluid rhinorrhea (349.81)

388.69 Other
Otorrhagia

⑤ **388.7 Otalgia**

388.70 Otalgia, unspecified
Earache NOS

388.71 Otogenic pain

388.72 Referred pain

388.8 Other disorders of ear

388.9 Unspecified disorder of ear

389 Hearing loss

⑤ **389.0 Conductive hearing loss**
Conductive deafness

389.00 Conductive hearing loss, unspecified

389.01 Conductive hearing loss, external ear

389.02 Conductive hearing loss, tympanic membrane

389.03 Conductive hearing loss, middle ear

389.04 Conductive hearing loss, inner ear

389.08 Conductive hearing loss of combined types

⑤ **389.1 Sensorineural hearing loss**
Perceptive hearing loss or deafness
Excludes: abnormal auditory perception (388.40-388.44)
psychogenic deafness (306.7)

389.10 Sensorineural hearing loss, unspecified

389.11 Sensory hearing loss, bilateral

389.12 Neural hearing loss, bilateral

389.14 Central hearing loss, bilateral

● **389.15 Sensorineural hearing loss, unilateral**

● **389.16 Sensorineural hearing loss, asymmetrical**

389.18 Sensorineural hearing loss of combined types, bilateral

389.2 Mixed conductive and sensorineural hearing loss
Deafness or hearing loss of type classifiable to 389.0 with type classifiable to 389.1

389.7 Deaf mutism, not elsewhere classifiable
Deaf, nonspeaking

389.8 Other specified forms of hearing loss

389.9 Unspecified hearing loss
Deafness NOS

   ● Code new
to this edition   ▲ Revision of
existing code   ④ ⑤ Fourth or fifth
digit required

7.   DISEASES OF THE CIRCULATORY SYSTEM (390-459)

ACUTE RHEUMATIC FEVER (390-392)

390 Rheumatic fever without mention of heart involvement
Arthritis, rheumatic, acute or subacute
Rheumatic fever (active) (acute)
Rheumatism, articular, acute or subacute

> *Excludes:* *that with heart involvement (391.0-391.9)*

391 Rheumatic fever with heart involvement

> *Excludes:* *chronic heart diseases of rheumatic origin (393.0-398.9) unless rheumatic fever is also present or there is evidence of recrudescence or activity of the rheumatic process*

391.0 Acute rheumatic pericarditis
Rheumatic:
fever (active) (acute) with pericarditis
pericarditis (acute)
Any condition classifiable to 390 with pericarditis

> *Excludes:* *that not specified as rheumatic (420.0-420.9)*

391.1 Acute rheumatic endocarditis
Rheumatic:
endocarditis, acute
fever (active) (acute) with endocarditis or valvulitis
valvulitis acute
Any condition classifiable to 390 with endocarditis or valvulitis

391.2 Acute rheumatic myocarditis
Rheumatic fever (active) (acute) with myocarditis
Any condition classifiable to 390 with myocarditis

391.8 Other acute rheumatic heart disease
Rheumatic:
fever (active) (acute) with other or multiple types of heart involvement
pancarditis, acute
Any condition classifiable to 390 with other or multiple types of heart involvement

391.9 Acute rheumatic heart disease, unspecified
Rheumatic:
carditis, acute
fever (active) (acute) with unspecified type of heart involvement
heart disease, active or acute
Any condition classifiable to 390 with unspecified type of heart involvement

392 Rheumatic chorea
Includes: Sydenham's chorea

> *Excludes:* *chorea:*
> *NOS (333.5)*
> *Huntington's (333.4)*

392.0 With heart involvement
Rheumatic chorea with heart involvement of any type classifiable to 391

392.9 Without mention of heart involvement

CHRONIC RHEUMATIC HEART DISEASE (393-398)

393 Chronic rheumatic pericarditis
Adherent pericardium, rheumatic
Chronic rheumatic:
mediastinopericarditis
myopericarditis

> *Excludes:* *pericarditis NOS or not specified as rheumatic (423.0-423.9)*

394 Diseases of mitral valve

> *Excludes:* *that with aortic valve involvement (396.0-396.9)*

394.0 Mitral stenosis
Mitral (valve):
obstruction (rheumatic)
stenosis NOS

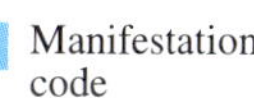

	Add 4th or 5th digit		Nonspecific code		Unspecified code		Manifestation code

394.1 Rheumatic mitral insufficiency
Rheumatic mitral:
   incompetence
   regurgitation

| Excludes: | that not specified as rheumatic (424.0) |

394.2 Mitral stenosis with insufficiency
Mitral stenosis with incompetence or regurgitation

394.9 Other and unspecified mitral valve diseases
Mitral (valve):
   disease (chronic)
   failure

395 Diseases of aortic valve

| Excludes: | that not specified as rheumatic (424.1) |
| | that with mitral valve involvement (396.0-396.9) |

395.0 Rheumatic aortic stenosis
Rheumatic aortic (valve) obstruction

395.1 Rheumatic aortic insufficiency
Rheumatic aortic:
   incompetence
   regurgitation

395.2 Rheumatic aortic stenosis with insufficiency
Rheumatic aortic stenosis with incompetence or regurgitation

395.9 Other and unspecified rheumatic aortic diseases
Rheumatic aortic (valve) disease

396 Diseases of mitral and aortic valves
Includes: involvement of both mitral and aortic valves, whether specified as rheumatic or
      not

396.0 Mitral valve stenosis and aortic valve stenosis
Atypical aortic (valve) stenosis
Mitral and aortic (valve) obstruction (rheumatic)

396.1 Mitral valve stenosis and aortic valve insufficiency

396.2 Mitral valve insufficiency and aortic valve stenosis

396.3 Mitral valve insufficiency and aortic valve insufficiency
Mitral and aortic (valve):
   incompetence
   regurgitation

396.8 Multiple involvement of mitral and aortic valves
Stenosis and insufficiency of mitral or aortic valve with stenosis or insufficiency, or
    both, of the other valve

396.9 Mitral and aortic valve diseases, unspecified

397 Diseases of other endocardial structures

397.0 Diseases of tricuspid valve
Tricuspid (valve) (rheumatic):
   disease
   insufficiency
   obstruction
   regurgitation
   stenosis

397.1 Rheumatic diseases of pulmonary valve

| Excludes: | that not specified as rheumatic (424.3) |

397.9 Rheumatic diseases of endocardium, valve unspecified
Rheumatic:
   endocarditis (chronic)
   valvulitis (chronic)

| Excludes: | that not specified as rheumatic (424.90-424.99) |

398 Other rheumatic heart disease

398.0 Rheumatic myocarditis
Rheumatic degeneration of myocardium

| Excludes: | myocarditis not specified as rheumatic (429.0) |

⑤ **398.9 Other and unspecified rheumatic heart diseases**

  ● Code new
    to this edition
  ▲ Revision of
    existing code
  ④ ⑤ Fourth or fifth
      digit required

398.90 Rheumatic heart disease, unspecified
    Rheumatic:
      carditis
      heart disease NOS

Excludes:	*carditis not specified as rheumatic (429.89)*
	heart disease NOS not specified as rheumatic (429.9)

398.91 Rheumatic heart failure (congestive)
    Rheumatic left ventricular failure

398.99 Other

HYPERTENSIVE DISEASE (401-405)

Excludes:	*that complicating pregnancy, childbirth, or the puerperium (642.0-642.9)*
	that involving coronary vessels (410.00-414.9)

401 Essential hypertension
    Includes: high blood pressure
                hyperpiesia
                hyperpiesis
                hypertension (arterial) (essential) (primary) (systemic)
                hypertensive vascular:
                    degeneration
                    disease

Excludes:	*elevated blood pressure without diagnosis of hypertension (796.2)*
	pulmonary hypertension (416.0-416.9)
	that involving vessels of:
	brain (430-438)
	eye (362.11)

401.0 Malignant

401.1 Benign

401.9 Unspecified

402 Hypertensive heart disease
Use additional code to specify type of heart failure (428.0-428.43), if known
    Includes: hypertensive:
                cardiomegaly
                cardiopathy
                cardiovascular disease
                heart (disease) (failure)
                any condition classifiable to 429.0-429.3, 429.8, 429.9 due to hypertension

⑤ **402.0 Malignant**

    402.00 Without heart failure

    402.01 With heart failure

⑤ **402.1 Benign**

    402.10 Without heart failure

    402.11 With heart failure

⑤ **402.9 Unspecified**

    402.90 Without heart failure

    402.91 With heart failure

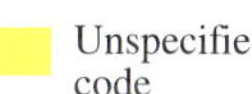

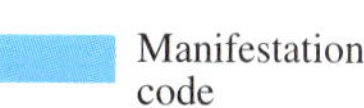

▲ **403** **Hypertensive chronic kidney disease**

The following fifth-digit subclassification is for use with category 403:

    0 **with chronic kidney disease stage I through stage IV, or unspecified**

       Use additional code to identify the stage of chronic kidney disease (585.1-585.4, 585.9)

    1 **with chronic kidney disease stage V or end stage renal disease**

       Use additional code to identify the stage of chronic kidney disease (585.5, 585.6)

Includes: arteriolar nephritis
         arteriosclerosis of:
           kidney
           renal arterioles
         arteriosclerotic nephritis (chronic) (interstitial)
         hypertensive:
           nephropathy
           renal failure
           uremia (chronic)
         nephrosclerosis
         renal sclerosis with hypertension
         any condition classifiable to 585, 586, or 587 with any condition classifiable to
           401

Excludes: *acute renal failure (584.5-584.9)*
         renal disease stated as not due to hypertension
         renovascular hypertension (405.0-405.9 with fifth-digit 1)

⑤ **403.0** **Malignant**

⑤ **403.1** **Benign**

⑤ **403.9** **Unspecified**

▲ **404** **Hypertensive heart and chronic kidney disease**

Use additional code to specify type of heart failure (428.0-428.43), if known

The following fifth-digit subclassification is for use with category 404:

    0 **without heart failure and with chronic kidney disease stage I through stage IV, or unspecified**

       Use additional code to identify the stage of chronic kidney disease (585.1-585.4, 585.9)

    1 **with heart failure and with chronic kidney disease stage I through stage IV, or unspecified**

       Use additional code to identify the stage of chronic kidney disease (585.1-585.4, 585.9)

    2 **without heart failure and with chronic kidney disease stage V or end stage renal disease**

       Use additional code to identify the stage of chronic kidney disease (585.5, 585.6)

    3 **with heart failure and chronic kidney disease stage V or end stage renal disease**

       Use additional code to identify the stage of chronic kidney disease (585.5-585.6)

Includes: disease:
         cardiornal
         cardiovascular renal
       any condition classifiable to 402 with any condition classifiable to 403

⑤ **404.0** **Malignant**

⑤ **404.1** **Benign**

⑤ **404.9** **Unspecified**

405 **Secondary hypertension**

⑤ **405.0** **Malignant**

    405.01 **Renovascular**

    405.09 **Other**

⑤ **405.1** **Benign**

    405.11 **Renovascular**

    405.19 **Other**

⑤ **405.9** **Unspecified**

    405.91 **Renovascular**

    405.99 **Other**

● Code new
to this edition
    ▲ Revision of
existing code
    ④ ⑤ Fourth or fifth
digit required

ISCHEMIC HEART DISEASE (410-414)

Includes: that with mention of hypertension

Use additional code, if desired, to identify presence of hypertension (401.0-405.9)

⑤ **410 Acute myocardial infarction**
ST elevation (STEMI) and non-ST elevation (NSTEMI) myocardial infarction
Includes: cardiac infarction
coronary (artery):
embolism
occlusion
rupture
thrombosis
infarction of heart, myocardium, or ventricle
rupture of heart, myocardium, or ventricle
any condition classifiable to 414.1-414.9 specified as acute or with a stated
duration of 8 weeks or less

The following fifth-digit subclassification is for use with category 410:

0 episode of care unspecified
Use when the source document does not contain sufficient information for the
assignment of fifth digit 1 or 2.

1 initial episode of care
Use fifth digit 1 to designate the first episode of care (regardless of facility site) for a
newly diagnosed myocardial infarction. The fifth digit 1 is assigned regardless of
the number of times a patient may be transferred during the initial episode of care

2 subsequent episode of care
Use fifth digit 2 to designate an episode of care following the initial episode when the
patient is admitted for further observation, evaluation, or treatment for a
myocardial infarction that has received initial treatment, but is still less than 8
weeks old.

⑤ **410.0 Of anterolateral wall**
ST elevation myocardial infarction (STEMI) of anterolateral wall

⑤ **410.1 Of other anterior wall**
ST elevation myocardial infarction (STEMI) of other anterior wall
Infarction:
anterior (wall) NOS (with contiguous portion of intraventricular septum)
anteroapical (with contiguous portion of intraventricular septum)
anteroseptal (with contiguous portion of intraventricular septum)

⑤ **410.2 Of inferolateral wall**
ST elevation myocardial infarction (STEMI) of inferolateral wall

⑤ **410.3 Of inferoposterior wall**
ST elevation myocardial infarction (STEMI) of inferoposterior wall

⑤ **410.4 Of other inferior wall**
ST elevation myocardial infarction (STEMI) of other inferior wall
Infarction:
diaphragmatic wall NOS (with contiguous portion of intraventricular septum)
inferior (wall) NOS (with contiguous portion of intraventricular septum)

⑤ **410.5 Of other lateral wall**
ST elevation myocardial infarction (STEMI) of other lateral wall

Infarction:	Infarction:
apical-lateral	high lateral
basal-lateral	posterolateral

⑤ **410.6 True posterior wall infarction**
ST elevation myocardial infarction (STEMI) of true posterior wall
Infarction:
posterobasal
strictly posterior

⑤ **410.7 Subendocardial infarction**
Non-ST elevation myocardial infarction (NSTEMI)
Nontransmural infarction

⑤ **410.8 Other specified sites**
ST elevation myocardial infarction (STEMI) of other specified sites
Infarction of:
atrium
papillary muscle
septum alone

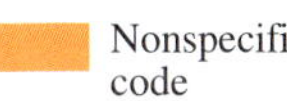
Add 4th or
5th digit

Nonspecific
code

Unspecified
code

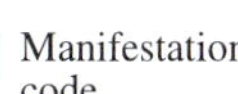
Manifestation
code

⑤ **410.9** **Unspecified site**
Acute myocardial infarction NOS
Coronary occlusion NOS
Myocardial infarction NOS

411 **Other acute and subacute forms of ischemic heart disease**

411.0 **Postmyocardial infarction syndrome**
Dressler's syndrome

411.1 **Intermediate coronary syndrome**

Impending infarction   Preinfarction syndrome
Preinfarction angina   Unstable angina

Excludes: *angina (pectoris) (413.9)*
decubitus (413.0)

⑤ **411.8** **Other**

411.81 **Acute coronary occlusion without myocardial infarction**
Acute coronary (artery):
embolism without or not resulting in myocardial infarction
obstruction without or not resulting in myocardial infarction
occlusion without or not resulting in myocardial infarction
thrombosis without or not resulting in myocardial infarction

Excludes: *obstruction without infarction due to atherosclerosis (414.00-414.07)*
occlusion without infarction due to atherosclerosis (414.00-414.07)

411.89 **Other**
Coronary insufficiency (acute)
Subendocardial ischemia

412 **Old myocardial infarction**
Healed myocardial infarction
Past myocardial infarction diagnosed on ECG [EKG] or other special investigation, but
currently presenting no symptoms

413 **Angina pectoris**

413.0 **Angina decubitus**
Nocturnal angina

413.1 **Prinzmetal angina**
Variant angina pectoris

413.9 **Other and unspecified angina pectoris**

Angina: Anginal syndrome
  NOS   Status anginosus
  cardiac   Stenocardia
  of effort   Syncope anginosa

Excludes: *preinfarction angina (411.1)*

414 **Other forms of chronic ischemic heart disease**

Excludes: *arteriosclerotic cardiovascular disease [ASCVD] (429.2)*
cardiovascular:
arteriosclerosis or sclerosis (429.2)
degeneration or disease (429.2)

⑤ **414.0** **Coronary atherosclerosis**
Arteriosclerotic heart disease [ASHD]
Atherosclerotic heart disease
Coronary (artery):
arteriosclerosis
arteritis or endarteritis
atheroma
sclerosis
stricture

Excludes: *embolism of graft (996.72)*
occlusion NOS of graft (996.72)
thrombus of graft (996.72)

414.00 **Of unspecified type of vessel, native or graft**

414.01 **Of native coronary artery**

414.02 **Of autologous vein bypass graft**

414.03 **Of nonautologous biological bypass graft**

414.04 **Of artery bypass graft**
Internal mammary artery

● Code new
to this edition

▲ Revision of
existing code

④ ⑤ Fourth or fifth
digit required

414.05 **Of unspecified type of bypass graft**
Bypass graft NOS

414.06 **Of native coronary artery of transplanted heart**

414.07 **Of bypass graft (artery) (vein) of transplanted heart**

⑤ **414.1** **Aneurysm and dissection of heart**

414.10 **Aneurysm of heart (wall)**
Aneurysm (arteriovenous):
mural
ventricular

414.11 **Aneurysm of coronary vessels**
Aneurysm (arteriovenous) of coronary vessels

414.12 **Dissection of coronary artery**

414.19 **Other aneurysm of heart**
Arteriovenous fistula, acquired, of heart

414.8 **Other specified forms of chronic ischemic heart disease**
Chronic coronary insufficiency
Ischemia, myocardial (chronic)
Any condition classifiable to 410 specified as chronic, or presenting with symptoms
after 8 weeks from date of infarction

Excludes: *coronary insufficiency (acute) (411.89)*

414.9 **Chronic ischemic heart disease, unspecified**
Ischemic heart disease NOS

DISEASES OF PULMONARY CIRCULATION (415-417)

415 **Acute pulmonary heart disease**

415.0 **Acute cor pulmonale**

Excludes: *cor pulmonale NOS (416.9)*

⑤ **415.1** **Pulmonary embolism and infarction**
Pulmonary (artery) (vein):
apoplexy
embolism
infarction (hemorrhagic)
thrombosis

Excludes: *that complicating:*
abortion (634-638 with .6, 639.6)
ectopic or molar pregnancy (639.6)
pregnancy, childbirth, or the puerperium (673.0-673.8)

415.11 **Iatrogenic pulmonary embolism and infarction**

415.19 **Other**

416 **Chronic pulmonary heart disease**

416.0 **Primary pulmonary hypertension**
Idiopathic pulmonary arteriosclerosis
Pulmonary hypertension (essential) (idiopathic) (primary)

416.1 **Kyphoscoliotic heart disease**

416.8 **Other chronic pulmonary heart diseases**
Pulmonary hypertension, secondary

416.9 **Chronic pulmonary heart disease, unspecified**
Chronic cardiopulmonary disease
Cor pulmonale (chronic) NOS

417 **Other diseases of pulmonary circulation**

417.0 **Arteriovenous fistula of pulmonary vessels**

Excludes: *congenital arteriovenous fistula (747.3)*

417.1 **Aneurysm of pulmonary artery**

Excludes: *congenital aneurysm (747.3)*

417.8 **Other specified diseases of pulmonary circulation**
Pulmonary:
arteritis
endarteritis
Rupture of pulmonary vessel
Stricture of pulmonary vessel

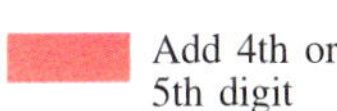

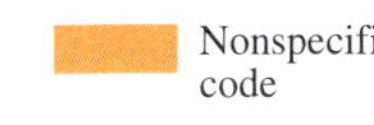

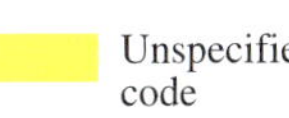

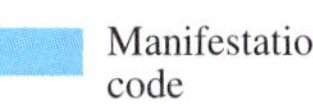

417.9 **Unspecified disease of pulmonary circulation**

OTHER FORMS OF HEART DISEASE (420-429)

420 **Acute pericarditis**
Includes: acute:
mediastinopericarditis
myopericarditis
pericardial effusion
pleuropericarditis
pneumopericarditis

Excludes: *acute rheumatic pericarditis (391.0)*

postmyocardial infarction syndrome [Dressler's] (411.0)

420.0 ***Acute pericarditis in diseases classified elsewhere***
Code first underlying disease, as:
actinomycosis (039.8)
amebiasis (006.8)
chronic uremia (585.9)
nocardiosis (039.8)
tuberculosis (017.9)
uremia NOS (586)

Excludes: *pericarditis (acute) (in):*
Coxsackie (virus) (074.21)
gonococcal (098.83)
histoplasmosis (115.0-115.9 with fifth-digit 3)
meningococcal infection (036.41)
syphilitic (093.81)

⑤ **420.9** **Other and unspecified acute pericarditis**

420.90 **Acute pericarditis, unspecified**
Pericarditis (acute):
NOS
infective NOS
sicca

420.91 **Acute idiopathic pericarditis**
Pericarditis, acute:
benign
nonspecific
viral

420.99 **Other**

Pericarditis (acute):	Pericarditis (acute):
pneumococcal	streptococcal
purulent	suppurative
staphylococcal	Pneumopyopericardium
	Pyopericardium

Excludes: *pericarditis in diseases classified elsewhere (420.0)*

421 **Acute and subacute endocarditis**

421.0 **Acute and subacute bacterial endocarditis**

Endocarditis (acute) (chronic) (subacute):	Endocarditis (acute) (chronic) (subacute):
bacterial	septic
infective NOS	ulcerative
lenta	vegetative
malignant	Infective aneurysm
purulent	Subacute bacterial endocarditis [SBE]

Use additional code, if desired, to identify infectious organism [e.g., Streptococcus 041.0, Staphylococcus 041.1]

● Code new
 to this edition

▲ Revision of
 existing code

④ ⑤ Fourth or fifth
 digit required

421.1 *Acute and subacute infective endocarditis in diseases classified elsewhere*
    Code first underlying disease, as:
      blastomycosis (116.0)
      Q fever (083.0)
      typhoid (fever) (002.0)

    Excludes: *endocarditis (in):*
        Coxsackie (virus) (074.22)
        gonococcal (098.84)
        histoplasmosis (115.0-115.9 with fifth-digit 4)
        meningococcal infection (036.42)
        monilial (112.81)

421.9 **Acute endocarditis, unspecified**
    Endocarditis, acute or subacute
    Myoendocarditis, acute or subacute
    Periendocarditis, acute or subacute

    Excludes: *acute rheumatic endocarditis (391.1)*

422 **Acute myocarditis**

    Excludes: *acute rheumatic myocarditis (391.2)*

422.0 *Acute myocarditis in diseases classified elsewhere*
    Code first underlying disease, as:
      myocarditis (acute):
        influenzal (487.8)
        tuberculous (017.9)

    Excludes: *myocarditis (acute) (due to):*
        aseptic, of newborn (074.23)
        Coxsackie (virus) (074.23)
        diphtheritic (032.82)
        meningococcal infection (036.43)
        syphilitic (093.82)
        toxoplasmosis (130.3)

⑤ **422.9** **Other and unspecified acute myocarditis**

    422.90 **Acute myocarditis, unspecified**
      Acute or subacute (interstitial) myocarditis

    422.91 **Idiopathic myocarditis**
      Myocarditis (acute or subacute):
        Fiedler's
        giant cell
        isolated (diffuse) (granulomatous)
        nonspecific granulomatous

    422.92 **Septic myocarditis**
      Myocarditis, acute or subacute:
        pneumococcal
        staphylococcal

    Use additional code, if desired, to identify infectious organism [e.g., Staphylococcus 041.1]

    Excludes: *myocarditis, acute or subacute:*
        in bacterial diseases classified elsewhere (422.0)
        streptococcal (391.2)

    422.93 **Toxic myocarditis**

    422.99 **Other**

423 **Other diseases of pericardium**

    Excludes: *that specified as rheumatic (393)*

423.0 **Hemopericardium**

423.1 **Adhesive pericarditis**
    Adherent pericardium   Pericarditis:
    Fibrosis of pericardium   adhesive
    Milk spots   obliterative
                    Soldiers' patches

423.2 **Constrictive pericarditis**
    Concato's disease
    Pick's disease of heart (and liver)

423.8 **Other specified diseases of pericardium**
    Calcification of pericardium
    Fistula of pericardium

423.9 **Unspecified disease of pericardium**

424 **Other diseases of endocardium**

> *Excludes:* *bacterial endocarditis (421.0-421.9)*
> *rheumatic endocarditis (391.1, 394.0-397.9)*
> *syphilitic endocarditis (093.20-093.24)*

424.0 Mitral valve disorders

Mitral (valve):
incompetence NOS of specified cause, except rheumatic
insufficiency NOS of specified cause, except rheumatic
regurgitation NOS of specified cause, except rheumatic

> *Excludes:* *mitral (valve):*
> *disease (394.9)*
> *failure (394.9)*
> *stenosis (394.0)*
> *the listed conditions:*
> *specified as rheumatic (394.1)*
> *unspecified as to cause but with mention of:*
> *diseases of aortic valve (396.0-396.9)*
> *mitral stenosis or obstruction (394.2)*

424.1 Aortic valve disorders

Aortic (valve):
incompetence NOS of specified cause, except rheumatic
insufficiency NOS of specified cause, except rheumatic
regurgitation NOS of specified cause, except rheumatic
stenosis NOS of specified cause, except rheumatic

> *Excludes:* *hypertrophic subaortic stenosis (425.1)*
> *that specified as rheumatic (395.0-395.9)*
> *that of unspecified cause but with mention of diseases of mitral valve*
> *(396.0-396.9)*

424.2 Tricuspid valve disorders, specified as nonrheumatic

Tricuspid valve:
incompetence of specified cause, except rheumatic
insufficiency of specified cause, except rheumatic
regurgitation of specified cause, except rheumatic
stenosis of specified cause, except rheumatic

> *Excludes:* *rheumatic or of unspecified cause (397.0)*

424.3 Pulmonary valve disorders

Pulmonic:
incompetence NOS
insufficiency NOS

Pulmonic:
regurgitation NOS
stenosis NOS

> *Excludes:* *that specified as rheumatic (397.1)*

⑤ **424.9 Endocarditis, valve unspecified**

424.90 **Endocarditis, valve unspecified, unspecified cause**
Endocarditis (chronic):
NOS
nonbacterial thrombotic
Valvular:
incompetence of unspecified valve, unspecified cause
insufficiency of unspecified valve, unspecified cause
regurgitation of unspecified valve, unspecified cause
stenosis of unspecified valve, unspecified cause
Valvulitis (chronic)

424.91 ***Endocarditis in diseases classified elsewhere***
Code first underlying disease, as:
atypical verrucous endocarditis [Libman-Sacks] (710.0)
disseminated lupus erythematosus (710.0)
tuberculosis (017.9)

> *Excludes:* *syphilitic (093.20-093.24)*

424.99 **Other**
Any condition classifiable to 424.90 with specified cause, except rheumatic

> *Excludes:* *endocardial fibroelastosis (425.3)*
> *that specified as rheumatic (397.9)*

425 **Cardiomyopathy**
Includes: myocardiopathy

● Code new
to this edition

▲ Revision of
existing code

④ ⑤ Fourth or fifth
digit required

425.0 **Endomyocardial fibrosis**

425.1 **Hypertrophic obstructive cardiomyopathy**
Hypertrophic subaortic stenosis (idiopathic)

425.2 **Obscure cardiomyopathy of Africa**
Becker's disease
Idiopathic mural endomyocardial disease

425.3 **Endocardial fibroelastosis**
Elastomyofibrosis

425.4 **Other primary cardiomyopathies**

Cardiomyopathy:
  NOS
  congestive
  constrictive
  familial
  hypertrophic

Cardiomyopathy:
  idiopathic
  nonobstructive
  obstructive
  restrictive
Cardiovascular collagenosis

425.5 **Alcoholic cardiomyopathy**

425.7 *Nutritional and metabolic cardiomyopathy*
Code first underlying disease, as:
  amyloidosis (277.30-277.39)
  beriberi (265.0)
  cardiac glycogenosis (271.0)
  mucopolysaccharidosis (277.5)
  thyrotoxicosis (242.0-242.9)

Excludes: *gouty tophi of heart (274.82)*

425.8 *Cardiomyopathy in other diseases classified elsewhere*
Code first underlying disease, as:
  Friedreich's ataxia (334.0)
  myotonia atrophica (359.2)
  progressive muscular dystrophy (359.1)
  sarcoidosis (135)

Excludes: *cardiomyopathy in Chagas' disease (086.0)*

425.9 **Secondary cardiomyopathy, unspecified**

426 **Conduction disorders**

426.0 **Atrioventricular block, complete**
Third degree atrioventricular block

⑤ **426.1** **Atrioventricular block, other and unspecified**

426.10 **Atrioventricular block, unspecified**
Atrioventricular [AV] block (incomplete) (partial)

426.11 **First degree atrioventricular block**
Incomplete atrioventricular block, first degree
Prolonged P-R interval NOS

426.12 **Mobitz (type) II atrioventricular block**
Incomplete atrioventricular block:
  Mobitz (type) II
  second degree, Mobitz (type) II

426.13 **Other second degree atrioventricular block**
Incomplete atrioventricular block:
  Mobitz (type) I [Wenckebach's]
  second degree:
    NOS
    Mobitz (type) I
  with 2:1 atrioventricular response [block]
Wenckebach's phenomenon

426.2 **Left bundle branch hemiblock**
Block:
  left anterior fascicular
  left posterior fascicular

426.3 **Other left bundle branch block**
Left bundle branch block:
  NOS
  anterior fascicular with posterior fascicular
  complete
  main stem

426.4 **Right bundle branch block**

⑤ **426.5 Bundle branch block, other and unspecified**

    426.50 Bundle branch block, unspecified

    426.51 Right bundle branch block and left posterior fascicular block

    426.52 Right bundle branch block and left anterior fascicular block

    426.53 Other bilateral bundle branch block
        Bifascicular block NOS
        Bilateral bundle branch block NOS
        Right bundle branch with left bundle branch block (incomplete) (main stem)

    426.54 Trifascicular block

426.6 Other heart block
    Intraventricular block: Sinoatrial block
      NOS   Sinoauricular block
      diffuse
      myofibrillar

426.7 Anomalous atrioventricular excitation
    Atrioventricular conduction:
      accelerated
      accessory
      pre-excitation
    Ventricular pre-excitation
    Wolff-Parkinson-White syndrome

⑤ **426.8 Other specified conduction disorders**

    426.81 Lown-Ganong-Levine syndrome
        Syndrome of short P-R interval, normal QRS complexes, and supraventricular tachycardias

    426.82 Long QT syndrome

    426.89 Other
        Dissociation:
          atrioventricular [AV]
          interference
          isorhythmic
        Nonparoxysmal AV nodal tachycardia

426.9 Conduction disorder, unspecified
    Heart block NOS
    Stokes-Adams syndrome

427 Cardiac dysrhythmias
    Excludes: *that complicating:*
        abortion (634-638 with .7, 639.8)
        ectopic or molar pregnancy (639.8)
        labor or delivery (668.1, 669.4)

427.0 Paroxysmal supraventricular tachycardia
    Paroxysmal tachycardia:
      atrial [PAT]
      atrioventricular [AV]
      junctional
      nodal

427.1 Paroxysmal ventricular tachycardia
    Ventricular tachycardia (paroxysmal)

427.2 Paroxysmal tachycardia, unspecified
    Bouveret-Hoffmann syndrome
    Paroxysmal tachycardia:
      NOS
      essential

⑤ **427.3 Atrial fibrillation and flutter**

    427.31 Atrial fibrillation

    427.32 Atrial flutter

⑤ **427.4 Ventricular fibrillation and flutter**

    427.41 Ventricular fibrillation

    427.42 Ventricular flutter

427.5 Cardiac arrest
    Cardiorespiratory arrest

⑤ **427.6 Premature beats**

● Code new to this edition   ▲ Revision of existing code   ④ ⑤ Fourth or fifth digit required

427.60 **Premature beats, unspecified**
Ectopic beats
Extrasystoles
Extrasystolic arrhythmia
Premature contractions or systoles NOS

427.61 **Supraventricular premature beats**
Atrial premature beats, contractions, or systoles

427.69 **Other**
Ventricular premature beats, contractions, or systoles

⑤ **427.8** **Other specified cardiac dysrhythmias**

427.81 **Sinoatrial node dysfunction**
Sinus bradycardia: Syndrome:
   persistent   sick sinus
   severe   tachycardia-bradycardia

Excludes: *sinus bradycardia NOS (427.89)*

427.89 **Other**
Rhythm disorder: Rhythm disorder:
   coronary sinus   nodal
   ectopic   Wandering (atrial) pacemaker

Excludes: *carotid sinus syncope (337.0)*
neonatal bradycardia (779.81)
neonatal tachycardia (779.82)
reflex bradycardia (337.0)
tachycardia (785.0)

427.9 **Cardiac dysrhythmia, unspecified**
Arrhythmia (cardiac) NOS

428 **Heart failure**
Code, if applicable, heart failure due to hypertension first (402.0-402.9, with fifth-digit 1 or
404.0-404.9 with fifth digit 1 or 3)

Excludes: *following cardiac surgery (429.4)*
rheumatic (398.91)
that complicating:
abortion (634-638 with .7, 639.8)
ectopic or molar pregnancy (639.8)
labor or delivery (668.1, 669.4)

428.0 **Congestive heart failure, unspecified**
Congestive heart disease
Right heart failure (secondary to left heart failure)

Excludes: *fluid overload NOS (276.6)*

428.1 **Left heart failure**
Acute edema of lung with heart disease NOS or heart failure
Acute pulmonary edema with heart disease NOS or heart failure
Cardiac asthma
Left ventricular failure

⑤ **428.2** **Systolic heart failure**

Excludes: *combined systolic and diastolic heart failure (428.40-428.43)*

428.20 **Unspecified**

428.21 **Acute**

428.22 **Chronic**

428.23 **Acute on chronic**

⑤ **428.3** **Diastolic heart failure**

Excludes: *combined systolic and diastolic heart failure (428.40-428.43)*

428.30 **Unspecified**

428.31 **Acute**

428.32 **Chronic**

428.33 **Acute on chronic**

⑤ **428.4** **Combined systolic and diastolic heart failure**

428.40 **Unspecified**

428.41 **Acute**

428.42 **Chronic**

Add 4th or 5th digit   Nonspecific code   Unspecified code   Manifestation code

428.43 Acute on chronic

428.9 Heart failure, unspecified
Cardiac failure NOS
Heart failure NOS
Myocardial failure NOS
Weak heart

429 Ill-defined descriptions and complications of heart disease

429.0 Myocarditis, unspecified
Myocarditis:
NOS (with mention of arteriosclerosis)
chronic (interstitial) (with mention of arteriosclerosis)
fibroid (with mention of arteriosclerosis)
senile (with mention of arteriosclerosis)
Use additional code, if desired, to identify presence of arteriosclerosis
Excludes: acute or subacute (422.0-422.9)
rheumatic (398.0)
acute (391.2)
that due to hypertension (402.0-402.9)

429.1 Myocardial degeneration
Degeneration of heart or myocardium:
fatty (with mention of arteriosclerosis)
mural (with mention of arteriosclerosis)
muscular (with mention of arteriosclerosis)
Myocardial:
degeneration (with mention of arteriosclerosis)
disease (with mention of arteriosclerosis)
Use additional code, if desired, to identify presence of arteriosclerosis
Excludes: that due to hypertension (402.0-402.9)

429.2 Cardiovascular disease, unspecified
Arteriosclerotic cardiovascular disease [ASCVD]
Cardiovascular arteriosclerosis
Cardiovascular:
degeneration (with mention of arteriosclerosis)
disease (with mention of arteriosclerosis)
sclerosis (with mention of arteriosclerosis)
Use additional code, if desired, to identify presence of arteriosclerosis
Excludes: that due to hypertension (402.0-402.9)

429.3 Cardiomegaly
Cardiac:
dilatation
hypertrophy
Ventricular dilatation
Excludes: that due to hypertension (402.0-402.9)

429.4 Functional disturbances following cardiac surgery
Cardiac insufficiency following cardiac surgery or due to prosthesis
Heart failure following cardiac surgery or due to prosthesis
Postcardiotomy syndrome
Postvalvulotomy syndrome
Excludes: cardiac failure in the immediate postoperative period (997.1)

429.5 Rupture of chordae tendineae

429.6 Rupture of papillary muscle

⑤ **429.7 Certain sequelae of myocardial infarction, not elsewhere classified**
Use additional code to identify the associated myocardial infarction:
with onset of 8 weeks or less (410.00-410.92)
with onset of more than 8 weeks (414.8)
Excludes: congenital defects of heart (745, 746)
coronary aneurysm (414.11)
disorders of papillary muscle (429.6, 429.81)
postmyocardial infarction syndrome (411.0)
rupture of chordae tendineae (429.5)

429.71 Acquired cardiac septal defect
Excludes: acute septal infarction (410.00-410.92)

429.79 Other
Mural thrombus (atrial) (ventricular), acquired, following myocardial infarction

⑤ **429.8 Other ill-defined heart diseases**

● Code new
to this edition

▲ Revision of
existing code

④ ⑤ Fourth or fifth
digit required

429.81 Other disorders of papillary muscle
Papillary muscle:
  atrophy
  degeneration
  dysfunction
Papillary muscle:
  incompetence
  incoordination
  scarring

429.82 Hyperkinetic heart disease

● **429.83 Takotsubo syndrome**
  Broken heart syndrome
  Reversible left ventricular dysfunction following sudden emotional stress
  Stress induced cardiomyopathy
  Transient left ventricular apical ballooning syndrome

429.89 Other
  Carditis
Excludes: *that due to hypertension (402.0-402.9)*

429.9 Heart disease, unspecified
  Heart disease (organic) NOS
  Morbus cordis NOS
Excludes: *that due to hypertension (402.0-402.9)*

CEREBROVASCULAR DISEASE (430-438)

Includes: with mention of hypertension (conditions classifiable to 401-405)

Use additional code, if desired, to identify presence of hypertension

Excludes: *any condition classifiable to 430-434, 436, 437 occurring during pregnancy,*
childbirth, or the puerperium, or specified as puerperal (674.0)
iatrogenic cerebrovascular infarction or hemorrhage (997.02)

430 Subarachnoid hemorrhage
Meningeal hemorrhage
Ruptured:
  berry aneurysm
  (congenital) cerebral aneurysm NOS
Excludes: *syphilitic ruptured cerebral aneurysm (094.87)*

431 Intracerebral hemorrhage
Hemorrhage (of):
  basilar
  bulbar
  cerebellar
  cerebral
  cerebromeningeal
  cortical
  internal capsule
Hemorrhage (of):
  intrapontine
  pontine
  subcortical
  ventricular
  Rupture of blood vessel in brain

432 Other and unspecified intracranial hemorrhage

432.0 Nontraumatic extradural hemorrhage
  Nontraumatic epidural hemorrhage

432.1 Subdural hemorrhage
  Subdural hematoma, nontraumatic

432.9 Unspecified intracranial hemorrhage
  Intracranial hemorrhage NOS

⑤ **433 Occlusion and stenosis of precerebral arteries**
The following fifth-digit subclassification is for use with category 433:

  0 without mention of cerebral infarction

  1 with cerebral infarction

Includes: embolism of basilar, carotid, and vertebral arteries
  narrowing of basilar, carotid, and vertebral arteries
  obstruction of basilar, carotid, and vertebral arteries
  thrombosis of basilar, carotid, and vertebral arteries
Excludes: *insufficiency NOS of precerebral arteries (435.0-435.9)*

⑤ **433.0 Basilar artery**

⑤ **433.1 Carotid artery**

⑤ **433.2 Vertebral artery**

⑤ **433.3 Multiple and bilateral**

⑤ **433.8 Other specified precerebral artery**

⑤ **433.9 Unspecified precerebral artery**
    Precerebral artery NOS

⑤ **434 Occlusion of cerebral arteries**
    The following fifth-digit subclassification is for use with category 434:

> **0 without mention of cerebral infarction**
>
> **1 with cerebral infarction**

⑤ **434.0 Cerebral thrombosis**
    Thrombosis of cerebral arteries

⑤ **434.1 Cerebral embolism**

⑤ **434.9 Cerebral artery occlusion, unspecified**

435 Transient cerebral ischemia
    Includes: cerebrovascular insufficiency (acute) with transient focal neurological signs and
                symptoms
              insufficiency of basilar, carotid, and vertebral arteries
              spasm of cerebral arteries

> Excludes: *acute cerebrovascular insufficiency NOS (437.1)*
>   *that due to any condition classifiable to 433 (433.0-433.9)*

435.0 Basilar artery syndrome

435.1 Vertebral artery syndrome

435.2 Subclavian steal syndrome

435.3 Vertebrobasilar artery syndrome

435.8 Other specified transient cerebral ischemias

435.9 Unspecified transient cerebral ischemia
    Impending cerebrovascular accident
    Intermittent cerebral ischemia
    Transient ischemic attack [TIA]

436 Acute, but ill-defined, cerebrovascular disease
    Apoplexy, apoplectic:
      NOS
      attack
      cerebral
      seizure
    Cerebral seizure

> Excludes: *any condition classifiable to categories 430-435*
>   *cerebrovascular accident (434.91)*
>   *CVA (ischemic) (434.91)*
>   *embolic (434.11)*
>   *hemorrhagic (430, 431, 432.0-432.9)*
>   *thrombotic (434.01)*
>   *postoperative cerebrovascular accident (997.02)*
>   *stroke (ischemic) (434.91)*
>   *embolic (434.11)*
>   *hemorrhagic (430, 431, 432.0-432.9)*
>   *thrombotic (434.01)*

437 Other and ill-defined cerebrovascular disease

437.0 Cerebral atherosclerosis
    Atheroma of cerebral arteries
    Cerebral arteriosclerosis

437.1 Other generalized ischemic cerebrovascular disease
    Acute cerebrovascular insufficiency NOS
    Cerebral ischemia (chronic)

437.2 Hypertensive encephalopathy

437.3 Cerebral aneurysm, nonruptured
    Internal carotid artery, intracranial portion
    Internal carotid artery NOS

> Excludes: *congenital cerebral aneurysm, nonruptured (747.81)*
>   *internal carotid artery, extracranial portion (442.81)*

437.4 Cerebral arteritis

437.5 Moyamoya disease

437.6 Nonpyogenic thrombosis of intracranial venous sinus

> Excludes: *pyogenic (325)*

● Code new   ▲ Revision of   ④ ⑤ Fourth or fifth
  to this edition   existing code   digit required

437.7 Transient global amnesia

437.8 Other

437.9 Unspecified
Cerebrovascular disease or lesion NOS

438 Late effects of cerebrovascular disease
Note: This category is to be used to indicate conditions in 430-437 as the cause of late effects. The "late effects" include conditions specified as such, as sequelae, which may occur at any time after the onset of the causal condition.

438.0 Cognitive deficits

⑤ **438.1 Speech and language deficits**

438.10 Speech and language deficit, unspecified

438.11 Aphasia

438.12 Dysphasia

438.19 Other speech and language deficits

⑤ **438.2 Hemiplegia/hemiparesis**

438.20 Hemiplegia affecting unspecified side

438.21 Hemiplegia affecting dominant side

438.22 Hemiplegia affecting nondominant side

⑤ **438.3 Monoplegia of upper limb**

438.30 Monoplegia of upper limb affecting unspecified side

438.31 Monoplegia of upper limb affecting dominant side

438.32 Monoplegia of upper limb affecting nondominant side

⑤ **438.4 Monoplegia of lower limb**

438.40 Monoplegia of lower limb affecting unspecified side

438.41 Monoplegia of lower limb affecting dominant side

438.42 Monoplegia of lower limb affecting nondominant side

⑤ **438.5 Other paralytic syndrome**
Use additional code to identify type of paralytic syndrome, such as:
locked-in state (344.81)
quadriplegia (344.00-344.09)

Excludes: *late effects of cerebrovascular accident with:*
hemiplegia/hemiparesis (438.20-438.22)
monoplegia of lower limb (438.40-438.42)
monoplegia of upper limb (438.30-438.32)

438.50 Other paralytic syndrome affecting unspecified side

438.51 Other paralytic syndrome affecting dominant side

438.52 Other paralytic syndrome affecting nondominant side

438.53 Other paralytic syndrome, bilateral

438.6 Alterations of sensations
Use additional code to identify the altered sensation

438.7 Disturbances of vision
Use additional code to identify the visual disturbance

⑤ **438.8 Other late effects of cerebrovascular disease**

438.81 Apraxia

438.82 Dysphagia

438.83 Facial weakness
Facial droop

438.84 Ataxia

438.85 Vertigo

438.89 Other late effects of cerebrovascular disease
Use additional code to identify the late effect

438.9 Unspecified late effects of cerebrovascular disease

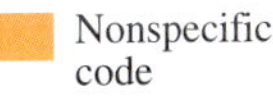

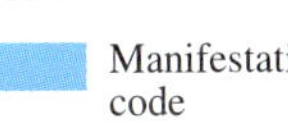

DISEASES OF ARTERIES, ARTERIOLES, AND CAPILLARIES (440-448)

440 Atherosclerosis

Includes: arteriolosclerosis
arteriosclerosis (obliterans) (senile)
arteriosclerotic vascular disease
atheroma
degeneration:
  arterial
  arteriovascular
  vascular
endarteritis deformans or obliterans
senile arteritis
senile endarteritis

Excludes: *atheroembolism (445.01-445.89)*
atherosclerosis of bypass graft of the extremities (440.30-440.32)

440.0 Of aorta

440.1 Of renal artery

Excludes: *atherosclerosis of renal arterioles (403.00-403.91)*

⑤ **440.2 Of native arteries of the extremities**

Excludes: *atherosclerosis of bypass graft of the extremities (440.30-440.32)*

440.20 Atherosclerosis of the extremities, unspecified

440.21 Atherosclerosis of the extremities with intermittent claudication

440.22 Atherosclerosis of the extremities with rest pain
Any condition classifiable to 440.21

440.23 Atherosclerosis of the extremities with ulceration
Any condition classifiable to 440.21 and 440.22
Use additional code for any associated ulceration (707.10-707.9)

440.24 Atherosclerosis of the extremities with gangrene
Any condition classifiable to 440.21, 440.22, and 440.23 with ischemic gangrene 785.4
Use additional code for any associated ulceration (707.10-707.9)

Excludes: *gas gangrene 040.0*

440.29 Other

⑤ **440.3 Of bypass graft of the extremities**

Excludes: *atherosclerosis of native artery of the extremity (440.21-440.24)*
embolism [occlusion NOS] [thrombus]
of graft (996.74)

440.30 Of unspecified graft

440.31 Of autologous vein bypass graft

440.32 Of nonautologous biological bypass graft

440.8 Of other specified arteries

Excludes: *basilar (433.0)*

carotid (433.1)
cerebral (437.0)
coronary (414.00-414.07)
mesenteric (557.1)
precerebral (433.0-433.9)
pulmonary (416.0)
vertebral (433.2)

440.9 Generalized and unspecified atherosclerosis
Arteriosclerotic vascular disease NOS

Excludes: *arteriosclerotic cardiovascular disease [ASCVD] (429.2)*

441 Aortic aneurysm and dissection

Excludes: *syphilitic aortic aneurysm (093.0)*
traumatic aortic aneurysm (901.0, 902.0)

⑤ **441.0 Dissection of aorta**

441.00 Unspecified site

441.01 Thoracic

441.02 Abdominal

● Code new to this edition   ▲ Revision of existing code   ④ ⑤ Fourth or fifth digit required

441.03   Thoracoabdominal

441.1   Thoracic aneurysm, ruptured

441.2   Thoracic aneurysm without mention of rupture

441.3   Abdominal aneurysm, ruptured

441.4   Abdominal aneurysm without mention of rupture

441.5   Aortic aneurysm of unspecified site, ruptured
Rupture of aorta NOS

441.6   Thoracoabdominal aneurysm, ruptured

441.7   Thoracoabdominal aneurysm, without mention of rupture

441.9   Aortic aneurysm of unspecified site without mention of rupture
Aneurysm
Dilatation of aorta
Hyaline necrosis of aorta

442   Other aneurysm
Includes: aneurysm (ruptured) (cirsoid) (false) (varicose)
aneurysmal varix

Excludes: *arteriovenous aneurysm or fistula:*
acquired (447.0)
congenital (747.60-747.69)
traumatic (900.0-904.9)

442.0   Of artery of upper extremity

442.1   Of renal artery

442.2   Of iliac artery

442.3   Of artery of lower extremity
Aneurysm:
femoral artery
popliteal artery

⑤ **442.8   Of other specified artery**

442.81   Artery of neck
Aneurysm of carotid artery (common) (external) (internal, extracranial portion)

Excludes: *internal carotid artery, intracranial portion (437.3)*

442.82   Subclavian artery

442.83   Splenic artery

442.84   Other visceral artery
Aneurysm:
celiac artery
gastroduodenal artery
gastroepiploic artery
hepatic artery
pancreaticoduodenal artery
superior mesenteric artery

442.89   Other
Aneurysm:
mediastinal artery
spinal artery

Excludes: *cerebral (nonruptured) (437.3)*
congenital (747.81)
ruptured (430)
coronary (414.11)
heart (414.10)
pulmonary (417.1)

442.9   Of unspecified site

443   Other peripheral vascular disease

443.0   Raynaud's syndrome
Raynaud's:
disease
phenomenon (secondary)
Use additional code, if desired, to identify gangrene (785.4)

443.1   Thromboangiitis obliterans [Buerger's disease]
Presenile gangrene

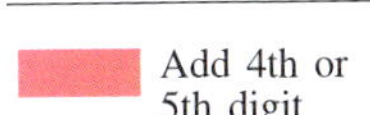

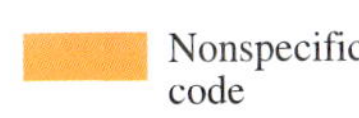

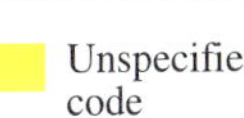

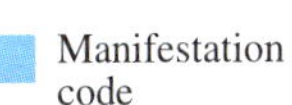

⑤ **443.2 Other arterial dissection**

Excludes: *dissection of aorta (441.00-441.03)*
dissection of coronary arteries (414.12)

443.21 Dissection of carotid artery

443.22 Dissection of iliac artery

443.23 Dissection of renal artery

443.24 Dissection of vertebral artery

443.29 Dissection of other artery

⑤ **443.8 Other specified peripheral vascular diseases**

443.81 *Peripheral angiopathy in diseases classified elsewhere*
Code first underlying disease, as:
diabetes mellitus (250.7)

443.82 Erythromelalgia

443.89 Other
Acrocyanosis
Acroparesthesia:
simple [Schultze's type]
vasomotor [Nothnagel's type]
Erythrocyanosis

Excludes: *chilblains (991.5)*
frostbite (991.0-991.3)
immersion foot (991.4)

443.9 Peripheral vascular disease, unspecified
Intermittent claudication NOS
Peripheral:
angiopathy NOS
vascular disease NOS
Spasm of artery

Excludes: *atherosclerosis of the arteries of the extremities (440.20-440.22)*
spasm of cerebral artery (435.0-435.9)

444 Arterial embolism and thrombosis
Includes: infarction:
embolic
thrombotic
occlusion

Excludes: *atheroembolism (445.01-445.89)*
that complicating:
abortion (634-638 with .6, 639.6)
ectopic or molar pregnancy (639.6)
pregnancy, childbirth, or the puerperium (673.0-673.8)

444.0 Of abdominal aorta
Aortic bifurcation syndrome   Leriche's syndrome
Aortoiliac obstruction   Saddle embolus

444.1 Of thoracic aorta
Embolism or thrombosis of aorta (thoracic)

⑤ **444.2 Of arteries of the extremities**

444.21 Upper extremity

444.22 Lower extremity
Arterial embolism or thrombosis:
femoral
peripheral NOS
popliteal

Excludes: *iliofemoral (444.81)*

⑤ **444.8 Of other specified artery**

444.81 Iliac artery

● Code new
to this edition

▲ Revision of
existing code

④ ⑤ Fourth or fifth
digit required

444.89 **Other**

> *Excludes:* *basilar (433.0)*
> *carotid (433.1)*
> *cerebral (434.0-434.9)*
> *coronary (410.00-410.92)*
> *mesenteric (557.0)*
> *ophthalmic (362.30-362.34)*
> *precerebral (433.0-433.9)*
> *pulmonary (415.19)*
> *renal (593.81)*
> *retinal (362.30-362.34)*
> *vertebral (433.2)*

444.9 **Of unspecified artery**

445 **Atheroembolism**
Includes: Atherothrombotic microembolism
Cholesterol embolism

⑤ **445.0** **Of extremities**

445.01 **Upper extremity**

445.02 **Lower extremity**

⑤ **445.8** **Of other sites**

445.81 **Kidney**

Use additional code for any associated acute renal failure or chronic kidney disease (584, 585)

445.89 **Other site**

446 **Polyarteritis nodosa and allied conditions**

446.0 **Polyarteritis nodosa**
Disseminated necrotizing periarteritis
Necrotizing angiitis
Panarteritis (nodosa)
Periarteritis (nodosa)

446.1 **Acute febrile mucocutaneous lymph node syndrome [MLNS]**
Kawasaki disease

⑤ **446.2** **Hypersensitivity angiitis**

> *Excludes:* *antiglomerular basement membrane disease without pulmonary hemorrhage*
> *(583.89)*

446.20 **Hypersensitivity angiitis, unspecified**

446.21 **Goodpasture's syndrome**
Antiglomerular basement membrane antibody-mediated nephritis with pulmonary hemorrhage

Use additional code, if desired, to identify renal disease (583.81)

446.29 **Other specified hypersensitivity angiitis**

446.3 **Lethal midline granuloma**
Malignant granuloma of face

446.4 **Wegener's granulomatosis**
Necrotizing respiratory granulomatosis
Wegener's syndrome

446.5 **Giant cell arteritis**
Cranial arteritis   Temporal arteritis
Horton's disease

446.6 **Thrombotic microangiopathy**
Moschcowitz's syndrome
Thrombotic thrombocytopenic purpura

446.7 **Takayasu's disease**
Aortic arch arteritis
Pulseless disease

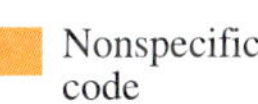

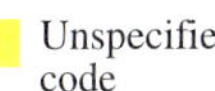

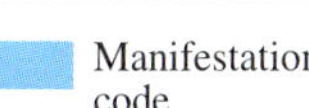

Manifestation
code

447 **Other disorders of arteries and arterioles**

447.0 **Arteriovenous fistula, acquired**
Arteriovenous aneurysm, acquired

Excludes: *cerebrovascular (437.3)*
coronary (414.19)
pulmonary (417.0)
surgically created arteriovenous shunt or fistula:
complication (996.1, 996.61-996.62)
status or presence (V45.1)
traumatic (900.0-904.9)

447.1 **Stricture of artery**

447.2 **Rupture of artery**
Erosion of artery
Fistula, except arteriovenous of artery
Ulcer of artery

Excludes: *traumatic rupture of artery (900.0-904.9)*

447.3 **Hyperplasia of renal artery**
Fibromuscular hyperplasia of renal artery

447.4 **Celiac artery compression syndrome**
Celiac axis syndrome
Marable's syndrome

447.5 **Necrosis of artery**

447.6 **Arteritis, unspecified**
Aortitis NOS
Endarteritis NOS

Excludes: *arteritis, endarteritis:*
aortic arch (446.7)
cerebral (437.4)
coronary (414.00-414.07)
deformans (440.0-440.9)
obliterans (440.0-440.9)
pulmonary (417.8)
senile (440.0-440.9)
polyarteritis NOS (446.0)
syphilitic aortitis (093.1)

447.8 **Other specified disorders of arteries and arterioles**
Fibromuscular hyperplasia of arteries, except renal

447.9 **Unspecified disorders of arteries and arterioles**

448 **Disease of capillaries**

448.0 **Hereditary hemorrhagic telangiectasia**
Rendu-Osler-Weber disease

448.1 **Nevus, non-neoplastic**

Nevus: Nevus:
  araneus   spider
  senile   stellar

Excludes: *neoplastic (216.0-216.9)*
port wine (757.32)
strawberry (757.32)

448.9 **Other and unspecified capillary diseases**
Capillary:
  hemorrhage
  hyperpermeability
  thrombosis

Excludes: *capillary fragility (hereditary) (287.8)*

● Code new
to this edition

▲ Revision of
existing code

④ ⑤ Fourth or fifth
digit required

DISEASES OF VEINS AND LYMPHATICS, AND OTHER DISEASES OF CIRCULATORY SYSTEM (451-459)

451 Phlebitis and thrombophlebitis
Includes: endophlebitis
inflammation, vein
periphlebitis
suppurative phlebitis

Use additional E Code, if desired, to identify drug, if drug-induced

Excludes: *that complicating:*
abortion (634-638 with .7, 639.8)
ectopic or molar pregnancy (639.8)
pregnancy, childbirth, or the puerperium (671.0-671.9)
that due to or following:
implant or catheter device (996.61-996.62)
infusion, perfusion, or transfusion (999.2)

451.0 Of superficial vessels of lower extremities
Saphenous vein (greater) (lesser)

⑤ **451.1 Of deep vessels of lower extremities**

451.11 Femoral vein (deep) (superficial)

451.19 Other
Femoropopliteal vein
Popliteal vein
Tibial vein

451.2 Of lower extremities, unspecified

⑤ **451.8 Of other sites**

Excludes: *intracranial venous sinus (325)*
nonpyogenic (437.6)
portal (vein) (572.1)

451.81 Iliac vein

451.82 Of superficial veins of upper extremities
Antecubital vein
Basilic vein
Cephalic vein

451.83 Of deep veins of upper extremities
Brachial vein
Radial vein
Ulnar vein

451.84 Of upper extremities, unspecified

451.89 Other
Axillary vein
Jugular vein
Subclavian vein
Thrombophlebitis of breast (Mondor's disease)

451.9 Of unspecified site

452 Portal vein thrombosis
Portal (vein) obstruction

Excludes: *hepatic vein thrombosis (453.0)*
phlebitis of portal vein (572.1)

453 Other venous embolism and thrombosis

Excludes: *that complicating:*
abortion (634-638 with .7, 639.8)
ectopic or molar pregnancy (639.8)
pregnancy, childbirth, or the puerperium (671.0-671.9)
that with inflammation, phlebitis, and thrombophlebitis (451.0-451.9)

453.0 Budd-Chiari syndrome
Hepatic vein thrombosis

453.1 Thrombophlebitis migrans

453.2 Of vena cava

453.3 Of renal vein

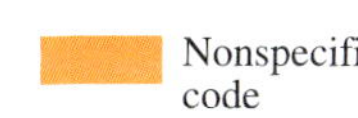

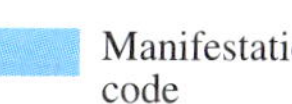

⑤ **453.4 Venous embolism and thrombosis of deep vessels of lower extremity**

453.40 Venous embolism and thrombosis of unspecified deep vessels of lower extremity
Deep vein thrombosis NOS
DVT NOS

453.41 Venous embolism and thrombosis of deep vessels of proximal lower extremity
Femoral
Iliac
Popliteal
Thigh
Upper leg NOS

453.42 Venous embolism and thrombosis of deep vessels of distal lower extremity
Calf
Lower leg NOS
Peroneal
Tibial

453.8 Of other specified veins
Excludes: *cerebral (434.0-434.9)*
coronary (410.00-410.92)
intracranial venous sinus (325)
nonpyogenic (437.6)
mesenteric (557.0)
portal (452)
precerebral (433.0-433.9)
pulmonary (415.19)

453.9 Of unspecified site
Embolism of vein
Thrombosis (vein)

454 Varicose veins of lower extremities
Excludes: *that complicating pregnancy, childbirth, or the puerperium (671.0)*

454.0 With ulcer
Varicose ulcer (lower extremity, any part)
Varicose veins with ulcer of lower extremity [any part] or of unspecified site
Any condition classifiable to 454.9 with ulcer or specified as ulcerated

454.1 With inflammation
Stasis dermatitis
Varicose veins with inflammation of lower extremity [any part] or of unspecified site
Any condition classifiable to 454.9 with inflammation or specified as inflamed

454.2 With ulcer and inflammation
Varicose veins with ulcer and inflammation of lower extremity [any part] or of unspecified site
Any condition classifiable to 454.9 with ulcer and inflammation

454.8 With other complications
Edema
Pain
Swelling

454.9 Asymptomatic varicose veins
Phlebectasia of lower extremity [any part] or of unspecified site
Varicose veins NOS
Varicose veins of lower extremity [any part] or of unspecified site
Varix of lower extremity [any part] or of unspecified site

455 Hemorrhoids
Includes: hemorrhoids (anus) (rectum)
piles
varicose veins, anus or rectum

Excludes: *that complicating pregnancy, childbirth or the puerperium (671.8)*

455.0 Internal hemorrhoids without mention of complication

455.1 Internal thrombosed hemorrhoids

455.2 Internal hemorrhoids with other complication
Internal hemorrhoids:
bleeding
prolapsed
Internal hemorrhoids:
strangulated
ulcerated

455.3 External hemorrhoids without mention of complication

● Code new to this edition   ▲ Revision of existing code   ④ ⑤ Fourth or fifth digit required

455.4 **External thrombosed hemorrhoids**

455.5 **External hemorrhoids with other complication**
External hemorrhoids:
  bleeding
  prolapsed
External hemorrhoids:
  strangulated
  ulcerated

455.6 **Unspecified hemorrhoids without mention of complication**
Hemorrhoids NOS

455.7 **Unspecified thrombosed hemorrhoids**
Thrombosed hemorrhoids, unspecified whether internal or external

455.8 **Unspecified hemorrhoids with other complication**
Hemorrhoids, unspecified whether internal or external:
  bleeding
  prolapsed
  strangulated
  ulcerated

455.9 **Residual hemorrhoidal skin tags**
Skin tags, anus or rectum

456 **Varicose veins of other sites**

456.0 **Esophageal varices with bleeding**

456.1 **Esophageal varices without mention of bleeding**

⑤ **456.2** *Esophageal varices in diseases classified elsewhere*
Code first underlying cause, as:
  cirrhosis of liver (571.0-571.9)
  portal hypertension (572.3)

456.20 *With bleeding*

456.21 *Without mention of bleeding*

456.3 **Sublingual varices**

456.4 **Scrotal varices**
Varicocele

456.5 **Pelvic varices**
Varices of broad ligament

456.6 **Vulval varices**
Varices of perineum

Excludes: *that complicating pregnancy, childbirth, or the puerperium (671.1)*

456.8 **Varices of other sites**
Varicose veins of nasal septum (with ulcer)

Excludes: *placental varices (656.7)*
retinal varices (362.17)
varicose ulcer of unspecified site (454.0)
varicose veins of unspecified site (454.9)

457 **Noninfectious disorders of lymphatic channels**

457.0 **Postmastectomy lymphedema syndrome**
Elephantiasis due to mastectomy
Obliteration of lymphatic vessel due to mastectomy

457.1 **Other lymphedema**
Elephantiasis (nonfilarial) NOS
Lymphangiectasis
Lymphedema:
  acquired (chronic)
  praecox
  secondary
Obliteration, lymphatic vessel

Excludes: *elephantiasis (nonfilarial):*
congenital (757.0)
eyelid (374.83)
vulva (624.8)

457.2 **Lymphangitis**
Lymphangitis:
  NOS
  chronic
  subacute

Excludes: *acute lymphangitis (682.0-682.9)*

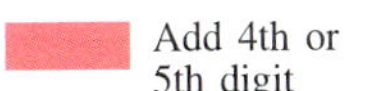

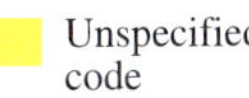

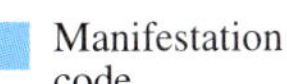

457.8 Other noninfectious disorders of lymphatic channels
Chylocele (nonfilarial) Lymph node or vessel:
Chylous: fistula
  ascites infarction
  cyst rupture

Excludes: chylocele:
filarial (125.0-125.9)
tunica vaginalis (nonfilarial) (608.84)

457.9 Unspecified noninfectious disorder of lymphatic channels

458 Hypotension
Includes: hypopiesis

Excludes: cardiovascular collapse (785.50)
maternal hypotension syndrome (669.2)
shock (785.50-785.59)
Shy-Drager syndrome (333.0)

458.0 Orthostatic hypotension
Hypotension:
  orthostatic (chronic)
  postural

458.1 Chronic hypotension
Permanent idiopathic hypotension

⑤ **458.2 Iatrogenic hypotension**

458.21 Hypotension of hemodialysis
Intra-dialytic hypotension

458.29 Other iatrogenic hypotension
Postoperative hypotension

458.8 Other specified hypotension

458.9 Hypotension, unspecified
Hypotension (arterial) NOS

459 Other disorders of circulatory system

459.0 Hemorrhage, unspecified
Rupture of blood vessel NOS
Spontaneous hemorrhage NEC

Excludes: hemorrhage:

gastrointestinal NOS (578.9)
in newborn NOS (772.9)
secondary or recurrent following trauma (958.2)
traumatic rupture of blood vessel (900.0-904.9)

⑤ **459.1 Postphlebitic syndrome**
Chronic venous hypertension due to deep vein thrombosis

Excludes: chronic venous hyptertension without deep vein thrombosis (459.30-459.39)

459.10 Postphlebetic syndrome without complications
Asymptomatic postphlebetic syndrome
Postphlebetic syndrome NOS

459.11 Postphlebetic syndrome with ulcer

459.12 Postphlebetic syndrome with inflammation

459.13 Postphlebetic syndrome with ulcer and inflammation

459.19 Postphlebetic syndrome with other complication

459.2 Compression of vein
Stricture of vein
Vena cava syndrome (inferior) (superior)

⑤ **459.3 Chronic venous hypertension (idiopathic)**
Statis edema

Excludes: chronic venous hypertension due to deep vein thrombosis (459.10-459.19)
varicose veins (454.0-454.9)

459.30 Chronic venous hypertension without complications
Asymptomatic chronic venous hypertension
Chronic venous hypertension NOS

459.31 Chronic venous hypertension with ulcer

459.32 Chronic venous hypertension with inflammation

  ● Code new   ▲ Revision of   ④ ⑤ Fourth or fifth
  to this edition   existing code   digit required

459.33   **Chronic venous hypertension with ulcer and inflammation**

459.39   **Chronic venous hypertension with other complication**

⑤ **459.8**   **Other specified disorders of circulatory system**

459.81   **Venous (peripheral) insufficiency, unspecified**
Chronic venous insufficiency NOS

Use additional code for any associated ulceration (707.10-707.9)

459.89   **Other**
Collateral circulation (venous), any site
Phlebosclerosis
Venofibrosis

459.9   **Unspecified circulatory system disorder**

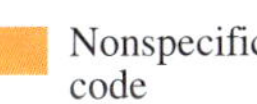

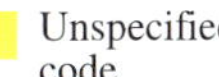

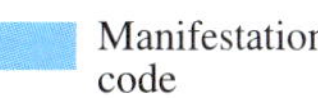

● Code new
to this edition

▲ Revision of
existing code

④ ⑤ Fourth or fifth
digit required

8. DISEASES OF THE RESPIRATORY SYSTEM (460-519)

Use additional code, if desired, to identify infectious organism

ACUTE RESPIRATORY INFECTIONS (460-466)

Excludes: *pneumonia and influenza (480.0-487.8)*

460 Acute nasopharyngitis [common cold]

Coryza (acute)
Nasal catarrh, acute
Nasopharyngitis:
  NOS
  acute
  infective NOS

Rhinitis:
  acute
  infective

Excludes: *nasopharyngitis, chronic (472.2)*
  pharyngitis:
    acute or unspecified (462)
    chronic (472.1)
  rhinitis:
    allergic (477.0-477.9)
    chronic or unspecified (472.0)
  sore throat:
    acute or unspecified (462)
    chronic (472.1)

461 Acute sinusitis

Includes: abscess acute, of sinus (accessory) (nasal)
  empyema acute, of sinus (accessory) (nasal)
  infection acute, of sinus (accessory) (nasal)
  inflammation acute, of sinus (accessory) (nasal)
  suppuration acute, of sinus (accessory) (nasal)

Excludes: *chronic or unspecified sinusitis (473.0-473.9)*

461.0 Maxillary
Acute antritis

461.1 Frontal

461.2 Ethmoidal

461.3 Sphenoidal

461.8 Other acute sinusitis
Acute pansinusitis

461.9 Acute sinusitis, unspecified
Acute sinusitis NOS

462 Acute pharyngitis

Acute sore throat NOS
Pharyngitis (acute):
  NOS
  gangrenous
  infective
  phlegmonous
  pneumococcal

Pharyngitis (acute):
  staphylococcal
  suppurative
  ulcerative
Sore throat (viral) NOS
Viral pharyngitis

Excludes: *abscess:*

  peritonsillar [quinsy] (475)
  pharyngeal NOS (478.29)
  retropharyngeal (478.24)
chronic pharyngitis (472.1)
infectious mononucleosis (075)
that specified as (due to):
  Coxsackie (virus) (074.0)
  gonococcus (098.6)
  herpes simplex (054.79)
  influenza (487.1)
  septic (034.0)
  streptococcal (034.0)

Add 4th or 5th digit | Nonspecific code | Unspecified code | Manifestation code

463 Acute tonsillitis

Tonsillitis (acute):
 NOS
 follicular
 gangrenous
 infective
 pneumococcal

Tonsillitis (acute):
 septic
 staphylococcal
 suppurative
 ulcerative
 viral

Excludes: *chronic tonsillitis (474.0)*
  hypertrophy of tonsils (474.1)
  peritonsillar abscess [quinsy] (475)
  sore throat:
   acute or NOS (462)
   septic (034.0)
  streptococcal tonsillitis (034.0)

464 Acute laryngitis and tracheitis

Excludes: *that associated with influenza (487.1)*
  that due to Streptococcus (034.0)

⑤ **464.0 Acute laryngitis**

Laryngitis (acute):
 NOS
 edematous
 Hemophilus influenza
  [H. influenzae]

Laryngitis (acute):
 pneumococcal
 septic
 suppurative
 ulcerative

Excludes: *chronic laryngitis (476.0-476.1)*
  influenzal laryngitis (487.1)

  464.00 Without mention of obstruction

  464.01 With obstruction

⑤ **464.1 Acute tracheitis**

Tracheitis (acute):
 NOS
 catarrhal
 viral

Excludes: *chronic tracheitis (491.8)*

  464.10 Without mention of obstruction

  464.11 With obstruction

⑤ **464.2 Acute laryngotracheitis**

Laryngotracheitis (acute)
Tracheitis (acute) with laryngitis (acute)

Excludes: *chronic laryngotracheitis (476.1)*

  464.20 Without mention of obstruction

  464.21 With obstruction

⑤ **464.3 Acute epiglottitis**

Viral epiglottitis

Excludes: *epiglottitis, chronic (476.1)*

  464.30 Without mention of obstruction

  464.31 With obstruction

 464.4 Croup

Croup syndrome

⑤ **464.5 Supraglottitis, unspecified**

  464.50 Without mention of obstruction

  464.51 With obstruction

465 Acute upper respiratory infections of multiple or unspecified sites

Excludes: *upper respiratory infection due to:*
  influenza (487.1)
  Streptococcus (034.0)

 465.0 Acute laryngopharyngitis

 465.8 Other multiple sites

Multiple URI

● Code new to this edition   ▲ Revision of existing code   ④ ⑤ Fourth or fifth digit required

465.9 **Unspecified site**
Acute URI NOS
Upper respiratory infection (acute)

466 **Acute bronchitis and bronchiolitis**
Includes: that with:
bronchospasm
obstruction

466.0 **Acute bronchitis**
Bronchitis, acute or subacute:
fibrinous
membranous
pneumococcal
purulent
septic
viral
with tracheitis
Croupous bronchitis
Tracheobronchitis, acute

Excludes: *acute bronchitis with chronic obstructive pulmonary disease (491.22)*

⑤ **466.1** **Acute bronchiolitis**
Bronchiolitis (acute)
Capillary pneumonia

466.11 **Acute bronchiolitis due to respiratory syncytial virus (RSV)**

466.19 **Acute bronchiolitis due to other infectious organisms**
Use additional code to identify organism

OTHER DISEASES OF THE UPPER RESPIRATORY TRACT (470-478)

470 **Deviated nasal septum**
Deflected septum (nasal) (acquired)

Excludes: *congenital (754.0)*

471 **Nasal polyps**

Excludes: *adenomatous polyps (212.0)*

471.0 **Polyp of nasal cavity**
Polyp:
choanal
nasopharyngeal

471.1 **Polypoid sinus degeneration**
Woakes' syndrome or ethmoiditis

471.8 **Other polyp of sinus**
Polyp of sinus: Polyp of sinus:
accessory   maxillary
ethmoidal   sphenoidal

471.9 **Unspecified nasal polyp**
Nasal polyp NOS

472 **Chronic pharyngitis and nasopharyngitis**

472.0 **Chronic rhinitis**
Ozena   Rhinitis:
Rhinitis: hypertrophic
NOS   obstructive
atrophic   purulent
granulomatous   ulcerative

Excludes: *allergic rhinitis (477.0-477.9)*

472.1 **Chronic pharyngitis**
Chronic sore throat
Pharyngitis:
atrophic
granular (chronic)
hypertrophic

472.2 **Chronic nasopharyngitis**

Excludes: *acute or unspecified nasopharyngitis (460)*

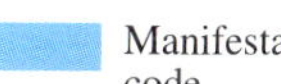

473 Chronic sinusitis
Includes: abscess (chronic) of sinus (accessory) (nasal)
empyema (chronic) of sinus (accessory) (nasal)
infection (chronic) of sinus (accessory) (nasal)
suppuration (chronic) of sinus (accessory) (nasal)

Excludes: *acute sinusitis (461.0-461.9)*

473.0 Maxillary
Antritis (chronic)

473.1 Frontal

473.2 Ethmoidal
Excludes: *Woakes' ethmoiditis (471.1)*

473.3 Sphenoidal

473.8 Other chronic sinusitis
Pansinusitis (chronic)

473.9 Unspecified sinusitis (chronic)
Sinusitis (chronic) NOS

474 Chronic disease of tonsils and adenoids

⑤ **474.0 Chronic tonsillitis and adenoiditis**
Excludes: *acute or unspecified tonsillitis (463)*

474.00 Chronic tonsillitis

474.01 Chronic adenoiditis

474.02 Chronic tonsillitis and adenoiditis

⑤ **474.1 Hypertrophy of tonsils and adenoids**
Enlargement of tonsils or adenoids
Hyperplasia of tonsils or adenoids
Hypertrophy of tonsils or adenoids

Excludes: *that with adenoiditis (474.01)*
that with adenoiditis and tonsillitis (474.02)
that with tonsillitis (474.00)

474.10 Tonsils with adenoids

474.11 Tonsils alone

474.12 Adenoids alone

474.2 Adenoid vegetations

474.8 Other chronic disease of tonsils and adenoids
Amygdalolith
Calculus, tonsil
Cicatrix of tonsil (and adenoid)
Tonsillar tag
Ulcer, tonsil

474.9 Unspecified chronic disease of tonsils and adenoids
Disease (chronic) of tonsils (and adenoids)

475 Peritonsillar abscess
Abscess of tonsil
Peritonsillar cellulitis
Quinsy

Excludes: *tonsillitis:*
acute or NOS (463)
chronic (474.0)

476 Chronic laryngitis and laryngotracheitis

476.0 Chronic laryngitis
Laryngitis:
catarrhal
hypertrophic
Sicca

476.1 Chronic laryngotracheitis
Laryngitis, chronic, with tracheitis (chronic)
Tracheitis, chronic, with laryngitis

Excludes: *chronic tracheitis (491.8)*
laryngitis and tracheitis, acute or unspecified (464.00-464.51)

      ● Code new   ▲ Revision of   ④ ⑤ Fourth or fifth
to this edition   existing code   digit required

477 Allergic rhinitis
    Includes: allergic rhinitis (nonseasonal) (seasonal)
              hay fever
              spasmodic rhinorrhea
    Excludes: *allergic rhinitis with asthma (bronchial) (493.0)*

477.0 Due to pollen
      Pollinosis

477.1 Due to food

477.2 Due to animal (cat) (dog) hair and dander

477.8 Due to other allergen

477.9 Cause unspecified

478 Other diseases of upper respiratory tract

478.0 Hypertrophy of nasal turbinates

⑤ **478.1 Other diseases of nasal cavity and sinuses**
      Excludes: *varicose ulcer of nasal septum (456.8)*

    ● **478.11 Nasal mucositis (ulcerative)**
Use additional E code to identify adverse effects of therapy, such as:
          antineoplastic and immunosuppressive drugs (E930.7, E933.1)
          radiation therapy (E879.2)

    ● **478.19 Other disease of nasal cavity and sinuses**
            Abscess of nose (septum)
            Necrosis of nose (septum)
            Ulcer of nose (septum)
            Cyst or mucocele of sinus (nasal)
            Rhinolith

⑤ **478.2 Other diseases of pharynx, not elsewhere classified**
      478.20 Unspecified disease of pharynx

      478.21 Cellulitis of pharynx or nasopharynx

      478.22 Parapharyngeal abscess

      478.24 Retropharyngeal abscess

      478.25 Edema of pharynx or nasopharynx

      478.26 Cyst of pharynx or nasopharynx

      478.29 Other
            Abscess of pharynx or nasopharynx
      Excludes: *ulcerative pharyngitis (462)*

⑤ **478.3 Paralysis of vocal cords or larynx**
      478.30 Paralysis, unspecified
            Laryngoplegia
            Paralysis of glottis

      478.31 Unilateral, partial

      478.32 Unilateral, complete

      478.33 Bilateral, partial

      478.34 Bilateral, complete

478.4 Polyp of vocal cord or larynx
      Excludes: *adenomatous polyps (212.1)*

478.5 Other diseases of vocal cords
            Abscess of vocal cords
            Cellulitis of vocal cords
            Granuloma of vocal cords
            Leukoplakia of vocal cords
            Chorditis (fibrinous) (nodosa) (tuberosa)
            Singers' nodes

478.6 Edema of larynx
            Edema (of):
              glottis
              subglottic
              supraglottic

⑤ **478.7 Other diseases of larynx, not elsewhere classified**
      478.70 Unspecified disease of larynx

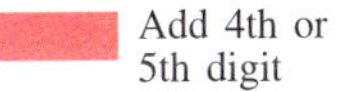

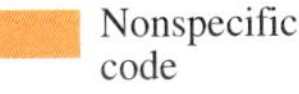

Unspecified
code

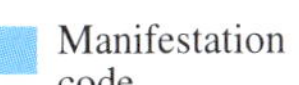

478.71   **Cellulitis and perichondritis of larynx**

478.74   **Stenosis of larynx**

478.75   **Laryngeal spasm**
      Laryngismus (stridulus)

478.79   **Other**
      Abscess of larynx
      Necrosis of larynx
      Obstruction of larynx
      Pachyderma of larynx
      Ulcer of larynx

Excludes: *ulcerative laryngitis (464.00-464.01)*

478.8   **Upper respiratory tract hypersensitivity reaction, site unspecified**
Excludes: *hypersensitivity reaction of lower respiratory tract, as:*
      extrinsic allergic alveolitis (495.0-495.9)
      pneumoconiosis (500-505)

478.9   **Other and unspecified diseases of upper respiratory tract**
      Abscess of trachea
      Cicatrix of trachea

PNEUMONIA AND INFLUENZA (480-487)

Excludes: *pneumonia:*
      allergic or eosinophilic (518.3)
      aspiration:
        NOS (507.0)
        newborn (770.18)
        solids and liquids (507.0-507.8)
      congenital (770.0)
      lipoid (507.1)
      passive (514)
      rheumatic (390)

480 **Viral pneumonia**

480.0   **Pneumonia due to adenovirus**

480.1   **Pneumonia due to respiratory syncytial virus**

480.2   **Pneumonia due to parainfluenza virus**

480.3   **Pneumonia due to SARS-associated coronavirus**

480.8   **Pneumonia due to other virus not elsewhere classified**
Excludes: *congenital rubella pneumonitis (771.0)*
      influenza with pneumonia, any form (487.0)
      pneumonia complicating viral diseases classified elsewhere (484.1-484.8)

480.9   **Viral pneumonia, unspecified**

481 **Pneumococcal pneumonia [*Streptococcus pneumoniae* pneumonia]**
      Lobar pneumonia, organism unspecified

482 **Other bacterial pneumonia**

482.0   **Pneumonia due to Klebsiella pneumoniae**

482.1   **Pneumonia due to Pseudomonas**

482.2   **Pneumonia due to Hemophilus influenzae [H. influenzae]**

⑤ **482.3**   **Pneumonia due to Streptococcus**
Excludes: *Streptococcus pneumoniae pneumonia (481)*

    482.30   **Streptococcus, unspecified**

    482.31   **Group A**

    482.32   **Group B**

    482.39   **Other Streptococcus**

⑤ **482.4**   **Pneumonia due to Staphylococcus**

    482.40   **Pneumonia due to Staphylococcus, unspecified**

    482.41   **Pneumonia due to Staphylococcus aureus**

    482.49   **Other Staphylococcus pneumonia**

⑤ **482.8**   **Pneumonia due to other specified bacteria**
Excludes: *pneumonia complicating infectious disease classified elsewhere (484.1-484.8)*

● Code new to this edition   ▲ Revision of existing code   ④ ⑤ Fourth or fifth digit required

482.81 Anaerobes
Bacteroides (melaninogenicus)
Gram-negative anaerobes

482.82 Escherichia coli [E. coli]

482.83 Other gram-negative bacteria
Gram-negative pneumonia NOS
Proteus
Serratia marcescens

Excludes: *Gram-negative anaerobes (482.81)*
Legionnaires' disease (482.84)

482.84 Legionnaires' disease

482.89 Other specified bacteria

482.9 Bacterial pneumonia unspecified

483 Pneumonia due to other specified organism

483.0 Mycoplasma pneumoniae
Eaton's agent
Pleuropneumonia-like organism [PPLO]

483.1 Chlamydia

483.8 Other specified organism

484 Pneumonia in infectious diseases classified elsewhere

Excludes: *influenza with pneumonia, any form (487.0)*

484.1 Pneumonia in cytomegalic inclusion disease
Code first underlying disease (078.5)

484.3 Pneumonia in whooping cough
Code first underlying disease (033.0-033.9)

484.5 Pneumonia in anthrax
Code first underlying disease (022.1)

484.6 Pneumonia in aspergillosis
Code first underlying disease (117.3)

484.7 Pneumonia in other systemic mycoses
Code first underlying disease

Excludes: *pneumonia in:*

candidiasis (112.4)
coccidioidomycosis (114.0)
histoplasmosis (115.0-115.9 with fifth-digit 5)

484.8 Pneumonia in other infectious diseases classified elsewhere
Code first underlying disease, as:
Q fever (083.0)
typhoid fever (002.0)

Excludes: *pneumonia in:*

actinomycosis (039.1)
measles (055.1)
nocardiosis (039.1)
ornithosis (073.0)
Pneumocystis carinii (136.3)
salmonellosis (003.22)
toxoplasmosis (130.4)
tuberculosis (011.6)
tularemia (021.2)
varicella (052.1)

485 Bronchopneumonia, organism unspecified

Bronchopneumonia:	Pneumonia:
hemorrhagic	lobular
terminal	segmental
Pleurobronchopneumonia	

Excludes: *bronchiolitis (acute) (466.11-466.19)*
chronic (491.8)
lipoid pneumonia (507.1)

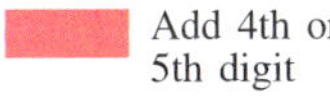

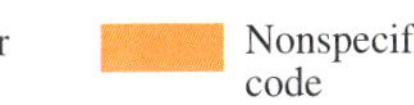

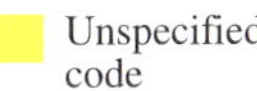

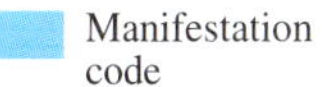

486 Pneumonia, organism unspecified

> *Excludes:* *hypostatic or passive pneumonia (514)*
>
> *influenza with pneumonia, any form (487.0)*
> *inhalation or aspiration pneumonia due to foreign materials (507.0-507.8)*
> *pneumonitis due to fumes and vapors (506.0)*

487 Influenza

> *Excludes:* *Hemophilus influenzae [H. influenzae]:*
>
> *infection NOS (041.5)*
> *laryngitis (464.00-464.01)*
> *meningitis (320.0)*

487.0 With pneumonia

Influenza with pneumonia, any form
Influenzal:
  bronchopneumonia
  pneumonia
Use additional code to identify the type of pneumonia (480.0-480.9, 481, 482.0-482.9, 483.0-483.8, 485)

487.1 With other respiratory manifestations

Influenza NOS
Influenzal:
  laryngitis
  pharyngitis
  respiratory infection (upper) (acute)

487.8 With other manifestations

Encephalopathy due to influenza
Influenza with involvement of gastrointestinal tract

> *Excludes:* *"intestinal flu" [viral gastroenteritis] (008.8)*

CHRONIC OBSTRUCTIVE PULMONARY DISEASE AND ALLIED CONDITIONS (490-496)

490 Bronchitis, not specified as acute or chronic

Bronchitis NOS: Tracheobronchitis NOS
  catarrhal
with tracheitis NOS

> *Excludes:* *bronchitis:*
>
> *allergic NOS (493.9)*
> *asthmatic NOS (493.9)*
> *due to fumes and vapors (506.0)*

491 Chronic bronchitis

> *Excludes:* *chronic obstructive asthma (493.2)*

491.0 Simple chronic bronchitis

Catarrhal bronchitis, chronic
Smokers' cough

491.1 Mucopurulent chronic bronchitis

Bronchitis (chronic) (recurrent):
  fetid
  mucopurulent
  purulent

⑤ **491.2 Obstructive chronic bronchitis**

Bronchitis: Bronchitis with:
  emphysematous   chronic airway obstruction
  obstructive (chronic) (diffuse) emphysema

> *Excludes:* *asthmatic bronchitis (acute) NOS (493.9)*
>
> *chronic obstructive asthma (493.2)*

491.20 Without exacerbation

Emphysema with chronic bronchitis

491.21 With (acute) exacerbation

Acute exacerbation of chronic obstructive pulmonary disease [COPD]
Decompensated chronic obstructive pulmonary disease [COPD]
Decompensated chronic obstructive pulmonary disease [COPD] with exacerbation

> *Excludes:* *chronic obstructive asthma with acute exacerbation (493.22)*

491.22 With acute bronchitis

● Code new
  to this edition

▲ Revision of
  existing code

④ ⑤ Fourth or fifth
  digit required

491.8 Other chronic bronchitis
Chronic:
tracheitis
tracheobronchitis

491.9 Unspecified chronic bronchitis

492 Emphysema

492.0 Emphysematous bleb
Giant bullous emphysema
Ruptured emphysematous bleb
Tension pneumatocele
Vanishing lung

492.8 Other emphysema

Emphysema (lung or pulmonary):
NOS
centriacinar
centrilobular
obstructive
panacinar

Emphysema (lung or pulmonary):
panlobular
unilateral
vesicular
MacLeod's syndrome
Swyer-James syndrome
Unilateral hyperlucent lung

Excludes: *emphysema:*

compensatory (518.2)
due to fumes and vapors (506.4)
interstitial (518.1)
newborn (770.2)
mediastinal (518.1)
surgical (subcutaneous) (998.81)
traumatic (958.7)
with chronic bronchitis (491.20-491.22)

493 Asthma

Excludes: *wheezing NOS (786.07)*

The following fifth-digit subclassification is for use with codes 493.0-493.2, 493.9:

0 unspecified

1 with status asthmaticus

2 with (acute) exacerbation

⑤ **493.0 extrinsic asthma**
Asthma:
allergic with stated cause
atopic
childhood
hay
platinum
Hay fever with asthma

Excludes: *asthma:*

allergic NOS (493.9)
detergent (507.8)
miners' (500)
wood (495.8)

⑤ **493.1 Intrinsic asthma**
Late-onset asthma

⑤ **493.2 Chronic obstructive asthma**
Asthma with chronic obstructive pulmonary disease [COPD]
Chronic asthmatic bronchitis

Excludes: *chronic obstructive bronchitis (491.20-491.22)*
acute bronchitis (466.0)

⑤ **493.8 Other forms of asthma**

493.81 Exercise induced bronchospasm

493.82 Cough variant asthma

⑤ **493.9 Asthma, unspecified**
Asthma (bronchial) (allergic NOS)
Bronchitis:
allergic
asthmatic

Add 4th or 5th digit	Nonspecific code	Unspecified code	Manifestation code

494 Bronchiectasis
Bronchiectasis (fusiform) (postinfectious) (recurrent)
Bronchiolectasis

> Excludes: congenital (748.61)
> tuberculous bronchiectasis (current disease) (011.5)

494.0 Bronchiectasis without acute exacerbation

494.1 Bronchiectasis with acute exacerbation

495 Extrinsic allergic alveolitis
Includes: allergic alveolitis and pneumonitis due to inhaled organic dust particles of fungal,
thermophilic actinomycete, or other origin

495.0 Farmers' lung

495.1 Bagassosis

495.2 Bird-fanciers' lung
Budgerigar-fanciers' disease or lung
Pigeon-fanciers' disease or lung

495.3 Suberosis
Cork-handlers' disease or lung

495.4 Malt workers' lung
Alveolitis due to Aspergillus clavatus

495.5 Mushroom workers' lung

495.6 Maple bark-strippers' lung
Alveolitis due to Cryptostroma corticale

495.7 "Ventilation" pneumonitis
Allergic alveolitis due to fungal, thermophilic actinomycete, and other organisms
growing in ventilation [air conditioning] systems

495.8 Other specified allergic alveolitis and pneumonitis

Cheese-washers' lung	Pituitary snuff-takers' disease
Coffee workers' lung	Sequoiosis or red-cedar asthma
Fish-meal workers' lung	Wood asthma
Furriers' lung	
Grain-handlers' disease or lung	

495.9 Unspecified allergic alveolitis and pneumonitis
Alveolitis, allergic (extrinsic)
Hypersensitivity pneumonitis

496 Chronic airway obstruction, not elsewhere classified
Note: This code is not to be used with any code from categories 491-493
Chronic:
nonspecific lung disease
obstructive lung disease
obstructive pulmonary disease [COPD] NOS

> Excludes: chronic obstructive lung disease [COPD] specified (as) (with):
> allergic alveolitis (495.0-495.9)
> asthma (493.2)
> bronchiectasis (494.0-494.1)
> bronchitis (491.20-491.22)
> with emphysema (491.20-491.22)
> decompensated (491.21)
> emphysema (492.0-492.8)

PNEUMOCONIOSES AND OTHER LUNG DISEASES DUE TO EXTERNAL AGENTS (500-508)

500 Coal workers' pneumoconiosis

Anthracosilicosis	Coal workers' lung
Anthracosis	Miner's asthma
Black lung disease	

501 Asbestosis

502 Pneumoconiosis due to other silica or silicates
Pneumoconiosis due to talc
Silicotic fibrosis (massive) of lung
Silicosis (simple) (complicated)

503 Pneumoconiosis due to other inorganic dust

Aluminosis (of lung)	Graphite fibrosis (of lung)
Bauxite fibrosis (of lung)	Siderosis
Berylliosis	Stannosis

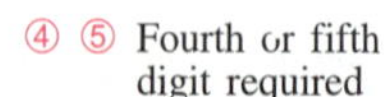

● Code new
to this edition

▲ Revision of
existing code

④ ⑤ Fourth or fifth
digit required

504 Pneumonopathy due to inhalation of other dust
   Byssinosis   Flax-dressers' disease
   Cannabinosis

   Excludes: *allergic alveolitis (495.0-495.9)*
               asbestosis (501)
               bagassosis (495.1)
               farmers' lung (495.0)

505 Pneumoconiosis, unspecified

506 Respiratory conditions due to chemical fumes and vapors
   Use additional E code, if desired, to identify cause

   506.0 Bronchitis and pneumonitis due to fumes and vapors
        Chemical bronchitis (acute)

   506.1 Acute pulmonary edema due to fumes and vapors
        Chemical pulmonary edema (acute)

        Excludes: *acute pulmonary edema NOS (518.4)*
                    chronic or unspecified pulmonary edema (514)

   506.2 Upper respiratory inflammation due to fumes and vapors

   506.3 Other acute and subacute respiratory conditions due to fumes and vapors

   506.4 Chronic respiratory conditions due to fumes and vapors
        Emphysema (diffuse) (chronic) due to inhalation of chemical fumes and vapors
        Obliterative bronchiolitis (chronic) (subacute) due to inhalation of chemical fumes and
            vapors
        Pulmonary fibrosis (chronic) due to inhalation of chemical fumes and vapors

   506.9 Unspecified respiratory conditions due to fumes and vapors
        Silo-fillers' disease

507 Pneumonitis due to solids and liquids

        Excludes: *fetal aspiration pneumonitis (770.18)*

   507.0 Due to inhalation of food or vomitus
        Aspiration pneumonia (due to):
          NOS
          food (regurgitated)
          gastric secretions
          milk
          saliva
          vomitus

   507.1 Due to inhalation of oils and essences
        Lipoid pneumonia (exogenous)

        Excludes: *endogenous lipoid pneumonia (516.8)*

   507.8 Due to other solids and liquids
        Detergent asthma

508 Respiratory conditions due to other and unspecified external agents
   Use additional E code, if desired, to identify cause

   508.0 Acute pulmonary manifestations due to radiation
        Radiation pneumonitis

   508.1 Chronic and other pulmonary manifestations due to radiation
        Fibrosis of lung following radiation

   508.8 Respiratory conditions due to other specified external agents

   508.9 Respiratory conditions due to unspecified external agent

OTHER DISEASES OF RESPIRATORY SYSTEM (510-519)

510 Empyema
   Use additional code, if desired, to identify infectious organism (041.0-041.9)

        Excludes: *abscess of lung (513.0)*

   510.0 With fistula
        Fistula: Fistula:
          bronchocutaneous   mediastinal
          bronchopleural   pleural
          hepatopleural   thoracic
        Any condition classifiable to 510.9 with fistula

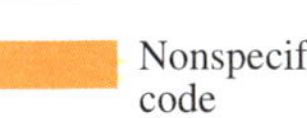

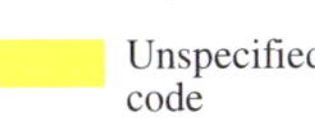

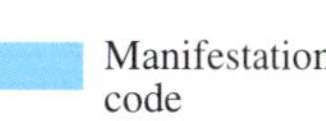

Manifestation
code

510.9 Without mention of fistula

Abscess:
  pleura
  thorax
Empyema (chest) (lung)
  (pleura)
Fibrinopurulent pleurisy

Pleurisy:
  purulent
  septic
  seropurulent
  suppurative
Pyopneumothorax
Pyothorax

511 Pleurisy

> Excludes: malignant pleural effusion (197.2)
>   pleurisy with mention of tuberculosis, current disease (012.0)

511.0 Without mention of effusion or current tuberculosis

Adhesion, lung or pleura
Calcification of pleura
Pleurisy (acute) (sterile):
  diaphragmatic
  fibrinous
  interlobar

Pleurisy:
  NOS
  pneumococcal
  staphylococcal
  streptococcal
Thickening of pleura

511.1 With effusion, with mention of a bacterial cause other than tuberculosis

Pleurisy with effusion (exudative) (serous):
  pneumococcal
  staphylococcal
  streptococcal
  other specified nontuberculous bacterial cause

511.8 Other specified forms of effusion, except tuberculous

Encysted pleurisy
Hemopneumothorax
Hemothorax

Hydropneumothorax
Hydrothorax

> Excludes: traumatic (860.2-860.5, 862.29, 862.39)

511.9 Unspecified pleural effusion

Pleural effusion NOS
Pleurisy:
  exudative
  serofibrinous

Pleurisy:
  serous
  with effusion NOS

512 Pneumothorax

512.0 Spontaneous tension pneumothorax

512.1 Iatrogenic pneumothorax

Postoperative pneumothorax

512.8 Other spontaneous pneumothorax

Pneumothorax:
  NOS
  acute
  chronic

> Excludes: pneumothorax:
>   congenital (770.2)
>   traumatic (860.0-860.1, 860.4-860.5)
>   tuberculous, current disease (011.7)

513 Abscess of lung and mediastinum

513.0 Abscess of lung

Abscess (multiple) of lung
Gangrenous or necrotic pneumonia
Pulmonary gangrene or necrosis

513.1 Abscess of mediastinum

● Code new
to this edition

▲ Revision of
existing code

④ ⑤ Fourth or fifth
digit required

514 Pulmonary congestion and hypostasis
Hypostatic:
  bronchopneumonia
  pneumonia
Passive pneumonia
Pulmonary congestion (chronic) (passive)
Pulmonary edema:
  NOS
  chronic

Excludes: *acute pulmonary edema:*
  NOS (518.4)
  with mention of heart disease or failure (428.1)
hypostatic pneumonia due to or specified as a specific type of pneumonia – code
  to the type of pneumonia (480.0-480.9, 481, 482.0-482.49, 483.0-483.8, 485,
  486, 487.0)

515 Postinflammatory pulmonary fibrosis
Cirrhosis of lung, chronic or unspecified
Fibrosis of lung (atrophic) (confluent) (massive) (perialveolar) (peribronchial), chronic or
  unspecified
Induration of lung, chronic or unspecified

516 Other alveolar and parietoalveolar pneumonopathy

516.0 Pulmonary alveolar proteinosis

516.1 Idiopathic pulmonary hemosiderosis
  Essential brown induration of lung
  Code first underlying disease (275.0)

516.2 Pulmonary alveolar microlithiasis

516.3 Idiopathic fibrosing alveolitis
  Alveolar capillary block
  Diffuse (idiopathic) (interstitial) pulmonary fibrosis
  Hamman-Rich syndrome

516.8 Other specified alveolar and parietoalveolar pneumonopathies
  Endogenous lipoid pneumonia
  Interstitial pneumonia (desquamative) (lymphoid)
  Excludes: *lipoid pneumonia, exogenous or unspecified (507.1)*

516.9 Unspecified alveolar and parietoalveolar pneumonopathy

517 Lung involvement in conditions classified elsewhere
  Excludes: *rheumatoid lung (714.81)*

517.1 Rheumatic pneumonia
  Code first underlying disease (390)

517.2 Lung involvement in systemic sclerosis
  Code first underlying disease (710.1)

517.3 Acute chest syndrome
  Code first sickle-cell disease in crisis (282.42, 282.62, 282.64, 282.69)

517.8 Lung involvement in other diseases classified elsewhere
  Code first underlying disease, as:
    amyloidosis (277.30-277.39)
    polymyositis (710.4)
    sarcoidosis (135)
    Sjögren's disease (710.2)
    systemic lupus erythematosus (710.0)
  Excludes: *syphilis (095.1)*

518 Other diseases of lung

518.0 Pulmonary collapse
  Atelectasis
  Collapse of lung
  Middle lobe syndrome
  Excludes: *atelectasis:*
    congenital (partial) (770.5)
      primary (770.4)
    tuberculous, current disease (011.8)

	Add 4th or 5th digit		Nonspecific code		Unspecified code		Manifestation code

518.1 Interstitial emphysema
Mediastinal emphysema

Excludes: *surgical (subcutaneous) emphysema (998.81)*
that in fetus or newborn (770.2)
traumatic emphysema (958.7)

518.2 Compensatory emphysema

518.3 Pulmonary eosinophilia
Eosinophilic asthma   Tropical eosinophilia
Löffler's syndrome
Pneumonia:
 allergic
 eosinophilic

518.4 Acute edema of lung, unspecified
Acute pulmonary edema NOS
Pulmonary edema, postoperative

Excludes: *pulmonary edema:*
acute, with mention of heart disease or failure (428.1)
chronic or unspecified (514)
due to external agents (506.0-508.9)

518.5 Pulmonary insufficiency following trauma and surgery
Adult respiratory distress syndrome
Pulmonary insufficiency following:
 shock
 surgery
 trauma
Shock lung

Excludes: *adult respiratory distress syndrome associated with other conditions (518.82)*
pneumonia:
aspiration (507.0)
hypostatic (514)
respiratory failure in other conditions (518.81, 518.83-518.84)

518.6 Allergic bronchopulmonary aspergillosis

● **518.7 Transfusion related acute lung injury (TRALI)**

⑤ **518.8 Other diseases of lung**

518.81 Acute respiratory failure
Respiratory failure NOS

Excludes: *acute and chronic respiratory failure (518.84)*
acute respiratory distress (518.82)
chronic respiratory failure (518.83)
respiratory arrest (799.1)
respiratory failure, newborn (770.84)

518.82 Other pulmonary insufficiency, not elsewhere classified
Acute respiratory distress
Acute respiratory insufficiency
Adult respiratory distress syndrome NEC

Excludes: *adult respiratory distress syndrome associated with trauma and surgery (518.5)*
pulmonary insufficiency following trauma and surgery (518.5)
respiratory distress:
NOS (786.09)
newborn (770.89)
syndrome, newborn (769)
shock lung (518.5)

518.83 Chronic respiratory failure

518.84 Acute and chronic respiratory failure
Acute or chronic respiratory failure

518.89 Other diseases of lung, not elsewhere classified
Broncholithiasis   Lung disease NOS
Calcification of lung   Pulmolithiasis

519 Other diseases of respiratory system

⑤ **519.0 Tracheostomy complications**

519.00 Tracheostomy complication, unspecified

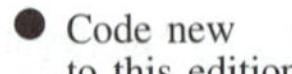

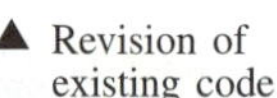

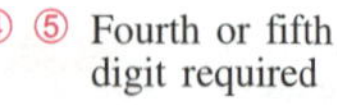

519.01   Infection of tracheostomy

Use additional code to identify type of infection, such as:
    abscess or cellulitis of neck (682.1)
    septicemia (038.0-038.9)

Use additional code to identify organism (041.00-041.9)

519.02   Mechanical complication of tracheostomy
    Tracheal stenosis due to tracheostomy

519.09   Other tracheostomy complications
    Hemorrhage due to tracheostomy
    Tracheoesophageal fistula due to tracheostomy

⑤ **519.1   Other diseases of trachea and bronchus, not elsewhere classified**

● **519.11   Acute bronchospasm**
    Bronchospasm NOS

Excludes: *acute bronchitis with bronchospasm (466.0)*
    asthma (493.00-493.92)
    exercise induced bronchospasm (493.81)

● **519.19   Other diseases of trachea and bronchus**
    Calcification of bronchus or trachea
    Stenosis of bronchus or trachea
    Ulcer of bronchus or trachea

519.2   Mediastinitis

519.3   Other diseases of mediastinum, not elsewhere classified
    Fibrosis of mediastinum
    Hernia of mediastinum
    Retraction of mediastinum

519.4   Disorders of diaphragm
    Diaphragmitis
    Paralysis of diaphragm
    Relaxation of diaphragm

Excludes: *congenital defect of diaphragm (756.6)*
    diaphragmatic hernia (551-553 with .3)
    congenital (756.6)

519.8   Other diseases of respiratory system, not elsewhere classified

519.9   Unspecified disease of respiratory system
    Respiratory disease (chronic) NOS

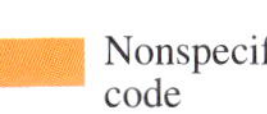

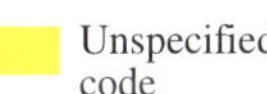

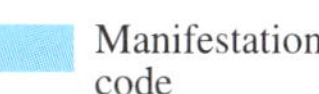

● Code new
to this edition

▲ Revision of
existing code

④ ⑤ Fourth or fifth
digit required

9.   DISEASES OF THE DIGESTIVE SYSTEM (520-579)

DISEASES OF ORAL CAVITY, SALIVARY GLANDS, AND JAWS (520-529)

520 Disorders of tooth development and eruption

520.0 Anodontia
Absence of teeth (complete) (congenital) (partial)
Hypodontia
Oligodontia

Excludes: *acquired absence of teeth (525.10-525.19)*

520.1 Supernumerary teeth
Distomolar   Paramolar
Fourth molar   Supplemental teeth
Mesiodens

Excludes: *supernumerary roots (520.2)*

520.2 Abnormalities of size and form
Concrescence of teeth   Macrodontia
Fusion of teeth   Microdontia
Gemination of teeth   Peg-shaped [conical] teeth
Dens evaginatus   Supernumerary roots
Dens in dente   Taurodontism
Dens invaginatus   Tuberculum paramolare
Enamel pearls

Excludes: *that due to congenital syphilis (090.5)*
tuberculum Carabelli, which is regarded as a normal variation

520.3 Mottled teeth
Dental fluorosis
Mottling of enamel
Nonfluoride enamel opacities

520.4 Disturbances of tooth formation
Aplasia and hypoplasia of cementum   Horner's teeth
Dilaceration of tooth   Hypocalcification of teeth
Enamel hypoplasia (neonatal) (postnatal) Regional odontodysplasia
(prenatal)   Turner's tooth

Excludes: *Hutchinson's teeth and mulberry molars in congenital syphilis (090.5)*
mottled teeth (520.3)

520.5 Hereditary disturbances in tooth structure, not elsewhere classified
Amelogenesis imperfecta
Dentinogenesis imperfecta
Odontogenesis imperfecta
Dentinal dysplasia
Shell teeth

520.6 Disturbances of tooth eruption
Teeth: Tooth eruption:
  embedded   late
  impacted   obstructed
  natal   premature
  neonatal
  prenatal
  primary [deciduous]:
    persistent
    shedding, premature

Excludes: *exfoliation of teeth (attributable to disease of surrounding tissues) (525.0-525.19)*

520.7 Teething syndrome

520.8 Other specified disorders of tooth development and eruption
Color changes during tooth formation
Pre-eruptive color changes

Excludes: *posteruptive color changes (521.7)*

520.9 Unspecified disorder of tooth development and eruption

521 Diseases of hard tissue of teeth

⑤ **521.0 Dental caries**

521.00   Dental caries, unspecified

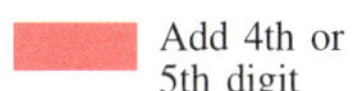

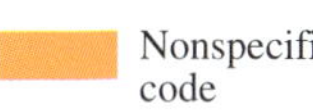

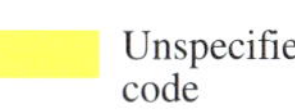

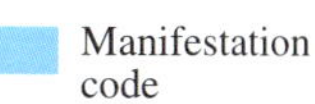

521.01 Dental caries limited to enamel
Initial caries
White spot lesion

521.02 Dental caries extending into dentine

521.03 Dental caries extending into pulp

521.04 Arrested dental caries

521.05 Odontoclasia
Infantile melanodontia
Melanodontoclasia

Excludes: internal and external resorption of teeth (521.40-521.49)

521.06 Dental caries pit and fissure
Primary dental caries, pit and fissure origin

521.07 Dental caries of smooth surface
Primary dental caries, smooth surface origin

521.08 Dental caries of root surface
Primary dental caries, root surface

521.09 Other dental caries

⑤ **521.1 Excessive attrition (approximal wear) (occlusal wear)**

521.10 Excessive attrition, unspecified

521.11 Excessive attrition, limited to enamel

521.12 Excessive attrition, extending into dentine

521.13 Excessive attrition, extending into pulp

521.14 Excessive attrition, localized

521.15 Excessive attrition, generalized

⑤ **521.2 Abrasion**
Abrasion of teeth:
dentifrice
habitual
occupational
ritual
traditional
Wedge defect NOS of teeth

521.20 Abrasion, unspecified

521.21 Abrasion, limited to enamel

521.22 Abrasion, extending into dentine

521.23 Abrasion, extending into pulp

521.24 Abrasion, localized

521.25 Abrasion, generalized

⑤ **521.3 Erosion**
Erosion of teeth: Erosion of teeth:
NOS idiopathic
due to: occupational
medicine
persistent vomiting

521.30 Erosion, unspecified

521.31 Erosion, limited to enamel

521.32 Erosion, extending into dentine

521.33 Erosion, extending into pulp

521.34 Erosion, localized

521.35 Erosion, generalized

⑤ **521.4 Pathological resorption**

521.40 Pathological resorption, unspecified

521.41 Pathological resorption, internal

521.42 Pathological resorption, external

521.49 Other pathological resorption
Internal granuloma of pulp

521.5 Hypercementosis
Cementation hyperplasia

● Code new
to this edition
▲ Revision of
existing code
④ ⑤ Fourth or fifth
digit required

521.6 Ankylosis of teeth

521.7 Intrinsic posteruptive color changes
Staining [discoloration] of teeth:
   NOS
   due to:
     drugs
     metals
     pulpal bleeding

Excludes: *accretions [deposits] on teeth (523.6)*
     extrinsic color changes (523.6)
     pre-eruptive color changes (520.8)

⑤ **521.8 Other specific diseases of hard tissues of teeth**

● **521.81 Cracked tooth**

Excludes: *asymptomatic craze lines in enamel – omit code*
     broken tooth due to trauma (873.63, 873.73)
     fractured tooth due to trauma (873.63, 873.73)

● **521.89 Other specific diseases of hard tissues of teeth**
     Irradiated enamel
     Sensitive dentin

521.9 Unspecified disease of hard tissues of teeth

522 Diseases of pulp and periapical tissues

522.0 Pulpitis

Pulpal:	Pulpitis:
abscess	acute
polyp	chronic (hyperplastic) (ulcerative)
	suppurative

522.1 Necrosis of the pulp
Pulp gangrene

522.2 Pulp degeneration
Denticles
Pulp calcifications
Pulp stones

522.3 Abnormal hard tissue formation in pulp
Secondary or irregular dentin

522.4 Acute apical periodontitis of pulpal origin

522.5 Periapical abscess without sinus
Abscess:
  dental
  dentoalveolar

Excludes: *periapical abscess with sinus (522.7)*

522.6 Chronic apical periodontitis
Apical or periapical granuloma
Apical periodontitis NOS

522.7 Periapical abscess with sinus
Fistula:
  alveolar process
  dental

522.8 Radicular cyst
Cyst:
  apical (periodontal)
  periapical
  radiculodental
  residual radicular

Excludes: *lateral developmental or lateral periodontal cyst (526.0)*

522.9 Other and unspecified diseases of pulp and periapical tissues

523 Gingival and periodontal diseases

⑤ **523.0 Acute gingivitis**

Excludes: *acute necrotizing ulcerative gingivitis (101)*
     herpetic gingivostomatitis (054.2)

● **523.00 Acute gingivitis, plaque induced**
     Acute gingivitis NOS

● **523.01 Acute gingivitis, non-plaque induced**

Add 4th or 5th digit	Nonspecific code	Unspecified code	Manifestation code

⑤ **523.1** **Chronic gingivitis**
    Gingivitis (chronic):   Gingivitis (chronic):
      desquamative   simple marginal
      hyperplastic   ulcerative

Excludes: *herpetic gingivostomatitis (054.2)*

● **523.10** **Chronic gingivitis, plaque induced**
    Chronic gingivitis NOS
    Gingivitis NOS

● **523.11** **Chronic gingivitis, non-plaque induced**

⑤ **523.2** **Gingival recession**
    Gingival recession (postinfective) (postoperative)

    523.20 **Gingival recession, unspecified**

    523.21 **Gingival recession, minimal**

    523.22 **Gingival recession, moderate**

    523.23 **Gingival recession, severe**

    523.24 **Gingival recession, localized**

    523.25 **Gingival recession, generalized**

⑤ **523.3** **Aggressive and acute periodontitis**
    Acute:
      pericementitis
      pericoronitis

Excludes: *acute apical periodontitis (522.4)*
             periapical abscess (522.5, 522.7)

● **523.30** **Aggressive periodontitis, unspecified**

● **523.31** **Aggressive periodontitis, localized**
    Periodontal abscess

● **523.32** **Aggressive periodontitis, generalized**

● **523.33** **Aggressive periodontitis**

⑤ **523.4** **Chronic periodontitis**
    Chronic pericoronitis
    Pericementitis (chronic)
    Periodontitis:
      NOS
      complex
      simplex

Excludes: *chronic apical periodontitis (522.6)*

● **523.40** **Chronic periodontitis, unspecified**

● **523.41** **Chronic periodontitis, localized**

● **523.42** **Chronic periodontitis, generalized**

523.5 **Periodontosis**

523.6 **Accretions on teeth**
    Dental calculus:
      subgingival
      supragingival
    Deposits on teeth:
      betel
      materia alba
      soft
      tartar
      tobacco
    Extrinsic discoloration of teeth

Excludes: *intrinsic discoloration of teeth (521.7)*

    ● Code new   ▲ Revision of   ④ ⑤ Fourth or fifth
       to this edition   existing code   digit required

523.8 Other specified periodontal diseases

Giant cell:	Gingival polyp
epulis	Periodontal lesions due to traumatic occlusion
peripheral granuloma	Peripheral giant cell granuloma
Gingival:	
cysts	
enlargement NOS	
fibromatosis	

Excludes: *leukoplakia of gingiva (528.6)*

523.9 Unspecified gingival and periodontal disease

524 Dentofacial anomalies, including malocclusion

⑤ **524.0 Major anomalies of jaw size**

Excludes: *hemifacial atrophy or hypertrophy (754.0)*
unilateral condylar hyperplasia or hypoplasia of mandible (526.89)

524.00 Unspecified anomaly

524.01 Maxillary hyperplasia

524.02 Mandibular hyperplasia

524.03 Maxillary hypoplasia

524.04 Mandibular hypoplasia

524.05 Macrogenia

524.06 Microgenia

524.07 Excessive tuberosity of jaw
Entire maxillary tuberosity

524.09 Other specified anomaly

⑤ **524.1 Anomalies of relationship of jaw to cranial base**

524.10 Unspecified anomaly
prognathism
retrognathism

524.11 Maxillary asymmetry

524.12 Other jaw asymmetry

524.19 Other specified anomaly

⑤ **524.2 Anomalies of dental arch relationship**
Anomaly of dental arch

Excludes: *hemifacial atrophy or hypertrophy (754.0)*
soft tissue impingement (524.81-524.82)
unilateral condylar hyperplasia or hypoplasia of mandible (526.89)

524.20 Unspecified anomaly of dental arch relationship

▲ **524.21 Malocclusion, Angle's class I**
Neutro-occlusion

▲ **524.22 Malocclusion, Angle's class II**
Disto-occlusion Division I
Disto-occlusion Division II

▲ **524.23 Malocclusion, Angle's class III**
Mesio-occlusion

524.24 Open anterior occlusal relationship
Anterior open bite

524.25 Open posterior occlusal relationship
Posterior open bite

524.26 Excessive horizontal overlap
Excessive horizontal overjet

524.27 Reverse articulation
Anterior articulation
Crossbite
Posterior articulation

524.28 Anomalies of interarch distance
Excessive interarch distance
Inadequate interarch distance

524.29 Other anomalies of dental arch relationship
Other anomalies of dental arch

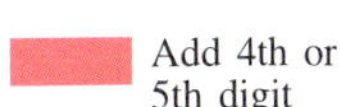

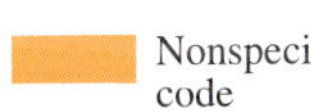

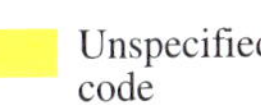

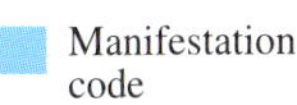

⑤ **524.3 Anomalies of tooth position of fully erupted teeth**

> *Excludes:* *impacted or embedded teeth with abnormal position of such teeth or adjacent teeth (520.6)*

524.30 Unspecified anomaly of tooth position
Diastema of teeth NOS
Displacement of teeth NOS
Transposition of teeth NOS

524.31 Crowding of teeth

524.32 Excessive spacing of teeth

524.33 Horizontal displacement of teeth
Tipped teeth
Tipping of teeth

524.34 Vertical displacement of teeth
Extruded tooth
Infraeruption of teeth
Intruded tooth
Supraeruption of teeth

524.35 Rotation of tooth/teeth

524.36 Insufficient interocclusal distance of teeth (ridge)
Lack of adequate intermaxillary vertical dimension

524.37 Excessive interocclusal distance of teeth
Excessive intermaxillary vertical dimension
Loss of occlusal vertical dimension

524.39 Other anomalies of tooth position

524.4 Malocclusion, unspecified

⑤ **524.5 Dentofacial functional abnormalities**

524.50 Dentofacial functional abnormality, unspecified

524.51 Abnormal jaw closure

524.52 Limited mandibular range of motion

524.53 Deviation in opening and closing of the mandible

524.54 Insufficient anterior guidance
Insufficient anterior occlusal guidance

524.55 Centric occlusion maximum intercuspation discrepancy
Centric occlusion of teeth discrepancy

524.56 Non-working side interference
Balancing side interference

524.57 Lack of posterior occlusal support

524.59 Other dentofacial functional abnormalities
Abnormal swallowing
Mouth breathing
Sleep postures
Tongue, lip, or finger habits

⑤ **524.6 Temporomandibular joint disorders**

> *Excludes:* *current temporomandibular joint:*
> *dislocation (830.0-830.1)*
> *strain (848.1)*

524.60 Temporomandibular joint disorders, unspecified
Temporomandibular joint-pain-dysfunction syndrome [TMJ]

524.61 Adhesions and ankylosis (bony or fibrous)

524.62 Arthralgia of temporomandibular joint

524.63 Articular disc disorder (reducing or non-reducing)

524.64 Temporomandibular joint sounds on opening and/or closing the jaw

524.69 Other specified temporomandibular joint disorders

⑤ **524.7 Dental alveolar anomalies**

524.70 Unspecified alveolar anomaly

524.71 Alveolar maxillary hyperplasia

524.72 Alveolar mandibular hyperplasia

524.73 Alveolar maxillary hypoplasia

524.74 Alveolar mandibular hypoplasia

   ● Code new to this edition   ▲ Revision of existing code   ④ ⑤ Fourth or fifth digit required

524.75 Vertical displacement of alveolus and teeth
Extrusion of alveolus and teeth

524.76 Occlusal plane deviation

524.79 Other specified alveolar anomaly

⑤ **524.8 Other specified dentofacial anomalies**

524.81 Anterior soft tissue impingement

524.82 Posterior soft tissue impingement

524.89 Other specified dentofacial anomalies

524.9 Unspecified dentofacial anomalies

525 Other diseases and conditions of the teeth and supporting structures

525.0 Exfoliation of teeth due to systemic causes

⑤ **525.1 Loss of teeth due to trauma, extraction, or periodontal disease**
Code first class of edentulism (525.40-525.44, 525.50-525.54)

525.10 Acquired absence of teeth, unspecified
Tooth extraction status, NOS

525.11 Loss of teeth due to trauma

525.12 Loss of teeth due to periodontal disease

525.13 Loss of teeth due to caries

525.19 Other loss of teeth

⑤ **525.2 Atrophy of edentulous alveolar ridge**

525.20 Unspecified atrophy of edentulous alveolar ridge
Atrophy of the mandible NOS
Atrophy of the maxilla NOS

525.21 Minimal atrophy of the mandible

525.22 Moderate atrophy of the mandible

525.23 Severe atrophy of the mandible

525.24 Minimal atrophy of the maxilla

525.25 Moderate atrophy of the maxilla

525.26 Severe atrophy of the maxilla

525.3 Retained dental root

⑤ **525.4 Complete edentulism**
Use additional code to identify cause of edentulism (525.10-525.19)

525.40 Complete edentulism, unspecified
Edentulism NOS

525.41 Complete edentulism, class I

525.42 Complete edentulism, class II

525.43 Complete edentulism, class III

525.44 Complete edentulism, class IV

⑤ **525.5 Partial edentulism**
Use additional code to identify cause of edentulism (525.10-525.19)

525.50 Partial edentulism, unspecified

525.51 Partial edentulism, class I

525.52 Partial edentulism, class II

525.53 Partial edentulism, class III

525.54 Partial edentulism, class IV

● **525.6 Unsatisfactory restoration of tooth**
Defective bridge, crown, fillings
Defective dental restoration

Excludes: *dental restoration status (V45.84)*
unsatisfactory endodontic treatment (526.61-526.69)

● **525.60 Unspecified unsatisfactory restoration of tooth**
Unspecified defective dental restoration

● **525.61 Open restoration margins**
Dental restoration failure of marginal integrity
Open margin on tooth restoration

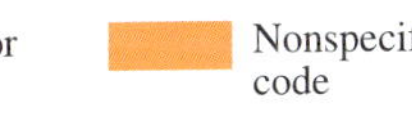

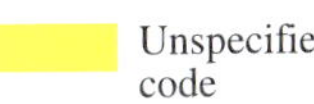

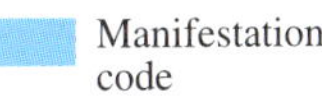

● **525.62 Unrepairable overhanging of dental restorative materials**
Overhanging of tooth restoration

● **525.63 Fractured dental restorative material without loss of material**
Excludes: *cracked tooth (521.81)*
fractured tooth (873.63, 873.73)

● **525.64 Fractured dental restorative material with loss of material**
Excludes: *cracked tooth (521.81)*
fractured tooth (873.63, 873.73)

● **525.65 Contour of existing restoration of tooth biologically incompatible with oral health**
Dental restoration failure of periodontal anatomical integrity
Unacceptable contours of existing restoration
Unacceptable morphology of existing restoration

● **525.66 Allergy to existing dental restorative material**
Use additional code to identify the specific type of allergy

● **525.67 Poor aesthetics of existing restoration**
Dental restoration aesthetically inadequate or displeasing

● **525.69 Other unsatisfactory restoration of existing tooth**

525.8 Other specified disorders of the teeth and supporting structures
Enlargement of alveolar ridge NOS
Irregular alveolar process

525.9 Unspecified disorder of the teeth and supporting structures

526 Diseases of the jaws

526.0 Developmental odontogenic cysts

Cyst:
dentigerous
eruption
follicular
lateral developmental

Cyst:
lateral periodontal
primordial
Keratocyst

Excludes: *radicular cyst (522.8)*

526.1 Fissural cysts of jaw
Cyst:
globulomaxillary
incisor canal
median anterior maxillary
median palatal
nasopalatine
palatine of papilla
Excludes: *cysts of oral soft tissues (528.4)*

526.2 Other cysts of jaws

Cyst of jaw:
NOS
aneurysmal

Cyst of jaw:
hemorrhagic
traumatic

526.3 Central giant cell (reparative) granuloma
Excludes: *peripheral giant cell granuloma (523.8)*

526.4 Inflammatory conditions
Abscess of jaw (acute) (chronic) (suppurative)
Osteitis of jaw (acute) (chronic) (suppurative)
Osteomyelitis (neonatal) of jaw (acute) (chronic) (suppurative)
Periostitis of jaw (acute) (chronic) (suppurative)
Sequestrum of jaw bone
Excludes: *alveolar osteitis (526.5)*

526.5 Alveolitis of jaw
Alveolar osteitis
Dry socket

● **526.6 Periradicular pathology associated with previous endodontic treatment**

● **526.61 Perforation of root canal space**

● **526.62 Endodontic overfill**

● **526.63 Endodontic underfill**

● **526.69 Other periradicular pathology associated with previous endodontic treatment**

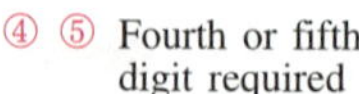

● Code new
to this edition

▲ Revision of
existing code

④ ⑤ Fourth or fifth
digit required

⑤ **526.8 Other specified diseases of the jaws**

    526.81 Exostosis of jaw
        Torus mandibularis
        Torus palatinus

    526.89 Other
        Cherubism of jaw(s)
        Fibrous dysplasia of jaw(s)
        Latent bone cyst of jaw(s)
        Osteoradionecrosis of jaw(s)
        Unilateral condylar hyperplasia or hypoplasia of mandible

526.9 Unspecified disease of the jaws

527 Diseases of the salivary glands

527.0 Atrophy

527.1 Hypertrophy

527.2 Sialoadenitis
    Parotitis: Sialoangitis
      NOS   Sialodochitis
      allergic
      toxic

    Excludes: *epidemic or infectious parotitis (072.0-072.9)*
                uveoparotid fever (135)

527.3 Abscess

527.4 Fistula
    Excludes: *congenital fistula of salivary glands (750.24)*

527.5 Sialolithiasis
    Calculus of salivary gland or duct
    Stone of salivary gland or duct
    Sialodocholithiasis

527.6 Mucocele
    Mucous:
      extravasation cyst of salivary gland
      retention cyst of salivary gland
    Ranula

527.7 Disturbance of salivary secretion
    Hyposecretion   Sialorrhea
    Ptyalism   Xerostomia

527.8 Other specified diseases of the salivary glands
    Benign lymphoepithelial lesion of salivary gland
    Sialectasia
    Sialosis
    Stenosis of salivary duct
    Stricture of salivary duct

527.9 Unspecified disease of the salivary glands

528 Diseases of the oral soft tissues, excluding lesions specific for gingiva and tongue

▲ **528.0 Stomatitis and mucositis (ulcerative)**
    Excludes: *cellulitis and abscess of mouth (528.3)*
             diphtheritic stomatitis (032.0)
             epizootic stomatitis (078.4)
             gingivitis (523.0-523.1)
             oral thrush (112.0)
             Stevens-Johnson syndrome (695.1)
             stomatitis:
               acute necrotizing ulcerative (101)
               aphthous (528.2)
               gangrenous (528.1)
               herpetic (054.2)
               Vincent's (101)

    ● **528.00 Stomatitis and mucositis, unspecified**
        Mucositis NOS
        Ulcerative mucositis NOS
        Ulcerative stomatitis NOS
        Vesicular stomatitis NOS

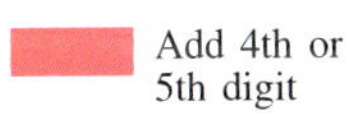

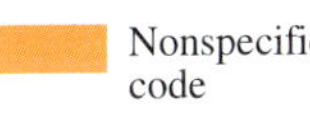

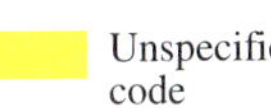

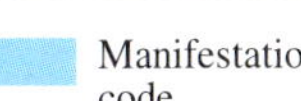

● **528.01 Mucositis (ulcerative) due to antineoplastic therapy**

Use additional E code to identify adverse effects of therapy, such as:
>> antineoplastic and immunosuppressive drugs (E930.7, E933.1)
>> radiation therapy (E879.2)

● `528.02` **Mucositis (ulcerative) due to other drugs**

Use additional E code to identify drug

● `528.09` **Other stomatitis and mucositis (ulcerative)**

528.1 Cancrum oris
>> Gangrenous stomatitis
>> Noma

528.2 Oral aphthae

Aphthous stomatitis	Recurrent aphthous ulcer
Canker sore	Stomatitis herpetiformis
Periadenitis mucosa necrotica recurrens	

> *Excludes:* *herpetic stomatitis (054.2)*

528.3 Cellulitis and abscess
>> Cellulitis of mouth (floor)
>> Ludwig's angina
>> Oral fistula

> *Excludes:* *abscess of tongue (529.0)*
>> *cellulitis or abscess of lip (528.5)*
>> *fistula (of):*
>>> *dental (522.7)*
>>> *lip (528.5)*
>> *gingivitis (523.00-523.11)*

528.4 Cysts
>> Dermoid cyst of mouth
>> Epidermoid cyst of mouth
>> Epstein's pearl of mouth
>> Lymphoepithelial cyst of mouth
>> Nasoalveolar cyst of mouth
>> Nasolabial cyst of mouth

> *Excludes:* *cyst:*
>> *gingiva (523.8)*
>> *tongue (529.8)*

528.5 Diseases of lips

Abscess of lip(s)	Cheilitis:
Cellulitis of lip(s)	NOS
Fistula of lip(s)	angular
Hypertrophy of lip(s)	Cheilodynia
	Cheilosis

> *Excludes:* *actinic cheilitis (692.79)*
>> *congenital fistula of lip (750.25)*
>> *leukoplakia of lips (528.6)*

528.6 Leukoplakia of oral mucosa, including tongue
>> Leukokeratosis of oral mucosa
>> Leukoplakia of:
>>> gingiva
>>> lips
>>> tongue

> *Excludes:* *carcinoma in situ (230.0, 232.0)*
>> *leukokeratosis nicotina palati (528.79)*

⑤ **528.7 Other disturbances of oral epithelium, including tongue**

> *Excludes:* *carcinoma in situ (230.0, 232.0)*
>> *leukokeratosis NOS (702)*

>> **528.71 Minimal keratinized residual ridge mucosa**
>>> Minimal keratinization of alveolar ridge mucosa

>> **528.72 Excessive keratinized residual ridge mucosa**
>>> Excessive keratinization of alveolar ridge mucosa

● Code new to this edition	▲ Revision of existing code	④ ⑤ Fourth or fifth digit required

528.79 **Other disturbances of oral epithelium, including tongue**
Erythroplakia of mouth or tongue
Focal epithelial hyperplasia of mouth or tongue
Leukoedema of mouth or tongue
Leukokeratosis nicotina palate
Other oral epithelium disturbances

528.8 **Oral submucosal fibrosis, including of tongue**

528.9 **Other and unspecified diseases of the oral soft tissues**
Cheek and lip biting
Denture sore mouth
Denture stomatitis
Melanoplakia
Papillary hyperplasia of palate
Eosinophilic granuloma of oral mucosa
Irritative hyperplasia of oral mucosa
Pyogenic granuloma of oral mucosa
Ulcer (traumatic) of oral mucosa

529 **Diseases and other conditions of the tongue**

529.0 **Glossitis**
Abscess of tongue
Ulceration (traumatic) of tongue

> *Excludes:* *glossitis:*
> *benign migratory (529.1)*
> *Hunter's (529.4)*
> *median rhomboid (529.2)*
> *Moeller's (529.4)*

529.1 **Geographic tongue**
Benign migratory glossitis
Glossitis areata exfoliativa

529.2 **Median rhomboid glossitis**

529.3 **Hypertrophy of tongue papillae**
Black hairy tongue
Coated tongue
Hypertrophy of foliate papillae
Lingua villosa nigra

529.4 **Atrophy of tongue papillae**
Bald tongue
Glazed tongue
Glossitis:
Hunter's
Moeller's
Glossodynia exfoliativa
Smooth atrophic tongue

529.5 **Plicated tongue**
Fissured tongue
Furrowed tongue
Scrotal tongue

> *Excludes:* *fissure of tongue, congenital (750.13)*

529.6 **Glossodynia**
Glossopyrosis
Painful tongue

> *Excludes:* *glossodynia exfoliativa (529.4)*

529.8 **Other specified conditions of the tongue**
Atrophy (of) tongue
Crenated (of) tongue
Enlargement (of) tongue
Hypertrophy (of) tongue
Glossocele
Glossoptosis

> *Excludes:* *erythroplasia of tongue (528.79)*
> *leukoplakia of tongue (528.6)*
> *macroglossia (congenital) (750.15)*
> *microglossia (congenital) (750.16)*
> *oral submucosal fibrosis (528.8)*

529.9 **Unspecified condition of the tongue**

Add 4th or 5th digit | Nonspecific code | Unspecified code | Manifestation code

DISEASES OF ESOPHAGUS, STOMACH, AND DUODENUM (530-538)

530 **Diseases of esophagus**

> *Excludes:* esophageal varices (456.0-456.2)

530.0 Achalasia and cardiospasm
Achalasia (of cardia)
Aperistalsis of esophagus
Megaesophagus

> *Excludes:* congenital cardiospasm (750.7)

⑤ **530.1 Esophagitis**
Abscess of esophagus
Esophagitis:
  NOS
  chemical
  peptic
Esophagitis:
  postoperative
  regurgitant

Use additional E code, if desired, to identify cause, if induced by chemical

> *Excludes:* tuberculous esophagitis (017.8)

    530.10 **Esophagitis, unspecified**

    530.11 **Reflux esophagitis**

    530.12 **Acute esophagitis**

    530.19 **Other esophagitis**

⑤ **530.2 Ulcer of esophagus**
Ulcer of esophagus
  fungal
  peptic
Ulcer of esophagus due to ingestion of:
  aspirin
  chemicals
  medicines

Use additional E code, if desired, to identify cause, if induced by chemical or drug

    530.20 **Ulcer of esophagus without bleeding**
    Ulcer of esophagus NOS

    530.21 **Ulcer of esophagus with bleeding**

> *Excludes:* bleeding esophageal varices (456.0, 456.20)

530.3 Stricture and stenosis of esophagus
Compression of esophagus
Obstruction of esophagus

> *Excludes:* congenital stricture of esophagus (750.3)

530.4 Perforation of esophagus
Rupture of esophagus

> *Excludes:* traumatic perforation of esophagus (862.22, 862.32, 874.4-874.5)

530.5 Dyskinesia of esophagus
Corkscrew esophagus
Curling esophagus
Esophagospasm
Spasm of esophagus

> *Excludes:* cardiospasm (530.0)

530.6 Diverticulum of esophagus, acquired
Diverticulum, acquired:
  epiphrenic
  pharyngoesophageal
  pulsion
  subdiaphragmatic
  traction
  Zenker's (hypopharyngeal)
Esophageal pouch, acquired
Esophagocele, acquired

> *Excludes:* congenital diverticulum of esophagus (750.4)

530.7 Gastroesophageal laceration-hemorrhage syndrome
Mallory-Weiss syndrome

⑤ **530.8 Other specified disorders of esophagus**

● Code new
to this edition

▲ Revision of
existing code

④ ⑤ Fourth or fifth
digit required

530.81 **Esophageal reflux**
Gastroesophageal reflux
| *Excludes:* | *reflux esophagitis (530.11)* |

530.82 **Esophageal hemorrhage**
| *Excludes:* | *hemorrhage due to esophageal varices (456.0-456.2)* |

530.83 **Esophageal leukoplakia**

530.84 **Tracheoesophageal fistula**
| *Excludes:* | *congenital tracheoesophageal fistula (750.3)* |

530.85 **Barrett's esophagus**

530.86 **Infection of esophagostomy**
Use additional code to specify infection

530.87 **Mechanical complication of esophagostomy**
Malfunction of esophagostomy

530.89 **Other**
| *Excludes:* | *Paterson-Kelly syndrome (280.8)* |

530.9 **Unspecified disorder of esophagus**

531 **Gastric ulcer**
Includes: ulcer (peptic):
prepyloric
pylorus
stomach

Use additional E code, if desired, to identify drug, if drug-induced
| *Excludes:* | *peptic ulcer NOS (533.0-533.9)* |
The following fifth-digit subclassification is for use with category 531:

0 **without mention of obstruction**

1 **with obstruction**

531.0 **Acute with hemorrhage**

531.1 **Acute with perforation**

531.2 **Acute with hemorrhage and perforation**

531.3 **Acute without mention of hemorrhage or perforation**

531.4 **Chronic or unspecified with hemorrhage**

531.5 **Chronic or unspecified with perforation**

531.6 **Chronic or unspecified with hemorrhage and perforation**

531.7 **Chronic without mention of hemorrhage or perforation**

531.9 **Unspecified as acute or chronic, without mention of hemorrhage or perforation**

532 **Duodenal ulcer**
Includes: erosion (acute) of duodenum
ulcer (peptic):
duodenum
postpyloric

Use additional E code, if desired, to identify drug, if drug-induced
| *Excludes:* | *peptic ulcer NOS (533.0-533.9)* |
The following fifth-digit subclassification is for use with category 532:

0 **without mention of obstruction**

1 **with obstruction**

532.0 **Acute with hemorrhage**

532.1 **Acute with perforation**

532.2 **Acute with hemorrhage and perforation**

532.3 **Acute without mention of hemorrhage or perforation**

532.4 **Chronic or unspecified with hemorrhage**

532.5 **Chronic or unspecified with perforation**

532.6 **Chronic or unspecified with hemorrhage and perforation**

532.7 **Chronic without mention of hemorrhage or perforation**

532.9 **Unspecified as acute or chronic, without mention of hemorrhage or perforation**

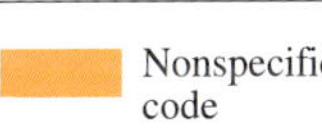

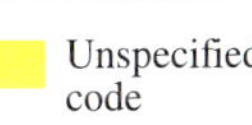

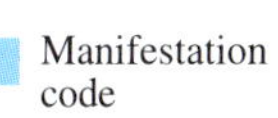

Manifestation
code

⑤ **533 Peptic ulcer, site unspecified**
    Includes: gastroduodenal ulcer NOS
             peptic ulcer NOS
             stress ulcer NOS

Use additional E code, if desired, to identify drug, if drug-induced

    |Excludes:| *peptic ulcer:*
             duodenal (532.0-532.9)
             gastric (531.0-531.9)

The following fifth-digit subclassification is for use with category 533:

    0 without mention of obstruction

    1 with obstruction

⑤ **533.0 Acute with hemorrhage**

⑤ **533.1 Acute with perforation**

⑤ **533.2 Acute with hemorrhage and perforation**

⑤ **533.3 Acute without mention of hemorrhage and perforation**

⑤ **533.4 Chronic or unspecified with hemorrhage**

⑤ **533.5 Chronic or unspecified with perforation**

⑤ **533.6 Chronic or unspecified with hemorrhage and perforation**

⑤ **533.7 Chronic without mention of hemorrhage or perforation**

⑤ **533.9 Unspecified as acute or chronic, without mention of hemorrhage or perforation**

⑤ **534 Gastrojejunal ulcer**
    Includes: ulcer (peptic) or erosion:
             anastomotic
             gastrocolic
             gastrointestinal
             gastrojejunal
             jejunal
             marginal
             stomal

    |Excludes:| *primary ulcer of small intestine (569.82)*
The following fifth-digit subclassification is for use with category 534:

    0 without mention of obstruction

    1 with obstruction

⑤ **534.0 Acute with hemorrhage**

⑤ **534.1 Acute with perforation**

⑤ **534.2 Acute with hemorrhage and perforation**

⑤ **534.3 Acute without mention of hemorrhage or perforation**

⑤ **534.4 Chronic or unspecified with hemorrhage**

⑤ **534.5 Chronic or unspecified with perforation**

⑤ **534.6 Chronic or unspecified with hemorrhage and perforation**

⑤ **534.7 Chronic without mention of hemorrhage or perforation**

⑤ **534.9 Unspecified as acute or chronic, without mention of hemorrhage or perforation**

⑤ **535 Gastritis and duodenitis**
The following fifth-digit subclassification is for use with category 535

    0 without mention of hemorrhage

    1 with hemorrhage

⑤ **535.0 Acute gastritis**

⑤ **535.1 Atrophic gastritis**
    Gastritis:
      atrophic-hyperplastic
      chronic (atrophic)

⑤ **535.2 Gastric mucosal hypertrophy**
    Hypertrophic gastritis

⑤ **535.3 Alcoholic gastritis**

● Code new
  to this edition
    ▲ Revision of
      existing code
    ④ ⑤ Fourth or fifth
         digit required

⑤ **535.4** **Other specified gastritis**
  Gastritis: Gastritis:
    allergic   superficial
    bile induced   toxic
    irritant

⑤ **535.5** **Unspecified gastritis and gastroduodenitis**

⑤ **535.6** **Duodenitis**

536 **Disorders of function of stomach**
  Excludes: functional disorders of stomach specified as psychogenic (306.4)

536.0 **Achlorhydria**

536.1 **Acute dilatation of stomach**
  Acute distention of stomach

536.2 **Persistent vomiting**
  Habit vomiting
  Persistent vomiting [not of pregnancy]
  Uncontrollable vomiting

  Excludes: excessive vomiting in pregnancy (643.0-643.9)
            vomiting NOS (787.0)

536.3 **Gastroparesis**
  Gastroparalysis

⑤ **536.4** **Gastrostomy complications**

  536.40 **Gastrostomy complications, unspecified**

  536.41 **Infection of gastrostomy**
  Use additional code to specify type of infection, such as:
            abscess or cellulitis of abdomen (682.2)
            septicemia (038.0-038.9)

  Use additional code to identify organism (041.00-041.9)

  536.42 **Mechanical complication of gastrostomy**

  536.49 **Other gastrostomy complications**

536.8 **Dyspepsia and other specified disorders of function of stomach**
  Achylia gastrica   Hyperchlorhydria
  Hourglass contraction of   Hypochlorhydria
    stomach   Indigestion
  Hyperacidity   Tachygastria

  Excludes: achlorhydria (536.0)
            heartburn (787.1)

536.9 **Unspecified functional disorder of stomach**
  Functional gastrointestinal:
    disorder
    disturbance
    irritation

537 **Other disorders of stomach and duodenum**

537.0 **Acquired hypertrophic pyloric stenosis**
  Constriction of pylorus, acquired or adult
  Obstruction of pylorus, acquired or adult
  Stricture of pylorus, acquired or adult

  Excludes: congenital or infantile pyloric stenosis (750.5)

537.1 **Gastric diverticulum**
  Excludes: congenital diverticulum of stomach (750.7)

537.2 **Chronic duodenal ileus**

537.3 **Other obstruction of duodenum**
  Cicatrix of duodenum
  Stenosis of duodenum
  Stricture of duodenum
  Volvulus of duodenum

  Excludes: congenital obstruction of duodenum (751.1)

537.4 **Fistula of stomach or duodenum**
  Gastrocolic fistula
  Gastrojejunocolic fistula

537.5 **Gastroptosis**

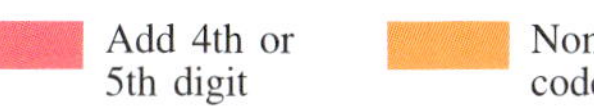

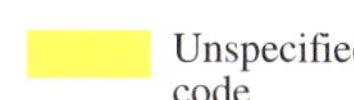

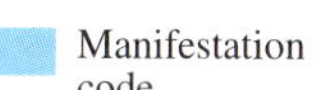

Manifestation
code

537.6 Hourglass stricture or stenosis of stomach
Cascade stomach

Excludes: *congenital hourglass stomach (750.7)*
hourglass contraction of stomach (536.8)

⑤ **537.8 Other specified disorders of stomach and duodenum**

537.81 Pylorospasm

Excludes: *congenital pylorospasm (750.5)*

537.82 Angiodysplasia of stomach and duodenum without mention of hemorrhage

537.83 Angiodysplasia of stomach and duodenum with hemorrhage

537.84 Dieulafoy lesion (hemorrhagic) of stomach and duodenum

537.89 Other
Gastric or duodenal:
prolapse
rupture
Intestinal metaplasia of gastric mucosa
Passive congestion of stomach

Excludes: *diverticula of duodenum (562.00-562.01)*
gastrointestinal hemorrhage (578.0-578.9)

537.9 Unspecified disorder of stomach and duodenum

● **538 Gastrointestinal mucositis (ulcerative)**
Use additional E code to identify adverse effects of therapy, such as:
antineoplastic and immunosuppressive drugs (E930.7, E933.1)
radiation therapy (E879.2)

Excludes: *mucositis (ulcerative) of mouth and oral soft tissue (528.00-528.09)*

APPENDICITIS (540-543)

540 Acute appendicitis

540.0 With generalized peritonitis
Appendicitis (acute):
fulminating with: perforation, peritonitis (generalized), rupture
gangrenous with: perforation, peritonitis (generalized), rupture
obstructive with: perforation, peritonitis (generalized), rupture
Cecitis (acute) with: perforation peritonitis (generalized) rupture
Rupture of appendix

Excludes: *acute appendicitis with peritoneal abscess (540.1)*

540.1 With peritoneal abscess
Abscess of appendix
With generalized peritonitis

540.9 Without mention of peritonitis
Acute:
appendicitis:
fulminating without mention of perforation, peritonitis, or rupture
gangrenous without mention of perforation, peritonitis, or rupture
inflamed without mention of perforation, peritonitis, or rupture
obstructive without mention of perforation, peritonitis, or rupture
cecitis without mention of perforation, peritonitis, or rupture

541 Appendicitis, unqualified

542 Other appendicitis
Appendicitis: Appendicitis:
chronic   relapsing
recurrent   subacute

Excludes: *hyperplasia (lymphoid) of appendix (543.0)*

543 Other diseases of appendix

543.0 Hyperplasia of appendix (lymphoid)

● Code new
to this edition

▲ Revision of
existing code

④ ⑤ Fourth or fifth
digit required

543.9 **Other and unspecified diseases of appendix**
    Appendicular or appendiceal:
      colic
      concretion
      fistula
    Diverticulum of appendix
    Fecalith of appendix
    Intussusception of appendix
    Mucocele of appendix
    Stercolith of appendix

HERNIA OF ABDOMINAL CAVITY (550-553)

    Includes: hernia:
        acquired
        congenital, except diaphragmatic or hiatal

⑤ **550** **Inguinal hernia**
    Includes: bubonocele
        inguinal hernia (direct) (double) (indirect) (oblique) (sliding)
        scrotal hernia

The following fifth-digit subclassification is for use with category 550:

    0 **unilateral or unspecified (not specified as recurrent)**
       Unilateral NOS

    1 **unilateral or unspecified, recurrent**

    2 **bilateral (not specified as recurrent)**
       Bilateral NOS

    3 **bilateral, recurrent**

⑤ **550.0** **Inguinal hernia, with gangrene**
    Inguinal hernia with gangrene (and obstruction)

⑤ **550.1** **Inguinal hernia, with obstruction, without mention of gangrene**
    Inguinal hernia with mention of incarceration, irreducibility, or strangulation

⑤ **550.9** **Inguinal hernia, without mention of obstruction or gangrene**
    Inguinal hernia NOS

551 **Other hernia of abdominal cavity, with gangrene**
    Includes: that with gangrene (and obstruction)

⑤ **551.0** **Femoral hernia with gangrene**

    551.00 **Unilateral or unspecified (not specified as recurrent)**
       Femoral hernia NOS with gangrene

    551.01 **Unilateral or unspecified, recurrent**

    551.02 **Bilateral (not specified as recurrent)**

    551.03 **Bilateral, recurrent**

  551.1 **Umbilical hernia with gangrene**
    Parumbilical hernia specified as gangrenous

⑤ **551.2** **Ventral hernia with gangrene**

    551.20 **Ventral, unspecified, with gangrene**

    551.21 **Incisional, with gangrene**
       Hernia:
         postoperative specified as gangrenous
         recurrent, ventral specified as gangrenous

    551.29 **Other**
       Epigastric hernia specified as gangrenous

  551.3 **Diaphragmatic hernia with gangrene**
    Hernia:
      hiatal (esophageal) (sliding) specified as gangrenous
      paraesophageal specified as gangrenous
    Thoracic stomach specified as gangrenous

    Excludes: *congenital diaphragmatic hernia (756.6)*

551.8 **Hernia of other specified sites, with gangrene**
    Any condition classifiable to 553.8 if specified as gangrenous

551.9 **Hernia of unspecified site, with gangrene**
    Any condition classifiable to 553.9 if specified as gangrenous

552 **Other hernia of abdominal cavity, with obstruction, but without mention of gangrene**

    Excludes: *that with mention of gangrene (551.0-551.9)*

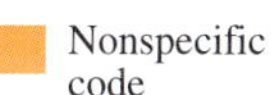
Add 4th or
5th digit

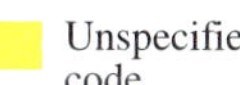
Nonspecific
code

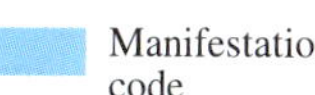
Unspecified
code

Manifestation
code

⑤ **552.0 Femoral hernia with obstruction**
Femoral hernia specified as incarcerated, irreducible, strangulated, or causing obstruction

552.00 Unilateral or unspecified (not specified as recurrent)

552.01 Unilateral or unspecified, recurrent

552.02 Bilateral (not specified as recurrent)

552.03 Bilateral, recurrent

552.1 Umbilical hernia with obstruction
Parumbilical hernia specified as incarcerated, irreducible, strangulated, or causing obstruction

⑤ **552.2 Ventral hernia with obstruction**
Ventral hernia specified as incarcerated, irreducible, strangulated, or causing obstruction

552.20 Ventral, unspecified, with obstruction

552.21 Incisional, with obstruction
Hernia:
postoperative specified as incarcerated, irreducible, strangulated, or causing obstruction
recurrent, ventral specified as incarcerated, irreducible, strangulated, or causing obstruction

552.29 Other
Epigastric hernia specified as incarcerated, irreducible, strangulated, or causing obstruction

552.3 Diaphragmatic hernia with obstruction
Hernia:
hiatal (esophageal) (sliding), specified as incarcerated, irreducible, strangulated, or causing obstruction
paraesophageal, specified as incarcerated, irreducible, strangulated, or causing obstruction
Thoracic stomach, specified as incarcerated, irreducible, strangulated, or causing obstruction

Excludes: *congenital diaphragmatic hernia (756.6)*

552.8 Hernia of other specified sites, with obstruction
Any condition classifiable to 553.8 if specified as incarcerated, irreducible, strangulated, or causing obstruction

Excludes: *hernia due to adhesion with obstruction (560.81)*

552.9 Hernia of unspecified site, with obstruction
Any condition classifiable to 553.9 if specified as incarcerated, irreducible, strangulated, or causing obstruction

553 Other hernia of abdominal cavity without mention of obstruction or gangrene

Excludes: *the listed conditions with mention of:*
gangrene (and obstruction) (551.0-551.9)
obstruction (552.0-552.9)

⑤ **553.0 Femoral hernia**

553.00 Unilateral or unspecified (not specified as recurrent)
Femoral hernia NOS

553.01 Unilateral or unspecified, recurrent

553.02 Bilateral (not specified as recurrent)

553.03 Bilateral, recurrent

553.1 Umbilical hernia
Parumbilical hernia

⑤ **553.2 Ventral hernia**

553.20 Ventral, unspecified

553.21 Incisional
Hernia:
postoperative
recurrent, ventral

553.29 Other
Hernia:
epigastric
spigelian

● Code new to this edition   ▲ Revision of existing code   ④ ⑤ Fourth or fifth digit required

553.3 Diaphragmatic hernia
Hernia:
hiatal (esophageal) (sliding)
paraesophageal
Thoracic stomach

Excludes: congenital:
diaphragmatic hernia (756.6)
hiatal hernia (750.6)
esophagocele (530.6)

553.8 Hernia of other specified sites

Hernia:
ischiatic
ischiorectal
lumbar
obturator
pudendal

Hernia:
retroperitoneal
sciatic
Other abdominal hernia of specified site

Excludes: vaginal enterocele (618.6)

553.9 Hernia of unspecified site

Enterocele
Epiplocele
Hernia:
NOS
interstitial

Hernia:
intestinal
intra-abdominal
Rupture (nontraumatic)
Sarcoepiplocele

NONINFECTIOUS ENTERITIS AND COLITIS (555-558)

555 Regional enteritis
Includes: Crohn's disease
Granulomatous enteritis

Excludes: ulcerative colitis (556)

555.0 Small intestine

Ileitis:
regional
segmental
terminal

Regional enteritis or Crohn's disease of:
duodenum
ileum
jejunum

555.1 Large intestine

Colitis:
granulomatous
regional
transmural

Regional enteritis or Crohn's disease of:
colon
large bowel
rectum

555.2 Small intestine with large intestine
Regional ileocolitis

555.9 Unspecified site
Crohn's disease NOS
Regional enteritis NOS

556 Ulcerative colitis

556.0 Ulcerative (chronic) enterocolitis

556.1 Ulcerative (chronic) ileocolitis

556.2 Ulcerative (chronic) proctitis

556.3 Ulcerative (chronic) proctosigmoiditis

556.4 Pseudopolyposis of colon

556.5 Left-sided ulcerative (chronic) colitis

556.6 Universal ulcerative (chronic) colitis
Pancolitis

556.8 Other ulcerative colitis

556.9 Ulcerative colitis, unspecified
Ulcerative enteritis NOS

557 Vascular insufficiency of intestine

Excludes: necrotizing enterocolitis of the newborn (777.5)

Add 4th or 5th digit   Nonspecific code   Unspecified code   Manifestation code

557.0 Acute vascular insufficiency of intestine
> Acute:
>> hemorrhagic enterocolitis
>> ischemic colitis, enteritis, or enterocolitis
>> massive necrosis of intestine
> Bowel infarction
> Embolism of mesenteric artery
> Fulminant enterocolitis
> Hemorrhagic necrosis of intestine
> Infarction of appendices epiploicae
> Intestinal gangrene
> Intestinal infarction (acute) (agnogenic) (hemorrhagic) (nonocclusive)
> Mesenteric infarction (embolic) (thrombotic)
> Necrosis of intestine
> Terminal hemorrhagic enteropathy
> Thrombosis of mesenteric artery

557.1 Chronic vascular insufficiency of intestine
> Angina, abdominal
> Chronic ischemic colitis, enteritis, or enterocolitis
> Ischemic stricture of intestine
> Mesenteric:
>> angina
>> artery syndrome (superior)
>> vascular insufficiency

557.9 Unspecified vascular insufficiency of intestine
> Alimentary pain due to vascular insufficiency
> Ischemic colitis, enteritis, or enterocolitis NOS

558 Other and unspecified noninfectious gastroenteritis and colitis
> Excludes: *infectious:*
>> *colitis, enteritis, or gastroenteritis (009.0-009.1)*
>> *diarrhea (009.2-009.3)*

558.1 Gastroenteritis and colitis due to radiation
> Radiation enterocolitis

558.2 Toxic gastroenteritis and colitis
Use additional E code, if desired, to identify cause

558.3 Allergic gastroenteritis and colitis
Use additional code to identify type of food allergy (V15.01-V15.05)

558.9 Other and unspecified noninfectious gastroenteritis and colitis
> Colitis NOS, dietetic, or noninfectious
> Enteritis NOS, dietetic, or noninfectious
> Gastroenteritis NOS, dietetic, or noninfectious
> Ileitis NOS, dietetic, or noninfectious
> Jejunitis NOS, dietetic, or noninfectious
> Sigmoiditis NOS, dietetic, or noninfectious

OTHER DISEASES OF INTESTINES AND PERITONEUM (560-569)

560 Intestinal obstruction without mention of hernia
> Excludes: *duodenum (537.2-537.3)*
>> *inguinal hernia with obstruction (550.1)*
>> *intestinal obstruction complicating hernia (552.0-552.9)*
>> *mesenteric:*
>>> *embolism (557.0)*
>>> *infarction (557.0)*
>>> *thrombosis (557.0)*
>> *neonatal intestinal obstruction (277.01, 777.1-777.2, 777.4)*

560.0 Intussusception
> Intussusception (colon) (intestine) (rectum)
> Invagination of intestine or colon
> Excludes: *intussusception of appendix (543.9)*

560.1 Paralytic ileus
> Adynamic ileus
> Ileus (of intestine) (of bowel) (of colon)
> Paralysis of intestine or colon
> Excludes: *gallstone ileus (560.31)*

● Code new to this edition   ▲ Revision of existing code   ④ ⑤ Fourth or fifth digit required

560.2 Volvulus
    Knotting of intestine, bowel, or colon
    Strangulation of intestine, bowel, or colon
    Torsion of intestine, bowel, or colon
    Twist of intestine, bowel, or colon

⑤ **560.3 Impaction of intestine**

    560.30 Impaction of intestine, unspecified
        Impaction of colon

    560.31 Gallstone ileus
        Obstruction of intestine by gallstone

    560.39 Other
        Concretion of intestine
        Enterolith
        Fecal impaction

⑤ **560.8 Other specified intestinal obstruction**

    560.81 Intestinal or peritoneal adhesions with obstruction (postoperative) (postinfection)

    Excludes: *adhesions without obstruction (568.0)*

    560.89 Other
        Acute pseudo-obstruction of intestine
        Mural thickening causing obstruction

    Excludes: *ischemic stricture of intestine (557.1)*

560.9 Unspecified intestinal obstruction
    Enterostenosis
    Obstruction of intestine or colon
    Occlusion of intestine or colon
    Stenosis of intestine or colon
    Stricture of intestine or colon

    Excludes: *congenital stricture or stenosis of intestine (751.1-751.2)*

562 Diverticula of intestine
Use additional code, if desired, to identify any associated:
    peritonitis (567.0-567.9)

    Excludes: *congenital diverticulum of colon (751.5)*
            diverticulum of appendix (543.9)
            Meckel's diverticulum (751.0)

⑤ **562.0 Small intestine**

    562.00 Diverticulosis of small intestine (without mention of hemorrhage)
        Diverticulosis:
           duodenum without mention of diverticulitis
           ileum without mention of diverticulitis
           jejunum without mention of diverticulitis

    562.01 Diverticulitis of small intestine (without mention of hemorrhage)
        Diverticulitis (with diverticulosis):
           duodenum
           ileum
           jejunum
           small intestine

    562.02 Diverticulosis of small intestine with hemorrhage

    562.03 Diverticulitis of small intestine with hemorrhage

⑤ **562.1 Colon**

    562.10 Diverticulosis of colon (without mention of hemorrhage)
        Diverticulosis:
           NOS without mention of diverticulitis
           intestine (large) without mention of diverticulitis
        Diverticular disease (colon) without mention of diverticulitis

    562.11 Diverticulitis of colon (without mention of hemorrhage)
        Diverticulitis (with diverticulosis):
           NOS
           colon
           intestine (large)

    562.12 Diverticulosis of colon with hemorrhage

    562.13 Diverticulitis of colon with hemorrhage

Add 4th or 5th digit	Nonspecific code	Unspecified code	Manifestation code

564 Functional digestive disorders, not elsewhere classified
Excludes: *functional disorders of stomach (536.0-536.9)*
those specified as psychogenic (306.4)

⑤ **564.0 Constipation**

564.00 Constipation, unspecified

564.01 Slow transit constipation

564.02 Outlet dysfunction constipation

564.09 Other constipation

564.1 Irritable bowel syndrome
Irritable colon   Spastic colon

564.2 Postgastric surgery syndromes
Dumping syndrome   Postgastrectomy syndrome
Jejunal syndrome   Postvagotomy syndrome

Excludes: *malnutrition following gastrointestinal surgery (579.3)*
postgastrojejunostomy ulcer (534.0-534.9)

564.3 Vomiting following gastrointestinal surgery
Vomiting (bilious) following gastrointestinal surgery

564.4 Other postoperative functional disorders
Diarrhea following gastrointestinal surgery

Excludes: *colostomy and enterostomy complications (569.60-569.69)*

564.5 Functional diarrhea
Excludes: *diarrhea:*
NOS (787.91)
psychogenic (306.4)

564.6 Anal spasm
Proctalgia fugax

564.7 Megacolon, other than Hirschsprung's
Dilatation of colon

Excludes: *megacolon:*
congenital [Hirschsprung's] (751.3)
toxic (556)

⑤ **564.8 Other specified functional disorders of intestine**
Excludes: *malabsorption (579.0-579.9)*

564.81 Neurogenic bowel

564.89 Other functional disorders of intestine
Atony of colon

564.9 Unspecified functional disorder of intestine

565 Anal fissure and fistula

565.0 Anal fissure
Tear of anus, nontraumatic

Excludes: *traumatic (863.89, 863.99)*

565.1 Anal fistula
Fistula:
anorectal
rectal
rectum to skin

Excludes: *fistula of rectum to internal organs—see Alphabetic Index*
ischiorectal fistula (566)
rectovaginal fistula (619.1)

566 Abscess of anal and rectal regions
Abscess: Cellulitis:
ischiorectal   anal
perianal   perirectal
perirectal   rectal
     Ischiorectal fistula

● Code new to this edition   ▲ Revision of existing code   ④ ⑤ Fourth or fifth digit required

567 Peritonitis and retroperitoneal infections

    | Excludes: | *peritonitis:*

benign paroxysmal (277.31)
pelvic, female (614.5, 614.7)
periodic familial (277.31)
puerperal (670)
with or following:
  abortion (634-638 with .0, 639.0)
  appendicitis (540.0-540.1)
  ectopic or molar pregnancy (639.0)

567.0 *Peritonitis in infectious diseases classified elsewhere*
    Code first underlying disease

    | Excludes: | *peritonitis:*

gonococcal (098.86)
syphilitic (095.2)
tuberculous (014.0)

567.1 Pneumococcal peritonitis

⑤ **567.2 Other suppurative peritonitis**

    567.21 Peritonitis (acute) generalized
      Pelvic peritonitis, male

    567.22 Peritoneal abscess

Abscess (of):   Abscess (of):
  abdominopelvic   retrocecal
  mesenteric   subdiaphragmatic
  omentum   subhepatic
  peritoneum   subphrenic

    567.23 Spontaneous bacterial peritonitis

    | Excludes: | *bacterial peritonitis NOS (567.29)*

    567.29 Other suppurative peritonitis
      Subphrenic peritonitis

⑤ **567.3 Retroperitoneal infections**

    567.31 Psoas muscle abscess

    567.38 Other retroperitoneal abscess

    567.39 Other retroperitoneal infections

⑤ **567.8 Other specified peritonitis**

    567.81 Choleperitonitis
      Peritonitis due to bile

    567.82 Sclerosing mesenteritis
      Fat necrosis of peritoneum
      (Idiopathic) sclerosing mesenteric fibrosis
      Mesenteric lipodystrophy
      Mesenteric panniculitis
      Retractile mesenteritis

    567.89 Other specified peritonitis
      Chronic proliferative peritonitis
      Mesenteric saponification
      Peritonitis due to urine

567.9 Unspecified peritonitis
    Peritonitis:
      NOS
      of unspecified cause

568 Other disorders of peritoneum

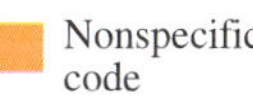

| | Add 4th or 5th digit | | Nonspecific code | | Unspecified code | | Manifestation code |

568.0 Peritoneal adhesions (postoperative) (postinfection)

Adhesions (of):
  abdominal (wall)
  diaphragm
  intestine
  male pelvis

Adhesions (of):
  mesenteric
  omentum
  stomach
Adhesive bands

Excludes: *adhesions:*

  pelvic, female (614.6)
  with obstruction:
    duodenum (537.3)
    intestine (560.81)

⑤ **568.8 Other specified disorders of peritoneum**

  568.81 Hemoperitoneum (nontraumatic)

  568.82 Peritoneal effusion (chronic)

Excludes: *ascites NOS (789.5)*

  568.89 Other

    Peritoneal:
      cyst
      granuloma

568.9 Unspecified disorder of peritoneum

569 Other disorders of intestine

569.0 Anal and rectal polyp

  Anal and rectal polyp NOS

Excludes: *adenomatous anal and rectal polyp (211.4)*

569.1 Rectal prolapse

Procidentia:
  anus (sphincter)
  rectum (sphincter)
Proctoptosis

Prolapse:
  anal canal
  rectal mucosa

Excludes: *prolapsed hemorrhoids (455.2, 455.5)*

569.2 Stenosis of rectum and anus

  Stricture of anus (sphincter)

569.3 Hemorrhage of rectum and anus

Excludes: *gastrointestinal bleeding NOS (578.9)*

    melena (578.1)

⑤ **569.4 Other specified disorders of rectum and anus**

  569.41 Ulcer of anus and rectum

    Solitary ulcer of anus (sphincter) or rectum (sphincter)
    Stercoral ulcer of anus (sphincter) or rectum (sphincter)

  569.42 Anal or rectal pain

  569.49 Other

    Granuloma of rectum (sphincter)
    Rupture of rectum (sphincter)
    Hypertrophy of anal papillae
    Proctitis NOS

Excludes: *fistula of rectum to:*

  internal organs—see Alphabetic Index
  skin (565.1)
hemorrhoids (455.0-455.9)
incontinence of sphincter ani (787.6)

569.5 Abscess of intestine

Excludes: *appendiceal abscess (540.1)*

⑤ **569.6 Colostomy and enterostomy complications**

  569.60 Colostomy and enterostomy complication, unspecified

  569.61 Infection of colostomy or enterostomy

Use additional code to specify type of infection, such as:
    abscess or cellulitis of abdomen (682.2)
    septicemia (038.0-038.9)

Use additional code to identify organism (041.00-041.9)

● Code new to this edition   ▲ Revision of existing code   ④ ⑤ Fourth or fifth digit required

569.62 Mechanical complication of colostomy and enterostomy
Malfunction of colostomy and enterostomy

569.69 Other complication
Fistula
Hernia
Prolapse

⑤ **569.8 Other specified disorders of intestine**

569.81 Fistula of intestine, excluding rectum and anus
Fistula: Fistula:
  abdominal wall   enteroenteric
  enterocolic   ileorectal

Excludes: fistula of intestine to internal organs —see Alphabetic Index
persistent postoperative fistula (998.6)

569.82 Ulceration of intestine
Primary ulcer of intestine
Ulceration of colon

Excludes: that with perforation (569.83)

569.83 Perforation of intestine

569.84 Angiodysplasia of intestine (without mention of hemorrhage)

569.85 Angiodysplasia of intestine with hemorrhage

569.86 Dieulafoy lesion (hemorrhagic) of intestine

569.89 Other
Enteroptosis
Granuloma of intestine
Prolapse of intestine
Pericolitis
Perisigmoiditis
Visceroptosis

Excludes: gangrene of intestine, mesentery, or omentum (557.0)
hemorrhage of intestine NOS (578.9)
obstruction of intestine (560.0-560.9)

569.9 Unspecified disorder of intestine

OTHER DISEASES OF DIGESTIVE SYSTEM (570-579)

570 Acute and subacute necrosis of liver
Acute hepatic failure
Acute or subacute hepatitis, not specified as infective
Necrosis of liver (acute) (diffuse) (massive) (subacute)
Parenchymatous degeneration of liver
Yellow atrophy (liver) (acute) (subacute)

Excludes: icterus gravis of newborn (773.0-773.2)
serum hepatitis (070.2-070.3)
that with:
  abortion (634-638 with .7, 639.8)
  ectopic or molar pregnancy (639.8)
  pregnancy, childbirth, or the puerperium (646.7)
viral hepatitis (070.0-070.9)

571 Chronic liver disease and cirrhosis

571.0 Alcoholic fatty liver

571.1 Acute alcoholic hepatitis
Acute alcoholic liver disease

571.2 Alcoholic cirrhosis of liver
Florid cirrhosis
Laennec's cirrhosis (alcoholic)

571.3 Alcoholic liver damage, unspecified

⑤ **571.4 Chronic hepatitis**

Excludes: viral hepatitis (acute) (chronic) (070.0-070.9)

571.40 Chronic hepatitis, unspecified

571.41 Chronic persistent hepatitis

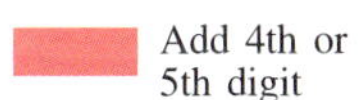

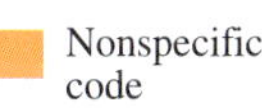

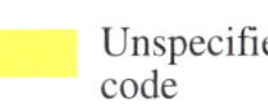

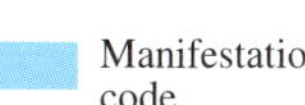

571.49 Other
Chronic hepatitis:
  active
  aggressive
Recurrent hepatitis

571.5 Cirrhosis of liver without mention of alcohol

Cirrhosis of liver:
  NOS
  cryptogenic
  macronodular
  micronodular

Cirrhosis of liver:
  posthepatitic
  postnecrotic
  Healed yellow atrophy (liver)
  Portal cirrhosis

571.6 Biliary cirrhosis
Chronic nonsuppurative destructive cholangitis
Cirrhosis:
  cholangitic
  cholestatic

571.8 Other chronic nonalcoholic liver disease
Chronic yellow atrophy (liver)
Fatty liver, without mention of alcohol

571.9 Unspecified chronic liver disease without mention of alcohol

572 Liver abscess and sequelae of chronic liver disease

572.0 Abscess of liver

Excludes: amebic liver abscess (006.3)

572.1 Portal pyemia
Phlebitis of portal vein   Pylephlebitis
Portal thrombophlebitis   Pylethrombophlebitis

572.2 Hepatic coma
Hepatic encephalopathy
Hepatocerebral intoxication
Portal-systemic encephalopathy

572.3 Portal hypertension

572.4 Hepatorenal syndrome

Excludes: that following delivery (674.8)

572.8 Other sequelae of chronic liver disease

573 Other disorders of liver

Excludes: amyloid or lardaceous degeneration of liver (277.39)
  congenital cystic disease of liver (751.62)
  glycogen infiltration of liver (271.0)
  hepatomegaly NOS (789.1)
  portal vein obstruction (452)

573.0 Chronic passive congestion of liver

573.1 Hepatitis in viral diseases classified elsewhere
Code first underlying disease as:
  Coxsackie virus disease (074.8)
  cytomegalic inclusion virus disease (078.5)
  infectious mononucleosis (075)

Excludes: hepatitis (in):
  mumps (072.71)
  viral (070.0-070.9)
  yellow fever (060.0-060.9)

573.2 Hepatitis in other infectious diseases classified elsewhere
Code first underlying disease, as:
  malaria (084.9)

Excludes: hepatitis in:
  late syphilis (095.3)
  secondary syphilis (091.62)
  toxoplasmosis (130.5)

573.3 Hepatitis, unspecified
Toxic (noninfectious) hepatitis
Use additional E code, if desired, to identify cause

573.4 Hepatic infarction

● Code new
  to this edition   ▲ Revision of
  existing code   ④ ⑤ Fourth or fifth
  digit required

573.8 **Other specified disorders of liver**
Hepatoptosis

573.9 **Unspecified disorder of liver**

574 **Cholelithiasis**

The following fifth-digit subclassification is for use with category 574:

0 **without mention of obstruction**

1 **with obstruction**

574.0 **Calculus of gallbladder with acute cholecystitis**
Biliary calculus with acute cholecystitis
Calculus of cystic duct with acute cholecystitis
Cholelithiasis with acute cholecystitis
Any condition classifiable to 574.2 with acute cholecystitis

574.1 **Calculus of gallbladder with other cholecystitis**
Biliary calculus with cholecystitis
Calculus of cystic duct with cholecystitis
Cholelithiasis with cholecystitis
Cholecystitis with cholelithiasis NOS
Any condition classifiable to 574.2 with cholecystitis (chronic)

574.2 **Calculus of gallbladder without mention of cholecystitis**

Biliary:	Cholelithiasis NOS
calculus NOS	Colic (recurrent) of gallbladder
colic NOS	Gallstone (impacted)
Calculus of cystic duct	

574.3 **Calculus of bile duct with acute cholecystitis**
Calculus of bile duct [any] with acute cholecystitis
Choledocholithiasis with acute cholecystitis
Any condition classifiable to 574.5 with acute cholecystitis

574.4 **Calculus of bile duct with other cholecystitis**
Calculus of bile duct [any] with cholecystitis (chronic)
Choledocholithiasis with cholecystitis (chronic)
Any condition classifiable to 574.5 with cholecystitis (chronic)

574.5 **Calculus of bile duct without mention of cholecystitis**

Calculus of:	Choledocholithiasis
bile duct [any]	Hepatic:
common duct	colic (recurrent)
hepatic duct	lithiasis

574.6 **Calculus of gallbladder and bile duct with acute cholecystitis**
Any condition classifiable to 574.0 and 574.3

574.7 **Calculus of gallbladder and bile duct with other cholecystitis**
Any condition classifiable to 574.1 and 574.4

574.8 **Calculus of gallbladder and bile duct with acute and chronic cholecystitis**
Any condition classifiable to 574.6 and 574.7

574.9 **Calculus of gallbladder and bile duct without cholecystitis**
Any condition classifiable to 574.2 and 574.5

575 **Other disorders of gallbladder**

575.0 **Acute cholecystitis**
Abscess of gallbladder without mention of calculus
Angiocholecystitis without mention of calculus
Cholecystitis without mention of calculus:
emphysematous (acute)
gangrenous
suppurative
Empyema of gallbladder without mention of calculus
Gangrene of gallbladder without mention of calculus

Excludes: *that with:*
acute and chronic cholecystitis (575.12)
choledocholithiasis (574.3)
choledocholithiasis and cholelithiasis (574.6)
cholelithiasis (574.0)

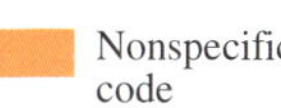

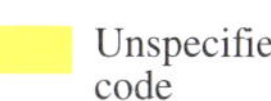

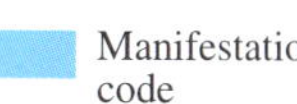

Manifestation
code

⑤ **575.1 Other cholecystitis**
Cholecystitis:
  NOS without mention of calculus
  chronic without mention of calculus

Excludes: *that with:*
    choledocholithiasis (574.4)
    choledocholithiasis and cholelithiasis (574.8)
    cholelithiasis (574.1)

575.10 Cholecystitis, unspecified
Cholecystitis NOS

575.11 Chronic cholecystitis

575.12 Acute and chronic cholecystits

575.2 Obstruction of gallbladder
Occlusion of cystic duct or gallbladder without mention of calculus
Stenosis of cystic duct or gallbladder without mention of calculus
Stricture of cystic duct or gallbladder without mention of calculus

Excludes: *that with calculus (574.0-574.2 with fifth-digit 1)*

575.3 Hydrops of gallbladder
Mucocele of gallbladder

575.4 Perforation of gallbladder
Rupture of cystic duct or gallbladder

575.5 Fistula of gallbladder
Fistula:
  cholecystoduodenal
  cholecystoenteric

575.6 Cholesterolosis of gallbladder
Strawberry gallbladder

575.8 Other specified disorders of gallbladder
Adhesions (of) cystic duct or gallbladder
Atrophy (of) cystic duct or gallbladder
Cyst (of) cystic duct or gallbladder
Hypertrophy (of) cystic duct or gallbladder
Nonfunctioning (of) cystic duct or gallbladder
Ulcer (of) cystic duct or gallbladder
Biliary dyskinesia

Excludes: *nonvisualization of gallbladder (793.3)*
    Hartmann's pouch of intestine (V44.3)

575.9 Unspecified disorder of gallbladder

576 Other disorders of biliary tract
Excludes: *that involving the:*
    cystic duct (575.0-575.9)
    gallbladder (575.0-575.9)

576.0 Postcholecystectomy syndrome

576.1 Cholangitis
Cholangitis: Cholangitis:
  NOS   recurrent
  acute   sclerosing
  ascending   secondary
  chronic   stenosing
  primary   suppurative

576.2 Obstruction of bile duct
Occlusion of bile duct, except cystic duct, without mention of calculus
Stenosis of bile duct, except cystic duct, without mention of calculus
Stricture of bile duct, except cystic duct, without mention of calculus

Excludes: *congenital (751.61)*
    that with calculus (574.3-574.5 with fifth-digit 1)

576.3 Perforation of bile duct
Rupture of bile duct, except cystic duct

576.4 Fistula of bile duct
Choledochoduodenal fistula

576.5 Spasm of sphincter of Oddi

● Code new   ▲ Revision of   ④ ⑤ Fourth or fifth
  to this edition   existing code   digit required

576.8 Other specified disorders of biliary tract
Adhesions of bile duct [any]
Atrophy of bile duct [any]
Cyst of bile duct [any]
Hypertrophy of bile duct [any]
Stasis of bile duct [any]
Ulcer of bile duct [any]

Excludes: *congenital choledochal cyst (751.69)*

576.9 Unspecified disorder of biliary tract

577 Diseases of pancreas

577.0 Acute pancreatitis
Abscess of pancreas
Necrosis of pancreas:
  acute
  infective
Pancreatitis:
  NOS
  acute (recurrent)
  apoplectic
  hemorrhagic
  subacute
  suppurative

Excludes: *mumps pancreatitis (072.3)*

577.1 Chronic pancreatitis
Chronic pancreatitis:
  NOS
  infectious
  interstitial
Pancreatitis:
  painless
  recurrent
  relapsing

577.2 Cyst and pseudocyst of pancreas

577.8 Other specified diseases of pancreas
Atrophy of pancreas
Calculus of pancreas
Cirrhosis of pancreas
Fibrosis of pancreas
Pancreatic:
  infantilism
  necrosis:
    NOS
    aseptic
    fat
Pancreatolithiasis

Excludes: *fibrocystic disease of pancreas (277.00-277.09)*
islet cell tumor of pancreas (211.7)
pancreatic steatorrhea (579.4)

577.9 Unspecified disease of pancreas

578 Gastrointestinal hemorrhage
Excludes: *that with mention of:*
angiodysplasia of stomach and duodenum (537.83)
angiodysplasia of intestine (569.85)
diverticulitis, intestine:
  large (562.13)
  small (562.03)
diverticulosis, intestine:
  large (562.12)
  small (562.02)
gastritis and duodenitis (535.0-535.6)
ulcer:
  duodenal (532.0-532.9)
  gastric (531.0-531.9)
  gastrojejunal (534.0-534.9)
  peptic (533.0-533.9)

578.0 Hematemesis
Vomiting of blood

578.1 Blood in stool
Melena

Excludes: *occult blood (792.1)*

578.9 Hemorrhage of gastrointestinal tract, unspecified
Gastric hemorrhage
Intestinal hemorrhage

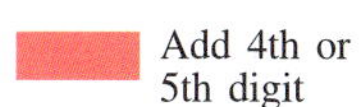
Add 4th or
5th digit

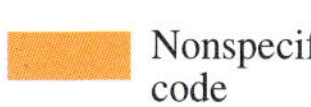
Nonspecific
code

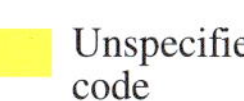
Unspecified
code

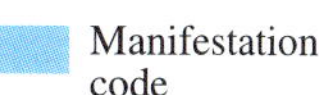
Manifestation
code

579 Intestinal malabsorption

  579.0 Celiac disease

Celiac:	Gee (-Herter) disease
crisis	Gluten enteropathy
infantilism	Idiopathic steatorrhea
rickets	Nontropical sprue

  579.1 Tropical sprue

Sprue:	Tropical steatorrhea
NOS	
tropical	

  579.2 Blind loop syndrome

    Postoperative blind loop syndrome

  579.3 Other and unspecified postsurgical nonabsorption

    Hypoglycemia following gastrointestinal surgery
    Malnutrition following gastrointestinal surgery

  579.4 Pancreatic steatorrhea

  579.8 Other specified intestinal malabsorption

Enteropathy:	Steatorrhea (chronic)
exudative	
protein-losing	

  579.9 Unspecified intestinal malabsorption

    Malabsorption syndrome NOS

● Code new
to this edition

▲ Revision of
existing code

④ ⑤ Fourth or fifth
digit required

10.   DISEASES OF THE GENITOURINARY SYSTEM (580-629)

NEPHRITIS, NEPHROTIC SYNDROME, AND NEPHROSIS (580-589)

Excludes: *hypertensive chronic kidney disease (403.00-403.91, 404.00-404.93)*

580   Acute glomerulonephritis
Includes: acute nephritis

580.0   With lesion of proliferative glomerulonephritis
Acute (diffuse) proliferative glomerulonephritis
Acute poststreptococcal glomerulonephritis

580.4   With lesion of rapidly progressive glomerulonephritis
Acute nephritis with lesion of necrotizing glomerulitis

⑤ **580.8   With other specified pathological lesion in kidney**

580.81   Acute glomerulonephritis in diseases classified elsewhere
Code first underlying disease, as:
infectious hepatitis (070.0-070.9)
mumps (072.79)
subacute bacterial endocarditis (421.0)
typhoid fever (002.0)

580.89   Other
Glomerulonephritis, acute, with lesion of:
exudative nephritis
interstitial (diffuse) (focal) nephritis

580.9   Acute glomerulonephritis with unspecified pathological lesion in kidney
Glomerulonephritis:
NOS specified as acute
hemorrhagic specified as acute
Nephritis specified as acute
Nephropathy specified as acute

581   Nephrotic syndrome

581.0   With lesion of proliferative glomerulonephritis

581.1   With lesion of membranous glomerulonephritis
Epimembranous nephritis
Idiopathic membranous glomerular disease
Nephrotic syndrome with lesion of:
focal glomerulosclerosis
sclerosing membranous glomerulonephritis
segmental hyalinosis

581.2   With lesion of membranoproliferative glomerulonephritis
Nephrotic syndrome with lesion (of):
endothelial glomerulonephritis
hypocomplementemic persistent glomerulonephritis
lobular glomerulonephritis
mesangiocapillary glomerulonephritis
mixed membranous and proliferative glomerulonephritis

581.3   With lesion of minimal change glomerulonephritis
Foot process disease   Minimal change:
Lipoid nephrosis   glomerular disease
                                                        glomerulitis
                                                        nephrotic syndrome

⑤ **581.8   With other specified pathological lesion in kidney**

581.81   Nephrotic syndrome in diseases classified elsewhere
Code first underlying disease, as:
amyloidosis (277.30-277.39)
diabetes mellitus (250.4)
malaria (084.9)
polyarteritis (446.0)
systemic lupus erythematosus (710.0)

Excludes: *nephrosis in epidemic hemorrhagic fever (078.6)*

581.89   Other
Glomerulonephritis with edema and lesion of:
exudative nephritis
interstitial (diffuse) (focal) nephritis

| Add 4th or 5th digit | Nonspecific code | Unspecified code | Manifestation code |

581.9 Nephrotic syndrome with unspecified pathological lesion in kidney
Glomerulonephritis with edema NOS
Nephritis:
 nephrotic NOS
 with edema NOS
Nephrosis NOS
Renal disease with edema NOS

582 Chronic glomerulonephritis
Includes: chronic nephritis

582.0 With lesion of proliferative glomerulonephritis
Chronic (diffuse) proliferative glomerulonephritis

582.1 With lesion of membranous glomerulonephritis
Chronic glomerulonephritis:
 membranous
 sclerosing
Focal glomerulosclerosis
Segmental hyalinosis

582.2 With lesion of membranoproliferative glomerulonephritis
Chronic glomerulonephritis:
 endothelial
 hypocomplementemic persistent
 lobular
 membranoproliferative
 mesangiocapillary
 mixed membranous and proliferative

582.4 With lesion of rapidly progressive glomerulonephritis
Chronic nephritis with lesion of necrotizing glomerulitis

⑤ **582.8 With other specified pathological lesion in kidney**

  582.81 *Chronic glomerulonephritis in diseases classified elsewhere*
  Code first underlying disease, as:
   amyloidosis (277.30-277.39)
   systemic lupus erythematosus (710.0)

  582.89 Other
  Chronic glomerulonephritis with lesion of:
   exudative nephritis
   interstitial (diffuse) (focal) nephritis

582.9 Chronic glomerulonephritis with unspecified pathological lesion in kidney
Glomerulonephritis:
 NOS specified as chronic
 hemorrhagic specified as chronic
Nephritis specified as chronic
Nephropathy specified as chronic

583 Nephritis and nephropathy, not specified as acute or chronic
Includes: "renal disease" so stated, not specified as acute or chronic but with stated
 pathology or cause

583.0 With lesion of proliferative glomerulonephritis
Proliferative:
 glomerulonephritis (diffuse) NOS
 nephritis NOS
 nephropathy NOS

583.1 With lesion of membranous glomerulonephritis
Membranous: Membranous nephropathy NOS
 glomerulonephritis NOS
 nephritis NOS

583.2 With lesion of membranoproliferative glomerulonephritis
Membranoproliferative:
 glomerulonephritis NOS
 nephritis NOS
 nephropathy NOS
Nephritis NOS, with lesion of:
 hypocomplementemic persistent glomerulonephritis
 lobular glomerulonephritis
 mesangiocapillary glomerulonephritis
 mixed membranous and proliferative glomerulonephritis

● Code new   ▲ Revision of   ④ ⑤ Fourth or fifth
  to this edition   existing code   digit required

583.4 **With lesion of rapidly progressive glomerulonephritis**
Necrotizing or rapidly progressive:
glomerulitis NOS
glomerulonephritis NOS
nephritis NOS
nephropathy NOS
Nephritis, unspecified, with lesion of necrotizing glomerulitis

583.6 **With lesion of renal cortical necrosis**
Nephritis NOS with (renal) cortical necrosis
Nephropathy NOS with (renal) cortical necrosis
Renal cortical necrosis NOS

583.7 **With lesion of renal medullary necrosis**
Nephritis NOS with (renal) medullary [papillary] necrosis
Nephropathy NOS with (renal) medullary [papillary] necrosis

⑤ **583.8** **With other specified pathological lesion in kidney**

583.81 *Nephritis and nephropathy, not specified as acute or chronic, in diseases classified elsewhere*
Code first underlying disease, as:
amyloidosis (277.30-277.39)
diabetes mellitus (250.4)
gonococcal infection (098.19)
Goodpasture's syndrome (446.21)
systemic lupus erythematosus (710.0)
tuberculosis (016.0)

Excludes: *gouty nephropathy (274.10)*
syphilitic nephritis (095.4)

583.89 **Other**
Glomerulitis with lesion of:
exudative nephritis
interstitial nephritis
Glomerulonephritis with lesion of:
exudative nephritis
interstitial nephritis
Nephritis with lesion of:
exudative nephritis
interstitial nephritis
Nephropathy with lesion of:
exudative nephritis
interstitial nephritis
Renal disease with lesion of:
exudative nephritis
interstitial nephritis

583.9 **With unspecified pathological lesion in kidney**
Glomerulitis NOS
Glomerulonephritis NOS
Nephritis NOS
Nephropathy NOS

Excludes: *nephropathy complicating pregnancy, labor, or the puerperium (642.0-642.9, 646.2)*
renal disease NOS with no stated cause (593.9)

584 **Acute renal failure**

Excludes: *following labor and delivery (669.3)*
posttraumatic (958.5)
that complicating:
abortion (634-638 with .3, 639.3)
ectopic or molar pregnancy (639.3)

584.5 **With lesion of tubular necrosis**
Lower nephron nephrosis
Renal failure with (acute) tubular necrosis
Tubular necrosis:
NOS
acute

584.6 **With lesion of renal cortical necrosis**

584.7 **With lesion of renal medullary [papillary] necrosis**
Necrotizing renal papillitis

584.8 **With other specified pathological lesion in kidney**

584.9 **Acute renal failure, unspecified**

Add 4th or 5th digit	Nonspecific code	Unspecified code	Manifestation code

585 Chronic kidney disease (CKD)
Code first hypertensive chronic kidney disease, if applicable, (403.00-403.91, 404.00-404.94)
Use additional code to identify kidney transplant status, if applicable (V42.0)

585.1 Chronic kidney disease, Stage I

585.2 Chronic kidney disease, Stage II (mild)

585.3 Chronic kidney disease, Stage III (moderate)

585.4 Chronic kidney disease, Stage IV (severe)

585.5 Chronic kidney disease, Stage V
Excludes: chronic kidney disease, stage V requiring chronic dialysis (585.6)

585.6 End stage renal disease
Chronic kidney disease requiring chronic dialysis

585.9 Chronic kidney disease, unspecified
Chronic renal disease
Chronic renal failure NOS
Chronic renal insufficiency

586 Renal failure, unspecified
Uremia NOS
Excludes: following labor and delivery (669.3)
posttraumatic renal failure (958.5)
that complicating:
abortion (634-638 with .3, 639.3)
ectopic or molar pregnancy (639.3)
uremia:
extrarenal (788.9)
prerenal (788.9)
with any condition classifiable to 401 (403.0-403.9 with fifth-digit 1)

587 Renal sclerosis, unspecified
Atrophy of kidney
Contracted kidney
Renal:
cirrhosis
fibrosis

Excludes: nephrosclerosis (arteriolar) (arteriosclerotic) (403.00-403.92)
with hypertension (403.00-403.92)

588 Disorders resulting from impaired renal function

588.0 Renal osteodystrophy
Azotemic osteodystrophy
Phosphate-losing tubular
disorders
Renal:
dwarfism
infantilism
rickets

588.1 Nephrogenic diabetes insipidus
Excludes: diabetes insipidus NOS (253.5)

⑤ **588.8 Other specified disorders resulting from impaired renal function**
Excludes: secondary hypertension (405.0-405.9)

588.81 Secondary hyperparathyroidism (of renal origin)
Secondary hyperparathyroidism NOS

588.89 Other specified disorders resulting from impaired renal function
Hypokalemic nephropathy

588.9 Unspecified disorder resulting from impaired renal function

589 Small kidney of unknown cause

589.0 Unilateral small kidney

589.1 Bilateral small kidneys

589.9 Small kidney, unspecified

OTHER DISEASES OF URINARY SYSTEM (590-599)

590 Infections of kidney
Use additional code, if desired, to identify organism, such as Escherichia coli [E. coli] (041.4)

⑤ **590.0 Chronic pyelonephritis**
Chronic pyelitis
Chronic pyonephrosis

Code, if applicable, any causal condition first

590.00 Without lesion of renal medullary necrosis

● Code new
to this edition

▲ Revision of
existing code

④ ⑤ Fourth or fifth
digit required

590.01   With lesion of renal medullary necrosis

⑤ **590.1   Acute pyelonephritis**
Acute pyelitis
Acute pyonephrosis

590.10   Without lesion of renal medullary necrosis

590.11   With lesion of renal medullary necrosis

590.2   Renal and perinephric abscess
Abscess: Carbuncle of kidney
  kidney
  nephritic
  perirenal

590.3   Pyeloureteritis cystica
Infection of renal pelvis and ureter
Ureteritis cystica

⑤ **590.8   Other pyelonephritis or pyonephrosis, not specified as acute or chronic**

590.80   Pyelonephritis, unspecified
Pyelitis NOS
Pyelonephritis NOS

590.81   *Pyelitis or pyelonephritis in diseases classified elsewhere*
Code first underlying disease, as:
tuberculosis (016.0)

590.9   Infection of kidney, unspecified

Excludes: *urinary tract infection NOS (599.0)*

591   Hydronephrosis
Hydrocalycosis   Hydroureteronephrosis
Hydronephrosis

Excludes: *congenital hydronephrosis (753.29)*
hydroureter (593.5)

592   Calculus of kidney and ureter

Excludes: *nephrocalcinosis (275.4)*

592.0   Calculus of kidney
Nephrolithiasis NOS   Staghorn calculus
Renal calculus or stone   Stone in kidney

Excludes: *uric acid nephrolithiasis (274.11)*

592.1   Calculus of ureter
Ureteric stone
Ureterolithiasis

592.9   Urinary calculus, unspecified

593   Other disorders of kidney and ureter

593.0   Nephroptosis
Floating kidney
Mobile kidney

593.1   Hypertrophy of kidney

593.2   Cyst of kidney, acquired
Cyst (multiple) (solitary) of kidney, not congenital
Peripelvic (lymphatic) cyst

Excludes: *calyceal or pyelogenic cyst of kidney (591)*
congenital cyst of kidney (753.1)
polycystic (disease of) kidney (753.1)

593.3   Stricture or kinking of ureter
Angulation of ureter (postoperative)
Constriction of ureter (postoperative)
Stricture of pelviureteric junction

593.4   Other ureteric obstruction
Idiopathic retroperitoneal fibrosis
Occlusion NOS of ureter

Excludes: *that due to calculus (592.1)*

593.5   Hydroureter

Excludes: *congenital hydroureter (753.22)*
hydroureteronephrosis (591)

<table>
<tr><td>Add 4th or 5th digit</td><td>Nonspecific code</td><td>Unspecified code</td><td>Manifestation code</td></tr>
</table>

593.6 Postural proteinuria
Benign postural proteinuria
Orthostatic proteinuria

Excludes: *proteinuria NOS (791.0)*

⑤ **593.7 Vesicoureteral reflux**

593.70 Unspecified or without reflux nephropathy

593.71 With reflux nephropathy, unilateral

593.72 With reflux nephropathy, bilateral

593.73 With reflux nephropathy NOS

⑤ **593.8 Other specified disorders of kidney and ureter**

593.81 Vascular disorders of kidney
Renal (artery):   Renal infarction
  embolism
  hemorrhage
  thrombosis

593.82 Ureteral fistula
Intestinoureteral fistula

Excludes: *fistula between ureter and female genital tract (619.0)*

593.89 Other
Adhesions, kidney or ureter
Periureteritis
Polyp of ureter
Pyelectasia
Ureterocele

Excludes: *tuberculosis of ureter (016.2)*
ureteritis cystica (590.3)

593.9 Unspecified disorder of kidney and ureter
Acute renal disease
Acute renal insufficiency
Renal disease NOS
Salt-losing nephritis or syndrome

Excludes: *chronic renal insufficiency (585.9)*
cystic kidney disease (753.1)
nephropathy, so stated (583.0-583.9)
renal disease:
  arising in pregnancy or the puerperium (642.1-642.2, 642.4-642.7, 646.2)
  not specified as acute or chronic, but with stated pathology or cause (583.0-583.9)

594 Calculus of lower urinary tract

594.0 Calculus in diverticulum of bladder

594.1 Other calculus in bladder
Urinary bladder stone

Excludes: *staghorn calculus (592.0)*

594.2 Calculus in urethra

594.8 Other lower urinary tract calculus

594.9 Calculus of lower urinary tract, unspecified

Excludes: *calculus of urinary tract NOS (592.9)*

595 Cystitis

Excludes: *prostatocystitis (601.3)*
Use additional code, if desired, to identify organism, such as Escherichia coli [E. coli] (041.4)

595.0 Acute cystitis

Excludes: *trigonitis (595.3)*

595.1 Chronic interstitial cystitis
Hunner's ulcer   Submucous cystitis
Panmural fibrosis of bladder

595.2 Other chronic cystitis
Chronic cystitis NOS
Subacute cystitis

Excludes: *trigonitis (595.3)*

● Code new   ▲ Revision of   ④ ⑤ Fourth or fifth
   to this edition   existing code   digit required

595.3 Trigonitis
Follicular cystitis
Trigonitis (acute) (chronic)
Urethrotrigonitis

595.4 *Cystitis in diseases classified elsewhere*
Code first underlying disease, as:
actinomycosis (039.8)
amebiasis (006.8)
bilharziasis (120.0-120.9)
Echinococcus infestation (122.3, 122.6)

Excludes: cystitis:

diphtheritic (032.84)
gonococcal (098.11, 098.31)
monilial (112.2)
trichomonal (131.09)
tuberculous (016.1)

⑤ **595.8 Other specified types of cystitis**

595.81 Cystitis cystica

595.82 Irradiation cystitis
Use additional E code, if desired, to identify cause

595.89 Other
Abscess of bladder
Cystitis:
bullous
emphysematous
glandularis

595.9 Cystitis, unspecified

596 Other disorders of bladder
Use additional code, if desired, to identify urinary incontinence (625.6, 788.30-788.39)

596.0 Bladder neck obstruction
Contracture (acquired) of bladder neck or vesicourethral orifice
Obstruction (acquired) of bladder neck or vesicourethral orifice
Stenosis (acquired) of bladder neck or vesicourethral orifice

Excludes: congenital (753.6)

596.1 Intestinovesical fistula
Fistula:　　　　　　　　　Fistula:
enterovesical　　　　　　vesicoenteric
vesicocolic　　　　　　　vesicorectal

596.2 Vesical fistula, not elsewhere classified
Fistula:　　　　　　　　　Fistula:
bladder NOS　　　　　　vesicocutaneous
urethrovesical　　　　　vesicoperineal

Excludes: fistula between bladder and female genital tract (619.0)

596.3 Diverticulum of bladder
Diverticulitis of bladder
Diverticulum (acquired) (false) of bladder

Excludes: that with calculus in diverticulum of bladder (594.0)

596.4 Atony of bladder
High compliance bladder, of bladder
Hypotonicity of bladder
Inertia of bladder

Excludes: neurogenic bladder (596.54)

⑤ **596.5 Other functional disorders of bladder**

Excludes: cauda equina syndrome
with neurogenic bladder (344.61)

596.51 Hypertonicity of bladder
Hyperactivity
Overactive bladder

596.52 Low bladder compliance

596.53 Paralysis of bladder

596.54 Neurogenic bladder NOS

Add 4th or 5th digit	Nonspecific code	Unspecified code	Manifestation code

596.55   Detrusor sphincter dyssynergia

596.59   Other functional disorder of bladder
Detrusor instability

596.6   Rupture of bladder, nontraumatic

596.7   Hemorrhage into bladder wall
Hyperemia of bladder

Excludes: *acute hemorrhagic cystitis (595.0)*

596.8   Other specified disorders of bladder

Bladder:	Bladder:
calcified	hemorrhage
contracted	hypertrophy

Excludes: *cystocele, female (618.01-618.02, 618.09, 618.2-618.4)*
hernia or prolapse of bladder, female (618.01-618.02, 618.09, 618.2-618.4)

596.9   Unspecified disorder of bladder

597   Urethritis, not sexually transmitted, and urethral syndrome

Excludes: *nonspecific urethritis, so stated (099.4)*

597.0   Urethral abscess

Abscess of:	Abscess:
bulbourethral gland	periurethral
Cowper's gland	urethral (gland)
Littré's gland	Periurethral cellulitis

Excludes: *urethral caruncle (599.3)*

⑤ **597.8   Other urethritis**

597.80   Urethritis, unspecified

597.81   Urethral syndrome NOS

597.89   Other

Adenitis, Skene's	Meatitis, urethral
glands	Ulcer, urethra (meatus)
Cowperitis	Verumontanitis

Excludes: *trichomonal (131.02)*

598   Urethral stricture
Includes: pinhole meatus
stricture of urinary meatus

Excludes: *congenital stricture of urethra and urinary meatus (753.6)*
Use additional code to identify urinary incontinence (625.6, 788.30-788.39)

⑤ **598.0   Urethral stricture due to infection**

598.00   Due to unspecified infection

598.01   *Due to infective diseases classified elsewhere*
Code first underlying disease, as:
gonococcal infection (098.2)
schistosomiasis (120.0-120.9)
syphilis (095.8)

598.1   Traumatic urethral stricture
Stricture of urethra:
late effect of injury
postobstetric

Excludes: *postoperative following surgery on genitourinary tract (598.2)*

598.2   Postoperative urethral stricture
Postcatheterization stricture of urethra

598.8   Other specified causes of urethral stricture

598.9   Urethral stricture, unspecified

599   Other disorders of urethra and urinary tract

599.0   Urinary tract infection, site not specified
Pyuria

Excludes: *candidiasis of urinary tract (112.2)*
urinary tract infection of newborn (771.82)

Use additional code to identify organism, such as Escherichia coli [E. coli] (041.4)

   ● Code new
to this edition   ▲ Revision of
existing code   ④ ⑤ Fourth or fifth
digit required

599.1 Urethral fistula
Fistula:
urethroperineal
urethrorectal

Urinary fistula NOS

Excludes: *fistula:*
urethroscrotal (608.89)
urethrovaginal (619.0)
urethrovesicovaginal (619.0)

599.2 Urethral diverticulum

599.3 Urethral caruncle
Polyp of urethra

599.4 Urethral false passage

599.5 Prolapsed urethral mucosa
Prolapse of urethra
Urethrocele

Excludes: *urethrocele, female (618.03, 618.09, 618.2-618.4)*

⑤ **599.6 Urinary obstruction**

599.60 Urinary obstruction, unspecified
Obstructive uropathy NOS
Urinary (tract) obstruction NOS

599.69 Urinary obstruction, not elsewhere classified
Code, if applicable, any causal condition first, such as:
hyperplasia of prostate (600.0-600.9 with fifth-digit 1)

599.7 Hematuria
Hematuria (benign) (essential)

Excludes: *hemoglobinuria (791.2)*

⑤ **599.8 Other specified disorders of urethra and urinary tract**
Excludes: *symptoms and other conditions classifiable to 788.0-788.9, 791.0-791.9*
Use additional code, if desired, to identify urinary incontinence (625.6, 788.30-788.39)

599.81 Urethral hypermobility

599.82 Intrinsic (urethral) sphincter deficiency [ISD]

599.83 Urethral instability

599.84 Other specified disorders of urethra
Rupture of urethra (nontraumatic)
Urethral:
cyst
granuloma

599.89 Other specified disorders of urinary tract

599.9 Unspecified disorder of urethra and urinary tract

DISEASES OF MALE GENITAL ORGANS (600-608)

600 Hyperplasia of prostate
Includes: enlarged prostate

⑤ **600.0 Hypertrophy (benign) of prostate**
Benign prostatic hypertrophy
Enlargement of prostate
Smooth enlarged prostate
Soft enlarged prostate

▲ **600.00 Hypertrophy (benign) of prostate without urinary obstruction and other lower urinary tract symptoms (LUTS)**
Hypertrophy (benign) of prostate NOS

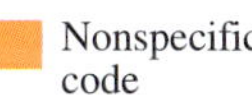

Add 4th or 5th digit	Nonspecific code	Unspecified code	Manifestation code

▲ **600.01** **Hypertrophy (benign) of prostate with urinary obstruction and other lower urinary tract symptoms (LUTS)**
Hypertrophy (benign) of prostate with urinary retention

Use additional code to identify symptoms:
incomplete bladder emptying (788.21)
nocturia (788.43)
straining on urination (788.65)
urinary frequency (788.41)
urinary hesitancy (788.64)
urinary incontinence (788.30-788.39)
urinary obstruction (599.69)
urinary retention (788.20)
urinary urgency (788.63)
weak urinary stream (788.62)

⑤ **600.1** **Nodular prostate**
Hard, firm prostate
Multinodular prostate

Excludes: *malignant neoplasm of prostate (185)*

600.10 **Nodular prostate without urinary obstruction**
Nodular prostate NOS

600.11 **Nodular prostate with urinary obstruction**
Nodular prostate with urinary retention

⑤ **600.2** **Benign localized hyperplasia of prostate**
Adenofibromatous hypertrophy of prostate
Adenoma of prostate
Fibroadenoma of prostate
Fibroma of prostate
Myoma of prostate
Polyp of prostate

Excludes: *benign neoplasms of prostate (222.2)*
hypertrophy of prostate (600.00-600.01)
malignant neoplasm of prostate (185)

▲ **600.20** **Benign localized hyperplasia of prostate without urinary obstruction and other lower urinary tract symptoms (LUTS)**
Benign localized hyperplasia of prostate NOS

▲ **600.21** **Benign localized hyperplasia of prostate with urinary obstruction and other lower urinary tract symptoms (LUTS)**
Benign localized hyperplasia of prostate with urinary retention

Use additional code to identify symptoms:
incomplete bladder emptying (788.21)
nocturia (788.43)
straining on urination (788.65)
urinary frequency (788.41)
urinary hesitancy (788.64)
urinary incontinence (788.30-788.39)
urinary obstruction (599.69)
urinary retention (788.20)
urinary urgency (788.63)
weak urinary stream (788.62)

600.3 **Cyst of prostate**

⑤ **600.9** **Hyperplasia of prostate, unspecified**
Median bar
Prostatic obstruction NOS

▲ **600.90** **Hyperplasia of prostate, unspecified, without urinary obstruction and other lower urinary symptoms (LUTS)**
Hyperplasia of prostate NOS

   ● Code new
to this edition   ▲ Revision of
existing code   ④ ⑤ Fourth or fifth
digit required

▲ **600.91 Hyperplasia of prostate, unspecified, with urinary obstruction and other lower urinary symptoms (LUTS)**
Hyperplasia of prostate, unspecified, with urinary retention

Use additional code to identify symptoms:
incomplete bladder emptying (788.21)
nocturia (788.43)
straining on urination (788.65)
urinary frequency (788.41)
urinary hesitancy (788.64)
urinary incontinence (788.30-788.39)
urinary obstruction (599.69)
urinary retention (788.20)
urinary urgency (788.63)
weak urinary stream (788.62)

601 Inflammatory diseases of prostate
Use additional code, if desired, to identify organism, such as Staphylococcus (041.1), or Streptococcus (041.0)

601.0 Acute prostatitis

601.1 Chronic prostatitis

601.2 Abscess of prostate

601.3 Prostatocystitis

601.4 Prostatitis in diseases classified elsewhere
Code first underlying disease, as:
actinomycosis (039.8)
blastomycosis (116.0)
syphilis (095.8)
tuberculosis (016.5)

Excludes: prostatitis:
gonococcal (098.12, 098.32)
monilial (112.2)
trichomonal (131.03)

601.8 Other specified inflammatory diseases of prostate
Prostatitis:
cavitary
diverticular
granulomatous

601.9 Prostatitis, unspecified
Prostatitis NOS

602 Other disorders of prostate

602.0 Calculus of prostate
Prostatic stone

602.1 Congestion or hemorrhage of prostate

602.2 Atrophy of prostate

602.3 Dysplasia of prostate
Prostatic intraepithelial neoplasia I (PIN I)
Prostatic intraepithelial neoplasia II (PIN II)

Excludes: Prostatic intraepithelial neoplasia III (PIN III) (233.4)

602.8 Other specified disorders of prostate
Fistula of prostate
Infarction of prostate
Stricture of prostate
Periprostatic adhesions

602.9 Unspecified disorder of prostate

603 Hydrocele
Includes: hydrocele of spermatic cord, testis, or tunica vaginalis

Excludes: congenital (778.6)

603.0 Encysted hydrocele

603.1 Infected hydrocele
Use additional code, if desired, to identify organism

603.8 Other specified types of hydrocele

603.9 Hydrocele, unspecified

	Add 4th or 5th digit		Nonspecific code		Unspecified code		Manifestation code

604 **Orchitis and epididymitis**
Use additional code, if desired, to identify organism, such as Escherichia coli [E. coli] (041.4),
Staphylococcus (041.1), or Streptococcus (041.0)

604.0 **Orchitis, epididymitis, and epididymo-orchitis, with abscess**
Abscess of epididymis or testis

⑤ **604.9** **Other orchitis, epididymitis, and epididymo-orchitis, without mention of abscess**

604.90 **Orchitis and epididymitis, unspecified**

604.91 *Orchitis and epididymitis in diseases classified elsewhere*
Code first underlying disease, as:
diphtheria (032.89)
filariasis (125.0-125.9)
syphilis (095.8)

Excludes: *orchitis:*
gonococcal (098.13, 098.33)
mumps (072.0)
tuberculous (016.5)
tuberculous epididymitis (016.4)

604.99 **Other**

605 **Redundant prepuce and phimosis**
Adherent prepuce   Phimosis (congenital)
Paraphimosis   Tight foreskin

606 **Infertility, male**

606.0 **Azoospermia**
Absolute infertility
Infertility due to:
germinal (cell) aplasia
spermatogenic arrest (complete)

606.1 **Oligospermia**
Infertility due to:
germinal cell desquamation
hypospermatogenesis
incomplete spermatogenic arrest

606.8 **Infertility due to extratesticular causes**
Infertility due to:
drug therapy
infection
obstruction of efferent ducts
radiation
systemic disease

606.9 **Male infertility, unspecified**

607 **Disorders of penis**
Excludes: *phimosis (605)*

607.0 **Leukoplakia of penis**
Kraurosis of penis
Excludes: *carcinoma in situ of penis (233.5)*
erythroplasia of Queyrat (233.5)

607.1 **Balanoposthitis**
Balanitis
Use additional code, if desired, to identify organism

607.2 **Other inflammatory disorders of penis**
Abscess of corpus cavernosum or penis
Boil of corpus cavernosum or penis
Carbuncle of corpus cavernosum or penis
Cellulitis of corpus cavernosum or penis
Cavernitis (penis)
Use additional code, if desired, to identify organism
Excludes: *herpetic infection (054.13)*

607.3 **Priapism**
Painful erection

⑤ **607.8** **Other specified disorders of penis**

607.81 **Balanitis xerotica obliterans**
Induratio penis plastica

   ● Code new   ▲ Revision of   ④ ⑤ Fourth or fifth
to this edition   existing code   digit required

607.82 Vascular disorders of penis
 Embolism of corpus cavernosum or penis
 Hematoma (nontraumatic) of corpus cavernosum or penis
 Hemorrhage of corpus cavernosum or penis
 Thrombosis of corpus cavernosum or penis

607.83 Edema of penis

607.84 Impotence of organic origin
Excludes: nonorganic (302.72)

607.85 Peyronie's disease

607.89 Other
 Atrophy of corpus cavernosum or penis
 Fibrosis of corpus cavernosum or penis
 Hypertrophy of corpus cavernosum or penis
 Ulcer (chronic) of corpus cavernosum or penis

607.9 Unspecified disorder of penis

608 Other disorders of male genital organs

608.0 Seminal vesiculitis
 Abscess of seminal vesicle
 Cellulitis of seminal vesicle
 Vesiculitis (seminal)

Use additional code, if desired, to identify organism
Excludes: gonococcal infection (098.14, 098.34)

608.1 Spermatocele

⑤ **608.2 Torsion of testis**

● **608.20 Torsion of testis, unspecified**

● **608.21 Extravaginal torsion of spermatic cord**

● **608.22 Intravaginal torsion of spermatic cord**

● **608.23 Torsion of appendix testis**

● **608.24 Torsion of appendix epididymis**

608.3 Atrophy of testis

608.4 Other inflammatory disorders of male genital organs
 Abscess of scrotum, spermatic cord, testis [except abscess], tunica vaginalis, or vas deferens
 Boil of scrotum, spermatic cord, testis [except abscess], tunica vaginalis, or vas deferens
 Carbuncle of scrotum, spermatic cord, testis [except abscess], tunica vaginalis, or vas deferens
 Cellulitis of scrotum, spermatic cord, testis [except abscess], tunica vaginalis, or vas deferens
 Vasitis

Use additional code, if desired, to identify organism
Excludes: abscess of testis (604.0)

⑤ **608.8 Other specified disorders of male genital organs**

608.81 *Disorders of male genital organs in diseases classified elsewhere*
 Code first underlying disease, as:
  filariasis (125.0-125.9)
  tuberculosis (016.5)

608.82 Hematospermia

608.83 Vascular disorders
 Hematoma (nontraumatic) of seminal vesicle, spermatic cord, testis, scrotum, tunica vaginalis, or vas deferens
 Hemorrhage of seminal vesicle, spermatic cord, testis, scrotum, tunica vaginalis, or vas deferens
 Thrombosis of seminal vesicle, spermatic cord, testis, scrotum, tunica vaginalis, or vas deferens
 Hematocele NOS, male

608.84 Chylocele of tunica vaginalis

608.85 Stricture
 Stricture of:
  spermatic cord
  tunica vaginalis
  vas deferens

608.86 Edema

608.87 Retrograde ejaculation

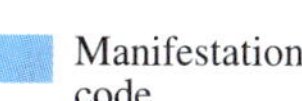

	Add 4th or 5th digit		Nonspecific code		Unspecified code		Manifestation code

608.89 Other
Atrophy of seminal vesicle, spermatic cord, testis, scrotum, tunica vaginalis, or vas deferens
Fibrosis of seminal vesicle, spermatic cord, testis, scrotum, tunica vaginalis, or vas deferens
Hypertrophy of seminal vesicle, spermatic cord, testis, scrotum, tunica vaginalis, or vas deferens
Ulcer of seminal vesicle, spermatic cord, testis, scrotum, tunica vaginalis, or vas deferens

Excludes: atrophy of testis (608.3)

608.9 Unspecified disorder of male genital organs

DISORDERS OF BREAST (610-611)

610 Benign mammary dysplasias

610.0 Solitary cyst of breast
Cyst (solitary) of breast

610.1 Diffuse cystic mastopathy
Chronic cystic mastitis   Fibrocystic disease of breast
Cystic breast

610.2 Fibroadenosis of breast
Fibroadenosis of breast: Fibroadenosis of breast:
  NOS   diffuse
  chronic   periodic
  cystic   segmental

610.3 Fibrosclerosis of breast

610.4 Mammary duct ectasia
Comedomastitis   Mastitis:
Dust ectasia   periductal
                      plasma cell

610.8 Other specified benign mammary dysplasias
Mazoplasia
Sebaceous cyst of breast

610.9 Benign mammary dysplasia, unspecified

611 Other disorders of breast
Excludes: that associated with lactation or the puerperium (675.0-676.9)

611.0 Inflammatory disease of breast
Abscess (acute) (chronic) (nonpuerperal) of:
  areola
  breast
Mammillary fistula
Mastitis (acute) (subacute) (nonpuerperal):
  NOS
  infective
  retromammary
  submammary

Excludes: carbuncle of breast (680.2)
  chronic cystic mastitis (610.1)
  neonatal infective mastitis (771.5)
  thrombophlebitis of breast [Mondor's disease] (451.89)

611.1 Hypertrophy of breast
Gynecomastia
Hypertrophy of breast:
  NOS
  massive pubertal

611.2 Fissure of nipple

611.3 Fat necrosis of breast
Fat necrosis (segmental) of breast

611.4 Atrophy of breast

611.5 Galactocele

611.6 Galactorrhea not associated with childbirth

⑤ **611.7 Signs and symptoms in breast**

611.71 Mastodynia
Pain in breast

● Code new to this edition   ▲ Revision of existing code   ④ ⑤ Fourth or fifth digit required

611.72 Lump or mass in breast

611.79 Other
Induration of breast   Nipple discharge
Inversion of nipple   Retraction of nipple

611.8 Other specified disorders of breast
Hematoma (nontraumatic) of breast
Infarction of breast
Occlusion of breast duct
Subinvolution of breast (postlactational) (postpartum)

611.9 Unspecified breast disorder

INFLAMMATORY DISEASE OF FEMALE PELVIC ORGANS (614-616)

Use additional code, if desired, to identify organism, such as Staphylococcus (041.1), or
Streptococcus (041.0)

Excludes: *that associated with pregnancy, abortion, childbirth, or the puerperium (630-676.9)*

614 Inflammatory disease of ovary, fallopian tube, pelvic cellular tissue, and peritoneum

Excludes: *endometritis (615.0-615.9)*

major infection following delivery (670)
that complicating:
abortion (634-638 with .0, 639.0)
ectopic or molar pregnancy (639.0)
pregnancy or labor (646.6)

614.0 Acute salpingitis and oophoritis
Any condition classifiable to 614.2, specified as acute or subacute

614.1 Chronic salpingitis and oophoritis
Hydrosalpinx
Salpingitis:
follicularis
isthmica nodosa
Any condition classifiable to 614.2, specified as chronic

614.2 Salpingitis and oophoritis not specified as acute, subacute, or chronic

Abscess (of):   Perisalpingitis
    fallopian tube   Pyosalpinx
    ovary   Salpingitis
    tubo-ovarian   Salpingo-oophoritisRTubo-ovarian inflammatory disease
Oophoritis
Perioophoritis

Excludes: *gonococcal infection (chronic) (098.37)*

acute (098.17)
tuberculous (016.6)

614.3 Acute parametritis and pelvic cellulitis
Acute inflammatory pelvic disease
Any condition classifiable to 614.4, specified as acute

614.4 Chronic or unspecified parametritis and pelvic cellulitis
Abscess (of):
broad ligament, chronic or NOS
parametrium, chronic or NOS
pelvis, female, chronic or NOS
pouch of Douglas, chronic or NOS
Chronic inflammatory pelvic disease
Pelvic cellulitis, female

Excludes: *tuberculous (016.7)*

614.5 Acute or unspecified pelvic peritonitis, female

614.6 Pelvic peritoneal adhesions, female (postoperative) (postinfection)
Adhesions:
peritubal
tubo-ovarian

Use additional code, if desired, to identify any associated infertility (628.2)

614.7 Other chronic pelvic peritonitis, female

Excludes: *tuberculous (016.7)*

614.8 Other specified inflammatory disease of female pelvic organs and tissues

<table>
<tr><td>Add 4th or
5th digit</td><td>Nonspecific
code</td><td>Unspecified
code</td><td>Manifestation
code</td></tr>
</table>

614.9 Unspecified inflammatory disease of female pelvic organs and tissues
Pelvic infection or inflammation, female NOS
Pelvic inflammatory disease [PID]

615 Inflammatory diseases of uterus, except cervix
Excludes: *following delivery (670)*
hyperplastic endometritis (621.30-621.33)
that complicating:
abortion (634-638 with .0, 639.0)
ectopic or molar pregnancy (639.0)
pregnancy or labor (646.6)

615.0 Acute
Any condition classifiable to 615.9, specified as acute or subacute

615.1 Chronic
Any condition classifiable to 615.9, specified as chronic

615.9 Unspecified inflammatory disease of uterus

Endometritis	Perimetritis
Endomyometritis	Pyometra
Metritis	Uterine abscess
Myometritis	

616 Inflammatory disease of cervix, vagina, and vulva
Excludes: *that complicating:*
abortion (634-638 with .0, 639.0)
ectopic or molar pregnancy (639.0)
pregnancy, childbirth, or the puerperium (646.6)

616.0 Cervicitis and endocervicitis
Cervicitis with or without mention of erosion or ectropion
Endocervicitis with or without mention of erosion or ectropion
Nabothian (gland) cyst or follicle

Excludes: *erosion or ectropion without mention of cervicitis (622.0)*

⑤ **616.1 Vaginitis and vulvovaginitis**

616.10 Vaginitis and vulvovaginitis, unspecified
Vaginitis:
NOS
postirradiation
Vulvitis NOS
Vulvovaginitis NOS

Use additional code, if desired, to identify organism, such as Escherichia coli [E. coli]
(041.4), Staphylococcus (041.1), or Streptococcus (041.0)

Excludes: *noninfective leukorrhea (623.5)*

postmenopausal or senile vaginitis (627.3)

616.11 Vaginitis and vulvovaginitis in diseases classified elsewhere
Code first underlying disease, as:
pinworm vaginitis (127.4)

Excludes: *herpetic vulvovaginitis (054.11)*
monilial vulvovaginitis (112.1)
trichomonal vaginitis or vulvovaginitis (131.01)

616.2 Cyst of Bartholin's gland
Bartholin's duct cyst

616.3 Abscess of Bartholin's gland
Vulvovaginal gland abscess

616.4 Other abscess of vulva
Abscess of vulva
Carbuncle of vulva
Furuncle of vulva

⑤ **616.5 Ulceration of vulva**

616.50 Ulceration of vulva, unspecified
Ulcer NOS of vulva

● Code new to this edition	▲ Revision of existing code	④ ⑤ Fourth or fifth digit required

616.51 Ulceration of vulva in diseases classified elsewhere
Code first underlying disease, as:
Behçet's syndrome (136.1)
tuberculosis (016.7)

Excludes: *vulvar ulcer (in):*
gonococcal (098.0)
herpes simplex (054.12)
syphilitic (091.0)

⑤ **616.8 Other specified inflammatory diseases of cervix, vagina, and vulva**

Excludes: *noninflammatory disorders of:*
cervix (622.0-622.9)
vagina (623.0-623.9)
vulva (624.0-624.9)

● **616.81 Mucositis (ulcerative) of cervix, vagina, and vulva**
Use additional E code to identify adverse effects of therapy, such as:
antineoplastic and immunosuppressive drugs (E930.7, E933.1)
radiation therapy (E879.2)

● **616.89 Other inflammatory disease of cervix, vagina and vulva**
Caruncle, vagina or labium
Ulcer, vagina

616.9 Unspecified inflammatory disease of cervix, vagina, and vulva

OTHER DISORDERS OF FEMALE GENITAL TRACT (617-629)

617 Endometriosis

617.0 Endometriosis of uterus
Adenomyosis
Endometriosis:
cervix
internal
myometrium

Excludes: *stromal endometriosis (236.0)*

617.1 Endometriosis of ovary
Chocolate cyst of ovary
Endometrial cystoma of ovary

617.2 Endometriosis of fallopian tube

617.3 Endometriosis of pelvic peritoneum
Endometriosis: Endometriosis:
broad ligament   parametrium
cul-de-sac (Douglas')   round ligament

617.4 Endometriosis of rectovaginal septum and vagina

617.5 Endometriosis of intestine
Endometriosis:
appendix
colon
rectum

617.6 Endometriosis in scar of skin

617.8 Endometriosis of other specified sites
Endometriosis: Endometriosis:
bladder   umbilicus
lung   vulva

617.9 Endometriosis, site unspecified

618 Genital prolapse
Use additional code, if desired, to identify urinary incontinence (625.6, 788.31, 788.33-788.39)

Excludes: *that complicating pregnancy, labor, or delivery (654.4)*

⑤ **618.0 Prolapse of vaginal walls without mention of uterine prolapse**

Excludes: *that with uterine prolapse (618.2-618.4)*
enterocele (618.6)
vaginal vault prolapse following hysterectomy (618.5)

618.00 Unspecified prolapse of vaginal walls
Vaginal prolapse NOS

618.01 Cystocele, midline
Cystocele NOS

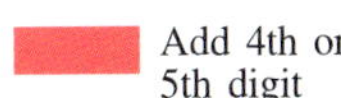

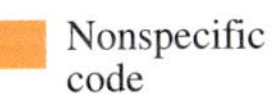

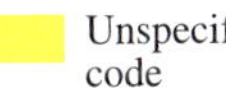

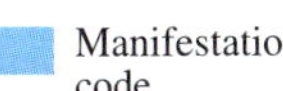

618.02 Cystocele, lateral
    Paravaginal

618.03 Urethrocele

618.04 Rectocele
    Proctocele

618.05 Perineocele

618.09 Other prolapse of vaginal walls without mention of uterine prolapse
    Cystourethrocele

618.1 Uterine prolapse without mention of vaginal wall prolapse

Descensus uteri	Uterine prolapse:
Uterine prolapse:	first degree
NOS	second degree
complete	third degree

Excludes: *that with mention of cystocele, urethrocele, or rectocele (618.2-618.4)*

618.2 Uterovaginal prolapse, incomplete

618.3 Uterovaginal prolapse, complete

618.4 Uterovaginal prolapse, unspecified

618.5 Prolapse of vaginal vault after hysterectomy

618.6 Vaginal enterocele, congenital or acquired
    Pelvic enterocele, congenital or acquired

618.7 Old laceration of muscles of pelvic floor

⑤ **618.8 Other specified genital prolapse**

618.81 Incompetence or weakening of pubocervical tissue

618.82 Incompetence or weakening of rectovaginal tissue

618.83 Pelvic muscle wasting
    Disuse atrophy of pelvic muscles and anal sphincter

● **618.84 Cervical stump prolapse**

618.89 Other specified genital prolapse

618.9 Unspecified genital prolapse

619 Fistula involving female genital tract

Excludes: *vesicorectal and intestinovesical fistula (596.1)*

619.0 Urinary-genital tract fistula, female

Fistula:	Fistula:
cervicovesical	uteroureteric
ureterovaginal	uterovesical
urethrovaginal	vesicocervicovaginal
urethrovesicovaginal	vesicovaginal

619.1 Digestive-genital tract fistula, female

Fistula:	Fistula:
intestinouterine	rectovulval
intestinovaginal	sigmoidovaginal
rectovaginal	uterorectal

619.2 Genital tract-skin fistula, female
    Fistula:
      uterus to abdominal wall
      vaginoperinea

619.8 Other specified fistulas involving female genital tract

Fistula:	Fistula:
cervix	uterus
cul-de-sac (Douglas')	vagina

619.9 Unspecified fistula involving female genital tract

620 Noninflammatory disorders of ovary, fallopian tube, and broad ligament

Excludes: *hydrosalpinx (614.1)*

620.0 Follicular cyst of ovary
    Cyst of graafian follicle

620.1 Corpus luteum cyst or hematoma
    Corpus luteum hemorrhage or rupture
    Lutein cyst

● Code new to this edition   ▲ Revision of existing code   ④ ⑤ Fourth or fifth digit required

620.2 Other and unspecified ovarian cyst
Cyst of ovary:
  NOS
  corpus albicans
  retention NOS
  serous
  theca-lutein
Simple cystoma of ovary

Excludes: *cystadenoma (benign) (serous) (220)*
    developmental cysts (752.0)
    neoplastic cysts (220)
    polycystic ovaries (256.4)
    Stein-Leventhal syndrome (256.4)

620.3 Acquired atrophy of ovary and fallopian tube
Senile involution of ovary

620.4 Prolapse or hernia of ovary and fallopian tube
Displacement of ovary and fallopian tube
Salpingocele

620.5 Torsion of ovary, ovarian pedicle, or fallopian tube
Torsion:
  accessory tube
  hydatid of Morgagni

620.6 Broad ligament laceration syndrome
Masters-Allen syndrome

620.7 Hematoma of broad ligament
Hematocele, broad ligament

620.8 Other noninflammatory disorders of ovary, fallopian tube, and broad ligament
Cyst of broad ligament or fallopian tube
Polyp of broad ligament or fallopian tube
Infarction of ovary or fallopian tube
Rupture of ovary or fallopian tube
Hematosalpinx of ovary or fallopian tube

Excludes: *hematosalpinx in ectopic pregnancy (639.2)*
    peritubal adhesions (614.6)
    torsion of ovary, ovarian pedicle, or fallopian tube (620.5)

620.9 Unspecified noninflammatory disorder of ovary, fallopian tube, and broad ligament

621 Disorders of uterus, not elsewhere classified

621.0 Polyp of corpus uteri
Polyp:
  endometrium
  uterus NOS

Excludes: *cervical polyp NOS (622.7)*

621.1 Chronic subinvolution of uterus

Excludes: *puerperal (674.8)*

621.2 Hypertrophy of uterus
Bulky or enlarged uterus

Excludes: *puerperal (674.8)*

⑤ **621.3 Endometrial hyperplasia**
Hyperplasia (adenomatous) (cystic) (glandular) of endometrium
Hyperplastic endometritis

  621.30 Endometrial hyperplasia, unspecified
    Endometrial hyperplasia NOS

  621.31 Simple endometrial hyperplasia without atypia

  621.32 Complex endometrial hyperplasia without atypia

  621.33 Endometrial hyperplasia with atypia

621.4 Hematometra
Hemometra

Excludes: *that in congenital anomaly (752.2-752.3)*

621.5 Intrauterine synechiae
Adhesions of uterus
Band(s) of uterus

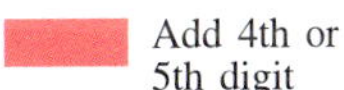

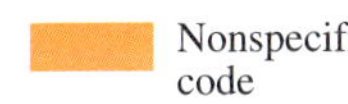

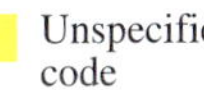

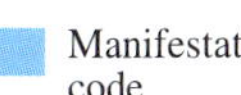

621.6 Malposition of uterus
Anteversion of uterus
Retroflexion of uterus
Retroversion of uterus

Excludes: *malposition complicating pregnancy, labor, or delivery (654.3-654.4)*
prolapse of uterus (618.1-618.4)

621.7 Chronic inversion of uterus

Excludes: *current obstetrical trauma (665.2)*
prolapse of uterus (618.1-618.4)

621.8 Other specified disorders of uterus, not elsewhere classified
Atrophy, acquired of uterus
Cyst of uterus
Fibrosis NOS of uterus
Old laceration (postpartum) of uterus
Ulcer of uterus

Excludes: *bilharzial fibrosis (120.0-120.9)*
endometriosis (617.0)
fistulas (619.0-619.8)
inflammatory diseases (615.0-615.9)

621.9 Unspecified disorder of uterus

622 Noninflammatory disorders of cervix

Excludes: *abnormality of cervix complicating pregnancy, labor, or delivery (654.5-654.6)*
fistula (619.0-619.8)

622.0 Erosion and ectropion of cervix
Eversion of cervix
Ulcer of cervix

Excludes: *that in chronic cervicitis (616.0)*

⑤ **622.1 Dysplasia of cervix (uteri)**

Excludes: *abnormal results from cervical cytologic examination without histologic*
confirmation (795.00-795.09)
carcinoma in situ of cervix (233.1)
cervical intraepithelial neoplasia III [CIN III] (233.1)

622.10 Dysplasia of cervix, unspecified
Anaplasia of cervix
Cervical atypism
Cervical dysplasia NOS

622.11 Mild dysplasia of cervix
Cervical intraepithelial neoplasia I [CIN I]

622.12 Moderate dysplasia of cervix
Cervical intraepithelial neoplasia II [CIN II]

Excludes: *carcinoma in situ of cervix (233.1)*
cervical intraepithelial neoplasia III [CIN III] (233.1)
severe dysplasia (233.1)

622.2 Leukoplakia of cervix (uteri)

Excludes: *carcinoma in situ of cervix (233.1)*

622.3 Old laceration of cervix
Adhesions of cervix
Band(s) of cervix
Cicatrix (postpartum) of cervix

Excludes: *current obstetrical trauma (665.3)*

622.4 Stricture and stenosis of cervix
Atresia (acquired) of cervix
Contracture of cervix
Occlusion of cervix
Pinpoint os uteri

Excludes: *congenital (752.49)*
that complicating labor (654.6)

622.5 Incompetence of cervix

Excludes: *complicating pregnancy (654.5)*
that affecting fetus or newborn (761.0)

● Code new
to this edition

▲ Revision of
existing code

④ ⑤ Fourth or fifth
digit required

622.6 Hypertrophic elongation of cervix

622.7 Mucous polyp of cervix
Polyp NOS of cervix

Excludes: *adenomatous polyp of cervix (219.0)*

622.8 Other specified noninflammatory disorders of cervix
Atrophy (senile) of cervix
Cyst of cervix
Fibrosis of cervix
Hemorrhage of cervix

Excludes: *endometriosis (617.0)*
fistula (619.0-619.8)
inflammatory diseases (616.0)

622.9 Unspecified noninflammatory disorder of cervix

623 Noninflammatory disorders of vagina

Excludes: *abnormality of vagina complicating pregnancy, labor, or delivery (654.7)*
congenital absence of vagina (752.49)
congenital diaphragm or bands (752.49)
fistulas involving vagina (619.0-619.8)

623.0 Dysplasia of vagina

Excludes: *carcinoma in situ of vagina (233.3)*

623.1 Leukoplakia of vagina

623.2 Stricture or atresia of vagina
Adhesions (postoperative) (postradiation) of vagina
Occlusion of vagina
Stenosis, vagina

Use additional E code, if desired, to identify any external cause

Excludes: *congenital atresia or stricture (752.49)*

623.3 Tight hymenal ring
Rigid hymen acquired or congenital
Tight hymenal ring acquired or congenital
Tight introitus acquired or congenital

Excludes: *imperforate hymen (752.42)*

623.4 Old vaginal laceration

Excludes: *old laceration involving muscles of pelvic floor (618.7)*

623.5 Leukorrhea, not specified as infective
Leukorrhea NOS of vagina
Vaginal discharge NOS

Excludes: *trichomonal (131.00)*

623.6 Vaginal hematoma

Excludes: *current obstetrical trauma (665.7)*

623.7 Polyp of vagina

623.8 Other specified noninflammatory disorders of vagina
Cyst of vagina
Hemorrhage of vagina

623.9 Unspecified noninflammatory disorder of vagina

624 Noninflammatory disorders of vulva and perineum

Excludes: *abnormality of vulva and perineum complicating pregnancy, labor, or delivery (654.8)*
condyloma acuminatum (078.1)
fistulas involving:
perineum—see Alphabetic Index
vulva (619.0-619.8)
vulval varices (456.6)
vulvar involvement in skin conditions (690-709.9)

624.0 Dystrophy of vulva
Kraurosis of vulva
Leukoplakia of vulva

Excludes: *carcinoma in situ of vulva (233.3)*

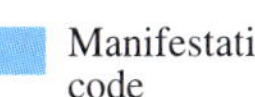

	Add 4th or 5th digit		Nonspecific code		Unspecified code		Manifestation code

624.1 Atrophy of vulva

624.2 Hypertrophy of clitoris
Excludes: *that in endocrine disorders (255.2, 256.1)*

624.3 Hypertrophy of labia
Hypertrophy of vulva NOS

624.4 Old laceration or scarring of vulva

624.5 Hematoma of vulva
Excludes: *that complicating delivery (664.5)*

624.6 Polyp of labia and vulva

624.8 Other specified noninflammatory disorders of vulva and perineum
Cyst of vulva
Edema of vulva
Stricture of vulva

624.9 Unspecified noninflammatory disorder of vulva and perineum

625 Pain and other symptoms associated with female genital organs

625.0 Dyspareunia
Excludes: *psychogenic dyspareunia (302.76)*

625.1 Vaginismus
Colpospasm
Vulvismus
Excludes: *psychogenic vaginismus (306.51)*

625.2 Mittelschmerz
Intermenstrual pain
Ovulation pain

625.3 Dysmenorrhea
Painful menstruation
Excludes: *psychogenic dysmenorrhea (306.52)*

625.4 Premenstrual tension syndromes
Menstrual: Premenstrual dysphoric disorder
  migraine   Premenstrual syndrome
  molimen   Premenstrual tension NOS

625.5 Pelvic congestion syndrome
Congestion-fibrosis syndrome
Taylor's syndrome

625.6 Stress incontinence, female
Excludes: *mixed incontinence (788.33)*
stress incontinence, male (788.32)

625.8 Other specified symptoms associated with female genital organs

625.9 Unspecified symptom associated with female genital organs

626 Disorders of menstruation and other abnormal bleeding from female genital tract
Excludes: *menopausal and premenopausal bleeding (627.0)*
pain and other symptoms associated with menstrual cycle (625.2-625.4)
postmenopausal bleeding (627.1)

626.0 Absence of menstruation
Amenorrhea (primary) (secondary)

626.1 Scanty or infrequent menstruation
Hypomenorrhea
Oligomenorrhea

626.2 Excessive or frequent menstruation
Heavy periods   Menorrhagia
Menometrorrhagia   Polymenorrhea
Excludes: *premenopausal (627.0)*
that in puberty (626.3)

626.3 Puberty bleeding
Excessive bleeding associated with onset of menstrual periods
Pubertal menorrhagia

● Code new
  to this edition
▲ Revision of
  existing code
④ ⑤ Fourth or fifth
  digit required

626.4 Irregular menstrual cycle
Irregular:
    bleeding NOS
    menstruation
    periods

626.5 Ovulation bleeding
Regular intermenstrual bleeding

626.6 Metrorrhagia
Bleeding unrelated to menstrual cycle
Irregular intermenstrual bleeding

626.7 Postcoital bleeding

626.8 Other
Dysfunctional or functional uterine hemorrhage NOS
Menstruation:
    retained
    suppression of

626.9 Unspecified

627 Menopausal and postmenopausal disorders

Excludes: *asymptomatic age-related (natural) postmenopausal status (V49.81)*

627.0 Premenopausal menorrhagia
Excessive bleeding associated with onset of menopause
Menorrhagia:
    climacteric
    menopausal
    preclimacteric

627.1 Postmenopausal bleeding

627.2 Symptomatic menopausal or female climacteric states
Symptoms, such as flushing, sleeplessness, headache, lack of concentration, associated
    with the menopause

627.3 Postmenopausal atrophic vaginitis
Senile (atrophic) vaginitis

627.4 Symptomatic states associated with artificial menopause
Postartificial menopause syndromes
Any condition classifiable to 627.1, 627.2, or 627.3 which follows induced menopause

627.8 Other specified menopausal and postmenopausal disorders

Excludes: *premature menopause NOS (256.31)*

627.9 Unspecified menopausal and postmenopausal disorder

628 Infertility, female
Includes: primary and secondary sterility

628.0 Associated with anovulation
Anovulatory cycle

Use additional code for any associated Stein-Leventhal syndrome (256.4)

628.1 *Of pituitary-hypothalamic origin*
Code first underlying cause, as:
    adiposogenital dystrophy (253.8)
    anterior pituitary disorder (253.0-253.4)

628.2 Of tubal origin
Infertility associated with congenital anomaly of tube
Tubal:
    block
    occlusion
    stenosis

Use additional code for any associated peritubal adhesions (614.6)

628.3 Of uterine origin
Infertility associated with congenital anomaly of uterus
Nonimplantation

Use additional code for any associated tuberculous endometritis (016.7)

628.4 Of cervical or vaginal origin
Infertility associated with:
    anomaly of cervical mucus
    congenital structural anomaly
    dysmucorrhea

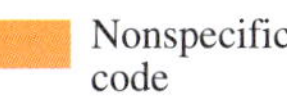

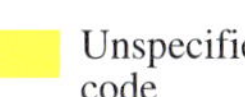

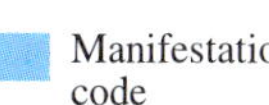

628.8 **Of other specified origin**

628.9 **Of unspecified origin**

629 **Other disorders of female genital organs**

629.0 Hematocele, female, not elsewhere classified
Excludes: hematocele or hematoma:
broad ligament (620.7)
fallopian tube (620.8)
that associated with ectopic pregnancy (633.00-633.91)
uterus (621.4)
vagina (623.6)
vulva (624.5)

629.1 Hydrocele, canal of Nuck
Cyst of canal of Nuck (acquired)
Excludes: congenital (752.41)

⑤ **629.2 Female genital mutilation status**
Female circumcision status
Female genital cutting

629.20 Female genital mutilation status, unspecified
Female genital cutting status, unspecified
Female genital mutilation status NOS
Female genital mutilation status, type 4

629.21 Female genital mutilation Type I status
Clitorectomy status
Female genital cutting Type I status

629.22 Female genital mutilation Type II status
Clitorectomy with excision of labia minor status
Female genital cutting Type II status

629.23 Female genital mutilation Type III status
Female genital cutting Type III status
Infibulation status

● **629.29 Other female genital mutilation status**
Female genital cutting Type IV status
Female genital mutilation Type IV status
Other female genital cutting status

⑤ **629.8 Other specified disorders of female genital organs**

● **629.81 Habitual aborter without current pregnancy**
Excludes: habitual aborter with current pregnancy (646.3)

● **629.89 Other specified disorders of female genital organs**

629.9 Unspecified disorder of female genital organs

● Code new to this edition   ▲ Revision of existing code   ④ ⑤ Fourth or fifth digit required

11. COMPLICATIONS OF PREGNANCY, CHILDBIRTH, AND THE PUERPERIUM (630-677)

ECTOPIC AND MOLAR PREGNANCY (630-633)

Use additional code from category 639 to identify any complications

630 Hydatidiform mole
Trophoblastic disease NOS
Vesicular mole

> *Excludes:* *chorioadenoma (destruens) (236.1)*
> *chorionepithelioma (181)*
> *malignant hydatidiform mole (236.1)*

631 Other abnormal product of conception

Blighted ovum	Mole:
Mole:	fleshy
NOS	stone
carneous	

632 Missed abortion
Early fetal death before completion of 22 weeks' gestation with retention of dead fetus
Retained products of conception, not following spontaneous or induced abortion or delivery

> *Excludes:* *failed induced abortion (638.0-638.9)*
> *fetal death (intrauterine) (late) (656.4)*
> *missed delivery (656.4)*
> *that with abnormal product of conception (630, 631)*

633 Ectopic pregnancy
Includes: ruptured ectopic pregnancy

⑤ **633.0 Abdominal pregnancy**
Intraperitoneal pregnancy

    633.00   Abdominal pregnancy without intrauterine pregnancy

    633.01   Abdominal pregnancy with intrauterine pregnancy

⑤ **633.1 Tubal pregnancy**
Fallopian pregnancy
Rupture of (fallopian) tube due to pregnancy
Tubal abortion

    633.10   Tubal pregnancy without intrauterine pregnancy

    633.11   Tubal pregnancy with intrauterine pregnancy

⑤ **633.2 Ovarian pregnancy**

    633.20   Ovarian pregnancy without intrauterine pregnancy

    633.21   Ovarian pregnancy with intrauterine pregnancy

⑤ **633.8 Other ectopic pregnancy**

Pregnancy:	Pregnancy:
cervical	intraligamentous
combined	mesometric
cornual	mural

    633.80   Other ectopic pregnancy without intrauterine pregnancy

    633.81   Other ectopic pregnancy with intrauterine pregnancy

⑤ **633.9 Unspecified ectopic pregnancy**

    633.90   Unspecified ectopic pregnancy without intrauterine pregnancy

    633.91   Unspecified ectopic pregnancy with intrauterine pregnancy

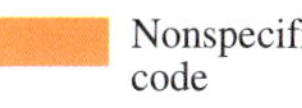

	Add 4th or 5th digit		Nonspecific code		Unspecified code		Manifestation code

OTHER PREGNANCY WITH ABORTIVE OUTCOME (634-639)

Note: Use the following fifth-digit subclassification with categories 634-637:

   0 **Unspecified**

   1 **Incomplete**

   2 **Complete**

The following fourth-digit subdivisions are for use with categories 634-638:

.0 **Complicated by genital tract and pelvic infection**
     Endometritis
     Salpingo-oophoritis
     Sepsis NOS
     Septicemia NOS
     Any condition classifiable to 639.0, with condition classifiable to 634-638

    Excludes: *urinary tract infection (634-638 with .7)*

.1 **Complicated by delayed or excessive hemorrhage**
     Afibrinogenemia
     Defibrination syndrome
     Intravascular hemolysis
     Any condition classifiable to 639.1, with condition classifiable to 634-638

.2 **Complicated by damage to pelvic organs and tissues**
     Laceration, perforation, or tear of:
      bladder
      uterus
     Any condition classifiable to 639.2, with condition classifiable to 634-638

.3 **Complicated by renal failure**
     Oliguria
     Uremia
     Any condition classifiable to 639.3, with condition classifiable to 634-638

.4 **Complicated by metabolic disorder**
     Electrolyte imbalance with conditions classifiable to 634-638

.5 **Complicated by shock**
     Circulatory collapse
     Shock (postoperative) (septic)
     Any condition classifiable to 639.5, with condition classifiable to 634-638

.6 **Complicated by embolism**
     Embolism:
      NOS
      amniotic fluid
      pulmonary
     Any condition classifiable to 639.6, with condition classifiable to 634-638

.7 **With other specified complications**
     Cardiac arrest or failure
     Urinary tract infection
     Any condition classifiable to 639.8, with condition classifiable to 634-638

.8 **With unspecified complication**

.9 **Without mention of complication**

⑤ **634** **Abortion**
     Includes: miscarriage
               spontaneous abortion

  ⑤ **634.0** **Complicated by genital tract and pelvic infection**

  ⑤ **634.1** **Complicated by delayed or excessive hemorrhage**

  ⑤ **634.2** **Complicated by damage to pelvic organs or tissues**

  ⑤ **634.3** **Complicated by renal failure**

  ⑤ **634.4** **Complicated by metabolic disorder**

  ⑤ **634.5** **Complicated by shock**

  ⑤ **634.6** **Complicated by embolism**

  ⑤ **634.7** **With other specified complications**

  ⑤ **634.8** **With unspecified complication**

  ⑤ **634.9** **Without mention of complication**

● Code new to this edition   ▲ Revision of existing code   ④ ⑤ Fourth or fifth digit required

⑤ **635 Legally induced abortion**
Includes: abortion or termination of pregnancy:
elective
legal
therapeutic

Excludes: *menstrual extraction or regulation (V25.3)*

⑤ **635.0 Complicated by genital tract and pelvic infection**
⑤ **635.1 Complicated by delayed or excessive hemorrhage**
⑤ **635.2 Complicated by damage to pelvic organs or tissues**
⑤ **635.3 Complicated by renal failure**
⑤ **635.4 Complicated by metabolic disorder**
⑤ **635.5 Complicated by shock**
⑤ **635.6 Complicated by embolism**
⑤ **635.7 With other specified complications**
⑤ **635.8 With unspecified complication**
⑤ **635.9 Without mention of complication**

⑤ **636 Illegally induced abortion**
Includes: abortion:
criminal
illegal
self-induced

⑤ **636.0 Complicated by genital tract and pelvic infection**
⑤ **636.1 Complicated by delayed or excessive hemorrhage**
⑤ **636.2 Complicated by damage to pelvic organs or tissues**
⑤ **636.3 Complicated by renal failure**
⑤ **636.4 Complicated by metabolic disorder**
⑤ **636.5 Complicated by shock**
⑤ **636.6 Complicated by embolism**
⑤ **636.7 With other specified complications**
⑤ **636.8 With unspecified complication**
⑤ **636.9 Without mention of complication**

⑤ **637 Unspecified abortion**
Includes: abortion NOS
retained products of conception following abortion, not classifiable elsewhere

⑤ **637.0 Complicated by genital tract and pelvic infection**
⑤ **637.1 Complicated by delayed or excessive hemorrhage**
⑤ **637.2 Complicated by damage to pelvic organs or tissues**
⑤ **637.3 Complicated by renal failure**
⑤ **637.4 Complicated by metabolic disorder**
⑤ **637.5 Complicated by shock**
⑤ **637.6 Complicated by embolism**
⑤ **637.7 With other specified complications**
⑤ **637.8 With unspecified complication**
⑤ **637.9 Without mention of complication**

638 Failed attempted abortion
Includes: failure of attempted induction of (legal) abortion

Excludes: *incomplete abortion (634.0-637.9)*

638.0 Complicated by genital tract and pelvic infection
638.1 Complicated by delayed or excessive hemorrhage
638.2 Complicated by damage to pelvic organs or tissues
638.3 Complicated by renal failure
638.4 Complicated by metabolic disorder
638.5 Complicated by shock
638.6 Complicated by embolism
638.7 With other specified complications

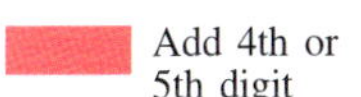

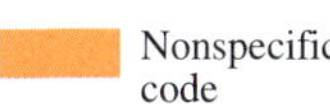

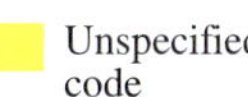

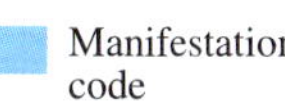

638.8 **With unspecified complication**

638.9 **Without mention of complication**

639 **Complications following abortion and ectopic and molar pregnancies**
Note: This category is provided for use when it is required to classify separately the
complications classifiable to the fourth-digit level in categories 634-638; for example:
- a) when the complication itself was responsible for an episode of medical care, the
  abortion, ectopic or molar pregnancy itself having been dealt with at a previous
  episode
- b) when these conditions are immediate complications of ectopic or molar pregnancies
  classifiable to 630-633 where they cannot be identified at fourth-digit level.

639.0 **Genital tract and pelvic infection**
Endometritis following conditions classifiable to 630-638
Parametritis following conditions classifiable to 630-638
Pelvic peritonitis following conditions classifiable to 630-638
Salpingitis following conditions classifiable to 630-638
Salpingo-oophoritis following conditions classifiable to 630-638
Sepsis NOS following conditions classifiable to 630-638
Septicemia NOS following conditions classifiable to 630-638

> *Excludes:* *urinary tract infection (639.8)*

639.1 **Delayed or excessive hemorrhage**
Afibrinogenemia following conditions classifiable to 630-638
Defibrination syndrome following conditions classifiable to 630-638
Intravascular hemolysis following conditions classifiable to 630-638

639.2 **Damage to pelvic organs and tissues**
Laceration, perforation, or tear of:
    bladder following conditions classifiable to 630-638
    bowel following conditions classifiable to 630-638
    broad ligament following conditions classifiable to 630-638
    cervix following conditions classifiable to 630-638
    periurethral tissue following conditions classifiable to 630-638
    uterus following conditions classifiable to 630-638
    vagina following conditions classifiable to 630-638

639.3 **Renal failure**
Oliguria following conditions classifiable to 630-638
Renal:
    failure (acute) following conditions classifiable to 630-638
    shutdown following conditions classifiable to 630-638
    tubular necrosis following conditions classifiable to 630-638
Uremia following conditions classifiable to 630-638

639.4 **Metabolic disorders**
Electrolyte imbalance following conditions classifiable to 630-638

639.5 **Shock**
Circulatory collapse following conditions classifiable to 630-638
Shock (postoperative) (septic) following conditions classifiable to 630-638

639.6 **Embolism**
Embolism:
    NOS following conditions classifiable to 630-638
    air following conditions classifiable to 630-638
    amniotic fluid following conditions classifiable to 630-638
    blood-clot following conditions classifiable to 630-638
    fat following conditions classifiable to 630-638
    pulmonary following conditions classifiable to 630-638
    pyemic following conditions classifiable to 630-638
    septic following conditions classifiable to 630-638
    soap following conditions classifiable to 630-638

639.8 **Other specified complications following abortion or ectopic and molar pregnancy**
Acute yellow atrophy or necrosis of liver following conditions classifiable to 630-638
Cardiac arrest or failure following conditions classifiable to 630-638
Cerebral anoxia following conditions classifiable to 630-638
Urinary tract infection following conditions classifiable to 630-638

639.9 **Unspecified complication following abortion or ectopic and molar pregnancy**
Complication(s) not further specified following conditions classifiable to 630-638

● Code new
  to this edition

▲ Revision of
  existing code

④ ⑤ Fourth or fifth
  digit required

COMPLICATIONS MAINLY RELATED TO PREGNANCY (640-649)

Includes: the listed conditions even if they arose or were present during labor, delivery, or the puerperium

The following fifth-digit subclassification is for use with categories 640-649 to denote the current episode of care:

0 **unspecified as to episode of care or not applicable**

1 **delivered, with or without mention of antepartum condition**
Antepartum condition with delivery
Delivery NOS (with mention of antepartum complication during current episode of care)
Intrapartum obstetric condition (with mention of antepartum complication during current episode of care)
Pregnancy, delivered (with mention of antepartum complication during current episode of care)

2 **delivered, with mention of postpartum complication**
Delivery with mention of puerperal complication during current episode of care

3 **antepartum condition or complication**
Antepartum obstetric condition, not delivered during the current episode of care

4 **postpartum condition or complication**
Postpartum or puerperal obstetric condition or complication following delivery that occurred:
during previous episode of care
outside hospital, with subsequent admission for observation or care

⑤ **640** **Hemorrhage in early pregnancy**
Includes: hemorrhage before completion of 22 weeks' gestation

⑤ **640.0** **Threatened abortion**
[0,1,3]

⑤ **640.8** **Other specified hemorrhage in early pregnancy**
[0,1,3]

⑤ **640.9** **Unspecified hemorrhage in early pregnancy**
[0,1,3]

⑤ **641** **Antepartum hemorrhage, abruptio placentae, and placenta previa**

⑤ **641.0** **Placenta previa without hemorrhage**
[0,1,3]   Low implantation of placenta without hemorrhage
Placenta previa noted:
during pregnancy without hemorrhage
before labor (and delivered by cesarean delivery) without hemorrhage

⑤ **641.1** **Hemorrhage from placenta previa**
[0,1,3]   Low-lying placenta NOS or with hemorrhage (intrapartum)
Placenta previa:
incomplete NOS or with hemorrhage (intrapartum)
marginal NOS or with hemorrhage (intrapartum)
partial NOS or with hemorrhage (intrapartum)
total NOS or with hemorrhage (intrapartum)

Excludes: *hemorrhage from vasa previa (663.5)*

⑤ **641.2** **Premature separation of placenta**
[0,1,3]   Ablatio placentae
Abruptio placentae
Accidental antepartum hemorrhage
Couvelaire uterus
Detachment of placenta (premature)
Premature separation of normally implanted placenta

⑤ **641.3** **Antepartum hemorrhage associated with coagulation defects**
[0,1,3]   Antepartum or intrapartum hemorrhage associated with:
afibrinogenemia
hyperfibrinolysis
hypofibrinogenemia

Excludes: *coagulation defects not associated with antepartum hemorrhage (649.3)*

⑤ **641.8** **Other antepartum hemorrhage**
[0,1,3]   Antepartum or intrapartum hemorrhage associated with:
trauma
uterine leiomyoma

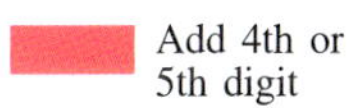

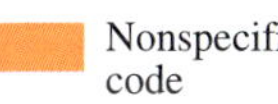

Unspecified
code

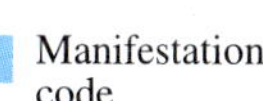

⑤ **641.9 Unspecified antepartum hemorrhage**
[0,1,3]   Hemorrhage:
                antepartum NOS
                intrapartum NOS
                of pregnancy NOS

⑤ **642 Hypertension complicating pregnancy, childbirth, and the puerperium**

⑤ **642.0 Benign essential hypertension complicating pregnancy, childbirth, and the puerperium**
[0-4]   Hypertension:
                benign essential specified as complicating, or as a reason for obstetric care during
                    pregnancy, childbirth, or the puerperium
                chronic NOS specified as complicating, or as a reason for obstetric care during
                    pregnancy, childbirth, or the puerperium
                essential specified as complicating, or as a reason for obstetric care during
                    pregnancy, childbirth, or the puerperium
                pre-existing NOS specified as complicating, or as a reason for obstetric care during
                    pregnancy, childbirth, or the puerperium

⑤ **642.1 Hypertension secondary to renal disease, complicating pregnancy, childbirth, and the
        puerperium**
[0-4]   Hypertension secondary to renal disease, specified as complicating, or as a reason for
                obstetric care during pregnancy, childbirth, or the puerperium

⑤ **642.2 Other pre-existing hypertension complicating pregnancy, childbirth, and the puerperium**
[0-4]   Hypertensive:
                chronic kidney disease specified as complicating, or as a reason for obstetric care
                    during pregnancy, childbirth, or the puerperium
                heart and chronic kidney disease specified as complicating, or as a reason for obstetric
                    care during pregnancy, childbirth, or the puerperium
                heart disease specified as complicating, or as a reason for obstetric care during
                    pregnancy, childbirth, or the puerperium
            Malignant hypertension specified as complicating, or as a reason for obstetric care
                during pregnancy, childbirth, or the puerperium

⑤ **642.3 Transient hypertension of pregnancy**
[0-4]   Gestational hypertension
            Transient hypertension, so described, in pregnancy, childbirth, or the puerperium

⑤ **642.4 Mild or unspecified pre-eclampsia**
[0-4]   Hypertension in pregnancy, childbirth, or the puerperium, not specified as pre-existing,
                with either albuminuria or edema, or both; mild or unspecified
            Pre-eclampsia: Toxemia (pre-eclamptic):
            NOS   NOS
            mild   mild

> Excludes: *albuminuria in pregnancy, without mention of hypertension (646.2)*
>   *edema in pregnancy, without mention of hypertension (646.1)*

⑤ **642.5 Severe pre-eclampsia**
[0-4]   Hypertension in pregnancy, childbirth, or the puerperium, not specified as pre-existing,
                with either albuminuria or edema, or both; specified as severe
            Pre-eclampsia, severe
            Toxemia (pre-eclamptic), severe

⑤ **642.6 Eclampsia**
[0-4]   Toxemia:
                eclamptic
                with convulsions

⑤ **642.7 Pre-eclampsia or eclampsia superimposed on pre-existing hypertension**
[0-4]   Conditions classifiable to 642.4-642.6, with conditions classifiable to 642.0-642.2

⑤ **642.9 Unspecified hypertension complicating pregnancy, childbirth, or the puerperium**
[0-4]   Hypertension NOS, without mention of albuminuria or edema, complicating pregnancy,
                childbirth, or the puerperium

⑤ **643 Excessive vomiting in pregnancy**
        Includes: hyperemesis arising during pregnancy
                    vomiting:
                        persistent arising during pregnancy
                        vicious arising during pregnancy
                    hyperemesis gravidarum

⑤ **643.0 Mild hyperemesis gravidarum**
[0,1,3]   Hyperemesis gravidarum, mild or unspecified, starting before the end of the 22nd week
                of gestation

        ● Code new   ▲ Revision of   ④ ⑤ Fourth or fifth
              to this edition   existing code   digit required

⑤ **643.1 Hyperemesis gravidarum with metabolic disturbance**
[0,1,3]   Hyperemesis gravidarum, starting before the end of the 22nd week of gestation, with metabolic disturbance, such as:
  carbohydrate depletion
  dehydration
  electrolyte imbalance

⑤ **643.2 Late vomiting of pregnancy**
[0,1,3]   Excessive vomiting starting after 22 completed weeks of gestation

⑤ **643.8 Other vomiting complicating pregnancy**
[0,1,3]   Vomiting due to organic disease or other cause, specified as complicating pregnancy, or as a reason for obstetric care during pregnancy
Use additional code, if desired, to specify cause

⑤ **643.9 Unspecified vomiting of pregnancy**
[0,1,3]   Vomiting as a reason for care during pregnancy, length of gestation unspecified

⑤ **644 Early or threatened labor**

⑤ **644.0 Threatened premature labor**
[0,3]   Premature labor after 22 weeks, but before 37 completed weeks of gestation without delivery

  Excludes: *that occurring before 22 completed weeks of gestation (640.0)*

⑤ **644.1 Other threatened labor**
[0,3]   False labor:
  NOS without delivery
  after 37 completed weeks of gestation without delivery
 Threatened labor NOS without delivery

⑤ **644.2 Early onset of delivery**
[0,1]   Onset (spontaneous) of delivery before 37 completed weeks of gestation
 Premature labor with onset of delivery before 37 completed weeks of gestation

⑤ **645 Late pregnancy**

⑤ **645.1 Post term pregnancy**
[0,1,3]   Pregnancy over 40 completed weeks to 42 completed weeks gestation

⑤ **645.2 Prolonged pregnancy**
[0,1,3]   Pregnancy which has advanced beyond 42 completed weeks gestation

⑤ **646 Other complications of pregnancy, not elsewhere classified**
Use additional code(s) to further specify complication

⑤ **646.0 Papyraceous fetus**
[0,1,3]

⑤ **646.1 Edema or excessive weight gain in pregnancy, without mention of hypertension**
[0-4]   Gestational edema
 Maternal obesity syndrome

  Excludes: *that with mention of hypertension (642.0-642.9)*

⑤ **646.2 Unspecified renal disease in pregnancy, without mention of hypertension**
[0-4]   Albuminuria in pregnancy or the puerperium, without mention of hypertension
 Nephropathy NOS in pregnancy or the puerperium, without mention of hypertension
 Renal disease NOS in pregnancy or the puerperium, without mention of hypertension
 Uremia in pregnancy or the puerperium, without mention of hypertension
 Gestational proteinuria in pregnancy or the puerperium, without mention of hypertension

  Excludes: *that with mention of hypertension (642.0-642.9)*

⑤ **646.3 Habitual aborter**
[0,1,3]

  Excludes: *with current abortion (634.0-634.9)*
   without current pregnancy (629.9)

⑤ **646.4 Peripheral neuritis in pregnancy**
[0-4]

⑤ **646.5 Asymptomatic bacteriuria in pregnancy**
[0-4]

⑤ **646.6 Infections of genitourinary tract in pregnancy**
[0-4]   Conditions classifiable to 590, 595, 597, 599.0, 616 complicating pregnancy, childbirth, or the puerperium
 Conditions classifiable to (614.0-614.5, 617.7-614.9, 615) complicating pregnancy or labor

  Excludes: *major puerperal infection (670)*

	Add 4th or 5th digit		Nonspecific code		Unspecified code		Manifestation code

⑤ **646.7 Liver disorders in pregnancy**
[0,1,3]   Acute yellow atrophy of liver (obstetric) (true) of pregnancy
Icterus gravis of pregnancy
Necrosis of liver of pregnancy

Excludes: *hepatorenal syndrome following delivery (674.8)*
viral hepatitis (647.6)

⑤ **646.8 Other specified complications of pregnancy**
[0-4]   Fatigue during pregnancy
Herpes gestationis
Insufficient weight gain of pregnancy

⑤ **646.9 Unspecified complication of pregnancy**
[0,1,3]

⑤ **647 Infectious and parasitic conditions in the mother classifiable elsewhere, but complicating pregnancy, childbirth, or the puerperium**
Includes: the listed conditions when complicating the pregnant state, aggravated by the pregnancy, or when a main reason for obstetric care

Excludes: *those conditions in the mother known or suspected to have affected the fetus (655.0-655.9)*

Use additional code(s) to further specify complication

⑤ **647.0 Syphilis**
[0-4]   Conditions classifiable to 090-097

⑤ **647.1 Gonorrhea**
[0-4]   Conditions classifiable to 098

⑤ **647.2 Other venereal diseases**
[0-4]   Conditions classifiable to 099

⑤ **647.3 Tuberculosis**
[0-4]   Conditions classifiable to 010-018

⑤ **647.4 Malaria**
[0-4]   Conditions classifiable to 084

⑤ **647.5 Rubella**
[0-4]   Conditions classifiable to 056

⑤ **647.6 Other viral diseases**
[0-4]   Conditions classifiable to 042 and 050-079, except 056

⑤ **647.8 Other specified infectious and parasitic diseases**
[0-4]

⑤ **647.9 Unspecified infection or infestation**
[0-4]

⑤ **648 Other current conditions in the mother classifiable elsewhere, but complicating pregnancy, childbirth, or the puerperium**
Includes: the listed conditions when complicating the pregnant state, aggravated by the pregnancy, or when a main reason for obstetric care

Excludes: *those conditions in the mother known or suspected to have affected the fetus (655.0-655.9)*

Use additional code(s) to identify the condition

⑤ **648.0 Diabetes mellitus**
[0-4]   Conditions classifiable to 250

Excludes: *gestational diabetes (648.8)*

⑤ **648.1 Thyroid dysfunction**
[0-4]   Conditions classifiable to 240-246

⑤ **648.2 Anemia**
[0-4]   Conditions classifiable to 280-285

⑤ **648.3 Drug dependence**
[0-4]   Conditions classifiable to 304

⑤ **648.4 Mental disorders**
[0-4]   Conditions classifiable to 290-303, 305.0, 305.2-305.9, 306-316, 317-319

⑤ **648.5 Congenital cardiovascular disorders**
[0-4]   Conditions classifiable to 745-747

      ● Code new   ▲ Revision of   ④ ⑤ Fourth or fifth
to this edition   existing code   digit required

⑤ **648.6 Other cardiovascular diseases**
[0-4]   Conditions classifiable to 390-398, 410-429

> Excludes: *cerebrovascular disorders in the puerperium (674.0)*
> *peripartum cardiomyopathy (674.5)*
> *venous complications (671.0-671.9)*

⑤ **648.7 Bone and joint disorders of back, pelvis, and lower limbs**
[0-4]   Conditions classifiable to 720-724, and those classifiable to 711-719 or 725-738, specified as affecting the lower limbs

⑤ **648.8 Abnormal glucose tolerance**
[0-4]   Conditions classifiable to 790.21-790.29
Gestational diabetes
Use additional code, if applicable, for associated long-term (current) insulin use (V58.67)

⑤ **648.9 Other current conditions classifiable elsewhere**
[0-4]   Conditions classifiable to 440-459
Nutritional deficiencies [conditions classifiable to 260-269]

● **649 Other conditions or status of the mother complicating pregnancy, childbirth, or the puerperium**

The following fifth-digit subclassification is for use with categories 640-649 to denote the current episode of care:

0 **unspecified as to episode of care or not applicable**

1 **delivered, with or without mention of antepartum condition**
Antepartum condition with delivery
Delivery NOS (with mention of antepartum complication during current episode of care)
Intrapartum obstetric condition (with mention of antepartum complication during current episode of care)
Pregnancy, delivered (with mention of antepartum complication during current episode of care)

2 **delivered, with mention of postpartum complication**
Delivery with mention of puerperal complication during current episode of care

3 **antepartum condition or complication**
Antepartum obstetric condition, not delivered during the current episode of care

4 **postpartum condition or complication**
Postpartum or puerperal obstetric condition or complication following delivery that occurred:
during previous episode of care
outside hospital, with subsequent admission for observation or care

● **649.0 Tobacco use disorder complicating pregnancy, childbirth, or the puerperium**
[0-4]   Smoking complicating pregnancy, childbirth, or the puerperium

● **649.1 Obesity complicating pregnancy, childbirth, or the puerperium**
[0-4]
Use additional code to identify the obesity (278.00, 278.01)

● **649.2 Bariatric surgery status complicating pregnancy, childbirth, or the puerperium**
[0-4]   Gastric banding status complicating pregnancy, childbirth, or the puerperium
Gastric bypass status for obesity complicating pregnancy, childbirth, or the puerperium
Obesity surgery status complicating pregnancy, childbirth, or the puerperium

● **649.3 Coagulation defects complicating pregnancy, childbirth, or the puerperium**
[0-4]   Conditions classifiable to 286
Use additional code to identify the specific coagulation defect (286.0-286.9)

> Excludes: *coagulation defects causing antepartum hemorrhage (641.3)*
> *postpartum coagulation defects (666.3)*

● **649.4 Epilepsy complicating pregnancy, childbirth, or the puerperium**
[0-4]   Conditions classifiable to 345
Use additional code to identify the specific type of epilepsy (345.00-345.91)

> Excludes: *eclampsia (642.6)*

● **649.5 Spotting complicating pregnancy**
[0,1,3]

> Excludes: *antepartum hemorrhage (641.0-641.9)*
> *hemorrhage in early pregnancy (640.0-640.9)*

● **649.6 Uterine size date discrepancy**
[0-4]

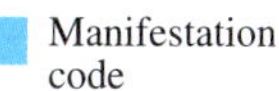

NORMAL DELIVERY, AND OTHER INDICATIONS FOR CARE IN PREGNANCY, LABOR, AND DELIVERY (650-659)

650 Normal delivery

Delivery requiring minimal or no assistance, with or without episiotomy, without fetal manipulation [e.g., rotation version] or instrumentation [forceps] of spontaneous, cephalic, vaginal, full-term, single, live born infant. This code is for use as a single diagnosis code and is not to be used with any other code in the range 630-676.

> *Excludes:* *breech delivery (assisted) (spontaneous) NOS (652.2)*
> *delivery by vacuum extractor, forceps, cesarean section, or breech extraction, without specified complication (669.5-669.7)*

Use additional code to indicate outcome of delivery (V27.0)

The following fifth-digit subclassification is for use with categories 651-659 to denote the current episode of care:

   0   unspecified as to episode of care or not applicable

   1   delivered, with or without mention of antepartum condition

   2   delivered, with mention of postpartum complication

   3   antepartum condition or complication

   4   postpartum condition or complication

⑤ **651 Multiple gestation**

⑤ **651.0 Twin pregnancy**
[0,1,3]

⑤ **651.1 Triplet pregnancy**
[0,1,3]

⑤ **651.2 Quadruplet pregnancy**
[0,1,3]

⑤ **651.3 Twin pregnancy with fetal loss and retention of one fetus**
[0,1,3]

⑤ **651.4 Triplet pregnancy with fetal loss and retention of one or more fetus(es)**
[0,1,3]

⑤ **651.5 Quadruplet pregnancy with fetal loss and retention of one or more fetus(es)**
[0,1,3]

⑤ **651.6 Other multiple pregnancy with fetal loss and retention of one or more fetus(es)**
[0,1,3]

⑤ **651.7 Multiple gestation following (elective) fetal reduction**
[0,1,3]   Fetal reduction of multiple fetuses reduced to single fetus

   651.70 Multiple gestation following (elective) fetal reduction, unspecified as to episode of care or not applicable

   651.71 Multiple gestation following (elective) fetal reduction, delivered, with or without mention of antepartum condition

   651.73 Multiple gestation following (elective) fetal reduction, antepartum condition or complication

⑤ **651.8 Other specified multiple gestation**
[0,1,3]

⑤ **651.9 Unspecified multiple gestation**
[0,1,3]

⑤ **652 Malposition and malpresentation of fetus**
Code first any associated obstructed labor (660.0)

⑤ **652.0 Unstable lie**
[0,1,3]

⑤ **652.1 Breech or other malpresentation successfully converted to cephalic presentation**
[0,1,3]   Cephalic version NOS

⑤ **652.2 Breech presentation without mention of version**
[0,1,3]   Breech delivery (assisted) (spontaneous) NOS
   Buttocks presentation
   Complete breech
   Frank breech

> *Excludes:* *footling presentation (652.8)*
> *incomplete breech (652.8)*

● Code new to this edition   ▲ Revision of existing code   ④ ⑤ Fourth or fifth digit required

⑤ **652.3 Transverse or oblique presentation**
[0,1,3]   Oblique lie   Transverse lie

    Excludes: transverse arrest of fetal head (660.3)

⑤ **652.4 Face or brow presentation**
[0,1,3]   Mentum presentation

⑤ **652.5 High head at term**
[0,1,3]   Failure of head to enter pelvic brim

⑤ **652.6 Multiple gestation with malpresentation of one fetus or more**
[0,1,3]

⑤ **652.7 Prolapsed arm**
[0,1,3]

⑤ **652.8 Other specified malposition or malpresentation**
[0,1,3]   Compound presentation

⑤ **652.9 Unspecified malposition or malpresentation**
[0,1,3]

⑤ **653 Disproportion**
    Code first any associated obstructed labor (660.1)

⑤ **653.0 Major abnormality of bony pelvis, not further specified**
[0,1,3]   Pelvic deformity NOS

⑤ **653.1 Generally contracted pelvis**
[0,1,3]   Contracted pelvis NOS

⑤ **653.2 Inlet contraction of pelvis**
[0,1,3]   Inlet contraction (pelvis)

⑤ **653.3 Outlet contraction of pelvis**
[0,1,3]   Outlet contraction (pelvis)

⑤ **653.4 Fetopelvic disproportion**
[0,1,3]   Cephalopelvic disproportion NOS
       Disproportion of mixed maternal and fetal origin, with normally formed fetus

⑤ **653.5 Unusually large fetus causing disproportion**
[0,1,3]   Disproportion of fetal origin with normally formed fetus
       Fetal disproportion NOS

    Excludes: that when the reason for medical care was concern for the fetus (656.6)

⑤ **653.6 Hydrocephalic fetus causing disproportion**
[0,1,3]

    Excludes: that when the reason for medical care was concern for the fetus (655.0)

⑤ **653.7 Other fetal abnormality causing disproportion**
[0,1,3]   Conjoined twins   Fetal:
       Fetal: myelomeningocele
        ascites   sacral teratoma
        hydrops   tumor

⑤ **653.8 Disproportion of other origin**
[0,1,3]

    Excludes: shoulder (girdle) dystocia (660.4)

⑤ **653.9 Unspecified disproportion**
[0,1,3]

⑤ **654 Abnormality of organs and soft tissues of pelvis**
    Includes: the listed conditions during pregnancy, childbirth, or the puerperium
    Code first any associated obstructed labor (660.2)

⑤ **654.0 Congenital abnormalities of uterus**
[0-4]   Double uterus   Uterus bicornis

⑤ **654.1 Tumors of body of uterus**
[0-4]   Uterine fibroids

⑤ **654.2 Previous cesarean delivery NOS**
[0,1,3]   Uterine scar from previous cesarean delivery

⑤ **654.3 Retroverted and incarcerated gravid uterus**
[0-4]

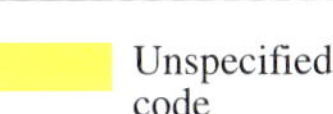

⑤ **654.4** **Other abnormalities in shape or position of gravid uterus and of neighboring structures**
[0-4] Cystocele
Pelvic floor repair
Pendulous abdomen
Prolapse of gravid uterus
Rectocele
Rigid pelvic floor

⑤ **654.5** **Cervical incompetence**
[0-4] Presence of Shirodkar suture with or without mention of cervical incompetence

⑤ **654.6** **Other congenital or acquired abnormality of cervix**
[0-4] Cicatricial cervix
Polyp of cervix
Previous surgery to cervix
Rigid cervix (uteri)
Stenosis or stricture of cervix
Tumor of cervix

⑤ **654.7** **Congenital or acquired abnormality of vagina**
[0-4] Previous surgery to vagina
Septate vagina
Stenosis of vagina (acquired) (congenital)
Stricture of vagina
Tumor of vagina

⑤ **654.8** **Congenital or acquired abnormality of vulva**
[0-4] Fibrosis of perineum
Persistent hymen
Previous surgery to perineum or vulva
Rigid perineum
Tumor of vulva

> *Excludes:* *varicose veins of vulva (671.1)*

⑤ **654.9** **Other and unspecified**
[0-4] Uterine scar NEC

⑤ **655** **Known or suspected fetal abnormality affecting management of mother**
Includes: the listed conditions in the fetus as a reason for observation or obstetrical care of the mother, or for termination of pregnancy

⑤ **655.0** **Central nervous system malformation in fetus**
[0,1,3] Fetal or suspected fetal:
anencephaly
hydrocephalus
spina bifida (with myelomeningocele)

⑤ **655.1** **Chromosomal abnormality in fetus**
[0,1,3]

⑤ **655.2** **Hereditary disease in family possibly affecting fetus**
[0,1,3]

⑤ **655.3** **Suspected damage to fetus from viral disease in the mother**
[0,1,3] Suspected damage to fetus from maternal rubella

⑤ **655.4** **Suspected damage to fetus from other disease in the mother**
[0,1,3] Suspected damage to fetus from maternal:
alcohol addiction
listeriosis
toxoplasmosis

⑤ **655.5** **Suspected damage to fetus from drugs**
[0,1,3]

⑤ **655.6** **Suspected damage to fetus from radiation**
[0,1,3]

⑤ **655.7** **Decreased fetal movements**
[0,1,3]

⑤ **655.8** **Other known or suspected fetal abnormality, not elsewhere classified**
[0,1,3] Suspected damage to fetus from:
environmental toxins
intrauterine contraceptive device

⑤ **655.9** **Unspecified**
[0,1,3]

● Code new to this edition   ▲ Revision of existing code   ④ ⑤ Fourth or fifth digit required

⑤ **656** **Other fetal and placental problems affecting management of mother**

⑤ **656.0** **Fetal-maternal hemorrhage**
[0,1,3]   Leakage (microscopic) of fetal blood into maternal circulation

⑤ **656.1** **Rhesus isoimmunization**
[0,1,3]   Anti-D [Rh] antibodies
Rh incompatibility

⑤ **656.2** **Isoimmunization from other and unspecified blood-group incompatibility**
[0,1,3]   ABO isoimmunization

⑤ **656.3** **Fetal distress**
[0,1,3]   Fetal metabolic acidemia

> *Excludes:* *abnormal fetal acid-base balance (656.8)*
> *abnormality in fetal heart rate or rhythm (659.7)*
> *fetal bradycardia (659.7)*
> *fetal tachycardia (659.7)*
> *meconium in liquor (656.8)*

⑤ **656.4** **Intrauterine death**
[0,1,3]   Fetal death:
NOS
after completion of 22 weeks' gestation
late
Missed delivery

> *Excludes:* *missed abortion (632)*

⑤ **656.5** **Poor fetal growth**
[0,1,3]   "Light-for-dates"   "Small-for-dates"
"Placental insufficiency"

⑤ **656.6** **Excessive fetal growth**
[0,1,3]   "Large-for-dates"

⑤ **656.7** **Other placental conditions**
[0,1,3]   Abnormal placenta   Placental infarct

> *Excludes:* *placental polyp (674.4)*
> *placentitis (658.4)*

⑤ **656.8** **Other specified fetal and placental problems**
[0,1,3]   Abnormal acid-base balance
Intrauterine acidosis
Lithopedian
Meconium in liquor

⑤ **656.9** **Unspecified fetal and placental problem**
[0,1,3]

⑤ **657** **Polyhydramnios**
[0,1,3]   Hydramnios
Use 0 as fourth-digit for this category

⑤ **658** **Other problems associated with amniotic cavity and membranes**

> *Excludes:* *amniotic fluid embolism (673.1)*

⑤ **658.0** **Oligohydramnios**
[0,1,3]   Oligohydramnios without mention of rupture of membranes

⑤ **658.1** **Premature rupture of membranes**
[0,1,3]   Rupture of amniotic sac less than 24 hours prior to the onset of labor

⑤ **658.2** **Delayed delivery after spontaneous or unspecified rupture of membranes**
[0,1,3]   Prolonged rupture of membranes NOS
Rupture of amniotic sac 24 hours or more prior to the onset of labor

⑤ **658.3** **Delayed delivery after artificial rupture of membranes**
[0,1,3]

⑤ **658.4** **Infection of amniotic cavity**
[0,1,3]   Amnionitis
Chorioamnionitis
Membranitis
Placentitis

⑤ **658.8** **Other**
[0,1,3]   Amnion nodosum
Amniotic cyst

⑤ **658.9 Unspecified**
[0,1,3]

⑤ **659 Other indications for care or intervention related to labor and delivery, not elsewhere classified**

⑤ **659.0 Failed mechanical induction**
[0,1,3]   Failure of induction of labor by surgical or other instrumental methods

⑤ **659.1 Failed medical or unspecified induction**
[0,1,3]   Failed induction NOS
Failure of induction of labor by medical methods, such as oxytocic drugs

⑤ **659.2 Maternal pyrexia during labor, unspecified**
[0,1,3]

⑤ **659.3 Generalized infection during labor**
[0,1,3]   Septicemia during labor

⑤ **659.4 Grand multiparity**
[0,1,3]

> *Excludes:* supervision only, in pregnancy (V23.3)
> without current pregnancy (V61.5)

⑤ **659.5 Elderly primigravida**
[0,1,3]   First pregnancy in a woman who will be 35 years of age or older at expected date of delivery

> *Excludes:* supervision only, in pregnancy (V23.81)

⑤ **659.6 Elderly multigravida**
[0,1,3]   Second or more pregnancy in a woman who will be 35 years of age or older at expected date of delivery

> *Excludes:* elderly primigravida 659.5
> supervision only, in pregnancy (V23.82)

⑤ **659.7 Abnormality in fetal heart rate or rhythm**
[0,1,3]   Depressed fetal heart tones
Fetal:
  bradycardia
  tachycardia
Fetal heart rate decelerations
Non-reassuring fetal heart rate or rhythm

⑤ **659.8 Other specified indications for care or intervention related to labor and delivery**
[0,1,3]   Pregnancy in female less than 16 years old at expected date of delivery
Very young maternal age

⑤ **659.9 Unspecified indication for care or intervention related to labor and delivery**
[0,1,3]

● Code new to this edition   ▲ Revision of existing code   ④ ⑤ Fourth or fifth digit required

COMPLICATIONS OCCURRING MAINLY IN THE COURSE OF LABOR AND DELIVERY (660-669)

The following fifth-digit subclassification is for use with categories 660-669 to denote the current episode of care:

0 **unspecified as to episode of care or not applicable**

1 **delivered, with or without mention of antepartum condition**

2 **delivered, with mention of postpartum complication**

3 **antepartum condition or complication**

4 **postpartum condition or complication**

⑤ **660** **Obstructed labor**

⑤ **660.0** **Obstruction caused by malposition of fetus at onset of labor**
[0,1,3] Any condition classifiable to 652, causing obstruction during labor
Use additional code from 652.0-652.9, if desired, to identify condition

⑤ **660.1** **Obstruction by bony pelvis**
[0,1,3] Any condition classifiable to 653, causing obstruction during labor
Use additional code from 653.0-653.9, if desired, to identify condition

⑤ **660.2** **Obstruction by abnormal pelvic soft tissues**
[0,1,3] Prolapse of anterior lip of cervix
Any condition classifiable to 654, causing obstruction during labor
Use additional code from 654.0-654.9, if desired, to identify condition

⑤ **660.3** **Deep transverse arrest and persistent occipitoposterior position**
[0,1,3]

⑤ **660.4** **Shoulder (girdle) dystocia**
[0,1,3] Impacted shoulders

⑤ **660.5** **Locked twins**
[0,1,3]

⑤ **660.6** **Failed trial of labor, unspecified**
[0,1,3] Failed trial of labor, without mention of condition or suspected condition

⑤ **660.7** **Failed forceps or vacuum extractor, unspecified**
[0,1,3] Application of ventouse or forceps, without mention of condition

⑤ **660.8** **Other causes of obstructed labor**
[0,1,3] Use additional code to identify condition

⑤ **660.9** **Unspecified obstructed labor**
[0,1,3] Dystocia:
NOS
fetal NOS
maternal NOS

⑤ **661** **Abnormality of forces of labor**

⑤ **661.0** **Primary uterine inertia**
[0,1,3] Failure of cervical dilation
Hypotonic uterine dysfunction, primary
Prolonged latent phase of labor

⑤ **661.1** **Secondary uterine inertia**
[0,1,3] Arrested active phase of labor
Hypotonic uterine dysfunction, secondary

⑤ **661.2** **Other and unspecified uterine inertia**
[0,1,3] Desultory labor   Poor contractions
Irregular labor   Slow slope active phase of labor

⑤ **661.3** **Precipitate labor**
[0,1,3]

⑤ **661.4** **Hypertonic, incoordinate, or prolonged uterine contractions**
[0,1,3] Cervical spasm
Contraction ring (dystocia)
Dyscoordinate labor
Hourglass contraction of uterus
Hypertonic uterine dysfunction
Incoordinate uterine action
Retraction ring (Bandl's) (pathological)
Tetanic contractions
Uterine dystocia NOS
Uterine spasm

	Add 4th or 5th digit		Nonspecific code		Unspecified code		Manifestation code

⑤ **661.9 Unspecified abnormality of labor**
[0,1,3]

⑤ **662** **Long labor**

⑤ **662.0 Prolonged first stage**
[0,1,3]

⑤ **662.1 Prolonged labor, unspecified**
[0,1,3]

⑤ **662.2 Prolonged second stage**
[0,1,3]

⑤ **662.3 Delayed delivery of second twin, triplet, etc.**
[0,1,3]

⑤ **663** **Umbilical cord complications**

⑤ **663.0 Prolapse of cord**
[0,1,3]   Presentation of cord

⑤ **663.1 Cord around neck, with compression**
[0,1,3]   Cord tightly around neck

⑤ **663.2 Other and unspecified cord entanglement, with compression**
[0,1,3]   Entanglement of cords of twins in mono-amniotic sac
           Knot in cord (with compression)

⑤ **663.3 Other and unspecified cord entanglement, without mention of compression**
[0,1,3]

⑤ **663.4 Short cord**
[0,1,3]

⑤ **663.5 Vasa previa**
[0,1,3]

⑤ **663.6 Vascular lesions of cord**
[0,1,3]   Bruising of cord
           Hematoma of cord
           Thrombosis of vessels of cord

⑤ **663.8 Other umbilical cord complications**
[0,1,3]   Velamentous insertion of umbilical cord

⑤ **663.9 Unspecified umbilical cord complication**
[0,1,3]

⑤ **664** **Trauma to perineum and vulva during delivery**
           Includes: damage from instruments
                      that from extension of episiotomy

⑤ **664.0 First-degree perineal laceration**
[0,1,4]   Perineal laceration, rupture, or tear involving:
               fourchette
               hymen
               labia
               skin
               vagina
               vulva

⑤ **664.1 Second-degree perineal laceration**
[0,1,4]   Perineal laceration, rupture, or tear (following episiotomy) involving:
               pelvic floor
               perineal muscles
               vaginal muscles

           | *Excludes:* | *that involving anal sphincter (664.2)* |

⑤ **664.2 Third-degree perineal laceration**
[0,1,4]   Perineal laceration, rupture, or tear (following episiotomy) involving:
               anal sphincter
               rectovaginal septum
               sphincter NOS

           | *Excludes:* | *that with anal or rectal mucosal laceration (664.3)* |

⑤ **664.3 Fourth-degree perineal laceration**
[0,1,4]   Perineal laceration, rupture, or tear as classifiable to 664.2 and involving also:
               anal mucosa
               rectal mucosa

● Code new   ▲ Revision of   ④ ⑤ Fourth or fifth
  to this edition   existing code   digit required

⑤ **664.4** **Unspecified perineal laceration**
[0,1,4]   Central laceration

⑤ **664.5** **Vulval and perineal hematoma**
[0,1,4]

⑤ **664.8** **Other specified trauma to perineum and vulva**
[0,1,4]

⑤ **664.9** **Unspecified trauma to perineum and vulva**
[0,1,4]

⑤ **665** **Other obstetrical trauma**
           Includes: damage from instruments

⑤ **665.0** **Rupture of uterus before onset of labor**
[0,1,3]

⑤ **665.1** **Rupture of uterus during labor**
[0,1]   Rupture of uterus NOS

⑤ **665.2** **Inversion of uterus**
[0,2,4]

⑤ **665.3** **Laceration of cervix**
[0,1,4]

⑤ **665.4** **High vaginal laceration**
[0,1,4]   Laceration of vaginal wall or sulcus without mention of perineal laceration

⑤ **665.5** **Other injury to pelvic organs**
[0,1,4]   Injury to:
              bladder
              urethra

⑤ **665.6** **Damage to pelvic joints and ligaments**
[0,1,4]   Avulsion of inner symphyseal cartilage
            Damage to coccyx
            Separation of symphysis (pubis)

⑤ **665.7** **Pelvic hematoma**
[0,1,2,4]   Hematoma of vagina

⑤ **665.8** **Other specified obstetrical trauma**
[0-4]

⑤ **665.9** **Unspecified obstetrical trauma**
[0-4]

⑤ **666** **Postpartum hemorrhage**

⑤ **666.0** **Third-stage hemorrhage**
[0,2,4]   Hemorrhage associated with retained, trapped, or adherent placenta
            Retained placenta NOS

⑤ **666.1** **Other immediate postpartum hemorrhage**
[0,2,4]   Atony of uterus with hemorrhage
            Hemorrhage within the first 24 hours following delivery of placenta
            Postpartum hemorrhage (atonic) NOS

            | *Excludes:* | atony of uterus without hemorrhage (669.8) |

⑤ **666.2** **Delayed and secondary postpartum hemorrhage**
[0,2,4]   Hemorrhage:
              after the first 24 hours following delivery
              associated with retained portions of placenta or membranes
            Postpartum hemorrhage specified as delayed or secondary
            Retained products of conception NOS, following delivery

⑤ **666.3** **Postpartum coagulation defects**
[0,2,4]   Postpartum afibrinogenemia
            Postpartum fibrinolysis

⑤ **667** **Retained placenta or membranes, without hemorrhage**

⑤ **667.0** **Retained placenta without hemorrhage**
[0,2,4]   Placenta accreta without hemorrhage
            Retained placenta: without hemorrhage
              NOS without hemorrhage
              total without hemorrhage

⑤ **667.1** **Retained portions of placenta or membranes, without hemorrhage**
[0,2,4]   Retained products of conception following delivery, without hemorrhage

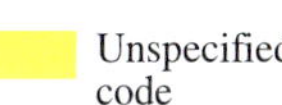

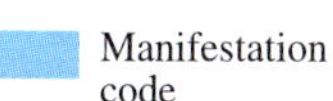

| | Add 4th or 5th digit | | Nonspecific code |

⑤ **668** **Complications of the administration of anesthetic or other sedation in labor and delivery**
Includes: complications arising from the administration of a general or local anesthetic, analgesic, or other sedation in labor and delivery

Excludes: *reaction to spinal or lumbar puncture (349.0)*
spinal headache (349.0)

Use additional code(s) to further specify complication

⑤ **668.0** **Pulmonary complications**
[0-4] Inhalation [aspiration] of stomach contents or secretions following anesthesia or other sedation in labor or delivery
Mendelson's syndrome following anesthesia or other sedation in labor or delivery
Pressure collapse of lung following anesthesia or other sedation in labor or delivery

⑤ **668.1** **Cardiac complications**
[0-4] Cardiac arrest or failure following anesthesia or other sedation in labor and delivery

⑤ **668.2** **Central nervous system complications**
[0-4] Cerebral anoxia following anesthesia or other sedation in labor and delivery

⑤ **668.8** **Other complications of anesthesia or other sedation in labor and delivery**
[0-4]

⑤ **668.9** **Unspecified complication of anesthesia and other sedation**
[0-4]

⑤ **669** **Other complications of labor and delivery, not elsewhere classified**

⑤ **669.0** **Maternal distress**
[0-4] Metabolic disturbance in labor and delivery

⑤ **669.1** **Shock during or following labor and delivery**
[0-4] Obstetric shock

⑤ **669.2** **Maternal hypotension syndrome**
[0-4]

⑤ **669.3** **Acute renal failure following labor and delivery**
[0,2,4]

⑤ **669.4** **Other complications of obstetrical surgery and procedures**
[0-4] Cardiac:
arrest following cesarean or other obstetrical surgery or procedure, including delivery NOS
failure following cesarean or other obstetrical surgery or procedure, including delivery NOS
Cerebral anoxia following cesarean or other obstetrical surgery or procedure, including delivery NOS

Excludes: *complications of obstetrical surgical wounds (674.1-674.3)*

⑤ **669.5** **Forceps or vacuum extractor delivery without mention of indication**
[0,1] Delivery by ventouse, without mention of indication

⑤ **669.6** **Breech extraction, without mention of indication**
[0,1]

Excludes: *breech delivery NOS (652.2)*

⑤ **669.7** **Cesarean delivery, without mention of indication**
[0,1]

⑤ **669.8** **Other complications of labor and delivery**
[0-4]

⑤ **669.9** **Unspecified complication of labor and delivery**
[0-4]

● Code new to this edition   ▲ Revision of existing code   ④ ⑤ Fourth or fifth digit required

COMPLICATIONS OF THE PUERPERIUM (670-677)

Note: Categories 671 and 673-676 include the listed conditions even if they occur during pregnancy or childbirth.

The following fifth-digit subclassification is for use with categories 670-676 to denote the current episode of care:

0   **unspecified as to episode of care or not applicable**

1   **delivered, with or without mention of antepartum condition**

2   **delivered, with mention of postpartum complication**

3   **antepartum condition or complication**

4   **postpartum condition or complication**

⑤ **670** **Major puerperal infection**
[0,2,4]

Puerperal:	Puerperal:
endometritis	peritonitis
fever (septic)	pyemia
pelvic:	salpingitis
cellulitis	septicemia
sepsis	

Use 0 as fourth-digit for this category

> *Excludes:* *infection following abortion (639.0)*
> *minor genital tract infection following delivery (646.6)*
> *puerperal pyrexia NOS (672)*
> *puerperal fever NOS (672)*
> *puerperal pyrexia of unknown origin (672)*
> *urinary tract infection following delivery (646.6)*

⑤ **671** **Venous complications in pregnancy and the puerperium**

⑤ **671.0** **Varicose veins of legs**
[0-4]   Varicose veins NOS

⑤ **671.1** **Varicose veins of vulva and perineum**
[0-4]

⑤ **671.2** **Superficial thrombophlebitis**
[0-4]   Thrombophlebitis (superficial)

⑤ **671.3** **Deep phlebothrombosis, antepartum**
[0,1,3]   Deep-vein thrombosis, antepartum

⑤ **671.4** **Deep phlebothrombosis, postpartum**
[0,2,4]   Deep-vein thrombosis, postpartum
       Pelvic thrombophlebitis, postpartum
       Phlegmasia alba dolens (puerperal)

⑤ **671.5** **Other phlebitis and thrombosis**
[0-4]   Cerebral venous thrombosis
       Thrombosis of intracranial venous sinus

⑤ **671.8** **Other venous complications**
[0-4]   Hemorrhoids

⑤ **671.9** **Unspecified venous complication**
[0-4]   Phlebitis NOS
       Thrombosis NOS

⑤ **672** **Pyrexia of unknown origin during the puerperium**
[0,2,4]   Puerperal fever NOS
       Postpartum fever NOS

Use 0 as fourth-digit for this category

⑤ **673** **Obstetrical pulmonary embolism**
Includes: pulmonary emboli in pregnancy, childbirth, or the puerperium, or specified as puerperal

> *Excludes:* *embolism following abortion (639.6)*

⑤ **673.0** **Obstetrical air embolism**
[0-4]

⑤ **673.1** **Amniotic fluid embolism**
[0-4]

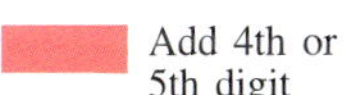

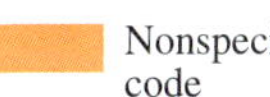

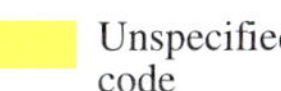

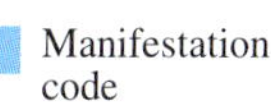

⑤ **673.2 Obstetrical blood-clot embolism**
[0-4] Puerperal pulmonary embolism NOS

⑤ **673.3 Obstetrical pyemic and septic embolism**
[0-4]

⑤ **673.8 Other pulmonary embolism**
[0-4] Fat embolism

⑤ **674 Other and unspecified complications of the puerperium, not elsewhere classified**

⑤ **674.0 Cerebrovascular disorders in the puerperium**
[0-4] Any condition classifiable to 430-434, 436-437 occurring during pregnancy, childbirth, or the puerperium, or specified as puerperal

Excludes: *intracranial venous sinus thrombosis (671.5)*

⑤ **674.1 Disruption of cesarean wound**
[0,2,4] Dehiscence or disruption of uterine wound

Excludes: *uterine rupture before onset of labor (665.0)*
uterine rupture during labor (665.1)

⑤ **674.2 Disruption of perineal wound**
[0,2,4] Breakdown of perineum
Disruption of wound of:
  episiotomy
  perineal laceration
Secondary perineal tear

⑤ **674.3 Other complications of obstetrical surgical wounds**
[0,2,4] Hematoma of cesarean section or perineal wound
Hemorrhage of cesarean section or perineal wound
Infection of cesarean section or perineal wound

Excludes: *damage from instruments in delivery (664.0-665.9)*

⑤ **674.4 Placental polyp**
[0,2,4]

⑤ **674.5 Peripartum cardiomyopathy**
[0-4] Postpartum cardiomyopathy

⑤ **674.8 Other**
[0,2,4] Hepatorenal syndrome, following delivery
Postpartum:
  subinvolution of uterus
  uterine hypertrophy

⑤ **674.9 Unspecified**
[0,2,4] Sudden death of unknown cause during the puerperium

⑤ **675 Infections of the breast and nipple associated with childbirth**
Includes: the listed conditions during pregnancy, childbirth, or the puerperium

⑤ **675.0 Infections of nipple**
[0-4] Abscess of nipple

⑤ **675.1 Abscess of breast**
[0-4] Abscess:
  mammary
  subareolar
  submammary
Mastitis:
  purulent
  retromammary
  submammary

⑤ **675.2 Nonpurulent mastitis**
[0-4] Lymphangitis of breast
Mastitis:
  NOS
  interstitial
  parenchymatous

⑤ **675.8 Other specified infections of the breast and nipple**
[0-4]

⑤ **675.9 Unspecified infection of the breast and nipple**
[0-4]

● Code new to this edition   ▲ Revision of existing code   ④ ⑤ Fourth or fifth digit required

⑤ **676 Other disorders of the breast associated with childbirth and disorders of lactation**
Includes: the listed conditions during pregnancy, the puerperium, or lactation

⑤ **676.0 Retracted nipple**
[0-4]

⑤ **676.1 Cracked nipple**
[0-4]   Fissure of nipple

⑤ **676.2 Engorgement of breasts**
[0-4]

⑤ **676.3 Other and unspecified disorder of breast**
[0-4]

⑤ **676.4 Failure of lactation**
[0-4]   Agalactia

⑤ **676.5 Suppressed lactation**
[0-4]

⑤ **676.6 Galactorrhea**
[0-4]

> Excludes: *galactorrhea not associated with childbirth (611.6)*

⑤ **676.8 Other disorders of lactation**
[0-4]   Galactocele

⑤ **676.9 Unspecified disorder of lactation**
[0-4]

677 Late effect of complication of pregnancy, childbirth, and the puerperium
Note: This category is to be used to indicate conditions in 632-648.9 and 651-676.9 as the cause of the late effect, themselves classifiable elsewhere. The "late effects" include conditions specified as such, or as sequelae, which may occur at any time after the puerperium.
Code first any sequelae

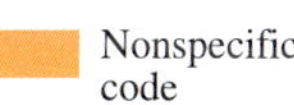

● Code new
to this edition

▲ Revision of
existing code

④ ⑤ Fourth or fifth
digit required

12. DISEASES OF THE SKIN AND SUBCUTANEOUS TISSUE (680-709)

INFECTIONS OF SKIN AND SUBCUTANEOUS TISSUE (680-686)

Excludes: certain infections of skin classified under "Infectious and Parasitic Diseases," such
as:
erysipelas (035)
erysipeloid of Rosenbach (027.1)
herpes:
simplex (054.0-054.9)
zoster (053.0-053.9)
molluscum contagiosum (078.0)
viral warts (078.1)

680 Carbuncle and furuncle
Includes: boil
furunculosis

680.0 Face
Ear [any part]
Face [any part, except eye]
Nose (septum)
Temple (region)

Excludes: eyelid (373.13)
lacrimal apparatus (375.31)
orbit (376.01)

680.1 Neck

680.2 Trunk

Abdominal wall	Flank
Back [any part, except buttocks]	Groin
	Pectoral region
Breast	Perineum
Chest wall	Umbilicus

Excludes: buttocks (680.5)
external genital organs:
female (616.4)
male (607.2, 608.4)

680.3 Upper arm and forearm
Arm [any part, except hand]
Axilla
Shoulder

680.4 Hand

Finger [any]	Wrist
Thumb	

680.5 Buttock
Anus
Gluteal region

680.6 Leg, except foot

Ankle	Knee
Hip	Thigh

680.7 Foot
Heel
Toe

680.8 Other specified sites
Head [any part, except face]
Scalp

Excludes: external genital organs:
female (616.4)
male (607.2, 608.4)

680.9 Unspecified site

Boil NOS	Furuncle NOS
Carbuncle NOS	

681 Cellulitis and abscess of finger and toe
Includes: that with lymphangitis
Use additional code, if desired, to identify organism, such as Staphylococcus (041.1)

⑤ **681.0 Finger**

681.00 Cellulitis and abscess, unspecified

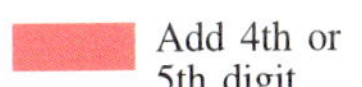
Add 4th or
5th digit

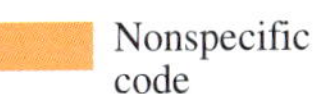
Nonspecific
code

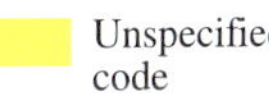
Unspecified
code

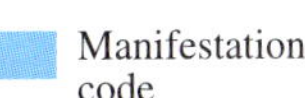
Manifestation
code

    681.01 **Felon**
          Pulp abscess
          Whitlow

    Excludes: *herpetic whitlow (054.6)*

    681.02 **Onychia and paronychia of finger**
          Panaritium of finger
          Perionychia of finger

⑤ **681.1** **Toe**

    681.10 **Cellulitis and abscess, unspecified**

    681.11 **Onychia and paronychia of toe**
          Panaritium of toe
          Perionychia of toe

681.9 **Cellulitis and abscess of unspecified digit**
      Infection of nail NOS

682 **Other cellulitis and abscess**
    Includes: abscess (acute) (with lymphangitis) except of finger or toe
              cellulitis (diffuse) (with lymphangitis) except of finger or toe
              lymphangitis, acute (with lymphangitis) except of finger or toe

Use additional code, if desired, to identify organism, such as Staphylococcus (041.1)

    Excludes: *lymphangitis (chronic) (subacute) (457.2)*

682.0 **Face**
    Cheek, external   Nose, external
    Chin   Submandibular
    Forehead   Temple (region)

    Excludes: *ear [any part] (380.10-380.16)*
             eyelid (373.13)
             lacrimal apparatus (375.31)
             lip (528.5)
             mouth (528.3)
             nose (internal) (478.1)
             orbit (376.01)

682.1 **Neck**

682.2 **Trunk**
    Abdominal wall   Groin
    Back [any part, except   Pectoral region
       buttock]   Perineum
    Chest wall   Umbilicus, except newborn
    Flank

    Excludes: *anal and rectal regions (566)*
             breast:
               NOS (611.0)
               puerperal (675.1)
             external genital organs:
               female (616.3-616.4)
               male (604.0, 607.2, 608.4)
             umbilicus, newborn (771.4)

682.3 **Upper arm and forearm**
    Arm [any part, except hand]
    Axilla
    Shoulder

    Excludes: *hand (682.4)*

682.4 **Hand, except fingers and thumb**
    Wrist

    Excludes: *finger and thumb (681.00-681.02)*

682.5 **Buttock**
    Gluteal region

    Excludes: *anal and rectal regions (566)*

682.6 **Leg, except foot**
    Ankle   Knee
    Hip   Thigh

   ● Code new   ▲ Revision of   ④ ⑤ Fourth or fifth
     to this edition   existing code   digit required

682.7 Foot, except toes
Heel

Excludes: toe (681.10-681.11)

682.8 Other specified sites
Head [except face]
Scalp

Excludes: face (682.0)

682.9 Unspecified site
Abscess NOS
Cellulitis NOS

Lymphangitis, acute NOS

Excludes: lymphangitis NOS (457.2)

683 Acute lymphadenitis
Abscess (acute), lymph gland or node, except mesenteric
Adenitis, acute, lymph gland or node, except mesenteric
Lymphadenitis, acute, lymph gland or node, except mesenteric

Use additional code, if desired, to identify organism, such as Staphylococcus (041.1)

Excludes: enlarged glands NOS (785.6)

lymphadenitis:
chronic or subacute, except mesenteric (289.1)
mesenteric (acute) (chronic) (subacute) (289.2)
unspecified (289.3)

684 Impetigo
Impetiginization of other dermatoses
Impetigo (contagiosa) [any site] [any organism]:
bullous
circinate
neonatorum
simplex
Pemphigus neonatorum

Excludes: impetigo herpetiformis (694.3)

685 Pilonidal cyst
Includes:

fistula, coccygeal or pilonidal
sinus, coccygeal or pilonidal

685.0 With abscess

685.1 Without mention of abscess

686 Other local infections of skin and subcutaneous tissue
Use additional code, if desired, to identify any infectious organism (041.0-041.8)

⑤ **686.0 Pyoderma**
Dermatitis:
purulent
septic
suppurative

686.00   Pyoderma, unspecified

686.01   Pyoderma gangrenosum

686.09   Other pyoderma

686.1 Pyogenic granuloma
Granuloma:
septic
suppurative
telangiectaticum

Excludes: pyogenic granuloma of oral mucosa (528.9)

686.8 Other specified local infections of skin and subcutaneous tissue
Bacterid (pustular)
Dermatitis vegetans

Ecthyma
Perlèche

Excludes: dermatitis infectiosa eczematoides (690.8)
panniculitis (729.30-729.39)

686.9 Unspecified local infection of skin and subcutaneous tissue
Fistula of skin NOS
Skin infection NOS

Excludes: fistula to skin from internal organs—see Alphabetic Index

Add 4th or 5th digit	Nonspecific code	Unspecified code	Manifestation code

OTHER INFLAMMATORY CONDITIONS OF SKIN AND SUBCUTANEOUS TISSUE (690-698)

Excludes: *panniculitis (729.30-729.39)*

690 Erythematosquamous dermatosis

Excludes: *eczematous dermatitis of eyelid (373.31)*
parakeratosis variegata (696.2)
psoriasis (696.0-696.1)
seborrheic keratosis (702.11-702.19)

⑤ **690.1 Seborrheic dermatitis**

690.10 Seborrheic dermatitis, unspecified
Seborrheic dermatitis NOS

690.11 Seborrhea capitis
Cradle cap

690.12 Seborrheic infantile dermatitis

690.18 Other seborrheic dermatitis

690.8 Other erythematosquamous dermatosis

691 Atopic dermatitis and related conditions

691.0 Diaper or napkin rash
Ammonia dermatitis
Diaper or napkin:
  dermatitis
  erythema
  rash
Psoriasiform napkin eruption

691.8 Other atopic dermatitis and related conditions

Atopic dermatitis
Besnier's prurigo
Eczema:
  atopic
  flexural
  intrinsic (allergic)

Neurodermatitis:
  atopic
  diffuse (of Brocq)

692 Contact dermatitis and other eczema
Includes:

dermatitis:
  NOS
  contact
  occupational
  venenata

eczema (acute) (chronic):
  NOS
  allergic
  erythematous
  occupational

Excludes: *allergy NOS (995.3)*
contact dermatitis of eyelids (373.32)
dermatitis due to substances taken internally (693.0-693.9)
eczema of external ear (380.22)
perioral dermatitis (695.3)
urticarial reactions (708.0-708.9, 995.1)

692.0 Due to detergents

692.1 Due to oils and greases

692.2 Due to solvents
Dermatitis due to solvents of:
  chlorocompound group
  cyclohexane group
  ester group
  glycol group
  hydrocarbon group
  ketone group

● Code new
to this edition

▲ Revision of
existing code

④ ⑤ Fourth or fifth
digit required

692.3 Due to drugs and medicines in contact with skin

Dermatitis (allergic) (contact) due to:
arnica
fungicides
iodine
keratolytics
mercurials
neomycin
pediculocides
phenols
scabicides
any drug applied to skin
Dermatitis medicamentosa due to drug applied to skin

Use additional E code, if desired, to identify drug

Excludes: *allergy NOS due to drugs (995.27)*
dermatitis due to ingested drugs (693.0)
dermatitis medicamentosa NOS (693.0)

692.4 Due to other chemical products

Dermatitis due to:
acids
adhesive plaster
alkalis
caustics
dichromate

Dermatitis due to:
insecticide
nylon
plastic
rubber

692.5 Due to food in contact with skin

Dermatitis, contact, due to:
cereals
fish
flour

Dermatitis, contact, due to:
fruit
meat
milk

Excludes: *dermatitis due to:*
dyes (692.89)
ingested foods (693.1)
preservatives (692.89)

692.6 Due to plants [except food]

Dermatitis due to:
lacquer tree [Rhus verniciflua]
poison ivy [Rhus toxicodendron]
poison oak [Rhus diversiloba]
poison sumac [Rhus venenata]
poison vine [Rhus radicans]
primrose [Primula]
ragweed [Senecio jacobae]
other plants in contact with the skin

Excludes: *allergy NOS due to pollen (477.0)*
nettle rash (708.8)

⑤ **692.7 Due to solar radiation**

Excludes: *sunburn due to other ultraviolet radiation exposure (692.82)*

692.70 Unspecified dermatitis due to sun

692.71 Sunburn
First degree sunburn
Sunburn NOS

692.72 Acute dermatitis due to solar radiation
Berloque dermatitis
Photoallergic response
Phototoxic response
Polymorphus light eruption
Acute solar skin damage NOS

Excludes: *sunburn (692.71, 692.76-692.77)*
Use additional E code, if desired, to identify drug, if drug induced

692.73 Actinic reticuloid and actinic granuloma

692.74 Other chronic dermatitis due to solar radiation
Solar elastosis
Chronic solar skin damage NOS

Excludes: *actinic [solar] keratosis (702.0)*

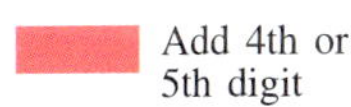

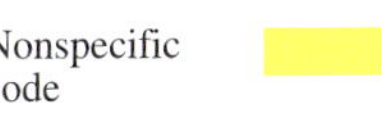

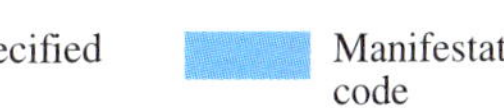

692.75   **Disseminated superficial actinic porokeratosis (DSAP)**

692.76   **Sunburn of second degree**

692.77   **Sunburn of third degree**

692.79   **Other dermatitis due to solar radiation**
Hydroa aestivale
Photodermatitis due to sun
Photosensitiveness due to sun
Solar skin damage NOS

⑤ **692.8**   **Due to other specified agents**

692.81   **Dermatitis due to cosmetics**

692.82   **Dermatitis due to other radiation**
Infrared rays
Light, except from sun
Radiation NOS
Ultraviolet rays, except from sun
X-rays
Tanning bed

Excludes: that due to solar radiation (692.70-692.79)

692.83   **Dermatitis due to metals**
Jewelry

692.84   **Due to animal (cat) (dog) dander**
Due to animal (cat) (dog) hair

692.89   **Other**
Dermatitis due to:
  cold weather
  dyes
  hot weather
  preservatives

Excludes: allergy (NOS) (rhinitis) due to animal hair or dander (477.2)
    allergy to dust (477.8)
    sunburn (692.71, 692.76-692.77)

692.9   **Unspecified cause**
Dermatitis: Eczema NOS
  NOS
  contact NOS
  venenata NOS

693   **Dermatitis due to substances taken internally**

Excludes: adverse effect NOS of drugs and medicines (995.20)
    allergy NOS (995.3)
    contact dermatitis (692.0-692.9)
    urticarial reactions (708.0-708.9, 995.1)

693.0   **Due to drugs and medicines**
Dermatitis medicamentosa NOS

Use additional E code, if desired, to identify drug

Excludes: that due to drugs in contact with skin (692.3)

693.1   **Due to food**

693.8   **Due to other specified substances taken internally**

693.9   **Due to unspecified substance taken internally**

Excludes: dermatitis NOS (692.9)

694   **Bullous dermatoses**

694.0   **Dermatitis herpetiformis**
Dermatosis herpetiformis
Duhring's disease
Hydroa herpetiformis

Excludes: herpes gestationis (646.8)
    dermatitis herpetiformis:
     juvenile (694.2)
     senile (694.5)

694.1   **Subcorneal pustular dermatosis**
Sneddon-Wilkinson disease or syndrome

● Code new
to this edition

▲ Revision of
existing code

④ ⑤ Fourth or fifth
digit required

694.2 Juvenile dermatitis herpetiformis
Juvenile pemphigoid

694.3 Impetigo herpetiformis

694.4 Pemphigus

Pemphigus:
  NOS
  erythematosus
  foliaceus

Pemphigus:
  malignant
  vegetans
  vulgaris

Excludes: *pemphigus neonatorum (684)*

694.5 Pemphigoid
Benign pemphigus NOS
Bullous pemphigoid
Herpes circinatus bullosus
Senile dermatitis herpetiformis

⑤ **694.6 Benign mucous membrane pemphigoid**
Cicatricial pemphigoid
Mucosynechial atrophic bullous dermatitis

694.60 Without mention of ocular involvement

694.61 With ocular involvement
Ocular pemphigus

694.8 Other specified bullous dermatoses

Excludes: *herpes gestationis (646.8)*

694.9 Unspecified bullous dermatoses

695 Erythematous conditions

695.0 Toxic erythema
Erythema venenatum

695.1 Erythema multiforme

Erythema iris
Herpes iris
Lyell's syndrome

Scalded skin syndrome
Stevens-Johnson syndrome
Toxic epidermal necrolysis

695.2 Erythema nodosum

Excludes: *tuberculous erythema nodosum (017.1)*

695.3 Rosacea

Acne:
  erythematosa
  rosacea

Perioral dermatitis
Rhinophyma

695.4 Lupus erythematosus
Lupus:
  erythematodes (discoid)
  erythematosus (discoid), not disseminated

Excludes: *lupus (vulgaris) NOS (017.0)*
          systemic [disseminated] lupus erythematosus (710.0)

⑤ **695.8 Other specified erythematous conditions**

695.81 Ritter's disease
Dermatitis exfoliativa neonatorum

695.89 Other
Erythema intertrigo
Intertrigo
Pityriasis rubra (Hebra)

Excludes: *mycotic intertrigo (111.0-111.9)*

695.9 Unspecified erythematous condition
Erythema NOS
Erythroderma (secondary)

696 Psoriasis and similar disorders

696.0 Psoriatic arthropathy

696.1 Other psoriasis
Acrodermatitis continua
Dermatitis repens
Psoriasis:
  NOS
  any type, except arthropathic

Excludes: *psoriatic arthropathy (696.0)*

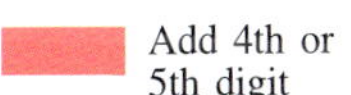

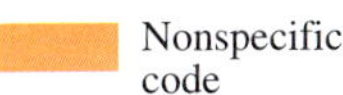

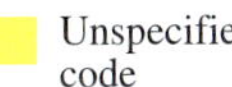

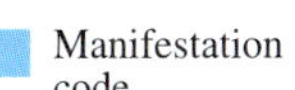

696.2 Parapsoriasis
  Parakeratosis variegata
  Parapsoriasis lichenoides chronica
  Pityriasis lichenoides et varioliformis

696.3 Pityriasis rosea
  Pityriasis circinata (et maculata)

696.4 Pityriasis rubra pilaris
  Devergie's disease
  Lichen ruber acuminatus

  Excludes: *pityriasis rubra (Hebra) (695.89)*

696.5 Other and unspecified pityriasis
  Pityriasis:
    NOS
    alba
    streptogenes

  Excludes: *pityriasis simplex (690.18)*
       pityriasis versicolor (111.0)

696.8 Other

697 Lichen

  Excludes: *lichen:*

       obtusus corneus (698.3)
       pilaris (congenital) (757.39)
       ruber acuminatus (696.4)
       sclerosus et atrophicus (701.0)
       scrofulosus (017.0)
       simplex chronicus (698.3)
       spinulosus (congenital) (757.39)
       urticatus (698.2)

697.0 Lichen planus
  Lichen:
    planopilaris
    ruber planus

697.1 Lichen nitidus
  Pinkus' disease

697.8 Other lichen, not elsewhere classified
  Lichen:
    ruber moniliforme
    striata

697.9 Lichen, unspecified

698 Pruritus and related conditions

  Excludes: *pruritus specified as psychogenic (306.3)*

698.0 Pruritus ani
  Perianal itch

698.1 Pruritus of genital organs

698.2 Prurigo
  Lichen urticatus
  Prurigo:
    NOS
    Hebra's
    mitis
    simplex
  Urticaria papulosa (Hebra)

  Excludes: *prurigo nodularis (698.3)*

698.3 Lichenification and lichen simplex chronicus
  Hyde's disease
  Neurodermatitis (circumscripta) (local)
  Prurigo nodularis

  Excludes: *neurodermatitis, diffuse (of Brocq) (691.8)*

698.4 Dermatitis factitia [artefacta]
  Dermatitis ficta
  Neurotic excoriation

Use additional code, if desired, to identify any associated mental disorder

● Code new
  to this edition

▲ Revision of
  existing code

④ ⑤ Fourth or fifth
  digit required

698.8 **Other specified pruritic conditions**
Pruritus:
  hiemalis
  senilis
Winter itch

698.9 **Unspecified pruritic disorder**
Itch NOS
Pruritus NOS

OTHER DISEASES OF SKIN AND SUBCUTANEOUS TISSUE (700-709)

Excludes: *conditions confined to eyelids (373.0-374.9)*
         congenital conditions of skin, hair, and nails (757.0-757.9)

700 **Corns and callosities**
Callus
Clavus

701 **Other hypertrophic and atrophic conditions of skin**

Excludes: *dermatomyositis (710.3)*
         hereditary edema of legs (757.0)
         scleroderma (generalized) (710.1)

701.0 **Circumscribed scleroderma**
Addison's keloid
Dermatosclerosis, localized
Lichen sclerosus et atrophicus
Morphea
Scleroderma, circumscribed or localized

701.1 **Keratoderma, acquired**
Acquired:
  ichthyosis
  keratoderma palmaris et plantaris
Elastosis perforans serpiginosa
Hyperkeratosis:
  NOS
  follicularis in cutem penetrans
  palmoplantaris climacterica
Keratoderma:
  climactericum
  tylodes, progressive
Keratosis (blennorrhagica)

Excludes: *Darier's disease [keratosis follicularis] (congenital) (757.39)*
         keratosis:
           arsenical (692.4)
           gonococcal (098.81)

701.2 **Acquired acanthosis nigricans**
Keratosis nigricans

701.3 **Striae atrophicae**
Atrophic spots of skin
Atrophoderma maculatum
Atrophy blanche (of Milian)
Degenerative colloid atrophy
Senile degenerative atrophy
Striae distensae

701.4 **Keloid scar**
Cheloid
Hypertrophic scar
Keloid

701.5 **Other abnormal granulation tissue**
Excessive granulation

701.8 **Other specified hypertrophic and atrophic conditions of skin**
Acrodermatitis atrophicans chronica
Atrophia cutis senilis
Atrophoderma neuriticum
Confluent and reticulate papillomatosis
Cutis laxa senilis
Elastosis senilis
Folliculitis ulerythematosa reticulata
Gougerot-Carteaud syndrome or disease

Add 4th or 5th digit	Nonspecific code	Unspecified code	Manifestation code

701.9 **Unspecified hypertrophic and atrophic conditions of skin**
Atrophoderma

702 **Other dermatoses**

Excludes: carcinoma in situ (232.0-232.9)

702.0 **Actinic keratosis**

⑤ **702.1** **Seborrheic keratosis**

702.11 **Inflamed seborrheic keratosis**

702.19 **Other seborrheic keratosis**
Seborrheic keratosis NOS

702.8 **Other specified dermatoses**

703 **Diseases of nail**

Excludes: congenital anomalies (757.5)
onychia and paronychia (681.02, 681.11)

703.0 **Ingrowing nail**
Ingrowing nail with infection
Unguis incarnatus

Excludes: infection, nail NOS (681.9)

703.8 **Other specified diseases of nail**
Dystrophia unguium
Hypertrophy of nail
Koilonychia
Leukonychia (punctata) (striata)
Onychauxis
Onychogryposis
Onycholysis

703.9 **Unspecified disease of nail**

704 **Diseases of hair and hair follicles**

Excludes: congenital anomalies (757.4)

⑤ **704.0** **Alopecia**

Excludes: madarosis (374.55)
syphilitic alopecia (091.82)

704.00 **Alopecia, unspecified**
Baldness
Loss of hair

704.01 **Alopecia areata**
Ophiasis

704.02 **Telogen effluvim**

704.09 **Other**
Folliculitis decalvans
Hypotrichosis:
NOS
postinfectional NOS
Pseudopelade

704.1 **Hirsutism**
Hypertrichosis:
NOS
lanuginosa, acquired
Polytrichia

Excludes: hypertrichosis of eyelid (374.54)

704.2 **Abnormalities of the hair**
Atrophic hair
Clastothrix
Fragilitas crinium
Trichiasis:
NOS
cicatrical
Trichorrhexis (nodosa)

Excludes: trichiasis of eyelid (374.05)

704.3 **Variations in hair color**
Canities (premature)
Grayness, hair (premature)
Heterochromia of hair
Poliosis:
NOS
circumscripta, acquired

● Code new
to this edition
▲ Revision of
existing code
④ ⑤ Fourth or fifth
digit required

704.8 Other specified diseases of hair and hair follicles
Folliculitis:
  NOS
  abscedens et suffodiens
  pustular
Perifolliculitis:
  NOS
  capitis abscedens et suffodiens
  scalp
Sycosis:
  NOS
  barbae [not parasitic]
  lupoid
  vulgaris

704.9 Unspecified disease of hair and hair follicles

705 Disorders of sweat glands

705.0 Anhidrosis
Hypohidrosis
Oligohidrosis

705.1 Prickly heat
Heat rash
Miliaria rubra (tropicalis)
Sudamina

⑤ **705.2 Focal hyperhidrosis**

Excludes: generalized (secondary) hyperhidrosis (780.8)

705.21 Primary focal hyperhidrosis
Focal hyperhidrosis NOS
Hyperhidrosis NOS
Hyperhidrosis of:
  axilla
  face
  palms
  soles

705.22 Secondary focal hyperhidrosis
Frey's syndrome

⑤ **705.8 Other specified disorders of sweat glands**

705.81 Dyshidrosis
Cheiropompholyx
Pompholyx

705.82 Fox-Fordyce disease

705.83 Hidradenitis
Hidradenitis suppurativa

705.89 Other
Bromhidrosis
Chromhidrosis
Granulosis rubra nasi
Urhidrosis

Excludes: generalized hyperhidrosis (780.8)
  hidrocystoma (216.0-216.9)

705.9 Unspecified disorder of sweat glands
Disorder of sweat glands NOS

706 Diseases of sebaceous glands

706.0 Acne varioliformis
Acne:
  frontalis
  necrotica

706.1 Other acne
Acne:
  NOS
  conglobata
  cystic
  pustular
  vulgaris
Blackhead
Comedo

Excludes: acne rosacea (695.3)

706.2 Sebaceous cyst
Atheroma, skin
Keratin cyst
Wen

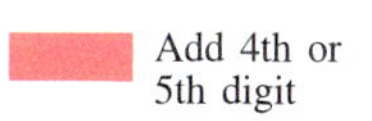

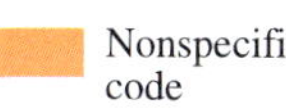

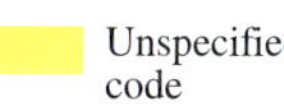

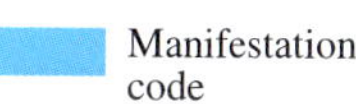

706.3 Seborrhea
Excludes: *seborrhea:*
      capitis (690.11)
      sicca (690.18)
      seborrheic dermatitis (690.11)
      seborrheic keratosis (702.11-702.19)

706.8 Other specified diseases of sebaceous glands
Asteatosis (cutis)
Xerosis cutis

706.9 Unspecified disease of sebaceous glands

707 Chronic ulcer of skin
Includes: non-infected sinus of skin
          non-healing ulcer

Excludes: *specific infections classified under "Infectious and Parasitic Diseases"*
      (001.0-136.9)
      varicose ulcer (454.0, 454.2)

⑤ **707.0 Decubitus ulcer**
Bed sore   Plaster ulcer
Decubitus ulcer [any site]   Pressure ulcer

    707.00 Unspecified site

    707.01 Elbow

    707.02 Upper back
           Shoulder blades

    707.03 Lower back
           Sacrum

    707.04 Hip

    707.05 Buttock

    707.06 Ankle

    707.07 Heel

    707.09 Other site
           Head

⑤ **707.1 Ulcer of lower limbs, except decubitus**
Ulcer, chronic, of lower limb:
   neurogenic of lower limb
   trophic of lower limb

Code, if applicable, any causal condition first:
   atherosclerosis of the extremities with ulceration (440.23)
   chronic venous hypertension with ulcer (459.31)
   chronic venous hypertension with ulcer and inflammation (459.33)
   diabetes mellitus (250.80-250.83)
   postphlebetic syndrome with ulcer (459.11)
   postphlebetic syndrome with ulcer and inflammation (459.13)

    707.10 Ulcer of lower limb, unspecified

    707.11 Ulcer of thigh

    707.12 Ulcer of calf

    707.13 Ulcer of ankle

    707.14 Ulcer of heel and midfoot
           Plantar surface of midfoot

    707.15 Ulcer of other part of foot
           Toes

    707.19 Ulcer of other part of lower limb

707.8 Chronic ulcer of other specified sites
Ulcer, chronic, of other specified sites:
   neurogenic of other specified sites
   trophic of other specified sites

707.9 Chronic ulcer of unspecified site
Chronic ulcer NOS   Tropical ulcer NOS
Trophic ulcer NOS   Ulcer of skin NOS

● Code new   ▲ Revision of   ④ ⑤ Fourth or fifth
   to this edition   existing code   digit required

708 Urticaria

Excludes: edema:
>   angioneurotic (995.1)
>   Quincke's (995.1)
> hereditary angioedema (277.6)
> urticaria:
>   giant (995.1)
>   papulosa (Hebra) (698.2)
>   pigmentosa (juvenile) (congenital) (757.33)

708.0 Allergic urticaria

708.1 Idiopathic urticaria

708.2 Urticaria due to cold and heat
Thermal urticaria

708.3 Dermatographic urticaria
Dermatographia
Factitial urticaria

708.4 Vibratory urticaria

708.5 Cholinergic urticaria

708.8 Other specified urticaria
Nettle rash
Urticaria:
  chronic
  recurrent periodic

708.9 Urticaria, unspecified
Hives NOS

709 Other disorders of skin and subcutaneous tissue

⑤ **709.0 Dyschromia**

Excludes: albinism (270.2)
>   pigmented nevus (216.0-216.9)
> that of eyelid (374.52-374.53)

709.00 Dyschromia, unspecified

709.01 Vitiligo

709.09 Other

709.1 Vascular disorders of skin
Angioma serpiginosum
Purpura (primary) annularis telangiectodes

709.2 Scar conditions and fibrosis of skin
Adherent scar (skin)
Cicatrix
Disfigurement (due to scar)
Fibrosis, skin NOS
Scar NOS

Excludes: keloid scar (701.4)

709.3 Degenerative skin disorders

Calcinosis: Degeneration, skin
  circumscripta   Deposits, skin
  cutis   Senile dermatosis NOS
Colloid milium   Subcutaneous calcification

709.4 Foreign body granuloma of skin and subcutaneous tissue

Excludes: residual foreign body without granuloma of skin and subcutaneous tissue (729.6)
> that of muscle (728.82)

709.8 Other specified disorders of skin
Epithelial hyperplasia
Menstrual dermatosis
Vesicular eruption

709.9 Unspecified disorder of skin and subcutaneous tissue
Dermatosis NOS

13. DISEASES OF THE MUSCULOSKELETAL SYSTEM AND CONNECTIVE TISSUE (710-739)

The following fifth-digit subclassification is for use with categories 711-712, 715-716, 718-719, and 730:

0   **site unspecified**

1   **shoulder region**
    Acromioclavicular joint(s)
    Glenohumeral joint(s)
    Sternoclavicular joint(s)
    Clavicle
    Scapula

2   **upper arm**
    Elbow joint   Humerus

3   **forearm**
    Radius   Wrist joint
    Ulna

4   **hand**
    Carpus   Phalanges [fingers]
    Metacarpus

5   **pelvic region and thigh**
    Buttock   Hip (joint)
    Femur

6   **lower leg**
    Fibula   Patella
    Knee joint   Tibia

7   **ankle and foot**
    Ankle joint   Phalanges, foot
    Digits [toes]   Tarsus
    Metatarsus   Other joints in foot

8   **other specified sites**
    Head   Skull
    Neck   Trunk
    Ribs   Vertebral column

9   **multiple sites**

ARTHROPATHIES AND RELATED DISORDERS (710-719)

> *Excludes:* disorders of spine (720.0-724.9)

710 **Diffuse diseases of connective tissue**
    Includes: all collagen diseases whose effects are not mainly confined to a single system

> *Excludes:* those affecting mainly the cardiovascular system, i.e., polyarteritis nodosa and allied conditions (446.0-446.7)

710.0 **Systemic lupus erythematosus**
    Disseminated lupus erythematosus
    Libman-Sacks disease

Use additional code, if desired, to identify manifestation, as:
       endocarditis (424.91)
       nephritis (583.81)
         chronic (582.81)
       nephrotic syndrome (581.81)

> *Excludes:* lupus erythematosus (discoid) NOS (695.4)

710.1 **Systemic sclerosis**
    Acrosclerosis
    CRST syndrome
    Progressive systemic sclerosis
    Scleroderma

Use additional code, if desired, to identify manifestation, as:
       lung involvement (517.2)
       myopathy (359.6)

> *Excludes:* circumscribed scleroderma (701.0)

710.2 **Sicca syndrome**
    Keratoconjunctivitis sicca
    Sjögren's disease

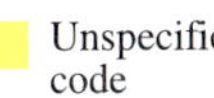
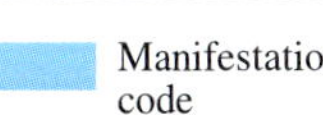

710.3 Dermatomyositis
Poikilodermatomyositis
Polymyositis with skin involvement

710.4 Polymyositis

710.5 Eosinophilia myalgia syndrome
Toxic oil syndrome

Use additional E code, if desired, to identify drug, if drug induced

710.8 Other specified diffuse diseases of connective tissue
Multifocal fibrosclerosis (idiopathic) NEC
Systemic fibrosclerosing syndrome

710.9 Unspecified diffuse connective tissue disease
Collagen disease NOS

⑤ 711 Arthropathy associated with infections
Includes: arthritis associated with conditions classifiable below
arthropathy associated with conditions classifiable below
polyarthritis associated with conditions classifiable below
polyarthropathy associated with conditions classifiable below

Excludes:	rheumatic fever (390)

The following fifth-digit subclassification is for use with category 711; valid digits are in [brackets] under each code. For definitions, see the beginning of this chapter:

0 site unspecified

1 shoulder region

2 upper arm

3 forearm

4 hand

5 pelvic region and thigh

6 lower leg

7 ankle and foot

8 other specified sites

9 multiple sites

⑤ 711.0 Pyogenic arthritis
[0-9]   Arthritis or polyarthritis (due to):
coliform [Escherichia coli]
Hemophilus influenzae [H. influenzae]
pneumococcal
Pseudomonas
staphylococcal
streptococcal
Pyarthrosis

Use additional code, if desired, to identify infectious organism (041.0-041.8)

⑤ *711.1 Arthropathy associated with Reiter's disease and nonspecific urethritis*
[0-9]   *Code first underlying disease, as:*
nonspecific urethritis (099.4)
Reiter's disease (099.3)

⑤ *711.2 Arthropathy in Behçet's syndrome*
[0-9]   *Code first underlying disease (136.1)*

⑤ *711.3 Postdysenteric arthropathy*
[0-9]   *Code first underlying disease, as:*
dysentery (009.0)
enteritis, infectious (008.0-009.3)
paratyphoid fever (002.1-002.9)
typhoid fever (002.0)

Excludes:	salmonella arthritis (003.23)

⑤ *711.4 Arthropathy associated with other bacterial diseases*
[0-9]   *Code first underlying disease, as:*
diseases classifiable to 010-040, 090-099, except as in 711.1, 711.3, and 713.5
leprosy (030.0-030.9)
tuberculosis (015.0-015.9)

Excludes:	gonococcal arthritis (098.50)
	meningococcal arthritis (036.82)

● Code new to this edition   ▲ Revision of existing code   ④ ⑤ Fourth or fifth digit required

⑤ **711.5** *Arthropathy associated with other viral diseases*
[0-9]   *Code first underlying disease, as:*
   diseases classifiable to 045-049, 050-079, 480, 487
   O'nyong nyong (066.3)

Excludes: *that due to rubella (056.71)*

⑤ **711.6** *Arthropathy associated with mycoses*
[0-9]   *Code first underlying disease (110.0-118)*

⑤ **711.7** *Arthropathy associated with helminthiasis*
[0-9]   *Code first underlying disease, as:*
   filariasis (125.0-125.9)

⑤ **711.8** *Arthropathy associated with other infectious and parasitic diseases*
[0-9]   *Code first underlying disease, as:*
   diseases classifiable to 080-088, 100-104, 130-136

Excludes: *arthropathy associated with sarcoidosis (713.7)*

⑤ **711.9** **Unspecified infective arthritis**
[0-9]   Infective arthritis or polyarthritis (acute) (chronic) (subacute) NOS

⑤ **712** **Crystal arthropathies**
   Includes: crystal-induced arthritis and synovitis

Excludes: *gouty arthropathy (274.0)*

The following fifth-digit subclassification is for use with category 712; valid digits are in [brackets] under each code. See beginning of this chapter for definitions:

   0 **site unspecified**
   1 **shoulder region**
   2 **upper arm**
   3 **forearm**
   4 **hand**
   5 **pelvic region and thigh**
   6 **lower leg**
   7 **ankle and foot**
   8 **other specified sites**
   9 **multiple sites**

⑤ **712.1** *Chondrocalcinosis due to dicalcium phosphate crystals*
[0-9]   Chondrocalcinosis due to dicalcium phosphate crystals (with other crystals)
   Code first underlying disease (275.4)

⑤ **712.2** *Chondrocalcinosis due to pyrophosphate crystals*
[0-9]   *Code first underlying disease (275.4)*

⑤ **712.3** *Chondrocalcinosis, unspecified*
[0-9]   *Code first underlying disease (275.4)*

⑤ **712.8** **Other specified crystal arthropathies**
[0-9]

⑤ **712.9** **Unspecified crystal arthropathy**
[0-9]

713 **Arthropathy associated with other disorders classified elsewhere**
   Includes: arthritis associated with conditions classifiable below
   arthropathy associated with conditions classifiable below
   polyarthritis associated with conditions classifiable below
   polyarthropathy associated with conditions classifiable below

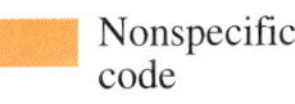

Add 4th or 5th digit	Nonspecific code	Unspecified code	Manifestation code

713.0 Arthropathy associated with other endocrine and metabolic disorders
 Code first underlying disease, as:
  acromegaly (253.0)
  hemochromatosis (275.0)
  hyperparathyroidism (252.00-252.08)
  hypogammaglobulinemia (279.00-279.09)
  hypothyroidism (243-244.9)
  lipoid metabolism disorder (272.0-272.9)
  ochronosis (270.2)

 Excludes: *arthropathy associated with:*
   amyloidosis (713.7)
   crystal deposition disorders, except gout (712.1-712.9)
   diabetic neuropathy (713.5)
   gouty arthropathy (274.0)

713.1 Arthropathy associated with gastrointestinal conditions other than infections
 Code first underlying disease, as:
  regional enteritis (555.0-555.9)
  ulcerative colitis (556)

713.2 Arthropathy associated with hematological disorders
 Code first underlying disease, as:
  hemoglobinopathy (282.4-282.7)
  hemophilia (286.0-286.2)
  leukemia (204.0-208.9)
  malignant reticulosis (202.3)
  multiple myelomatosis (203.0)

 Excludes: *arthropathy associated with Henoch-Schönlein purpura (713.6)*

713.3 Arthropathy associated with dermatological disorders
 Code first underlying disease, as:
  erythema multiforme (695.1)
  erythema nodosum (695.2)

 Excludes: *psoriatic arthropathy (696.0)*

713.4 Arthropathy associated with respiratory disorders
 Code first underlying disease, as:
  diseases classifiable to 490-519

 Excludes: *arthropathy associated with respiratory infections (711.0, 711.4-711.8)*

713.5 Arthropathy associated with neurological disorders
  Charcot's arthropathy associated with diseases classifiable elsewhere
  Neuropathic arthritis associated with diseases classifiable elsewhere
 Code first underlying disease, as:
  neuropathic joint disease [Charcot's joints]:
   NOS (094.0)
   diabetic (250.6)
   syringomyelic (336.0)
   tabetic [syphilitic] (094.0)

713.6 Arthropathy associated with hypersensitivity reaction
 Code first underlying disease, as:
  Henoch (-Schönlein) purpura (287.0)
  serum sickness (999.5)

 Excludes: *allergic arthritis NOS (716.2)*

713.7 Other general diseases with articular involvement
 Code first underlying disease, as:
  amyloidosis (277.30-277.39)
  familial Mediterranean fever (277.31)
  sarcoidosis (135)

713.8 Arthropathy associated with other conditions classifiable elsewhere
 Code first underlying disease, as:
  conditions classifiable elsewhere except as in 711.1-711.8, 712, and 713.0-713.7

714 Rheumatoid arthritis and other inflammatory polyarthropathies
 Excludes: *rheumatic fever (390)*
   rheumatoid arthritis of spine NOS (720.0)

● Code new to this edition ▲ Revision of existing code ④ ⑤ Fourth or fifth digit required

714.0 Rheumatoid arthritis
Arthritis or polyarthritis:
atrophic
rheumatic (chronic)
Use additional code, if desired, to identify manifestation, as:
myopathy (359.6)
polyneuropathy (357.1)
Excludes: *juvenile rheumatoid arthritis NOS (714.30)*

714.1 Felty's syndrome
Rheumatoid arthritis with splenoadenomegaly and leukopenia

714.2 Other rheumatoid arthritis with visceral or systemic involvement
Rheumatoid carditis

⑤ **714.3 Juvenile chronic polyarthritis**

    714.30 Polyarticular juvenile rheumatoid arthritis, chronic or unspecified
      Juvenile rheumatoid arthritis NOS
      Still's disease

    714.31 Polyarticular juvenile rheumatoid arthritis, acute

    714.32 Pauciarticular juvenile rheumatoid arthritis

    714.33 Monoarticular juvenile rheumatoid arthritis

714.4 Chronic postrheumatic arthropathy
Chronic rheumatoid nodular fibrositis
Jaccoud's syndrome

⑤ **714.8 Other specified inflammatory polyarthropathies**

    714.81 Rheumatoid lung
      Caplan's syndrome
      Diffuse interstitial rheumatoid disease of lung
      Fibrosing alveolitis, rheumatoid

    714.89 Other

714.9 Unspecified inflammatory polyarthropathy
Inflammatory polyarthropathy or polyarthritis NOS
Excludes: *polyarthropathy NOS (716.5)*

⑤ **715 Osteoarthrosis and allied disorders**
Note: Localized, in the subcategories below, includes bilateral involvement of the same site.
Includes: arthritis or polyarthritis:
degenerative
hypertrophic
degenerative joint disease
osteoarthritis
Excludes: *Marie-Strümpell spondylitis (720.0)*
osteoarthrosis [osteoarthritis] of spine (721.0-721.9)

The following fifth-digit subclassification is for use with category 715; valid digits are in [brackets] under each code. See beginning of this chapter for definitions:

0 site unspecified

1 shoulder region

2 upper arm

3 forearm

4 hand

5 pelvic region and thigh

6 lower leg

7 ankle and foot

8 other specified sites

9 multiple sites

⑤ **715.0 Osteoarthrosis, generalized**
[0,4,9]   Degenerative joint disease, involving multiple joints
      Primary generalized hypertrophic osteoarthrosis

⑤ **715.1 Osteoarthrosis, localized, primary**
[0-8]   Localized osteoarthropathy, idiopathic

⑤ **715.2 Osteoarthrosis, localized, secondary**
[0-8]   Coxae malum senilis

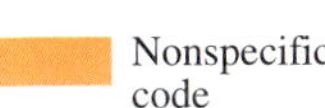

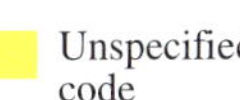

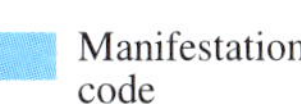

Manifestation
code

⑤ **715.3 Osteoarthrosis, localized, not specified whether primary or secondary**
[0-8] Otto's pelvis

⑤ **715.8 Osteoarthrosis involving, or with mention of more than one site, but not specified as**
[0,9] **generalized**

⑤ **715.9 Osteoarthrosis, unspecified whether generalized or localized**
[0-8]

⑤ **716 Other and unspecified arthropathies**
⎵ *Excludes:* cricoarytenoid arthropathy (478.79)⎵

The following fifth-digit subclassification is for use with category 716; valid digits are in [brackets] under each code. See beginning of this chapter for definitions:

0 **site unspecified**
1 **shoulder region**
2 **upper arm**
3 **forearm**
4 **hand**
5 **pelvic region and thigh**
6 **lower leg**
7 **ankle and foot**
8 **other specified sites**
9 **multiple sites**

⑤ **716.0 Kaschin-Beck disease**
[0-9] Endemic polyarthritis

⑤ **716.1 Traumatic arthropathy**
[0-9]

⑤ **716.2 Allergic arthritis**
[0-9]

⎵ *Excludes:* arthritis associated with Henoch-Schönlein purpura or serum sickness (713.6)⎵

⑤ **716.3 Climacteric arthritis**
[0-9] Menopausal arthritis

⑤ **716.4 Transient arthropathy**
[0-9]

⎵ *Excludes:* palindromic rheumatism (719.3)⎵

⑤ **716.5 Unspecified polyarthropathy or polyarthritis**
[0-9]

⑤ **716.6 Unspecified monoarthritis**
[0-8] Coxitis

⑤ **716.8 Other specified arthropathy**
[0-9]

⑤ **716.9 Arthropathy, unspecified**
[0-9] Arthritis (acute) (chronic) (subacute)
Arthropathy (acute) (chronic) (subacute)
Articular rheumatism (chronic)
Inflammation of joint NOS

717 Internal derangement of knee
Includes: degeneration of articular cartilage or meniscus of knee
rupture, old, of articular cartilage or meniscus of knee
tear, old, of articular cartilage or meniscus of knee

⎵ *Excludes:* acute derangement of knee (836.0-836.6)⎵
ankylosis (718.5)
contracture (718.4)
current injury (836.0-836.6)
deformity (736.4-736.6)
recurrent dislocation (718.3)

717.0 Old bucket handle tear of medial meniscus
Old bucket handle tear of unspecified cartilage

717.1 Derangement of anterior horn of medial meniscus

717.2 Derangement of posterior horn of medial meniscus

717.3 Other and unspecified derangement of medial meniscus
Degeneration of internal semilunar cartilage

● Code new to this edition   ▲ Revision of existing code   ④ ⑤ Fourth or fifth digit required

⑤ **717.4   Derangement of lateral meniscus**

      717.40   Derangement of lateral meniscus, unspecified

      717.41   Bucket handle tear of lateral meniscus

      717.42   Derangement of anterior horn of lateral meniscus

      717.43   Derangement of posterior horn of lateral meniscus

      717.49   Other

717.5   Derangement of meniscus, not elsewhere classified
    Congenital discoid meniscus
    Cyst of semilunar cartilage
    Derangement of semilunar cartilage NOS

717.6   Loose body in knee
    Joint mice, knee
    Rice bodies, knee (joint)

717.7   Chondromalacia of patella
    Chondromalacia patellae
    Degeneration [softening] of articular cartilage of patella

⑤ **717.8   Other internal derangement of knee**

      717.81   Old disruption of lateral collateral ligament

      717.82   Old disruption of medial collateral ligament

      717.83   Old disruption of anterior cruciate ligament

      717.84   Old disruption of posterior cruciate ligament

      717.85   Old disruption of other ligaments of knee
        Capsular ligament of knee

      717.89   Other
        Old disruption of ligaments of knee NOS

717.9   Unspecified internal derangement of knee
    Derangement NOS of knee

⑤ **718   Other derangement of joint**

    Excludes: *current injury (830.0-848.9)*
             jaw (524.60-524.69)

The following fifth-digit subclassification is for use with category 718; valid digits are in [brackets] under each code. See beginning of this chapter for definitions:

    0   site unspecified

    1   shoulder region

    2   upper arm

    3   forearm

    4   hand

    5   pelvic region and thigh

    6   lower leg

    7   ankle and foot

    8   other specified sites

    9   multiple sites

⑤ **718.0   Articular cartilage disorder**
   [0-5, 7-9] Meniscus:
        disorder
        rupture, old
        tear, old
      Old rupture of ligament(s) of joint NOS

    Excludes: *articular cartilage disorder:*
          in ochronosis (270.2)
          knee (717.0-717.9)
       chondrocalcinosis (275.4)
       metastatic calcification (275.4)

⑤ **718.1   Loose body in joint**
   [0-5, 7-9] Joint mice

    Excludes: *knee (717.6)*

⑤ **718.2   Pathological dislocation**
   [0-9]   Dislocation or displacement of joint, not recurrent and not current injury
        Spontaneous dislocation (joint)

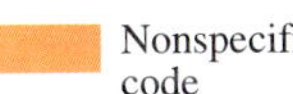

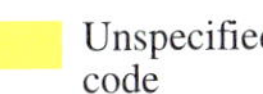

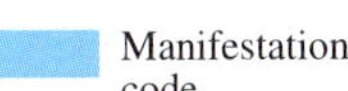

Manifestation
code

⑤ **718.3 Recurrent dislocation of joint**
[0-9]

⑤ **718.4 Contracture of joint**
[0-9]

⑤ **718.5 Ankylosis of joint**
[0-9]   Ankylosis of joint (fibrous) (osseous)
  Excludes: *spine (724.9)*
    stiffness of joint without mention of ankylosis (719.5)

⑤ **718.6 Unspecified intrapelvic protrusion of acetabulum**
[0, 5]   Protrusio acetabuli, unspecified

⑤ **718.7 Developmental dislocation of joint**
[0-9]
  Excludes: *congenital dislocation of joint (754.0-755.8)*
    traumatic dislocation of joint (830-839)

⑤ **718.8 Other joint derangement, not elsewhere classified**
[0-9]   Flail joint (paralytic)   Instability of joint
  Excludes: *deformities classifiable to 736 (736.0-736.9)*

⑤ **718.9 Unspecified derangement of joint**
[0-5, 7-9]
  Excludes: *knee (717.9)*

719 **Other and unspecified disorders of joint**
  Excludes: *jaw (524.60-524.69)*
The following fifth-digit subclassification is for use with codes 719.0-719.6, 719.8-719.9; valid
  digits are in [brackets] under each code. See list at beginning of chapter for definitions:

  0 **site unspecified**
  1 **shoulder region**
  2 **upper arm**
  3 **forearm**
  4 **hand**
  5 **pelvic region and thigh**
  6 **lower leg**
  7 **ankle and foot**
  8 **other specified sites**
  9 **multiple sites**

⑤ **719.0 Effusion of joint**
[0-9]   Hydrarthrosis
    Swelling of joint, with or without pain
  Excludes: *intermittent hydrarthrosis (719.3)*

⑤ **719.1 Hemarthrosis**
[0-9]
  Excludes: *current injury (840.0-848.9)*

⑤ **719.2 Villonodular synovitis**
[0-9]

⑤ **719.3 Palindromic rheumatism**
[0-9]   Hench-Rosenberg syndrome
    Intermittent hydrarthrosis

⑤ **719.4 Pain in joint**
[0-9]   Arthralgia

⑤ **719.5 Stiffness of joint, not elsewhere classified**
[0-9]

⑤ **719.6 Other symptoms referable to joint**
[0-9]   Joint crepitus   Snapping hip

719.7 Difficulty in walking
  Excludes: *abnormality of gait (781.2)*

● Code new
  to this edition

▲ Revision of
  existing code

④ ⑤ Fourth or fifth
  digit required

⑤ **719.8 Other specified disorders of joint**
[0-9]   Calcification of joint   Fistula of joint

Excludes: *temporomandibular joint-pain-dysfunction syndrome [Costen's syndrome] (524.60)*

⑤ **719.9 Unspecified disorder of joint**
[0-9]

DORSOPATHIES (720-724)

Excludes: *curvature of spine (737.0-737.9)*
osteochondrosis of spine (juvenile) (732.0)
adult (732.8)

720 Ankylosing spondylitis and other inflammatory spondylopathies

720.0 Ankylosing spondylitis
Rheumatoid arthritis of spine NOS
Spondylitis:
Marie-Strümpell
rheumatoid

720.1 Spinal enthesopathy
Disorder of peripheral ligamentous or muscular attachments of spine
Romanus lesion

720.2 Sacroiliitis, not elsewhere classified
Inflammation of sacroiliac joint NOS

⑤ **720.8 Other inflammatory spondylopathies**

720.81 Inflammatory spondylopathies in diseases classified elsewhere
Code first underlying disease, as:
tuberculosis (015.0)

720.89 Other

720.9 Unspecified inflammatory spondylopathy
Spondylitis NOS

721 Spondylosis and allied disorders

721.0 Cervical spondylosis without myelopathy
Cervical or cervicodorsal:
arthritis
osteoarthritis
spondylarthritis

721.1 Cervical spondylosis with myelopathy
Anterior spinal artery compression syndrome
Spondylogenic compression of cervical spinal cord
Vertebral artery compression syndrome

721.2 Thoracic spondylosis without myelopathy
Thoracic:
arthritis
osteoarthritis
spondylarthritis

721.3 Lumbosacral spondylosis without myelopathy
Lumbar or lumbosacral:
arthritis
osteoarthritis
spondylarthritis

⑤ **721.4 Thoracic or lumbar spondylosis with myelopathy**

721.41 Thoracic region
Spondylogenic compression of thoracic spinal cord

721.42 Lumbar region
Spondylogenic compression of lumbar spinal cord

721.5 Kissing spine
Baastrup's syndrome

721.6 Ankylosing vertebral hyperostosis

721.7 Traumatic spondylopathy
Kümmell's disease or spondylitis

721.8 Other allied disorders of spine

⑤ **721.9 Spondylosis of unspecified site**

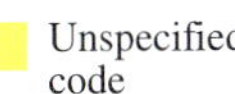

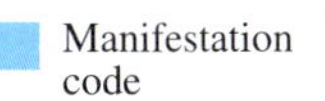

721.90 **Without mention of myelopathy**
    Spinal:
      arthritis (deformans) (degenerative) (hypertrophic)
      osteoarthritis NOS
    Spondylarthrosis NOS

721.91 **With myelopathy**
    Spondylogenic compression of spinal cord NOS

722 **Intervertebral disc disorders**

722.0 **Displacement of cervical intervertebral disc without myelopathy**
    Neuritis (brachial) or radiculitis due to displacement or rupture of cervical intervertebral disc
    Any condition classifiable to 722.2 of the cervical or cervicothoracic intervertebral disc

⑤ **722.1** **Displacement of thoracic or lumbar intervertebral disc without myelopathy**

    722.10 **Lumbar intervertebral disc without myelopathy**
      Lumbago or sciatica due to displacement of intervertebral disc
      Neuritis or radiculitis due to displacement or rupture of lumbar intervertebral disc
      Any condition classifiable to 722.2 of the lumbar or lumbosacral intervertebral disc

    722.11 **Thoracic intervertebral disc without myelopathy**
      Any condition classifiable to 722.2 of thoracic intervertebral disc

722.2 **Displacement of intervertebral disc, site unspecified, without myelopathy**
    Discogenic syndrome NOS
    Herniation of nucleus pulposus NOS
    Intervertebral disc NOS:
      extrusion
      prolapse
      protrusion
      rupture
    Neuritis or radiculitis due to displacement or rupture of intervertebral disc

⑤ **722.3** **Schmorl's nodes**

    722.30 **Unspecified region**

    722.31 **Thoracic region**

    722.32 **Lumbar region**

    722.39 **Other**

722.4 **Degeneration of cervical intervertebral disc**
    Degeneration of cervicothoracic intervertebral disc

⑤ **722.5** **Degeneration of thoracic or lumbar intervertebral disc**

    722.51 **Thoracic or thoracolumbar intervertebral disc**

    722.52 **Lumbar or lumbosacral intervertebral disc**

722.6 **Degeneration of intervertebral disc, site unspecified**
    Degenerative disc disease NOS
    Narrowing of intervertebral disc or space NOS

⑤ **722.7** **Intervertebral disc disorder with myelopathy**

    722.70 **Unspecified region**

    722.71 **Cervical region**

    722.72 **Thoracic region**

    722.73 **Lumbar region**

⑤ **722.8** **Postlaminectomy syndrome**

    722.80 **Unspecified region**

    722.81 **Cervical region**

    722.82 **Thoracic region**

    722.83 **Lumbar region**

⑤ **722.9** **Other and unspecified disc disorder**
    Calcification of intervertebral cartilage or disc
    Discitis

    722.90 **Unspecified region**

    722.91 **Cervical region**

    722.92 **Thoracic region**

    722.93 **Lumbar region**

● Code new to this edition   ▲ Revision of existing code   ④ ⑤ Fourth or fifth digit required

723 **Other disorders of cervical region**

> *Excludes:* *conditions due to:*
> *intervertebral disc disorders (722.0-722.9)*
> *spondylosis (721.0-721.9)*

723.0 **Spinal stenosis in cervical region**

723.1 **Cervicalgia**
Pain in neck

723.2 **Cervicocranial syndrome**
Barré-Liéou syndrome
Posterior cervical sympathetic syndrome

723.3 **Cervicobrachial syndrome (diffuse)**

723.4 **Brachial neuritis or radiculitis NOS**
Cervical radiculitis
Radicular syndrome of upper limbs

723.5 **Torticollis, unspecified**
Contracture of neck

> *Excludes:* *congenital (754.1)*
> *due to birth injury (767.8)*
> *hysterical (300.11)*
> *ocular torticollis (781.93)*
> *psychogenic (306.0)*
> *spasmodic (333.83)*
> *traumatic, current (847.0)*

723.6 **Panniculitis specified as affecting neck**

723.7 **Ossification of posterior longitudinal ligament in cervical region**

723.8 **Other syndromes affecting cervical region**
Cervical syndrome NEC
Klippel's disease
Occipital neuralgia

723.9 **Unspecified musculoskeletal disorders and symptoms referable to neck**
Cervical (region) disorder NOS

724 **Other and unspecified disorders of back**

> *Excludes:* *collapsed vertebra (code to cause, e.g., osteoporosis, 733.00-733.09)*
> *conditions due to:*
> *intervertebral disc disorders (722.0-722.9)*
> *spondylosis (721.0-721.9)*

⑤ **724.0** **Spinal stenosis, other than cervical**

    724.00 **Spinal stenosis, unspecified region**

    724.01 **Thoracic region**

    724.02 **Lumbar region**

    724.09 **Other**

724.1 **Pain in thoracic spine**

724.2 **Lumbago**
Low back pain
Low back syndrome
Lumbalgia

724.3 **Sciatica**
Neuralgia or neuritis of sciatic nerve

> *Excludes:* *specified lesion of sciatic nerve (355.0)*

724.4 **Thoracic or lumbosacral neuritis or radiculitis, unspecified**
Radicular syndrome of lower limbs

724.5 **Backache, unspecified**
Vertebrogenic (pain) syndrome NOS

724.6 **Disorders of sacrum**
Ankylosis, lumbosacral or sacroiliac (joint)
Instability, lumbosacral or sacroiliac (joint)

⑤ **724.7** **Disorders of coccyx**

    724.70 **Unspecified disorder of coccyx**

    724.71 **Hypermobility of coccyx**

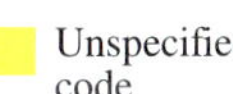

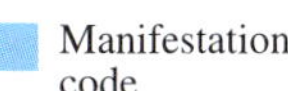

724.79 **Other**
Coccygodynia

724.8 **Other symptoms referable to back**
Ossification of posterior longitudinal ligament NOS
Panniculitis specified as sacral or affecting back

724.9 **Other unspecified back disorders**
Ankylosis of spine NOS
Compression of spinal nerve root NEC
Spinal disorder NOS

Excludes: sacroiliitis (720.2)

RHEUMATISM, EXCLUDING THE BACK (725-729)

Includes: disorders of muscles and tendons and their attachments, and of other soft tissues

725 **Polymyalgia rheumatica**

726 **Peripheral enthesopathies and allied syndromes**
Note: Enthesopathies are disorders of peripheral ligamentous or muscular attachments.

Excludes: spinal enthesopathy (720.1)

726.0 **Adhesive capsulitis of shoulder**

⑤ 726.1 **Rotator cuff syndrome of shoulder and allied disorders**

726.10 **Disorders of bursae and tendons in shoulder region, unspecified**
Rotator cuff syndrome NOS
Supraspinatus syndrome NOS

726.11 **Calcifying tendinitis of shoulder**

726.12 **Bicipital tenosynovitis**

726.19 **Other specified disorders**

Excludes: complete rupture of rotator cuff, nontraumatic (727.61)

726.2 **Other affections of shoulder region, not elsewhere classified**
Periarthritis of shoulder
Scapulohumeral fibrositis

⑤ 726.3 **Enthesopathy of elbow region**

726.30 **Enthesopathy of elbow, unspecified**

726.31 **Medial epicondylitis**

726.32 **Lateral epicondylitis**
Epicondylitis NOS
Golfers' elbow
Tennis elbow

726.33 **Olecranon bursitis**
Bursitis of elbow

726.39 **Other**

726.4 **Enthesopathy of wrist and carpus**
Bursitis of hand or wrist
Periarthritis of wrist

726.5 **Enthesopathy of hip region**
Bursitis of hip   Psoas tendinitis
Gluteal tendinitis   Trochanteric tendinitis
Iliac crest spur

⑤ 726.6 **Enthesopathy of knee**

726.60 **Enthesopathy of knee, unspecified**
Bursitis of knee NOS

726.61 **Pes anserinus tendinitis or bursitis**

726.62 **Tibial collateral ligament bursitis**
Pellegrini-Stieda syndrome

726.63 **Fibular collateral ligament bursitis**

726.64 **Patellar tendinitis**

726.65 **Prepatellar bursitis**

726.69 **Other**
Bursitis:
infrapatellar
subpatellar

   ● Code new
to this edition   ▲ Revision of
existing code   ④ ⑤ Fourth or fifth
digit required

⑤ **726.7 Enthesopathy of ankle and tarsus**

    726.70 Enthesopathy of ankle and tarsus, unspecified
        Metatarsalgia NOS

    Excludes: *Morton's metatarsalgia (355.6)*

    726.71 Achilles bursitis or tendinitis

    726.72 Tibialis tendinitis
        Tibialis (anterior) (posterior) tendinitis

    726.73 Calcaneal spur

    726.79 Other
        Peroneal tendinitis

726.8 Other peripheral enthesopathies

⑤ **726.9 Unspecified enthesopathy**

    726.90 Enthesopathy of unspecified site
        Capsulitis NOS
        Periarthritis NOS
        Tendinitis NOS

    726.91 Exostosis of unspecified site
        Bone spur NOS

727 Other disorders of synovium, tendon, and bursa

⑤ **727.0 Synovitis and tenosynovitis**

    727.00 Synovitis and tenosynovitis, unspecified
        Synovitis NOS
        Tenosynovitis NOS

    727.01 *Synovitis and tenosynovitis in diseases classified elsewhere*
        Code first underlying disease, as:
            tuberculosis (015.0-015.9)

    Excludes: *crystal-induced (275.4)*
          gonococcal (098.51)
          gouty (274.0)
          syphilitic (095.7)

    727.02 Giant cell tumor of tendon sheath

    727.03 Trigger finger (acquired)

    727.04 Radial styloid tenosynovitis
        de Quervain's disease

    727.05 Other tenosynovitis of hand and wrist

    727.06 Tenosynovitis of foot and ankle

    727.09 Other

727.1 Bunion

727.2 Specific bursitides often of occupational origin
    Beat:
      elbow
      hand
      knee
    Chronic crepitant synovitis of wrist
    Miners':
      elbow
      knee

727.3 Other bursitis
    Bursitis NOS

    Excludes: *bursitis:*
          gonococcal (098.52)
          subacromial (726.19)
          subcoracoid (726.19)
          subdeltoid (726.19)
          syphilitic (095.7)
          "frozen shoulder" (726.0)

⑤ **727.4 Ganglion and cyst of synovium, tendon, and bursa**

    727.40 Synovial cyst, unspecified

    Excludes: *that of popliteal space (727.51)*

    727.41 Ganglion of joint

727.42	**Ganglion of tendon sheath**
727.43	**Ganglion, unspecified**
727.49	**Other**

Cyst of bursa

⑤ **727.5 Rupture of synovium**

727.50	**Rupture of synovium, unspecified**
727.51	**Synovial cyst of popliteal space**

Baker's cyst (knee)

727.59	**Other**

⑤ **727.6 Rupture of tendon, nontraumatic**

727.60	**Nontraumatic rupture of unspecified tendon**
727.61	**Complete rupture of rotator cuff**
727.62	**Tendons of biceps (long head)**
727.63	**Extensor tendons of hand and wrist**
727.64	**Flexor tendons of hand and wrist**
727.65	**Quadriceps tendon**
727.66	**Patellar tendon**
727.67	**Achilles tendon**
727.68	**Other tendons of foot and ankle**
727.69	**Other**

⑤ **727.8 Other disorders of synovium, tendon, and bursa**

727.81 **Contracture of tendon (sheath)**
Short Achilles tendon (acquired)

727.82 **Calcium deposits in tendon and bursa**
Calcification of tendon NOS
Calcific tendinitis NOS

Excludes: peripheral ligamentous or muscular attachments (726.0-726.9)

727.83 **Plica syndrome**
Plica knee

727.89 **Other**
Abscess of bursa or tendon

Excludes: xanthomatosis localized to tendons (272.7)

727.9 Unspecified disorder of synovium, tendon, and bursa

728 Disorders of muscle, ligament, and fascia

Excludes: enthesopathies (726.0-726.9)
muscular dystrophies (359.0-359.1)
myoneural disorders (358.00-358.9)
myopathies (359.2-359.9)
old disruption of ligaments of knee (717.81-717.89)

728.0 Infective myositis
Myositis:
purulent
suppurative

Excludes: myositis:
epidemic (074.1)
interstitial (728.81)
syphilitic (095.6)
tropical (040.81)

⑤ **728.1 Muscular calcification and ossification**

728.10 **Calcification and ossification, unspecified**
Massive calcification (paraplegic)

728.11 **Progressive myositis ossificans**

728.12 **Traumatic myositis ossificans**
Myositis ossificans (circumscripta)

728.13 **Postoperative heterotopic calcification**

728.19 **Other**
Polymyositis ossificans

● Code new
to this edition   ▲ Revision of
existing code   ④ ⑤ Fourth or fifth
digit required

728.2 Muscular wasting and disuse atrophy, not elsewhere classified
Amyotrophia NOS
Myofibrosis

Excludes: *neuralgic amyotrophy (353.5)*
pelvic muscle wasting and disuse atrophy (618.83)
progressive muscular atrophy (335.0-335.9)

728.3 Other specific muscle disorders
Arthrogryposis
Immobility syndrome (paraplegic)

Excludes: *arthrogryposis multiplex congenita (754.89)*
stiff-man syndrome (333.91)

728.4 Laxity of ligament

728.5 Hypermobility syndrome

728.6 Contracture of palmar fascia
Dupuytren's contracture

⑤ **728.7 Other fibromatoses**

728.71 Plantar fascial fibromatosis
Contracture of plantar fascia
Plantar fasciitis (traumatic)

728.79 Other
Garrod's or knuckle pads
Nodular fasciitis
Pseudosarcomatous fibromatosis (proliferative) (subcutaneous)

⑤ **728.8 Other disorders of muscle, ligament, and fascia**

728.81 Interstitial myositis

728.82 Foreign body granuloma of muscle
Talc granuloma of muscle

728.83 Rupture of muscle, nontraumatic

728.84 Diastasis of muscle
Diastasis recti (abdomen)

Excludes: *diastasis recti complicating pregnancy, labor, and delivery (665.8)*

728.85 Spasm of muscle

728.86 Necrotizing fasciitis
Use additional code to identify:
infectious organism (041.00 - 041.89)
gangrene (785.4), if applicable

728.87 Muscle weakness (generalized)

Excludes: *generalized weakness (780.79)*

728.88 Rhabdomyolysis

728.89 Other
Eosinophilic fasciitis

Use additional E code, if desired, to identify drug, if drug induced

728.9 Unspecified disorder of muscle, ligament, and fascia

729 Other disorders of soft tissues

Excludes: *acroparesthesia (443.89)*
carpal tunnel syndrome (354.0)
disorders of the back (720.0-724.9)
entrapment syndromes (354.0-355.9)
palindromic rheumatism (719.3)
periarthritis (726.0-726.9)
psychogenic rheumatism (306.0)

729.0 Rheumatism, unspecified and fibrositis

729.1 Myalgia and myositis, unspecified
Fibromyositis NOS

Add 4th or 5th digit | Nonspecific code | Unspecified code | Manifestation code

729.2 Neuralgia, neuritis, and radiculitis, unspecified

> *Excludes:* *brachial radiculitis (723.4)*
> *cervical radiculitis (723.4)*
> *lumbosacral radiculitis (724.4)*
> *mononeuritis (354.0-355.9)*
> *radiculitis due to intervertebral disc involvement (722.0-722.2, 722.7)*
> *sciatica (724.3)*

⑤ **729.3 Panniculitis, unspecified**

    729.30 Panniculitis, unspecified site
        Weber-Christian disease

    729.31 Hypertrophy of fat pad, knee
        Hypertrophy of infrapatellar fat pad

    729.39 Other site

> *Excludes:* *panniculitis specified as (affecting):*
> *back (724.8)*
> *neck (723.6)*
> *sacral (724.8)*

729.4 Fasciitis, unspecified

> *Excludes:* *necrotizing fasciitis (728.86)*
> *nodular fasciitis (728.79)*

729.5 Pain in limb

729.6 Residual foreign body in soft tissue

> *Excludes:* *foreign body granuloma:*
> *muscle (728.82)*
> *skin and subcutaneous tissue (709.4)*

● **729.7 Nontraumatic compartment syndrome**

> *Excludes:* *compartment syndrome NOS (958.90)*
> *traumatic compartment syndrome (958.90-958.99)*

  ● **729.71 Nontraumatic compartment syndrome of upper extremity**
        Nontraumatic compartment syndrome of shoulder, arm, forearm, wrist, hand
        and fingers

  ● **729.72 Nontraumatic compartment syndrome of lower extremity**
        Nontraumatic compartment syndrome of hip, buttock, thigh, leg, foot and toes

  ● **729.73 Nontraumatic compartment syndrome of abdomen**

  ● **729.79 Nontraumatic compartment syndrome of other sites**

⑤ **729.8 Other musculoskeletal symptoms referable to limbs**

    729.81 Swelling of limb

    729.82 Cramp

    729.89 Other

> *Excludes:* *abnormality of gait (781.2)*
> *tetany (781.7)*
> *transient paralysis of limb (781.4)*

729.9 Other and unspecified disorders of soft tissue
    Polyalgia

● Code new to this edition   ▲ Revision of existing code   ④ ⑤ Fourth or fifth digit required

OSTEOPATHIES, CHONDROPATHIES, AND ACQUIRED MUSCULOSKELETAL DEFORMITIES (730-739)

⑤ **730 Osteomyelitis, periostitis, and other infections involving bone**

> Excludes: jaw (526.4-526.5)
>> petrous bone (383.2)

Use additional code, if desired, to identify organism, such as Staphylococcus (041.1)

The following fifth-digit subclassification is for use with category 730; valid digits are in [brackets] under each code. See beginning of this chapter for definitions:

0 site unspecified

1 shoulder region

2 upper arm

3 forearm

4 hand

5 pelvic region and thigh

6 lower leg

7 ankle and foot

8 other specified sites

9 multiple sites

⑤ **730.0 Acute osteomyelitis**
[0-9] Abscess of any bone except accessory sinus, jaw, or mastoid
Acute or subacute osteomyelitis, with or without mention of periostitis

Use additional code to identify major osseous defect, if applicable (731.3)

⑤ **730.1 Chronic osteomyelitis**
[0-9] Brodie's abscess
Chronic or old osteomyelitis, with or without mention of periostitis
Sequestrum of bone
Sclerosing osteomyelitis of Garré

Use additional code to identify major osseous defect, if applicable (731.3)

> Excludes: aseptic necrosis of bone (733.40-733.49)

⑤ **730.2 Unspecified osteomyelitis**
[0-9] Osteitis or osteomyelitis NOS, with or without mention of periostitis
Use additional code to identify major osseous defect, if applicable (731.3)

⑤ **730.3 Periostitis without mention of osteomyelitis**
[0-9] Abscess of periosteum without mention of osteomyelitis
Periostosis without mention of osteomyelitis

> Excludes: that in secondary syphilis (091.61)

⑤ ***730.7 Osteopathy resulting from poliomyelitis***
[0-9] *Code first underlying disease (045.0-045.9)*

⑤ ***730.8 Other infections involving bone in diseases classified elsewhere***
[0-9] *Code first underlying disease, as:*
tuberculosis (015.0-015.9)
typhoid fever (002.0)

> Excludes: syphilis of bone NOS (095.5)

⑤ **730.9 Unspecified infection of bone**
[0-9]

731 Osteitis deformans and osteopathies associated with other disorders classified elsewhere

731.0 Osteitis deformans without mention of bone tumor
Paget's disease of bone

731.1 Osteitis deformans in diseases classified elsewhere
Code first underlying disease, as:
malignant neoplasm of bone (170.0-170.9)

731.2 Hypertrophic pulmonary osteoarthropathy
Bamberger-Marie disease

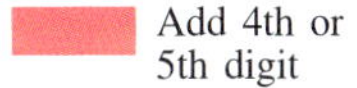

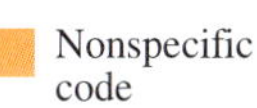

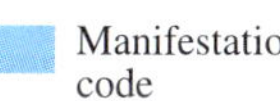

● **731.3 Major osseous defects**
    Code first underlying disease, if known, such as:
      aseptic necrosis (733.40-733.49)
      malignant neoplasm of bone (170.0-170.9)
      osteomyelitis (730.00-730.29)
      osteoporosis (733.00-733.09)
      peri-prosthetic osteolysis (996.45)

731.8 *Other bone involvement in diseases classified elsewhere*
    Code first underlying disease, as:
      diabetes mellitus (250.8)
    Use additional code to specify bone condition, such as:
      acute osteomyelitis (730.00-730.09)

732 Osteochondropathies

732.0 Juvenile osteochondrosis of spine
    Juvenile osteochondrosis (of):
      marginal or vertebral epiphysis (of Scheuermann)
      spine NOS
    Vertebral epiphysitis

    Excludes: adolescent postural kyphosis (737.0)

732.1 Juvenile osteochondrosis of hip and pelvis
    Coxa plana
    Ischiopubic synchondrosis (of van Neck)
    Osteochondrosis (juvenile) of:
      acetabulum
      head of femur (of Legg-Calvé-Perthes)
      iliac crest (of Buchanan)
      symphysis pubis (of Pierson)
    Pseudocoxalgia

732.2 Nontraumatic slipped upper femoral epiphysis
    Slipped upper femoral epiphysis NOS

732.3 Juvenile osteochondrosis of upper extremity
    Osteochondrosis (juvenile) of:
      capitulum of humerus (of Panner)
      carpal lunate (of Kienbock)
      hand NOS
      head of humerus (of Haas)
      heads of metacarpals (of Mauclaire)
      lower ulna (of Burns)
      radial head (of Brailsford)
      upper extremity NOS

732.4 Juvenile osteochondrosis of lower extremity, excluding foot
    Osteochondrosis (juvenile) of:
      lower extremity NOS
      primary patellar center (of Köhler)
      proximal tibia (of Blount)
      secondary patellar center (of Sinding-Larsen)
      tibial tubercle (of Osgood-Schlatter)
    Tibia vara

732.5 Juvenile osteochondrosis of foot
    Calcaneal apophysitis
    Epiphysitis, os calcis
    Osteochondrosis (juvenile) of:
      astragalus (of Diaz)
      calcaneum (of Sever)
      foot NOS
      metatarsal
        second (of Freiberg)
        fifth (of Iselin)
      os tibiale externum (Haglund)
      tarsal navicular (of Köhler)

732.6 Other juvenile osteochondrosis
    Apophysitis specified as juvenile, of other site, or site NOS
    Epiphysitis specified as juvenile, of other site, or site NOS
    Osteochondritis specified as juvenile, of other site, or site NOS
    Osteochondrosis specified as juvenile, of other site, or site NOS

732.7 Osteochondritis dissecans

● Code new to this edition   ▲ Revision of existing code   ④ ⑤ Fourth or fifth digit required

732.8 **Other specified forms of osteochondropathy**
Adult osteochondrosis of spine

732.9 **Unspecified osteochondropathy**
Apophysitis
NOS
not specified as adult or juvenile, of unspecified site
Epiphysitis
NOS
not specified as adult or juvenile, of unspecified site
Osteochondritis
NOS
not specified as adult or juvenile, of unspecified site
Osteochondrosis
NOS
not specified as adult or juvenile, of unspecified site

733 **Other disorders of bone and cartilage**
Excludes: *bone spur (726.91)*

cartilage of, or loose body in, joint (717.0-717.9, 718.0-718.9)
giant cell granuloma of jaw (526.3)
osteitis fibrosa cystica generalisata (252.01)
osteomalacia (268.2)
polyostotic fibrous dysplasia of bone (756.54)
prognathism, retrognathism (524.1)
xanthomatosis localized to bone (272.7)

⑤ **733.0** **Osteoporosis**
Use additional code to identify major osseous defect, if applicable (731.3)

733.00 **Osteoporosis, unspecified**
Wedging of vertebra NOS

733.01 **Senile osteoporosis**
Postmenopausal osteoporosis

733.02 **Idiopathic osteoporosis**

733.03 **Disuse osteoporosis**

733.09 **Other**
Drug-induced osteoporosis
Use additional E code, if desired, to identify drug

⑤ **733.1** **Pathologic fracture**
Spontaneous fracture
Excludes: *traumatic fracture (800-829)*

stress fracture (733.93-733.95)

733.10 **Pathologic fracture, unspecified site**

733.11 **Pathologic fracture of humerus**

733.12 **Pathologic fracture of distal radius and ulna**
Wrist NOS

733.13 **Pathologic fracture of vertebrae**
Collapse of vertebra NOS

733.14 **Pathologic fracture of neck of femur**
Femur NOS
Hip NOS

733.15 **Pathologic fracture of other specified part of femur**

733.16 **Pathologic fracture of tibia or fibula**
Ankle NOS

733.19 **Pathologic fracture of other specified site**

⑤ **733.2** **Cyst of bone**

733.20 **Cyst of bone (localized), unspecified**

733.21 **Solitary bone cyst**
Unicameral bone cyst

733.22 **Aneurysmal bone cyst**

733.29 **Other**
Fibrous dysplasia (monostotic)
Excludes: *cyst of jaw (526.0-526.2, 526.89)*

osteitis fibrosa cystica (252.01)
polyostotic fibrous dysplasia of bone (756.54)

Add 4th or 5th digit	Nonspecific code	Unspecified code	Manifestation code

733.3 Hyperostosis of skull
Hyperostosis interna frontalis
Leontiasis ossium

⑤ **733.4 Aseptic necrosis of bone**
Use additional code to identify major osseous defect, if applicable (731.3)

Excludes: osteochondropathies (732.0-732.9)

733.40 Aseptic necrosis of bone, site unspecified

733.41 Head of humerus

733.42 Head and neck of femur
Femur NOS

Excludes: Legg-Calvé-Perthes disease (732.1)

733.43 Medial femoral condyle

733.44 Talus

733.49 Other

733.5 Osteitis condensans
Piriform sclerosis of ilium

733.6 Tietze's disease
Costochondral junction syndrome
Costochondritis

733.7 Algoneurodystrophy
Disuse atrophy of bone
Sudeck's atrophy

⑤ **733.8 Malunion and nonunion of fracture**

733.81 Malunion of fracture

733.82 Nonunion of fracture
Pseudoarthrosis (bone)

⑤ **733.9 Other and unspecified disorders of bone and cartilage**

733.90 Disorder of bone and cartilage, unspecified

733.91 Arrest of bone development or growth
Epiphyseal arrest

733.92 Chondromalacia
Chondromalacia:
NOS
localized, except patella
systemic
tibial plateau

Excludes: chondromalacia of patella (717.7)

733.93 Stress fracture of tibia or fibula
Stress reaction of tibia or fibula

733.94 Stress fracture of the metatarsals
Stress reaction of metatarsals

733.95 Stress fracture of other bone
Stress reaction of other bone

733.99 Other
Diaphysitis
Hypertrophy of bone
Relapsing polychondritis

734 Flat foot
Pes planus (acquired)
Talipes planus (acquired)

Excludes: congenital (754.61)
rigid flat foot (754.61)
spastic (everted) flat foot (754.61)

735 Acquired deformities of toe

Excludes: congenital (754.60-754.69, 755.65-755.66)

735.0 Hallux valgus (acquired)

735.1 Hallux varus (acquired)

735.2 Hallux rigidus

735.3 Hallux malleus

● Code new to this edition   ▲ Revision of existing code   ④ ⑤ Fourth or fifth digit required

735.4 Other hammer toe (acquired)

735.5 Claw toe (acquired)

735.8 Other acquired deformities of toe

735.9 Unspecified acquired deformity of toe

736 Other acquired deformities of limbs

> *Excludes:* congenital (754.3-755.9)

⑤ 736.0 **Acquired deformities of forearm, excluding fingers**

    736.00 Unspecified deformity
        Deformity of elbow, forearm, hand, or wrist (acquired) NOS

    736.01 Cubitus valgus (acquired)

    736.02 Cubitus varus (acquired)

    736.03 Valgus deformity of wrist (acquired)

    736.04 Varus deformity of wrist (acquired)

    736.05 Wrist drop (acquired)

    736.06 Claw hand (acquired)

    736.07 Club hand, acquired

    736.09 Other

736.1 **Mallet finger**

⑤ 736.2 **Other acquired deformities of finger**

    736.20 Unspecified deformity
        Deformity of finger (acquired) NOS

    736.21 Boutonniere deformity

    736.22 Swan-neck deformity

    736.29 Other

> *Excludes:* trigger finger (727.03)

⑤ 736.3 **Acquired deformities of hip**

    736.30 Unspecified deformity
        Deformity of hip (acquired) NOS

    736.31 Coxa valga (acquired)

    736.32 Coxa vara (acquired)

    736.39 Other

⑤ 736.4 **Genu valgum or varum (acquired)**

    736.41 Genu valgum (acquired)

    736.42 Genu varum (acquired)

736.5 **Genu recurvatum (acquired)**

736.6 Other acquired deformities of knee
    Deformity of knee (acquired) NOS

⑤ 736.7 **Other acquired deformities of ankle and foot**

> *Excludes:* deformities of toe (acquired) (735.0-735.9)
>
>   pes planus (acquired) (734)

    736.70 Unspecified deformity of ankle and foot, acquired

    736.71 Acquired equinovarus deformity
        Clubfoot, acquired

> *Excludes:* clubfoot not specified as acquired (754.5-754.7)

    736.72 Equinus deformity of foot, acquired

    736.73 Cavus deformity of foot

> *Excludes:* that with claw foot (736.74)

    736.74 Claw foot, acquired

    736.75 Cavovarus deformity of foot, acquired

    736.76 Other calcaneus deformity

    736.79 Other
        Acquired:
          pes not elsewhere classified
          talipes not elsewhere classified

⑤ **736.8　Acquired deformities of other parts of limbs**

　　　736.81　Unequal leg length (acquired)

　　　736.89　Other
　　　　　Deformity (acquired):
　　　　　　arm or leg, not elsewhere classified
　　　　　　shoulder

736.9　Acquired deformity of limb, site unspecified

737　Curvature of spine
　　Excludes: congenital (754.2)

737.0　Adolescent postural kyphosis
　　Excludes: osteochondrosis of spine (juvenile) (732.0)
　　　　　　adult (732.8)

⑤ **737.1　Kyphosis (acquired)**

　　　737.10　Kyphosis (acquired) (postural)

　　　737.11　Kyphosis due to radiation

　　　737.12　Kyphosis, postlaminectomy

　　　737.19　Other
　　Excludes: that associated with conditions classifiable elsewhere (737.41)

⑤ **737.2　Lordosis (acquired)**

　　　737.20　Lordosis (acquired) (postural)

　　　737.21　Lordosis, postlaminectomy

　　　737.22　Other postsurgical lordosis

　　　737.29　Other
　　Excludes: that associated with conditions classifiable elsewhere (737.42)

⑤ **737.3　Kyphoscoliosis and scoliosis**

　　　737.30　Scoliosis [and kyphoscoliosis], idiopathic

　　　737.31　Resolving infantile idiopathic scoliosis

　　　737.32　Progressive infantile idiopathic scoliosis

　　　737.33　Scoliosis due to radiation

　　　737.34　Thoracogenic scoliosis

　　　737.39　Other
　　Excludes: that associated with conditions classifiable elsewhere (737.43)
　　　　　　that in kyphoscoliotic heart disease (416.1)

⑤ **737.4　Curvature of spine associated with other conditions**
　　　Code first associated condition, as:
　　　　Charcot-Marie-Tooth disease (356.1)
　　　　mucopolysaccharidosis (277.5)
　　　　neurofibromatosis (237.7)
　　　　osteitis deformans (731.0)
　　　　osteitis fibrosa cystica (252.01)
　　　　osteoporosis (733.00-733.09)
　　　　poliomyelitis (138)
　　　　tuberculosis [Pott's curvature] (015.0)

　　　737.40　Curvature of spine, unspecified

　　　737.41　Kyphosis

　　　737.42　Lordosis

　　　737.43　Scoliosis

737.8　Other curvatures of spine

737.9　Unspecified curvature of spine
　　　Curvature of spine (acquired) (idiopathic) NOS
　　　Hunchback, acquired
　　Excludes: deformity of spine NOS (738.5)

738　Other acquired deformity
　　Excludes: congenital (754.0-756.9, 758.0-759.9)
　　　　　　dentofacial anomalies (524.0-524.9)

● Code new
　to this edition

▲ Revision of
　existing code

④ ⑤ Fourth or fifth
　　digit required

738.0 Acquired deformity of nose
Deformity of nose (acquired)
Overdevelopment of nasal bones
Excludes: *deflected or deviated nasal septum (470)*

⑤ **738.1 Other acquired deformity of head**
    738.10 Unspecified deformity
    738.11 Zygomatic hyperplasia
    738.12 Zygomatic hypoplasia
    738.19 Other specified deformity

738.2 Acquired deformity of neck

738.3 Acquired deformity of chest and rib
Deformity: Pectus:
  chest (acquired)   carinatum, acquired
  rib (acquired)   excavatum, acquired

738.4 Acquired spondylolisthesis
Degenerative spondylolisthesis
Spondylolysis, acquired
Excludes: *congenital (756.12)*

738.5 Other acquired deformity of back or spine
Deformity of spine NOS
Excludes: *curvature of spine (737.0-737.9)*

738.6 Acquired deformity of pelvis
Pelvic obliquity
Excludes: *intrapelvic protrusion of acetabulum (718.6)*
        that in relation to labor and delivery (653.0-653.4, 653.8-653.9)

738.7 Cauliflower ear

738.8 Acquired deformity of other specified site
Deformity of clavicle

738.9 Acquired deformity of unspecified site

739 Nonallopathic lesions, not elsewhere classified
Includes: segmental dysfunction
         somatic dysfunction

739.0 Head region
Occipitocervical region

739.1 Cervical region
Cervicothoracic region

739.2 Thoracic region
Thoracolumbar region

739.3 Lumbar region
Lumbosacral region

739.4 Sacral region
Sacrococcygeal region
Sacroiliac region

739.5 Pelvic region
Hip region
Pubic region

739.6 Lower extremities

739.7 Upper extremities
Acromioclavicular region
Sternoclavicular region

739.8 Rib cage
Costochondral region   Sternochondral region
Costovertebral region

739.9 Abdomen and other

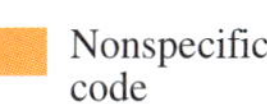

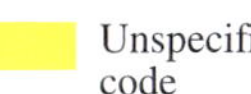

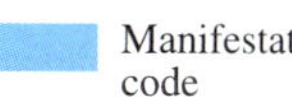

Manifestation
code

● Code new
to this edition

▲ Revision of
existing code

④ ⑤ Fourth or fifth
digit required

14. CONGENITAL ANOMALIES (740-759)

740 Anencephalus and similar anomalies

740.0 Anencephalus

Acrania	Hemianencephaly
Amyelencephalus	Hemicephaly

740.1 Craniorachischisis

740.2 Iniencephaly

741 Spina bifida

> Excludes: spina bifida occulta (756.17)

The following fifth-digit subclassification is for use with category 741:

   0   **unspecified region**

   1   **cervical region**

   2   **dorsal [thoracic] region**

   3   **lumbar region**

741.0 With hydrocephalus
Arnold-Chiari syndrome, type II
Any condition classifiable to 741.9 with any condition classifiable to 742.3
Chiari malformation, type II

741.9 Without mention of hydrocephalus

Hydromeningocele (spinal)	Myelocystocele
Hydromyelocele	Rachischisis
Meningocele (spinal)	Spina bifida (aperta)
Meningomyelocele	Syringomyelocele
Myelocele	

742 Other congenital anomalies of nervous system

> Excludes: congenital central alveolar hypoventilation syndrome (327.25)

742.0 Encephalocele

Encephalocystocele	Meningocele, cerebral
Encephalomyelocele	Meningoencephalocele
Hydroencephalocele	
Hydromeningocele, cranial	

742.1 Microcephalus
Hydromicrocephaly
Micrencephaly

742.2 Reduction deformities of brain
Absence of part of brain
Agenesis of part of brain
Agyria
Aplasia of part of brain
Arhinencephaly
Hypoplasia of part of brain
Holoprosencephaly
Microgyria

742.3 Congenital hydrocephalus
Aqueduct of Sylvius:
  anomaly
  obstruction, congenital
  stenosis
Atresia of foramina of Magendie and Luschka
Hydrocephalus in newborn

> Excludes: hydrocephalus:
>   acquired (331.3-331.4)
>   due to congenital toxoplasmosis (771.2)
>   with any condition classifiable to 741.9 (741.0)

742.4 Other specified anomalies of brain

Congenital cerebral cyst	Multiple anomalies of brain NOS
Macroencephaly	Porencephaly
Macrogyria	Ulegyria
Megalencephaly	

742.5 Other specified anomalies of spinal cord

    742.51 Diastematomyelia

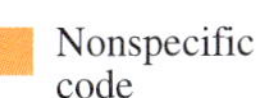

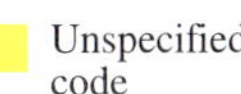

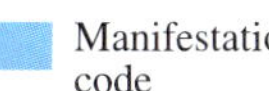

Manifestation
code

742.53 Hydromyelia
Hydrorhachis

742.59 Other
Amyelia
Atelomyelia
Congenital anomaly of spinal meninges
Defective development of cauda equina
Hypoplasia of spinal cord
Myelatelia
Myelodysplasia

742.8 Other specified anomalies of nervous system

Agenesis of nerve	Jaw-winking syndrome
Displacement of brachial plexus	Marcus-Gunn syndrome
	Riley-Day syndrome
Familial dysautonomia	

Excludes: *neurofibromatosis (237.7)*

742.9 Unspecified anomaly of brain, spinal cord, and nervous system
Anomaly of brain, nervous system, and spinal cord
Congenital:
disease of brain, nervous system, and spinal cord
lesion of brain, nervous system, and spinal cord
Deformity of brain, nervous system, and spinal cord

743 Congenital anomalies of eye

⑤ **743.0 Anophthalmos**

743.00 Clinical anophthalmos, unspecified
Agenesis of eye
Congenital absence of eye
Anophthalmos NOS

743.03 Cystic eyeball, congenital

743.06 Cryptophthalmos

⑤ **743.1 Microphthalmos**
Dysplasia of eye
Hypoplasia of eye
Rudimentary eye

743.10 Microphthalmos, unspecified

743.11 Simple microphthalmos

743.12 Microphthalmos associated with other anomalies of eye and adnexa

⑤ **743.2 Buphthalmos**

Glaucoma:	Hydrophthalmos
congenital	
newborn	

Excludes: *glaucoma of childhood (365.14)*
traumatic glaucoma due to birth injury (767.8)

743.20 Buphthalmos, unspecified

743.21 Simple buphthalmos

743.22 Buphthalmos associated with other ocular anomalies
Keratoglobus, congenital associated with buphthalmos
Megalocornea associated with buphthalmos

⑤ **743.3 Congenital cataract and lens anomalies**
Excludes: *infantile cataract (366.00-366.09)*

743.30 Congenital cataract, unspecified

743.31 Capsular and subcapsular cataract

743.32 Cortical and zonular cataract

743.33 Nuclear cataract

743.34 Total and subtotal cataract, congenital

743.35 Congenital aphakia
Congenital absence of lens

743.36 Anomalies of lens shape
Microphakia
Spherophakia

743.37 Congenital ectopic lens

● Code new to this edition   ▲ Revision of existing code   ④ ⑤ Fourth or fifth digit required

743.39　Other

⑤ **743.4**　**Coloboma and other anomalies of anterior segment**

743.41　**Anomalies of corneal size and shape**
Microcornea

Excludes: that associated with buphthalmos (743.22)

743.42　**Corneal opacities, interfering with vision, congenital**

743.43　**Other corneal opacities, congenital**

743.44　**Specified anomalies of anterior chamber, chamber angle, and related structures**
Anomaly:
　Axenfeld's
　Peters'
　Rieger's

743.45　**Aniridia**

743.46　**Other specified anomalies of iris and ciliary body**
Anisocoria, congenital
Atresia of pupil
Coloboma of iris
Corectopia

743.47　**Specified anomalies of sclera**

743.48　**Multiple and combined anomalies of anterior segment**

743.49　**Other**

⑤ **743.5**　**Congenital anomalies of posterior segment**

743.51　**Vitreous anomalies**
Congenital vitreous opacity

743.52　**Fundus coloboma**

743.53　**Chorioretinal degeneration, congenital**

743.54　**Congenital folds and cysts of posterior segment**

743.55　**Congenital macular changes**

743.56　**Other retinal changes, congenital**

743.57　**Specified anomalies of optic disc**
Coloboma of optic disc (congenital)

743.58　**Vascular anomalies**
Congenital retinal aneurysm

743.59　**Other**

⑤ **743.6**　**Congenital anomalies of eyelids, lacrimal system, and orbit**

743.61　**Congenital ptosis**

743.62　**Congenital deformities of eyelids**
Ablepharon　　　　Congenital:
Absence of eyelid　　ectropion
Accessory eyelid　　entropion

743.63　**Other specified congenital anomalies of eyelid**
Absence, agenesis, of cilia

743.64　**Specified congenital anomalies of lacrimal gland**

743.65　**Specified congenital anomalies of lacrimal passages**
Absence, agenesis of:
　lacrimal apparatus
　punctum lacrimale
Accessory lacrimal canal

743.66　**Specified congenital anomalies of orbit**

743.69　**Other**
Accessory eye muscles

743.8　**Other specified anomalies of eye**

Excludes: congenital nystagmus (379.51)
　　ocular albinism (270.2)
　　optic nerve hypoplasia (377.43)
　　retinitis pigmentosa (362.74)

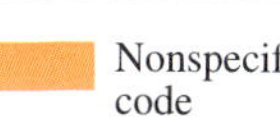
Add 4th or 5th digit

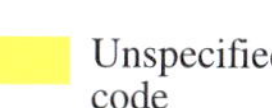
Nonspecific code

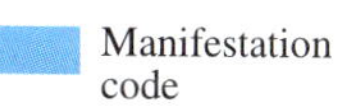
Unspecified code　　Manifestation code

743.9 **Unspecified anomaly of eye**
Congenital:
anomaly NOS of eye [any part]
deformity NOS of eye [any part]

744 **Congenital anomalies of ear, face, and neck**
Excludes: *anomaly of:*
cervical spine (754.2, 756.10-756.19)
larynx (748.2-748.3)
nose (748.0-748.1)
parathyroid gland (759.2)
thyroid gland (759.2)
cleft lip (749.10-749.25)

⑤ **744.0** **Anomalies of ear causing impairment of hearing**
Excludes: *congenital deafness without mention of cause (389.0-389.9)*

744.00 **Unspecified anomaly of ear with impairment of hearing**

744.01 **Absence of external ear**
Absence of:
auditory canal (external)
auricle (ear) (with stenosis or atresia of auditory canal)

744.02 **Other anomalies of external ear with impairment of hearing**
Atresia or stricture of auditory canal (external)

744.03 **Anomaly of middle ear, except ossicles**
Atresia or stricture of osseous meatus (ear)

744.04 **Anomalies of ear ossicles**
Fusion of ear ossicles

744.05 **Anomalies of inner ear**
Congenital anomaly of:
membranous labyrinth
organ of Corti

744.09 **Other**
Absence of ear, congenital

744.1 **Accessory auricle**
Accessory tragus   Supernumerary:
Polyotia   ear
Preauricular appendage   lobule

⑤ **744.2** **Other specified anomalies of ear**
Excludes: *that with impairment of hearing (744.00-744.09)*

744.21 **Absence of ear lobe, congenital**

744.22 **Macrotia**

744.23 **Microtia**

744.24 **Specified anomalies of Eustachian tube**
Absence of Eustachian tube

744.29 **Other**
Bat ear   Prominence of auricle
Darwin's tubercle   Ridge ear
Pointed ear

Excludes: *preauricular sinus (744.46)*

744.3 **Unspecified anomaly of ear**
Congenital:
anomaly NOS of ear, not elsewhere classified
deformity NOS of ear, not elsewhere classified

⑤ **744.4** **Branchial cleft cyst or fistula; preauricular sinus**

744.41 **Branchial cleft sinus or fistula**
Branchial:
sinus (external) (internal)
vestige

744.42 **Branchial cleft cyst**

744.43 **Cervical auricle**

744.46 **Preauricular sinus or fistula**

744.47 **Preauricular cyst**

● Code new   ▲ Revision of   ④ ⑤ Fourth or fifth
to this edition   existing code   digit required

744.49 **Other**
Fistula (of):
auricle, congenital
cervicoaural

744.5 **Webbing of neck**
Pterygium colli

⑤ **744.8** **Other specified anomalies of face and neck**

744.81 **Macrocheilia**
Hypertrophy of lip, congenital

744.82 **Microcheilia**

744.83 **Macrostomia**

744.84 **Microstomia**

744.89 **Other**

Excludes: *congenital fistula of lip (750.25)*
musculoskeletal anomalies (754.0-754.1, 756.0)

744.9 **Unspecified anomalies of face and neck**
Congenital:
anomaly NOS of face [any part] or neck [any part]
deformity NOS of face [any part] or neck [any part]

745 **Bulbus cordis anomalies and anomalies of cardiac septal closure**

745.0 **Common truncus**
Absent septum between aorta and pulmonary artery
Communication (abnormal) between aorta and pulmonary artery
Aortic septal defect
Common aortopulmonary trunk
Persistent truncus arteriosus

⑤ **745.1** **Transposition of great vessels**

745.10 **Complete transposition of great vessels**
Transposition of great vessels:
NOS
classical

745.11 **Double outlet right ventricle**
Dextratransposition of aorta
Incomplete transposition of great vessels
Origin of both great vessels from right ventricle
Taussig-Bing syndrome or defect

745.12 **Corrected transposition of great vessels**

745.19 **Other**

745.2 **Tetralogy of Fallot**
Fallot's pentalogy
Ventricular septal defect with pulmonary stenosis or atresia, dextraposition of aorta, and
hypertrophy of right ventricle

Excludes: *Fallot's triad (746.09)*

745.3 **Common ventricle**
Cor triloculare biatriatum
Single ventricle

745.4 **Ventricular septal defect**
Eisenmenger's defect or complex
Gerbode defect
Interventricular septal defect
Left ventricular-right atrial communication
Roger's disease

Excludes: *common atrioventricular canal type (745.69)*
single ventricle (745.3)

745.5 **Ostium secundum type atrial septal defect**
Defect: Patent or persistent:
atrium secundum   foramen ovale
fossa ovalis   ostium secundum
Lutembacher's syndrome

⑤ **745.6** **Endocardial cushion defects**

745.60 **Endocardial cushion defect, unspecified type**

745.61 Ostium primum defect
Persistent ostium primum

745.69 Other
Absence of atrial septum
Atrioventricular canal type ventricular septal defect
Common atrioventricular canal
Common atrium

745.7 Cor biloculare
Absence of atrial and ventricular septa

745.8 Other

745.9 Unspecified defect of septal closure
Septal defect NOS

746 Other congenital anomalies of heart

    |Excludes:| *endocardial fibroelastosis (425.3)*

⑤ **746.0 Anomalies of pulmonary valve**

    |Excludes:| *infundibular or subvalvular pulmonic stenosis (746.83)*
                  tetralogy of Fallot (745.2)

746.00 Pulmonary valve anomaly, unspecified

746.01 Atresia, congenital
Congenital absence of pulmonary valve

746.02 Stenosis, congenital

746.09 Other
Congenital insufficiency of pulmonary valve
Fallot's triad or trilogy

746.1 Tricuspid atresia and stenosis, congenital
Absence of tricuspid valve

746.2 Ebstein's anomaly

746.3 Congenital stenosis of aortic valve
Congenital aortic stenosis

    |Excludes:| *congenital:*
                  subaortic stenosis (746.81)
                  supravalvular aortic stenosis (747.22)

746.4 Congenital insufficiency of aortic valve
Bicuspid aortic valve
Congenital aortic insufficiency

746.5 Congenital mitral stenosis
Fused commissure of mitral valve
Parachute deformity of mitral valve
Supernumerary cusps of mitral valve

746.6 Congenital mitral insufficiency

746.7 Hypoplastic left heart syndrome
Atresia, or marked hypoplasia, of aortic orifice or valve, with hypoplasia of ascending
aorta and defective development of left ventricle (with mitral valve atresia)

⑤ **746.8 Other specified anomalies of heart**

746.81 Subaortic stenosis

746.82 Cor triatriatum

746.83 Infundibular pulmonic stenosis
Subvalvular pulmonic stenosis

746.84 Obstructive anomalies of heart, not elsewhere classified
Uhl's disease

746.85 Coronary artery anomaly
Anomalous origin or communication of coronary artery
Arteriovenous malformation of coronary artery
Coronary artery:
  absence
  arising from aorta or pulmonary trunk
  single

746.86 Congenital heart block
Complete or incomplete atrioventricular [AV] block

● Code new
to this edition
   ▲ Revision of
existing code
   ④ ⑤ Fourth or fifth
digit required

746.87 Malposition of heart and cardiac apex
Abdominal heart   Levocardia (isolated)
Dextrocardia   Mesocardia
Ectopia cordis

Excludes: *dextrocardia with complete transposition of viscera (759.3)*

746.89 Other
Atresia of cardiac vein
Hypoplasia of cardiac vein
Congenital:
 cardiomegaly
 diverticulum, left ventricle
 pericardial defect

746.9 Unspecified anomaly of heart
Congenital:
 anomaly of heart NOS
 heart disease NOS

747 Other congenital anomalies of circulatory system

747.0 Patent ductus arteriosus
Patent ductus Botalli
Persistent ductus arteriosus

⑤ **747.1 Coarctation of aorta**

747.10 Coarctation of aorta (preductal) (postductal)
Hypoplasia of aortic arch

747.11 Interruption of aortic arch

⑤ **747.2 Other anomalies of aorta**

747.20 Anomaly of aorta, unspecified

747.21 Anomalies of aortic arch
Anomalous origin, right subclavian artery
Dextraposition of aorta
Double aortic arch
Kommerell's diverticulum
Overriding aorta
Persistent:
 convolutions, aortic arch
 right aortic arch
Vascular ring

Excludes: *hypoplasia of aortic arch (747.10)*

747.22 Atresia and stenosis of aorta
Absence of aorta
Aplasia of aorta
Hypoplasia of aorta
Stricture of aorta
Supra (valvular)-aortic stenosis

Excludes: *congenital aortic (valvular) stenosis or stricture, so stated (746.3)*
hypoplasia of aorta in hypoplastic left heart syndrome (746.7)

747.29 Other
Aneurysm of sinus of Valsalva
Congenital:
 aneurysm of aorta
 dilation of aorta

747.3 Anomalies of pulmonary artery
Agenesis of pulmonary artery
Anomaly of pulmonary artery
Atresia of pulmonary artery
Coarctation of pulmonary artery
Hypoplasia of pulmonary artery
Stenosis of pulmonary artery
Pulmonary arteriovenous aneurysm

⑤ **747.4 Anomalies of great veins**

747.40 Anomaly of great veins, unspecified
Anomaly NOS of:
 pulmonary veins
 vena cava

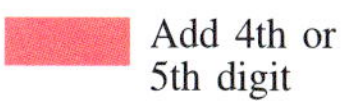

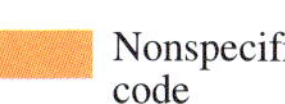

Unspecified
code

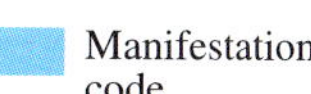

747.41　Total anomalous pulmonary venous connection
Total anomalous pulmonary venous return [TAPVR]:
　subdiaphragmatic
　supradiaphragmatic

747.42　Partial anomalous pulmonary venous connection
Partial anomalous pulmonary venous return

747.49　Other anomalies of great veins
Absence of vena cava (inferior) (superior)
Congenital stenosis of vena cava (inferior) (superior)
Persistent:
　left posterior cardinal vein
　left superior vena cava
Scimitar syndrome
Transposition of pulmonary veins NOS

747.5　Absence or hypoplasia of umbilical artery
Single umbilical artery

⑤ **747.6　Other anomalies of peripheral vascular system**
Absence of artery or vein, not elsewhere classified
Anomaly of artery or vein, not elsewhere classified
Atresia of artery or vein, not elsewhere classified
Arteriovenous aneurysm (peripheral)
Arteriovenous malformation of the peripheral vascular system
Congenital:
　aneurysm (peripheral)
　phlebectasia
　stricture, artery
　varix
Multiple renal arteries

Excludes: *anomalies of:*
*　　cerebral vessels (747.81)*
*　　pulmonary artery (747.3)*
*　congenital retinal aneurysm (743.58)*
*　hemangioma (228.00-228.09)*
*　lymphangioma (228.1)*

747.60　Anomaly of the peripheral vascular system, unspecified site

747.61　Gastrointestinal vessel anomaly

747.62　Renal vessel anomaly

747.63　Upper limb vessel anomaly

747.64　Lower limb vessel anomaly

747.69　Anomalies of other specified sites of peripheral vascular system

⑤ **747.8　Other specified anomalies of circulatory system**

747.81　Anomalies of cerebrovascular system
Arteriovenous malformation of brain
Cerebral arteriovenous aneurysm, congenital
Congenital anomalies of cerebral vessels

Excludes: *ruptured cerebral (arteriovenous) aneurysm (430)*

747.82　Spinal vessel anomaly
Arteriovenous malformation of spinal vessel

747.83　Persistent fetal circulation
Persistent pulmonary hypertension
Primary pulmonary hypertension of newborn

747.89　Other
Aneurysm, congenital, specified site not elsewhere classified

Excludes: *congenital aneurysm:*
*　coronary (746.85)*
*　peripheral (747.6)*
*　pulmonary (747.3)*
*　retinal (743.58)*

747.9　Unspecified anomaly of circulatory system

748　Congenital anomalies of respiratory system

Excludes: *congenital central alveolar hypoventilation syndrome (327.25)*
*　congenital defect of diaphragm (756.6)*

● Code new
　to this edition
▲ Revision of
　existing code
④ ⑤ Fourth or fifth
　digit required

748.0 Choanal atresia
Atresia of nares (anterior) (posterior)
Congenital stenosis of nares (anterior) (posterior)

748.1 Other anomalies of nose

Absent nose
Accessory nose
Cleft nose
Deformity of wall of nasal
   sinus

Congenital:
   deformity of nose
   notching of tip of nose
   perforation of wall of nasal sinus

Excludes: *congenital deviation of nasal septum (754.0)*

748.2 Web of larynx
Web of larynx:
   NOS
   glottic
   subglottic

748.3 Other anomalies of larynx, trachea, and bronchus

Absence or agenesis of:
   bronchus
   larynx
   trachea
Anomaly (of):
   cricoid cartilage
   epiglottis
   thyroid cartilage
   tracheal cartilage
Atresia (of):
   epiglottis
   glottis
   larynx
   trachea
Cleft thyroid, cartilage,
   congenital

Congenital:
   dilation, trachea
   stenosis:
     larynx
     trachea
   tracheocele
Diverticulum:
   bronchus
   trachea
Fissure of epiglottis
Laryngocele
Posterior cleft of cricoid cartilage (congenital)
Rudimentary tracheal bronchus
Stridor, laryngeal, congenital

748.4 Congenital cystic lung

Disease, lung:
   cystic, congenital
   polycystic, congenital

Honeycomb lung, congenital

Excludes: *acquired or unspecified cystic lung (518.89)*

748.5 Agenesis, hypoplasia, and dysplasia of lung
Absence of lung (fissures) (lobe)
Aplasia of lung
Hypoplasia of lung (lobe)
Sequestration of lung

⑤ **748.6 Other anomalies of lung**

   748.60 Anomaly of lung, unspecified

   748.61 Congenital bronchiectasis

   748.69 Other
      Accessory lung (lobe)
      Azygos lobe (fissure), lung

748.8 Other specified anomalies of respiratory system
Abnormal communication between pericardial and pleural sacs
Anomaly, pleural folds
Atresia of nasopharynx
Congenital cyst of mediastinum

748.9 Unspecified anomaly of respiratory system
Anomaly of respiratory system NOS

749 Cleft palate and cleft lip

⑤ **749.0 Cleft palate**

   749.00 Cleft palate, unspecified

   749.01 Unilateral, complete

   749.02 Unilateral, incomplete
      Cleft uvula

   749.03 Bilateral, complete

   749.04 Bilateral, incomplete

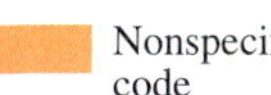

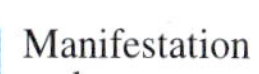

⑤ **749.1 Cleft lip**
    Cheiloschisis   Harelip
    Congenital fissure of lip   Labium leporinum

    749.10 Cleft lip, unspecified
    749.11 Unilateral, complete
    749.12 Unilateral, incomplete
    749.13 Bilateral, complete
    749.14 Bilateral, incomplete

⑤ **749.2 Cleft palate with cleft lip**
    Cheilopalatoschisis

    749.20 Cleft palate with cleft lip, unspecified
    749.21 Unilateral, complete
    749.22 Unilateral, incomplete
    749.23 Bilateral, complete
    749.24 Bilateral, incomplete
    749.25 Other combinations

750 Other congenital anomalies of upper alimentary tract
    Excludes: *dentofacial anomalies (524.0-524.9)*

    750.0 Tongue tie
        Ankyloglossia

⑤ **750.1 Other anomalies of tongue**
    750.10 Anomaly of tongue, unspecified
    750.11 Aglossia
    750.12 Congenital adhesions of tongue
    750.13 Fissure of tongue
        Bifid tongue
        Double tongue
    750.15 Macroglossia
        Congenital hypertrophy of tongue
    750.16 Microglossia
        Hypoplasia of tongue
    750.19 Other

⑤ **750.2 Other specified anomalies of mouth and pharynx**
    750.21 Absence of salivary gland
    750.22 Accessory salivary gland
    750.23 Atresia, salivary duct
        Imperforate salivary duct
    750.24 Congenital fistula of salivary gland
    750.25 Congenital fistula of lip
        Congenital (mucus) lip pits
    750.26 Other specified anomalies of mouth
        Absence of uvula
    750.27 Diverticulum of pharynx
        Pharyngeal pouch
    750.29 Other specified anomalies of pharynx
        Imperforate pharynx

    750.3 Tracheoesophageal fistula, esophageal atresia and stenosis
    Absent esophagus   Congenital fistula:
    Atresia of esophagus   esophagobronchial
    Congenital: esophagotracheal
      esophageal ring   Imperforate esophagus
      stenosis of esophagus   Webbed esophagus
      stricture of esophagus

● Code new to this edition   ▲ Revision of existing code   ④ ⑤ Fourth or fifth digit required

750.4 Other specified anomalies of esophagus
Dilatation, congenital (of) esophagus
Displacement, congenital (of) esophagus
Diverticulum (of) esophagus
Duplication (of) esophagus
Giant esophagus
Esophageal pouch

Excludes: congenital hiatus hernia (750.6)

750.5 Congenital hypertrophic pyloric stenosis
Congenital or infantile:
constriction of pylorus
hypertrophy of pylorus
spasm of pylorus
stenosis of pylorus
stricture of pylorus

750.6 Congenital hiatus hernia
Displacement of cardia through esophageal hiatus

Excludes: congenital diaphragmatic hernia (756.6)

750.7 Other specified anomalies of stomach
Congenital: Duplication of stomach
  cardiospasm   Megalogastria
  hourglass stomach   Microgastria
Displacement of stomach   Transposition of stomach
Diverticulum of stomach,
  congenital

750.8 Other specified anomalies of upper alimentary tract

750.9 Unspecified anomaly of upper alimentary tract
Congenital:
anomaly NOS of upper alimentary tract [any part, except tongue]
deformity NOS of upper alimentary tract [any part, except tongue]

751 Other congenital anomalies of digestive system

751.0 Meckel's diverticulum
Meckel's diverticulum (displaced) (hypertrophic)
Persistent:
omphalomesenteric duct
vitelline duct

751.1 Atresia and stenosis of small intestine
Atresia of:
duodenum
ileum
intestine NOS
Congenital:
absence of small intestine or intestine NOS
obstruction of small intestine or intestine NOS
stenosis of small intestine or intestine NOS
stricture of small intestine or intestine NOS
Imperforate jejunum

751.2 Atresia and stenosis of large intestine, rectum, and anal canal
Absence: Congenital or infantile:
  anus (congenital)   obstruction of large intestine
  appendix, congenital   occlusion of anus
  large intestine, congenital   stricture of anus
  rectum   Imperforate:
Atresia of: anus
  anus   rectum
  colon   Stricture of rectum, congenital
  rectum

751.3 Hirschsprung's disease and other congenital functional disorders of colon
Aganglionosis   Congenital megacolon
Congenital dilation of colon   Macrocolon

751.4 Anomalies of intestinal fixation
Congenital adhesions: Rotation of cecum or colon:
  omental, anomalous   failure of
  peritoneal   incomplete
Jackson's membrane   insufficient
Malrotation of colon   Universal mesentery

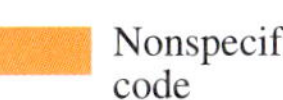
Add 4th or
5th digit

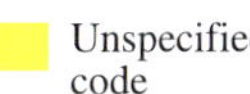
Nonspecific
code

Unspecified
code

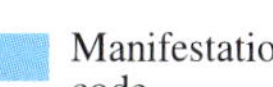
Manifestation
code

751.5   Other anomalies of intestine

Congenital diverticulum,
   colon
Dolichocolon
Duplication of:
   anus
   appendix
   cecum
   intestine
Ectopic anus

Megaloappendix
Megaloduodenum
Microcolon
Persistent cloaca
Transposition of:
   appendix
   colon
   intestine

⑤ **751.6   Anomalies of gallbladder, bile ducts, and liver**

751.60   Unspecified anomaly of gallbladder, bile ducts, and liver

751.61   Biliary atresia
Congenital:
   absence of bile duct (common) or passage
   hypoplasia of bile duct (common) or passage
   obstruction of bile duct (common) or passage
   stricture of bile duct (common) or passage

751.62   Congenital cystic disease of liver
Congenital polycystic disease of liver
Fibrocystic disease of liver

751.69   Other anomalies of gallbladder, bile ducts, and liver

Absence of:
   gallbladder, congenital
   liver (lobe)
Accessory:
   hepatic ducts
   liver
Congenital:
   choledochal cyst
   hepatomegaly

Duplication of:
   biliary duct
   cystic duct
   gallbladder
   liver
Floating:
   gallbladder
   liver
Intrahepatic gallbladder

751.7   Anomalies of pancreas
Absence of pancreas
Accessory pancreas
Agenesis of pancreas
Annular pancreas
Ectopic pancreatic tissue
Hypoplasia of pancreas
Pancreatic heterotopia

Excludes:	*diabetes mellitus:*
	congenital (250.0-250.9)
	neonatal (775.1)
	fibrocystic disease of pancreas (277.00-277.09)

751.8   Other specified anomalies of digestive system
Absence (complete) (partial) of alimentary tract NOS
Duplication of digestive organs NOS
Malposition, congenital of digestive organs NOS

Excludes:	*congenital diaphragmatic hernia (756.6)*
	congenital hiatus hernia (750.6)

751.9   Unspecified anomaly of digestive system
Congenital:
   anomaly NOS of digestive system NOS
   deformity NOS of digestive system NOS

752   Congenital anomalies of genital organs

Excludes:	*syndromes associated with anomalies in the number and form of chromosomes (758.0-758.9)*
	testicular feminization syndrome (259.5)

752.0   Anomalies of ovaries
Absence, congenital (of) ovary
Accessory ovary
Ectopic ovary
Streak of ovary

⑤ **752.1   Anomalies of fallopian tubes and broad ligaments**

752.10   Unspecified anomaly of fallopian tubes and broad ligaments

---

● Code new
   to this edition

▲ Revision of
   existing code

④ ⑤ Fourth or fifth
   digit required

752.11 Embryonic cyst of fallopian tubes and broad ligaments
Cyst:
epoophoron
fimbrial
parovarian

752.19 Other
Absence of fallopian tube or broad ligament
Accessory fallopian tube or broad ligament
Atresia of fallopian tube or broad ligament

752.2 Doubling of uterus
Didelphic uterus
Doubling of uterus [any degree] (associated with doubling of cervix and vagina)

752.3 Other anomalies of uterus
Absence, congenital, of uterus
Agenesis of uterus
Aplasia of uterus
Bicornuate uterus
Uterus unicornis
Uterus with only one functioning horn

⑤ **752.4 Anomalies of cervix, vagina, and external female genitalia**

752.40 Unspecified anomaly of cervix, vagina, and external female genitalia

752.41 Embryonic cyst of cervix, vagina, and external female genitalia
Cyst of:
canal of Nuck, congenital
Gartner's duct
Cyst of:
vagina, embryonal
vulva, congenital

752.42 Imperforate hymen

752.49 Other anomalies of cervix, vagina, and external female genitalia
Absence of cervix, clitoris, vagina, or vulva
Agenesis of cervix, clitoris, vagina, or vulva
Congenital stenosis or stricture of:
cervical canal
vagina

Excludes: *double vagina associated with total duplication (752.2)*

⑤ **752.5 Undescended and retractile testicle**

752.51 Undescended testis
Cryptorchism
Ectopic testis

752.52 Retractile testis

⑤ **752.6 Hypospadias and epispadias and other penile anomalies**

752.61 Hypospadias

752.62 Epispadias
Anaspadias

752.63 Congenital chordee

752.64 Micropenis

752.65 Hidden penis

752.69 Other penile anomalies

752.7 Indeterminate sex and pseudohermaphroditism
Gynandrism
Hermaphroditism
Ovotestis
Pseudohermaphroditism (male) (female)
Pure gonadal dysgenesis

Excludes: *pseudohermaphroditism:*
female, with adrenocortical disorder (255.2)
male, with gonadal disorder (257.8)
with specified chromosomal anomaly (758.0-758.9)
testicular feminization syndrome (259.5)

⑤ **752.8 Other specified anomalies of genital organs**
Excludes: *congenital hydrocele (778.6)*
penile anomalies (752.61-752.69)
phimosis or paraphimosis (605)

752.81 Scrotal transposition

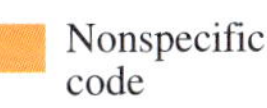

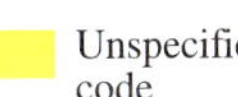

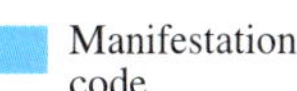

Manifestation
code

752.89 Other specified anomalies of genital organs
Absence of:
  prostate
  spermatic cord
  vas deferens
Anorchism
Aplasia (congenital) of:
  prostate
  round ligament
  testicle
Atresia of:
  ejaculatory duct
  vas deferens
Fusion of testes
Hypoplasia of testes
Monorchism
Polyorchism

752.9 Unspecified anomaly of genital organs
Congenital:
  anomaly NOS of genital organ, NEC
  deformity NOS of genital organ, NEC

753 Congenital anomalies of urinary system

753.0 Renal agenesis and dysgenesis
Atrophy of kidney: Congenital absence of kidney(s)
  congenital   Hypoplasia of kidney(s)
  infantile

⑤ **753.1 Cystic kidney disease**
Excludes: acquired cyst of kidney (593.2)

753.10 Cystic kidney disease, unspecified

753.11 Congenital single renal cyst

753.12 Polycystic kidney, unspecified type

753.13 Polycystic kidney, autosomal dominant

753.14 Polycystic kidney, autosomal recessive

753.15 Renal dysplasia

753.16 Medullary cystic kidney
Nephronopthisis

753.17 Medullary sponge kidney

753.19 Other specified cystic kidney disease
Multicystic kidney

⑤ **753.2 Obstructive defects of renal pelvis and ureter**

753.20 Unspecified obstructive defect of renal pelvis and ureter

753.21 Congenital obstruction of ureteropelvic junction

753.22 Congenital obstruction of ureterovesical junction
Adynamic ureter
Congenital hydroureter

753.23 Congenital ureterocele

753.29 Other

753.3 Other specified anomalies of kidney
Accessory kidney   Fusion of kidneys
Congenital: Giant kidney
  calculus of kidney   Horseshoe kidney
  displaced kidney   Hyperplasia of kidney
Discoid kidney   Lobulation of kidney
Double kidney with double   Malrotation of kidney
  pelvis   Trifid kidney (pelvis)
Ectopic kidney

753.4 Other specified anomalies of ureter
Absent ureter   Double ureter
Accessory ureter   Ectopic ureter
Deviation of ureter   Implantation, anomalous of ureter
Displaced ureteric orifice

753.5 Exstrophy of urinary bladder
Ectopia vesicae   Extroversion of bladder

● Code new   ▲ Revision of   ④ ⑤ Fourth or fifth
  to this edition   existing code   digit required

753.6 Atresia and stenosis of urethra and bladder neck
Congenital obstruction: Imperforate urinary meatus
  bladder neck Impervious urethra
  urethra Urethral valve formation
Congenital stricture of:
  urethra (valvular)
  urinary meatus
  vesicourethral orifice

753.7 Anomalies of urachus
Cyst (of) urachus Persistent umbilical sinus
Fistula (of) urachus
Patent (of) urachus

753.8 Other specified anomalies of bladder and urethra
Absence, congenital of: Congenital urethrorectal fistula
  bladder Congenital prolapse of:
  urethra   bladder (mucosa)
Accessory: urethra
  bladder Double:
  urethra   urethra
Congenital: urinary meatus
  diverticulum of bladder
  hernia of bladder

753.9 Unspecified anomaly of urinary system
Congenital:
  anomaly NOS of urinary system [any part, except urachus]
  deformity NOS of urinary system [any part, except urachus]

754 Certain congenital musculoskeletal deformities
Includes: nonteratogenic deformities which are considered to be due to intrauterine
  malposition and pressure

754.0 Of skull, face, and jaw
Asymmetry of face Dolichocephaly
Compression facies Plagiocephaly
Depressions in skull Potter's facies
Deviation of nasal Squashed or bent nose, congenital
  septum, congenital

Excludes: *dentofacial anomalies (524.0-524.9)*
    syphilitic saddle nose (090.5)

754.1 Of sternocleidomastoid muscle
Congenital sternomastoid torticollis
Congenital wryneck
Contracture of sternocleidomastoid (muscle)
Sternomastoid tumor

754.2 Of spine
Congenital postural:
  lordosis
  scoliosis

⑤ **754.3 Congenital dislocation of hip**

  754.30 Congenital dislocation of hip, unilateral
    Congenital dislocation of hip NOS

  754.31 Congenital dislocation of hip, bilateral

  754.32 Congenital subluxation of hip, unilateral
    Congenital flexion deformity, hip or thigh
    Predislocation status of hip at birth
    Preluxation of hip, congenital

  754.33 Congenital subluxation of hip, bilateral

  754.35 Congenital dislocation of one hip with subluxation of other hip

⑤ **754.4 Congenital genu recurvatum and bowing of long bones of leg**

  754.40 Genu recurvatum

  754.41 Congenital dislocation of knee (with genu recurvatum)

  754.42 Congenital bowing of femur

  754.43 Congenital bowing of tibia and fibula

  754.44 Congenital bowing of unspecified long bones of leg

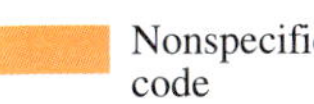

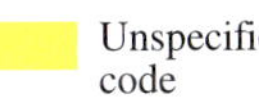

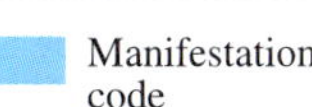

Manifestation
code

⑤ **754.5 Varus deformities of feet**
Excludes: acquired (736.71, 736.75, 736.79)

754.50 Talipes varus
Congenital varus deformity of foot, unspecified
Pes varus

754.51 Talipes equinovarus
Equinovarus (congenital)

754.52 Metatarsus primus varus

754.53 Metatarsus varus

754.59 Other
Talipes calcaneovarus

⑤ **754.6 Valgus deformities of feet**
Excludes: valgus deformity of foot (acquired) (736.79)

754.60 Talipes valgus
Congenital valgus deformity of foot, unspecified

754.61 Congenital pes planus
Congenital rocker bottom flat foot
Flat foot, congenital

Excludes: pes planus (acquired) (734)

754.62 Talipes calcaneovalgus

754.69 Other
Talipes:
   equinovalgus
   planovalgus

⑤ **754.7 Other deformities of feet**
Excludes: acquired (736.70-736.79)

754.70 Talipes, unspecified
Congenital deformity of foot NOS

754.71 Talipes cavus
Cavus foot (congenital)

754.79 Other
Asymmetric talipes
Talipes:
   calcaneus
   equinus

⑤ **754.8 Other specified nonteratogenic anomalies**

754.81 Pectus excavatum
Congenital funnel chest

754.82 Pectus carinatum
Congenital pigeon chest [breast]

754.89 Other
Club hand (congenital)
Congenital:
   deformity of chest wall
   dislocation of elbow
Generalized flexion contractures of lower limb joints, congenital
Spade-like hand (congenital)

755 Other congenital anomalies of limbs
Excludes: those deformities classifiable to 754.0-754.8

⑤ **755.0 Polydactyly**

755.00 Polydactyly, unspecified digits
Supernumerary digits

755.01 Of fingers
Accessory fingers

755.02 Of toes
Accessory toes

⑤ **755.1 Syndactyly**
Symphalangy
Webbing of digits

755.10 Of multiple and unspecified sites

● Code new to this edition   ▲ Revision of existing code   ④ ⑤ Fourth or fifth digit required

755.11   **Of fingers without fusion of bone**

755.12   **Of fingers with fusion of bone**

755.13   **Of toes without fusion of bone**

755.14   **Of toes with fusion of bone**

⑤ **755.2**   **Reduction deformities of upper limb**

755.20   **Unspecified reduction deformity of upper limb**
Ectromelia NOS of upper limb
Hemimelia NOS of upper limb
Shortening of arm, congenital

755.21   **Transverse deficiency of upper limb**
Amelia of upper limb
Congenital absence of:
   fingers, all (complete or partial)
   forearm, including hand and fingers
   upper limb, complete
Congenital amputation of upper limb
Transverse hemimelia of upper limb

755.22   **Longitudinal deficiency of upper limb, not elsewhere classified**
Phocomelia NOS of upper limb
Rudimentary arm

755.23   **Longitudinal deficiency, combined, involving humerus, radius, and ulna (complete or incomplete)**
Congenital absence of arm and forearm (complete or incomplete) with or
   without metacarpal deficiency and/or phalangeal deficiency, incomplete
Phocomelia, complete, of upper limb

755.24   **Longitudinal deficiency, humeral, complete or partial (with or without distal deficiencies, incomplete)**
Congenital absence of humerus (with or without absence of some [but not all]
   distal elements)
Proximal phocomelia of upper limb

755.25   **Longitudinal deficiency, radioulnar, complete or partial (with or without distal deficiencies, incomplete)**
Congenital absence of radius and ulna (with or without absence of some [but
   not all] distal elements)
Distal phocomelia of upper limb

755.26   **Longitudinal deficiency, radial, complete or partial (with or without distal deficiencies, incomplete)**
Agenesis of radius
Congenital absence of radius (with or without absence of some [but not all]
   distal elements)

755.27   **Longitudinal deficiency, ulnar, complete or partial (with or without distal deficiencies, incomplete)**
Agenesis of ulna
Congenital absence of ulna (with or without absence of some [but not all]
   distal elements)

755.28   **Longitudinal deficiency, carpals or metacarpals, complete or partial (with or without incomplete phalangeal deficiency)**

755.29   **Longitudinal deficiency, phalanges, complete or partial**
Absence of finger, congenital
Aphalangia of upper limb, terminal, complete or partial

> *Excludes:*   *terminal deficiency of all five digits (755.21)*
> *transverse deficiency of phalanges (755.21)*

⑤ **755.3**   **Reduction deformities of lower limb**

755.30   **Unspecified reduction deformity of lower limb**
Ectromelia NOS of lower limb
Hemimelia NOS of lower limb
Shortening of leg, congenital

755.31   **Transverse deficiency of lower limb**
Amelia of lower limb
Congenital absence of:
   foot
   leg, including foot and toes
   lower limb, complete
   toes, all, complete
Transverse hemimelia of lower limb

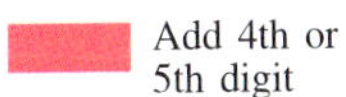 Add 4th or 5th digit

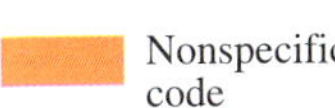 Nonspecific code

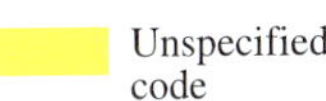 Unspecified code

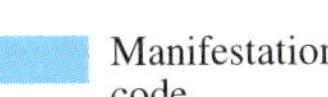 Manifestation code

755.32 Longitudinal deficiency of lower limb, not elsewhere classified
Phocomelia NOS of lower limb

755.33 Longitudinal deficiency, combined, involving femur, tibia, and fibula (complete or incomplete)
Congenital absence of thigh and (lower) leg (complete or incomplete) with or without metacarpal deficiency and/or phalangeal deficiency, incomplete
Phocomelia, complete, of lower limb

755.34 Longitudinal deficiency, femoral, complete or partial (with or without distal deficiencies, incomplete)
Congenital absence of femur (with or without absence of some [but not all] distal elements)
Proximal phocomelia of lower limb

755.35 Longitudinal deficiency, tibiofibular, complete or partial (with or without distal deficiencies, incomplete)
Congenital absence of tibia and fibula (with or without absence of some [but not all] distal elements)
Distal phocomelia of lower limb

755.36 Longitudinal deficiency, tibia, complete or partial (with or without distal deficiencies, incomplete)
Agenesis of tibia
Congenital absence of tibia (with or without absence of some [but not all] distal elements)

755.37 Longitudinal deficiency, fibular, complete or partial (with or without distal deficiencies, incomplete)
Agenesis of fibula
Congenital absence of fibula (with or without absence of some [but not all] distal elements)

755.38 Longitudinal deficiency, tarsals or metatarsals, complete or partial (with or without incomplete phalangeal deficiency)

755.39 Longitudinal deficiency, phalanges, complete or partial
Absence of toe, congenital
Aphalangia of lower limb, terminal, complete or partial

Excludes: *terminal deficiency of all five digits (755.31)*
transverse deficiency of phalanges (755.31)

755.4 Reduction deformities, unspecified limb
Absence, congenital (complete or partial) of limb NOS
Amelia of unspecified limb
Ectromelia of unspecified limb
Hemimelia of unspecified limb
Phocomelia of unspecified limb

⑤ **755.5 Other anomalies of upper limb, including shoulder girdle**

755.50 Unspecified anomaly of upper limb

755.51 Congenital deformity of clavicle

755.52 Congenital elevation of scapula
Sprengel's deformity

755.53 Radioulnar synostosis

755.54 Madelung's deformity

755.55 Acrocephalosyndactyly
Apert's syndrome

755.56 Accessory carpal bones

755.57 Macrodactylia (fingers)

755.58 Cleft hand, congenital
Lobster-claw hand

755.59 Other
Cleidocranial dysostosis
Cubitus:
valgus, congenital
varus, congenital

Excludes: *club hand (congenital) (754.89)*
congenital dislocation of elbow (754.89)

⑤ **755.6 Other anomalies of lower limb, including pelvic girdle**

755.60 Unspecified anomaly of lower limb

755.61 Coxa valga, congenital

● Code new to this edition　　　▲ Revision of existing code　　　④ ⑤ Fourth or fifth digit required

755.62   **Coxa vara, congenital**

755.63   **Other congenital deformity of hip (joint)**
Congenital anteversion of femur (neck)

Excludes: *congenital dislocation of hip (754.30-754.35)*

755.64   **Congenital deformity of knee (joint)**
Congenital:
   absence of patella
   genu valgum [knock-knee]
   genu varum [bowleg]
   Rudimentary patella

755.65   **Macrodactylia of toes**

755.66   **Other anomalies of toes**
Congenital:
   hallux valgus
   hallux varus
   hammer toe

755.67   **Anomalies of foot, not elsewhere classified**
Astragaloscaphoid synostosis
Calcaneonavicular bar
Coalition of calcaneus
Talonavicular synostosis
Tarsal coalitions

755.69   **Other**
Congenital:
   angulation of tibia
   deformity (of):
     ankle (joint)
     sacroiliac (joint)
   fusion of sacroiliac joint

755.8   **Other specified anomalies of unspecified limb**

755.9   **Unspecified anomaly of unspecified limb**
Congenital:
   anomaly NOS of unspecified limb
   deformity NOS of unspecified limb

Excludes: *reduction deformity of unspecified limb (755.4)*

756   **Other congenital musculoskeletal anomalies**

Excludes: *those deformities classifiable to 754.0-754.8*

756.0   **Anomalies of skull and face bones**
Absence of skull bones
Acrocephaly
Congenital deformity of
   forehead
Craniosynostosis
Crouzon's disease
Hypertelorism
Imperfect fusion of skull
Oxycephaly
Platybasia
Premature closure of cranial sutures
Tower skull
Trigonocephaly

Excludes: *acrocephalosyndactyly [Apert's syndrome] (755.55)*
dentofacial anomalies (524.0-524.9)
skull defects associated with brain anomalies, such as:
   anencephalus (740.0)
   encephalocele (742.0)
   hydrocephalus (742.3)
   microcephalus (742.1)

⑤ **756.1**   **Anomalies of spine**

756.10   **Anomaly of spine, unspecified**

756.11   **Spondylolysis, lumbosacral region**
Prespondylolisthesis (lumbosacral)

756.12   **Spondylolisthesis**

756.13   **Absence of vertebra, congenital**

756.14   **Hemivertebra**

756.15   **Fusion of spine [vertebra], congenital**

756.16   **Klippel-Feil syndrome**

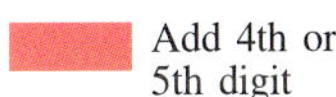

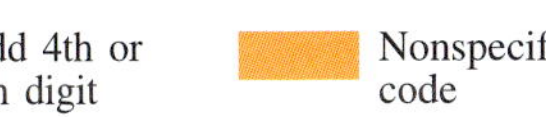

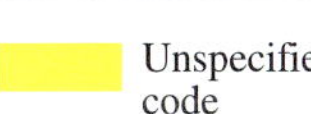

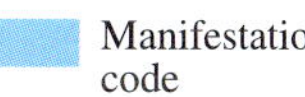

756.17 Spina bifida occulta

Excludes: *spina bifida (aperta) (741.0-741.9)*

756.19 Other
Platyspondylia
Supernumerary vertebra

756.2 Cervical rib
Supernumerary rib in the cervical region

756.3 Other anomalies of ribs and sternum
Congenital absence of:
  rib
  sternum
Congenital:
  fissure of sternum
  fusion of ribs
Sternum bifidum

Excludes: *nonteratogenic deformity of chest wall (754.81-754.89)*

756.4 Chondrodystrophy
Achondroplasia
Chondrodystrophia (fetalis)
Dyschondroplasia
Enchondromatosis
Ollier's disease

Excludes: *lipochondrodystrophy [Hurler's syndrome] (277.5)*
Morquio's disease (277.5)

⑤ **756.5 Osteodystrophies**

756.50 Osteodystrophy, unspecified

756.51 Osteogenesis imperfecta
Fragilitas ossium
Osteopsathyrosis

756.52 Osteopetrosis

756.53 Osteopoikilosis

756.54 Polyostotic fibrous dysplasia of bone

756.55 Chondroectodermal dysplasia
Ellis-van Creveld syndrome

756.56 Multiple epiphyseal dysplasia

756.59 Other
Albright (-McCune)-Sternberg syndrome

756.6 Anomalies of diaphragm
Absence of diaphragm
Congenital hernia:
  diaphragmatic
  foramen of Morgagni
Eventration of diaphragm

Excludes: *congenital hiatus hernia (750.6)*

⑤ **756.7 Anomalies of abdominal wall**

756.70 Anomaly of abdominal wall, unspecified

756.71 Prune belly syndrome
Eagle-Barrett syndrome
Prolapse of bladder mucosa

756.79 Other congenital anomalies of abdominal wall
Exomphalos
Gastroschisis
Omphalocele

Excludes: *umbilical hernia (551-553 with .1)*

⑤ **756.8 Other specified anomalies of muscle, tendon, fascia, and connective tissue**

756.81 Absence of muscle and tendon
Absence of muscle (pectoral)

756.82 Accessory muscle

756.83 Ehlers-Danlos syndrome

● Code new
to this edition

▲ Revision of
existing code

④ ⑤ Fourth or fifth
digit required

756.89 **Other**
Amyotrophia congenita
Congenital shortening of tendon

756.9 **Other and unspecified anomalies of musculoskeletal system**
Congenital:
anomaly NOS of musculoskeletal system, not elsewhere classified
deformity NOS of musculoskeletal system, not elsewhere classified

757 **Congenital anomalies of the integument**
Includes: anomalies of skin, subcutaneous tissue, hair, nails, and breast

Excludes: hemangioma (228.00-228.09)

pigmented nevus (216.0-216.9)

757.0 **Hereditary edema of legs**
Congenital lymphedema   Milroy's disease
Hereditary trophedema

757.1 **Ichthyosis congenita**
Congenital ichthyosis
Harlequin fetus
Ichthyosiform erythroderma

757.2 **Dermatoglyphic anomalies**
Abnormal palmar creases

⑤ **757.3** **Other specified anomalies of skin**

757.31 **Congenital ectodermal dysplasia**

757.32 **Vascular hamartomas**
Birthmarks
Port-wine stain
Strawberry nevus

757.33 **Congenital pigmentary anomalies of skin**
Congenital poikiloderma
Urticaria pigmentosa
Xeroderma pigmentosum

Excludes: albinism (270.2)

757.39 **Other**
Accessory skin tags, congenital
Congenital scar
Epidermolysis bullosa
Keratoderma (congenital)

Excludes: pilonidal cyst (685.0-685.1)

757.4 **Specified anomalies of hair**
Congenital: Congenital:
alopecia   hypertrichosis
atrichosis   monilethrix
beaded hair   Persistent lanugo

757.5 **Specified anomalies of nails**
Anonychia   Congenital:
Congenital: leukonychia
clubnail   onychauxis
koilonychia   pachyonychia

757.6 **Specified anomalies of breast**
Absent breast or nipple
Accessory breast or nipple
Supernumerary breast or nipple
Hypoplasia of breast

Excludes: absence of pectoral muscle (756.81)

757.8 **Other specified anomalies of the integument**

757.9 **Unspecified anomaly of the integument**
Congenital:
anomaly NOS of integument
deformity NOS of integument

758 **Chromosomal anomalies**
Includes: syndromes associated with anomalies in the number and form of chromosomes
Use additional codes for conditions associated with the chromosomal anomalies

758.0 Down's syndrome
Mongolism
Translocation Down's
syndrome

Trisomy:
21 or 22
G

758.1 Patau's syndrome
Trisomy:
13
D_1

758.2 Edwards' syndrome
Trisomy:
18
E_3

⑤ **758.3 Autosomal deletion syndromes**

758.31 Cri-du-chat syndrome
Deletion 5p

758.32 Velo-cardio-facial syndrome
Deletion 22q11.2

758.33 Other microdeletions
Miller-Dieker syndrome
Smith-Magenis syndrome

758.39 Other autosomal deletions

758.4 Balanced autosomal translocation in normal individual

758.5 Other conditions due to autosomal anomalies
Accessory autosomes NEC

758.6 Gonadal dysgenesis
Ovarian dysgenesis
Turner's syndrome
XO syndrome

| Excludes: | pure gonadal dysgenesis (752.7) |

758.7 Klinefelter's syndrome
XXY syndrome

⑤ **758.8 Other conditions due to chromosome anomalies**

758.81 Other conditions due to sex chromosome anomalies

758.89 Other

758.9 Conditions due to anomaly of unspecified chromosome

759 Other and unspecified congenital anomalies

759.0 Anomalies of spleen
Aberrant spleen
Absent spleen
Accessory spleen

Congenital splenomegaly
Ectopic spleen
Lobulation of spleen

759.1 Anomalies of adrenal gland
Aberrant adrenal gland
Absent adrenal gland
Accessory adrenal gland

| Excludes: | adrenogenital disorders (255.2) |
| | congenital disorders of steroid metabolism (255.2) |

759.2 Anomalies of other endocrine glands
Absent parathyroid gland
Accessory thyroid gland
Persistent thyroglossal or thyrolingual duct
Thyroglossal (duct) cyst

Excludes:	congenital:
	goiter (246.1)
	hypothyroidism (243)

759.3 Situs inversus
Situs inversus or transversus:
abdominalis
thoracis
Transposition of viscera:
abdominal
thoracic

| Excludes: | dextrocardia without mention of complete transposition (746.87) |

● Code new
to this edition

▲ Revision of
existing code

④ ⑤ Fourth or fifth
digit required

759.4 Conjoined twins
    Craniopagus   Thoracopagus
    Dicephalus   Xiphopagus
    Pygopagus

759.5 Tuberous sclerosis
    Bourneville's disease
    Epiloia

759.6 Other hamartoses, not elsewhere classified
    Syndrome:
        Peutz-Jeghers
        Sturge-Weber (-Dimitri)
        von Hippel-Lindau

    Excludes: *neurofibromatosis (237.7)*

759.7 Multiple congenital anomalies, so described
    Congenital:
        anomaly, multiple NOS
        deformity, multiple NOS

⑤ **759.8 Other specified anomalies**

   759.81 Prader-Willi syndrome

   759.82 Marfan syndrome

   759.83 Fragile X syndrome

   759.89 Other
        Congenital malformation syndromes affecting multiple systems, not elsewhere
            classified
        Laurence-Moon-Biedl syndrome

759.9 Congenital anomaly, unspecified

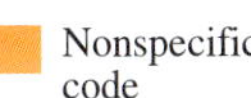
Add 4th or
5th digit

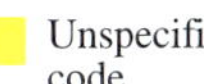
Nonspecific
code

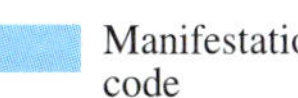
Unspecified
code

Manifestation
code

● Code new
to this edition

▲ Revision of
existing code

④ ⑤ Fourth or fifth
digit required

15. CERTAIN CONDITIONS ORIGINATING IN THE PERINATAL PERIOD (760-779)

Includes: conditions which have their origin in the perinatal period, before birth through the first 28 days after birth, even though death or morbidity occurs later

Use additional code(s) to further specify condition

MATERNAL CAUSES OF PERINATAL MORBIDITY AND MORTALITY (760-763)

760 Fetus or newborn affected by maternal conditions which may be unrelated to present pregnancy
Includes: the listed maternal conditions only when specified as a cause of mortality or morbidity of the fetus or newborn

Excludes: *maternal endocrine and metabolic disorders affecting fetus or newborn (775.0-775.9)*

760.0 Maternal hypertensive disorders
Fetus or newborn affected by maternal conditions classifiable to 642

760.1 Maternal renal and urinary tract diseases
Fetus or newborn affected by maternal conditions classifiable to 580-599

760.2 Maternal infections
Fetus or newborn affected by maternal infectious disease classifiable to 001-136 and 487, but fetus or newborn not manifesting that disease

Excludes: *congenital infectious diseases (771.0-771.8)*
maternal genital tract and other localized infections (760.8)

760.3 Other chronic maternal circulatory and respiratory diseases
Fetus or newborn affected by chronic maternal conditions classifiable to 390-459, 490-519, 745-748

760.4 Maternal nutritional disorders
Fetus or newborn affected by:
maternal disorders classifiable to 260-269
maternal malnutrition NOS

Excludes: *fetal malnutrition (764.10-764.29)*

760.5 Maternal injury
Fetus or newborn affected by maternal conditions classifiable to 800-995

760.6 Surgical operation on mother

Excludes: *cesarean section for present delivery (763.4)*
damage to placenta from amniocentesis, cesarean section, or surgical induction (762.1)
previous surgery to uterus or pelvic organs (763.89)

⑤ 760.7 Noxious influences affecting fetus or newborn via placenta or breast milk
Fetus or newborn affected by noxious substance transmitted via placenta or breast milk

Excludes: *anesthetic and analgesic drugs administered during labor and delivery (763.5)*
drug withdrawal syndrome in newborn (779.5)

760.70 Unspecified noxious substance
Fetus or newborn affected by:
Drug NEC

760.71 Alcohol
Fetal alcohol syndrome

760.72 Narcotics

760.73 Hallucinogenic agents

760.74 Anti-infectives
Antibiotics
Antifungals

760.75 Cocaine

760.76 Diethylstilbestrol (DES)

760.77 Anticonvulsants
Carbamazepine
Phenobarbital
Phenytoin
Valproic acid

760.78 Antimetabolic agents
Methotrexate
Retinoic acid
Statins

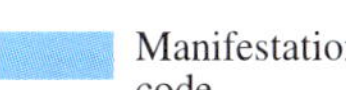

760.79 Other
Fetus or newborn affected by:
immune sera transmitted via placenta or breast milk
medicinal agents NEC transmitted via placenta or breast milk
toxic substance NEC transmitted via placenta or breast milk

760.8 Other specified maternal conditions affecting fetus or newborn
Maternal genital tract and other localized infection affecting fetus or newborn, but fetus
or newborn not manifesting that disease

Excludes: *maternal urinary tract infection affecting fetus or newborn (760.1)*

760.9 Unspecified maternal condition affecting fetus or newborn

761 Fetus or newborn affected by maternal complications of pregnancy
Includes: the listed maternal conditions only when specified as a cause of mortality or
morbidity of the fetus or newborn

761.0 Incompetent cervix

761.1 Premature rupture of membranes

761.2 Oligohydramnios

Excludes: *that due to premature rupture of membranes (761.1)*

761.3 Polyhydramnios
Hydramnios (acute) (chronic)

761.4 Ectopic pregnancy
Pregnancy:
abdominal
intraperitoneal
tubal

761.5 Multiple pregnancy
Triplet (pregnancy)
Twin (pregnancy)

761.6 Maternal death

761.7 Malpresentation before labor
Breech presentation before labor
External version before labor
Oblique lie before labor
Transverse lie before labor
Unstable lie before labor

761.8 Other specified maternal complications of pregnancy affecting fetus or newborn
Spontaneous abortion, fetus

761.9 Unspecified maternal complication of pregnancy affecting fetus or newborn

762 Fetus or newborn affected by complications of placenta, cord, and membranes
Includes: the listed maternal conditions only when specified as a cause of mortality or
morbidity in the fetus or newborn

762.0 Placenta previa

762.1 Other forms of placental separation and hemorrhage
Abruptio placentae
Antepartum hemorrhage
Damage to placenta from amniocentesis, cesarean section, or surgical induction
Maternal blood loss
Premature separation of placenta
Rupture of marginal sinus

762.2 Other and unspecified morphological and functional abnormalities of placenta
Placental:
dysfunction
infarction
insufficiency

762.3 Placental transfusion syndromes
Placental and cord abnormality resulting in twin-to-twin or other transplacental
transfusion
Use additional code, if desired, to indicate resultant condition in fetus or newborn:
fetal blood loss (772.0)
polycythemia neonatorum (776.4)

762.4 Prolapsed cord
Cord presentation

● Code new
to this edition
▲ Revision of
existing code
④ ⑤ Fourth or fifth
digit required

762.5 Other compression of umbilical cord
    Cord around neck   Knot in cord
    Entanglement of cord   Torsion of cord

762.6 Other and unspecified conditions of umbilical cord
    Short umbilical cord
    Thrombosis of umbilical cord
    Varices of umbilical cord
    Velamentous insertion of umbilical cord
    Vasa previa

    Excludes: *infection of umbilical cord (771.4)*
        single umbilical artery (747.5)

762.7 Chorioamnionitis
    Amnionitis
    Membranitis
    Placentitis

762.8 Other specified abnormalities of chorion and amnion

762.9 Unspecified abnormality of chorion and amnion

763 Fetus or newborn affected by other complications of labor and delivery
    Includes: the listed conditions only when specified as a cause of mortality or morbidity in
        the fetus or newborn

763.0 Breech delivery and extraction

763.1 Other malpresentation, malposition, and disproportion during labor and delivery
    Fetus or newborn affected by:
        abnormality of bony pelvis
        contracted pelvis
        persistent occipitoposterior position
        shoulder presentation
        transverse lie
        conditions classifiable to 652, 653, and 660

763.2 Forceps delivery
    Fetus or newborn affected by forceps extraction

763.3 Delivery by vacuum extractor

763.4 Cesarean delivery
    Excludes: *placental separation or hemorrhage from cesarean section (762.1)*

763.5 Maternal anesthesia and analgesia
    Reactions and intoxications from maternal opiates and tranquilizers during labor and
        delivery
    Excludes: *drug withdrawal syndrome in newborn (779.5)*

763.6 Precipitate delivery
    Rapid second stage

763.7 Abnormal uterine contractions
    Fetus or newborn affected by:
        contraction ring
        hypertonic labor
        hypotonic uterine dysfunction
        uterine inertia or dysfunction
        conditions classifiable to 661, except 661.3

⑤ **763.8 Other specified complications of labor and delivery affecting fetus or newborn**

    763.81 Abnormality in fetal heart rate or rhythm before the onset of labor

    763.82 Abnormality in fetal heart rate or rhythm during labor

    763.83 Abnormality in fetal heart rate or rhythm, unspecified as to time of onset

    763.84 Meconium passage during delivery
    Excludes: *meconium aspiration (770.11, 770.12)*
        meconium staining (779.84)

763.89   Other specified complications of labor and delivery affecting fetus or newborn
Fetus or newborn affected by:
abnormality of maternal soft tissues
destructive operation on live fetus to facilitate delivery
induction of labor (medical)
previous surgery to uterus or pelvic organs
other conditions classifiable to 650-669
other procedures used in labor and delivery

763.9   Unspecified complication of labor and delivery affecting fetus or newborn

OTHER CONDITIONS ORIGINATING IN THE PERINATAL PERIOD (764-779)

The following fifth-digit subclassification is for use with categories 764 and codes 765.0 and 765.1 to denote birthweight:

0   unspecified [weight]

1   less than 500 grams

2   500-749 grams

3   750-999 grams

4   1,000- 1,249 grams

5   1,250-1,499 grams

6   1,500-1,749 grams

7   1,750-1,999 grams

8   2,000-2,499 grams

9   2,500 grams and over

⑤ **764   Slow fetal growth and fetal malnutrition**

⑤ **764.0   "Light-for-dates" without mention of fetal malnutrition**
Infants underweight for gestational age
"Small-for-dates"

⑤ **764.1   "Light-for-dates" with signs of fetal malnutrition**
Infants "light-for-dates" classifiable to 764.0, who in addition show signs of fetal malnutrition, such as dry peeling skin and loss of subcutaneous tissue

⑤ **764.2   Fetal malnutrition without mention of "light-for-dates"**
Infants, not underweight for gestational age, showing signs of fetal malnutrition, such as dry peeling skin and loss of subcutaneous tissue
Intrauterine malnutrition

⑤ **764.9   Fetal growth retardation, unspecified**
Intrauterine growth retardation

765   Disorders relating to short gestation and low birthweight
Includes: the listed conditions, without further specification, as causes of mortality, morbidity, or additional care, in fetus or newborn

⑤ **765.0   Extreme immaturity**
Note: Usually implies a birthweight of less than 1000 grams
Use additional code for weeks of gestation (765.20-765.29)

⑤ **765.1   Other preterm infants**
Prematurity NOS
Prematurity or small size, not classifiable to 765.0 or as "light-for-dates" in 764
Note: Usually implies a birthweight of 1000-2499 grams
Use additional code for weeks of gestation (765.20-765.29)

⑤ **765.2   Weeks of gestation**

765.20   Unspecified weeks of gestation

765.21   Less than 24 completed weeks of gestation

765.22   24 completed weeks of gestation

765.23   25-26 completed weeks of gestation

765.24   27-28 completed weeks of gestation

765.25   29-30 completed weeks of gestation

765.26   31-32 completed weeks of gestation

765.27   33-34 completed weeks of gestation

765.28   35-36 completed weeks of gestation

765.29   37 or more completed weeks of gestation

● Code new to this edition   ▲ Revision of existing code   ④ ⑤ Fourth or fifth digit required

766 Disorders relating to long gestation and high birthweight
Includes: the listed conditions, without further specification, as causes of mortality, morbidity, or additional care, in fetus or newborn

766.0 Exceptionally large baby
Note: Usually implies a birthweight of 4500 grams or more.

766.1 Other "heavy-for-dates" infants
Other fetus or infant "heavy-" or "large-for-dates" regardless of period of gestation

⑤ **766.2 Late infant, not "heavy-for-dates"**

766.21 Post-term infant
Infant with gestation period over 40 completed weeks to 42 completed weeks

766.22 Prolonged gestation of infant
Infant with gestation period over 42 completed weeks
Postmaturity NOS

767 Birth trauma

767.0 Subdural and cerebral hemorrhage
Subdural and cerebral hemorrhage, whether described as due to birth trauma or to intrapartum anoxia or hypoxia
Subdural hematoma (localized)
Tentorial tear
Use additional code, if desired, to identify cause

> *Excludes:* *intraventricular hemorrhage (772.10-772.14)*
> *subarachnoid hemorrhage (772.2)*

⑤ **767.1 Injuries to scalp**

767.11 Epicranial subaponeurotic hemorrhage (massive)
Subgaleal hemorrhage

767.19 Other injuries to scalp
Caput succedaneum
Cephalhematoma
Chignon (from vacuum extraction)

767.2 Fracture of clavicle

767.3 Other injuries to skeleton
Fracture of:
long bones
skull

> *Excludes:* *congenital dislocation of hip (754.30-754.35)*
> *fracture of spine, congenital (767.4)*

767.4 Injury to spine and spinal cord
Dislocation of spine or spinal cord due to birth trauma
Fracture of spine or spinal cord due to birth trauma
Laceration of spine or spinal cord due to birth trauma
Rupture of spine or spinal cord due to birth trauma

767.5 Facial nerve injury
Facial palsy

767.6 Injury to brachial plexus
Palsy or paralysis:
brachial
Erb (-Duchenne)
Klumpke (-Déjérine)

767.7 Other cranial and peripheral nerve injuries
Phrenic nerve paralysis

767.8 Other specified birth trauma

Eye damage	Rupture of:
Hematoma of:	liver
liver (subcapsular)	spleen
testes	Scalpel wound
vulva	Traumatic glaucoma

> *Excludes:* *hemorrhage classifiable to 772.0-772.9*

767.9 Birth trauma, unspecified
Birth injury NOS

768 Intrauterine hypoxia and birth asphyxia
Use only when associated with newborn morbidity classifiable elsewhere

> *Excludes:* *acidemia NOS of newborn (775.81)*
> *acidosis NOS of newborn (775.81)*
> *cerebral ischemia NOS (779.2)*
> *hypoxia NOS of newborn (770.88)*
> *mixed metabolic and respiratory acidosis of newborn (775.81)*
> *respiratory arrest of newborn (770.87)*

768.0 Fetal death from asphyxia or anoxia before onset of labor or at unspecified time

768.1 Fetal death from asphyxia or anoxia during labor

768.2 Fetal distress before onset of labor, in liveborn infant
Fetal metabolic acidemia before onset of labor, in liveborn infant

▲ **768.3 Fetal distress first noted during labor and delivery, in liveborn infant**
Fetal metabolic acidemia first noted during labor and delivery, in liveborn infant

768.4 Fetal distress, unspecified as to time of onset, in liveborn infant
Fetal metabolic acidemia unspecified as to time of onset, in liveborn infant

768.5 Severe birth asphyxia
Birth asphyxia with neurologic involvement

> *Excludes:* *hypoxic-ischemic encephalopathy (HIE) (768.7)*

768.6 Mild or moderate birth asphyxia
Other specified birth asphyxia (without mention of neurologic involvement)

> *Excludes:* *hypoxic-ischemic encephalopathy (HIE) (768.7)*

● **768.7 Hypoxic-ischemic encephalopathy (HIE)**

768.9 Unspecified birth asphyxia in liveborn infant
Anoxia NOS, in liveborn infant
Asphyxia NOS, in liveborn infant

769 Respiratory distress syndrome
Cardiorespiratory distress syndrome of newborn
Hyaline membrane disease (pulmonary)
Idiopathic respiratory distress syndrome [IRDS or RDS] of newborn
Pulmonary hypoperfusion syndrome

> *Excludes:* *transient tachypnea of newborn (770.6)*

770 Other respiratory conditions of fetus and newborn

770.0 Congenital pneumonia
Infective pneumonia acquired prenatally

> *Excludes:* *pneumonia from infection acquired after birth (480.0-486)*

⑤ **770.1 Fetal and newborn aspiration**

> *Excludes:* *aspiration of postnatal stomach contents (770.85, 770.86)*
> *meconium passage during delivery (763.84)*
> *meconium staining (779.84)*

770.10 Fetal and newborn aspiration, unspecified

770.11 Meconium aspiration without respiratory symptoms
Meconium aspiration NOS

770.12 Meconium aspiration with respiratory symptoms
Meconium aspiration pneumonia
Meconium aspiration pneumonitis
Meconium aspiration syndrome NOS
Use additional code to identify any secondary pulmonary hypertension (416.8), if applicable

770.13 Aspiration of clear amniotic fluid without respiratory symptoms
Aspiration of clear amniotic fluid NOS

770.14 Aspiration of clear amniotic fluid with respiratory symptoms
Aspiration of clear amniotic fluid with pneumonia
Aspiration of clear amniotic fluid with pneumonitis
Use additional code to identify any secondary pulmonary hypertension (416.8), if applicable

770.15 Aspiration of blood without respiratory symptoms
Aspiration of blood NOS

● Code new
to this edition

▲ Revision of
existing code

④ ⑤ Fourth or fifth
digit required

770.16 Aspiration of blood with respiratory symptoms
Aspiration of blood with pneumonia
Aspiration of blood with pneumonitis
Use additional code to identify any secondary pulmonary hypertension (416.8), if applicable

770.17 Other fetal and newborn aspiration without respiratory symptoms

770.18 Other fetal and newborn aspiration with respiratory symptoms
Other aspiration pneumonia
Other aspiration pneumonitis
Use additional code to identify any secondary pulmonary hypertension (416.8), if applicable

770.2 Interstitial emphysema and related conditions
Pneumomediastinum originating in the perinatal period
Pneumopericardium originating in the perinatal period
Pneumothorax originating in the perinatal period

770.3 Pulmonary hemorrhage
Hemorrhage:
alveolar (lung) originating in the perinatal period
intra-alveolar (lung) originating in the perinatal period
massive pulmonary originating in the perinatal period

770.4 Primary atelectasis
Pulmonary immaturity NOS

770.5 Other and unspecified atelectasis
Atelectasis:
NOS, originating in the perinatal period
partial, originating in the perinatal period
secondary, originating in the perinatal period
Pulmonary collapse, originating in the perinatal period

770.6 Transitory tachypnea of newborn
Idiopathic tachypnea of newborn
Wet lung syndrome

Excludes: *respiratory distress syndrome (769)*

770.7 Chronic respiratory disease arising in the perinatal period
Bronchopulmonary dysplasia
Interstitial pulmonary fibrosis of prematurity
Wilson-Mikity syndrome

⑤ **770.8 Other respiratory problems after birth**

Excludes: *mixed metabolic and respiratory acidosis of newborn (775.81)*

770.81 Primary apnea of newborn
Apneic spells of newborn NOS
Essential apnea of newborn
Sleep apnea of newborn

770.82 Other apnea of newborn
Obstructure apnea of newborn

770.83 Cyanotic attacks of newborn

770.84 Respiratory failure of newborn

Excludes: *respiratory distress syndrome (769)*

770.85 Aspiration of postnatal stomach contents without respiratory symptoms
Aspiration of postnatal stomach contents NOS

770.86 Aspiration of postnatal stomach contents with respiratory symptoms
Aspiration of postnatal stomach contents with pneumonia
Aspiration of postnatal stomach contents with pneumonitis
Use additional code to identify any secondary pulmonary hypertension (416.8), if applicable

● **770.87 Respiratory arrest of newborn**

● **770.88 Hypoxemia of newborn**
Hypoxia NOS of newborn

770.89 Other respiratory problems after birth

770.9 Unspecified respiratory condition of fetus and newborn

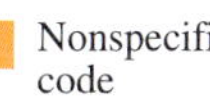

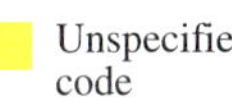

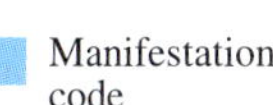

771 Infections specific to the perinatal period
Includes: infections acquired before or during birth via the umbilicus or during the first 28 days after birth

Excludes: *congenital pneumonia (770.0)*
congenital syphilis (090.0-090.9)
maternal infectious disease as a cause of mortality or morbidity in fetus or newborn, but fetus or newborn not manifesting the disease (760.2)
ophthalmia neonatorum due to gonococcus (098.40)
other infections not specifically classified to this category

771.0 Congenital rubella
Congenital rubella pneumonitis

771.1 Congenital cytomegalovirus infection
Congenital cytomegalic inclusion disease

771.2 Other congenital infections

Congenital:
  herpes simplex
  listeriosis
  malaria

Congenital:
  toxoplasmosis
  tuberculosis

771.3 Tetanus neonatorum
Tetanus omphalitis

Excludes: *hypocalcemic tetany (775.4)*

771.4 Omphalitis of the newborn
Infection:
  navel cord
  umbilical stump

Excludes: *tetanus omphalitis (771.3)*

771.5 Neonatal infective mastitis

Excludes: *noninfective neonatal mastitis (778.7)*

771.6 Neonatal conjunctivitis and dacryocystitis
Ophthalmia neonatorum NOS

Excludes: *ophthalmia neonatorum due to gonococcus (098.40)*

771.7 Neonatal Candida infection
Neonatal moniliasis
Thrush in newborn

⑤ **771.8 Other infection specific to the perinatal period**
Use additional code to identify organism (041.00-041.9)

771.81 Septicemia [sepsis] of newborn

771.82 Urinary tract infection of newborn

771.83 Bacteremia of newborn

771.89 Other infections specific to the perinatal period
Intra-amniotic infection of fetus NOS
Infection of newborn NOS

772 Fetal and neonatal hemorrhage

Excludes: *hematological disorders of fetus and newborn (776.0-776.9)*

772.0 Fetal blood loss

Fetal blood loss from:
  cut end of co-twin's cord
  placenta
  ruptured cord
  vasa previa

Fetal exsanguination
Fetal hemorrhage into:
  co-twin
  mother's circulation

⑤ **772.1 Intraventricular hemorrhage**
Intraventricular hemorrhage from any perinatal cause

772.10 Unspecified grade

772.11 Grade I
Bleeding into germinal matrix

772.12 Grade II
Bleeding into ventricle

772.13 Grade III
Bleeding with enlargement of ventricle

● Code new
to this edition

▲ Revision of
existing code

④ ⑤ Fourth or fifth
digit required

    772.14   Grade IV
           Bleeding into cerebral cortex

772.2 Subarachnoid hemorrhage
      Subarachnoid hemorrhage from any perinatal cause

    | Excludes: | *subdural and cerebral hemorrhage (767.0)*

772.3 Umbilical hemorrhage after birth
      Slipped umbilical ligature

772.4 Gastrointestinal hemorrhage

    | Excludes: | *swallowed maternal blood (777.3)*

772.5 Adrenal hemorrhage

772.6 Cutaneous hemorrhage
      Bruising in fetus or newborn
      Ecchymoses in fetus or newborn
      Petechiae in fetus or newborn
      Superficial hematoma in fetus or newborn

772.8 Other specified hemorrhage of fetus or newborn

    | Excludes: | *hemorrhagic disease of newborn (776.0)*
                pulmonary hemorrhage (770.3)

772.9 Unspecified hemorrhage of newborn

773 Hemolytic disease of fetus or newborn, due to isoimmunization

773.0 Hemolytic disease due to Rh isoimmunization
      Anemia due to RH:
        antibodies
        isoimmunization
        maternal/fetal incompatibility
      Erythroblastosis (fetalis) due to RH:
        antibodies
        isoimmunization
        maternal/fetal incompatibility
      Hemolytic disease (fetus) (newborn) due to RH:
        antibodies
        isoimmunization
        maternal/fetal incompatibility
      Jaundice due to RH:
        antibodies
        isoimmunization
        maternal/fetal incompatibility
      Rh hemolytic disease
      Rh isoimmunization

773.1 Hemolytic disease due to ABO isoimmunization
      ABO hemolytic disease
      ABO isoimmunization
      Anemia due to ABO: antibodies, isoimmunization, or maternal/fetal incompatibility
      Erythroblastosis (fetalis) due to ABO:
        antibodies
        isoimmunization
        maternal/fetal incompatibility
      Hemolytic disease (fetus) (newborn) due to ABO:
        antibodies
        isoimmunization
        maternal/fetal incompatibility
      Jaundice due to ABO:
        antibodies
        isoimmunization
        maternal/fetal incompatibility

773.2 Hemolytic disease due to other and unspecified isoimmunization
      Erythroblastosis (fetalis) (neonatorum) NOS
      Hemolytic disease (fetus) (newborn) NOS
      Jaundice or anemia due to other and unspecified blood-group incompatibility

773.3 Hydrops fetalis due to isoimmunization
Use additional code, if desired, to identify type of isoimmunization (773.0-773.2)

773.4 Kernicterus due to isoimmunization
Use additional code, if desired, to identify type of isoimmunization (773.0-773.2)

773.5 Late anemia due to isoimmunization

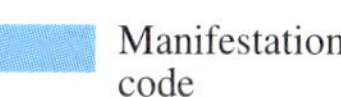

774 **Other perinatal jaundice**

774.0 *Perinatal jaundice from hereditary hemolytic anemias*
Code first underlying disease (282.0-282.9)

774.1 **Perinatal jaundice from other excessive hemolysis**
Fetal or neonatal jaundice from:
bruising
drugs or toxins transmitted from mother
infection
polycythemia
swallowed maternal blood

Use additional code, if desired, to identify cause

Excludes: *jaundice due to isoimmunization (773.0-773.2)*

774.2 **Neonatal jaundice associated with preterm delivery**
Hyperbilirubinemia of prematurity
Jaundice due to delayed conjugation associated with preterm delivery

⑤ **774.3** **Neonatal jaundice due to delayed conjugation from other causes**

774.30 **Neonatal jaundice due to delayed conjugation, cause unspecified**

774.31 *Neonatal jaundice due to delayed conjugation in diseases classified elsewhere*
Code first underlying diseases, as:
congenital hypothyroidism (243)
Crigler-Najjar syndrome (277.4)
Gilbert's syndrome (277.4)

774.39 **Other**
Jaundice due to delayed conjugation from causes, such as:
breast milk inhibitors
delayed development of conjugating system

774.4 **Perinatal jaundice due to hepatocellular damage**
Fetal or neonatal hepatitis
Giant cell hepatitis
Inspissated bile syndrome

774.5 *Perinatal jaundice from other causes*
Code first underlying cause, as:
congenital obstruction of bile duct (751.61)
galactosemia (271.1)
mucoviscidosis (277.00-277.09)

774.6 **Unspecified fetal and neonatal jaundice**
Icterus neonatorum
Neonatal hyperbilirubinemia (transient)
Physiologic jaundice NOS in newborn

Excludes: *that in preterm infants (774.2)*

774.7 **Kernicterus not due to isoimmunization**
Bilirubin encephalopathy
Kernicterus of newborn NOS

Excludes: *kernicterus due to isoimmunization (773.4)*

775 **Endocrine and metabolic disturbances specific to the fetus and newborn**
Includes: transitory endocrine and metabolic disturbances caused by the infant's response to maternal endocrine and metabolic factors, its removal from them, or its adjustment to extrauterine existence

775.0 **Syndrome of "infant of a diabetic mother"**
Maternal diabetes mellitus affecting fetus or newborn (with hypoglycemia)

775.1 **Neonatal diabetes mellitus**
Diabetes mellitus syndrome in newborn infant

775.2 **Neonatal myasthenia gravis**

775.3 **Neonatal thyrotoxicosis**
Neonatal hyperthyroidism (transient)

775.4 **Hypocalcemia and hypomagnesemia of newborn**
Cow's milk hypocalcemia
Hypocalcemic tetany, neonatal
Neonatal hypoparathyroidism
Phosphate-loading hypocalcemia

775.5 **Other transitory neonatal electrolyte disturbances**
Dehydration, neonatal

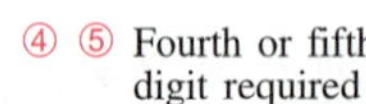

● Code new
to this edition

▲ Revision of
existing code

④ ⑤ Fourth or fifth
digit required

775.6 Neonatal hypoglycemia

> Excludes: *infant of mother with diabetes mellitus (775.0)*

775.7 Late metabolic acidosis of newborn

▲ **775.8 Other neonatal endocrine and metabolic disturbances**

● **775.81 Other acidosis of newborn**
Acidemia NOS of newborn
Acidosis of newborn NOS
Mixed metabolic and respiratory acidosis of newborn

● **775.89 Other neonatal endocrine and metabolic disturbances**
Amino-acid metabolic disorders described as transitory

775.9 Unspecified endocrine and metabolic disturbances specific to the fetus and newborn

776 Hematological disorders of fetus and newborn
Includes: disorders specific to the fetus or newborn

776.0 Hemorrhagic disease of newborn
Hemorrhagic diathesis of newborn
Vitamin K deficiency of newborn

> Excludes: *fetal or neonatal hemorrhage (772.0-772.9)*

776.1 Transient neonatal thrombocytopenia
Neonatal thrombocytopenia due to:
exchange transfusion
idiopathic maternal thrombocytopenia
isoimmunization

776.2 Disseminated intravascular coagulation in newborn

776.3 Other transient neonatal disorders of coagulation
Transient coagulation defect, newborn

776.4 Polycythemia neonatorum
Plethora of newborn
Polycythemia due to:
donor twin transfusion
maternal-fetal transfusion

776.5 Congenital anemia
Anemia following fetal blood loss

> Excludes: *anemia due to isoimmunization (773.0-773.2, 773.5)*
> *hereditary hemolytic anemias (282.0-282.9)*

776.6 Anemia of prematurity

776.7 Transient neonatal neutropenia
Isoimmune neutropenia
Maternal transfer neutropenia

> Excludes: *congenital neutropenia (nontransient) (288.01)*

776.8 Other specified transient hematological disorders

776.9 Unspecified hematological disorder specific to fetus or newborn

777 Perinatal disorders of digestive system
Includes: disorders specific to the fetus and newborn

> Excludes: *intestinal obstruction classifiable to 560.0-560.9*

777.1 Meconium obstruction
Congenital fecaliths
Delayed passage of meconium
Meconium ileus NOS
Meconium plug syndrome

> Excludes: *meconium ileus in cystic fibrosis (277.01)*

777.2 Intestinal obstruction due to inspissated milk

777.3 Hematemesis and melena due to swallowed maternal blood
Swallowed blood syndrome in newborn

> Excludes: *that not due to swallowed maternal blood (772.4)*

777.4 Transitory ileus of newborn

> Excludes: *Hirschsprung's disease (751.3)*

777.5 Necrotizing enterocolitis in fetus or newborn
Pseudomembranous enterocolitis in newborn

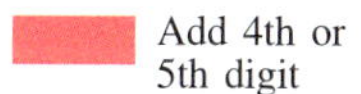

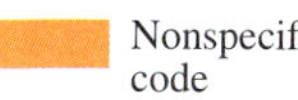

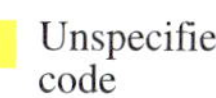

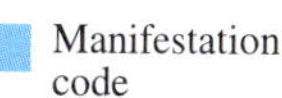

777.6 Perinatal intestinal perforation
Meconium peritonitis

777.8 Other specified perinatal disorders of digestive system

777.9 Unspecified perinatal disorder of digestive system

778 Conditions involving the integument and temperature regulation of fetus and newborn

778.0 Hydrops fetalis not due to isoimmunization
Idiopathic hydrops

| Excludes: | hydrops fetalis due to isoimmunization (773.3) |

778.1 Sclerema neonatorum
Subcutaneous fat necrosis

778.2 Cold injury syndrome of newborn

778.3 Other hypothermia of newborn

778.4 Other disturbances of temperature regulation of newborn
Dehydration fever in newborn
Environmentally-induced pyrexia
Hyperthermia in newborn
Transitory fever of newborn

778.5 Other and unspecified edema of newborn
Edema neonatorum

778.6 Congenital hydrocele
Congenital hydrocele of tunica vaginalis

778.7 Breast engorgement in newborn
Noninfective mastitis of newborn

| Excludes: | infective mastitis of newborn (771.5) |

778.8 Other specified conditions involving the integument of fetus and newborn
Urticaria neonatorum

| Excludes: | impetigo neonatorum (684) |
| | pemphigus neonatorum (684) |

778.9 Unspecified condition involving the integument and temperature regulation of fetus and newborn

779 Other and ill-defined conditions originating in the perinatal period

779.0 Convulsions in newborn
Fits in newborn
Seizures in newborn

779.1 Other and unspecified cerebral irritability in newborn

779.2 Cerebral depression, coma, and other abnormal cerebral signs
Cerebral ischemia NOS of newborn
CNS dysfunction in newborn NOS

Excludes:	cerebral ischemia due to birth trauma (767.0)
	intrauterine cerebral ischemia (768.2-768.9)
	intraventricular hemorrhage (772.10-772.14)

779.3 Feeding problems in newborn
Regurgitation of food in newborn
Slow feeding in newborn
Vomiting in newborn

779.4 Drug reactions and intoxications specific to newborn
Gray syndrome from chloramphenicol administration in newborn

| Excludes: | fetal alcohol syndrome (760.71) |
| | reactions and intoxications from maternal opiates and tranquilizers (763.5) |

779.5 Drug withdrawal syndrome in newborn
Drug withdrawal syndrome in infant of dependent mother

| Excludes: | fetal alcohol syndrome (760.71) |

779.6 Termination of pregnancy (fetus)
Fetus death due to:
induced abortion
termination of pregnancy

| Excludes: | spontaneous abortion (fetus) (761.8) |

779.7 Periventricular leukomalacia

⑤ **779.8 Other specified conditions originating in the perinatal period**

● Code new
to this edition

▲ Revision of
existing code

④ ⑤ Fourth or fifth
digit required

779.81 Neonatal bradycardia

Excludes: *abnormality in fetal heart rate or rhythm complicating labor and delivery*
(763.81-763.83)
bradycardia due to birth asphyxia (768.5-768.9)

779.82 Neonatal tachycardia

Excludes: *abnormality in fetal heart rate or rhythm complicating labor and delivery*
(763.81-763.83)

779.83 Delayed separation of umbilical cord

779.84 Meconium staining

Excludes: *meconium aspiration (770.11, 770.12)*
meconium passage during delivery (763.84)

● **779.85 Cardiac arrest of newborn**

779.89 Other specified conditions originating in the perinatal period

Use additional code to specify condition

779.9 Unspecified condition originating in the perinatal period
Congenital debility NOS
Stillbirth NEC

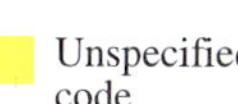

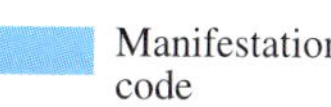

● Code new
to this edition

▲ Revision of
existing code

④ ⑤ Fourth or fifth
digit required

16. SYMPTOMS, SIGNS, AND ILL-DEFINED CONDITIONS (780-799)

This section includes symptoms, signs, abnormal results of laboratory or other investigative procedures, and ill-defined conditions regarding which no diagnosis classifiable elsewhere is recorded.

Signs and symptoms that point rather definitely to a given diagnosis are assigned to some category in the preceding part of the classification. In general, categories 780-796 include the more ill-defined conditions and symptoms that point with perhaps equal suspicion to two or more diseases or to two or more systems of the body, and without the necessary study of the case to make a final diagnosis. Practically all categories in this group could be designated as "not otherwise specified," or as "unknown etiology," or as "transient." The Alphabetic Index should be consulted to determine which symptoms and signs are to be allocated here and which to more specific sections of the classification; the residual subcategories numbered .9 are provided for other relevant symptoms which cannot be allocated elsewhere in the classification.

The conditions and signs or symptoms included in categories 780-796 consist of: (a) cases for which no more specific diagnosis can be made even after all facts bearing on the case have been investigated; (b) signs or symptoms existing at the time of initial encounter that proved to be transient and whose causes could not be determined; (c) provisional diagnoses in a patient who failed to return for further investigation or care; (d) cases referred elsewhere for investigation or treatment before the diagnosis was made; (e) cases in which a more precise diagnosis was not available for any other reason; (f) certain symptoms which represent important problems in medical care and which it might be desired to classify in addition to a known cause.

SYMPTOMS (780-789)

780 **General symptoms**

⑤ **780.0 Alteration of consciousness**

> *Excludes:* *coma:*
>> *diabetic (250.2-250.3)*
>> *hepatic (572.2)*
>> *originating in the perinatal period (779.2)*

780.01 Coma

780.02 Transient alteration of awareness

780.03 Persistent vegetative state

780.09 Other
Drowsiness   Somnolence
Semicoma   Stupor
Unconsciousness

780.1 Hallucinations
Hallucinations: Hallucinations:
  NOS   olfactory
  auditory   tactile
  gustatory

> *Excludes:* *those associated with mental disorders, as functional psychoses (295.0-298.9)*
>> *organic brain syndromes (290.0-294.9, 310.0-310.9)*
>> *visual hallucinations (368.16)*

780.2 Syncope and collapse
Blackout   (Near) (Pre) syncope
Fainting   Vasovagal attack

> *Excludes:* *carotid sinus syncope (337.0)*
>> *heat syncope (992.1)*
>> *neurocirculatory asthenia (306.2)*
>> *orthostatic hypotension (458.0)*
>> *shock NOS (785.50)*

⑤ **780.3 Convulsions**

> *Excludes:* *convulsions:*
>> *epileptic (345.10-345.91)*
>> *in newborn (779.0)*

▲ **780.31 Febrile convulsions (simple), unspecified**
Febrile seizure NOS

● **780.32 Complex febrile convulsions**
Febrile seizure:
  atypical
  complex
  complicated

> *Excludes:* *status epilepticus (345.3)*

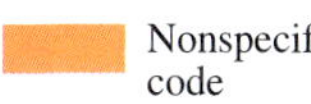

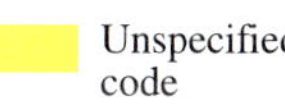

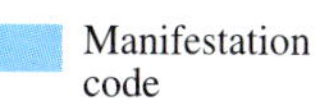

Manifestation
code

780.39 Other convulsions
      Convulsive disorder NOS
      Fit NOS
      Recurrent convulsions NOS
      Seizure NOS

780.4 Dizziness and giddiness
      Light-headedness
      Vertigo NOS

Excludes: *Ménière's disease and other specified vertiginous syndromes (386.0-386.9)*

⑤ **780.5 Sleep disturbances**

Excludes: *circadian rhythm sleep disorders (327.30-327.39)*
      organic hypersomnia (327.10-327.19)
      organic insomnia (327.00-327.09)
      organic sleep apnea (327.20-327.29)
      organic sleep related movement disorders (327.51-327.59)
      parasomnias (327.40-327.49)
      that of nonorganic origin (307.40-307.49)

780.50 Sleep disturbance, unspecified

780.51 Insomnia with sleep apnea, unspecified

780.52 Insomnia, unspecified

780.53 Hypersomnia with sleep apnea, unspecified

780.54 Hypersomnia, unspecified

780.55 Disruption of 24 hour sleep wake cycle, unspecified

780.56 Dysfunctions associated with sleep stages or arousal from sleep

780.57 Unspecified sleep apnea

780.58 Sleep related movement disorder, unspecified

Excludes: *restless legs syndrome (333.94)*

780.59 Other

780.6 Fever
      Chills with fever   Hyperpyrexia NOS
      Fever NOS   Pyrexia NOS
      Fever of unknown origin   Pyrexia of unknown origin
      (FUO)

Code first underlying condition when associated fever is present,
    such as with:
      leukemia (codes from categories 204-208)
      neutropenia (288.00-288.09)
      sickle-cell disease (282.60-282.69)

Excludes: *pyrexia of unknown origin (during):*
      in newborn (778.4)
      labor (659.2)
      the puerperium (672)

⑤ **780.7 Malaise and fatigue**

Excludes: *debility, unspecified (799.3)*
      fatigue (during):
        combat (308.0-308.9)
        heat (992.6)
        pregnancy (646.8)
      neurasthenia (300.5)
      senile asthenia (797.5)

780.71 Chronic fatigue syndrome

780.79 Other malaise and fatigue
      Asthenia NOS
      Lethargy
      Postviral (asthenic) syndrome
      Tiredness

780.8 Generalized hyperhidrosis
      Diaphoresis
      Excessive sweating
      Secondary hyperhidrosis

Excludes: *focal (localized) (primary) (secondary) hyperhidrosis (705.21-705.22)*
      Frey's syndrome (705.22)

  ● Code new   ▲ Revision of   ④ ⑤ Fourth or fifth
     to this edition   existing code   digit required

⑤ **780.9 Other general symptoms**

> *Excludes:* *hypothermia:*
> *NOS (accidental) (991.6)*
> *due to anesthesia (995.89)*
> *of newborn (778.2-778.3)*
> *memory disturbance as part of a pattern of mental disorder*

780.91 Fussy infant (baby)

780.92 Excessive crying of infant (baby)

> *Excludes:* *excessive crying of child, adolescent or adult (780.95)*

780.93 Memory loss
Amnesia (retrograde)
Memory loss NOS

> *Excludes:* *mild memory disturbance due to organic brain damage (310.1)*
> *transient global amnesia (437.7)*

780.94 Early satiety

▲ **780.95 Excessive crying of child, adolescent, or adult**

> *Excludes:* *excessive crying of infant (baby) (780.92)*

● **780.96 Generalized pain**
Pain NOS

● **780.97 Altered mental status**
Change in mental status

> *Excludes:* *altered level of consciousness (780.01-780.09)*
> *altered mental status due to known condition — code to condition*
> *delirium NOS (780.09)*

780.99 Other general symptoms
Chill(s) NOS
Hypothermia, not associated with low environmental temperature

781 Symptoms involving nervous and musculoskeletal systems

> *Excludes:* *depression NOS (311)*
> *disorders specifically relating to:*
> *back (724.0-724.9)*
> *hearing (388.0-389.9)*
> *joint (718.0-719.9)*
> *limb (729.0-729.9)*
> *neck (723.0-723.9)*
> *vision (368.0-369.9)*
> *pain in limb (729.5)*

781.0 Abnormal involuntary movements
Abnormal head movements
Fasciculation
Spasms NOS
Tremor NOS

> *Excludes:* *abnormal reflex (796.1)*
> *chorea NOS (333.5)*
> *infantile spasms (345.60-345.61)*
> *spastic paralysis (342.1, 343.0-344.9)*
> *specified movement disorders classifiable to 333 (333.0-333.9)*
> *that of nonorganic origin (307.2-307.3)*

781.1 Disturbances of sensation of smell and taste
Anosmia   Parosmia
Parageusia

781.2 Abnormality of gait
Gait: Gait:
  ataxic   spastic
  paralytic   staggering

> *Excludes:* *ataxia:*
> *NOS (781.3)*
> *locomotor (progressive) (094.0)*
> *difficulty in walking (719.7)*

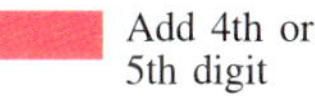

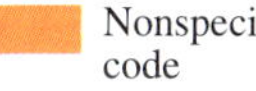

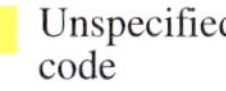

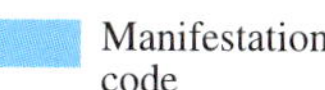

781.3 Lack of coordination
Ataxia NOS
Muscular incoordination

Excludes: *ataxic gait (781.2)*
cerebellar ataxia (334.0-334.9)
difficulty in walking (719.7)
vertigo NOS (780.4)

781.4 Transient paralysis of limb
Monoplegia, transient NOS

Excludes: *paralysis (342.0-344.9)*

781.5 Clubbing of fingers

781.6 Meningismus
Dupré's syndrome
Meningism

781.7 Tetany
Carpopedal spasm

Excludes: *tetanus neonatorum (771.3)*

tetany:
hysterical (300.11)
newborn (hypocalcemic) (775.4)
parathyroid (252.1)
psychogenic (306.0)

781.8 Neurologic neglect syndrome

Asomatognosia	Left-sided neglect
Hemi-akinesia	Sensory extinction
Hemi-inattention	Sensory neglect
Hemispatial neglect	Visuospatial neglect

⑤ **781.9 Other symptoms involving nervous and musculoskeletal systems**

781.91 Loss of height

Excludes: *osteoporosis (733.00-733.09)*

781.92 Abnormal posture

781.93 Ocular torticollis

781.94 Facial weakness
Facial droop

Excludes: *facial weakness due to late effect of cerebrovascular accident (438.83)*

781.99 Other symptoms involving nervous and musculoskeletal systems

782 Symptoms involving skin and other integumentary tissue

Excludes: *symptoms relating to breast (611.71-611.79)*

782.0 Disturbance of skin sensation

Anesthesia of skin	Hypoesthesia
Burning or prickling	Numbness
sensation	Paresthesia
Hyperesthesia	Tingling

782.1 Rash and other nonspecific skin eruption
Exanthem

Excludes: *vesicular eruption (709.8)*

782.2 Localized superficial swelling, mass, or lump
Subcutaneous nodules

Excludes: *localized adiposity (278.1)*

782.3 Edema

Anasarca	Localized edema NOS
Dropsy	

Excludes: *ascites (789.5)*
edema of:
newborn NOS (778.5)
pregnancy (642.0-642.9, 646.1)
fluid retention (276.6)
hydrops fetalis (773.3, 778.0)
hydrothorax (511.8)
nutritional edema (260, 262)

● Code new
to this edition

▲ Revision of
existing code

④ ⑤ Fourth or fifth
digit required

782.4 Jaundice, unspecified, not of newborn
Cholemia NOS
Icterus NOS

> *Excludes:* *jaundice in newborn (774.0-774.7)*
> *due to isoimmunization (773.0-773.2, 773.4)*

782.5 Cyanosis

> *Excludes:* *newborn (770.83)*

⑤ **782.6 Pallor and flushing**

782.61 Pallor

782.62 Flushing
Excessive blushing

782.7 Spontaneous ecchymoses
Petechiae

> *Excludes:* *ecchymosis in fetus or newborn (772.6)*
> *purpura (287.0-287.9)*

782.8 Changes in skin texture
Induration of skin
Thickening of skin

782.9 Other symptoms involving skin and integumentary tissues

783 Symptoms concerning nutrition, metabolism, and development

783.0 Anorexia
Loss of appetite

> *Excludes:* *anorexia nervosa (307.1)*
> *loss of appetite of nonorganic origin (307.59)*

783.1 Abnormal weight gain

> *Excludes:* *excessive weight gain in pregnancy (646.1)*
> *obesity (278.00)*
> *morbid (278.01)*

⑤ **783.2 Abnormal loss of weight and underweight**
Use additional code to identify Body Mass Index (BMI), if known (V85.0-V85.54)

783.21 Loss of weight

783.22 Underweight

783.3 Feeding difficulties and mismanagement
Feeding problem (elderly) (infant)

> *Excludes:* *feeding disturbance or problems:*
> *in newborn (779.3)*
> *of nonorganic origin (307.50-307.59)*

⑤ **783.4 Lack of expected normal physiological development in childhood**

> *Excludes:* *delay in sexual development and puberty (259.0)*
> *gonadal dysgenesis (758.6)*
> *pituitary dwarfism (253.3)*
> *slow fetal growth and fetal malnutrition (764.00-764.99)*
> *specific delays in mental development (315.0-315.9)*

783.40 Lack of normal physiological development, unspecified
Inadequate development
Lack of development

783.41 Failure to thrive
Failure to gain weight

783.42 Delayed milestones
Late talker
Late walker

783.43 Short stature
Growth failure
Growth retardation
Lack of growth
Physical retardation

783.5 Polydipsia
Excessive thirst

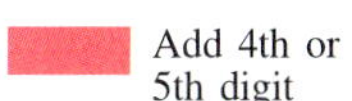

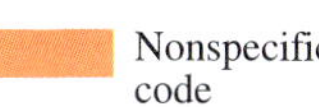

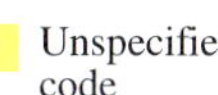

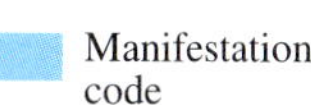

783.6 Polyphagia
Excessive eating
Hyperalimentation NOS

Excludes: *disorders of eating of nonorganic origin (307.50-307.59)*

783.7 Adult failure to thrive

783.9 Other symptoms concerning nutrition, metabolism, and development
Hypometabolism

Excludes: *abnormal basal metabolic rate (794.7)*
dehydration (276.51)
other disorders of fluid, electrolyte, and acid-base balance (276.0-276.9)

784 Symptoms involving head and neck

Excludes: *encephalopathy NOS (348.30)*
specific symptoms involving neck classifiable to 723 (723.0-723.9)

784.0 Headache
Facial pain
Pain in head NOS

Excludes: *atypical face pain (350.2)*
migraine (346.0-346.9)
tension headache (307.81)

784.1 Throat pain

Excludes: *dysphagia (787.2)*
neck pain (723.1)
sore throat (462)
chronic (472.1)

784.2 Swelling, mass, or lump in head and neck
Space-occupying lesion, intracranial NOS

784.3 Aphasia

Excludes: *aphasia due to late effects of cerebrovascular disease (438.11)*
developmental aphasia (315.31)

⑤ **784.4 Voice disturbance**

784.40 Voice disturbance, unspecified

784.41 Aphonia
Loss of voice

784.49 Other
Change in voice   Hypernasality
Dysphonia   Hyponasality
Hoarseness

784.5 Other speech disturbance
Dysarthria   Slurred speech
Dysphasia

Excludes: *stammering and stuttering (307.0)*
that of nonorganic origin (307.0, 307.9)

⑤ **784.6 Other symbolic dysfunction**

Excludes: *developmental learning delays (315.0-315.9)*

784.60 Symbolic dysfunction, unspecified

784.61 Alexia and dyslexia
Alexia (with agraphia)

784.69 Other
Acalculia   Agraphia NOS
Agnosia   Apraxia

784.7 Epistaxis
Hemorrhage from nose
Nosebleed

784.8 Hemorrhage from throat

Excludes: *hemoptysis (786.3)*

⑤ **784.9 Other symptoms involving head and neck**

● **784.91 Postnasal drip**

● **784.99   Other symptoms involving head and neck**
  Choking sensation
  Halitosis
  Mouth breathing
  Sneezing

785   Symptoms involving cardiovascular system

  Excludes: *heart failure NOS (428.9)*

785.0   Tachycardia, unspecified
  Rapid heart beat

  Excludes: *neonatal tachycardia (779.82)*

  paroxysmal tachycardia (427.0-427.2)

785.1   Palpitations
  Awareness of heart beat

  Excludes: *specified dysrhythmias (427.0-427.9)*

785.2   Undiagnosed cardiac murmurs
  Heart murmur NOS

785.3   Other abnormal heart sounds
  Cardiac dullness, increased or decreased
  Friction fremitus, cardiac
  Precordial friction

785.4   Gangrene
  Gangrene NOS
  Gangrene spreading cutaneous
  Gangrenous cellulitis
  Phagedena

Code first any associated underlying condition, as:
  diabetes (250.7)
  Raynaud's syndrome (443.0)

  Excludes: *gangrene of certain sites—see Alphabetic Index*

  gangrene with atherosclerosis of the extremities (440.24)
  gas gangrene (040.0)

⑤ **785.5   Shock without mention of trauma**

  785.50   Shock, unspecified
    Failure of peripheral circulation

  785.51   Cardiogenic shock

  785.52   *Septic shock*
    endotoxic
    gram-negative

Code first systemic inflammatory response syndrome due to infectious process with organ dysfunction (995.92)

  785.59   Other
    Shock:
      hypovolemic

  Excludes: *shock (due to):*

    anesthetic (995.4)
    anaphylactic (995.0)
      due to serum (999.4)
    electric (994.8)
    following abortion (639.5)
    lightning (994.0)
    obstetrical (669.1)
    postoperative (998.0)
    traumatic (958.4)

785.6   Enlargement of lymph nodes
  Lymphadenopathy
  "Swollen glands"

  Excludes: *lymphadenitis (chronic) (289.1-289.3)*

    acute (683)

785.9   Other symptoms involving cardiovascular system
  Bruit (arterial)
  Weak pulse

786   Symptoms involving respiratory system and other chest symptoms

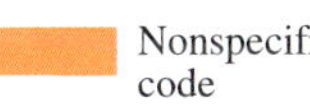

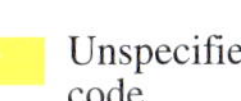

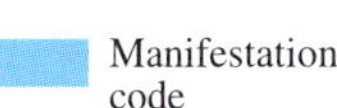

⑤ **786.0 Dyspnea and respiratory abnormalities**

786.00 Respiratory abnormality, unspecified

786.01 Hyperventilation

Excludes: *hyperventilation, psychogenic (306.1)*

786.02 Orthopnea

786.03 Apnea

Excludes: *apnea of newborn (770.81, 770.82)*
        sleep apnea (780.51, 780.53, 780.57)

786.04 Cheyne-Stokes respiration

786.05 Shortness of breath

786.06 Tachypnea

Excludes: *transitory tachypnea of newborn (770.6)*

786.07 Wheezing

Excludes: *asthma (493.00-493.92)*

786.09 Other
        Respiratory:
            distress
            insufficiency

Excludes: *respiratory distress:*
            following trauma and surgery (518.5)
            newborn (770.89)
            syndrome (newborn) (769)
                adult (518.5)
        respiratory failure (518.81, 518.83-518.84)
            newborn (770.84)

786.1 Stridor

Excludes: *congenital laryngeal stridor (748.3)*

786.2 Cough

Excludes: *cough:*
            psychogenic (306.1)
            smokers' (491.0)
            with hemorrhage (786.3)

786.3 Hemoptysis
        Cough with hemorrhage
        Pulmonary hemorrhage NOS

Excludes: *pulmonary hemorrhage of newborn (770.3)*

786.4 Abnormal sputum
        Abnormal:
            amount (of) sputum
            color (of) sputum
            odor (of) sputum
        Excessive sputum

⑤ **786.5 Chest pain**

786.50 Chest pain, unspecified

786.51 Precordial pain

786.52 Painful respiration
        Pain:
            anterior chest wall
            pleuritic
        Pleurodynia

Excludes: *epidemic pleurodynia (074.1)*

786.59 Other
        Discomfort in chest
        Pressure in chest
        Tightness in chest

Excludes: *pain in breast (611.71)*

786.6 Swelling, mass, or lump in chest

Excludes: *lump in breast (611.72)*

● Code new   ▲ Revision of   ④ ⑤ Fourth or fifth
to this edition   existing code   digit required

786.7 Abnormal chest sounds
Abnormal percussion, chest   Rales
Friction sounds, chest   Tympany, chest

Excludes: *wheezing (786.07)*

786.8 Hiccough

Excludes: *psychogenic hiccough (306.1)*

786.9 Other symptoms involving respiratory system and chest
Breath-holding spell

787 Symptoms involving digestive system

Excludes: *constipation (564.00-564.09)*
pylorospasm (537.81)
congenital (750.5)

⑤ **787.0 Nausea and vomiting**
Emesis

Excludes: *hematemesis NOS (578.0)*
vomiting:
bilious, following gastrointestinal surgery (564.3)
cyclical (536.2)
psychogenic (306.4)
excessive, in pregnancy (643.0-643.9)
habit (536.2)
of newborn (779.3)
psychogenic NOS (307.54)

787.01 Nausea with vomiting

787.02 Nausea alone

787.03 Vomiting alone

787.1 Heartburn
Pyrosis
Waterbrash

Excludes: *dyspepsia or indigestion (536.8)*

787.2 Dysphagia
Difficulty in swallowing

787.3 Flatulence, eructation, and gas pain
Abdominal distention (gaseous)
Bloating
Tympanites (abdominal) (intestinal)

Excludes: *aerophagy (306.4)*

787.4 Visible peristalsis
Hyperperistalsis

787.5 Abnormal bowel sounds
Absent bowel sounds
Hyperactive bowel sounds

787.6 Incontinence of feces
Encopresis NOS
Incontinence of sphincter ani

Excludes: *that of nonorganic origin (307.7)*

787.7 Abnormal feces
Bulky stools

Excludes: *abnormal stool content (792.1)*
melena:
NOS (578.1)
newborn (772.4, 777.3)

⑤ **787.9 Other symptoms involving digestive system**

Excludes: *gastrointestinal hemorrhage (578.0-578.9)*
intestinal obstruction (560.0-560.9)
specific functional digestive disorders:
esophagus (530.0-530.9)
stomach and duodenum (536.0-536.9)
those not elsewhere classified (564.00-564.9)

787.91 Diarrhea
Diarrhea NOS

787.99 Other
Change in bowel habits
Tenesmus (rectal)

788 Symptoms involving urinary system

Excludes: *hematuria (599.7)*
nonspecific findings on examination of the urine (791.0-791.9)
small kidney of unknown cause (589.0-589.9)
uremia NOS (586)
urinary obstruction (599.60, 599.69)

788.0 Renal colic
Colic (recurrent) of:
kidney
ureter

788.1 Dysuria
Painful urination
Strangury

⑤ **788.2 Retention of urine**
Code, if applicable, any causal condition first, such as:
hyperplasia of prostate (600.0-600.9 with fifth-digit 1)

788.20 Retention of urine, unspecified

788.21 Incomplete bladder emptying

788.29 Other specified retention of urine

⑤ **788.3 Urinary incontinence**

Excludes: *that of nonorganic origin (307.6)*
Code, if applicable, any causal condition first, such as:
congenital ureterocele (753.23)
genital prolapse (618.00-618.9)
hyperplasia of prostate (600.0-600.9 with fifth-digit 1)

788.30 Urinary incontinence, unspecified
Enuresis NOS

788.31 Urge incontinence

788.32 Stress incontinence, male

Excludes: *stress incontinence (female) (625.6)*

788.33 Mixed incontinence (male) (female)
Urge and stress

788.34 Incontinence without sensory awareness

788.35 Post-void dribbling

788.36 Nocturnal enuresis

788.37 Continuous leakage

788.38 Overflow incontinence

788.39 Other urinary incontinence

⑤ **788.4 Frequency of urination and polyuria**
Code, if applicable, any causal condition first, such as:
hyperplasia of prostate (600.0-600.9 with fifth-digit 1)

788.41 Urinary frequency
Frequency of micturition

788.42 Polyuria

788.43 Nocturia

788.5 Oliguria and anuria
Deficient secretion of urine
Suppression of urinary secretion

Excludes: *that complicating:*
abortion (634-638 with .3, 639.3)
ectopic or molar pregnancy (639.3)
pregnancy, childbirth, or the puerperium (642.0-642.9, 646.2)

⑤ **788.6 Other abnormality of urination**
Code, if applicable, any causal condition first, such as:
hyperplasia of prostate (600.0-600.9 with fifth-digit 1)

788.61 Splitting of urinary stream
Intermittent urinary stream

● Code new
to this edition

▲ Revision of
existing code

④ ⑤ Fourth or fifth
digit required

788.62 Slowing of urinary stream
Weak stream

788.63 Urgency of urination

Excludes: *urge incontinence (788.31, 788.33)*

● **788.64 Urinary hesitancy**

● **788.65 Straining on urination**

788.69 **Other**

788.7 Urethral discharge
Penile discharge
Urethrorrhea

788.8 Extravasation of urine

788.9 Other symptoms involving urinary system
Extrarenal uremia
Vesical:
pain
tenesmus

789 Other symptoms involving abdomen and pelvis
The following fifth-digit subclassification is to be used for codes 789.0, 789.3, 789.4, 789.6

0 **unspecified site**

1 **right upper quadrant**

2 **left upper quadrant**

3 **right lower quadrant**

4 **left lower quadrant**

5 **periumbilic**

6 **epigastric**

7 **generalized**

9 **other specified site**
multiple sites

Excludes: *symptoms referable to genital organs:*
female (625.0-625.9)
male (607.0-608.9)
psychogenic (302.70-302.79)

⑤ **789.0 Abdominal pain**
Colic:
NOS
infantile
Cramps, abdominal

Excludes: *renal colic (788.0)*

789.1 Hepatomegaly
Enlargement of liver

789.2 Splenomegaly
Enlargement of spleen

⑤ **789.3 Abdominal or pelvic swelling, mass, or lump**
Diffuse or generalized swelling or mass:
abdominal NOS
umbilical

Excludes: *abdominal distention (gaseous) (787.3)*
ascites (789.5)

⑤ **789.4 Abdominal rigidity**

789.5 Ascites
Fluid in peritoneal cavity

⑤ **789.6 Abdominal tenderness**
Rebound tenderness

789.9 Other symptoms involving abdomen and pelvis
Umbilical:
bleeding
discharge

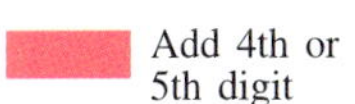

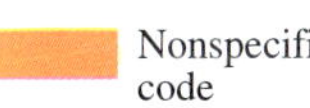

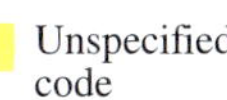

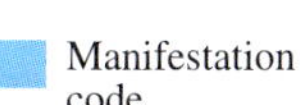

NONSPECIFIC ABNORMAL FINDINGS (790-796)

790 Nonspecific findings on examination of blood

Excludes: abnormalities of:
platelets (287.0-287.9)
thrombocytes (287.0-287.9)
white blood cells (288.00-288.9)

⑤ **790.0 Abnormality of red blood cells**

Excludes: anemia:
congenital (776.5)
newborn, due to isoimmunization (773.0-773.2, 773.5)
of premature infant (776.6)
other specified types (280.0-285.9)
hemoglobin disorders (282.5-282.7)
polycythemia:
familial (289.6)
neonatorum (776.4)
secondary (289.0)
vera (238.4)

790.01 Precipitous drop in hematocrit
Drop in hematocrit

790.09 Other abnormality of red blood cells
Abnormal red cell morphology NOS
Abnormal red cell volume NOS
Anisocytosis
Poikilocytosis

790.1 Elevated sedimentation rate

⑤ **790.2 Abnormal glucose**

Excludes: diabetes mellitus (250.00-250.93)
dysmetabolic syndrome X (277.7)
gestational diabetes (648.8)
glycosuria (791.5)
hypoglycemia (251.2)
that complicating pregnancy, childbirth, or the puerperium (648.8)

790.21 Impaired fasting glucose
Elevated fasting glucose

790.22 Impaired glucose tolerance test (oral)
Elevated glucose tolerance test

790.29 Other abnormal glucose
Abnormal glucose NOS
Abnormal non-fasting glucose
Hyperglycemia NOS
Pre-diabetes NOS

790.3 Excessive blood level of alcohol
Elevated blood-alcohol

790.4 Nonspecific elevation of levels of transaminase or lactic acid dehydrogenase [LDH]

790.5 Other nonspecific abnormal serum enzyme levels
Abnormal serum level of:
acid phosphatase
alkaline phosphatase
Abnormal serum level of:
amylase
lipase

Excludes: deficiency of circulating enzymes (277.6)

790.6 Other abnormal blood chemistry
Abnormal blood level of:
cobalt
copper
iron
lead
Abnormal blood level of:
lithium
magnesium
mineral
zinc

Excludes: abnormality of electrolyte or acid-base balance (276.0-276.9)
hypoglycemia NOS (251.2)
lead poisoning (984.0-984.9)
specific finding indicating abnormality of:
amino-acid transport and metabolism (270.0-270.9)
carbohydrate transport and metabolism (271.0-271.9)
lipid metabolism (272.0-272.9)
uremia NOS (586)

● Code new to this edition　　▲ Revision of existing code　　④ ⑤ Fourth or fifth digit required

790.7 Bacteremia

> *Excludes:* *bacteremia of newborn (771.83)*
> *septicemia (038)*

Use additional code, if desired, to identify organism (041)

790.8 Viremia, unspecified

⑤ **790.9 Other nonspecific findings on examination of blood**

790.91 Abnormal arterial blood gases

790.92 Abnormal coagulation profile
Abnormal or prolonged:
bleeding time
coagulation time
partial thromboplastin time [PTT]
prothrombin time [PT]

> *Excludes:* *coagulation (hemorrhagic) disorders (286.0-286.9)*

790.93 Elevated prostate specific antigen (PSA)

790.94 Euthyroid sick syndrome

790.95 Elevated C-reactive protein (CRP)

790.99 Other

791 Nonspecific findings on examination of urine

> *Excludes:* *hematuria NOS (599.7)*
> *specific findings indicating abnormality of:*
> *amino-acid transport and metabolism (270.0-270.9)*
> *carbohydrate transport and metabolism (271.0-271.9)*

791.0 Proteinuria
Albuminuria
Bence-Jones proteinuria

> *Excludes:* *postural proteinuria (593.6)*
> *that arising during pregnancy or the puerperium (642.0-642.9, 646.2)*

791.1 Chyluria

> *Excludes:* *filarial (125.0-125.9)*

791.2 Hemoglobinuria

791.3 Myoglobinuria

791.4 Biliuria

791.5 Glycosuria

> *Excludes:* *renal glycosuria (271.4)*

791.6 Acetonuria
Ketonuria

791.7 Other cells and casts in urine

791.9 Other nonspecific findings on examination of urine
Crystalluria
Elevated urine levels of:
17-ketosteroids
catecholamines
indolacetic acid
vanillylmandelic acid [VMA]
Melanuria

792 Nonspecific abnormal findings in other body substances

> *Excludes:* *that in chromosomal analysis (795.2)*

792.0 Cerebrospinal fluid

792.1 Stool contents
Abnormal stool color
Fat in stool   Occult blood
Mucus in stool   Pus in stool

> *Excludes:* *blood in stool [melena] (578.1)*
> *newborn (772.4, 777.3)*

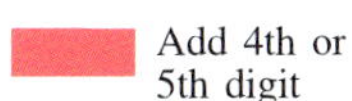

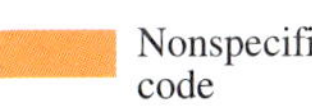

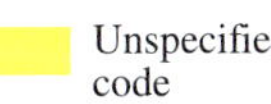

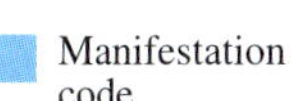

792.2 Semen
Abnormal spermatozoa
Excludes: *azoospermia (606.0)*
oligospermia (606.1)

792.3 Amniotic fluid

792.4 Saliva
Excludes: *that in chromosomal analysis (795.2)*

792.5 Cloudy (hemodialysis) (peritoneal) dialysis effluent

792.9 Other nonspecific abnormal findings in body substances
Peritoneal fluid   Synovial fluid
Pleural fluid   Vaginal fluids

793 Nonspecific abnormal findings on radiological and other examinations of body structure
Includes: nonspecific abnormal findings of:
thermography
ultrasound examination [echogram]
x-ray examination
Excludes: *abnormal results of function studies and radioisotope scans (794.0-794.9)*

793.0 Skull and head
Excludes: *nonspecific abnormal echoencephalogram (794.01)*

793.1 Lung field
Coin lesion of lung
Shadow, lung

793.2 Other intrathoracic organ
Abnormal: Mediastinal shift
echocardiogram
heart shadow
ultrasound cardiogram

793.3 Biliary tract
Nonvisualization of gallbladder

793.4 Gastrointestinal tract

793.5 Genitourinary organs
Filling defect:
bladder
kidney
ureter

793.6 Abdominal area, including retroperitoneum

793.7 Musculoskeletal system

⑤ **793.8 Breast**

793.80 Abnormal mammogram, unspecified

793.81 Mammographic microcalcification
Excludes: *mammographic calcification (793.89)*
mammographic calculus (793.89)

793.89 Other abnormal findings on radiological examination of breast
Mammographic calcification
Mammographic calculus

⑤ **793.9 Other**
Excludes: *abnormal finding by radioisotope localization of placenta (794.9)*

● **793.91 Image test inconclusive due to excess body fat**
Use additional code to identify Body Mass Index (BMI), if known
(V85.0-V85.54)

● **793.99 Other nonspecific abnormal findings on radiological and other examinations of body structure**
Abnormal:
placental finding by x-ray or ultrasound method
radiological findings in skin and subcutaneous tissue

794 Nonspecific abnormal results of function studies
Includes: radioisotope:
scans
uptake studies
scintiphotography

          ● Code new   ▲ Revision of   ④ ⑤ Fourth or fifth
to this edition   existing code   digit required

⑤ **794.0 Brain and central nervous system**

  794.00 Abnormal function study, unspecified

  794.01 Abnormal echoencephalogram

  794.02 Abnormal electroencephalogram [EEG]

  794.09 Other
  Abnormal brain scan

⑤ **794.1 Peripheral nervous system and special senses**

  794.10 Abnormal response to nerve stimulation, unspecified

  794.11 Abnormal retinal function studies
  Abnormal electroretinogram [ERG]

  794.12 Abnormal electro-oculogram [EOG]

  794.13 Abnormal visually evoked potential

  794.14 Abnormal oculomotor studies

  794.15 Abnormal auditory function studies

  794.16 Abnormal vestibular function studies

  794.17 Abnormal electromyogram [EMG]

  Excludes: *that of eye (794.14)*

  794.19 Other

794.2 Pulmonary
  Abnormal lung scan
  Reduced:
    ventilatory capacity
    vital capacity

⑤ **794.3 Cardiovascular**

  794.30 Abnormal function study, unspecified

  794.31 Abnormal electrocardiogram [ECG] [EKG]

  Excludes: *long QT syndrome (426.82)*

  794.39 Other
  Abnormal:
    ballistocardiogram
    phonocardiogram
    vectorcardiogram

794.4 Kidney
  Abnormal renal function test

794.5 Thyroid
  Abnormal thyroid:
    scan
    uptake

794.6 Other endocrine function study

794.7 Basal metabolism
  Abnormal basal metabolic rate [BMR]

794.8 Liver
  Abnormal liver scan

794.9 Other
  Bladder
  Pancreas
  Placenta
  Spleen

795 Other and nonspecific abnormal cytological, histological, immunological and DNA test findings

  Excludes: *nonspecific abnormalities of red blood cells (790.01-790.09)*

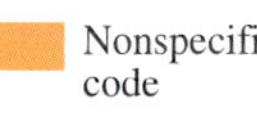

Add 4th or 5th digit	Nonspecific code	Unspecified code	Manifestation code

⑤ **795.0 Abnormal Papanicolaou smear of cervix and cervical HPV**
Abnormal thin preparation smear of cervix
Abnormal cervical cytology

Excludes: *carcinoma in-situ of cervix (233.1)*
cervical intraepithelial neoplasia I [CIN I] (622.11)
cervical intraepithelial neoplasia II [CIN II] (622.12)
cervical intraepithelial neoplasia III [CIN III] (233.1)
dysplasia (histologically confirmed) of cervix (uteri) NOS (622.10)
mild dysplasia (histologically confirmed) (622.11)
moderate dysplasia (histologically confirmed) (622.12)
severe dysplasia (histologically confirmed) (233.1)

795.00 Abnormal glandular Papanicolaou smear of cervix
Atypical endocervical cells NOS
Atypical endometrial cells NOS
Atypical glandular cells NOS

795.01 Papanicolaou smear of cervix with atypical squamous cells of undetermined significance (ASC-US)

795.02 Papanicolaou smear of cervix with atypical squamous cells cannot exclude high grade squamous intraepithelial lesion (ASC-H)

795.03 Papanicolaou smear of cervix with low grade squamous intraepithelial lesion (LGSIL)

795.04 Papanicolaou smear of cervix with high grade squamous intraepithelial lesion (HGSIL)

795.05 Cervical high risk human papillomavirus (HPV) DNA test positive

● **795.06 Papanicolaou smear of cervix with cytologic evidence of malignancy**

795.08 Unsatisfactory smear
Inadequate sample

795.09 Other abnormal Papanicolaou smear of cervix and cervical HPV
Cervical low risk human papillomavirus (HPV) DNA test positive
Papanicolaou smear of cervix with low risk human papillomavirus (HPV) DNA test positive

Use additional code for associated human papillomavirus (HPV) (079.4)

Excludes: *encounter for Papanicolaou cervical smear to confirm findings of recent normal smear following initial abnormal smear (V72.32)*

795.1 Nonspecific abnormal Papanicolaou smear of other site

795.2 Nonspecific abnormal findings on chromosomal analysis
Abnormal karyotype

⑤ **795.3 Nonspecific positive culture findings**
Positive culture findings in:
nose
sputum
throat
wound

Excludes: *that of:*
blood (790.7-790.8)
urine (791.9)

795.31 Nonspecific positive findings for anthrax
Positive findings by nasal swab

795.39 Other nonspecific positive culture findings

795.4 Other nonspecific abnormal histological findings

795.5 Nonspecific reaction to tuberculin skin test without active tuberculosis
Abnormal result of Mantoux test
PPD positive
Tuberculin (skin test):
positive
reactor

795.6 False positive serological test for syphilis
False positive Wassermann reaction

● Code new
to this edition

▲ Revision of
existing code

④ ⑤ Fourth or fifth
digit required

⑤ **795.7   Other nonspecific immunological findings**

     Excludes: *abnormal tumor markers (795.81-795.89)*

        elevated prostate specific antigen [PSA] (790.93)
        elevated tumor associated antigens (795.81-795.89)
        isoimmunization, in pregnancy (656.1-656.2)
          affecting fetus or newborn (773.0-773.2)

    795.71   Nonspecific serologic evidence of human immunodeficiency virus [HIV]
        Inconclusive human immunodeficiency virus [HIV] test (adult) (infant)

Note: This code is ONLY to be used when a test finding is reported as nonspecific. Asymptomatic positive findings are coded to V08. If any HIV infection symptom or condition is present, see code 042. Negative findings are not coded.

     Excludes: *acquired immunodeficiency syndrome [AIDS] (042)*

        asymptomatic human immunodeficiency virus, [HIV] infection status (V08)
        HIV infection, symptomatic (042)
        human immunodeficiency virus [HIV] disease (042)
          positive (status) NOS (V08)

    795.79   Other and unspecified nonspecific immunological findings
        Raised antibody titer
        Raised level of immunoglobulins

● **795.8   Abnormal tumor markers**
        Elevated tumor associated antigens [TAA]
        Elevated tumor specific antigens [TSA]

     Excludes: *elevated prostate specific antigen [PSA] (790.93)*

   ● **795.81   Elevated carcinoembryonic antigen (CEA)**
   ● **795.82   Elevated cancer antigen 125 (CA 125)**
   ● **795.89   Other abnormal tumor markers**

796   Other nonspecific abnormal findings

    796.0   Nonspecific abnormal toxicological findings
        Abnormal levels of heavy metals or drugs in blood, urine, or other tissue

     Excludes: *excessive blood level of alcohol (790.3)*

    796.1   Abnormal reflex

    796.2   Elevated blood pressure reading without diagnosis of hypertension

Note: This category is to be used to record an episode of elevated blood pressure in a patient in whom no formal diagnosis of hypertension has been made, or as an incidental finding.

    796.3   Nonspecific low blood pressure reading

    796.4   Other abnormal clinical findings

    796.5   Abnormal finding on antenatal screening

    796.6   Abnormal findings on neonatal screening

     Excludes: *nonspecific serologic evidence of human immunodeficiency virus [HIV] (795.71)*

    796.9   Other

ILL-DEFINED AND UNKNOWN CAUSES OF MORBIDITY AND MORTALITY (797-799)

797   Senility without mention of psychosis
        Old age
        Senescence
        Senile asthenia
        Senile debility
        Senile exhaustion

     Excludes: *senile psychoses (290.0-290.9)*

798   Sudden death, cause unknown

    798.0   Sudden infant death syndrome
        Cot death
        Crib death
        Sudden death of nonspecific cause in infancy

    798.1   Instantaneous death

    798.2   Death occurring in less than 24 hours from onset of symptoms, not otherwise explained
        Death known not to be violent or instantaneous, for which no cause could be discovered
        Died without sign of disease

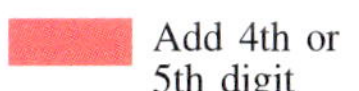

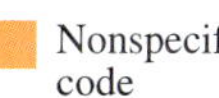

Unspecified
code

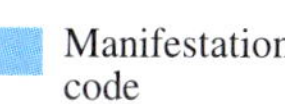

798.9 Unattended death
Death in circumstances where the body of the deceased was found and no cause could be discovered
Found dead

799 Other ill-defined and unknown causes of morbidity and mortality

⑤ **799.0 Asphyxia and hypoxemia**

Excludes: *asphyxia and hypoxemia (due to)*
  hypercapnia (786.09)

  799.01 Asphyxia

  799.02 Hypoxemia

799.1 Respiratory arrest
Cardiorespiratory failure

Excludes: *cardiac arrest (427.5)*
  failure of peripheral circulation (785.50)
  respiratory distress:
    NOS (786.09)
    acute (518.82)
    following trauma and surgery (518.5)
    newborn (770.89)
    syndrome (newborn) (769)
      adult (following trauma and surgery) (518.5)
      other (518.82)
    respiratory failure (518.81, 518.83-518.84)
    newborn (770.84)
    respiratory insufficiency (786.09)
    acute (518.82)

799.2 Nervousness
"Nerves"

799.3 Debility, unspecified

Excludes: *asthenia (780.79)*
  nervous debility (300.5)
  neurasthenia (300.5)
  senile asthenia (797)

799.4 Cachexia
Wasting disease

Code first underlying condition, if known

⑤ **799.8 Other ill-defined conditions**

  799.81 Decreased libido
  Decreased sexual desire

Excludes: *psychosexual dysfunction with inhibited sexual desire (302.71)*

  799.89 Other ill-defined conditions

799.9 Other unknown and unspecified cause
Undiagnosed disease, not specified as to site or system involved
Unknown cause of morbidity or mortality

     ● Code new
      to this edition   ▲ Revision of
        existing code   ④ ⑤ Fourth or fifth
          digit required

17. INJURY AND POISONING (800-999)

Use E code(s) to identify the cause and intent of the injury or poisoning (E800-E999)

Note:

1. The principle of multiple coding of injuries should be followed wherever possible. Combination categories for multiple injuries are provided for use when there is insufficient detail as to the nature of the individual conditions, or for primary tabulation purposes when it is more convenient to record a single code; otherwise, the component injuries should be coded separately.

   Where multiple sites of injury are specified in the titles, the word "with" indicates involvement of both sites, and the word "and" indicates involvement of either or both sites. The word "finger" includes thumb.

2. Categories for "late effect" of injuries are to be found at 905-909.

FRACTURES (800-829)

> Excludes: malunion (733.81)
> nonunion (733.82)
> pathologic or spontaneous fracture (733.10-733.19)
> stress fractures (733.93-733.95)

The terms "condyle," "coronoid process," "ramus," and "symphysis" indicate the portion of the bone fractured, not the name of the bone involved.

The descriptions "closed" and "open" used in the fourth-digit subdivisions include the following terms:

closed (with or without delayed healing):

comminuted	impacted
depressed	linear
elevated	simple
fissured	slipped epiphysis
fracture NOS	spiral
greenstick	

open (with or without delayed healing):

compound	puncture
infected	with foreign body
missile	

A fracture not indicated as closed or open should be classified as closed.

FRACTURE OF SKULL (800-804)

The following fifth-digit subclassification is for use with the appropriate codes in categories 800, 801, 803, and 804:

0 **unspecified state of consciousness**

1 **with no loss of consciousness**

2 **with brief [less than one hour] loss of consciousness**

3 **with moderate [1-24 hours] loss of consciousness and return to pre-existing conscious level**

4 **with prolonged [more than 24 hours] loss of consciousness and return to pre-existing conscious level**

5 **with prolonged [more than 24 hours] loss of consciousness, without return to pre-existing conscious level**
   Use fifth-digit 5 to designate when a patient is unconscious and dies before regaining consciousness, regardless of the duration of the loss of consciousness

6 **with loss of consciousness of unspecified duration**

9 **with concussion, unspecified**

⑤ **800** **Fracture of vault of skull**
   Includes: frontal bone
   parietal bone

⑤ **800.0** **Closed without mention of intracranial injury**

⑤ **800.1** **Closed with cerebral laceration and contusion**

⑤ **800.2** **Closed with subarachnoid, subdural, and extradural hemorrhage**

⑤ **800.3** **Closed with other and unspecified intracranial hemorrhage**

⑤ **800.4** **Closed with intracranial injury of other and unspecified nature**

⑤ **800.5** **Open without mention of intracranial injury**

⑤ **800.6** **Open with cerebral laceration and contusion**

⑤ **800.7** **Open with subarachnoid, subdural, and extradural hemorrhage**

Add 4th or 5th digit	Nonspecific code	Unspecified code	Medicare secondary payer (MSP) alert

⑤ **800.8** **Open with other and unspecified intracranial hemorrhage**

⑤ **800.9** **Open with intracranial injury of other and unspecified nature**

⑤ **801** **Fracture of base of skull**
Includes:

fossa:	sinus:
anterior	ethmoid
middle	frontal
posterior	sphenoid bone
occiput bone	temporal bone
orbital roof	

⑤ **801.0** **Closed without mention of intracranial injury**

⑤ **801.1** **Closed with cerebral laceration and contusion**

⑤ **801.2** **Closed with subarachnoid, subdural, and extradural hemorrhage**

⑤ **801.3** **Closed with other and unspecified intracranial hemorrhage**

⑤ **801.4** **Closed with intracranial injury of other and unspecified nature**

⑤ **801.5** **Open without mention of intracranial injury**

⑤ **801.6** **Open with cerebral laceration and contusion**

⑤ **801.7** **Open with subarachnoid, subdural, and extradural hemorrhage**

⑤ **801.8** **Open with other and unspecified intracranial hemorrhage**

⑤ **801.9** **Open with intracranial injury of other and unspecified nature**

802 **Fracture of face bones**

802.0 **Nasal bones, closed**

802.1 **Nasal bones, open**

⑤ **802.2** **Mandible, closed**
Inferior maxilla
Lower jaw (bone)

802.20 **Unspecified site**

802.21 **Condylar process**

802.22 **Subcondylar**

802.23 **Coronoid process**

802.24 **Ramus, unspecified**

802.25 **Angle of jaw**

802.26 **Symphysis of body**

802.27 **Alveolar border of body**

802.28 **Body, other and unspecified**

802.29 **Multiple sites**

⑤ **802.3** **Mandible, open**

802.30 **Unspecified site**

802.31 **Condylar process**

802.32 **Subcondylar**

802.33 **Coronoid process**

802.34 **Ramus, unspecified**

802.35 **Angle of jaw**

802.36 **Symphysis of body**

802.37 **Alveolar border of body**

802.38 **Body, other and unspecified**

802.39 **Multiple sites**

802.4 **Malar and maxillary bones, closed**

Superior maxilla	Zygoma
Upper jaw (bone)	Zygomatic arch

802.5 **Malar and maxillary bones, open**

802.6 **Orbital floor (blow-out), closed**

802.7 **Orbital floor (blow-out), open**

● Code new to this edition ▲ Revision of existing code ④ ⑤ Fourth or fifth digit required

802.8 **Other facial bones, closed**
    Alveolus
    Orbit:
      NOS
      part other than roof or floor
    Palate
    Excludes: *orbital:*
        floor (802.6)
        roof (801.0-801.9)

802.9 **Other facial bones, open**

⑤ **803** **Other and unqualified skull fractures**
    Includes: skull NOS
              skull multiple NOS

⑤ **803.0** **Closed without mention of intracranial injury**

⑤ **803.1** **Closed with cerebral laceration and contusion**

⑤ **803.2** **Closed with subarachnoid, subdural, and extradural hemorrhage**

⑤ **803.3** **Closed with other and unspecified intracranial hemorrhage**

⑤ **803.4** **Closed with intracranial injury of other and unspecified nature**

⑤ **803.5** **Open without mention of intracranial injury**

⑤ **803.6** **Open with cerebral laceration and contusion**

⑤ **803.7** **Open with subarachnoid, subdural, and extradural hemorrhage**

⑤ **803.8** **Open with other and unspecified intracranial hemorrhage**

⑤ **803.9** **Open with intracranial injury of other and unspecified nature**

⑤ **804** **Multiple fractures involving skull or face with other bones**

⑤ **804.0** **Closed without mention of intracranial injury**

⑤ **804.1** **Closed with cerebral laceration and contusion**

⑤ **804.2** **Closed with subarachnoid, subdural, and extradural hemorrhage**

⑤ **804.3** **Closed with other and unspecified intracranial hemorrhage**

⑤ **804.4** **Closed with intracranial injury of other and unspecified nature**

⑤ **804.5** **Open without mention of intracranial injury**

⑤ **804.6** **Open with cerebral laceration and contusion**

⑤ **804.7** **Open with subarachnoid, subdural, and extradural hemorrhage**

⑤ **804.8** **Open with other and unspecified intracranial hemorrhage**

⑤ **804.9** **Open with intracranial injury of other and unspecified nature**

FRACTURE OF NECK AND TRUNK (805-809)

805 **Fracture of vertebral column without mention of spinal cord injury**
    Includes: neural arch
              spine
              spinous process
              transverse process
              vertebra

The following fifth-digit subclassification is for use with codes 805.0-805.1:

    0 **cervical vertebra, unspecified level**

    1 **first cervical vertebra**

    2 **second cervical vertebra**

    3 **third cervical vertebra**

    4 **fourth cervical vertebra**

    5 **fifth cervical vertebra**

    6 **sixth cervical vertebra**

    7 **seventh cervical vertebra**

    8 **multiple cervical vertebrae**

⑤ **805.0** **Cervical, closed**
    Atlas
    Axis

⑤ **805.1** **Cervical, open**

805.2 **Dorsal [thoracic], closed**

805.3 **Dorsal [thoracic], open**

805.4 **Lumbar, closed**

805.5 **Lumbar, open**

805.6 **Sacrum and coccyx, closed**

805.7 **Sacrum and coccyx, open**

805.8 **Unspecified, closed**

805.9 **Unspecified, open**

806 **Fracture of vertebral column with spinal cord injury**
   Includes: any condition classifiable to 805 with:
            complete or incomplete transverse lesion (of cord)
            hematomyelia
         injury to:
            cauda equina
            nerve
         paralysis
         paraplegia
         quadriplegia
         spinal concussion

⑤ **806.0** **Cervical, closed**

   806.00 **C_1-C_4 level with unspecified spinal cord injury**
      Cervical region NOS with spinal cord injury NOS

   806.01 **C_1-C_4 level with complete lesion of cord**

   806.02 **C_1-C_4 level with anterior cord syndrome**

   806.03 **C_1-C_4 level with central cord syndrome**

   806.04 **C_1-C_4 level with other specified spinal cord injury**
      C_1-C_4 level with:
         incomplete spinal cord lesion NOS
         posterior cord syndrome

   806.05 **C_5-C_7 level with unspecified spinal cord injury**

   806.06 **C_5-C_7 level with complete lesion of cord**

   806.07 **C_5-C_7 level with anterior cord syndrome**

   806.08 **C_5-C_7 level with central cord syndrome**

   806.09 **C_5-C_7 level with other specified spinal cord injury**
      C_5-C_7 level with:
         incomplete spinal cord lesion NOS
         posterior cord syndrome

⑤ **806.1** **Cervical, open**

   806.10 **C_1-C_4 level with unspecified spinal cord injury**

   806.11 **C_1-C_4 level with complete lesion of cord**

   806.12 **C_1-C_4 level with anterior cord syndrome**

   806.13 **C_1-C_4 level with central cord syndrome**

   806.14 **C_1-C_4 level with other specified spinal cord injury**
      C_1-C_4 level with:
         incomplete spinal cord lesion NOS
         posterior cord syndrome

   806.15 **C_5-C_7 level with unspecified spinal cord injury**

   806.16 **C_5-C_7 level with complete lesion of cord**

   806.17 **C_5-C_7 level with anterior cord syndrome**

   806.18 **C_5-C_7 level with central cord syndrome**

   806.19 **C_5-C_7 level with other specified spinal cord injury**
      C_5-C_7 level with:
         incomplete spinal cord lesion NOS
         posterior cord syndrome

⑤ **806.2** **Dorsal [thoracic], closed**

   806.20 **T_1-T_6 level with unspecified spinal cord injury**
      Thoracic region NOS with spinal cord injury NOS

   806.21 **T_1-T_6 level with complete lesion of cord**

   806.22 **T_1-T_6 level with anterior cord syndrome**

   806.23 **T_1-T_6 level with central cord syndrome**

● Code new
to this edition

▲ Revision of
existing code

④ ⑤ Fourth or fifth
digit required

806.24 T_1-T_6 level with other specified spinal cord injury
T_1-T_6 level with:
    incomplete spinal cord lesion NOS
    posterior cord syndrome

806.25 T_7-T_{12} level with unspecified spinal cord injury

806.26 T_7-T_{12} level with complete lesion of cord

806.27 T_7-T_{12} level with anterior cord syndrome

806.28 T_7-T_{12} level with central cord syndrome

806.29 T_7-T_{12} level with other specified spinal cord injury
T_7-T_{12} level with:
    incomplete spinal cord lesion NOS
    posterior cord syndrome

⑤ **806.3 Dorsal [thoracic], open**

806.30 T_1-T_6 level with unspecified spinal cord injury

806.31 T_1-T_6 level with complete lesion of cord

806.32 T_1-T_6 level with anterior cord syndrome

806.33 T_1-T_6 level with central cord syndrome

806.34 T_1-T_6 level with other specified spinal cord injury
T_1-T_6 level with:
    incomplete spinal cord lesion NOS
    posterior cord syndrome

806.35 T_7-T_{12} level with unspecified spinal cord injury

806.36 T_7-T_{12} level with complete lesion of cord

806.37 T_7-T_{12} level with anterior cord syndrome

806.38 T_7-T_{12} level with central cord syndrome

806.39 T_7-T_{12} level with other specified spinal cord injury
T_7-T_{12} level with:
    incomplete spinal cord lesion NOS
    posterior cord syndrome

806.4 Lumbar, closed

806.5 Lumbar, open

⑤ **806.6 Sacrum and coccyx, closed**

806.60 With unspecified spinal cord injury

806.61 With complete cauda equina lesion

806.62 With other cauda equina injury

806.69 With other spinal cord injury

⑤ **806.7 Sacrum and coccyx, open**

806.70 With unspecified spinal cord injury

806.71 With complete cauda equina lesion

806.72 With other cauda equina injury

806.79 With other spinal cord injury

806.8 Unspecified, closed

806.9 Unspecified, open

807 Fracture of rib(s), sternum, larynx, and trachea
The following fifth-digit subclassification is for use with codes 807.0-807.1:

0 rib(s), unspecified

1 one rib

2 two ribs

3 three ribs

4 four ribs

5 five ribs

6 six ribs

7 seven ribs

8 eight or more ribs

9 multiple ribs, unspecified

⑤ **807.0 Rib(s), closed**

⑤ **807.1 Rib(s), open**

807.2 Sternum, closed

807.3 Sternum, open

807.4 Flail chest

807.5 Larynx and trachea, closed
    Hyoid bone   Trachea
    Thyroid cartilage

807.6 Larynx and trachea, open

808 Fracture of pelvis

808.0 Acetabulum, closed

808.1 Acetabulum, open

808.2 Pubis, closed

808.3 Pubis, open

⑤ **808.4 Other specified part, closed**

    808.41 Ilium

    808.42 Ischium

    808.43 Multiple pelvic fractures with disruption of pelvic circle

    808.49 Other
        Innominate bone
        Pelvic rim

⑤ **808.5 Other specified part, open**

    808.51 Ilium

    808.52 Ischium

    808.53 Multiple pelvic fractures with disruption of pelvic circle

    808.59 Other

808.8 Unspecified, closed

808.9 Unspecified, open

809 Ill-defined fractures of bones of trunk
    Includes: bones of trunk with other bones except those of skull and face
              multiple bones of trunk

    | *Excludes:* | *multiple fractures of:* |

        pelvic bones alone (808.0-808.9)
        ribs alone (807.0-807.1, 807.4)
        ribs or sternum with limb bones (819.0-819.1, 828.0-828.1)
        skull or face with other bones (804.0-804.9)

809.0 Fracture of bones of trunk, closed

809.1 Fracture of bones of trunk, open

FRACTURE OF UPPER LIMB (810-819)

⑤ **810 Fracture of clavicle**
    Includes: collar bone
              interligamentous part of clavicle

The following fifth-digit subclassification is for use with category 810:

    0 unspecified part
        Clavicle NOS

    1 sternal end of clavicle

    2 shaft of clavicle

    3 acromial end of clavicle

⑤ **810.0 Closed**

⑤ **810.1 Open**

● Code new   ▲ Revision of   ④ ⑤ Fourth or fifth
   to this edition   existing code   digit required

⑤ **811** **Fracture of scapula**
    Includes: shoulder blade
The following fifth-digit subclassification is for use with category 811:

    0 **unspecified part**

    1 **acromial process**
        Acromion (process)

    2 **coracoid process**

    3 **glenoid cavity and neck of scapula**

    9 **other**
        Scapula body

⑤ **811.0** **Closed**

⑤ **811.1** **Open**

812 **Fracture of humerus**

  ⑤ **812.0** **Upper end, closed**

    812.00 **Upper end, unspecified part**
        Proximal end
        Shoulder

    812.01 **Surgical neck**
        Neck of humerus NOS

    812.02 **Anatomical neck**

    812.03 **Greater tuberosity**

    812.09 **Other**
        Head
        Upper epiphysis

  ⑤ **812.1** **Upper end, open**

    812.10 **Upper end, unspecified part**

    812.11 **Surgical neck**

    812.12 **Anatomical neck**

    812.13 **Greater tuberosity**

    812.19 **Other**

  ⑤ **812.2** **Shaft or unspecified part, closed**

    812.20 **Unspecified part of humerus**
        Humerus NOS
        Upper arm NOS

    812.21 **Shaft of humerus**

  ⑤ **812.3** **Shaft or unspecified part, open**

    812.30 **Unspecified part of humerus**

    812.31 **Shaft of humerus**

  ⑤ **812.4** **Lower end, closed**
    Distal end of humerus
    Elbow

    812.40 **Lower end, unspecified part**

    812.41 **Supracondylar fracture of humerus**

    812.42 **Lateral condyle**
        External condyle

    812.43 **Medial condyle**
        Internal epicondyle

    812.44 **Condyle(s), unspecified**
        Articular process NOS
        Lower epiphysis NOS

    812.49 **Other**
        Multiple fractures of lower end
        Trochlea

  ⑤ **812.5** **Lower end, open**

    812.50 **Lower end, unspecified part**

    812.51 **Supracondylar fracture of humerus**

    812.52 **Lateral condyle**

    812.53 **Medial condyle**

	Add 4th or 5th digit		Nonspecific code		Unspecified code		Medicare secondary payer (MSP) alert

812.54 **Condyle(s), unspecified**

812.59 **Other**

813 **Fracture of radius and ulna**

⑤ **813.0** **Upper end, closed**
Proximal end

813.00 **Upper end of forearm, unspecified**

813.01 **Olecranon process of ulna**

813.02 **Coronoid process of ulna**

813.03 **Monteggia's fracture**

813.04 **Other and unspecified fractures of proximal end of ulna (alone)**
Multiple fractures of ulna, upper end

813.05 **Head of radius**

813.06 **Neck of radius**

813.07 **Other and unspecified fractures of proximal end of radius (alone)**
Multiple fractures of radius, upper end

813.08 **Radius with ulna, upper end [any part]**

⑤ **813.1** **Upper end, open**

813.10 **Upper end of forearm, unspecified**

813.11 **Olecranon process of ulna**

813.12 **Coronoid process of ulna**

813.13 **Monteggia's fracture**

813.14 **Other and unspecified fractures of proximal end of ulna (alone)**

813.15 **Head of radius**

813.16 **Neck of radius**

813.17 **Other and unspecified fractures of proximal end of radius (alone)**

813.18 **Radius with ulna, upper end [any part]**

⑤ **813.2** **Shaft, closed**

813.20 **Shaft, unspecified**

813.21 **Radius (alone)**

813.22 **Ulna (alone)**

813.23 **Radius with ulna**

⑤ **813.3** **Shaft, open**

813.30 **Shaft, unspecified**

813.31 **Radius (alone)**

813.32 **Ulna (alone)**

813.33 **Radius with ulna**

⑤ **813.4** **Lower end, closed**
Distal end

813.40 **Lower end of forearm, unspecified**

813.41 **Colles' fracture**
Smith's fracture

813.42 **Other fractures of distal end of radius (alone)**
Dupuytren's fracture, radius
Radius, lower end

813.43 **Distal end of ulna (alone)**
Ulna: Ulna:
  head   lower epiphysis
  lower end   styloid process

813.44 **Radius with ulna, lower end**

813.45 **Torus fracture of radius**

⑤ **813.5** **Lower end, open**

813.50 **Lower end of forearm, unspecified**

813.51 **Colles' fracture**

813.52 **Other fractures of distal end of radius (alone)**

813.53 **Distal end of ulna (alone)**

● Code new
to this edition

▲ Revision of
existing code

④ ⑤ Fourth or fifth
digit required

813.54 Radius with ulna, lower end

⑤ **813.8** Unspecified part, closed

813.80 Forearm, unspecified

813.81 Radius (alone)

813.82 Ulna (alone)

813.83 Radius with ulna

⑤ **813.9** Unspecified part, open

813.90 Forearm, unspecified

813.91 Radius (alone)

813.92 Ulna (alone)

813.93 Radius with ulna

⑤ **814** Fracture of carpal bone(s)

The following fifth-digit subclassification is for use with category 814:

0 carpal bone, unspecified
Wrist NOS

1 navicular [scaphoid] of wrist

2 lunate [semilunar] bone of wrist

3 triquetral [cuneiform] bone of wrist

4 pisiform

5 trapezium bone [larger multangular]

6 trapezoid bone [smaller multangular]

7 capitate bone [os magnum]

8 hamate [unciform] bone

9 other

⑤ **814.0** Closed

⑤ **814.1** Open

⑤ **815** Fracture of metacarpal bone(s)
Includes: hand [except finger]
          metacarpus

The following fifth-digit subclassification is for use with category 815:

0 metacarpal bone(s), site unspecified

1 base of thumb [first] metacarpal
Bennett's fracture

2 base of other metacarpal bone(s)

3 shaft of metacarpal bone(s)

4 neck of metacarpal bone(s)

9 multiple sites of metacarpus

⑤ **815.0** Closed

⑤ **815.1** Open

⑤ **816** Fracture of one or more phalanges of hand
Includes: finger(s)
          thumb

The following fifth-digit subclassification is for use with category 816:

0 phalanx or phalanges, unspecified

1 middle or proximal phalanx or phalanges

2 distal phalanx or phalanges

3 multiple sites

⑤ **816.0** Closed

⑤ **816.1** Open

817 Multiple fractures of hand bones
Includes: metacarpal bone(s) with phalanx or phalanges of same hand

817.0 Closed

817.1 Open

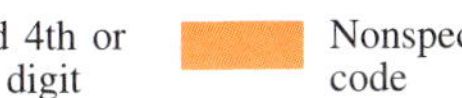

Add 4th or 5th digit	Nonspecific code	Unspecified code	Medicare secondary payer (MSP) alert

818 **Ill-defined fractures of upper limb**
Includes: arm NOS
multiple bones of same upper limb

Excludes: *multiple fractures of:*
metacarpal bone(s) with phalanx or phalanges (817.0-817.1)
phalanges of hand alone (816.0-816.1)
radius with ulna (813.0-813.9)

818.0 **Closed**

818.1 **Open**

819 **Multiple fractures involving both upper limbs, and upper limb with rib(s) and sternum**
Includes: arm(s) with rib(s) or sternum
both arms [any bones]

819.0 **Closed**

819.1 **Open**

FRACTURE OF LOWER LIMB (820-829)

820 **Fracture of neck of femur**

⑤ **820.0** **Transcervical fracture, closed**

820.00 **Intracapsular section, unspecified**

820.01 **Epiphysis (separation) (upper)**
Transepiphyseal

820.02 **Midcervical section**
Transcervical NOS

820.03 **Base of neck**
Cervicotrochanteric section

820.09 **Other**
Head of femur
Subcapital

⑤ **820.1** **Transcervical fracture, open**

820.10 **Intracapsular section, unspecified**

820.11 **Epiphysis (separation) (upper)**

820.12 **Midcervical section**

820.13 **Base of neck**

820.19 **Other**

⑤ **820.2** **Pertrochanteric fracture, closed**

820.20 **Trochanteric section, unspecified**
Trochanter:
NOS
greater
lesser

820.21 **Intertrochanteric section**

820.22 **Subtrochanteric section**

⑤ **820.3** **Pertrochanteric fracture, open**

820.30 **Trochanteric section, unspecified**

820.31 **Intertrochanteric section**

820.32 **Subtrochanteric section**

820.8 **Unspecified part of neck of femur, closed**
Hip NOS
Neck of femur NOS

820.9 **Unspecified part of neck of femur, open**

821 **Fracture of other and unspecified parts of femur**

⑤ **821.0** **Shaft or unspecified part, closed**

821.00 **Unspecified part of femur**
Thigh
Upper leg

Excludes: *hip NOS (820.8)*

821.01 **Shaft**

⑤ **821.1** **Shaft or unspecified part, open**

● Code new
to this edition   ▲ Revision of
existing code   ④ ⑤ Fourth or fifth
digit required

    821.10   **Unspecified part of femur**

    821.11   **Shaft**

⑤ **821.2**   **Lower end, closed**
    Distal end

    821.20   **Lower end, unspecified part**

    821.21   **Condyle, femoral**

    821.22   **Epiphysis, lower (separation)**

    821.23   **Supracondylar fracture of femur**

    821.29   **Other**
      Multiple fractures of lower end

⑤ **821.3**   **Lower end, open**

    821.30   **Lower end, unspecified part**

    821.31   **Condyle, femoral**

    821.32   **Epiphysis, lower (separation)**

    821.33   **Supracondylar fracture of femur**

    821.39   **Other**

822   **Fracture of patella**

    822.0   **Closed**

    822.1   **Open**

⑤ **823**   **Fracture of tibia and fibula**

    | Excludes: | *Dupuytren's fracture (824.4-824.5)*
                ankle (824.4-824.5)
                radius (813.42, 813.52)
           Pott's fracture (824.4-824.5)
           that involving ankle (824.0-824.9)

The following fifth-digit subclassification is for use with category 823:

    0   **tibia alone**

    1   **fibula alone**

    2   **fibula with tibia**

⑤ **823.0**   **Upper end, closed**
    Head   Tibia:
    Proximal end   condyles
                            tuberosity

⑤ **823.1**   **Upper end, open**

⑤ **823.2**   **Shaft, closed**

⑤ **823.3**   **Shaft, open**

⑤ **823.4**   **Torus fracture**

⑤ **823.8**   **Unspecified part, closed**
    Lower leg NOS

⑤ **823.9**   **Unspecified part, open**

824   **Fracture of ankle**

    824.0   **Medial malleolus, closed**
      Tibia involving:
        ankle
        malleolus

    824.1   **Medial malleolus, open**

    824.2   **Lateral malleolus, closed**
      Fibula involving:
        ankle
        malleolus

    824.3   **Lateral malleolus, open**

    824.4   **Bimalleolar, closed**
      Dupuytren's fracture, fibula
      Pott's fracture

    824.5   **Bimalleolar, open**

    824.6   **Trimalleolar, closed**
      Lateral and medial malleolus with anterior or posterior lip of tibia

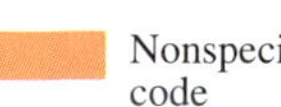

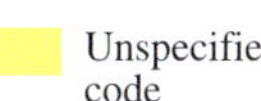

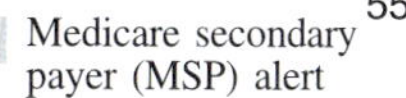

Medicare secondary
payer (MSP) alert

824.7 Trimalleolar, open

824.8 Unspecified, closed
Ankle NOS

824.9 Unspecified, open

825 Fracture of one or more tarsal and metatarsal bones

825.0 Fracture of calcaneus, closed
Heel bone
Os calcis

825.1 Fracture of calcaneus, open

⑤ **825.2 Fracture of other tarsal and metatarsal bones, closed**

825.20 Unspecified bone(s) of foot [except toes]
Instep

825.21 Astragalus
Talus

825.22 Navicular [scaphoid], foot

825.23 Cuboid

825.24 Cuneiform, foot

825.25 Metatarsal bone(s)

825.29 Other
Tarsal with metatarsal bone(s) only

Excludes: calcaneus (825.0)

⑤ **825.3 Fracture of other tarsal and metatarsal bones, open**

825.30 Unspecified bone(s) of foot [except toes]

825.31 Astragalus

825.32 Navicular [scaphoid], foot

825.33 Cuboid

825.34 Cuneiform, foot

825.35 Metatarsal bone(s)

825.39 Other

826 Fracture of one or more phalanges of foot
Includes: toe(s)

826.0 Closed

826.1 Open

827 Other, multiple, and ill-defined fractures of lower limb
Includes: leg NOS
multiple bones of same lower limb

Excludes: multiple fractures of:
ankle bones alone (824.4-824.9)
phalanges of foot alone (826.0-826.1)
tarsal with metatarsal bones (825.29, 825.39)
tibia with fibula (823.0-823.9 with fifth-digit 2)

827.0 Closed

827.1 Open

828 Multiple fractures involving both lower limbs, lower with upper limb, and lower limb(s) with rib(s) and sternum
Includes: arm(s) with leg(s) [any bones]
both legs [any bones]
leg(s) with rib(s) or sternum

828.0 Closed

828.1 Open

829 Fracture of unspecified bones

829.0 Unspecified bone, closed

829.1 Unspecified bone, open

● Code new
to this edition

▲ Revision of
existing code

④ ⑤ Fourth or fifth
digit required

DISLOCATION (830-839)

Includes: displacement
           subluxation

Excludes: *congenital dislocation (754.0-755.8)*
pathological dislocation (718.2)
recurrent dislocation (718.3)

The descriptions "closed" and "open", used in the fourth-digit subdivisions, include the following terms:

closed:	open:
complete	compound
dislocation NOS	infected
partial	with foreign body
simple	
uncomplicated	

A dislocation not indicated as closed or open should be classified as closed.

830 Dislocation of jaw
Includes: jaw (cartilage) (meniscus)
           mandible
           maxilla (inferior)
           temporomandibular (joint)

830.0 Closed dislocation

830.1 Open dislocation

831 Dislocation of shoulder

Excludes: *sternoclavicular joint (839.61, 839.71)*
sternum (839.61, 839.71)

The following fifth-digit subclassification is for use with category 831:

0 shoulder, unspecified
Humerus NOS

1 anterior dislocation of humerus

2 posterior dislocation of humerus

3 inferior dislocation of humerus

4 acromioclavicular (joint)
Clavicle

9 other
Scapula

831.0 Closed dislocation

831.1 Open dislocation

832 Dislocation of elbow
The following fifth-digit subclassification is for use with category 832:

0 elbow unspecified

1 anterior dislocation of elbow

2 posterior dislocation of elbow

3 medial dislocation of elbow

4 lateral dislocation of elbow

9 other

832.0 Closed dislocation

832.1 Open dislocation

833 Dislocation of wrist
The following fifth-digit subclassification is for use with category 833:

0 wrist, unspecified part
Carpal (bone)   Radius, distal end

1 radioulnar (joint), distal

2 radiocarpal (joint)

3 midcarpal (joint)

4 carpometacarpal (joint)

5 metacarpal (bone), proximal end

9 other
Ulna, distal end

Add 4th or 5th digit	Nonspecific code	Unspecified code	Medicare secondary payer (MSP) alert

⑤ **833.0 Closed dislocation**

⑤ **833.1 Open dislocation**

⑤ **834 Dislocation of finger**
Includes: finger(s)
            phalanx of hand
            thumb

The following fifth-digit subclassification is for use with category 834:

0 finger, unspecified part

1 metacarpophalangeal (joint)
     Metacarpal (bone), distal end

2 interphalangeal (joint), hand

⑤ **834.0 Closed dislocation**

⑤ **834.1 Open dislocation**

⑤ **835 Dislocation of hip**
The following fifth-digit subclassification is for use with category 835:

0 dislocation of hip, unspecified

1 posterior dislocation

2 obturator dislocation

3 other anterior dislocation

⑤ **835.0 Closed dislocation**

⑤ **835.1 Open dislocation**

836 Dislocation of knee

Excludes: *dislocation of knee:*
            old or pathological (718.2)
            recurrent (718.3)
            internal derangement of knee joint (717.0-717.5, 717.8-717.9)
            old tear of cartilage or meniscus of knee (717.0-717.5, 717.8-717.9)

836.0 Tear of medial cartilage or meniscus of knee, current
     Bucket handle tear:
       NOS current injury
     medial meniscus current injury

836.1 Tear of lateral cartilage or meniscus of knee, current

836.2 Other tear of cartilage or meniscus of knee, current
     Tear of:
       cartilage (semilunar) current injury, not specified as medial or lateral
       meniscus current injury, not specified as medial or lateral

836.3 Dislocation of patella, closed

836.4 Dislocation of patella, open

⑤ **836.5 Other dislocation of knee, closed**

   836.50 Dislocation of knee, unspecified

   836.51 Anterior dislocation of tibia, proximal end
          Posterior dislocation of femur, distal end

   836.52 Posterior dislocation of tibia, proximal end
          Anterior dislocation of femur, distal end

   836.53 Medial dislocation of tibia, proximal end

   836.54 Lateral dislocation of tibia, proximal end

   836.59 Other

⑤ **836.6 Other dislocation of knee, open**

   836.60 Dislocation of knee, unspecified

   836.61 Anterior dislocation of tibia, proximal end

   836.62 Posterior dislocation of tibia, proximal end

   836.63 Medial dislocation of tibia, proximal end

   836.64 Lateral dislocation of tibia, proximal end

   836.69 Other

● Code new to this edition   ▲ Revision of existing code   ④ ⑤ Fourth or fifth digit required

837 Dislocation of ankle
    Includes: astragalus
                fibula, distal end
                navicular, foot
                scaphoid, foot
                tibia, distal end

837.0 Closed dislocation

837.1 Open dislocation

⑤ **838 Dislocation of foot**
The following fifth-digit subclassification is for use with category 838:

    0 **foot, unspecified**

    1 **tarsal (bone), joint unspecified**

    2 **midtarsal (joint)**

    3 **tarsometatarsal (joint)**

    4 **metatarsal (bone), joint unspecified**

    5 **metatarsophalangeal (joint)**

    6 **interphalangeal (joint), foot**

    9 **other**
        Phalanx of foot
        Toe(s)

⑤ **838.0 Closed dislocation**

⑤ **838.1 Open dislocation**

839 Other, multiple, and ill-defined dislocations

⑤ **839.0 Cervical vertebra, closed**
    Cervical spine
    Neck

    839.00 Cervical vertebra, unspecified

    839.01 First cervical vertebra

    839.02 Second cervical vertebra

    839.03 Third cervical vertebra

    839.04 Fourth cervical vertebra

    839.05 Fifth cervical vertebra

    839.06 Sixth cervical vertebra

    839.07 Seventh cervical vertebra

    839.08 Multiple cervical vertebrae

⑤ **839.1 Cervical vertebra, open**

    839.10 Cervical vertebra, unspecified

    839.11 First cervical vertebra

    839.12 Second cervical vertebra

    839.13 Third cervical vertebra

    839.14 Fourth cervical vertebra

    839.15 Fifth cervical vertebra

    839.16 Sixth cervical vertebra

    839.17 Seventh cervical vertebra

    839.18 Multiple cervical vertebrae

⑤ **839.2 Thoracic and lumbar vertebra, closed**

    839.20 Lumbar vertebra

    839.21 Thoracic vertebra
        Dorsal [thoracic] vertebra

⑤ **839.3 Thoracic and lumbar vertebra, open**

    839.30 Lumbar vertebra

    839.31 Thoracic vertebra

⑤ **839.4 Other vertebra, closed**

    839.40 Vertebra, unspecified site
        Spine NOS

▮ Add 4th or 5th digit	▮ Nonspecific code	▮ Unspecified code	▮ Medicare secondary payer (MSP) alert

839.41 **Coccyx**

839.42 **Sacrum**
Sacroiliac (joint)

839.49 **Other**

⑤ **839.5** **Other vertebra, open**

839.50 **Vertebra, unspecified site**

839.51 **Coccyx**

839.52 **Sacrum**

839.59 **Other**

⑤ **839.6** **Other location, closed**

839.61 **Sternum**
Sternoclavicular joint

839.69 **Other**
Pelvis

⑤ **839.7** **Other location, open**

839.71 **Sternum**

839.79 **Other**

839.8 **Multiple and ill-defined, closed**
Arm
Back
Hand
Multiple locations, except fingers or toes alone
Other ill-defined locations
Unspecified location

839.9 **Multiple and ill-defined, open**

SPRAINS AND STRAINS OF JOINTS AND ADJACENT MUSCLES (840-848)

Includes: avulsion of: joint capsule, ligament, muscle, tendon
hemarthrosis of: joint capsule, ligament, muscle, tendon
laceration of: joint capsule, ligament, muscle, tendon
rupture of: joint capsule, ligament, muscle, tendon
sprain of: joint capsule, ligament, muscle, tendon
strain of: joint capsule, ligament, muscle, tendon
tear of: joint capsule, ligament, muscle, tendon

Excludes: *laceration of tendon in open wounds (880-884 and 890-894 with .2)*

840 **Sprains and strains of shoulder and upper arm**

840.0 **Acromioclavicular (joint) (ligament)**

840.1 **Coracoclavicular (ligament)**

840.2 **Coracohumeral (ligament)**

840.3 **Infraspinatus (muscle) (tendon)**

840.4 **Rotator cuff (capsule)**

Excludes: *complete rupture of rotator cuff, nontraumatic (727.61)*

840.5 **Subscapularis (muscle)**

840.6 **Supraspinatus (muscle) (tendon)**

840.7 **Superior glenoid labrum lesion**
SLAP lesion

840.8 **Other specified sites of shoulder and upper arm**

840.9 **Unspecified site of shoulder and upper arm**
Arm NOS
Shoulder NOS

841 **Sprains and strains of elbow and forearm**

841.0 **Radial collateral ligament**

841.1 **Ulnar collateral ligament**

841.2 **Radiohumeral (joint)**

841.3 **Ulnohumeral (joint)**

841.8 **Other specified sites of elbow and forearm**

841.9 **Unspecified site of elbow and forearm**
Elbow NOS

● Code new
to this edition
▲ Revision of
existing code
④ ⑤ Fourth or fifth
digit required

842 Sprains and strains of wrist and hand

⑤ 842.0 Wrist

842.00 Unspecified site

842.01 Carpal (joint)

842.02 Radiocarpal (joint) (ligament)

842.09 Other
Radioulnar joint, distal

⑤ 842.1 Hand

842.10 Unspecified site

842.11 Carpometacarpal (joint)

842.12 Metacarpophalangeal (joint)

842.13 Interphalangeal (joint)

842.19 Other
Midcarpal (joint)

843 Sprains and strains of hip and thigh

843.0 Iliofemoral (ligament)

843.1 Ischiocapsular (ligament)

843.8 Other specified sites of hip and thigh

843.9 Unspecified site of hip and thigh
Hip NOS
Thigh NOS

844 Sprains and strains of knee and leg

844.0 Lateral collateral ligament of knee

844.1 Medial collateral ligament of knee

844.2 Cruciate ligament of knee

844.3 Tibiofibular (joint) (ligament), superior

844.8 Other specified sites of knee and leg

844.9 Unspecified site of knee and leg
Knee NOS
Leg NOS

845 Sprains and strains of ankle and foot

⑤ 845.0 Ankle

845.00 Unspecified site

845.01 Deltoid (ligament), ankle
Internal collateral (ligament), ankle

845.02 Calcaneofibular (ligament)

845.03 Tibiofibular (ligament), distal

845.09 Other
Achilles tendon

⑤ 845.1 Foot

845.10 Unspecified site

845.11 Tarsometatarsal (joint) (ligament)

845.12 Metatarsophalangeal (joint)

845.13 Interphalangeal (joint), toe

845.19 Other

846 Sprains and strains of sacroiliac region

846.0 Lumbosacral (joint) (ligament)

846.1 Sacroiliac ligament

846.2 Sacrospinatus (ligament)

846.3 Sacrotuberous (ligament)

846.8 Other specified sites of sacroiliac region

846.9 Unspecified site of sacroiliac region

847 Sprains and strains of other and unspecified parts of back

> Excludes: lumbosacral (846.0)

Add 4th or 5th digit	Nonspecific code	Unspecified code	Medicare secondary payer (MSP) alert

847.0 Neck
Anterior longitudinal (ligament), cervical
Atlanto-axial (joints)
Atlanto-occipital (joints)
Whiplash injury

> *Excludes:* *neck injury NOS (959.0)*
> *thyroid region (848.2)*

847.1 Thoracic

847.2 Lumbar

847.3 Sacrum
Sacrococcygeal (ligament)

847.4 Coccyx

847.9 Unspecified site of back
Back NOS

848 Other and ill-defined sprains and strains

848.0 Septal cartilage of nose

848.1 Jaw
Temporomandibular (joint) (ligament)

848.2 Thyroid region
Cricoarytenoid (joint) (ligament)
Cricothyroid (joint) (ligament)
Thyroid cartilage

848.3 Ribs
Chondrocostal (joint) without mention of injury to sternum
Costal cartilage without mention of injury to sternum

⑤ **848.4 Sternum**

> **848.40 Unspecified site**

> **848.41 Sternoclavicular (joint) (ligament)**

> **848.42 Chondrosternal (joint)**

> **848.49 Other**
> Xiphoid cartilage

848.5 Pelvis
Symphysis pubis

> *Excludes:* *that in childbirth (665.6)*

848.8 Other specified sites of sprains and strains

848.9 Unspecified site of sprain and strain

INTRACRANIAL INJURY, EXCLUDING THOSE WITH SKULL FRACTURE (850-854)

> *Excludes:* *intracranial injury with skull fracture (800-801 and 803-804, except .0 and .5)*
> *open wound of head without intracranial injury (870.0-873.9)*
> *skull fracture alone (800-801 and 803-804 with .0, .5)*

The description "with open intracranial wound," used in the fourth-digit subdivisions, includes those specified as open or with mention of infection or foreign body.

The following fifth-digit subclassification is for use with categories 851-854:

0 unspecified state of consciousness

1 with no loss of consciousness

2 with brief [less than one hour] loss of consciousness

3 with moderate [1-24 hours] loss of consciousness

4 with prolonged [more than 24 hours] loss of consciousness and return to pre-existing conscious level

5 with prolonged [more than 24 hours] loss of consciousness, without return to pre-existing conscious level

> **Use fifth-digit 5 to designate when a patient is unconscious and dies before regaining consciousness, regardless of the duration of the loss of consciousness**

6 with loss of consciousness of unspecified duration

9 with concussion, unspecified

 Code new
to this edition

▲ Revision of
existing code

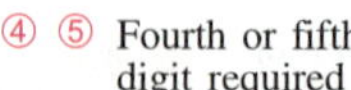 Fourth or fifth
digit required

850 **Concussion**
    Includes: commotio cerebri
    Excludes: *concussion with:*
        cerebral laceration or contusion (851.0-851.9)
        cerebral hemorrhage (852-853)
      head injury NOS (959.01)

850.0 **With no loss of consciousness**
    Concussion with mental confusion or disorientation, without loss of consciousness

⑤ **850.1** **With brief loss of consciousness**
    Loss of consciousness for less than one hour

    850.11 **With loss of consciousness of 30 minutes or less**

    850.12 **With loss of consciousness from 31 to 59 minutes**

850.2 **With moderate loss of consciousness**
    Loss of consciousness for 1-24 hours

850.3 **With prolonged loss of consciousness and return to pre-existing conscious level**
    Loss of consciousness for more than 24 hours with complete recovery

850.4 **With prolonged loss of consciousness, without return to pre-existing conscious level**

850.5 **With loss of consciousness of unspecified duration**

850.9 **Concussion, unspecified**

⑤ **851** **Cerebral laceration and contusion**

⑤ **851.0** **Cortex (cerebral) contusion without mention of open intracranial wound**

⑤ **851.1** **Cortex (cerebral) contusion with open intracranial wound**

⑤ **851.2** **Cortex (cerebral) laceration without mention of open intracranial wound**

⑤ **851.3** **Cortex (cerebral) laceration with open intracranial wound**

⑤ **851.4** **Cerebellar or brain stem contusion without mention of open intracranial wound**

⑤ **851.5** **Cerebellar or brain stem contusion with open intracranial wound**

⑤ **851.6** **Cerebellar or brain stem laceration without mention of open intracranial wound**

⑤ **851.7** **Cerebellar or brain stem laceration with open intracranial wound**

⑤ **851.8** **Other and unspecified cerebral laceration and contusion, without mention of open intracranial wound**
    Brain (membrane) NOS

⑤ **851.9** **Other and unspecified cerebral laceration and contusion, with open intracranial wound**

⑤ **852** **Subarachnoid, subdural, and extradural hemorrhage, following injury**
    Excludes: *Cerebral contusion or laceration (with hemorrhage) (851.0-851.9)*

⑤ **852.0** **Subarachnoid hemorrhage following injury without mention of open intracranial wound**
    Middle meningeal hemorrhage following injury

⑤ **852.1** **Subarachnoid hemorrhage following injury with open intracranial wound**

⑤ **852.2** **Subdural hemorrhage following injury without mention of open intracranial wound**

⑤ **852.3** **Subdural hemorrhage following injury with open intracranial wound**

⑤ **852.4** **Extradural hemorrhage following injury without mention of open intracranial wound**
    Epidural hematoma following injury

⑤ **852.5** **Extradural hemorrhage following injury with open intracranial wound**

⑤ **853** **Other and unspecified intracranial hemorrhage following injury**

⑤ **853.0** **Without mention of open intracranial wound**
    Cerebral compression due to injury
    Intracranial hematoma following injury
    Traumatic cerebral hemorrhage

⑤ **853.1** **With open intracranial wound**

⑤ **854** **Intracranial injury of other and unspecified nature**
    Includes: brain injury NOS
        cavernous sinus
        intracranial injury
    Excludes: *any condition classifiable to 850-853*
        head injury NOS (959.01)

⑤ **854.0** **Without mention of open intracranial wound**

⑤ **854.1** **With open intracranial wound**

INTERNAL INJURY OF THORAX, ABDOMEN, AND PELVIS (860-869)

Includes:
blast injuries of internal organs
blunt trauma of internal organs
bruise of internal organs
concussion injuries (except cerebral) of internal organs
crushing of internal organs
hematoma of internal organs
laceration of internal organs
puncture of internal organs
tear of internal organs
traumatic rupture of internal organs

Excludes: *concussion NOS (850.0-850.9)*
flail chest (807.4)
foreign body entering through orifice (930.0-939.9)
injury to blood vessels (901.0-902.9)

The description "with open wound," used in the fourth-digit subdivisions, includes those with mention of infection or foreign body.

860 **Traumatic pneumothorax and hemothorax**

860.0 **Pneumothorax without mention of open wound into thorax**

860.1 **Pneumothorax with open wound into thorax**

860.2 **Hemothorax without mention of open wound into thorax**

860.3 **Hemothorax with open wound into thorax**

860.4 **Pneumohemothorax without mention of open wound into thorax**

860.5 **Pneumohemothorax with open wound into thorax**

861 **Injury to heart and lung**

Excludes: *injury to blood vessels of thorax (901.0-901.9)*

⑤ **861.0** **Heart, without mention of open wound into thorax**

861.00 **Unspecified injury**

861.01 **Contusion**
Cardiac contusion
Myocardial contusion

861.02 **Laceration without penetration of heart chambers**

861.03 **Laceration with penetration of heart chambers**

⑤ **861.1** **Heart, with open wound into thorax**

861.10 **Unspecified injury**

861.11 **Contusion**

861.12 **Laceration without penetration of heart chambers**

861.13 **Laceration with penetration of heart chambers**

⑤ **861.2** **Lung, without mention of open wound into thorax**

861.20 **Unspecified injury**

861.21 **Contusion**

861.22 **Laceration**

⑤ **861.3** **Lung, with open wound into thorax**

861.30 **Unspecified injury**

861.31 **Contusion**

861.32 **Laceration**

862 **Injury to other and unspecified intrathoracic organs**

Excludes: *injury to blood vessels of thorax (901.0-901.9)*

862.0 **Diaphragm, without mention of open wound into cavity**

862.1 **Diaphragm, with open wound into cavity**

⑤ **862.2** **Other specified intrathoracic organs, without mention of open wound into cavity**

862.21 **Bronchus**

862.22 **Esophagus**

● Code new
to this edition

▲ Revision of
existing code

④ ⑤ Fourth or fifth
digit required

862.29 Other
Pleura
Thymus gland

⑤ **862.3** Other specified intrathoracic organs, with open wound into cavity

862.31 Bronchus

862.32 Esophagus

862.39 Other

862.8 Multiple and unspecified intrathoracic organs, without mention of open wound into cavity
Crushed chest
Multiple intrathoracic organs

862.9 Multiple and unspecified intrathoracic organs, with open wound into cavity

863 Injury to gastrointestinal tract

Excludes: *anal sphincter laceration during delivery (664.2)*
bile duct (868.0-868.1 with fifth-digit 2)
gallbladder (868.0-868.1 with fifth-digit 2)

863.0 Stomach, without mention of open wound into cavity

863.1 Stomach, with open wound into cavity

⑤ **863.2** Small intestine, without mention of open wound into cavity

863.20 Small intestine, unspecified site

863.21 Duodenum

863.29 Other

⑤ **863.3** Small intestine, with open wound into cavity

863.30 Small intestine, unspecified site

863.31 Duodenum

863.39 Other

⑤ **863.4** Colon or rectum, without mention of open wound into cavity

863.40 Colon, unspecified site

863.41 Ascending [right] colon

863.42 Transverse colon

863.43 Descending [left] colon

863.44 Sigmoid colon

863.45 Rectum

863.46 Multiple sites in colon and rectum

863.49 Other

⑤ **863.5** Colon or rectum, with open wound into cavity

863.50 Colon, unspecified site

863.51 Ascending [right] colon

863.52 Transverse colon

863.53 Descending [left] colon

863.54 Sigmoid colon

863.55 Rectum

863.56 Multiple sites in colon and rectum

863.59 Other

⑤ **863.8** Other and unspecified gastrointestinal sites, without mention of open wound into cavity

863.80 Gastrointestinal tract, unspecified site

863.81 Pancreas, head

863.82 Pancreas, body

863.83 Pancreas, tail

863.84 Pancreas, multiple and unspecified sites

863.85 Appendix

863.89 Other
Intestine NOS

Add 4th or 5th digit	Nonspecific code	Unspecified code	Medicare secondary payer (MSP) alert

⑤ **863.9 Other and unspecified gastrointestinal sites, with open wound into cavity**

863.90 **Gastrointestinal tract, unspecified site**

863.91 **Pancreas, head**

863.92 **Pancreas, body**

863.93 **Pancreas, tail**

863.94 **Pancreas, multiple and unspecified sites**

863.95 **Appendix**

863.99 **Other**

⑤ 864 **Injury to liver**

The following fifth-digit subclassification is for use with category 864:

0 **unspecified injury**

1 **hematoma and contusion**

2 **laceration, minor**
Laceration involving capsule only, or without significant involvement of hepatic parenchyma [i.e., less than 1 cm deep]

3 **laceration, moderate**
Laceration involving parenchyma but without major disruption of parenchyma [i.e., less than 10 cm long and less than 3 cm deep]

4 **laceration, major**
Laceration with significant disruption of hepatic parenchyma [i.e., 10 cm long and 3 cm deep]
Multiple moderate lacerations, with or without hematoma
Stellate lacerations of liver

5 **laceration, unspecified**

9 **other**

⑤ **864.0 Without mention of open wound into cavity**

⑤ **864.1 With open wound into cavity**

⑤ 865 **Injury to spleen**

The following fifth-digit subclassification is for use with category 865:

0 **unspecified injury**

1 **hematoma without rupture of capsule**

2 **capsular tears, without major disruption of parenchyma**

3 **laceration extending into parenchyma**

4 **massive parenchymal disruption**

9 **other**

⑤ **865.0 Without mention of open wound into cavity**

⑤ **865.1 With open wound into cavity**

⑤ 866 **Injury to kidney**

The following fifth-digit subclassification is for use with category 866:

0 **unspecified injury**

1 **hematoma without rupture of capsule**

2 **laceration**

3 **complete disruption of kidney parenchyma**

⑤ **866.0 Without mention of open wound into cavity**

⑤ **866.1 With open wound into cavity**

867 **Injury to pelvic organs**

Excludes: *injury during delivery (664.0-665.9)*

867.0 **Bladder and urethra, without mention of open wound into cavity**

867.1 **Bladder and urethra, with open wound into cavity**

867.2 **Ureter, without mention of open wound into cavity**

867.3 **Ureter, with open wound into cavity**

867.4 **Uterus, without mention of open wound into cavity**

867.5 **Uterus, with open wound into cavity**

● Code new to this edition   ▲ Revision of existing code   ④ ⑤ Fourth or fifth digit required

867.6 **Other specified pelvic organs, without mention of open wound into cavity**
Fallopian tube   Seminal vesicle
Ovary   Vas deferens
Prostate

867.7 **Other specified pelvic organs, with open wound into cavity**

867.8 **Unspecified pelvic organs, without mention of open wound into cavity**

867.9 **Unspecified pelvic organ, with open wound into cavity**

868 **Injury to other intra-abdominal organs**
The following fifth-digit subclassification is for use with category 868:

  0   unspecified intra-abdominal organ

  1   adrenal gland

  2   bile duct and gallbladder

  3   peritoneum

  4   retroperitoneum

  9   other and multiple intra-abdominal organs

868.0 **Without mention of open wound into cavity**

868.1 **With open wound into cavity**

869 **Internal injury to unspecified or ill-defined organs**
Includes: internal injury NOS
            multiple internal injury NOS

869.0 **Without mention of open wound into cavity**

869.1 **With open wound into cavity**

OPEN WOUND (870-897)

Includes: animal bite
            avulsion
            cut
            laceration
            puncture wound
            traumatic amputation

Excludes: *burn (940.0-949.5)*
crushing (925-929.9)
puncture of internal organs (860.0-869.1)
superficial injury (910.0-919.9)
that incidental to:
dislocation (830.0-839.9)
fracture (800.0-829.1)
internal injury (860.0-869.1)
intracranial injury (851.0-854.1)

Note: The description "complicated" used in the fourth-digit subdivisions includes those with mention of delayed healing, delayed treatment, foreign body, or infection.

Use additional code to identify infection.

OPEN WOUND OF HEAD, NECK, AND TRUNK (870-879)

870 **Open wound of ocular adnexa**

870.0 **Laceration of skin of eyelid and periocular area**

870.1 **Laceration of eyelid, full-thickness, not involving lacrimal passages**

870.2 **Laceration of eyelid involving lacrimal passages**

870.3 **Penetrating wound of orbit, without mention of foreign body**

870.4 **Penetrating wound of orbit with foreign body**
Excludes: *retained (old) foreign body in orbit (376.6)*

870.8 **Other specified open wounds of ocular adnexa**

870.9 **Unspecified open wound of ocular adnexa**

871 **Open wound of eyeball**
Excludes: *2nd cranial nerve [optic] injury (950.0-950.9)*
3rd cranial nerve [oculomotor] injury (951.0)

871.0 **Ocular laceration without prolapse of intraocular tissue**

871.1 **Ocular laceration with prolapse or exposure of intraocular tissue**

871.2 **Rupture of eye with partial loss of intraocular tissue**

871.3 Avulsion of eye
    Traumatic enucleation

871.4 Unspecified laceration of eye

871.5 Penetration of eyeball with magnetic foreign body
    Excludes: retained (old) magnetic foreign body in globe (360.50-360.59)

871.6 Penetration of eyeball with (nonmagnetic) foreign body
    Excludes: retained (old) (nonmagnetic) foreign body in globe (360.60-360.69)

871.7 Unspecified ocular penetration

871.9 Unspecified open wound of eyeball

872 Open wound of ear
  ⑤ **872.0 External ear, without mention of complication**

      872.00 External ear, unspecified site

      872.01 Auricle, ear
        Pinna

      872.02 Auditory canal

  ⑤ **872.1 External ear, complicated**

      872.10 External ear, unspecified site

      872.11 Auricle, ear

      872.12 Auditory canal

  ⑤ **872.6 Other specified parts of ear, without mention of complication**

      872.61 Ear drum
        Drumhead
        Tympanic membrane

      872.62 Ossicles

      872.63 Eustachian tube

      872.64 Cochlea

      872.69 Other and multiple sites

  ⑤ **872.7 Other specified parts of ear, complicated**

      872.71 Ear drum

      872.72 Ossicles

      872.73 Eustachian tube

      872.74 Cochlea

      872.79 Other and multiple sites

  872.8 Ear, part unspecified, without mention of complication
    Ear NOS

  872.9 Ear, part unspecified, complicated

873 Other open wound of head
  873.0 Scalp, without mention of complication

  873.1 Scalp, complicated

  ⑤ **873.2 Nose, without mention of complication**

      873.20 Nose, unspecified site

      873.21 Nasal septum

      873.22 Nasal cavity

      873.23 Nasal sinus

      873.29 Multiple sites

  ⑤ **873.3 Nose, complicated**

      873.30 Nose, unspecified site

      873.31 Nasal septum

      873.32 Nasal cavity

      873.33 Nasal sinus

      873.39 Multiple sites

  ⑤ **873.4 Face, without mention of complication**

      873.40 Face, unspecified site

● Code new to this edition   ▲ Revision of existing code   ④ ⑤ Fourth or fifth digit required

    873.41 **Cheek**

    873.42 **Forehead**
       Eyebrow

    873.43 **Lip**

    873.44 **Jaw**

    `873.49` **Other and multiple sites**

⑤ **873.5 Face, complicated**

    `873.50` **Face, unspecified site**

    873.51 **Cheek**

    873.52 **Forehead**

    873.53 **Lip**

    873.54 **Jaw**

    `873.59` **Other and multiple sites**

⑤ **873.6 Internal structures of mouth, without mention of complication**

    `873.60` **Mouth, unspecified site**

    873.61 **Buccal mucosa**

    873.62 **Gum (alveolar process)**

  ▲ 873.63 **Tooth (broken) (fractured) (due to trauma)**
   Excludes: *cracked tooth (521.81)*

    873.64 **Tongue and floor of mouth**

    873.65 **Palate**

    `873.69` **Other and multiple sites**

⑤ **873.7 Internal structures of mouth, complicated**

    `873.70` **Mouth, unspecified site**

    873.71 **Buccal mucosa**

    873.72 **Gum (alveolar process)**

  ▲ 873.73 **Tooth (broken) (fractured) (due to trauma)**
   Excludes: *cracked tooth (521.81)*

    873.74 **Tongue and floor of mouth**

    873.75 **Palate**

    `873.79` **Other and multiple sites**

`873.8` **Other and unspecified open wound of head without mention of complication**
    Head NOS

`873.9` **Other and unspecified open wound of head, complicated**

`874` **Open wound of neck**

⑤ **874.0 Larynx and trachea, without mention of complication**

    874.00 **Larynx with trachea**

    874.01 **Larynx**

    874.02 **Trachea**

⑤ **874.1 Larynx and trachea, complicated**

    874.10 **Larynx with trachea**

    874.11 **Larynx**

    874.12 **Trachea**

  874.2 **Thyroid gland, without mention of complication**

  874.3 **Thyroid gland, complicated**

  874.4 **Pharynx, without mention of complication**
    Cervical esophagus

  874.5 **Pharynx, complicated**

`874.8` **Other and unspecified parts, without mention of complication**
    Nape of neck   Throat NOS
    Supraclavicular region

`874.9` **Other and unspecified parts, complicated**

🟥	Add 4th or 5th digit	🟧 Nonspecific code	🟨 Unspecified code	▨ Medicare secondary payer (MSP) alert

875 Open wound of chest (wall)
> *Excludes:* *open wound into thoracic cavity (860.0-862.9)*
> *traumatic pneumothorax and hemothorax (860.1, 860.3, 860.5)*

875.0 Without mention of complication

875.1 Complicated

876 Open wound of back
Includes: loin
lumbar region
> *Excludes:* *open wound into thoracic cavity (860.0-862.9)*
> *traumatic pneumothorax and hemothorax (860.1, 860.3, 860.5)*

876.0 Without mention of complication

876.1 Complicated

877 Open wound of buttock
Includes: sacroiliac region

877.0 Without mention of complication

877.1 Complicated

878 Open wound of genital organs (external), including traumatic amputation
> *Excludes:* *injury during delivery (664.0-665.9)*
> *internal genital organs (867.0-867.9)*

878.0 Penis, without mention of complication

878.1 Penis, complicated

878.2 Scrotum and testes, without mention of complication

878.3 Scrotum and testes, complicated

878.4 Vulva, without mention of complication
Labium (majus) (minus)

878.5 Vulva, complicated

878.6 Vagina, without mention of complication

878.7 Vagina, complicated

878.8 Other and unspecified parts, without mention of complication

878.9 Other and unspecified parts, complicated

879 Open wound of other and unspecified sites, except limbs

879.0 Breast, without mention of complication

879.1 Breast, complicated

879.2 Abdominal wall, anterior, without mention of complication
Abdominal wall NOS   Pubic region
Epigastric region   Umbilical region
Hypogastric region

879.3 Abdominal wall, anterior, complicated

879.4 Abdominal wall, lateral, without mention of complication
Flank   Iliac (region)
Groin   Inguinal region
Hypochondrium

879.5 Abdominal wall, lateral, complicated

879.6 Other and unspecified parts of trunk, without mention of complication
Pelvic region   Trunk NOS
Perineum

879.7 Other and unspecified parts of trunk, complicated

879.8 Open wound(s) (multiple) of unspecified site(s) without mention of complication
Multiple open wounds NOS
Open wound NOS

879.9 Open wound(s) (multiple) of unspecified site(s), complicated

● Code new
to this edition   ▲ Revision of
existing code   ④ ⑤ Fourth or fifth
digit required

OPEN WOUND OF UPPER LIMB (880-887)

⑤ **880** Open wound of shoulder and upper arm
The following fifth-digit subclassification is for use with category 880:

    0 shoulder region
    1 scapular region
    2 axillary region
    3 upper arm
    9 multiple sites

⑤ **880.0** Without mention of complication

⑤ **880.1** Complicated

⑤ **880.2** With tendon involvement

⑤ **881** Open wound of elbow, forearm, and wrist
The following fifth-digit subclassification is for use with category 881:

    0 forearm
    1 elbow
    2 wrist

⑤ **881.0** Without mention of complication

⑤ **881.1** Complicated

⑤ **881.2** With tendon involvement

882 Open wound of hand except finger(s) alone

882.0 Without mention of complication

882.1 Complicated

882.2 With tendon involvement

883 Open wound of finger(s)
Includes: fingernail
          thumb (nail)

883.0 Without mention of complication

883.1 Complicated

883.2 With tendon involvement

884 Multiple and unspecified open wound of upper limb
Includes: arm NOS
          multiple sites of one upper limb
          upper limb NOS

884.0 Without mention of complication

884.1 Complicated

884.2 With tendon involvement

885 Traumatic amputation of thumb (complete) (partial)
Includes: thumb(s) (with finger(s) of either hand)

885.0 Without mention of complication

885.1 Complicated

886 Traumatic amputation of other finger(s) (complete) (partial)
Includes: finger(s) of one or both hands, without mention of thumb(s)

886.0 Without mention of complication

886.1 Complicated

887 Traumatic amputation of arm and hand (complete) (partial)

887.0 Unilateral, below elbow, without mention of complication

887.1 Unilateral, below elbow, complicated

887.2 Unilateral, at or above elbow, without mention of complication

887.3 Unilateral, at or above elbow, complicated

887.4 Unilateral, level not specified, without mention of complication

887.5 Unilateral, level not specified, complicated

887.6 Bilateral [any level], without mention of complication
    One hand and other arm

887.7 Bilateral [any level], complicated

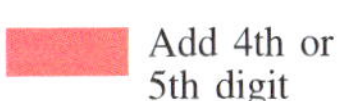

Nonspecific
code

Unspecified
code

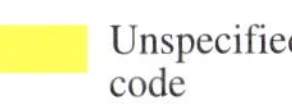

OPEN WOUND OF LOWER LIMB (890-897)

890 Open wound of hip and thigh

    890.0 Without mention of complication

    890.1 Complicated

    890.2 With tendon involvement

891 Open wound of knee, leg [except thigh], and ankle
    Includes: leg NOS
            multiple sites of leg, except thigh

    Excludes: *that of thigh (890.0-890.2)*
            with multiple sites of lower limb (894.0-894.2)

    891.0 Without mention of complication

    891.1 Complicated

    891.2 With tendon involvement

892 Open wound of foot except toe(s) alone
    Includes: heel

    892.0 Without mention of complication

    892.1 Complicated

    892.2 With tendon involvement

893 Open wound of toe(s)
    Includes: toenail

    893.0 Without mention of complication

    893.1 Complicated

    893.2 With tendon involvement

894 Multiple and unspecified open wound of lower limb
    Includes: lower limb NOS
            multiple sites of one lower limb, with thigh

    894.0 Without mention of complication

    894.1 Complicated

    894.2 With tendon involvement

895 Traumatic amputation of toe(s) (complete) (partial)
    Includes: toe(s) of one or both feet

    895.0 Without mention of complication

    895.1 Complicated

896 Traumatic amputation of foot (complete) (partial)

    896.0 Unilateral, without mention of complication

    896.1 Unilateral, complicated

    896.2 Bilateral, without mention of complication

        Excludes: *one foot and other leg (897.6-897.7)*

    896.3 Bilateral, complicated

897 Traumatic amputation of leg(s) (complete) (partial)

    897.0 Unilateral, below knee, without mention of complication

    897.1 Unilateral, below knee, complicated

    897.2 Unilateral, at or above knee, without mention of complication

    897.3 Unilateral, at or above knee, complicated

    897.4 Unilateral, level not specified, without mention of complication

    897.5 Unilateral, level not specified, complicated

    897.6 Bilateral [any level], without mention of complication
        One foot and other leg

    897.7 Bilateral [any level], complicated

● Code new to this edition   ▲ Revision of existing code   ④ ⑤ Fourth or fifth digit required

INJURY TO BLOOD VESSELS (900-904)

Includes: arterial hematoma of blood vessel, secondary to other injuries e.g., fracture or
open wound
avulsion of blood vessel, secondary to other injuries e.g., fracture or open wound
cut of blood vessel, secondary to other injuries e.g., fracture or open wound
laceration of blood vessel, secondary to other injuries e.g., fracture or open wound
rupture of blood vessel, secondary to other injuries e.g., fracture or open wound
traumatic aneurysm or fistula (arteriovenous) of blood vessel, secondary to other
injuries e.g., fracture or open wound

Excludes: *accidental puncture or laceration during medical procedure (998.2)*
intracranial hemorrhage following injury (851.0-854.1)

900 Injury to blood vessels of head and neck

⑤ **900.0 Carotid artery**

900.00 Carotid artery, unspecified

900.01 Common carotid artery

900.02 External carotid artery

900.03 Internal carotid artery

900.1 Internal jugular vein

⑤ **900.8 Other specified blood vessels of head and neck**

900.81 External jugular vein
Jugular vein NOS

900.82 Multiple blood vessels of head and neck

900.89 Other

900.9 Unspecified blood vessel of head and neck

901 Injury to blood vessels of thorax

Excludes: *traumatic hemothorax (860.2-860.5)*

901.0 Thoracic aorta

901.1 Innominate and subclavian arteries

901.2 Superior vena cava

901.3 Innominate and subclavian veins

⑤ **901.4 Pulmonary blood vessels**

901.40 Pulmonary vessel(s), unspecified

901.41 Pulmonary artery

901.42 Pulmonary vein

⑤ **901.8 Other specified blood vessels of thorax**

901.81 Intercostal artery or vein

901.82 Internal mammary artery or vein

901.83 Multiple blood vessels of thorax

901.89 Other
Azygos vein
Hemiazygos vein

901.9 Unspecified blood vessel of thorax

902 Injury to blood vessels of abdomen and pelvis

902.0 Abdominal aorta

⑤ **902.1 Inferior vena cava**

902.10 Inferior vena cava, unspecified

902.11 Hepatic veins

902.19 Other

⑤ **902.2 Celiac and mesenteric arteries**

902.20 Celiac and mesenteric arteries, unspecified

902.21 Gastric artery

902.22 Hepatic artery

902.23 Splenic artery

902.24 Other specified branches of celiac axis

902.25 Superior mesenteric artery (trunk)

Add 4th or 5th digit	Nonspecific code	Unspecified code	Medicare secondary payer (MSP) alert

902.26 Primary branches of superior mesenteric artery
Ileo-colic artery

902.27 Inferior mesenteric artery

902.29 Other

⑤ **902.3 Portal and splenic veins**

902.31 Superior mesenteric vein and primary subdivisions
Ileo-colic vein

902.32 Inferior mesenteric vein

902.33 Portal vein

902.34 Splenic vein

902.39 Other
Cystic vein
Gastric vein

⑤ **902.4 Renal blood vessels**

902.40 Renal vessel(s), unspecified

902.41 Renal artery

902.42 Renal vein

902.49 Other
Suprarenal arteries

⑤ **902.5 Iliac blood vessels**

902.50 Iliac vessel(s), unspecified

902.51 Hypogastric artery

902.52 Hypogastric vein

902.53 Iliac artery

902.54 Iliac vein

902.55 Uterine artery

902.56 Uterine vein

902.59 Other

⑤ **902.8 Other specified blood vessels of abdomen and pelvis**

902.81 Ovarian artery

902.82 Ovarian vein

902.87 Multiple blood vessels of abdomen and pelvis

902.89 Other

902.9 Unspecified blood vessel of abdomen and pelvis

903 Injury to blood vessels of upper extremity

⑤ **903.0 Axillary blood vessels**

903.00 Axillary vessel(s), unspecified

903.01 Axillary artery

903.02 Axillary vein

903.1 Brachial blood vessels

903.2 Radial blood vessels

903.3 Ulnar blood vessels

903.4 Palmar artery

903.5 Digital blood vessels

903.8 Other specified blood vessels of upper extremity
Multiple blood vessels of upper extremity

903.9 Unspecified blood vessel of upper extremity

904 Injury to blood vessels of lower extremity and unspecified sites

904.0 Common femoral artery
Femoral artery above profunda origin

904.1 Superficial femoral artery

904.2 Femoral veins

904.3 Saphenous veins
Saphenous vein (greater) (lesser)

⑤ **904.4 Popliteal blood vessels**

● Code new
to this edition

▲ Revision of
existing code

④ ⑤ Fourth or fifth
digit required

      904.40 Popliteal vessel(s), unspecified

      904.41 Popliteal artery

      904.42 Popliteal vein

⑤ **904.5** Tibial blood vessels

      904.50 Tibial vessel(s), unspecified

      904.51 Anterior tibial artery

      904.52 Anterior tibial vein

      904.53 Posterior tibial artery

      904.54 Posterior tibial vein

904.6 Deep plantar blood vessels

904.7 Other specified blood vessels of lower extremity
    Multiple blood vessels of lower extremity

904.8 Unspecified blood vessel of lower extremity

904.9 Unspecified site
    Injury to blood vessel NOS

LATE EFFECTS OF INJURIES, POISONINGS, TOXIC EFFECTS, AND OTHER EXTERNAL CAUSES (905-909)

Note: These categories are to be used to indicate conditions classifiable to 800-999 as the cause of late effects, which are themselves classified elsewhere. The "late effects" include those specified as such, or as sequelae, which may occur at any time after the acute injury.

905 Late effects of musculoskeletal and connective tissue injuries

905.0 Late effect of fracture of skull and face bones
    Late effect of injury classifiable to 800-804

905.1 Late effect of fracture of spine and trunk without mention of spinal cord lesion
    Late effect of injury classifiable to 805, 807-809

905.2 Late effect of fracture of upper extremities
    Late effect of injury classifiable to 810-819

905.3 Late effect of fracture of neck of femur
    Late effect of injury classifiable to 820

905.4 Late effect of fracture of lower extremities
    Late effect of injury classifiable to 821-827

905.5 Late effect of fracture of multiple and unspecified bones
    Late effect of injury classifiable to 828-829

905.6 Late effect of dislocation
    Late effect of injury classifiable to 830-839

905.7 Late effect of sprain and strain without mention of tendon injury
    Late effect of injury classifiable to 840-848, except tendon injury

905.8 Late effect of tendon injury
    Late effect of tendon injury due to:
      open wound [injury classifiable to 880-884 with .2, 890-894 with .2]
      sprain and strain [injury classifiable to 840-848]

905.9 Late effect of traumatic amputation
    Late effect of injury classifiable to 885-887, 895-897

    Excludes: *late amputation stump complication (997.60-997.69)*

906 Late effects of injuries to skin and subcutaneous tissues

906.0 Late effect of open wound of head, neck, and trunk
    Late effect of injury classifiable to 870-879

906.1 Late effect of open wound of extremities without mention of tendon injury
    Late effect of injury classifiable to 880-884, 890-894 except .2

906.2 Late effect of superficial injury
    Late effect of injury classifiable to 910-919

906.3 Late effect of contusion
    Late effect of injury classifiable to 920-924

906.4 Late effect of crushing
    Late effect of injury classifiable to 925-929

906.5 Late effect of burn of eye, face, head, and neck
    Late effect of injury classifiable to 940-941

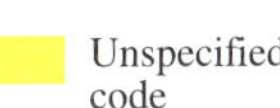

Add 4th or 5th digit   Nonspecific code   Unspecified code   Medicare secondary payer (MSP) alert

906.6 Late effect of burn of wrist and hand
Late effect of injury classifiable to 944

906.7 Late effect of burn of other extremities
Late effect of injury classifiable to 943 or 945

906.8 Late effect of burns of other specified sites
Late effect of injury classifiable to 942, 946-947

906.9 Late effect of burn of unspecified site
Late effect of injury classifiable to 948-949

907 Late effects of injuries to the nervous system

907.0 Late effect of intracranial injury without mention of skull fracture
Late effect of injury classifiable to 850-854

907.1 Late effect of injury to cranial nerve
Late effect of injury classifiable to 950-951

907.2 Late effect of spinal cord injury
Late effect of injury classifiable to 806, 952

907.3 Late effect of injury to nerve root(s), spinal plexus(es), and other nerves of trunk
Late effect of injury classifiable to 953-954

907.4 Late effect of injury to peripheral nerve of shoulder girdle and upper limb
Late effect of injury classifiable to 955

907.5 Late effect of injury to peripheral nerve of pelvic girdle and lower limb
Late effect of injury classifiable to 956

907.9 Late effect of injury to other and unspecified nerve
Late effect of injury classifiable to 957

908 Late effects of other and unspecified injuries

908.0 Late effect of internal injury to chest
Late effect of injury classifiable to 860-862

908.1 Late effect of internal injury to intra-abdominal organs
Late effect of injury classifiable to 863-866, 868

908.2 Late effect of internal injury to other internal organs
Late effect of injury classifiable to 867 or 869

908.3 Late effect of injury to blood vessel of head, neck, and extremities
Late effect of injury classifiable to 900, 903-904

908.4 Late effect of injury to blood vessel of thorax, abdomen, and pelvis
Late effect of injury classifiable to 901-902

908.5 Late effect of foreign body in orifice
Late effect of injury classifiable to 930-939

908.6 Late effect of certain complications of trauma
Late effect of complications classifiable to 958

908.9 Late effect of unspecified injury
Late effect of injury classifiable to 959

909 Late effects of other and unspecified external causes

909.0 Late effect of poisoning due to drug, medicinal or biological substance
Late effect of conditions classifiable to 960-979

Excludes: *late effect of adverse effect of drug, medicinal or biological substance (909.5)*

909.1 Late effect of toxic effects of nonmedical substances
Late effect of conditions classifiable to 980-989

909.2 Late effect of radiation
Late effect of conditions classifiable to 990

909.3 Late effect of complications of surgical and medical care
Late effect of conditions classifiable to 996-999

909.4 Late effect of certain other external causes
Late effect of conditions classifiable to 991-994

909.5 Late effect of adverse effect of drug, medicinal or biological substance

Excludes: *late effect of poisoning due to drug, medicinal or biological substance (909.0)*

909.9 Late effect of other and unspecified external causes

   ● Code new
to this edition   ▲ Revision of
existing code   ④ ⑤ Fourth or fifth
digit required

SUPERFICIAL INJURY (910-919)

> *Excludes:* burn (blisters) (940.0-949.5)
> contusion (920-924.9)
> foreign body:
>   granuloma (728.82)
>   inadvertently left in operative wound (998.4)
>   residual, in soft tissue (729.6)
> insect bite, venomous (989.5)
> open wound with incidental foreign body (870.0-897.7)

910 Superficial injury of face, neck, and scalp except eye
Includes: cheek
ear
gum
lip
nose
throat

> *Excludes:* eye and adnexa (918.0-918.9)

910.0 Abrasion or friction burn without mention of infection

910.1 Abrasion or friction burn, infected

910.2 Blister without mention of infection

910.3 Blister, infected

910.4 Insect bite, nonvenomous, without mention of infection

910.5 Insect bite, nonvenomous, infected

910.6 Superficial foreign body (splinter) without major open wound and without mention of infection

910.7 Superficial foreign body (splinter) without major open wound, infected

910.8 Other and unspecified superficial injury of face, neck, and scalp without mention of infection

910.9 Other and unspecified superficial injury of face, neck, and scalp, infected

911 Superficial injury of trunk
Includes:

abdominal wall	interscapular region
anus	labium (majus) (minus)
back	penis
breast	perineum
buttock	scrotum
chest wall	testis
flank	vagina
groin	vulva

> *Excludes:* hip (916.0-916.9)
> scapular region (912.0-912.9)

911.0 Abrasion or friction burn without mention of infection

911.1 Abrasion or friction burn, infected

911.2 Blister without mention of infection

911.3 Blister, infected

911.4 Insect bite, nonvenomous, without mention of infection

911.5 Insect bite, nonvenomous, infected

911.6 Superficial foreign body (splinter) without major open wound and without mention of infection

911.7 Superficial foreign body (splinter) without major open wound, infected

911.8 Other and unspecified superficial injury of trunk without mention of infection

911.9 Other and unspecified superficial injury of trunk, infected

912 Superficial injury of shoulder and upper arm
Includes: axilla   scapular region

912.0 Abrasion or friction burn without mention of infection

912.1 Abrasion or friction burn, infected

912.2 Blister without mention of infection

912.3 Blister, infected

912.4 Insect bite, nonvenomous, without mention of infection

Add 4th or 5th digit   Nonspecific code   Unspecified code   Medicare secondary payer (MSP) alert

912.5 Insect bite, nonvenomous, infected

912.6 Superficial foreign body (splinter) without major open wound and without mention of infection

912.7 Superficial foreign body (splinter) without major open wound, infected

912.8 Other and unspecified superficial injury of shoulder and upper arm without mention of infection

912.9 Other and unspecified superficial injury of shoulder and upper arm, infected

913 Superficial injury of elbow, forearm, and wrist

913.0 Abrasion or friction burn without mention of infection

913.1 Abrasion or friction burn, infected

913.2 Blister without mention of infection

913.3 Blister, infected

913.4 Insect bite, nonvenomous, without mention of infection

913.5 Insect bite, nonvenomous, infected

913.6 Superficial foreign body (splinter) without major open wound and without mention of infection

913.7 Superficial foreign body (splinter) without major open wound, infected

913.8 Other and unspecified superficial injury of elbow, forearm, and wrist without mention of infection

913.9 Other and unspecified superficial injury of elbow, forearm, and wrist, infected

914 Superficial injury of hand(s) except finger(s) alone

914.0 Abrasion or friction burn without mention of infection

914.1 Abrasion or friction burn, infected

914.2 Blister without mention of infection

914.3 Blister, infected

914.4 Insect bite, nonvenomous, without mention of infection

914.5 Insect bite, nonvenomous, infected

914.6 Superficial foreign body (splinter) without major open wound and without mention of infection

914.7 Superficial foreign body (splinter) without major open wound, infected

914.8 Other and unspecified superficial injury of hand without mention of infection

914.9 Other and unspecified superficial injury of hand, infected

915 Superficial injury of finger(s)

    Includes: fingernail   thumb (nail)

915.0 Abrasion or friction burn without mention of infection

915.1 Abrasion or friction burn, infected

915.2 Blister without mention of infection

915.3 Blister, infected

915.4 Insect bite, nonvenomous, without mention of infection

915.5 Insect bite, nonvenomous, infected

915.6 Superficial foreign body (splinter) without major open wound and without mention of infection

915.7 Superficial foreign body (splinter) without major open wound, infected

915.8 Other and unspecified superficial injury of fingers without mention of infection

915.9 Other and unspecified superficial injury of fingers, infected

916 Superficial injury of hip, thigh, leg, and ankle

916.0 Abrasion or friction burn without mention of infection

916.1 Abrasion or friction burn, infected

916.2 Blister without mention of infection

916.3 Blister, infected

916.4 Insect bite, nonvenomous, without mention of infection

916.5 Insect bite, nonvenomous, infected

916.6 Superficial foreign body (splinter) without major open wound and without mention of infection

● Code new to this edition   ▲ Revision of existing code   ④ ⑤ Fourth or fifth digit required

916.7 Superficial foreign body (splinter) without major open wound, infected

916.8 Other and unspecified superficial injury of hip, thigh, leg, and ankle without mention of infection

916.9 Other and unspecified superficial injury of hip, thigh, leg, and ankle, infected

917 Superficial injury of foot and toe(s)
Includes: heel   toenail

917.0 Abrasion or friction burn without mention of infection

917.1 Abrasion or friction burn, infected

917.2 Blister without mention of infection

917.3 Blister, infected

917.4 Insect bite, nonvenomous, without mention of infection

917.5 Insect bite, nonvenomous, infected

917.6 Superficial foreign body (splinter) without major open wound and without mention of infection

917.7 Superficial foreign body (splinter) without major open wound, infected

917.8 Other and unspecified superficial injury of foot and toes without mention of infection

917.9 Other and unspecified superficial injury of foot and toes, infected

918 Superficial injury of eye and adnexa
Excludes: burn (940.0-940.9)
foreign body on external eye (930.0-930.9)

918.0 Eyelids and periocular area
Abrasion   Superficial foreign body (splinter)
Insect bite

918.1 Cornea
Corneal abrasion
Superficial laceration
Excludes: corneal injury due to contact lens (371.82)

918.2 Conjunctiva

918.9 Other and unspecified superficial injuries of eye
Eye (ball) NOS

919 Superficial injury of other, multiple, and unspecified sites
Excludes: multiple sites classifiable to the same three-digit category (910.0-918.9)

919.0 Abrasion or friction burn without mention of infection

919.1 Abrasion or friction burn, infected

919.2 Blister without mention of infection

919.3 Blister, infected

919.4 Insect bite, nonvenomous, without mention of infection

919.5 Insect bite, nonvenomous, infected
919.6 Superficial foreign body (splinter) without major open wound and without mention of infection
919.7 Superficial foreign body (splinter) without major open wound, infected
919.8 Other and unspecified superficial injury without mention of infection

919.9 Other and unspecified superficial injury, infected

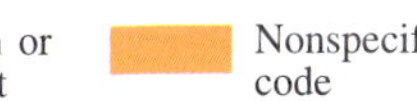

Add 4th or 5th digit   Nonspecific code   Unspecified code   Medicare secondary payer (MSP) alert

CONTUSION WITH INTACT SKIN SURFACE (920-924)

Includes: bruise without fracture or open wound
hematoma without fracture or open wound

Excludes: *concussion (850.0-850.9)*
hemarthrosis (840.0-848.9)
internal organs (860.0-869.1)
that incidental to:
crushing injury (925-929.9)
dislocation (830.0-839.9)
fracture (800.0-829.1)
internal injury (860.0-869.1)
intracranial injury (850.0-854.1)
nerve injury (950.0-957.9)
open wound (870.0-897.7)

920 Contusion of face, scalp, and neck except eye(s)

Cheek	Mandibular joint area
Ear (auricle)	Nose
Gum	Throat
Lip	

921 Contusion of eye and adnexa

921.0 Black eye, not otherwise specified

921.1 Contusion of eyelids and periocular area

921.2 Contusion of orbital tissues

921.3 Contusion of eyeball

921.9 Unspecified contusion of eye
Injury of eye NOS

922 Contusion of trunk

922.0 Breast

922.1 Chest wall

922.2 Abdominal wall
Flank
Groin

⑤ **922.3 Back**

Excludes: *scapular region (923.01)*

922.31 Back

Excludes: *interscapular region (922.33)*

922.32 Buttock

922.33 Interscapular region

922.4 Genital organs

Labium (majus) (minus)	Testis
Penis	Vagina
Perineum	Vulva
Scrotum	

922.8 Multiple sites of trunk

922.9 Unspecified part
Trunk NOS

923 Contusion of upper limb

⑤ **923.0 Shoulder and upper arm**

923.00 Shoulder region

923.01 Scapular region

923.02 Axillary region

923.03 Upper arm

923.09 Multiple sites

⑤ **923.1 Elbow and forearm**

923.10 Forearm

923.11 Elbow

⑤ **923.2 Wrist and hand(s), except finger(s) alone**

923.20 Hand(s)

● Code new
to this edition

▲ Revision of
existing code

④ ⑤ Fourth or fifth
digit required

923.21 Wrist

923.3 Finger
Fingernail
Thumb (nail)

923.8 Multiple sites of upper limb

923.9 Unspecified part of upper limb
Arm NOS

924 Contusion of lower limb and of other and unspecified sites

⑤ **924.0 Hip and thigh**

924.00 Thigh

924.01 Hip

⑤ **924.1 Knee and lower leg**

924.10 Lower leg

924.11 Knee

⑤ **924.2 Ankle and foot, excluding toe(s)**

924.20 Foot
Heel

924.21 Ankle

924.3 Toe
Toenail

924.4 Multiple sites of lower limb

924.5 Unspecified part of lower limb
Leg NOS

924.8 Multiple sites, not elsewhere classified

924.9 Unspecified site

CRUSHING INJURY (925-929)

Use additional code to identify any associated injuries, such as:
fractures (800-829)
internal injuries (860.0-869.1)
intracranial injury (850.0-854.1)

925 Crushing injury of face, scalp, and neck
Cheek   Pharynx
Ear   Throat
Larynx

925.1 Crushing injury of face and scalp
Cheek   Ear

925.2 Crushing injury of neck
Larynx   Throat
Pharynx

926 Crushing injury of trunk

926.0 External genitalia
Labium (majus) (minus)   Testis
Penis   Vulva
Scrotum

⑤ **926.1 Other specified sites**

926.11 Back

926.12 Buttock

926.19 Other
Breast

926.8 Multiple sites of trunk

926.9 Unspecified site
Trunk NOS

927 Crushing injury of upper limb

⑤ **927.0 Shoulder and upper arm**

927.00 Shoulder region

927.01 Scapular region

927.02 Axillary region

Add 4th or 5th digit	Nonspecific code	Unspecified code	Medicare secondary payer (MSP) alert

927.03   **Upper arm**

927.09   **Multiple sites**

⑤ 927.1   **Elbow and forearm**

927.10   **Forearm**

927.11   **Elbow**

⑤ 927.2   **Wrist and hand(s), except finger(s) alone**

927.20   **Hand(s)**

927.21   **Wrist**

927.3   **Finger(s)**

927.8   **Multiple sites of upper limb**

927.9   **Unspecified site**
Arm NOS

928   **Crushing injury of lower limb**

⑤ 928.0   **Hip and thigh**

928.00   **Thigh**

928.01   **Hip**

⑤ 928.1   **Knee and lower leg**

928.10   **Lower leg**

928.11   **Knee**

⑤ 928.2   **Ankle and foot, excluding toe(s) alone**

928.20   **Foot**
Heel

928.21   **Ankle**

928.3   **Toe(s)**

928.8   **Multiple sites of lower limb**

928.9   **Unspecified site**
Leg NOS

929   **Crushing injury of multiple and unspecified sites**

929.0   **Multiple sites, not elsewhere classified**

929.9   **Unspecified site**

EFFECTS OF FOREIGN BODY ENTERING THROUGH ORIFICE (930-939)

Excludes: *foreign body:*
granuloma (728.82)
inadvertently left in operative wound (998.4, 998.7)
in open wound (800-839, 851-897)
residual, in soft tissues (729.6)
superficial without major open wound (910-919 with .6 or .7)

930   **Foreign body on external eye**

Excludes: *foreign body in penetrating wound of:*
eyeball (871.5-871.6)
retained (old) (360.5-360.6)
ocular adnexa (870.4)
retained (old) (376.6)

930.0   **Corneal foreign body**

930.1   **Foreign body in conjunctival sac**

930.2   **Foreign body in lacrimal punctum**

930.8   **Other and combined sites**

930.9   **Unspecified site**
External eye NOS

931   **Foreign body in ear**
Auditory canal
Auricle

932   **Foreign body in nose**
Nasal sinus
Nostril

933   **Foreign body in pharynx and larynx**

   ● Code new
to this edition   ▲ Revision of
existing code   ④ ⑤ Fourth or fifth
digit required

933.0 Pharynx
Nasopharynx
Throat NOS

933.1 Larynx
Asphyxia due to foreign body
Choking due to:
food (regurgitated)
phlegm

934 Foreign body in trachea, bronchus, and lung

934.0 Trachea

934.1 Main bronchus

934.8 Other specified parts
Bronchioles
Lung

934.9 Respiratory tree, unspecified
Inhalation of liquid or vomitus, lower respiratory tract NOS

935 Foreign body in mouth, esophagus, and stomach

935.0 Mouth

935.1 Esophagus

935.2 Stomach

936 Foreign body in intestine and colon

937 Foreign body in anus and rectum
Rectosigmoid (junction)

938 Foreign body in digestive system, unspecified
Alimentary tract NOS
Swallowed foreign body

939 Foreign body in genitourinary tract

939.0 Bladder and urethra

939.1 Uterus, any part

Excludes: *intrauterine contraceptive device:*
complications from (996.32, 996.65)
presence of (V45.51)

939.2 Vulva and vagina

939.3 Penis

939.9 Unspecified site

BURNS (940-949)

Includes: burns from:
electrical heating appliance
electricity
flame
hot object
lightning
radiation
chemical burns (external) (internal)
scalds

Excludes: *friction burns (910-919 with .0, .1)*
sunburn (692.71, 692.76-692.77)

940 Burn confined to eye and adnexa

940.0 Chemical burn of eyelids and periocular area

940.1 Other burns of eyelids and periocular area

940.2 Alkaline chemical burn of cornea and conjunctival sac

940.3 Acid chemical burn of cornea and conjunctival sac

940.4 Other burn of cornea and conjunctival sac

940.5 Burn with resulting rupture and destruction of eyeball

940.9 Unspecified burn of eye and adnexa

⑤ **941** **Burn of face, head, and neck**

Excludes: mouth (947.0)

The following fifth-digit subclassification is for use with category 941:

0 **face and head, unspecified site**

1 ear [any part]

2 eye (with other parts of face, head, and neck)

3 lip(s)

4 chin

5 nose (septum)

6 scalp [any part]
Temple (region)

7 forehead and cheek

8 neck

9 **multiple sites [except with eye] of face, head, and neck**

⑤ **941.0** **Unspecified degree**

⑤ 941.1 **Erythema [first degree]**

⑤ 941.2 **Blisters, epidermal loss [second degree]**

⑤ 941.3 **Full-thickness skin loss [third degree NOS]**

⑤ 941.4 **Deep necrosis of underlying tissues [deep third degree] without mention of loss of a body part**

⑤ 941.5 **Deep necrosis of underlying tissues [deep third degree] with loss of a body part**

⑤ **942** **Burn of trunk**

Excludes: scapular region (943.0-943.5 with fifth-digit 6)

The following fifth-digit subclassification is for use with category 942:

0 **trunk, unspecified site**

1 **breast**

2 **chest wall, excluding breast and nipple**

3 **abdominal wall**
Flank   Groin

4 **back [any part]**
Buttock   Interscapular region

5 **genitalia**
Labium (majus) (minus)   Scrotum
Penis   Testis
Perineum   Vulva

9 **other and multiple sites of trunk**

⑤ **942.0** **Unspecified degree**

⑤ 942.1 **Erythema [first degree]**

⑤ 942.2 **Blisters, epidermal loss [second degree]**

⑤ 942.3 **Full-thickness skin loss [third degree NOS]**

⑤ 942.4 **Deep necrosis of underlying tissues [deep third degree] without mention of loss of a body part**

⑤ 942.5 **Deep necrosis of underlying tissues [deep third degree] with loss of a body part**

⑤ **943** **Burn of upper limb, except wrist and hand**

The following fifth-digit subclassification is for use with category 943:

0 **upper limb, unspecified site**

1 **forearm**

2 **elbow**

3 **upper arm**

4 **axilla**

5 **shoulder**

6 **scapular region**

9 **multiple sites of upper limb, except wrist and hand**

⑤ **943.0** **Unspecified degree**

⑤ 943.1 **Erythema [first degree]**

● Code new to this edition   ▲ Revision of existing code   ④ ⑤ Fourth or fifth digit required

⑤ **943.2 Blisters, epidermal loss [second degree]**

⑤ **943.3 Full-thickness skin loss [third degree NOS]**

⑤ **943.4 Deep necrosis of underlying tissues [deep third degree] without mention of loss of a body part**

⑤ **943.5 Deep necrosis of underlying tissues [deep third degree] with loss of a body part**

⑤ **944 Burn of wrist(s) and hand(s)**

The following fifth-digit subclassification is for use with category 944:

   0 hand, unspecified site

   1 single digit [finger (nail)] other than thumb

   2 thumb (nail)

   3 two or more digits, not including thumb

   4 two or more digits including thumb

   5 palm

   6 back of hand

   7 wrist

   8 multiple sites of wrist(s) and hand(s)

⑤ **944.0 Unspecified degree**

⑤ **944.1 Erythema [first degree]**

⑤ **944.2 Blisters, epidermal loss [second degree]**

⑤ **944.3 Full-thickness skin loss [third degree NOS]**

⑤ **944.4 Deep necrosis of underlying tissues [deep third degree] without mention of loss of a body part**

⑤ **944.5 Deep necrosis of underlying tissues [deep third degree] with loss of a body part**

⑤ **945 Burn of lower limb(s)**

The following fifth-digit subclassification is for use with category 945:

   0 lower limb [leg], unspecified site

   1 toe(s) (nail)

   2 foot

   3 ankle

   4 lower leg

   5 knee

   6 thigh [any part]

   9 multiple sites of lower limb(s)

⑤ **945.0 Unspecified degree**

⑤ **945.1 Erythema [first degree]**

⑤ **945.2 Blisters, epidermal loss [second degree]**

⑤ **945.3 Full-thickness skin loss [third degree NOS]**

⑤ **945.4 Deep necrosis of underlying tissues [deep third degree] without mention of loss of a body part**

⑤ **945.5 Deep necrosis of underlying tissues [deep third degree] with loss of a body part**

946 Burns of multiple specified sites

Includes: burns of sites classifiable to more than one three-digit category in 940-945

Excludes: *multiple burns NOS (949.0-949.5)*

946.0 Unspecified degree

946.1 Erythema [first degree]

946.2 Blisters, epidermal loss [second degree]

946.3 Full-thickness skin loss [third degree NOS]

946.4 Deep necrosis of underlying tissues [deep third degree] without mention of loss of a body part

946.5 Deep necrosis of underlying tissues [deep third degree] with loss of a body part

947 Burn of internal organs

Includes: burns from chemical agents (ingested)

947.0 Mouth and pharynx

   Gum

   Tongue

Add 4th or 5th digit	Nonspecific code	Unspecified code	Medicare secondary payer (MSP) alert

947.1 Larynx, trachea, and lung

947.2 Esophagus

947.3 Gastrointestinal tract
Colon Small intestine
Rectum Stomach

947.4 Vagina and uterus

947.8 Other specified sites

947.9 Unspecified site

⑤ **948 Burns classified according to extent of body surface involved**

Excludes: *sunburn (692.71, 692.76-692.77)*

Note: This category is to be used when the site of the burn is unspecified, or with categories 940-947 when the site is specified.

The following fifth-digit subclassification is for use with category 948 to indicate the percent of *body surface* with *third degree burn*; valid digits are in [brackets] under each code:

0   less than 10 percent or unspecified

1   10-19%

2   20-29%

3   30-39%

4   40-49%

5   50-59%

6   60-69%

7   70-79%

8   80-89%

9   90% or more of body surface

⑤ **948.0 Burn [any degree] involving less than 10 percent of body surface**
[0]

⑤ **948.1 10-19 percent of body surface**
[0-1]

⑤ **948.2 20-29 percent of body surface**
[0-2]

⑤ **948.3 30-39 percent of body surface**
[0-3]

⑤ **948.4 40-49 percent of body surface**
[0-4]

⑤ **948.5 50-59 percent of body surface**
[0-5]

⑤ **948.6 60-69 percent of body surface**
[0-6]

⑤ **948.7 70-79 percent of body surface**
[0-7]

⑤ **948.8 80-89 percent of body surface**
[0-8]

⑤ **948.9 90 percent or more of body surface**
[0-9]

949 Burn, unspecified
Includes: burn NOS
multiple burns NOS

Excludes: *burn of unspecified site but with statement of the extent of body surface involved (948.0-948.9)*

949.0 Unspecified degree

949.1 Erythema [first degree]

949.2 Blisters, epidermal loss [second degree]

949.3 Full-thickness skin loss [third degree NOS]

949.4 Deep necrosis of underlying tissues [deep third degree] without mention of loss of a body part

949.5 Deep necrosis of underlying tissues [deep third degree] with loss of a body part

● Code new to this edition   ▲ Revision of existing code   ④ ⑤ Fourth or fifth digit required

INJURY TO NERVES AND SPINAL CORD (950-957)

Includes:
> division of nerve (with open wound)
> lesion in continuity (with open wound)
> traumatic neuroma (with open wound)
> traumatic transient paralysis (with open wound)

Excludes: *accidental puncture or laceration during medical procedure (998.2)*

950 Injury to optic nerve and pathways

950.0 Optic nerve injury
Second cranial nerve

950.1 Injury to optic chiasm

950.2 Injury to optic pathways

950.3 Injury to visual cortex

950.9 Unspecified
Traumatic blindness NOS

951 Injury to other cranial nerve(s)

951.0 Injury to oculomotor nerve
Third cranial nerve

951.1 Injury to trochlear nerve
Fourth cranial nerve

951.2 Injury to trigeminal nerve
Fifth cranial nerve

951.3 Injury to abducens nerve
Sixth cranial nerve

951.4 Injury to facial nerve
Seventh cranial nerve

951.5 Injury to acoustic nerve
Auditory nerve   Traumatic deafness NOS
Eighth cranial nerve

951.6 Injury to accessory nerve
Eleventh cranial nerve

951.7 Injury to hypoglossal nerve
Twelfth cranial nerve

951.8 Injury to other specified cranial nerves
Glossopharyngeal [9th cranial] nerve
Olfactory [1st cranial] nerve
Pneumogastric [10th cranial] nerve
Traumatic anosmia NOS
Vagus [10th cranial] nerve

951.9 Injury to unspecified cranial nerve

952 Spinal cord injury without evidence of spinal bone injury

⑤ **952.0 Cervical**

    952.00 C_1-C_4 level with unspecified spinal cord injury
    Spinal cord injury, cervical region NOS

    952.01 C_1-C_4 level with complete lesion of spinal cord

    952.02 C_1-C_4 level with anterior cord syndrome

    952.03 C_1-C_4 level with central cord syndrome

    952.04 C_1-C_4 level with other specified spinal cord injury
    Incomplete spinal cord lesion at C_1-C_4 level:
      NOS
      with posterior cord syndrome

    952.05 C_5-C_7 level with unspecified spinal cord injury

    952.06 C_5-C_7 level with complete lesion of spinal cord

    952.07 C_5-C_7 level with anterior cord syndrome

    952.08 C_5-C_7 level with central cord syndrome

    952.09 C_5-C_7 level with other specified spinal cord injury
    Incomplete spinal cord lesion at C_5-C_7 level:
      NOS
      with posterior cord syndrome

⑤ **952.1 Dorsal [thoracic]**

952.10 T$_1$-T$_6$ level with unspecified spinal cord injury
Spinal cord injury, thoracic region NOS

952.11 T$_1$-T$_6$ level with complete lesion of spinal cord

952.12 T$_1$-T$_6$ level with anterior cord syndrome

952.13 T$_1$-T$_6$ level with central cord syndrome

952.14 T$_1$-T$_6$ level with other specified spinal cord injury
Incomplete spinal cord lesion at T$_1$-T$_6$ level:
   NOS
   with posterior cord syndrome

952.15 T$_7$-T$_{12}$ level with unspecified spinal cord injury

952.16 T$_7$-T$_{12}$ level with complete lesion of spinal cord

952.17 T$_7$-T$_{12}$ level with anterior cord syndrome

952.18 T$_7$-T$_{12}$ level with central cord syndrome

952.19 T$_7$-T$_{12}$ level with other specified spinal cord injury
Incomplete spinal cord lesion at T$_7$-T$_{12}$ level:
   NOS
   with posterior cord syndrome

952.2 **Lumbar**

952.3 **Sacral**

952.4 **Cauda equina**

952.8 Multiple sites of spinal cord

952.9 Unspecified site of spinal cord

953 Injury to nerve roots and spinal plexus

953.0 **Cervical root**

953.1 **Dorsal root**

953.2 **Lumbar root**

953.3 **Sacral root**

953.4 **Brachial plexus**

953.5 **Lumbosacral plexus**

953.8 Multiple sites

953.9 Unspecified site

954 Injury to other nerve(s) of trunk, excluding shoulder and pelvic girdles

954.0 **Cervical sympathetic**

954.1 Other sympathetic
   Celiac ganglion or plexus   Splanchnic nerve(s)
   Inferior mesenteric plexus   Stellate ganglion

954.8 Other specified nerve(s) of trunk

954.9 Unspecified nerve of trunk

955 Injury to peripheral nerve(s) of shoulder girdle and upper limb

955.0 **Axillary nerve**

955.1 **Median nerve**

955.2 **Ulnar nerve**

955.3 **Radial nerve**

955.4 **Musculocutaneous nerve**

955.5 **Cutaneous sensory nerve, upper limb**

955.6 **Digital nerve**

955.7 Other specified nerve(s) of shoulder girdle and upper limb

955.8 Multiple nerves of shoulder girdle and upper limb

955.9 Unspecified nerve of shoulder girdle and upper limb

956 Injury to peripheral nerve(s) of pelvic girdle and lower limb

956.0 **Sciatic nerve**

956.1 **Femoral nerve**

956.2 **Posterior tibial nerve**

956.3 **Peroneal nerve**

956.4 **Cutaneous sensory nerve, lower limb**

● Code new
to this edition   ▲ Revision of
existing code   ④ ⑤ Fourth or fifth
digit required

956.5 Other specified nerve(s) of pelvic girdle and lower limb

956.8 Multiple nerves of pelvic girdle and lower limb

956.9 Unspecified nerve of pelvic girdle and lower limb

957 Injury to other and unspecified nerves

    957.0 Superficial nerves of head and neck

    957.1 Other specified nerve(s)

    957.8 Multiple nerves in several parts
        Multiple nerve injury NOS

    957.9 Unspecified site
        Nerve injury NOS

CERTAIN TRAUMATIC COMPLICATIONS AND UNSPECIFIED INJURIES (958-959)

958 Certain early complications of trauma
    Excludes: *adult respiratory distress syndrome (518.5)*
        flail chest (807.4)
        shock lung (518.5)
        that occurring during or following medical procedures (996.0-999.9)

    958.0 Air embolism
        Pneumathemia
    Excludes: *that complicating:*
        abortion (634-638 with .6, 639.6)
        ectopic or molar pregnancy (639.6)
        pregnancy, childbirth, or the puerperium (673.0)

    958.1 Fat embolism
    Excludes: *that complicating:*
        abortion (634-638 with .6, 639.6)
        pregnancy, childbirth, or the puerperium (673.8)

    958.2 Secondary and recurrent hemorrhage

    958.3 Posttraumatic wound infection, not elsewhere classified
    Excludes: *infected open wounds—code to complicated open wound of site*

    958.4 Traumatic shock
        Shock (immediate) (delayed) following injury
    Excludes: *shock:*
        anaphylactic (995.0)
          due to serum (999.4)
        anesthetic (995.4)
        electric (994.8)
        following abortion (639.5)
        lightning (994.0)
        nontraumatic NOS (785.50)
        obstetric (669.1)
        postoperative (998.0)

    958.5 Traumatic anuria
        Crush syndrome
        Renal failure following crushing
    Excludes: *that due to a medical procedure (997.5)*

    958.6 Volkmann's ischemic contracture
        Posttraumatic muscle contracture

    958.7 Traumatic subcutaneous emphysema
    Excludes: *subcutaneous emphysema resulting from a procedure (998.81)*

    958.8 Other early complications of trauma

    ● **958.9** Traumatic compartment syndrome
    Excludes: *nontraumatic compartment syndrome (729.71-729.79)*

        ● **958.90** Compartment syndrome, unspecified

        ● **958.91** Traumatic compartment syndrome of upper extremity
            Traumatic compartment syndrome of shoulder, arm, forearm, wrist, hand, and fingers

        ● **958.92** Traumatic compartment syndrome of lower extremity
            Traumatic compartment syndrome of hip, buttock, thigh, leg, foot, and toes

● **958.93**   **Traumatic compartment syndrome of abdomen**

● **958.99**   **Traumatic compartment syndrome of other sites**

959   **Injury, other and unspecified**
Includes: injury NOS

Excludes: *injury NOS of:*

blood vessels (900.0-904.9)
eye (921.0-921.9)
internal organs (860.0-869.1)
intracranial sites (854.0-854.1)
nerves (950.0-951.9, 953.0-957.9)
spinal cord (952.0-952.9)

⑤ **959.0**   **Head, face and neck**

Cheek	Mouth
Ear	Nose
Eyebrow	Throat
Lip	

959.01   **Head injury, unspecified**

Excludes: *concussion (850.1-850.9)*

with head injury NOS (850.1-850.9)
head injury NOS with loss of consciousness (850.1-850.5)
specified intracranial injuries (850.0-854.1)

959.09   **Injury of face and neck**

⑤ **959.1**   **Trunk**

Excludes: *scapular region (959.2)*

959.11   **Other injury of chest wall**

959.12   **Other injury of abdomen**

959.13   **Fracture of corpus cavernosum penis**

959.14   **Other injury of external genitals**

959.19   **Other injury of other sites of trunk**
Injury of trunk NOS

959.2   **Shoulder and upper arm**
Axilla
Scapular region

959.3   **Elbow, forearm, and wrist**

959.4   **Hand, except finger**

959.5   **Finger**
Fingernail
Thumb (nail)

959.6   **Hip and thigh**
Upper leg

959.7   **Knee, leg, ankle, and foot**

959.8   **Other specified sites, including multiple**

Excludes: *multiple sites classifiable to the same four-digit category (959.0-959.7)*

959.9   **Unspecified site**

● Code new
to this edition   ▲ Revision of
existing code   ④ ⑤ Fourth or fifth
digit required

POISONING BY DRUGS, MEDICINAL AND BIOLOGICAL SUBSTANCES (960-979)

Includes: overdose of these substances
wrong substances given or taken in error

Excludes: *adverse effects ["hypersensitivity," "reaction," etc.] of correct substance properly administered. Such cases are to be classified according to the nature of the adverse effect, such as:*

adverse effect NOS (995.20)
allergic lymphadenitis (289.3)
aspirin gastritis (535.4)
blood disorders (280.0-289.9)
dermatitis:
  contact (692.0-692.9)
  due to ingestion (693.0-693.9)
nephropathy (583.9)
[The drug giving rise to the adverse effect may be identified by use of categories E930-E949]
drug dependence (304.0-304.9)
drug reaction and poisoning affecting the newborn (760.0-779.9)
nondependent abuse of drugs (305.0-305.9)
pathological drug intoxication (292.2)

Use additional code to specify the effects of the poisoning

960 Poisoning by antibiotics

Excludes: *antibiotics:*

  ear, nose, and throat (976.6)
  eye (976.5)
  local (976.0)

960.0 Penicillins

Ampicillin	Cloxacillin
Carbenicillin	Penicillin G

960.1 Antifungal antibiotics

Amphotericin B	Nystatin
Griseofulvin	Trichomycin

Excludes: *preparations intended for topical use (976.0-976.9)*

960.2 Chloramphenicol group

Chloramphenicol
Thiamphenicol

960.3 Erythromycin and other macrolides

Oleandomycin
Spiramycin

960.4 Tetracycline group

Doxycycline	Oxytetracycline
Minocycline	

960.5 Cephalosporin group

Cephalexin	Cephaloridine
Cephaloglycin	Cephalothin

960.6 Antimycobacterial antibiotics

Cycloserine	Rifampin
Kanamycin	Streptomycin

960.7 Antineoplastic antibiotics

Actinomycin such as:	Bleomycin
Cactinomycin	Daunorubicin
Dactinomycin	Mitomycin

960.8 Other specified antibiotics

960.9 Unspecified antibiotic

961 Poisoning by other anti-infectives

Excludes: *anti-infectives:*

  ear, nose, and throat (976.6)
  eye (976.5)
  local (976.0)

961.0 Sulfonamides

Sulfadiazine	Sulfamethoxazole
Sulfafurazole	

961.1 Arsenical anti-infectives

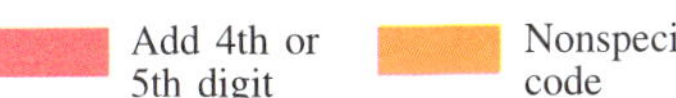

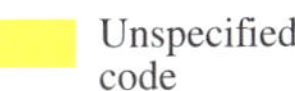

961.2 Heavy metal anti-infectives
Compounds of: Compounds of:
antimony lead
bismuth mercury

Excludes: mercurial diuretics (974.0)

961.3 Quinoline and hydroxyquinoline derivatives
Chiniofon
Diiodohydroxyquin

Excludes: antimalarial drugs (961.4)

961.4 Antimalarials and drugs acting on other blood protozoa
Chloroquine Proguanil [chloroguanide]
Cycloguanil Pyrimethamine
Primaquine Quinine

961.5 Other antiprotozoal drugs
Emetine

961.6 Anthelmintics
Hexylresorcinol Thiabendazole
Piperazine

961.7 Antiviral drugs
Methisazone

Excludes: amantadine (966.4)
cytarabine (963.1)
idoxuridine (976.5)

961.8 Other antimycobacterial drugs
Ethambutol Para-aminosalicylic acid derivatives
Ethionamide Sulfones
Isoniazid

961.9 Other and unspecified anti-infectives
Flucytosine
Nitrofuran derivatives

962 Poisoning by hormones and synthetic substitutes

Excludes: oxytocic hormones (975.0)

962.0 Adrenal cortical steroids
Cortisone derivatives
Desoxycorticosterone derivatives
Fluorinated corticosteroids

962.1 Androgens and anabolic congeners
Methandriol Oxymetholone
Nandrolone Testosterone

962.2 Ovarian hormones and synthetic substitutes
Contraceptives, oral
Estrogens
Estrogens and progestogens, combined
Progestogens

962.3 Insulins and antidiabetic agents
Acetohexamide Insulin
Biguanide derivatives, oral Phenformin
Chlorpropamide Sulfonylurea derivatives, oral
Glucagon Tolbutamide

962.4 Anterior pituitary hormones
Corticotropin
Gonadotropin
Somatotropin [growth hormone]

962.5 Posterior pituitary hormones
Vasopressin

Excludes: oxytocic hormones (975.0)

962.6 Parathyroid and parathyroid derivatives

962.7 Thyroid and thyroid derivatives
Dextrothyroxin Liothyronine
Levothyroxine sodium Thyroglobulin

● Code new to this edition   ▲ Revision of existing code   ④ ⑤ Fourth or fifth digit required

962.8 Antithyroid agents
Iodides
Thiouracil
Thiourea

962.9 Other and unspecified hormones and synthetic substitutes

963 Poisoning by primarily systemic agents

963.0 Antiallergic and antiemetic drugs
Antihistamines
Chlorpheniramine
Diphenhydramine
Diphenylpyraline
Thonzylamine
Tripelennamine

Excludes: phenothiazine-based tranquilizers (969.1)

963.1 Antineoplastic and immunosuppressive drugs
Azathioprine
Busulfan
Chlorambucil
Cyclophosphamide
Cytarabine
Fluorouracil
Mercaptopurine
thio-TEPA

Excludes: antineoplastic antibiotics (960.7)

963.2 Acidifying agents

963.3 Alkalizing agents

963.4 Enzymes, not elsewhere classified
Penicillinase

963.5 Vitamins, not elsewhere classified
Vitamin A
Vitamin D

Excludes: nicotinic acid (972.2)
vitamin K (964.3)

963.8 Other specified systemic agents
Heavy metal antagonists

963.9 Unspecified systemic agent

964 Poisoning by agents primarily affecting blood constituents

964.0 Iron and its compounds
Ferric salts
Ferrous sulfate and other ferrous salts

964.1 Liver preparations and other antianemic agents
Folic acid

964.2 Anticoagulants
Coumarin
Heparin
Phenindione
Warfarin sodium

964.3 Vitamin K [phytonadione]

964.4 Fibrinolysis-affecting drugs
Aminocaproic acid
Streptodornase
Streptokinase
Urokinase

964.5 Anticoagulant antagonists and other coagulants
Hexadimethrine
Protamine sulfate

964.6 Gamma globulin

964.7 Natural blood and blood products
Blood plasma
Human fibrinogen
Packed red cells
Whole blood

Excludes: transfusion reactions (999.4-999.8)

964.8 Other specified agents affecting blood constituents
Macromolecular blood substitutes
Plasma expanders

964.9 Unspecified agent affecting blood constituents

965 Poisoning by analgesics, antipyretics, and antirheumatics

Excludes: drug dependence (304.0-304.9)
nondependent abuse (305.0-305.9)

⑤ **965.0 Opiates and related narcotics**

965.00 Opium (alkaloids), unspecified

Add 4th or 5th digit | Nonspecific code | Unspecified code | Medicare secondary payer (MSP) alert

965.01 Heroin
Diacetylmorphine

965.02 Methadone

965.09 Other
Codeine [methylmorphine]
Meperidine [pethidine]
Morphine

965.1 Salicylates
Acetylsalicylic acid [aspirin]
Salicylic acid salts

965.4 Aromatic analgesics, not elsewhere classified
Acetanilid
Paracetamol [acetaminophen]
Phenacetin [acetophenetidin]

965.5 Pyrazole derivatives
Aminophenazone [aminopyrine]
Phenylbutazone

⑤ **965.6 Antirheumatics [antiphlogistics]**

Excludes: *salicylates (965.1)*
steroids (962.0-962.9)

965.61 Propionic acid derivatives
Fenoprofen	Ketoprofen
Flurbiprofen	Naproxen
Ibuprofen	Oxaprozin

965.69 Other antirheumatics
Gold salts
Indomethacin

965.7 Other non-narcotic analgesics
Pyrabital

965.8 Other specified analgesics and antipyretics
Pentazocine

965.9 Unspecified analgesic and antipyretic

966 Poisoning by anticonvulsants and anti-Parkinsonism drugs

966.0 Oxazolidine derivatives
Paramethadione
Trimethadione

966.1 Hydantoin derivatives
Phenytoin

966.2 Succinimides
Ethosuximide
Phensuximide

966.3 Other and unspecified anticonvulsants
Primidone

Excludes: *barbiturates (967.0)*
sulfonamides (961.0)

966.4 Anti-Parkinsonism drugs
Amantadine
Ethopropazine [profenamine]
Levodopa [L-dopa]

967 Poisoning by sedatives and hypnotics

Excludes: *drug dependence (304.0-304.9)*
nondependent abuse (305.0-305.9)

967.0 Barbiturates
Amobarbital [amylobarbitone]
Barbital [barbitone]
Butabarbital [butabarbitone]
Pentobarbital [pentobarbitone]
Phenobarbital [phenobarbitone]
Secobarbital [quinalbarbitone]

Excludes: *thiobarbiturate anesthetics (968.3)*

967.1 Chloral hydrate group

967.2 Paraldehyde

● Code new to this edition ▲ Revision of existing code ④ ⑤ Fourth or fifth digit required

967.3 Bromine compounds
Bromide
Carbromal (derivatives)

967.4 Methaqualone compounds

967.5 Glutethimide group

967.6 Mixed sedatives, not elsewhere classified

967.8 Other sedatives and hypnotics

967.9 Unspecified sedative or hypnotic
Sleeping:
drug NOS
pill NOS
tablet NOS

968 Poisoning by other central nervous system depressants and anesthetics
Excludes: *drug dependence (304.0-304.9)*
nondependent abuse (305.0-305.9)

968.0 Central nervous system muscle-tone depressants
Chlorphenesin (carbamate)   Methocarbamol
Mephenesin

968.1 Halothane

968.2 Other gaseous anesthetics
Ether
Halogenated hydrocarbon derivatives, except halothane
Nitrous oxide

968.3 Intravenous anesthetics
Excludes: *Methohexital [methohexitone]*
Thiobarbiturates, such as thiopental sodium

968.4 Other and unspecified general anesthetics

968.5 Surface [topical] and infiltration anesthetics
Cocaine   Procaine
Lidocaine [lignocaine]   Tetracaine

968.6 Peripheral nerve and plexus-blocking anesthetics

968.7 Spinal anesthetics

968.9 Other and unspecified local anesthetics

969 Poisoning by psychotropic agents
Excludes: *drug dependence (304.0-304.9)*
nondependent abuse (305.0-305.9)

969.0 Antidepressants
Amitriptyline   Monoamine oxidase [MAO] inhibitors
Imipramine

969.1 Phenothiazine-based tranquilizers
Chlorpromazine   Prochlorperazine
Fluphenazine   Promazine

969.2 Butyrophenone-based tranquilizers
Haloperidol   Trifluperidol
Spiperone

969.3 Other antipsychotics, neuroleptics, and major tranquilizers

969.4 Benzodiazepine-based tranquilizers
Chlordiazepoxide   Lorazepam
Diazepam   Medazepam
Flurazepam   Nitrazepam

969.5 Other tranquilizers
Hydroxyzine
Meprobamate

969.6 Psychodysleptics [hallucinogens]
Cannabis (derivatives)   Mescaline
Lysergide [LSD]   Psilocin
Marihuana (derivatives)   Psilocybin

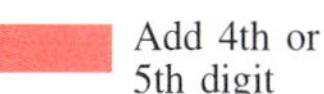
Add 4th or
5th digit

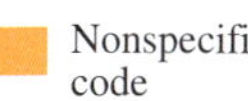
Nonspecific
code

Unspecified
code

Medicare secondary
payer (MSP) alert

969.7 Psychostimulants
Amphetamine
Caffeine

Excludes: central appetite depressants (977.0)

969.8 Other specified psychotropic agents

969.9 Unspecified psychotropic agent

970 Poisoning by central nervous system stimulants

970.0 Analeptics
Lobeline
Nikethamide

970.1 Opiate antagonists
Levallorphan   Naloxone
Nalorphine

970.8 Other specified central nervous system stimulants

970.9 Unspecified central nervous system stimulant

971 Poisoning by drugs primarily affecting the autonomic nervous system

971.0 Parasympathomimetics [cholinergics]
Acetylcholine   Pilocarpine
Anticholinesterase:
  organophosphorus
  reversible

971.1 Parasympatholytics [anticholinergics and antimuscarinics] and spasmolytics
Atropine   Hyoscine [scopolamine]
Homatropine   Quaternary ammonium derivatives

Excludes: papaverine (972.5)

971.2 Sympathomimetics [adrenergics]
Epinephrine [adrenalin]
Levarterenol [noradrenalin]

971.3 Sympatholytics [antiadrenergics]
Phenoxybenzamine
Tolazoline hydrochloride

971.9 Unspecified drug primarily affecting autonomic nervous system

972 Poisoning by agents primarily affecting the cardiovascular system

972.0 Cardiac rhythm regulators
Practolol   Propranolol
Procainamide   Quinidine

Excludes: lidocaine (968.5)

972.1 Cardiotonic glycosides and drugs of similar action
Digitalis glycosides   Strophanthins
Digoxin

972.2 Antilipemic and antiarteriosclerotic drugs
Clofibrate
Nicotinic acid derivatives

972.3 Ganglion-blocking agents
Pentamethonium bromide

972.4 Coronary vasodilators
Dipyridamole   Nitrites
Nitrates [nitroglycerin]

972.5 Other vasodilators
Cyclandelate   Papaverine
Diazoxide

Excludes: nicotinic acid (972.2)

972.6 Other antihypertensive agents
Clonidine   Rauwolfia alkaloids
Guanethidine   Reserpine

972.7 Antivaricose drugs, including sclerosing agents
Sodium morrhuate
Zinc salts

● Code new to this edition   ▲ Revision of existing code   ④ ⑤ Fourth or fifth digit required

972.8 Capillary-active drugs
Adrenochrome derivatives
Metaraminol

972.9 Other and unspecified agents primarily affecting the cardiovascular system

973 Poisoning by agents primarily affecting the gastrointestinal system

973.0 Antacids and antigastric secretion drugs
Aluminum hydroxide
Magnesium trisilicate

973.1 Irritant cathartics
Bisacodyl   Phenolphthalein
Castor oil

973.2 Emollient cathartics
Dioctyl sulfosuccinates

973.3 Other cathartics, including intestinal atonia drugs
Magnesium sulfate

973.4 Digestants
Pancreatin   Pepsin
Papain

973.5 Antidiarrheal drugs
Kaolin
Pectin

> *Excludes:* *anti-infectives (960.0-961.9)*

973.6 Emetics

973.8 Other specified agents primarily affecting the gastrointestinal system

973.9 Unspecified agent primarily affecting the gastrointestinal system

974 Poisoning by water, mineral, and uric acid metabolism drugs

974.0 Mercurial diuretics
Chlormerodrin   Mersalyl
Mercaptomerin

974.1 Purine derivative diuretics
Theobromine
Theophylline

> *Excludes:* *aminophylline [theophylline ethylenediamine] (975.7)*
> *caffeine (969.7)*

974.2 Carbonic acid anhydrase inhibitors
Acetazolamide

974.3 Saluretics
Benzothiadiazides
Chlorothiazide group

974.4 Other diuretics
Ethacrynic acid
Furosemide

974.5 Electrolytic, caloric, and water-balance agents

974.6 Other mineral salts, not elsewhere classified

974.7 Uric acid metabolism drugs
Allopurinol   Probenecid
Colchicine

975 Poisoning by agents primarily acting on the smooth and skeletal muscles and respiratory system

975.0 Oxytocic agents
Ergot alkaloids   Prostaglandins
Oxytocin

975.1 Smooth muscle relaxants
Adiphenine
Metaproterenol [orciprenaline]

> *Excludes:* *papaverine (972.5)*

975.2 Skeletal muscle relaxants

975.3 Other and unspecified drugs acting on muscles

Add 4th or 5th digit	Nonspecific code	Unspecified code	Medicare secondary payer (MSP) alert

975.4 Antitussives
Dextromethorphan
Pipazethate

975.5 Expectorants
Acetylcysteine   Terpin hydrate
Guaifenesin

975.6 Anti-common cold drugs

975.7 Antiasthmatics
Aminophylline [theophylline ethylenediamine]

975.8 Other and unspecified respiratory drugs

976 Poisoning by agents primarily affecting skin and mucous membrane, ophthalmological, otorhinolaryngological, and dental drugs

976.0 Local anti-infectives and anti-inflammatory drugs

976.1 Antipruritics

976.2 Local astringents and local detergents

976.3 Emollients, demulcents, and protectants

976.4 Keratolytics, keratoplastics, other hair treatment drugs and preparations

976.5 Eye anti-infectives and other eye drugs
Idoxuridine

976.6 Anti-infectives and other drugs and preparations for ear, nose, and throat

976.7 Dental drugs topically applied

Excludes: *anti-infectives (976.0)*
local anesthetics (968.5)

976.8 Other agents primarily affecting skin and mucous membrane
Spermicides [vaginal contraceptives]

976.9 Unspecified agent primarily affecting skin and mucous membrane

977 Poisoning by other and unspecified drugs and medicinal substances

977.0 Dietetics
Central appetite depressants

977.1 Lipotropic drugs

977.2 Antidotes and chelating agents, not elsewhere classified

977.3 Alcohol deterrents

977.4 Pharmaceutical excipients
Pharmaceutical adjuncts

977.8 Other specified drugs and medicinal substances
Contrast media used for diagnostic x-ray procedures
Diagnostic agents and kits

977.9 Unspecified drug or medicinal substance

978 Poisoning by bacterial vaccines

978.0 BCG

978.1 Typhoid and paratyphoid

978.2 Cholera

978.3 Plague

978.4 Tetanus

978.5 Diphtheria

978.6 Pertussis vaccine, including combinations with a pertussis component

978.8 Other and unspecified bacterial vaccines

978.9 Mixed bacterial vaccines, except combinations with a pertussis component

979 Poisoning by other vaccines and biological substances

Excludes: *gamma globulin (964.6)*

979.0 Smallpox vaccine

979.1 Rabies vaccine

979.2 Typhus vaccine

979.3 Yellow fever vaccine

979.4 Measles vaccine

● Code new
to this edition

▲ Revision of
existing code

④ ⑤ Fourth or fifth
digit required

979.5 Poliomyelitis vaccine

979.6 Other and unspecified viral and rickettsial vaccines
    Mumps vaccine

979.7 Mixed viral-rickettsial and bacterial vaccines, except combinations with a pertussis component

> *Excludes:* *combinations with a pertussis component (978.6)*

979.9 Other and unspecified vaccines and biological substances

TOXIC EFFECTS OF SUBSTANCES CHIEFLY NONMEDICINAL AS TO SOURCE (980-989)

> *Excludes:* *burns from chemical agents (ingested) (947.0-947.9)*
> *localized toxic effects indexed elsewhere (001.0-799.9)*
> *respiratory conditions due to external agents (506.0-508.9)*

Use additional code to specify the nature of the toxic effect

980 Toxic effect of alcohol

980.0 Ethyl alcohol
    Denatured alcohol
    Ethanol
    Grain alcohol

Use additional code to identify any associated:
    acute alcohol intoxication (305.0)
      in alcoholism (303.0)
    drunkenness (simple) (305.0)
      pathological (291.4)

980.1 Methyl alcohol
    Methanol   Wood alcohol

980.2 Isopropyl alcohol
    Dimethyl carbinol   Rubbing alcohol
    Isopropanol

980.3 Fusel oil
    Alcohol:
      amyl
      butyl
      propyl

980.8 Other specified alcohols

980.9 Unspecified alcohol

981 Toxic effect of petroleum products
    Benzine   Petroleum:
    Gasoline   ether
    Kerosene   naphtha
    Paraffin wax   spirit

982 Toxic effect of solvents other than petroleum-based

982.0 Benzene and homologues

982.1 Carbon tetrachloride

982.2 Carbon disulfide
    Carbon bisulfide

982.3 Other chlorinated hydrocarbon solvents
    Tetrachloroethylene
    Trichloroethylene

> *Excludes:* *chlorinated hydrocarbon preparations other than solvents (989.2)*

982.4 Nitroglycol

982.8 Other nonpetroleum-based solvents
    Acetone

983 Toxic effect of corrosive aromatics, acids, and caustic alkalis

983.0 Corrosive aromatics
    Carbolic acid or phenol
    Cresol

983.1 Acids
    Acid:
      hydrochloric
      nitric
      sulfuric

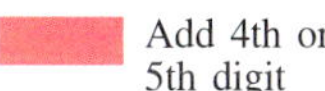

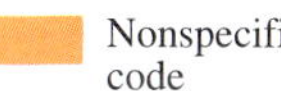

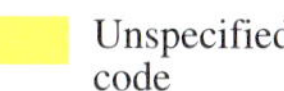

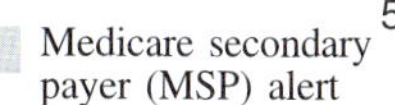

983.2 Caustic alkalis
    Lye   Sodium hydroxide
    Potassium hydroxide

983.9 Caustic, unspecified

984 Toxic effect of lead and its compounds (including fumes)
    Includes: that from all sources except medicinal substances

984.0 Inorganic lead compounds
    Lead dioxide
    Lead salts

984.1 Organic lead compounds
    Lead acetate
    Tetraethyl lead

984.8 Other lead compounds

984.9 Unspecified lead compound

985 Toxic effect of other metals
    Includes: that from all sources except medicinal substances

985.0 Mercury and its compounds
    Minamata disease

985.1 Arsenic and its compounds

985.2 Manganese and its compounds

985.3 Beryllium and its compounds

985.4 Antimony and its compounds

985.5 Cadmium and its compounds

985.6 Chromium

985.8 Other specified metals
    Brass fumes   Iron compounds
    Copper salts   Nickel compounds

985.9 Unspecified metal

986 Toxic effect of carbon monoxide
    Carbon monoxide from any source

987 Toxic effect of other gases, fumes, or vapors

987.0 Liquefied petroleum gases
    Butane
    Propane

987.1 Other hydrocarbon gas

987.2 Nitrogen oxides
    Nitrogen dioxide
    Nitrous fumes

987.3 Sulfur dioxide

987.4 Freon
    Dichloromonofluoromethane

987.5 Lacrimogenic gas
    Bromobenzyl cyanide   Ethyliodoacetate
    Chloroacetophenone

987.6 Chlorine gas

987.7 Hydrocyanic acid gas

987.8 Other specified gases, fumes, or vapors
    Phosgene
    Polyester fumes

987.9 Unspecified gas, fume, or vapor

988 Toxic effect of noxious substances eaten as food
    Excludes: *allergic reaction to food, such as:*
          gastroenteritis (558.3)
          rash (692.5, 693.1)
          food poisoning (bacterial) (005.0-005.9)
          toxic effects of food contaminants, such as:
             aflatoxin and other mycotoxin (989.7)
             mercury (985.0)

988.0 Fish and shellfish

● Code new to this edition   ▲ Revision of existing code   ④ ⑤ Fourth or fifth digit required

988.1　Mushrooms

988.2　Berries and other plants

988.8　Other specified noxious substances eaten as food

988.9　Unspecified noxious substance eaten as food

989　Toxic effect of other substances, chiefly nonmedicinal as to source

989.0　Hydrocyanic acid and cyanides
　　　　Potassium cyanide
　　　　Sodium cyanide

　　Excludes: gas and fumes (987.7)

989.1　Strychnine and salts

989.2　Chlorinated hydrocarbons
　　　　Aldrin　　　　　　　　DDT
　　　　Chlordane　　　　　　Dieldrin

　　Excludes: chlorinated hydrocarbon solvents (982.0-982.3)

989.3　Organophosphate and carbamate
　　　　Carbaryl　　　　　　　Parathion
　　　　Dichlorvos　　　　　　Phorate
　　　　Malathion　　　　　　Phosdrin

989.4　Other pesticides, not elsewhere classified
　　　　Mixtures of insecticides

989.5　Venom
　　　　Bites of venomous snakes, lizards, and spiders
　　　　Tick paralysis

989.6　Soaps and detergents

989.7　Aflatoxin and other mycotoxin [food contaminants]

⑤ 989.8　Other substances, chiefly nonmedicinal as to source

　　989.81　Asbestos

　　Excludes: asbestosis (501)
　　　　　　　　exposure to asbestos (V15.84)

　　989.82　Latex

　　989.83　Silicone

　　Excludes: silicone used in medical devices, implants and grafts (996.00-996.79)

　　989.84　Tobacco

　　989.89　Other

989.9　Unspecified substance, chiefly nonmedicinal as to source

OTHER AND UNSPECIFIED EFFECTS OF EXTERNAL CAUSES (990-995)

990　Effects of radiation, unspecified
　　　Complication of phototherapy　　　　Radiation sickness
　　　Complication of radiation therapy

　　Excludes: specified adverse effects of radiation
　　　　　　　Such conditions are to be classified according to the nature of the adverse effect,
　　　　　　　　　as:
　　　　　　　　burns (940.0-949.5)
　　　　　　　　dermatitis (692.7-692.8)
　　　　　　　　leukemia (204.0-208.9)
　　　　　　　　pneumonia (508.0)
　　　　　　　　sunburn (692.71, 692.76-692.77)
　　　　　　　[The type of radiation giving rise to the adverse effect may be identified by use
　　　　　　　　of the E codes.]

991　Effects of reduced temperature

991.0　Frostbite of face

991.1　Frostbite of hand

991.2　Frostbite of foot

991.3　Frostbite of other and unspecified sites

991.4　Immersion foot
　　　　Trench foot

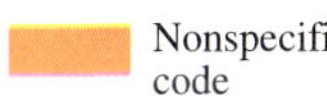
Add 4th or
5th digit

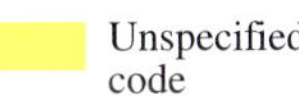
Nonspecific
code

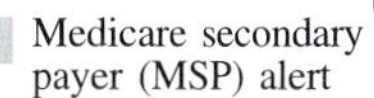
Unspecified
code

Medicare secondary
payer (MSP) alert

991.5 Chilblains
Erythema pernio
Perniosis

991.6 Hypothermia
Hypothermia (accidental)

Excludes: *hypothermia following anesthesia (995.89)*
hypothermia not associated with low environmental temperature (780.99)

991.8 Other specified effects of reduced temperature

991.9 Unspecified effect of reduced temperature
Effects of freezing or excessive cold NOS

992 Effects of heat and light

Excludes: *burns (940.0-949.5)*
diseases of sweat glands due to heat (705.0-705.9)
malignant hyperpyrexia following anesthesia (995.86)
sunburn (692.71, 692.76-692.77)

992.0 Heat stroke and sunstroke

Heat apoplexy	Siriasis
Heat pyrexia	Thermoplegia
Ictus solaris	

992.1 Heat syncope
Heat collapse

992.2 Heat cramps

992.3 Heat exhaustion, anhydrotic
Heat prostration due to water depletion

Excludes: *that associated with salt depletion (992.4)*

992.4 Heat exhaustion due to salt depletion
Heat prostration due to salt (and water) depletion

992.5 Heat exhaustion, unspecified
Heat prostration NOS

992.6 Heat fatigue, transient

992.7 Heat edema

992.8 Other specified heat effects

992.9 Unspecified

993 Effects of air pressure

993.0 Barotrauma, otitic
Aero-otitis media
Effects of high altitude on ears

993.1 Barotrauma, sinus
Aerosinusitis
Effects of high altitude on sinuses

993.2 Other and unspecified effects of high altitude

Alpine sickness	Hypobaropathy
Andes disease	Mountain sickness
Anoxia due to high altitude	

993.3 Caisson disease

Bends	Decompression sickness
Compressed-air disease	Divers' palsy or paralysis

993.4 Effects of air pressure caused by explosion

993.8 Other specified effects of air pressure

993.9 Unspecified effect of air pressure

994 Effects of other external causes

Excludes: *certain adverse effects not elsewhere classified (995.0-995.8)*

994.0 Effects of lightning
Shock from lightning
Struck by lightning NOS

Excludes: *burns (940.0-949.5)*

994.1 Drowning and nonfatal submersion
Bathing cramp
Immersion

● Code new
to this edition

▲ Revision of
existing code

④ ⑤ Fourth or fifth
digit required

994.2 Effects of hunger
Deprivation of food
Starvation

994.3 Effects of thirst
Deprivation of water

994.4 Exhaustion due to exposure

994.5 Exhaustion due to excessive exertion
Overexertion

994.6 Motion sickness

Air sickness   Travel sickness
Seasickness

994.7 Asphyxiation and strangulation

Suffocation (by):   Suffocation (by):
  bedclothes   plastic bag
  cave-in   pressure
  constriction   strangulation
  mechanical

Excludes: *asphyxia from:*

> *carbon monoxide (986)*
> *inhalation of food or foreign body (932-934.9)*
> *other gases, fumes, and vapors (987.0-987.9)*

994.8 Electrocution and nonfatal effects of electric current
Shock from electric current

Excludes: *electric burns (940.0-949.5)*

994.9 Other effects of external causes
Effects of:
  abnormal gravitational [G] forces or states
  weightlessness

995 Certain adverse effects not elsewhere classified

Excludes: *complications of surgical and medical care (996.0-999.9)*

995.0 Other anaphylactic shock
Allergic shock NOS or due to adverse effect of correct medicinal substance properly
  administered
Anaphylactic reaction NOS or due to adverse effect of correct medicinal substance
  properly administered
Anaphylaxis NOS or due to adverse effect of correct medicinal substance properly
  administered

Excludes: *anaphylactic reaction to serum (999.4)*
> *anaphylactic shock due to adverse food reaction (995.60-995.69)*

Use additional E code, if desired, to identify external cause, such as:
  adverse effects of correct medicinal substance properly administered (E930-E949)

995.1 Angioneurotic edema
Giant urticaria

Excludes: *Urticaria:*
> *due to serum (999.5)*
> *other specified (698.2, 708.0-708.9, 757.33)*

▲ **995.2 Other and unspecified adverse effect of drug, medicinal and biological substance**
Adverse effect to correct medicinal substance properly administered
Allergic reaction to correct medicinal substance properly administered
Hypersensitivity to correct medicinal substance properly administered
Idiosyncrasy due to correct medicinal substance properly administered
Drug:
  hypersensitivity NOS
  reaction NOS

Excludes: *pathological drug intoxication (292.2)*

● **995.20 Unspecified adverse effect of unspecified drug, medicinal and biological
substance**

● **995.21 Arthus phenomenon**
Arthus reaction

● **995.22 Unspecified adverse effect of anesthesia**

● **995.23 Unspecified adverse effect of insulin**

● **995.27** **Other drug allergy**
Drug allergy NOS
Drug hypersensitivity NOS

● **995.29** **Unspecified adverse effect of other drug, medicinal and biological substance**

995.3 **Allergy, unspecified**
Allergic reaction NOS   Idiosyncrasy NOS
Hypersensitivity NOS

Excludes: *allergic reaction NOS to correct medicinal substance properly administered*
(995.27)
allergy to existing dental restorative materials (525.66)
specific types of allergic reaction, such as:
allergic diarrhea (558.3)
dermatitis (691.0-693.9)
hay fever (477.0-477.9)

995.4 **Shock due to anesthesia**
Shock due to anesthesia in which the correct substance was properly administered

Excludes: *complications of anesthesia in labor or delivery (668.0-668.9)*
overdose or wrong substance given (968.0-969.9)
postoperative shock NOS (998.0)
specified adverse effects of anesthesia classified elsewhere, such as:
anoxic brain damage (348.1)
hepatitis (070.0-070.9), etc.
unspecified adverse effect of anesthesia (995.22)

⑤ **995.5** **Child maltreatment syndrome**
Use additional code(s), if applicable, to identify any associated injuries
Use additional E code to identify:
nature of abuse (E960-E968)
perpetrator (E967.0-E967.9)

995.50 **Child abuse, unspecified**

995.51 **Child emotional/psychological abuse**

995.52 **Child neglect (nutritional)**

995.53 **Child sexual abuse**

995.54 **Child physical abuse**
Battered baby or child syndrome

Excludes: *Shaken infant syndrome (995.55)*

995.55 **Shaken infant syndrome**
Use additional code(s) to identify any associated injuries

995.59 **Other child abuse and neglect**
Multiple forms of abuse

⑤ **995.6** **Anaphylactic shock due to adverse food reaction**
Anaphylactic shock due to nonpoisonous foods

995.60 **Due to unspecified food**

995.61 **Due to peanuts**

995.62 **Due to crustaceans**

995.63 **Due to fruits and vegetables**

995.64 **Due to tree nuts and seeds**

995.65 **Due to fish**

995.66 **Due to food additives**

995.67 **Due to milk products**

995.68 **Due to eggs**

995.69 **Due to other specified food**

● Code new   ▲ Revision of   ④ ⑤ Fourth or fifth
to this edition   existing code   digit required

995.7 **Other adverse food reactions, not elsewhere classified**

Use additional code to identify the type of reaction, such as:
    hives (708.0)
    wheezing (786.07)

Excludes: *anaphylactic shock due to adverse food reaction (995.60-995.69)*
    asthma (493.0, 493.9)
    dermatitis due to food (693.1)
     in contact with the skin (692.5)
    gastroenteritis and colitis due to food (558.3)
    rhinitis due to food (477.1)

⑤ **995.8** **Other specified adverse effects, not elsewhere classified**

995.80 **Adult maltreatment, unspecified**
    Abused person NOS

Use additional code to identify:
    any associated injury
    perpetrator (E967.0-E967.9)

995.81 **Adult physical abuse**
    Battered:
        person syndrome NEC
        man
        spouse
        woman

Use additional code to identify:
    any associated injury
    nature of abuse (E960-E968)
    perpetrator (E967.0-E967.9)

995.82 **Adult emotional/psychological abuse**

Use additional E code to identify perpetrator (E967.0-E967.9)

995.83 **Adult sexual abuse**

Use additional code to identify:
    any associated injury
    perpetrator (E967.0-E967.9)

995.84 **Adult neglect (nutritional)**

Use additional code to identify:
    intent of neglect (E904.0, E968.4)
    perpetrator (E967.0-967.9)

995.85 **Other adult abuse and neglect**
    Multiple forms of abuse and neglect

Use additional code to identify:
    any associated injury
    intent of neglect (E904.0, E968.4)
    nature of abuse (E960-E968)
    perpetrator (E967.0-E967.9)

995.86 **Malignant hyperthermia**
    Malignant hyperpyrexia due to anesthesia

995.89 **Other**
    Hypothermia due to anesthesia

⑤ **995.9** **Systemic inflammatory response syndrome (SIRS)**

995.90 **Systemic inflammatory response syndrome, unspecified**
    SIRS NOS

▲ **995.91** **Sepsis**
    Systemic inflammatory response syndrome due to infectious process without
        acute organ dysfunction

Code first underlying infection

Excludes: *sepsis with acute organ dysfunction (995.92)*
    sepsis with multiple organ dysfunction (995.92)
    severe sepsis (995.92)

	Add 4th or 5th digit		Nonspecific code		Unspecified code		Medicare secondary payer (MSP) alert

▲ **995.92   Severe sepsis**
Sepsis with acute organ dysfunction
Sepsis with multiple organ dysfunction (MOD)
Systemic inflammatory response syndrome due to infectious process with acute organ dysfunction

Code first underlying infection

Use additional code to specify acute organ dysfunction, such as:
acute renal failure (584.5-584.9)
acute respiratory failure (518.81)
critical illness myopathy (359.81)
critical illness polyneuropathy (357.82)
disseminated intravascular coagulopathy (DIC) syndrome (286.6)
encephalopathy (348.31)
hepatic failure (570)
septic shock (785.52)

▲ **995.93   Systemic inflammatory response syndrome due to noninfectious process without acute organ dysfunction**

Code first underlying conditions, such as:
acute pancreatitis (577.0)
trauma

| Excludes: | *systemic inflammatory response syndrome due to noninfectious process with acute organ dysfunction (995.94)* |

▲ **995.94   Systemic inflammatory response syndrome due to noninfectious process with acute organ dysfunction**

Code first underlying condition, such as:
acute pancreatitis (577.0)
trauma

Use additional code to specify acute organ dysfunction, such as:
acute renal failure (584.5-584.9)
acute respiratory failure (518.81)
critical illness myopathy (359.81)
critical illness polyneuropathy (357.82)
disseminated intravascular coagulopathy (DIC) syndrome (286.6)
encephalopathy (348.31)
hepatic failure (570)

| Excludes: | *severe sepsis (995.92)* |

COMPLICATIONS OF SURGICAL AND MEDICAL CARE, NOT ELSEWHERE CLASSIFIED (996-999)

| Excludes: | *adverse effects of medicinal agents (001.0-799.9, 995.0-995.8)* |

burns from local applications and irradiation (940.0-949.5)
complications of:
conditions for which the procedure was performed
surgical procedures during abortion, labor, and delivery (630-676.9)
poisoning and toxic effects of drugs and chemicals (960.0-989.9)
postoperative conditions in which no complications are present, such as:
artificial opening status (V44.0-V44.9)
closure of external stoma (V55.0-V55.9)
fitting of prosthetic device (V52.0-V52.9)
specified complications classified elsewhere
anesthetic shock (995.4)
electrolyte imbalance (276.0-276.9)
postlaminectomy syndrome (772.80-722.83)
postmastectomy lymphedema syndrome (457.0)
postoperative psychosis (293.0-293.9)
any other condition classified elsewhere in the Alphabetic Index when described as due to a procedure

● Code new
to this edition

▲ Revision of
existing code

④ ⑤ Fourth or fifth
digit required

996 **Complications peculiar to certain specified procedures**

    Includes: complications, not elsewhere classified, in the use of artificial substitutes [e.g., Dacron, metal, Silastic, Teflon] or natural sources [e.g., bone] involving:

        anastomosis (internal)
        graft (bypass) (patch)
        implant
        internal device:
          catheter
          electronic
          fixation
          prosthetic
        reimplant
        transplant

    Excludes: *accidental puncture or laceration during procedure (998.2)*
        complications of internal anastomosis of:
          gastrointestinal tract (997.4)
          urinary tract (997.5)
        mechanical complication of respirator (V46.14)
        other specified complications classified elsewhere, such as:
          hemolytic anemia (283.1)
          functional cardiac disturbances (429.4)
          serum hepatitis (070.2-070.3)

⑤ **996.0** **Mechanical complication of cardiac device, implant, and graft**

    Breakdown (mechanical)   Obstruction, mechanical
    Displacement   Perforation
    Leakage   Protrusion

    996.00 **Unspecified device, implant, and graft**

    996.01 **Due to cardiac pacemaker (electrode)**

    996.02 **Due to heart valve prosthesis**

    996.03 **Due to coronary bypass graft**

    Excludes: *atherosclerosis of graft (414.02, 414.03)*
        embolism [occlusion NOS] [thrombus] of graft (996.72)

    996.04 **Due to automatic implantable cardiac defibrillator**

    996.09 **Other**

996.1 **Mechanical complication of other vascular device, implant, and graft**

    Mechanical complications involving:
      aortic (bifurcation) graft (replacement)
      arteriovenous:
        dialysis catheter
        fistula surgically created
        shunt surgicall created
      balloon (counterpulsation) device, intra-aortic
      carotid artery bypass graft
      femoral-popliteal bypass graft
      umbrella device, vena cava

    Excludes: *atherosclerosis of biological graft (440.30-440.32)*
        embolism [occlusion NOS] [thrombus] of (biological) (synthetic) graft (996.74)
        peritoneal dialysis catheter (996.56)

996.2 **Mechanical complication of nervous system device, implant, and graft**

    Mechanical complications involving:
      dorsal column stimulator
      electrodes implanted in brain [brain "pacemaker"]
      peripheral nerve graft
      ventricular (communicating) shunt

⑤ **996.3** **Mechanical complication of genitourinary device, implant, and graft**

    996.30 **Unspecified device, implant, and graft**

    996.31 **Due to urethral [indwelling] catheter**

    996.32 **Due to intrauterine contraceptive device**

996.39 **Other**
  Cystostomy catheter
  Prosthetic reconstruction of vas deferens
  Repair (graft) of ureter without mention of resection

Excludes: *complications due to:*
  external stoma of urinary tract (997.5)
  internal anastomosis of urinary tract (997.5)

⑤ **996.4** **Mechanical complication of internal orthopedic device, implant, and graft**
Use additional code to identify prosthetic joint with mechanical complication (V43.60-V43.69)

996.40 **Unspecified mechanical complication of internal orthopedic device, implant, and graft**

996.41 **Mechanical loosening of prosthetic joint**
  Aseptic loosening

996.42 **Dislocation of prosthetic joint**
  Instability of prosthetic joint
  Subluxation of prosthetic joint

996.43 **Prosthetic joint implant failure**
  Breakage (fracture) of prosthetic joint

996.44 **Peri-prosthetic fracture around prosthetic joint**

996.45 **Peri-prosthetic osteolysis**
Use additional code to identify major osseous defect, if applicable (731.3)

996.46 **Articular bearing surface wear of prosthetic joint**

996.47 **Other mechanical complication of prosthetic joint implant**
  Mechanical complication of prosthetic joint NOS

996.49 **Other mechanical complication of other internal orthopedic device, implant, and graft**

Excludes: *mechanical complication of prosthetic joint implant (996.41-996.47)*

⑤ **996.5** **Mechanical complication of other specified prosthetic device, implant, and graft**
  Mechanical complications involving:
    prosthetic implant in:
      bile duct
      breast
      chin
      orbit of eye
    nonabsorbable surgical material NOS
    other graft, implant, and internal device, not elsewhere classified

996.51 **Due to corneal graft**

996.52 **Due to graft of other tissue, not elsewhere classified**
  Skin graft failure or rejection

Excludes: *failure of artificial skin graft (996.55)*
  failure of decellularized allodermis (996.55)
  sloughing of temporary skin allografts or xenografts (pigskin)—omit code

996.53 **Due to ocular lens prosthesis**

Excludes: *contact lenses—code to condition*

996.54 **Due to breast prosthesis**
  Breast capsule (prosthesis)
  Mammary implant

996.55 **Due to artificial skin graft and decellularized allodermis**
  Dislodgement   Displacement
  Failure   Non-adherence
  Poor incorporation   Shearing

996.56 **Due to peritoneal dialysis catheter**

Excludes: *mechanical complication of arteriovenous dialysis catheter (996.1)*

996.57 **Due to insulin pump**

996.59 **Due to other implant and internal device, not elsewhere classified**
  Nonabsorbable surgical material NOS
  Prosthetic implant in:
    bile duct
    chin
    orbit of eye

● Code new   ▲ Revision of   ④ ⑤ Fourth or fifth
  to this edition   existing code   digit required

⑤ **996.6   Infection and inflammatory reaction due to internal prosthetic device, implant, and graft**

> Infection (causing obstruction) due to (presence of) any device, implant and graft classifiable to 996.0-996.5
>
> Inflammation due to (presence of) any device, implant and graft classifiable to 996.0-996.5

Use additional code to identify specified infections

996.60   Due to unspecified device, implant, and graft

996.61   Due to cardiac device, implant, and graft
> Cardiac pacemaker or defibrillator:
>   electrode(s), lead(s)
>   pulse generator
>   subcutaneous pocket
> Coronary artery bypass graft
> Heart valve prosthesis

996.62   Due to other vascular device, implant, and graft
> Arterial graft
> Arteriovenous fistula or shunt
> Infusion pump
> Vascular catheter (arterial) (dialysis) (venous)

996.63   Due to nervous system device, implant, and graft
> Electrodes implanted in brain
> Peripheral nerve graft
> Spinal canal catheter
> Ventricular (communicating) shunt (catheter)

996.64   Due to indwelling urinary catheter

Use additional code to identify specified infections, such as:
> Cystitis (595.0-595.9)
> Sepsis (038.0-038.9)

996.65   Due to other genitourinary device, implant, and graft
> Intrauterine contraceptive device

996.66   Due to internal joint prosthesis

Use additional code to identify infected prosthetic joint (V43.60-V43.69)

996.67   Due to other internal orthopedic device, implant, and graft
> Bone growth stimulator (electrode)
> Internal fixation device (pin) (rod) (screw)

996.68   Due to peritoneal dialysis catheter
> Exit-site infection or inflammation

996.69   Due to other internal prosthetic device, implant, and graft
> Breast prosthesis
> Ocular lens prosthesis
> Prosthetic orbital implant

⑤ **996.7   Other complications of internal (biological) (synthetic) prosthetic device, implant, and graft**

> Complication NOS due to (presence of) any device, implant, and graft classifiable to 996.0-996.5
>   occlusion NOS
> Embolism due to (presence of) any device, implant, and graft classifiable to 996.0-996.5
> Fibrosis due to (presence of) any device, implant, and graft classifiable to 996.0-996.5
> Hemorrhage due to (presence of) any device, implant, and graft classifiable to 996.0-996.5
> Pain due to (presence of) any device, implant, and graft classifiable to 996.0-996.5
> Stenosis due to (presence of) any device, implant, and graft classifiable to 996.0-996.5
> Thrombus due to (presence of) any device, implant, and graft classifiable to 996.0-996.5

Use additional code to identify complication, such as:
> pain due to presence of device, implant or graft (338.18-338.19,338.28-338.29)

Excludes: *transplant rejection (996.8)*

996.70   Due to unspecified device, implant, and graft

996.71   Due to heart valve prosthesis

996.72   Due to other cardiac device, implant, and graft
> Cardiac pacemaker or defibrillator:
>   electrode(s), lead(s)
>   subcutaneous pocket
> Coronary artery bypass (graft)

Excludes: *occlusion due to atherosclerosis (414.02-414.06)*

	Add 4th or 5th digit		Nonspecific code		Unspecified code		Medicare secondary payer (MSP) alert

996.73 Due to renal dialysis device, implant, and graft

996.74 Due to other vascular device, implant, and graft

Excludes: *occlusion of biological graft due to atherosclerosis (440.30-440.32)*

996.75 Due to nervous system device, implant, and graft

996.76 Due to genitourinary device, implant, and graft

996.77 Due to internal joint prosthesis

996.78 Due to other internal orthopedic device, implant, and graft

996.79 Due to other internal prosthetic device, implant, and graft

⑤ **996.8 Complications of transplanted organ**

Use additional code, if desired, to identify nature of complication, such as:
  Cytomegalovirus (CMV) infection (078.5)
  Transplant failure or rejection

996.80 Transplanted organ, unspecified

996.81 Kidney

996.82 Liver

996.83 Heart

996.84 Lung

996.85 Bone Marrow
  Graft-versus-host disease (acute) (chronic)

996.86 Pancreas

996.87 Intestine

996.89 Other specified transplanted organ

⑤ **996.9 Complications of reattached extremity or body part**

996.90 Unspecified extremity

996.91 Forearm

996.92 Hand

996.93 Finger(s)

996.94 Upper extremity, other and unspecified

996.95 Foot and toe(s)

996.96 Lower extremity, other and unspecified

996.99 Other specified body part

997 Complications affecting specified body systems, not elsewhere classified

Use additional code to identify complication

Excludes: *the listed conditions when specified as:*

  causing shock (998.0)
  complications of:
    anesthesia:
      adverse effect (001.0-799.9, 995.0-995.8)
      in labor or delivery (668.0-668.9)
      poisoning (968.0-969.9)
    implanted device or graft (996.0-996.9)
    obstetrical procedures (669.0-669.4)
    reattached extremity (996.90-996.96)
    transplanted organ (996.80-996.89)

⑤ **997.0 Nervous system complications**

997.00 Nervous system complication, unspecified

997.01 Central nervous system complication
  Anoxic brain damage
  Cerebral hypoxia

Excludes: *cerebrovascular hemorrhage or infarction (997.02)*

997.02 Iatrogenic cerebrovascular infarction or hemorrhage
  Postoperative stroke

997.09 Other nervous system complications

● Code new
  to this edition

▲ Revision of
  existing code

④ ⑤ Fourth or fifth
  digit required

997.1 Cardiac complications
    Cardiac arrest during or resulting from a procedure
    Cardiac insufficiency during or resulting from a procedure
    Cardiorespiratory failure during or resulting from a procedure
    Heart failure during or resulting from a procedure
    Excludes: *the listed conditions as long-term effects of cardiac surgery or due to the presence of cardiac prosthetic device (429.4)*

997.2 Peripheral vascular complications
    Phlebitis or thrombophlebitis during or resulting from a procedure
    Excludes: *the listed conditions due to:*
        implant or catheter device (996.62)
        infusion, perfusion, or transfusion (999.2)
        complications affecting blood vessels (997.71-997.79)

997.3 Respiratory complications
    Mendelson's syndrome resulting from a procedure
    Pneumonia (aspiration) resulting from a procedure
    Excludes: *iatrogenic [postoperative] pneumothorax (512.1)*
        iatrogenic pulmonary embolism (415.11)
        Mendelson's syndrome in labor and delivery (668.0)
        specified complications classified elsewhere, such as:
          adult respiratory distress syndrome (518.5)
          pulmonary edema, postoperative (518.4)
          respiratory insufficiency, acute, postoperative (518.5)
          shock lung (518.5)
          tracheostomy complications (519.00-519.09)
        transfusion related acute lung injury (TRALI) (518.7)

997.4 Digestive system complications
    Complications of intestinal (internal) anastomosis and bypass, not elsewhere classified, except that involving urinary tract
    Hepatic failure specified as due to a procedure
    Hepatorenal syndrome specified as due to a procedure
    Intestinal obstruction NOS specified as due to a procedure
    Excludes: *specified gastrointestinal complications classified elsewhere, such as:*
        blind loop syndrome (579.2)
        colostomy or enterostomy complications (569.60-569.69)
        gastrostomy complications (536.40-536.49)
        gastrojejunal ulcer (534.0-534.9)
        infection of esophagostomy (530.86)
        infection of external stoma (569.61)
        mechanical complication of esophagostomy (530.87)
        pelvic peritoneal adhesions, female (614.6)
        peritoneal adhesions (568.0)
        peritoneal adhesions with obstruction (560.81)
       postcholecystectomy syndrome (576.0)
        postgastric surgery syndromes (564.2)
        vomiting following gastrointestinal surgery (564.3)

997.5 Urinary complications
    Complications of:
      external stoma of urinary tract
      internal anastomosis and bypass of urinary tract, including that involving intestinal tract
    Oliguria or anuria specified as due to procedure
    Renal:
      failure (acute) specified as due to procedure
      insufficiency (acute) specified as due to procedure
    Tubular necrosis (acute) specified as due to procedure
    Excludes: *specified complications classified elsewhere, such as:*
        postoperative stricture of:
          ureter (593.3)
          urethra (598.2)

⑤ **997.6 Amputation stump complication**
    Excludes: *admission for treatment for a current traumatic amputation; code to complicated traumatic amputation*
        phantom limb (syndrome) (353.6)

      997.60   **Unspecified complication**

      997.61   **Neuroma of amputation stump**

	Add 4th or 5th digit		Nonspecific code		Unspecified code		Medicare secondary payer (MSP) alert

997.62   Infection (chronic)
Use additional code to identify the organism

997.69   Other

⑤ **997.7   Vascular complications of other vessels**

Excludes: *peripheral vascular complications (997.2)*

997.71   Vascular complications of mesenteric artery

997.72   Vascular complications of renal artery

997.79   Vascular complications of other vessels

⑤ **997.9   Complications affecting other specified body systems, not elsewhere classified**

Excludes: *specified complications classified elsewhere, such as:*
broad ligament laceration syndrome (620.6)
postartificial menopause syndrome (627.4)
postoperative stricture of vagina (623.2)

997.91   Hypertension

Excludes: *essential hypertension (401.0-401.9)*

997.99   Other
Vitreous touch syndrome

998   Other complications of procedures, NEC

998.0   Postoperative shock
Collapse NOS during or resulting from a surgical procedure
Shock (endotoxic) (hypovolemic) (septic) during or resulting from a surgical procedure

Excludes: *shock:*
anaphylactic due to serum (999.4)
anesthetic (995.4)
electric (994.8)
following abortion (639.5)
obstetric (669.1)
traumatic (958.4)

⑤ **998.1   Hemorrhage or hematoma or seroma complicating a procedure**

Excludes: *hemorrhage due to implanted device or graft (996.70-996.79)*
hemorrhage, hematoma or seroma complicating cesarean section or puerperal
perineal wound (674.3)

998.11   Hemorrhage complicating a procedure

998.12   Hematoma complicating a procedure

998.13   Seroma complicating a procedure

998.2   Accidental puncture or laceration during a procedure
Accidental perforation by catheter or other instrument during a procedure on:
blood vessel
nerve
organ

Excludes: *iatrogenic [postoperative] pneumothorax (512.1)*
puncture or laceration caused by implanted device intentionally left in operation
wound (996.0-996.5)
specified complications classified elsewhere, such as:
broad ligament laceration syndrome (620.6)
trauma from instruments during delivery (664.0-665.9)

⑤ **998.3   Disruption of operation wound**
Dehiscence of operation wound
Rupture of operation wound

Excludes: *disruption of:*
cesarean wound (674.1)
perineal wound, puerperal (674.2)

998.31   Disruption of internal operation wound

998.32   Disruption of external operation wound
Disruption of operation wound NOS

   ● Code new
to this edition   ▲ Revision of
existing code   ④ ⑤ Fourth or fifth
digit required

998.4 Foreign body accidentally left during a procedure
Adhesions due to foreign body accidentally left in operative wound or body cavity during a procedure
Obstruction due to foreign body accidentally left in operative wound or body cavity during a procedure
Perforation due to foreign body accidentally left in operative wound or body cavity during a procedure

Excludes: *obstruction or perforation caused by implanted device intentionally left in body (996.0-996.5)*

⑤ **998.5 Postoperative infection**

Excludes: *bleb associated endophthalmitis (379.63)*

infection due to:
implanted device (996.60-996.69)
infusion, perfusion, or transfusion (999.3)
postoperative obstetrical wound infection (674.3)

998.51   Infected postoperative seroma
Use additional code to identify organism

998.59   Other postoperative infection
Abscess: postoperative
intra-abdominal postoperative
stitch postoperative
subphrenic postoperative
wound postoperative
Septicemia postoperative
Use additional code to identify infection

998.6 Persistent postoperative fistula

998.7 Acute reaction to foreign substance accidentally left during a procedure
Peritonitis:
aseptic
chemical

⑤ **998.8 Other specified complications of procedures, not elsewhere classified**

998.81   Emphysema (subcutaneous) (surgical) resulting from a procedure

998.82   Cataract fragments in eye following cataract surgery

998.83   Non-healing surgical wound

998.89   Other specified complications

998.9 Unspecified complication of procedure, not elsewhere classified
Postoperative complication NOS

Excludes: *complication NOS of obstetrical surgery or procedure (669.4)*

999 Complications of medical care, not elsewhere classified
Includes: complications, not elsewhere classified, of:
dialysis (hemodialysis) (peritoneal) (renal)
extracorporeal circulation
hyperalimentation therapy
immunization
infusion
inhalation therapy
injection
inoculation
perfusion
transfusion
vaccination
ventilation therapy

Excludes: *specified complications classified elsewhere such as:*

complications of implanted device (996.0-996.9)
contact dermatitis due to drugs (692.3)
dementia dialysis (294.8)
transient (293.9)
dialysis disequilibrium syndrome (276.0-276.9)
poisoning and toxic effects of drugs and chemicals (960.0-989.9)
postvaccinal encephalitis (323.51)
water and electrolyte imbalance (276.0-276.9)

999.0 Generalized vaccinia

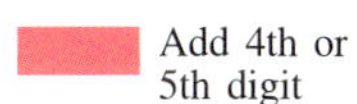

999.1 Air embolism
Air embolism to any site following infusion, perfusion, or transfusion

> *Excludes:* *embolism specified as:*
> *complicating:*
> *abortion (634-638 with .6, 639.6)*
> *ectopic or molar pregnancy (639.6)*
> *pregnancy, childbirth, or the puerperium (673.0)*
> *due to implanted device (996.7)*
> *traumatic (958.0)*

999.2 Other vascular complications
Phlebitis following infusion, perfusion, or transfusion
Thromboembolism following infusion, perfusion, or transfusion
Thrombophlebitis following infusion, perfusion, or transfusion

> *Excludes:* *the listed conditions when specified as:*
> *due to implanted device (996.61-996.62, 996.72-996.74)*
> *postoperative NOS (997.2, 997.71-997.79)*

999.3 Other infection
Infection following infusion, injection, transfusion, or vaccination
Sepsis following infusion, injection, transfusion, or vaccination
Septicemia following infusion, injection, transfusion, or vaccination

> *Excludes:* *the listed conditions when specified as:*
> *due to implanted device (996.60-996.69)*
> *postoperative NOS (998.51-998.59)*

999.4 Anaphylactic shock due to serum

> *Excludes:* *shock:*
> *allergic NOS (995.0)*
> *anaphylactic:*
> *NOS (995.0)*
> *due to drugs and chemicals (995.0)*

999.5 Other serum reaction

Intoxication by serum	Serum sickness
Protein sickness	Urticaria due to serum
Serum rash	

> *Excludes:* *serum hepatitis (070.2-070.3)*

999.6 ABO incompatibility reaction
Incompatible blood transfusion
Reaction to blood group incompatibility in infusion or transfusion

999.7 Rh incompatibility reaction
Reactions due to Rh factor in infusion or transfusion

999.8 Other transfusion reaction
Septic shock due to transfusion
Transfusion reaction NOS

> *Excludes:* *postoperative shock (998.0)*
> *transfusion related acute lung injury (TRALI) (518.7)*

999.9 Other and unspecified complications of medical care, not elsewhere classified
Complications, not elsewhere classified, of:
electroshock therapy
inhalation therapy
ultrasound therapy
ventilation therapy
Unspecified misadventure of medical care

> *Excludes:* *unspecified complication of:*
> *phototherapy (990)*
> *radiation therapy (990)*

● Code new to this edition	▲ Revision of existing code	④ ⑤ Fourth or fifth digit required

SUPPLEMENTARY CLASSIFICATION OF FACTORS INFLUENCING HEALTH STATUS AND CONTACT WITH HEALTH SERVICES (V01-V86)

This classification is provided to deal with occasions when circumstances other than a disease or injury classifiable to categories 001-999 (the main part of ICD) are recorded as "diagnoses" or "problems." This can arise mainly in three ways:

a) When a person who is not currently sick encounters the health services for some specific purpose, such as to act as a donor of an organ or tissue, to receive prophylactic vaccination, or to discuss a problem which is in itself not a disease or injury. This will be a fairly rare occurrence among hospital inpatients, but will be relatively more common among hospital outpatients and patients of family practitioners, health clinics, etc.

b) When a person with a known disease or injury, whether it is current or resolving, encounters the health care system for a specific treatment of that disease or injury (e.g., dialysis for renal disease; chemotherapy for malignancy; cast change).

c) When some circumstance or problem is present which influences the person's health status but is not in itself a current illness or injury. Such factors may be elicited during population surveys, when the person may or may not be currently sick, or be recorded as an additional factor to be borne in mind when the person is receiving care for some current illness or injury classifiable to categories 001-999.

In the latter circumstances the V code should be used only as a supplementary code and should not be the one selected for use in primary, single cause tabulations. Examples of these circumstances are a personal history of certain diseases, or a person with an artificial heart valve in situ.

PERSONS WITH POTENTIAL HEALTH HAZARDS RELATED TO COMMUNICABLE DISEASES (V01-V06)

> Excludes: *family history of infectious and parasitic diseases (V18.8)*
> *personal history of infectious and parasitic diseases (V12.0)*

V01 Contact with or exposure to communicable diseases

V01.0 Cholera
Conditions classifiable to 001

V01.1 Tuberculosis
Conditions classifiable to 010-018

V01.2 Poliomyelitis
Conditions classifiable to 045

V01.3 Smallpox
Conditions classifiable to 050

V01.4 Rubella
Conditions classifiable to 056

V01.5 Rabies
Conditions classifiable to 071

V01.6 Venereal diseases
Conditions classifiable to 090-099

⑤ **V01.7 Other viral diseases**
Conditions classifiable to 042-078 and V08, except as above

V01.71 Varicella

V01.79 Other viral diseases

⑤ **V01.8 Other communicable diseases**
Conditions classifiable to 001-136, except as above

V01.81 Anthrax

V01.82 Exposure to SARS-associated coronavirus

V01.83 Escherichia coli (E. coli)

V01.84 Meningococcus

V01.89 Other communicable diseases

V01.9 Unspecified communicable disease

V02 Carrier or suspected carrier of infectious diseases

V02.0 Cholera

V02.1 Typhoid

V02.2 Amebiasis

V02.3 Other gastrointestinal pathogens

V02.4 Diphtheria

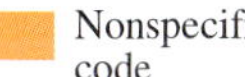

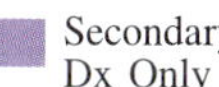

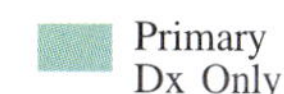

Secondary
Dx Only

Primary
Dx Only

⑤ **V02.5 Other specified bacterial diseases**

    V02.51 Group B streptococcus

    V02.52 Other streptococcus

    V02.59 Other specified bacterial diseases
        Meningococcal
        Staphylococcal

⑤ **V02.6 Viral hepatitis**
    Hepatitis Australian-antigen [HAA] [SH] carrier
    Serum hepatitis carrier

    V02.60 Viral hepatitis carrier, unspecified

    V02.61 Hepatitis B carrier

    V02.62 Hepatitis C carrier

    V02.69 Other viral hepatitis carrier

V02.7 Gonorrhea

V02.8 Other venereal diseases

V02.9 Other specified infectious organism

V03 Need for prophylactic vaccination and inoculation against bacterial diseases
    Excludes: *vaccination not carried out (V64.00-V64.09)*
        vaccines against combinations of diseases (V06.0-V06.9)

V03.0 Cholera alone

V03.1 Typhoid-paratyphoid alone [TAB]

V03.2 Tuberculosis [BCG]

V03.3 Plague

V03.4 Tularemia

V03.5 Diphtheria alone

V03.6 Pertussis alone

V03.7 Tetanus toxoid alone

⑤ **V03.8 Other specified vaccinations against single bacterial diseases**

    V03.81 Hemophilus influenza, type B [Hib]

    V03.82 Streptococcus pneumoniae [pneumococcus]

    V03.89 Other specified vaccination

V03.9 Unspecified single bacterial disease

V04 Need for prophylactic vaccination and inoculation against certain viral diseases
    Excludes: *vaccines against combinations of diseases (V06.0-V06.9)*

V04.0 Poliomyelitis

V04.1 Smallpox

V04.2 Measles alone

V04.3 Rubella alone

V04.4 Yellow fever

V04.5 Rabies

V04.6 Mumps alone

V04.7 Common cold

⑤ **V04.8 Other viral diseases**

    V04.81 Influenza

    V04.82 Respiratory syncytial virus (RSV)

    V04.89 Other viral diseases

V05 Need for other prophylactic vaccination and inoculation against single diseases
    Excludes: *vaccines against combinations of diseases (V06.0-V06.9)*

V05.0 Arthropod-borne viral encephalitis

V05.1 Other arthropod-borne viral diseases

V05.2 Leishmaniasis

V05.3 Viral hepatitis

● Code new to this edition   ▲ Revision of existing code   ④ ⑤ Fourth or fifth digit required

V05.4 Varicella
  Chickenpox

V05.8 Other specified disease

V05.9 Unspecified single disease

V06 Need for prophylactic vaccination and inoculation against combinations of diseases
  Note: Use additional single vaccination codes from categories V03-V05 to identify any
    vaccinations not included in a combination code.

V06.0 Cholera with typhoid-paratyphoid [cholera + TAB]

V06.1 Diphtheria-tetanus-pertussis, combined [DTP] [DTaP]

V06.2 Diphtheria-tetanus-pertussis with typhoid-paratyphoid [DTP + TAB]

V06.3 Diphtheria-tetanus-pertussis with poliomyelitis [DTP + polio]

V06.4 Measles-mumps-rubella [MMR]

V06.5 Tetanus-diphtheria [Td] [DT]

V06.6 Streptococcus pneumoniae [pneumococcus] and influenza

V06.8 Other combinations
  Excludes: *multiple single vaccination codes (V03.0-V05.9)*

V06.9 Unspecified combined vaccine

PERSONS WITH NEED FOR ISOLATION, OTHER POTENTIAL HEALTH HAZARDS AND PROPHYLACTIC MEASURES (V07-V09)

V07 Need for isolation and other prophylactic measures
  Excludes: *prophylactic organ removal (V50.41-V50.49)*

V07.0 Isolation
  Admission to protect the individual from his surroundings or for isolation of individual
    after contact with infectious diseases

V07.1 Desensitization to allergens

V07.2 Prophylactic immunotherapy
  Administration of:
    antivenin
    immune sera [gamma globulin]
    RhoGAM
    tetanus antitoxin

⑤ **V07.3 Other prophylactic chemotherapy**

  V07.31 Prophylactic fluoride administration

  V07.39 Other prophylactic chemotherapy
  Excludes: *maintenance chemotherapy following disease (V58.11)*

V07.4 Hormone replacement therapy (postmenopausal)

V07.8 Other specified prophylactic measure

V07.9 Unspecified prophylactic measure

V08 Asymptomatic human immunodeficiency virus [HIV] infection status
  HIV positive NOS
  Note: This code is ONLY to be used when NO HIV infection symptoms or conditions are
    present. If any HIV infection symptoms or conditions are present, see code 042.
  Excludes: *AIDS (042)*
       human immunodeficiency virus [HIV] disease (042)
       exposure to HIV (V01.79)
       nonspecific serologic evidence of HIV (795.71)
       symptomatic human immunodeficiency virus [HIV] infection (042)

V09 Infection with drug-resistant microorganisms
  Note: This category is intended for use as an additional code for infectious conditions classified
    elsewhere to indicate the presence of drug-resistance of the infectious organism.

V09.0 Infection with microorganisms resistant to penicillins
  Methicillin-resistant staphylococcus aureus (MRSA)

V09.1 Infection with microorganisms resistant to cephalosporins and other B-lactam antibiotics

V09.2 Infection with microorganisms resistant to macrolides

V09.3 Infection with microorganisms resistant to tetracyclines

V09.4 Infection with microorganisms resistant to aminoglycosides

Add 4th or 5th digit | Nonspecific code | Unspecific code | Secondary Dx Only | Primary Dx Only

⑤ **V09.5** **Infection with microorganisms resistant to quinolones and fluoroquinolones**

V09.50 Without mention of resistance to multiple quinolones and fluoroquinolones

V09.51 With resistance to multiple quinolones and fluoroquinolones

V09.6 Infection with microorganisms resistant to sulfonamides

⑤ **V09.7** **Infection with microorganisms resistant to other specified antimycobacterial agents**

Excludes: *Amikacin (V09.4)*
Kanamycin (V09.4)
Streptomycin [SM] (V09.4)

V09.70 Without mention of resistance to multiple antimycobacterial agents

V09.71 With resistance to multiple antimycobacterial agents

⑤ **V09.8** **Infection with microorganisms resistant to other specified drugs**
Vancomycin (glycopeptide) intermediate staphylococcus aureus (VISA/GISA)
Vancomycin (glycopeptide) resistant enterococcus (VRE)
Vancomycin (glycopeptide) resistant staphylococcus aureus (VRSA/GRSA)

V09.80 Without mention of resistance to multiple drugs

V09.81 With resistance to multiple drugs

⑤ **V09.9** **Infection with drug-resistant microorganisms, unspecified**
Drug resistance NOS

V09.90 Without mention of multiple drug resistance

V09.91 With multiple drug resistance
Multiple drug resistance NOS

PERSONS WITH POTENTIAL HEALTH HAZARDS RELATED TO PERSONAL AND FAMILY HISTORY (V10-V19)

Excludes: *obstetric patients where the possibility that the fetus might be affected is the reason for observation or management during pregnancy (655.0-655.9)*

V10 **Personal history of malignant neoplasm**

⑤ **V10.0** **Gastrointestinal tract**
History of conditions classifiable to 140-159

V10.00 Gastrointestinal tract, unspecified

V10.01 Tongue

V10.02 Other and unspecified oral cavity and pharynx

V10.03 Esophagus

V10.04 Stomach

V10.05 Large intestine

V10.06 Rectum, rectosigmoid junction, and anus

V10.07 Liver

V10.09 Other

⑤ **V10.1** **Trachea, bronchus, and lung**
History of conditions classifiable to 162

V10.11 Bronchus and lung

V10.12 Trachea

⑤ **V10.2** **Other respiratory and intrathoracic organs**
History of conditions classifiable to 160, 161, 163-165

V10.20 Respiratory organ, unspecified

V10.21 Larynx

V10.22 Nasal cavities, middle ear, and accessory sinuses

V10.29 Other

V10.3 **Breast**
History of conditions classifiable to 174 and 175

⑤ **V10.4** **Genital organs**
History of conditions classifiable to 179-187

V10.40 Female genital organ, unspecified

V10.41 Cervix uteri

V10.42 Other parts of uterus

V10.43 Ovary

● Code new to this edition   ▲ Revision of existing code   ④ ⑤ Fourth or fifth digit required

V10.44 Other female genital organs

V10.45 Male genital organ, unspecified

V10.46 Prostate

V10.47 Testis

V10.48 Epididymis

V10.49 Other male genital organs

⑤ V10.5 **Urinary organs**
History of conditions classifiable to 188 and 189

V10.50 Urinary organ, unspecified

V10.51 Bladder

V10.52 Kidney

Excludes: renal pelvis (V10.53)

V10.53 Renal pelvis

V10.59 Other

⑤ V10.6 **Leukemia**
Conditions classifiable to 204-208

Excludes: leukemia in remission (204-208)

V10.60 Leukemia, unspecified

V10.61 Lymphoid leukemia

V10.62 Myeloid leukemia

V10.63 Monocytic leukemia

V10.69 Other

⑤ V10.7 **Other lymphatic and hematopoietic neoplasms**
Conditions classifiable to 200-203

Excludes: listed conditions in 200-203 in remission

V10.71 Lymphosarcoma and reticulosarcoma

V10.72 Hodgkin's disease

V10.79 Other

⑤ V10.8 **Personal history of malignant neoplasm of other sites**
History of conditions classifiable to 170-173, 190-195

V10.81 Bone

V10.82 Malignant melanoma of skin

V10.83 Other malignant neoplasm of skin

V10.84 Eye

V10.85 Brain

V10.86 Other parts of nervous system

Excludes: peripheral, sympathetic, and parasympathetic nerves (V10.89)

V10.87 Thyroid

V10.88 Other endocrine glands and related structures

V10.89 Other

V10.9 Unspecified personal history of malignant neoplasm

V11 Personal history of mental disorder

V11.0 Schizophrenia

Excludes: that in remission (295.0-295.9 with fifth-digit 5)

V11.1 Affective disorders
Personal history of manic-depressive psychosis

Excludes: that in remission (296.0-296.6 with fifth-digit 5, 6)

V11.2 Neurosis

V11.3 Alcoholism

V11.8 Other mental disorders

V11.9 Unspecified mental disorder

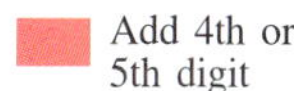

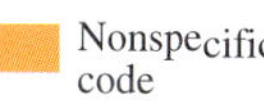

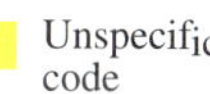

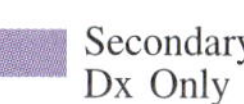

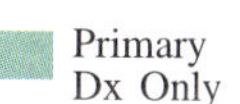

V12 Personal history of certain other diseases

⑤ V12.0 Infectious and parasitic diseases

> *Excludes:* *personal history of infectious diseases specific to a body system*

V12.00 Unspecified infectious and parasitic disease

V12.01 Tuberculosis

V12.02 Poliomyelitis

V12.03 Malaria

V12.09 Other

V12.1 Nutritional deficiency

V12.2 Endocrine, metabolic, and immunity disorders

> *Excludes:* *history of allergy (V14.0-V14.9, V15.01-V15.09)*

V12.3 Diseases of blood and blood-forming organs

⑤ V12.4 Disorders of nervous system and sense organs

V12.40 Unspecified disorder of nervous system and sense organs

V12.41 Benign neoplasm of the brain

V12.42 Infections of the central nervous system
Encephalitis
Meningitis

V12.49 Other disorders of nervous system and sense organs

> *Excludes:* *old myocardial infarction (412)*
> *postmyocardial infarction syndrome (411.0)*

V12.50 Unspecified circulatory disease

V12.51 Venous thrombosis and embolism
Pulmonary embolism

V12.52 Thrombophlebitis

V12.59 Other
Note: Assign code V12.59 (and not a code from category 438) as an additional code for history of cerebrovascular disease when no neurologic deficits are present.

⑤ V12.6 Diseases of respiratory system

> *Excludes:* *tuberculosis (V12.01)*

V12.60 Unspecified disease of respiratory system

V12.61 Pneumonia (recurrent)

V12.69 Other diseases of respiratory system

⑤ V12.7 Diseases of digestive system

V12.70 Unspecified digestive disease

V12.71 Peptic ulcer disease

V12.72 Colonic polyps

V12.79 Other

V13 Personal history of other diseases

⑤ V13.0 Disorders of urinary system

V13.00 Unspecified urinary disorder

V13.01 Urinary calculi

V13.02 Urinary (tract) infection

V13.03 Nephrotic syndrome

V13.09 Other

V13.1 Trophoblastic disease

> *Excludes:* *supervision during a current pregnancy (V23.1)*

⑤ V13.2 Other genital system and obstetric disorders

> *Excludes:* *supervision during a current pregnancy of a woman with poor obstetric history (V23.0-V23.9)*
> *habitual aborter (646.3)*
> *without current history (629.9)*

V13.21 Personal history of pre-term labor

> *Excludes:* *current pregnancy with history of pre-term labor (V23.41)*

　● Code new to this edition　▲ Revision of existing code　④ ⑤ Fourth or fifth digit required

V13.29 Other genital system and obstetric disorders

V13.3 Diseases of skin and subcutaneous tissue

V13.4 Arthritis

V13.5 Other musculoskeletal disorders

⑤ **V13.6** Congenital malformations

V13.61 Hypospadias

V13.69 Other congenital malformations

V13.7 Perinatal problems

Excludes: *low birth weight status (V21.30-V21.35)*

V13.8 Other specified diseases

V13.9 Unspecified disease

V14 Personal history of allergy to medicinal agents

V14.0 Penicillin

V14.1 Other antibiotic agent

V14.2 Sulfonamides

V14.3 Other anti-infective agent

V14.4 Anesthetic agent

V14.5 Narcotic agent

V14.6 Analgesic agent

V14.7 Serum or vaccine

V14.8 Other specified medicinal agents

V14.9 Unspecified medicinal agent

V15 Other personal history presenting hazards to health

⑤ **V15.0** Allergy, other than to medicinal agents

Excludes: *allergy to food substance used as base for medicinal agent (V14.0-V14.9)*

V15.01 Allergy to peanuts

V15.02 Allergy to milk products

Excludes: *lactose intolerance (271.3)*

V15.03 Allergy to eggs

V15.04 Allergy to seafood
Seafood (octopus) (squid) ink
Shellfish

V15.05 Allergy to other foods
Food additives
Nuts other than peanuts

V15.06 Allergy to insects
Bugs
Insect bites and stings
Spiders

V15.07 Allergy to latex
Latex sensitivity

V15.08 Allergy to radiographic dye
Contrast media used for diagnostic x-ray procedures

V15.09 Other allergy, other than to medicinal agents

V15.1 Surgery to heart and great vessels

Excludes: *replacement by transplant or other means (V42.1-V42.2, V43.2-V43.4)*

V15.2 Surgery to other major organs

Excludes: *replacement by transplant or other means (V42.0-V43.8)*

V15.3 Irradiation
Previous exposure to therapeutic or other ionizing radiation

⑤ **V15.4** Psychological trauma

Excludes: *history of condition classifiable to 290-316 (V11.0-V11.9)*

V15.41 History of physical abuse
Rape

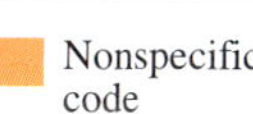

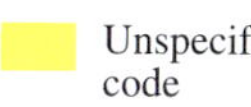

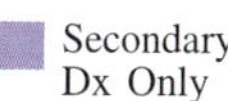

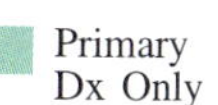

V15.42 **History of emotional abuse**
    Neglect

V15.49 **Other**

V15.5 **Injury**

V15.6 **Poisoning**

V15.7 **Contraception**

    Excludes: *current contraceptive management (V25.0-V25.4)*
                presence of intrauterine contraceptive device as incidental finding (V45.5)

⑤ **V15.8 Other specified personal history presenting hazards to health**

V15.81 **Noncompliance with medical treatment**

V15.82 **History of tobacco use**

    Excludes: *tobacco dependence (305.1)*

V15.84 **Exposure to asbestos**

V15.85 **Exposure to potentially hazardous body fluids**

V15.86 **Exposure to lead**

V15.87 **History of extracorporeal membrane oxygenation [ECMO]**

V15.88 **History of fall**
    At risk for falling

V15.89 **Other**

V15.9 **Unspecified personal history presenting hazards to health**

V16 **Family history of malignant neoplasm**

V16.0 **Gastrointestinal tract**
    Family history of condition classifiable to 140-159

V16.1 **Trachea, bronchus, and lung**
    Family history of condition classifiable to 162

V16.2 **Other respiratory and intrathoracic organs**
    Family history of condition classifiable to 160-161, 163-165

V16.3 **Breast**
    Family history of condition classifiable to 174

⑤ **V16.4** **Genital organs**
    Family history of condition classifiable to 179-187

V16.40 **Genital organ, unspecified**

V16.41 **Ovary**

V16.42 **Prostate**

V16.43 **Testis**

V16.49 **Other**

⑤ **V16.5** **Urinary organs**
    Family history of condition classifiable to 189

V16.51 **Kidney**

V16.59 **Other**

V16.6 **Leukemia**
    Family history of condition classifiable to 204-208

V16.7 **Other lymphatic and hematopoietic neoplasms**
    Family history of condition classifiable to 200-203

V16.8 **Other specified malignant neoplasm**
    Family history of other condition classifiable to 140-199

V16.9 **Unspecified malignant neoplasm**

V17 **Family history of certain chronic disabling diseases**

V17.0 **Psychiatric condition**
    Excludes: *family history of mental retardation (V18.4)*

V17.1 **Stroke (cerebrovascular)**

V17.2 **Other neurological diseases**
    Epilepsy
    Huntington's chorea

V17.3 **Ischemic heart disease**

● Code new to this edition   ▲ Revision of existing code   ④ ⑤ Fourth or fifth digit required

V17.4 Other cardiovascular diseases

V17.5 Asthma

V17.6 Other chronic respiratory conditions

V17.7 Arthritis

⑤ V17.8 Other musculoskeletal diseases

     V17.81 Osteoporosis

     V17.89 Other musculoskeletal diseases

V18 Family history of certain other specific conditions

V18.0 Diabetes mellitus

V18.1 Other endocrine and metabolic diseases

V18.2 Anemia

V18.3 Other blood disorders

V18.4 Mental retardation

⑤ V18.5 Digestive disorders

    ● V18.51 Colonic polyps

    Excludes: *family history of malignant neoplasm of gastrointestinal tract (V16.0)*

    ● **V18.59** Other digestive disorders

⑤ V18.6 Kidney diseases

     V18.61 Polycystic kidney

     V18.69 Other kidney diseases

V18.7 Other genitourinary diseases

V18.8 Infectious and parasitic diseases

V18.9 Genetic disease carrier

V19 Family history of other conditions

V19.0 Blindness or visual loss

V19.1 Other eye disorders

V19.2 Deafness or hearing loss

V19.3 Other ear disorders

V19.4 Skin conditions

V19.5 Congenital anomalies

V19.6 Allergic disorders

V19.7 Consanguinity

V19.8 Other condition

PERSONS ENCOUNTERING HEALTH SERVICES IN CIRCUMSTANCES RELATED TO REPRODUCTION AND DEVELOPMENT (V20-V29)

V20 Health supervision of infant or child

   V20.0 Foundling

   V20.1 Other healthy infant or child receiving care

      Medical or nursing care supervision of healthy infant in cases of:

        maternal illness, physical or psychiatric

        socioeconomic adverse condition at home

        too many children at home preventing or interfering with normal care

   V20.2 Routine infant or child health check

      Developmental testing of infant or child

      Immunizations appropriate for age

      Initial and subsequent routine newborn check

      Routine vision and hearing testing

      Excludes: *special screening for developmental handicaps (V79.3)*

   Use additional code(s) to identify:

      Special screening examination(s) performed (V73.0-V82.9)

V21 Constitutional states in development

   V21.0 Period of rapid growth in childhood

   V21.1 Puberty

   V21.2 Other adolescence

⑤ **V21.3 Low birth weight status**
> Excludes: *history of perinatal problems (V13.7)*

  V21.30 Low birth weight status, unspecified
  V21.31 Low birth weight status, less than 500 grams
  V21.32 Low birth weight status, 500-999 grams
  V21.33 Low birth weight status, 1000-1499 grams
  V21.34 Low birth weight status, 1500-1999 grams
  V21.35 Low birth weight status, 2000-2500 grams

V21.8 Other specified constitutional states in development

V21.9 Unspecified constitutional state in development

V22 Normal pregnancy
> Excludes: *pregnancy examination or test, pregnancy unconfirmed (V72.40)*

V22.0 Supervision of normal first pregnancy

V22.1 Supervision of other normal pregnancy

V22.2 Pregnant state, incidental
  Pregnant state NOS

V23 Supervision of high-risk pregnancy

V23.0 Pregnancy with history of infertility

V23.1 Pregnancy with history of trophoblastic disease
  Pregnancy with history of:
    hydatidiform mole
    vesicular mole
> Excludes: *that without current pregnancy (V13.1)*

V23.2 Pregnancy with history of abortion
  Pregnancy with history of conditions classifiable to 634-638
> Excludes: *habitual aborter:*
> *care during pregnancy (646.3)*
> *that without current pregnancy (629.9)*

V23.3 Grand multiparity
> Excludes: *care in relation to labor and delivery (659.4)*
> *that without current pregnancy (V61.5)*

⑤ **V23.4 Pregnancy with other poor obstetric history**
  Pregnancy with history of other conditions classifiable to 630-676

  V23.41 Pregnancy with history of pre-term labor
  V23.49 Pregnancy with other poor obstetric history

V23.5 Pregnancy with other poor reproductive history
  Pregnancy with history of stillbirth or neonatal death

V23.7 Insufficient prenatal care
  History of little or no prenatal care

⑤ **V23.8 Other high-risk pregnancy**

  V23.81 Elderly primigravida
    First pregnancy in a woman who will be 35 years of age or older at expected date of delivery
> Excludes: *elderly primigravida complicating pregnancy (659.5)*

  V23.82 Elderly multigravida
    Second or more pregnancy in a woman who will be 35 years of age or older at expected date of delivery
> Excludes: *elderly multigravida complicating pregnancy (659.6)*

  V23.83 Young primigravida
    First pregnancy in a female less than 16 years old at expected date of delivery
> Excludes: *young primigravida complicating pregnancy (659.8)*

  V23.84 Young multigravida
    Second or more pregnancy in a female less than 16 years old at expected date of delivery
> Excludes: *young multigravida complicating pregnancy (659.8)*

  V23.89 Other high-risk pregnancy

● Code new to this edition   ▲ Revision of existing code   ④ ⑤ Fourth or fifth digit required

V23.9 Unspecified high-risk pregnancy

V24 Postpartum care and examination

V24.0 Immediately after delivery
Care and observation in uncomplicated cases

V24.1 Lactating mother
Supervision of lactation

V24.2 Routine postpartum follow-up

V25 Encounter for contraceptive management

⑤ **V25.0 General counseling and advice**

V25.01 Prescription of oral contraceptives

V25.02 Initiation of other contraceptive measures
Fitting of diaphragm
Prescription of foams, creams, or other agents

V25.03 Encounter for emergency contraceptive counseling and prescription
Encounter for postcoital contraceptive counseling and prescription

V25.09 Other
Family planning advice

V25.1 Insertion of intrauterine contraceptive device

V25.2 Sterilization
Admission for interruption of fallopian tubes or vas deferens

V25.3 Menstrual extraction
Menstrual regulation

⑤ **V25.4 Surveillance of previously prescribed contraceptive methods**
Checking, reinsertion, or removal of contraceptive device
Repeat prescription for contraceptive method
Routine examination in connection with contraceptive maintenance

Excludes: *presence of intrauterine contraceptive device as incidental finding (V45.5)*

V25.40 Contraceptive surveillance, unspecified

V25.41 Contraceptive pill

V25.42 Intrauterine contraceptive device
Checking, reinsertion, or removal of intrauterine device

V25.43 Implantable subdermal contraceptive

V25.49 Other contraceptive method

V25.5 Insertion of implantable subdermal contraceptive

V25.8 Other specified contraceptive management
Postvasectomy sperm count

Excludes: *sperm count following sterilization reversal (V26.22)*
sperm count for fertility testing (V26.21)

V25.9 Unspecified contraceptive management

V26 Procreative management

V26.0 Tuboplasty or vasoplasty after previous sterilization

V26.1 Artificial insemination

⑤ **V26.2 Investigation and testing**

Excludes: *postvasectomy sperm count (V25.8)*

V26.21 Fertility testing
Fallopian insufflation
Sperm count for fertility testing

Excludes: *genetic counseling and testing (V26.31-V26.39)*

V26.22 Aftercare following sterilization reversal
Fallopian insufflation following sterilization reversal
Sperm count following sterilization reversal

V26.29 Other investigation and testing

⑤ **V26.3 Genetic counseling and testing**

Excludes: *nonprocreative genetic screening (V82.71, V82.79)*

▲ **V26.31 Testing of female for genetic disease carrier status**

▲ **V26.32 Other genetic testing of female**
Use additional code to identify habitual aborter (629.81, 646.3)

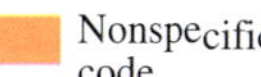

V26.33 Genetic counseling

● V26.34 Testing of male for genetic disease carrier status

● V26.35 Encounter for testing of male partner of habitual aborter

● V26.39 Other genetic testing of male

V26.4 General counseling and advice

⑤ V26.5 Sterilization status

V26.51 Tubal ligation status

Excludes: *infertility not due to previous tubal ligation (628.0-628.9)*

V26.52 Vasectomy status

V26.8 Other specified procreative management

V26.9 Unspecified procreative management

V27 Outcome of delivery

Note: This category is intended for the coding of the outcome of delivery on the mother's record.

V27.0 Single liveborn

V27.1 Single stillborn

V27.2 Twins, both liveborn

V27.3 Twins, one liveborn and one stillborn

V27.4 Twins, both stillborn

V27.5 Other multiple birth, all liveborn

V27.6 Other multiple birth, some liveborn

V27.7 Other multiple birth, all stillborn

V27.9 Unspecified outcome of delivery
Single birth, outcome to infant unspecified
Multiple birth, outcome to infant unspecified

▲ V28 Encounter for antenatal screening of mother

Excludes: *abnormal findings on screening—code to findings*
routine prenatal care (V22.0-V23.9)

V28.0 Screening for chromosomal anomalies by amniocentesis

V28.1 Screening for raised alpha-fetoprotein levels in amniotic fluid

V28.2 Other screening based on amniocentesis

V28.3 Screening for malformation using ultrasonics

V28.4 Screening for fetal growth retardation using ultrasonics

V28.5 Screening for isoimmunization

V28.6 Screening for Streptococcus B

V28.8 Other specified antenatal screening

V28.9 Unspecified antenatal screening

V29 Observation and evaluation of newborns for suspected condition not found

Note: This category is to be used for newborns, within the neonatal period, (the first 28 days of life) who are suspected of having an abnormal condition resulting from exposure from the mother or the birth process, but without signs or symptoms, and, which after examination and observation, is found not to exist.

V29.0 Observation for suspected infectious condition

V29.1 Observation for suspected neurological condition

V29.2 Observation for suspected respiratory condition

V29.3 Observation for suspected genetic or metabolic condition

V29.8 Observation for other specified suspected condition

V29.9 Observation for unspecified suspected condition

● Code new
to this edition

▲ Revision of
existing code

④ ⑤ Fourth or fifth
digit required

LIVEBORN INFANTS ACCORDING TO TYPE OF BIRTH (V30-V39)

Note: These categories are intended for the coding of liveborn infants who are consuming health care [e.g., crib or bassinet occupancy].

The following fourth-digit subdivisions are for use with categories V30-V39:

⑤ **.0 Born in hospital**

.1 Born before admission to hospital

.2 Born outside hospital and not hospitalized

The following two fifth-digits are for use with the fourth-digit .0, Born in hospital:

0   delivered without mention of cesarean delivery

1   delivered by cesarean delivery

④ **V30 Single liveborn**

④ **V31 Twin, mate liveborn**

④ **V32 Twin, mate stillborn**

④ **V33 Twin, unspecified**

④ **V34 Other multiple, mates all liveborn**

④ **V35 Other multiple, mates all stillborn**

④ **V36 Other multiple, mates live- and stillborn**

④ **V37 Other multiple, unspecified**

④ **V39 Unspecified**

PERSONS WITH A CONDITION INFLUENCING THEIR HEALTH STATUS (V40-V49)

Note: These categories are intended for use when these conditions are recorded as "diagnoses" or "problems."

V40 Mental and behavioral problems

    V40.0 Problems with learning

    V40.1 Problems with communication [including speech]

    V40.2 Other mental problems

    V40.3 Other behavioral problems

    V40.9 Unspecified mental or behavioral problem

V41 Problems with special senses and other special functions

    V41.0 Problems with sight

    V41.1 Other eye problems

    V41.2 Problems with hearing

    V41.3 Other ear problems

    V41.4 Problems with voice production

    V41.5 Problems with smell and taste

    V41.6 Problems with swallowing and mastication

    V41.7 Problems with sexual function

        Excludes: *marital problems (V61.10)*
                psychosexual disorders (302.0-302.9)

    V41.8 Other problems with special functions

    V41.9 Unspecified problem with special function

V42 Organ or tissue replaced by transplant
    Includes: homologous or heterologous (animal) (human) transplant organ status

    V42.0 Kidney

    V42.1 Heart

    V42.2 Heart valve

    V42.3 Skin

    V42.4 Bone

    V42.5 Cornea

    V42.6 Lung

    V42.7 Liver

⑤ **V42.8 Other specified organ or tissue**

        V42.81   Bone marrow

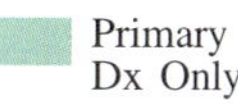

Add 4th or 5th digit	Nonspecific code	Unspecific code	Secondary Dx Only	Primary Dx Only

V42.82 **Peripheral stem cells**

V42.83 **Pancreas**

V42.84 **Intestines**

V42.89 **Other**

V42.9 **Unspecified organ or tissue**

V43 **Organ or tissue replaced by other means**
   Includes: organ or tissue assisted by other means
              replacement of organ by:
                 artificial device
                 mechanical device
                 prosthesis

   Excludes: *cardiac pacemaker in situ (V45.01)*
              fitting and adjustment of prosthetic device (V52.0-V52.9)
              renal dialysis status (V45.1)

V43.0 **Eye globe**

V43.1 **Lens**
   Pseudophakos

⑤ V43.2 **Heart**

V43.21 **Heart assist device**

V43.22 **Fully implantable artificial heart**

V43.3 **Heart valve**

V43.4 **Blood vessel**

V43.5 **Bladder**

⑤ V43.6 **Joint**

V43.60 **Unspecified joint**

V43.61 **Shoulder**

V43.62 **Elbow**

V43.63 **Wrist**

V43.64 **Hip**

V43.65 **Knee**

V43.66 **Ankle**

V43.69 **Other**

V43.7 **Limb**

⑤ V43.8 **Other organ or tissue**

V43.81 **Larynx**

V43.82 **Breast**

V43.83 **Artificial skin**

V43.89 **Other**

V44 **Artificial opening status**
   Excludes: *artificial openings requiring attention or management (V55.0-V55.9)*

V44.0 **Tracheostomy**

V44.1 **Gastrostomy**

V44.2 **Ileostomy**

V44.3 **Colostomy**

V44.4 **Other artificial opening of gastrointestinal tract**

⑤ V44.5 **Cystostomy**

V44.50 **Cystostomy, unspecified**

V44.51 **Cutaneous-vesicostomy**

V44.52 **Appendico-vesicostomy**

V44.59 **Other cystostomy**

V44.6 **Other artificial opening of urinary tract**
   Nephrostomy
   Ureterostomy
   Urethrostomy

V44.7 **Artificial vagina**

● Code new   ▲ Revision of   ④ ⑤ Fourth or fifth
to this edition   existing code   digit required

V44.8 **Other artificial opening status**

V44.9 **Unspecified artificial opening status**

V45 **Other postprocedural states**

Excludes: *aftercare management (V51-V58.9)*
malfunction or other complication—code to condition

⑤ **V45.0 Cardiac device in situ**

Excludes: *artificial heart (V43.22)*
heart assist device (V43.21)

   V45.00 **Unspecified cardiac device**

   V45.01 **Cardiac pacemaker**

   V45.02 **Automatic implantable cardiac defibrillator**

   V45.09 **Other specified cardiac device**
Carotid sinus pacemaker in situ

V45.1 **Renal dialysis status**
Hemodialysis status
Peritoneal dialysis status
Patient requiring intermittent renal dialysis
Presence of arterial-venous shunt (for dialysis)

Excludes: *admission for dialysis treatment, or session (V56.0)*

V45.2 **Presence of cerebrospinal fluid drainage device**
Cerebral ventricle (communicating) shunt, valve, or device in situ

Excludes: *malfunction (996.2)*

V45.3 **Intestinal bypass or anastomosis status**

Excludes: *bariatric surgery status (V45.86)*
gastric bypass status (V45.86)
obesity surgery status (V45.86)

V45.4 **Arthrodesis status**

⑤ **V45.5 Presence of contraceptive device**

Excludes: *checking, reinsertion, or removal of device (V25.42)*
complication from device (996.32)
insertion of device (V25.1)

   V45.51 **Intrauterine contraceptive device**

   V45.52 **Subdermal contraceptive implant**

   V45.59 **Other**

⑤ **V45.6 States following surgery of eye and adnexa**
Cataract extraction state following eye surgery
Filtering bleb state following eye surgery
Surgical eyelid adhesion state following eye surgery

Excludes: *aphakia (379.31)*
artificial eye globe (V43.0)

   V45.61 **Cataract extraction status**
Use additional code for associated artificial lens status (V43.1)

   V45.69 **Other states following surgery of eye and adnexa**

⑤ **V45.7 Acquired absence of organ**

   V45.71 **Acquired absence of breast**

   V45.72 **Acquired absence of intestine (large) (small)**

   V45.73 **Acquired absence of kidney**

   V45.74 **Other parts of urinary tract**
Bladder

   V45.75 **Stomach**

   V45.76 **Lung**

   V45.77 **Genital organs**

Excludes: *female genital mutilation status (629.20-629.29)*

   V45.78 **Eye**

   V45.79 **Other acquired absence of organ**

⑤ **V45.8 Other postprocedural status**

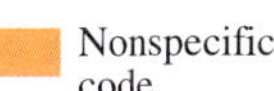

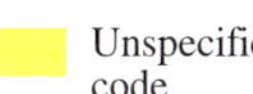

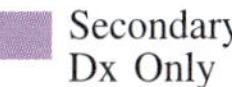

Secondary
Dx Only

Primary
Dx Only

V45.81 **Aortocoronary bypass status**

V45.82 **Percutaneous transluminal coronary angioplasty status**

V45.83 **Breast implant removal status**

V45.84 **Dental restoration status**
Dental crowns status
Dental fillings status

● **V45.86** **Bariatric surgery status**
Gastric banding status
Gastric bypass status for obesity
Obesity surgery status

Excludes: *bariatric surgery status complicating pregnancy, childbirth or the puerperium (649.2)*
intestinal bypass or anastomosis status (V45.3)

V45.89 **Other**
Presence of neuropacemaker or other electronic device

Excludes: *artificial heart valve in situ (V43.3)*
vascular prosthesis in situ (V43.4)

V46 **Other dependence on machines**

V46.0 **Aspirator**

⑤ **V46.1** **Respirator [Ventilator]**
Iron lung

V46.11 **Dependence on respirator, status**

V46.12 **Encounter for respirator dependence during power failure**

V46.13 **Encounter for weaning from respirator [ventilator]**

V46.14 **Mechanical complication of respirator [ventilator]**
Mechanical failure of respirator [ventilator]

V46.2 **Supplemental oxygen**
Long-term oxygen therapy

V46.8 **Other enabling machines**
Hyperbaric chamber
Possum [Patient-Operated-Selector-Mechanism]

Excludes: *cardiac pacemaker (V45.0)*
kidney dialysis machine (V45.1)

V46.9 **Unspecified machine dependence**

V47 **Other problems with internal organs**

V47.0 **Deficiencies of internal organs**

V47.1 **Mechanical and motor problems with internal organs**

V47.2 **Other cardiorespiratory problems**
Cardiovascular exercise intolerance with pain (with):
at rest
less than ordinary activity
ordinary activity

V47.3 **Other digestive problems**

V47.4 **Other urinary problems**

V47.5 **Other genital problems**

V47.9 **Unspecified**

V48 **Problems with head, neck, and trunk**

V48.0 **Deficiencies of head**

Excludes: *deficiencies of ears, eyelids, and nose (V48.8)*

V48.1 **Deficiencies of neck and trunk**

V48.2 **Mechanical and motor problems with head**

V48.3 **Mechanical and motor problems with neck and trunk**

V48.4 **Sensory problem with head**

V48.5 **Sensory problem with neck and trunk**

V48.6 **Disfigurements of head**

V48.7 **Disfigurements of neck and trunk**

V48.8 **Other problems with head, neck, and trunk**

● Code new to this edition　　▲ Revision of existing code　　④ ⑤ Fourth or fifth digit required

V48.9 Unspecified problem with head, neck, or trunk

V49 Other conditions influencing health status

V49.0 Deficiencies of limbs

V49.1 Mechanical problems with limbs

V49.2 Motor problems with limbs

V49.3 Sensory problems with limbs

V49.4 Disfigurements of limbs

V49.5 Other problems of limbs

⑤ V49.6 Upper limb amputation status

    V49.60 Unspecified level

    V49.61 Thumb

    V49.62 Other finger(s)

    V49.63 Hand

    V49.64 Wrist
       Disarticulation of wrist

    V49.65 Below elbow

    V49.66 Above elbow
       Disarticulation of elbow

    V49.67 Shoulder
       Disarticulation of shoulder

⑤ V49.7 Lower limb amputation status

    V49.70 Unspecified level

    V49.71 Great toe

    V49.72 Other toe(s)

    V49.73 Foot

    V49.74 Ankle
       Disarticulation of ankle

    V49.75 Below knee

    V49.76 Above knee
       Disarticulation of knee

    V49.77 Hip
       Disarticulation of hip

⑤ V49.8 Other specified conditions influencing health status

    V49.81 Asymptomatic postmenopausal status (age-related) (natural)

    Excludes: *menopausal and premenopausal disorders (627.0-627.9)*

       postsurgical menopause (256.2)
       premature menopause (256.31)
       symptomatic menopause (627.0-627.9)

    V49.82 Dental sealant status

    V49.83 Awaiting organ transplant status

    V49.84 Bed confinement status

    V49.89 Other specified conditions influencing health status

V49.9 Unspecified

PERSONS ENCOUNTERING HEALTH SERVICES FOR SPECIFIC PROCEDURES AND AFTERCARE (V50-V59)

Note: Categories V51-V58 are intended for use to indicate a reason for care in patients who may have already been treated for some disease or injury not now present, but who are receiving care to consolidate the treatment, to deal with residual states, or to prevent recurrence.

    Excludes: *follow-up examination for medical surveillance following treatment (V67.0-V67.9)*

V50 Elective surgery for purposes other than remedying health states

V50.0 Hair transplant

V50.1 Other plastic surgery for unacceptable cosmetic appearance
    Breast augmentation or reduction
    Face-lift

    Excludes: *plastic surgery following healed injury or operation (V51)*

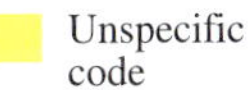

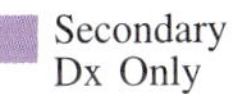

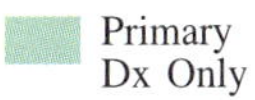

V50.2 Routine or ritual circumcision
Circumcision in the absence of significant medical indication

V50.3 Ear piercing

⑤ **V50.4 Prophylactic organ removal**
Excludes: *organ donations (V59.0-V59.9)*
therapeutic organ removal—code to condition

    V50.41 Breast

    V50.42 Ovary

    V50.49 Other

V50.8 Other

V50.9 Unspecified

V51 Aftercare involving the use of plastic surgery
Plastic surgery following healed injury or operation
Excludes: *cosmetic plastic surgery (V50.1)*
plastic surgery as treatment for current injury—code to condition
repair of scarred tissue—code to scar

V52 Fitting and adjustment of prosthetic device and implant
Includes: removal of device
Excludes: *malfunction or complication of prosthetic device (996.0-996.7)*
status only, without need for care (V43.0-V43.8)

V52.0 Artificial arm (complete) (partial)

V52.1 Artificial leg (complete) (partial)

V52.2 Artificial eye

V52.3 Dental prosthetic device

V52.4 Breast prosthesis and implant
Excludes: *admission for implant insertion (V50.1)*

V52.8 Other specified prosthetic device

V52.9 Unspecified prosthetic device

V53 Fitting and adjustment of other device
Includes: removal of device
replacement of device
Excludes: *status only, without need for care (V45.0-V45.8)*

⑤ **V53.0 Devices related to nervous system and special senses**

    V53.01 Fitting and adjustment of cerebral ventricular (communicating) shunt

    V53.02 Neuropacemaker (brain) (peripheral nerve) (spinal cord)

    V53.09 Fitting and adjustment of other devices related to nervous system and special senses
Auditory substitution device
Visual substitution device

V53.1 Spectacles and contact lenses

V53.2 Hearing aid

⑤ **V53.3 Cardiac device**
Reprogramming

    V53.31 Cardiac pacemaker
Excludes: *mechanical complication of cardiac pacemaker (996.01)*

    V53.32 Automatic implantable cardiac defibrillator

    V53.39 Other cardiac device

V53.4 Orthodontic devices

V53.5 Other intestinal appliance
Excludes: *colostomy (V55.3)*
ileostomy (V55.2)
other artificial opening of digestive tract (V55.4)

● Code new
to this edition

▲ Revision of
existing code

④ ⑤ Fourth or fifth
digit required

V53.6 Urinary devices
Urinary catheter
Excludes: *cystostomy (V55.5)*
nephrostomy (V55.6)
ureterostomy (V55.6)
urethrostomy (V55.6)

V53.7 Orthopedic devices

Orthopedic:
brace
cast

Orthopedic:
corset
shoes

Excludes: *other orthopedic aftercare (V54)*

V53.8 Wheelchair

⑤ **V53.9 Other and unspecified device**

V53.90 **Unspecified device**

V53.91 **Fitting and adjustment of insulin pump**
Insulin pump titration

V53.99 **Other device**

V54 **Other orthopedic aftercare**
Excludes: *fitting and adjustment of orthopedic devices (V53.7)*
malfunction of internal orthopedic device (996.40-996.49)
other complication of nonmechanical nature (996.60-996.79)

⑤ **V54.0 Aftercare involving internal fixation device**
Excludes: *malfunction of internal orthopedic device (996.40-996.49)*
removal of external fixation device (V54.89)

V54.01 **Encounter for removal of internal fixation device**

V54.02 **Encounter for lengthening/adjustment of growth rod**

V54.09 **Other aftercare involving internal fixation device**

⑤ **V54.1 Aftercare for healing traumatic fracture**
Excludes: *aftercare for amputation stump (V54.89)*

V54.10 **Aftercare for healing traumatic fracture of arm, unspecified**

V54.11 **Aftercare for healing traumatic fracture of upper arm**

V54.12 **Aftercare for healing traumatic fracture of lower arm**

V54.13 **Aftercare for healing traumatic fracture of hip**

V54.14 **Aftercare for healing traumatic fracture of leg, unspecified**

V54.15 **Aftercare for healing traumatic fracture of upper leg**
Excludes: *aftercare for healing traumatic fracture of hip (V54.13)*

V54.16 **Aftercare for healing traumatic fracture of lower leg**

V54.17 **Aftercare for healing traumatic fracture of vertebrae**

V54.19 **Aftercare for healing traumatic fracture of other bone**

⑤ **V54.2 Aftercare for healing pathologic fracture**

V54.20 **Aftercare for healing pathologic fracture of arm, unspecified**

V54.21 **Aftercare for healing pathologic fracture of upper arm**

V54.22 **Aftercare for healing pathologic fracture of lower arm**

V54.23 **Aftercare for healing pathologic fracture of hip**

V54.24 **Aftercare for healing pathologic fracture of leg, unspecified**

V54.25 **Aftercare for healing pathologic fracture of upper leg**
Excludes: *aftercare for healing pathologic fracture of hip (V54.23)*

V54.26 **Aftercare for healing pathologic fracture of lower leg**

V54.27 **Aftercare for healing pathologic fracture of vertebrae**

V54.29 **Aftercare for healing pathologic fracture of other bone**

⑤ **V54.8 Other orthopedic aftercare**

V54.81 **Aftercare following joint replacement**
Use additional code to identify joint replacement site (V43.60-V43.69)

V54.89 **Other orthopedic aftercare**
Aftercare for healing fracture NOS

Add 4th or 5th digit	Nonspecific code	Unspecific code	Secondary Dx Only	Primary Dx Only

V54.9 Unspecified orthopedic aftercare

V55 Attention to artificial openings
Includes: adjustment or repositioning of catheter
closure
passage of sounds or bougies
reforming
removal or replacement of catheter
toilet or cleansing

Excludes: *complications of external stoma (519.00-519.09, 569.60-569.69, 997.4, 997.5)*
status only, without need for care (V44.0-V44.9)

V55.0 Tracheostomy

V55.1 Gastrostomy

V55.2 Ileostomy

V55.3 Colostomy

V55.4 Other artificial opening of digestive tract

V55.5 Cystostomy

V55.6 Other artificial opening of urinary tract
Nephrostomy   Urethrostomy
Ureterostomy

V55.7 Artificial vagina

V55.8 Other specified artificial opening

V55.9 Unspecified artificial opening

V56 Encounter for dialysis and dialysis catheter care
Use additional code to identify the associated condition

Excludes: *dialysis preparation—code to condition*

V56.0 Extracorporeal dialysis
Dialysis (renal) NOS

Excludes: *dialysis status (V45.1)*

V56.1 Fitting and adjustment of extracorporeal dialysis catheter
Removal or replacement of catheter
Toilet or cleansing

Use additional code for any concurrent extracorporeal dialysis (V56.0)

V56.2 Fitting and adjustment of peritoneal dialysis catheter
Use additional code for any concurrent peritoneal dialysis (V56.8)

⑤ **V56.3 Encounter for adequacy testing for dialysis**

  V56.31 Encounter for adequacy testing for hemodialysis

  V56.32 Encounter for adequacy testing for peritoneal dialysis
  Peritoneal equilibration test

V56.8 Other dialysis
Peritoneal dialysis

V57 Care involving use of rehabilitation procedures
Use additional code to identify underlying condition

V57.0 Breathing exercises

V57.1 Other physical therapy
Therapeutic and remedial exercises, except breathing

⑤ **V57.2 Occupational therapy and vocational rehabilitation**

  V57.21 Encounter for occupational therapy

  V57.22 Encounter for vocational therapy

V57.3 Speech therapy

V57.4 Orthoptic training

⑤ **V57.8 Other specified rehabilitation procedure**

  V57.81 Orthotic training
  Gait training in the use of artificial limbs

  V57.89 Other
  Multiple training or therapy

V57.9 Unspecified rehabilitation procedure

● Code new   ▲ Revision of   ④ ⑤ Fourth or fifth
to this edition   existing code   digit required

V58 Encounter for other and unspecified procedures and aftercare

> *Excludes:* convalescence and palliative care (V66)

V58.0 Radiotherapy
Encounter or admission for radiotherapy

> *Excludes:* encounter for radioactive implant—code to condition
> radioactive iodine therapy—code to condition

⑤ **V58.1 Encounter for antineoplastic chemotherapy and immunotherapy**
Encounter or admission for chemotherapy

> *Excludes:* chemotherapy and immunotherapy for nonneoplastic conditions—code to condition
> prophylactic chemotherapy against disease which has never been present (V03.0-V07.9)

V58.11 Encounter for antineoplastic chemotherapy

V58.12 Encounter for antineoplastic immunotherapy

V58.2 Blood transfusion, without reported diagnosis

▲ **V58.3 Attention to dressings and sutures**
Change or removal of wound packing

> *Excludes:* attention to drains (V58.49)
> planned postoperative wound closure (V58.41)

● **V58.30 Encounter for change or removal of nonsurgical wound dressing**
Encounter for change or removal of wound dressing NOS

● **V58.31 Encounter for change or removal of surgical wound dressing**

● **V58.32 Encounter for removal of sutures**
Encounter for removal of staples

⑤ **V58.4 Other aftercare following surgery**
Note: Codes from this subcategory should be used in conjunction with other aftercare codes to fully identify the reason for the aftercare encounter

> *Excludes:* aftercare following sterilization reversal surgery (V26.22)
> attention to artificial openings (V55.0-V55.9)
> orthopedic aftercare (V54.0-V54.9)

V58.41 Encounter for planned postoperative wound closure

> *Excludes:* disruption of operative wound (998.3)
> encounter for dressings and suture aftercare (V58.30-V58.32)

V58.42 Aftercare following surgery for neoplasm
Conditions classifiable to 140-239

V58.43 Aftercare following surgery for injury and trauma
Conditions classifiable to 800-999

> *Excludes:* aftercare for healing traumatic fracture (V54.10-V54.19)

V58.44 Aftercare following organ transplant
Use additional code to identify the organ transplanted (V42.0-V42.9)

V58.49 Other specified aftercare following surgery
Change or removal of drains

V58.5 Orthodontics

> *Excludes:* fitting and adjustment of orthodontic device (V53.4)

⑤ **V58.6 Long-term (current) drug use**

> *Excludes:* drug abuse (305.00-305.93)
> drug dependence (304.00-304.93)
> hormone replacement therapy (postmenopausal) (V07.4)

V58.61 Long-term (current) use of anticoagulants

> *Excludes:* long-term (current) use of aspirin (V58.66)

V58.62 Long-term (current) use of antibiotics

V58.63 Long-term (current) use of antiplatelets/antithrombotics

> *Excludes:* long-term (current) use of aspirin (V58.66)

V58.64 Long-term (current) use of non-steroidal anti-inflammatories (NSAID)

> *Excludes:* long-term (current) use of aspirin (V58.66)

V58.65 Long-term (current) use of steroids

V58.66 Long-term (current) use of aspirin

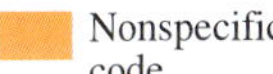

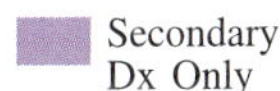

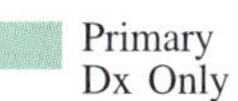

V58.67 **Long-term (current) use of insulin**

V58.69 **Long-term (current) use of other medications**
High-risk medications

⑤ **V58.7** **Aftercare following surgery to specified body systems, not elsewhere classified**
Note: Codes from this subcategory should be used in conjunction with other aftercare codes to fully identify the reason for the aftercare encounter

Excludes: *aftercare following organ transplant (V58.44)*

aftercare following surgery for neoplasm (V58.42)

V58.71 **Aftercare following surgery of the sense organs, NEC**
Conditions classifiable to 360-379, 380-389

V58.72 **Aftercare following surgery of the nervous system, NEC**
Conditions classifiable to 320-359

Excludes: *aftercare following surgery of the sense organs, NEC (V58.71)*

V58.73 **Aftercare following surgery of the circulatory system, NEC**
Conditions classifiable to 390-459

V58.74 **Aftercare following surgery of the respiratory system, NEC**
Conditions classifiable to 460-519

V58.75 **Aftercare following surgery of the teeth, oral cavity and digestive system, NEC**
Conditions classifiable to 520-579

V58.76 **Aftercare following surgery of the genitourinary system, NEC**
Conditions classifiable to 580-629

Excludes: *aftercare following sterilization reversal (V26.22)*

V58.77 **Aftercare following surgery of the skin and subcutaneous tissue, NEC**
Conditions classifiable to 680-709

V58.78 **Aftercare following surgery of the musculoskeletal system, NEC**
Conditions classifiable to 710-739

⑤ **V58.8** **Other specified procedures and aftercare**

V58.81 **Fitting and adjustment of vascular catheter**
Removal or replacement of catheter
Toilet or cleansing

Excludes: *complication of renal dialysis catheter (996.73)*

complication of vascular catheter (996.74)
dialysis preparation — code to condition
encounter for dialysis (V56.0-V56.8)
fitting and adjustment of dialysis catheter (V56.1)

V58.82 **Fitting and adjustment of non-vascular catheter NEC**
Removal or replacement of catheter
Toilet or cleansing

Excludes: *fitting and adjustment of peritoneal dialysis catheter (V56.2)*

fitting and adjustment of urinary catheter (V53.6)

V58.83 **Encounter for therapeutic drug monitoring**
Use additional code for any associated long-term (current) drug use (V58.61-V58.69)

Excludes: *blood-drug testing for medicolegal reasons (V70.4)*

V58.89 **Other specified aftercare**

V58.9 **Unspecified aftercare**

V59 **Donors**

Excludes: *examination of potential donor (V70.8)*

self-donation of organ or tissue—code to condition

⑤ **V59.0** **Blood**

V59.01 **Whole blood**

V59.02 **Stem cells**

V59.09 **Other**

V59.1 **Skin**

V59.2 **Bone**

V59.3 **Bone marrow**

V59.4 **Kidney**

V59.5 **Cornea**

● Code new
to this edition

▲ Revision of
existing code

④ ⑤ Fourth or fifth
digit required

V59.6 Liver

⑤ **V59.7 Egg (oocyte) (ovum)**

V59.70 Egg (oocyte) (ovum) donor, unspecified

V59.71 Egg (oocyte) (ovum) donor, under age 35, anonymous recipient
Egg donor, under age 35 NOS

V59.72 Egg (oocyte) (ovum) donor, under age 35, designated recipient

V59.73 Egg (oocyte) (ovum) donor, age 35 and over, anonymous recipient
Egg donor, age 35 and over NOS

V59.74 Egg (oocyte) (ovum) donor, age 35 and over, designated recipient

V59.8 Other specified organ or tissue

V59.9 Unspecified organ or tissue

PERSONS ENCOUNTERING HEALTH SERVICES IN OTHER CIRCUMSTANCES (V60-V69)

V60 Housing, household, and economic circumstances

V60.0 Lack of housing
Hobos
Social migrants
Tramps
Transients
Vagabonds

V60.1 Inadequate housing
Lack of heating
Restriction of space
Technical defects in home preventing adequate care

V60.2 Inadequate material resources
Economic problem
Poverty NOS

V60.3 Person living alone

V60.4 No other household member able to render care
Person requiring care (has) (is):
family member too handicapped, ill, or otherwise unsuited to render care
partner temporarily away from home
temporarily away from usual place of abode

| Excludes: | *holiday relief care (V60.5)* |

V60.5 Holiday relief care
Provision of health care facilities to a person normally cared for at home, to enable relatives to take a vacation

V60.6 Person living in residential institution
Boarding school resident

V60.8 Other specified housing or economic circumstances

V60.9 Unspecified housing or economic circumstance

V61 Other family circumstances
Includes: when these circumstances or fear of them, affecting the person directly involved or others, are mentioned as the reason, justified or not, for seeking or receiving medical advice or care

V61.0 Family disruption
Divorce
Estrangement

⑤ **V61.1 Counseling for marital and partner problems**

| Excludes: | *problems related to:* |

psychosexual disorders (302.0-302.9)
sexual function (V41.7)

V61.10 Counseling for marital and partner problems, unspecified
Marital conflict
Marital relationship problem
Partner conflict
Partner relationship problem

V61.11 Counseling for victim of spousal and partner abuse

| Excludes: | *encounter for treatment of current injuries due to abuse (995.80-995.85)* |

V61.12 Counseling for perpetrator of spousal and partner abuse

⑤ **V61.2 Parent-child problems**

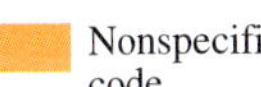

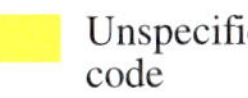

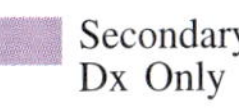

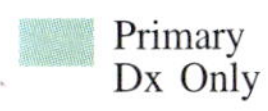

V61.20   **Counseling for parent-child problem, unspecified**
Concern about behavior of child
Parent-child conflict
Parent-child relationship problem

V61.21   **Counseling for victim of child abuse**
Child battering
Child neglect

Excludes: *current injuries due to abuse (995.50-995.59)*

V61.22   **Counseling for perpetrator of parental child abuse**

Excludes: *counseling for non-parental abuser (V62.83)*

V61.29   **Other**
Problem concerning adopted or foster child

V61.3 Problems with aged parents or in-laws

⑤ **V61.4 Health problems within family**

V61.41   **Alcoholism in family**

V61.49   **Other**
Care of sick or handicapped person in family or household
Presence of sick or handicapped person in family or household

V61.5 Multiparity

V61.6 Illegitimacy or illegitimate pregnancy

V61.7 Other unwanted pregnancy

V61.8 Other specified family circumstances
Problems with family members NEC
Sibling relationship problem

V61.9 Unspecified family circumstance

V62 Other psychosocial circumstances
Includes: those circumstances or fear of them, affecting the person directly involved or others, mentioned as the reason, justified or not, for seeking or receiving medical advice or care

Excludes: *previous psychological trauma (V15.41-V15.49)*

V62.0 Unemployment

Excludes: *circumstances when main problem is economic inadequacy or poverty (V60.2)*

V62.1 Adverse effects of work environment

V62.2 Other occupational circumstances or maladjustment
Career choice problem
Dissatisfaction with employment
Occupational problem

V62.3 Educational circumstances
Academic problem
Dissatisfaction with school environment
Educational handicap

V62.4 Social maladjustment
Acculturation problem
Cultural deprivation
Political, religious, or sex discrimination
Social: isolation, persecution

V62.5 Legal circumstances
Imprisonment   Litigation
Legal investigation   Prosecution

V62.6 Refusal of treatment for reasons of religion or conscience

⑤ **V62.8 Other psychological or physical stress, not elsewhere classified**

V62.81   **Interpersonal problems, not elsewhere classified**
Relational problem NOS

V62.82   **Bereavement, uncomplicated**

Excludes: *bereavement as adjustment reaction (309.0)*

V62.83   **Counseling for perpetrator of physical/sexual abuse**

Excludes: *counseling for perpetrator of parental child abuse (V61.22)*
counseling for perpetrator of spousal and partner abuse (V61.12)

● Code new to this edition   ▲ Revision of existing code   ④ ⑤ Fourth or fifth digit required

V62.84 Suicidal ideation
> *Excludes:* suicidal tendencies (300.9)

    V62.89 Other
        Borderline intellectual functioning
        Life circumstance problems
        Phase of life problems
        Religious or spiritual problem

V62.9 Unspecified psychosocial circumstance

V63 Unavailability of other medical facilities for care

V63.0 Residence remote from hospital or other health care facility

V63.1 Medical services in home not available
> *Excludes:* no other household member able to render care (V60.4)

V63.2 Person awaiting admission to adequate facility elsewhere

V63.8 Other specified reasons for unavailability of medical facilities
    Person on waiting list undergoing social agency investigation

V63.9 Unspecified reason for unavailability of medical facilities

V64 Persons encountering health services for specific procedures, not carried out

⑤ **V64.0 Vaccination not carried out**

    V64.00 Vaccination not carried out, unspecified reason

    V64.01 Vaccination not carried out because of acute illness

    V64.02 Vaccination not carried out because of chronic illness or condition

    V64.03 Vaccination not carried out because of immune compromised state

    V64.04 Vaccination not carried out because of allergy to vaccine or component

    V64.05 Vaccination not carried out because of caregiver refusal

    V64.06 Vaccination not carried out because of patient refusal

    V64.07 Vaccination not carried out for religious reasons

    V64.08 Vaccination not carried out because patient had disease being vaccinated against

    V64.09 Vaccination not carried out for other reason

V64.1 Surgical or other procedure not carried out because of contraindication

V64.2 Surgical or other procedure not carried out because of patient's decision

V64.3 Procedure not carried out for other reasons

⑤ **V64.4 Closed surgical procedure converted to open procedure**

    V64.41 Laparoscopic surgical procedure converted to open procedure

    V64.42 Thoracoscopic surgical procedure converted to open procedure

    V64.43 Arthroscopic surgical procedure converted to open procedure

V65 Other persons seeking consultation

V65.0 Healthy person accompanying sick person
    Boarder

⑤ **V65.1 Person consulting on behalf of another person**
    Advice or treatment for nonattending third party

> *Excludes:* concern (normal) about sick person in family (V61.41-V61.49)

    V65.11 Pediatric pre-birth visit for expectant mother

    V65.19 Other person consulting on behalf of another person

V65.2 Person feigning illness
    Malingerer
    Peregrinating patient

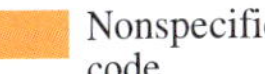

Nonspecific code

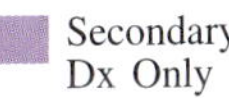

Secondary Dx Only

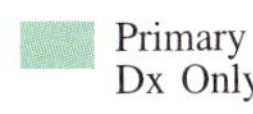

V65.3 Dietary surveillance and counseling
    Dietary surveillance and counseling (in):
      NOS
      colitis
      diabetes mellitus
      food allergies or intolerance
      gastritis
      hypercholesterolemia
      hypoglycemia
      obesity
   Use additional code to identify Body Mass Index (BMI), if known (V85.0-V85.54)

⑤ **V65.4 Other counseling, not elsewhere classified**
    Health:
      advice
      education
      instruction
    Excludes: *counseling (for):*
        contraception (V25.40-V25.49)
        genetic (V26.31-V26.39)
        on behalf of third party (V65.11, V65.19)
        procreative management (V26.4)

   V65.40 Counseling NOS

   V65.41 Exercise counseling

   V65.42 Counseling on substance use and abuse

   V65.43 Counseling on injury prevention

   V65.44 Human immunodeficiency virus [HIV] counseling

   V65.45 Counseling on other sexually transmitted diseases

   V65.46 Encounter for insulin pump training

   V65.49 Other specified counseling

V65.5 Person with feared complaint in whom no diagnosis was made
    Feared condition not demonstrated
    Problem was normal state
    "Worried well"

V65.8 Other reasons for seeking consultation
    Excludes: *specified symptoms*

V65.9 Unspecified reason for consultation

V66 Convalescence and palliative care

   V66.0 Following surgery

   V66.1 Following radiotherapy

   V66.2 Following chemotherapy

   V66.3 Following psychotherapy and other treatment for mental disorder

   V66.4 Following treatment of fracture

   V66.5 Following other treatment

   V66.6 Following combined treatment

   V66.7 Encounter for palliative care
    End-of-life care
    Hospice care
    Terminal care

   Code first underlying disease

   V66.9 Unspecified convalescence

V67 Follow-up examination
    Includes: surveillance only following completed treatment
    Excludes: *surveillance of contraception (V25.40-V25.49)*

⑤ **V67.0 Following surgery**

   V67.00 Following surgery, unspecified

● Code new to this edition   ▲ Revision of existing code   ④ ⑤ Fourth or fifth digit required

> **V67.01 Follow-up vaginal pap smear**
> Vaginal pap smear, status-post hysterectomy for malignant condition

Use additional code to identify:
>> acquired absence of uterus (V45.77)
>> personal history of malignant neoplasm (V10.40-V10.44)

> *Excludes:* *vaginal pap smear status-post hysterectomy for non-malignant condition (V76.47)*

> **V67.09 Following other surgery**

> *Excludes:* *sperm count following sterilization reversal (V26.22)*
>> *sperm count for fertility testing (V26.21)*

V67.1 Following radiotherapy

V67.2 Following chemotherapy
> Cancer chemotherapy follow-up

V67.3 Following psychotherapy and other treatment for mental disorder

V67.4 Following treatment of healed fracture

> *Excludes:* *current (healing) fracture aftercare (V54.0-V54.9)*

(5) **V67.5 Following other treatment**

> **V67.51 Following completed treatment with high-risk medication, NEC**

> *Excludes:* *long-term (current) drug use (V58.61-V58.69)*

> **V67.59 Other**

V67.6 Following combined treatment

V67.9 Unspecified follow-up examination

V68 Encounters for administrative purposes

V68.0 Issue of medical certificates
> Issue of medical certificate of:
>> cause of death
>> fitness
>> incapacity

> *Excludes:* *encounter for general medical examination (V70.0-V70.9)*

V68.1 Issue of repeat prescriptions
> Issue of repeat prescription for:
>> appliance
>> glasses
>> medications

> *Excludes:* *repeat prescription for contraceptives (V25.41-V25.49)*

V68.2 Request for expert evidence

(5) **V68.8 Other specified administrative purpose**

> **V68.81 Referral of patient without examination or treatment**

> **V68.89 Other**

V68.9 Unspecified administrative purpose

V69 Problems related to lifestyle

V69.0 Lack of physical exercise

V69.1 Inappropriate diet and eating habits

> *Excludes:* *anorexia nervosa (307.1)*
>> *bulimia (783.6)*
>> *malnutrition and other nutritional deficiencies (260-269.9)*
>> *other and unspecified eating disorders (307.50-307.59)*

V69.2 High-risk sexual behavior

V69.3 Gambling and betting

> *Excludes:* *pathological gambling (312.31)*

V69.4 Lack of adequate sleep
> Sleep deprivation

> *Excludes:* *insomnia (780.52)*

V69.5 Behavioral insomnia of childhood

V69.8 Other problems related to lifestyle
> Self-damaging behavior

V69.9 Problem related to lifestyle, unspecified

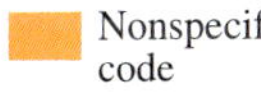

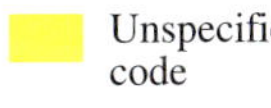

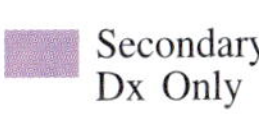

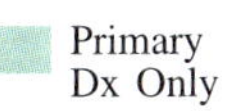

PERSONS WITHOUT REPORTED DIAGNOSIS ENCOUNTERED DURING EXAMINATION AND INVESTIGATION OF INDIVIDUALS AND POPULATIONS (V70-V82)

Note: Nonspecific abnormal findings disclosed at the time of these examinations are classifiable to categories 790-796.

V70 **General medical examination**

Use additional code(s) to identify any special screening examination(s) performed (V73.0-V82.9)

V70.0 **Routine general medical examination at a health care facility**
Health checkup

Excludes: *health checkup of infant or child (V20.2)*
pre-procedural general physical examination (V72.83)

V70.1 **General psychiatric examination, requested by the authority**

V70.2 **General psychiatric examination, other and unspecified**

V70.3 **Other medical examination for administrative purposes**
General medical examination for:

admission to old age home   marriage
adoption   prison
camp   school admission
driving license   sports competition
immigration and naturalization
insurance certification

Excludes: *attendance for issue of medical certificates (V68.0)*
pre-employment screening (V70.5)

V70.4 **Examination for medicolegal reasons**
Blood-alcohol tests
Blood-drug tests
Paternity testing

Excludes: *examination and observation following:*
accidents (V71.3, V71.4)
assault (V71.6)
rape (V71.5)

V70.5 **Health examination of defined subpopulations**
Armed forces personnel   Preschool children
Inhabitants of institutions   Prisoners
Occupational health   Prostitutes
examinations   Refugees
Pre-employment screening   School children
Students

V70.6 **Health examination in population surveys**

Excludes: *special screening (V73.0-V82.9)*

V70.7 **Examination of participant in clinical trial**
Examination of participant or control in clinical research

V70.8 **Other specified general medical examinations**
Examination of potential donor of organ or tissue

V70.9 **Unspecified general medical examination**

V71 **Observation and evaluation for suspected conditions not found**

Note: This category is to be used when persons without a diagnosis are suspected of having an abnormal condition, without signs or symptoms, which requires study, but after examination and observation, is found not to exist. This category is also for use for administrative and legal observation status.

⑤ **V71.0** **Observation for suspected mental condition**

V71.01 **Adult antisocial behavior**
Dyssocial behavior or gang activity in adult without manifest psychiatric disorder

V71.02 **Childhood or adolescent antisocial behavior**
Dyssocial behavior or gang activity in child or adolescent without manifest psychiatric disorder

V71.09 **Other suspected mental condition**

V71.1 **Observation for suspected malignant neoplasm**

V71.2 **Observation for suspected tuberculosis**

V71.3 **Observation following accident at work**

● Code new
to this edition

▲ Revision of
existing code

④ ⑤ Fourth or fifth
digit required

V71.4 **Observation following other accident**
Examination of individual involved in motor vehicle traffic accident

V71.5 **Observation following alleged rape or seduction**
Examination of victim or culprit

V71.6 **Observation following other inflicted injury**
Examination of victim or culprit

V71.7 **Observation for suspected cardiovascular disease**

⑤ **V71.8** **Observation and evaluation for other specified suspected conditions**

V71.81 **Abuse and neglect**

Excludes: adult abuse and neglect (995.80-995.85)
child abuse and neglect (995.50-995.59)

V71.82 **Observation and evaluation for suspected exposure to anthrax**

V71.83 **Observation and evaluation for suspected exposure to other biological agent**

V71.89 **Other specified suspected conditions**

V71.9 **Observation for unspecified suspected condition**

V72 **Special investigations and examinations**
Includes: routine examination of specific system

Excludes: general medical examination (V70.0-V70.4)
general screening examination of defined population groups (V70.5, V70.6, V70.7)
routine examination of infant or child (V20.2)

Use additional code(s) to identify any special screening examination(s) performed (V73.0-V82.9)

V72.0 **Examination of eyes and vision**

⑤ **V72.1** **Examination of ears and hearing**

● **V72.11** **Encounter for hearing examination following failed hearing screening**

● **V72.19** **Other examination of ears and hearing**

V72.2 **Dental examination**

⑤ **V72.3** **Gynecological examination**

Excludes: cervical Papanicolaou smear without general gynecological examination (V76.2)
routine examination in contraceptive management (V25.40-V25.49)

V72.31 **Routine gynecological examination**
General gynecological examination with or without Papanicolaou cervical smear
Pelvic examination (annual) (periodic)

Use additional code to identify routine vaginal Papanicolaou smear (V76.47)

V72.32 **Encounter for Papanicolaou cervical smear to confirm findings of recent normal smear following initial abnormal smear**

⑤ **V72.4** **Pregnancy examination or test**

V72.40 **Pregnancy examination or test, pregnancy unconfirmed**
Possible pregnancy, not (yet) confirmed

V72.41 **Pregnancy examination or test, negative result**

V72.42 **Pregnancy examination or test, positive result**

V72.5 **Radiological examination, not elsewhere classified**
Routine chest x-ray

Excludes: examination for suspected tuberculosis (V71.2)

V72.6 **Laboratory examination**

Excludes: that for suspected disorder (V71.0-V71.9)

V72.7 **Diagnostic skin and sensitization tests**
Allergy tests
Skin tests for hypersensitivity

Excludes: diagnostic skin tests for bacterial diseases (V74.0-V74.9)

⑤ **V72.8** **Other specified examinations**

V72.81 **Pre-operative cardiovascular examination**
Pre-procedural cardiovascular examination

V72.82 **Pre-operative respiratory examination**
Pre-procedural respiratory examination

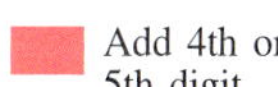

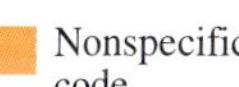

Unspecific
code

Secondary
Dx Only

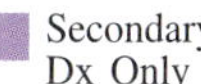

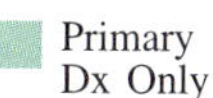

V72.83 **Other specified pre-operative examination**
Other pre-procedural examination
Pre-procedural general physical examination

Excludes: *routine general medical examination (V70.0)*

V72.84 **Pre-operative examination, unspecified**
Pre-procedural examination, unspecified

V72.85 **Other specified examination**

V72.86 **Encounter for blood typing**

V72.9 **Unspecified examination**

V73 **Special screening examination for viral and chlamydial diseases**

V73.0 **Poliomyelitis**

V73.1 **Smallpox**

V73.2 **Measles**

V73.3 **Rubella**

V73.4 **Yellow fever**

V73.5 **Other arthropod-borne viral diseases**
Dengue fever   Viral encephalitis:
Hemorrhagic fever   mosquito-borne
                          tick-borne

V73.6 **Trachoma**

⑤ V73.8 **Other specified viral and chlamydial diseases**

V73.88 **Other specified chlamydial diseases**

V73.89 **Other specified viral diseases**

⑤ V73.9 **Unspecified viral and chlamydial disease**

V73.98 **Unspecified chlamydial disease**

V73.99 **Unspecified viral disease**

V74 **Special screening examination for bacterial and spirochetal diseases**
Includes: diagnostic skin tests for these diseases

V74.0 **Cholera**

V74.1 **Pulmonary tuberculosis**

V74.2 **Leprosy [Hansen's disease]**

V74.3 **Diphtheria**

V74.4 **Bacterial conjunctivitis**

V74.5 **Venereal disease**

V74.6 **Yaws**

V74.8 **Other specified bacterial and spirochetal diseases**
Brucellosis   Tetanus
Leptospirosis   Whooping cough
Plague

V74.9 **Unspecified bacterial and spirochetal disease**

V75 **Special screening examination for other infectious diseases**

V75.0 **Rickettsial diseases**

V75.1 **Malaria**

V75.2 **Leishmaniasis**

V75.3 **Trypanosomiasis**
Chagas' disease
Sleeping sickness

V75.4 **Mycotic infections**

V75.5 **Schistosomiasis**

V75.6 **Filariasis**

V75.7 **Intestinal helminthiasis**

V75.8 **Other specified parasitic infections**

V75.9 **Unspecified infectious disease**

V76 **Special screening for malignant neoplasms**

V76.0 **Respiratory organs**

● Code new   ▲ Revision of   ④ ⑤ Fourth or fifth
to this edition   existing code   digit required

⑤ **V76.1 Breast**

      V76.10 Breast screening, unspecified

      V76.11 Screening mammogram for high-risk patient

      V76.12 Other screening mammogram

      V76.19 Other screening breast examination

V76.2 Cervix
    Routine cervical Papanicolaou smear

    Excludes: *that as part of a general gynecological examination (V72.31)*

V76.3 Bladder

⑤ **V76.4 Other sites**

      V76.41 Rectum

      V76.42 Oral cavity

      V76.43 Skin

      V76.44 Prostate

      V76.45 Testis

      V76.46 Ovary

      V76.47 Vagina
        Vaginal pap smear status-post hysterectomy for non-malignant condition
    Use additional code to identify acquired absence of uterus (V45.77)

    Excludes: *vaginal pap smear status-post hysterectomy for malignant condition (V67.01)*

      V76.49 Other sites

⑤ **V76.5 Intestine**

      V76.50 Intestine, unspecified

      V76.51 Colon

    Excludes: *rectum (V76.41)*

      V76.52 Small intestine

⑤ **V76.8 Other neoplasm**

      V76.81 Nervous system

      V76.89 Other neoplasm

V76.9 Unspecified

V77 Special screening for endocrine, nutritional, metabolic, and immunity disorders

V77.0 Thyroid disorders

V77.1 Diabetes mellitus

V77.2 Malnutrition

V77.3 Phenylketonuria [PKU]

V77.4 Galactosemia

V77.5 Gout

V77.6 Cystic fibrosis
    Screening for mucoviscidosis

V77.7 Other inborn errors of metabolism

V77.8 Obesity

⑤ **V77.9 Other and unspecified endocrine, nutritional, metabolic, and immunity disorders**

      V77.91 Screening for lipoid disorders
        Screening cholesterol level
        Screening for hypercholesterolemia
        Screening for hyperlipidemia

      V77.99 Other and unspecified endocrine, nutritional, metabolic, and immunity disorders

V78 Special screening for disorders of blood and blood-forming organs

V78.0 Iron deficiency anemia

V78.1 Other and unspecified deficiency anemia

V78.2 Sickle-cell disease or trait

V78.3 Other hemoglobinopathies

V78.8 Other disorders of blood and blood-forming organs

Add 4th or 5th digit	Nonspecific code	Unspecific code	Secondary Dx Only	Primary Dx Only

V78.9 Unspecified disorder of blood and blood-forming organs

V79 Special screening for mental disorders and developmental handicaps

V79.0 Depression

V79.1 Alcoholism

V79.2 Mental retardation

V79.3 Developmental handicaps in early childhood

V79.8 Other specified mental disorders and developmental handicaps

V79.9 Unspecified mental disorder and developmental handicap

V80 Special screening for neurological, eye, and ear diseases

V80.0 Neurological conditions

V80.1 Glaucoma

V80.2 Other eye conditions
Screening for:
cataract
congenital anomaly of eye
senile macular lesions

| Excludes: | general vision examination (V72.0) |

V80.3 Ear diseases
| Excludes: | general hearing examination (V72.1) |

V81 Special screening for cardiovascular, respiratory, and genitourinary diseases

V81.0 Ischemic heart disease

V81.1 Hypertension

V81.2 Other and unspecified cardiovascular conditions

V81.3 Chronic bronchitis and emphysema

V81.4 Other and unspecified respiratory conditions
| Excludes: | screening for: |
lung neoplasm (V76.0)
pulmonary tuberculosis (V74.1)

V81.5 Nephropathy
Screening for asymptomatic bacteriuria

V81.6 Other and unspecified genitourinary conditions

V82 Special screening for other conditions

V82.0 Skin conditions

V82.1 Rheumatoid arthritis

V82.2 Other rheumatic disorders

V82.3 Congenital dislocation of hip

V82.4 Maternal postnatal screening for chromosomal anomalies
| Excludes: | antenatal screening by amniocentesis (V28.0) |

V82.5 Chemical poisoning and other contamination
Screening for:
heavy metal poisoning
ingestion of radioactive substance
poisoning from contaminated water supply
radiation exposure

V82.6 Multiphasic screening

● **V82.7** Genetic screening
| Excludes: | genetic testing for procreative management (V26.31-V26.32) |

● **V82.71** Screening for genetic disease carrier status

● **V82.79** Other genetic screening

⑤ **V82.8** Other specified conditions

V82.81 Osteoporosis
Use additional code to identify:
hormone replacement therapy (postmenopausal) status (V07.4)
postmenopausal (natural) status (V49.81)

V82.89 Other specified conditions

  ● Code new
to this edition   ▲ Revision of
existing code   ④ ⑤ Fourth or fifth
digit required

V82.9 Unspecified condition

GENETICS (V83-V84)

V83 Genetic carrier status

⑤ **V83.0** Hemophilia A carrier

    V83.01 Asymptomatic hemophilia A carrier

    V83.02 Symptomatic hemophilia A carrier

⑤ **V83.8** Other genetic carrier status

    V83.81 Cystic fibrosis gene carrier

    V83.89 Other genetic carrier status

V84 Genetic susceptibility to disease

    Includes: Confirmed abnormal gene

Use additional code, if applicable, for any associated family history of the disease (V16-V19)

⑤ **V84.0** Genetic susceptibility to malignant neoplasm

    Code first, if applicable, any current malignant neoplasms (140.0-195.8, 200.0-208.9, 230.0-234.9)

Use additional code, if applicable, for any personal history of malignant neoplasm (V10.0-V10.9)

    V84.01 Genetic susceptibility to malignant neoplasm of breast

    V84.02 Genetic susceptibility to malignant neoplasm of ovary

    V84.03 Genetic susceptibility to malignant neoplasm of prostate

    V84.04 Genetic susceptibility to malignant neoplasm of endometrium

    V84.09 Genetic susceptibility to other malignant neoplasm

V84.8 Genetic susceptibility to other disease

BODY MASS INDEX (V85)

V85 Body Mass Index [BMI]

    Kilograms per meters squared

Note: BMI adult codes are for use for persons over 20 years old

V85.0 Body Mass Index less than 19, adult

V85.1 Body Mass Index between 19-24, adult

⑤ **V85.2** Body Mass Index between 25-29, adult

    V85.21 Body Mass Index 25.0-25.9, adult

    V85.22 Body Mass Index 26.0-26.9, adult

    V85.23 Body Mass Index 27.0-27.9, adult

    V85.24 Body Mass Index 28.0-28.9, adult

    V85.25 Body Mass Index 29.0-29.9, adult

⑤ **V85.3** Body Mass Index between 30-39, adult

    V85.30 Body Mass Index 30.0-30.9, adult

    V85.31 Body Mass Index 31.0-31.9, adult

    V85.32 Body Mass Index 32.0-32.9, adult

    V85.33 Body Mass Index 33.0-33.9, adult

    V85.34 Body Mass Index 34.0-34.9, adult

    V85.35 Body Mass Index 35.0-35.9, adult

    V85.36 Body Mass Index 36.0-36.9, adult

    V85.37 Body Mass Index 37.0-37.9, adult

    V85.38 Body Mass Index 38.0-38.9, adult

    V85.39 Body Mass Index 39.0-39.9, adult

V85.4 Body Mass Index 40 and over, adult

● **85.5** Body Mass Index, pediatric

    Note:BMI pediatric codes are for use for persons age 2-20 years old. These percentiles are based on the growth charts published by the Centers for Disease Control and Prevention (CDC)

    ● **V85.51** Body Mass Index, pediatric, less than 5th percentile for age

    ● **V85.52** Body Mass Index, pediatric, 5th percentile to less than 85th percentile for age

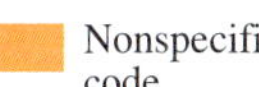 Add 4th or 5th digit   Nonspecific code   Unspecific code   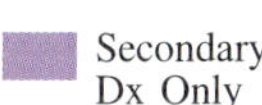 Secondary Dx Only   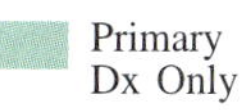 Primary Dx Only

- ● **V85.53** Body Mass Index, pediatric, 85th percentile to less than 95th percentile for age
- ● **V85.54** Body Mass Index, pediatric, greater than or equal to 95th percentile for age

ESTROGEN RECEPTOR STATUS (V86)

● **V86** Estrogen receptor status
  Code first malignant neoplasm of breast (174.0-174.9, 175.0-175.9)

  - ● V86.0 Estrogen receptor positive status (ER+)
  - ● V86.1 Estrogen receptor negative status (ER−)

● Code new
to this edition

▲ Revision of
existing code

④ ⑤ Fourth or fifth
digit required

SUPPLEMENTARY CLASSIFICATION OF EXTERNAL CAUSES OF INJURY AND POISONING (E800-E999)

This section is provided to permit the classification of environmental events, circumstances, and conditions as the cause of injury, poisoning, and other adverse effects. Where a code from this section is applicable, it is intended that it shall be used in addition to a code from one of the main chapters of *ICD-9-CM*, indicating the nature of the condition. Certain other conditions which may be stated to be due to external causes are classified in Chapters 1 to 16 of *ICD-9-CM*. For these, the "E" code classification should be used for more detailed analysis.

Machinery accidents [other than those connected with transport] are classifiable to category E919, in which the fourth-digit allows a broad classification of the type of machinery involved. If a more detailed classification of type of machinery is required, it is suggested that the "Classification of Industrial Accidents according to Agency," prepared by the International Labor Office, be used in addition. This is reproduced in Appendix D, for optional use.

Categories for "late effects" of accidents and other external causes are to be found at E929, E959, E969, E977, E989, and E999.

Definitions and examples related to transport accidents

    (a) A **transport accident** (E800-E848) is any accident involving a device designed primarily for, or being used at the time primarily for, conveying persons or goods from one place to another.

        Includes: accidents involving:
                aircraft and spacecraft (E840-E845)
                watercraft (E830-E838)
                motor vehicle (E810-E825)
                railway (E800-E807)
                other road vehicles (E826-E829)

      In classifying accidents which involve more than one kind of transport, the above order of precedence of transport accidents should be used.

      Accidents involving agriculture and construction machines, such as tractors, cranes, and bulldozers, are regarded as transport accidents only when these vehicles are under their own power on a highway [otherwise the vehicles are regarded as machinery]. Vehicles which can travel on land or water, such as hovercraft and other amphibious vehicles, are regarded as watercraft when on the water, as motor vehicles when on the highway, and as off-road motor vehicles when on land, but off the highway.

        | *Excludes:* | *accidents:*

            in sports which involve the use of transport but where the transport vehicle itself was not involved in the accident
            involving vehicles which are part of industrial equipment used entirely on industrial premises
            occurring during transportation but unrelated to the hazards associated with the means of transportation [e.g., injuries received in a fight on board ship; transport vehicle involved in a cataclysm such as an earthquake]
            to persons engaged in the maintenance or repair of transport equipment or vehicle not in motion, unless injured by another vehicle in motion

    (b) A **railway accident** is a transport accident involving a railway train or other railway vehicle operated on rails, whether in motion or not.

        | *Excludes:* | *accidents:*

            in repair shops
            in roundhouse or on turntable
            on railway premises but not involving a train or other railway vehicle

    (c) A **railway train** or **railway vehicle** is any device with or without cars coupled to it, designed for traffic on a railway.

        Includes: interurban:
                electric car (operated chiefly on its own right-of-way, not open to other traffic)
                streetcar (operated chiefly on its own right-of-way, not open to other traffic)
             railway train, any power [diesel] [electric] [steam]
                funicular
                monorail or two-rail
                subterranean or elevated
             other vehicle designed to run on a railway track

        | *Excludes:* | *interurban electric cars [streetcars] specified to be operating on a right-of-way that forms part of the public street or highway [definition (n)]*

    (d) A **railway** or **railroad** is a right-of-way designed for traffic on rails, which is used by carriages or wagons transporting passengers or freight, and by other rolling stock, and which is not open to other public vehicular traffic.

�—▬ Add 4th or 5th digit   ▬ Nonspecific code   Unspecified code   ▬ Manifestation code

(e) A **motor vehicle accident** is a transport accident involving a motor vehicle. It is defined as a motor vehicle traffic accident or as a motor vehicle nontraffic accident according to whether the accident occurs on a public highway or elsewhere.

Excludes: *injury or damage due to cataclysm*

injury or damage while a motor vehicle, not under its own power, is being loaded on, or unloaded from, another conveyance

(f) A **motor vehicle traffic accident** is any motor vehicle accident occurring on a public highway [i.e., originating, terminating, or involving a vehicle partially on the highway]. A motor vehicle accident is assumed to have occurred on the highway unless another place is specified, except in the case of accidents involving only off-road motor vehicles which are classified as nontraffic accidents unless the contrary is stated.

(g) A **motor vehicle nontraffic accident** is any motor vehicle accident which occurs entirely in any place other than a public highway.

(h) A **public highway [trafficway]** or **street** is the entire width between property lines [or other boundary lines] of every way or place, of which any part is open to the use of the public for purposes of vehicular traffic as a matter of right or custom. A roadway is that part of the public highway designed, improved, and ordinarily used, for vehicular travel.

Includes: approaches (public) to:
docks
public building
station

Excludes: *driveway (private)*

parking lot
ramp
roads in:
airfield
farm
industrial premises
mine
private grounds
quarry

(i) A **motor vehicle** is any mechanically or electrically powered device, not operated on rails, upon which any person or property may be transported or drawn upon a highway. Any object such as a trailer, coaster, sled, or wagon being towed by a motor vehicle is considered a part of the motor vehicle.

Includes: automobile [any type]
bus
construction machinery, farm and industrial machinery, steam roller, tractor, army tank, highway grader, or similar vehicle on wheels or treads, while in transport under own power
fire engine (motorized)
motorcycle
motorized bicycle [moped] or scooter
trolley bus not operating on rails
truck
van

Excludes: *devices used solely to move persons or materials within the confines of a building and its premises, such as:*
building elevator
coal car in mine
electric baggage or mail truck used solely within a railroad station
electric truck used solely within an industrial plant
moving overhead crane

(j) A **motorcycle** is a two-wheeled motor vehicle having one or two riding saddles and sometimes having a third wheel for the support of a sidecar. The sidecar is considered part of the motorcycle.

Includes: motorized:
bicycle [moped]
scooter
tricycle

(k) An **off-road motor vehicle** is a motor vehicle of special design, to enable it to negotiate rough or soft terrain or snow. Examples of special design are high construction, special wheels and tires, driven by treads, or support on a cushion of air.

Includes: all terrain vehicle [ATV]
army tank
hovercraft, on land or swamp
snowmobile

(l) A **driver** of a motor vehicle is the occupant of the motor vehicle operating it or intending to operate it. A **motorcyclist** is the driver of a motorcycle. Other authorized occupants of a motor vehicle are **passengers.**

(m) An **other road vehicle** is any device, except a motor vehicle, in, on, or by which any person or property may be transported on a highway.

    Includes: animal carrying a person or goods
                  animal-drawn vehicle
                  animal harnessed to conveyance
                  bicycle [pedal cycle]
                  streetcar
                  tricycle (pedal)

    Excludes: *pedestrian conveyance [definition (q)]*

(n) A **streetcar** is a device designed and used primarily for transporting persons within a municipality, running on rails, usually subject to normal traffic control signals, and operated principally on a right-of-way that forms part of the traffic way. A trailer being towed by a streetcar is considered a part of the streetcar.

    Includes: interurban or intraurban electric or streetcar, when specified to be operating on a street or public highway
                  tram (car)
                  trolley (car)

(o) A **pedal cycle** is any road transport vehicle operated solely by pedals.

    Includes: bicycle
                  pedal cycle
                  tricycle

    Excludes: *motorized bicycle [definition (i)]*

(p) A **pedal cyclist** is any person riding on a pedal cycle or in a sidecar attached to such a vehicle.

(q) A **pedestrian conveyance** is any human powered device by which a pedestrian may move other than by walking or by which a walking person may move another pedestrian.

    Includes:

baby carriage	roller skates
coaster wagon	scooter
ice skates	skateboard
perambulator	skis
pushcart	sled
pushchair	wheelchair

(r) A **pedestrian** is any person involved in an accident who was not at the time of the accident riding in or on a motor vehicle, railroad train, streetcar, animal-drawn or other vehicle, or on a bicycle or animal.

    Includes: person:
                      changing tire of vehicle
                      in or operating a pedestrian conveyance
                      making adjustment to motor of vehicle
                      on foot

(s) A **watercraft** is any device for transporting passengers or goods on the water.

(t) A **small boat** is any watercraft propelled by paddle, oars, or small motor, with a passenger capacity of less than ten.

    Includes:

boat NOS	rowboat
canoe	rowing shell
coble	scull
dinghy	skiff
punt	small motorboat
raft	

    Excludes: *barge*
                  lifeboat (used after abandoning ship)
                  raft (anchored) being used as diving platform
                  yacht

(u) An **aircraft** is any device for transporting passengers or goods in the air.

    Includes: airplane [any type]
                  balloon
                  bomber
                  dirigible
                  glider (hang)
                  military aircraft
                  parachute

(v) A **commercial transport aircraft** is any device for collective passenger or freight transportation by air, whether run on commercial lines for profit or by government authorities, with the exception of military craft.

Add 4th or 5th digit	Nonspecific code	Unspecified code	Manifestation code

RAILWAY ACCIDENTS (E800-E807)

Note: For definitions of railway accident and related terms see definitions (a) to (d).

Excludes: *accidents involving railway train and:*

> *aircraft (E840.0-E845.9)*
> *motor vehicle (E810.0-E825.9)*
> *watercraft (E830.0-E838.9)*

The following fourth-digit subdivisions are for use with categories E800-E807 to identify the injured person:

.0 Railway employee
Any person who by virtue of his employment in connection with a railway, whether by the railway company or not, is at increased risk of involvement in a railway accident, such as:
catering staff of train
driver
guard
porter
postal staff on train
railway fireman
shunter
sleeping car attendant

.1 Passenger on railway
Any authorized person traveling on a train, except a railway employee.

Excludes: *intending passenger waiting at station (.8)*

> *unauthorized rider on railway vehicle (.8)*

.2 Pedestrian
See definition (r)

.3 Pedal cyclist
See definition (p)

.8 Other specified person
Intending passenger or bystander waiting at station
Unauthorized rider on railway vehicle

.9 Unspecified person

④ **E800 Railway accident involving collision with rolling stock**
Includes: collision between railway trains or railway vehicles, any kind
collision NOS on railway
derailment with antecedent collision with rolling stock or NOS

④ **E801 Railway accident involving collision with other object**
Includes: collision of railway train with:
buffers
fallen tree on railway
gates
platform
rock on railway
streetcar
other nonmotor vehicle
other object

Excludes: *collision with:*

> *aircraft (E840.0-E842.9)*
> *motor vehicle (E810.0-E810.9, E820.0-E822.9)*

④ **E802 Railway accident involving derailment without antecedent collision**

④ **E803 Railway accident involving explosion, fire, or burning**

Excludes: *explosion or fire, with antecedent derailment (E802.0-E802.9)*

> *explosion or fire, with mention of antecedent collision (E800.0-E801.9)*

④ **E804 Fall in, on, or from railway train**
Includes: fall while alighting from or boarding railway train

Excludes: *fall related to collision, derailment, or explosion of railway train (E800.0-E803.9)*

④ **E805 Hit by rolling stock**
Includes: crushed by railway train or part
injured by railway train or part
killed by railway train or part
knocked down by railway train or part
run over by railway train or part

Excludes: *pedestrian hit by object set in motion by railway train (E806.0-E806.9)*

● Code new to this edition   ▲ Revision of existing code   ④ ⑤ Fourth or fifth digit required

④ **E806** **Other specified railway accident**
       Includes: hit by object falling in railway train
                  injured by door or window on railway train
                  nonmotor road vehicle or pedestrian hit by object set in motion by railway train
                  railway train hit by falling:
                    earth NOS
                    rock
                    tree
                  other object

Excludes:	*railway accident due to cataclysm (E908-E909)*

④ **E807** **Railway accident of unspecified nature**
       Includes:
                  found dead on railway right-of-way NOS
                  injured on railway right-of-way NOS
                  railway accident NOS

MOTOR VEHICLE TRAFFIC ACCIDENTS (E810-E819)

Note: For definitions of motor vehicle traffic accident, and related terms, see definitions (e) to (k).

Excludes:	*accidents involving motor vehicle and aircraft (E840.0-E845.9)*

The following fourth-digit subdivisions are for use with categories E810-E819 to identify the injured person:

.0 Driver of motor vehicle other than motorcycle
    See definition (l)

.1 Passenger in motor vehicle other than motorcycle
    See definition (l)

.2 Motorcyclist
    See definition (l)

.3 Passenger on motorcycle
    See definition (l)

.4 Occupant of streetcar

.5 Rider of animal; occupant of animal-drawn vehicle

.6 Pedal cyclist
    See definition (p)

.7 Pedestrian
    See definition (r)

.8 Other specified person
    Occupant of vehicle other than above
    Person in railway train involved in accident
    Unauthorized rider of motor vehicle

.9 Unspecified person

④ **E810** **Motor vehicle traffic accident involving collision with train**

Excludes:	*motor vehicle collision with object set in motion by railway train (E815.0-E815.9)*
	railway train hit by object set in motion by motor vehicle (E818.0-E818.9)

④ **E811** **Motor vehicle traffic accident involving re-entrant collision with another motor vehicle**
       Includes: collision between motor vehicle which accidentally leaves the roadway then
                  re-enters the same roadway, or the opposite roadway on a divided highway, and
                  another motor vehicle

Excludes:	*collision on the same roadway when none of the motor vehicles involved have left*
	and re-entered the roadway (E812.0-E812.9)

④ **E812** **Other motor vehicle traffic accident involving collision with motor vehicle**
       Includes: collision with another motor vehicle parked, stopped, stalled, disabled, or
                  abandoned on the highway
                  motor vehicle collision NOS

Excludes:	*collision with object set in motion by another motor vehicle (E815.0-E815.9)*
	re-entrant collision with another motor vehicle (E811.0-E811.9)

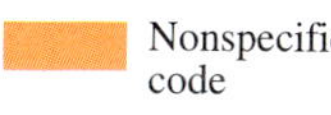

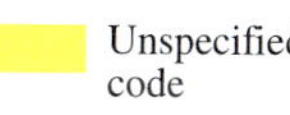

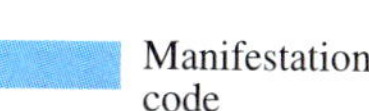

④**E813** **Motor vehicle traffic accident involving collision with other vehicle**
Includes: collision between motor vehicle, any kind, and:
    other road (nonmotor transport) vehicle, such as:
        animal carrying a person
        animal-drawn vehicle
        pedal cycle
    streetcar

Excludes: *collision with:*
    object set in motion by nonmotor road vehicle (E815.0-E815.9)
    pedestrian (E814.0-E814.9)
    nonmotor road vehicle hit by object set in motion by motor vehicle
        (E818.0-E818.9)

④**E814** **Motor vehicle traffic accident involving collision with pedestrian**
Includes: collision between motor vehicle, any kind, and pedestrian
    pedestrian dragged, hit, or run over by motor vehicle, any kind

Excludes: *pedestrian hit by object set in motion by motor vehicle (E818.0-E818.9)*

④**E815** **Other motor vehicle traffic accident involving collision on the highway**
Includes: collision (due to loss of control) (on highway) between motor vehicle, any kind, and:
    abutment (bridge) (overpass)
    animal (herded) (unattended)
    fallen stone, traffic sign, tree, utility pole
    guard rail or boundary fence
    interhighway divider
    landslide (not moving)
    object set in motion by railway train or road vehicle (motor) (nonmotor)
    object thrown in front of motor vehicle
    safety island
    temporary traffic sign or marker
    wall of cut made for road
    other object, fixed, movable, or moving

Excludes: *collision with:*
    any object off the highway (resulting from loss of control) (E816.0-E816.9)
    any object which normally would have been off the highway and is not stated to
        have been on it (E816.0-E816.9)
    motor vehicle parked, stopped, stalled, disabled, or abandoned on highway
        (E812.0-E812.9)
    moving landslide (E909)
    motor vehicle hit by object:
    set in motion by railway train or road vehicle (motor) (nonmotor)
        (E818.0-E818.9)
    thrown into or on vehicle (E818.0-E818.9)

    ● Code new   ▲ Revision of   ④ ⑤ Fourth or fifth
       to this edition   existing code   digit required

④ **E816** **Motor vehicle traffic accident due to loss of control, without collision on the highway**
  Includes: motor vehicle:
    failing to make curve and:
      colliding with object off the highway
      overturning
      stopping abruptly off the highway
    going out of control (due to):
      blowout and:
        colliding with object off the highway
        overturning
        stopping abruptly off the highway
      burst tire and:
        colliding with object off the highway
        overturning
        stopping abruptly off the highway
      driver falling asleep and:
        colliding with object off the highway
        overturning
        stopping abruptly off the highway
      driver inattention and:
        colliding with object off the highway
        overturning
        stopping abruptly off the highway
      excessive speed and:
        colliding with object off the highway
        overturning
        stopping abruptly off the highway
      failure of mechanical part and:
        colliding with object off the highway
        overturning
        stopping abruptly off the highway

    Excludes: *collision on highway following loss of control (E810.0-E815.9)*
          loss of control of motor vehicle following collision on the highway
            (E810.0-E815.9)

④ **E817** **Noncollision motor vehicle traffic accident while boarding or alighting**
  Includes: fall down stairs of motor bus while boarding or alighting
    fall from car in street while boarding or alighting
    injured by moving part of the vehicle while boarding or alighting
    trapped by door of motor bus while boarding or alighting

④ **E818** **Other noncollision motor vehicle traffic accident**
  Includes: accidental poisoning from exhaust gas generated by motor vehicle while in motion
    breakage of any part of motor vehicle while in motion
    explosion of any part of motor vehicle while in motion
    fall, jump, or being accidentally pushed from motor vehicle while in motion
    fire starting in motor vehicle while in motion
    hit by object thrown into or on motor vehicle while in motion
    injured by being thrown against some part of, or object in motor vehicle while in
      motion
    injury from moving part of motor vehicle while in motion
    object falling in or on motor vehicle while in motion
    object thrown on motor vehicle while in motion
    collision of railway train or road vehicle except motor vehicle, with object set in
      motion by motor vehicle
    motor vehicle hit by object set in motion by railway train or road vehicle (motor)
      (nonmotor)
    pedestrian, railway train, or road vehicle (motor) (nonmotor) hit by object set in
      motion by motor vehicle

    Excludes: *collision between motor vehicle and:*
         object set in motion by railway train or road vehicle (motor) (nonmotor)
           (E815.0-E815.9)
         object thrown towards the motor vehicle (E815.0-E815.9)
       person overcome by carbon monoxide generated by stationary motor vehicle off
         the roadway with motor running (E868.2)

④ **E819** **Motor vehicle traffic accident of unspecified nature**
  Includes: motor vehicle traffic accident NOS
    traffic accident NOS

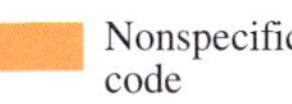

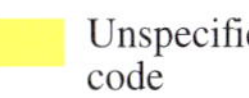

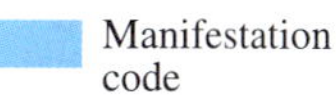

MOTOR VEHICLE NONTRAFFIC ACCIDENTS (E820-E825)

Note: For definitions of motor vehicle nontraffic accident and related terms see definitions (a) to (k).

Includes: accidents involving motor vehicles being used in recreational or sporting activities off the highway

collision and noncollision motor vehicle accidents occurring entirely off the highway

Excludes: *accidents involving motor vehicle and:*

aircraft (E840.0-E845.9)
watercraft (E830.0-E838.9)
accidents, not on the public highway, involving agricultural and construction machinery but not involving another motor vehicle (E919.0, E919.2, E919.7)

The following fourth-digit subdivisions are for use with categories E820-E825 to identify the injured person:

.0 Driver of motor vehicle other than motorcycle
See definition (l)

.1 Passenger in motor vehicle other than motorcycle
See definition (l)

.2 Motorcyclist
See definition (l)

.3 Passenger on motorcycle
See definition (l)

.4 Occupant of streetcar

.5 Rider of animal; occupant of animal-drawn vehicle

.6 Pedal cyclist
See definition (p)

.7 Pedestrian
See definition (r)

.8 Other specified person
Occupant of vehicle other than above
Person on railway train involved in accident
Unauthorized rider of motor vehicle

.9 Unspecified person

④ **E820** **Nontraffic accident involving motor-driven snow vehicle**
Includes: breakage of part of motor-driven snow vehicle (not on public highway)
fall from motor-driven snow vehicle (not on public highway)
hit by motor-driven snow vehicle (not on public highway)
overturning of motor-driven snow vehicle (not on public highway)
run over or dragged by motor-driven snow vehicle (not on public highway)
collision of motor-driven snow vehicle with:
animal (being ridden) (-drawn vehicle)
another off-road motor vehicle
other motor vehicle, not on public highway
railway train
other object, fixed or movable
injury caused by rough landing of motor-driven snow vehicle (after leaving ground on rough terrain)

Excludes: *accident on the public highway involving motor driven snow vehicle*
(E810.0-E819.9)

● Code new to this edition   ▲ Revision of existing code   ④ ⑤ Fourth or fifth digit required

④ **E821 Nontraffic accident involving other off-road motor vehicle**
      Includes: breakage of part of off-road motor vehicle, except snow vehicle (not on public highway)
                 fall from off-road motor vehicle, except snow vehicle (not on public highway)
                 hit by off-road motor vehicle, except snow vehicle (not on public highway)
                 overturning of off-road motor vehicle, except snow vehicle (not on public highway)
                 run over or dragged by off-road motor vehicle, except snow vehicle (not on public highway)
                 thrown against some part of or object in off-road motor vehicle, except snow vehicle (not on public highway)
                 collision with:
                   animal (being ridden) (-drawn vehicle)
                   another off-road motor vehicle, except snow vehicle
                   other motor vehicle, not on public highway
                   other object, fixed or movable

      Excludes: *accident on public highway involving off-road motor vehicle (E810.0-E819.9)*
                 collision between motor driven snow vehicle and other off-road motor vehicle (E820.0-E820.9)
                 hovercraft accident on water (E830.0-E838.9)

④ **E822 Other motor vehicle nontraffic accident involving collision with moving object**
      Includes: collision, not on public highway, between motor vehicle, except off-road motor vehicle and:
                 animal
                 nonmotor vehicle
                 other motor vehicle, except off-road motor vehicle
                 pedestrian
                 railway train
                 other moving object

      Excludes: *collision with:*
                 motor-driven snow vehicle (E820.0-E820.9)
                 other off-road motor vehicle (E821.0-E821.9)

④ **E823 Other motor vehicle nontraffic accident involving collision with stationary object**
      Includes: collision, not on public highway, between motor vehicle, except off-road motor vehicle, and any object, fixed or movable, but not in motion

④ **E824 Other motor vehicle nontraffic accident while boarding and alighting**
      Includes: fall while boarding or alighting from motor vehicle, except off-road motor vehicle, not on public highway
                 injury from moving part of motor vehicle while boarding or alighting from motor vehicle, except off-road motor vehicle, not on public highway
                 trapped by door of motor vehicle while boarding or alighting from motor vehicle, except off-road motor vehicle, not on public highway

④ **E825 Other motor vehicle nontraffic accident of other and unspecified nature**
      Includes: accidental poisoning from carbon monoxide generated by motor vehicle while in motion, not on public highway
                 breakage of any part of motor vehicle while in motion, not on public highway
                 explosion of any part of motor vehicle while in motion, not on public highway
                 fall, jump, or being accidentally pushed from motor vehicle while in motion, not on public highway
                 fire starting in motor vehicle while in motion, not on public highway
                 hit by object thrown into, towards, or on motor vehicle while in motion, not on public highway
                 injured by being thrown against some part of, or object in motor vehicle while in motion, not on public highway
                 injury from moving part of motor vehicle while in motion, not on public highway
                 object falling in or on motor vehicle while in motion, not on public highway
                 motor vehicle nontraffic accident NOS

      Excludes: *fall from or in stationary motor vehicle (E884.9, E885.9)*
                 overcome by carbon monoxide or exhaust gas generated by stationary motor vehicle off the roadway with motor running (E868.2)
                 struck by falling object from or in stationary motor vehicle (E916)

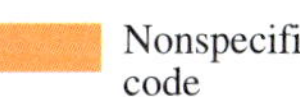

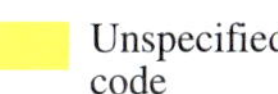

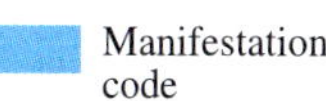

OTHER ROAD VEHICLE ACCIDENTS (E826-E829)

Note: Other road vehicle accidents are transport accidents involving road vehicles other than motor vehicles. For definitions of other road vehicle and related terms see definitions (m) to (o).

Includes: accidents involving other road vehicles being used in recreational or sporting activities

Excludes: *collision of other road vehicle [any] with:*
  aircraft (E840.0-E845.9)
  motor vehicle (E813.0-E813.9, E820.0-E822.9)
  railway train (E801.0-E801.9)

The following fourth-digit subdivisions are for use with categories E826-E829 to identify the injured person:

.0 Pedestrian
   See definition (r)

.1 Pedal cyclist
   See definition (p)

.2 Rider of animal

.3 Occupant of animal-drawn vehicle

.4 Occupant of streetcar

.8 Other specified person

.9 Unspecified person

④ **E826 Pedal cycle accident**
[0-9]

Includes: breakage of any part of pedal cycle
collision between pedal cycle and:
   animal (being ridden) (herded) (unattended)
   another pedal cycle
   nonmotor road vehicle, any
   pedestrian
   other object, fixed, movable, or moving, not set in motion by motor vehicle,
      railway train, or aircraft
entanglement in wheel of pedal cycle
fall from pedal cycle
hit by object falling or thrown on the pedal cycle
pedal cycle accident NOS
pedal cycle overturned

④ **E827 Animal-drawn vehicle accident**
[0,2-4,8,9]

Includes: breakage of any part of vehicle
collision between animal-drawn vehicle and:
   animal (being ridden) (herded) (unattended)
   nonmotor road vehicle, except pedal cycle
   pedestrian, pedestrian conveyance, or pedestrian vehicle
   other object, fixed, movable, or moving, not set in motion by motor vehicle,
      railway train, or aircraft
fall from animal-drawn vehicle
knocked down by animal-drawn vehicle
overturning of animal-drawn vehicle
run over by animal-drawn vehicle
thrown from animal-drawn vehicle

Excludes: *collision of animal-drawn vehicle with pedal cycle (E826.0-E826.9)*

● Code new
to this edition

▲ Revision of
existing code

④ ⑤ Fourth or fifth
digit required

④ **E828** **Accident involving animal being ridden**
[0,2,4,8,9]

    Includes: collision between animal being ridden and:
      another animal
      nonmotor road vehicle, except pedal cycle, and animal-drawn vehicle
      pedestrian, pedestrian conveyance, or pedestrian vehicle
      other object, fixed, movable, or moving, not set in motion by motor vehicle,
        railway train, or aircraft
    fall from animal being ridden
    knocked down by animal being ridden
    thrown from animal being ridden
    trampled by animal being ridden
    ridden animal stumbled and fell

    Excludes: *collision of animal being ridden with:*
      animal-drawn vehicle (E827.0-E827.9)
      pedal cycle (E826.0-E826.9)

④ **E829** **Other road vehicle accidents**
[0,4,8,9]

    Includes: accident while boarding or alighting from:
      streetcar
      nonmotor road vehicle not classifiable to E826-E828
    blow from object in:
      streetcar
      nonmotor road vehicle not classifiable to E826-E828
    breakage of any part of:
      streetcar
      nonmotor road vehicle not classifiable to E826-E828
    caught in door of:
      streetcar
      nonmotor road vehicle not classifiable to E826-E828
    derailment of:
      streetcar
      nonmotor road vehicle not classifiable to E826-E828
    fall in, on, or from:
      streetcar
      nonmotor road vehicle not classifiable to E826-E828
    fire in:
      streetcar
      nonmotor road vehicle not classifiable to E826-E828
    collision between streetcar or nonmotor road vehicle, except as in E826-E828, and:
      animal (not being ridden)
      another nonmotor road vehicle not classifiable to E826-E828
      pedestrian
      other object, fixed, movable, or moving, not set in motion by motor vehicle,
        railway train, or aircraft
    nonmotor road vehicle accident NOS
    streetcar accident NOS

    Excludes: *collision with:*
      animal being ridden (E828.0-E828.9)
      animal-drawn vehicle (E827.0-E827.9)
      pedal cycle (E826.0-E826.9)

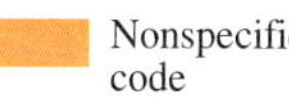
Add 4th or 5th digit

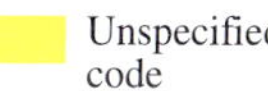
Nonspecific code

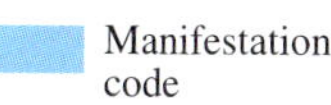
Unspecified code

Manifestation code

WATER TRANSPORT ACCIDENTS (E830-E838)

Note: For definitions of water transport accident and related terms see definitions (a), (s), and (t).

Includes: watercraft accidents in the course of recreational activities

Excludes: *accidents involving both aircraft, including objects set in motion by aircraft, and watercraft (E840.0-E845.9)*

The following fourth-digit subdivisions are for use with categories E830-E838 to identify the injured person:

.0 Occupant of small boat, unpowered

.1 Occupant of small boat, powered
See definition (t)

Excludes: *water skier (.4)*

.2 Occupant of other watercraft—crew
Persons:
engaged in operation of watercraft
providing passenger services [cabin attendants, ship's physician, catering personnel]
working on ship during voyage in other capacity [musician in band, operators of shops and beauty parlors]

.3 Occupant of other watercraft—other than crew
Passenger
Occupant of lifeboat, other than crew, after abandoning ship

.4 Water skier

.5 Swimmer

.6 Dockers, stevedores
Longshoreman employed on the dock in loading and unloading ships

.8 Other specified person
Immigration and custom officials on board ship
Person:
accompanying passenger or member of crew
visiting boat
Pilot (guiding ship into port)

.9 Unspecified person

④ **E830 Accident to watercraft causing submersion**
Includes: submersion and drowning due to:
boat overturning
boat submerging
falling or jumping from burning ship
falling or jumping from crushed watercraft
ship sinking
other accident to watercraft

④ **E831 Accident to watercraft causing other injury**
Includes: any injury, except submersion and drowning, as a result of an accident to watercraft
burned while ship on fire
crushed between ships in collision
crushed by lifeboat after abandoning ship
fall due to collision or other accident to watercraft
hit by falling object due to accident to watercraft
injured in watercraft accident involving collision
struck by boat or part thereof after fall or jump from damaged boat

Excludes: *burns from localized fire or explosion on board ship (E837.0-E837.9)*

④ **E832 Other accidental submersion or drowning in water transport accident**
Includes: submersion or drowning as a result of an accident other than accident to the watercraft, such as:
fall:
from gangplank
from ship
overboard
thrown overboard by motion of ship
washed overboard

Excludes: *submersion or drowning of swimmer or diver who voluntarily jumps from boat not involved in an accident (E910.0-E910.9)*

④ **E833 Fall on stairs or ladders in water transport**

Excludes: *fall due to accident to watercraft (E831.0-E831.9)*

● Code new to this edition   ▲ Revision of existing code   ④ ⑤ Fourth or fifth digit required

④ **E834** **Other fall from one level to another in water transport**
> *Excludes:* fall due to accident to watercraft (E831.0-E831.9)

④ **E835** **Other and unspecified fall in water transport**
> *Excludes:* fall due to accident to watercraft (E831.0-E831.9)

④ **E836** **Machinery accident in water transport**
Includes: injuries in water transport caused by:
        deck machinery
        engine room machinery
        galley machinery
        laundry machinery
        loading machinery

④ **E837** **Explosion, fire, or burning in watercraft**
Includes: explosion of boiler on steamship
        localized fire on ship

> *Excludes:* burning ship (due to collision or explosion) resulting in:
>   submersion or drowning (E830.0-E830.9)
>   other injury (E831.0-E831.9)

④ **E838** **Other and unspecified water transport accident**
Includes: accidental poisoning by gases or fumes on ship
        atomic power plant malfunction in watercraft
        crushed between ship and stationary object [wharf]
        crushed between ships without accident to watercraft
        crushed by falling object on ship or while loading or unloading
        hit by boat while water skiing
        struck by boat or part thereof (after fall from boat)
        watercraft accident NOS

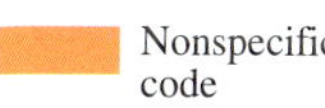

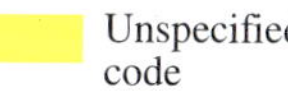

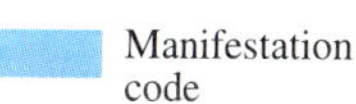

Manifestation
code

AIR AND SPACE TRANSPORT ACCIDENTS (E840-E845)

Note: For definition of aircraft and related terms see definitions (u) and (v).

The following fourth-digit subdivisions are for use with categories E840-E845 to identify the injured person:

.0 Occupant of spacecraft

.1 Occupant of military aircraft, any
Crew in military aircraft [air force] [army] [national guard] [navy]
Passenger (civilian) (military) in military aircraft [air force] [army] [national guard] [navy]
Troops in military aircraft [air force] [army] [national guard] [navy]

Excludes: *occupants of aircraft operated under jurisdiction of police departments (.5)*
parachutist (.7)

.2 Crew of commercial aircraft (powered) in surface to surface transport

.3 Other occupant of commercial aircraft (powered) in surface to surface transport
Flight personnel:
  not part of crew
  on familiarization flight
Passenger on aircraft (powered) NOS

.4 Occupant of commercial aircraft (powered) in surface to air transport
Occupant [crew] [passenger] of aircraft (powered) engaged in activities, such as:
  aerial spraying (crops) (fire retardants)
  air drops of emergency supplies
  air drops of parachutists, except from military craft
  crop dusting
  lowering of construction material [bridge or telephone pole]
  sky writing

.5 Occupant of other powered aircraft
Occupant [crew] [passenger] of aircraft [powered] engaged in activities, such as:
  aerobatic flying
  aircraft racing
  rescue operation
  storm surveillance
  traffic surveillance
Occupant of private plane NOS

.6 Occupant of unpowered aircraft, except parachutist
Occupant of aircraft classifiable to E842

.7 Parachutist (military) (other)
Person making voluntary descent

Excludes: *person making descent after accident to aircraft (.1-.6)*

.8 Ground crew, airline employee
Persons employed at airfields (civil) (military) or launching pads, not occupants of aircraft

.9 Other person

④**E840 Accident to powered aircraft at takeoff or landing**
Includes: collision of aircraft with any object, fixed, movable, or moving while taking off or landing
crash while taking off or landing
explosion on aircraft while taking off or landing
fire on aircraft while taking off or landing
forced landing

④**E841 Accident to powered aircraft, other and unspecified**
Includes: aircraft accident NOS
aircraft crash or wreck NOS
any accident to powered aircraft while in transit or when not specified whether in transit, taking off, or landing
collision of aircraft with another aircraft, bird, or any object, while in transit
explosion on aircraft while in transit
fire on aircraft while in transit

● Code new
to this edition

▲ Revision of
existing code

④ ⑤ Fourth or fifth
digit required

④ **E842** **Accident to unpowered aircraft**
[6-9]

      Includes: any accident, except collision with powered aircraft, to:
              balloon
              glider
              hang glider
              kite carrying a person
              hit by object falling from unpowered aircraft

④ **E843** **Fall in, on, or from aircraft**
[0-9]

      Includes: accident in boarding or alighting from aircraft, any kind
              fall in, on, or from aircraft [any kind], while in transit, taking off, or landing,
                  except when as a result of an accident to aircraft

④ **E844** **Other specified air transport accidents**
[0-9]

      Includes: hit by:
              aircraft without accident to aircraft
              object falling from aircraft without accident to aircraft
            injury by or from:
              machinery on aircraft without accident to aircraft
              rotating propeller without accident to aircraft
              voluntary parachute descent without accident to aircraft
            poisoning by carbon monoxide from aircraft while in transit without accident to
                aircraft
            sucked into jet without accident to aircraft
            any accident involving other transport vehicle (motor) (nonmotor) due to being hit
                by object set in motion by aircraft (powered)

       Excludes: *air sickness (E903)*
              effects of:
                high altitude (E902.0-E902.1)
                pressure change (E902.0-E902.1)
              injury in parachute descent due to accident to aircraft (840.0-E842.9)

④ **E845** **Accident involving spacecraft**
[0,8,9]

      Includes: launching pad accident
       Excludes: *effects of weightlessness in spacecraft (E928.0)*

VEHICLE ACCIDENTS NOT ELSEWHERE CLASSIFIABLE (E846-E848)

E846 **Accidents involving powered vehicles used solely within the buildings and premises of industrial or commercial establishment**
      Accident to, on, or involving:
          battery powered airport passenger vehicle
          battery powered trucks (baggage) (mail)
          coal car in mine
          logging car
          self propelled truck, industrial
          station baggage truck (powered)
          tram, truck, or tub (powered) in mine or quarry
      Breakage of any part of vehicle
      Collision with:
          pedestrian
          other vehicle or object within premises
      Explosion of powered vehicle, industrial or commercial
      Fall from powered vehicle, industrial or commercial
      Overturning of powered vehicle, industrial or commercial
      Struck by powered vehicle, industrial or commercial

       Excludes: *accidental poisoning by exhaust gas from vehicle not elsewhere classifiable*
               (E868.2)
              injury by crane, lift (fork), or elevator (E919.2)

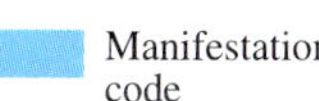

E847 Accidents involving cable cars not running on rails
 Accident to, on, or involving:
  cable car, not on rails
  ski chair-lift
  ski-lift with gondola
  téléférique
 Breakage of cable
 Caught or dragged by cable car, not on rails
 Fall or jump from cable car, not on rails
 Object thrown from or in cable car, not on rails

E848 Accidents involving other vehicles, not elsewhere classifiable
 Accident to, on, or involving:
  ice yacht
  land yacht
  nonmotor, nonroad vehicle NOS

E849 Place of occurrence
 The following category is for use to denote the place where the injury or poisoning occurred.

E849.0 Home

Apartment	Private:
Boarding house	driveway
Farm house	garage
Home premises	garden
House (residential)	home
Noninstitutional place	walk
of residence	Swimming pool in private house or garden
	Yard of home

 Excludes: *home under construction but not yet occupied (E849.3)*
   institutional place of residence (E849.7)

E849.1 Farm
 Farm:
  buildings
  land under cultivation

 Excludes: *farm house and home premises of farm (E849.0)*

E849.2 Mine and quarry

Gravel pit	Tunnel under construction
Sand pit	

E849.3 Industrial place and premises

Building under	Industrial yard
construction	Loading platform (factory) (store)
Dockyard	Plant, industrial
Dry dock	Railway yard
Factory	Shop (place of work)
building	Warehouse
premises	Workhouse
Garage (place of work)	

E849.4 Place for recreation and sport

Amusement park	Public park
Baseball field	Racecourse
Basketball court	Resort NOS
Beach resort	Riding school
Cricket ground	Rifle range
Fives court	Seashore resort
Football field	Skating rink
Golf course	Sports ground
Gymnasium	Sports palace
Hockey field	Stadium
Holiday camp	Swimming pool, public
Ice palace	Tennis court
Lake resort	Vacation resort
Mountain resort	
Playground, including	
school playground	

 Excludes: *that in private house or garden (E849.0)*

E849.5 Street and highway

● Code new
   to this edition   ▲ Revision of
   existing code   ④ ⑤ Fourth or fifth
   digit required

E849.6 Public building

Building (including adjacent grounds) used by the general public or by a particular group of the public, such as:

airport	nightclub
bank	office
café	office building
casino	opera house
church	post office
cinema	public hall
clubhouse	radio broadcasting station
courthouse	restaurant
dance hall	school (state) (public) (private)
garage building (for car storage)	shop, commercial
	station (bus) (railway)
hotel	store
market (grocery or other commodity)	theater
movie house	
music hall	

Excludes: *home garage (E849.0)*
industrial building or workplace (E849.3)

E849.7 Residential institution

Children's home	Old people's home
Dormitory	Orphanage
Hospital	Prison
Jail	Reform school

E849.8 Other specified places

Beach NOS	Pond or pool (natural)
Canal	Prairie
Caravan site NOS	Public place NOS
Derelict house	Railway line
Desert	Reservoir
Dock	River
Forest	Sea
Harbor	Seashore NOS
Hill	Stream
Lake NOS	Swamp
Mountain	Trailer court
Parking lot	Woods
Parking place	

E849.9 Unspecified place

ACCIDENTAL POISONING BY DRUGS, MEDICINAL SUBSTANCES, AND BIOLOGICALS (E850-E858)

Includes: accidental overdose of drug, wrong drug given or taken in error, and drug taken inadvertently

accidents in the use of drugs and biologicals in medical and surgical procedures

Excludes: *administration with suicidal or homicidal intent or intent to harm, or in circumstances classifiable to E980-E989 (E950.0-E950.5, E962.0, E980.0-E980.5)*

correct drug properly administered in therapeutic or prophylactic dosage, as the cause of adverse effect (E930.0-E949.9)

See Alphabetic Index for more complete list of specific drugs to be classified under the fourth-digit subdivisions. The American Hospital Formulary numbers can be used to classify new drugs listed by the American Hospital Formulary Service (AHFS). See appendix C.

E850 Accidental poisoning by analgesics, antipyretics, and antirheumatics

E850.0 Heroin

Diacetylmorphine

E850.1 Methadone

E850.2 Other opiates and related narcotics

Codeine [methylmorphine]	Morphine
Meperidine [pethidine]	Opium (alkaloids)

E850.3 Salicylates

Acetylsalicylic acid [aspirin]
Amino derivatives of salicylic acid
Salicylic acid salts

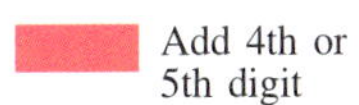

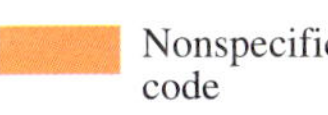

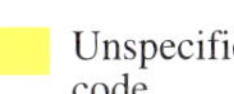

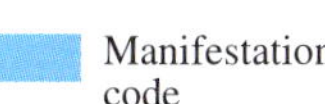

E850.4 Aromatic analgesics, not elsewhere classified
Acetanilid
Paracetamol [acetaminophen]
Phenacetin [acetophenetidin]

E850.5 Pyrazole derivatives
Aminophenazone [amidopyrine]
Phenylbutazone

E850.6 Antirheumatics [antiphlogistics]
Gold salts   Indomethacin

> *Excludes:* *salicylates (E850.3)*
>   *steroids (E858.0)*

E850.7 Other non-narcotic analgesics
Pyrabital

E850.8 Other specified analgesics and antipyretics
Pentazocine

E850.9 Unspecified analgesic or antipyretic

E851 Accidental poisoning by barbiturates
Amobarbital [amylobarbitone]
Barbital [barbitone]
Butabarbital [butabarbitone]
Pentobarbital [pentobarbitone]
Phenobarbital [phenobarbitone]
Secobarbital [quinalbarbitone]

> *Excludes:* *thiobarbiturates (E855.1)*

E852 Accidental poisoning by other sedatives and hypnotics

E852.0 Chloral hydrate group

E852.1 Paraldehyde

E852.2 Bromine compounds
Bromides   Carbromal (derivatives)

E852.3 Methaqualone compounds

E852.4 Glutethimide group

E852.5 Mixed sedatives, not elsewhere classified

E852.8 Other specified sedatives and hypnotics

E852.9 Unspecified sedative or hypnotic
Sleeping:
  drug NOS
  pill NOS
  tablet NOS

E853 Accidental poisoning by tranquilizers

E853.0 Phenothiazine-based tranquilizers
Chlorpromazine   Prochlorperazine
Fluphenazine   Promazine

E853.1 Butyrophenone-based tranquilizers
Haloperidol   Trifluperidol
Spiperone

E853.2 Benzodiazepine-based tranquilizers
Chlordiazepoxide   Lorazepam
Diazepam   Medazepam
Flurazepam   Nitrazepam

E853.8 Other specified tranquilizers
Hydroxyzine   Meprobamate

E853.9 Unspecified tranquilizer

E854 Accidental poisoning by other psychotropic agents

E854.0 Antidepressants
Amitriptyline   Monoamine oxidase [MAO] inhibitors
Imipramine

E854.1 Psychodysleptics [hallucinogens]
Cannabis derivatives   Mescaline
Lysergide [LSD]   Psilocin
Marihuana (derivatives) Psilocybin

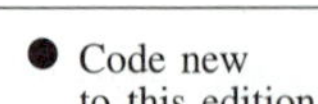
Code new
to this edition

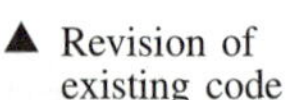
Revision of
existing code

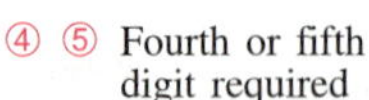
Fourth or fifth
digit required

E854.2 **Psychostimulants**
Amphetamine   Caffeine

Excludes: central appetite depressants (E858.8)

E854.3 **Central nervous system stimulants**
Analeptics   Opiate antagonists

E854.8 **Other psychotropic agents**

E855 **Accidental poisoning by other drugs acting on central and autonomic nervous system**

E855.0 **Anticonvulsant and anti-Parkinsonism drugs**
Amantadine
Hydantoin derivatives
Levodopa [L-dopa]
Oxazolidine derivatives [paramethadione] [trimethadione]
Succinimides

E855.1 **Other central nervous system depressants**
Ether   Intravenous anesthetics
Gaseous anesthetics   Thiobarbiturates, such as thiopental sodium
Halogenated hydrocarbon
 derivatives

E855.2 **Local anesthetics**
Cocaine   Procaine
Lidocaine [lignocaine]   Tetracaine

E855.3 **Parasympathomimetics [cholinergics]**
Acetylcholine   Pilocarpine
Anticholinesterase:
 organophosphorus
 reversible

E855.4 **Parasympatholytics [anticholinergics and antimuscarinics] and spasmolytics**
Atropine   Hyoscine [scopolamine]
Homatropine   Quaternary ammonium derivatives

E855.5 **Sympathomimetics [adrenergics]**
Epinephrine [adrenalin]
Levarterenol [noradrenalin]

E855.6 **Sympatholytics [antiadrenergics]**
Phenoxybenzamine   Tolazoline hydrochloride

E855.8 **Other specified drugs acting on central and autonomic nervous systems**

E855.9 **Unspecified drug acting on central and autonomic nervous systems**

E856 **Accidental poisoning by antibiotics**

E857 **Accidental poisoning by other anti-infectives**

E858 **Accidental poisoning by other drugs**

E858.0 **Hormones and synthetic substitutes**

E858.1 **Primarily systemic agents**

E858.2 **Agents primarily affecting blood constituents**

E858.3 **Agents primarily affecting cardiovascular system**

E858.4 **Agents primarily affecting gastrointestinal system**

E858.5 **Water, mineral, and uric acid metabolism drugs**

E858.6 **Agents primarily acting on the smooth and skeletal muscles and respiratory system**

E858.7 **Agents primarily affecting skin and mucous membrane, ophthalmological, otorhinolaryngological, and dental drugs**

E858.8 **Other specified drugs**
Central appetite depressants

E858.9 **Unspecified drug**

ACCIDENTAL POISONING BY OTHER SOLID AND LIQUID SUBSTANCES, GASES, AND VAPORS (E860-E869)

Note: Categories in this section are intended primarily to indicate the external cause of poisoning states classifiable to 980-989. They may also be used to indicate external causes of localized effects classifiable to 001-799.

E860 **Accidental poisoning by alcohol, not elsewhere classified**

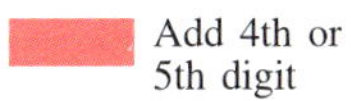

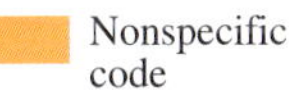

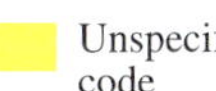

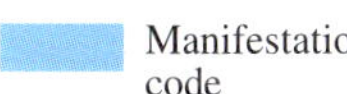

E860.0 Alcoholic beverages
Alcohol in preparations intended for consumption

E860.1 Other and unspecified ethyl alcohol and its products
Denatured alcohol   Grain alcohol NOS
Ethanol NOS   Methylated spirit

E860.2 Methyl alcohol
Methanol   Wood alcohol

E860.3 Isopropyl alcohol
Dimethyl carbinol   Secondary propyl alcohol
Isopropanol
Rubbing alcohol substitute

E860.4 Fusel oil
Alcohol:
  amyl
  butyl
  propyl

E860.8 Other specified alcohols

E860.9 Unspecified alcohol

E861 Accidental poisoning by cleansing and polishing agents, disinfectants, paints, and varnishes

E861.0 Synthetic detergents and shampoos

E861.1 Soap products

E861.2 Polishes

E861.3 Other cleansing and polishing agents
Scouring powders

E861.4 Disinfectants
Household and other disinfectants not ordinarily used on the person
> *Excludes:* carbolic acid or phenol (E864.0)

E861.5 Lead paints

E861.6 Other paints and varnishes
Lacquers   Paints, other than lead
Oil colors   White washes

E861.9 Unspecified

E862 Accidental poisoning by petroleum products, other solvents and their vapors, not elsewhere classified

E862.0 Petroleum solvents
Petroleum:
  ether
  benzine
  naphtha

E862.1 Petroleum fuels and cleaners
Antiknock additives to petroleum fuels
Gas oils
Gasoline or petrol
Kerosene
> *Excludes:* kerosene insecticides (E863.4)

E862.2 Lubricating oils

E862.3 Petroleum solids
Paraffin wax

E862.4 Other specified solvents
Benzene

E862.9 Unspecified solvent

E863 Accidental poisoning by agricultural and horticultural chemical and pharmaceutical preparations other than plant foods and fertilizers
> *Excludes:* plant foods and fertilizers (E866.5)

E863.0 Insecticides of organochlorine compounds
Benzene hexachloride   Dieldrin
Chlordane   Endrine
DDT   Toxaphene

● Code new to this edition   ▲ Revision of existing code   ④ ⑤ Fourth or fifth digit required

E863.1 Insecticides of organophosphorus compounds
    Demeton   Parathion
    Diazinon   Phenylsulphthion
    Dichlorvos   Phorate
    Malathion   Phosdrin
    Methyl parathion

E863.2 Carbamates
    Aldicarb   Propoxur
    Carbaryl

E863.3 Mixtures of insecticides

E863.4 Other and unspecified insecticides
    Kerosene insecticides

E863.5 Herbicides
    2, 4-Dichlorophenoxyacetic acid [2, 4-D]
    2, 4, 5-Trichlorophenoxyacetic acid [2, 4, 5-T]
    Chlorates
    Diquat
    Mixtures of plant food and fertilizers with herbicides
    Paraquat

E863.6 Fungicides
    Organic mercurials (used in seed dressing)
    Pentachlorophenols

E863.7 Rodenticides
    Fluoroacetates   Warfarin
    Squill and derivatives   Zinc phosphide
    Thallium

E863.8 Fumigants
    Cyanides   Phosphine
    Methyl bromide

E863.9 Other and unspecified

E864 Accidental poisoning by corrosives and caustics, not elsewhere classified
    Excludes: *those as components of disinfectants (E861.4)*

E864.0 Corrosive aromatics
    Carbolic acid or phenol

E864.1 Acids
    Acid:
      hydrochloric
      nitric
      sulfuric

E864.2 Caustic alkalis
    Lye

E864.3 Other specified corrosives and caustics

E864.4 Unspecified corrosives and caustics

E865 Accidental poisoning from poisonous foodstuffs and poisonous plants
    Includes: any meat, fish, or shellfish
              plants, berries, and fungi eaten as, or in mistake for, food, or by a child
    Excludes: *anaphylactic shock due to adverse food reaction (995.6)*
              food poisoning (bacterial) (005.0-005.9)
              poisoning and toxic reactions to venomous plants (E905.6-E905.7)

E865.0 Meat

E865.1 Shellfish

E865.2 Other fish

E865.3 Berries and seeds

E865.4 Other specified plants

E865.5 Mushrooms and other fungi

E865.8 Other specified foods

E865.9 Unspecified foodstuff or poisonous plant

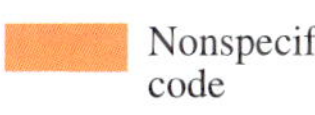
Add 4th or 5th digit

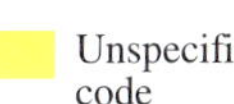
Nonspecific code

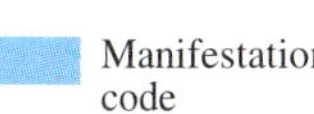
Unspecified code

Manifestation code

E866 Accidental poisoning by other and unspecified solid and liquid substances

> *Excludes:* *these substances as a component of:*
> *medicines (E850.0-E858.9)*
> *paints (E861.5-E861.6)*
> *pesticides (E863.0-E863.9)*
> *petroleum fuels (E862.1)*

E866.0 Lead and its compounds and fumes

E866.1 Mercury and its compounds and fumes

E866.2 Antimony and its compounds and fumes

E866.3 Arsenic and its compounds and fumes

E866.4 Other metals and their compounds and fumes

Beryllium (compounds)   Iron (compounds)
Brass fumes   Manganese (compounds)
Cadmium (compounds)   Nickel (compounds)
Copper salts   Thallium (compounds)

E866.5 Plant foods and fertilizers

> *Excludes:* *mixtures with herbicides (E863.5)*

E866.6 Glues and adhesives

E866.7 Cosmetics

E866.8 Other specified solid or liquid substances

E866.9 Unspecified solid or liquid substance

E867 Accidental poisoning by gas distributed by pipeline

Carbon monoxide from incomplete combustion of piped gas
Coal gas NOS
Liquefied petroleum gas distributed through pipes (pure or mixed with air)
Piped gas (natural) (manufactured)

E868 Accidental poisoning by other utility gas and other carbon monoxide

E868.0 Liquefied petroleum gas distributed in mobile containers

Butane or carbon monoxide from incomplete combustion of this gas
Liquefied hydrocarbon gas NOS or carbon monoxide from incomplete combustion of this gas
Propane or carbon monoxide from incomplete combustion of this gas

E868.1 Other and unspecified utility gas

Acetylene or or carbon monoxide from incomplete combustion of these gases
Gas NOS used for lighting, heating, cooking, or carbon monoxide from incomplete combustion of these gases
Water gas or carbon monoxide from incomplete combustion of these gases

E868.2 Motor vehicle exhaust gas

Exhaust gas from:
  farm tractor, not in transit
  gas engine
  motor pump
  motor vehicle, not in transit
  any type of combustion engine not in watercraft

> *Excludes:* *poisoning by carbon monoxide from:*
> *aircraft while in transit (E844.0-E844.9)*
> *motor vehicle while in transit (E818.0-E818.9)*
> *watercraft whether or not in transit (E838.0-E838.9)*

E868.3 Carbon monoxide from incomplete combustion of other domestic fuels

Carbon monoxide from incomplete combustion of:
  coal in domestic stove or fireplace
  coke in domestic stove or fireplace
  kerosene in domestic stove or fireplace
  wood in domestic stove or fireplace

> *Excludes:* *carbon monoxide from smoke and fumes due to conflagration (E890.0-E893.9)*

E868.8 Carbon monoxide from other sources

Carbon monoxide from:
  blast furnace gas
  incomplete combustion of fuels in industrial use
  kiln vapor

E868.9 Unspecified carbon monoxide

● Code new   ▲ Revision of   ④ ⑤ Fourth or fifth
  to this edition   existing code   digit required

E869 **Accidental poisoning by other gases and vapors**

> *Excludes:* *effects of gases used as anesthetics (E855.1, E938.2)*
> *fumes from heavy metals (E866.0-E866.4)*
> *smoke and fumes due to conflagration or explosion (E890.0-E899)*

E869.0 **Nitrogen oxides**

E869.1 **Sulfur dioxide**

E869.2 **Freon**

E869.3 **Lacrimogenic gas [tear gas]**
Bromobenzyl cyanide   Ethyliodoacetate
Chloroacetophenone

E869.4 **Second-hand tobacco smoke**

E869.8 **Other specified gases and vapors**
Chlorine   Hydrocyanic acid gas

E869.9 **Unspecified gases and vapors**

MISADVENTURES TO PATIENTS DURING SURGICAL AND MEDICAL CARE (E870-E876)

> *Excludes:* *accidental overdose of drug and wrong drug given in error (E850.0-E858.9)*
> *surgical and medical procedures as the cause of abnormal reaction by the patient,*
> *without mention of misadventure at the time of procedure (E878.0-E879.9)*

E870 **Accidental cut, puncture, perforation, or hemorrhage during medical care**

E870.0 **Surgical operation**

E870.1 **Infusion or transfusion**

E870.2 **Kidney dialysis or other perfusion**

E870.3 **Injection or vaccination**

E870.4 **Endoscopic examination**

E870.5 **Aspiration of fluid or tissue, puncture, and catheterization**
Abdominal paracentesis Lumbar puncture
Aspirating needle biopsy Thoracentesis
Blood sampling

> *Excludes:* *heart catheterization (E870.6)*

E870.6 **Heart catheterization**

E870.7 **Administration of enema**

E870.8 **Other specified medical care**

E870.9 **Unspecified medical care**

E871 **Foreign object left in body during procedure**

E871.0 **Surgical operation**

E871.1 **Infusion or transfusion**

E871.2 **Kidney dialysis or other perfusion**

E871.3 **Injection or vaccination**

E871.4 **Endoscopic examination**

E871.5 **Aspiration of fluid or tissue, puncture, and catheterization**
Abdominal paracentesis Lumbar puncture
Aspiration needle biopsy Thoracentesis
Blood sampling

> *Excludes:* *heart catheterization (E871.6)*

E871.6 **Heart catheterization**

E871.7 **Removal of catheter or packing**

E871.8 **Other specified procedures**

E871.9 **Unspecified procedure**

E872 **Failure of sterile precautions during procedure**

E872.0 **Surgical operation**

E872.1 **Infusion or transfusion**

E872.2 **Kidney dialysis and other perfusion**

E872.3 **Injection or vaccination**

E872.4 **Endoscopic examination**

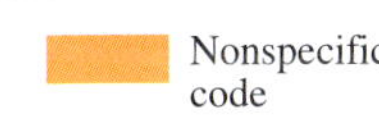

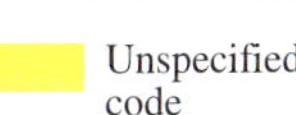

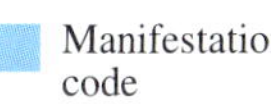

Manifestation
code

E872.5 **Aspiration of fluid or tissue, puncture, and catheterization**
Abdominal paracentesis   Lumbar puncture
Aspirating needle biopsy   Thoracentesis
Blood sampling

Excludes: *heart catheterization (E872.6)*

E872.6 **Heart catheterization**

E872.8 **Other specified procedures**

E872.9 **Unspecified procedure**

E873 **Failure in dosage**

Excludes: *accidental overdose of drug, medicinal or biological substance (E850.0-E858.9)*

E873.0 **Excessive amount of blood or other fluid during transfusion or infusion**

E873.1 **Incorrect dilution of fluid during infusion**

E873.2 **Overdose of radiation in therapy**

E873.3 **Inadvertent exposure of patient to radiation during medical care**

E873.4 **Failure in dosage in electroshock or insulin-shock therapy**

E873.5 **Inappropriate [too hot or too cold] temperature in local application and packing**

E873.6 **Nonadministration of necessary drug or medicinal substance**

E873.8 **Other specified failure in dosage**

E873.9 **Unspecified failure in dosage**

E874 **Mechanical failure of instrument or apparatus during procedure**

E874.0 **Surgical operation**

E874.1 **Infusion and transfusion**
Air in system

E874.2 **Kidney dialysis and other perfusion**

E874.3 **Endoscopic examination**

E874.4 **Aspiration of fluid or tissue, puncture, and catheterization**
Abdominal paracentesis   Lumbar puncture
Aspirating needle biopsy   Thoracentesis
Blood sampling

Excludes: *heart catheterization (E874.5)*

E874.5 **Heart catheterization**

E874.8 **Other specified procedures**

E874.9 **Unspecified procedure**

E875 **Contaminated or infected blood, other fluid, drug, or biological substance**
Includes: presence of:
bacterial pyrogens
endotoxin-producing bacteria
serum hepatitis-producing agent

E875.0 **Contaminated substance transfused or infused**

E875.1 **Contaminated substance injected or used for vaccination**

E875.2 **Contaminated drug or biological substance administered by other means**

E875.8 **Other**

E875.9 **Unspecified**

E876 **Other and unspecified misadventures during medical care**

E876.0 **Mismatched blood in transfusion**

E876.1 **Wrong fluid in infusion**

E876.2 **Failure in suture and ligature during surgical operation**

E876.3 **Endotracheal tube wrongly placed during anesthetic procedure**

E876.4 **Failure to introduce or to remove other tube or instrument**

Excludes: *foreign object left in body during procedure (E871.0-E871.9)*

E876.5 **Performance of inappropriate operation**

E876.8 **Other specified misadventures during medical care**
Performance of inappropriate treatment NEC

E876.9 **Unspecified misadventure during medical care**

    ● Code new
to this edition   ▲ Revision of
existing code   ④ ⑤ Fourth or fifth
digit required

SURGICAL AND MEDICAL PROCEDURES AS THE CAUSE OF ABNORMAL REACTION OF PATIENT OR LATER COMPLICATION, WITHOUT MENTION OF MISADVENTURE AT THE TIME OF PROCEDURE (E878-E879)

Includes: procedures as the cause of abnormal reaction, such as:
    displacement or malfunction of prosthetic device
    hepatorenal failure, postoperative
    malfunction of external stoma
    postoperative intestinal obstruction
    rejection of transplanted organ

Excludes: *anesthetic management properly carried out as the cause of adverse effect (E937.0-E938.9)*
infusion and transfusion, without mention of misadventure in the technique of procedure (E930.0-E949.9)

E878 **Surgical operation and other surgical procedures as the cause of abnormal reaction of patient, or of later complication, without mention of misadventure at the time of operation**

E878.0 **Surgical operation with transplant of whole organ**
Transplantation of:
  heart
  kidney
  liver

E878.1 **Surgical operation with implant of artificial internal device**
Cardiac pacemaker   Heart valve prosthesis
Electrodes implanted in brain   Internal orthopedic device

E878.2 **Surgical operation with anastomosis, bypass, or graft, with natural or artificial tissues used as implant**
Anastomosis: Graft of blood vessel, tendon, or skin
  arteriovenous
  gastrojejunal

Excludes: *external stoma (E878.3)*

E878.3 **Surgical operation with formation of external stoma**
Colostomy   Gastrostomy
Cystostomy   Ureterostomy
Duodenostomy

E878.4 **Other restorative surgery**

E878.5 **Amputation of limb(s)**

E878.6 **Removal of other organ (partial) (total)**

E878.8 **Other specified surgical operations and procedures**

E878.9 **Unspecified surgical operations and procedures**

E879 **Other procedures, without mention of misadventure at the time of procedure, as the cause of abnormal reaction of patient, or of later complication**

E879.0 **Cardiac catheterization**

E879.1 **Kidney dialysis**

E879.2 **Radiological procedure and radiotherapy**

Excludes: *radio-opaque dyes for diagnostic x-ray procedures (E947.8)*

E879.3 **Shock therapy**
Electroshock therapy   Insulin-shock therapy

E879.4 **Aspiration of fluid**
Lumbar puncture   Thoracentesis

E879.5 **Insertion of gastric or duodenal sound**

E879.6 **Urinary catheterization**

E879.7 **Blood sampling**

E879.8 **Other specified procedures**
Blood transfusion

E879.9 **Unspecified procedure**

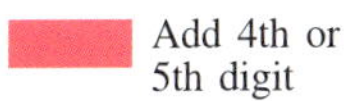

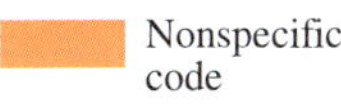

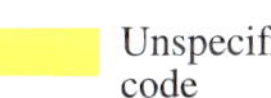

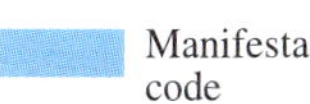

ACCIDENTAL FALLS (E880-E888)

> *Excludes:* *falls (in or from):*
> *burning building (E890.8, E891.8)*
> *into fire (E890.0-E899)*
> *into water (with submersion or drowning) (E910.0-E910.9)*
> *machinery (in operation) (E919.0-E919.9)*
> *on edged, pointed, or sharp object (E920.0-E920.9)*
> *transport vehicle (E800.0-E845.9)*
> *vehicle not elsewhere classifiable (E846-E848)*

E880 Fall on or from stairs or steps

E880.0 Escalator

E880.1 Fall on or from sidewalk curb

> *Excludes:* *fall from moving sidewalk (E885.9)*

E880.9 Other stairs or steps

E881 Fall on or from ladders or scaffolding

E881.0 Fall from ladder

E881.1 Fall from scaffolding

E882 Fall from or out of building or other structure

Fall from:
balcony
bridge
building
flagpole
tower

Fall from:
turret
viaduct
wall
window
Fall through roof

> *Excludes:* *collapse of a building or structure (E916)*
> *fall or jump from burning building (E890.8, E891.8)*

E883 Fall into hole or other opening in surface

Includes:

fall into:
cavity
dock
hole
pit
quarry

fall into:
shaft
swimming pool
tank
well

> *Excludes:* *fall into water NOS (E910.9)*
> *that resulting in drowning or submersion without mention of injury (E910.0-E910.9)*

E883.0 Accident from diving or jumping into water [swimming pool]

Strike or hit:
against bottom when jumping or diving into water
wall or board of swimming pool
water surface

> *Excludes:* *diving with insufficient air supply (E913.2)*
> *effects of air pressure from diving (E902.2)*

E883.1 Accidental fall into well

E883.2 Accidental fall into storm drain or manhole

E883.9 Fall into other hole or other opening in surface

E884 Other fall from one level to another

E884.0 Fall from playground equipment

> *Excludes:* *recreational machinery (E919.8)*

E884.1 Fall from cliff

E884.2 Fall from chair

E884.3 Fall from wheelchair

E884.4 Fall from bed

E884.5 Fall from other furniture

E884.6 Fall from commode
Toilet

● Code new to this edition ▲ Revision of existing code ④ ⑤ Fourth or fifth digit required

E884.9 **Other fall from one level to another**
Fall from:
  embankment
  haystack
Fall from:
  stationary vehicle
  tree

E885 **Fall on same level from slipping, tripping, or stumbling**

E885.0 **Fall from (nonmotorized) scooter**

E885.1 **Fall from roller skates**
In-line skates

E885.2 **Fall from skateboard**

E885.3 **Fall from skis**

E885.4 **Fall from snowboard**

E885.9 **Fall from other slipping, tripping or stumbling**
Fall on moving sidewalk

E886 **Fall on same level from collision, pushing, or shoving, by or with other person**
Excludes: *crushed or pushed by a crowd or human stampede (E917.1, E917.6)*

E886.0 **In sports**
Tackles in sports
Excludes: *kicked, stepped on, struck by object, in sports (E917.0, E917.5)*

E886.9 **Other and unspecified**
Fall from collision of pedestrian (conveyance) with another pedestrian (conveyance)

E887 **Fracture, cause unspecified**

E888 **Other and unspecified fall**
Accidental fall NOS
Fall on same level NOS

E888.0 **Fall resulting in striking against sharp object**
Use additional external cause code to identify object (E920)

E888.1 **Fall resulting in striking against other object**

E888.8 **Other fall**

E888.9 **Unspecified fall**
Fall NOS

ACCIDENTS CAUSED BY FIRE AND FLAMES (E890-E899)

Includes: asphyxia or poisoning due to conflagration or ignition
         burning by fire
         secondary fires resulting from explosion

Excludes: *arson (E968.0)*

    fire in or on:
      machinery (in operation) (E919.0-E919.9)
      transport vehicle other than stationary vehicle (E800.0-E845.9)
      vehicle not elsewhere classifiable (E846-E848)

E890 **Conflagration in private dwelling**
Includes: conflagration in:
     apartment
     boarding house
     camping place
     caravan
     farmhouse
     house
     lodging house
     mobile home
     private garage
     rooming house
     tenement
    conflagration originating from sources classifiable to E893-E898 in the above
      buildings

E890.0 **Explosion caused by conflagration**

E890.1 **Fumes from combustion of polyvinylchloride [PVC] and similar material in conflagration**

E890.2 **Other smoke and fumes from conflagration**
Carbon monoxide from conflagration in private building
Fumes NOS from conflagration in private building
Smoke NOS from conflagration in private building

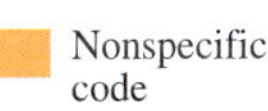

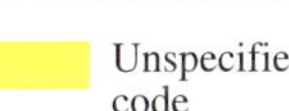

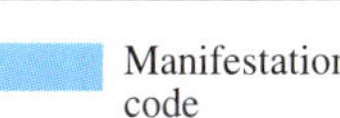

Manifestation
code

E890.3 **Burning caused by conflagration**

E890.8 **Other accident resulting from conflagration**
 Collapse of burning private building
 Fall from burning private building
 Hit by object falling from burning private building
 Jump from burning private building

E890.9 **Unspecified accident resulting from conflagration in private dwelling**

E891 **Conflagration in other and unspecified building or structure**

Conflagration in:
 barn
 church
 convalescent and other
  residential home
 dormitory of educational
  institution
 factory

Conflagration in:
 farm outbuildings
 hospital
 hotel
 school
 store
 theater

Conflagration originating from sources classifiable to E893-E898, in the above buildings

E891.0 **Explosion caused by conflagration**

E891.1 **Fumes from combustion of polyvinylchloride [PVC] and similar material in conflagration**

E891.2 **Other smoke and fumes from conflagration**
 Carbon monoxide from conflagration in building or structure
 Fumes NOS from conflagration in building or structure
 Smoke NOS from conflagration in building or structure

E891.3 **Burning caused by conflagration**

E891.8 **Other accident resulting from conflagration**
 Collapse of burning building or structure
 Fall from burning building or structure
 Hit by object falling from burning building or structure
 Jump from burning building or structure

E891.9 **Unspecified accident resulting from conflagration of other and unspecified building or structure**

E892 **Conflagration not in building or structure**
Fire (uncontrolled) (in) (of):
 forest
 grass
 hay
 lumber
 mine
 prairie
 transport vehicle [any], except while in transit
 tunnel

E893 **Accident caused by ignition of clothing**

 Excludes: *ignition of clothing:*
  from highly inflammable material (E894)
  with conflagration (E890.0-E892)

E893.0 **From controlled fire in private dwelling**
 Ignition of clothing from:
  normal fire (charcoal) (coal) (electric) (gas) (wood) in:
   brazier in private dwelling (as listed in E890)
   fireplace in private dwelling (as listed in E890)
   furnace in private dwelling (as listed in E890)
   stove in private dwelling (as listed in E890)

E893.1 **From controlled fire in other building or structure**
 Ignition of clothing from:
  normal fire (charcoal) (coal) (electric) (gas) (wood) in:
   brazier in other building or structure (as listed in E891)
   fireplace in other building or structure (as listed in E891)
   furnace in other building or structure (as listed in E891)
   stove in other building or structure (as listed in E891)

E893.2   From controlled fire not in building or structure
Ignition of clothing from:
  bonfire (controlled)
  brazier fire (controlled), not in building or structure
  trash fire (controlled)

Excludes: *conflagration not in building (E892)*
  trash fire out of control (E892)

E893.8   From other specified sources
Ignition of clothing from: Ignition of clothing from:
  blowlamp   cigarette
  blowtorch   lighter
  burning bedspread   matches
  candle   pipe
  cigar   welding torch

E893.9   Unspecified source
Ignition of clothing (from controlled fire NOS) (in building NOS) NOS

E894   Ignition of highly inflammable material
Ignition of:
  benzine (with ignition of clothing)
  gasoline (with ignition of clothing)
  fat (with ignition of clothing)
  kerosene (with ignition of clothing)
  paraffin (with ignition of clothing)
  petrol (with ignition of clothing)

Excludes: *ignition of highly inflammable material with:*
  conflagration (E890.0-E892)
  explosion (E923.0-E923.9)

E895   Accident caused by controlled fire in private dwelling
Burning by (flame of) normal fire (charcoal) (coal) (electric) (gas) (wood) in:
  brazier in private dwelling (as listed in E890)
  fireplace in private dwelling (as listed in E890)
  furnace in private dwelling (as listed in E890)
  stove in private dwelling (as listed in E890)

Excludes: *burning by hot objects not producing fire or flames (E924.0-E924.9)*
  ignition of clothing from these sources (E893.0)
  poisoning by carbon monoxide from incomplete combustion of fuel (E867-E868.9)
  that with conflagration (E890.0-E890.9)

E896   Accident caused by controlled fire in other and unspecified building or structure
Burning by (flame of) normal fire (charcoal) (coal) (electric) (gas) (wood) in:
  brazier in other building or structure (as listed in E891)
  fireplace in other building or structure (as listed in E891)
  furnace in other building or structure (as listed in E891)
  stove in other building or structure (as listed in E891)

Excludes: *burning by hot objects not producing fire or flames (E924.0-E924.9)*
  ignition of clothing from these sources (E893.1)
  poisoning by carbon monoxide from incomplete combustion of fuel (E867-E868.9)
  that with conflagration (E891.0-E891.9)

E897   Accident caused by controlled fire not in building or structure
Burns from flame of:
  bonfire (controlled)
  brazier fire (controlled), not in building or structure
  trash fire (controlled)

Excludes: *ignition of clothing from these sources (E893.2)*
  trash fire out of control (E892)
  that with conflagration (E892)

E898   Accident caused by other specified fire and flames
Excludes: *conflagration (E890.0-E892)*
  that with ignition of:
    clothing (E893.0-E893.9)
    highly inflammable material (E894)

E898.0   Burning bedclothes
Bed set on fire NOS

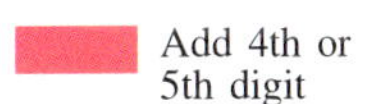

Nonspecific
code

Unspecified
code

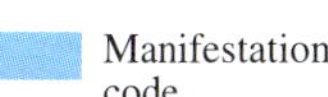

E898.1   **Other**

Burning by:
  blowlamp
  blowtorch
  candle
  cigar
  cigarette
  fire in room NOS

Burning by:
  lamp
  lighter
  matches
  pipe
  welding torch

E899   **Accident caused by unspecified fire**

Burning NOS

ACCIDENTS DUE TO NATURAL AND ENVIRONMENTAL FACTORS (E900-E909)

E900   **Excessive heat**

E900.0   **Due to weather conditions**

Excessive heat as the external cause of:
  ictus solaris
  siriasis
  sunstroke

E900.1   **Of man-made origin**

Heat (in):
  boiler room
  drying room
  factory
  furnace room

Heat (in):
  generated in transport vehicle
  kitchen

E900.9   **Of unspecified origin**

E901   **Excessive cold**

E901.0   **Due to weather conditions**

Excessive cold as the cause of:
  chilblains NOS
  immersion foot

E901.1   **Of man-made origin**

Contact with or inhalation of:
  dry ice
  liquid air
  liquid hydrogen
  liquid nitrogen
Prolonged exposure in:
  deep freeze unit
  refrigerator

E901.8   **Other specified origin**

E901.9   **Of unspecified origin**

E902   **High and low air pressure and changes in air pressure**

E902.0   **Residence or prolonged visit at high altitude**

Residence or prolonged visit at high altitude as the cause of:
  Acosta syndrome
  Alpine sickness
  altitude sickness
  Andes disease
  anoxia, hypoxia
  barotitis, barodontalgia, barosinusitis, otitic barotrauma
  hypobarism, hypobaropathy
  mountain sickness
  range disease

E902.1   **In aircraft**

Sudden change in air pressure in aircraft during ascent or descent as the cause of:
  aeroneurosis
  aviators' disease

● Code new
  to this edition

▲ Revision of
  existing code

④ ⑤ Fourth or fifth
   digit required

E902.2 **Due to diving**
High air pressure from rapid descent in water as the cause of:
  caisson disease
  divers' disease
  divers' palsy or paralysis
Reduction in atmospheric pressure while surfacing from deep water diving as the
  cause of:
  caisson disease
  divers' disease
  divers' palsy or paralysis

E902.8 **Due to other specified causes**
Reduction in atmospheric pressure while surfacing from underground

E902.9 **Unspecified cause**

E903 Travel and motion

E904 Hunger, thirst, exposure, and neglect

Excludes: *any condition resulting from homicidal intent (E968.0-E968.9)*

*hunger, thirst, and exposure resulting from accidents connected with transport
(E800.0-E848)*

E904.0 **Abandonment or neglect of infants and helpless persons**
Exposure to weather conditions resulting from abandonment or neglect
Hunger or thirst resulting from abandonment or neglect
Desertion of newborn
Inattention at or after birth
Lack of care (helpless person) (infant)

Excludes: *criminal [purposeful] neglect (E968.4)*

E904.1 **Lack of food**
Lack of food as the cause of:
  inanition
  insufficient nourishment
  starvation

Excludes: *hunger resulting from abandonment or neglect (E904.0)*

E904.2 **Lack of water**
Lack of water as the cause of:
  dehydration
  inanition

Excludes: *dehydration due to acute fluid loss (276.51)*

E904.3 **Exposure (to weather conditions), not elsewhere classifiable**
Exposure NOS   Struck by hailstones
Humidity

Excludes: *struck by lightning (E907)*

E904.9 **Privation, unqualified**
Destitution

E905 Venomous animals and plants as the cause of poisoning and toxic reactions
Includes: chemical released by animal
  insects
  release of venom through fangs, hairs, spines, tentacles, and other venom
    apparatus

Excludes: *eating of poisonous animals or plants (E865.0-E865.9)*

E905.0 **Venomous snakes and lizards**
Cobra   Mamba
Copperhead snake   Rattlesnake
Coral snake   Sea snake
Fer de lance   Snake (venomous)
Gila monster   Viper
Krait   Water moccasin

Excludes: *bites of snakes and lizards known to be nonvenomous (E906.2)*

E905.1 **Venomous spiders**
Black widow spider   Tarantula (venomous)
Brown spider

E905.2 **Scorpion**

E905.3 **Hornets, wasps, and bees**
Yellow jacket

E905.4   **Centipede and venomous millipede (tropical)**

E905.5   **Other venomous arthropods**
Sting of:
  ant
  caterpillar

E905.6   **Venomous marine animals and plants**
Puncture by sea urchin spine   Sting of:
Sting of: nematocysts
  coral   sea anemone
  jelly fish   sea cucumber
                                                         other marine animal or plant

Excludes:	*bites and other injuries caused by nonvenomous marine animal (E906.2-E906.8)*
	bite of sea snake (venomous) (E905.0)

E905.7   **Poisoning and toxic reactions caused by other plants**
Injection of poisons or toxins into or through skin by plant thorns, spines, or other
  mechanisms

Excludes:	*puncture wound NOS by plant thorns or spines (E920.8)*

E905.8   **Other specified**

E905.9   **Unspecified**
Sting NOS   Venomous bite NOS

E906   **Other injury caused by animals**

Excludes:	*poisoning and toxic reactions caused by venomous animals and insects (E905.0-E905.9)*
	road vehicle accident involving animals (E827.0-E828.9)
	tripping or falling over an animal (E885.9)

E906.0   **Dog bite**

E906.1   **Rat bite**

E906.2   **Bite of nonvenomous snakes and lizards**

E906.3   **Bite of other animal except arthropod**
Cats   Rodents, except rats
Moray eel   Shark

E906.4   **Bite of nonvenomous arthropod**
Insect bite NOS

E906.5   **Bite by unspecified animal**
Animal bite NOS

E906.8   **Other specified injury caused by animal**
Butted by animal
Fallen on by horse or other animal, not being ridden
Gored by animal
Implantation of quills of porcupine
Pecked by bird
Run over by animal, not being ridden
Stepped on by animal, not being ridden

Excludes:	*injury by animal being ridden (E828.0-E828.9)*

E906.9   **Unspecified injury caused by animal**

E907   **Lightning**

Excludes:	*injury from:*
	fall of tree or other object caused by lightning (E916)
	fire caused by lightning (E890.0-E892)

E908   **Cataclysmic storms, and floods resulting from storms**

Excludes:	*collapse of dam or man-made structure causing flood (E909.3)*

E908.0   **Hurricane**
Storm surge
"Tidal wave" caused by storm action
Typhoon

E908.1   **Tornado**
Cyclone
Twisters

● Code new
  to this edition   ▲ Revision of
                             existing code   ④ ⑤ Fourth or fifth
                                                          digit required

E908.2 Floods
Torrential rainfall
Flash flood

Excludes: collapse of dam or man-made structure causing flood (909.3)

E908.3 Blizzard (snow) (ice)

E908.4 Dust storm

E908.8 Other cataclysmic storms

E908.9 Unspecified cataclysmic storms, and floods resulting from storms
Storm NOS

E909 Cataclysmic earth surface movements and eruptions

Excludes: "tidal wave" caused by storm action (E908.0)

transport accident involving collision with avalanche or landslide not in motion
(E800.0-E848)

E909.0 Earthquakes

E909.1 Volcanic eruptions
Burns from lava
Ash inhalation

E909.2 Avalanche, landslide, or mudslide

E909.3 Collapse of dam or man-made structure

E909.4 Tidal wave caused by earthquake
Tidal wave NOS
Tsunami

Excludes: tidal wave caused by tropical storm (E908.0)

E909.8 Other cataclysmic earth surface movements and eruptions

E909.9 Unspecified cataclysmic earth surface movements and eruptions

ACCIDENTS CAUSED BY SUBMERSION, SUFFOCATION, AND FOREIGN BODIES (E910-E915)

E910 Accidental drowning and submersion
Includes: immersion
swimmers' cramp

Excludes: diving accident (NOS) (resulting in injury except drowning) (E883.0)

diving with insufficient air supply (E913.2)
drowning and submersion due to:
cataclysm (E908-E909)
machinery accident (E919.0-E919.9)
transport accident (E800.0-E845.9)
effect of high and low air pressure (E902.2)
injury from striking against objects while in running water (E917.2)

E910.0 While water-skiing
Fall from water skis with submersion or drowning

Excludes: accident to water-skier involving a watercraft and resulting in submersion or other
injury (E830.4, E831.4)

E910.1 While engaged in other sport or recreational activity with diving equipment
Scuba diving NOS
Skin diving NOS
Underwater spear fishing NOS

E910.2 While engaged in other sport or recreational activity without diving equipment
Fishing or hunting, except from boat or with diving equipment
Ice skating
Playing in water
Surfboarding
Swimming NOS
Voluntarily jumping from boat, not involved in accident, for swim NOS
Wading in water

Excludes: jumping into water to rescue another person (E910.3)

E910.3 While swimming or diving for purposes other than recreation or sport
Marine salvage (with diving equipment)
Pearl diving (with diving equipment)
Placement of fishing nets (with diving equipment)
Rescue (attempt) of another person (with diving equipment)
Underwater construction or repairs (with diving equipment)

E910.4   **In bathtub**

E910.8   **Other accidental drowning or submersion**
Drowning in:
quenching tank
swimming pool

E910.9   **Unspecified accidental drowning or submersion**
Accidental fall into water NOS
Drowning NOS

E911   **Inhalation and ingestion of food causing obstruction of respiratory tract or suffocation**
Aspiration and inhalation of food [any] (into respiratory tract) NOS
Asphyxia by food [including bone, seed in food, regurgitated food]
Choked on food [including bone, seed in food, regurgitated food]
Suffocation by food [including bone, seed in food, regurgitated food]
Compression of trachea by food lodged in esophagus
Interruption of respiration by food lodged in esophagus
Obstruction of respiration by food lodged in esophagus
Obstruction of pharynx by food (bolus)

Excludes: *injury, except asphyxia and obstruction of respiratory passage, caused by food*
(E915)
obstruction of esophagus by food without mention of asphyxia or obstruction of
respiratory passage (E915)

E912   **Inhalation and ingestion of other object causing obstruction of respiratory tract or**
suffocation
Aspiration and inhalation of foreign body except food (into respiratory tract) NOS
Foreign object [bean] [marble] in nose
Obstruction of pharynx by foreign body
Compression by foreign body in esophagus
Interruption of respiration by foreign body in esophagus
Obstruction of respiration by foreign body in esophagus

Excludes: *injury, except asphyxia and obstruction of respiratory passage, caused by foreign*
body (E915)
obstruction of esophagus by foreign body without mention of asphyxia or
obstruction in respiratory passage (E915)

E913   **Accidental mechanical suffocation**

Excludes: *mechanical suffocation from or by:*
accidental inhalation or ingestion of:
food (E911)
foreign object (E912)
cataclysm (E908-E909)
explosion (E921.0-E921.9, E923.0-E923.9)
machinery accident (E919.0-E919.9)

E913.0   **In bed or cradle**

Excludes: *suffocation by plastic bag (E913.1)*

E913.1   **By plastic bag**

E913.2   **Due to lack of air (in closed place)**
Accidentally closed up in refrigerator or other airtight enclosed space
Diving with insufficient air supply

Excludes: *suffocation by plastic bag (E913.1)*

E913.3   **By falling earth or other substance**
Cave-in NOS

Excludes: *cave-in caused by cataclysmic earth surface movements and eruptions (E909)*
struck by cave-in without asphyxiation or suffocation (E916)

E913.8   **Other specified means**
Accidental hanging, except in bed or cradle

E913.9   **Unspecified means**
Asphyxia, mechanical NOS
Strangulation NOS
Suffocation NOS

E914   **Foreign body accidentally entering eye and adnexa**
Excludes: *corrosive liquid (E924.1)*

E915   **Foreign body accidentally entering other orifice**
Excludes: *aspiration and inhalation of foreign body, any, (into respiratory tract) NOS*
(E911-E912)

   ● Code new   ▲ Revision of   ④ ⑤ Fourth or fifth
to this edition   existing code   digit required

OTHER ACCIDENTS (E916-E928)

E916 Struck accidentally by falling object

Collapse of building, except on fire | Object falling from:
Falling: | machine, not in operation
  rock | stationary vehicle
  snowslide NOS
  stone
  tree

    Code first: collapse of building on fire (E890.0-E891.9)
          falling object in:
            cataclysm (E908-E909)
            machinery accidents (E919.0-E919.9)
            transport accidents (E800.0-E845.9)
            vehicle accidents not elsewhere classifiable (E846-E848)
          object set in motion by:
            explosion (E921.0-E921.9, E923.0-E923.9)
            firearm (E922.0-E922.9)
          projected object (E917.0-E917.9)

E917 Striking against or struck accidentally by objects or persons

    Includes: bumping into or against:
          object (moving) (projected) (stationary)
          pedestrian conveyance
          person
        colliding with:
          object (moving) (projected) (stationary)
          pedestrian conveyance
          person
        kicking against:
          object (moving) (projected) (stationary)
          pedestrian conveyance
          person
        stepping on:
          object (moving) (projected) (stationary)
          pedestrian conveyance
          person
        struck by:
          object (moving) (projected) (stationary)
          pedestrian conveyance
          person

   Excludes: *fall from collision with another person, except when caused by a crowd*
      (E886.0-E886.9)
    fall from stumbling over object (E885.9)
    fall resulting in striking against object (E888.0, E888.1)
    injury caused by:
      assault (E960.0-E960.1, E967.0-E967.9)
      cutting or piercing instrument (E920.0-E920.9)
      explosion (E921.0-E921.9, E923.0-E923.9)
      firearm (E922.0-E922.9)
      machinery (E919.0-E919.9)
      transport vehicle (E800.0-E845.9)
      vehicle not elsewhere classifiable (E846-E848)

E917.0 In sports without subsequent fall
    Kicked or stepped on during game (football) (rugby)
    Struck by hit or thrown ball
    Struck by hockey stick or puck

E917.1 Caused by a crowd, by collective fear or panic without subsequent fall
    Crushed by crown or human stampede
    Pushed by crown or human stampede
    Stepped on by crown or human stampede

E917.2 In running water without subsequent fall
   Excludes: *drowning or submersion (E910.0-E910.9)*
      that in sports (E917.0, E917.5)

E917.3 Furniture without subsequent fall
   Excludes: *fall from furniture (E884.2, E884.4-E884.5)*

E917.4 Other stationary object without subsequent fall
    Bath tub
    Fence
    Lamp-post

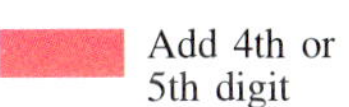

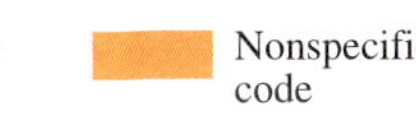

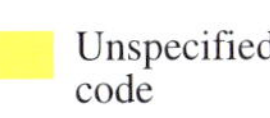

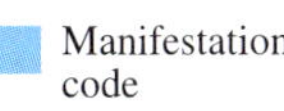

E917.5   **Object in sports with subsequent fall**
Knocked down while boxing

E917.6   **Caused by a crowd, by collective fear or panic with subsequent fall**

E917.7   **Furniture with subsequent fall**
Excludes: *fall from furniture (E884.2, E884.4-E884.5)*

E917.8   **Other stationary object with subsequent fall**
Bath tub
Fence
Lamp-post

E917.9   **Other striking against with or without subsequent fall**

E918   Caught accidentally in or between objects
Caught, crushed, jammed, or pinched in or between moving or stationary objects, such as:
escalator
folding object
hand tools, appliances, or implements
sliding door and door frame
under packing crate
washing machine wringer

Excludes: *injury caused by:*

cutting or piercing instrument (E920.0-E920.9)
machinery (E919.0-E919.9)
transport vehicle (E800.0-E845.9)
vehicle not elsewhere classifiable (E846-E848)
struck accidentally by:
falling object (E916)
object (moving) (projected) (E917.0-E917.9)

E919   Accidents caused by machinery
Includes:
burned by machinery (accident)
caught in (moving parts of) machinery (accident)
collapse of machinery (accident)
crushed by machinery (accident)
cut or pierced by machinery (accident)
drowning or submersion caused by machinery (accident)
explosion of, on, in machinery (accident)
fall from or into moving part of machinery (accident)
fire starting in or on machinery (accident)
mechanical suffocation caused by machinery (accident)
object falling from, on, in motion by machinery (accident)
overturning of machinery (accident)
pinned under machinery (accident)
run over by machinery (accident)
struck by machinery (accident)
thrown from machinery (accident)
caught between machinery and other object
machinery accident NOS

Excludes: *accidents involving machinery, not in operation (E884.9, E916-E918)*

injury caused by:
electric current in connection with machinery (E925.0-E925.9)
escalator (E880.0, E918)
explosion of pressure vessel in connection with machinery (E921.0-E921.9)
moving sidewalk (E885.9)
powered hand tools, appliances, and implements (E916-E918, E920.0-E921.9, E923.0-E926.9)
transport vehicle accidents involving machinery (E800.0-E848.9)
poisoning by carbon monoxide generated by machine (E868.8)

E919.0   **Agriculture machines**

Animal-powered agricultural machine	Farm tractor
	Harvester
Combine	Hay mower or rake
Derrick, hay	Reaper
Farm machinery NOS	Thresher

Excludes: *that in transport under own power on the highway (E810.0-E819.9)*
that being towed by another vehicle on the highway (E810.0-E819.9, E827.0-E827.9, E829.0-E829.9)
that involved in accident classifiable to E820-E829 (E820.0-E829.9)

● Code new
to this edition

▲ Revision of
existing code

④ ⑤ Fourth or fifth
digit required

E919.1   **Mining and earth-drilling machinery**
    Bore or drill (land)   Shaft lift
    (seabed)   Under-cutter
    Shaft hoist

    Excludes: *coal car, tram, truck, and tub in mine (E846)*

E919.2   **Lifting machines and appliances**
    Chain hoist except in agricultural or mining operations
    Crane except in agricultural or mining operations
    Derrick except in agricultural or mining operations
    Elevator (building) (grain) except in agricultural or mining operations
    Forklift truck except in agricultural or mining operations
    Lift except in agricultural or mining operations
    Pulley block except in agricultural or mining operations
    Winch except in agricultural or mining operations

    Excludes: *that being towed by another vehicle on the highway (E810.0-E819.9,*
        E827.0-E827.9, E829.0-E829.9)
        that in transport under own power on the highway (E810.0-E819.9)
        that involved in accident classifiable to E820-E829 (E820.0-E829.9)

E919.3   **Metalworking machines**
    Abrasive wheel   Metal:
    Forging machine   drilling machine
    Lathe   milling machine
    Mechanical shears   power press
        rolling-mill
        sawing machine

E919.4   **Woodworking and forming machines**
    Band saw   Powered saw
    Bench saw   Radial saw
    Circular saw   Sander
    Molding machine
    Overhead plane

    Excludes: *hand saw (E920.1)*

E919.5   **Prime movers, except electrical motors**
    Gas turbine   Steam engine
    Internal combustion engine   Water driven turbine

    Excludes: *that being towed by other vehicle on the highway (E810.0-E819.9, E827.0-E827.9,*
        E829.0-E829.9)
        that in transport under own power on the highway (E810.0-E819.9)

E919.6   **Transmission machinery**
    Transmission: Transmission:
     belt   pinion
     cable   pulley
     chain   shaft
     gear

E919.7   **Earth moving, scraping, and other excavating machines**
    Bulldozer   Steam shovel
    Road scraper

    Excludes: *that being towed by other vehicle on the highway (E810.0-E819.9, E827.0-E827.9,*
        E829.0-E829.9)
        that in transport under own power on the highway (E810.0-E819.9)

E919.8   **Other specified machinery**
    Machines for manufacture of: Printing machine
     clothing   Recreational machinery
     foodstuffs and beverages   Spinning, weaving, and textile machines
     paper

E919.9   **Unspecified machinery**

E920   **Accidents caused by cutting and piercing instruments or objects**
    Includes: accidental injury (by) object:
        edged
        pointed
        sharp

E920.0   **Powered lawn mower**

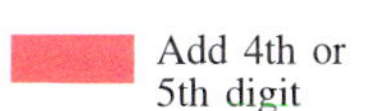

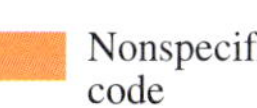

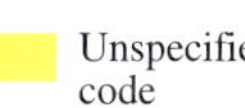

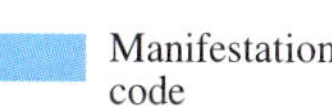

E920.1 Other powered hand tools

Any powered hand tool [compressed air] [electric] [explosive cartridge] [hydraulic power], such as:

drill	rivet gun
hand saw	snow blower
hedge clipper	staple gun

Excludes: *band saw (E919.4)*
bench saw (E919.4)

E920.2 Powered household appliances and implements

Blender	Electric:
Electric:	knife
beater or mixer	sewing machine
can opener	Garbage disposal appliance
fan	

E920.3 Knives, swords, and daggers

E920.4 Other hand tools and implements

Axe	Paper cutter
Can opener NOS	Pitchfork
Chisel	Rake
Fork	Scissors
Hand saw	Screwdriver
Hoe	Sewing machine, not powered
Ice pick	Shovel
Needle (sewing)	

E920.5 Hypodermic needle

Contaminated needle
Needle stick

E920.8 Other specified cutting and piercing instruments or objects

Arrow	Nail
Broken glass	Plant thorn
Dart	Splinter
Edge of stiff paper	Tin can lid
Lathe turnings	

Excludes: *animal spines or quills (E906.8)*
flying glass due to explosion (E921.0-E923.9)

E920.9 Unspecified cutting and piercing instrument or object

E921 Accident caused by explosion of pressure vessel

Includes: accidental explosion of pressure vessels, whether or not part of machinery

Excludes: *explosion of pressure vessel on transport vehicle (E800.0-E845.9)*

E921.0 Boilers

E921.1 Gas cylinders

Air tank	Pressure gas tank

E921.8 Other specified pressure vessels

Aerosol can	Pressure cooker
Automobile tire	

E921.9 Unspecified pressure vessel

E922 Accident caused by firearm and air gun missile

E922.0 Handgun

Pistol	Revolver

Excludes: *Verey pistol (E922.8)*

E922.1 Shotgun (automatic)

E922.2 Hunting rifle

E922.3 Military firearms

Army rifle	Machine gun

E922.4 Air gun

BB gun	Pellet gun

E922.5 Paintball gun

E922.8 Other specified firearm missile

Verey pistol [flare]

E922.9 Unspecified firearm missile

Gunshot wound NOS	Shot NOS

● Code new to this edition   ▲ Revision of existing code   ④ ⑤ Fourth or fifth digit required

E923 Accident caused by explosive material
    Includes: flash burns and other injuries resulting from explosion of explosive material
             ignition of highly explosive material with explosion

Excludes: *explosion:*
    in or on machinery (E919.0-E919.9)
    on any transport vehicle, except stationary motor vehicle (E800.0-E848)
    with conflagration (E890.0, E891.0, E892)
    secondary fires resulting from explosion (E890.0-E899)

E923.0 Fireworks

E923.1 Blasting materials
    Blasting cap   Explosive [any] used in blasting operations
    Detonator
    Dynamite

E923.2 Explosive gases
    Acetylene   Fire damp
    Butane   Gasoline fumes
    Coal gas   Methane
    Explosion in mine NOS   Propane

E923.8 Other explosive materials
    Bomb   Torpedo
    Explosive missile   Explosion in munitions:
    Grenade   dump
    Mine   factory
    Shell

E923.9 Unspecified explosive material
    Explosion NOS

E924 Accident caused by hot substance or object, caustic or corrosive material, and steam

Excludes: *burning NOS (E899)*
    chemical burn resulting from swallowing a corrosive substance (E860.0-E864.4)
    fire caused by these substances and objects (E890.0-E894)
    radiation burns (E926.0-E926.9)
    therapeutic misadventures (E870.0-E876.9)

E924.0 Hot liquids and vapors, including steam
    Burning or scalding by:
        boiling water
        hot or boiling liquids not primarily caustic or corrosive
        liquid metal
        steam
        other hot vapor

Excludes: *hot (boiling) tap water (E924.2)*

E924.1 Caustic and corrosive substances
    Burning by:
        acid [any kind]
        ammonia
        caustic oven cleaner or other substance
        corrosive substance
        lye
        vitriol

E924.2 Hot (boiling) tap water

E924.8 Other
    Burning by:
        heat from electric heating appliance
        hot object NOS
        light bulb
        steam pipe

E924.9 Unspecified

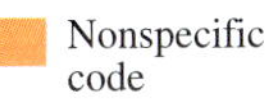

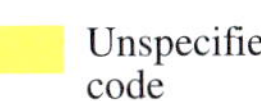

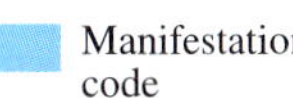

E925 Accident caused by electric current
Includes: electric current from exposed wire, faulty appliance, high voltage cable, live rail,
or open electric socket as the cause of:
burn
cardiac fibrillation
convulsion
electric shock
electrocution
puncture wound
respiratory paralysis

Excludes: *burn by heat from electrical appliance (E924.8)*
lightning (E907)

E925.0 Domestic wiring and appliances

E925.1 Electric power generating plants, distribution stations, transmission lines
Broken power line

E925.2 Industrial wiring, appliances, and electrical machinery
Conductors
Control apparatus
Electrical equipment and machinery
Transformers

E925.8 Other electric current
Wiring and appliances in or on:
farm [not farmhouse]
outdoors
public building
residential institutions
schools

E925.9 Unspecified electric current
Burns or other injury from electric current NOS
Electric shock NOS
Electrocution NOS

E926 Exposure to radiation
Excludes: *abnormal reaction to or complication of treatment without mention of*
misadventure (E879.2)
atomic power plant malfunction in water transport (E838.0-E838.9)
misadventure to patient in surgical and medical procedures (E873.2-E873.3)
use of radiation in war operations (E996-E997.9)

E926.0 Radiofrequency radiation
Overexposure to:
microwave radiation from:
high-powered radio and television transmitters
industrial radiofrequency induction heaters
radar installations
radar radiation from:
high-powered radio and television transmitters
industrial radiofrequency induction heaters
radar installations
radiofrequency from:
high-powered radio and television transmitters
industrial radiofrequency induction heaters
radar installations
radiofrequency radiation [any] from:
high-powered radio and television transmitters
industrial radiofrequency induction heaters
radar installations

E926.1 Infra-red heaters and lamps
Exposure to infra-red radiation from heaters and lamps as the cause of:
blistering
burning
charring
inflammatory change

Excludes: *physical contact with heater or lamp (E924.8)*

● Code new
to this edition

▲ Revision of
existing code

④ ⑤ Fourth or fifth
digit required

E926.2   Visible and ultraviolet light sources
Arc lamps
Black light sources
Electrical welding arc
Oxygas welding torch
Sun rays
Tanning bed

Excludes: excessive heat from these sources (E900.1-E900.9)

E926.3   X-rays and other electromagnetic ionizing radiation
Gamma rays
X-rays (hard) (soft)

E926.4   Lasers

E926.5   Radioactive isotopes
Radiobiologicals
Radiopharmaceuticals

E926.8   Other specified radiation
Artificially accelerated beams of ionized particles generated by:
betatrons
synchrotrons

E926.9   Unspecified radiation
Radiation NOS

E927   Overexertion and strenuous movements
Excessive physical exercise   Strenuous movements in:
Overexertion (from):   recreational activities
lifting   other activities
pulling
pushing

E928   Other and unspecified environmental and accidental causes

E928.0   Prolonged stay in weightless environment
Weightlessness in spacecraft (simulator)

E928.1   Exposure to noise
Noise (pollution)
Sound waves
Supersonic waves

E928.2   Vibration

E928.3   Human bite

E928.4   External constriction caused by hair

E928.5   External constriction caused by other object

E928.8   Other

E928.9   Unspecified accident
Accident NOS stated as accidentally inflicted
Blow NOS stated as accidentally inflicted
Casualty (not due to war), stated as accidentally inflicted, but not otherwise specified
Decapitation, stated as accidentally inflicted, but not otherwise specified
Injury [any part of body, or unspecified], stated as accidentally inflicted, but not
otherwise specified
Killed, stated as accidentally inflicted, but not otherwise specified
Knocked down, stated as accidentally inflicted, but not otherwise specified
Mangled, stated as accidentally inflicted, but not otherwise specified
Wound, stated as accidentally inflicted, but not otherwise specified

Excludes: fracture, cause unspecified (E887)
injuries undetermined whether accidentally or purposely inflicted (E980.0-E989)

LATE EFFECTS OF ACCIDENTAL INJURY (E929)

Note: This category is to be used to indicate accidental injury as the cause of death or disability
from late effects, which are themselves classifiable elsewhere. The "late effects" include
conditions reported as such or as sequelae which may occur at any time after the acute
injury.

E929   Late effects of accidental injury

Excludes: late effects of:
surgical and medical procedures (E870.0-E879.9)
therapeutic use of drugs and medicines (E930.0-E949.9)

E929.0   Late effects of motor vehicle accident
Late effects of accidents classifiable to E810-E825

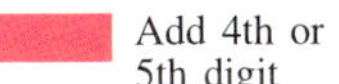
Add 4th or
5th digit

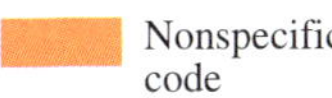
Nonspecific
code

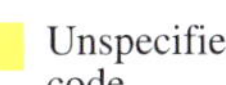
Unspecified
code

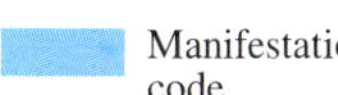
Manifestation
code

E929.1 Late effects of other transport accident
Late effects of accidents classifiable to E800-E807, E826-E838, E840-E848

E929.2 Late effects of accidental poisoning
Late effects of accidents classifiable to E850-E858, E860-E869

E929.3 Late effects of accidental fall
Late effects of accidents classifiable to E880-E888

E929.4 Late effects of accident caused by fire
Late effects of accidents classifiable to E890-E899

E929.5 Late effects of accident due to natural and environmental factors
Late effects of accidents classifiable to E900-E909

E929.8 Late effects of other accidents
Late effects of accidents classifiable to E910-E928.8

E929.9 Late effects of unspecified accident
Late effects of accidents classifiable to E928.9

DRUGS, MEDICINAL AND BIOLOGICAL SUBSTANCES CAUSING ADVERSE EFFECTS IN THERAPEUTIC USE (E930-E949)

Includes: correct drug properly administered in therapeutic or prophylactic dosage, as the cause of any adverse effect including allergic or hypersensitivity reactions

Excludes: *accidental overdose of drug and wrong drug given or taken in error (E850.0-E858.9)*
accidents in the technique of administration of drug or biological substance, such as accidental puncture during injection, or contamination of drug (E870.0-E876.9)
administration with suicidal or homicidal intent or intent to harm, or in circumstances classifiable to E980-E989 (E950.0-E950.5, E962.0, E980.0-E980.5)

See Alphabetic Index for more complete list of specific drugs to be classified under the fourth-digit subdivisions. The American Hospital Formulary numbers can be used to classify new drugs listed by the American Hospital Formulary Service (AHFS). See appendix C.

E930 Antibiotics

Excludes: *that used as eye, ear, nose, and throat [ENT], and local anti-infectives (E946.0-E946.9)*

E930.0 Penicillins
Natural
Synthetic
Semisynthetic, such as:
ampicillin
cloxacillin
nafcillin
oxacillin

E930.1 Antifungal antibiotics
Amphotericin B
Griseofulvin
Hachimycin [trichomycin]
Nystatin

E930.2 Chloramphenicol group
Chloramphenicol
Thiamphenicol

E930.3 Erythromycin and other macrolides
Oleandomycin
Spiramycin

E930.4 Tetracycline group
Doxycycline
Minocycline
Oxytetracycline

E930.5 Cephalosporin group
Cephalexin
Cephaloglycin
Cephaloridine
Cephalothin

● Code new to this edition　　▲ Revision of existing code　　④ ⑤ Fourth or fifth digit required

E930.6 Antimycobacterial antibiotics
Cycloserine
Kanamycin
Rifampin
Streptomycin

E930.7 Antineoplastic antibiotics
Actinomycins, such as:
Cactinomycin
Dactinomycin
Bleomycin
Daunorubicin
Mitomycin

Excludes: other antineoplastic drugs (E933.1)

E930.8 Other specified antibiotics

E930.9 Unspecified antibiotic

E931 Other anti-infectives

Excludes: ENT, and local anti-infectives (E946.0-E946.9)

E931.0 Sulfonamides
Sulfadiazine
Sulfafurazole
Sulfamethoxazole

E931.1 Arsenical anti-infectives

E931.2 Heavy metal anti-infectives
Compounds of:
antimony
bismuth
lead
mercury

Excludes: mercurial diuretics (E944.0)

E931.3 Quinoline and hydroxyquinoline derivatives
Chiniofon
Diiodohydroxyquin

Excludes: antimalarial drugs (E931.4)

E931.4 Antimalarials and drugs acting on other blood protozoa
Chloroquine phosphate   Proguanil [chloroguanide]
Cycloguanil   Pyrimethamine
Primaquine   Quinine (sulphate)

E931.5 Other antiprotozoal drugs
Emetine

E931.6 Anthelmintics
Hexylresorcinol   Piperazine
Male fern oleoresin   Thiabendazole

E931.7 Antiviral drugs
Methisazone

Excludes: amantadine (E936.4)

cytarabine (E933.1)
idoxuridine (E946.5)

E931.8 Other antimycobacterial drugs
Ethambutol   Para-aminosalicylic acid derivatives
Ethionamide   Sulfones
Isoniazid

E931.9 Other and unspecified anti-infectives
Flucytosine   Nitrofuran derivatives

E932 Hormones and synthetic substitutes

E932.0 Adrenal cortical steroids
Cortisone derivatives
Desoxycorticosterone derivatives
Fluorinated corticosteroids

E932.1 Androgens and anabolic congeners
Nandrolone phenpropionate
Oxymetholone
Testosterone and preparations

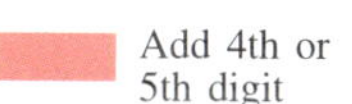

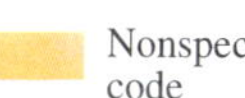

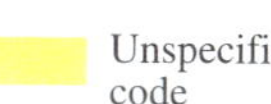

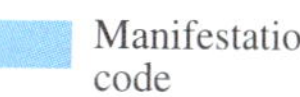

E932.2 Ovarian hormones and synthetic substitutes
Contraceptives, oral
Estrogens
Estrogens and progestogens combined
Progestogens

E932.3 Insulins and antidiabetic agents
Acetohexamide
Biguanide derivatives, oral
Chlorpropamide
Glucagon
Insulin
Phenformin
Sulfonylurea derivatives, oral
Tolbutamide

Excludes: *adverse effect of insulin administered for shock therapy (E879.3)*

E932.4 Anterior pituitary hormones
Corticotropin
Gonadotropin
Somatotropin [growth hormone]

E932.5 Posterior pituitary hormones
Vasopressin

Excludes: *oxytocic agents (E945.0)*

E932.6 Parathyroid and parathyroid derivatives

E932.7 Thyroid and thyroid derivatives
Dextrothyroxine
Levothyroxine sodium
Liothyronine
Thyroglobulin

E932.8 Antithyroid agents
Iodides
Thiouracil
Thiourea

E932.9 Other and unspecified hormones and synthetic substitutes

E933 Primarily systemic agents

E933.0 Antiallergic and antiemetic drugs
Antihistamines
Chlorpheniramine
Diphenhydramine
Diphenylpyraline
Thonzylamine
Tripelennamine

Excludes: *phenothiazine-based tranquilizers (E939.1)*

E933.1 Antineoplastic and immunosuppressive drugs
Azathioprine
Busulfan
Chlorambucil
Cyclophosphamide
Cytarabine
Fluorouracil
Mechlorethamine hydrochloride
Mercaptopurine
Triethylenethiophosphoramide [thio-TEPA]

Excludes: *antineoplastic antibiotics (E930.7)*

E933.2 Acidifying agents

E933.3 Alkalizing agents

E933.4 Enzymes, not elsewhere classified
Penicillinase

E933.5 Vitamins, not elsewhere classified
Vitamin A
Vitamin D

Excludes: *nicotinic acid (E942.2)*
vitamin K (E934.3)

E933.8 Other systemic agents, not elsewhere classified
Heavy metal antagonists

E933.9 Unspecified systemic agent

E934 Agents primarily affecting blood constituents

E934.0 Iron and its compounds
Ferric salts
Ferrous sulphate and other ferrous salts

E934.1 Liver preparations and other antianemic agents
Folic acid

E934.2 Anticoagulants
Coumarin
Heparin
Phenindione
Prothrombin synthesis inhibitor
Warfarin sodium

● Code new to this edition   ▲ Revision of existing code   ④ ⑤ Fourth or fifth digit required

E934.3 **Vitamin K [phytonadione]**

E934.4 **Fibrinolysis-affecting drugs**
Aminocaproic acid   Streptokinase
Streptodornase   Urokinase

E934.5 **Anticoagulant antagonists and other coagulants**
Hexadimethrine bromide   Protamine sulfate

E934.6 **Gamma globulin**

E934.7 **Natural blood and blood products**
Blood plasma   Packed red cells
Human fibrinogen   Whole blood

E934.8 **Other agents affecting blood constituents**
Macromolecular blood substitutes

E934.9 **Unspecified agent affecting blood constituents**

E935 **Analgesics, antipyretics, and antirheumatics**

E935.0 **Heroin**
Diacetylmorphine

E935.1 **Methadone**

E935.2 **Other opiates and related narcotics**
Codeine [methylmorphine]   Opium (alkaloids)
Morphine   Meperidine [pethidine]

E935.3 **Salicylates**
Acetylsalicylic acid [aspirin]
Amino derivatives of salicylic acid
Salicylic acid salts

E935.4 **Aromatic analgesics, not elsewhere classified**
Acetanilid
Paracetamol [acetaminophen]
Phenacetin [acetophenetidin]

E935.5 **Pyrazole derivatives**
Aminophenazone [aminopyrine]
Phenylbutazone

E935.6 **Antirheumatics [antiphlogistics]**
Gold salts   Indomethacin

Excludes: *salicylates (E935.3)*
steroids (E932.0)

E935.7 **Other non-narcotic analgesics**
Pyrabital

E935.8 **Other specified analgesics and antipyretics**
Pentazocine

E935.9 **Unspecified analgesic and antipyretic**

E936 **Anticonvulsants and anti-Parkinsonism drugs**

E936.0 **Oxazolidine derivatives**
Paramethadione
Trimethadione

E936.1 **Hydantoin derivatives**
Phenytoin

E936.2 **Succinimides**
Ethosuximide
Phensuximide

E936.3 **Other and unspecified anticonvulsants**
Beclamide
Primidone

E936.4 **Anti-Parkinsonism drugs**
Amantadine
Ethopropazine [profenamine]
Levodopa [L-dopa]

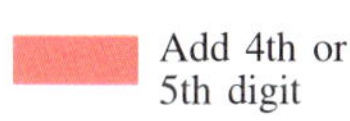

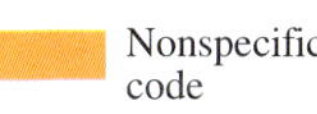

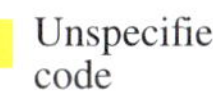

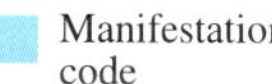

E937 **Sedatives and hypnotics**

   E937.0 **Barbiturates**
       Amobarbital [amylobarbitone]
       Barbital [barbitone]
       Butabarbital [butabarbitone]
       Pentobarbital [pentobarbitone]
       Phenobarbital [phenobarbitone]
       Secobarbital [quinalbarbitone]

       | Excludes: | thiobarbiturates (E938.3)

   E937.1 **Chloral hydrate group**

   E937.2 **Paraldehyde**

   E937.3 **Bromine compounds**
       Bromide
       Carbromal (derivatives)

   E937.4 **Methaqualone compounds**

   E937.5 **Glutethimide group**

   E937.6 **Mixed sedatives, not elsewhere classified**

   E937.8 **Other sedatives and hypnotics**

   E937.9 **Unspecified**
       Sleeping:
         drug NOS
         pill NOS
         tablet NOS

E938 **Other central nervous system depressants and anesthetics**

   E938.0 **Central nervous system muscle-tone depressants**
       Chlorphenesin (carbamate)   Methocarbamol
       Mephenesin

   E938.1 **Halothane**

   E938.2 **Other gaseous anesthetics**
       Ether
       Halogenated hydrocarbon derivatives, except halothane
       Nitrous oxide

   E938.3 **Intravenous anesthetics**
       Ketamine   Thiobarbiturates, such as thiopental sodium
       Methohexital
       [methohexitone]

   E938.4 **Other and unspecified general anesthetics**

   E938.5 **Surface and infiltration anesthetics**
       Cocaine   Procaine
       Lidocaine [lignocaine]   Tetracaine

   E938.6 **Peripheral nerve- and plexus-blocking anesthetics**

   E938.7 **Spinal anesthetics**

   E938.9 **Other and unspecified local anesthetics**

E939 **Psychotropic agents**

   E939.0 **Antidepressants**
       Amitriptyline   Monoamine oxidase [MAO] inhibitors
       Imipramine

   E939.1 **Phenothiazine-based tranquilizers**
       Chlorpromazine   Prochlorperazine
       Fluphenazine   Promazine
       Phenothiazine

   E939.2 **Butyrophenone-based tranquilizers**
       Haloperidol   Trifluperidol
       Spiperone

   E939.3 **Other antipsychotics, neuroleptics, and major tranquilizers**

   E939.4 **Benzodiazepine-based tranquilizers**
       Chlordiazepoxide   Lorazepam
       Diazepam   Medazepam
       Flurazepam   Nitrazepam

   E939.5 **Other tranquilizers**
       Hydroxyzine   Meprobamate

  ● Code new
     to this edition   ▲ Revision of
                 existing code   ④ ⑤ Fourth or fifth
                                         digit required

E939.6	**Psychodysleptics [hallucinogens]**	
	Cannabis (derivatives)	Mescaline
	Lysergide [LSD]	Psilocin
	Marihuana (derivatives)	Psilocybin

E939.7 Psychostimulants
Amphetamine   Caffeine

Excludes: central appetite depressants (E947.0)

E939.8 Other psychotropic agents

E939.9 Unspecified psychotropic agent

E940 Central nervous system stimulants

E940.0 Analeptics
Lobeline
Nikethamide

E940.1 Opiate antagonists
Levallorphan
Nalorphine
Naloxone

E940.8 Other specified central nervous system stimulants

E940.9 Unspecified central nervous system stimulant

E941 Drugs primarily affecting the autonomic nervous system

E941.0 Parasympathomimetics [cholinergics]
Acetylcholine   Pilocarpine
Anticholinesterase:
  organophosphorus
  reversible

E941.1 Parasympatholytics [anticholinergics and antimuscarinics] and spasmolytics
Atropine   Hyoscine [scopolamine]
Homatropine   Quaternary ammonium derivatives

Excludes: papaverine (E942.5)

E941.2 Sympathomimetics [adrenergics]
Epinephrine [adrenalin]
Levarterenol [noradrenalin]

E941.3 Sympatholytics [antiadrenergics]
Phenoxybenzamine
Tolazoline hydrochloride

E941.9 Unspecified drug primarily affecting the autonomic nervous system

E942 Agents primarily affecting the cardiovascular system

E942.0 Cardiac rhythm regulators
Practolol   Propranolol
Procainamide   Quinidine

E942.1 Cardiotonic glycosides and drugs of similar action
Digitalis glycosides   Strophanthins
Digoxin

E942.2 Antilipemic and antiarteriosclerotic drugs
Cholestyramine   Nicotinic acid derivatives
Clofibrate   Sitosterols

Excludes: dextrothyroxine (E932.7)

E942.3 Ganglion-blocking agents
Pentamethonium bromide

E942.4 Coronary vasodilators
Dipyridamole   Nitrites
Nitrates [nitroglycerin]   Prenylamine

E942.5 Other vasodilators
Cyclandelate   Hydralazine
Diazoxide   Papaverine

E942.6 Other antihypertensive agents
Clonidine   Rauwolfia alkaloids
Guanethidine   Reserpine

E942.7 Antivaricose drugs, including sclerosing agents
Monoethanolamine   Zinc salts

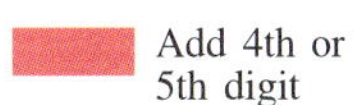

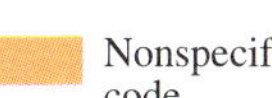

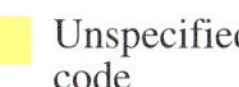

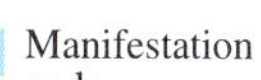

E942.8 **Capillary-active drugs**
    Adrenochrome derivatives   Metaraminol
    Bioflavonoids

E942.9 **Other and unspecified agents primarily affecting the cardiovascular system**

E943 **Agents primarily affecting gastrointestinal system**

E943.0 **Antacids and antigastric secretion drugs**
    Aluminum hydroxide   Magnesium trisilicate

E943.1 **Irritant cathartics**
    Bisacodyl   Phenolphthalein
    Castor oil

E943.2 **Emollient cathartics**
    Sodium dioctyl sulfosuccinate

E943.3 **Other cathartics, including intestinal atonia drugs**
    Magnesium sulfate

E943.4 **Digestants**
    Pancreatin   Pepsin
    Papain

E943.5 **Antidiarrheal drugs**
    Bismuth subcarbonate   Pectin
    Kaolin

    Excludes: *anti-infectives (E930.0-E931.9)*

E943.6 **Emetics**

E943.8 **Other specified agents primarily affecting the gastrointestinal system**

E943.9 **Unspecified agent primarily affecting the gastrointestinal system**

E944 **Water, mineral, and uric acid metabolism drugs**

E944.0 **Mercurial diuretics**
    Chlormerodrin   Mercurophylline
    Mercaptomerin   Mersalyl

E944.1 **Purine derivative diuretics**
    Theobromine   Theophylline

    Excludes: *aminophylline [theophylline ethylenediamine] (E945.7)*

E944.2 **Carbonic acid anhydrase inhibitors**
    Acetazolamide

E944.3 **Saluretics**
    Benzothiadiazides
    Chlorothiazide group

E944.4 **Other diuretics**
    Ethacrynic acid
    Furosemide

E944.5 **Electrolytic, caloric, and water-balance agents**

E944.6 **Other mineral salts, not elsewhere classified**

E944.7 **Uric acid metabolism drugs**
    Cinchophen and congeners   Phenoquin
    Colchicine   Probenecid

E945 **Agents primarily acting on the smooth and skeletal muscles and respiratory system**

E945.0 **Oxytocic agents**
    Ergot alkaloids
    Prostaglandins

E945.1 **Smooth muscle relaxants**
    Adiphenine
    Metaproterenol [orciprenaline]

    Excludes: *papaverine (E942.5)*

E945.2 **Skeletal muscle relaxants**
    Alcuronium chloride
    Suxamethonium chloride

E945.3 **Other and unspecified drugs acting on muscles**

E945.4 **Antitussives**
    Dextromethorphan
    Pipazethate hydrochloride

    ● Code new   ▲ Revision of   ④ ⑤ Fourth or fifth
    to this edition   existing code   digit required

E945.5 **Expectorants**
Acetylcysteine
Cocillana
Guaifenesin [glyceryl guaiacolate]
Ipecacuanha
Terpin hydrate

E945.6 **Anti-common cold drugs**

E945.7 **Antiasthmatics**
Aminophylline [theophylline ethylenediamine]

E945.8 **Other and unspecified respiratory drugs**

E946 **Agents primarily affecting skin and mucous membrane, ophthalmological, otorhinolaryngological, and dental drugs**

E946.0 **Local anti-infectives and anti-inflammatory drugs**

E946.1 **Antipruritics**

E946.2 **Local astringents and local detergents**

E946.3 **Emollients, demulcents, and protectants**

E946.4 **Keratolytics, keratoplastics, other hair treatment drugs and preparations**

E946.5 **Eye anti-infectives and other eye drugs**
Idoxuridine

E946.6 **Anti-infectives and other drugs and preparations for ear, nose, and throat**

E946.7 **Dental drugs topically applied**

E946.8 **Other agents primarily affecting skin and mucous membrane**
Spermicides

E946.9 **Unspecified agent primarily affecting skin and mucous membrane**

E947 **Other and unspecified drugs and medicinal substances**

E947.0 **Dietetics**

E947.1 **Lipotropic drugs**

E947.2 **Antidotes and chelating agents, not elsewhere classified**

E947.3 **Alcohol deterrents**

E947.4 **Pharmaceutical excipients**

E947.8 **Other drugs and medicinal substances**
Contrast media used for diagnostic x-ray procedures
Diagnostic agents and kits

E947.9 **Unspecified drug or medicinal substance**

E948 **Bacterial vaccines**

E948.0 **BCG vaccine**

E948.1 **Typhoid and paratyphoid**

E948.2 **Cholera**

E948.3 **Plague**

E948.4 **Tetanus**

E948.5 **Diphtheria**

E948.6 **Pertussis vaccine, including combinations with a pertussis component**

E948.8 **Other and unspecified bacterial vaccines**

E948.9 **Mixed bacterial vaccines, except combinations with a pertussis component**

E949 **Other vaccines and biological substances**
Excludes: *gamma globulin (E934.6)*

E949.0 **Smallpox vaccine**

E949.1 **Rabies vaccine**

E949.2 **Typhus vaccine**

E949.3 **Yellow fever vaccine**

E949.4 **Measles vaccine**

E949.5 **Poliomyelitis vaccine**

E949.6 **Other and unspecified viral and rickettsial vaccines**
Mumps vaccine

E949.7 **Mixed viral-rickettsial and bacterial vaccines, except combinations with a pertussis component**
Excludes: *combinations with a pertussis component (E948.6)*

Add 4th or 5th digit — Nonspecific code — Unspecified code — Manifestation code

E949.9 Other and unspecified vaccines and biological substances

SUICIDE AND SELF-INFLICTED INJURY (E950-E959)

Includes: injuries in suicide and attempted suicide
self-inflicted injuries specified as intentional

E950 Suicide and self-inflicted poisoning by solid or liquid substances

E950.0 Analgesics, antipyretics, and antirheumatics

E950.1 Barbiturates

E950.2 Other sedatives and hypnotics

E950.3 Tranquilizers and other psychotropic agents

E950.4 Other specified drugs and medicinal substances

E950.5 Unspecified drug or medicinal substances

E950.6 Agricultural and horticultural chemical and pharmaceutical preparations other than plant foods and fertilizers

E950.7 Corrosive and caustic substances
Suicide and self-inflicted poisoning by substances classifiable to E864

E950.8 Arsenic and its compounds

E950.9 Other and unspecified solid and liquid substances

E951 Suicide and self-inflicted poisoning by gases in domestic use

E951.0 Gas distributed by pipeline

E951.1 Liquefied petroleum gas distributed in mobile containers

E951.8 Other utility gas

E952 Suicide and self-inflicted poisoning by other gases and vapors

E952.0 Motor vehicle exhaust gas

E952.1 Other carbon monoxide

E952.8 Other specified gases and vapors

E952.9 Unspecified gases and vapors

E953 Suicide and self-inflicted injury by hanging, strangulation, and suffocation

E953.0 Hanging

E953.1 Suffocation by plastic bag

E953.8 Other specified means

E953.9 Unspecified means

E954 Suicide and self-inflicted injury by submersion [drowning]

E955 Suicide and self-inflicted injury by firearms, air guns and explosives

E955.0 Handgun

E955.1 Shotgun

E955.2 Hunting rifle

E955.3 Military firearms

E955.4 Other and unspecified firearm
Gunshot NOS
Shot NOS

E955.5 Explosives

E955.6 Air gun
BB gun
Pellet gun

E955.7 Paintball gun

E955.9 Unspecified

E956 Suicide and self-inflicted injury by cutting and piercing instrument

E957 Suicide and self-inflicted injuries by jumping from high place

E957.0 Residential premises

E957.1 Other man-made structures

E957.2 Natural sites

E957.9 Unspecified

E958 Suicide and self-inflicted injury by other and unspecified means

E958.0 Jumping or lying before moving object

● Code new
to this edition   ▲ Revision of
existing code   ④ ⑤ Fourth or fifth
digit required

E958.1   **Burns, fire**

E958.2   **Scald**

E958.3   **Extremes of cold**

E958.4   **Electrocution**

E958.5   **Crashing of motor vehicle**

E958.6   **Crashing of aircraft**

E958.7   **Caustic substances, except poisoning**

> *Excludes:* *poisoning by caustic substance (E950.7)*

E958.8   **Other specified means**

E958.9   **Unspecified means**

E959 Late effects of self-inflicted injury

Note: This category is to be used to indicate circumstances classifiable to E950-E958 as the cause of death or disability from late effects, which are themselves classifiable elsewhere. The "late effects" include conditions reported as such or as sequelae which may occur at any time after the attempted suicide or self-inflicted injury.

HOMICIDE AND INJURY PURPOSELY INFLICTED BY OTHER PERSONS (E960-E969)

Includes: injuries inflicted by another person with intent to injure or kill, by any means

> *Excludes:* *injuries due to:*
>> *legal intervention (E970-E978)*
>> *operations of war (E990-E999)*
>> *terrorism (E979)*

E960 Fight, brawl, rape

E960.0   **Unarmed fight or brawl**

    Beatings NOS
    Brawl or fight with hands, fists, feet
    Injured or killed in fight NOS

> *Excludes:* *homicidal:*
>> *injury by weapons (E965.0-E966, E969)*
>> *strangulation (E963)*
>> *submersion (E964)*

E960.1   **Rape**

E961 Assault by corrosive or caustic substance, except poisoning

Injury or death purposely caused by corrosive or caustic substance, such as:
    acid [any]
    corrosive substance
    vitriol

> *Excludes:* *burns from hot liquid (E968.3)*
>> *chemical burns from swallowing a corrosive substance (E962.0-E962.9)*

E962 Assault by poisoning

E962.0   **Drugs and medicinal substances**

    Homicidal poisoning by any drug or medicinal substance

E962.1   **Other solid and liquid substances**

E962.2   **Other gases and vapors**

E962.9   **Unspecified poisoning**

E963 Assault by hanging and strangulation

Homicidal (attempt):
    garrotting or ligature
    hanging
    strangulation
    suffocation

E964 Assault by submersion [drowning]

E965 Assault by firearms and explosives

E965.0   **Handgun**

    Pistol
    Revolver

E965.1   **Shotgun**

E965.2   **Hunting rifle**

E965.3   **Military firearms**

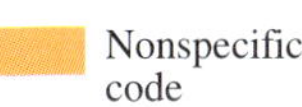
Add 4th or 5th digit   Nonspecific code

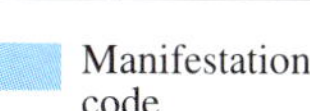
Unspecified code   Manifestation code

E965.4 **Other and unspecified firearm**

E965.5 **Antipersonnel bomb**

E965.6 **Gasoline bomb**

E965.7 **Letter bomb**

E965.8 **Other specified explosive**
　　　Bomb NOS (placed in) car
　　　Bomb NOS (placed in) house
　　　Dynamite

E965.9 **Unspecified explosive**

E966 **Assault by cutting and piercing instrument**
　　　Assassination (attempt), homicide (attempt) by any instrument classifiable under E920
　　　Homicidal cut, any part of the body
　　　Homicidal puncture, any part of the body
　　　Homicidal stab, any part of the body
　　　Stabbed, any part of the body

E967 **Perpetrator of child and adult abuse**
　　　Note: selection of the correct perpetrator code is based on the relationship between the
　　　　perpetrator and the victim

E967.0 **By father, stepfather or boyfriend**
　　　Male partner of child's parent or guardian

E967.1 **By other specified person**

E967.2 **By mother, stepmother or girlfriend**
　　　Female partner of child's parent or guardian

E967.3 **By spouse or partner**
　　　Abuse of spouse or partner by ex-spouse or ex-partner

E967.4 **By child**

E967.5 **By sibling**

E967.6 **By grandparent**

E967.7 **By other relative**

E967.8 **By non-related caregiver**

E967.9 **By unspecified person**

E968 **Assault by other and unspecified means**

E968.0 **Fire**
　　　Arson
　　　Homicidal burns NOS

　　　| Excludes: | burns from hot liquid (E968.3)

E968.1 **Pushing from a high place**

E968.2 **Striking by blunt or thrown object**

E968.3 **Hot liquid**
　　　Homicidal burns by scalding

E968.4 **Criminal neglect**
　　　Abandonment of child, infant, or other helpless person with intent to injure or kill

E968.5 **Transport vehicle**
　　　Being struck by other vehicle or run down with intent to injure
　　　Pushed in front of, thrown from, or dragged by moving vehicle with intent to injure

E968.6 **Air gun**
　　　BB gun
　　　Pellet gun

E968.7 **Human bite**

E968.8 **Other specified means**

E968.9 **Unspecified means**
　　　Assassination (attempt) NOS　　　Manslaughter (nonaccidental)
　　　Homicidal (attempt):　　　　　　Murder (attempt) NOS
　　　　injury NOS　　　　　　　　　Violence, non-accidental
　　　　wound NOS

E969 **Late effects of injury purposely inflicted by other person**
　　　Note: This category is to be used to indicate circumstances classifiable to E960-E968 as the
　　　　cause of death or disability from late effects, which are themselves classifiable elsewhere.
　　　　The "late effects" include conditions reported as such, or as sequelae which may occur at
　　　　any time after the acute injury.

　　● Code new　　　　　　▲ Revision of　　　　　④ ⑤ Fourth or fifth
　　　to this edition　　　　　　existing code　　　　　digit required

LEGAL INTERVENTION (E970-E978)

Includes: injuries inflicted by the police or other law-enforcing agents, including military on duty, in the course of arresting or attempting to arrest lawbreakers, suppressing disturbances, maintaining order, and other legal action
legal execution

Excludes: *injuries caused by civil insurrections (E990.0-E999)*

E970 Injury due to legal intervention by firearms
Gunshot wound
Injury by:
    machine gun
    revolver
    rifle pellet or rubber bullet
    shot NOS

E971 Injury due to legal intervention by explosives
Injury by:
    dynamite
    explosive shell
    grenade
    mortar bomb

E972 Injury due to legal intervention by gas
Asphyxiation by gas
Injury by tear gas
Poisoning by gas

E973 Injury due to legal intervention by blunt object
Hit, struck by:
    baton (nightstick)
    blunt object
    stave

E974 Injury due to legal intervention by cutting and piercing instrument
Cut
Incised wound
Injured by bayonet
Stab wound

E975 Injury due to legal intervention by other specified means
Blow
Manhandling

E976 Injury due to legal intervention by unspecified means

E977 Late effects of injuries due to legal intervention
Note: This category is to be used to indicate circumstances classifiable to E970-E976 as the cause of death or disability from late effects, which are themselves classifiable elsewhere. The "late effects" include conditions reported as such, or as sequelae which may occur at any time after the acute injury due to legal intervention.

E978 Legal execution
All executions performed at the behest of the judiciary or ruling authority [whether permanent or temporary] as:

asphyxiation by gas
beheading, decapitation
    (by guillotine)
capital punishment
electrocution

hanging
poisoning
shooting
other specified means

TERRORISM (E979)

E979 Terrorism
Injuries resulting from the unlawful use of force or violence against persons or property to intimidate or coerce a Government, the civilian population, or any segment thereof, in furtherance of political or social objective

E979.0 Terrorism involving explosion of marine weapons
Depth-charge
Marine mine
Mine NOS, at sea or in harbor
Sea-based artillery shell
Torpedo
Underwater blast

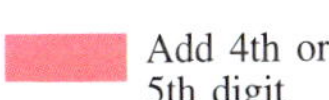

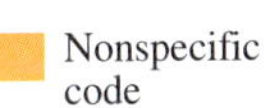

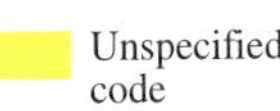

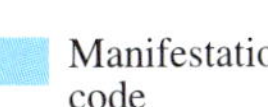

E979.1 Terrorism involving destruction of aircraft
Aircraft used as a weapon
Aircraft:
  burned
  exploded
  shot down
Crushed by falling aircraft

E979.2 Terrorism involving other explosions and fragments
Antipersonnel bomb (fragments)
Blast NOS
Explosion (of):
  artillery shell
  breech-block
  cannon block
  mortar bomb
  munitions being used in terrorism
  NOS
Fragments from:
  artillery shell
  bomb
  grenade
  guided missile
  land-mine
  rocket
  shell
  shrapnel
Mine NOS

E979.3 Terrorism involving fires, conflagration and hot substances
Burning building or structure:
  collapse of
  fall from
  hit by falling object in
  jump from
Conflagration NOS
Fire (causing):
  asphyxia
  burns
  NOS
  other injury
Melting of fittings and furniture in burning
Petrol bomb
Smouldering building or structure

E979.4 Terrorism involving firearms
Bullet:
  carbine
  machine gun
  pistol
  rifle
  rubber (rifle)
Pellets (shotgun)

E979.5 Terrorism involving nuclear weapons
Blast effects
Exposure to ionizing radiation from nuclear weapon
Fireball effects
Heat from nuclear weapon
Other direct and secondary effects of nuclear weapons

E979.6 Terrorism involving biological weapons
Anthrax
Cholera
Smallpox

E979.7 Terrorism involving chemical weapons
Gases, fumes, chemicals
Hydrogen cyanide
Phosgene
Sarin

● Code new
to this edition   ▲ Revision of
existing code   ④ ⑤ Fourth or fifth
digit required

E979.8 **Terrorism involving other means**
Drowning and submersion
Lasers
Piercing or stabbing instruments
Terrorism NOS

E979.9 **Terrorism, secondary effects**
Note: This code is for use to identify conditions occuring subsequent to a terrorist attack not those that are due to the intial terrorist act

> *Excludes:* *late effect of terroist attack (E999.1)*

INJURY UNDETERMINED WHETHER ACCIDENTALLY OR PURPOSELY INFLICTED (E980-E989)

Note: Categories E980-E989 are for use when it is unspecified or it cannot be determined whether the injuries are accidental (unintentional), suicide (attempted), or assault.

E980 **Poisoning by solid or liquid substances, undetermined whether accidentally or purposely inflicted**

E980.0 **Analgesics, antipyretics, and antirheumatics**

E980.1 **Barbiturates**

E980.2 **Other sedatives and hypnotics**

E980.3 **Tranquilizers and other psychotropic agents**

E980.4 **Other specified drugs and medicinal substances**

E980.5 **Unspecified drug or medicinal substance**

E980.6 **Corrosive and caustic substances**
Poisoning, undetermined whether accidental or purposeful, by substances classifiable to E864

E980.7 **Agricultural and horticultural chemical and pharmaceutical preparations other than plant foods and fertilizers**

E980.8 **Arsenic and its compounds**

E980.9 **Other and unspecified solid and liquid substances**

E981 **Poisoning by gases in domestic use, undetermined whether accidentally or purposely inflicted**

E981.0 **Gas distributed by pipeline**

E981.1 **Liquefied petroleum gas distributed in mobile containers**

E981.8 **Other utility gas**

E982 **Poisoning by other gases, undetermined whether accidentally or purposely inflicted**

E982.0 **Motor vehicle exhaust gas**

E982.1 **Other carbon monoxide**

E982.8 **Other specified gases and vapors**

E982.9 **Unspecified gases and vapors**

E983 **Hanging, strangulation, or suffocation, undetermined whether accidentally or purposely inflicted**

E983.0 **Hanging**

E983.1 **Suffocation by plastic bag**

E983.8 **Other specified means**

E983.9 **Unspecified means**

E984 **Submersion [drowning], undetermined whether accidentally or purposely inflicted**

E985 **Injury by firearms, air guns and explosives, undetermined whether accidentally or purposely inflicted**

E985.0 **Handgun**

E985.1 **Shotgun**

E985.2 **Hunting rifle**

E985.3 **Military firearms**

E985.4 **Other and unspecified firearm**

E985.5 **Explosives**

E985.6 **Air gun**
BB gun
Pellet gun

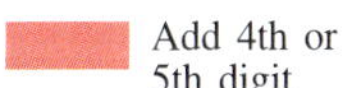

E985.7 **Paintball gun**

E986 **Injury by cutting and piercing instruments, undetermined whether accidentally or purposely inflicted**

E987 **Falling from high place, undetermined whether accidentally or purposely inflicted**

    E987.0 **Residential premises**

    E987.1 **Other man-made structures**

    E987.2 **Natural sites**

    E987.9 **Unspecified site**

E988 **Injury by other and unspecified means, undetermined whether accidentally or purposely inflicted**

    E988.0 **Jumping or lying before moving object**

    E988.1 **Burns, fire**

    E988.2 **Scald**

    E988.3 **Extremes of cold**

    E988.4 **Electrocution**

    E988.5 **Crashing of motor vehicle**

    E988.6 **Crashing of aircraft**

    E988.7 **Caustic substances, except poisoning**

    E988.8 **Other specified means**

    E988.9 **Unspecified means**

E989 **Late effects of injury, undetermined whether accidentally or purposely inflicted**

    Note: This category is to be used to indicate circumstances classifiable to E980-E988 as the cause of death or disability from late effects, which are themselves classifiable elsewhere. The "late effects" include conditions reported as such or as sequelae which may occur at any time after the acute injury, undetermined whether accidentally or purposely inflicted.

INJURY RESULTING FROM OPERATIONS OF WAR (E990-E999)

    Includes: injuries to military personnel and civilians caused by war and civil insurrections and occurring during the time of war and insurrection

    Excludes: *accidents during training of military personnel, manufacture of war material and transport, unless attributable to enemy action*

E990 **Injury due to war operations by fires and conflagrations**
    Includes: asphyxia, burns, or other injury originating from fire caused by a fire-producing device or indirectly by any conventional weapon

    E990.0 **From gasoline bomb**

    E990.9 **From other and unspecified source**

E991 **Injury due to war operations by bullets and fragments**

    E991.0 **Rubber bullets (rifle)**

    E991.1 **Pellets (rifle)**

    E991.2 **Other bullets**
        Bullet [any, except rubber bullets and pellets]
          carbine
          machine gun
          pistol
          rifle
          shotgun

    E991.3 **Antipersonnel bomb (fragments)**

    E991.9 **Other and unspecified fragments**
        Fragments from: Fragments from:
          artillery shell   land mine
          bombs, except antipersonnel rockets
          grenade   shell
          guided missile   Shrapnel

E992 **Injury due to war operations by explosion of marine weapons**
    Depth charge   Sea-based artillery shell
    Marine mines   Torpedo
    Mine NOS, at sea or in harbor Underwater blast

● Code new   ▲ Revision of   ④ ⑤ Fourth or fifth
  to this edition   existing code   digit required

E993 Injury due to war operations by other explosion
Accidental explosion of munitions
   being used in war
Accidental explosion of own weapons
Air blast NOS
Blast NOS
Explosion NOS
Explosion of:
  artillery shell
  breech block
  cannon block
  mortar bomb
Injury by weapon burst

E994 Injury due to war operations by destruction of aircraft
Airplane:
  burned
  exploded
  shot down
Crushed by falling airplane

E995 Injury due to war operations by other and unspecified forms of conventional warfare
Battle wounds
Bayonet injury
Drowned in war operations

E996 Injury due to war operations by nuclear weapons
Blast effects
Exposure to ionizing radiation from nuclear weapons
Fireball effects
Heat
Other direct and secondary effects of nuclear weapons

E997 Injury due to war operations by other forms of unconventional warfare

E997.0 Lasers

E997.1 Biological warfare

E997.2 Gases, fumes, and chemicals

E997.8 Other specified forms of unconventional warfare

E997.9 Unspecified form of unconventional warfare

E998 Injury due to war operations but occurring after cessation of hostilities
Injuries due to operations of war but occurring after cessation of hostilities by any means classifiable under E990-E997
Injuries by explosion of bombs or mines placed in the course of operations of war, if the explosion occurred after cessation of hostilities

E999 Late effect of injury due to war operations and terrorism
Note: This category is to be used to indicate circumstances classifiable to E979, E990-E998 as the cause of death or disability from late effects, which are themselves classifiable elsewhere. The "late effects" include conditions reported as such or as sequelae which may occur at any time after the acute injury, resulting from operations of war or terrorism.

E999.0 Late effect of injury due to war operations

E999.1 Late effect of injury due to terrorism

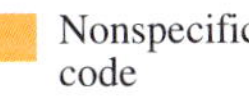 Add 4th or 5th digit

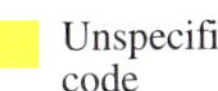 Nonspecific code

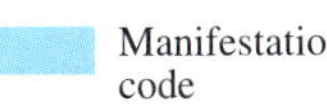 Unspecified code

Manifestation code

APPENDIX A:
MORPHOLOGY OF NEOPLASMS

The World Health Organization has published an adaptation of the International Classification of Diseases for oncology (ICD-O). It contains a coded nomenclature for the morphology of neoplasms, which is reproduced here for those who wish to use it in conjunction with Chapter 2 of the *International Classification of Diseases, 9th Revision, Clinical Modification.*

The morphology code numbers consist of five digits; the first four identify the histological type of the neoplasm and the fifth indicates its behavior. The one-digit behavior code is as follows:

/0 Benign

/1 Uncertain whether benign or malignant
    Borderline malignancy

/2 Carcinoma in situ
    Intraepithelial
    Noninfiltrating
    Noninvasive

/3 Malignant, primary site

/6 Malignant, metastatic site
    Secondary site

/9 Malignant, uncertain whether primary or metastatic site

In the nomenclature below, the morphology code numbers include the behavior code appropriate to the histological type of neoplasm, but this behavior code should be changed if other reported information makes this necessary. For example, "chordoma (M9370/3)" is assumed to be malignant; the term "benign chordoma" should be coded M9370/0. Similarly, "superficial spreading adenocarcinoma (M8143/3)" described as "noninvasive" should be coded M8143/2 and "melanoma (M8720/3)" described as "secondary" should be coded M8720/6.

The following table shows the correspondence between the morphology code and the different sections of Chapter 2:

Morphology code Histology/Behavior			ICD-9-CM Chapter 2
Any	0	210-229	Benign neoplasms
M8000-M8004	1	239	Neoplasms of unspecified nature
M8010+	1	235-238	Neoplasms of uncertain behavior
Any	2	230-234	Carcinoma in situ
Any	3	140-195 200-208	Malignant neoplasms, stated or presumed to be primary
Any	6	196-198	Malignant neoplasms, stated or presumed to be secondary

The ICD-O behavior digit /9 is inapplicable in an ICD context, since all malignant neoplasms are presumed to be primary (/3) or secondary (/6) according to other information on the medical record.

Only the first-listed term of the full ICD-O morphology nomenclature appears against each code number in the list below. The ICD-9-CM Alphabetical Index (Volume 2), however, includes all the ICD-O synonyms as well as a number of other morphological names still likely to be encountered on medical records but omitted from ICD-O as outdated or otherwise undesirable.

A coding difficulty sometimes arises where a morphological diagnosis contains two qualifying adjectives that have different code numbers. An example is "transitional cell epidermoid carcinoma." "Transitional cell carcinoma NOS" is M8120/3 and "epidermoid carcinoma NOS" is M8070/3. In such circumstances, the higher number (M8120/3 in this example) should be used, as it is usually more specific.

CODED NOMENCLATURE FOR MORPHOLOGY OF NEOPLASMS

M800   **Neoplasms NOS**
M8000/0   *Neoplasm, benign*
M8000/1   *Neoplasm, uncertain whether benign or malignant*
M8000/3   *Neoplasm, malignant*
M8000/6   *Neoplasm, metastatic*
M8000/9   *Neoplasm, malignant, uncertain whether primary or metastatic*
M8001/0   *Tumor cells, benign*
M8001/1   *Tumor cells, uncertain whether benign or malignant*
M8001/3   *Tumor cells, malignant*
M8002/3   *Malignant tumor, small cell type*
M8003/3   *Malignant tumor, giant cell type*
M8004/3   *Malignant tumor, fusiform cell type*

M801-M804 Epithelial neoplasms NOS
M8010/0   *Epithelial tumor, benign*
M8010/2   *Carcinoma in situ NOS*
M8010/3   *Carcinoma NOS*
M8010/6   *Carcinoma, metastatic NOS*
M8010/9   *Carcinomatosis*
M8011/0   *Epithelioma, benign*
M8011/3   *Epithelioma, malignant*
M8012/3   *Large cell carcinoma NOS*
M8020/3   *Carcinoma, undifferentiated type NOS*
M8021/3   *Carcinoma, anaplastic type NOS*
M8022/3   *Pleomorphic carcinoma*
M8030/3   *Giant cell and spindle cell carcinoma*
M8031/3   *Giant cell carcinoma*
M8032/3   *Spindle cell carcinoma*
M8033/3   *Pseudosarcomatous carcinoma*
M8034/3   *Polygonal cell carcinoma*
M8035/3   *Spheroidal cell carcinoma*
M8040/1   *Tumorlet*
M8041/3   *Small cell carcinoma NOS*
M8042/3   *Oat cell carcinoma*
M8043/3   *Small cell carcinoma, fusiform cell type*

M805-M808 Papillary and squamous cell neoplasms
M8050/0   *Papilloma NOS (except Papilloma of urinary bladder M8120/1)*
M8050/2   *Papillary carcinoma in situ*
M8050/3   *Papillary carcinoma NOS*
M8051/0   *Verrucous papilloma*
M8051/3   *Verrucous carcinoma NOS*
M8052/0   *Squamous cell papilloma*
M8052/3   *Papillary squamous cell carcinoma*
M8053/0   *Inverted papilloma*
M8060/0   *Papillomatosis NOS*
M8070/2   *Squamous cell carcinoma in situ NOS*
M8070/3   *Squamous cell carcinoma NOS*
M8070/6   *Squamous cell carcinoma, metastatic NOS*
M8071/3   *Squamous cell carcinoma, keratinizing type NOS*
M8072/3   *Squamous cell carcinoma, large cell, nonkeratinizing type*
M8073/3   *Squamous cell carcinoma, small cell, nonkeratinizing type*
M8074/3   *Squamous cell carcinoma, spindle cell type*
M8075/3   *Adenoid squamous cell carcinoma*
M8076/2   *Squamous cell carcinoma in situ with questionable stromal invasion*
M8076/3   *Squamous cell carcinoma, microinvasive*
M8080/2   *Queyrat's erythroplasia*
M8081/2   *Bowen's disease*
M8082/3   *Lymphoepithelial carcinoma*

M809-M811 Basal cell neoplasms
M8090/1   *Basal cell tumor*
M8090/3   *Basal cell carcinoma NOS*
M8091/3   *Multicentric basal cell carcinoma*
M8092/3   *Basal cell carcinoma, morphea type*
M8093/3   *Basal cell carcinoma, fibroepithelial type*
M8094/3   *Basosquamous carcinoma*
M8095/3   *Metatypical carcinoma*
M8096/0   *Intraepidermal epithelioma of Jadassohn*
M8100/0   *Trichoepithelioma*
M8101/0   *Trichofolliculoma*

M8102/0	*Tricholemmoma*
M8110/0	*Pilomatrixoma*

M812-M813 Transitional cell papillomas and carcinomas

M8120/0	*Transitional cell papilloma NOS*
M8120/1	*Urothelial papilloma*
M8120/2	*Transitional cell carcinoma in situ*
M8120/3	*Transitional cell carcinoma NOS*
M8121/0	*Schneiderian papilloma*
M8121/1	*Transitional cell papilloma, inverted type*
M8121/3	*Schneiderian carcinoma*
M8122/3	*Transitional cell carcinoma, spindle cell type*
M8123/3	*Basaloid carcinoma*
M8124/3	*Cloacogenic carcinoma*
M8130/3	*Papillary transitional cell carcinoma*

M814-M838 Adenomas and adenocarcinomas

M8140/0	*Adenoma NOS*
M8140/1	*Bronchial adenoma NOS*
M8140/2	*Adenocarcinoma in situ*
M8140/3	*Adenocarcinoma NOS*
M8140/6	*Adenocarcinoma, metastatic NOS*
M8141/3	*Scirrhous adenocarcinoma*
M8142/3	*Linitis plastica*
M8143/3	*Superficial spreading adenocarcinoma*
M8144/3	*Adenocarcinoma, intestinal type*
M8145/3	*Carcinoma, diffuse type*
M8146/0	*Monomorphic adenoma*
M8147/0	*Basal cell adenoma*
M8150/0	*Islet cell adenoma*
M8150/3	*Islet cell carcinoma*
M8151/0	*Insulinoma NOS*
M8151/3	*Insulinoma, malignant*
M8152/0	*Glucagonoma NOS*
M8152/3	*Glucagonoma, malignant*
M8153/1	*Gastrinoma NOS*
M8153/3	*Gastrinoma, malignant*
M8154/3	*Mixed islet cell and exocrine adenocarcinoma*
M8160/0	*Bile duct adenoma*
M8160/3	*Cholangiocarcinoma*
M8161/0	*Bile duct cystadenoma*
M8161/3	*Bile duct cystadenocarcinoma*
M8170/0	*Liver cell adenoma*
M8170/3	*Hepatocellular carcinoma NOS*
M8180/0	*Hepatocholangioma, benign*
M8180/3	*Combined hepatocellular carcinoma and cholangiocarcinoma*
M8190/0	*Trabecular adenoma*
M8190/3	*Trabecular adenocarcinoma*
M8191/0	*Embryonal adenoma*
M8200/0	*Eccrine dermal cylindroma*
M8200/3	*Adenoid cystic carcinoma*
M8201/3	*Cribriform carcinoma*
M8210/0	*Adenomatous polyp NOS*
M8210/3	*Adenocarcinoma in adenomatous polyp*
M8211/0	*Tubular adenoma NOS*
M8211/3	*Tubular adenocarcinoma*
M8220/0	*Adenomatous polyposis coli*
M8220/3	*Adenocarcinoma in adenomatous polyposis coli*
M8221/0	*Multiple adenomatous polyps*
M8230/3	*Solid carcinoma NOS*
M8231/3	*Carcinoma simplex*
M8240/1	*Carcinoid tumor NOS*
M8240/3	*Carcinoid tumor, malignant*
M8241/1	*Carcinoid tumor, argentaffin NOS*
M8241/3	*Carcinoid tumor, argentaffin, malignant*
M8242/1	*Carcinoid tumor, nonargentaffin NOS*
M8242/3	*Carcinoid tumor, nonargentaffin, malignant*
M8243/3	*Mucocarcinoid tumor, malignant*
M8244/3	*Composite carcinoid*
M8250/1	*Pulmonary adenomatosis*
M8250/3	*Bronchiolo-alveolar adenocarcinoma*
M8251/0	*Alveolar adenoma*

M8251/3	*Alveolar adenocarcinoma*
M8260/0	*Papillary adenoma NOS*
M8260/3	*Papillary adenocarcinoma NOS*
M8261/1	*Villous adenoma NOS*
M8261/3	*Adenocarcinoma in villous adenoma*
M8262/3	*Villous adenocarcinoma*
M8263/0	*Tubulovillous adenoma*
M8270/0	*Chromophobe adenoma*
M8270/3	*Chromophobe carcinoma*
M8280/0	*Acidophil adenoma*
M8280/3	*Acidophil carcinoma*
M8281/0	*Mixed acidophil-basophil adenoma*
M8281/3	*Mixed acidophil-basophil carcinoma*
M8290/0	*Oxyphilic adenoma*
M8290/3	*Oxyphilic adenocarcinoma*
M8300/0	*Basophil adenoma*
M8300/3	*Basophil carcinoma*
M8310/0	*Clear cell adenoma*
M8310/3	*Clear cell adenocarcinoma NOS*
M8311/1	*Hypernephroid tumor*
M8312/3	*Renal cell carcinoma*
M8313/0	*Clear cell adenofibroma*
M8320/3	*Granular cell carcinoma*
M8321/0	*Chief cell adenoma*
M8322/0	*Water-clear cell adenoma*
M8322/3	*Water-clear cell adenocarcinoma*
M8323/0	*Mixed cell adenoma*
M8323/3	*Mixed cell adenocarcinoma*
M8324/0	*Lipoadenoma*
M8330/0	*Follicular adenoma*
M8330/3	*Follicular adenocarcinoma NOS*
M8331/3	*Follicular adenocarcinoma, well differentiated type*
M8332/3	*Follicular adenocarcinoma, trabecular type*
M8333/0	*Microfollicular adenoma*
M8334/0	*Macrofollicular adenoma*
M8340/3	*Papillary and follicular adenocarcinoma*
M8350/3	*Nonencapsulated sclerosing carcinoma*
M8360/1	*Multiple endocrine adenomas*
M8361/1	*Juxtaglomerular tumor*
M8370/0	*Adrenal cortical adenoma NOS*
M8370/3	*Adrenal cortical carcinoma*
M8371/0	*Adrenal cortical adenoma, compact cell type*
M8372/0	*Adrenal cortical adenoma, heavily pigmented variant*
M8373/0	*Adrenal cortical adenoma, clear cell type*
M8374/0	*Adrenal cortical adenoma, glomerulosa cell type*
M8375/0	*Adrenal cortical adenoma, mixed cell type*
M8380/0	*Endometrioid adenoma NOS*
M8380/1	*Endometrioid adenoma, borderline malignancy*
M8380/3	*Endometrioid carcinoma*
M8381/0	*Endometrioid adenofibroma NOS*
M8381/1	*Endometrioid adenofibroma, borderline malignancy*
M8381/3	*Endometrioid adenofibroma, malignant*

M839-M842 Adnexal and skin appendage neoplasms

M8390/0	*Skin appendage adenoma*
M8390/3	*Skin appendage carcinoma*
M8400/0	*Sweat gland adenoma*
M8400/1	*Sweat gland tumor NOS*
M8400/3	*Sweat gland adenocarcinoma*
M8401/0	*Apocrine adenoma*
M8401/3	*Apocrine adenocarcinoma*
M8402/0	*Eccrine acrospiroma*
M8403/0	*Eccrine spiradenoma*
M8404/0	*Hidrocystoma*
M8405/0	*Papillary hydradenoma*
M8406/0	*Papillary syringadenoma*
M8407/0	*Syringoma NOS*
M8410/0	*Sebaceous adenoma*
M8410/3	*Sebaceous adenocarcinoma*
M8420/0	*Ceruminous adenoma*
M8420/3	*Ceruminous adenocarcinoma*

M843	**Mucoepidermoid neoplasms**
M8430/1	*Mucoepidermoid tumor*
M8430/3	*Mucoepidermoid carcinoma*
M844-M849	**Cystic, mucinous, and serous neoplasms**
M8440/0	*Cystadenoma NOS*
M8440/3	*Cystadenocarcinoma NOS*
M8441/0	*Serous cystadenoma NOS*
M8441/1	*Serous cystadenoma, borderline malignancy*
M8441/3	*Serous cystadenocarcinoma NOS*
M8450/0	*Papillary cystadenoma NOS*
M8450/1	*Papillary cystadenoma, borderline malignancy*
M8450/3	*Papillary cystadenocarcinoma NOS*
M8460/0	*Papillary serous cystadenoma NOS*
M8460/1	*Papillary serous cystadenoma, borderline malignancy*
M8460/3	*Papillary serous cystadenocarcinoma*
M8461/0	*Serous surface papilloma NOS*
M8461/1	*Serous surface papilloma, borderline malignancy*
M8461/3	*Serous surface papillary carcinoma*
M8470/0	*Mucinous cystadenoma NOS*
M8470/1	*Mucinous cystadenoma, borderline malignancy*
M8470/3	*Mucinous cystadenocarcinoma NOS*
M8471/0	*Papillary mucinous cystadenoma NOS*
M8471/1	*Papillary mucinous cystadenoma, borderline malignancy*
M8471/3	*Papillary mucinous cystadenocarcinoma*
M8480/0	*Mucinous adenoma*
M8480/3	*Mucinous adenocarcinoma*
M8480/6	*Pseudomyxoma peritonei*
M8481/3	*Mucin-producing adenocarcinoma*
M8490/3	*Signet ring cell carcinoma*
M8490/6	*Metastatic signet ring cell carcinoma*
M850-M854	**Ductal, lobular, and medullary neoplasms**
M8500/2	*Intraductal carcinoma, noninfiltrating NOS*
M8500/3	*Infiltrating duct carcinoma*
M8501/2	*Comedocarcinoma, noninfiltrating*
M8501/3	*Comedocarcinoma NOS*
M8502/3	*Juvenile carcinoma of the breast*
M8503/0	*Intraductal papilloma*
M8503/2	*Noninfiltrating intraductal papillary adenocarcinoma*
M8504/0	*Intracystic papillary adenoma*
M8504/2	*Noninfiltrating intracystic carcinoma*
M8505/0	*Intraductal papillomatosis NOS*
M8506/0	*Subareolar duct papillomatosis*
M8510/3	*Medullary carcinoma NOS*
M8511/3	*Medullary carcinoma with amyloid stroma*
M8512/3	*Medullary carcinoma with lymphoid stroma*
M8520/2	*Lobular carcinoma in situ*
M8520/3	*Lobular carcinoma NOS*
M8521/3	*Infiltrating ductular carcinoma*
M8530/3	*Inflammatory carcinoma*
M8540/3	*Paget's disease, mammary*
M8541/3	*Paget's disease and infiltrating duct carcinoma of breast*
M8542/3	*Paget's disease, extramammary (except Paget's disease of bone)*
M855	**Acinar cell neoplasms**
M8550/0	*Acinar cell adenoma*
M8550/1	*Acinar cell tumor*
M8550/3	*Acinar cell carcinoma*
M856-M858	**Complex epithelial neoplasms**
M8560/3	*Adenosquamous carcinoma*
M8561/0	*Adenolymphoma*
M8570/3	*Adenocarcinoma with squamous metaplasia*
M8571/3	*Adenocarcinoma with cartilaginous and osseous metaplasia*
M8572/3	*Adenocarcinoma with spindle cell metaplasia*
M8573/3	*Adenocarcinoma with apocrine metaplasia*
M8580/0	*Thymoma, benign*
M8580/3	*Thymoma, malignant*
M859-M867	**Specialized gonadal neoplasms**
M8590/1	*Sex cord-stromal tumor*
M8600/0	*Thecoma NOS*
M8600/3	*Theca cell carcinoma*

M8610/0	*Luteoma NOS*
M8620/1	*Granulosa cell tumor NOS*
M8620/3	*Granulosa cell tumor, malignant*
M8621/1	*Granulosa cell-theca cell tumor*
M8630/0	*Androblastoma, benign*
M8630/1	*Androblastoma NOS*
M8630/3	*Androblastoma, malignant*
M8631/0	*Sertoli-Leydig cell tumor*
M8632/1	*Gynandroblastoma*
M8640/0	*Tubular androblastoma NOS*
M8640/3	*Sertoli cell carcinoma*
M8641/0	*Tubular androblastoma with lipid storage*
M8650/0	*Leydig cell tumor, benign*
M8650/1	*Leydig cell tumor NOS*
M8650/3	*Leydig cell tumor, malignant*
M8660/0	*Hilar cell tumor*
M8670/0	*Lipid cell tumor of ovary*
M8671/0	*Adrenal rest tumor*

M868-M871 Paragangliomas and glomus tumors

M8680/1	*Paraganglioma NOS*
M8680/3	*Paraganglioma, malignant*
M8681/1	*Sympathetic paraganglioma*
M8682/1	*Parasympathetic paraganglioma*
M8690/1	*Glomus jugulare tumor*
M8691/1	*Aortic body tumor*
M8692/1	*Carotid body tumor*
M8693/1	*Extra-adrenal paraganglioma NOS*
M8693/3	*Extra-adrenal paraganglioma, malignant*
M8700/0	*Pheochromocytoma NOS*
M8700/3	*Pheochromocytoma, malignant*
M8710/3	*Glomangiosarcoma*
M8711/0	*Glomus tumor*
M8712/0	*Glomangioma*

M872-M879 Nevi and melanomas

M8720/0	*Pigmented nevus NOS*
M8720/3	*Malignant melanoma NOS*
M8721/3	*Nodular melanoma*
M8722/0	*Balloon cell nevus*
M8722/3	*Balloon cell melanoma*
M8723/0	*Halo nevus*
M8724/0	*Fibrous papule of the nose*
M8725/0	*Neuronevus*
M8726/0	*Magnocellular nevus*
M8730/0	*Nonpigmented nevus*
M8730/3	*Amelanotic melanoma*
M8740/0	*Junctional nevus*
M8740/3	*Malignant melanoma in junctional nevus*
M8741/2	*Precancerous melanosis NOS*
M8741/3	*Malignant melanoma in precancerous melanosis*
M8742/2	*Hutchinson's melanotic freckle*
M8742/3	*Malignant melanoma in Hutchinson's melanotic freckle*
M8743/3	*Superficial spreading melanoma*
M8750/0	*Intradermal nevus*
M8760/0	*Compound nevus*
M8761/1	*Giant pigmented nevus*
M8761/3	*Malignant melanoma in giant pigmented nevus*
M8770/0	*Epithelioid and spindle cell nevus*
M8771/3	*Epithelioid cell melanoma*
M8772/3	*Spindle cell melanoma NOS*
M8773/3	*Spindle cell melanoma, type A*
M8774/3	*Spindle cell melanoma, type B*
M8775/3	*Mixed epithelioid and spindle cell melanoma*
M8780/0	*Blue nevus NOS*
M8780/3	*Blue nevus, malignant*
M8790/0	*Cellular blue nevus*

M880 Soft tissue tumors and sarcomas NOS

M8800/0	*Soft tissue tumor, benign*
M8800/3	*Sarcoma NOS*
M8800/9	*Sarcomatosis NOS*
M8801/3	*Spindle cell sarcoma*

M8802/3	*Giant cell sarcoma (except of bone M9250/3)*
M8803/3	*Small cell sarcoma*
M8804/3	*Epithelioid cell sarcoma*

M881-M883 Fibromatous neoplasms

M8810/0	*Fibroma NOS*
M8810/3	*Fibrosarcoma NOS*
M8811/0	*Fibromyxoma*
M8811/3	*Fibromyxosarcoma*
M8812/0	*Periosteal fibroma*
M8812/3	*Periosteal fibrosarcoma*
M8813/0	*Fascial fibroma*
M8813/3	*Fascial fibrosarcoma*
M8814/3	*Infantile fibrosarcoma*
M8820/0	*Elastofibroma*
M8821/1	*Aggressive fibromatosis*
M8822/1	*Abdominal fibromatosis*
M8823/1	*Desmoplastic fibroma*
M8830/0	*Fibrous histiocytoma NOS*
M8830/1	*Atypical fibrous histiocytoma*
M8830/3	*Fibrous histiocytoma, malignant*
M8831/0	*Fibroxanthoma NOS*
M8831/1	*Atypical fibroxanthoma*
M8831/3	*Fibroxanthoma, malignant*
M8832/0	*Dermatofibroma NOS*
M8832/1	*Dermatofibroma protuberans*
M8832/3	*Dermatofibrosarcoma NOS*

M884 Myxomatous neoplasms

M8840/0	*Myxoma NOS*
M8840/3	*Myxosarcoma*

M885-M888 Lipomatous neoplasms

M8850/0	*Lipoma NOS*
M8850/3	*Liposarcoma NOS*
M8851/0	*Fibrolipoma*
M8851/3	*Liposarcoma, well differentiated type*
M8852/0	*Fibromyxolipoma*
M8852/3	*Myxoid liposarcoma*
M8853/3	*Round cell liposarcoma*
M8854/3	*Pleomorphic liposarcoma*
M8855/3	*Mixed type liposarcoma*
M8856/0	*Intramuscular lipoma*
M8857/0	*Spindle cell lipoma*
M8860/0	*Angiomyolipoma*
M8860/3	*Angiomyoliposarcoma*
M8861/0	*Angiolipoma NOS*
M8861/1	*Angiolipoma, infiltrating*
M8870/0	*Myelolipoma*
M8880/0	*Hibernoma*
M8881/0	*Lipoblastomatosis*

M889-M892 Myomatous neoplasms

M8890/0	*Leiomyoma NOS*
M8890/1	*Intravascular leiomyomatosis*
M8890/3	*Leiomyosarcoma NOS*
M8891/1	*Epithelioid leiomyoma*
M8891/3	*Epithelioid leiomyosarcoma*
M8892/1	*Cellular leiomyoma*
M8893/0	*Bizarre leiomyoma*
M8894/0	*Angiomyoma*
M8894/3	*Angiomyosarcoma*
M8895/0	*Myoma*
M8895/3	*Myosarcoma*
M8900/0	*Rhabdomyoma NOS*
M8900/3	*Rhabdomyosarcoma NOS*
M8901/3	*Pleomorphic rhabdomyosarcoma*
M8902/3	*Mixed type rhabdomyosarcoma*
M8903/0	*Fetal rhabdomyoma*
M8904/0	*Adult rhabdomyoma*
M8910/3	*Embryonal rhabdomyosarcoma*
M8920/3	*Alveolar rhabdomyosarcoma*

M893-M899 Complex mixed and stromal neoplasms
M8930/3 *Endometrial stromal sarcoma*
M8931/1 *Endolymphatic stromal myosis*
M8932/0 *Adenomyoma*
M8940/0 *Pleomorphic adenoma*
M8940/3 *Mixed tumor, malignant NOS*
M8950/3 *Mullerian mixed tumor*
M8951/3 *Mesodermal mixed tumor*
M8960/1 *Mesoblastic nephroma*
M8960/3 *Nephroblastoma NOS*
M8961/3 *Epithelial nephroblastoma*
M8962/3 *Mesenchymal nephroblastoma*
M8970/3 *Hepatoblastoma*
M8980/3 *Carcinosarcoma NOS*
M8981/3 *Carcinosarcoma, embryonal type*
M8982/0 *Myoepithelioma*
M8990/0 *Mesenchymoma, benign*
M8990/1 *Mesenchymoma, NOS*
M8990/3 *Mesenchymoma, malignant*
M8991/3 *Embryonal sarcoma*

M900-M903 Fibroepithelial neoplasms
M9000/0 *Brenner tumor NOS*
M9000/1 *Brenner tumor, borderline malignancy*
M9000/3 *Brenner tumor, malignant*
M9010/0 *Fibroadenoma NOS*
M9011/0 *Intracanalicular fibroadenoma NOS*
M9012/0 *Pericanalicular fibroadenoma*
M9013/0 *Adenofibroma NOS*
M9014/0 *Serous adenofibroma*
M9015/0 *Mucinous adenofibroma*
M9020/0 *Cellular intracanalicular fibroadenoma*
M9020/1 *Cystosarcoma phyllodes NOS*
M9020/3 *Cystosarcoma phyllodes, malignant*
M9030/0 *Juvenile fibroadenoma*

M904 Synovial neoplasms
M9040/0 *Synovioma, benign*
M9040/3 *Synovial sarcoma NOS*
M9041/3 *Synovial sarcoma, spindle cell type*
M9042/3 *Synovial sarcoma, epithelioid cell type*
M9043/3 *Synovial sarcoma, biphasic type*
M9044/3 *Clear cell sarcoma of tendons and aponeuroses*

M905 Mesothelial neoplasms
M9050/0 *Mesothelioma, benign*
M9050/3 *Mesothelioma, malignant*
M9051/0 *Fibrous mesothelioma, benign*
M9051/3 *Fibrous mesothelioma, malignant*
M9052/0 *Epithelioid mesothelioma, benign*
M9052/3 *Epithelioid mesothelioma, malignant*
M9053/0 *Mesothelioma, biphasic type, benign*
M9053/3 *Mesothelioma, biphasic type, malignant*
M9054/0 *Adenomatoid tumor NOS*

M906-M909 Germ cell neoplasms
M9060/3 *Dysgerminoma*
M9061/3 *Seminoma NOS*
M9062/3 *Seminoma, anaplastic type*
M9063/3 *Spermatocytic seminoma*
M9064/3 *Germinoma*
M9070/3 *Embryonal carcinoma NOS*
M9071/3 *Endodermal sinus tumor*
M9072/3 *Polyembryoma*
M9073/1 *Gonadoblastoma*
M9080/0 *Teratoma, benign*
M9080/1 *Teratoma NOS*
M9080/3 *Teratoma, malignant NOS*
M9081/3 *Teratocarcinoma*
M9082/3 *Malignant teratoma, undifferentiated type*
M9083/3 *Malignant teratoma, intermediate type*
M9084/0 *Dermoid cyst*
M9084/3 *Dermoid cyst with malignant transformation*

M9090/0	*Struma ovarii NOS*
M9090/3	*Struma ovarii, malignant*
M9091/1	*Strumal carcinoid*

M910 **Trophoblastic neoplasms**
M9100/0	*Hydatidiform mole NOS*
M9100/1	*Invasive hydatidiform mole*
M9100/3	*Choriocarcinoma*
M9101/3	*Choriocarcinoma combined with teratoma*
M9102/3	*Malignant teratoma, trophoblastic*

M911 **Mesonephromas**
M9110/0	*Mesonephroma, benign*
M9110/1	*Mesonephric tumor*
M9110/3	*Mesonephroma, malignant*
M9111/1	*Endosalpingioma*

M912-M916 **Blood vessel tumors**
M9120/0	*Hemangioma NOS*
M9120/3	*Hemangiosarcoma*
M9121/0	*Cavernous hemangioma*
M9122/0	*Venous hemangioma*
M9123/0	*Racemose hemangioma*
M9124/3	*Kupffer cell sarcoma*
M9130/0	*Hemangioendothelioma, benign*
M9130/1	*Hemangioendothelioma NOS*
M9130/3	*Hemangioendothelioma, malignant*
M9131/0	*Capillary hemangioma*
M9132/0	*Intramuscular hemangioma*
M9140/3	*Kaposi's sarcoma*
M9141/0	*Angiokeratoma*
M9142/0	*Verrucous keratotic hemangioma*
M9150/0	*Hemangiopericytoma, benign*
M9150/1	*Hemangiopericytoma NOS*
M9150/3	*Hemangiopericytoma, malignant*
M9160/0	*Angiofibroma NOS*
M9161/1	*Hemangioblastoma*

M917 **Lymphatic vessel tumors**
M9170/0	*Lymphangioma NOS*
M9170/3	*Lymphangiosarcoma*
M9171/0	*Capillary lymphangioma*
M9172/0	*Cavernous lymphangioma*
M9173/0	*Cystic lymphangioma*
M9174/0	*Lymphangiomyoma*
M9174/1	*Lymphangiomyomatosis*
M9175/0	*Hemolymphangioma*

M918-M920 **Osteomas and osteosarcomas**
M9180/0	*Osteoma NOS*
M9180/3	*Osteosarcoma NOS*
M9181/3	*Chondroblastic osteosarcoma*
M9182/3	*Fibroblastic osteosarcoma*
M9183/3	*Telangiectatic osteosarcoma*
M9184/3	*Osteosarcoma in Paget's disease of bone*
M9190/3	*Juxtacortical osteosarcoma*
M9191/0	*Osteoid osteoma NOS*
M9200/0	*Osteoblastoma*

M921-M924 **Chondromatous neoplasms**
M9210/0	*Osteochondroma*
M9210/1	*Osteochondromatosis NOS*
M9220/0	*Chondroma NOS*
M9220/1	*Chondromatosis NOS*
M9220/3	*Chondrosarcoma NOS*
M9221/0	*Juxtacortical chondroma*
M9221/3	*Juxtacortical chondrosarcoma*
M9230/0	*Chondroblastoma NOS*
M9230/3	*Chondroblastoma, malignant*
M9240/3	*Mesenchymal chondrosarcoma*
M9241/0	*Chondromyxoid fibroma*

M925 **Giant cell tumors**
M9250/1	*Giant cell tumor of bone NOS*
M9250/3	*Giant cell tumor of bone, malignant*

M9251/1	*Giant cell tumor of soft parts NOS*
M9251/3	*Malignant giant cell tumor of soft parts*

M926   **Miscellaneous bone tumors**
M9260/3	*Ewing's sarcoma*
M9261/3	*Adamantinoma of long bones*
M9262/0	*Ossifying fibroma*

M927-M934 **Odontogenic tumors**
M9270/0	*Odontogenic tumor, benign*
M9270/1	*Odontogenic tumor NOS*
M9270/3	*Odontogenic tumor, malignant*
M9271/0	*Dentinoma*
M9272/0	*Cementoma NOS*
M9273/0	*Cementoblastoma, benign*
M9274/0	*Cementifying fibroma*
M9275/0	*Gigantiform cementoma*
M9280/0	*Odontoma NOS*
M9281/0	*Compound odontoma*
M9282/0	*Complex odontoma*
M9290/0	*Ameloblastic fibro-odontoma*
M9290/3	*Ameloblastic odontosarcoma*
M9300/0	*Adenomatoid odontogenic tumor*
M9301/0	*Calcifying odontogenic cyst*
M9310/0	*Ameloblastoma NOS*
M9310/3	*Ameloblastoma, malignant*
M9311/0	*Odontoameloblastoma*
M9312/0	*Squamous odontogenic tumor*
M9320/0	*Odontogenic myxoma*
M9321/0	*Odontogenic fibroma NOS*
M9330/0	*Ameloblastic fibroma*
M9330/3	*Ameloblastic fibrosarcoma*
M9340/0	*Calcifying epithelial odontogenic tumor*

M935-M937 **Miscellaneous tumors**
M9350/1	*Craniopharyngioma*
M9360/1	*Pinealoma*
M9361/1	*Pineocytoma*
M9362/3	*Pineoblastoma*
M9363/0	*Melanotic neuroectodermal tumor*
M9370/3	*Chordoma*

M938-M948 **Gliomas**
M9380/3	*Glioma, malignant*
M9381/3	*Gliomatosis cerebri*
M9382/3	*Mixed glioma*
M9383/1	*Subependymal glioma*
M9384/1	*Subependymal giant cell astrocytoma*
M9390/0	*Choroid plexus papilloma NOS*
M9390/3	*Choroid plexus papilloma, malignant*
M9391/3	*Ependymoma NOS*
M9392/3	*Ependymoma, anaplastic type*
M9393/1	*Papillary ependymoma*
M9394/1	*Myxopapillary ependymoma*
M9400/3	*Astrocytoma NOS*
M9401/3	*Astrocytoma, anaplastic type*
M9410/3	*Protoplasmic astrocytoma*
M9411/3	*Gemistocytic astrocytoma*
M9420/3	*Fibrillary astrocytoma*
M9421/3	*Pilocytic astrocytoma*
M9422/3	*Spongioblastoma NOS*
M9423/3	*Spongioblastoma polare*
M9430/3	*Astroblastoma*
M9440/3	*Glioblastoma NOS*
M9441/3	*Giant cell glioblastoma*
M9442/3	*Glioblastoma with sarcomatous component*
M9443/3	*Primitive polar spongioblastoma*
M9450/3	*Oligodendroglioma NOS*
M9451/3	*Oligodendroglioma, anaplastic type*
M9460/3	*Oligodendroblastoma*
M9470/3	*Medulloblastoma NOS*
M9471/3	*Desmoplastic medulloblastoma*
M9472/3	*Medullomyoblastoma*

M9480/3	*Cerebellar sarcoma NOS*
M9481/3	*Monstrocellular sarcoma*

M949-M952 Neuroepitheliomatous neoplasms

M9490/0	*Ganglioneuroma*
M9490/3	*Ganglioneuroblastoma*
M9491/0	*Ganglioneuromatosis*
M9500/3	*Neuroblastoma NOS*
M9501/3	*Medulloepithelioma NOS*
M9502/3	*Teratoid medulloepithelioma*
M9503/3	*Neuroepithelioma NOS*
M9504/3	*Spongioneuroblastoma*
M9505/1	*Ganglioglioma*
M9506/0	*Neurocytoma*
M9507/0	*Pacinian tumor*
M9510/3	*Retinoblastoma NOS*
M9511/3	*Retinoblastoma, differentiated type*
M9512/3	*Retinoblastoma, undifferentiated type*
M9520/3	*Olfactory neurogenic tumor*
M9521/3	*Esthesioneurocytoma*
M9522/3	*Esthesioneuroblastoma*
M9523/3	*Esthesioneuroepithelioma*

M953 Meningiomas

M9530/0	*Meningioma NOS*
M9530/1	*Meningiomatosis NOS*
M9530/3	*Meningioma, malignant*
M9531/0	*Meningotheliomatous meningioma*
M9532/0	*Fibrous meningioma*
M9533/0	*Psammomatous meningioma*
M9534/0	*Angiomatous meningioma*
M9535/0	*Hemangioblastic meningioma*
M9536/0	*Hemangiopericytic meningioma*
M9537/0	*Transitional meningioma*
M9538/1	*Papillary meningioma*
M9539/3	*Meningeal sarcomatosis*

M954-M957 Nerve sheath tumor

M9540/0	*Neurofibroma NOS*
M9540/1	*Neurofibromatosis NOS*
M9540/3	*Neurofibrosarcoma*
M9541/0	*Melanotic neurofibroma*
M9550/0	*Plexiform neurofibroma*
M9560/0	*Neurilemmoma NOS*
M9560/1	*Neurinomatosis*
M9560/3	*Neurilemmoma, malignant*
M9570/0	*Neuroma NOS*

M958 Granular cell tumors and alveolar soft part sarcoma

M9580/0	*Granular cell tumor NOS*
M9580/3	*Granular cell tumor, malignant*
M9581/3	*Alveolar soft part sarcoma*

M959-M963 Lymphomas, NOS or diffuse

M9590/0	*Lymphomatous tumor, benign*
M9590/3	*Malignant lymphoma NOS*
M9591/3	*Malignant lymphoma, non Hodgkin's type*
M9600/3	*Malignant lymphoma, undifferentiated cell type NOS*
M9601/3	*Malignant lymphoma, stem cell type*
M9602/3	*Malignant lymphoma, convoluted cell type NOS*
M9610/3	*Lymphosarcoma NOS*
M9611/3	*Malignant lymphoma, lymphoplasmacytoid type*
M9612/3	*Malignant lymphoma, immunoblastic type*
M9613/3	*Malignant lymphoma, mixed lymphocytic-histiocytic NOS*
M9614/3	*Malignant lymphoma, centroblastic-centrocytic, diffuse*
M9615/3	*Malignant lymphoma, follicular center cell NOS*
M9620/3	*Malignant lymphoma, lymphocytic, well differentiated NOS*
M9621/3	*Malignant lymphoma, lymphocytic, intermediate differentiation NOS*
M9622/3	*Malignant lymphoma, centrocytic*
M9623/3	*Malignant lymphoma, follicular center cell, cleaved NOS*
M9630/3	*Malignant lymphoma, lymphocytic, poorly differentiated NOS*
M9631/3	*Prolymphocytic lymphosarcoma*
M9632/3	*Malignant lymphoma, centroblastic type NOS*
M9633/3	*Malignant lymphoma, follicular center cell, noncleaved NOS*

M964   **Reticulosarcomas**
M9640/3   *Reticulosarcoma NOS*
M9641/3   *Reticulosarcoma, pleomorphic cell type*
M9642/3   *Reticulosarcoma, nodular*

M965-M966 Hodgkin's disease
M9650/3   *Hodgkin's disease NOS*
M9651/3   *Hodgkin's disease, lymphocytic predominance*
M9652/3   *Hodgkin's disease, mixed cellularity*
M9653/3   *Hodgkin's disease, lymphocytic depletion NOS*
M9654/3   *Hodgkin's disease, lymphocytic depletion, diffuse fibrosis*
M9655/3   *Hodgkin's disease, lymphocytic depletion, reticular type*
M9656/3   *Hodgkin's disease, nodular sclerosis NOS*
M9657/3   *Hodgkin's disease, nodular sclerosis, cellular phase*
M9660/3   *Hodgkin's paragranuloma*
M9661/3   *Hodgkin's granuloma*
M9662/3   *Hodgkin's sarcoma*

M969   **Lymphomas, nodular or follicular**
M9690/3   *Malignant lymphoma, nodular NOS*
M9691/3   *Malignant lymphoma, mixed lymphocytic-histiocytic, nodular*
M9692/3   *Malignant lymphoma, centroblastic-centrocytic, follicular*
M9693/3   *Malignant lymphoma, lymphocytic, well differentiated, nodular*
M9694/3   *Malignant lymphoma, lymphocytic, intermediate differentiation, nodular*
M9695/3   *Malignant lymphoma, follicular center cell, cleaved, follicular*
M9696/3   *Malignant lymphoma, lymphocytic, poorly differentiated, nodular*
M9697/3   *Malignant lymphoma, centroblastic type, follicular*
M9698/3   *Malignant lymphoma, follicular center cell, noncleaved, follicular*

M970   **Mycosis fungoides**
M9700/3   *Mycosis fungoides*
M9701/3   *Sezary's disease*

M971-M972 Miscellaneous reticuloendothelial neoplasms
M9710/3   *Microglioma*
M9720/3   *Malignant histiocytosis*
M9721/3   *Histiocytic medullary reticulosis*
M9722/3   *Letterer-Siwe's disease*

M973   **Plasma cell tumors**
M9730/3   *Plasma cell myeloma*
M9731/0   *Plasma cell tumor, benign*
M9731/1   *Plasmacytoma NOS*
M9731/3   *Plasma cell tumor, malignant*

M974   **Mast cell tumors**
M9740/1   *Mastocytoma NOS*
M9740/3   *Mast cell sarcoma*
M9741/3   *Malignant mastocytosis*

M975   **Burkitt's tumor**
M9750/3   *Burkitt's tumor*

M980-M994 Leukemias

M980   **Leukemias NOS**
M9800/3   *Leukemia NOS*
M9801/3   *Acute leukemia NOS*
M9802/3   *Subacute leukemia NOS*
M9803/3   *Chronic leukemia NOS*
M9804/3   *Aleukemic leukemia NOS*

M981   **Compound leukemias**
M9810/3   *Compound leukemia*

M982   **Lymphoid leukemias**
M9820/3   *Lymphoid leukemia NOS*
M9821/3   *Acute lymphoid leukemia*
M9822/3   *Subacute lymphoid leukemia*
M9823/3   *Chronic lymphoid leukemia*
M9824/3   *Aleukemic lymphoid leukemia*
M9825/3   *Prolymphocytic leukemia*

M983   **Plasma cell leukemias**
M9830/3   *Plasma cell leukemia*

M984   **Erythroleukemias**
M9840/3   *Erythroleukemia*
M9841/3   *Acute erythremia*

M9842/3   *Chronic erythremia*

M985   **Lymphosarcoma cell leukemias**
M9850/3   *Lymphosarcoma cell leukemia*

M986   **Myeloid leukemias**
M9860/3   *Myeloid leukemia NOS*
M9861/3   *Acute myeloid leukemia*
M9862/3   *Subacute myeloid leukemia*
M9863/3   *Chronic myeloid leukemia*
M9864/3   *Aleukemic myeloid leukemia*
M9865/3   *Neutrophilic leukemia*
M9866/3   *Acute promyelocytic leukemia*

M987   **Basophilic leukemias**
M9870/3   *Basophilic leukemia*

M988   **Eosinophilic leukemias**
M9880/3   *Eosinophilic leukemia*

M989   **Monocytic leukemias**
M9890/3   *Monocytic leukemia NOS*
M9891/3   *Acute monocytic leukemia*
M9892/3   *Subacute monocytic leukemia*
M9893/3   *Chronic monocytic leukemia*
M9894/3   *Aleukemic monocytic leukemia*

M990-M994 **Miscellaneous leukemias**
M9900/3   *Mast cell leukemia*
M9910/3   *Megakaryocytic leukemia*
M9920/3   *Megakaryocytic myelosis*
M9930/3   *Myeloid sarcoma*
M9940/3   *Hairy cell leukemia*

M995-M997 **Miscellaneous myeloproliferative and lymphoproliferative disorders**
M9950/1   *Polycythemia vera*
M9951/1   *Acute panmyelosis*
M9960/1   *Chronic myeloproliferative disease*
M9961/1   *Myelosclerosis with myeloid metaplasia*
M9962/1   *Idiopathic thrombocythemia*
M9970/1   *Chronic lymphoproliferative disease*

APPENDIX B:
GLOSSARY OF MENTAL DISORDERS

Note: *Appendix B Glossary of Mental Disorders* has been removed from the official ICD-9-CM CD-Rom effective with the FY2005 update.

APPENDIX C:
CLASSIFICATION OF DRUGS BY AMERICAN HOSPITAL FORMULARY SERVICE LIST NUMBER AND THEIR ICD-9-CM EQUIVALENTS

The coding of adverse effects of drugs is keyed to the continually revised Hospital Formulary of the American Hospital Formulary Service (AHFS) published under the direction of the American Society of Hospital Pharmacists.

	AHFS*LIST	ICD-9-CM Diagnosis Code

The following section gives the ICD-9-CM diagnosis code for each AHFS list.

4:00	**ANTIHISTAMINE DRUGS**	963.0
8:00	**ANTI-INFECTIVE AGENTS**	
8:04	Amebacides	961.5
	hydroxyquinoline derivatives	961.3
	arsenical anti-infectives	961.1
8:08	Anthelmintics	961.6
	quinoline derivatives	961.3
8:12.04	Antifungal Antibiotics	960.1
	nonantibiotics	961.9
8:12.06	Cephalosporins	960.5
8:12.08	Chloramphenicol	960.2
8:12.12	The Erythromycins	960.3
8:12.16	The Penicillins	960.0
8:12.20	The Streptomycins	960.6
8:12.24	The Tetracyclines	960.4
8:12.28	Other Antibiotics	960.8
	antimycobacterial antibiotics	960.6
	macrolides	960.3
8:16	Antituberculars	961.8
	antibiotics	960.6
8:18	Antivirals	961.7
8:20	Plasmodicides (antimalarials)	961.4
8:24	Sulfonamides	961.0
8:26	The Sulfones	961.8
8:28	Treponemicides	961.2
8:32	Trichomonacides	961.5
	hydroxyquinoline derivatives	961.3
	nitrofuran derivatives	961.9
8:36	Urinary Germicides	961.9
	quinoline derivatives	961.3
8:40	Other Anti-Infectives	961.9
10:00	**ANTINEOPLASTIC AGENTS**	963.1
	antibiotics	960.7
	progestogens	962.2
12:00	**AUTONOMIC DRUGS**	
12:04	Parasympathomimetic (Cholinergic) Agents	971.0
12:08	Parasympatholytic (Cholinergic Blocking) Agents	971.1
12:12	Sympathomimetic (Adrenergic) Agents	971.2
12:16	Sympatholytic (Adrenergic Blocking) Agents	971.3

	AHFS*LIST	ICD-9-CM Diagnosis Code
12:20	Skeletal Muscle Relaxants	975.2
	central nervous system muscle-tone depressants	968.0
16:00	**BLOOD DERIVATIVES**	964.7
20:00	**BLOOD FORMATION AND COAGULATION**	
20:04	Antianemia Drugs	964.1
20:04.04	Iron Preparations	964.0
20:04.08	Liver and Stomach Preparations	964.1
20:12.04	Anticoagulants	964.2
20:12.08	Antiheparin agents	964.5
20:12.12	Coagulants	964.5
20:12.16	Hemostatics	964.5
	capillary-active drugs	972.8
	fibrinolysis-affecting agents	964.4
	natural products	964.7
24:00	**CARDIOVASCULAR DRUGS**	
24:04	Cardiac Drugs	972.9
	cardiotonic agents	972.1
	rhythm regulators	972.0
24:06	Antilipemic Agents	972.2
	thyroid derivatives	962.7
24:08	Hypotensive Agents	972.6
	adrenergic blocking agents	971.3
	ganglion-blocking agents	972.3
	vasodilators	972.5
24:12	Vasodilating Agents	972.5
	coronary	972.4
	nicotinic acid derivatives	972.2
24:16	Sclerosing Agents	972.7
28:00	**CENTRAL NERVOUS SYSTEM DRUGS**	
28:04	General Anesthetics	968.4
	gaseous anesthetics	968.2
	halothane	968.1
	intravenous anesthetics	968.3
28:08	Analgesics and Antipyretics	965.9
	antirheumatics	965.6
	aromatic analgesics	965.4
	non-narcotics NEC	965.7
	opium alkaloids	965.00
	heroin	965.01
	methadone	965.02
	specified type NEC	965.09
	pyrazole derivatives	965.5
	salicylates	965.1
	specified type NEC	965.8
28:10	Narcotic Antagonists	970.1
28:12	Anticonvulsants	966.3
	barbiturates	967.0
	benzodiazepine-based tranquilizers	969.4
	bromides	967.3
	hydantoin derivatives	966.1
	oxazolidine derivative	966.0
	succinimides	966.2
28:16.04	Antidepressants	969.0

	AHFS*LIST	ICD-9-CM Diagnosis Code
28:16.08	Tranquilizers	969.5
	benzodiazepine-based	969.4
	butyrophenone-based	969.2
	major NEC	969.3
	phenothiazine-based	969.1
28:16.12	Other Psychotherapeutic Agents	969.8
28:20	Respiratory and Cerebral Stimulants	970.9
	analeptics	970.0
	anorexigenic agents	977.0
	psychostimulants	969.7
	specified type NEC	970.8
28:24	Sedatives and Hypnotics	967.9
	barbiturates	967.0
	benzodiazepine-based tranquilizers	969.4
	chloral hydrate group	967.1
	glutethamide group	967.5
	intravenous anesthetics	968.3
	methaqualone	967.4
	paraldehyde	967.2
	phenothiazine-based tranquilizers	969.1
	specified type NEC	967.8
	thiobarbiturates	968.3
	tranquilizer NEC	969.5
36:00	**DIAGNOSTIC AGENTS**	977.8
40:00	**ELECTROLYTE, CALORIC, AND WATER BALANCE AGENTS NEC**	974.5
40:04	Acidifying Agents	963.2
40:08	Alkalinizing Agents	963.3
40:10	Ammonia Detoxicants	974.5
40:12	Replacement Solutions NEC	974.5
	plasma volume expanders	964.8
40:16	Sodium-Removing Resins	974.5
40:18	Potassium-Removing Resins	974.5
40:20	Caloric Agents	974.5
40:24	Salt and Sugar Substitutes	974.5
40:28	Diuretics NEC	974.4
	carbonic acid anhydrase inhibitors	974.2
	mercurials	974.0
	purine derivatives	974.1
	saluretics	974.3
40:36	Irrigating Solutions	974.5
40:40	Uricosuric Agents	974.7
44:00	**ENZYMES NEC**	963.4
	fibrinolysis-affecting agents	964.4
	gastric agents	973.4
48:00	**EXPECTORANTS AND COUGH PREPARATIONS**	
	antihistamine agents	963.0
	antitussives	975.4
	codeine derivatives	965.09
	expectorants	975.5
	narcotic agents NEC	965.09

	AHFS*LIST	ICD-9-CM Diagnosis Code
52:00	**EYE, EAR, NOSE, AND THROAT PREPARATIONS**	
52:04	Anti-Infectives	
	ENT	976.6
	ophthalmic	976.5
52:04.04	Antibiotics	
	ENT	976.6
	ophthalmic	976.5
52:04.06	Antivirals	
	ENT	976.6
	ophthalmic	976.5
52:04.08	Sulfonamides	
	ENT	976.6
	ophthalmic	976.5
52:04.12	Miscellaneous Anti-Infectives	
	ENT	976.6
	ophthalmic	976.5
52:08	Anti-Inflammatory Agents	
	ENT	976.6
	ophthalmic	976.5
52:10	Carbonic Anhydrase Inhibitors	974.2
52:12	Contact Lens Solutions	976.5
52:16	Local Anesthetics	968.5
52:20	Miotics	971.0
52:24	Mydriatics	
	adrenergics	971.2
	anticholinergics	971.1
	antimuscarinics	971.1
	parasympatholytics	971.1
	spasmolytics	971.1
	sympathomimetics	971.2
52:28	Mouth Washes and Gargles	976.6
52:32	Vasoconstrictors	971.2
52:36	Unclassified Agents	
	ENT	976.6
	ophthalmic	976.5
56:00	**GASTROINTESTINAL DRUGS**	
56:04	Antacids and Absorbants	973.0
56:08	Anti-Diarrhea Agents	973.5
56:10	Antiflatulents	973.8
56:12	Cathartics NEC	973.3
	emollients	973.2
	irritants	973.1
56:16	Digestants	973.4
56:20	Emetics and Antiemetics	
	antiemetics	963.0
	emetics	973.6
56:24	Lipotropic Agents	977.1
60:00	**GOLD COMPOUNDS**	965.6
64:00	**HEAVY METAL ANTAGONISTS**	963.8
68:00	**HORMONES AND SYNTHETIC SUBSTITUTES**	
68:04	Adrenals	962.0
68:08	Androgens	962.1

	AHFS*LIST	ICD-9-CM Diagnosis Code
68:12	Contraceptives	962.2
68:16	Estrogens	962.2
68:18	Gonadotropins	962.4
68:20	Insulins and Antidiabetic Agents	962.3
68:20.08	Insulins	962.3
68:24	Parathyroid	962.6
68:28	Pituitary	
	anterior	962.4
	posterior	962.5
68:32	Progestogens	962.2
68:34	Other Corpus Luteum Hormones	962.2
68:36	Thyroid and Antithyroid	
	antithyroid	962.8
	thyroid	962.7
72:00	**LOCAL ANESTHETICS NEC**	968.9
	topical (surface) agents	968.5
	infiltrating agents (intradermal) (subcutaneous)	
	(submucosal)	968.5
	nerve blocking agents (peripheral)	968.6
	(plexus)(regional)	
	spinal	968.7
76:00	**OXYTOCICS**	975.0
78:00	**RADIOACTIVE AGENTS**	990
80:00	**SERUMS, TOXOIDS, AND VACCINES**	
80:04	Serums	979.9
	immune globulin (gamma) (human)	964.6
80:08	Toxoids NEC	978.8
	diphtheria	978.5
	and tetanus	978.9
	with pertussis component	978.6
	tetanus	978.4
	and diphtheria	978.9
	with pertussis component	978.6
80:12	Vaccines NEC	979.9
	bacterial NEC	978.8
	with	
	other bacterial component	978.9
	pertussis component	978.6
	viral and rickettsial component	979.7
	rickettsial NEC	979.6
	with	
	bacterial component	979.7
	pertussis component	978.6
	viral component	979.7
	viral NEC	979.6
	with	
	bacterial component	979.7
	pertussis component	978.6
	rickettsial component	979.7
84:00	**SKIN AND MUCOUS MEMBRANE PREPARATIONS**	
84:04	Anti-Infectives	976.0
84:04.04	Antibiotics	976.0
84:04.08	Fungicides	976.0
84:04.12	Scabicides and Pediculicides	976.0
84:04.16	Miscellaneous Local Anti-Infectives	976.0

	AHFS*LIST	ICD-9-CM Diagnosis Code
84:06	Anti-Inflammatory Agents	976.0
84:08	Antipruritics and Local Anesthetics	
	antipruritics	976.1
	local anesthetics	968.5
84:12	Astringents	976.2
84:16	Cell Stimulants and Proliferants	976.8
84:20	Detergents	976.2
84:24	Emollients, Demulcents, and Protectants	976.3
84:28	Keratolytic Agents	976.4
84:32	Keratoplastic Agents	976.4
84:36	Miscellaneous Agents	976.8
86:00	**SPASMOLYTIC AGENTS**	975.1
	antiasthmatics	975.7
	papaverine	972.5
	theophyllin	974.1
88:00	**VITAMINS**	
88:04	Vitamin A	963.5
88:08	Vitamin B Complex	963.5
	hematopoietic vitamin	964.1
	nicotinic acid derivatives	972.2
88:12	Vitamin C	963.5
88:16	Vitamin D	963.5
88:20	Vitamin E	963.5
88:24	Vitamin K Activity	964.3
88:28	Multivitamin Preparations	963.5
92:00	**UNCLASSIFIED THERAPEUTIC AGENTS**	

APPENDIX D:
CLASSIFICATION OF INDUSTRIAL ACCIDENTS
ACCORDING TO AGENCY

Annex B to the Resolution concerning Statistics of Employment Injuries adopted by the Tenth International Conference of Labor Statisticians on 12 October 1962

1 MACHINES

11 Prime-Movers, except Electrical Motors
111 Steam engines
112 Internal combustion engines
119 Others

12 Transmission Machinery
121 Transmission shafts
122 Transmission belts, cables, pulleys, pinions, chains, gears
129 Others

13 Metalworking Machines
131 Power presses
132 Lathes
133 Milling machines
134 Abrasive wheels
135 Mechanical shears
136 Forging machines
137 Rolling-mills
139 Others

14 Wood and Assimilated Machines
141 Circular saws
142 Other saws
143 Molding machines
144 Overhand planes
149 Others

15 Agricultural Machines
151 Reapers (including combine reapers)
152 Threshers
159 Others

16 Mining Machinery
161 Under-cutters
169 Others

19 Other Machines Not Elsewhere Classified
191 Earth-moving machines, excavating and scraping machines, except means of transport
192 Spinning, weaving and other textile machines
193 Machines for the manufacture of foodstuffs and beverages
194 Machines for the manufacture of paper
195 Printing machines
199 Others

2 MEANS OF TRANSPORT AND LIFTING EQUIPMENT

21 Lifting Machines and Appliances
211 Cranes
212 Lifts and elevators
213 Winches
214 Pulley blocks
219 Others

22 Means of Rail Transport
221 Inter-urban railways
222 Rail transport in mines, tunnels, quarries, industrial establishments, docks, etc.
229 Others

23 Other Wheeled Means of Transport, Excluding Rail Transport
231 Tractors
232 Lorries

2 MEANS OF TRANSPORT AND LIFTING EQUIPMENT *continued*

233 Trucks
234 Motor vehicles, not elsewhere classified
235 Animal-drawn vehicles
236 Hand-drawn vehicles
239 Others

24 Means of Air Transport

25 Means of Water Transport
251 Motorized means of water transport
252 Non-motorized means of water transport

26 Other Means of Transport
261 Cable-cars
262 Mechanical conveyors, except cable-cars
269 Others

3 OTHER EQUIPMENT

31 Pressure Vessels
311 Boilers
312 Pressurized containers
313 Pressurized piping and accessories
314 Gas cylinders
315 Caissons, diving equipment
319 Others

32 Furnaces, Ovens, Kilns
321 Blast furnaces
322 Refining furnaces
323 Other furnaces
324 Kilns
325 Ovens

33 Refrigerating Plants

34 Electrical Installations, Including Electric Motors, but Excluding Electric Hand Tools
341 Rotating machines
342 Conductors
343 Transformers
344 Control apparatus
349 Others

35 Electric Hand Tools

36 Tools, Implements, and Appliances, Except Electric Hand Tools
361 Power-driven hand tools, except electric hand tools
362 Hand tools, not power-driven
369 Others

37 Ladders, Mobile Ramps

38 Scaffolding

39 Other Equipment, Not Elsewhere Classified

4 MATERIALS, SUBSTANCES AND RADIATIONS

41 Explosives

42 Dusts, Gases, Liquids and Chemicals, Excluding Explosives
421 Dusts
422 Gases, vapors, fumes
423 Liquids, not elsewhere classified
424 Chemicals, not elsewhere classified

43 Flying Fragments

44 Radiations
441 Ionizing radiations
449 Others

49 Other Materials and Substances Not Elsewhere Classified

5 WORKING ENVIRONMENT

51 Outdoor
511 Weather
512 Traffic and working surfaces
513 Water
519 Others

52 Indoor
521 Floors
522 Confined quarters
523 Stairs
524 Other traffic and working surfaces
525 Floor openings and wall openings
526 Environmental factors (lighting, ventilation, temperature, noise, etc.)
529 Others

53 Underground
531 Roofs and faces of mine roads and tunnels, etc.
532 Floors of mine roads and tunnels, etc.
533 Working-faces of mines, tunnels, etc.
534 Mine shafts
535 Fire
536 Water
539 Others

6 OTHER AGENCIES, NOT ELSEWHERE CLASSIFIED

61 Animals
611 Live animals
612 Animals products

69 Other Agencies, Not Elsewhere Classified

7 AGENCIES NOT CLASSIFIED FOR LACK OF SUFFICIENT DATA

APPENDIX E:
LIST OF THREE-DIGIT CATEGORIES

1. INFECTIOUS AND PARASITIC DISEASES

Intestinal infectious diseases (001-009)
    001   Cholera
    002   Typhoid and paratyphoid fevers
    003   Other salmonella infections
    004   Shigellosis
    005   Other food poisoning (bacterial)
    006   Amebiasis
    007   Other protozoal intestinal diseases
    008   Intestinal infections due to other organisms
    009   Ill-defined intestinal infections

Tuberculosis (010-018)
    010   Primary tuberculous infection
    011   Pulmonary tuberculosis
    012   Other respiratory tuberculosis
    013   Tuberculosis of meninges and central nervous system
    014   Tuberculosis of intestines, peritoneum, and mesenteric glands
    015   Tuberculosis of bones and joints
    016   Tuberculosis of genitourinary system
    017   Tuberculosis of other organs
    018   Miliary tuberculosis

Zoonotic bacterial diseases (020-027)
    020   Plague
    021   Tularemia
    022   Anthrax
    023   Brucellosis
    024   Glanders
    025   Melioidosis
    026   Rat-bite fever
    027   Other zoonotic bacterial diseases

Other bacterial diseases (030-041)
    030   Leprosy
    031   Diseases due to other mycobacteria
    032   Diphtheria
    033   Whooping cough
    034   Streptococcal sore throat and scarlet fever
    035   Erysipelas
    036   Meningococcal infection
    037   Tetanus
    038   Septicemia
    039   Actinomycotic infections
    040   Other bacterial diseases
    041   Bacterial infection in conditions classified elsewhere and of unspecified site

Human immunodeficiency virus (HIV) infection (042)
    042   Human immunodeficiency virus [HIV] disease

Poliomyelitis and other non-arthropod-borne viral diseases of central nervous system (045-049)
    045   Acute poliomyelitis
    046   Slow virus infection of central nervous system
    047   Meningitis due to enterovirus
    048   Other enterovirus diseases of central nervous system
    049   Other non-arthropod-borne viral diseases of central nervous system

Viral diseases accompanied by exanthem (050-057)
    050   Smallpox
    051   Cowpox and paravaccinia
    052   Chickenpox
    053   Herpes zoster
    054   Herpes simplex
    055   Measles
    056   Rubella

1. INFECTIOUS AND PARASITIC DISEASES *continued*

057   Other viral exanthemata

Arthropod-borne viral diseases (060-066)

060   Yellow fever
061   Dengue
062   Mosquito-borne viral encephalitis
063   Tick-borne viral encephalitis
064   Viral encephalitis transmitted by other and unspecified arthropods
065   Arthropod-borne hemorrhagic fever
066   Other arthropod-borne viral diseases

Other diseases due to viruses and Chlamydiae (070-079)

070   Viral hepatitis
071   Rabies
072   Mumps
073   Ornithosis
074   Specific diseases due to Coxsackie virus
075   Infectious mononucleosis
076   Trachoma
077   Other diseases of conjunctiva due to viruses and Chlamydiae
078   Other diseases due to viruses and Chlamydiae
079   Viral and Chlamydial infection in conditions classified elsewhere and of unspecified
        site

Rickettsioses and other arthropod-borne diseases (080-088)

080   Louse-borne [epidemic] typhus
081   Other typhus
082   Tick-borne rickettsioses
083   Other rickettsioses
084   Malaria
085   Leishmaniasis
086   Trypanosomiasis
087   Relapsing fever
088   Other arthropod-borne diseases

Syphilis and other venereal diseases (090-099)

090   Congenital syphilis
091   Early syphilis, symptomatic
092   Early syphilis, latent
093   Cardiovascular syphilis
094   Neurosyphilis
095   Other forms of late syphilis, with symptoms
096   Late syphilis, latent
097   Other and unspecified syphilis
098   Gonococcal infections
099   Other venereal diseases

Other spirochetal diseases (100-104)

100   Leptospirosis
101   Vincent's angina
102   Yaws
103   Pinta
104   Other spirochetal infection

Mycoses (110-118)

110   Dermatophytosis
111   Dermatomycosis, other and unspecified
112   Candidiasis
114   Coccidioidomycosis
115   Histoplasmosis
116   Blastomycotic infection
117   Other mycoses
118   Opportunistic mycoses

Helminthiases (120-129)

120   Schistosomiasis [bilharziasis]
121   Other trematode infections
122   Echinococcosis

1. INFECTIOUS AND PARASITIC DISEASES *continued*

123   Other cestode infection
124   Trichinosis
125   Filarial infection and dracontiasis
126   Ancylostomiasis and necatoriasis
127   Other intestinal helminthiases
128   Other and unspecified helminthiases
129   Intestinal parasitism, unspecified

Other infectious and parasitic diseases (130-136)

130   Toxoplasmosis
131   Trichomoniasis
132   Pediculosis and phthirus infestation
133   Acariasis
134   Other infestation
135   Sarcoidosis
136   Other and unspecified infectious and parasitic diseases

Late effects of infectious and parasitic diseases (137-139)

137   Late effects of tuberculosis
138   Late effects of acute poliomyelitis
139   Late effects of other infectious and parasitic diseases

2. NEOPLASMS

Malignant neoplasm of lip, oral cavity, and pharynx (140-149)

140   Malignant neoplasm of lip
141   Malignant neoplasm of tongue
142   Malignant neoplasm of major salivary glands
143   Malignant neoplasm of gum
144   Malignant neoplasm of floor of mouth
145   Malignant neoplasm of other and unspecified parts of mouth
146   Malignant neoplasm of oropharynx
147   Malignant neoplasm of nasopharynx
148   Malignant neoplasm of hypopharynx
149   Malignant neoplasm of other and ill-defined sites within the lip, oral cavity, and pharynx

Malignant neoplasm of digestive organs and peritoneum (150-159)

150   Malignant neoplasm of esophagus
151   Malignant neoplasm of stomach
152   Malignant neoplasm of small intestine, including duodenum
153   Malignant neoplasm of colon
154   Malignant neoplasm of rectum, rectosigmoid junction, and anus
155   Malignant neoplasm of liver and intrahepatic bile ducts
156   Malignant neoplasm of gallbladder and extrahepatic bile ducts
157   Malignant neoplasm of pancreas
158   Malignant neoplasm of retroperitoneum and peritoneum
159   Malignant neoplasm of other and ill-defined sites within the digestive organs and peritoneum

Malignant neoplasm of respiratory and intrathoracic organs (160-165)

160   Malignant neoplasm of nasal cavities, middle ear, and accessory sinuses
161   Malignant neoplasm of larynx
162   Malignant neoplasm of trachea, bronchus, and lung
163   Malignant neoplasm of pleura
164   Malignant neoplasm of thymus, heart, and mediastinum
165   Malignant neoplasm of other and ill-defined sites within the respiratory system and intrathoracic organs

Malignant neoplasm of bone, connective tissue, skin, and breast (170-176)

170   Malignant neoplasm of bone and articular cartilage
171   Malignant neoplasm of connective and other soft tissue
172   Malignant melanoma of skin
173   Other malignant neoplasm of skin
174   Malignant neoplasm of female breast
175   Malignant neoplasm of male breast
176   Kaposi's sarcoma

2. NEOPLASMS *continued*

Malignant neoplasm of genitourinary organs (179-189)

179	Malignant neoplasm of uterus, part unspecified
180	Malignant neoplasm of cervix uteri
181	Malignant neoplasm of placenta
182	Malignant neoplasm of body of uterus
183	Malignant neoplasm of ovary and other uterine adnexa
184	Malignant neoplasm of other and unspecified female genital organs
185	Malignant neoplasm of prostate
186	Malignant neoplasm of testis
187	Malignant neoplasm of penis and other male genital organs
188	Malignant neoplasm of bladder
189	Malignant neoplasm of kidney and other and unspecified urinary organs

Malignant neoplasm of other and unspecified sites (190-199)

190	Malignant neoplasm of eye
191	Malignant neoplasm of brain
192	Malignant neoplasm of other and unspecified parts of nervous system
193	Malignant neoplasm of thyroid gland
194	Malignant neoplasm of other endocrine glands and related structures
195	Malignant neoplasm of other and ill-defined sites
196	Secondary and unspecified malignant neoplasm of lymph nodes
197	Secondary malignant neoplasm of respiratory and digestive systems
198	Secondary malignant neoplasm of other specified sites
199	Malignant neoplasm without specification of site

Malignant neoplasm of lymphatic and hematopoietic tissue (200-208)

200	Lymphosarcoma and reticulosarcoma
201	Hodgkin's disease
202	Other malignant neoplasm of lymphoid and histiocytic tissue
203	Multiple myeloma and immunoproliferative neoplasms
204	Lymphoid leukemia
205	Myeloid leukemia
206	Monocytic leukemia
207	Other specified leukemia
208	Leukemia of unspecified cell type

Benign neoplasms (210-229)

210	Benign neoplasm of lip, oral cavity, and pharynx
211	Benign neoplasm of other parts of digestive system
212	Benign neoplasm of respiratory and intrathoracic organs
213	Benign neoplasm of bone and articular cartilage
214	Lipoma
215	Other benign neoplasm of connective and other soft tissue
216	Benign neoplasm of skin
217	Benign neoplasm of breast
218	Uterine leiomyoma
219	Other benign neoplasm of uterus
220	Benign neoplasm of ovary
221	Benign neoplasm of other female genital organs
222	Benign neoplasm of male genital organs
223	Benign neoplasm of kidney and other urinary organs
224	Benign neoplasm of eye
225	Benign neoplasm of brain and other parts of nervous system
226	Benign neoplasm of thyroid gland
227	Benign neoplasm of other endocrine glands and related structures
228	Hemangioma and lymphangioma, any site
229	Benign neoplasm of other and unspecified sites

Carcinoma in situ (230-234)

230	Carcinoma in situ of digestive organs
231	Carcinoma in situ of respiratory system
232	Carcinoma in situ of skin
233	Carcinoma in situ of breast and genitourinary system
234	Carcinoma in situ of other and unspecified sites

Neoplasms of uncertain behavior (235-238)

235	Neoplasm of uncertain behavior of digestive and respiratory systems

2. NEOPLASMS *continued*

236 Neoplasm of uncertain behavior of genitourinary organs
237 Neoplasm of uncertain behavior of endocrine glands and nervous system
238 Neoplasm of uncertain behavior of other and unspecified sites and tissues

Neoplasm of unspecified nature (239)

239 Neoplasm of unspecified nature

3. ENDOCRINE, NUTRITIONAL AND METABOLIC DISEASES, AND IMMUNITY DISORDERS

Disorders of thyroid gland (240-246)

240 Simple and unspecified goiter
241 Nontoxic nodular goiter
242 Thyrotoxicosis with or without goiter
243 Congenital hypothyroidism
244 Acquired hypothyroidism
245 Thyroiditis
246 Other disorders of thyroid

Diseases of other endocrine glands (250-259)

250 Diabetes mellitus
251 Other disorders of pancreatic internal secretion
252 Disorders of parathyroid gland
253 Disorders of the pituitary gland and its hypothalamic control
254 Diseases of thymus gland
255 Disorders of adrenal glands
256 Ovarian dysfunction
257 Testicular dysfunction
258 Polyglandular dysfunction and related disorders
259 Other endocrine disorders

Nutritional deficiencies (260-269)

260 Kwashiorkor
261 Nutritional marasmus
262 Other severe protein-calorie malnutrition
263 Other and unspecified protein-calorie malnutrition
264 Vitamin A deficiency
265 Thiamine and niacin deficiency states
266 Deficiency of B-complex components
267 Ascorbic acid deficiency
268 Vitamin D deficiency
269 Other nutritional deficiencies

Other metabolic and immunity disorders (270-279)

270 Disorders of amino-acid transport and metabolism
271 Disorders of carbohydrate transport and metabolism
272 Disorders of lipoid metabolism
273 Disorders of plasma protein metabolism
274 Gout
275 Disorders of mineral metabolism
276 Disorders of fluid, electrolyte, and acid-base balance
277 Other and unspecified disorders of metabolism
278 Overweight, obesity and other hyperalimentation
279 Disorders involving the immune mechanism

4. DISEASES OF THE BLOOD AND BLOOD-FORMING ORGANS

Diseases of blood and blood-forming organs (280-289)

280 Iron deficiency anemias
281 Other deficiency anemias
282 Hereditary hemolytic anemias
283 Acquired hemolytic anemias
284 Aplastic anemia and other bone marrow failure syndromes
285 Other and unspecified anemias
286 Coagulation defects
287 Purpura and other hemorrhagic conditions
288 Diseases of white blood cells
289 Other diseases of blood and blood-forming organs

5. MENTAL DISORDERS

Organic psychotic conditions (290-294)
- 290 Dementias
- 291 Alcohol-induced mental disorders
- 292 Drug-induced mental disorders
- 293 Transient mental disorders due to conditions classified elsewhere
- 294 Persistent mental disorders due to conditions classified elsewhere

Other psychoses (295-299)
- 295 Schizophrenic disorders
- 296 Episodic mood disorders
- 297 Delusional disorders
- 298 Other nonorganic psychoses
- 299 Pervasive developmental disorders

Neurotic disorders, personality disorders, and other nonpsychotic mental disorders (300-316)
- 300 Anxiety, dissociative and somatoform disorders
- 301 Personality disorders
- 302 Sexual and gender identity disorders
- 303 Alcohol dependence syndrome
- 304 Drug dependence
- 305 Nondependent abuse of drugs
- 306 Physiological malfunction arising from mental factors
- 307 Special symptoms or syndromes, not elsewhere classified
- 308 Acute reaction to stress
- 309 Adjustment reaction
- 310 Specific nonpsychotic mental disorders due to brain damage
- 311 Depressive disorder, not elsewhere classified
- 312 Disturbance of conduct, not elsewhere classified
- 313 Disturbance of emotions specific to childhood and adolescence
- 314 Hyperkinetic syndrome of childhood
- 315 Specific delays in development
- 316 Psychic factors associated with diseases classified elsewhere

Mental retardation (317-319)
- 317 Mild mental retardation
- 318 Other specified mental retardation
- 319 Unspecified mental retardation

6. DISEASES OF THE NERVOUS SYSTEM AND SENSE ORGANS

Inflammatory diseases of the central nervous system (320-326)
- 320 Bacterial meningitis
- 321 Meningitis due to other organisms
- 322 Meningitis of unspecified cause
- 323 Encephalitis, myelitis, and encephalomyelitis
- 324 Intracranial and intraspinal abscess
- 325 Phlebitis and thrombophlebitis of intracranial venous sinuses
- 326 Late effects of intracranial abscess or pyogenic infection

Organic sleep disorders (327)
- 327 Organic sleep disorders

Hereditary and degenerative diseases of the central nervous system (330-337)
- 330 Cerebral degenerations usually manifest in childhood
- 331 Other cerebral degenerations
- 332 Parkinson's disease
- 333 Other extrapyramidal disease and abnormal movement disorders
- 334 Spinocerebellar disease
- 335 Anterior horn cell disease
- 336 Other diseases of spinal cord
- 337 Disorders of the autonomic nervous system

Pain (338)
- 338 Pain, not elsewhere classified

Other disorders of the central nervous system (340-349)
- 340 Multiple sclerosis
- 341 Other demyelinating diseases of central nervous system
- 342 Hemiplegia and hemiparesis

6. DISEASES OF THE NERVOUS SYSTEM AND SENSE ORGANS *continued*

343 Infantile cerebral palsy
344 Other paralytic syndromes
345 Epilepsy and recurrent seizures
346 Migraine
347 Cataplexy and narcolepsy
348 Other conditions of brain
349 Other and unspecified disorders of the nervous system

Disorders of the peripheral nervous system (350-359)

350 Trigeminal nerve disorders
351 Facial nerve disorders
352 Disorders of other cranial nerves
353 Nerve root and plexus disorders
354 Mononeuritis of upper limb and mononeuritis multiplex
355 Mononeuritis of lower limb and unspecified site
356 Hereditary and idiopathic peripheral neuropathy
357 Inflammatory and toxic neuropathy
358 Myoneural disorders
359 Muscular dystrophies and other myopathies

Disorders of the eye and adnexa (360-379)

360 Disorders of the globe
361 Retinal detachments and defects
362 Other retinal disorders
363 Chorioretinal inflammations, scars and other disorders of choroid
364 Disorders of iris and ciliary body
365 Glaucoma
366 Cataract
367 Disorders of refraction and accommodation
368 Visual disturbances
369 Blindness and low vision
370 Keratitis
371 Corneal opacity and other disorders of cornea
372 Disorders of conjunctiva
373 Inflammation of eyelids
374 Other disorders of eyelids
375 Disorders of lacrimal system
376 Disorders of the orbit
377 Disorders of optic nerve and visual pathways
378 Strabismus and other disorders of binocular eye movements
379 Other disorders of eye

Diseases of the ear and mastoid process (380-389)

380 Disorders of external ear
381 Nonsuppurative otitis media and Eustachian tube disorders
382 Suppurative and unspecified otitis media
383 Mastoiditis and related conditions
384 Other disorders of tympanic membrane
385 Other disorders of middle ear and mastoid
386 Vertiginous syndromes and other disorders of vestibular system
387 Otosclerosis
388 Other disorders of ear
389 Hearing loss

7. DISEASES OF THE CIRCULATORY SYSTEM

Acute rheumatic fever (390-392)

390 Rheumatic fever without mention of heart involvement
391 Rheumatic fever with heart involvement
392 Rheumatic chorea

Chronic rheumatic heart disease (393-398)

393 Chronic rheumatic pericarditis
394 Diseases of mitral valve
395 Diseases of aortic valve
396 Diseases of mitral and aortic valves
397 Diseases of other endocardial structures

7. **DISEASES OF THE CIRCULATORY SYSTEM** *continued*

    398   Other rheumatic heart disease

Hypertensive disease (401-405)

    401   Essential hypertension
    402   Hypertensive heart disease
    403   Hypertensive chronic kidney disease
    404   Hypertensive heart and chronic kidney disease
    405   Secondary hypertension

Ischemic heart disease (410-414)

    410   Acute myocardial infarction
    411   Other acute and subacute form of ischemic heart disease
    412   Old myocardial infarction
    413   Angina pectoris
    414   Other forms of chronic ischemic heart disease

Diseases of pulmonary circulation (415-417)

    415   Acute pulmonary heart disease
    416   Chronic pulmonary heart disease
    417   Other diseases of pulmonary circulation

Other forms of heart disease (420-429)

    420   Acute pericarditis
    421   Acute and subacute endocarditis
    422   Acute myocarditis
    423   Other diseases of pericardium
    424   Other diseases of endocardium
    425   Cardiomyopathy
    426   Conduction disorders
    427   Cardiac dysrhythmias
    428   Heart failure
    429   Ill-defined descriptions and complications of heart disease

Cerebrovascular disease (430-438)

    430   Subarachnoid hemorrhage
    431   Intracerebral hemorrhage
    432   Other and unspecified intracranial hemorrhage
    433   Occlusion and stenosis of precerebral arteries
    434   Occlusion of cerebral arteries
    435   Transient cerebral ischemia
    436   Acute but ill-defined cerebrovascular disease
    437   Other and ill-defined cerebrovascular disease
    438   Late effects of cerebrovascular disease

Diseases of arteries, arterioles, and capillaries (440-448)

    440   Atherosclerosis
    441   Aortic aneurysm and dissection
    442   Other aneurysm
    443   Other peripheral vascular disease
    444   Arterial embolism and thrombosis
    445   Atheroembolism
    446   Polyarteritis nodosa and allied conditions
    447   Other disorders of arteries and arterioles
    448   Diseases of capillaries

Diseases of veins and lymphatics, and other diseases of circulatory system (451-459)

    451   Phlebitis and thrombophlebitis
    452   Portal vein thrombosis
    453   Other venous embolism and thrombosis
    454   Varicose veins of lower extremities
    455   Hemorrhoids
    456   Varicose veins of other sites
    457   Noninfective disorders of lymphatic channels
    458   Hypotension
    459   Other disorders of circulatory system

8. DISEASES OF THE RESPIRATORY SYSTEM

Acute respiratory infections (460-466)
- 460 Acute nasopharyngitis [common cold]
- 461 Acute sinusitis
- 462 Acute pharyngitis
- 463 Acute tonsillitis
- 464 Acute laryngitis and tracheitis
- 465 Acute upper respiratory infections of multiple or unspecified sites
- 466 Acute bronchitis and bronchiolitis

Other diseases of upper respiratory tract (470-478)
- 470 Deviated nasal septum
- 471 Nasal polyps
- 472 Chronic pharyngitis and nasopharyngitis
- 473 Chronic sinusitis
- 474 Chronic disease of tonsils and adenoids
- 475 Peritonsillar abscess
- 476 Chronic laryngitis and laryngotracheitis
- 477 Allergic rhinitis
- 478 Other diseases of upper respiratory tract

Pneumonia and influenza (480-487)
- 480 Viral pneumonia
- 481 Pneumococcal pneumonia [*Streptococcus pneumoniae* pneumonia]
- 482 Other bacterial pneumonia
- 483 Pneumonia due to other specified organism
- 484 Pneumonia in infectious diseases classified elsewhere
- 485 Bronchopneumonia, organism unspecified
- 486 Pneumonia, organism unspecified
- 487 Influenza

Chronic obstructive pulmonary disease and allied conditions (490-496)
- 490 Bronchitis, not specified as acute or chronic
- 491 Chronic bronchitis
- 492 Emphysema
- 493 Asthma
- 494 Bronchiectasis
- 495 Extrinsic allergic alveolitis
- 496 Chronic airway obstruction, not elsewhere classified

Pneumoconioses and other lung diseases due to external agents (500-508)
- 500 Coal workers' pneumoconiosis
- 501 Asbestosis
- 502 Pneumoconiosis due to other silica or silicates
- 503 Pneumoconiosis due to other inorganic dust
- 504 Pneumopathy due to inhalation of other dust
- 505 Pneumoconiosis, unspecified
- 506 Respiratory conditions due to chemical fumes and vapors
- 507 Pneumonitis due to solids and liquids
- 508 Respiratory conditions due to other and unspecified external agents

Other diseases of respiratory system (510-519)
- 510 Empyema
- 511 Pleurisy
- 512 Pneumothorax
- 513 Abscess of lung and mediastinum
- 514 Pulmonary congestion and hypostasis
- 515 Postinflammatory pulmonary fibrosis
- 516 Other alveolar and parietoalveolar pneumopathy
- 517 Lung involvement in conditions classified elsewhere
- 518 Other diseases of lung
- 519 Other diseases of respiratory system

9. DISEASES OF THE DIGESTIVE SYSTEM

Diseases of oral cavity, salivary glands, and jaws (520-529)
- 520 Disorders of tooth development and eruption
- 521 Diseases of hard tissues of teeth
- 522 Diseases of pulp and periapical tissues

9. DISEASES OF THE DIGESTIVE SYSTEM *continued*

523 Gingival and periodontal diseases
524 Dentofacial anomalies, including malocclusion
525 Other diseases and conditions of the teeth and supporting structures
526 Diseases of the jaws
527 Diseases of the salivary glands
528 Diseases of the oral soft tissues, excluding lesions specific for gingiva and tongue
529 Diseases and other conditions of the tongue

Diseases of esophagus, stomach, and duodenum (530-538)

530 Diseases of esophagus
531 Gastric ulcer
532 Duodenal ulcer
533 Peptic ulcer, site unspecified
534 Gastrojejunal ulcer
535 Gastritis and duodenitis
536 Disorders of function of stomach
537 Other disorders of stomach and duodenum
538 Gastrointestinal mucositis (ulcerative)

Appendicitis (540-543)

540 Acute appendicitis
541 Appendicitis, unqualified
542 Other appendicitis
543 Other diseases of appendix

Hernia of abdominal cavity (550-553)

550 Inguinal hernia
551 Other hernia of abdominal cavity, with gangrene
552 Other hernia of abdominal cavity, with obstruction, but without mention of gangrene
553 Other hernia of abdominal cavity without mention of obstruction or gangrene

Noninfectious enteritis and colitis (555-558)

555 Regional enteritis
556 Ulcerative colitis
557 Vascular insufficiency of intestine
558 Other and unspecified noninfectious gastroenteritis and colitis

Other diseases of intestines and peritoneum (560-569)

560 Intestinal obstruction without mention of hernia
562 Diverticula of intestine
564 Functional digestive disorders, not elsewhere classified
565 Anal fissure and fistula
566 Abscess of anal and rectal regions
567 Peritonitis and retroperitoneal infections
568 Other disorders of peritoneum
569 Other disorders of intestine

Other diseases of digestive system (570-579)

570 Acute and subacute necrosis of liver
571 Chronic liver disease and cirrhosis
572 Liver abscess and sequelae of chronic liver disease
573 Other disorders of liver
574 Cholelithiasis
575 Other disorders of gallbladder
576 Other disorders of biliary tract
577 Diseases of pancreas
578 Gastrointestinal hemorrhage
579 Intestinal malabsorption

10. DISEASES OF THE GENITOURINARY SYSTEM

Nephritis, nephrotic syndrome, and nephrosis (580-589)

580 Acute glomerulonephritis
581 Nephrotic syndrome
582 Chronic glomerulonephritis
583 Nephritis and nephropathy, not specified as acute or chronic
584 Acute renal failure
585 Chronic kidney disease (CKD)

10. DISEASES OF THE GENITOURINARY SYSTEM *continued*

586 Renal failure, unspecified
587 Renal sclerosis, unspecified
588 Disorders resulting from impaired renal function
589 Small kidney of unknown cause

Other diseases of urinary system (590-599)
590 Infections of kidney
591 Hydronephrosis
592 Calculus of kidney and ureter
593 Other disorders of kidney and ureter
594 Calculus of lower urinary tract
595 Cystitis
596 Other disorders of bladder
597 Urethritis, not sexually transmitted, and urethral syndrome
598 Urethral stricture
599 Other disorders of urethra and urinary tract

Diseases of male genital organs (600-608)
600 Hyperplasia of prostate
601 Inflammatory diseases of prostate
602 Other disorders of prostate
603 Hydrocele
604 Orchitis and epididymitis
605 Redundant prepuce and phimosis
606 Infertility, male
607 Disorders of penis
608 Other disorders of male genital organs

Disorders of breast (610-611)
610 Benign mammary dysplasias
611 Other disorders of breast

Inflammatory disease of female pelvic organs (614-616)
614 Inflammatory disease of ovary, fallopian tube, pelvic cellular tissue, and peritoneum
615 Inflammatory diseases of uterus, except cervix
616 Inflammatory disease of cervix, vagina, and vulva

Other disorders of female genital tract (617-629)
617 Endometriosis
618 Genital prolapse
619 Fistula involving female genital tract
620 Noninflammatory disorders of ovary, fallopian tube, and broad ligament
621 Disorders of uterus, not elsewhere classified
622 Noninflammatory disorders of cervix
623 Noninflammatory disorders of vagina
624 Noninflammatory disorders of vulva and perineum
625 Pain and other symptoms associated with female genital organs
626 Disorders of menstruation and other abnormal bleeding from female genital tract
627 Menopausal and postmenopausal disorders
628 Infertility, female
629 Other disorders of female genital organs

11. COMPLICATIONS OF PREGNANCY, CHILDBIRTH AND THE PUERPERIUM

Ectopic and molar pregnancy (630-633)
630 Hydatidiform mole
631 Other abnormal product of conception
632 Missed abortion
633 Ectopic pregnancy

Other pregnancy with abortive outcome (634-639)
634 Abortion
635 Legally induced abortion
636 Illegally induced abortion
637 Unspecified abortion
638 Failed attempted abortion
639 Complications following abortion and ectopic and molar pregnancies

11. COMPLICATIONS OF PREGNANCY, CHILDBIRTH AND THE PUERPERIUM *continued*

Complications mainly related to pregnancy (640-649)

640	Hemorrhage in early pregnancy
641	Antepartum hemorrhage, abruptio placentae, and placenta previa
642	Hypertension complicating pregnancy, childbirth, and the puerperium
643	Excessive vomiting in pregnancy
644	Early or threatened labor
645	Late pregnancy
646	Other complications of pregnancy, not elsewhere classified
647	Infectious and parasitic conditions in the mother classifiable elsewhere but complicating pregnancy, childbirth, and the puerperium
648	Other current conditions in the mother classifiable elsewhere but complicating pregnancy, childbirth, and the puerperium
649	Other conditions or status of the mother complicating pregnancy, childbirth or the puerperium

Normal delivery, and other indications for care in pregnancy, labor, and delivery (650-659)

650	Normal delivery
651	Multiple gestation
652	Malposition and malpresentation of fetus
653	Disproportion
654	Abnormality of organs and soft tissues of pelvis
655	Known or suspected fetal abnormality affecting management of mother
656	Other fetal and placental problems affecting management of mother
657	Polyhydramnios
658	Other problems associated with amniotic cavity and membranes
659	Other indications for care or intervention related to labor and delivery and not elsewhere classified

Complications occurring mainly in the course of labor and delivery (660-669)

660	Obstructed labor
661	Abnormality of forces of labor
662	Long labor
663	Umbilical cord complications
664	Trauma to perineum and vulva during delivery
665	Other obstetrical trauma
666	Postpartum hemorrhage
667	Retained placenta or membranes, without hemorrhage
668	Complications of the administration of anesthetic or other sedation in labor and delivery
669	Other complications of labor and delivery, not elsewhere classified

Complications of the puerperium (670-677)

670	Major puerperal infection
671	Venous complications in pregnancy and the puerperium
672	Pyrexia of unknown origin during the puerperium
673	Obstetrical pulmonary embolism
674	Other and unspecified complications of the puerperium, not elsewhere classified
675	Infections of the breast and nipple associated with childbirth
676	Other disorders of the breast associated with childbirth, and disorders of lactation
677	Late effect of complication of pregnancy, childbirth, and the puerperium

12. DISEASES OF THE SKIN AND SUBCUTANEOUS TISSUE

Infections of skin and subcutaneous tissue (680-686)

680	Carbuncle and furuncle
681	Cellulitis and abscess of finger and toe
682	Other cellulitis and abscess
683	Acute lymphadenitis
684	Impetigo
685	Pilonidal cyst
686	Other local infections of skin and subcutaneous tissue

Other inflammatory conditions of skin and subcutaneous tissue (690-698)

690	Erythematosquamous dermatosis
691	Atopic dermatitis and related conditions
692	Contact dermatitis and other eczema
693	Dermatitis due to substances taken internally
694	Bullous dermatoses

12. DISEASES OF THE SKIN AND SUBCUTANEOUS TISSUE *continued*

- 695 Erythematous conditions
- 696 Psoriasis and similar disorders
- 697 Lichen
- 698 Pruritus and related conditions

Other diseases of skin and subcutaneous tissue (700-709)

- 700 Corns and callosities
- 701 Other hypertrophic and atrophic conditions of skin
- 702 Other dermatoses
- 703 Diseases of nail
- 704 Diseases of hair and hair follicles
- 705 Disorders of sweat glands
- 706 Diseases of sebaceous glands
- 707 Chronic ulcer of skin
- 708 Urticaria
- 709 Other disorders of skin and subcutaneous tissue

13. DISEASES OF THE MUSCULOSKELETAL SYSTEM AND CONNECTIVE TISSUE

Arthropathies and related disorders (710-719)

- 710 Diffuse diseases of connective tissue
- 711 Arthropathy associated with infections
- 712 Crystal arthropathies
- 713 Arthropathy associated with other disorders classified elsewhere
- 714 Rheumatoid arthritis and other inflammatory polyarthropathies
- 715 Osteoarthrosis and allied disorders
- 716 Other and unspecified arthropathies
- 717 Internal derangement of knee
- 718 Other derangement of joint
- 719 Other and unspecified disorder of joint

Dorsopathies (720-724)

- 720 Ankylosing spondylitis and other inflammatory spondylopathies
- 721 Spondylosis and allied disorders
- 722 Intervertebral disc disorders
- 723 Other disorders of cervical region
- 724 Other and unspecified disorders of back

Rheumatism, excluding the back (725-729)

- 725 Polymyalgia rheumatica
- 726 Peripheral enthesopathies and allied syndromes
- 727 Other disorders of synovium, tendon, and bursa
- 728 Disorders of muscle, ligament, and fascia
- 729 Other disorders of soft tissues

Osteopathies, chondropathies, and acquired musculoskeletal deformities (730-739)

- 730 Osteomyelitis, periostitis, and other infections involving bone
- 731 Osteitis deformans and osteopathies associated with other disorders classified elsewhere
- 732 Osteochondropathies
- 733 Other disorders of bone and cartilage
- 734 Flat foot
- 735 Acquired deformities of toe
- 736 Other acquired deformities of limbs
- 737 Curvature of spine
- 738 Other acquired deformity
- 739 Nonallopathic lesions, not elsewhere classified

14. CONGENITAL ANOMALIES

- 740 Anencephalus and similar anomalies
- 741 Spina bifida
- 742 Other congenital anomalies of nervous system
- 743 Congenital anomalies of eye
- 744 Congenital anomalies of ear, face, and neck
- 745 Bulbus cordis anomalies and anomalies of cardiac septal closure
- 746 Other congenital anomalies of heart
- 747 Other congenital anomalies of circulatory system

14. CONGENITAL ANOMALIES *continued*

748   Congenital anomalies of respiratory system
749   Cleft palate and cleft lip
750   Other congenital anomalies of upper alimentary tract
751   Other congenital anomalies of digestive system
752   Congenital anomalies of genital organs
753   Congenital anomalies of urinary system
754   Certain congenital musculoskeletal deformities
755   Other congenital anomalies of limbs
756   Other congenital musculoskeletal anomalies
757   Congenital anomalies of the integument
758   Chromosomal anomalies
759   Other and unspecified congenital anomalies

15. CERTAIN CONDITIONS ORIGINATING IN THE PERINATAL PERIOD

Maternal causes of perinatal morbidity and mortality (760-763)

760   Fetus or newborn affected by maternal conditions which may be unrelated to present pregnancy
761   Fetus or newborn affected by maternal complications of pregnancy
762   Fetus or newborn affected by complications of placenta, cord, and membranes
763   Fetus or newborn affected by other complications of labor and delivery

Other conditions originating in the perinatal period (764-779)

764   Slow fetal growth and fetal malnutrition
765   Disorders relating to short gestation and low birthweight
766   Disorders relating to long gestation and high birthweight
767   Birth trauma
768   Intrauterine hypoxia and birth asphyxia
769   Respiratory distress syndrome
770   Other respiratory conditions of fetus and newborn
771   Infections specific to the perinatal period
772   Fetal and neonatal hemorrhage
773   Hemolytic disease of fetus or newborn, due to isoimmunization
774   Other perinatal jaundice
775   Endocrine and metabolic disturbances specific to the fetus and newborn
776   Hematological disorders of fetus and newborn
777   Perinatal disorders of digestive system
778   Conditions involving the integument and temperature regulation of fetus and newborn
779   Other and ill-defined conditions originating in the perinatal period

16. SYMPTOMS, SIGNS, AND ILL-DEFINED CONDITIONS

Symptoms (780-789)

780   General symptoms
781   Symptoms involving nervous and musculoskeletal systems
782   Symptoms involving skin and other integumentary tissue
783   Symptoms concerning nutrition, metabolism, and development
784   Symptoms involving head and neck
785   Symptoms involving cardiovascular system
786   Symptoms involving respiratory system and other chest symptoms
787   Symptoms involving digestive system
788   Symptoms involving urinary system
789   Other symptoms involving abdomen and pelvis

Nonspecific abnormal findings (790-796)

790   Nonspecific findings on examination of blood
791   Nonspecific findings on examination of urine
792   Nonspecific abnormal findings in other body substances
793   Nonspecific abnormal findings on radiological and other examination of body structure
794   Nonspecific abnormal results of function studies
795   Other and nonspecific abnormal cytological, histological, immunological and DNA test findings
796   Other nonspecific abnormal findings

Ill-defined and unknown causes of morbidity and mortality (797-799)

797   Senility without mention of psychosis
798   Sudden death, cause unknown
799   Other ill-defined and unknown causes of morbidity and mortality

17. INJURY AND POISONING

Fracture of skull (800-804)

800 Fracture of vault of skull
801 Fracture of base of skull
802 Fracture of face bones
803 Other and unqualified skull fractures
804 Multiple fractures involving skull or face with other bones

Fracture of neck and trunk (805-809)

805 Fracture of vertebral column without mention of spinal cord injury
806 Fracture of vertebral column with spinal cord injury
807 Fracture of rib(s), sternum, larynx, and trachea
808 Fracture of pelvis
809 Ill-defined fractures of bones of trunk

Fracture of upper limb (810-819)

810 Fracture of clavicle
811 Fracture of scapula
812 Fracture of humerus
813 Fracture of radius and ulna
814 Fracture of carpal bone(s)
815 Fracture of metacarpal bone(s)
816 Fracture of one or more phalanges of hand
817 Multiple fractures of hand bones
818 Ill-defined fractures of upper limb
819 Multiple fractures involving both upper limbs, and upper limb with rib(s) and sternum

Fracture of lower limb (820-829)

820 Fracture of neck of femur
821 Fracture of other and unspecified parts of femur
822 Fracture of patella
823 Fracture of tibia and fibula
824 Fracture of ankle
825 Fracture of one or more tarsal and metatarsal bones
826 Fracture of one or more phalanges of foot
827 Other, multiple, and ill-defined fractures of lower limb
828 Multiple fractures involving both lower limbs, lower with upper limb, and lower
     limb(s) with rib(s) and sternum
829 Fracture of unspecified bones

Dislocation (830-839)

830 Dislocation of jaw
831 Dislocation of shoulder
832 Dislocation of elbow
833 Dislocation of wrist
834 Dislocation of finger
835 Dislocation of hip
836 Dislocation of knee
837 Dislocation of ankle
838 Dislocation of foot
839 Other, multiple, and ill-defined dislocations

Sprains and strains of joints and adjacent muscles (840-848)

840 Sprains and strains of shoulder and upper arm
841 Sprains and strains of elbow and forearm
842 Sprains and strains of wrist and hand
843 Sprains and strains of hip and thigh
844 Sprains and strains of knee and leg
845 Sprains and strains of ankle and foot
846 Sprains and strains of sacroiliac region
847 Sprains and strains of other and unspecified parts of back
848 Other and ill-defined sprains and strains

Intracranial injury, excluding those with skull fracture (850-854)

850 Concussion
851 Cerebral laceration and contusion
852 Subarachnoid, subdural, and extradural hemorrhage, following injury
853 Other and unspecified intracranial hemorrhage following injury
854 Intracranial injury of other and unspecified nature

17. INJURY AND POISONING *continued*

Internal injury of thorax, abdomen, and pelvis (860-869)

860 Traumatic pneumothorax and hemothorax
861 Injury to heart and lung
862 Injury to other and unspecified intrathoracic organs
863 Injury to gastrointestinal tract
864 Injury to liver
865 Injury to spleen
866 Injury to kidney
867 Injury to pelvic organs
868 Injury to other intra-abdominal organs
869 Internal injury to unspecified or ill-defined organs

Open wound of head, neck, and trunk (870-879)

870 Open wound of ocular adnexa
871 Open wound of eyeball
872 Open wound of ear
873 Other open wound of head
874 Open wound of neck
875 Open wound of chest (wall)
876 Open wound of back
877 Open wound of buttock
878 Open wound of genital organs (external), including traumatic amputation
879 Open wound of other and unspecified sites, except limbs

Open wound of upper limb (880-887)

880 Open wound of shoulder and upper arm
881 Open wound of elbow, forearm, and wrist
882 Open wound of hand except finger(s) alone
883 Open wound of finger(s)
884 Multiple and unspecified open wound of upper limb
885 Traumatic amputation of thumb (complete) (partial)
886 Traumatic amputation of other finger(s) (complete) (partial)
887 Traumatic amputation of arm and hand (complete) (partial)

Open wound of lower limb (890-897)

890 Open wound of hip and thigh
891 Open wound of knee, leg [except thigh], and ankle
892 Open wound of foot except toe(s) alone
893 Open wound of toe(s)
894 Multiple and unspecified open wound of lower limb
895 Traumatic amputation of toe(s) (complete) (partial)
896 Traumatic amputation of foot (complete) (partial)
897 Traumatic amputation of leg(s) (complete) (partial)

Injury to blood vessels (900-904)

900 Injury to blood vessels of head and neck
901 Injury to blood vessels of thorax
902 Injury to blood vessels of abdomen and pelvis
903 Injury to blood vessels of upper extremity
904 Injury to blood vessels of lower extremity and unspecified sites

Late effects of injuries, poisonings, toxic effects, and other external causes (905-909)

905 Late effects of musculoskeletal and connective tissue injuries
906 Late effects of injuries to skin and subcutaneous tissues
907 Late effects of injuries to the nervous system
908 Late effects of other and unspecified injuries
909 Late effects of other and unspecified external causes

Superficial injury (910-919)

910 Superficial injury of face, neck, and scalp except eye
911 Superficial injury of trunk
912 Superficial injury of shoulder and upper arm
913 Superficial injury of elbow, forearm, and wrist
914 Superficial injury of hand(s) except finger(s) alone
915 Superficial injury of finger(s)
916 Superficial injury of hip, thigh, leg, and ankle
917 Superficial injury of foot and toe(s)

17. INJURY AND POISONING *continued*

918 Superficial injury of eye and adnexa
919 Superficial injury of other, multiple, and unspecified sites

Contusion with intact skin surface (920-924)
920 Contusion of face, scalp, and neck except eye(s)
921 Contusion of eye and adnexa
922 Contusion of trunk
923 Contusion of upper limb
924 Contusion of lower limb and of other and unspecified sites

Crushing injury (925-929)
925 Crushing injury of face, scalp, and neck
926 Crushing injury of trunk
927 Crushing injury of upper limb
928 Crushing injury of lower limb
929 Crushing injury of multiple and unspecified sites

Effects of foreign body entering through orifice (930-939)
930 Foreign body on external eye
931 Foreign body in ear
932 Foreign body in nose
933 Foreign body in pharynx and larynx
934 Foreign body in trachea, bronchus, and lung
935 Foreign body in mouth, esophagus, and stomach
936 Foreign body in intestine and colon
937 Foreign body in anus and rectum
938 Foreign body in digestive system, unspecified
939 Foreign body in genitourinary tract

Burns (940-949)
940 Burn confined to eye and adnexa
941 Burn of face, head, and neck
942 Burn of trunk
943 Burn of upper limb, except wrist and hand
944 Burn of wrist(s) and hand(s)
945 Burn of lower limb(s)
946 Burns of multiple specified sites
947 Burn of internal organs
948 Burns classified according to extent of body surface involved
949 Burn, unspecified

Injury to nerves and spinal cord (950-957)
950 Injury to optic nerve and pathways
951 Injury to other cranial nerve(s)
952 Spinal cord injury without evidence of spinal bone injury
953 Injury to nerve roots and spinal plexus
954 Injury to other nerve(s) of trunk excluding shoulder and pelvic girdles
955 Injury to peripheral nerve(s) of shoulder girdle and upper limb
956 Injury to peripheral nerve(s) of pelvic girdle and lower limb
957 Injury to other and unspecified nerves

Certain traumatic complications and unspecified injuries (958-959)
958 Certain early complications of trauma
959 Injury, other and unspecified

Poisoning by drugs, medicinal and biological substances (960-979)
960 Poisoning by antibiotics
961 Poisoning by other anti-infectives
962 Poisoning by hormones and synthetic substitutes
963 Poisoning by primarily systemic agents
964 Poisoning by agents primarily affecting blood constituents
965 Poisoning by analgesics, antipyretics, and antirheumatics
966 Poisoning by anticonvulsants and anti-Parkinsonism drugs
967 Poisoning by sedatives and hypnotics
968 Poisoning by other central nervous system depressants and anesthetics
969 Poisoning by psychotropic agents
970 Poisoning by central nervous system stimulants
971 Poisoning by drugs primarily affecting the autonomic nervous system

17. INJURY AND POISONING *continued*

972 Poisoning by agents primarily affecting the cardiovascular system
973 Poisoning by agents primarily affecting the gastrointestinal system
974 Poisoning by water, mineral, and uric acid metabolism drugs
975 Poisoning by agents primarily acting on the smooth and skeletal muscles and respiratory system
976 Poisoning by agents primarily affecting skin and mucous membrane, ophthalmological, otorhinolaryngological, and dental drugs
977 Poisoning by other and unspecified drugs and medicinals
978 Poisoning by bacterial vaccines
979 Poisoning by other vaccines and biological substances

Toxic effects of substances chiefly nonmedicinal as to source (980-989)

980 Toxic effect of alcohol
981 Toxic effect of petroleum products
982 Toxic effect of solvents other than petroleum-based
983 Toxic effect of corrosive aromatics, acids, and caustic alkalis
984 Toxic effect of lead and its compounds (including fumes)
985 Toxic effect of other metals
986 Toxic effect of carbon monoxide
987 Toxic effect of other gases, fumes, or vapors
988 Toxic effect of noxious substances eaten as food
989 Toxic effect of other substances, chiefly nonmedicinal as to source

Other and unspecified effects of external causes (990-995)

990 Effects of radiation, unspecified
991 Effects of reduced temperature
992 Effects of heat and light
993 Effects of air pressure
994 Effects of other external causes
995 Certain adverse effects, not elsewhere classified

Complications of surgical and medical care, not elsewhere classified (996-999)

996 Complications peculiar to certain specified procedures
997 Complications affecting specified body systems, not elsewhere classified
998 Other complications of procedures, not elsewhere classified
999 Complications of medical care, not elsewhere classified

SUPPLEMENTARY CLASSIFICATION OF FACTORS INFLUENCING HEALTH STATUS AND CONTACT WITH HEALTH SERVICES

Persons with potential health hazards related to communicable diseases (V01-V06)

V01 Contact with or exposure to communicable diseases
V02 Carrier or suspected carrier of infectious diseases
V03 Need for prophylactic vaccination and inoculation against bacterial diseases
V04 Need for prophylactic vaccination and inoculation against certain viral diseases
V05 Need for other prophylactic vaccination and inoculation against single diseases
V06 Need for prophylactic vaccination and inoculation against combinations of diseases

Persons with need for isolation, other potential health hazards and prophylactic measures (V07-V09)

V07 Need for isolation and other prophylactic measures
V08 Asymptomatic human immunodeficiency virus (HIV) infection status
V09 Infection with drug-resistant microorganisms

Persons with potential health hazards related to personal and family history (V10-V19)

V10 Personal history of malignant neoplasm
V11 Personal history of mental disorder
V12 Personal history of certain other diseases
V13 Personal history of other diseases
V14 Personal history of allergy to medicinal agents
V15 Other personal history presenting hazards to health
V16 Family history of malignant neoplasm
V17 Family history of certain chronic disabling diseases
V18 Family history of certain other specific conditions
V19 Family history of other conditions

Persons encountering health services in circumstances related to reproduction and development (V20-V29)

V20 Health supervision of infant or child
V21 Constitutional states in development

SUPPLEMENTARY CLASSIFICATION...HEALTH STATUS/HEALTH SERVICES *continued*

V22 Normal pregnancy
V23 Supervision of high-risk pregnancy
V24 Postpartum care and examination
V25 Encounter for contraceptive management
V26 Procreative management
V27 Outcome of delivery
V28 Encounter for antenatal screening of mother
V29 Observation and evaluation of newborns and infants for suspected condition not found

Liveborn infants according to type of birth (V30-V39)
V30 Single liveborn
V31 Twin, mate liveborn
V32 Twin, mate stillborn
V33 Twin, unspecified
V34 Other multiple, mates all liveborn
V35 Other multiple, mates all stillborn
V36 Other multiple, mates live- and stillborn
V37 Other multiple, unspecified
V39 Unspecified

Persons with a condition influencing their health status (V40-V49)
V40 Mental and behavioral problems
V41 Problems with special senses and other special functions
V42 Organ or tissue replaced by transplant
V43 Organ or tissue replaced by other means
V44 Artificial opening status
V45 Other postprocedural states
V46 Other dependence on machines
V47 Other problems with internal organs
V48 Problems with head, neck, and trunk
V49 Other conditions influencing health status

Persons encountering health services for specific procedures and aftercare (V50-V59)
V50 Elective surgery for purposes other than remedying health states
V51 Aftercare involving the use of plastic surgery
V52 Fitting and adjustment of prosthetic device and implant
V53 Fitting and adjustment of other device
V54 Other orthopedic aftercare
V55 Attention to artificial openings
V56 Encounter for dialysis and dialysis catheter care
V57 Care involving use of rehabilitation procedures
V58 Encounter for other and unspecified procedures and aftercare
V59 Donors

Persons encountering health services in other circumstances (V60-V69)
V60 Housing, household, and economic circumstances
V61 Other family circumstances
V62 Other psychosocial circumstances
V63 Unavailability of other medical facilities for care
V64 Persons encountering health services for specific procedures, not carried out
V65 Other persons seeking consultation
V66 Convalescence and palliative care
V67 Follow-up examination
V68 Encounters for administrative purposes
V69 Problems related to lifestyle

Persons without reported diagnosis encountered during examination and investigation of individuals and populations (V70-V86)
V70 General medical examination
V71 Observation and evaluation for suspected conditions not found
V72 Special investigations and examinations
V73 Special screening examination for viral and chlamydial diseases
V74 Special screening examination for bacterial and spirochetal diseases
V75 Special screening examination for other infectious diseases
V76 Special screening for malignant neoplasms
V77 Special screening for endocrine, nutritional, metabolic, and immunity disorders
V78 Special screening for disorders of blood and blood-forming organs

SUPPLEMENTARY CLASSIFICATION...HEALTH STATUS/HEALTH SERVICES *continued*

V79 Special screening for mental disorders and developmental handicaps
V80 Special screening for neurological, eye, and ear diseases
V81 Special screening for cardiovascular, respiratory, and genitourinary diseases
V82 Special screening for other conditions
V83 Genetic carrier status
V84 Genetic susceptibility to disease
V85 Body mass index
V86 Estrogen receptor status

SUPPLEMENTARY CLASSIFICATION OF EXTERNAL CAUSES OF INJURY AND POISONING

Railway accidents (E800-E807)

E800 Railway accident involving collision with rolling stock
E801 Railway accident involving collision with other object
E802 Railway accident involving derailment without antecedent collision
E803 Railway accident involving explosion, fire, or burning
E804 Fall in, on, or from railway train
E805 Hit by rolling stock
E806 Other specified railway accident
E807 Railway accident of unspecified nature

Motor vehicle traffic accidents (E810-E819)

E810 Motor vehicle traffic accident involving collision with train
E811 Motor vehicle traffic accident involving re-entrant collision with another motor vehicle
E812 Other motor vehicle traffic accident involving collision with another motor vehicle
E813 Motor vehicle traffic accident involving collision with other vehicle
E814 Motor vehicle traffic accident involving collision with pedestrian
E815 Other motor vehicle traffic accident involving collision on the highway
E816 Motor vehicle traffic accident due to loss of control, without collision on the highway
E817 Noncollision motor vehicle traffic accident while boarding or alighting
E818 Other noncollision motor vehicle traffic accident
E819 Motor vehicle traffic accident of unspecified nature

Motor vehicle nontraffic accidents (E820-E825)

E820 Nontraffic accident involving motor-driven snow vehicle
E821 Nontraffic accident involving other off-road motor vehicle
E822 Other motor vehicle nontraffic accident involving collision with moving object
E823 Other motor vehicle nontraffic accident involving collision with stationary object
E824 Other motor vehicle nontraffic accident while boarding and alighting
E825 Other motor vehicle nontraffic accident of other and unspecified nature

Other road vehicle accidents (E826-E829)

E826 Pedal cycle accident
E827 Animal-drawn vehicle accident
E828 Accident involving animal being ridden
E829 Other road vehicle accidents

Water transport accidents (E830-E838)

E830 Accident to watercraft causing submersion
E831 Accident to watercraft causing other injury
E832 Other accidental submersion or drowning in water transport accident
E833 Fall on stairs or ladders in water transport
E834 Other fall from one level to another in water transport
E835 Other and unspecified fall in water transport
E836 Machinery accident in water transport
E837 Explosion, fire, or burning in watercraft
E838 Other and unspecified water transport accident

Air and space transport accidents (E840-E845)

E840 Accident to powered aircraft at takeoff or landing
E841 Accident to powered aircraft, other and unspecified
E842 Accident to unpowered aircraft
E843 Fall in, on, or from aircraft
E844 Other specified air transport accidents
E845 Accident involving spacecraft

SUPPLEMENTARY CLASSIFICATION...INJURY AND POISONING *continued*

Vehicle accidents, not elsewhere classifiable (E846-E849)

E846 Accidents involving powered vehicles used solely within the buildings and premises of an industrial or commercial establishment

E847 Accidents involving cable cars not running on rails

E848 Accidents involving other vehicles, not elsewhere classifiable

E849 Place of occurrence

Accidental poisoning by drugs, medicinal substances, and biologicals (E850-E858)

E850 Accidental poisoning by analgesics, antipyretics, and antirheumatics

E851 Accidental poisoning by barbiturates

E852 Accidental poisoning by other sedatives and hypnotics

E853 Accidental poisoning by tranquilizers

E854 Accidental poisoning by other psychotropic agents

E855 Accidental poisoning by other drugs acting on central and autonomic nervous systems

E856 Accidental poisoning by antibiotics

E857 Accidental poisoning by other anti-infectives

E858 Accidental poisoning by other drugs

Accidental poisoning by other solid and liquid substances, gases, and vapors (E860-E869)

E860 Accidental poisoning by alcohol, not elsewhere classified

E861 Accidental poisoning by cleansing and polishing agents, disinfectants, paints, and varnishes

E862 Accidental poisoning by petroleum products, other solvents and their vapors, not elsewhere classified

E863 Accidental poisoning by agricultural and horticultural chemical and pharmaceutical preparations other than plant foods and fertilizers

E864 Accidental poisoning by corrosives and caustics, not elsewhere classified

E865 Accidental poisoning from poisonous foodstuffs and poisonous plants

E866 Accidental poisoning by other and unspecified solid and liquid substances

E867 Accidental poisoning by gas distributed by pipeline

E868 Accidental poisoning by other utility gas and other carbon monoxide

E869 Accidental poisoning by other gases and vapors

Misadventures to patients during surgical and medical care (E870-E876)

E870 Accidental cut, puncture, perforation, or hemorrhage during medical care

E871 Foreign object left in body during procedure

E872 Failure of sterile precautions during procedure

E873 Failure in dosage

E874 Mechanical failure of instrument or apparatus during procedure

E875 Contaminated or infected blood, other fluid, drug, or biological substance

E876 Other and unspecified misadventures during medical care

Surgical and medical procedures as the cause of abnormal reaction of patient or later complication, without mention of misadventure at the time of procedure (E878-E879)

E878 Surgical operation and other surgical procedures as the cause of abnormal reaction of patient, or of later complication, without mention of misadventure at the time of operation

E879 Other procedures, without mention of misadventure at the time of procedure, as the cause of abnormal reaction of patient, or of later complication

Accidental falls (E880-E888)

E880 Fall on or from stairs or steps

E881 Fall on or from ladders or scaffolding

E882 Fall from or out of building or other structure

E883 Fall into hole or other opening in surface

E884 Other fall from one level to another

E885 Fall on same level from slipping, tripping, or stumbling

E886 Fall on same level from collision, pushing or shoving, by or with other person

E887 Fracture, cause unspecified

E888 Other and unspecified fall

Accidents caused by fire and flames (E890-E899)

E890 Conflagration in private dwelling

E891 Conflagration in other and unspecified building or structure

E892 Conflagration not in building or structure

E893 Accident caused by ignition of clothing

E894 Ignition of highly inflammable material

E895 Accident caused by controlled fire in private dwelling

E896 Accident caused by controlled fire in other and unspecified building or structure

SUPPLEMENTARY CLASSIFICATION...INJURY AND POISONING *continued*

E897 Accident caused by controlled fire not in building or structure
E898 Accident caused by other specified fire and flames
E899 Accident caused by unspecified fire

Accidents due to natural and environmental factors (E900-E909)

E900 Excessive heat
E901 Excessive cold
E902 High and low air pressure and changes in air pressure
E903 Travel and motion
E904 Hunger, thirst, exposure, and neglect
E905 Venomous animals and plants as the cause of poisoning and toxic reactions
E906 Other injury caused by animals
E907 Lightning
E908 Cataclysmic storms, and floods resulting from storms
E909 Cataclysmic earth surface movements and eruptions

Accidents caused by submersion, suffocation, and foreign bodies (E910-E915)

E910 Accidental drowning and submersion
E911 Inhalation and ingestion of food causing obstruction of respiratory tract or suffocation
E912 Inhalation and ingestion of other object causing obstruction of respiratory tract or
     suffocation
E913 Accidental mechanical suffocation
E914 Foreign body accidentally entering eye and adnexa
E915 Foreign body accidentally entering other orifice

Other accidents (E916-E928)

E916 Struck accidentally by falling object
E917 Striking against or struck accidentally by objects or persons
E918 Caught accidentally in or between objects
E919 Accidents caused by machinery
E920 Accidents caused by cutting and piercing instruments or objects
E921 Accident caused by explosion of pressure vessel
E922 Accident caused by firearm and air gun missile
E923 Accident caused by explosive material
E924 Accident caused by hot substance or object, caustic or corrosive material, and steam
E925 Accident caused by electric current
E926 Exposure to radiation
E927 Overexertion and strenuous movements
E928 Other and unspecified environmental and accidental causes

Late effects of accidental injury (E929)

E929 Late effects of accidental injury

Drugs, medicinal and biological substances causing adverse effects in therapeutic use (E930-E949)

E930 Antibiotics
E931 Other anti-infectives
E932 Hormones and synthetic substitutes
E933 Primarily systemic agents
E934 Agents primarily affecting blood constituents
E935 Analgesics, antipyretics, and antirheumatics
E936 Anticonvulsants and anti-Parkinsonism drugs
E937 Sedatives and hypnotics
E938 Other central nervous system depressants and anesthetics
E939 Psychotropic agents
E940 Central nervous system stimulants
E941 Drugs primarily affecting the autonomic nervous system
E942 Agents primarily affecting the cardiovascular system
E943 Agents primarily affecting gastrointestinal system
E944 Water, mineral, and uric acid metabolism drugs
E945 Agents primarily acting on the smooth and skeletal muscles and respiratory system
E946 Agents primarily affecting skin and mucous membrane, ophthalmological,
     otorhinolaryngological, and dental drugs
E947 Other and unspecified drugs and medicinal substances
E948 Bacterial vaccines
E949 Other vaccines and biological substances

SUPPLEMENTARY CLASSIFICATION...INJURY AND POISONING *continued*

Suicide and self-inflicted injury (E950-E959)

E950 Suicide and self-inflicted poisoning by solid or liquid substances
E951 Suicide and self-inflicted poisoning by gases in domestic use
E952 Suicide and self-inflicted poisoning by other gases and vapors
E953 Suicide and self-inflicted injury by hanging, strangulation, and suffocation
E954 Suicide and self-inflicted injury by submersion [drowning]
E955 Suicide and self-inflicted injury by firearms, air guns and explosives
E956 Suicide and self-inflicted injury by cutting and piercing instruments
E957 Suicide and self-inflicted injuries by jumping from high place
E958 Suicide and self-inflicted injury by other and unspecified means
E959 Late effects of self-inflicted injury

Homicide and injury purposely inflicted by other persons (E960-E969)

E960 Fight, brawl, and rape
E961 Assault by corrosive or caustic substance, except poisoning
E962 Assault by poisoning
E963 Assault by hanging and strangulation
E964 Assault by submersion [drowning]
E965 Assault by firearms and explosives
E966 Assault by cutting and piercing instrument
E967 Perpetrator of child and adult abuse
E968 Assault by other and unspecified means
E969 Late effects of injury purposely inflicted by other person

Legal intervention (E970-E978)

E970 Injury due to legal intervention by firearms
E971 Injury due to legal intervention by explosives
E972 Injury due to legal intervention by gas
E973 Injury due to legal intervention by blunt object
E974 Injury due to legal intervention by cutting and piercing instruments
E975 Injury due to legal intervention by other specified means
E976 Injury due to legal intervention by unspecified means
E977 Late effects of injuries due to legal intervention
E978 Legal execution
E979 Terrorism

Injury undetermined whether accidentally or purposely inflicted (E980-E989)

E980 Poisoning by solid or liquid substances, undetermined whether accidentally or
   purposely inflicted
E981 Poisoning by gases in domestic use, undetermined whether accidentally or purposely
   inflicted
E982 Poisoning by other gases, undetermined whether accidentally or purposely inflicted
E983 Hanging, strangulation, or suffocation, undetermined whether accidentally or
   purposely inflicted
E984 Submersion [drowning], undetermined whether accidentally or purposely inflicted
E985 Injury by firearms, air guns and explosives, undetermined whether accidentally or
   purposely inflicted
E986 Injury by cutting and piercing instruments, undetermined whether accidentally or
   purposely inflicted
E987 Falling from high place, undetermined whether accidentally or purposely inflicted
E988 Injury by other and unspecified means, undetermined whether accidentally or
   purposely inflicted
E989 Late effects of injury, undetermined whether accidentally or purposely inflicted

Injury resulting from operations of war (E990-E999)

E990 Injury due to war operations by fires and conflagrations
E991 Injury due to war operations by bullets and fragments
E992 Injury due to war operations by explosion of marine weapons
E993 Injury due to war operations by other explosion
E994 Injury due to war operations by destruction of aircraft
E995 Injury due to war operations by other and unspecified forms of conventional warfare
E996 Injury due to war operations by nuclear weapons
E997 Injury due to war operations by other forms of unconventional warfare
E998 Injury due to war operations but occurring after cessation of hostilities
E999 Late effects of injury due to war operations and terrorism

DISEASES: ALPHABETIC INDEX

VOLUME 2

A

AAT (alpha-1 antitrypsin) deficiency 273.4
AAV (disease) (illness) (infection)—*see* Human
    immunodeficiency virus (disease) (illness)
    (infection)
Abactio —*see* Abortion, induced
Abactus venter —*see* Abortion, induced
Abarognosis 781.99
Abasia (-astasia) 307.9
    atactica 781.3
    choreic 781.3
    hysterical 300.11
    paroxysmal trepidant 781.3
    spastic 781.3
    trembling 781.3
    trepidans 781.3
Abderhalden-Kaufmann-Lignac syndrome
    (cystinosis) 270.0
Abdomen, abdominal —*see also* condition
    accordion 306.4
    acute 789.0
    angina 557.1
    burst 868.00
    convulsive equivalent (*see also* Epilepsy) 345.5
    heart 746.87
    muscle deficiency syndrome 756.79
    obstipum 756.79
Abdominalgia 789.0
    periodic 277.31
Abduction contracture, hip or other joint —*see*
    Contraction, joint
Abercrombie's syndrome (amyloid
    degeneration) 277.39
Aberrant (congenital)—*see also* Malposition,
    congenital
    adrenal gland 759.1
    blood vessel NEC 747.60
        arteriovenous NEC 747.60
        cerebrovascular 747.81
        gastrointestinal 747.61
        lower limb 747.64
        renal 747.62
        spinal 747.82
        upper limb 747.63
    breast 757.6
    endocrine gland NEC 759.2
    gastrointestinal vessel (peripheral) 747.61
    hepatic duct 751.69
    lower limb vessel (peripheral) 747.64
    pancreas 751.7
    parathyroid gland 759.2
    peripheral vascular vessel NEC 747.60
    pituitary gland (pharyngeal) 759.2
    renal blood vessel 747.62
    sebaceous glands, mucous membrane, mouth
        750.26
    spinal vessel 747.82
    spleen 759.0
    testis (descent) 752.51
    thymus gland 759.2
    thyroid gland 759.2
    upper limb vessel (peripheral) 747.63
Aberratio
    lactis 757.6
    testis 752.51
Aberration —*see also* Anomaly
    chromosome—*see* Anomaly, chromosome(s)
    distantial 368.9

Aberration—*continued*
    mental (*see also* Disorder, mental,
        nonpsychotic) 300.9
Abetalipoproteinemia 272.5
Abionarce 780.79
Abiotrophy 799.89
Ablatio
    placentae—*see* Placenta, ablatio
    retinae (*see also* Detachment, retina) 361.9
Ablation
    pituitary (gland) (with hypofunction) 253.7
    placenta—*see* Placenta, ablatio
    uterus 621.8
Ablepharia, ablepharon, ablephary 743.62
Ablepsia —*see* Blindness
Ablepsy —*see* Blindness
Ablutomania 300.3
Abnormal, abnormality, abnormalities —*see*
    also Anomaly
    acid-base balance 276.4
        fetus or newborn—*see* Distress, fetal
    adaptation curve, dark 368.63
    alveolar ridge 525.9
    amnion 658.9
        affecting fetus or newborn 762.9
    anatomical relationship NEC 759.9
    apertures, congenital, diaphragm 756.6
    auditory perception NEC 388.40
    autosomes NEC 758.5
        13 758.1
        18 758.2
        21 or 22 758.0
        D_1 758.1
        E_3 758.2
        G 758.0
    ballistocardiogram 794.39
    basal metabolic rate (BMR) 794.7
    biosynthesis, testicular androgen 257.2
    blood level (of)
        cobalt 790.6
        copper 790.6
        iron 790.6
        lead 790.6
        lithium 790.6
        magnesium 790.6
        mineral 790.6
        zinc 790.6
    blood pressure
        elevated (without diagnosis of hypertension)
            796.2
        low (*see also* Hypotension) 458.9
            reading (incidental) (isolated) (nonspecific)
                796.3
    bowel sounds 787.5
    breathing behavior—*see* Respiration
    caloric test 794.19
    cervix (acquired) NEC 622.9
        congenital 752.40
        in pregnancy or childbirth 654.6
            causing obstructed labor 660.2
                affecting fetus or newborn 763.1
    chemistry, blood NEC 790.6
    chest sounds 786.7
    chorion 658.9
        affecting fetus or newborn 762.9
    chromosomal NEC 758.89
        analysis, nonspecific result 795.2

Abnormal, abnormality —*continued*
  movement 781.0
    disorder, NEC 333.90
      sleep related, unspecified 780.58
      specified, NEC 333.99
    head 781.0
    involuntary 781.0
    specified type NEC 333.99
  muscle contraction, localized 728.85
  myoglobin (Aberdeen) (Annapolis) 289.9
  narrowness, eyelid 743.62
  optokinetic response 379.57
  organs or tissues of pelvis NEC
    in pregnancy or childbirth 654.9
      affecting fetus or newborn 763.89
      causing obstructed labor 660.2
        affecting fetus or newborn 763.1
  origin—*see* Malposition, congenital
  palmar creases 757.2
  Papanicolaou (smear)
    cervix 795.00
      with
        atypical squamous cell
          cannot exclude high grade squamous
              intraepithelial lesion (ASC-H)
              795.02
          of undetermined significance (ASC-US)
              795.01
        cytologic evidence of malignancy 795.06
        favor benign (ASCUS favor benign)
            795.01
        favor dysplasia (ASCUS favor dysplasia)
            795.02
        high grade squamous intraepithelial lesion
            (HGSIL) 795.04
        low grade squamous intraepithelial lesion
            (LGSIL) 795.03
      nonspecific finding NEC 795.09
    other site 795.1
  parturition
    affecting fetus or newborn 763.9
    mother—*see* Delivery, complicated
  pelvis (bony)—*see* Deformity, pelvis
  percussion, chest 786.7
  periods (grossly) (*see also* Menstruation) 626.9
  phonocardiogram 794.39
  placenta—*see* Placenta, abnormal
  plantar reflex 796.1
  plasma protein—*see* Deficiency, plasma, protein
  pleural folds 748.8
  position—*see also* Malposition
    gravid uterus 654.4
      causing obstructed labor 660.2
        affecting fetus or newborn 763.1
  posture NEC 781.92
  presentation (fetus)—*see* Presentation, fetus,
      abnormal
  product of conception NEC 631
  puberty—*see* Puberty
  pulmonary
    artery 747.3
    function, newborn 770.89
    test results 794.2
    ventilation, newborn 770.89
      hyperventilation 786.01
  pulsations in neck 785.1
  pupil reflexes 379.40
  quality of milk 676.8
  radiological examination 793.99
    abdomen NEC 793.6
    biliary tract 793.3

Abnormal, abnormality —*continued*
  breast 793.89
    mammogram NOS 793.80
    mammographic
      calcification 793.89
      calculus 793.89
      microcalcification 793.81
  gastrointestinal tract 793.4
  genitourinary organs 793.5
  head 793.0
  image test inconclusive due to excess body fat
      793.91
  intrathoracic organ NEC 793.2
  lung (field) 793.1
  musculoskeletal system 793.7
  retroperitoneum 793.6
  skin and subcutaneous tissue 793.99
  skull 793.0
  red blood cells 790.09
    morphology 790.09
    volume 790.09
  reflex NEC 796.1
  renal function test 794.4
  respiration signs—*see* Respiration
  response to nerve stimulation 794.10
  retinal correspondence 368.34
  rhythm, heart—*see also* Arrhythmia fetus—*see*
      Distress, fetal
  saliva 792.4
  scan
    brain 794.09
    kidney 794.4
    liver 794.8
    lung 794.2
    thyroid 794.5
  secretion
    gastrin 251.5
    glucagon 251.4
  semen 792.2
  serum level (of)
    acid phosphatase 790.5
    alkaline phosphatase 790.5
    amylase 790.5
    enzymes NEC 790.5
    lipase 790.5
  shape
    cornea 743.41
    gallbladder 751.69
    gravid uterus 654.4
      affecting fetus or newborn 763.89
      causing obstructed labor 660.2
        affecting fetus or newborn 763.1
    head (*see also* Anomaly, skull) 756.0
    organ or site, congenital NEC—*see* Distortion
  sinus venosus 747.40
  size
    fetus, complicating delivery 653.5
      causing obstructed labor 660.1
    gallbladder 751.69
    head (*see also* Anomaly, skull) 756.0
    organ or site, congenital NEC—*see* Distortion
    teeth 520.2
  skin and appendages, congenital NEC 757.9
  soft parts of pelvis—*see* Abnormal, organs or
      tissues of pelvis
  spermatozoa 792.2
  sputum (amount) (color) (excessive) (odor)
      (purulent) 786.4
  stool NEC 787.7
    bloody 578.1
      occult 792.1

Abscess—*continued*
  extradural 324.9
    brain 324.0
    late effect—*see* category 326
    spinal cord 324.1
  extraperitoneal—*see* Abscess, peritoneum
  eye 360.00
  eyelid 373.13
  face (any part, except eye) 682.0
  fallopian tube (*see also* Salpingo-oophoritis)
    614.2
  fascia 728.89
  fauces 478.29
  fecal 569.5
  femoral (region) 682.6
  filaria, filarial (*see also* Infestation, filarial)
    125.9
  finger (any) (intrathecal) (periosteal)
    (subcutaneous) (subcuticular) 681.00
  fistulous NEC 682.9
  flank 682.2
  foot (except toe) 682.7
  forearm 682.3
  forehead 682.0
  frontal (sinus) (chronic) (*see also* Sinusitis,
    frontal) 473.1
  gallbladder (*see also* Cholecystitis, acute) 575.0
  gastric 535.0
  genital organ or tract NEC
    female 616.9
      with
        abortion—*see* Abortion, by type, with
          sepsis
        ectopic pregnancy (*see also* categories
          633.0-633.9) 639.0
        molar pregnancy (*see also* categories
          630-632) 639.0
      following
        abortion 639.0
        ectopic or molar pregnancy 639.0
      puerperal, postpartum, childbirth 670
    male 608.4
  genitourinary system, tuberculous (*see also*
    Tuberculosis) 016.9
  gingival 523.30
  gland, glandular (lymph) (acute) NEC 683
  glottis 478.79
  gluteal (region) 682.5
  gonorrheal NEC (*see also* Gonococcus) 098.0
  groin 682.2
  gum 523.30
  hand (except finger or thumb) 682.4
  head (except face) 682.8
  heart 429.89
  heel 682.7
  helminthic (*see also* Infestation, by specific
    parasite) 128.9
  hepatic 572.0
    amebic (*see also* Abscess, liver, amebic) 006.3
    duct 576.8
  hip 682.6
    tuberculous (active) (*see also* Tuberculosis)
      015.1
  ileocecal 540.1
  ileostomy (bud) 569.6
  iliac (region) 682.2
    fossa 540.1
  iliopsoas 567.31
    tuberculous (see also Tuberculosis) 015.0
      [730.88]
  infraclavicular (fossa) 682.3

Abscess—*continued*
  inguinal (region) 682.2
    lymph gland or node 683
  intersphincteric (anus) 566
  intestine, intestinal 569.5
    rectal 566
  intra-abdominal (*see also* Abscess, peritoneum)
    567.22
    postoperative 998.59
  intracranial 324.0
    late effect—*see* category 326
  intramammary—*see* Abscess, breast
  intramastoid (*see also* Mastoiditis, acute) 383.00
  intraorbital 376.01
  intraperitoneal 567.22
  intraspinal 324.1
    late effect—*see* category 326
  intratonsillar 475
  iris 364.3
  ischiorectal 566
  jaw (bone) (lower) (upper) 526.4
    skin 682.0
  joint (*see also* Arthritis, pyogenic) 711.0
    vertebral (tuberculous) (*see also* Tuberculosis)
      015.0 *[730.88]*
      nontuberculous 724.8
  kidney 590.2
    with
      abortion—*see* Abortion, by type, with
        urinary tract infection
      calculus 592.0
      ectopic pregnancy (*see also* categories
        633.0-633.9) 639.8
      molar pregnancy (*see also* categories
        630-632) 639.8
    complicating pregnancy or puerperium 646.6
      affecting fetus or newborn 760.1
    following
      abortion 639.8
      ectopic or molar pregnancy 639.8
  knee 682.6
    joint 711.06
    tuberculous (active) (*see also* Tuberculosis)
      015.2
  labium (majus) (minus) 616.4
    complicating pregnancy, childbirth, or
      puerperium 646.6
  lacrimal (passages) (sac) (*see also*
    Dacryocystitis) 375.30
    caruncle 375.30
    gland (*see also* Dacryoadenitis) 375.00
  lacunar 597.0
  larynx 478.79
  lateral (alveolar) 522.5
    with sinus 522.7
  leg, except foot 682.6
  lens 360.00
  lid 373.13
  lingual 529.0
    tonsil 475
  lip 528.5
  Littre's gland 597.0
  liver 572.0
    amebic 006.3
      with
        brain abscess (and lung abscess) 006.5
        lung abscess 006.4
      due to Entamoeba histolytica 006.3
      dysenteric (*see also* Abscess, liver, amebic)
        006.3
    pyogenic 572.0

Abscess—*continued*
    with
        abortion—*see* Abortion, by type, with sepsis
        appendicitis 540.1
        ectopic pregnancy (*see also* categories
          633.0-633.9) 639.0
        molar pregnancy (*see also* categories
          630-632) 639.0
    following
        abortion 639.0
        ectopic or molar pregnancy 639.0
    pelvic, female (*see also* Disease, pelvis,
        inflammatory) 614.4
        acute 614.3
    postoperative 998.59
    puerperal, postpartum, childbirth 670
    tuberculous (*see also* Tuberculosis) 014.0
  peritonsillar 475
  perityphlic 540.1
  periureteral 593.89
  periurethral 597.0
    gonococcal (acute) 098.0
      chronic or duration of 2 months or over
        098.2
  periuterine (*see also* Disease, pelvis,
    inflammatory) 614.4
    acute 614.3
  perivesical 595.89
  pernicious NEC 682.9
  petrous bone—*see* Petrositis
  phagedenic NEC 682.9
    chancroid 099.0
  pharynx, pharyngeal (lateral) 478.29
  phlegmonous NEC 682.9
  pilonidal 685.0
  pituitary (gland) 253.8
  pleura 510.9
    with fistula 510.0
  popliteal 682.6
  postanal 566
  postcecal 540.1
  postlaryngeal 478.79
  postnasal 478.19
  postpharyngeal 478.24
  posttonsillar 475
  posttyphoid 002.0
  Pott's (*see also* Tuberculosis) 015.0 *[730.88]*
  pouch of Douglas (chronic) (*see also* Disease,
    pelvis, inflammatory) 614.4
  premammary—*see* Abscess, breast
  prepatellar 682.6
  prostate (*see also* Prostatitis) 601.2
    gonococcal (acute) 098.12
      chronic or duration of 2 months or over 098.32
  psoas 567.31
    tuberculous (*see also* Tuberculosis) 015.0
      [730.88]
  pterygopalatine fossa 682.8
  pubis 682.2
  puerperal—Puerperal, abscess, by site
  pulmonary—*see* Abscess, lung
  pulp, pulpal (dental) 522.0
    finger 681.01
    toe 681.10
  pyemic—*see* Septicemia
  pyloric valve 535.0
  rectovaginal septum 569.5
  rectovesical 595.89
  rectum 566
  regional NEC 682.9
  renal (*see also* Abscess, kidney) 590.2

Abscess—*continued*
  retina 363.00
  retrobulbar 376.01
  retrocecal 567.22
  retrolaryngeal 478.79
  retromammary—*see* Abscess, breast
  retroperineal 682.2
  retroperitoneal 567.38
    postprocedural 998.59
  retropharyngeal 478.24
    tuberculous (*see also* Tuberculosis) 012.8
  retrorectal 566
  retrouterine (*see also* Disease, pelvis,
    inflammatory) 614.4
    acute 614.3
  retrovesical 595.89
  root, tooth 522.5
    with sinus (alveolar) 522.7
  round ligament (*see also* Disease, pelvis,
    inflammatory) 614.4
    acute 614.3
  rupture (spontaneous) NEC 682.9
  sacrum (tuberculous) (*see also* Tuberculosis)
    015.0 *[730.88]*
    nontuberculous 730.08
  salivary duct or gland 527.3
  scalp (any part) 682.8
  scapular 730.01
  sclera 379.09
  scrofulous (*see also* Tuberculosis) 017.2
  scrotum 608.4
  seminal vesicle 608.0
    amebic 006.8
  septal, dental 522.5
    with sinus (alveolar) 522.7
  septum (nasal) 478.19
  serous (*see also* Periostitis) 730.3
  shoulder 682.3
  side 682.2
  sigmoid 569.5
  sinus (accessory) (chronic) (nasal) (*see also*
    Sinusitis) 473.9
    intracranial venous (any) 324.0
    late effect—*see* category 326
  Skene's duct or gland 597.0
  skin NEC 682.9
    tuberculous (primary) (*see also* Tuberculosis)
      017.0
  sloughing NEC 682.9
  specified site NEC 682.8
    amebic 006.8
  spermatic cord 608.4
  sphenoidal (sinus) (*see also* Sinusitis,
    sphenoidal) 473.3
  spinal
    cord (any part) (staphylococcal) 324.1
      tuberculous (*see also* Tuberculosis) 013.5
    epidural 324.1
  spine (column) (tuberculous) (*see also*
    Tuberculosis) 015.0 *[730.88]*
    nontuberculous 730.08
  spleen 289.59
    amebic 006.8
  staphylococcal NEC 682.9
  stitch 998.59
  stomach (wall) 535.0
  strumous (tuberculous) (*see also* Tuberculosis)
    017.2
  subarachnoid 324.9
    brain 324.0
    cerebral 324.0

Abscess—*continued*
late effect—*see* category 326
spinal cord 324.1
subareolar—*see also* Abscess, breast
puerperal, postpartum 675.1
subcecal 540.1
subcutaneous NEC 682.9
subdiaphragmatic 567.22
subdorsal 682.2
subdural 324.9
brain 324.0
late effect—*see* category 326
spinal cord 324.1
subgaleal 682.8
subhepatic 567.22
sublingual 528.3
gland 527.3
submammary—*see* Abscess, breast
submandibular (region) (space) (triangle) 682.0
gland 527.3
submaxillary (region) 682.0
gland 527.3
submental (pyogenic) 682.0
gland 527.3
subpectoral 682.2
subperiosteal—*see* Abscess, bone
subperitoneal 567.22
subphrenic—*see also* Abscess, peritoneum
567.22
postoperative 998.59
subscapular 682.2
subungual 681.9
suburethral 597.0
sudoriparous 705.89
suppurative NEC 682.9
supraclavicular (fossa) 682.3
suprahepatic 567.22
suprapelvic (*see also* Disease, pelvis,
inflammatory) 614.4
acute 614.3
suprapubic 682.2
suprarenal (capsule) (gland) 255.8
sweat gland 705.89
syphilitic 095.8
teeth, tooth (root) 522.5
with sinus (alveolar) 522.7
supporting structures NEC 523.30
temple 682.0
temporal region 682.0
temporosphenoidal 324.0
late effect—*see* category 326
tendon (sheath) 727.89
testicle—*see* Orchitis
thecal 728.89
thigh (acquired) 682.6
thorax 510.9
with fistula 510.0
throat 478.29
thumb (intrathecal) (periosteal) (subcutaneous)
(subcuticular) 681.00
thymus (gland) 254.1
thyroid (gland) 245.0
toe (any) (intrathecal) (periosteal)
(subcutaneous) (subcuticular) 681.10
tongue (staphylococcal) 529.0
tonsil(s) (lingual) 475
tonsillopharyngeal 475
tooth, teeth (root) 522.5
with sinus (alveolar) 522.7
supporting structure NEC 523.30
trachea 478.9

Abscess—*continued*
trunk 682.2
tubal (*see also* Salpingo-oophoritis) 614.2
tuberculous—*see* Tuberculosis, abscess
tubo-ovarian (*see also* Salpingo-oophoritis)
614.2
tunica vaginalis 608.4
umbilicus NEC 682.2
newborn 771.4
upper arm 682.3
upper respiratory 478.9
urachus 682.2
urethra (gland) 597.0
urinary 597.0
uterus, uterine (wall) (*see also* Endometritis)
615.9
ligament (*see also* Disease, pelvis,
inflammatory) 614.4
acute 614.3
neck (*see also* Cervicitis) 616.0
uvula 528.3
vagina (wall) (*see also* Vaginitis) 616.10
vaginorectal (*see also* Vaginitis) 616.10
vas deferens 608.4
vermiform appendix 540.1
vertebra (column) (tuberculous) (*see also*
Tuberculosis) 015.0 *[730.88]*
nontuberculous 730.0
vesical 595.89
vesicouterine pouch (*see also* Disease, pelvis,
inflammatory) 614.4
vitreous (humor) (pneumococcal) 360.04
vocal cord 478.5
von Bezold's 383.01
vulva 616.4
complicating pregnancy, childbirth, or
puerperium 646.6
vulvovaginal gland (*see also* Vaginitis) 616.3
web-space 682.4
wrist 682.4
Absence (organ or part) (complete or partial)
acoustic nerve 742.8
adrenal (gland) (congenital) 759.1
acquired V45.79
albumin (blood) 273.8
alimentary tract (complete) (congenital) (partial)
751.8
lower 751.5
upper 750.8
alpha-fucosidase 271.8
alveolar process (acquired) 525.8
congenital 750.26
anus, anal (canal) (congenital) 751.2
aorta (congenital) 747.22
aortic valve (congenital) 746.89
appendix, congenital 751.2
arm (acquired) V49.60
above elbow V49.66
below elbow V49.65
congenital (*see also* Deformity, reduction,
upper limb) 755.20
lower—*see* Absence, forearm, congenital
upper (complete) (partial) (with absence of
distal elements, incomplete) 755.24
with
complete absence of distal elements
755.21
forearm (incomplete) 755.23
artery (congenital) (peripheral) NEC (*see also*
Anomaly, peripheral vascular system)
747.60

Absence—*continued*
   brain 747.81
     cerebral 747.81
     coronary 746.85
     pulmonary 747.3
     umbilical 747.5
   atrial septum 745.69
   auditory canal (congenital) (external) 744.01
   auricle (ear) (with stenosis or atresia of auditory
     canal), congenital 744.01
   bile, biliary duct (common) or passage
     (congenital) 751.61
     bladder (acquired) V45.74
     congenital 753.8
   bone (congenital) NEC 756.9
     marrow 284.9
       acquired (secondary) 284.8
       congenital 284.09
       hereditary 284.09
       idiopathic 284.9
     skull 756.0
   bowel sounds 787.5
   brain 740.0
     specified part 742.2
   breast(s) (acquired) V45.71
     congenital 757.6
   broad ligament (congenital) 752.19
   bronchus (congenital) 748.3
   calvarium, calvaria (skull) 756.0
   canaliculus lacrimalis, congenital 743.65
   carpal(s) (congenital) (complete) (partial) (with
     absence of distal elements, incomplete) (*see
     also* Deformity, reduction, upper limb)
     755.28
     with complete absence of distal elements
      755.21
   cartilage 756.9
   caudal spine 756.13
   cecum (acquired) (postoperative)
     (posttraumatic) V45.72
     congenital 751.2
   cementum 520.4
   cerebellum (congenital) (vermis) 742.2
   cervix (acquired) (uteri) V45.77
     congenital 752.49
   chin, congenital 744.89
   cilia (congenital) 743.63
     acquired 374.89
   circulatory system, part NEC 747.89
   clavicle 755.51
   clitoris (congenital) 752.49
   coccyx, congenital 756.13
   cold sense (*see also* Disturbance, sensation)
     782.0
   colon (acquired) (postoperative) V45.72
     congenital 751.2
   congenital
     lumen—*see* Atresia
     organ or site NEC—*see* Agenesis
     septum—*see* Imperfect, closure
   corpus callosum (congenital) 742.2
   cricoid cartilage 748.3
   diaphragm (congenital) (with hernia) 756.6
     with obstruction 756.6
   digestive organ(s) or tract, congenital (complete)
     (partial) 751.8
     acquired V45.79
     lower 751.5
     upper 750.8
   ductus arteriosus 747.89

Absence—*continued*
   duodenum (acquired) (postoperative) V45.72
     congenital 751.1
   ear, congenital 744.09
     acquired V45.79
     auricle 744.01
     external 744.01
     inner 744.05
     lobe, lobule 744.21
     middle, except ossicles 744.03
       ossicles 744.04
     ossicles 744.04
   ejaculatory duct (congenital) 752.89
   endocrine gland NEC (congenital) 759.2
   epididymis (congenital) 752.89
     acquired V45.77
   epiglottis, congenital 748.3
   epileptic (atonic) (typical) (*see also* Epilepsy)
     345.0
   erythrocyte 284.9
   erythropoiesis 284.9
     congenital 284.01
   esophagus (congenital) 750.3
   Eustachian tube (congenital) 744.24
   extremity (acquired)
     congenital (*see also* Deformity, reduction)
      755.4
     lower V49.70
     upper V49.60
   extrinsic muscle, eye 743.69
   eye (acquired) V45.78
     adnexa (congenital) 743.69
     congenital 743.00
     muscle (congenital) 743.69
   eyelid (fold), congenital 743.62
     acquired 374.89
   face
     bones NEC 756.0
     specified part NEC 744.89
   fallopian tube(s) (acquired) V45.77
     congenital 752.19
   femur, congenital (complete) (partial) (with
     absence of distal elements, incomplete) (*see
     also* Deformity, reduction, lower limb)
     755.34
     with
       complete absence of distal elements 755.31
       tibia and fibula (incomplete) 755.33
   fibrin 790.92
     fibrinogen (congenital) 286.3
     acquired 286.6
   fibula, congenital (complete) (partial) (with
     absence of distal elements, incomplete) (*see
     also* Deformity, reduction, lower limb)
     755.37
     with
       complete absence of distal elements 755.31
       tibia 755.35
         with
           complete absence of distal elements
            755.31
           femur (incomplete) 755.33
             with complete absence of distal
               elements 755.31
   finger (acquired) V49.62
     congenital (complete) (partial) (*see also*
      Deformity, reduction, upper limb) 755.29
     meaning all fingers (complete) (partial)
      755.21
     transverse 755.21
   fissures of lungs (congenital) 748.5

Absence—*continued*
  organ
    of Corti (congenital) 744.05
    or site
      acquired V45.79
      congenital NEC 759.89
  osseous meatus (ear) 744.03
  ovary (acquired) V45.77
    congenital 752.0
  oviduct (acquired) V45.77
    congenital 752.19
  pancreas (congenital) 751.7
    acquired (postoperative) (posttraumatic)
        V45.79
  parathyroid gland (congenital) 759.2
  parotid gland(s) (congenital) 750.21
  patella, congenital 755.64
  pelvic girdle (congenital) 755.69
  penis (congenital) 752.69
    acquired V45.77
  pericardium (congenital) 746.89
  perineal body (congenital) 756.81
  phalange(s), congenital 755.4
    lower limb (complete) (intercalary) (partial)
        (terminal) (*see also* Deformity, reduction,
        lower limb) 755.39
      meaning all toes (complete) (partial) 755.31
      transverse 755.31
    upper limb (complete) (intercalary) (partial)
        (terminal) (*see also* Deformity, reduction,
        upper limb) 755.29
      meaning all digits (complete) (partial)
          755.21
      transverse 755.21
  pituitary gland (congenital) 759.2
  postoperative—*see* Absence, by site, acquired
  prostate (congenital) 752.89
    acquired V45.77
  pulmonary
    artery 747.3
    trunk 747.3
    valve (congenital) 746.01
    vein 747.49
  punctum lacrimale (congenital) 743.65
  radius, congenital (complete) (partial) (with
      absence of distal elements, incomplete)
      755.26
    with
      complete absence of distal elements 755.21
      ulna 755.25
        with
          complete absence of distal elements
              755.21
          humerus (incomplete) 755.23
  ray, congenital 755.4
    lower limb (complete) (partial) (*see also*
        Deformity, reduction, lower limb) 755.38
      meaning all rays 755.31
      transverse 755.31
    upper limb (complete) (partial) (*see also*
        Deformity, reduction, upper limb) 755.28
      meaning all rays 755.21
      transverse 755.21
  rectum (congenital) 751.2
    acquired V45.79
  red cell 284.9
    acquired (secondary) 284.8
    congenital 284.01
    hereditary 284.01
    idiopathic 284.9
  respiratory organ (congenital) NEC 748.9

Absence—*continued*
  rib (acquired) 738.3
    congenital 756.3
  roof of orbit (congenital) 742.0
  round ligament (congenital) 752.89
  sacrum, congenital 756.13
  salivary gland(s) (congenital) 750.21
  scapula 755.59
  scrotum, congenital 752.89
  seminal tract or duct (congenital) 752.89
    acquired V45.77
  septum (congenital)—*see also* Imperfect,
      closure, septum
    atrial 745.69
    and ventricular 745.7
    between aorta and pulmonary artery 745.0
    ventricular 745.3
      and atrial 745.7
  sex chromosomes 758.81
  shoulder girdle, congenital (complete) (partial)
      755.59
  skin (congenital) 757.39
  skull bone 756.0
    with
      anencephalus 740.0
      encephalocele 742.0
      hydrocephalus 742.3
        with spina bifida (*see also* Spina bifida)
            741.0
      microcephalus 742.1
  spermatic cord (congenital) 752.89
  spinal cord 742.59
  spine, congenital 756.13
  spleen (congenital) 759.0
    acquired V45.79
  sternum, congenital 756.3
  stomach (acquired) (partial) (postoperative)
      V45.75
    congenital 750.7
    with postgastric surgery syndrome 564.2
  submaxillary gland(s) (congenital) 750.21
  superior vena cava (congenital) 747.49
  tarsal(s), congenital (complete) (partial) (with
      absence of distal elements, incomplete) (*see
      also* Deformity, reduction, lower limb)
      755.38
  teeth, tooth (congenital) 520.0
    with abnormal spacing 524.30
    acquired 525.10
      due to
        caries 525.13
        extraction 525.10
        periodontal disease 525.12
        trauma 525.11
      with malocclusion 524.30
  tendon (congenital) 756.81
  testis (congenital) 752.89
    acquired V45.77
  thigh (acquired) 736.89
  thumb (acquired) V49.61
    congenital 755.29
  thymus gland (congenital) 759.2
  thyroid (gland) (surgical) 246.8
    with hypothyroidism 244.0
    cartilage, congenital 748.3
    congenital 243
  tibia, congenital (complete) (partial) (with absence
      of distal elements, incomplete) (*see also*
      Deformity, reduction, lower limb) 755.36

Abulia 799.89
Abulomania 301.6
Abuse
  adult 995.80
    emotional 995.82
    multiple forms 995.85
    neglect (nutritional) 995.84
    physical 995.81
    psychological 995.82
    sexual 995.83
  alcohol (*see also* Alcoholism) 305.0
    dependent 303.9
    non-dependent 305.0
  child 995.50
    counseling
      perpetrator
        non-parent V62.83
          parent V61.22
        victim V61.21
    emotional 995.51
    multiple forms 995.59
    neglect (nutritional) 995.52
    physical 995.54
      shaken infant syndrome 995.55
    psychological 995.51
    sexual 995.53
  drugs, nondependent 305.9

> *Note—Use the following fifth-digit*
> *subclassification with the following codes:*
> *305.0, 305.2-305.9:*
>
> *0 unspecifidd*
> *1 continuous*
> *2 episodic*
> *3 in remission*

    amphetamine type 305.7
    antidepressants 305.8
    anxiolytic 305.4
    barbiturates 305.4
    caffeine 305.9
    cannabis 305.2
    cocaine type 305.6
    hallucinogens 305.3
    hashish 305.2
    hypnotic 305.4
    inhalant 305.9
    LSD 305.3
    marijuana 305.2
    mixed 305.9
    morphine type 305.5
    opioid type 305.5
    phencyclidine (PCP) 305.9
    sedative 305.4
    specified NEC 305.9
    tranquilizers 305.4
  spouse 995.80
  tobacco 305.1
Acalcerosis 275.40
Acalcicosis 275.40
Acalculia 784.69
  developmental 315.1
Acanthocheilonemiasis 125.4
Acanthocytosis 272.5
Acanthokeratodermia 701.1
Acantholysis 701.8
  bullosa 757.39
Acanthoma (benign) (M8070/0)—*see also*
    Neoplasm, by site, benign
  malignant (M8070/3)—*see* Neoplasm, by site,
    malignant

Acanthosis (acquired) (nigricans) 701.2
  adult 701.2
  benign (congenital) 757.39
  congenital 757.39
  glycogenic
    esophagus 530.8
  juvenile 701.2
  tongue 529.8
Acanthrocytosis 272.5
Acapnia 276.3
Acarbia 276.2
Acardia 759.89
Acardiacus amorphus 759.89
Acardiotrophia 429.1
Acardius 759.89
Acariasis 133.9
  sarcoptic 133.0
Acaridiasis 133.9
Acarinosis 133.9
Acariosis 133.9
Acarodermatitis 133.9
  urticarioides 133.9
Acarophobia 300.29
Acatalasemia 277.89
Acatalasia 277.89
Acatamathesia 784.69
Acataphasia 784.5
Acathisia 781.0
  due to drugs 333.99
Acceleration, accelerated
  atrioventricular conduction 426.7
  idioventricular rhythm 427.89
Accessory (congenital)
  adrenal gland 759.1
  anus 751.5
  appendix 751.5
  atrioventricular conduction 426.7
  auditory ossicles 744.04
  auricle (ear) 744.1
  autosome(s) NEC 758.5
    21 or 22 758.0
  biliary duct or passage 751.69
  bladder 753.8
  blood vessels (peripheral) (congenital) NEC (*see*
      also Anomaly, peripheral vascular system)
      747.60
    cerebral 747.81
    coronary 746.85
  bone NEC 756.9
    foot 755.67
  breast tissue, axilla 757.6
  carpal bones 755.56
  cecum 751.5
  cervix 752.49
  chromosome(s) NEC 758.5
    13-15 758.1
    16-18 758.2
    21 or 22 758.0
    autosome(s) NEC 758.5
    D_1 758.1
    E_3 758.2
    G 758.0
    sex 758.81
  coronary artery 746.85
  cusp(s), heart valve NEC 746.89
    pulmonary 746.09
  cystic duct 751.69
  digits 755.00
  ear (auricle) (lobe) 744.1
  endocrine gland NEC 759.2

Accessory—*continued*
external os 752.49
eyelid 743.62
eye muscle 743.69
face bone(s) 756.0
fallopian tube (fimbria) (ostium) 752.19
fingers 755.01
foreskin 605
frontonasal process 756.0
gallbladder 751.69
genital organ(s)
  female 752.89
    external 752.49
    internal NEC 752.89
  male NEC 752.89
    penis 752.69
genitourinary organs NEC 752.89
heart 746.89
  valve NEC 746.89
    pulmonary 746.09
hepatic ducts 751.69
hymen 752.49
intestine (large) (small) 751.5
kidney 753.3
lacrimal canal 743.65
leaflet, heart valve NEC 746.89
  pulmonary 746.09
ligament, broad 752.19
liver (duct) 751.69
lobule (ear) 744.1
lung (lobe) 748.69
muscle 756.82
navicular of carpus 755.56
nervous system, part NEC 742.8
nipple 757.6
nose 748.1
organ or site NEC—*see* Anomaly, specified
  type NEC
ovary 752.0
oviduct 752.19
pancreas 751.7
parathyroid gland 759.2
parotid gland (and duct) 750.22
pituitary gland 759.2
placental lobe—*see* Placenta, abnormal
preauricular appendage 744.1
prepuce 605
renal arteries (multiple) 747.62
rib 756.3
  cervical 756.2
roots (teeth) 520.2
salivary gland 750.22
sesamoids 755.8
sinus—*see* condition
skin tags 757.39
spleen 759.0
sternum 756.3
submaxillary gland 750.22
tarsal bones 755.67
teeth, tooth 520.1
  causing crowding 524.31
tendon 756.89
thumb 755.01
thymus gland 759.2
thyroid gland 759.2
toes 755.02
tongue 750.13
tragus 744.1
ureter 753.4
urethra 753.8
urinary organ or tract NEC 753.8

Accessory—*continued*
uterus 752.2
vagina 752.49
valve, heart NEC 746.89
  pulmonary 746.09
vertebra 756.19
vocal cords 748.3
vulva 752.49
Accident, accidental —*see also* condition
birth NEC 767.9
cardiovascular (*see also* Disease,
    cardiovascular) 429.2
cerebral (*see also* Disease, cerebrovascular,
    acute) 434.91
cerebrovascular (current) (CVA) (*see also*
    Disease, cerebrovascular, acute) 434.91
  embolic 434.11
  healed or old V12.59
  hemorrhagic—*see* Hemorrhage, brain
  impending 435.9
  ischemic 434.91
  late effect—*see* Late effect(s) (of)
      cerebrovascular disease
  postoperative 997.02
  thrombotic 434.01
coronary (*see also* Infarct, myocardium) 410.9
craniovascular (*see also* Disease,
    cerebrovascular, acute) 436
during pregnancy, to mother
  affecting fetus or newborn 760.5
heart, cardiac (*see also* Infarct, myocardium)
    410.9
intrauterine 779.89
vascular—*see* Disease, cerebrovascular, acute
Accommodation
disorder of 367.51
  drug-induced 367.89
  toxic 367.89
insufficiency of 367.4
paralysis of 367.51
  hysterical 300.11
spasm of 367.53
Accouchement —*see* Delivery
Accreta placenta (without hemorrhage) 667.0
with hemorrhage 666.0
Accretio cordis (nonrheumatic) 423.1
Accretions on teeth 523.6
Accumulation secretion, prostate 602.8
Acephalia, acephalism, acephaly 740.0
Acephalic monster 740.0
Acephalobrachia monster 759.89
Acephalocardia 759.89
Acephalocardius 759.89
Acephalochiria 759.89
Acephalochirus monster 759.89
Acephalogaster 759.89
Acephalostomus monster 759.89
Acephalothorax 759.89
Acephalus 740.0
Acetonemia 790.6
diabetic 250.1
Acetonglycosuria 982.8
Acetonuria 791.6
Achalasia 530.0
cardia 530.0
digestive organs congenital NEC 751.8
esophagus 530.0
pelvirectal 751.3
psychogenic 306.4
pylorus 750.5
sphincteral NEC 564.89

Achard-Thiers syndrome (adrenogenital) 255.2
Ache (s)—*see* Pain
Acheilia 750.26
Acheiria 755.21
Achillobursitis 726.71
Achillodynia 726.71
Achlorhydria, achlorhydric 536.0
  anemia 280.9
  diarrhea 536.0
  neurogenic 536.0
  postvagotomy 564.2
  psychogenic 306.4
  secondary to vagotomy 564.2
Achloroblepsia 368.52
Achloropsia 368.52
Acholia 575.8
Acholuric jaundice (familial) (splenomegalic)
    (*see also* Spherocytosis) 282.0
  acquired 283.9
Achondroplasia 756.4
Achrestic anemia 281.8
Achroacytosis, lacrimal gland 375.00
  tuberculous (*see also* Tuberculosis) 017.3
Achroma, cutis 709.00
Achromate (congenital) 368.54
Achromatopia 368.54
Achromatopsia (congenital) 368.54
Achromia
  congenital 270.2
  parasitica 111.0
  unguium 703.8
Achylia
  gastrica 536.8
    neurogenic 536.3
      psychogenic 306.4
  pancreatica 577.1
Achylosis 536.8
Acid
  burn—*see also* Burn, by site
    from swallowing acid—*see* Burn, internal
      organs
  deficiency
    amide nicotinic 265.2
    amino 270.9
    ascorbic 267
    folic 266.2
    nicotinic (amide) 265.2
    pantothenic 266.2
  intoxication 276.2
  peptic disease 536.8
  stomach 536.8
    psychogenic 306.4
Acidemia 276.2
  arginosuccinic 270.6
  fetal
    affecting management of pregnancy 656.3
    before onset of labor, in liveborn infant 768.2
    during labor and delivery, in liveborn infant
      768.3
    intrauterine—*see* Distress, fetal 656.3
    unspecified as to time of onset, in liveborn
      infant 768.4
  newborn 775.81
  pipecolic 270.7
Acidity, gastric (high) (low) 536.8
  psychogenic 306.4
Acidocytopenia 288.59
Acidocytosis 288.3
Acidopenia 288.59

Acidosis 276.2
  diabetic 250.1
  fetal, affecting management of pregnancy 656.8
  fetal, affecting newborn 775.81
  kidney tubular 588.89
  lactic 276.2
  metabolic NEC 276.2
    with respiratory acidosis 276.4
      of newborn 775.81
    late, of newborn 775.7
  newborn 775.81
  renal
    hyperchloremic 588.89
    tubular (distal) (proximal) 588.89
  respiratory 276.2
    complicated by
      metabolic acidosis 276.4
        of newborn 775.81
      metabolic alkalosis 276.4
Aciduria 791.9
  arginosuccinic 270.6
  beta-aminoisobutyric (BAIB) 277.2
  glutaric
    type I 270.7
    type II (type IIA, IIB, IIC) 277.85
    type III 277.86
  glycolic 271.8
  methylmalonic 270.3
    with glycinemia 270.7
  organic 270.9
  orotic (congenital) (hereditary) (pyrimidine
      deficiency) 281.4
Acladiosis 111.8
  skin 111.8
Aclasis
  diaphyseal 756.4
  tarsoepiphyseal 756.59
Acleistocardia 745.5
Aclusion 524.4
Acmesthesia 782.0
Acne (pustular) (vulgaris) 706.1
  agminata (*see also* Tuberculosis) 017.0
  artificialis 706.1
  atrophica 706.0
  cachecticorum (Hebra) 706.1
  conglobata 706.1
  conjunctiva 706.1
  cystic 706.1
  decalvans 704.09
  erythematosa 695.3
  eyelid 706.1
  frontalis 706.0
  indurata 706.1
  keloid 706.1
  lupoid 706.0
  necrotic, necrotica 706.0
    miliaris 704.8
  neonatal 706.1
  nodular 706.1
  occupational 706.1
  papulosa 706.1
  rodens 706.0
  rosacea 695.3
  scorbutica 267
  scrofulosorum (Bazin) (*see also* Tuberculosis)
      017.0
  summer 692.72
  tropical 706.1
  varioliformis 706.0
Acneiform drug eruptions 692.3
Acnitis (primary) (*see also* Tuberculosis) 017.0
Acomia 704.00

Addiction —*see also* Dependence
  absinthe 304.6
  alcoholic (ethyl) (methyl) (wood) 303.9
    complicating pregnancy, childbirth, or
        puerperium 648.4
      affecting fetus or newborn 760.71
    suspected damage to fetus affecting
        management of pregnancy 655.4
  drug (*see also* Dependence) 304.9
  ethyl alcohol 303.9
  heroin 304.0
  hospital 301.51
  methyl alcohol 303.9
  methylated spirit 303.9
  morphine (-like substances) 304.0
  nicotine 305.1
  opium 304.0
  tobacco 305.1
  wine 303.9
Addison's
  anemia (pernicious) 281.0
  disease (bronze) (primary adrenal insufficiency)
      255.4
    tuberculous (*see also* Tuberculosis) 017.6
  keloid (morphea) 701.0
  melanoderma (adrenal cortical hypofunction)
      255.4
Addison-Biermer anemia (pernicious) 281.0
Addison-Gull disease —*see* Xanthoma
Addisonian crisis or melanosis (acute
    adrenocortical insufficiency) 255.4
Additional —*see also* Accessory
  chromosome(s) 758.5
    13-15 758.1
    16-18 758.2
    21 758.0
    autosome(s) NEC 758.5
    sex 758.81
Adduction contracture, hip or other joint —*see*
    Contraction, joint
**ADEM (acute disseminated encephalomyelitis)
    (postinfectious)** 136.9 *[323.61]*
  infectious 136.9 *[323.61]*
  noninfectious 323.81
Adenasthenia gastrica 536.0
Aden fever 061
Adenitis (*see also* Lymphadenitis) 289.3
  acute, unspecified site 683
    epidemic infectious 075
  axillary 289.3
    acute 683
    chronic or subacute 289.1
  Bartholin's gland 616.89
  bulbourethral gland (*see also* Urethritis) 597.89
  cervical 289.3
    acute 683
    chronic or subacute 289.1
  chancroid (Ducrey's bacillus) 099.0
  chronic (any lymph node, except mesenteric)
      289.1
    mesenteric 289.2
  Cowper's gland (*see also* Urethritis) 597.89
  epidemic, acute 075
  gangrenous 683
  gonorrheal NEC 098.89
  groin 289.3
    acute 683
    chronic or subacute 289.1
  infectious 075
  inguinal (region) 289.3
    acute 683

Adenitis—*continued*
    chronic or subacute 289.1
  lymph gland or node, except mesenteric 289.3
    acute 683
    chronic or subacute 289.1
    mesenteric (acute) (chronic) (nonspecific)
        (subacute) 289.2
    mesenteric (acute) (chronic) (nonspecific)
        (subacute) 289.2
    due to Pasteurella multocida (P. septica) 027.2
  parotid gland (suppurative) 527.2
  phlegmonous 683
  salivary duct or gland (any) (recurring)
      (suppurative) 527.2
  scrofulous (*see also* Tuberculosis) 017.2
  septic 289.3
  Skene's duct or gland (*see also* Urethritis)
      597.89
  strumous, tuberculous (*see also* Tuberculosis)
      017.2
  subacute, unspecified site 289.1
  sublingual gland (suppurative) 527.2
  submandibular gland (suppurative) 527.2
  submaxillary gland (suppurative) 527.2
  suppurative 683
  tuberculous—*see* Tuberculosis, lymph gland
  urethral gland (*see also* Urethritis) 597.89
  venereal NEC 099.8
  Wharton's duct (suppurative) 527.2
Adenoacanthoma (M8570/3)—*see* Neoplasm, by
    site, malignant
Adenoameloblastoma (M9300/0) 213.1
  upper jaw (bone) 213.0
Adenocarcinoma (M8140/3)—*see also*
    Neoplasm, by site, malignant

> *Note—The list of adjectival modifiers below is
> not exhaustive. A description of
> adenocarcinoma that does not appear in this list
> should be coded in the same manner as
> carcinoma with that description. Thus, "mixed
> acidophil-basophil adenocarcinoma," should be
> coded in the same manner as "mixed
> acidophil-basophil carcinoma," which appears
> in the list under "Carcinoma."*
>
> *Except where otherwise indicated, the
> morphological varieties of adenocarcinoma in
> the list below should be coded by site as for
> "Neoplasm, malignant."*

  with
    apocrine metaplasia (M8573/3)
    cartilaginous (and osseous) metaplasia
        (M8571/3)
    osseous (and cartilaginous) metaplasia
        (M8571/3)
    spindle cell metaplasia (M8572/3)
    squamous metaplasia (M8570/3)
  acidophil (M8280/3)
    specified site—*see* Neoplasm, by site,
        malignant
    unspecified site 194.3
  acinar (M8550/3)
  acinic cell (M8550/3)
  adrenal cortical (M8370/3) 194.0
  alveolar (M8251/3)
  and
    epidermoid carcinoma, mixed (M8560/3)
    squamous cell carcinoma, mixed (M8560/3)
  apocrine (M8401/3)
    breast—*see* Neoplasm, breast, malignant

Adenofibroma (M9013/0)
  clear cell (M8313/0)—*see* Neoplasm, by site,
    benign
  endometrioid (M8381/0) 220
    borderline malignancy (M8381/1) 236.2
    malignant (M8381/3) 183.0
  mucinous (M9015/0)
    specified site—*see* Neoplasm, by site, benign
    unspecified site 220
  prostate 600.20
    with
      other lower urinary tract symptoms (LUTS)
        600.21
      urinary
        obstruction 600.21
        retention 600.21
  serous (M9014/0)
    specified site—*see* Neoplasm, by site, benign
    unspecified site 220
  specified site—*see* Neoplasm, by site, benign
  unspecified site 220
Adenofibrosis
  breast 610.2
  endometrioid 617.0
Adenoiditis 474.01
  acute 463
  chronic 474.01
    with chronic tonsillitis 474.02
Adenoids (congenital) (of nasal fossa) 474.9
  hypertrophy 474.12
  vegetations 474.2
Adenolipomatosis (symmetrical) 272.8
Adenolymphoma (M8561/0)
  specified site—*see* Neoplasm, by site, benign
  unspecified 210.2
Adenoma (sessile) (M8140/0)—*see also*
  Neoplasm, by site, benign

> *Note—Except where otherwise indicated, the*
> *morphological varieties of adenoma in the list*
> *below should be coded by site as for*
> *"Neoplasm, benign."*

  acidophil (M8280/0)
    specified site—*see* Neoplasm, by site, benign
    unspecified site 227.3
  acinar (cell) (M8550/0)
  acinic cell (M8550/0)
  adrenal (cortex) (cortical) (functioning)
    (M8370/0) 227.0
    clear cell type (M8373/0) 227.0
    compact cell type (M8371/0) 227.0
    glomerulosa cell type (M8374/0) 227.0
    heavily pigmented variant (M8372/0) 227.0
    mixed cell type (M8375/0) 227.0
  alpha cell (M8152/0)
    pancreas 211.7
    specified site NEC—*see* Neoplasm, by site,
      benign
    unspecified site 211.7
  alveolar (M8251/0)
  apocrine (M8401/0)
    breast 217
    specified site NEC—*see* Neoplasm, skin,
      benign
    unspecified site 216.9
  basal cell (M8147/0)
  basophil (M8300/0)
    specified site—*see* Neoplasm, by site, benign
    unspecified site 227.3
  beta cell (M8151/0)
    pancreas 211.7

Adenoma—*continued*
    specified site NEC—*see* Neoplasm, by site,
      benign
    unspecified site 211.7
  bile duct (M8160/0) 211.5
  black (M8372/0) 227.0
  bronchial (M8140/1) 235.7
    carcinoid type (M8240/3)—*see* Neoplasm,
      lung, malignant
    cylindroid type (M8200/3)—*see* Neoplasm,
      lung, malignant
  ceruminous (M8420/0) 216.2
  chief cell (M8321/0) 227.1
    chromophobe (M8270/0)
    (specified site—*see* Neoplasm, by site, benign
    unspecified site 227.3
  clear cell (M8310/0)
  colloid (M8334/0)
    specified site—*see* Neoplasm, by site, benign
    unspecified site 226
  cylindroid type, bronchus (M8200/3)—*see*
    Neoplasm, lung, malignant
  duct (M8503/0)
  embryonal (M8191/0)
  endocrine, multiple (M8360/1)
    single specified site—*see* Neoplasm, by site,
      uncertain behavior
    two or more specified sites 237.4
    unspecified site 237.4
  endometrioid (M8380/0)—*see also* Neoplasm,
    by site, benign
    borderline malignancy (M8380/1)—*see*
      Neoplasm, by site, uncertain behavior
  eosinophil (M8280/0)
    specified site—*see* Neoplasm, by site, benign
    unspecified site 227.3
  fetal (M8333/0)
    specified site—*see* Neoplasm, by site, benign
    unspecified site 226
  follicular (M8330/0)
    specified site—*see* Neoplasm, by site, benign
    unspecified site 226
  hepatocellular (M8170/0) 211.5
  Hürthle cell (M8290/0) 226
  intracystic papillary (M8504/0)
  islet cell (functioning) (M8150/0)
    pancreas 211.7
    specified site NEC—*see* Neoplasm, by site,
      benign
    unspecified site 211.7
  liver cell (M8170/0) 211.5
  macrofollicular (M8334/0)
    specified site NEC—*see* Neoplasm, by site,
      benign
    unspecified site 226
  malignant, malignum (M8140/3)—*see*
    Neoplasm, by site, malignant
  mesonephric (M9110/0)
  microfollicular (M8333/0)
    specified site—*see* Neoplasm, by site, benign
    unspecified site 226
  mixed cell (M8323/0)
  monomorphic (M8146/0)
  mucinous (M8480/0)
  mucoid cell (M8300/0)
    specified site—*see* Neoplasm, by site, benign
    unspecified site 227.3
  multiple endocrine (M8360/1)
    single specified site—*see* Neoplasm, by site,
      uncertain behavior
    two or more specified sites 237.4

Adenoma—*continued*
   unspecified site 237.4
  nipple (M8506/0) 217
  oncocytic (M8290/0)
  oxyphilic (M8290/0)
  papillary (M8260/0)—*see also* Neoplasm, by
    site, benign
   intracystic (M8504/0)
  papillotubular (M8263/0)
  Pick's tubular (M8640/0)
   specified site—*see* Neoplasm, by site, benign
   unspecified site
    female 220
    male 222.0
  pleomorphic (M8940/0)
  polypoid (M8210/0)
  prostate (benign) 600.20
   with
    other lower urinary tract symptoms (LUTS)
     600.21
    urinary
     obstruction 600.21
     retention 600.21
  rete cell 222.0
  sebaceous, sebaceum (gland) (senile)
    (M8410/0)—*see also* Neoplasm, skin,
    benign
   disseminata 759.5
  Sertoli cell (M8640/0)
   specified site—*see* Neoplasm, by site, benign
   unspecified site
    female 220
    male 222.0
  skin appendage (M8390/0)—*see* Neoplasm,
    skin, benign
  sudoriferous gland (M8400/0)—*see* Neoplasm,
    skin, benign
  sweat gland or duct (M8400/0)—*see* Neoplasm,
    skin, benign
  testicular (M8640/0)
   specified site—*see* Neoplasm, by site, benign
   unspecified site
    female 220
    male 222.0
  thyroid 226
  trabecular (M8190/0)
  tubular (M8211/0)—*see also* Neoplasm, by site,
    benign
   papillary (M8460/3)
   Pick's (M8640/0)
    specified site—*see* Neoplasm, by site,
     benign
    unspecified site
     female 220
     male 222.0
  tubulovillous (M8263/0)
  villoglandular (M8263/0)
  villous (M8261/1)—*see* Neoplasm, by site,
    uncertain behavior
  water-clear cell (M8322/0) 227.1
  wolffian duct (M9110/0)
Adenomatosis (M8220/0)
  endocrine (multiple) (M8360/1)
   single specified site—*see* Neoplasm, by site,
    uncertain behavior
   two or more specified sites 237.4
   unspecified site 237.4
  erosive of nipple (M8506/0) 217
  pluriendocrine—*see* Adenomatosis, endocrine

Adenomatosis—*continued*
  pulmonary (M8250/1) 235.7
   malignant (M8250/3)—*see* Neoplasm, lung,
    malignant
  specified site—*see* Neoplasm, by site, benign
  unspecified site 211.3
Adenomatous
  cyst, thyroid (gland)—*see* Goiter, nodular
  goiter (nontoxic) (*see also* Goiter, nodular)
    241.9
  toxic or with hyperthyroidism 242.3
Adenomyoma (M8932/0)—*see also* Neoplasm,
   by site, benign
  prostate 600.20
   with
    other lower urinary tract symptoms (LUTS)
     600.21
    urinary
     obstruction 600.21
     retention 600.21
Adenomyometritis 617.0
Adenomyosis (uterus) (internal) 617.0
Adenopathy (lymph gland) 785.6
  inguinal 785.6
  mediastinal 785.6
  mesentery 785.6
  syphilitic (secondary) 091.4
   tracheobronchial 785.6
   tuberculous (*see also* Tuberculosis) 012.1
    primary, progressive 010.8
  tuberculous (*see also* Tuberculosis, lymph
    gland) 017.2
   tracheobronchial 012.1
    primary, progressive 010.8
Adenopharyngitis 462
Adenophlegmon 683
Adenosalpingitis 614.1
Adenosarcoma (M8960/3) 189.0
Adenosclerosis 289.3
Adenosis
  breast (sclerosing) 610.2
  vagina, congenital 752.49
Adentia (complete) (partial) (*see also* Absence,
   teeth) 520.0
Adherent
  labium (minus) 624.4
  pericardium (nonrheumatic) 423.1
   rheumatic 393
  placenta 667.0
   with hemorrhage 666.0
  prepuce 605
  scar (skin) NEC 709.2
  tendon in scar 709.2
**Adhesion(s), adhesive (postinfectional)(postop-
   erative)**
  abdominal (wall) (*see also* Adhesions,
    peritoneum) 568.0
  amnion to fetus 658.8
   affecting fetus or newborn 762.8
  appendix 543.9
  arachnoiditis—*see* Meningitis
  auditory tube (Eustachian) 381.89
  bands—*see also* Adhesions, peritoneum
   cervix 622.3
   uterus 621.5
  bile duct (any) 576.8
  bladder (sphincter) 596.8
  bowel (*see also* Adhesions, peritoneum) 568.0
  cardiac 423.1
   rheumatic 398.99
  cecum (*see also* Adhesions, peritoneum) 568.0

Adhesion(s)—*continued*
  postoperative (gastrointestinal tract) (*See also*
    Adhesions, peritoneum) 568.0
    eyelid 997.99
      surgically created V45.69
    urethra 598.2
  postpartal, old 624.4
  preputial, prepuce 605
  pulmonary 511.0
  pylorus (*see also* Adhesions, peritoneum) 568.0
  Rosenmüller's fossa 478.29
  sciatic nerve 355.0
  seminal vesicle 608.89
  shoulder (joint) 726.0
  sigmoid flexure (*see also* Adhesions,
    peritoneum) 568.0
  spermatic cord (acquired) 608.89
    congenital 752.89
  spinal canal 349.2
    nerve 355.9
      root 724.9
        cervical NEC 723.4
        lumbar NEC 724.4
        lumbosacral 724.4
        thoracic 724.4
  stomach (*see also* Adhesions, peritoneum) 568.0
  subscapular 726.2
  tendonitis 726.90
    shoulder 726.0
  testicle 608.89
  tongue (congenital) (to gum or roof of mouth)
    750.12
    acquired 529.8
  trachea 519.19
  tubo-ovarian 614.6
  tunica vaginalis 608.89
  ureter 593.89
  uterus 621.5
    to abdominal wall 614.6
      in pregnancy or childbirth 654.4
        affecting fetus or newborn 763.89
  vagina (chronic) (postoperative) (postradiation)
    623.2
  vaginitis (congenital) 752.49
  vesical 596.8
  vitreous 379.29
Adie (-Holmes) syndrome (tonic pupillary
  reaction) 379.46
Adiponecrosis neonatorum 778.1
Adiposa dolorosa 272.8
Adiposalgia 272.8
Adiposis 278.0
  cerebralis 253.8
  dolorosa 272.8
  tuberosa simplex 272.8
Adiposity 278.02
  heart (*see also* Degeneration, myocardial) 429.1
  localized 278.1
Adiposogenital dystrophy 253.8
Adjustment
  prosthesis or other device—*see* Fitting of
  reaction—*see* Reaction, adjustment
Administration, prophylactic
  antibiotics V07.39
  antitoxin, any V07.2
  antivenin V07.2
  chemotherapeutic agent NEC V07.39
  chemotherapy NEC V07.39
  diphtheria antitoxin V07.2
  fluoride V07.31
  gamma globulin V07.2

Administration, prophylactic—*continued*
  immune sera (gamma globulin) V07.2
  passive immunization agent V07.2
  RhoGAM V07.2
Admission (encounter)
  as organ donor—*see* Donor
  by mistake V68.9
  for
    adequacy testing (for)
      hemodialysis V56.31
      peritoneal dialysis V56.32
    adjustment (of)
      artificial
        arm (complete) (partial) V52.0
        eye V52.2
        leg (complete) (partial) V52.1
      brain neuropacemaker V53.02
      breast
        implant V52.4
        prosthesis V52.4
      cardiac device V53.39
        defibrillator, automatic implantable
          V53.32
        pacemaker V53.31
          carotid sinus V53.39
      catheter
        non-vascular V58.82
        vascular V58.81
      cerebral ventricle (communicating) shunt
        V53.01
      colostomy belt V53.5
      contact lenses V53.1
      cystostomy device V53.6
      dental prosthesis V52.3
      device, unspecified type V53.90
        abdominal V53.5
        cardiac V53.39
          defibrillator, automatic implantable
            V53.32
          pacemaker V53.31
            carotid sinus V53.39
        cerebral ventricle (communicating) shunt
          V53.01
        insulin pump V53.91
        intrauterine contraceptive V25.1
        nervous system V53.09
        orthodontic V53.4
        other device V53.99
        prosthetic V52.9
          breast V52.4
          dental V52.3
          eye V52.2
          specified type NEC V52.8
        special senses V53.09
        substitution
          auditory V53.09
          nervous system V53.09
          visual V53.09
        urinary V53.6
      dialysis catheter
        extracorporeal V56.1
        peritoneal V56.2
      diaphragm (contraceptive) V25.02
      growth rod V54.02
      hearing aid V53.2
      ileostomy device V53.5
      intestinal appliance or device NEC V53.5
      intrauterine contraceptive device V25.1
      neuropacemaker (brain) (peripheral nerve)
        (spinal cord) V53.02
      orthodontic device V53.4

Admission—*continued*
 for —*continued*
  Dick V74.8
  Kveim V82.89
  Mantoux V74.1
  mycotic infection NEC V75.4
  parasitic disease NEC V75.8
  Schick V74.3
  Schultz-Charlton V74.8
  social service (agency) referral or evaluation
   V63.8
  speech therapy V57.3
  sterilization V25.2
  suspected disorder (ruled out) (without need
   for further care)—*see* Observation
  terminal care V66.7
  tests only—*see* Test
  therapeutic drug monitoring V58.83
  therapy
   blood transfusion, without reported
    diagnosis V58.2
   breathing exercises V57.0
   chemotherapy, antineoplastic V58.11
    prophylactic NEC V07.39
     fluoride V07.31
   dialysis (intermittent) (treatment)
    extracorporeal V56.0
    peritoneal V56.8
    renal V56.0
    specified type NEC V56.8
    exercise (remedial) NEC V57.1
    breathing V57.0
   immunotherapy, antineoplastic V58.12
   long-term (current) drug use NEC V58.69
    antibiotics V58.62
    anticoagulants V58.61
    anti-inflammatories, non-steroidal
     (NSAID) V58.64
    antiplatelets V58.63
    antithrombotics V58.63
    aspirin V58.66
    insulin V58.67
    steroids V58.65
   occupational V57.21
   orthoptic V57.4
   physical NEC V57.1
   radiation V58.0
   speech V57.3
   vocational V57.22
  toilet or cleaning
   of artificial opening — *see* Attention to,
    artificial, opening
   of non-vascular catheter V58.82
   of vascular catheter V58.81
  tubal ligation V25.2
  tuboplasty for previous sterilization V26.0
  vaccination, prophylactic (against)
   arthropod-borne virus, viral NEC V05.1
    disease NEC V05.1
    encephalitis V05.0
   Bacille Calmette Guérin (BCG) V03.2
   BCG V03.2
   chickenpox V05.4
   cholera alone V03.0
    with typhoid-paratyphoid (cholera + TAB)
     V06.0
   common cold V04.7
   dengue V05.1
   diphtheria alone V03.5
   diphtheria-tetanus-pertussis (DTP) (DTaP)
    V06.1

Admission—*continued*
 for —*continued*
  with
   poliomyelitis (DTP + polio) V06.3
   typhoid-paratyphoid (DTP + TAB)
    V06.2
  diphtheria-tetanus [Td] [DT] without
   pertussis V06.5
  disease (single) NEC V05.9
   bacterial NEC V03.9
    specified type NEC V03.89
   combinations NEC V06.9
    specified type NEC V06.8
   specified type NEC V05.8
   viral NEC V04.89
  encephalitis, viral, arthropod-borne V05.0
  Hemophilus influenzae, type B [Hib]
   V03.81
  hepatitis, viral V05.3
  immune sera (gamma globulin) V07.2
  influenza V04.81
   with
    Streptococcus pneumoniae
     [pneumococcus] V06.6
  Leishmaniasis V05.2
  measles alone V04.2
  measles-mumps-rubella (MMR) V06.4
  mumps alone V04.6
   with measles and rubella (MMR) V06.4
  not done because of contraindication V64.09
  pertussis alone V03.6
  plague V03.3
  pneumonia V03.82
  poliomyelitis V04.0
   with diphtheria-tetanus-pertussis (DTP +
    polio) V06.3
  rabies V04.5
  respiratory syncytial virus (RSV) V04.82
  rubella alone V04.3
   with measles and mumps (MMR) V06.4
  smallpox V04.1
  specified type NEC V05.8
   Streptococcus pneumoniae
    [pneumococcus] V03.82
   with
    influenza V06.6
  tetanus toxoid alone V03.7
   with diphtheria [Td] [DT] V06.5
   and pertussis (DTP) (DTaP) V06.1
  tuberculosis (BCG) V03.2
  tularemia V03.4
  typhoid alone V03.1
   with diphtheria-tetanus-pertussis (TAB +
    DTP) V06.2
  typhoid-paratyphoid alone (TAB) V03.1
  typhus V05.8
  varicella V05.4
  viral encephalitis, arthropod-borne V05.0
  viral hepatitis V05.3
  yellow fever V04.4
 vasectomy V25.2
 vasoplasty for previous sterilization V26.0
 vision examination V72.0
 vocational therapy V57.22
 waiting period for admission to other facility
  V63.2
  undergoing social agency investigation
   V63.8
 well baby and child care V20.2
 x-ray of chest
  for suspected tuberculosis V71.2
  routine V72.5

Adnexitis (suppurative) (*see also*
   Salpingo-oophoritis) 614.2
Adolescence NEC V21.2
Adoption
   agency referral V68.89
   examination V70.3
   held for V68.89
Adrenal gland —*see* condition
Adrenalism 255.9
   tuberculous (*see also* Tuberculosis) 017.6
Adrenalitis, adrenitis 255.8
   meningococcal hemorrhagic 036.3
Adrenarche, precocious 259.1
Adrenocortical syndrome 255.2
Adrenogenital syndrome (acquired) (congenital)
   255.2
   iatrogenic, fetus or newborn 760.79
Adrenoleukodystrophy 277.86
   neonatal 277.86
   x-linked 277.86
Adrenomyeloneuropathy 277.86
Adventitious bursa —*see* Bursitis
Adynamia (episodica) (hereditary) (periodic)
   359.3
Adynamic
   ileus or intestine (*see also* ileus) 560.1
   ureter 753.22
Aeration lung imperfect, newborn 770.5
Aerobullosis 993.3
Aerocele —*see* Embolism, air
Aerodermectasia
   subcutaneous (traumatic) 958.7
      surgical 998.81
   surgical 998.81
Aerodontalgia 993.2
Aeroembolism 993.3
Aerogenes capsulatus infection (*see also*
   Gangrene, gas) 040.0
Aero-otitis media 993.0
Aerophagy, aerophagia 306.4
   psychogenic 306.4
Aerosinusitis 993.1
Aerotitis 993.0
Affection, affections —*see also* Disease
   sacroiliac (joint), old 724.6
   shoulder region NEC 726.2
Afibrinogenemia 286.3
   acquired 286.6
   congenital 286.3
   postpartum 666.3
African
   sleeping sickness 086.5
   tick fever 087.1
   trypanosomiasis 086.5
      Gambian 086.3
      Rhodesian 086.4
Aftercare V58.9
   amputation stump V54.89
   artificial openings—*see* Attention to, artificial,
      opening
   blood transfusion without reported diagnosis
      V58.2
   breathing exercise V57.0
   cardiac device V53.39
      defibrillator, automatic implantable V53.32
      pacemaker V53.31
         carotid sinus V53.39
   carotid sinus pacemaker V53.39
   cerebral ventricle (communicating) shunt
      V53.01

Aftercare—*continued*
   chemotherapy session (adjunctive)
      (maintenance) V58.11
   defibrillator, automatic implantable cardiac
      V53.32
   exercise (remedial) (therapeutic) V57.1
      breathing V57.0
   extracorporeal dialysis (intermittent) (treatment)
      V56.0
   following surgery NEC V58.49
      wound closure, planned V58.41
      for
         injury V58.43
         neoplasm V58.42
         organ transplant V58.44
         trauma V58.43
      joint replacement V54.81
      of
         circulatory system V58.73
         digestive system V58.75
         genital organs V58.76
         genitourinary system V58.76
         musculoskeletal system V58.78
         nervous system V58.72
         oral cavity V58.75
         respiratory system V58.74
         sense organs V58.71
         skin V58.77
         subcutaneous tissue V58.77
         teeth V58.75
         urinary system V58.76
   fracture V54.9
      healing V54.89
         pathologic
            ankle V54.29
            arm V54.20
               lower V54.22
               upper V54.21
            finger V54.29
            foot V54.29
            hand V54.29
            hip V54.23
            leg V54.24
               lower V54.26
               upper V54.25
            pelvis V54.29
            specified site NEC V54.29
            toe(s) V54.29
            vertebrae V54.27
            wrist V54.29
         traumatic
            ankle V54.19
            arm V54.10
               lower V54.12
               upper V54.11
            finger V54.19
            foot V54.19
            hand V54.19
            hip V54.13
            leg V54.14
               lower V54.16
               upper V54.15
            pelvis V54.19
            specified site NEC V54.19
            toe(s) V54.19
            vertebrae V54.17
            wrist V54.19
   removal of
      external fixation device V54.89
      internal fixation device V54.01
   specified care NEC V54.89

Aftercare—*continued*
  gait training V57.1
    for use of artificial limb(s) V57.81
  internal fixation device V54.09
  involving
    dialysis (intermittent) (treatment)
      extracorporeal V56.0
      peritoneal V56.8
      renal V56.0
    gait training V57.1
      for use of artificial limb(s) V57.81
    growth rod
      adjustment V54.02
      lengthening V54.02
    internal fixation device V54.09
    orthoptic training V57.4
    orthotic training V57.81
    radiotherapy session V58.0
    removal of
      drains V58.49
      dressings
        wound V58.30
          nonsurgical V58.30
          surgical V58.31
      fixation device
        external V54.89
        internal V54.01
      fracture plate V54.01
      nonsurgical wound dressing V58.30
      pins V54.01
      plaster cast V54.89
      rods V54.01
      screws V54.01
      staples V58.32
      surgical wound dressings V58.31
      sutures V58.32
      traction device, external V54.89
      wound packing V58.30
        nonsurgical V58.30
        surgical V58.31
  neuropacemaker (brain) (peripheral nerve)
      (spinal cord) V53.02
  occupational therapy V57.21
  orthodontic V58.5
  orthopedic V54.9
    change of external fixation or traction device
        V54.8
    following joint replacement V54.81
    internal fixation device V54.09
    removal of fixation device
      external V54.89
      internal V54.01
    specified care NEC V54.89
  orthoptic training V57.4
  orthotic training V57.81
  pacemaker
    brain V53.02
    cardiac V53.31
    carotid sinus V53.39
    peripheral nerve V53.02
    spinal cord V53.02
  peritoneal dialysis (intermittent) (treatment)
      V56.8
  physical therapy NEC V57.1
    breathing exercises V57.0
  radiotherapy session V58.0
  rehabilitation procedure V57.9
    breathing exercises V57.0
    multiple types V57.89
    occupational V57.21
    orthoptic V57.4

Aftercare—*continued*
    orthotic V57.81
    physical therapy NEC V57.1
    remedial exercises V57.1
    specified type NEC V57.89
    speech V57.3
    therapeutic exercises V57.1
    vocational V57.22
  renal dialysis (intermittent) (treatment) V56.0
  specified type NEC V58.89
    removal of non-vascular catheter V58.82
    removal of vascular catheter V58.81
  speech therapy V57.3
  stump, amputation V54.89
  vocational rehabilitation V57.22
After-cataract 366.50
  obscuring vision 366.53
  specified type, not obscuring vision 366.52
Agalactia 676.4
Agammaglobulinemia 279.00
  with lymphopenia 279.2
  acquired (primary) (secondary) 279.06
  Bruton's X-linked 279.04
  infantile sex-linked (Bruton's) (congenital)
      279.04
  Swiss-type 279.2
Aganglionosis (bowel) (colon) 751.3
Age (old) (*see also* Senile) 797
Agenesis —*see also* Absence, by site, congenital
  acoustic nerve 742.8
  adrenal (gland) 759.1
  alimentary tract (complete) (partial) NEC 751.8
    lower 751.2
    upper 750.8
  anus, anal (canal) 751.2
  aorta 747.22
  appendix 751.2
  arm (complete) (partial) (*see also* Deformity,
      reduction, upper limb) 755.20
  artery (peripheral) NEC (*see also* Anomaly,
      peripheral vascular system) 747.60
    brain 747.81
    coronary 746.85
    pulmonary 747.3
    umbilical 747.5
  auditory (canal) (external) 744.01
  auricle (ear) 744.01
  bile, biliary duct or passage 751.61
  bone NEC 756.9
  brain 740.0
    specified part 742.2
  breast 757.6
  bronchus 748.3
  canaliculus lacrimalis 743.65
  carpus NEC (*see also* Deformity, reduction,
      upper limb) 755.28
  cartilage 756.9
  cecum 751.2
  cerebellum 742.2
  cervix 752.49
  chin 744.89
  cilia 743.63
  circulatory system, part NEC 747.89
  clavicle 755.51
  clitoris 752.49
  coccyx 756.13
  colon 751.2
  corpus callosum 742.2
  cricoid cartilage 748.3
  diaphragm (with hernia) 756.6

Agenesis—*continued*
  digestive organ(s) or tract (complete) (partial)
      NEC 751.8
    lower 751.2
    upper 750.8
  ductus arteriosus 747.89
  duodenum 751.1
  ear NEC 744.09
    auricle 744.01
    lobe 744.21
  ejaculatory duct 752.89
  endocrine (gland) NEC 759.2
  epiglottis 748.3
  esophagus 750.3
  Eustachian tube 744.24
  extrinsic muscle, eye 743.69
  eye 743.00
    adnexa 743.69
  eyelid (fold) 743.62
  face
    bones NEC 756.0
    specified part NEC 744.89
  fallopian tube 752.19
  femur NEC (*see also* Absence, femur,
      congenital) 755.34
  fibula NEC (*see also* Absence, fibula,
      congenital) 755.37
  finger NEC (*see also* Absence, finger,
      congenital) 755.29
  foot (complete) (*see also* Deformity, reduction,
      lower limb) 755.31
  gallbladder 751.69
  gastric 750.8
  genitalia, genital (organ)
    female 752.89
      external 752.49
      internal NEC 752.89
    male 752.89
      penis 752.69
  glottis 748.3
  gonadal 758.6
  hair 757.4
  hand (complete) (*see also* Deformity, reduction,
      upper limb) 755.21
  heart 746.89
    valve NEC 746.89
      aortic 746.89
      mitral 746.89
      pulmonary 746.01
  hepatic 751.69
  humerus NEC (*see also* Absence, humerus,
      congenital) 755.24
  hymen 752.49
  ileum 751.1
  incus 744.04
  intestine (small) 751.1
    large 751.2
  iris (dilator fibers) 743.45
  jaw 524.09
  jejunum 751.1
  kidney(s) (partial) (unilateral) 753.0
  labium (majus) (minus) 752.49
  labyrinth, membranous 744.05
  lacrimal apparatus (congenital) 743.65
  larynx 748.3
  leg NEC (*see also* Deformity, reduction, lower
      limb) 755.30
  lens 743.35

Agenesis—*continued*
  limb (complete) (partial) (*see also* Deformity,
      reduction) 755.4
    lower NEC 755.30
    upper 755.20
  lip 750.26
  liver 751.69
  lung (bilateral) (fissures) (lobe) (unilateral)
      748.5
  mandible 524.09
  maxilla 524.09
  metacarpus NEC 755.28
  metatarsus NEC 755.38
  muscle (any) 756.81
  musculoskeletal system NEC 756.9
  nail(s) 757.5
  neck, part 744.89
  nerve 742.8
  nervous system, part NEC 742.8
  nipple 757.6
  nose 748.1
  nuclear 742.8
  organ
    of Corti 744.05
    or site not listed—*see* Anomaly, specified type
        NEC
  osseous meatus (ear) 744.03
  ovary 752.0
  oviduct 752.19
  pancreas 751.7
  parathyroid (gland) 759.2
  patella 755.64
  pelvic girdle (complete) (partial) 755.69
  penis 752.69
  pericardium 746.89
  perineal body 756.81
  pituitary (gland) 759.2
  prostate 752.89
  pulmonary
    artery 747.3
    trunk 747.3
    vein 747.49
  punctum lacrimale 743.65
  radioulnar NEC (*see also* Absence, forearm,
      congenital) 755.25
  radius NEC (*see also* Absence, radius,
      congenital) 755.26
  rectum 751.2
  renal 753.0
  respiratory organ NEC 748.9
  rib 756.3
  roof of orbit 742.0
  round ligament 752.89
  sacrum 756.13
  salivary gland 750.21
  scapula 755.59
  scrotum 752.89
  seminal duct or tract 752.89
  septum
    atrial 745.69
    between aorta and pulmonary artery 745.0
    ventricular 745.3
  shoulder girdle (complete) (partial) 755.59
  skull (bone) 756.0
    with
      anencephalus 740.0
      encephalocele 742.0
      hydrocephalus 742.3
        with spina bifida (*see also* Spina bifida)
            741.0

Akathisia, acathisia 781.0
  due to drugs 333.99
  neuroleptic-induced acute 333.99
Akinesia algeria 352.6
Akiyami 100.89
Akureyri disease (epidemic neuromyasthenia)
    049.8
Alacrima (congenital) 743.65
Alactasia (hereditary) 271.3
Alagille syndrome 759.89
Alalia 784.3
  developmental 315.31
    receptive-expressive 315.32
  secondary to organic lesion 784.3
Alaninemia 270.8
Alastrim 050.1
Albarrán's disease (colibacilluria) 791.9
Albers-Schönberg's disease (marble bones)
    756.52
Albert's disease 726.71
Albinism, albino (choroid) (cutaneous) (eye)
    (generalized) (isolated) (ocular)
    (oculocutaneous) (partial) 270.2
Albinismus 270.2
Albright (-Martin) (-Bantam) disease
    (pseudohypoparathyroidism) 275.49
Albright (-McCune) (-Sternberg) syndrome
    (osteitis fibrosa disseminata) 756.59
Albuminous —*see* condition
Albuminuria, albuminuric (acute) (chronic)
    (subacute) 791.0
  Bence-Jones 791.0
  cardiac 785.9
  complicating pregnancy, childbirth, or
      puerperium 646.2
    with hypertension—*see* Toxemia, of
        pregnancy
    affecting fetus or newborn 760.1
  cyclic 593.6
  gestational 646.2
  gravidarum 646.2
    with hypertension—*see* Toxemia, of
        pregnancy
    affecting fetus or newborn 760.1
  heart 785.9
  idiopathic 593.6
  orthostatic 593.6
  postural 593.6
  pre-eclamptic (mild) 642.4
    affecting fetus or newborn 760.0
    severe 642.5
      affecting fetus or newborn 760.0
  recurrent physiologic 593.6
  scarlatinal 034.1
Albumosuria 791.0
  Bence-Jones 791.0
  myelopathic (M9730/3) 203.0
Alcaptonuria 270.2
Alcohol, alcoholic
  abstinance 291.81
  acute intoxication 305.0
    with dependence 303.0
  addiction (*see also* Alcoholism) 303.9
    maternal
      with suspected fetal damage affecting
          management of pregnancy 655.4
      affecting fetus or newborn 760.71
  amnestic disorder, persisting 291.1
  anxiety 291.89
  brain syndrome, chronic 291.2

Alcohol, alcoholic—*continued*
  cardiopathy 425.5
  chronic (*see also* Alcoholism) 303.9
  cirrhosis (liver) 571.2
  delirium 291.0
    acute 291.0
    chronic 291.1
    tremens 291.0
    withdrawal 291.0
  dementia NEC 291.2
  deterioration 291.2
  drunkenness (simple) 305.0
  hallucinosis (acute) 291.3
  induced
    circadian rhythm sleep disorder 291.82
    hypersomnia 291.82
    insomnia 291.82
    mental disorder 291.9
      anxiety 291.89
      mood 291.89
      sexual 291.89
      sleep 291.82
      specified type 291.89
    parasomnia 291.82
    persisting
      amnestic disorder 291.1
      dementia 291.2
    psychotic disorder
      with
        delusions 291.5
        hallucinations 291.3
    sleep disorder 291.82
  insanity 291.9
  intoxication (acute) 305.0
    with dependence 303.0
    pathological 291.4
  jealousy 291.5
  Korsakoff's, Korsakov's, Korsakow's 291.1
  liver NEC 571.3
    acute 571.1
    chronic 571.2
  mania (acute) (chronic) 291.9
  mood 291.89
  paranoia 291.5
  paranoid (type) psychosis 291.5
  pellagra 265.2
  poisoning, accidental (acute) NEC 980.9
    specified type of alcohol—*see* Table of drugs
        and chemicals
  psychosis (*see also* Psychosis, alcoholic) 291.9
    Korsakoff's, Korsakov's, Korsakow's 291.1
    polyneuritic 291.1
      with
        delusions 291.5
        hallucinations 291.3
  related disorder 291.9
  withdrawal symptoms, syndrome NEC 291.81
    delirium 291.0
    hallucinosis 291.3
Alcoholism 303.9

*Note—Use the following fifth-digit
subclassification with category 303:*

0 unspecifhed
1 continuous
2 episodic
3 in remission

  with psychosis (*see also* Psychosis, alcoholic)
      291.9
  acute 303.0

Allergy, allergic—*continued*
  rose 477.0
  Senecio jacobae 477.0
  serum (prophylactic) (therapeutic) 999.5
    anaphylactic shock 999.4
  shock (anaphylactic)
    due to
      adverse effect of correct medicinal substance
          properly administered 995.0
      food—*see* Anaphylactic shock, due to, food
    from serum or immunization 999.5
      anaphylactic 999.4
  sinusitis (*see also* Fever, hay) 477.9
  skin reaction 692.9
    specified substance—*see* Dermatitis, due to
  tree (any) (hay fever) (pollen) 477.0
    asthma (*see also* Asthma) 493.0
  upper respiratory (*see also* Fever, hay) 477.9
  urethritis 597.89
  urticaria 708.0
  vaccine—*see* Allergy, serum
Allescheriosis 117.6
Alligator skin disease (ichthyosis congenita)
    757.1
  acquired 701.1
Allocheiria, allochiria (*see also* Disturbance,
    sensation) 782.0
Almeida's disease (Brazilian blastomycosis) 116.1
Alopecia (atrophicans) (pregnancy) (premature)
    (senile) 704.00
  adnata 757.4
  areata 704.01
  celsi 704.01
  cicatrisata 704.09
  circumscripta 704.01
  congenital, congenitalis 757.4
  disseminata 704.01
  effluvium (telogen) 704.02
  febrile 704.09
  generalisata 704.09
  hereditaria 704.09
  marginalis 704.01
  mucinosa 704.09
  postinfectional 704.09
  seborrheica 704.09
  specific 091.82
  syphilitic (secondary) 091.82
  telogen effluvium 704.02
  totalis 704.09
  toxica 704.09
  universalis 704.09
  x-ray 704.09
Alper's disease 330.8
Alpha-lipoproteinemia 272.4
Alpha thalassemia 282.49
Alphos 696.1
Alpine sickness 993.2
Alport's syndrome (hereditary
    hematuria-nephropathy-deafness) 759.89
Alteration (of), altered
  awareness 780.09
    transient 780.02
  consciousness 780.09
    persistent vegetative state 780.03
    transient 780.02
  mental status 780.97
    amnesia (retrograde) 780.93
    memory loss 780.93
Alternaria (infection) 118
Alternating —*see* condition

Altitude, high (effects)—*see* Effect, adverse,
    high altitude
Aluminosis (of lung) 503
Alvarez syndrome (transient cerebral ischemia)
    435.9
Alveolar capillary block syndrome 516.3
Alveolitis
  allergic (extrinsic) 495.9
    due to organisms (fungal, thermophilic
        actinomycete, other) growing in
        ventilation (air conditioning systems)
        495.7
    specified type NEC 495.8
  due to
    Aspergillus clavatus 495.4
    Cryptostroma corticale 495.6
  fibrosing (chronic) (cryptogenic) (lung) 516.3
    idiopathic 516.3
    rheumatoid 714.81
  jaw 526.5
  sicca dolorosa 526.5
Alveolus, alveolar —*see* condition
Alymphocytosis (pure) 279.2
Alymphoplasia, thymic 279.2
Alzheimer's
  dementia (senile)
    with behavioral disturbance 331.0 *[294.11]*
    without behavioral disturbance 331.0 *[294.10]*
  disease or sclerosis 331.0
    with dementia—*see* Alzheimer's, dementia
Amastia (*see also* Absence, breast) 611.8
Amaurosis (acquired) (congenital) (*see also*
    Blindness) 369.00
  fugax 362.34
  hysterical 300.11
  Leber's (congenital) 362.76
  tobacco 377.34
  uremic—*see* Uremia
Amaurotic familial idiocy (infantile) (juvenile)
    (late) 330.1
Ambisexual 752.7
Amblyopia (acquired) (congenital) (partial) 368.00
  color 368.59
    acquired 368.55
  deprivation 368.02
  ex anopsia 368.00
  hysterical 300.11
  nocturnal 368.60
    vitamin A deficiency 264.5
  refractive 368.03
  strabismic 368.01
  suppression 368.01
  tobacco 377.34
  toxic NEC 377.34
  uremic—*see* Uremia
Ameba, amebic (histolytica)–*see also* Amebiasis
  abscess 006.3
    bladder 006.8
    brain (with liver and lung abscess) 006.5
    liver 006.3
      with
        brain abscess (and lung abscess) 006.5
        lung abscess 006.4
    lung (with liver abscess) 006.4
      with brain abscess 006.5
    seminal vesicle 006.8
    spleen 006.8
  carrier (suspected of) V02.2
  meningoencephalitis
    due to Naegleria (gruberi) 136.2
    primary 136.2

Amebiasis NEC 006.9
  with
    brain abscess (with liver or lung abscess) 006.5
    liver abscess (without mention of brain or lung
      abscess) 006.3
    lung abscess (with liver abscess) 006.4
      with brain abscess 006.5
  acute 006.0
  bladder 006.8
  chronic 006.1
  cutaneous 006.6
  cutis 006.6
  due to organism other than Entamoeba
    histolytica 007.8
  hepatic (*see also* Abscess, liver, amebic) 006.3
  nondysenteric 006.2
  seminal vesicle 006.8
  specified
    organism NEC 007.8
    site NEC 006.8
Ameboma 006.8
Amelia 755.4
  lower limb 755.31
  upper limb 755.21
Ameloblastoma (M9310/0) 213.1
  jaw (bone) (lower) 213.1
    upper 213.0
  long bones (M9261/3)—*see* Neoplasm, bone,
    malignant
  malignant (M9310/3) 170.1
    jaw (bone) (lower) 170.1
      upper 170.0
  mandible 213.1
  tibial (M9261/3) 170.7
Amelogenesis imperfecta 520.5
  nonhereditaria (segmentalis) 520.4
Amenorrhea (primary) (secondary) 626.0
  due to ovarian dysfunction 256.8
  hyperhormonal 256.8
Amentia (*see also* Retardation, mental) 319
  Meynert's (nonalcoholic) 294.0
    alcoholic 291.1
  nevoid 759.6
American
  leishmaniasis 085.5
  mountain tick fever 066.1
  trypanosomiasis—*see* Trypanosomiasis,
    American
Ametropia (*see also* Disorder, accommodation)
  367.9
Amianthosis 501
Amimia 784.69
Amino acid
  deficiency 270.9
    anemia 281.4
  metabolic disorder (*see also* Disorder, amino
    acid) 270.9
Aminoaciduria 270.9
  imidazole 270.5
Amnesia (retrograde) 780.93
  auditory 784.69
    developmental 315.31
    secondary to organic lesion 784.69
  dissociative 300.12
  hysterical or dissociative type 300.12
  psychogenic 300.12
  transient global 437.7
Amnestic (confabulatory) syndrome 294.0
  alcohol-induced persisting 291.1
  drug-induced persisting 292.83
  posttraumatic 294.0

Amniocentesis screening (for) V28.2
  alphafetoprotein level, raised V28.1
  chromosomal anomalies V28.0
Amnion, amniotic —*see also* condition
  nodosum 658.8
Amnionitis (complicating pregnancy) 658.4
  affecting fetus or newborn 762.7
Amoral trends 301.7
Amotio retinae (*see also* Detachment, retina) 361.9
Ampulla
  lower esophagus 530.89
  phrenic 530.89
Amputation
  any part of fetus, to facilitate delivery 763.89
  cervix (supravaginal) (uteri) 622.8
    in pregnancy or childbirth 654.6
      affecting fetus or newborn 763.89
  clitoris—*see* Wound, open, clitoris
  congenital
    lower limb 755.31
    upper limb 755.21
  neuroma (traumatic)—*see also* Injury, nerve, by
    site
    surgical complications (late) 997.61
  penis—*see* Amputation, traumatic, penis
  status (without complication)—*see* Absence, by
    site, acquired
  stump (surgical)(posttraumatic)
    abnormal, painful, or with complication (late)
      997.60
    healed or old NEC —*see also* Absence, by
      site, acquired
      lower V49.70
      upper V49.60
  traumatic (complete) (partial)

> *Note—"Complicated" includes traumatic*
> *amputation with delayed healing, delayed*
> *treatment, foreign body, or infection.*

    arm 887.4
      at or above elbow 887.2
        complicated 887.3
      below elbow 887.0
        complicated 887.1
      both (bilateral) (any level(s)) 887.6
        complicated 887.7
      complicated 887.5
    finger(s) (one or both hands) 886.0
      with thumb(s) 885.0
        complicated 885.1
      complicated 886.1
    foot (except toe(s) only) 896.0
      and other leg 897.6
        complicated 897.7
      both (bilateral) 896.2
        complicated 896.3
      complicated 896.1
      toe(s) only (one or both feet) 895.0
        complicated 895.1
    genital organ(s) (external) NEC 878.8
      complicated 878.9
    hand (except finger(s) only) 887.0
      and other arm 887.6
        complicated 887.7
      both (bilateral) 887.6
        complicated 887.7
      complicated 887.1
      finger(s) (one or both hands) 886.0
        with thumb(s) 885.0
          complicated 885.1
        complicated 886.1

Androblastoma (M8630/1)
  benign (M8630/0)
    specified site—*see* Neoplasm, by site, benign
    unspecified site
      female 220
      male 222.0
  malignant (M8630/3)
    specified site—*see* Neoplasm, by site,
      malignant
    unspecified site
      female 183.0
      male 186.9
  specified site—*see* Neoplasm, by site, uncertain
    behavior
  tubular (M8640/0)
    with lipid storage (M8641/0)
      specified site—*see* Neoplasm, by site,
        benign
      unspecified site
        female 220
        male 222.0
    specified site—*see* Neoplasm, by site, benign
    unspecified site
      female 220
      male 222.0
  unspecified site
    female 236.2
    male 236.4
Android pelvis 755.69
  with disproportion (fetopelvic) 653.3
    affecting fetus or newborn 763.1
    causing obstructed labor 660.1
      affecting fetus or newborn 763.1
Anectasis, pulmonary (newborn or fetus) 770.5
Anemia 285.9
  in
    chronic illness NEC 285.29
    chronic kidney disease 285.21
    end-stage renal disease 285.21
    neoplastic disease 285.22
  with
    disorder of
      anaerobic glycolysis 282.3
      pentose phosphate pathway 282.2
    koilonychia 280.9
  6-phosphogluconic dehydrogenase deficiency
    282.2
  achlorhydric 280.9
  achrestic 281.8
  Addison's (pernicious) 281.0
  Addison-Biermer (pernicious) 281.0
  agranulocytic 288.09
  amino acid deficiency 281.4
  aplastic 284.9
    acquired (secondary) 284.8
    congenital 284.01
    constitutional 284.01
    due to
      chronic systemic disease 284.8
      drugs 284.8
      infection 284.8
      radiation 284.8
    idiopathic 284.9
    myxedema 244.9
    of or complicating pregnancy 648.2
    red cell (acquired) (with thymoma) 284.8
      congenital 284.01
      pure 284.01
    specified type NEC 284.8
    toxic (paralytic) 284.8

Anemia—*continued*
  aregenerative 284.9
    congenital 284.01
  asiderotic 280.9
  atypical (primary) 285.9
  autohemolysis of Selwyn and Dacie (type I)
    282.2
  autoimmune hemolytic 283.0
  Baghdad Spring 282.2
  Balantidium coli 007.0
  Biermer's (pernicious) 281.0
  blood loss (chronic) 280.0
    acute 285.1
  bothriocephalus 123.4
  brickmakers' (*see also* Ancylostomiasis) 126.9
  cerebral 437.8
  childhood 282.9
  chlorotic 280.9
  chronica congenita aregenerativa 284.01
  chronic simple 281.9
  combined system disease NEC 281.0 *[336.2]*
    due to dietary deficiency 281.1 *[336.2]*
  complicating pregnancy or childbirth 648.2
  congenital (following fetal blood loss) 776.5
    aplastic 284.01
    due to isoimmunization NEC 773.2
    Heinz-body 282.7
    hereditary hemolytic NEC 282.9
    nonspherocytic
      Type I 282.2
      Type II 282.3
    pernicious 281.0
    spherocytic (*see also* Spherocytosis) 282.0
  Cooley's (erythroblastic) 282.49
  crescent—*see* Disease, sickle-cell
  cytogenic 281.0
  Dacie's (nonspherocytic)
    Type I 282.2
    Type II 282.3
  Davidson's (refractory) 284.9
  deficiency 281.9
    2, 3 diphosphoglycurate mutase 282.3
    2, 3 PG 282.3
    6-PGD 282.2
    6-phosphogluronic dehydrogenase 282.2
    amino acid 281.4
    combined B_{12} and folate 281.3
    enzyme, drug-induced (hemolytic) 282.2
    erythrocytic glutathione 282.2
    folate 281.2
      dietary 281.2
      drug-induced 281.2
    folic acid 281.2
      dietary 281.2
      drug-induced 281.2
    G-6-PD 282.2
    GGS-R 282.2
    glucose-6-phosphate dehydrogenase (G-6-PD)
      282.2
    glucose-phosphate isomerase 282.3
    glutathione peroxidase 282.2
    glutathione reductase 282.2
    glyceraldehyde phosphate dehydrogenase
      282.3
    GPI 282.3
    G SH 282.2
    hexokinase 282.3
    iron (Fe) 280.9
      specified NEC 280.8

Aneurysm—*continued*
    thoracic 441.01
      thoracoabdominal 441.03
   syphilitic 093.9
  ductus arteriosus 747.0
  embolic—*see* Embolism, artery
  endocardial, infective (any valve) 421.0
  femoral 442.3
  gastroduodenal 442.84
  gastroepiploic 442.84
  heart (chronic or with a stated duration of over 8
      weeks) (infectional) (wall) 414.10
    acute or with a stated duration of 8 weeks or
       less (*see also* Infarct, myocardium) 410.9
    congenital 746.89
    valve—*see* Endocarditis
  hepatic 442.84
  iliac (common) 442.2
  infective (any valve) 421.0
  innominate (nonsyphilitic) 442.89
    syphilitic 093.89
  interauricular septum (*see also* Aneurysm, heart)
    414.10
  interventricular septum (*see also* Aneurysm,
    heart) 414.10
  intracranial—*see* Aneurysm, brain
  intrathoracic (nonsyphilitic) 441.2
    ruptured 441.1
    syphilitic 093.0
  jugular vein 453.8
  lower extremity 442.3
  lung (pulmonary artery) 417.1
  malignant 093.9
  mediastinal (nonsyphilitic) 442.89
    syphilitic 093.89
  miliary (congenital) (ruptured) (*see also*
    Hemorrhage, subarachnoid) 430
  mitral (heart) (valve) 424.0
  mural (arteriovenous) (heart) (*see also*
    Aneurysm, heart) 414.10
  mycotic, any site 421.0
    ruptured, brain (*see also* Hemorrhage,
      subarachnoid) 430
    without endocarditis —*see* Aneurysm, by site
  myocardium (*see also* Aneurysm, heart) 414.10
  neck 442.81
  pancreaticoduodenal 442.84
  patent ductus arteriosus 747.0
  peripheral NEC 442.89
    congenital NEC (*see also* Aneurysm,
      congenital) 747.60
  popliteal 442.3
  pulmonary 417.1
    arteriovenous 747.3
      acquired 417.0
    syphilitic 093.89
    valve (heart) (*see also* Endocarditis,
      pulmonary) 424.3
  racemose 442.9
    congenital (peripheral) NEC 747.60
  radial 442.0
  Rasmussen's (*see also* Tuberculosis) 011.2
  renal 442.1
  retinal (acquired) 362.17
    congenital 743.58
    diabetic 250.5 *[362.01]*
  sinus, aortic (of Valsalva) 747.29
  specified site NEC 442.89
  spinal (cord) 442.89
    congenital 747.82
    syphilitic (hemorrhage) 094.89

Aneurysm—*continued*
 spleen, splenic 442.83
 subclavian 442.82
   syphilitic 093.89
 superior mesenteric 442.84
 syphilitic 093.9
   aorta 093.0
   central nervous system 094.89
   congenital 090.5
   spine, spinal 094.89
 thoracoabdominal 441.7
   ruptured 441.6
 thorax, thoracic (arch) (nonsyphilitic) 441.2
   dissecting 441.01
   ruptured 441.1
   syphilitic 093.0
 traumatic (complication) (early)—*see* Injury,
   blood vessel, by site
 tricuspid (heart) (valve)—*see* Endocarditis,
   tricuspid
 ulnar 442.0
 upper extremity 442.0
 valve, valvular—*see* Endocarditis
 venous 456.8
   congenital NEC (*see also* Aneurysm,
    congenital) 747.60
 ventricle (arteriovenous) (*see also* Aneurysm,
   heart) 414.10
 visceral artery NEC 442.84
Angiectasis 459.89
Angiectopia 459.9
Angiitis 447.6
 allergic granulomatous 446.4
 hypersensitivity 446.20
   Goodpasture's syndrome 446.21
   specified NEC 446.29
 necrotizing 446.0
 Wegener's (necrotizing respiratory
   granulomatosis) 446.4
Angina (attack) (cardiac) (chest) (effort) (heart)
   (pectoris) (syndrome) (vasomotor) 413.9
 abdominal 557.1
 accelerated 411.1
 agranulocytic 288.03
 aphthous 074.0
 catarrhal 462
 crescendo 411.1
 croupous 464.4
 cruris 443.9
   due to atherosclerosis NEC (*see also*
    Arteriosclerosis, extremities) 440.20
 decubitus 413.0
 diphtheritic (membranous) 032.0
 erysipelatous 034.0
 erythematous 462
 exudative, chronic 476.0
 faucium 478.29
 gangrenous 462
   diphtheritic 032.0
 infectious 462
 initial 411.1
 intestinal 557.1
 ludovici 528.3
 Ludwig's 528.3
 malignant 462
   diphtheritic 032.0
 membranous 464.4
   diphtheritic 032.0
 mesenteric 557.1
 monocytic 075
 nocturnal 413.0

Angina—*continued*
  phlegmonous 475
    diphtheritic 032.0
  preinfarctional 411.1
  Prinzmetal's 413.1
  progressive 411.1
  pseudomembranous 101
  psychogenic 306.2
  pultaceous, diphtheritic 032.0
  scarlatinal 034.1
  septic 034.0
  simple 462
  stable NEC 413.9
  staphylococcal 462
  streptococcal 034.0
  stridulous, diphtheritic 032.3
  syphilitic 093.9
    congenital 090.5
  tonsil 475
  trachealis 464.4
  unstable 411.1
  variant 413.1
  Vincent's 101
Angioblastoma (M9161/1)—*see* Neoplasm,
    connective tissue, uncertain behavior
Angiocholecystitis (*see also* Cholecystitis, acute)
    575.0
Angiocholitis (*see also* Cholecystitis, acute)
    576.1
Angiodysgensis spinalis 336.1
Angiodysplasia (intestinalis) (intestine) 569.84
  with hemorrhage 569.85
  duodenum 537.82
    with hemorrhage 537.83
  stomach 537.82
    with hemorrhage 537.83
Angioedema (allergic) (any site) (with urticaria)
    995.1
  hereditary 277.6
Angioendothelioma (M9130/1)—*see also*
    Neoplasm, by site, uncertain behavior
  benign (M9130/0) (*see also* Hemangioma, by
    site) 228.00
  bone (M9260/3)—*see* Neoplasm, bone,
    malignant
  Ewing's (M9260/3)—*see* Neoplasm, bone,
    malignant
  nervous system (M9130/0) 228.09
Angiofibroma (M9160/0)—*see also* Neoplasm,
    by site, benign
  juvenile (M9160/0) 210.7
    specified site—*see* Neoplasm, by site, benign
    unspecified site 210.7
Angiohemophilia (A) (B) 286.4
Angioid streaks (choroid) (retina) 363.43
Angiokeratoma (M9141/0)—*see also* Neoplasm,
    skin, benign
  corporis diffusum 272.7
Angiokeratosis
  diffuse 272.7
Angioleiomyoma (M8894/0)—*see* Neoplasm,
    connective tissue, benign
Angioleucitis 683
Angiolipoma (M8861/0) (*see also* Lipoma, by
    site) 214.9
  infiltrating (M8861/1)—*see* Neoplasm,
    connective tissue, uncertain behavior
Angioma (M9120/0) (*see also* Hemangioma, by
    site) 228.00
  capillary 448.1
  hemorrhagicum hereditaria 448.0

Angioma—*continued*
  malignant (M9120/3)—*see* Neoplasm,
    connective tissue, malignant
  pigmentosum et atrophicum 757.33
  placenta—*see* Placenta, abnormal
  plexiform (M9131/0)—*see* Hemangioma, by
    site
  senile 448.1
  serpiginosum 709.1
  spider 448.1
  stellate 448.1
Angiomatosis 757.32
  bacillary 083.8
  corporis diffusum universale 272.7
  cutaneocerebral 759.6
  encephalocutaneous 759.6
  encephalofacial 759.6
  encephalotrigeminal 759.6
  hemorrhagic familial 448.0
  hereditary familial 448.0
  heredofamilial 448.0
  meningo-oculofacial 759.6
  multiple sites 228.09
  neuro-oculocutaneous 759.6
  retina (Hippel's disease) 759.6
  retinocerebellosa 759.6
  retinocerebral 759.6
  systemic 228.09
Angiomyolipoma (M8860/0)
  specified site—*see* Neoplasm, connective tissue,
    benign
  unspecified site 223.0
Angiomyoliposarcoma (M8860/3)—*see*
    Neoplasm, connective tissue, malignant
Angiomyoma (M8894/0)—*see* Neoplasm,
    connective tissue, benign
Angiomyosarcoma (M8894/3)—*see* Neoplasm,
    connective tissue, malignant
Angioneurosis 306.2
Angioneurotic edema (allergic) (any site) (with
    urticaria) 995.1
  hereditary 277.6
Angiopathia, angiopathy 459.9
  diabetic (peripheral) 250.7 *[443.81]*
  peripheral 443.9
    diabetic 250.7 *[443.81]*
    specified type NEC 443.89
  retinae syphilitica 093.89
  retinalis (juvenilis) 362.18
    background 362.10
    diabetic 250.5 *[362.01]*
    proliferative 362.29
    tuberculous (*see also* Tuberculosis) 017.3
      [362.18]
Angiosarcoma (M9120/3)—*see* Neoplasm,
    connective tissue, malignant
Angiosclerosis —*see* Arteriosclerosis
Angioscotoma, enlarged 368.42
Angiospasm 443.9
  brachial plexus 353.0
  cerebral 435.9
  cervical plexus 353.2
  nerve
    arm 354.9
      axillary 353.0
      median 354.1
      ulnar 354.2
    autonomic (*see also* Neuropathy, peripheral,
      autonomic) 337.9
    axillary 353.0

Angiospasm—*continued*
  leg 355.8
    plantar 355.6
    lower extremity—*see* Angiospasm, nerve, leg
    median 354.1
    peripheral NEC 355.9
    spinal NEC 355.9
    sympathetic (*see also* Neuropathy, peripheral,
        autonomic) 337.9
    ulnar 354.2
    upper extremity—*see* Angiospasm, nerve, arm
  peripheral NEC 443.9
  traumatic 443.9
    foot 443.9
    leg 443.9
  vessel 443.9
Angiospastic disease or edema 443.9
Angle's
  class I 524.21
  class II 524.22
  class III 524.23
Anguillulosis 127.2
Angulation
  cecum (*see also* Obstruction, intestine) 560.9
  coccyx (acquired) 738.6
    congenital 756.19
  femur (acquired) 736.39
    congenital 755.69
  intestine (large) (small) (*see also* Obstruction,
      intestine) 560.9
  sacrum (acquired) 738.5
    congenital 756.19
  sigmoid (flexure) (*see also* Obstruction,
      intestine) 560.9
  spine (*see also* Curvature, spine) 737.9
  tibia (acquired) 736.89
    congenital 755.69
  ureter 593.3
  wrist (acquired) 736.09
    congenital 755.59
Angulus infectiosus 686.8
Anhedonia 302.72
Anhidrosis (lid) (neurogenic) (thermogenic)
    705.0
Anhydration 276.51
  with
    hypernatremia 276.0
    hyponatremia 276.1
Anhydremia 276.52
  with
    hypernatremia 276.0
    hyponatremia 276.1
Anidrosis 705.0
Aniridia (congenital) 743.45
Anisakiasis (infection) (infestation) 127.1
Anisakis larva infestation 127.1
Aniseikonia 367.32
Anisocoria (pupil) 379.41
  congenital 743.46
Anisocytosis 790.09
Anisometropia (congenital) 367.31
Ankle —*see* condition
Ankyloblepharon (acquired) (eyelid) 374.46
  filiforme (adnatum) (congenital) 743.62
  total 743.62
Ankylodactly (*see also* Syndactylism) 755.10
Ankyloglossia 750.0

Ankylosis (fibrous) (osseous) 718.50
  ankle 718.57
  any joint, produced by surgical fusion V45.4
  cricoarytenoid (cartilage) (joint) (larynx) 478.79
  dental 521.6
  ear ossicle NEC 385.22
    malleus 385.21
  elbow 718.52
  finger 718.54
  hip 718.55
  incostapedial joint (infectional) 385.22
  joint, produced by surgical fusion NEC V45.4
  knee 718.56
  lumbosacral (joint) 724.6
  malleus 385.21
  multiple sites 718.59
  postoperative (status) V45.4
  sacroiliac (joint) 724.6
  shoulder 718.51
  specified site NEC 718.58
  spine NEC 724.9
  surgical V45.4
  teeth, tooth (hard tissues) 521.6
  temporomandibular joint 524.61
  wrist 718.53
Ankylostoma —*see* Ancylostoma
Ankylostomiasis (intestinal)—*see*
    Ancylostomiasis
Ankylurethria (*see also* Stricture, urethra) 598.9
Annular —*see also* condition
  detachment, cervix 622.8
  organ or site, congenital NEC—*see* Distortion
  pancreas (congenital) 751.7
Anodontia (complete) (partial) (vera) 520.0
  with abnormal spacing 524.30
  acquired 525.10
    causing malocclusion 524.30
    due to
      caries 525.13
      extraction 525.10
      periodontal disease 525.12
      trauma 525.11
Anomaly, anomalous (congenital) (unspecified
    type) 759.9
  abdomen 759.9
  abdominal wall 756.70
  acoustic nerve 742.9
  adrenal (gland) 759.1
  Alder (-Reilly) (leukocyte granulation) 288.2
  alimentary tract 751.9
    lower 751.5
    specified type NEC 751.8
    upper (any part, except tongue) 750.9
      tongue 750.10
        specified type NEC 750.19
  alveolar 524.70
    ridge (process) 525.8
    specified NEC 524.79
  ankle (joint) 755.69
  anus, anal (canal) 751.5
  aorta, aortic 747.20
    arch 747.21
    coarctation (postductal) (preductal) 747.10
    cusp or valve NEC 746.9
    septum 745.0
    specified type NEC 747.29
  aorticopulmonary septum 745.0
  apertures, diaphragm 756.6
  appendix 751.5
  aqueduct of Sylvius 742.3
    with spina bifida (*see also* Spina bifida) 741.0

Anomaly, anomalous—*continued*
  chest (wall) 756.3
  chin 744.9
    specified type NEC 744.89
  chordae tendineae 746.9
  choroid 743.9
    plexus 742.9
  chromosomes, chromosomal 758.9
    13 (13-15) 758.1
    18 (16-l8) 758.2
    21 or 22 758.0
    autosomes NEC (*see also* Abnormality,
        autosomes) 758.5
      deletion 758.39
    Christchurch 758.39
    D₁ 758.1
    E₃ 758.2
    G 758.0
    mitochondrial 758.9
    mosaics 758.89
    sex 758.81
      complement, XO 758.6
      complement, XXX 758.81
      complement, XYY 758.81
      gonadal dysgenesis 758.6
      Klinefelter's 758.7
      Turner's 758.6
    trisomy 21 758.0
  cilia 743.9
  circulatory system 747.9
    specified type NEC 747.89
  clavicle 755.51
  clitoris 752.40
  coccyx 756.10
  colon 751.5
  common duct 751.60
  communication
    coronary artery 746.85
    left ventricle with right atrium 745.4
  concha (ear) 744.3
  connection
    renal vessels with kidney 747.62
    total pulmonary venous 747.41
  connective tissue 756.9
    specified type NEC 756.89
  cornea 743.9
    shape 743.41
    size 743.41
    specified type NEC 743.49
  coronary
    artery 746.85
    vein 746.89
  cranium—*see* Anomaly, skull
  cricoid cartilage 748.3
  cushion, endocardial 745.60
    specified type NEC 745.69
  cystic duct 751.60
  dental arch 524.20
    specified NEC 524.29
  dental arch relationship 524.20
    angle's class I 524.21
    angle's class II 524.22
    angle's class III 524.23
    articulation
      anterior 524.27
      posterior 524.27
      reverse 524.27
    disto-occlusion 524.22
      division I 524.22
      division II 524.22
    excessive horizontal overlap 524.26

Anomaly, anomalous—*continued*
  interarch distance (excessive) (inadequate)
      524.28
  mesio-occlusion 524.23
  neutro-occlusion 524.21
  open
    anterior occlusal relationship 524.24
    posterior occlusal relationship 524.25
  specified NEC 524.29
  dentition 520.6
  dentofacial NEC 524.9
    functional 524.50
    specified type NEC 524.89
  dermatoglyphic 757.2
  Descemet's membrane 743.9
    specified type NEC 743.49
  development
    cervix 752.40
    vagina 752.40
    vulva 752.40
  diaphragm, diaphragmatic (apertures) NEC
      756.6
  digestive organ(s) or system 751.9
    lower 751.5
    specified type NEC 751.8
    upper 750.9
  distribution, coronary artery 746.85
  ductus
    arteriosus 747.0
    Botalli 747.0
  duodenum 751.5
  dura 742.9
    brain 742.4
    spinal cord 742.59
  ear 744.3
    causing impairment of hearing 744.00
      specified type NEC 744.09
    external 744.3
      causing impairment of hearing 744.02
      specified type NEC 744.29
    inner (causing impairment of hearing) 744.05
    middle, except ossicles (causing impairment
        of hearing) 744.03
      ossicles 744.04
    ossicles 744.04
    prominent auricle 744.29
    specified type NEC 744.29
      with hearing impairment 744.09
  Ebstein's (heart) 746.2
    tricuspid valve 746.2
  ectodermal 757.9
  Eisenmenger's (ventricular septal defect) 745.4
  ejaculatory duct 752.9
    specified type NEC 752.89
  elbow (joint) 755.50
  endocardial cushion 745.60
    specified type NEC 745.69
  endocrine gland NEC 759.2
  epididymis 752.9
  epiglottis 748.3
  esophagus 750.9
    specified type NEC 750.4
  Eustachian tube 744.3
    specified type NEC 744.24
  eye (any part) 743.9
    adnexa 743.9
      specified type NEC 743.69
    anophthalmos 743.00

Anomaly, anomalous—*continued*
    subvalvular 746.83
      tricuspid 746.9
        atresia 746.1
        stenosis 746.1
      ventricle 746.9
  heel 755.67
  Hegglin's 288.2
  hemianencephaly 740.0
  hemicephaly 740.0
  hemicrania 740.0
  hepatic duct 751.60
  hip (joint) 755.63
  hourglass
    bladder 753.8
    gallbladder 751.69
    stomach 750.7
  humerus 755.50
  hymen 752.40
  hypersegmentation of neutrophils, hereditary
    288.2
  hypophyseal 759.2
  ileocecal (coil) (valve) 751.5
  ileum (intestine) 751.5
  ilium 755.60
  integument 757.9
    specified type NEC 757.8
  interarch distance (excessive) (inadequate)
    524.28
  intervertebral cartilage or disc 756.10
  intestine (large) (small) 751.5
    fixational type 751.4
  iris 743.9
    specified type NEC 743.46
  ischium 755.60
  jaw NEC 524.9
    closure 524.51
    size NEC 524.00
    specified type NEC 524.89
  jaw-cranial base relationship 524.10
    specified NEC 524.19
  jejunum 751.5
  joint 755.9
    hip
      dislocation (*see also* Dislocation, hip,
        congenital) 754.30
      predislocation (*see also* Subluxation,
        congenital, hip) 754.32
      preluxation (*see also* Subluxation,
        congenital, hip) 754.32
      subluxation (*see also* Subluxation,
        congenital, hip) 754.32
    lumbosacral 756.10
      spondylolisthesis 756.12
      spondylosis 756.11
    multiple arthrogryposis 754.89
    sacroiliac 755.69
  Jordan's 288.2
  kidney(s) (calyx) (pelvis) 753.9
    vessel 747.62
  Klippel-Feil (brevicollis) 756.16
  knee (joint) 755.64
  labium (majus) (minus) 752.40
  labyrinth, membranous (causing impairment of
    hearing) 744.05
  lacrimal
    apparatus, duct or passage 743.9
      specified type NEC 743.65
    gland 743.9
      specified type NEC 743.64
  Langdon Down (mongolism) 758.0

Anomaly, anomalous—*continued*
  larynx, laryngeal (muscle) 748.3
    web, webbed 748.2
  leg (lower) (upper) 755.60
    reduction NEC (*see also* Deformity, reduction,
      lower limb) 755.30
  lens 743.9
    shape 743.36
    specified type NEC 743.39
  leukocytes, genetic 288.2
    granulation (constitutional) 288.2
  lid (fold) 743.9
  ligament 756.9
    broad 752.10
    round 752.9
  limb, except reduction deformity 755.9
    lower 755.60
      reduction deformity (*see also* Deformity,
        reduction, lower limb) 755.30
      specified type NEC 755.69
    upper 755.50
      reduction deformity (*see also* Deformity,
        reduction, upper limb) 755.20
      specified type NEC 755.59
  lip 750.9
    harelip (*see also* Cleft, lip) 749.10
    specified type NEC 750.26
  liver (duct) 751.60
    atresia 751.69
  lower extremity 755.60
    vessel 747.64
  lumbosacral (joint) (region) 756.10
  lung (fissure) (lobe) NEC 748.60
    agenesis 748.5
    specified type NEC 748.69
  lymphatic system 759.9
  Madelung's (radius) 755.54
  mandible 524.9
    size NEC 524.00
  maxilla 524.9
    size NEC 524.00
  May (-Hegglin) 288.2
  meatus urinarius 753.9
    specified type NEC 753.8
  meningeal bands or folds, constriction of 742.8
  meninges 742.9
    brain 742.4
    spinal 742.59
  meningocele (*see also* Spina bifida) 741.9
  mesentery 751.9
  metacarpus 755.50
  metatarsus 755.67
  middle ear, except ossicles (causing impairment
    of hearing) 744.03
    ossicles 744.04
  mitral (leaflets) (valve) 746.9
    atresia 746.89
    insufficiency 746.6
    specified type NEC 746.89
    stenosis 746.5
  mouth 750.9
    specified type NEC 750.26
  multiple NEC 759.7
    specified type NEC 759.89
  muscle 756.9
    eye 743.9
      specified type NEC 743.69
    specified type NEC 756.89
  musculoskeletal system, except limbs 756.9
    specified type NEC 756.9

Anomaly, anomalous—*continued*
  nail 757.9
    specified type NEC 757.5
  narrowness, eyelid 743.62
  nasal sinus or septum 748.1
  neck (any part) 744.9
    specified type NEC 744.89
  nerve 742.9
    acoustic 742.9
      specified type NEC 742.8
    optic 742.9
    specified type NEC 742.8
    specified type NEC 742.8
  nervous system NEC 742.9
    brain 742.9
      specified type NEC 742.4
    specified type NEC 742.8
  neurological 742.9
  nipple 757.6
  nonteratogenic NEC 754.89
  nose, nasal (bone) (cartilage) (septum) (sinus)
    748.1
  ocular muscle 743.9
  omphalomesenteric duct 751.0
  opening, pulmonary veins 747.49
  optic
    disc 743.9
      specified type NEC 743.57
    nerve 742.9
  opticociliary vessels 743.9
  orbit (eye) 743.9
    specified type NEC 743.66
  organ
    of Corti (causing impairment of hearing)
      744.05
    or site 759.9
      specified type NEC 759.89
  origin
    both great arteries from same ventricle 745.11
    coronary artery 746.85
    innominate artery 747.69
    left coronary artery from pulmonary artery
      746.85
    pulmonary artery 747.3
    renal vessels 747.62
    subclavian artery (left) (right) 747.21
  osseous meatus (ear) 744.03
  ovary 752.0
  oviduct 752.10
  palate (hard) (soft) 750.9
    cleft (*see also* Cleft, palate) 749.00
  pancreas (duct) 751.7
  papillary muscles 746.9
  parathyroid gland 759.2
  paraurethral ducts 753.9
  parotid (gland) 750.9
  patella 755.64
  Pelger-Huët (hereditary hyposegmentation)
    288.2
  pelvic girdle 755.60
    specified type NEC 755.69
  pelvis (bony) 755.60
    complicating delivery 653.0
    rachitic 268.1
      fetal 756.4
  penis (glans) 752.69
  pericardium 746.89
  peripheral vascular system NEC 747.60
    gastrointestinal 747.61
    lower limb 747.64
    renal 747.62

Anomaly, anomalous—*continued*
    specified site NEC 747.69
    spinal 747.82
    upper limb 747.63
  Peter's 743.44
  pharynx 750.9
    branchial cleft 744.41
    specified type NEC 750.29
  Pierre Robin 756.0
  pigmentation NEC 709.00
    congenital 757.33
  pituitary (gland) 759.2
  pleural folds 748.8
  portal vein 747.40
  position tooth, teeth 524.30
    crowding 524.31
    displacement 524.30
      horizontal 524.33
      vertical 524.34
    distance
      interocclusal
        excessive 524.37
        insufficient 524.36
    excessive spacing 524.32
    rotation 524.35
    specified NEC 524.39
  preauricular sinus 744.46
  prepuce 752.9
  prostate 752.9
  pulmonary 748.60
    artery 747.3
    circulation 747.3
    specified type NEC 748.69
    valve 746.00
      atresia 746.01
      insufficiency 746.09
      specified type NEC 746.09
      stenosis 746.02
        infundibular 746.83
        subvalvular 746.83
    vein 747.40
    venous
      connection 747.49
        partial 747.42
        total 747.41
      return 747.49
        partial 747.42
        total (TAPVR) (complete)
          (subdiaphragmatic)
          (supradiaphragmatic) 747.41
  pupil 743.9
  pylorus 750.9
    hypertrophy 750.5
    stenosis 750.5
  rachitic, fetal 756.4
  radius 755.50
  rectovaginal (septum) 752.40
  rectum 751.5
  refraction 367.9
  renal 753.9
    vessel 747.62
  respiratory system 748.9
    specified type NEC 748.8
  rib 756.3
    cervical 756.2
  Rieger's 743.44
  rings, trachea 748.3
  rotation—*see also* Malrotation
    hip or thigh (*see also* Subluxation, congenital,
      hip) 754.32
  round ligament 752.9

Anomaly, anomalous—*continued*
  submaxillary gland 750.9
  superior vena cava 747.40
  talipes—*see* Talipes
  tarsus 755.67
    with complete absence of distal elements 755.31
  teeth, tooth NEC 520.9
    position 524.30
      crowding 524.31
      displacement 524.30
        horizontal 524.33
        vertical 524.34
      distance
        interocclusal
          excessive 524.37
          insufficient 524.36
      excessive spacing 524.32
      rotation 524.35
      specified NEC 524.39
    spacing 524.30
  tendon 756.9
    specified type NEC 756.89
  termination
    coronary artery 746.85
  testis 752.9
  thebesian valve 746.9
  thigh 755.60
    flexion (*see also* Subluxation, congenital, hip) 754.32
  thorax (wall) 756.3
  throat 750.9
  thumb 755.50
    supernumerary 755.01
  thymus gland 759.2
  thyroid (gland) 759.2
    cartilage 748.3
  tibia 755.60
    saber 090.5
  toe 755.66
    supernumerary 755.02
    webbed (*see also* Syndactylism, toes) 755.13
  tongue 750.10
    specified type NEC 750.19
  trachea, tracheal 748.3
    cartilage 748.3
    rings 748.3
  tragus 744.3
  transverse aortic arch 747.21
  trichromata 368.59
  trichromatopsia 368.59
  tricuspid (leaflet) (valve) 746.9
    atresia 746.1
    Ebstein's 746.2
    specified type NEC 746.89
    stenosis 746.1
  trunk 759.9
  Uhl's (hypoplasia of myocardium, right ventricle) 746.84
  ulna 755.50
  umbilicus 759.9
    artery 747.5
  union, trachea with larynx 748.3
  unspecified site 759.9
  upper extremity 755.50
    vessel 747.63
  urachus 753.7
    specified type NEC 753.7

Anomaly, anomalous—*continued*
  ureter 753.9
    obstructive 753.20
    specified type NEC 753.4
      obstructive 753.29
  urethra (valve) 753.9
    obstructive 753.6
    specified type NEC 753.8
  urinary tract or system (any part, except urachus) 753.9
    specified type NEC 753.8
    urachus 753.7
  uterus 752.3
    with only one functioning horn 752.3
    in pregnancy or childbirth 654.0
      affecting fetus or newborn 763.89
      causing obstructed labor 660.2
        affecting fetus or newborn 763.1
  uvula 750.9
  vagina 752.40
  valleculae 748.3
  valve (heart) NEC 746.9
    formation, ureter 753.29
    pulmonary 746.00
    specified type NEC 746.89
  vascular NEC (*see also* Anomaly, peripheral vascular system) 747.60
    ring 747.21
  vas deferens 752.9
  vein(s) (peripheral) NEC (*see also* Anomaly, peripheral vascular system) 747.60
    brain 747.81
    cerebral 747.81
    coronary 746.89
    great 747.40
      specified type NEC 747.49
    portal 747.40
    pulmonary 747.40
    retina 743.9
  vena cava (inferior) (superior) 747.40
  venous return (pulmonary) 747.49
    partial 747.42
    total 747.41
  ventricle, ventricular (heart) 746.9
    bands 746.9
    folds 746.9
    septa 745.4
  vertebra 756.10
  vesicourethral orifice 753.9
  vessels NEC (*see also* Anomaly, peripheral vascular system) 747.60
    optic papilla 743.9
  vitelline duct 751.0
  vitreous humor 743.9
    specified type NEC 743.51
  vulva 752.40
  wrist (joint) 755.50
Anomia 784.69
Anonychia 757.5
  acquired 703.8
Anophthalmos, anophthalmus (clinical) (congenital) (globe) 743.00
  acquired V45.78
Anopsia (altitudinal) (quadrant) 368.46
Anorchia 752.89
Anorchism, anorchidism 752.89
Anorexia 783.0
  hysterical 300.11
  nervosa 307.1

Anuria—*continued*
  due to a procedure 997.5
  following
    abortion 639.3
    ectopic or molar pregnancy 639.3
  newborn 753.3
  postrenal 593.4
  puerperal, postpartum, childbirth 669.3
  specified as due to a procedure 997.5
  sulfonamide
    correct substance properly administered 788.5
    overdose or wrong substance given or taken
      961.0
  traumatic (following crushing) 958.5
Anus, anal —*see* condition
Anusitis 569.49
Anxiety (neurosis) (reaction) (state) 300.00
  alcohol-induced 291.89
  depression 300.4
  drug-induced 292.89
  due to or associated with physical condition
    293.84
  generalized 300.02
  hysteria 300.20
  in
    acute stress reaction 308.0
    transient adjustment reaction 309.24
  panic type 300.01
  separation, abnormal 309.21
  syndrome (organic) (transient) 293.84
Aorta, aortic —*see* condition
Aortectasia 441.9
Aortitis (nonsyphilitic) 447.6
  arteriosclerotic 440.0
  calcific 447.6
  Döhle-Heller 093.1
  luetic 093.1
  rheumatic (*see also* Endocarditis, acute,
    rheumatic) 391.1
  rheumatoid—*see* Arthritis, rheumatoid
  specific 093.1
  syphilitic 093.1
    congenital 090.5
Apathetic thyroid storm (*see also*
  Thyrotoxicosis) 242.9
Apepsia 536.8
  achlorhydric 536.0
  psychogenic 306.4
Aperistalsis, esophagus 530.0
Apert's syndrome (acrocephalosyndactyly)
  755.55
Apert-Gallais syndrome (adrenogenital) 255.2
Apertognathia 524.20
Aphagia 787.2
  psychogenic 307.1
Aphakia (acquired) (bilateral) (postoperative)
  (unilateral) 379.31
  congenital 743.35
Aphalangia (congenital) 755.4
  lower limb (complete) (intercalary) (partial)
    (terminal) 755.39
    meaning all digits (complete) (partial) 755.31
    transverse 755.31
  upper limb (complete) (intercalary) (partial)
    (terminal) 755.29
    meaning all digits (complete) (partial) 755.21
    transverse 755.21

Aphasia (amnestic) (ataxic) (auditory) (Broca's)
  (choreatic) (classic) (expressive) (global)
  (ideational) (ideokinetic) (ideomotor) (jargon)
  (motor) (nominal) (receptive) (semantic)
  (sensory) (syntactic) (verbal) (visual)
  (Wernicke's) 784.3
  developmental 315.31
  syphilis, tertiary 094.89
  uremic—*see* Uremia
Aphemia 784.3
  uremic—*see* Uremia
Aphonia 784.41
  clericorum 784.49
  hysterical 300.11
  organic 784.41
  psychogenic 306.1
Aphthae, aphthous —*see also* condition
  Bednar's 528.2
  cachectic 529.0
  epizootic 078.4
  fever 078.4
  oral 528.2
  stomatitis 528.2
  thrush 112.0
  ulcer (oral) (recurrent) 528.2
    genital organ(s) NEC
      female 629.89
      male 608.89
    larynx 478.79
Apical —*see* condition
Apical ballooning syndrome 429.83
Aplasia —*see also* Agenesis
  alveolar process (acquired) 525.8
    congenital 750.26
  aorta (congenital) 747.22
  aortic valve (congenital) 746.89
  axialis extracorticalis (congenital) 330.0
  bone marrow (myeloid) 284.9
    acquired (secondary) 284.8
    congenital 284.01
    idiopathic 284.9
  brain 740.0
    specified part 742.2
  breast 757.6
  bronchus 748.3
  cementum 520.4
  cerebellar 742.2
  congenital (pure) red cell 284.01
  corpus callosum 742.2
  erythrocyte 284.8
    congenital 284.01
  extracortical axial 330.0
  eye (congenital) 743.00
  fovea centralis (congenital) 743.55
  germinal (cell) 606.0
  iris 743.45
  labyrinth, membranous 744.05
  limb (congenital) 755.4
    lower NEC 755.30
    upper NEC 755.20
  lung (bilateral) (congenital) (unilateral) 748.5
  nervous system NEC 742.8
  nuclear 742.8
  ovary 752.0
  Pelizaeus-Merzbacher 330.0
  prostate (congenital) 752.89

Aplasia—*continued*
red cell (with thymoma) 284.8
acquired (secondary) 284.8
congenital 284.01
hereditary 284.01
of infants 284.01
primary 284.01
pure 284.01
round ligament (congenital) 752.89
salivary gland 750.21
skin (congenital) 757.39
spinal cord 742.59
spleen 759.0
testis (congenital) 752.89
thymic, with immunodeficiency 279.2
thyroid 243
uterus 752.3
ventral horn cell 742.59
Apleuria 756.3
Apnea, apneic (spells) 786.03
newborn, neonatorum 770.81
essential 770.81
obstructive 770.82
primary 770.81
sleep 770.81
specified NEC 770.82
psychogenic 306.1
sleep, unspecified 780.57
with
hypersomnia, unspecified 780.53
hyposomnia, unspecified 780.51
insomnia, unspecified 780.51
sleep disturbance 780.57
central, in conditions classified elsewhere 327.27
obstructive (adult) (pediatric) 327.23
organic 327.20
other 327.29
primary central 327.21
Apneumatosis newborn 770.4
Apodia 755.31
Apophysitis (bone) (*see also* Osteochondrosis) 732.9
calcaneus 732.5
juvenile 732.6
Apoplectiform convulsions (*see also* Disease, cerebrovascular, acute) 436
Apoplexia, apoplexy, apoplectic (*see also* Disease, cerebrovascular, acute) 436
abdominal 569.89
adrenal 036.3
attack 436
basilar (*see also* Disease, cerebrovascular, acute) 436
brain (*see also* Disease, cerebrovascular, acute) 436
bulbar (*see also* Disease, cerebrovascular, acute) 436
capillary (*see also* Disease, cerebrovascular, acute) 436
cardiac (*see also* Infarct, myocardium) 410.9
cerebral (*see also* Disease, cerebrovascular, acute) 436
chorea (*see also* Disease, cerebrovascular, acute) 436
congestive (*see also* Disease, cerebrovascular, acute) 436
newborn 767.4
embolic (*see also* Embolism, brain) 434.1
fetus 767.0
fit (*see also* Disease, cerebrovascular, acute) 436

Apoplexia, apoplexy, apoplectic—*continued*
healed or old V12.59
heart (auricle) (ventricle) (*see also* Infarct, myocardium) 410.9
heat 992.0
hemiplegia (*see also* Disease, cerebrovascular, acute) 436
hemorrhagic (stroke) (*see also* Hemorrhage, brain) 432.9
ingravescent (*see also* Disease, cerebrovascular, acute) 436
late effect—*see* Late effect(s) (of) cerebrovascular disease
lung—*see* Embolism, pulmonary
meninges, hemorrhagic (*see also* Hemorrhage, subarachnoid) 430
neonatorum 767.0
newborn 767.0
pancreatitis 577.0
placenta 641.2
progressive (*see also* Disease, cerebrovascular, acute) 436
pulmonary (artery) (vein)—*see* Embolism, pulmonary
sanguineous (*see also* Disease, cerebrovascular, acute) 436
seizure (*see also* Disease, cerebrovascular, acute) 436
serous (*see also* Disease, cerebrovascular, acute) 436
spleen 289.59
stroke (*see also* Disease, cerebrovascular, acute) 436
thrombotic (*see also* Thrombosis, brain) 434.0
uremic—*see* Uremia
uteroplacental 641.2
Appendage
fallopian tube (cyst of Morgagni) 752.11
intestine (epiploic) 751.5
preauricular 744.1
testicular (organ of Morgagni) 752.89
Appendicitis 541
with
perforation, peritonitis (generalized), or rupture 540.0
with peritoneal abscess 540.1
peritoneal abscess 540.1
acute (catarrhal) (fulminating) (gangrenous) (inflammatory) (obstructive) (retrocecal) (suppurative) 540.9
with
perforation, peritonitis, or rupture 540.0
with peritoneal abscess 540.1
peritoneal abscess 540.1
amebic 006.8
chronic (recurrent) 542
exacerbation—*see* Appendicitis, acute
fulminating—*see* Appendicitis, acute
gangrenous—*see* Appendicitis, acute
healed (obliterative) 542
interval 542
neurogenic 542
obstructive 542
pneumococcal 541
recurrent 542
relapsing 542
retrocecal 541
subacute (adhesive) 542
subsiding 542
suppurative—*see* Appendicitis, acute
tuberculous (*see also* Tuberculosis) 014.8

Arrhenoblastoma (M8630.1)
  benign (M8630/0)
    specified site—*see* Neoplasm, by site, benign
    unspecified site
      female 220
      male 222.0
  malignant (M8630/3)
    specified site— *see* Neoplasm, by site,
      malignant
    unspecified site
      female 183.0
      male 186.9
  specified site—*see* Neoplasm, by site, uncertain
    behavior
  unspecified site
    female 236.2
    male 236.4
Arrhinencephaly 742.2
  due to
    trisomy 13 (13-15) 758.1
    trisomy 18 (16-18) 758.2
Arrhythmia (auricle) (cardiac) (cordis) (gallop
    rhythm) (juvenile) (nodal) (reflex) (sinus)
    (supraventricular) (transitory) (ventricle) 427.9
  bigeminal rhythm 427.89
  block 426.9
  bradycardia 427.89
  contractions, premature 427.60
  coronary sinus 427.89
  ectopic 427.89
  extrasystolic 427.60
  postoperative 997.1
  psychogenic 306.2
  vagal 780.2
Arrillaga-Ayerza syndrome (pulmonary artery
    sclerosis with pulmonary hypertension) 416.0
Arsenical
  dermatitis 692.4
  keratosis 692.4
  pigmentation 985.1
    from drug or medicinal agent
      correct substance properly administered
        709.09
      overdose or wrong substance given or taken
        961.1
Arsenism 985.1
  from drug or medicinal agent
    correct substance properly administered 692.4
    overdose or wrong substance given or taken
      961.1
Arterial —*see* condition
Arteriectasis 447.8
Arteriofibrosis —*see* Arteriosclerosis
Arteriolar sclerosis —*see* Arteriosclerosis
Arteriolith —*see* Arteriosclerosis
Arteriolitis 447.6
  necrotizing, kidney 447.5
  renal—*see* Hypertension, kidney
Arteriolosclerosis —*see* Arteriosclerosis
Arterionephrosclerosis (*see also* Hypertension,
    kidney) 403.90
Arteriopathy 447.9
Arteriosclerosis, arteriosclerotic (artery)
    (deformans) (diffuse) (disease) (endarteritis)
    (general) (obliterans) (obliterative) (occlusive)
    (senile) (with calcification) 440.9
  with
    gangrene 440.24
    psychosis (*see also* Psychosis, arteriosclerotic)
      290.40
    ulceration 440.23

Arteriosclerosis, arteriosclerotic—*continued*
  aorta 440.0
  arteries of extremities NEC — *see*
    Arteriosclerosis, extremities
  basilar (artery) (*see also* Occlusion, artery,
    basilar) 433.0
  brain 437.0
  bypass graft
    coronary artery 414.05
      autologous artery (gastroepiploic) (internal
        mammary) 414.04
      autologous vein 414.02
      nonautologous biological 414.03
      of transplanted heart 414.07
    extremity 440.30
      autologous vein 440.31
      nonautologous biological 440.32
  cardiac — *see* Arteriosclerosis, coronary
  cardiopathy — *see* Arteriosclerosis, coronary
  cardiorenal (*see* also Hypertension, cardiorenal)
    404.90
  cardiovascular (*see also* Disease,
    cardiovascular) 429.2
  carotid (artery) (common) (internal) (*see also*
    Occlusion, artery, carotid) 433.1
  central nervous system 437.0
  cerebral 437.0
    late effect—*see* Late effect(s) (of)
      cerebrovascular disease
  cerebrospinal 437.0
  cerebrovascular 437.0
  coronary (artery) 414.00
    graft—*see* Arteriosclerosis, bypass graft
    native artery 414.01
    of transplanted heart 414.06
    of transplanted heart 414.06
  extremities (native artery) 440.20
    bypass graft 440.30
      autologous vein 440.31
      nonautologous biological 440.32
    claudication (intermittent) 440.21
    and
      gangrene 440.24
      rest pain 440.22
      and
        gangrene 440.24
        ulceration 440.23
          and gangrene 440.24
      ulceration 440.23
        and gangrene 440.24
    gangrene 440.24
    rest pain 440.22
    and
      gangrene 440.24
      ulceration 440.23
        and gangrene 440.24
    specified site NEC 440.29
    ulceration 440.23
      and gangrene 440.24
  heart (disease) — *see also* Arteriosclerosis,
    coronary
    valve 424.99
      aortic 424.1
      mitral 424.0
      pulmonary 424.3
      tricuspid 424.2
  kidney (*see also* Hypertension, kidney) 403.90
  labyrinth, labyrinthine 388.00
  medial NEC 440.20
  mesentery (artery) 557.1
  Mönckeberg's 440.20

Arteriosclerosis, arteriosclerotic—*continued*
  myocarditis 429.0
  nephrosclerosis (*see also* Hypertension, kidney) 403.90
  peripheral (of extremities) *see* Arteriosclerosis, extremities
  precerebral 433.9
    specified artery NEC 433.8
  pulmonary (idiopathic) 416.0
  renal (*see also* Hypertension, kidney) 403.90
    arterioles (*see also* Hypertension, kidney) 403.90
    artery 440.1
  retinal (vascular) 440.8 *[362.13]*
  specified artery NEC 440.8
    with gangrene 440.8 *[785.4]*
  spinal (cord) 437.0
  vertebral (artery) (*see also* Occlusion, artery, vertebral) 433.2
Arteriospasm 443.9
Arteriovenous —*see* condition
Arteritis 447.6
  allergic (*see also* Angiitis, hypersensitivity) 446.20
  aorta (nonsyphilitic) 447.6
    syphilitic 093.1
  aortic arch 446.7
  brachiocephalica 446.7
  brain 437.4
    syphilitic 094.89
  branchial 446.7
  cerebral 437.4
    late effect—*see* Late effect(s) (of) cerebrovascular disease
    syphilitic 094.89
  coronary (artery) —*see also* Arteriosclerosis, coronary
    rheumatic 391.9
      chronic 398.99
    syphilitic 093.89
  cranial (left) (right) 446.5
  deformans—*see* Arteriosclerosis
  giant cell 446.5
  necrosing or necrotizing 446.0
  nodosa 446.0
  obliterans—*see also* Arteriosclerosis
    subclaviocarotica 446.7
  pulmonary 417.8
  retina 362.18
  rheumatic—*see* Fever, rheumatic
  senile—*see* Arteriosclerosis
  suppurative 447.2
  syphilitic (general) 093.89
    brain 094.89
    coronary 093.89
    spinal 094.89
  temporal 446.5
  young female, syndrome 446.7
Artery, arterial —*see* condition
Arthralgia (*see also* Pain, joint) 719.4
  allergic (*see also* Pain, joint) 719.4
  in caisson disease 993.3
  psychogenic 307.89
  rubella 056.71
  Salmonella 003.23
  temporomandibular joint 524.62

Arthritis, arthritic (acute) (chronic) (subacute) 716.9

Note—Use the following fifth-digit subclassification with categories 711-712, 715-716:

0 *site unspecified*
1 *shoulder region*
2 *upper arm*
3 *forearm*
4 *hand*
5 *pelvic region and thigh*
6 *lower leg*
7 *ankle and foot*
8 *other specified sites*
9 *multiple sites*

---

  allergic 716.2
  ankylosing (crippling) (spine) 720.0
    sites other than spine 716.9
  atrophic 714.0
    spine 720.9
  back (*see also* Arthritis, spine) 721.90
  Bechterew's (ankylosing spondylitis) 720.0
  blennorrhagic 098.50
  cervical, cervicodorsal (*see also* Spondylosis, cervical) 721.0
  Charcot's 094.0 *[713.5]*
    diabetic 250.6 *[713.5]*
    syringomyelic 336.0 *[713.5]*
    tabetic 094.0 *[713.5]*
  chylous (*see also* Filariasis) 125.9 *[711.7]*
  climacteric NEC 716.3
  coccyx 721.8
  cricoarytenoid 478.79
  crystal (-induced)—*see* Arthritis, due to crystals
  deformans (*see also* Osteoarthrosis) 715.9
    spine 721.90
      with myelopathy 721.91
  degenerative (*see also* Osteoarthrosis) 715.9
    idiopathic 715.09
    polyarticular 715.09
    spine 721.90
      with myelopathy 721.91
  dermatoarthritis, lipoid 272.8 *[713.0]*
  due to or associated with
    acromegaly 253.0 *[713.0]*
    actinomycosis 039.8 *[711.4]*
    amyloidosis 277.39 *[713.7]*
    bacterial disease NEC 040.89 *[711.4]*
    Behçet's syndrome 136.1 *[711.2]*
    blastomycosis 116.0 *[711.6]*
    brucellosis (*see also* Brucellosis) 023.9 *[711.4]*
    caisson disease 993.3
    coccidioidomycosis 114.3 *[711.6]*
    coliform (Escherichia coli) 711.0
    colitis, ulcerative (*see also* Colitis, ulcerative) 556.9 *[713.1]*
    cowpox 051.0 *[711.5]*
    crystals (*see also* Gout)
      dicalcium phosphate 275.49 *[712.1]*
      pyrophosphate 275.49 *[712.2]*
      specified NEC 275.49 *[712.8]*
    dermatoarthritis, lipoid 272.8 *[713.0]*
    dermatological disorder NEC 709.9 *[713.3]*
    diabetes 250.6 *[713.5]*
    diphtheria 032.89 *[711.4]*
    dracontiasis 125.7 *[711.7]*
    dysentery 009.0 *[711.3]*
    endocrine disorder NEC 259.9 *[713.0]*

Arthritis, arthritic—*continued*
  enteritis NEC 009.1 *[711.3]*
    infectious (*see also* Enteritis, infectious)
      009.0 *[711.3]*
      specified organism NEC 008.8 *[711.3]*
    regional (*see also* Enteritis, regional) 555.9
      [713.1]
    specified organism NEC 008.8 *[711.3]*
  epiphyseal slip, nontraumatic (old) 716.8
  erysipelas 035 *[711.4]*
  erythema
    epidemic 026.1
    multiforme 695.1 *[713.3]*
    nodosum 695.2 *[713.3]*
  Escherichia coli 711.0
  filariasis NEC 125.9 *[711.7]*
  gastrointestinal condition NEC 569.9 *[713.1]*
  glanders 024 *[711.4]*
  Gonococcus 098.50
  gout 274.0
  H. influenzae 711.0
  helminthiasis NEC 128.9 *[711.7]*
  hematological disorder NEC 289.9 *[713.2]*
  hemochromatosis 275.0 *[713.0]*
  hemoglobinopathy NEC (*see also* Disease,
    hemoglobin) 282.7 *[713.2]*
  hemophilia (*see also* Hemophilia) 286.0
    [713.2]
  Hemophilus influenzae (H. influenzae) 711.0
  Henoch (-Schönlein) purpura 287.0 *[713.6]*
  histoplasmosis NEC (*see also* Histoplasmosis)
    115.99 *[711.6]*
  hyperparathyroidism 252.00 *[713.0]*
  hypersensitivity reaction NEC 995.3 *[713.6]*
  hypogammaglobulinemia (*see also*
    Hypogammaglobulinemia) 279.00 *[713.0]*
  hypothyroidism NEC 244.9 *[713.0]*
  infection (*see also* Arthritis, infectious) 711.9
  infectious disease NEC 136.9 *[711.8]*
  leprosy (*see also* Leprosy) 030.9 *[711.4]*
  leukemia NEC (M9800/3) 208.9 *[713.2]*
  lipoid dermatoarthritis 272.8 *[713.0]*
  Lyme disease 088.81 *[711.8]*
  meaning Osteoarthritis—*see* Osteoarthrosis
  Mediterranean fever, familial 277.31 *[713.7]*
  meningococcal infection 036.82
  metabolic disorder NEC 277.9 *[713.0]*
  multiple myelomatosis (M9730/3) 203.0
    [713.2]
  mumps 072.79 *[711.5]*
  mycobacteria 031.8 *[711.4]*
  mycosis NEC 117.9 *[711.6]*
  neurological disorder NEC 349.9 *[713.5]*
  ochronosis 270.2 *[713.0]*
  O'Nyong Nyong 066.3 *[711.5]*
  parasitic disease NEC 136.9 *[711.8]*
  paratyphoid fever (*see also* Fever,
    paratyphoid) 002.9 *[711.3]*
  Pneumococcus 711.0
  poliomyelitis (*see also* Poliomyelitis) 045.9
    [711.5]
  Pseudomonas 711.0
  psoriasis 696.0
  pyogenic organism (E. coli) (H. influenzae)
    (Pseudomonas) (Streptococcus) 711.0
  rat-bite fever 026.1 *[711.4]*
  regional enteritis (*see also* Enteritis, regional)
    555.9 *[713.1]*
  Reiter's disease 099.3 *[711.1]*
  respiratory disorder NEC 519.9 *[713.4]*

Arthritis, arthritic—*continued*
  reticulosis, malignant (M9720/3) 202.3
    [713.2]
  rubella 056.71
  salmonellosis 003.23
  sarcoidosis 135 *[713.7]*
  serum sickness 999.5 *[713.6]*
  Staphylococcus 711.0
  Streptococcus 711.0
  syphilis (*see also* Syphilis) 094.0 *[711.4]*
  syringomyelia 336.0 *[713.5]*
  thalassemia 282.49 *[713.2]*
  tuberculosis (*see also* Tuberculosis, arthritis)
    015.9 *[711.4]*
  typhoid fever 002.0 *[711.3]*
  ulcerative colitis (*see also* Colitis, ulcerative)
    556.9 *[713.1]*
  urethritis
    nongonococcal (*see also* Urethritis,
      nongonococcal) 099.40 *[711.1]*
    nonspecific (*see also* Urethritis,
      nongonococcal) 099.40 *[711.1]*
    Reiter's 099.3 *[711.1]*
  viral disease NEC 079.99 *[711.5]*
 erythema epidemic 026.1
 gonococcal 098.50
 gouty (acute) 274.0
 hypertrophic (*see also* Osteoarthrosis) 715.9
  spine 721.90
    with myelopathy 721.91
 idiopathic, blennorrheal 099.3
 in caisson disease 993.3 *[713.8]*
 infectious or infective (acute) (chronic)
    (subacute) NEC 711.9
  nonpyogenic 711.9
  spine 720.9
 inflammatory NEC 714.9
 juvenile rheumatoid (chronic) (polyarticular)
    714.30
  acute 714.31
  monoarticular 714.33
  pauciarticular 714.32
 lumbar (*see also* Spondylosis, lumbar) 721.3
 meningococcal 036.82
 menopausal NEC 716.3
 migratory—*see* Fever, rheumatic
 neuropathic (Charcot's) 094.0 *[713.5]*
  diabetic 250.6 *[713.5]*
  nonsyphilitic NEC 349.9 *[713.5]*
  syringomyelic 336.0 *[713.5]*
  tabetic 094.0 *[713.5]*
 nodosa (*see also* Osteoarthrosis) 715.9
  spine 721.90
    with myelopathy 721.91
 nonpyogenic NEC 716.9
  spine 721.90
    with myelopathy 721.91
 ochronotic 270.2 *[713.0]*
 palindromic (*see also* Rheumatism,
    palindromic) 719.3
 pneumococcal 711.0
 postdysenteric 009.0 *[711.3]*
 postrheumatic, chronic (Jaccoud's) 714.4
 primary progressive 714.0
  spine 720.9
 proliferative 714.0
  spine 720.0
 psoriatic 696.0
 purulent 711.0
 pyogenic or pyemic 711.0

Arthritis, arthritic—*continued*
  rheumatic 714.0
    acute or subacute—*see* Fever, rheumatic
    chronic 714.0
    spine 720.9
  rheumatoid (nodular) 714.0
    with
      splenoadenomegaly and leukopenia 714.1
      visceral or systemic involvement 714.2
    aortitis 714.89
    carditis 714.2
    heart disease 714.2
    juvenile (chronic) (polyarticular) 714.30
      acute 714.31
        monoarticular 714.33
        pauciarticular 714.32
      spine 720.0
  rubella 056.71
  sacral, sacroiliac, sacrococcygeal (*see also*
    Spondylosis, sacral) 721.3
  scorbutic 267
  senile or senescent (*see also* Osteoarthrosis)
    715.9
    spine 721.90
      with myelopathy 721.91
  septic 711.0
  serum (nontherapeutic) (therapeutic) 999.5
    [713.6]
  specified form NEC 716.8
  spine 721.90
    with myelopathy 721.91
    atrophic 720.9
    degenerative 721.90
      with myelopathy 721.91
    hypertrophic (with deformity) 721.90
      with myelopathy 721.91
    infectious or infective NEC 720.9
    Marie-Strümpell 720.0
    nonpyogenic 721.90
      with myelopathy 721.91
    pyogenic 720.9
    rheumatoid 720.0
    traumatic (old) 721.7
    tuberculous (*see also* Tuberculosis) 015.0
      [720.81]
  staphylococcal 711.0
  streptococcal 711.0
  suppurative 711.0
  syphilitic 094.0 *[713.5]*
    congenital 090.49 *[713.5]*
  syphilitica deformans (Charcot) 094.0 *[713.5]*
  temporomandibular joint 524.69
  thoracic (*see also* Spondylosis, thoracic) 721.2
  toxic of menopause 716.3
  transient 716.4
  traumatic (chronic) (old) (post) 716.1
    current injury—*see* nature of injury
  tuberculous (*see also* Tuberculosis, arthritis)
    015.9 *[711.4]*
  urethritica 099.3 *[711.1]*
  urica, uratic 274.0
  venereal 099.3 *[711.1]*
  vertebral (*see also* Arthritis, spine) 721.90
  villous 716.8
  von Bechterew's 720.0
Arthrocele (*see also* Effusion, joint) 719.0
Arthrochondritis —*see* Arthritis
Arthrodesis status V45.4
Arthrodynia (*see also* Pain, joint) 719.4
  psychogenic 307.89

Arthrodysplasia 755.9
Arthrofibrosis, joint (*see also* Ankylosis) 718.5
Arthrogryposis 728.3
  multiplex, congenita 754.89
Arthrokatadysis 715.35
Arthrolithiasis 274.0
Arthro-onychodysplasia 756.89
Arthro-osteo-onychodysplasia 756.89
Arthropathy (*see also* Arthritis) 716.9

> *Note—Use the following fifth-digit*
> *subclassification with categories 711-712, 716:*
>
> *0 site unspecified*
> *1 shoulder region*
> *2 upper arm*
> *3 forearm*
> *4 hand*
> *5 pelvic region and thigh*
> *6 lower leg*
> *7 ankle and foot*
> *8 other specified sites*
> *9 multiple sites*

  Behçet's 136.1 *[711.2]*
  Charcot's 094.0 *[713.5]*
    diabetic 250.6 *[713.5]*
    syringomyelic 336.0 *[713.5]*
    tabetic 094.0 *[713.5]*
  crystal (-induced)—*see* Arthritis, due to crystals
  gouty 274.0
  neurogenic, neuropathic (Charcot's) (tabetic)
    094.0 *[713.5]*
    diabetic 250.6 *[713.5]*
    nonsyphilitic NEC 349.9 *[713.5]*
    syringomyelic 336.0 *[713.5]*
  postdysenteric NEC 009.0 *[711.3]*
  postrheumatic, chronic (Jaccoud's) 714.4
  psoriatic 696.0
  pulmonary 731.2
  specified NEC 716.8
  syringomyelia 336.0 *[713.5]*
  tabes dorsalis 094.0 *[713.5]*
  tabetic 094.0 *[713.5]*
  transient 716.4
  traumatic 716.1
  uric acid 274.0
Arthrophyte (*see also* Loose, body, joint) 718.1
Arthrophytis 719.80
  ankle 719.87
  elbow 719.82
  foot 719.87
  hand 719.84
  hip 719.85
  knee 719.86
  multiple sites 719.89
  pelvic region 719.85
  shoulder (region) 719.81
  specified site NEC 719.88
  wrist 719.83
Arthropyosis (*see also* Arthritis, pyogenic) 711.0
Arthroscopic surgical procedure converted to
  open procedure V64.43
Arthrosis (deformans) (degenerative) (*see also*
  Osteoarthrosis) 715.9
  Charcot's 094.0 *[713.5]*
  polyarticular 715.09
  spine (*see also* Spondylosis) 721.90

Arthus' phenomenon 995.21
　due to
　　correct substance properly administered
　　　995.21
　　overdose or wrong substance given or taken
　　　977.9
　　　specified drug—*see* Table of drugs and
　　　　chemicals
　serum 999.5
Articular —*see also* condition
　disc disorder (reducing or non-reducing) 524.63
　spondylolisthesis 756.12
Articulation
　anterior 524.27
　posterior 524.27
　reverse 524.27
Artificial
　device (prosthetic)—*see* Fitting, device
　insemination V26.1
　menopause (states) (symptoms) (syndrome)
　　627.4
　opening status (functioning) (without
　　complication) V44.9
　　anus (colostomy) V44.3
　　colostomy V44.3
　　cystostomy V44.50
　　　appendico-vesicostomy V44.52
　　　cutaneous-vesicostomy V44.51
　　　specified type NEC V44.59
　　enterostomy V44.4
　　gastrostomy V44.1
　　ileostomy V44.2
　　intestinal tract NEC V44.4
　　jejunostomy V44.4
　　nephrostomy V44.6
　　specified site NEC V44.8
　　tracheostomy V44.0
　　ureterostomy V44.6
　　urethrostomy V44.6
　　urinary tract NEC V44.6
　　vagina V44.7
　vagina status V44.7
ARV (disease) (illness) (infection)—*see* Human
　immunodeficiency virus (disease) (illness)
　(infection)
Arytenoid —*see* condition
Asbestosis (occupational) 501
Asboe-Hansen's disease (incontinentia pigmenti)
　757.33
Ascariasis (intestinal) (lung) 127.0
Ascaridiasis 127.0
Ascaridosis 127.0
Ascaris 127.0
　lumbricoides (infestation) 127.0
　pneumonia 127.0
Ascending —*see* condition
ASC-H (atypical squamous cells cannot exclude
　high grade squamous intraepithelial lesion)
　795.02
Aschoff's bodies (*see also* Myocarditis,
　rheumatic) 398.0
Ascites 789.5
　abdominal NEC 789.5
　cancerous (M8000/6) 197.6
　cardiac 428.0
　chylous (nonfilarial) 457.8
　　filarial (*see also* Infestation, filarial) 125.9
　congenital 778.0
　due to S. japonicum 120.2
　fetal, causing fetopelvic disproportion 653.7
　heart 428.0

Ascites—*continued*
　joint (*see also* Effusion, joint) 719.0
　malignant (M8000/6) 197.6
　pseudochylous 789.5
　syphilitic 095.2
　tuberculous (*see also* Tuberculosis) 014.0
Ascorbic acid (vitamin C) deficiency (scurvy)
　267
ASC-US (atypical squamous cells of
　undetermined significance) 795.01
ASCVD (arteriosclerotic cardiovascular disease)
　429.2
Aseptic —*see* condition
Asherman's syndrome 621.5
Asialia 527.7
Asiatic cholera (*see also* Cholera) 001.9
Asocial personality or trends 301.7
Asomatognosia 781.8
Aspergillosis 117.3
　with pneumonia 117.3 *[484.6]*
　allergic bronchopulmonary 518.6
　nonsyphilitic NEC 117.3
Aspergillus (flavus) (fumigatus) (infection)
　(terreus) 117.3
Aspermatogenesis 606.0
Aspermia (testis) 606.0
Asphyxia, asphyxiation (by) 799.01
　antenatal—*see* Distress, fetal
　bedclothes 994.7
　birth (*see also* Asphyxia, newborn) 768.9
　bunny bag 994.7
　carbon monoxide 986
　caul (*see also* Asphyxia, newborn) 768.9
　cave-in 994.7
　　crushing—*see* Injury, internal, intrathoracic
　　　organs
　constriction 994.7
　crushing—*see* Injury, internal, intrathoracic
　　organs
　drowning 994.1
　fetal, affecting newborn 768.9
　food or foreign body (in larynx) 933.1
　　bronchioles 934.8
　　bronchus (main) 934.1
　　lung 934.8
　　nasopharynx 933.0
　　nose, nasal passages 932
　　pharynx 933.0
　　respiratory tract 934.9
　　　specified part NEC 934.8
　　throat 933.0
　　trachea 934.0
　gas, fumes, or vapor NEC 987.9
　　specified—*see* Table of drugs and chemicals
　gravitational changes 994.7
　hanging 994.7
　inhalation—*see* Inhalation
　intrauterine
　　fetal death (before onset of labor) 768.0
　　　during labor 768.1
　　liveborn infant—*see* Distress, fetal, liveborn
　　　infant
　local 443.0
　mechanical 994.7
　　during birth (*see also* Distress, fetal) 768.9
　mucus 933.1
　　bronchus (main) 934.1
　　larynx 933.1
　　lung 934.8
　　nasal passages 932
　　newborn 770.18

Asthma, asthmatic (bronchial) (catarrh)
(spasmodic) 493.9

> *Note—The following fifth digit*
> *subclassification is for use with codes*
> *493.0-493.2, 493.9:*
>
> *0 unspecified*
> *1 with status asthmaticus*
> *2 with (acute) exacerbation*

with
  chronic obstructive pulmonary disease
    (COPD) 493.2
  hay fever 493.0
  rhinitis, allergic 493.0
allergic 493.9
  stated cause (external allergen) 493.0
atopic 493.0
cardiac (*see also* Failure, ventricular, left) 428.1
cardiobronchial (*see also* Failure, ventricular,
  left) 428.1
cardiorenal (*see also* Hypertension, cardiorenal)
  404.90
childhood 493.0
colliers' 500
cough variant 493.82
croup 493.9
detergent 507.8
due to
  detergent 507.8
  inhalation of fumes 506.3
  internal immunological process 493.0
endogenous (intrinsic) 493.1
eosinophilic 518.3
exercise induced bronchospasm 493.81
exogenous (cosmetics) (dander or dust) (drugs)
  (dust) (feathers) (food) (hay) (platinum)
  (pollen) 493.0
extrinsic 493.0
grinders' 502
hay 493.0
heart (*see also* Failure, ventricular, left) 428.1
IgE 493.0
infective 493.1
intrinsic 493.1
Kopp's 254.8
late-onset 493.1
meat-wrappers' 506.9
Millar's (laryngismus stridulus) 478.75
millstone makers' 502
miners' 500
Monday morning 504
New Orleans (epidemic) 493.0
platinum 493.0
pneumoconiotic (occupational) NEC 505
potters' 502
psychogenic 316 *[493.9]*
pulmonary eosinophilic 518.3
red cedar 495.8
Rostan's (*see also* Failure, ventricular, left)
  428.1
sandblasters' 502
sequoiosis 495.8
stonemasons' 502
thymic 254.8
tuberculous (*see also* Tuberculosis, pulmonary)
  011.9
Wichmann's (laryngismus stridulus) 478.75
wood 495.8
Astigmatism (compound) (congenital) 367.20
irregular 367.22
regular 367.21

Astroblastoma (M9430/3)
nose 748.1
specified site—*see* Neoplasm, by site,
  malignant
unspecified site 191.9
Astrocytoma (cystic) (M9400/3)
anaplastic type (M9401/3)
  specified site—*see* Neoplasm, by site,
    malignant
  unspecified site 191.9
fibrillary (M9420/3)
  specified site—*see* Neoplasm, by site,
    malignant
  unspecified site 191.9
fibrous (M9420/3)
  specified site—*see* Neoplasm, by site,
    malignant
  unspecified site 191.9
gemistocytic (M9411/3)
  specified site—*see* Neoplasm, by site,
    malignant
  unspecified site 191.9
juvenile (M9421/3)
  specified site—*see* Neoplasm, by site,
    malignant
  unspecified site 191.9
nose 748.1
pilocytic (M9421/3)
  specified site—*see* Neoplasm, by site,
    malignant
  unspecified site 191.9
piloid (M9421/3)
  specified site—*see* Neoplasm, by site, malignant
  unspecified site 191.9
protoplasmic (M9410/3)
  specified site—*see* Neoplasm, by site,
    malignant
  unspecified site 191.9
specified site—*see* Neoplasm, by site, malignant
subependymal (M9383/1) 237.5
  giant cell (M9384/1) 237.5
unspecified site 191.9
Astroglioma (M9400/3)
nose 748.1
specified site—*see* Neoplasm, by site, malignant
unspecified site 191.9
Asymbolia 784.60
Asymmetrical breathing 786.09
Asymmetry —*see also* Distortion
chest 786.9
face 754.0
jaw NEC 524.12
  maxillary 524.11
pelvis with disproportion 653.0
  affecting fetus or newborn 763.1
  causing obstructed labor 660.1
    affecting fetus or newborn 763.1
Asynergia 781.3
Asynergy 781.3
ventricular 429.89
Asystole (heart) (*see also* Arrest, cardiac) 427.5
At risk for falling V15.88
Ataxia, ataxy, ataxic 781.3
acute 781.3
brain 331.89
cerebellar 334.3
  hereditary (Marie's) 334.2
  in
    alcoholism 303.9 *[334.4]*
    myxedema (*see also* Myxedema) 244.9
      [334.4]

Atresia, atretic—*continued*
  artery NEC (*see also* Atresia, blood vessel)
    747.60
    cerebral 747.81
    coronary 746.85
    eye 743.58
    pulmonary 747.3
    umbilical 747.5
  auditory canal (external) 744.02
  bile, biliary duct (common) or passage 751.61
    acquired (*see also* Obstruction, biliary) 576.2
  bladder (neck) 753.6
  blood vessel (peripheral) NEC 747.60
    cerebral 747.81
    gastrointestinal 747.61
    lower limb 747.64
    pulmonary artery 747.3
    renal 747.62
    spinal 747.82
    upper limb 747.63
  bronchus 748.3
  canal, ear 744.02
  cardiac
    valve 746.89
      aortic 746.89
      mitral 746.89
      pulmonary 746.01
      tricuspid 746.1
  cecum 751.2
  cervix (acquired) 622.4
    congenital 752.49
    in pregnancy or childbirth 654.6
      affecting fetus or newborn 763.89
      causing obstructed labor 660.2
        affecting fetus or newborn 763.1
  choana 748.0
  colon 751.2
  cystic duct 751.61
    acquired 575.8
      with obstruction (*see also* Obstruction,
        gallbladder) 575.2
  digestive organs NEC 751.8
  duodenum 751.1
  ear canal 744.02
  ejaculatory duct 752.89
  epiglottis 748.3
  esophagus 750.3
  Eustachian tube 744.24
  fallopian tube (acquired) 628.2
    congenital 752.19
  follicular cyst 620.0
  foramen of
    Luschka 742.3
      with spina bifida (*see also* Spina bifida) 741.0
    Magendie 742.3
      with spina bifida (*see also* Spina bifida)
        741.0
  gallbladder 751.69
  genital organ
    external
      female 752.49
      male NEC 752.89
        penis 752.69
    internal
      female 752.89
      male 752.89
  glottis 748.3
  gullet 750.3
  heart
    valve NEC 746.89
      aortic 746.89

Atresia, atretic—*continued*
    mitral 746.89
    pulmonary 746.01
    tricuspid 746.1
  hymen 752.42
    acquired 623.3
    postinfective 623.3
  ileum 751.1
  intestine (small) 751.1
    large 751.2
  iris, filtration angle (*see also* Buphthalmia)
    743.20
  jejunum 751.1
  kidney 753.3
  lacrimal, apparatus 743.65
    acquired—*see* Stenosis, lacrimal
  larynx 748.3
  ligament, broad 752.19
  lung 748.5
  meatus urinarius 753.6
  mitral valve 746.89
    with atresia or hypoplasia of aortic orifice or
      valve, with hypoplasia of ascending aorta
      and defective development of left ventricle
      746.7
  nares (anterior) (posterior) 748.0
  nasolacrimal duct 743.65
  nasopharynx 748.8
  nose, nostril 748.0
    acquired 738.0
  organ or site NEC—*see* Anomaly, specified
    type NEC
  osseous meatus (ear) 744.03
  oviduct (acquired) 628.2
    congenital 752.19
  parotid duct 750.23
    acquired 527.8
  pulmonary (artery) 747.3
    valve 746.01
    vein 747.49
  pulmonic 746.01
  pupil 743.46
  rectum 751.2
  salivary duct or gland 750.23
    acquired 527.8
  sublingual duct 750.23
    acquired 527.8
  submaxillary duct or gland 750.23
    acquired 527.8
  trachea 748.3
  tricuspid valve 746.1
  ureter 753.29
  ureteropelvic junction 753.21
  ureterovesical orifice 753.22
  urethra (valvular) 753.6
  urinary tract NEC 753.29
  uterus 752.3
    acquired 621.8
  vagina (acquired) 623.2
    congenital 752.49
    postgonococcal (old) 098.2
    postinfectional 623.2
    senile 623.2
  vascular NEC (*see also* Atresia, blood vessel)
    747.60
    cerebral 747.81
  vas deferens 752.89
  vein NEC (*see also* Atresia, blood vessel)
    747.60
    cardiac 746.89
    great 747.49

Atrophy, atrophic—*continued*
  gastritis (chronic) 535.1
  gastrointestinal 569.89
  genital organ, male 608.89
  glandular 289.3
  globe (phthisis bulbi) 360.41
  gum (*see also* Recession, gingival) 523.20
  hair 704.2
  heart (brown) (senile) (*see also* Degeneration,
    myocardial) 429.1
  hemifacial 754.0
    Romberg 349.89
  hydronephrosis 591
  infantile 261
    paralysis, acute (*see also* Poliomyelitis, with
      paralysis) 045.1
  intestine 569.89
  iris (generalized) (postinfectional) (sector
    shaped) 364.59
    essential 364.51
    progressive 364.51
    sphincter 364.54
  kidney (senile) (*see also* Sclerosis, renal) 587
    with hypertension (*see also* Hypertension,
      kidney) 403.90
    congenital 753.0
    hydronephrotic 591
    infantile 753.0
  lacrimal apparatus (primary) 375.13
    secondary 375.14
  Landouzy-Déjérine 359.1
  laryngitis, infection 476.0
  larynx 478.79
  Leber's optic 377.16
  lip 528.5
  liver (acute) (subacute) (*see also* Necrosis, liver)
    570
    chronic (yellow) 571.8
    yellow (congenital) 570
      with
        abortion—*see* Abortion, by type, with
          specified complication NEC
        ectopic pregnancy (*see also* categories
          633.0-633.9) 639.8
        molar pregnancy (*see also* categories
          630-632) 639.8
      chronic 571.8
      complicating pregnancy 646.7
      following
        abortion 639.8
        ectopic or molar pregnancy 639.8
      from injection, inoculation or transfusion
        (onset within 8 months after
        administration)—*see* Hepatitis, viral
      healed 571.5
      obstetric 646.7
      postabortal 639.8
      postimmunization—*see* Hepatitis, viral
      posttransfusion—*see* Hepatitis, viral
      puerperal, postpartum 674.8
  lung (senile) 518.89
    congenital 748.69
  macular (dermatological) 701.3
    syphilitic, skin 091.3
      striated 095.8
  muscle, muscular 728.2
    disuse 728.2
    Duchenne-Aran 335.21
    extremity (lower) (upper) 728.2
    familial spinal 335.11
    general 728.2

Atrophy, atrophic—*continued*
  idiopathic 728.2
  infantile spinal 335.0
  myelopathic (progressive) 335.10
  myotonic 359.2
  neuritic 356.1
  neuropathic (peroneal) (progressive) 356.1
  peroneal 356.1
  primary (idiopathic) 728.2
  progressive (familial) (hereditary) (pure)
    335.21
    adult (spinal) 335.19
    infantile (spinal) 335.0
    juvenile (spinal) 335.11
    spinal 335.10
      adult 335.19
      hereditary or familial 335.11
      infantile 335.0
    pseudohypertrophic 359.1
      spinal (progressive) 335.10
    adult 335.19
    Aran-Duchenne 335.21
    familial 335.11
    hereditary 335.11
    infantile 335.0
      juvenile 335.11
    syphilitic 095.6
  myocardium (*see also* Degeneration,
    myocardial) 429.1
  myometrium (senile) 621.8
      cervix 622.8
  myotatic 728.2
  myotonia 359.2
  nail 703.8
    congenital 757.5
  nasopharynx 472.2
  nerve—*see also* Disorder, nerve
    abducens 378.54
    accessory 352.4
    acoustic or auditory 388.5
    cranial 352.9
      first (olfactory) 352.0
      second (optic) (*see also* Atrophy, optic
        nerve) 377.10
      third (oculomotor) (partial) 378.51
        total 378.52
      fourth (trochlear) 378.53
      fifth (trigeminal) 350.8
      sixth (abducens) 378.54
      seventh (facial) 351.8
      eighth (auditory) 388.5
      ninth (glossopharyngeal) 352.2
      tenth (pneumogastric) (vagus) 352.3
      eleventh (accessory) 352.4
      twelfth (hypoglossal) 352.5
    facial 351.8
    glossopharyngeal 352.2
    hypoglossal 352.5
    oculomotor (partial) 378.51
      total 378.52
    olfactory 352.0
    peripheral 355.9
    pneumogastric 352.3
    trigeminal 350.8
    trochlear 378.53
    vagus (pneumogastric) 352.3
  nervous system, congenital 742.8
  neuritic (*see also* Disorder, nerve) 355.9
  neurogenic NEC 355.9
    bone
      tabetic 094.0

 |

Avulsion—*continued*
  head (intracranial) NEC—*see also* Injury,
      intracranial, with open intracranial wound
    complete 874.9
     external site NEC 873.8
      complicated 873.9
  internal organ or site—*see* Injury, internal, by site
  joint—*see also* Dislocation, by site
    capsule—*see* Sprain, by site
  ligament—*see* Sprain, by site
  limb—*see also* Amputation, traumatic, by site
    skin and subcutaneous tissue—*see* Wound,
      open, by site
  muscle—*see* Sprain, by site
  nerve (root)—*see* Injury, nerve, by site
  scalp—*see* Wound, open, scalp
  skin and subcutaneous tissue—*see* Wound,
    open, by site
  symphyseal cartilage (inner), complicating
    delivery 665.6
  tendon—*see also* Sprain, by site
    with open wound—*see* Wound, open, by site
  toenail—*see* Wound, open, toe(s)
  tooth 873.63
    complicated 873.73
Awaiting organ transplant status V49.83
Awareness of heart beat 785.1
Axe grinders' disease 502
Axenfeld's anomaly or syndrome 743.44
Axilla, axillary —*see also* condition
  breast 757.6
Axonotmesis —*see* Injury, nerve, by site
Ayala's disease 756.89
Ayerza's disease or syndrome (pulmonary
    artery sclerosis with pulmonary hypertension)
    416.0
Azoospermia 606.0
Azorean disease (of the nervous system) 334.8
Azotemia 790.6
  meaning uremia (*see also* Uremia) 586
Aztec ear 744.29
Azygos lobe, lung (fissure) 748.69

B

Baader's syndrome (erythema multiforme exudativum) 695.1
Baastrup's syndrome 721.5
Babesiasis 088.82
Babesiosis 088.82
Babington's disease (familial hemorrhagic telangiectasia) 448.0
Babinski's syndrome (cardiovascular syphilis) 093.89
Babinski-Fröhlich syndrome (adiposogenital dystrophy) 253.8
Babinski-Nageotte syndrome 344.89
Bacillary —*see* condition
Bacilluria 791.9
  asymptomatic, in pregnancy or puerperium 646.5
  tuberculous (*see also* Tuberculosis) 016.9
Bacillus —*see also* Infection, bacillus
  abortus infection 023.1
  anthracis infection 022.9
  coli
    infection 041.4
      generalized 038.42
      intestinal 008.00
    pyemia 038.42
    septicemia 038.42
  Flexner's 004.1
  fusiformis infestation 101
  mallei infection 024
  Shiga's 004.0
  suipestifer infection (*see also* Infection, Salmonella) 003.9
Back —*see* condition
Backache (postural) 724.5
  psychogenic 307.89
  sacroiliac 724.6
Backflow (pyelovenous) (*see also* Disease, renal) 593.9
Backknee (*see also* Genu, recurvatum) 736.5
Bacteremia (*see also* Infection, bacillus) 790.7
  newborn 771.83
Bacteria
  in blood (*see also* Bacteremia) 790.7
  in urine (*see also* Bacteriuria) 599.0
Bacterial —*see* condition
Bactericholia (*see also* Cholecystitis, acute) 575.0
Bacterid, bacteride (Andrews' pustular) 686.8
Bacteriuria, bacteruria 791.9
  with
    urinary tract infection 599.0
  asymptomatic 791.9
    in pregnancy or puerperium 646.5
      affecting fetus or newborn 760.1
Bad
  breath 784.99
  heart—*see* Disease, heart
  trip (*see also* Abuse, drugs, nondependent) 305.3
Baehr-Schiffrin disease (thrombotic thrombocytopenic purpura) 446.6
Baelz's disease (cheilitis glandularis apostematosa) 528.5
Baerensprung's disease (eczema marginatum) 110.3
Bagassosis (occupational) 495.1
Baghdad boil 085.1

Bagratuni's syndrome (temporal arteritis) 446.5
Baker's
  cyst (knee) 727.51
    tuberculous (*see also* Tuberculosis) 015.2
  itch 692.89
Bakwin-Krida syndrome (craniometaphyseal dysplasia) 756.89
Balanitis (circinata) (gangraenosa) (infectious) (vulgaris) 607.1
  amebic 006.8
  candidal 112.2
  chlamydial 099.53
  due to Ducrey's bacillus 099.0
  erosiva circinata et gangraenosa 607.1
  gangrenous 607.1
  gonococcal (acute) 098.0
    chronic or duration of 2 months or over 098.2
  nongonococcal 607.1
  phagedenic 607.1
  venereal NEC 099.8
  xerotica obliterans 607.81
Balanoposthitis 607.1
  chlamydial 099.53
  gonococcal (acute) 098.0
    chronic or duration of 2 months or over 098.2
  ulcerative NEC 099.8
Balanorrhagia —*see* Balanitis
Balantidiasis 007.0
Balantidiosis 007.0
Balbuties, balbutio 307.0
Bald
  patches on scalp 704.00
  tongue 529.4
Baldness (*see also* Alopecia) 704.00
Balfour's disease (chloroma) 205.3
Balint's syndrome (psychic paralysis of visual fixation) 368.16
Balkan grippe 083.0
Ball
  food 938
  hair 938
Ballantyne (-Runge) syndrome (postmaturity) 766.22
Balloon disease (*see also* Effect, adverse, high altitude) 993.2
Ballooning posterior leaflet syndrome 424.0
Baló's disease or concentric sclerosis 341.1
Bamberger's disease (hypertrophic pulmonary osteoarthropathy) 731.2
Bamberger-Marie disease (hypertrophic pulmonary osteoarthropathy) 731.2
Bamboo spine 720.0
Bancroft's filariasis 125.0
Band(s)
  adhesive (*see also* Adhesions, peritoneum) 568.0
  amniotic 658.8
    affecting fetus or newborn 762.8
  anomalous or congenital—*see also* Anomaly, specified type NEC
    atrial 746.9
    heart 746.9
    intestine 751.4
    omentum 751.4
    ventricular 746.9
  cervix 622.3
  gallbladder (congenital) 751.69

Birth—*continued*
    radial nerve 767.6
    spinal (cord) (hemorrhage) (laceration)
      (rupture) 767.4
   rupture
    intracranial 767.0
    liver 767.8
    spinal cord 767.4
    spleen 767.8
    viscera 767.8
   scalp 767.19
   scalpel wound 767.8
   skeleton NEC 767.3
   specified NEC 767.8
   spinal cord 767.4
   spleen 767.8
   subdural hemorrhage 767.0
   tentorial, tear 767.0
   testes 767.8
   vulva 767.8
  instrumental, NEC, affecting fetus or newborn
    763.2
  lack of care, after or at 995.52
  multiple
   affected by maternal complications of
     pregnancy 761.5
   healthy liveborn—*see* Newborn, multiple
  neglect, after or at 995.52
  newborn—*see* Newborn
  palsy or paralysis NEC 767.7
  precipitate, fetus or newborn 763.6
  premature (infant) 765.1
  prolonged, affecting fetus or newborn 763.9
  retarded, fetus or newborn 763.9
  shock, newborn 779.89
  strangulation or suffocation
   due to aspiration of clear amniotic fluid 770.13
    with respiratory symptoms 770.14
   mechanical 767.8
  trauma NEC 767.9
  triplet
   affected by maternal complications of
     pregnancy 761.5
   healthy liveborn—*see* Newborn, multiple
  twin
   affected by maternal complications of
     pregnancy 761.5
   healthy liveborn—*see* Newborn, twin
  ventouse, affecting fetus or newborn 763.3
Birthmark 757.32
Bisalbuminemia 273.8
Biskra button 085.1
Bite(s)
  with intact skin surface—*see* Contusion
  animal—*see* Wound, open, by site
   intact skin surface—*see* Contusion
  centipede 989.5
  chigger 133.8
  fire ant 989.5
  flea—*see* Injury, superficial, by site
  human (open wound)—*see also* Wound, open,
    by site
   intact skin surface—*see* Contusion
  insect
   nonvenomous—*see* Injury, superficial, by site
   venomous 989.5
  mad dog (death from) 071
  open
   anterior 524.24
   posterior 524.25
  poisonous 989.5

Bite(s)—*continued*
  red bug 133.8
  reptile 989.5
   nonvenomous—*see* Wound, open, by site
  snake 989.5
   nonvenomous—*see* Wound, open, by site
  spider (venomous) 989.5
   nonvenomous—*see* Injury, superficial, by site
  venomous 989.5
Biting
  cheek or lip 528.9
  nail 307.9
Black
  death 020.9
  eye NEC 921.0
  hairy tongue 529.3
  heel 924.20
  lung disease 500
  palm 923.20
Blackfan-Diamond anemia or syndrome
  (congenital hypoplastic anemia) 284.01
Blackhead 706.1
Blackout 780.2
Blackwater fever 084.8
Bladder —*see* Condition
Blast
  blindness 921.3
  concussion—*see* Blast, injury
  injury 869.0
   with open wound into cavity 869.1
   abdomen or thorax—*see* Injury, internal, by
    site
   brain (*see also* Concussion, brain) 850.9
    with skull fracture—*see* Fracture, skull
   ear (acoustic nerve trauma) 951.5
    with perforation, tympanic membrane—*see*
     Wound, open, ear, drum
   lung (*see also* Injury, internal, lung) 861.20
   otitic (explosive) 388.11
Blastomycosis, blastomycotic (chronic)
  (cutaneous) (disseminated) (lung) (pulmonary)
  (systemic) 116.0
  Brazilian 116.1
  European 117.5
  keloidal 116.2
  North American 116.0
  primary pulmonary 116.0
  South American 116.1
Bleb(s) 709.8
  emphysematous (bullous) (diffuse) (lung)
   (ruptured) (solitary) 492.0
  filtering, eye (postglaucoma) (status) V45.69
   with complication 997.99
   postcataract extraction (complication) 997.99
  lung (ruptured) 492.0
   congenital 770.5
  subpleural (emphysematous) 492.0
Bleeder (familial) (hereditary) (*see also* Defect,
  coagulation) 286.9
  nonfamilial 286.9
Bleeding (*see also* Hemorrhage) 459.0
  anal 569.3
  anovulatory 628.0
  atonic, following delivery 666.1
  capillary 448.9
  due to subinvolution 621.1
   puerperal 666.2
  ear 388.69
  excessive, associated with menopausal onset
   627.0
  familial (*see also* Defect, coagulation) 286.9

Blindness—*continued*
  one eye 369.74
    with vision of other eye (specified as)
      near-normal 369.75
      normal 369.76
  near-total
    both eyes 369.04
      with impairment of lesser eye (specified as)
        blind, not further specified 369.02
        total 369.03
    one eye 369.64
      with vision of other eye (specified as)
        near-normal 369.65
        normal 369.66
  night 368.60
    acquired 368.62
    congenital (Japanese) 368.61
    hereditary 368.61
    specified type NEC 368.69
    vitamin A deficiency 264.5
  nocturnal—*see* Blindness, night
  one eye 369.60
    with low vision of other eye 369.10
  profound
    both eyes 369.08
      with impairment of lesser eye (specified as)
        blind, not further specified 369.05
        near-total 369.07
        total 369.06
    one eye 369.67
      with vision of other eye (specified as)
        near-normal 369.68
        normal 369.69
  psychic 784.69
  severe
    both eyes 369.22
      with impairment of lesser eye (specified as)
        blind, not further specified 369.11
        low vision, not further specified 369.21
        near-total 369.13
        profound 369.14
        total 369.12
    one eye 369.71
      with vision of other eye (specified as)
        near-normal 369.72
        normal 369.73
  snow 370.24
  sun 363.31
  temporary 368.12
  total
    both eyes 369.01
    one eye 369.61
      with vision of other eye (specified as)
        near-normal 369.62
        normal 369.63
  transient 368.12
  traumatic NEC 950.9
  word (developmental) 315.01
    acquired 784.61
    secondary to organic lesion 784.61
Blister —*see also* Injury, superficial, by site
  beetle dermatitis 692.89
  due to burn—*see* Burn, by site, second degree
  fever 054.9
  multiple, skin, nontraumatic 709.8
Bloating 787.3
Bloch-Siemens syndrome (incontinentia
  pigmenti) 757.33
Bloch-Stauffer dyshormonal dermatosis 757.33
Bloch-Sulzberger disease or syndrome
  (incontinentia pigmenti) (melanoblastosis)
  757.33

Block
  alveolar capillary 516.3
  arborization (heart) 426.6
  arrhythmic 426.9
  atrioventricular (AV) (incomplete) (partial)
    426.10
    with
      2:1 atrioventricular response block 426.13
      atrioventricular dissociation 426.0
    first degree (incomplete) 426.11
    second degree (Mobitz type I) 426.13
      Mobitz (type) II 426.12
    third degree 426.0
    complete 426.0
      congenital 746.86
    congenital 746.86
    Mobitz (incomplete)
      type I (Wenckebach's) 426.13
      type II 426.12
    partial 426.13
  auriculoventricular (*see also* Block,
    atrioventricular) 426.10
    complete 426.0
      congenital 746.86
    congenital 746.86
  bifascicular (cardiac) 426.53
  bundle branch (complete) (false) (incomplete)
    426.50
    bilateral 426.53
    left (complete) (main stem) 426.3
      with right bundle branch block 426.53
      anterior fascicular 426.2
        with
          posterior fascicular block 426.3
          right bundle branch block 426.52
      hemiblock 426.2
      incomplete 426.2
        with right bundle branch block 426.53
      posterior fascicular 426.2
        with
          anterior fascicular block 426.3
          right bundle branch block 426.51
    right 426.4
      with
        left bundle branch block (incomplete)
          (main stem) 426.53
        left fascicular block 426.53
          anterior 426.52
          posterior 426.51
    Wilson's type 426.4
  cardiac 426.9
  conduction 426.9
    complete 426.0
  Eustachian tube (*see also* Obstruction,
    Eustachian tube) 381.60
  fascicular (left anterior) (left posterior) 426.2
  foramen Magendie (acquired) 331.3
    congenital 742.3
      with spina bifida (*see also* Spina bifida)
        741.0
  heart 426.9
    first degree (atrioventricular) 426.11
    second degree (atrioventricular) 426.13
    third degree (atrioventricular) 426.0
    bundle branch (complete) (false) (incomplete)
      426.50
      bilateral 426.53
      left (*see also* Block, bundle branch, left)
        426.3
      right (*see also* Block, bundle branch, right)
        426.4

Block—*continued*
  complete (atrioventricular) 426.0
    congenital 746.86
  incomplete 426.13
  intra-atrial 426.6
  intraventricular NEC 426.6
  sinoatrial 426.6
  specified type NEC 426.6
  hepatic vein 453.0
  intraventricular (diffuse) (myofibrillar) 426.6
    bundle branch (complete) (false) (incomplete)
        426.50
      bilateral 426.53
      left (*see also* Block, bundle branch, left)
          426.3
      right (*see also* Block, bundle branch, right)
          426.4
  kidney (*see also* Disease, renal) 593.9
    postcystoscopic 997.5
  myocardial (*see also* Block, heart) 426.9
  nodal 426.10
  optic nerve 377.49
  organ or site (congenital) NEC—*see* Atresia
  parietal 426.6
  peri-infarction 426.6
  portal (vein) 452
  sinoatrial 426.6
  sinoauricular 426.6
  spinal cord 336.9
  trifascicular 426.54
  tubal 628.2
  vein NEC 453.9
Blocq's disease or syndrome (astasia-abasia)
    307.9
Blood
  constituents, abnormal NEC 790.6
  disease 289.9
    specified NEC 289.89
  donor V59.01
    other blood components V59.09
    stem cells V59.02
    whole blood V59.01
  dyscrasia 289.9
    with
      abortion—*see* Abortion, by type, with
          hemorrhage, delayed or excessive
      ectopic pregnancy (*see also* categories
          633.0-633.9) 639.1
      molar pregnancy (*see also* categories
          630-632) 639.1
    fetus or newborn NEC 776.9
    following
      abortion 639.1
      ectopic or molar pregnancy 639.1
    puerperal, postpartum 666.3
  flukes NEC (*see also* Infestation, Schistosoma)
      120.9
  in
    feces (*see also* Melena) 578.1
      occult 792.1
    urine (*see also* Hematuria) 599.7
  mole 631
  occult 792.1
  poisoning (*see also* Septicemia) 038.9
  pressure
    decreased, due to shock following injury 958.4
    fluctuating 796.4
    high (*see also* Hypertension) 401.9
      incidental reading (isolated) (nonspecific),
          without diagnosis of hypertension 796.2
    low (*see also* Hypotension) 458.9

Blood—*continued*
    incidental reading (isolated) (nonspecific),
        without diagnosis of hypotension 796.3
  spitting (*see also* Hemoptysis) 786.3
  staining cornea 371.12
  transfusion
    without reported diagnosis V58.2
    donor V59.01
      stem cells V59.02
    reaction or complication—*see* Complications,
        transfusion
  tumor—*see* Hematoma
  vessel rupture—*see* Hemorrhage
  vomiting (*see also* Hematemesis) 578.0
Blood-forming organ disease 289.9
Bloodgood's disease 610.1
Bloodshot eye 379.93
Bloom (-Machacek) (-Torre) syndrome 757.39
Blotch, palpebral 372.55
Blount's disease (tibia vara) 732.4
Blount-Barber syndrome (tibia vara) 732.4
Blue
  baby 746.9
  bloater 491.20
    with
      acute bronchitis 491.22
      exacerbation (acute) 491.21
  diaper syndrome 270.0
  disease 746.9
  dome cyst 610.0
  drum syndrome 381.02
  sclera 743.47
    with fragility of bone and deafness 756.51
  toe syndrome 445.02
Blueness 368.8
Blushing (abnormal) (excessive) 782.62
BMI (body mass index)
  adult
    25.0-25.9 V85.21
    26.0-26.9 V85.22
    27.0-27.9 V85.23
    28.0-28.9 V85.24
    29.0-29.9 V85.25
    30.0-30.9 V85.30
    31.0-31.9 V85.31
    32.0-32.9 V85.32
    33.0-33.9 V85.33
    34.0-34.9 V85.34
    35.0-35.9 V85.35
    36.0-36.9 V85.36
    37.0-37.9 V85.37
    38.0-38.9 V85.38
    39.0-39.9 V85.39
    40 and over V85.4
    between 19-24 V85.1
    less than 19 V85.0
  pediatric
    5th percentile to less than 85th percentile for
        age V85.52
    85th percentile to less than 95th percentile for
        age V85.53
    greater than or equal to 95th percentile for age
        V85.54
    less than 5th percentile for age V85.51
Boarder, hospital V65.0
  infant V65.0
Bockhart's impetigo (superficial folliculitis) 704.8
Bodechtel-Guttmann disease (subacute
    sclerosing panencephalitis) 046.2
Boder-Sedgwick syndrome (ataxia-
    telangiectasia) 334.8

Body, bodies
  Aschoff (*see also* Myocarditis, rheumatic) 398.0
  asteroid, vitreous 379.22
  choroid, colloid (degenerative) 362.57
    hereditary 362.77
  cytoid (retina) 362.82
  drusen (retina) (*see also* Drusen) 362.57
    optic disc 377.21
  fibrin, pleura 511.0
  foreign—*see* Foreign body
  Hassall-Henle 371.41
  loose
    joint (*see also* Loose, body, joint) 718.1
      knee 717.6
    knee 717.6
    sheath, tendon 727.82
  Mallory's 034.1
  mass index (BMI)
    adult
        25.0-25.9 V85.21
        26.0-26.9 V85.22
        27.0-27.9 V85.23
        28.0-28.9 V85.24
        29.0-29.9 V85.25
        30.0-30.9 V85.30
        31.0-31.9 V85.31
        32.0-32.9 V85.32
        33.0-33.9 V85.33
        34.0-34.9 V85.34
        35.0-35.9 V85.35
        36.0-36.9 V85.36
        37.0-37.9 V85.37
        38.0-38.9 V85.38
        39.0-39.9 V85.39
        40 and over V85.4
        between 19-24 V85.1
        less than 19 V85.0
    pediatric
        5th percentile to less than 85th percentile for
          age V85.52
        85th percentile to less than 95th percentile
          for age V85.53
        greater than or equal to 95th percentile for
          age V85.54
        less than 5th percentile for age V85.51
  Mooser 081.0
  Negri 071
  rice (joint) (*see also* Loose, body, joint) 718.1
    knee 717.6
  rocking 307.3
Boeck's
  disease (sarcoidosis) 135
  lupoid (miliary) 135
  sarcoid 135
Boerhaave's syndrome (spontaneous esophageal
    rupture) 530.4
Boggy
  cervix 622.8
  uterus 621.8
Boil (*see also* Carbuncle) 680.9
  abdominal wall 680.2
  Aleppo 085.1
  ankle 680.6
  anus 680.5
  arm (any part, above wrist) 680.3
  auditory canal, external 680.0
  axilla 680.3
  back (any part) 680.2
  Baghdad 085.1
  breast 680.2
  buttock 680.5

Boil —*continued*
  chest wall 680.2
  corpus cavernosum 607.2
  Delhi 085.1
  ear (any part) 680.0
  eyelid 373.13
  face (any part, except eye) 680.0
  finger (any) 680.4
  flank 680.2
  foot (any part) 680.7
  forearm 680.3
  Gafsa 085.1
  genital organ, male 608.4
  gluteal (region) 680.5
  groin 680.2
  hand (any part) 680.4
  head (any part, except face) 680.8
  heel 680.7
  hip 680.6
  knee 680.6
  labia 616.4
  lacrimal (*see also* Dacryocystitis) 375.30
    gland (*see also* Dacryoadenitis) 375.00
    passages (duct) (sac) (*see also* Dacryocystitis)
      375.30
  leg, any part except foot 680.6
  multiple sites 680.9
  Natal 085.1
  neck 680.1
  nose (external) (septum) 680.0
  orbit, orbital 376.01
  partes posteriores 680.5
  pectoral region 680.2
  penis 607.2
  perineum 680.2
  pinna 680.0
  scalp (any part) 680.8
  scrotum 608.4
  seminal vesicle 608.0
  shoulder 680.3
  skin NEC 680.9
  specified site NEC 680.8
  spermatic cord 608.4
  temple (region) 680.0
  testis 608.4
  thigh 680.6
  thumb 680.4
  toe (any) 680.7
  tropical 085.1
  trunk 680.2
  tunica vaginalis 608.4
  umbilicus 680.2
  upper arm 680.3
  vas deferens 608.4
  vulva 616.4
  wrist 680.4
Bold hives (*see also* Urticaria) 708.9
Bolivian hemorrhagic fever 078.7
Bombé, iris 364.74
Bomford-Rhoads anemia (refractory) 238.72
Bone —*see* condition
Bonnevie-Ullrich syndrome 758.6
Bonnier's syndrome 386.19
Bonvale Dam fever 780.79
Bony block of joint 718.80
  ankle 718.87
  elbow 718.82
  foot 718.87
  hand 718.84
  hip 718.85
  knee 718.86

Bony block of joint—*continued*
  multiple sites 718.89
  pelvic region 718.85
  shoulder (region) 718.81
  specified site NEC 718.88
  wrist 718.83
Borderline
  intellectual functioning V62.89
  pelvis 653.1
    with obstruction during labor 660.1
      affecting fetus or newborn 763.1
  psychosis (*see also* Schizophrenia) 295.5
    of childhood (*see also* Psychosis, childhood)
      299.8
  schizophrenia (*see also* Schizophrenia) 295.5
Borna disease 062.9
Bornholm disease (epidemic pleurodynia) 074.1
Borrelia vincentii (mouth) (pharynx) (tonsils) 101
Bostock's catarrh (*see also* Fever, hay) 477.9
Boston exanthem 048
Botalli, ductus (patent) (persistent) 747.0
Bothriocephalus latus infestation 123.4
Botulism 005.1
  wound—*see* Wound, open, by site, complicated
Bouba (*see also* Yaws) 102.9
Bouffée délirante 298.3
Bouillaud's disease or syndrome (rheumatic
  heart disease) 391.9
Bourneville's disease (tuberous sclerosis) 759.5
Boutonneuse fever 082.1
Boutonniere
  deformity (finger) 736.21
  hand (intrinsic) 736.21
Bouveret (-Hoffmann) disease or syndrome
  (paroxysmal tachycardia) 427.2
Bovine heart —*see* Hypertrophy, cardiac
Bowel —*see* condition
Bowen's
  dermatosis (precancerous) (M8081/2)—*see*
    Neoplasm, skin, in situ
  disease (M8081/2)—*see* Neoplasm, skin, in situ
  epithelioma (M8081/2)—*see* Neoplasm, skin, in
    situ
  type
    epidermoid carcinoma in situ (M8081/2)—*see*
      Neoplasm, skin, in situ
    intraepidermal squamous cell carcinoma
      (M8081/2)–*see* Neoplasm, skin, in situ
Bowing
  femur 736.89
    congenital 754.42
  fibula 736.89
    congenital 754.43
  forearm 736.09
    away from midline (cubitus valgus) 736.01
    toward midline (cubitus varus) 736.02
  leg(s), long bones, congenital 754.44
  radius 736.09
    away from midline (cubitus valgus) 736.01
    toward midline (cubitus varus) 736.02
  tibia 736.89
    congenital 754.43
Bowleg (s) 736.42
  congenital 754.44
  rachitic 268.1
Boyd's dysentery 004.2
Brachial —*see* condition
Brachman-de Lange syndrome (Amsterdam
  dwarf, mental retardation, and brachycephaly)
  759.89
Brachycardia 427.89

Brachycephaly 756.0
Brachymorphism and ectopia lentis 759.89
Bradley's disease (epidemic vomiting) 078.82
Bradycardia 427.89
  chronic (sinus) 427.81
  newborn 779.81
  nodal 427.89
  postoperative 997.1
  reflex 337.0
  sinoatrial 427.89
    with paroxysmal tachyarrhythmia or
      tachycardia 427.81
    chronic 427.81
  sinus 427.89
    with paroxysmal tachyarrhythmia or
      tachycardia 427.81
    chronic 427.81
    persistent 427.81
    severe 427.81
  tachycardia syndrome 427.81
  vagal 427.89
Bradypnea 786.09
Brailsford's disease 732.3
  radial head 732.3
  tarsal scaphoid 732.5
Brailsford-Morquio disease or syndrome
  (mucopolysaccharidosis IV) 277.5
Brain —*see also* condition
  death 348.8
  syndrome (acute) (chronic) (nonpsychotic)
    (organic) (with neurotic reaction) (with
    behavioral reaction) (*see also* Syndrome,
    brain) 310.9
    with
      presenile brain disease 290.10
      psychosis, psychotic reaction (*see also*
        Psychosis, organic) 294.9
    congenital (*see also* Retardation, mental) 319
Branched-chain amino-acid disease 270.3
Branchial —*see* condition
Brandt's syndrome (acrodermatitis
  enteropathica) 686.8
Brash (water) 787.1
Brass-founders' ague 985.8
Bravais-Jacksonian epilepsy (*see also* Epilepsy)
  345.5
Braxton Hicks contractions 644.1
Braziers' disease 985.8
Brazilian
  blastomycosis 116.1
  leishmaniasis 085.5
BRBPR (bright red blood per rectum) 569.3
Break
  cardiorenal—*see* Hypertension, cardiorenal
  retina (*see also* Defect, retina) 361.30
Breakbone fever 061
Breakdown
  device, implant, or graft—*see* Complications,
    mechanical
  nervous (*see also* Disorder, mental,
    nonpsychotic) 300.9
  perineum 674.2
Breast —*see* condition
Breast feeding difficulties 676.8
Breath
  foul 784.99
  holder, child 312.81
  holding spells 786.9
  shortness 786.05

Breathing
asymmetrical 786.09
bronchial 786.09
exercises V57.0
labored 786.09
mouth 784.99
   causing malocclusion 524.59
periodic 786.09
   high altitude 327.22
tic 307.20
Breathlessness 786.09
Breda's disease (*see also* Yaws) 102.9
Breech
delivery, affecting fetus or newborn 763.0
extraction, affecting fetus or newborn 763.0
presentation (buttocks) (complete) (frank) 652.2
   with successful version 652.1
      before labor, affecting fetus or newborn 761.7
      during labor, affecting fetus or newborn 763.0
Breisky's disease (kraurosis vulvae) 624.0
Brennemann's syndrome (acute mesenteric
   lymphadenitis) 289.2
Brenner's
tumor (benign) (M9000/0) 220
   borderline malignancy (M9000/1) 236.2
   malignant (M9000/3) 183.0
   proliferating (M9000/1) 236.2
Bretonneau's disease (diphtheritic malignant
   angina) 032.0
Breus' mole 631
Brevicollis 756.16
Bricklayers' itch 692.89
Brickmakers' anemia 126.9
Bridge
myocardial 746.85
Bright's
blindness—*see* Uremia
disease (*see also* Nephritis) 583.9
   arteriosclerotic (*see also* Hypertension,
      kidney) 403.90
Bright red blood per rectum (BRBPR) 569.3
Brill's disease (recrudescent typhus) 081.1
flea-borne 081.0
louse-borne 081.1
Brill-Symmers disease (follicular lymphoma)
   (M9690/3) 202.0
Brill-Zinsser disease (recrudescent typhus) 081.1
Brinton's disease (linitis plastica) (M8142/3)
   151.9
Brion-Kayser disease (*see also* Fever,
   paratyphoid) 002.9
Briquet's disorder or syndrome 300.81
Brissaud's
infantilism (infantile myxedema) 244.9
motor-verbal tic 307.23
Brissaud-Meige syndrome (infantile myxedema)
   244.9
Brittle
bones (congenital) 756.51
nails 703.8
   congenital 757.5
Broad —*see also* condition
beta disease 272.2
ligament laceration syndrome 620.6
Brock's syndrome (atelectasis due to enlarged
   lymph nodes) 518.0
Brocq's disease 691.8
atopic (diffuse) neurodermatitis 691.8
lichen simplex chronicus 698.3
parakeratosis psoriasiformis 696.2
parapsoriasis 696.2

Brocq-Duhring disease (dermatitis
   herpetiformis) 694.0
Brodie's
abscess (localized) (chronic) (*see also*
      Osteomyelitis) 730.1
disease (joint) (*see also* Osteomyelitis) 730.1
Broken
arches 734
   congenital 755.67
back—*see* Fracture, vertebra, by site
bone—*see* Fracture, by site
compensation—*see* Disease, heart
heart syndrome 429.83
implant or internal device—*see* listing under
      Complications, mechanical
neck—*see* Fracture, vertebra, cervical
nose 802.0
   open 802.1
tooth, teeth 873.63
   complicated 873.73
Bromhidrosis 705.89
Bromidism, bromism
acute 967.3
   correct substance properly administered
      349.82
   overdose or wrong substance given or taken
      967.3
chronic (*see also* Dependence) 304.1
Bromidrosiphobia 300.23
Bromidrosis 705.89
Bronchi, bronchial —*see* condition
Bronchiectasis (cylindrical) (diffuse) (fusiform)
   (localized) (moniliform) (postinfectious)
   (recurrent) (saccular) 494.0
with acute exacerbation 494.1
congenital 748.61
tuberculosis (*see also* Tuberculosis) 011.5
Bronchiolectasis —*see* Bronchiectasis
Bronchiolitis (acute) (infectious) (subacute)
   466.19
with
   bronchospasm or obstruction 466.19
   influenza, flu, or grippe 487.1
catarrhal (acute) (subacute) 466.19
chemical 506.0
   chronic 506.4
chronic (obliterative) 491.8
due to external agent—*see* Bronchitis, acute,
     due to
fibrosa obliterans 491.8
influenzal 487.1
obliterans 491.8
   status post lung transplant 996.84
   with organizing pneumonia (B.O.O.P.) 516.8
obliterative (chronic) (diffuse) (subacute) 491.8
   due to fumes or vapors 506.4
respiratory syncytial virus 466.11
vesicular—*see* Pneumonia, broncho-
Bronchitis (diffuse) (hypostatic) (infectious)
   (inflammatory) (simple) 490
with
   emphysema—*see* Emphysema
   influenza, flu, or grippe 487.1
   obstruction airway, chronic 491.20
     with
       acute bronchitis 491.22
       exacerbation (acute) 491.21
   tracheitis 490
     acute or subacute 466.0
       with bronchospasm or obstruction 466.0
     chronic 491.8

Bronchitis—*continued*
  acute or subacute 466.0
    with
      bronchospasm 466.0
      obstruction 466.0
      tracheitis 466.0
    chemical (due to fumes or vapors) 506.0
    due to
      fumes or vapors 506.0
      radiation 508.8
  allergic (acute) (*see also* Asthma) 493.9
  arachidic 934.1
  aspiration 507.0
    due to fumes or vapors 506.0
  asthmatic (acute) 493.90
    with
      acute exacerbation 493.92
      status asthmaticus 493.91
    chronic 493.2
  capillary 466.19
    with bronchospasm or obstruction 466.19
    chronic 491.8
  caseous (*see also* Tuberculosis) 011.3
  Castellani's 104.8
  catarrhal 490
    acute—*see* Bronchitis, acute
    chronic 491.0
  chemical (acute) (subacute) 506.0
    chronic 506.4
    due to fumes or vapors (acute) (subacute)
        506.0
      chronic 506.4
  chronic 491.9
    with
      tracheitis (chronic) 491.8
    asthmatic 493.2
    catarrhal 491.0
    chemical (due to fumes and vapors) 506.4
    due to
      fumes or vapors (chemical) (inhalation)
          506.4
      radiation 508.8
      tobacco smoking 491.0
    mucopurulent 491.1
    obstructive 491.20
      with
        acute bronchitis 491.22
        exacerbation (acute) 491.21
    purulent 491.1
    simple 491.0
    specified type NEC 491.8
  croupous 466.0
    with bronchospasm or obstruction 466.0
    due to fumes or vapors 506.0
  emphysematous 491.20
    with
      acute bronchitis 491.22
      exacerbation (acute) 491.21
  exudative 466.0
  fetid (chronic) (recurrent) 491.1
  fibrinous, acute or subacute 466.0
    with bronchospasm or obstruction 466.0
  grippal 487.1
  influenzal 487.1
  membranous, acute or subacute 466.0
    with bronchospasm or obstruction 466.0
  moulders' 502
  mucopurulent (chronic) (recurrent) 491.1
    acute or subacute 466.0
  non-obstructive 491.0
  obliterans 491.8

Bronchitis—*continued*
  obstructive (chronic) 491.20
    with
      acute bronchitis 491.22
      exacerbation (acute) 491.21
  pituitous 491.1
  plastic (inflammatory) 466.0
  pneumococcal, acute or subacute 466.0
    with bronchospasm or obstruction 466.0
  pseudomembranous 466.0
  purulent (chronic) (recurrent) 491.1
    acute or subacute 466.0
      with bronchospasm or obstruction 466.0
  putrid 491.1
  scrofulous (*see also* Tuberculosis) 011.3
  senile 491.9
  septic, acute or subacute 466.0
    with bronchospasm or obstruction 466.0
  smokers' 491.0
  spirochetal 104.8
  suffocative, acute or subacute 466.0
  summer (*see also* Asthma) 493.9
  suppurative (chronic) 491.1
    acute or subacute 466.0
  tuberculous (*see also* Tuberculosis) 011.3
  ulcerative 491.8
    Vincent's 101
  Vincent's 101
  viral, acute or subacute 466.0
    with bronchospasm or obstruction 466.0
Bronchoalveolitis 485
Bronchoaspergillosis 117.3
Bronchocele
  meaning
    dilatation of bronchus 519.19
    goiter 240.9
Bronchogenic carcinoma 162.9
Bronchohemisporosis 117.9
Broncholithiasis 518.89
  tuberculous (*see also* Tuberculosis) 011.3
Bronchomalacia 748.3
Bronchomoniliasis 112.89
Bronchomycosis 112.89
Bronchonocardiosis 039.1
Bronchopleuropneumonia —*see* Pneumonia,
  broncho-
Bronchopneumonia —*see* Pneumonia, broncho-
Bronchopneumonitis —*see* Pneumonia,
  broncho-
Bronchopulmonary —*see* condition
Bronchopulmonitis —*see* Pneumonia, broncho-
Bronchorrhagia 786.3
  newborn 770.3
  tuberculous (*see also* Tuberculosis) 011.3
Bronchorrhea (chronic) (purulent) 491.0
  acute 466.0
Bronchospasm 519.11
  with
    asthma—*see* Asthma
    bronchiolitis, acute 466.19
      due to respiratory syncytial virus 466.11
    bronchitis—*see* Bronchitis
    chronic obstructive pulmonary disease
        (COPD) 496
    emphysema—*see* Emphysema
      due to external agent—*see* Condition,
          respiratory, acture, due to
  acute 519.11
  due to external agent—*see* Condition,
      respiratory, acute, due to
  exercise induced 493.81

Bronchospirochetosis 104.8
Bronchostenosis 519.19
Bronchus *—see* condition
Bronze, bronzed
  diabetes 275.0
  disease (Addison's) (skin) 255.4
    tuberculous (*see also* Tuberculosis) 017.6
Brooke's disease or tumor (M8100/0)*—see*
  Neoplasm, skin, benign
Brow presentation complicating delivery 652.4
Brown's tendon sheath syndrome 378.61
Brown enamel of teeth (hereditary) 520.5
Brown-Séquard's paralysis (syndrome) 344.89
Brucella, brucellosis (infection) 023.9
  abortus 023.1
  canis 023.3
  dermatitis, skin 023.9
  melitensis 023.0
  mixed 023.8
  suis 023.2
Bruck's disease 733.99
Bruck-de Lange disease or syndrome
  (Amsterdam dwarf, mental retardation, and
  brachycephaly) 759.89
Brugada syndrome 746.89
Brug's filariasis 125.1
Brugsch's syndrome (acropachyderma) 757.39
Bruhl's disease (splenic anemia with fever)
  285.8
Bruise (skin surface intact)*—see also* Contusion
  with
    fracture*—see* Fracture, by site
    open wound*—see* Wound, open, by site
  internal organ (abdomen, chest, or pelvis)*—see*
    Injury, internal, by site
  umbilical cord 663.6
    affecting fetus or newborn 762.6
Bruit 785.9
  arterial (abdominal) (carotid) 785.9
  supraclavicular 785.9
Brushburn *—see* Injury, superficial, by site
Bruton's X-linked agammaglobulinemia
  279.04
Bruxism 306.8
  sleep related 327.53
Bubbly lung syndrome 770.7
Bubo 289.3
  blennorrhagic 098.89
  chancroidal 099.0
  climatic 099.1
  due to Hemophilus ducreyi 099.0
  gonococcal 098.89
  indolent NEC 099.8
  inguinal NEC 099.8
    chancroidal 099.0
    climatic 099.1
    due to H. ducreyi 099.0
  scrofulous (*see also* Tuberculosis) 017.2
  soft chancre 099.0
  suppurating 683
  syphilitic 091.0
    congenital 090.0
  tropical 099.1
  venereal NEC 099.8
  virulent 099.0

Bubonic plague 020.0
Bubonocele *—see* Hernia, inguinal
Buccal *—see* condition
Buchanan's disease (juvenile osteochondrosis of
  iliac crest) 732.1
Buchem's syndrome (hyperostosis corticalis)
  733.3
Buchman's disease (osteochondrosis, juvenile)
  732.1
Bucket handle fracture (semilunar cartilage)
  (*see also* Tear, meniscus) 836.2
Budd-Chiari syndrome (hepatic vein
  thrombosis) 453.0
Budgerigar-fanciers' disease or lung 495.2
Büdinger-Ludloff-Läwen disease 717.89
Buerger's disease (thromboangiitis obliterans)
  443.1
Bulbar *—see* condition
Bulbus cordis 745.9
  persistent (in left ventricle) 745.8
Bulging fontanels (congenital) 756.0
Bulimia 783.6
  nervosa 307.51
  nonorganic origin 307.51
Bulky uterus 621.2
Bulla(e) 709.8
  lung (emphysematous) (solitary) 492.0
Bullet wound *—see also* Wound, open, by site
  fracture*—see* Fracture, by site, open
  internal organ (abdomen, chest, or pelvis)*—see*
    Injury, internal, by site, with open wound
  intracranial*—see* Laceration, brain, with open
    wound
Bullis fever 082.8
Bullying (*see also* Disturbance, conduct) 312.0
Bundle
  branch block (complete) (false) (incomplete)
    426.50
    bilateral 426.53
    left (*see also* Block, bundle branch, left) 426.3
      hemiblock 426.2
    right (*see also* Block, bundle branch, right)
      426.4
  of His—*see* condition
  of Kent syndrome (anomalous atrioventricular
    excitation) 426.7
Bungpagga 040.81
Bunion 727.1
Bunionette 727.1
Bunyamwera fever 066.3
Buphthalmia, buphthalmos (congenital) 743.20
  associated with
    keratoglobus, congenital 743.22
    megalocornea 743.22
    ocular anomalies NEC 743.22
  isolated 743.21
  simple 743.21
Bürger-Grütz disease or syndrome (essential
  familial hyperlipemia) 272.3
Buried roots 525.3
Burke's syndrome 577.8
Burkitt's
  tumor (M9750/3) 200.2
  type malignant, lymphoma, lymphoblastic, or
    undifferentiated (M9750/3) 200.2

Burn (acid) (cathode ray) (caustic) (chemical)
(electric heating appliance) (electricity) (fire)
(flame) (hot liquid or object) (irradiation)
(lime) (radiation) (steam) (thermal) (x-ray)
949.0

> *Note—Use the following fifth-digit*
> *subclassification with category 948 to indicate*
> *the percent of body surface with third degree*
> *burn:*
>
> *0 less than 10% or unspecified*
> *1 10-19%*
> *2 20-29%*
> *3 30-39%*
> *4 40-49%*
> *5 50-59%*
> *6 60-69%*
> *7 70-79%*
> *8 80-89%*
> *9 90% or more of body surface*

  with
    blisters—*see* Burn, by site, second degree
    erythema—*see* Burn, by site, first degree
    skin loss (epidermal)—*see also* Burn, by site,
      second degree
      full thickness—*see also* Burn, by site, third
        degree
        with necrosis of underlying tissues—*see*
          Burn, by site, third degree, deep
    first degree—*see* Burn, by site, first degree
    second degree—*see* Burn, by site, second degree
    third degree—*see also* Burn, by site, third degree
    deep—*see* Burn, by site, third degree, deep
  abdomen, abdominal (muscle) (wall) 942.03
    with
      trunk—*see* Burn, trunk, multiple sites
    first degree 942.13
    second degree 942.23
    third degree 942.33
      deep 942.43
        with loss of body part 942.53
  ankle 945.03
    with
      lower limb(s)–*see* Burn, leg, multiple sites
    first degree 945.13
    second degree 945.23
    third degree 945.33
      deep 945.43
        with loss of body part 945.53
  anus—*see* Burn, trunk, specified site NEC
  arm(s) 943.00
    first degree 943.10
    second degree 943.20
    third degree 943.30
      deep 943.40
        with loss of body part 943.50
    lower—*see* Burn, forearm(s)
    multiple sites, except hand(s) or wrist(s) 943.09
      first degree 943.19
      second degree 943.29
      third degree 943.39
        deep 943.49
          with loss of body part 943.59
    upper 943.03
      first degree 943.13
      second degree 943.23
      third degree 943.33
        deep 943.43
          with loss of body part 943.53
  auditory canal (external)—*see* Burn, ear

Burn—*continued*
  auricle (ear)—*see* Burn, ear
  axilla 943.04
    with
      upper limb(s) except hand(s) or wrist(s)—*see*
        Burn, arm(s), multiple sites
    first degree 943.14
    second degree 943.24
    third degree 943.34
      deep 943.44
        with loss of body part 943.54
  back 942.04
    with
      trunk—*see* Burn, trunk, multiple sites
    first degree 942.14
    second degree 942.24
    third degree 942.34
      deep 942.44
        with loss of body part 942.54
  biceps
    brachii—*see* Burn, arm(s), upper
    femoris—*see* Burn, thigh
  breast(s) 942.01
    with
      trunk—*see* Burn, trunk, multiple sites
    first degree 942.11
    second degree 942.21
    third degree 942.31
      deep 942.41
        with loss of body part 942.51
  brow—*see* Burn, forehead
  buttock(s)—*see* Burn, back
  canthus (eye) 940.1
    chemical 940.0
  cervix (uteri) 947.4
  cheek (cutaneous) 941.07
    with
      face or head—*see* Burn, head, multiple sites
    first degree 941.17
    second degree 941.27
    third degree 941.37
      deep 941.47
        with loss of body part 941.57
  chest wall (anterior) 942.02
    with
      trunk—*see* Burn, trunk, multiple sites
    first degree 942.12
    second degree 942.22
    third degree 942.32
      deep 942.42
        with loss of body part 942.52
  chin 941.04
    with
      face or head—*see* Burn, head, multiple sites
    first degree 941.14
    second degree 941.24
    third degree 941.34
      deep 941.44
        with loss of body part 941.54
  clitoris—*see* Burn, genitourinary organs,
    external
  colon 947.3
  conjunctiva (and cornea) 940.4
    chemical
      acid 940.3
      alkaline 940.2
  cornea (and conjunctiva) 940.4
    chemical
      acid 940.3
      alkaline 940.2
  costal region—*see* Burn, chest wall

Burn—*continued*
 vagina 947.4
 vulva—*see* Burn, genitourinary organs, external
 wrist(s) 944.07
   with
     hand(s)—*see* Burn, hand(s), multiple sites
   first degree 944.17
   second degree 944.27
   third degree 944.37
     deep 944.47
       with loss of body part 944.57
Burnett's syndrome (milk-alkali) 275.42
Burnier's syndrome (hypophyseal dwarfism)
 253.3
Burning
 feet syndrome 266.2
 sensation (*see also* Disturbance, sensation)
   782.0
 tongue 529.6
Burns' disease (osteochondrosis, lower ulna)
 732.3
Bursa —*see also* condition
 pharynx 478.29
Bursitis NEC 727.3
 Achilles tendon 726.71
 adhesive 726.90
   shoulder 726.0
 ankle 726.79
 buttock 726.5
 calcaneal 726.79
 collateral ligament
   fibular 726.63
   tibial 726.62
 Duplay's 726.2
 elbow 726.33
 finger 726.8
 foot 726.79
 gonococcal 098.52
 hand 726.4
 hip 726.5
 infrapatellar 726.69
 ischiogluteal 726.5
 knee 726.60
 occupational NEC 727.2
 olecranon 726.33
 pes anserinus 726.61
 pharyngeal 478.29
 popliteal 727.51
 prepatellar 726.65
 radiohumeral 727.3
 scapulohumeral 726.19
   adhesive 726.0
 shoulder 726.10
   adhesive 726.0
 subacromial 726.19
   adhesive 726.0
 subcoracoid 726.19
 subdeltoid 726.19
   adhesive 726.0
 subpatellar 726.69
 syphilitic 095.7
 Thornwaldt's, Tornwaldt's (pharyngeal) 478.29
 toe 726.79
 trochanteric area 726.5
 wrist 726.4
Burst stitches or sutures (complication of
 surgery) (external) 998.32
 internal 998.31
Buruli ulcer 031.1
Bury's disease (erythema elevatum diutinum)
 695.89

Buschke's disease or scleredema (adultorum)
 710.1
Busquet's disease (osteoperiostitis) (*see also*
 Osteomyelitis) 730.1
Busse-Buschke disease (cryptococcosis) 117.5
Buttock —*see* condition
Button
 Biskra 085.1
 Delhi 085.1
 oriental 085.1
Buttonhole hand (intrinsic) 736.21
Bwamba fever (encephalitis) 066.3
Byssinosis (occupational) 504
Bywaters' syndrome 958.5

C

Cacergasia 300.9
Cachexia 799.4
  cancerous —*see also* Neoplasm, by site,
    malignant 799.4
  cardiac—*see* Disease, heart
  dehydration 276.51
    with
      hypernatremia 276.0
      hyponatremia 276.1
  due to malnutrition 799.4
  exophthalmic 242.0
  heart—*see* Disease, heart
  hypophyseal 253.2
  hypopituitary 253.2
  lead 984.9
    specified type of lead—*see* Table of drugs and
      chemicals
  malaria 084.9
  malignant —*see also* Neoplasm, by site,
    malignant 799.4
  marsh 084.9
  nervous 300.5
  old age 797
  pachydermic—*see* Hypothyroidism
  paludal 084.9
  pituitary (postpartum) 253.2
  renal (*see also* Disease, renal) 593.9
  saturnine 984.9
    specified type of lead—*see* Table of drugs and
      chemicals
  senile 797
  Simmonds' (pituitary cachexia) 253.2
  splenica 289.59
  strumipriva (*see also* Hypothyroidism) 244.9
  tuberculous NEC (*see also* Tuberculosis) 011.9
café au lait spots 709.09
Caffey's disease or syndrome (infantile cortical
  hyperostosis) 756.59
Caisson disease 993.3
Caked breast (puerperal, postpartum) 676.2
Cake kidney 753.3
Calabar swelling 125.2
Calcaneal spur 726.73
Calcaneoapophysitis 732.5
Calcaneonavicular bar 755.67
Calcareous —*see* condition
Calcicosis (occupational) 502
Calciferol (vitamin D) deficiency 268.9
  with
    osteomalacia 268.2
    rickets (*see also* Rickets) 268.0
Calcification
  adrenal (capsule) (gland) 255.4
    tuberculous (*see also* Tuberculosis) 017.6
  aorta 440.0
  artery (annular)—*see* Arteriosclerosis
  auricle (ear) 380.89
  bladder 596.8
    due to S. hematobium 120.0
  brain (cortex)—*see* Calcification, cerebral
  bronchus 519.19
  bursa 727.82
  cardiac (*see also* Degeneration, myocardial) 429.1
  cartilage (postinfectional) 733.99
  cerebral (cortex) 348.8
    artery 437.0
  cervix (uteri) 622.8

Calcification—*continued*
  choroid plexus 349.2
  conjunctiva 372.54
  corpora cavernosa (penis) 607.89
  cortex (brain)—*see* Calcification, cerebral
  dental pulp (nodular) 522.2
  dentinal papilla 520.4
  disc, intervertebral 722.90
    cervical, cervicothoracic 722.91
    lumbar, lumbosacral 722.93
    thoracic, thoracolumbar 722.92
  fallopian tube 620.8
  falx cerebri—*see* Calcification, cerebral
  fascia 728.89
  gallbladder 575.8
  general 275.40
  heart (*see also* Degeneration, myocardial) 429.1
    valve—*see* Endocarditis
  intervertebral cartilage or disc (postinfectional)
    722.90
    cervical, cervicothoracic 722.91
    lumbar, lumbosacral 722.93
    thoracic, thoracolumbar 722.92
  intracranial—*see* Calcification, cerebral
  intraspinal ligament 728.89
  joint 719.80
    ankle 719.87
    elbow 719.82
    foot 719.87
    hand 719.84
    hip 719.85
    knee 719.86
    multiple sites 719.89
    pelvic region 719.85
    shoulder (region) 719.81
    specified site NEC 719.88
    wrist 719.83
  kidney 593.89
    tuberculous (*see also* Tuberculosis) 016.0
  larynx (senile) 478.79
  lens 366.8
  ligament 728.89
    intraspinal 728.89
    knee (medial collateral) 717.89
  lung 518.89
    active 518.89
    postinfectional 518.89
    tuberculous (*see also* Tuberculosis,
      pulmonary) 011.9
  lymph gland or node (postinfectional) 289.3
    tuberculous (*see also* Tuberculosis, lymph
      gland) 017.2
  mammographic 793.89
  massive (paraplegic) 728.10
  medial NEC (*see also* Arteriosclerosis,
    extremities) 440.20
  meninges (cerebral) 349.2
  metastatic 275.40
  Mönckeberg's—*see* Arteriosclerosis
  muscle 728.10
    heterotopic, postoperative 728.13
  myocardium, myocardial (*see also*
    Degeneration, myocardial) 429.1
  ovary 620.8
  pancreas 577.8
  penis 607.99
  periarticular 728.89
  pericardium (*see also* Pericarditis) 423.8

Calcification—*continued*
  pineal gland 259.8
  pleura 511.0
    postinfectional 518.89
    tuberculous (*see also* Tuberculosis, pleura)
      012.0
  pulp (dental) (nodular) 522.2
  renal 593.89
  rider's bone 733.99
  sclera 379.16
  semilunar cartilage 717.89
  spleen 289.59
  subcutaneous 709.3
  suprarenal (capsule) (gland) 255.4
  tendon (sheath) 727.82
    with bursitis, synovitis or tenosynovitis 727.82
  trachea 519.19
  ureter 593.89
  uterus 621.8
  vitreous 379.29
Calcified —*see also* Calcification
  hematoma NEC 959.9
Calcinosis (generalized) (interstitial) (tumoral)
  (universalis) 275.49
  circumscripta 709.3
  cutis 709.3
  intervertebralis 275.49 *[722.90]*
  Raynaud's
    phenomenonsclerodactylytelangiectasis
    (CRST) 710.1
Calciphylaxis (*see also* Calcification, by site)
  275.49
Calcium
  blood
    high (*see also* Hypercalcemia) 275.42
    low (*see also* Hypocalcemia) 275.41
  deposits—*see also* Calcification, by site
    in bursa 727.82
    in tendon (sheath) 727.82
      with bursitis, synovitis or tenosynovitis
      727.82
  salts or soaps in vitreous 379.22
Calciuria 791.9
Calculi —*see* Calculus
Calculosis, intrahepatic —*see*
  Choledocholithiasis
Calculus, calculi, calculous 592.9
  ampulla of Vater—*see* Choledocholithiasis
  anuria (impacted) (recurrent) 592.0
  appendix 543.9
  bile duct (any)—*see* Choledocholithiasis
  biliary—*see* Cholelithiasis
  bilirubin, multiple—*see* Cholelithiasis
  bladder (encysted) (impacted) (urinary) 594.1
    diverticulum 594.0
  bronchus 518.89
  calyx (kidney) (renal) 592.0
    congenital 753.3
  cholesterol (pure) (solitary)—*see* Cholelithiasis
  common duct (bile)—*see* Choledocholithiasis
  conjunctiva 372.54
  cystic 594.1
    duct—*see* Cholelithiasis
  dental 523.6
    subgingival 523.6
    supragingival 523.6
  epididymis 608.89

Calculus, calculi, calculous—*continued*
  gallbladder—*see also* Cholelithiasis
    congenital 751.69
  hepatic (duct)—*see* Choledocholithiasis
  intestine (impaction) (obstruction) 560.39
  kidney (impacted) (multiple) (pelvis) (recurrent)
    (staghorn) 592.0
    congenital 753.3
  lacrimal (passages) 375.57
  liver (impacted)—*see* Choledocholithiasis
  lung 518.89
  mammographic 793.89
  nephritic (impacted) (recurrent) 592.0
  nose 478.19
  pancreas (duct) 577.8
  parotid gland 527.5
  pelvis, encysted 592.0
  prostate 602.0
  pulmonary 518.89
  renal (impacted) (recurrent) 592.0
    congenital 753.3
  salivary (duct) (gland) 527.5
  seminal vesicle 608.89
  staghorn 592.0
  Stensen's duct 527.5
  sublingual duct or gland 527.5
    congenital 750.26
  submaxillary duct, gland, or region 527.5
  suburethral 594.8
  tonsil 474.8
  tooth, teeth 523.6
  tunica vaginalis 608.89
  ureter (impacted) (recurrent) 592.1
  urethra (impacted) 594.2
  urinary (duct) (impacted) (passage) (tract) 592.9
    lower tract NEC 594.9
      specified site 594.8
  vagina 623.8
  vesical (impacted) 594.1
  Wharton's duct 527.5
Caliectasis 593.89
California
  disease 114.0
  encephalitis 062.5
Caligo cornea 371.03
Callositas, callosity (infected) 700
Callus (infected) 700
  bone 726.91
  excessive, following fracture—*see also* Late,
    effect (of), fracture
Calvé (-Perthes) disease (osteochondrosis,
  femoral capital) 732.1
Calvities (*see also* Alopecia) 704.00
Cameroon fever (*see also* Malaria) 084.6
Camptocormia 300.11
Camptodactyly (congenital) 755.59
Camurati-Engelmann disease (diaphyseal
  sclerosis) 756.59
Canal —*see* condition
Canaliculitis (lacrimal) (acute) 375.31
  Actinomyces 039.8
  chronic 375.41
Canavan's disease 330.0

Cancer (M8000/3)—*see also* Neoplasm, by site, malignant

> *Note—The term "cancer" when modified by an adjective or adjectival phrase indicating a morphological type should be coded in the same manner as "carcinoma" with that adjective or phrase. Thus, "squamous-cell cancer" should be coded in the same manner as "squamous-cell carcinoma," which appears in the list under "Carcinoma."*

   bile duct type (M8160/3), liver 155.1
   hepatocellular (M8170/3) 155.0
Cancerous (M8000/3)—*see* Neoplasm, by site, malignant
Cancerphobia 300.29
Cancrum oris 528.1
Candidiasis, candidal 112.9
   with pneumonia 112.4
   balanitis 112.2
   congenital 771.7
   disseminated 112.5
   endocarditis 112.81
   esophagus 112.84
   intertrigo 112.3
   intestine 112.85
   lung 112.4
   meningitis 112.83
   mouth 112.0
   nails 112.3
   neonatal 771.7
   onychia 112.3
   otitis externa 112.82
   otomycosis 112.82
   paronychia 112.3
   perionyxis 112.3
   pneumonia 112.4
   pneumonitis 112.4
   skin 112.3
   specified site NEC 112.89
   systemic 112.5
   urogenital site NEC 112.2
   vagina 112.1
   vulva 112.1
   vulvovaginitis 112.1
Candidiosis —*see* Candidiasis
Candiru infection or infestation 136.8
Canities (premature) 704.3
   congenital 757.4
Canker (mouth) (sore) 528.2
   rash 034.1
Cannabinosis 504
Canton fever 081.9
Cap
   cradle 690.11
Capillariasis 127.5
Capillary —*see* condition
Caplan's syndrome 714.81
Caplan-Colinet syndrome 714.81
Capsule —*see* condition
Capsulitis (joint) 726.90
   adhesive (shoulder) 726.0
   hip 726.5
   knee 726.60
   labyrinthine 387.8
   thyroid 245.9
   wrist 726.4
Caput
   crepitus 756.0
   medusae 456.8
   succedaneum 767.19

Carapata disease 087.1
Carate —*see* Pinta
Carbohydrate-deficient glycoprotein syndrome (CDGS) 271.8
Carboxyhemoglobinemia 986
Carbuncle 680.9
   abdominal wall 680.2
   ankle 680.6
   anus 680.5
   arm (any part, above wrist) 680.3
   auditory canal, external 680.0
   axilla 680.3
   back (any part) 680.2
   breast 680.2
   buttock 680.5
   chest wall 680.2
   corpus cavernosum 607.2
   ear (any part) (external) 680.0
   eyelid 373.13
   face (any part, except eye) 680.0
   finger (any) 680.4
   flank 680.2
   foot (any part) 680.7
   forearm 680.3
   genital organ (male) 608.4
   gluteal (region) 680.5
   groin 680.2
   hand (any part) 680.4
   head (any part, except face) 680.8
   heel 680.7
   hip 680.6
   kidney (*see also* Abscess, kidney) 590.2
   knee 680.6
   labia 616.4
   lacrimal
      gland (*see also* Dacryoadenitis) 375.00
      passages (duct) (sac) (*see also* Dacryocystitis) 375.30
   leg, any part except foot 680.6
   lower extremity, any part except foot 680.6
   malignant 022.0
   multiple sites 680.9
   neck 680.1
   nose (external) (septum) 680.0
   orbit, orbital 376.01
   partes posteriores 680.5
   pectoral region 680.2
   penis 607.2
   perineum 680.2
   pinna 680.0
   scalp (any part) 680.8
   scrotum 608.4
   seminal vesicle 608.0
   shoulder 680.3
   skin NEC 680.9
   specified site NEC 680.8
   spermatic cord 608.4
   temple (region) 680.0
   testis 608.4
   thigh 680.6
   thumb 680.4
   toe (any) 680.7
   trunk 680.2
   tunica vaginalis 608.4
   umbilicus 680.2
   upper arm 680.3
   urethra 597.0
   vas deferens 608.4
   vulva 616.4
   wrist 680.4
Carbunculus (*see also* Carbuncle) 680.9

Carcinoid (tumor) (M8240/1)—*see also*
Neoplasm, by site, uncertain behavior
and struma ovarii (M9091/1) 236.2
argentaffin (M8241/1)—*see* Neoplasm, by site
uncertain behavior
malignant (M8241/3)—*see* Neoplasm, by site,
malignant
benign (M9091/0) 220
composite (M8244/3)—*see* Neoplasm, by site,
malignant
goblet cell (M8243/3)—*see* Neoplasm, by site,
malignant
malignant (M8240/1)—*see* Neoplasm, by site,
uncertain behavior
nonargentaffin (M8242/1)—*see also* Neoplasm,
by site, uncertain behavior
malignant (M8242/3)—*see* Neoplasm, by site,
malignantstrumal (M9091/1) 236.2
syndrome (intestinal) (metastatic) 259.2
type bronchial adenoma (M8240/3)—*see*
Neoplasm, lung, malignant
Carcinoidosis 259.2
Carcinoma (M8010/3)—*see also* Neoplasm, by
site, malignant

> *Note—Except where otherwise indicated, the*
> *morphological varieties of carcinoma in the list*
> *below should be coded by site as for*
> *"Neoplasm, malignant."*

with
apocrine metaplasia (M8573/3)
cartilaginous (and osseous) metaplasia
(M8571/3)
osseous (and cartilaginous) metaplasia
(M8571/3)
productive fibrosis (M8141/3)
spindle cell metaplasia (M8572/3)
squamous metaplasia (M8570/3)
acidophil (M8280/3)
specified site—*see* Neoplasm, by site,
malignant
unspecified site 194.3
acidophil-basophil, mixed (M8281/3)
specified site—*see* Neoplasm, by site,
malignant
unspecified site 194.3
acinar (cell) (M8550/3)
acinic cell (M8550/3)
adenocystic (M8200/3)
adenoid
cystic (M8200/3)
squamous cell (M8075/3)
adenosquamous (M8560/3)
adnexal (skin) (M8390/3)—*see* Neoplasm, skin,
malignant
adrenal cortical (M8370/3) 194.0
alveolar (M8251/3)
cell (M8250/3)—*see* Neoplasm, lung,
malignant
anaplastic type (M8021/3)
apocrine (M8401/3)
breast—*see* Neoplasm, breast, malignant
specified site NEC—*see* Neoplasm, skin,
malignant
unspecified site 173.9
basal cell (pigmented) (M8090/3)—*see also*
Neoplasm, skin, malignant
fibro-epithelial type (M8093/3)—*see*
Neoplasm, skin, malignant
morphea type (M8092/3)—*see* Neoplasm,
skin, malignant

Carcinoma—*continued*
multicentric (M8091/3)—*see* Neoplasm, skin,
malignant
basaloid (M8123/3)
basal-squamous cell, mixed (M8094/3)—*see*
Neoplasm, skin, malignant
basophil (M8300/3)
specified site—*see* Neoplasm, by site,
malignant
unspecified site 194.3
basophil-acidophil, mixed (M8281/3)
specified site—*see* Neoplasm, by site,
malignant
unspecified site 194.3
basosquamous (M8094/3)—*see* Neoplasm, skin,
malignant
bile duct type (M8160/3)
and hepatocellular, mixed (M8180/3) 155.0
liver 155.1
specified site NEC—*see* Neoplasm, by site,
malignant
unspecified site 155.1
branchial or branchiogenic 146.8
bronchial or bronchogenic—*see* Neoplasm,
lung, malignant
bronchiolar (terminal) (M8250/3)—*see*
Neoplasm, lung, malignant
bronchiolo-alveolar (M8250/3)—*see* Neoplasm,
lung, malignant
bronchogenic (epidermoid) 162.9
C cell (M8510/3)
specified site—*see* Neoplasm, by site,
malignant
unspecified site 193
ceruminous (M8420/3) 173.2
chorionic (M9100/3)
specified site—*see* Neoplasm, by site,
malignant
unspecified site
female 181
male 186.9
chromophobe (M8270/3)
specified site—*see* Neoplasm, by site,
malignant
unspecified site 194.3
clear cell (mesonephroid type) (M8310/3)
cloacogenic (M8124/3)
specified site—*see* Neoplasm, by site,
malignant
unspecified site 154.8
colloid (M8480/3)
cribriform (M8201/3)
cylindroid type (M8200/3)
diffuse type (M8145/3)
specified site—*see* Neoplasm, by site,
malignant
unspecified site 151.9
duct (cell) (M8500/3)
with Paget's disease (M8541/3)—*see*
Neoplasm, breast, malignant
infiltrating (M8500/3)
specified site—*see* Neoplasm, by site,
malignant
unspecified site 174.9
ductal (M8500/3)
ductular, infiltrating (M8521/3)
embryonal (M9070/3)
and teratoma, mixed (M9081/3)
combined with choriocarcinoma
(M9101/3)—*see* Neoplasm, by site,
malignant

Carcinoma—*continued*
    infantile type (M9071/3)
    liver 155.0
    polyembryonal type (M9072/3)
    endometrioid (M8380/3)
    eosinophil (M8280/3)
      specified site—*see* Neoplasm, by site,
        malignant
      unspecified site 194.3
    epidermoid (M8070/3)—*see also* Carcinoma,
      squamous cell
      and adenocarcinoma, mixed (M8560/3)
      in situ, Bowen's type (M8081/2)—*see*
        Neoplasm, skin, in situ
    intradermal—*see* Neoplasm, skin, in situ
    fibroepithelial type basal cell (M8093/3)—*see*
      Neoplasm, skin, malignant
    follicular (M8330/3)
      and papillary (mixed) (M8340/3) 193
      moderately differentiated type (M8332/3) 193
      pure follicle type (M8331/3) 193
      specified site—*see* Neoplasm, by site,
        malignant
      trabecular type (M8332/3) 193
      unspecified site 193
      well differentiated type (M8331/3) 193
    gelatinous (M8480/3)
    giant cell (M8031/3)
      and spindle cell (M8030/3)
    granular cell (M8320/3)
    granulosa cell (M8620/3) 183.0
    hepatic cell (M8170/3) 155.0
    hepatocellular (M8170/3) 155.0
      and bile duct, mixed (M8180/3)
        155.0
    hepatocholangiolitic (M8180/3) 155.0
    Hurthle cell (thyroid) 193
    hypernephroid (M8311/3)
    in
      adenomatous
        polyp (M8210/3)
        polyposis coli (M8220/3) 153.9
      pleomorphic adenoma (M8940/3)
      polypoid adenoma (M8210/3)
      situ (M8010/3)—*see* Carcinoma,
        in situ
      tubular adenoma (M8210/3)
      villous adenoma (M8261/3)
    infiltrating duct (M8500/3)
      with Paget's disease (M8541/3)—*see*
        Neoplasm, breast, malignant
      specified site—*see* Neoplasm, by site,
        malignant
      unspecified site 174.9
    inflammatory (M8530/3)
      specified site—*see* Neoplasm, by site,
        malignant
      unspecified site 174.9
    in situ (M8010/2)—*see also* Neoplasm, by site,
      in situ
      epidermoid (M8070/2)—*see also* Neoplasm,
        by site, in situ
        with questionable stromal invasion
          (M8076/2)
          specified site—*see* Neoplasm, by site, in
            situ
          unspecified site 233.1
        Bowen's type (M8081/2)—*see* Neoplasm,
          skin, in situ

Carcinoma—*continued*
    intraductal (M8500/2)
      specified site—*see* Neoplasm, by site, in situ
      unspecified site 233.0
    lobular (M8520/2)
      specified site—*see* Neoplasm, by site, in situ
      unspecified site 233.0
    papillary (M8050/2)—*see* Neoplasm, by site,
      in situ
    squamous cell (M8070/2)—*see also*
      Neoplasm, by site, in situ
    with questionable stromal invasion (M8076/2)
      specified site—*see* Neoplasm, by site, in
        situ
      unspecified site 233.1
    transitional cell (M8120/2)—*see* Neoplasm,
      by site, in situ
    intestinal type (M8144/3)
      specified site—*see* Neoplasm, by site,
        malignant
      unspecified site 151.9
    intraductal (noninfiltrating) (M8500/2)
      papillary (M8503/2)
        specified site—*see* Neoplasm, by site, in situ
        unspecified site 233.0
      specified site—*see* Neoplasm, by site, in situ
      unspecified site 233.0
    intraepidermal (M8070/2)—*see also* Neoplasm,
      skin, in situ
      squamous cell, Bowen's type (M8081/2)—*see*
        Neoplasm, skin, in situ
    intraepithelial (M8010/2)—*see also* Neoplasm,
      by site, in situ
      squamous cell (M8072/2)—*see* Neoplasm, by
        site, in situ
    intraosseous (M9270/3) 170.1
      upper jaw (bone) 170.0
    islet cell (M8150/3)
      and exocrine, mixed (M8154/3)
        specified site—*see* Neoplasm, by site,
          malignant
        unspecified site 157.9
      pancreas 157.4
      specified site NEC—*see* Neoplasm, by site,
        malignant
      unspecified site 157.4
    juvenile, breast (M8502/3)—*see* Neoplasm,
      breast, malignant
    Kulchitsky's cell (carcinoid tumor of intestine)
      259.2
    large cell (M8012/3)
      squamous cell, nonkeratinizing type
        (M8072/3)
    Leydig cell (testis) (M8650/3)
      specified site—*see* Neoplasm, by site,
        malignant
      unspecified site 186.9
        female 183.0
        male 186.9
    liver cell (M8170/3) 155.0
    lobular (infiltrating) (M8520/3)
      non-infiltrating (M8520/3)
        specified site—*see* Neoplasm, by site, in situ
        unspecified site 233.0
      specified site—*see* Neoplasm, by site,
        malignant
      unspecified site 174.9
    lymphoepithelial (M8082/3)
    medullary (M8510/3)
      with
        amyloid stroma (M8511/3)

Carcinoma—*continued*
    specified site—*see* Neoplasm, by site,
      malignant
    unspecified site 193
   lymphoid stroma (M8512/3)
    specified site—*see* Neoplasm, by site,
      malignant
    unspecified site 174.9
  mesometanephric (M9110/3)
  mesonephric (M9110/3)
  metastatic (M8010/6)—*see* Metastasis, cancer
  metatypical (M8095/3)—*see* Neoplasm, skin,
    malignant
  morphea type basal cell (M8092/3)—*see*
    Neoplasm, skin, malignant
  mucinous (M8480/3)
  mucin-producing (M8481/3)
  mucin-secreting (M8481/3)
  mucoepidermoid (M8430/3)
  mucoid (M8480/3)
   cell (M8300/3)
    specified site—*see* Neoplasm, by site,
      malignant
    unspecified site 194.3
  mucous (M8480/3)
  nonencapsulated sclerosing (M8350/3) 193
  noninfiltrating
   intracystic (M8504/2)—*see* Neoplasm, by site,
    in situ
   intraductal (M8500/2)
    papillary (M8503/2)
     specified site—*see* Neoplasm, by site, in
      situ
      unspecified site 233.0
    specified site—*see* Neoplasm, by site, in situ
    unspecified site 233.0
   lobular (M8520/2)
    specified site—*see* Neoplasm, by site, in situ
    unspecified site 233.0
  oat cell (M8042/3)
   specified site—*see* Neoplasm, by site,
    malignant
   unspecified site 162.9
  odontogenic (M9270/3) 170.1
   upper jaw (bone) 170.0
  onocytic (M8290/3)
  oxyphilic (M8290/3)
  papillary (M8050/3)
   and follicular (mixed) (M8340/3) 193
   epidermoid (M8052/3)
   intraductal (noninfiltrating) (M8503/2)
    specified site—*see* Neoplasm, by site, in situ
    unspecified site 233.0
   serous (M8460/3)
    specified site—*see* Neoplasm, by site,
      malignant
    surface (M8461/3)
     specified site—*see* Neoplasm, by site,
      malignant
     unspecified site 183.0
    unspecified site 183.0
   squamous cell (M8052/3)
   transitional cell (M8130/3)
  papillocystic (M8450/3)
   specified site—*see* Neoplasm, by site,
    malignant
   unspecified site 183.0
  parafollicular cell (M8510/3)
   specified site—*see* Neoplasm, by site,
    malignant
   unspecified site 193

Carcinoma—*continued*
  pleomorphic (M8022/3)
  polygonal cell (M8034/3)
  prickle cell (M8070/3)
  pseudoglandular, squamous cell (M8075/3)
  pseudomucinous (M8470/3)
   specified site—*see* Neoplasm, by site,
    malignant
   unspecified site 183.0
  pseudosarcomatous (M8033/3)
  regaud type (M8082/3)—*see* Neoplasm,
    nasopharynx, malignant
  renal cell (M8312/3) 189.0
  reserve cell (M8041/3)
  round cell (M8041/3)
  Schmincke (M8082/3)—*see* Neoplasm,
    nasopharynx, malignant
  Schneiderian (M8121/3)
   specified site—*see* Neoplasm, by site,
    malignant
   unspecified site 160.0
  scirrhous (M8141/3)
  sebaceous (M8410/3)—*see* Neoplasm, skin,
    malignant
  secondary (M8010/6)—*see* Neoplasm, by site,
    malignant, secondary
  secretory, breast (M8502/3)—*see* Neoplasm,
    breast, malignant
  serous (M8441/3)
   papillary (M8460/3)
    specified site—*see* Neoplasm, by site,
      malignant
    unspecified site 183.0
   surface, papillary (M8461/3)
    specified site—*see* Neoplasm, by site,
      malignant
    unspecified site 183.0
  Sertoli cell (M8640/3)
   specified site—*see* Neoplasm, by site,
    malignant
   unspecified site 186.9
  signet ring cell (M8490/3)
   metastatic (M8490/6)—*see* Neoplasm, by site,
    secondary
  simplex (M8231/3)
  skin appendage (M8390/3)—*see* Neoplasm,
    skin, malignant
  small cell (M8041/3)
   fusiform cell type (M8043/3)
   squamous cell, non-keratinizing type
    (M8073/3)
  solid (M8230/3)
   with amyloid stroma (M8511/3)
    specified site—*see* Neoplasm, by site,
      malignant
    unspecified site 193
  spheroidal cell (M8035/3)
  spindle cell (M8032/3)
   and giant cell (M8030/3)
  spinous cell (M8070/3)
  squamous (cell) (M8070/3)
   adenoid type (M8075/3)
   and adenocarcinoma, mixed (M8560/3)
   intraepidermal, Bowen's type—*see* Neoplasm,
    skin, in situ
   keratinizing type (large cell) (M8071/3)
   large cell, non-keratinizing type (M8072/3)
   microinvasive (M8076/3)
    specified site—*see* Neoplasm, by site,
      malignant
    unspecified site 180.9

Carditis (acute) (bacterial) (chronic) (subacute) 429.89
  Coxsackie 074.20
  hypertensive (*see also* Hypertension, heart) 402.90
  meningococcal 036.40
  rheumatic—*see* Disease, heart, rheumatic
  rheumatoid 714.2
Care (of)
  child (routine) V20.1
  convalescent following V66.9
    chemotherapy V66.2
    medical NEC V66.5
    psychotherapy V66.3
    radiotherapy V66.1
    surgery V66.0
    surgical NEC V66.0
    treatment (for) V66.5
      combined V66.6
      fracture V66.4
      mental disorder NEC V66.3
      specified type NEC V66.5
  end-of-life care V66.7
  family member (handicapped) (sick)
    creating problem for family V61.49
    provided away from home for holiday relief V60.5
    unavailable, due to
      absence (person rendering care) (sufferer) V60.4
      inability (any reason) of person rendering care V60.4
  holiday relief V60.5
  hospice V66.7
  lack of (at or after birth) (infant) (child) 995.52
    adult 995.84
  lactation of mother V24.1
  palliative V66.7
  postpartum
    immediately after delivery V24.0
    routine follow-up V24.2
  prenatal V22.1
    first pregnancy V22.0
    high risk pregnancy V23.9
      specified problem NEC V23.8
  terminal V66.7
  unavailable, due to
    absence of person rendering care V60.4
    inability (any reason) of person rendering care V60.4
  well baby V20.1
Caries (bone) (*see also* Tuberculosis, bone) 015.9 *[730.8]*
  arrested 521.04
  cementum 521.03
  cerebrospinal (tuberculous) 015.0 *[730.88]*
  dental (acute) (chronic) (incipient) (infected) 521.00
    with pulp exposure 521.03
    extending to
      dentine 521.02
      pulp 521.03
    other specified NEC 521.09
    pit and fissure 521.06
    primary
      pit and fissure origin 521.06
      root surface 521.08
      smooth surface origin 521.07
    root surface 521.08
    smooth surface 521.07
  dentin (acute) (chronic) 521.02

Caries—*continued*
  enamel (acute) (chronic) (incipient) 521.01
  external meatus 380.89
  hip (*see also* Tuberculosis) 015.1 *[730.85]*
  initial 521.01
  knee 015.2 *[730.86]*
  labyrinth 386.8
  limb NEC 015.7 *[730.88]*
  mastoid (chronic) (process) 383.1
  middle ear 385.89
  nose 015.7 *[730.88]*
  orbit 015.7 *[730.88]*
  ossicle 385.24
  petrous bone 383.20
  sacrum (tuberculous) 015.0 *[730.88]*
  spine, spinal (column) (tuberculous) 015.0 *[730.88]*
  syphilitic 095.5
    congenital 090.0 *[730.8]*
  teeth (internal) 521.00
    initial 521.01
  vertebra (column) (tuberculous) 015.0 *[730.88]*
Carini's syndrome (ichthyosis congenita) 757.1
Carious teeth 521.00
Carneous mole 631
Carnosinemia 270.5
Carotid body or sinus syndrome 337.0
Carotidynia 337.0
Carotinemia (dietary) 278.3
Carotinosis (cutis) (skin) 278.3
Carpal tunnel syndrome 354.0
Carpenter's syndrome 759.89
Carpopedal spasm (*see also* Tetany) 781.7
Carpoptosis 736.05
Carrier (suspected) of
  amebiasis V02.2
  bacterial disease (meningococcal, staphylococcal, streptococcal) NEC V02.59
  cholera V02.0
  cystic fibrosis gene V83.81
  defective gene V83.89
  diphtheria V02.4
  dysentery (bacillary) V02.3
    amebic V02.2
  Endamoeba histolytica V02.2
  gastrointestinal pathogens NEC V02.3
  genetic defect V83.89
  gonorrhea V02.7
  group B streptococcus V02.51
  HAA (hepatitis Australian-antigen) V02.61
  hemophilia A (asymptomatic) V83.01
    symptomatic V83.02
  hepatitis V02.60
    Australian-antigen (HAA) V02.61
    B V02.61
    C V02.62
    serum V02.61
    specified type NEC V02.69
    viral V02.60
  infective organism NEC V02.9
  malaria V02.9
  paratyphoid V02.3
  Salmonella V02.3
    typhosa V02.1
  serum hepatitis V02.61
  Shigella V02.3
  Staphylococcus NEC V02.59
  Streptococcus NEC V02.52
    group B V02.51
  typhoid V02.1
  venereal disease NEC V02.8

Cell, cellular —*see also* condition
  anterior chamber (eye) (positive aqueous ray)
    364.04
Cellulitis (diffuse) (with lymphangitis) (*see also*
    Abscess) 682.9
  abdominal wall 682.2
  anaerobic (*see also* Gas gangrene) 040.0
  ankle 682.6
  anus 566
  areola 611.0
  arm (any part, above wrist) 682.3
  auditory canal (external) 380.10
  axilla 682.3
  back (any part) 682.2
  breast 611.0
    postpartum 675.1
  broad ligament (*see also* Disease, pelvis,
    inflammatory) 614.4
    acute 614.3
  buttock 682.5
  cervical (neck region) 682.1
  cervix (uteri) (*see also* Cervicitis) 616.0
  cheek, external 682.0
    internal 528.3
  chest wall 682.2
  chronic NEC 682.9
  colostomy 569.61
  corpus cavernosum 607.2
  digit 681.9
  Douglas' cul-de-sac or pouch (chronic) (*see also*
    Disease, pelvis, inflammatory) 614.4
    acute 614.3
  drainage site (following operation) 998.59
  ear, external 380.10
  enterostomy 569.61
  erysipelar (*see also* Erysipelas) 035
  esophagostomy 530.86
  eyelid 373.13
  face (any part, except eye) 682.0
  finger (intrathecal) (periosteal) (subcutaneous)
    (subcuticular) 681.00
  flank 682.2
  foot (except toe) 682.7
  forearm 682.3
  gangrenous (*see also* Gangrene) 785.4
  genital organ NEC
    female—*see* Abscess, genital organ, female
    male 608.4
  glottis 478.71
  gluteal (region) 682.5
  gonococcal NEC 098.0
  groin 682.2
  hand (except finger or thumb) 682.4
  head (except face) NEC 682.8
  heel 682.7
  hip 682.6
  jaw (region) 682.0
  knee 682.6
  labium (majus) (minus) (*see also* Vulvitis)
    616.10
  larynx 478.71
  leg, except foot 682.6
  lip 528.5
  mammary gland 611.0
  mouth (floor) 528.3
  multiple sites NEC 682.9
  nasopharynx 478.21
  navel 682.2
    newborn NEC 771.4
  neck (region) 682.1
  nipple 611.0

Cellulitis—*continued*
  nose 478.19
    external 682.0
  orbit, orbital 376.01
  palate (soft) 528.3
  pectoral (region) 682.2
  pelvis, pelvic
    with
      abortion—*see* Abortion, by type, with sepsis
      ectopic pregnancy (*see also* categories
        633.0-633.9) 639.0
      molar pregnancy (*see also* categories
        630-632) 639.0
    female (*see also* Disease, pelvis,
      inflammatory) 614.4
      acute 614.3
    following
      abortion 639.0
      ectopic or molar pregnancy 639.0
    male 567.21
    puerperal, postpartum, childbirth 670
  penis 607.2
  perineal, perineum 682.2
  perirectal 566
  peritonsillar 475
  periurethral 597.0
  periuterine (*see also* Disease, pelvis,
    inflammatory) 614.4
    acute 614.3
  pharynx 478.21
  phlegmonous NEC 682.9
  rectum 566
  retromammary 611.0
  retroperitoneal (*see also* Peritonitis) 567.238
  round ligament (*see also* Disease, pelvis,
    inflammatory) 614.4
    acute 614.3
  scalp (any part) 682.8
    dissecting 704.8
  scrotum 608.4
  seminal vesicle 608.0
  septic NEC 682.9
  shoulder 682.3
  specified sites NEC 682.8
  spermatic cord 608.4
  submandibular (region) (space) (triangle) 682.0
    gland 527.3
  submaxillary 528.3
    gland 527.3
  submental (pyogenic) 682.0
    gland 527.3
  suppurative NEC 682.9
  testis 608.4
  thigh 682.6
  thumb (intrathecal) (periosteal) (subcutaneous)
    (subcuticular) 681.00
  toe (intrathecal) (periosteal) (subcutaneous)
    (subcuticular) 681.10
  tonsil 475
  trunk 682.2
  tuberculous (primary) (*see also* Tuberculosis)
    017.0
  tunica vaginalis 608.4
  umbilical 682.2
    newborn NEC 771.4
  vaccinal 999.3
  vagina—*see* Vaginitis
  vas deferens 608.4
  vocal cords 478.5
  vulva (*see also* Vulvitis) 616.10
  wrist 682.4

Cementoblastoma, benign (M9273/0) 213.1
  upper jaw (bone) 213.0
Cementoma (M9273/0) 213.1
  gigantiform (M9276/0) 213.1
    upper jaw (bone) 213.0
  upper jaw (bone) 213.0
Cementoperiostitis 523.40
Cephalgia, cephalalgia (*see also* Headache) 784.0
  histamine 346.2
  nonorganic origin 307.81
  psychogenic 307.81
  tension 307.81
Cephalhematocele, cephalematocele
  due to birth injury 767.19
  fetus or newborn 767.19
  traumatic (*see also* Contusion, head) 920
Cephalhematoma, cephalematoma (calcified)
  due to birth injury 767.19
  fetus or newborn 767.19
  traumatic (*see also* Contusion, head) 920
Cephalic —*see* condition
Cephalitis —*see* Encephalitis
Cephalocele 742.0
Cephaloma —*see* Neoplasm, by site,
  malignant
Cephalomenia 625.8
Cephalopelvic —*see* condition
Cercomoniasis 007.3
Cerebellitis —*see* Encephalitis
Cerebellum (cerebellar)—*see* condition
Cerebral —*see* condition
Cerebritis —*see* Encephalitis
Cerebrohepatorenal syndrome 759.89
Cerebromacular degeneration 330.1
Cerebromalacia (*see also* Softening, brain) 434.9
Cerebrosidosis 272.7
Cerebrospasticity —*see* Palsy, cerebral
Cerebrospinal —*see* condition
Cerebrum —*see* condition
Ceroid storage disease 272.7
Cerumen (accumulation) (impacted) 380.4
Cervical —*see also* condition
  auricle 744.43
  high risk human papillomavirus (HPV) DNA
    test positive 795.05
  intraepithelial glandular neoplasia 233.1
  low rish human papillomavirus (Hpv) DNA test
    positive 795.09
  rib 756.2
Cervicalgia 723.1
Cervicitis (acute) (chronic) (nonvenereal)
    (subacute) (with erosion or ectropion) 616.0
  with
    abortion—*see* Abortion, by type, with sepsis
    ectopic pregnancy (*see also* categories
      633.0-633.9) 639.0
    molar pregnancy (*see also* categories 630-632)
      639.0
    ulceration 616.0
  chlamydial 099.53
  complicating pregnancy or puerperium 646.6
    affecting fetus or newborn 760.8
  following
    abortion 639.0
    ectopic or molar pregnancy 639.0
  gonococcal (acute) 098.15
    chronic or duration of 2 months or more 098.35
  senile (atrophic) 616.0
  syphilitic 095.8
  trichomonal 131.09
  tuberculous (*see also* Tuberculosis) 016.7

Cervicoaural fistula 744.49
Cervicocolpitis (emphysematosa) (*see also*
    Cervicitis) 616.0
Cervix —*see* condition
Cesarean delivery, operation or section NEC
    669.7
  affecting fetus or newborn 763.4
  post mortem, affecting fetus or newborn 761.6
  previous, affecting management of pregnancy
    654.2
Céstan's syndrome 344.89
Céstan-Chenais paralysis 344.89
Céstan-Raymond syndrome 433.8
Cestode infestation NEC 123.9
  specified type NEC 123.8
Cestodiasis 123.9
CGF (congenital generalized fibromatosis) 759.89
Chaberts' disease 022.9
Chacaleh 266.2
Chafing 709.8
Chagas' disease (*see also* Trypanosomiasis,
    American) 086.2
  with heart involvement 086.0
Chagres fever 084.0
Chalasia (cardiac sphincter) 530.81
Chalazion 373.2
Chalazoderma 757.39
Chalcosis 360.24
  cornea 371.15
  crystalline lens 360.24 [366.34]
  retina 360.24
Chalicosis (occupational) (pulmonum) 502
Chancre (any genital site) (hard) (indurated)
    (infecting) (primary) (recurrent) 091.0
  congenital 090.0
  conjunctiva 091.2
  Ducrey's 099.0
  extragenital 091.2
  eyelid 091.2
  Hunterian 091.0
  lip (syphilis) 091.2
  mixed 099.8
  nipple 091.2
  Nisbet's 099.0
  of
    carate 103.0
    pinta 103.0
    yaws 102.0
  palate, soft 091.2
  phagedenic 099.0
  Ricord's 091.0
  Rollet's (syphilitic) 091.0
  seronegative 091.0
  seropositive 091.0
  simple 099.0
  soft 099.0
    bubo 099.0
  urethra 091.0
  yaws 102.0
Chancriform syndrome 114.1
Chancroid 099.0
  anus 099.0
  penis (Ducrey's bacillus) 099.0
  perineum 099.0
  rectum 099.0
  scrotum 099.0
  urethra 099.0
  vulva 099.0
Chandipura fever 066.8
Chandler's disease (osteochondritis dissecans,
    hip) 732.7

> *Note—for malignant change occurring in a neoplasm, use the appropriate M code with behavior digit /3 e.g., malignant change in uterine fibroid—M8890/3. For malignant change occurring in a nonneoplastic condition (e.g., gastric ulcer) use the M code M8000/3.*

Chokes (resulting from bends) 993.3
Choking sensation 784.99
Cholangiectasis (*see also* Disease, gallbladder) 575.8
Cholangiocarcinoma (M8160/3)
  and hepatocellular carcinoma, combined (M8180/3) 155.0
  liver 155.1
  specified site NEC—*see* Neoplasm, by site, malignant
  unspecified site 155.1
Cholangiohepatitis 575.8
  due to fluke infestation 121.1
Cholangiohepatoma (M8180/3) 155.0
Cholangiolitis (acute) (chronic) (extrahepatic) (gangrenous) 576.1
  intrahepatic 575.8
  paratyphoidal (*see also* Fever, paratyphoid) 002.9
  typhoidal 002.0
Cholangioma (M8160/0) 211.5
  malignant—*see* Cholangiocarcinoma
Cholangitis (acute) (ascending) (catarrhal) (chronic) (infective) (malignant) (primary) (recurrent) (sclerosing) (secondary) (stenosing) (suppurative) 576.1
  chronic nonsuppurative destructive 571.6
  nonsuppurative destructive (chronic) 571.6
Cholecystdocholithiasis —*see* Choledocholithiasis
Cholecystitis 575.10
  with
    calculus, stones in
      bile duct (common) (hepatic)—*see* Choledocholithiasis
      gallbladder—*see* Cholelithiasis
  acute and chronic 575.12
  chronic 575.11
  emphysematous (acute) (*see also* Cholecystitis, acute) 575.0
  gangrenous (*see also* Cholecystitis, acute) 575.0
  paratyphoidal, current (*see also* Fever, paratyphoid) 002.9
  suppurative (*see also* Cholecystitis, acute) 575.0
  typhoidal 002.0
Choledochitis (suppurative) 576.1
Choledocholith —*see* Choledocholithiasis
Choledocholithiasis 574.5

> *Note—Use the following fifth-digit subclassification with category 574:*
>
> *0 without mention of obstruction*
> *1 with obstruction*

  with
    cholecystitis 574.4
      acute 574.3
      chronic 574.4
    cholelithiasis 574.9
      with
        cholecystitis 574.7
          acute 574.6
            and chronic 574.8
          chronic 574.7

Cholelithiasis (impacted) (multiple) 574.2

> *Note—Use the following fifth-digit subclassification with category 574:*
>
> *0 without mention of obstruction*
> *1 with obstruction*

  with
    cholecystitis 574.1
      acute 574.0
      chronic 574.1
    choledocholithiasis 574.9
      with
        cholecystitis 574.7
          acute 574.6
            and chronic 574.8
          chronic cholecystitis 574.7
Cholemia (*see also* Jaundice) 782.4
  familial 277.4
  Gilbert's (familial nonhemolytic) 277.4
Cholemic gallstone —*see* Cholelithiasis
Choleperitoneum, choleperitonitis (*see also* Disease, gallbladder) 567.81
Cholera (algid) (Asiatic) (asphyctic) (epidemic) (gravis) (Indian) (malignant) (morbus) (pestilential) (spasmodic) 001.9
  antimonial 985.4
  carrier (suspected) of V02.0
  classical 001.0
  contact V01.0
  due to
    Vibrio
      cholerae (Inaba, Ogawa, Hikojima serotypes) 001.0
      El Tor 001.1
  El Tor 001.1
  exposure to V01.0
  vaccination, prophylactic (against) V03.0
Cholerine (*see also* Cholera) 001.9
Cholestasis 576.8
  due to total parenteral nutrition (TPN) 573.8
Cholesteatoma (ear) 385.30
  attic (primary) 385.31
  diffuse 385.35
  external ear (canal) 380.21
  marginal (middle ear) 385.32
    with involvement of mastoid cavity 385.33
    secondary (with middle ear involvement) 385.33
  mastoid cavity 385.30
  middle ear (secondary) 385.32
    with involvement of mastoid cavity 385.33—
  postmastoidectomy cavity (recurrent) 383.32
  primary 385.31
  recurrent, postmastoidectomy cavity 383.32
  secondary (middle ear) 385.32
    with involvement of mastoid cavity 385.33
Cholesteatosis (middle ear) (*see also* Cholesteatoma) 385.30
  diffuse 385.35
Cholesteremia 272.0
Cholesterin
  granuloma, middle ear 385.82
  in vitreous 379.22
Cholesterol
  deposit
    retina 362.82
    vitreous 379.22
  imbibition of gallbladder (*see also* Disease, gallbladder) 575.6

Cholesterolemia 272.0
  essential 272.0
  familial 272.0
  hereditary 272.0
Cholesterosis, cholesterolosis (gallbladder) 575.6
  middle ear (*see also* Cholesteatoma) 385.30
  with
      cholecystitis—*see* Cholecystitis
      cholelithiasis—*see* Cholelithiasis
Cholocolic fistula (*see also* Fistula, gallbladder)
    575.5
Choluria 791.4
Chondritis (purulent) 733.99
  auricle 380.03
  costal 733.6
      Tietze's 733.6
  patella, posttraumatic 717.7
  pinna 380.03
  posttraumatica patellae 717.7
  tuberculous (active) (*see also* Tuberculosis) 015.9
      intervertebral 015.0 *[730.88]*
Chondroangiopathia calcarea seu punctate
    756.59
Chondroblastoma (M9230/0)—*see also*
    Neoplasm, bone, benign
  malignant (M9230/3)—*see* Neoplasm, bone,
      malignant
Chondrocalcinosis (articular) (crystal deposition)
    (dihydrate) (*see also* Arthritis, due to, crystals)
    275.49 *[712.3]*
  due to
      calcium pyrophosphate 275.49 *[712.2]*
      dicalcium phosphate crystals 275.49 *[712.1]*
      pyrophosphate crystals 275.4 *[712.2]*
Chondrodermatitis nodularis helicis 380.00
Chondrodysplasia 756.4
  angiomatose 756.4
  calcificans congenita 756.59
  epiphysialis punctata 756.59
  hereditary deforming 756.4
  rhizomelic punctata 277.86
Chondrodystrophia (fetalis) 756.4
  calcarea 756.4
  calcificans congenita 756.59
  fetalis hypoplastica 756.59
  hypoplastica calcinosa 756.59
  punctata 756.59
  tarda 277.5
Chondrodystrophy (familial) (hypoplastic) 756.4
Chondroectodermal dysplasia 756.55
Chondrolysis 733.99
Chondroma (M9220/0)—*see also* Neoplasm
    cartilage, benign
  juxtacortical (M9221/0)—*see* Neoplasm, bone,
      benign
  periosteal (M9221/0)—*see* Neoplasm, bone,
      benign
Chondromalacia 733.92
  epiglottis (congenital) 748.3
  generalized 733.92
  knee 717.7
  larynx (congenital) 748.3
  localized, except patella 733.92
  patella, patellae 717.7
  systemic 733.92
  tibial plateau 733.92
  trachea (congenital) 748.3
Chondromatosis (M9220/1)—*see* Neoplasm,
    cartilage, uncertain behavior
Chondromyxosarcoma (M9220/3)—*see*
    Neoplasm, cartilage, malignant

Chondro-osteodysplasia (Morquio-Brailsford
    type) 277.5
Chondro-osteodystrophy 277.5
Chondro-osteodystrophy 277.5
Chondro-osteoma (M9210/0)—*see* Neoplasm,
    bone, benign
Chondropathia tuberosa 733.6
Chondrosarcoma (M9220/3)—*see also*
    Neoplasm, cartilage, malignant
  juxtacortical (M9221/3)—*see* Neoplasm, bone,
      malignant
  mesenchymal (M9240/3)—*see* Neoplasm,
      connective tissue, malignant
Chordae tendineae rupture (chronic) 429.5
Chordee (nonvenereal) 607.89
  congenital 752.63
  gonococcal 098.2
Chorditis (fibrinous) (nodosa) (tuberosa) 478.5
Chordoma (M9370/3)—*see* Neoplasm, by site,
    malignant
Chorea (gravis) (minor) (spasmodic) 333.5
  with
      heart involvement—*see* Chorea with
          rheumatic heart disease
      rheumatic heart disease (chronic, inactive, or
          quiescent) (conditions classifiable to
          393-398)—*see also* Rheumatic heart
          condition involved
      active or acute (conditions classifiable to
          391) 392.0
  acute—*see* Chorea, Sydenham's
  apoplectic (*see also* Disease, cerebrovascular,
      acute) 436
  chronic 333.4
  electric 049.8
  gravidarum—*see* Eclampsia, pregnancy
  habit 307.22
  hereditary 333.4
  Huntington's 333.4
  posthemiplegic 344.89
  pregnancy—*see* Eclampsia, pregnancy
  progressive 333.4
      chronic 333.4
      hereditary 333.4
  rheumatic (chronic) 392.9
      with heart disease or involvement—*see*
          Chorea, with rheumatic heart disease
  senile 333.5
  Sydenham's 392.9
      with heart involvement—*see* Chorea, with
          rheumatic heart disease
      nonrheumatic 333.5
  variabilis 307.23
Choreoathetosis (paroxysmal) 333.5
Chorioadenoma (destruens) (M9100/1) 236.1
Chorioamnionitis 658.4
  affecting fetus or newborn 762.7
Chorioangioma (M9120/0) 219.8
Choriocarcinoma (M9100/3)
  combined with
      embryonal carcinoma (M9101/3)—*see*
          Neoplasm, by site, malignant
      teratoma (M9101/3)—*see* Neoplasm, by site,
          malignant
  specified site—*see* Neoplasm, by site, malignant
  unspecified site
      female 181
      male 186.9
Chorioencephalitis, lymphocytic (acute)
    (serous) 049.0

Cirrhosis, cirrhotic—*continued*
   congenital (due to failure of obliteration of
      umbilical vein) 777.8
   cryptogenic 571.5
     alcoholic 571.2
   fatty 571.8
     alcoholic 571.0
   macronodular 571.5
     alcoholic 571.2
   micronodular 571.5
     alcoholic 571.2
   nodular, diffuse 571.5
     alcoholic 571.2
   pigmentary 275.0
   portal 571.5
     alcoholic 571.2
   postnecrotic 571.5
     alcoholic 571.2
   syphilitic 095.3
  lung (chronic) (*see also* Fibrosis, lung) 515
  macronodular (of liver) 571.5
   alcoholic 571.2
  malarial 084.9
  metabolic NEC 571.5
  micronodular (of liver) 571.5
   alcoholic 571.2
  monolobular—*see* Cirrhosis, portal
  multilobular—*see* Cirrhosis, portal
  nephritis (*see also* Sclerosis, renal) 587
  nodular—*see* Cirrhosis, liver
  nutritional (fatty) 571.5
  obstructive (biliary) (extrahepatic)
    (intrahepatic)—*see* Cirrhosis, biliary
  ovarian 620.8
  paludal 084.9
  pancreas (duct) 577.8
  pericholangiolitic—*see* Cirrhosis, biliary
  periportal—*see* Cirrhosis, portal
  pigment, pigmentary (of liver) 275.0
  portal (of liver) 571.5
   alcoholic 571.2
  posthepatitic (*see also* Cirrhosis, postnecrotic)
    571.5
  postnecrotic (of liver) 571.5
   alcoholic 571.2
  primary (intrahepatic)—*see* Cirrhosis, biliary
  pulmonary (*see also* Fibrosis, lung) 515
  renal (*see also* Sclerosis, renal) 587
  septal (*see also* Cirrhosis, postnecrotic) 571.5
  spleen 289.51
  splenomegalic (of liver)—*see* Cirrhosis, liver
  stasis (liver)—*see* Cirrhosis, liver
  stomach 535.4
  Todd's (*see also* Cirrhosis, biliary) 571.6
  toxic (nodular)—*see* Cirrhosis, postnecrotic
  trabecular—*see* Cirrhosis, postnecrotic
  unilobar—*see* Cirrhosis, liver
  vascular (of liver)—*see* Cirrhosis, liver
  xanthomatous (biliary) (*see also* Cirrhosis,
    biliary) 571.6
   due to xanthomatosis (familial) (metabolic)
    (primary) 272.2
Cistern, subarachnoid 793.0
Citrullinemia 270.6
Citrullinuria 270.6
Ciuffini-Pancoast tumor (M8010/3) (carcinoma,
  pulmonary apex) 162.3
Civatte's disease or poikiloderma 709.09
Clam diggers' itch 120.3
Clap —*see* Gonorrhea
Clark's paralysis 343.9

Clarke-Hadfield syndrome (pancreatic
  infantilism) 577.8
Clastothrix 704.2
Claude's syndrome 352.6
Claude Bernard-Horner syndrome (*see also*
  Neuropathy, peripheral, autonomic) 337.9
Claudication, intermittent 443.9
  cerebral (artery) (*see also* Ischemia, cerebral,
    transient) 435.9
  due to atherosclerosis 440.21
  spinal cord (arteriosclerotic) 435.1
   syphilitic 094.89
  spinalis 435.1
  venous (axillary) 453.8
Claudicatio venosa intermittens 453.8
Claustrophobia 300.29
Clavus (infected) 700
Claw foot (congenital) 754.71
  acquired 736.74
Claw hand (acquired) 736.06
  congenital 755.59
Clawtoe (congenital) 754.71
  acquired 735.5
Clay eating 307.52
Clay shovelers' fracture —*see* Fracture,
  vertebra, cervical
Cleansing of artificial opening (*see also*
  Attention to artificial opening) V55.9
Cleft (congenital)—*see also* Imperfect, closure
  alveolar process 525.8
  branchial (persistent) 744.41
   cyst 744.42
  clitoris 752.49
  cricoid cartilage, posterior 748.3
  facial (*see also* Cleft, lip) 749.10
  lip 749.10
   with cleft palate 749.20
    bilateral (lip and palate) 749.24
     with unilateral lip or palate 749.25
     complete 749.23
     incomplete 749.24
    unilateral (lip and palate) 749.22
     with bilateral lip or palate 749.25
     complete 749.21
     incomplete 749.22
   bilateral 749.14
    with cleft palate, unilateral 749.25
    complete 749.13
    incomplete 749.14
   unilateral 749.12
    with cleft palate, bilateral 749.25
    complete 749.11
    incomplete 749.12
  nose 748.1
  palate 749.00
   with cleft lip 749.20
    bilateral (lip and palate) 749.24
     with unilateral lip or palate 749.25
     complete 749.23
     incomplete 749.24
    unilateral (lip and palate) 749.22
     with bilateral lip or palate 749.25
     complete 749.21
     incomplete 749.22
   bilateral 749.04
    with cleft lip, unilateral 749.25
    complete 749.03
    incomplete 749.04
   unilateral 749.02
    with cleft lip, bilateral 749.25
    complete 749.01

Coccidioidomycosis 114.9
  with pneumonia 114.0
  cutaneous (primary) 114.1
  disseminated 114.3
  extrapulmonary (primary) 114.1
  lung 114.5
    acute 114.0
    chronic 114.4
    primary 114.0
  meninges 114.2
  primary (pulmonary) 114.0
    acute 114.0
  prostate 114.3
  pulmonary 114.5
    acute 114.0
    chronic 114.4
    primary 114.0
  specified site NEC 114.3
Coccidioidosis 114.9
  lung 114.5
    acute 114.0
    chronic 114.4
    primary 114.0
  meninges 114.2
Coccidiosis (colitis) (diarrhea) (dysentery) 007.2
Cocciuria 791.9
Coccus in urine 791.9
Coccydynia 724.79
Coccygodynia 724.79
Coccyx —*see* condition
Cochin-China
  diarrhea 579.1
    anguilluliasis 127.2
  ulcer 085.1
Cock's peculiar tumor 706.2
Cockayne's disease or syndrome (microcephaly and dwarfism) 759.89
Cockayne-Weber syndrome (epidermolysis bullosa) 757.39
Cocked-up toe 735.2
Codman's tumor (benign chondroblastoma) (M9230/0)—*see* Neoplasm, bone, benign
Coenurosis 123.8
Coffee workers' lung 495.8
Cogan's syndrome 370.52
  congenital oculomotor apraxia 379.51
  nonsyphilitic interstitial keratitis 370.52
Coiling, umbilical cord —*see* Complications, umbilical cord
Coitus, painful (female) 625.0
  male 608.89
  psychogenic 302.76
Cold 460
  with influenza, flu, or grippe 487.1
  abscess—*see also* Tuberculosis, abscess
    articular—*see* Tuberculosis, joint
  agglutinin
    disease (chronic) or syndrome 283.0
    hemoglobinuria 283.0
      paroxysmal (cold) (nocturnal) 283.2
  allergic (*see also* Fever, hay) 477.9
  bronchus or chest—*see* Bronchitis
    with grippe or influenza 487.1
  common (head) 460
    vaccination, prophylactic (against) V04.7
  deep 464.10
  effects of 991.9
    specified effect NEC 991.8
  excessive 991.9
    specified effect NEC 991.8
  exhaustion from 991.8

Cold —*continued*
  exposure to 991.9
    specified effect NEC 991.8
  grippy 487.1
  head 460
  injury syndrome (newborn) 778.2
  intolerance 780.99
  on lung—*see* Bronchitis
  rose 477.0
  sensitivity, autoimmune 283.0
  virus 460
Coldsore (*see also* Herpes, simplex) 054.9
Colibacillosis 041.4
  generalized 038.42
Colibacilluria 791.9
Colic (recurrent) 789.0
  abdomen 789.0
    (recurrent)psychogenic 307.89
  appendicular 543.9
  appendix 543.9
  bile duct—*see* Choledocholithiasis
  biliary—*see* Cholelithiasis
  bilious—*see* Cholelithiasis
  common duct—*see* Choledocholithiasis
  Devonshire NEC 984.9
    specified type of lead—*see* Table of drugs and chemicals
  flatulent 787.3
  gallbladder or gallstone—*see* Cholelithiasis
  gastric 536.8
  hepatic (duct)—*see* Choledocholithiasis
  hysterical 300.11
  infantile 789.0
  intestinal 789.0
  kidney 788.0
  lead NEC 984.9
    specified type of lead—*see* Table of drugs and chemicals
  liver (duct)—*see* Choledocholithiasis
  mucous 564.9
    psychogenic 316 [564.9]
  nephritic 788.0
  painter's NEC 984.9
  pancreas 577.8
  psychogenic 306.4
  renal 788.0
  saturnine NEC 984.9
    specified type of lead—*see* Table of drugs and chemicals
  spasmodic 789.0
  ureter 788.0
  urethral 599.84
    due to calculus 594.2
  uterus 625.8
    menstrual 625.3
  vermicular 543.9
  virus 460
  worm NEC 128.9
Colicystitis (*see also* Cystitis) 595.9
Colitis (acute) (catarrhal) (croupous) (cystica superficialis) (exudative) (hemorrhagic) (noninfectious) (phlegmonous) (presumed noninfectious) 558.9
  adaptive 564.9
  allergic 558.3
  amebic (*see also* Amebiasis) 006.9
    nondysenteric 006.2
  anthrax 022.2
  bacillary (*see also* Infection, Shigella) 004.9
  balantidial 007.0

Colitis—*continued*
  chronic 558.9
    ulcerative (*see also* Colitis, ulcerative) 556.9
  coccidial 007.2
  dietetic 558.9
  due to radiation 558.1
  functional 558.9
  gangrenous 009.0
  giardial 007.1
  granulomatous 555.1
  gravis (*see also* Colitis, ulcerative) 556.9
  infectious (*see also* Enteritis, due to, specific
      organism) 009.0
    presumed 009.1
  ischemic 557.9
    acute 557.0
    chronic 557.1
    due to mesenteric artery insufficiency 557.1
  membranous 564.9
    psychogenic 316 *[564.9]*
  mucous 564.9
    psychogenic 316 *[564.9]*
  necrotic 009.0
  polyposa (*see also* Colitis, ulcerative) 556.9
  protozoal NEC 007.9
  pseudomembranous 008.45
  pseudomucinous 564.9
  regional 555.1
  segmental 555.1
  septic (*see also* Enteritis, due to, specific
      organism) 009.0
  spastic 564.9
    psychogenic 316 *[564.9]*
  staphylococcus 008.41
    food 005.0
  thromboulcerative 557.0
  toxic 558.2
  transmural 555.1
  trichomonal 007.3
  tuberculous (ulcerative) 014.8
  ulcerative (chronic) (idiopathic) (nonspecific)
      556.9
    entero- 556.0
    fulminant 557.0
    ileo- 556.1
    left-sided 556.5
    procto- 556.2
    proctosigmoid 556.3
    psychogenic 316 *[556]*
    specified NEC 556.8
    universal 556.6
Collagen disease NEC 710.9
  nonvascular 710.9
  vascular (allergic) (*see also* Angiitis,
      hypersensitivity) 446.20
Collagenosis (*see also* Collagen disease) 710.9
  cardiovascular 425.4
  mediastinal 519.3
Collapse 780.2
  adrenal 255.8
  cardiorenal (*see also* Hypertension, cardiorenal)
      404.90
  cardiorespiratory 785.51
    fetus or newborn 779.85
  cardiovascular (*see also* Disease, heart) 785.51
    fetus or newborn 779.85
  circulatory (peripheral) 785.59
    with
      abortion—*see* Abortion, by type, with shock
      ectopic pregnancy (*see also* categories
          633.0-633.9) 639.5

Collapse—*continued*
      molar pregnancy (*see also* categories
          630-632) 639.5
    during or after labor and delivery 669.1
    fetus or newborn 779.85
    following
      abortion 639.5
      ectopic or molar pregnancy 639.5
  during or after labor and delivery 669.1
    fetus or newborn 779.89
  external ear canal 380.50
    secondary to
      inflammation 380.53
      surgery 380.52
      trauma 380.51
  general 780.2
  heart—*see* Disease, heart
  heat 992.1
  hysterical 300.11
  labyrinth, membranous (congenital) 744.05
  lung (massive) (*see also* Atelectasis) 518.0
    pressure, during labor 668.0
  myocardial—*see* Disease, heart
  nervous (*see also* Disorder, mental,
      nonpsychotic) 300.9
  neurocirculatory 306.2
  nose 738.0
  postoperative (cardiovascular) 998.0
  pulmonary (*see also* Atelectasis) 518.0
    fetus or newborn 770.5
      partial 770.5
      primary 770.4
  thorax 512.8
    iatrogenic 512.1
    postoperative 512.1
  trachea 519.19
  valvular—*see* Endocarditis
  vascular (peripheral) 785.59
    with
      abortion—*see* Abortion, by type, with shock
      ectopic pregnancy (*see also* categories
          633.0-633.9) 639.5
      molar pregnancy (*see also* categories
          630-632) 639.5
    cerebral (*see also* Disease, cerebrovascular,
        acute) 436
    during or after labor and delivery 669.1
    fetus or newborn 779.89
    following
      abortion 639.5
      ectopic or molar pregnancy 639.5
  vasomotor 785.59
  vertebra 733.13
Collateral —*see also* condition
  circulation (venous) 459.89
  dilation, veins 459.89
Colles' fracture (closed) (reversed) (separation)
    813.41
  open 813.51
Collet's syndrome 352.6
Collet-Sicard syndrome 352.6
Colliculitis urethralis (*see also* Urethritis) 597.89
Colliers'
  asthma 500
  lung 500
  phthisis (*see also* Tuberculosis) 011.4
Collodion baby (ichthyosis congenita) 757.1
Colloid milium 709.3

Coloboma NEC 743.49
  choroid 743.59
  fundus 743.52
  iris 743.46
  lens 743.36
  lids 743.62
  optic disc (congenital) 743.57
    acquired 377.23
  retina 743.56
  sclera 743.47
Coloenteritis —*see* Enteritis
Colon —*see* condition
Coloptosis 569.89
Color
  amblyopia NEC 368.59
    acquired 368.55
  blindness NEC (congenital) 368.59
    acquired 368.55
Colostomy
  attention to V55.3
  fitting or adjustment V53.5
  malfunctioning 569.62
  status V44.3
Colpitis (*see also* Vaginitis) 616.10
Colpocele 618.6
Colpocystitis (*see also* Vaginitis) 616.10
Colporrhexis 665.4
Colpospasm 625.1
Column, spinal, vertebral —*see* condition
Coma 780.01
  apoplectic (*see also* Disease, cerebrovascular,
    acute) 436
  diabetic (with ketoacidosis) 250.3
    hyperosmolar 250.2
  eclamptic (*see also* Eclampsia) 780.39
  epileptic 345.3
  hepatic 572.2
  hyperglycemic 250.2
  hyperosmolar (diabetic) (nonketotic) 250.2
  hypoglycemic 251.0
    diabetic 250.3
  insulin 250.3
    hyperosmolar 250.2
    non-diabetic 251.0
    organic hyperinsulinism 251.0
  Kussmaul's (diabetic) 250.3
  liver 572.2
  newborn 779.2
  prediabetic 250.2
  uremic—*see* Uremia
Combat fatigue (*see also* Reaction, stress, acute)
  308.9
Combined —*see* condition
Comedo 706.1
Comedocarcinoma (M8501/3)—*see also*
  Neoplasm, breast, malignant
  noninfiltrating (M8501/2)
    specified site—*see* Neoplasm, by site, in situ
    unspecified site 233.0
Comedomastitis 610.4
Comedones 706.1
  lanugo 757.4
Comma bacillus, carrier (suspected) of V02.3
Comminuted fracture —*see* Fracture, by site
Common
  aortopulmonary trunk 745.0
  atrioventricular canal (defect) 745.69
  atrium 745.69
  cold (head) 460
    vaccination, prophylactic (against) V04.7
  truncus (arteriosus) 745.0
  ventricle 745.3

Commotio (current)
  cerebri (*see also* Concussion, brain) 850.9
    with skull fracture—*see* Fracture, skull, by site
  retinae 921.3
  spinalis—*see* Injury, spinal, by site
Commotion (current)
  brain (without skull fracture) (*see also*
    Concussion, brain) 850.9
    with skull fracture—*see* Fracture, skull, by site
  spinal cord—*see* Injury, spinal, by site
Communication
  abnormal—*see also* Fistula
    between
      base of aorta and pulmonary artery 745.0
      left ventricle and right atrium 745.4
      pericardial sac and pleural sac 748.8
      pulmonary artery and pulmonary vein 747.3
    congenital, between uterus and anterior
      abdominal wall 752.3
      bladder 752.3
      intestine 752.3
      rectum 752.3
  left ventricular-right atrial 745.4
  pulmonary artery-pulmonary vein 747.3
Compartment syndrome —*see* Syndrome,
  compartment
Compensation
  broken—*see* Failure, heart
  failure—*see* Failure, heart
  neurosis, psychoneurosis 300.11
Complaint —*see also* Disease
  bowel, functional 564.9
    psychogenic 306.4
  intestine, functional 564.9
    psychogenic 306.4
  kidney (*see also* Disease, renal) 593.9
  liver 573.9
  miners' 500
Complete —*see* condition
Complex
  cardiorenal (*see also* Hypertension, cardiorenal)
    404.90
  castration 300.9
  Costen's 524.60
  ego-dystonic homosexuality 302.0
  Eisenmenger's (ventricular septal defect) 745.4
  homosexual, ego-dystonic 302.0
  hypersexual 302.89
  inferiority 301.9
  jumped process
    spine—*see* Dislocation, vertebra
  primary, tuberculosis (*see also* Tuberculosis)
    010.0
  Taussig-Bing (transposition, aorta and
    overriding pulmonary artery) 745.11
Complications
  abortion NEC—*see* categories 634-639
  accidental puncture or laceration during a
    procedure 998.2
  amputation stump (late) (surgical) 997.60
    traumatic—*see* Amputation, traumatic
  anastomosis (and bypass)—*see also*
    Complications, due to (presence of) any
    device, implant, or graft classified to
    996.0-996.5 NEC
    hemorrhage NEC 998.11
    intestinal (internal) NEC 997.4
      involving urinary tract 997.5
    mechanical—*see* Complications, mechanical,
      graft
    urinary tract (involving intestinal tract) 997.5

Complications—*continued*
  genitourinary NEC 996.65
    indwelling urinary catheter 996.64
  heart assist device 996.61
  heart valve 996.61
  infusion pump 996.62
  insulin pump 996.69
  intrauterine contraceptive device 996.65
  joint prosthesis, internal 996.66
  ocular lens 996.69
  orbital (implant) 996.69
  orthopedic NEC 996.67
    joint, internal 996.66
  specified type NEC 996.69
  urinary catheter, indwelling 996.64
  ventricular shunt 996.63
infusion (procedure) 999.9
  blood—*see* Complications, transfusion
  infection NEC 999.3
  sepsis NEC 999.3
inhalation therapy NEC 999.9
injection (procedure) 999.9
  drug reaction (*see also* Reaction, drug) 995.27
  infection NEC 999.3
  sepsis NEC 999.3
  serum (prophylactic) (therapeutic)—*see*
    Complications, vaccination
  vaccine (any)—*see* Complications,
    vaccination
inoculation (any)—*see* Complications,
  vaccination
insulin pump 996.57
internal device (catheter) (electronic) (fixation)
    (prosthetic) NEC—*see also* Complications,
    due to (presence of) any device, implant, or
    graft classified to 996.0-996.5 NEC
  mechanical—*see* Complications, mechanical
intestinal transplant (immune or nonimmune
    cause) 996.87
intraoperative bleeding or hemorrhage 998.11
intrauterine contraceptive device (*see also*
    Complications, contraceptive device) 996.76
  infection or inflammation 996.65
  with fetal damage affecting management of
    pregnancy 655.8
jejunostomy 569.60
kidney transplant (immune or nonimmune
    cause) 996.81
labor 669.9
  specified condition NEC 669.8
liver transplant (immune or nonimmune cause)
    996.82
lumbar puncture 349.0
mechanical
  anastomosis—*see* Complications, mechanical,
    graft
  artificial heart 996.09
  bypass—*see* Complications, mechanical, graft
  catheter NEC 996.59
    cardiac 996.09
    cystostomy 996.39
    dialysis (hemodialysis) 996.1
      peritoneal 996.56
    during a procedure 998.2
    urethral, indwelling 996.31
  colostomy 569.62
  device NEC 996.59
    balloon (counterpulsation), intra-aortic 996.1
    cardiac 996.00
      automatic implantable defibrillator 996.04
      long-term effect 429.4

Complications—*continued*
  specified NEC 996.09
contraceptive, intrauterine 996.32
counterpulsation, intra-aortic 996.1
fixation, external, with internal components
    996.49
fixation, internal (nail, rod, plate) 996.40
genitourinary 996.30
  specified NEC 996.39
insulin pump 996.57
nervous system 996.2
orthopedic, internal 996.40
  prosthetic joint (*see also* Complications,
      mechanical device, orthopedic,
      prosthetic, joint) 996.47
prosthetic NEC 996.59
  joint (*see also* Complications, prosthetic
      joint) 996.47
    articular bearing surface wear 996.46
    aseptic loosening 996.41
    breakage 996.43
    dislocation 996.42
    failure 996.43
    fracture 996.43
      around prosthetic 996.44
      peri-prosthetic 996.44
    instability 996.42
    loosening 996.41
    peri-prosthetic osteolysis 996.45
    subluxation 996.42
    wear 996.46
  umbrella, vena cava 996.1
  vascular 996.1
dorsal column stimulator 996.2
electrode NEC 996.59
  brain 996.2
  cardiac 996.01
  spinal column 996.2
enterostomy 569.62
esophagostomy 530.87
fistula, arteriovenous, surgically created 996.1
gastrostomy 536.42
graft NEC 996.52
  aortic (bifurcation) 996.1
  aortocoronary bypass 996.03
  blood vessel NEC 996.1
  bone 996.49
  cardiac 996.00
  carotid artery bypass 996.1
  cartilage 996.49
  corneal 996.51
  coronary bypass 996.03
  decellularized allodermis 996.55
  genitourinary 996.30
    specified NEC 996.39
  muscle 996.49
  nervous system 996.2
  organ (immune or nonimmune cause) 996.80
    heart 996.83
    intestines 996.87
    kidney 996.81
    liver 996.82
    lung 996.84
    pancreas 996.86
    specified NEC 996.89
  orthopedic, internal 996.49
  peripheral nerve 996.2
  prosthetic NEC 996.59
  skin 996.52
    artificial 996.55
  specified NEC 996.59

Complications—*continued*
    renal artery 997.72
    wound infection 998.59
  therapeutic misadventure NEC 999.9
    surgical treatment 998.9
  tracheostomy 519.00
  transfusion (blood) (lymphocytes) (plasma)
    NEC 999.8
    acute lung injury (TRALI) 518.7
    atrophy, liver, yellow, subacute (within 8
      months of administration)—*see* Hepatitis,
      viral
    bone marrow 996.85
    embolism
      air 999.1
      thrombus 999.2
    hemolysis NEC 999.8
      bone marrow 996.85
    hepatitis (serum) (type B) (within 8 months
      after administration) *see* Hepatitis, viral
    incompatibility reaction (ABO) (blood group)
      999.6
      Rh (factor) 999.7
    infection 999.3
    jaundice (serum) (within 8 months after
      administration) *see* Hepatitis, viral
    sepsis 999.3
    shock or reaction NEC 999.8
      bone marrow 996.85
    subacute yellow atrophy of liver (within 8
      months after administration) *see* Hepatitis,
      viral
    thromboembolism 999.2
  transplant—*see also* Complications, due to
    (presence of) any device, implant, or graft
    classified to 996.0-996.5 NEC
    bone marrow 996.85
    organ (immune or nonimmune cause) (partial)
      (total) 996.80
      bone marrow 996.85
      heart 996.83
      intestines 996.87
      kidney 996.81
      liver 996.82
      lung 996.84
      pancreas 996.86
      specified NEC 996.89
  trauma NEC (early) 958.8
  ultrasound therapy NEC 999.9
  umbilical cord
    affecting fetus or newborn 762.6
    complicating delivery 663.9
      affecting fetus or newborn 762.6
      specified type NEC 663.8
  urethral catheter NEC 996.76
    infection or inflammation 996.64
    mechanical 996.31
  urinary, postoperative NEC 997.5
  vaccination 999.9
    anaphylaxis NEC 999.4
    cellulitis 999.3
    encephalitis or encephalomyelitis 323.51
    hepatitis (serum) (type B) (within 8 months
      after administration) *see* Hepatitis, viral
    infection (general) (local) NEC 999.3
    jaundice (serum) (within 8 months after
      administration) *see* Hepatitis, viral
    meningitis 997.09 *[321.8]*
    myelitis 323.52
    protein sickness 999.5
    reaction (allergic) 999.5

Complications—*continued*
    Herxheimer's 995.0
    serum 999.5
    sepsis 999.3
    serum intoxication, sickness, rash, or other
      serum reaction NEC 999.5
    shock (allergic) (anaphylactic) 999.4
    subacute yellow atrophy of liver (within 8
      months after administration) *see* Hepatitis,
      viral
    vaccinia (generalized) 999.0
    localized 999.3
  vascular
    device, implant, or graft NEC 996.74
      infection or inflammation 996.62
      mechanical NEC 996.1
        cardiac (*see also* Complications,
          mechanical, by type) 996.00
    following infusion, perfusion, or transfusion
      999.2
    postoperative NEC 997.2
      mesenteric artery 997.71
      other vessels 997.79
      peripheral vessels 997.2
      renal artery 997.72
  ventilation therapy NEC 999.9
  ventilator (respirator), mechanical V46.14
Compound presentation complicating delivery
  652.8
  causing obstructed labor 660.0
Compressed air disease 993.3
Compression
  with injury—*see* specific injury
  arm NEC 354.9
  artery 447.1
    celiac, syndrome 447.4
  brachial plexus 353.0
  brain (stem) 348.4
    due to
      contusion, brain—*see* Contusion, brain
      injury NEC—*see also* Hemorrhage, brain,
        traumatic
        birth—*see* Birth, injury, brain
      laceration, brain—*see* Laceration, brain
    osteopathic 739.0
  bronchus 519.19
  by cicatrix—*see* Cicatrix
  cardiac 423.9
  cauda equina 344.60
    with neurogenic bladder 344.61
  celiac (artery) (axis) 447.4
  cerebral—*see* Compression, brain
  cervical plexus 353.2
  cord (umbilical)—*see* Compression, umbilical
    cord
  cranial nerve 352.9
    second 377.49
    third (partial) 378.51
      total 378.52
    fourth 378.53
    fifth 350.8
    sixth 378.54
    seventh 351.8
  divers' squeeze 993.3
  duodenum (external) (*see also* Obstruction,
    duodenum) 537.3
  during birth 767.9
  esophagus 530.3
    congenital, external 750.3
  Eustachian tube 381.63
  facies (congenital) 754.0

Concussion—*continued*
    with loss of consciousness—*see* Concussion,
        with, loss of consciousness
  without loss of consciousness 850.0
  blast (air) (hydraulic) (immersion) (underwater)
    869.0
    with open wound into cavity 869.1
    abdomen or thorax—*see* Injury, internal, by
      site
    brain—*see* Concussion, brain
    ear (acoustic nerve trauma) 951.5
      with perforation, tympanic membrane—*see*
        Wound, open, ear drum
    thorax—*see* Injury, internal, intrathoracic
      organs NEC
  brain or cerebral (without skull fracture) 850.9
    with
      loss of consciousness 850.5
        brief (less than one hour)
          30 minutes or less 850.11
          31-59 minutes 850.12
        moderate (1-24 hours) 850.2
        prolonged (more than 24 hours) (with
          complete recovery) (with return to
          pre-existing conscious level) 850.3
          without return to pre-existing conscious
            level 850.4
      mental confusion or disorientation (without
        loss of consciousness) 850.0
        with loss of consciousness—*see*
          Concussion, brain, with, loss of
          consciousness
      skull fracture—*see* Fracture, skull, by site
    without loss of consciousness 850.0
  cauda equina 952.4
  cerebral—*see* Concussion, brain
  conus medullaris (spine) 952.4
  hydraulic—*see* Concussion, blast
  internal organs—*see* Injury, internal, by site
  labyrinth—*see* Injury, intracranial
  ocular 921.3
  osseous labyrinth—*see* Injury, intracranial
  spinal (cord)—*see also* Injury, spinal, by site
    due to
      broken
        back—*see* Fracture, vertebra, by site, with
          spinal cord injury
        neck—*see* Fracture, vertebra, cervical,
          with spinal cord injury
      fracture, fracture dislocation, or compression
        fracture of spine or vertebra—*see*
          Fracture, vertebra, by site, with spinal
          cord injury
  syndrome 310.2
  underwater blast—*see* Concussion, blast
Condition —*see also* Disease
  psychiatric 298.9
  respiratory NEC 519.9
    acute or subacute NEC 519.9
      due to
        external agent 508.9
          specified type NEC 508.8
        fumes or vapors (chemical) (inhalation)
          506.3
        radiation 508.0
    chronic NEC 519.9
      due to
        external agent 508.9
          specified type NEC 508.8
        fumes or vapors (chemical) (inhalation)
          506.4

Condition—*continued*
    radiation 508.1
  due to
    external agent 508.9
      specified type NEC 508.8
    fumes or vapors (chemical) (inhalation)
      506.9
Conduct disturbance (*see also* Disturbance,
    conduct) 312.9
  adjustment reaction 309.3
  hyperkinetic 314.2
Condyloma NEC 078.10
  acuminatum 078.11
  gonorrheal 098.0
  latum 091.3
  syphilitic 091.3
    congenital 090.0
  venereal, syphilitic 091.3
Confinement —*see* Delivery
Conflagration —*see also* Burn, by site
  asphyxia (by inhalation of smoke, gases, fumes,
    or vapors) 987.9
    specified agent—*see* Table of drugs and
      chemicals
Conflict
  family V61.9
    specified circumstance NEC V61.8
  interpersonal NEC V62.81
  marital V61.10
    involving divorce or estrangement V61.0
  parent-child V61.20
  partner V61.10
Confluent —*see* condition
Confusion, confused (mental) (state) (*see also*
    State, confusional) 298.9
  acute 293.0
  epileptic 293.0
  postoperative 293.9
  psychogenic 298.2
  reactive (from emotional stress, psychological
    trauma) 298.2
  subacute 293.1
Confusional arousals 327.41
Congelation 991.9
Congenital —*see also* condition
  aortic septum 747.29
  generalized fibromatosis (CGF) 759.89
  intrinsic factor deficiency 281.0
  malformation—*see* Anomaly
Congestion, congestive (chronic) (passive)
  asphyxia, newborn 768.9
  bladder 596.8
  bowel 569.89
  brain (*see also* Disease, cerebrovascular NEC)
    437.8
    malarial 084.9
  breast 611.79
  bronchi 519.19
  bronchial tube 519.19
  catarrhal 472.0
  cerebral—*see* Congestion, brain
  cerebrospinal—*see* Congestion, brain
  chest 514
  chill 780.99
    malarial (*see also* Malaria) 084.6
  circulatory NEC 459.9
  conjunctiva 372.71
  due to disturbance of circulation 459.9
  duodenum 537.3
  enteritis—*see* Enteritis
  eye 372.71

Congestion, congestive—*continued*
 fibrosis syndrome (pelvic) 625.5
 gastroenteritis—*see* Enteritis
 general 799.89
 glottis 476.0
 heart (*see also* Failure, heart) 428.0
 hepatic 573.0
 hypostatic (lung) 514
 intestine 569.89
 intracranial—*see* Congestion, brain
 kidney 593.89
 labyrinth 386.50
 larynx 476.0
 liver 573.0
 lung 514
   active or acute (*see also* Pneumonia) 486
     congenital 770.0
   chronic 514
   hypostatic 514
   idiopathic, acute 518.5
   passive 514
 malaria, malarial (brain) (fever) (*see also*
   Malaria) 084.6
 medulla—*see* Congestion, brain
 nasal 478.19
 orbit, orbital 376.33
   inflammatory (chronic) 376.10
     acute 376.00
 ovary 620.8
 pancreas 577.8
 pelvic, female 625.5
 pleural 511.0
 prostate (active) 602.1
 pulmonary—*see* Congestion, lung
 renal 593.89
 retina 362.89
 seminal vesicle 608.89
 spinal cord 336.1
 spleen 289.51
   chronic 289.51
 stomach 537.89
 trachea 464.11
 urethra 599.84
 uterus 625.5
   with subinvolution 621.1
 viscera 799.89
Congestive —*see* Congestion
Conical
 cervix 622.6
 cornea 371.60
 teeth 520.2
Conjoined twins 759.4
 causing disproportion (fetopelvic) 653.7
Conjugal maladjustment V61.10
 involving divorce or estrangement V61.0
Conjunctiva —*see* condition
Conjunctivitis (exposure) (infectious)
   (nondiphtheritic) (pneumococcal) (pustular)
   (staphylococcal) (streptococcal) NEC 372.30
 actinic 370.24
 acute 372.00
   atopic 372.05
   contagious 372.03
   follicular 372.02
   hemorrhagic (viral) 077.4
 adenoviral (acute) 077.3
 allergic (chronic) 372.14
   with hay fever 372.05
 anaphylactic 372.05
 angular 372.03
 Apollo (viral) 077.4

Conjunctivitis—*continued*
 atopic 372.05
 blennorrhagic (neonatorum) 098.40
 catarrhal 372.03
 chemical 372.01
   allergic 372.05
   meaning corrosion, *see* Burn, conjunctiva
 chlamydial 077.98
   due to
     Chlamydial trachomatis—*see* Trachoma
     paratrachoma 077.0
 chronic 372.10
   allergic 372.14
   follicular 372.12
   simple 372.11
   specified type NEC 372.14
   vernal 372.13
 diphtheritic 032.81
 due to
   dust 372.05
   enterovirus type 70 077.4
   erythema multiforme 695.1 *[372.33]*
   filariasis (*see also* Filariasis) 125.9 *[372.15]*
   mucocutaneous
     disease NEC 372.33
     leishmaniasis 085.5 *[372.15]*
   Reiter's disease 099.3 *[372.33]*
   syphilis 095.8 *[372.10]*
   toxoplasmosis (acquired) 130.1
     congenital (active) 771.2
   trachoma—*see* Trachoma
 dust 372.05
 eczematous 370.31
 epidemic 077.1
   hemorrhagic 077.4
 follicular (acute) 372.02
   adenoviral (acute) 077.3
   chronic 372.12
 glare 370.24
 gonococcal (neonatorum) 098.40
 granular (trachomatous) 076.1
   late effect 139.1
 hemorrhagic (acute) (epidemic) 077.4
 herpetic (simplex) 054.43
   zoster 053.21
 inclusion 077.0
 infantile 771.6
 influenzal 372.03
 Koch-Weeks 372.03
 light 372.05
 medicamentosa 372.05
 membranous 372.04
 meningococcic 036.89
 Morax-Axenfeld 372.02
 mucopurulent NEC 372.03
 neonatal 771.6
   gonococcal 098.40
 Newcastle's 077.8
 nodosa 360.14
 of Beal 077.3
 parasitic 372.15
   filariasis (*see also* Filariasis) 125.9 *[372.15]*
   mucocutaneous leishmaniasis 085.5 *[372.15]*
 Parinaud's 372.02
 petrificans 372.39
 phlyctenular 370.31
 pseudomembranous 372.04
   diphtheritic 032.81
 purulent 372.03
 Reiter's 099.3 *[372.33]*
 rosacea 695.3 *[372.31]*

Conjunctivitis—*continued*
  serous 372.01
    viral 077.99
  simple chronic 372.11
  specified NEC 372.39
  sunlamp 372.04
  swimming pool 077.0
  trachomatous (follicular) 076.1
    acute 076.0
    late effect 139.1
  traumatic NEC 372.39
  tuberculous (*see also* Tuberculosis) 017.3
    [370.31]
  tularemic 021.3
  tularensis 021.3
  vernal 372.13
    limbar 372.13 *[370.32]*
  viral 077.99
    acute hemorrhagic 077.4
    specified NEC 077.8
Conjunctivochalasis 372.81
Conjunctoblepharitis —*see* Conjunctivitis
Conn (-Louis) syndrome (primary aldosteronism)
  255.12
Connective tissue —*see* condition
Conradi (-Hünermann) syndrome or disease
  (chondrodysplasia calcificans congenita)
  756.59
Consanguinity V19.7
Consecutive —*see* condition
Consolidated lung (base)—*see* Pneumonia, lobar
Constipation 564.00
  atonic 564.09
  drug induced
    correct substance properly administered
      564.09
    overdose or wrong substance given or taken
      977.9
      specified drug—*see* Table of drugs and
        chemicals
  neurogenic 564.09
  other specified NEC 564.09
  outlet dysfunction 564.02
  psychogenic 306.4
  simple 564.00
  slow transit 564.01
  spastic 564.09
Constitutional —*see also* condition
  arterial hypotension (*see also* Hypotension)
    458.9
  obesity 278.00
    morbid 278.01
  psychopathic state 301.9
  short stature in childhood 783.43
  state, developmental V21.9
    specified development NEC V21.8
  substandard 301.6
Constitutionally substandard 301.6
Constriction
  anomalous, meningeal bands or folds 742.8
  aortic arch (congenital) 747.10
  asphyxiation or suffocation by 994.7
  bronchus 519.19
  canal, ear (*see also* Stricture, ear canal,
    acquired) 380.50
  duodenum 537.3
  gallbladder (*see also* Obstruction, gallbladder)
    575.2
    congenital 751.69
  intestine (*see also* Obstruction, intestine) 560.9

Constriction—*continued*
  larynx 478.74
    congenital 748.3
  meningeal bands or folds, anomalous 742.8
  organ or site, congenital NEC—*see* Atresia
  prepuce (congenital) 605
  pylorus 537.0
    adult hypertrophic 537.0
    congenital or infantile 750.5
    newborn 750.5
  ring (uterus) 661.4
    affecting fetus or newborn 763.7
  spastic—*see also* Spasm
    ureter 593.3
    urethra—*see* Stricture, urethra
  stomach 537.89
  ureter 593.3
  urethra—*see* Stricture, urethra
  visual field (functional) (peripheral) 368.45
Constrictive —*see* condition
Consultation V65.9
  medical—*see also* Counseling, medical
  specified reason NEC V65.8
  without complaint or sickness V65.9
    feared complaint unfounded V65.5
    specified reason NEC V65.8
Consumption —*see* Tuberculosis
Contact
  with
    AIDS virus V01.79
    anthrax V01.81
    cholera V01.0
    communicable disease V01.9
      specified type NEC V01.89
      viral NEC V01.79
    Escherichia coli (E. coli) V01.83
    German measles V01.4
    gonorrhea V01.6
    HIV V01.79
    human immunodeficiency virus V01.79
    meningococcus V01.84
    parasitic disease NEC V01.89
    poliomyelitis V01.2
    rabies V01.5
    rubella V01.4
    SARS-associated coronavirus V01.82
    smallpox V01.3
    syphilis V01.6
    tuberculosis V01.1
    varicella V01.71
    venereal disease V01.6
    viral disease NEC V01.79
  dermatitis—*see* Dermatitis
Contamination, food (*see also* Poisoning, food) 005.9
Contraception, contraceptive
  advice NEC V25.09
    family planning V25.09
    fitting of diaphragm V25.02
    prescribing or use of
      oral contraceptive agent V25.01
      specified agent NEC V25.02
  counseling NEC V25.09
    emergency V25.03
    family planning V25.09
    fitting of diaphragm V25.02
    prescribing or use of
      oral contraceptive agent V25.01
        emergency V25.03
        postcoital V25.03
      specified agent NEC V25.02

Contraception, contraceptive—*continued*
  device (in situ) V45.59
    causing menorrhagia 996.76
    checking V25.42
    complications 996.32
    insertion V25.1
    intrauterine V45.51
    reinsertion V25.42
    removal V25.42
    subdermal V45.52
  fitting of diaphragm V25.02
  insertion
    intrauterine contraceptive device V25.1
    subdermal implantable V25.5
  maintenance V25.40
    examination V25.40
      intrauterine device V25.42
      oral contraceptive V25.41
      specified method NEC V25.49
      subdermal implantable V25.43
    intrauterine device V25.42
    oral contraceptive V25.41
    specified method NEC V25.49
    subdermal implantable V25.43
  management NEC V25.49
  prescription
    oral contraceptive agent V25.01
      emergency V25.03
      postcoital V25.03
      repeat V25.41
    specified agent NEC V25.02
      repeat V25.49
  sterilization V25.2
  surveillance V25.40
    intrauterine device V25.42
    oral contraceptive agent V25.41
    specified method NEC V25.49
    subdermal implantable V25.43

Contraction, contracture, contracted
  Achilles tendon (*see also* Short, tendon,
    Achilles) 727.81
  anus 564.89
  axilla 729.9
  bile duct (*see also* Disease, biliary) 576.8
  bladder 596.8
    neck or sphincter 596.0
  bowel (*see also* Obstruction, intestine) 560.9
  Braxton Hicks 644.1
  bronchus 519.19
  burn (old)—*see* Cicatrix
  cecum (*see also* Obstruction, intestine) 560.9
  cervix (*see also* Stricture, cervix) 622.4
    congenital 752.49
  cicatricial—*see* Cicatrix
  colon (*see also* Obstruction, intestine) 560.9
  conjunctiva trachomatous, active 076.1
    late effect 139.1
  Dupuytren's 728.6
  eyelid 374.41
  eye socket (after enucleation) 372.64
  face 729.9
  fascia (lata) (postural) 728.89
    Dupuytren's 728.6
    palmar 728.6
    plantar 728.71
  finger NEC 736.29
    congenital 755.59
    joint (*see also* Contraction, joint) 718.44

Contraction—*continued*
  flaccid, paralytic
    joint (*see also* Contraction, joint) 718.4
    muscle 728.85
      ocular 378.50
  gallbladder (*see also* Obstruction, gallbladder)
    575.2
  hamstring 728.89
    tendon 727.81
  heart valve—*see* Endocarditis
  Hicks' 644.1
  hip (*see also* Contraction, joint) 718.4
  hourglass
    bladder 596.8
      congenital 753.8
    gallbladder (*see also* Obstruction, gallbladder)
      575.2
      congenital 751.69
    stomach 536.8
      congenital 750.7
      psychogenic 306.4
    uterus 661.4
      affecting fetus or newborn 763.7
  hysterical 300.11
  infantile (*see also* Epilepsy) 345.6
  internal os (*see also* Stricture, cervix) 622.4
  intestine (*see also* Obstruction, intestine) 560.9
  joint (abduction) (acquired) (adduction)
    (flexion) (rotation) 718.40
    ankle 718.47
    congenital NEC 755.8
      generalized or multiple 754.89
        lower limb joints 754.89
      hip (*see also* Subluxation, congenital, hip)
        754.32
      lower limb (including pelvic girdle) not
        involving hip 754.89
      upper limb (including shoulder girdle) 755.59
    elbow 718.42
    foot 718.47
    hand 718.44
    hip 718.45
    hysterical 300.11
    knee 718.46
    multiple sites 718.49
    pelvic region 718.45
    shoulder (region) 718.41
    specified site NEC 718.48
    wrist 718.43
  kidney (granular) (secondary) (*see also*
    Sclerosis, renal) 587
    congenital 753.3
    hydronephritic 591
    pyelonephritic (*see also* Pyelitis, chronic)
      590.00
    tuberculous (*see also* Tuberculosis) 016.0
  ligament 728.89
    congenital 756.89
  liver—*see* Cirrhosis, liver
  muscle (postinfectional) (postural) NEC 728.85
    congenital 756.89
      sternocleidomastoid 754.1
    extraocular 378.60
    eye (extrinsic) (*see also* Strabismus) 378.9
      paralytic (*see also* Strabismus, paralytic)
        378.50
    flaccid 728.85
    hysterical 300.11
    ischemic (Volkmann's) 958.6
    paralytic 728.85

Contraction—*continued*
　posttraumatic 958.6
　psychogenic 306.0
　　specified as conversion reaction 300.11
　myotonic 728.85
　neck (*see also* Torticollis) 723.5
　　congenital 754.1
　　psychogenic 306.0
　ocular muscle (*see also* Strabismus) 378.9
　　paralytic (*see also* Strabismus, paralytic) 378.50
　organ or site, congenital NEC—*see* Atresia
　outlet (pelvis)—*see* Contraction, pelvis
　palmar fascia 728.6
　paralytic
　　joint (*see also* Contraction, joint) 718.4
　　muscle 728.85
　　　ocular (*see also* Strabismus, paralytic) 378.50
　pelvis (acquired) (general) 738.6
　　affecting fetus or newborn 763.1
　　complicating delivery 653.1
　　　causing obstructed labor 660.1
　　　generally contracted 653.1
　　　　causing obstructed labor 660.1
　　　inlet 653.2
　　　　causing obstructed labor 660.1
　　　midpelvic 653.8
　　　　causing obstructed labor 660.1
　　　midplane 653.8
　　　　causing obstructed labor 660.1
　　　outlet 653.3
　　　　causing obstructed labor 660.1
　plantar fascia 728.71
　premature
　　atrial 427.61
　　auricular 427.61
　　auriculoventricular 427.61
　　heart (junctional) (nodal) 427.60
　　supraventricular 427.61
　　ventricular 427.69
　prostate 602.8
　pylorus (*see also* Pylorospasm) 537.81
　rectosigmoid (*see also* Obstruction, intestine) 560.9
　rectum, rectal (sphincter) 564.89
　　psychogenic 306.4
　ring (Bandl's) 661.4
　　affecting fetus or newborn 763.7
　scar—*see* Cicatrix
　sigmoid (*see also* Obstruction, intestine) 560.9
　socket, eye 372.64
　spine (*see also* Curvature, spine) 737.9
　stomach 536.8
　　hourglass 536.8
　　　congenital 750.7
　　　psychogenic 306.4
　　psychogenic 306.4
　tendon (sheath) (*see also* Short, tendon) 727.81
　toe 735.8
　ureterovesical orifice (postinfectional) 593.3
　urethra 599.84
　uterus 621.8
　　abnormal 661.9
　　　affecting fetus or newborn 763.7
　　clonic, hourglass or tetanic 661.4
　　　affecting fetus or newborn 763.7
　　dyscoordinate 661.4
　　　affecting fetus or newborn 763.7
　　hourglass 661.4
　　　affecting fetus or newborn 763.7
　　hypotonic NEC 661.2
　　　affecting fetus or newborn 763.7
　　incoordinate 661.4

Contraction—*continued*
　　affecting fetus or newborn 763.7
　　inefficient or poor 661.2
　　　affecting fetus or newborn 763.7
　　irregular 661.2
　　　affecting fetus or newborn 763.7
　　tetanic 661.4
　　　affecting fetus or newborn 763.7
　vagina (outlet) 623.2
　vesical 596.8
　　neck or urethral orifice 596.0
　visual field, generalized 368.45
　Volkmann's (ischemic) 958.6
Contusion (skin surface intact) 924.9
　with
　　crush injury—*see* Crush
　　dislocation—*see* Dislocation, by site
　　fracture—*see* Fracture, by site
　　internal injury—*see also* Injury, internal, by
　　　site
　　　heart—*see* Contusion, cardiac
　　　kidney—*see* Contusion, kidney
　　　liver—*see* Contusion, liver
　　　lung—*see* Contusion, lung
　　　spleen—*see* Contusion, spleen
　　intracranial injury—*see* Injury, intracranial
　　nerve injury—*see* Injury, nerve
　　open wound—*see* Wound, open, by site
　abdomen, abdominal (muscle) (wall) 922.2
　　organ(s) NEC 868.00
　adnexa, eye NEC 921.9
　ankle 924.21
　　with other parts of foot 924.20
　arm 923.9
　　lower (with elbow) 923.10
　　upper 923.03
　　　with shoulder or axillary region 923.09
　auditory canal (external) (meatus) (and other
　　part(s) of neck, scalp, or face, except eye)
　　920
　auricle, ear (and other part(s) of neck, scalp, or
　　face except eye) 920
　axilla 923.02
　　with shoulder or upper arm 923.09
　back 922.31
　bone NEC 924.9
　brain (cerebral) (membrane) (with hemorrhage)
　　851.8

---

*Note—Use the following fifth-digit
subclassification with categories 851-854:*

0　unspecified state of consciousness
1　with no loss of consciousness
*2　with brief [less than one hour] loss
　　of consciousness*
*3　with moderate [1-24 hours] loss of
　　consciousness*
*4　with prolonged [more than 24 hours] loss of
　　consciousness and return to pre-existing
　　conscious level*
*5　with prolonged [more than 24 hours] loss of
　　consciousness, without return to pre-existing
　　conscious level*
*Use fifth-digit 5 to designate when a patient is
unconscious and dies before regaining
conciousness, regardless of the duration of the
loss of conciousness*
*6　with loss of consciousness of unspecified
　　duration*
9　with concussion, unspecified

Contusion—*continued*
  pulmonary—*see* Contusion, lung
  quadriceps femoralis 924.00
  rib cage 922.1
  sacral region 922.32
  salivary ducts or glands (and other part(s) of
     neck, scalp, or face, except eye) 920
  scalp (and neck, or face any part, except eye)
     920
  scapular region 923.01
    with shoulder or upper arm 923.09
  sclera (eye) 921.3
  scrotum 922.4
  shoulder 923.00
    with upper arm or axillar regions 923.09
  skin NEC 924.9
  skull 920
  spermatic cord 922.4
  spinal cord—*see also* Injury, spinal, by site
    cauda equina 952.4
    conus medullaris 952.4
  spleen 865.01
    with open wound into cavity 865.11
  sternal region 922.1
  stomach—*see* Injury, internal, stomach
  subconjunctival 921.1
  subcutaneous NEC 924.9
  submaxillary region (and other part(s) of neck,
     scalp, or face, except eye) 920
  submental region (and other part(s) of neck,
     scalp, or face, except eye) 920
  subperiosteal NEC 924.9
  supraclavicular fossa (and other part(s) of neck,
     scalp, or face, except eye) 920
  supraorbital (and other part(s) of neck, scalp, or
     face, except eye) 920
  temple (region) (and other part(s) of neck, scalp,
     or face, except eye) 920
  testis 922.4
  thigh (and hip) 924.00
  thorax 922.1
    organ—*see* Injury, internal, intrathoracic
  throat (and other part(s) of neck, scalp, or face,
     except eye) 920
  thumb(s) (nail) (subungual) 923.3
  toe(s) (nail) (subungual) 924.3
  tongue (and other part(s) of neck, scalp, or face,
     except eye) 920
  trunk 922.9
    multiple sites 922.8
    specified site—*see* Contusion, by site
  tunica vaginalis 922.4
  tympanum (membrane) (and other part(s) of
     neck, scalp, or face, except eye) 920
  upper extremity 923.9
    multiple sites 923.8
  uvula (and other part(s) of neck, scalp, or face,
     except eye) 920
  vagina 922.4
  vocal cord(s) (and other part(s) of neck, scalp, or
     face, except eye) 920
  vulva 922.4
  wrist 923.21
    with hand(s), except finger(s) alone 923.20
Conus (any type) (congenital) 743.57
  acquired 371.60
  medullaris syndrome 336.8

Convalescence (following) V66.9
  chemotherapy V66.2
  medical NEC V66.5
  psychotherapy V66.3
  radiotherapy V66.1
  surgery NEC V66.0
  treatment (for) NEC V66.5
    combined V66.6
    fracture V66.4
    mental disorder NEC V66.3
    specified disorder NEC V66.5
Conversion
  closed surgical procedure to open procedure
    arthroscopic V64.43
    laparoscopic V64.41
    thoracoscopic V64.42
  hysteria, hysterical, any type 300.11
  neurosis, any 300.11
  reaction, any 300.11
Converter, tuberculosis (test reaction) 795.5
Convulsions (idiopathic) 780.39
  apoplectiform (*see also* Disease,
    cerebrovascular, acute) 436
  brain 780.39
  cerebral 780.39
  cerebrospinal 780.39
  due to trauma NEC—*see* Injury, intracranial
  eclamptic (*see also* Eclampsia) 780.39
  epileptic (*see also* Epilepsy) 345.9
  epileptiform (*see also* Seizure, epileptiform)
    780.39
  epileptoid (*see also* Seizure, epileptiform)
    780.39
  ether
    anesthetic
      correct substance properly administered
        780.39
      overdose or wrong substance given 968.2
    other specified type—*see* Table of drugs and
      chemicals
  febrile (simple) 780.31
    complex 780.32
  generalized 780.39
  hysterical 300.11
  infantile 780.39
    epilepsy—*see* Epilepsy
  internal 780.39
  jacksonian (*see also* Epilepsy) 345.5
  myoclonic 333.2
  newborn 779.0
  paretic 094.1
  pregnancy (nephritic) (uremic)—*see* Eclampsia,
    pregnancy
  psychomotor (*see also* Epilepsy) 345.4
  puerperal, postpartum—*see* Eclampsia,
    pregnancy
  recurrent 780.39
    epileptic—*see* Epilepsy
  reflex 781.0
  repetitive 780.39
    epileptic—*see* Epilepsy
    salaam (*see also* Epilepsy) 345.6
  scarlatinal 034.1
  spasmodic 780.39
  tetanus, tetanic (*see also* Tetanus) 037
  thymic 254.8
  uncinate 780.39
  uremic 586
Convulsive —*see also* Convulsions
  disorder or state 780.39
    epileptic—*see* Epilepsy
  equivalent, abdominal (*see also* Epilepsy) 345.5

Cooke-Apert-Gallais syndrome (adrenogenital) 255.2
Cooley's anemia (erythroblastic) 282.49
Coolie itch 126.9
Cooper's
disease 610.1
hernia—*see* Hernia, Cooper's
Coordination disturbance 781.3
Copper wire arteries, retina 362.13
Copra itch 133.8
Coprolith 560.39
Coprophilia 302.89
Coproporphyria, hereditary 277.1
Coprostasis 560.39
with hernia—*see also* Hernia, by site, with
obstruction
gangrenous—*see* Hernia, by site, with gangrene
Cor
biloculare 745.7
bovinum—*see* Hypertrophy, cardiac
bovis—*see also* Hypertrophy, cardiac
pulmonale (chronic) 416.9
acute 415.0
triatriatum, triatrium 746.82
triloculare 745.8
biatriatum 745.3
biventriculare 745.69
Corbus' disease 607.1
Cord —*see also* condition
around neck (tightly) (with compression)
affecting fetus or newborn 762.5
complicating delivery 663.1
without compression 663.3
affecting fetus or newborn 762.6
bladder NEC 344.61
tabetic 094.0
prolapse
affecting fetus or newborn 762.4
complicating delivery 663.0
Cord's angiopathy (*see also* Tuberculosis) 017.3
[362.18]
Cordis ectopia 746.87
Corditis (spermatic) 608.4
Corectopia 743.46
Cori type glycogen storage disease —*see*
Disease, glycogen storage
Cork-handlers' disease or lung 495.3
Corkscrew esophagus 530.5
Corlett's pyosis (impetigo) 684
Corn (infected) 700
Cornea—*see also* **condition**
donor V59.5
guttata (dystrophy) 371.57
plana 743.41
Cornelia de Lange's syndrome (Amsterdam
dwarf, mental retardation, and brachycephaly)
759.89
Cornual gestation or pregnancy —*see*
Pregnancy, cornual
Cornu cutaneum 702.8
Coronary (artery)—*see also* condition
arising from aorta or pulmonary trunk 746.85
Corpora —*see also* condition
amylacea (prostate) 602.8
cavernosa—*see* condition
Corpulence (*see also* Obesity) 278.0
Corpus —*see* condition
Corrigan's disease —*see* Insufficiency, aortic
Corrosive burn —*see* Burn, by site
Corsican fever (*see also* Malaria) 084.6

Cortical —*see also* condition
blindness 377.75
necrosis, kidney (bilateral) 583.6
Corticoadrenal —*see* condition
Corticosexual syndrome 255.2
Coryza (acute) 460
with grippe or influenza 487.1
syphilitic 095.8
congenital (chronic) 090.0
Costen's syndrome or complex 524.60
Costiveness (*see also* Constipation) 564.00
Costochondritis 733.6
Cotard's syndrome (paranoia) 297.1
Cot death 798.0
Cotungo's disease 724.3
Cough 786.2
with hemorrhage (*see also* Hemoptysis) 786.3
affected 786.2
bronchial 786.2
with grippe or influenza 487.1
chronic 786.2
epidemic 786.2
functional 306.1
hemorrhagic 786.3
hysterical 300.11
laryngeal, spasmodic 786.2
nervous 786.2
psychogenic 306.1
smokers' 491.0
tea tasters' 112.89
Counseling NEC V65.40
without complaint or sickness V65.49
abuse victim NEC V62.89
child V61.21
partner V61.11
spouse V61.11
child abuse, maltreatment, or neglect V61.21
contraceptive NEC V25.09
device (intrauterine) V25.02
maintenance V25.40
intrauterine contraceptive device V25.42
oral contraceptive (pill) V25.41
specified type NEC V25.49
subdermal implantable V25.43
management NEC V25.9
oral contraceptive (pill) V25.01
emergency V25.03
postcoital V25.03
prescription NEC V25.02
oral contraceptive (pill) V25.01
emergency V25.03
postcoital V25.03
repeat prescription V25.41
repeat prescription V25.40
subdermal implantable V25.43
surveillance V25.40
dietary V65.3
exercise V65.41
expectant mother, pediatric pre-birth visit
V65.11
explanation of
investigation finding NEC V65.49
medication NEC V65.49
family planning V25.09
for nonattending third party V65.19
genetic V26.33
gonorrhea V65.45
health (advice) (education) (instruction) NEC
V65.49
HIV V65.44
human immunodeficiency virus V65.44

Crush, crushed, crushing—*continued*
  finger(s) 927.3
    with hand(s) 927.20
      and wrist(s) 927.21
  flank 926.19
  foot, excluding toe(s) alone (with ankle) 928.20
  forearm (and elbow) 927.10
  genitalia, external (female) (male) 926.0
    internal—*see* Injury, internal, genital organ NEC
  hand, except finger(s) alone (and wrist) 927.20
  head—*see* Fracture, skull, by site
  heel 928.20
  hip 928.01
    with thigh 928.00
  internal organ (abdomen, chest, or pelvis)—*see*
    Injury, internal, by site
  knee 928.11
    with leg, lower 928.10
  labium (majus) (minus) 926.0
  larynx 925.2
  late effect—*see* Late, effects (of), crushing
  leg 928.9
    lower 928.10
      and knee 928.11
    upper 928.00
  limb
    lower 928.9
      multiple sites 928.8
    upper 927.9
      multiple sites 927.8
  multiple sites NEC 929.0
  neck 925.2
  nerve—*see* Injury, nerve, by site
  nose 802.0
    open 802.1
  penis 926.0
  pharynx 925.2
  scalp 925.2
  scapular region 927.01
    with shoulder or upper arm 927.09
  scrotum 926.0
  shoulder 927.00
    with upper arm or axillary region 927.09
  skull or cranium—*see* Fracture, skull, by site
  spinal cord—*see* Injury, spinal, by site
  syndrome (complication of trauma) 958.5
  testis 926.0
  thigh (with hip) 928.00
  throat 925.2
  thumb(s) (and fingers) 927.3
  toe(s) 928.3
    with foot 928.20
      and ankle 928.21
  tonsil 925.2
  trunk 926.9
    chest—*see* Injury, internal, intrathoracic
      organs NEC
    internal organ—*see* Injury, internal, by site
    multiple sites 926.8
    specified site NEC 926.19
  vulva 926.0
  wrist 927.21
    with hand(s), except fingers alone 927.20
Crusta lactea 690.11
Crusts 782.8
Crutch paralysis 953.4
Cruveilhier's disease 335.21
Cruveilhier-Baumgarten cirrhosis, disease, or
  syndrome 571.5
Cruz-Chagas disease (*see also* Trypanosomiasis)
  086.2

Crying
  constant, continuous
    adolescent 780.95
    adult 780.95
    baby 780.92
    child 780.95
    infant 780.92
    newborn 780.92
  excessive
    adolescent 780.95
    adult 780.95
    baby 780.92
    child 780.95
    infant 780.92
    newborn 780.92
Cryoglobulinemia (mixed) 273.2
Crypt (anal) (rectal) 569.49
Cryptitis (anal) (rectal) 569.49
Cryptococcosis (European) (pulmonary)
  (systemic) 117.5
Cryptococcus 117.5
  epidermicus 117.5
  neoformans, infection by 117.5
Cryptopapillitis (anus) 569.49
Cryptophthalmos (eyelid) 743.06
Cryptorchid, cryptorchism, cryptorchidism
  752.51
Cryptosporidiosis 007.4
Cryptotia 744.29
Crystallopathy
  calcium pyrophosphate (*see also* Arthritis)
    275.49 *[712.2]*
  dicalcium phosphate (*see also* Arthritis) 275.49
    [712.1]
  gouty 274.0
  pyrophosphate NEC (*see also* Arthritis) 275.49
    [712.2]
  uric acid 274.0
Crystalluria 791.9
Csillag's disease (lichen sclerosus et atrophicus)
  701.0
Cuban itch 050.1
Cubitus
  valgus (acquired) 736.01
    congenital 755.59
    late effect of rickets 268.1
  varus (acquired) 736.02
    congenital 755.59
    late effect of rickets 268.1
Cultural deprivation V62.4
Cupping of optic disc 377.14
Curling's ulcer —*see* Ulcer, duodenum
Curling esophagus 530.5
Curschmann (-Batten) (-Steinert) disease or
  syndrome 359.2
Curvature
  organ or site, congenital NEC—*see* Distortion
  penis (lateral) 752.69
  Pott's (spinal) (*see also* Tuberculosis) 015.0
    [737.43]
  radius, idiopathic, progressive (congenital)
    755.54
  spine (acquired) (angular) (idiopathic)
    (incorrect) (postural) 737.9
    congenital 754.2
    due to or associated with
      Charcot-Marie-Tooth disease 356.1 *[737.40]*
      mucopolysaccharidosis 277.5 *[737.40]*
      neurofibromatosis 237.71 *[737.40]*
      osteitis
        deformans 731.0 *[737.40]*

Curvature—*continued*
    fibrosa cystica 252.01 *[737.40]*
    osteoporosis (*see also* Osteoporosis) 733.00
      [737.40]
    poliomyelitis (*see also* Poliomyelitis) 138
      [737.40]
    tuberculosis (Pott's curvature) (*see also*
      Tuberculosis) 015.0 *[737.43]*
    kyphoscoliotic (*see also* Kyphoscoliosis)
      737.30
    kyphotic (*see also* Kyphosis) 737.10
    late effect of rickets 268.1 *[737.40]*
    Pott's 015.0 *[737.40]*
    scoliotic (*see also* Scoliosis) 737.30
    specified NEC 737.8
    tuberculous 015.0 *[737.40]*
Cushing's
  basophilism, disease, or syndrome (iatrogenic)
    (idiopathic) (pituitary basophilism) (pituitary
    dependent) 255.0
  ulcer—*see* Ulcer, peptic
Cushingoid due to steroid therapy
  correct substance properly administered 255.0
  overdose or wrong substance given or taken
    962.0
Cut (external)—*see* Wound, open, by site
Cutaneous —*see also* condition
  hemorrhage 782.7
  horn (cheek) (eyelid) (mouth) 702.8
  larva migrans 126.9
Cutis —*see also* condition
  hyperelastic 756.83
    acquired 701.8
  laxa 756.83
    senilis 701.8
  marmorata 782.61
  osteosis 709.3
  pendula 756.83
    acquired 701.8
  rhomboidalis nuchae 701.8
  verticis gyrata 757.39
    acquired 701.8
Cyanopathy, newborn 770.83
Cyanosis 782.5
  autotoxic 289.7
  common atrioventricular canal 745.69
  congenital 770.83
  conjunctiva 372.71
  due to
    endocardial cushion defect 745.60
    nonclosure, foramen botalli 745.5
    patent foramen botalli 745.5
    persistent foramen ovale 745.5
  enterogenous 289.7
  fetus or newborn 770.83
  ostium primum defect 745.61
  paroxysmal digital 443.0
  retina, retinal 362.10
Cycle
  anovulatory 628.0
  menstrual, irregular 626.4
Cyclencephaly 759.89
Cyclical vomiting 536.2
  psychogenic 306.4
Cyclitic membrane 364.74
Cyclitis (*see also* Iridocyclitis) 364.3
  acute 364.00
    primary 364.01
    recurrent 364.02

Cyclitis—*continued*
  chronic 364.10
    in
      sarcoidosis 135 *[364.11]*
      tuberculosis (*see also* Tuberculosis) 017.3
        [364.11]
  Fuchs' heterochromic 364.21
  granulomatous 364.10
  lens induced 364.23
  nongranulomatous 364.00
  posterior 363.21
  primary 364.01
  recurrent 364.02
  secondary (noninfectious) 364.04
    infectious 364.03
  subacute 364.00
    primary 364.01
    recurrent 364.02
Cyclokeratitis —*see* Keratitis
Cyclophoria 378.44
Cyclopia, cyclops 759.89
Cycloplegia 367.51
Cyclospasm 367.53
Cyclosporiasis 007.5
Cyclothymia 301.13
Cyclothymic personality 301.13
Cyclotropia 378.33
Cyesis —*see* Pregnancy
Cylindroma (M8200/3)—*see also* Neoplasm, by
  site, malignant
  eccrine dermal (M8200/0)—*see* Neoplasm, skin,
    benign
  skin (M8200/0)—*see* Neoplasm, skin, benign
Cylindruria 791.7
Cyllosoma 759.89
Cynanche
  diphtheritic 032.3
  tonsillaris 475
Cynorexia 783.6
Cyphosis —*see* Kyphosis
Cyprus fever (*see also* Brucellosis) 023.9
Cyriax's syndrome (slipping rib) 733.99
Cyst (mucus) (retention) (serous) (simple)

> *Note—In general, cysts are not neoplastic and
> are classified to the appropriate category for
> disease of the specified anatomical site. This
> generalization does not apply to certain types of
> cysts which are neoplastic in nature, for
> example, dermoid, nor does it apply to cysts of
> certain structures, for example, branchial cleft,
> which are classified as developmental
> anomalies. The following listing includes some
> of the most frequently reported sites of cysts as
> well as qualifiers which indicate the type of cyst.
> The latter qualifiers usually are not repeated
> under the anatomical sites. Since the code
> assignment for a given site may vary depending
> upon the type of cyst, the coder should refer to
> the listings under the specified type of cyst
> before consideration is given to the site.*

  accessory, fallopian tube 752.11
  adenoid (infected) 474.8
  adrenal gland 255.8
    congenital 759.1
  air, lung 518.89
  allantoic 753.7
  alveolar process (jaw bone) 526.2
  amnion, amniotic 658.8

Cyst —*continued*
  anterior chamber (eye) 364.60
    exudative 364.62
    implantation (surgical) (traumatic) 364.61
    parasitic 360.13
  anterior nasopalatine 526.1
  antrum 478.19
  anus 569.49
  apical (periodontal) (tooth) 522.8
  appendix 543.9
  arachnoid, brain 348.0
  arytenoid 478.79
  auricle 706.2
  Baker's (knee) 727.51
    tuberculous (*see also* Tuberculosis) 015.2
  Bartholin's gland or duct 616.2
  bile duct (*see also* Disease, biliary) 576.8
  bladder (multiple) (trigone) 596.8
  Blessig's 362.62
  blood, endocardial (*see also* Endocarditis) 424.90
  blue dome 610.0
  bone (local) 733.20
    aneurysmal 733.22
    jaw 526.2
      developmental (odontogenic) 526.0
      fissural 526.1
      latent 526.89
    solitary 733.21
    unicameral 733.21
  brain 348.0
    congenital 742.4
    hydatid (*see also* Echinococcus) 122.9
    third ventricle (colloid) 742.4
  branchial (cleft) 744.42
  branchiogenic 744.42
  breast (benign) (blue dome) (pedunculated) (solitary) (traumatic) 610.0
    involution 610.4
    sebaceous 610.8
  broad ligament (benign) 620.8
    embryonic 752.11
  bronchogenic (mediastinal) (sequestration) 518.89
    congenital 748.4
  buccal 528.4
  bulbourethral gland (Cowper's) 599.89
  bursa, bursal 727.49
    pharyngeal 478.26
  calcifying odontogenic (M9301/0) 213.1
    upper jaw (bone) 213.0
  canal of Nuck (acquired) (serous) 629.1
    congenital 752.41
  canthus 372.75
  carcinomatous (M8010/3)—*see* Neoplasm, by site, malignant
  cartilage (joint)—*see* Derangement, joint
  cauda equina 336.8
  cavum septi pellucidi NEC 348.0
  celomic (pericardium) 746.89
  cerebellopontine (angle)—*see* Cyst, brain
  cerebellum—*see* Cyst, brain
  cerebral—*see* Cyst, brain
  cervical lateral 744.42
  cervix 622.8
    embryonal 752.41
    nabothian (gland) 616.0
  chamber, anterior (eye) 364.60
    exudative 364.62
    implantation (surgical) (traumatic) 364.61
    parasitic 360.13

Cyst —*continued*
  chiasmal, optic NEC (*see also* Lesion, chiasmal) 377.54
  chocolate (ovary) 617.1
  choledochal (congenital) 751.69
    acquired 576.8
  choledochus 751.69
  chorion 658.8
  choroid plexus 348.0
  chyle, mesentery 457.8
  ciliary body 364.60
    exudative 364.64
    implantation 364.61
    primary 364.63
  clitoris 624.8
  coccyx (*see also* Cyst, bone) 733.20
  colloid
    third ventricle (brain) 742.4
    thyroid gland—*see* Goiter
  colon 569.89
  common (bile) duct (*see also* Disease, biliary) 576.8
  congenital NEC 759.89
    adrenal glands 759.1
    epiglottis 748.3
    esophagus 750.4
    fallopian tube 752.11
    kidney 753.10
      multiple 753.19
      single 753.11
    larynx 748.3
    liver 751.62
    lung 748.4
    mediastinum 748.8
    ovary 752.0
    oviduct 752.11
    pancreas 751.7
    periurethral (tissue) 753.8
    prepuce NEC 752.69
      penis 752.69
    sublingual 750.26
    submaxillary gland 750.26
    thymus (gland) 759.2
    tongue 750.19
    ureterovesical orifice 753.4
    vulva 752.41
  conjunctiva 372.75
  cornea 371.23
  corpora quadrigemina 348.0
  corpus
    albicans (ovary) 620.2
    luteum (ruptured) 620.1
  Cowper's gland (benign) (infected) 599.89
  cranial meninges 348.0
  craniobuccal pouch 253.8
  craniopharyngeal pouch 253.8
  cystic duct (*see also* Disease, gallbladder) 575.8
  Cysticercus (any site) 123.1
  Dandy-Walker 742.3
    with spina bifida (*see also* Spina bifida) 741.0
  dental 522.8
    developmental 526.0
    eruption 526.0
    lateral periodontal 526.0
    primordial (keratocyst) 526.0
    root 522.8
  dentigerous 526.0
    mandible 526.0
    maxilla 526.0
  dermoid (M9084/0)—*see also* Neoplasm, by site, benign

Cyst —*continued*
  with malignant transformation (M9084/3)
    183.0
   implantation
    external area or site (skin) NEC 709.8
    iris 364.61
    skin 709.8
    vagina 623.8
    vulva 624.8
   mouth 528.4
   oral soft tissue 528.4
   sacrococcygeal 685.1
    with abscess 685.0
  developmental of ovary, ovarian 752.0
  dura (cerebral) 348.0
   spinal 349.2
  ear (external) 706.2
  echinococcal (*see also* Echinococcus) 122.9
  embryonal
   cervix uteri 752.41
   genitalia, female external 752.41
   uterus 752.3
   vagina 752.41
  endometrial 621.8
   ectopic 617.9
  endometrium (uterus) 621.8
   ectopic—*see* Endometriosis
  enteric 751.5
  enterogenous 751.5
  epidermal (inclusion) (*see also* Cyst, skin) 706.2
  epidermoid (inclusion) (*see also* Cyst, skin)
   706.2
   mouth 528.4
   not of skin—*see* Cyst, by site
   oral soft tissue 528.4
  epididymis 608.89
  epiglottis 478.79
  epiphysis cerebri 259.8
  epithelial (inclusion) (*see also* Cyst, skin) 706.2
  epoophoron 752.11
  eruption 526.0
  esophagus 530.89
  ethmoid sinus 478.19
  eye (retention) 379.8
   congenital 743.03
   posterior segment, congenital 743.54
  eyebrow 706.2
  eyelid (sebaceous) 374.84
   infected 373.13
   sweat glands or ducts 374.84
  falciform ligament (inflammatory) 573.8
  fallopian tube 620.8
  female genital organs NEC 629.89
  fimbrial (congenital) 752.11
  fissural (oral region) 526.1
  follicle (atretic) (graafian) (ovarian) 620.0
   nabothian (gland) 616.0
  follicular (atretic) (ovarian) 620.0
   dentigerous 526.0
  frontal sinus 478.19
  gallbladder or duct 575.8
  ganglion 727.43
  Gartner's duct 752.41
  gas, of mesentery 568.89
  gingiva 523.8
  gland of moll 374.84
  globulomaxillary 526.1
  graafian follicle 620.0
  granulosal lutein 620.2

Cyst —*continued*
  hemangiomatous (M9121/0) (*see also*
   Hemangioma) 228.00
  hydatid (*see also* Echinococcus) 122.9
   fallopian tube (Morgagni) 752.11
   liver NEC 122.8
   lung NEC 122.9
   Morgagni 752.89
    fallopian tube 752.11
   specified site NEC 122.9
  hymen 623.8
   embryonal 752.41
  hypopharynx 478.26
  hypophysis, hypophyseal (duct) (recurrent)
   253.8
   cerebri 253.8
  implantation (dermoid)
   anterior chamber (eye) 364.61
   external area or site (skin) NEC 709.8
   iris 364.61
   vagina 623.8
   vulva 624.8
  incisor, incisive canal 526.1
  inclusion (epidermal) (epithelial) (epidermoid)
   (mucous) (squamous) (*see also* Cyst, skin)
   706.2
  not of skin—*see* Neoplasm, by site, benign
  intestine (large) (small) 569.89
  intracranial—*see* Cyst, brain
  intraligamentous 728.89
   knee 717.89
  intrasellar 253.8
  iris (idiopathic) 364.60
   exudative 364.62
   implantation (surgical) (traumatic) 364.61
   miotic pupillary 364.55
   parasitic 360.13
  Iwanoff's 362.62
  jaw (bone) (aneurysmal) (extravasation)
   (hemorrhagic) (traumatic) 526.2
   developmental (odontogenic) 526.0
   fissural 526.1
  keratin 706.2
  kidney (congenital) 753.10
   acquired 593.2
   calyceal (*see also* Hydronephrosis) 591
   multiple 753.19
   pyelogenic (*see also* Hydronephrosis) 591
   simple 593.2
   single 753.11
   solitary (not congenital) 593.2
  labium (majus) (minus) 624.8
   sebaceous 624.8
  lacrimal
   apparatus 375.43
   gland or sac 375.12
  larynx 478.79
  lens 379.39
   congenital 743.39
  lip (gland) 528.5
  liver 573.8
   congenital 751.62
   hydatid (*see also* Echinococcus) 122.8
    granulosis 122.0
    multilocularis 122.5
  lung 518.89
   congenital 748.4
   giant bullous 492.0

Cyst —*continued*
  popliteal 727.51
  porencephalic 742.4
    acquired 348.0
  postanal (infected) 685.1
    with abscess 685.0
  posterior segment of eye, congenital 743.54
  postmastoidectomy cavity 383.31
  preauricular 744.47
  prepuce 607.89
    congenital 752.69
  primordial (jaw) 526.0
  prostate 600.3
  pseudomucinous (ovary) (M8470/0) 220
  pudenda (sweat glands) 624.8
  pupillary, miotic 364.55
    sebaceous 624.8
  radicular (residual) 522.8
  radiculodental 522.8
  ranular 527.6
  Rathke's pouch 253.8
  rectum (epithelium) (mucous) 569.49
  renal—*see* Cyst, kidney
  residual (radicular) 522.8
  retention (ovary) 620.2
  retina 361.19
    macular 362.54
    parasitic 360.13
    primary 361.13
    secondary 361.14
  retroperitoneal 568.89
  sacrococcygeal (dermoid) 685.1
    with abscess 685.0
  salivary gland or duct 527.6
    mucous extravasation or retention 527.6
  Sampson's 617.1
  sclera 379.19
  scrotum (sebaceous) 706.2
    sweat glands 706.2
  sebaceous (duct) (gland) 706.2
    breast 610.8
    eyelid 374.84
    genital organ NEC
      female 629.89
      male 608.89
    scrotum 706.2
  semilunar cartilage (knee) (multiple) 717.5
  seminal vesicle 608.89
  serous (ovary) 620.2
  sinus (antral) (ethmoidal) (frontal) (maxillary)
    (nasal) (sphenoidal) 478.19
  Skene's gland 599.89
  skin (epidermal) (epidermoid, inclusion)
    (epithelial) (inclusion) (retention)
    (sebaceous) 706.2
    breast 610.8
    eyelid 374.84
    genital organ NEC
      female 629.89
      male 608.89
    neoplastic 216.3
    scrotum 706.2
    sweat gland or duct 705.89
  solitary
    bone 733.21
    kidney 593.2
  spermatic cord 608.89
  sphenoid sinus 478.19
  spinal meninges 349.2
  spine (*see also* Cyst, bone) 733.20
  spleen NEC 289.59

Cyst —*continued*
  congenital 759.0
    hydatid (*see also* Echinococcus) 122.9
  spring water (pericardium) 746.89
  subarachnoid 348.0
    intrasellar 793.0
  subdural (cerebral) 348.0
    spinal cord 349.2
  sublingual gland 527.6
    mucous extravasation or retention 527.6
  submaxillary gland 527.6
    mucous extravasation or retention 527.6
  suburethral 599.89
  suprarenal gland 255.8
  suprasellar—*see* Cyst, brain
  sweat gland or duct 705.89
  sympathetic nervous system 337.9
  synovial 727.40
    popliteal space 727.51
  Tarlov's 355.9
  tarsal 373.2
  tendon (sheath) 727.42
  testis 608.89
  theca-lutein (ovary) 620.2
  Thornwaldt's, Tornwaldt's 478.26
  thymus (gland) 254.8
  thyroglossal (duct) (infected) (persistent) 759.2
  thyroid (gland) 246.2
    adenomatous—*see* Goiter, nodular
    colloid (*see also* Goiter) 240.9
  thyrolingual duct (infected) (persistent) 759.2
  tongue (mucous) 529.8
  tonsil 474.8
  tooth (dental root) 522.8
  tubo-ovarian 620.8
    inflammatory 614.1
  tunica vaginalis 608.89
  turbinate (nose) (*see also* Cyst, bone) 733.20
  Tyson's gland (benign) (infected) 607.89
  umbilicus 759.89
  urachus 753.7
  ureter 593.89
  ureterovesical orifice 593.89
    congenital 753.4
  urethra 599.84
  urethral gland (Cowper's) 599.89
  uterine
    ligament 620.8
      embryonic 752.11
    tube 620.8
  uterus (body) (corpus) (recurrent) 621.8
    embryonal 752.3
  utricle (ear) 386.8
    prostatic 599.89
  utriculus masculinus 599.89
  vagina, vaginal (squamous cell) (wall) 623.8
    embryonal 752.41
    implantation 623.8
    inclusion 623.8
  vallecula, vallecular 478.79
  ventricle, neuroepithelial 348.0
  verumontanum 599.89
  vesical (orifice) 596.8
  vitreous humor 379.29
  vulva (sweat glands) 624.8
    congenital 752.41
    implantation 624.8
    inclusion 624.8
    sebaceous gland 624.8
  vulvovaginal gland 624.8
  wolffian 752.89

Cystadenocarcinoma (M8440/3)—*see also*
Neoplasm, by site, malignant
 bile duct type (M8161/3) 155.1
 endometrioid (M8380/3)—*see* Neoplasm, by
  site, malignant
 mucinous (M8470/3)
  papillary (M8471/3)
   specified site—*see* Neoplasm, by site,
    malignant
   unspecified site 183.0
  specified site—*see* Neoplasm, by site,
   malignant
  unspecified site 183.0
 papillary (M8450/3)
  mucinous (M8471/3)
   specified site—*see* Neoplasm, by site,
    malignant
   unspecified site 183.0
  pseudomucinous (M8471/3)
   specified site—*see* Neoplasm, by site,
    malignant
   unspecified site 183.0
  serous (M8460/3)
   specified site—*see* Neoplasm, by site,
    malignant
   unspecified site 183.0
  specified site—*see* Neoplasm, by site,
   malignant
  unspecified 183.0
 pseudomucinous (M8470/3)
  papillary (M8471/3)
   specified site—*see* Neoplasm, by site,
    malignant
   unspecified site 183.0
  specified site—*see* Neoplasm, by site,
   malignant
  unspecified site 183.0
 serous (M8441/3)
  papillary (M8460/3)
   specified site—*see* Neoplasm, by site,
    malignant
   unspecified site 183.0
  specified site—*see* Neoplasm, by site,
   malignant
  unspecified site 183.0
Cystadenofibroma (M9013/0)
 clear cell (M8313/0)—*see* Neoplasm, by site,
  benign
 endometrioid (M8381/0) 220
  borderline malignancy (M8381/1) 236.2
  malignant (M8381/3) 183.0
 mucinous (M9015/0)
  specified site—*see* Neoplasm, by site, benign
  unspecified site 220
 serous (M9014/0)
  specified site—*see* Neoplasm, by site, benign
  unspecified site 220
 specified site—*see* Neoplasm, by site, benign
 unspecified site 220
Cystadenoma (M8440/0)—*see also* Neoplasm,
 by site, benign
 bile duct (M8161/0) 211.5
 endometrioid (M8380/0)—*see also* Neoplasm,
  by site, benign
  borderline malignancy (M8380/1)—*see*
   Neoplasm, by site, uncertain behavior
 malignant (M8440/3)—*see* Neoplasm, by site,
  malignant
 mucinous (M8470/0)
  borderline malignancy (M8470/1)

Cystadenoma—*continued*
  specified site—*see* Neoplasm, uncertain
   behavior
  unspecified site 236.2
 papillary (M8471/0)
  borderline malignancy (M8471/1)
   specified site—*see* Neoplasm, by site,
    uncertain behavior
   unspecified site 236.2
  specified site—*see* Neoplasm, by site,
   benign
  unspecified site 220
 specified site—*see* Neoplasm, by site, benign
 unspecified site 220
 papillary (M8450/0)
  borderline malignancy (M8450/1)
   specified site—*see* Neoplasm, by site,
    uncertain behavior
   unspecified site 236.2
  lymphomatosum (M8561/0) 210.2
  mucinous (M8471/0)
   borderline malignancy (M8471/1)
    specified site—*see* Neoplasm, by site,
     uncertain behavior
    unspecified site 236.2
   specified site—*see* Neoplasm, by site,
    benign
   unspecified site 220
  pseudomucinous (M8471/0)
   borderline malignancy (M8471/1)
    specified site—*see* Neoplasm, by site,
     uncertain behavior
    unspecified site 236.2
   specified site—*see* Neoplasm, by site,
    benign
   unspecified site 220
  serous (M8460/0)
   borderline malignancy (M8460/1)
    specified site—*see* Neoplasm, by site,
     uncertain behavior
    unspecified site 236.2
   specified site—*see* Neoplasm, by site,
    benign
   unspecified site 220
  specified site—*see* Neoplasm, by site, benign
  unspecified site 220
 pseudomucinous (M8470/0)
  borderline malignancy (M8470/1)
   specified site—*see* Neoplasm, by site,
    uncertain behavior
   unspecified site 236.2
  papillary (M8471/0)
   borderline malignancy (M8471/1)
    specified site—*see* Neoplasm, by site,
     uncertain behavior
    unspecified site 236.2
   specified site—*see* Neoplasm, by site,
    benign
   unspecified site 220
  specified site—*see* Neoplasm, by site, benign
  unspecified site 220
 serous (M8441/0)
  borderline malignancy (M8441/1)
   specified site—*see* Neoplasm, by site,
    uncertain behavior
   unspecified site 236.2
  papillary (M8460/0)
   borderline malignancy (M8460/1)
    specified site—*see* Neoplasm, by site,
     uncertain behavior
    unspecified site 236.2

Cystolithiasis 594.1
Cystoma (M8440/0)—*see also* Neoplasm, by
   site, benign
  endometrial, ovary 617.1
  mucinous (M8470/0)
    specified site—*see* Neoplasm, by site, benign
    unspecified site 220
  serous (M8441/0)
    specified site—*see* Neoplasm, by site, benign
    unspecified site 220
  simple (ovary) 620.2
Cystoplegia 596.53
Cystoptosis 596.8
Cystopyelitis (*see also* Pyelitis) 590.80
Cystorrhagia 596.8
Cystosarcoma phyllodes (M9020/1) 238.3
  benign (M9020/0) 217
  malignant (M9020/3)—*see* Neoplasm, breast,
    malignant
Cystostomy status V44.50
  appendico-vesicostomy V44.52
  cutaneous-vesicostomy V44.51
  specified type NEC V44.59
  with complication 997.5
Cystourethritis (*see also* Urethritis) 597.89
Cystourethrocele (*see also* Cystocele)
  female (without uterine prolapse) 618.09
    with uterine prolapse 618.4
      complete 618.3
      incomplete 618.2
  male 596.8
Cytomegalic inclusion disease 078.5
  congenital 771.1
Cytomycosis, reticuloendothelial (*see also*
  Histoplasmosis, American) 115.00
Cytopenia 289.9
  refractory
    with
      multilineage dysplasia (RCMD) 238.72
        and ringed sideroblasts (RCMD-RS)
          238.72

D

Daae (-Finsen) disease (epidemic pleurodynia)
 074.1
Dabney's grip 074.1
Da Costa's syndrome (neurocirculatory asthenia)
 306.2
Dacryoadenitis, dacryadenitis 375.00
 acute 375.01
 chronic 375.02
Dacryocystitis 375.30
 acute 375.32
 chronic 375.42
 neonatal 771.6
 phlegmonous 375.33
 syphilitic 095.8
  congenital 090.0
 trachomatous, active 076.1
  late effect 139.1
 tuberculous (*see also* Tuberculosis) 017.3
Dacryocystoblennorrhea 375.42
Dacryocystocele 375.43
Dacryolith, dacryolithiasis 375.57
Dacryoma 375.43
Dacryopericystitis (acute) (subacute) 375.32
 chronic 375.42
Dacryops 375.11
Dacryosialadenopathy, atrophic 710.2
Dacryostenosis 375.56
 congenital 743.65
Dactylitis
 bone (*see also* Osteomyelitis) 730.2
 sickle-cell 282.62
  Hb-C 282.64
  Hb-SS 282.62
  specified NEC 282.69
 syphilitic 095.5
 tuberculous (*see also* Tuberculosis) 015.5
Dactylolysis spontanea 136.0
Dactylosymphysis (*see also* Syndactylism)
 755.10
Damage
 arteriosclerotic—*see* Arteriosclerosis
 brain 348.9
  anoxic, hypoxic 348.1
   during or resulting from a procedure 997.01
   ischemic, in newborn 768.7
  child NEC 343.9
  due to birth injury 767.0
  minimal (child) (*see also* Hyperkinesia) 314.9
  newborn 767.0
 cardiac—*see also* Disease, heart
 cardiorenal (vascular) (*see also* Hypertension,
  cardiorenal) 404.90
 central nervous system—*see* Damage, brain
 cerebral NEC—*see* Damage, brain
 coccyx, complicating delivery 665.6
 coronary (*see also* Ischemia, heart) 414.9
 eye, birth injury 767.8
 heart—*see also* Disease, heart
  valve—*see* Endocarditis
 hypothalamus NEC 348.9
 liver 571.9
  alcoholic 571.3
 myocardium (*see also* Degeneration,
  myocardial) 429.1

Damage—*continued*
 pelvic
  joint or ligament, during delivery 665.6
  organ NEC
   with
    abortion—*see* Abortion, by type, with
     damage to pelvic organs
    ectopic pregnancy (*see also* categories
     633.0-633.9) 639.2
    molar pregnancy (*see also* categories
     630-632) 639.2
   during delivery 665.5
   following
    abortion 639.2
    ectopic or molar pregnancy 639.2
 renal (*see also* Disease, renal) 593.9
 skin, solar 692.79
  acute 692.72
  chronic 692.74
 subendocardium, subendocardial (*see also*
  Degeneration, myocardial) 429.1
 vascular 459.9
Dameshek's syndrome (erythroblastic anemia)
 282.49
Dana-Putnam syndrome (subacute combined
 sclerosis with pernicious anemia) 281.0
 [336.2]
Danbolt (-Closs) syndrome (acrodermatitis
 enteropathica) 686.8
Dandruff 690.18
Dandy fever 061
Dandy-Walker deformity or syndrome (atresia,
 foramen of Magendie) 742.3
 with spina bifida (*see also* Spina bifida) 741.0
Dangle foot 736.79
Danielssen's disease (anesthetic leprosy) 030.1
Danlos' syndrome 756.83
Darier's disease (congenital) (keratosis
 follicularis) 757.39
 due to vitamin A deficiency 264.8
 meaning erythema annulare centrifugum 695.0
Darier-Roussy sarcoid 135
Darling's
 disease (*see also* Histoplasmosis, American)
  115.00
 histoplasmosis (*see also* Histoplasmosis,
  American) 115.00
Dartre 054.9
Darwin's tubercle 744.29
Davidson's anemia (refractory) 284.9
Davies' disease 425.0
Davies-Colley syndrome (slipping rib) 733.99
Dawson's encephalitis 046.2
Day blindness (*see also* Blindness, day) 368.60
Dead
 fetus
  retained (in utero) 656.4
   early pregnancy (death before 22 completed
    weeks gestation) 632
   late (death after 22 completed weeks
    gestation) 656.4
  syndrome 641.3
 labyrinth 386.50
 ovum, retained 631
Deaf and dumb NEC 389.7

Deciduoma malignum (M9100/3) 181
Deciduous tooth (retained) 520.6
Decline (general) (*see also* Debility) 799.3
Decompensation
  cardiac (acute) (chronic) (*see also* Disease,
      heart) 429.9
    failure—*see* Failure, heart
  cardiorenal (*see also* Hypertension, cardiorenal)
      404.90
  cardiovascular (*see also* Disease,
      cardiovascular) 429.2
  heart (*see also* Disease, heart) 429.9
    failure—*see* Failure, heart
  hepatic 572.2
  myocardial (acute) (chronic) (*see also* Disease,
      heart) 429.9
    failure—*see* Failure, heart
  respiratory 519.9
Decompression sickness 993.3
Decrease, decreased
  blood
    platelets (*see also* Thrombocytopenia) 287.5
    pressure 796.3
      due to shock following
        injury 958.4
        operation 998.0
    white cell count 288.50
      specified NEC 288.59
  cardiac reserve—*see* Disease, heart
  estrogen 256.39
    postablative 256.2
  fetal movements 655.7
  fragility of erythrocytes 289.89
  function
    adrenal (cortex) 255.4
      medulla 255.5
    ovary in hypopituitarism 253.4
    parenchyma of pancreas 577.8
    pituitary (gland) (lobe) (anterior) 253.2
      posterior (lobe) 253.8
  functional activity 780.99
  glucose 790.29
  haptoglobin (serum) NEC 273.8
  leukocytes 288.50
  libido 799.81
  lymphocytes 288.51
  platelets (*see also* Thrombocytopenia) 287.5
  pulse pressure 785.9
  respiration due to shock following injury 958.4
  sexual desire 799.81
  tear secretion NEC 375.15
  tolerance
    fat 579.8
    salt and water 276.9
  vision NEC 369.9
  white blood cell count 288.50
Decubital gangrene 707.00 *[785.4]*
Decubiti (*see also* Decubitus) 707.00
Decubitus (ulcer) 707.00
  with gangrene 707.00 *[785.4]*
  ankle 707.06
  back
    lower 707.03
    upper 707.02
  buttock 707.05
  elbow 707.01
  head 707.09
  heel 707.07
  hip 707.04
  other site 707.09
  sacrum 707.03
  shoulder blades 707.02

Deepening acetabulum 718.85
Defect, defective 759.9
  3-beta-hydroxysteroid dehydrogenase 255.2
  11-hydroxylase 255.2
  21-hydroxylase 255.2
  abdominal wall, congenital 756.70
  aorticopulmonary septum 745.0
  aortic septal 745.0
  atrial septal (ostium secundum type) 745.5
    acquired 429.71
      ostium primum type 745.61
      sinus venosus 745.8
  atrioventricular
    canal 745.69
    septum 745.4
      acquired 429.71
  atrium secundum 745.5
    acquired 429.71
  auricular septal 745.5
    acquired 429.71
  bilirubin excretion 277.4
  biosynthesis, testicular androgen 257.2
  bridge 525.60
  bulbar septum 745.0
  butanol-insoluble iodide 246.1
  chromosome—*see* Anomaly, chromosome
  circulation (acquired) 459.9
    congenital 747.9
    newborn 747.9
  clotting NEC (*see also* Defect, coagulation)
      286.9
  coagulation (factor) (*see also* Deficiency,
      coagulation factor) 286.9
    with
      abortion—*see* Abortion, by type, with
          hemorrhage
      ectopic pregnancy (*see also* categories
          634-638) 639.1
      molar pregnancy (*see also* categories
          630-632) 639.1
    acquired (any) 286.7
    antepartum or intrapartum 641.3
      affecting fetus or newborn 762.1
    causing hemorrhage of pregnancy or delivery
        641.3
    complicating pregnancy, childbirth, or the
        puerperium 649.3
    due to
      liver disease 286.7
      vitamin K deficiency 286.7
    newborn, transient 776.3
    postpartum 666.3
    specified type NEC 286.3
  conduction (heart) 426.9
    bone (*see also* Deafness, conductive) 389.00
  congenital, organ or site NEC—*see also*
      Anomaly
    circulation 747.9
    Descemet's membrane 743.9
      specified type NEC 743.49
    diaphragm 756.6
    ectodermal 757.9
    esophagus 750.9
    pulmonic cusps—*see* Anomaly, heart valve
    respiratory system 748.9
      specified type NEC 748.8
  crown 525.60
  cushion endocardial 745.60
  dental restoration 525.60
  dentin (hereditary) 520.5

Deficiency, deficient
  3-beta-hydroxysteroid dehydrogenase 255.2
  6-phosphogluconic dehydrogenase (anemia)
     282.2
  11-beta-hydroxylase 255.2
  17-alpha-hydroxylase 255.2
  18-hydroxysteroid dehydrogenase 255.2
  20-alpha-hydroxylase 255.2
  21-hydroxylase 255.2
  AAT (alpha-1 antitrypsin) 273.4
  abdominal muscle syndrome 756.79
  accelerator globulin (Ac G) (blood) (*see also*
     Defect, coagulation) 286.3
  AC globulin (congenital) (*see also* Defect,
     coagulation) 286.3
    acquired 286.7
  activating factor (blood) (*see also* Defect,
     coagulation) 286.3
  adenohypophyseal 253.2
  adenosine deaminase 277.2
  aldolase (hereditary) 271.2
  alpha-1-antitrypsin 273.4
  alpha-1-trypsin inhibitor 273.4
  alpha-fucosidase 271.8
  alpha-lipoprotein 272.5
  alpha-mannosidase 271.8
  amino acid 270.9
  anemia—*see* Anemia, deficiency
  aneurin 265.1
    with beriberi 265.0
  antibody NEC 279.00
  antidiuretic hormone 253.5
  antihemophilic
    factor (A) 286.0
      B 286.1
      C 286.2
    globulin (AHG) NEC 286.0
  antithrombin III 289.81
  antitrypsin 273.4
  argininosuccinate synthetase or lyase 270.6
  ascorbic acid (with scurvy) 267
  autoprothrombin
    I (*see also* Defect, coagulation) 286.3
    II 286.1
    C (*see also* Defect, coagulation) 286.3
  bile salt 579.8
  biotin 266.2
  biotinidase 277.6
  bradykinase-1 277.6
  brancher enzyme (amylopectinosis) 271.0
  calciferol 268.9
    with
      osteomalacia 268.2
      rickets (*see also* Rickets) 268.0
  calcium 275.40
    dietary 269.3
  calorie, severe 261
  carbamyl phosphate synthetase 270.6
  cardiac (*see also* Insufficiency, myocardial)
     428.0
  carnitine 277.81
    due to
      hemodialysis 277.83
      inborn errors of metabolism 277.82
      valproic acid therapy 277.83
    iatrogenic 277.83
    palmitoyltransferase (CPT1, CPT2) 277.85
    palmityl transferase (CPT1, CPT2) 277.85
    primary 277.81
    secondary 277.84
  carotene 264.9

Deficiency, deficient—*continued*
  Carr factor (*see also* Defect, coagulation) 286.9
  central nervous system 349.9
  ceruloplasmin 275.1
  cevitamic acid (with scurvy) 267
  choline 266.2
  Christmas factor 286.1
  chromium 269.3
  citrin 269.1
  clotting (blood) (*see also* Defect, coagulation)
     286.9
  coagulation factor NEC 286.9
    with
      abortion—*see* Abortion, by type, with
        hemorrhage
      ectopic pregnancy (*see also* categories
        634-638) 639.1
      molar pregnancy (*see also* categories
        630-632) 639.1
    acquired (any) 286.7
    antepartum or intrapartum 641.3
      affecting fetus or newborn 762.1
    complicating pregnancy, childbirth, or the
      puerperium 649.3
    due to
      liver disease 286.7
      vitamin K deficiency 286.7
    newborn, transient 776.3
    postpartum 666.3
    specified type NEC 286.3
  color vision (congenital) 368.59
    acquired 368.55
  combined, two or more coagulation factors (*see*
    also Defect, coagulation) 286.9
  complement factor NEC 279.8
  contact factor (*see also* Defect, coagulation)
     286.3
  copper NEC 275.1
  corticoadrenal 255.4
  craniofacial axis 756.0
  cyanocobalamin (vitamin B_{12}) 266.2
  debrancher enzyme (limit dextrinosis) 271.0
  desmolase 255.2
  diet 269.9
  dihydrofolate reductase 281.2
  dihydropteridine reductase 270.1
  disaccharidase (intestinal) 271.3
  disease NEC 269.9
  ear(s) V48.8
  edema 262
  endocrine 259.9
  enzymes, circulating NEC (*see also* Deficiency,
    by specific enzyme) 277.6
  ergosterol 268.9
    with
      osteomalacia 268.2
      rickets (*see also* Rickets) 268.0
  erythrocytic glutathione (anemia) 282.2
  eyelid(s) V48.8
  factor (*see also* Defect, coagulation) 286.9
    I (congenital) (fibrinogen) 286.3
      antepartum or intrapartum 641.3
        affecting fetus or newborn 762.1
      newborn, transient 776.3
      postpartum 666.3
    II (congenital) (prothrombin) 286.3
    V (congenital) (labile) 286.3
    VII (congenital) (stable) 286.3

Deficiency, deficient—*continued*
  VIII (congenital) (functional) 286.0
    with
      functional defect 286.0
      vascular defect 286.4
  IX (Christmas) (congenital) (functional) 286.1
  X (congenital) (Stuart-Prower) 286.3
  XI (congenital) (plasma thromboplastin
    antecedent) 286.2
  XII (congenital) (Hageman) 286.3
  XIII (congenital) (fibrin stabilizing) 286.3
  Hageman 286.3
  multiple (congenital) 286.9
    acquired 286.7
  fibrinase (*see also* Defect, coagulation) 286.3
  fibrinogen (congenital) (*see also* Defect,
    coagulation) 286.3
    acquired 286.6
  fibrin stabilizing factor (congenital) (*see also*
    Defect, coagulation) 286.3
    acquired 286.7
  finger—*see* Absence, finger
  Fletcher factor (*see also* Defect, coagulation)
    286.9
  fluorine 269.3
  folate, anemia 281.2
  folic acid (vitamin B$_c$) 266.2
    anemia 281.2
  follicle-stimulating hormone (FSH) 253.4
  fructokinase 271.2
  fructose-1, 6-diphosphate 271.2
  fructose-1-phosphate aldolase 271.2
  FSH (follicle-stimulating hormone) 253.4
  fucosidase 271.8
  galactokinase 271.1
  galactose-1-phosphate uridyl transferase 271.1
  gamma globulin in blood 279.00
  glass factor (*see also* Defect, coagulation) 286.3
  glucocorticoid 255.4
  glucose-6-phosphatase 271.0
  glucose-6-phosphate dehydrogenase anemia
    282.2
  glucuronyl transferase 277.4
  glutathione-reductase (anemia) 282.2
  glycogen synthetase 271.0
  growth hormone 253.3
  Hageman factor (congenital) (*see also* Defect,
    coagulation) 286.3
  head V48.0
  hemoglobin (*see also* Anemia) 285.9
  hepatophosphorylase 271.0
  hexose monophosphate (HMP) shunt 282.2
  HGH (human growth hormone) 253.3
  HG-PRT 277.2
  homogentisic acid oxidase 270.2
  hormone—*see also* Deficiency, by specific
    hormone
    anterior pituitary (isolated) (partial) NEC
      253.4
      growth (human) 253.3
    follicle-stimulating 253.4
    growth (human) (isolated) 253.3
    human growth 253.3
    interstitial cell-stimulating 253.4
    luteinizing 253.4
    melanocyte-stimulating 253.4
    testicular 257.2
  human growth hormone 253.3

Deficiency, deficient—*continued*
  humoral 279.00
    with
      hyper-IgM 279.05
        autosomal recessive 279.05
        X-linked 279.05
      increased IgM 279.05
    congenital hypogammaglobulinemia 279.04
    non-sex-linked 279.06
    selective immunoglobulin NEC 279.03
      IgA 279.01
      IgG 279.03
      IgM 279.02
        increased 279.05
    specified NEC 279.09
  hydroxylase 255.2
  hypoxanthine-guanine
    phosphoribosyltransferase (HG-PRT) 277.2
  ICSH (interstitial cell-stimulating hormone)
    253.4
  immunity NEC 279.3
    cell-mediated 279.10
      with
        hyperimmunoglobulinemia 279.2
        thrombocytopenia and eczema 279.12
      specified NEC 279.19
    combined (severe) 279.2
      syndrome 279.2
    common variable 279.06
    humoral NEC 279.00
    IgA (secretory) 279.01
    IgG 279.03
    IgM 279.02
  immunoglobulin, selective NEC 279.03
    IgA 279.01
    IgG 279.03
    IgM 279.02
  inositol (B complex) 266.2
  interferon 279.4
  internal organ V47.0
  interstitial cell-stimulating hormone (ICSH)
    253.4
  intrinsic (urethral) sphincter (ISD) 599.82
  intrinsic factor (Castle's) (congenital) 281.0
  invertase 271.3
  iodine 269.3
  iron, anemia 280.9
  labile factor (congenital) (*see also* Defect,
    coagulation) 286.3
    acquired 286.7
  lacrimal fluid (acquired) 375.15
    congenital 743.64
  lactase 271.3
  Laki-Lorand factor (*see also* Defect,
    coagulation) 286.3
  lecithin-cholesterol acyltranferase 272.5
  LH (luteinizing hormone) 253.4
  limb V49.0
    lower V49.0
      congenital (*see also* Deficiency, lower limb,
        congenital) 755.30
    upper V49.0
      congenital (*see also* Deficiency, upper limb,
        congenital) 755.20
  lipocaic 577.8
  lipoid (high-density) 272.5
  lipoprotein (familial) (high density) 272.5
  liver phosphorylase 271.0
  long chain 3-hydroxyacyl CoA dehydrogenase
    (LCHAD) 277.85

Deficiency, deficient—*continued*
  long chain/very long chain acyl CoA
    dehydrogenase (LCAD, VLCAD) 277.85
  lower limb V49.0
    congenital 755.30
      with complete absence of distal elements
        755.31
        longitudinal (complete) (partial) (with distal
          deficiencies, incomplete) 755.32
          with complete absence of distal elements
            755.31
          combined femoral, tibial, fibular
            (incomplete) 755.33
          femoral 755.34
          fibular 755.37
          metatarsal(s) 755.38
          phalange(s) 755.39
            meaning all digits 755.31
          tarsal(s) 755.38
          tibia 755.36
          tibiofibular 755.35
          transverse 755.31
  luteinizing hormone (LH) 253.4
  lysosomal alpha-1, 4 glucosidase 271.0
  magnesium 275.2
  mannosidase 271.8
  medium chain acyl CoA dehydrogenase
    (MCAD) 277.85
  melanocyte-stimulating hormone (MSH) 253.4
  menadione (vitamin K) 269.0
    newborn 776.0
  mental (familial) (hereditary) (*see also*
    Retardation, mental) 319
  mineral NEC 269.3
  molybdenum 269.3
  moral 301.7
  multiple, syndrome 260
  myocardial (*see also* Insufficiency myocardial)
    428.0
  myophosphorylase 271.0
  NADH (DPNH) -methemoglobin-reductase
    (congenital) 289.7
  NADH diaphorase or reductase (congenital)
    289.7
  neck V48.1
  niacin (amide) (-tryptophan) 265.2
  nicotinamide 265.2
  nicotinic acid (amide) 265.2
  nose V48.8
  number of teeth (*see also* Anodontia) 520.0
  nutrition, nutritional 269.9
    specified NEC 269.8
  ornithine transcarbamylase 270.6
  ovarian 256.39
  oxygen (*see also* Anoxia) 799.02
  pantothenic acid 266.2
  parathyroid (gland) 252.1
  phenylalanine hydroxylase 270.1
  phosphoenolpyruvate carboxykinase 271.8
  phosphofructokinase 271.2
  phosphoglucomutase 271.0
  phosphohexosisomerase 271.0
  phosphomannomutase 271.8
  phosphomannose isomerase 271.8
  phosphomannosyl mutase 271.8
  phosphorylase kinase, liver 271.0
  pituitary (anterior) 253.2
    posterior 253.5
  placenta—*see* Placenta, insufficiency

Deficiency, deficient—*continued*
  plasma
    cell 279.00
    protein (paraproteinemia) (pyroglobulinemia)
      273.8
      gamma globulin 279.00
    thromboplastin
      antecedent (PTA) 286.2
      component (PTC) 286.1
  platelet NEC 287.1
    constitutional 286.4
  polyglandular 258.9
  potassium (K) 276.8
  proaccelerin (congenital) (*see also* Defect,
    congenital) 286.3
    acquired 286.7
  proconvertin factor (congenital) (*see also*
    Defect, coagulation) 286.3
    acquired 286.7
  prolactin 253.4
  protein 260
    anemia 281.4
    C 289.81
    plasma—*see* Deficiency, plasma, protein
    S 289.81
  prothrombin (congenital) (*see also* Defect,
    coagulation) 286.3
    acquired 286.7
  Prower factor (*see also* Defect, coagulation)
    286.3
  PRT 277.2
  pseudocholinesterase 289.89
  psychobiological 301.6
  PTA 286.2
  PTC 286.1
  purine nucleoside phosphorylase 277.2
  pyracin (alpha) (beta) 266.1
  pyridoxal 266.1
  pyridoxamine 266.1
  pyridoxine (derivatives) 266.1
  pyruvate carboxylase 271.8
  pyruvate dehydrogenase 271.8
  pyruvate kinase (PK) 282.3
  riboflavin (vitamin B_2) 266.0
  saccadic eye movements 379.57
  salivation 527.7
  salt 276.1
  secretion
    ovary 256.39
    salivary gland (any) 527.7
    urine 788.5
  selenium 269.3
  serum
    antitrypsin, familial 273.4
    protein (congenital) 273.8
  short chain acyl CoA dehydrogenase (SCAD)
    277.85
  smooth pursuit movements (eye) 379.58
  sodium (Na) 276.1
  SPCA (*see also* Defect, coagulation) 286.3
  specified NEC 269.8
  stable factor (congenital) (*see also* Defect,
    coagulation) 286.3
    acquired 286.7
  Stuart (-Prower) factor (*see also* Defect,
    coagulation) 286.3
  sucrase 271.3
  sucrase-isomaltase 271.3
  sulfite oxidase 270.0
  syndrome, multiple 260
  thiamine, thiaminic (chloride) 265.1

Deficiency, deficient—*continued*
  thrombokinase (*see also* Defect, coagulation)
    286.3
    newborn 776.0
  thrombopoieten 287.39
  thymolymphatic 279.2
  thyroid (gland) 244.9
  tocopherol 269.1
  toe—*see* Absence, toe
  tooth bud (*see also* Anodontia) 520.0
  trunk V48.1
  UDPG-glycogen transferase 271.0
  upper limb V49.0
    congenital 755.20
      with complete absence of distal elements
        755.21
        longitudinal (complete) (partial) (with distal
          deficiencies, incomplete) 755.22
          carpal(s) 755.28
          combined humeral, radial, ulnar
            (incomplete) 755.23
          humeral 755.24
          metacarpal(s) 755.28
          phalange(s) 755.29
            meaning all digits 755.21
          radial 755.26
          radioulnar 755.25
          ulnar 755.27
        transverse (complete) (partial) 755.21
  vascular 459.9
  vasopressin 253.5
  viosterol (*see also* Deficiency, calciferol) 268.9
  vitamin (multiple) NEC 269.2
    A 264.9
      with
        Bitôt's spot 264.1
          corneal 264.2
            with corneal ulceration 264.3
        keratomalacia 264.4
        keratosis, follicular 264.8
        night blindness 264.5
        scar of cornea, xerophthalmic 264.6
        specified manifestation NEC 264.8
          ocular 264.7
        xeroderma 264.8
        xerophthalmia 264.7
        xerosis
          conjunctival 264.0
            with Bitôt's spot 264.1
          corneal 264.2
            with corneal ulceration 264.3
    B (complex) NEC 266.9
      with
        beriberi 265.0
        pellagra 265.2
      specified type NEC 266.2
    B_1 NEC 265.1
      beriberi 265.0
    B_2 266.0
    B_6 266.1
    B_{12} 266.2
    B_c (folic acid) 266.2
    C (ascorbic acid) (with scurvy) 267
    D (calciferol) (ergosterol) 268.9
      with
        osteomalacia 268.2
        rickets (*see also* Rickets) 268.0
    E 269.1
    folic acid 266.2
    G 266.0
    H 266.2

Deficiency, deficient—*continued*
  K 269.0
    of newborn 776.0
  nicotinic acid 265.2
  P 269.1
  PP 265.2
  specified NEC 269.1
  zinc 269.3
Deficient —*see also* Deficiency
  blink reflex 374.45
  craniofacial axis 756.0
  number of teeth (*see also* Anodontia) 520.0
  secretion of urine 788.5
Deficit
  neurologic NEC 781.99
    due to
      cerebrovascular lesion (*see also* Disease,
        cerebrovascular, acute) 436
        late effect—*see* Late effect(s) (of)
          cerebrovascular disease
      transient ischemic attack 435.9
  oxygen 799.02
Deflection
  radius 736.09
  septum (acquired) (nasal) (nose) 470
  spine—*see* Curvature, spine
  turbinate (nose) 470
Defluvium
  capillorum (*see also* Alopecia) 704.00
  ciliorum 374.55
  unguium 703.8
Deformity 738.9
  abdomen, congenital 759.9
  abdominal wall
    acquired 738.8
    congenital 756.70
    muscle deficiency syndrome 756.79
  acquired (unspecified site) 738.9
    specified site NEC 738.8
  adrenal gland (congenital) 759.1
  alimentary tract, congenital 751.9
    lower 751.5
    specified type NEC 751.8
    upper (any part, except tongue) 750.9
      specified type NEC 750.8
      tongue 750.10
        specified type NEC 750.19
  ankle (joint) (acquired) 736.70
    abduction 718.47
    congenital 755.69
    contraction 718.47
    specified NEC 736.79
  anus (congenital) 751.5
    acquired 569.49
  aorta (congenital) 747.20
    acquired 447.8
    arch 747.21
      acquired 447.8
    coarctation 747.10
  aortic
    arch 747.21
      acquired 447.8
    cusp or valve (congenital) 746.9
      acquired (*see also* Endocarditis, aortic)
        424.1
    ring 747.21
  appendix 751.5
  arm (acquired) 736.89
    congenital 755.50

Deformity—*continued*
  arteriovenous (congenital) (peripheral) NEC
      747.60
    gastrointestinal 747.61
    lower limb 747.64
    renal 747.62
    specified NEC 747.69
    spinal 747.82
    upper limb 747.63
  artery (congenital) (peripheral) NEC (*see also*
      Deformity, vascular) 747.60
    acquired 447.8
    cerebral 747.81
    coronary (congenital) 746.85
      acquired (*see also* Ischemia, heart) 414.9
    retinal 743.9
    umbilical 747.5
  atrial septal (congenital) (heart) 745.5
  auditory canal (congenital) (external) (*see also*
      Deformity, ear) 744.3
    acquired 380.50
  auricle
    ear (congenital) (*see also* Deformity, ear)
        744.3
      acquired 380.32
    heart (congenital) 746.9
  back (acquired)—*see* Deformity, spine
  Bartholin's duct (congenital) 750.9
  bile duct (congenital) 751.60
    acquired 576.8
      with calculus, choledocholithiasis, or
          stones—*see* Choledocholithiasis
  biliary duct or passage (congenital) 751.60
    acquired 576.8
      with calculus, choledocholithiasis, or
          stones—*see* Choledocholithiasis
  bladder (neck) (sphincter) (trigone) (acquired)
      596.8
    congenital 753.9
  bone (acquired) NEC 738.9
    congenital 756.9
    turbinate 738.0
  boutonniere (finger) 736.21
  brain (congenital) 742.9
    acquired 348.8
    multiple 742.4
    reduction 742.2
    vessel (congenital) 747.81
  breast (acquired) 611.8
    congenital 757.9
  bronchus (congenital) 748.3
    acquired 519.19
  bursa, congenital 756.9
  canal of Nuck 752.9
  canthus (congenital) 743.9
    acquired 374.89
  capillary (acquired) 448.9
    congenital NEC (*see also* Deformity, vascular)
        747.60
  cardiac—*see* Deformity, heart
  cardiovascular system (congenital) 746.9
  caruncle, lacrimal (congenital) 743.9
    acquired 375.69
  cascade, stomach 537.6
  cecum (congenital) 751.5
    acquired 569.89
  cerebral (congenital) 742.9
    acquired 348.8
  cervix (acquired) (uterus) 622.8
    congenital 752.40

Deformity—*continued*
  cheek (acquired) 738.19
    congenital 744.9
  chest (wall) (acquired) 738.3
    congenital 754.89
    late effect of rickets 268.1
  chin (acquired) 738.19
    congenital 744.9
  choroid (congenital) 743.9
    acquired 363.8
    plexus (congenital) 742.9
      acquired 349.2
  cicatricial—*see* Cicatrix
  cilia (congenital) 743.9
    acquired 374.89
  circulatory system (congenital) 747.9
  clavicle (acquired) 738.8
    congenital 755.51
  clitoris (congenital) 752.40
    acquired 624.8
  clubfoot—*see* Clubfoot
  coccyx (acquired) 738.6
    congenital 756.10
  colon (congenital) 751.5
    acquired 569.89
  concha (ear) (congenital) (*see also* Deformity,
      ear) 744.3
    acquired 380.32
  congenital, organ or site not listed (*see also*
      Anomaly) 759.9
  cornea (congenital) 743.9
    acquired 371.70
  coronary artery (congenital) 746.85
    acquired (*see also* Ischemia, heart) 414.9
  cranium (acquired) 738.19
    congenital (*see also* Deformity, skull,
        congenital) 756.0
  cricoid cartilage (congenital) 748.3
    acquired 478.79
  cystic duct (congenital) 751.60
    acquired 575.8
  Dandy-Walker 742.3
    with spina bifida (*see also* Spina bifida) 741.0
  diaphragm (congenital) 756.6
    acquired 738.8
  digestive organ(s) or system (congenital) NEC
      751.9
    specified type NEC 751.8
  ductus arteriosus 747.0
  duodenal bulb 537.89
  duodenum (congenital) 751.5
    acquired 537.89
  dura (congenital) 742.9
    brain 742.4
      acquired 349.2
    spinal 742.59
      acquired 349.2
  ear (congenital) 744.3
    acquired 380.32
    auricle 744.3
      causing impairment of hearing 744.02
    causing impairment of hearing 744.00
    external 744.3
      causing impairment of hearing 744.02
    internal 744.05
    lobule 744.3
    middle 744.03
      ossicles 744.04
    ossicles 744.04
  ectodermal (congenital) NEC 757.9
    specified type NEC 757.8

Deformity—*continued*
  ejaculatory duct (congenital) 752.9
    acquired 608.89
  elbow (joint) (acquired) 736.00
    congenital 755.50
    contraction 718.42
  endocrine gland NEC 759.2
  epididymis (congenital) 752.9
    acquired 608.89
    torsion 608.24
  epiglottis (congenital) 748.3
    acquired 478.79
  esophagus (congenital) 750.9
    acquired 530.89
  Eustachian tube (congenital) NEC 744.3
    specified type NEC 744.24
  extremity (acquired) 736.9
    congenital, except reduction deformity 755.9
      lower 755.60
      upper 755.50
    reduction—*see* Deformity, reduction
  eye (congenital) 743.9
    acquired 379.8
    muscle 743.9
  eyebrow (congenital) 744.89
  eyelid (congenital) 743.9
    acquired 374.89
    specified type NEC 743.62
  face (acquired) 738.19
    congenital (any part) 744.9
      due to intrauterine malposition and pressure 754.0
  fallopian tube (congenital) 752.10
    acquired 620.8
  femur (acquired) 736.89
    congenital 755.60
  fetal
    with fetopelvic disproportion 653.7
      affecting fetus or newborn 763.1
    causing obstructed labor 660.1
      affecting fetus or newborn 763.1
    known or suspected, affecting management of pregnancy 655.9
  finger (acquired) 736.20
    boutonniere type 736.21
    congenital 755.50
    flexion contracture 718.44
    swan neck 736.22
  flexion (joint) (acquired) 736.9
    congenital NEC 755.9
    hip or thigh (acquired) 736.39
      congenital (*see also* Subluxation, congenital, hip) 754.32
  foot (acquired) 736.70
    cavovarus 736.75
      congenital 754.59
    congenital NEC 754.70
      specified type NEC 754.79
    valgus (acquired) 736.79
      congenital 754.60
        specified type NEC 754.69
    varus (acquired) 736.79
      congenital 754.50
        specified type NEC 754.59
  forearm (acquired) 736.00
    congenital 755.50
  forehead (acquired) 738.19
    congenital (*see also* Deformity, skull, congenital) 756.0

Deformity—*continued*
  frontal bone (acquired) 738.19
    congenital (*see also* Deformity, skull, congenital) 756.0
  gallbladder (congenital) 751.60
    acquired 575.8
  gastrointestinal tract (congenital) NEC 751.9
    acquired 569.89
    specified type NEC 751.8
  genitalia, genital organ(s) or system NEC
    congenital 752.9
    female (congenital) 752.9
      acquired 629.89
      external 752.40
      internal 752.9
    male (congenital) 752.9
      acquired 608.89
  globe (eye) (congenital) 743.9
    acquired 360.89
  gum (congenital) 750.9
    acquired 523.9
  gunstock 736.02
  hand (acquired) 736.00
    claw 736.06
    congenital 755.50
    minus (and plus) (intrinsic) 736.09
    pill roller (intrinsic) 736.09
    plus (and minus) (intrinsic) 736.09
    swan neck (intrinsic) 736.09
  head (acquired) 738.10
    congenital (*see also* Deformity, skull, congenital) 756.0
    specified NEC 738.19
  heart (congenital) 746.9
    auricle (congenital) 746.9
    septum 745.9
      auricular 745.5
      specified type NEC 745.8
      ventricular 745.4
    valve (congenital) NEC 746.9
      acquired—*see* Endocarditis
      pulmonary (congenital) 746.00
      specified type NEC 746.89
    ventricle (congenital) 746.9
  heel (acquired) 736.76
    congenital 755.67
  hepatic duct (congenital) 751.60
    acquired 576.8
      with calculus, choledocholithiasis, or stones—*see* Choledocholithiasis
  hip (joint) (acquired) 736.30
    congenital NEC 755.63
    flexion 718.45
      congenital (*see also* Subluxation, congenital, hip) 754.32
  hourglass—*see* Contraction, hourglass
  humerus (acquired) 736.89
    congenital 755.50
  hymen (congenital) 752.40
  hypophyseal (congenital) 759.2
  ileocecal (coil) (valve) (congenital) 751.5
    acquired 569.89
  ileum (intestine) (congenital) 751.5
    acquired 569.89
  ilium (acquired) 738.6
    congenital 755.60
  integument (congenital) 757.9
  intervertebral cartilage or disc (acquired)—*see also* Displacement, intervertebral disc
    congenital 756.10

Deformity—*continued*
  intestine (large) (small) (congenital) 751.5
    acquired 569.89
  iris (acquired) 364.75
    congenital 743.9
    prolapse 364.8
  ischium (acquired) 738.6
    congenital 755.60
  jaw (acquired) (congenital) NEC 524.9
    due to intrauterine malposition and pressure
      754.0
  joint (acquired) NEC 738.8
    congenital 755.9
    contraction (abduction) (adduction)
      (extension) (flexion)—*see* Contraction,
      joint
  kidney(s) (calyx) (pelvis) (congenital) 753.9
    acquired 593.89
    vessel 747.62
      acquired 459.9
  Klippel-Feil (brevicollis) 756.16
  knee (acquired) NEC 736.6
    congenital 755.64
  labium (majus) (minus) (congenital) 752.40
    acquired 624.8
  lacrimal apparatus or duct (congenital) 743.9
    acquired 375.69
  larynx (muscle) (congenital) 748.3
    acquired 478.79
    web (glottic) (subglottic) 748.2
  leg (lower) (upper) (acquired) NEC 736.89
    congenital 755.60
    reduction—*see* Deformity, reduction, lower
      limb
  lens (congenital) 743.9
    acquired 379.39
  lid (fold) (congenital) 743.9
    acquired 374.89
  ligament (acquired) 728.9
    congenital 756.9
  limb (acquired) 736.9
    congenital, except reduction deformity 755.9
      lower 755.60
        reduction (*see also* Deformity, reduction,
          lower limb) 755.30
      upper 755.50
        reduction (*see also* Deformity, reduction,
          lower limb) 755.20
    specified NEC 736.89
  lip (congenital) NEC 750.9
    acquired 528.5
    specified type NEC 750.26
  liver (congenital) 751.60
    acquired 573.8
    duct (congenital) 751.60
      acquired 576.8
        with calculus, choledocholithiasis, or
          stones—*see* Choledocholithiasis
  lower extremity—*see* Deformity, leg
  lumbosacral (joint) (region) (congenital) 756.10
    acquired 738.5
  lung (congenital) 748.60
    acquired 518.89
    specified type NEC 748.69
  lymphatic system, congenital 759.9
  Madelung's (radius) 755.54
  maxilla (acquired) (congenital) 524.9
  meninges or membrane (congenital) 742.9
    brain 742.4
      acquired 349.2
    spinal (cord) 742.59

Deformity—*continued*
    acquired 349.2
  mesentery (congenital) 751.9
    acquired 568.89
  metacarpus (acquired) 736.00
    congenital 755.50
  metatarsus (acquired) 736.70
    congenital 754.70
  middle ear, except ossicles (congenital) 744.03
    ossicles 744.04
  mitral (leaflets) (valve) (congenital) 746.9
    acquired—*see* Endocarditis, mitral
    Ebstein's 746.89
    parachute 746.5
    specified type NEC 746.89
    stenosis, congenital 746.5
  mouth (acquired) 528.9
    congenital NEC 750.9
      specified type NEC 750.26
  multiple, congenital NEC 759.7
    specified type NEC 759.89
  muscle (acquired) 728.9
    congenital 756.9
      specified type NEC 756.89
      sternocleidomastoid (due to intrauterine
        malposition and pressure) 754.1
  musculoskeletal system, congenital NEC 756.9
    specified type NEC 756.9
  nail (acquired) 703.9
    congenital 757.9
  nasal—*see* Deformity, nose
  neck (acquired) NEC 738.2
    congenital (any part) 744.9
      sternocleidomastoid 754.1
  nervous system (congenital) 742.9
  nipple (congenital) 757.9
    acquired 611.8
  nose, nasal (cartilage) (acquired) 738.0
    bone (turbinate) 738.0
    congenital 748.1
      bent 754.0
      squashed 754.0
    saddle 738.0
      syphilitic 090.5
    septum 470
      congenital 748.1
    sinus (wall) (congenital) 748.1
      acquired 738.0
    syphilitic (congenital) 090.5
      late 095.8
  ocular muscle (congenital) 743.9
    acquired 378.60
  opticociliary vessels (congenital) 743.9
  orbit (congenital) (eye) 743.9
    acquired NEC 376.40
      associated with craniofacial deformities
        376.44
      due to
        bone disease 376.43
        surgery 376.47
        trauma 376.47
  organ of Corti (congenital) 744.05
  ovary (congenital) 752.0
    acquired 620.8
  oviduct (congenital) 752.10
    acquired 620.8
  palate (congenital) 750.9
    acquired 526.89
    cleft (congenital) (*see also* Cleft, palate)
      749.00
    hard, acquired 526.89

Deformity—*continued*
  soft, acquired 528.9
  pancreas (congenital) 751.7
    acquired 577.8
  parachute, mitral valve 746.5
  parathyroid (gland) 759.2
  parotid (gland) (congenital) 750.9
    acquired 527.8
  patella (acquired) 736.6
    congenital 755.64
  pelvis, pelvic (acquired) (bony) 738.6
    with disproportion (fetopelvic) 653.0
      affecting fetus or newborn 763.1
      causing obstructed labor 660.1
        affecting fetus or newborn 763.1
    congenital 755.60
    rachitic (late effect) 268.1
  penis (glans) (congenital) 752.9
    acquired 607.89
  pericardium (congenital) 746.9
    acquired—*see* Pericarditis
  pharynx (congenital) 750.9
    acquired 478.29
  Pierre Robin (congenital) 756.0
  pinna (acquired) 380.32
    congenital 744.3
  pituitary (congenital) 759.2
  pleural folds (congenital) 748.8
  portal vein (congenital) 747.40
  posture—*see* Curvature, spine
  prepuce (congenital) 752.9
    acquired 607.89
  prostate (congenital) 752.9
    acquired 602.8
  pulmonary valve—*see* Endocarditis, pulmonary
  pupil (congenital) 743.9
    acquired 364.75
  pylorus (congenital) 750.9
    acquired 537.89
  rachitic (acquired), healed or old 268.1
  radius (acquired) 736.00
    congenital 755.50
      reduction—*see* Deformity, reduction, upper
        limb
  rectovaginal septum (congenital) 752.40
    acquired 623.8
  rectum (congenital) 751.5
    acquired 569.49
  reduction (extremity) (limb) 755.4
    brain 742.2
    lower limb 755.30
      with complete absence of distal elements
        755.31
      longitudinal (complete) (partial) (with distal
        deficiencies, incomplete) 755.32
        with complete absence of distal elements
          755.31
        combined femoral, tibial, fibular
          (incomplete) 755.33
        femoral 755.34
        fibular 755.37
        metatarsal(s) 755.38
        phalange(s) 755.39
          meaning all digits 755.31
        tarsal(s) 755.38
        tibia 755.36
        tibiofibular 755.35
      transverse 755.31
    upper limb 755.20
      with complete absence of distal elements
        755.21

Deformity—*continued*
    longitudinal (complete) (partial) (with distal
      deficiencies, incomplete) 755.22
      with complete absence of distal elements
        755.21
      carpal(s) 755.28
      combined humeral, radial, ulnar
        (incomplete) 755.23
      humeral 755.24
      metacarpal(s) 755.28
      phalange(s) 755.29
        meaning all digits 755.21
      radial 755.26
      radioulnar 755.25
      ulnar 755.27
    transverse (complete) (partial) 755.21
  renal—*see* Deformity, kidney
  respiratory system (congenital) 748.9
    specified type NEC 748.8
  rib (acquired) 738.3
    congenital 756.3
      cervical 756.2
  rotation (joint) (acquired) 736.9
    congenital 755.9
    hip or thigh 736.39
      congenital (*see also* Subluxation, congenital,
        hip) 754.32
  sacroiliac joint (congenital) 755.69
    acquired 738.5
  sacrum (acquired) 738.5
    congenital 756.10
  saddle
    back 737.8
    nose 738.0
      syphilitic 090.5
  salivary gland or duct (congenital) 750.9
    acquired 527.8
  scapula (acquired) 736.89
    congenital 755.50
  scrotum (congenital) 752.9
    acquired 608.89
  sebaceous gland, acquired 706.8
  seminal tract or duct (congenital) 752.9
    acquired 608.89
  septum (nasal) (acquired) 470
    congenital 748.1
  shoulder (joint) (acquired) 736.89
    congenital 755.50
      specified type NEC 755.59
    contraction 718.41
  sigmoid (flexure) (congenital) 751.5
    acquired 569.89
  sinus of Valsalva 747.29
  skin (congenital) 757.9
    acquired NEC 709.8
  skull (acquired) 738.19
    congenital 756.0
      with
        anencephalus 740.0
        encephalocele 742.0
        hydrocephalus 742.3
          with spina bifida (*see also* Spina bifida)
            741.0
        microcephalus 742.1
      due to intrauterine malposition and pressure
        754.0
  soft parts, organs or tissues (of pelvis)
    in pregnancy or childbirth NEC 654.9
      affecting fetus or newborn 763.89
      causing obstructed labor 660.2
        affecting fetus or newborn 763.1

Deformity—*continued*
　spermatic cord (congenital) 752.9
　　acquired 608.89
　　　torsion 608.22
　　　　extravaginal 608.21
　　　　intravaginal 608.22
　spinal
　　column—*see* Deformity, spine
　　cord (congenital) 742.9
　　　acquired 336.8
　　　vessel (congenital) 747.82
　　nerve root (congenital) 742.9
　　　acquired 724.9
　　vessel 747.82
　spine (acquired) NEC 738.5
　　congenital 756.10
　　　due to intrauterine malposition and pressure
　　　　754.2
　　kyphoscoliotic (*see also* Kyphoscoliosis)
　　　737.30
　　kyphotic (*see also* Kyphosis) 737.10
　　lordotic (*see also* Lordosis) 737.20
　　rachitic 268.1
　　scoliotic (*see also* Scoliosis) 737.30
　spleen
　　acquired 289.59
　　congenital 759.0
　Sprengel's (congenital) 755.52
　sternum (acquired) 738.3
　　congenital 756.3
　stomach (congenital) 750.9
　　acquired 537.89
　submaxillary gland (congenital) 750.9
　　acquired 527.8
　swan neck (acquired)
　　finger 736.22
　　hand 736.09
　talipes—*see* Talipes
　teeth, tooth NEC 520.9
　testis (congenital) 752.9
　　acquired 608.89
　　　torsion 608.20
　thigh (acquired) 736.89
　　congenital 755.60
　thorax (acquired) (wall) 738.3
　　congenital 754.89
　　late effect of rickets 268.1
　thumb (acquired) 736.20
　　congenital 755.50
　thymus (tissue) (congenital) 759.2
　thyroid (gland) (congenital) 759.2
　　cartilage 748.3
　　　acquired 478.79
　tibia (acquired) 736.89
　　congenital 755.60
　　saber 090.5
　toe (acquired) 735.9
　　congenital 755.66
　　specified NEC 735.8
　tongue (congenital) 750.10
　　acquired 529.8
　tooth, teeth NEC 520.9
　trachea (rings) (congenital) 748.3
　　acquired 519.19
　transverse aortic arch (congenital) 747.21
　tricuspid (leaflets) (valve) (congenital) 746.9
　　acquired—*see* Endocarditis, tricuspid
　　atresia or stenosis 746.1
　　specified type NEC 746.89
　trunk (acquired) 738.3
　　congenital 759.9

Deformity—*continued*
　ulna (acquired) 736.00
　　congenital 755.50
　upper extremity—*see* Deformity, arm
　urachus (congenital) 753.7
　ureter (opening) (congenital) 753.9
　　acquired 593.89
　urethra (valve) (congenital) 753.9
　　acquired 599.84
　urinary tract or system (congenital) 753.9
　　urachus 753.7
　uterus (congenital) 752.3
　　acquired 621.8
　uvula (congenital) 750.9
　　acquired 528.9
　vagina (congenital) 752.40
　　acquired 623.8
　valve, valvular (heart) (congenital) 746.9
　　acquired—*see* Endocarditis
　　pulmonary 746.00
　　specified type NEC 746.89
　vascular (congenital) (peripheral) NEC 747.60
　　acquired 459.9
　　gastrointestinal 747.61
　　lower limb 747.64
　　renal 747.62
　　specified site NEC 747.69
　　spinal 747.82
　　upper limb 747.63
　vas deferens (congenital) 752.9
　　acquired 608.89
　vein (congenital) NEC (*see also* Deformity,
　　vascular) 747.60
　　brain 747.81
　　coronary 746.9
　　great 747.40
　vena cava (inferior) (superior) (congenital)
　　747.40
　vertebra—*see* Deformity, spine
　vesicourethral orifice (acquired) 596.8
　　congenital NEC 753.9
　　　specified type NEC 753.8
　vessels of optic papilla (congenital) 743.9
　visual field (contraction) 368.45
　vitreous humor (congenital) 743.9
　　acquired 379.29
　vulva (congenital) 752.40
　　acquired 624.8
　wrist (joint) (acquired) 736.00
　　congenital 755.50
　　contraction 718.43
　　valgus 736.03
　　　congenital 755.59
　　varus 736.04
　　　congenital 755.59
Degeneration, degenerative
　adrenal (capsule) (gland) 255.8
　　with hypofunction 255.4
　　fatty 255.8
　　hyaline 255.8
　　infectional 255.8
　　lardaceous 277.39
　amyloid (any site) (general) 277.39
　anterior cornua, spinal cord 336.8
　aorta, aortic 440.0
　　fatty 447.8
　　valve (heart) (*see also* Endocarditis, aortic)
　　　424.1
　arteriovascular—*see* Arteriosclerosis

Degeneration, degenerative—*continued*
  suprarenal (capsule) (gland) 255.8
    with hypofunction 255.4
  sweat gland 705.89
  synovial membrane (pulpy) 727.9
  tapetoretinal 362.74
    adult or presenile form 362.50
  testis (postinfectional) 608.89
  thymus (gland) 254.8
    fatty 254.8
    lardaceous 277.39
  thyroid (gland) 246.8
  tricuspid (heart) (valve)—*see* Endocarditis,
    tricuspid
  tuberculous NEC (*see also* Tuberculosis) 011.9
  turbinate 733.90
  uterus 621.8
    cystic 621.8
  vascular (senile)—*see also* Arteriosclerosis
    hypertensive—*see* Hypertension
  vitreoretinal (primary) 362.73
    secondary 362.66
  vitreous humor (with infiltration) 379.21
  wallerian NEC—*see* Disorder, nerve
  waxy (any site) 277.39
  Wilson's hepatolenticular 275.1
Deglutition
  paralysis 784.99
    hysterical 300.11
  pneumonia 507.0
Degos' disease or syndrome 447.8
Degradation disorder, branched-chain
  amino-acid 270.3
Dehiscence
  anastomosis—*see* Complications, anastomosis
  cesarean wound 674.1
  episiotomy 674.2
  operation wound 998.32
    internal 998.31
  perineal wound (postpartum) 674.2
  postoperative 998.32
    abdomen 998.32
      internal 998.31
    internal 998.31
  uterine wound 674.1
Dehydration (cachexia) 276.51
  newborn 775.5
  with
    hypernatremia 276.0
    hyponatremia 276.1
Deiters' nucleus syndrome 386.19
Déjérine's disease 356.0
Déjérine-Klumpke paralysis 767.6
Déjérine-Roussy syndrome 338.0
Déjérine-Sottas disease or neuropathy
  (hypertrophic) 356.0
Déjérine-Thomas atrophy or syndrome 333.0
de Lange's syndrome (Amsterdam dwarf, mental
  retardation, and brachycephaly) 759.89
Delay, delayed
  adaptation, cones or rods 368.63
  any plane in pelvis
    affecting fetus or newborn 763.1
    complicating delivery 660.1
  birth or delivery NEC 662.1
    affecting fetus or newborn 763.9
    second twin, triplet, or multiple mate 662.3
  closure—*see also* Fistula
    cranial suture 756.0
    fontanel 756.0
  coagulation NEC 790.92

Delay, delayed—*continued*
  conduction (cardiac) (ventricular) 426.9
  delivery NEC 662.1
    second twin, triplet, etc. 662.3
      affecting fetus or newborn 763.89
  development
    in childhood 783.40
      physiological 783.40
    intellectual NEC 315.9
    learning NEC 315.2
    reading 315.00
    sexual 259.0
    speech 315.39
      associated with hyperkinesis 314.1
    spelling 315.09
  gastric emptying 536.8
  menarche 256.39
    due to pituitary hypofunction 253.4
  menstruation (cause unknown) 626.8
  milestone in childhood 783.42
  motility—*see* Hypomotility
  passage of meconium (newborn) 777.1
  primary respiration 768.9
  puberty 259.0
  separation of umbilical cord 779.83
  sexual maturation, female 259.0
Del Castillo's syndrome (germinal aplasia) 606.0
Deleage's disease 359.89
Deletion syndrome
  5p 758.31
  22q11.2 758.32
  autosomal NEC 758.39
  constitutional 5q deletion 758.39
Delhi (boil) (button) (sore) 085.1
Delinquency (juvenile) 312.9
  group (*see also* Disturbance, conduct) 312.2
  neurotic 312.4
Delirium, delirious 780.09
  acute (psychotic) 293.0
  alcoholic 291.0
    acute 291.0
    chronic 291.1
  alcoholicum 291.0
  chronic (*see also* Psychosis) 293.89
    due to or associated with physical
      condition—*see* Psychosis, organic
  due to conditions classified elsewhere 293.0
  drug-induced 292.81
  eclamptic (*see also* Eclampsia) 780.39
  exhaustion (*see also* Reaction, stress, acute)
    308.9
  hysterical 300.11
  in
    presenile dementia 290.11
    senile dementia 290.3
  induced by drug 292.81
  manic, maniacal (acute) (*see also* Psychosis,
    affective) 296.0
    recurrent episode 296.1
    single episode 296.0
  puerperal 293.9
  senile 290.3
  subacute (psychotic) 293.1
  thyroid (*see also* Thyrotoxicosis) 242.9
  traumatic—*see also* Injury, intracranial
    with
      lesion, spinal cord—*see* Injury, spinal, by
        site
      shock, spinal—*see* Injury, spinal, by site
  tremens (impending) 291.0
  uremic—*see* Uremia

Delirium, delirious—*continued*
  withdrawal
    alcoholic (acute) 291.0
      chronic 291.1
    drug 292.0
Delivery

> *Note—Use the following fifth-digit*
> *subclassification with categories*
> *640-648, 651-676:*
>
> *0 unspecified as to episode of care*
> *1 delivered, with or without mention of*
> *   antepartum condition*
> *2 delivered, with mention of*
> *   postpartum complication*
> *3 antepartum condition or complication*
> *4 postpartum condition or*
> *   complication*

  breech (assisted) (spontaneous) 652.2
    affecting fetus or newborn 763.0
    extraction NEC 669.6
  cesarean (for) 669.7
    abnormal
      cervix 654.6
      pelvic organs or tissues 654.9
      pelvis (bony) (major) NEC 653.0
      presentation or position 652.9
        in multiple gestation 652.6
      size, fetus 653.5
      soft parts (of pelvis) 654.9
      uterus, congenital 654.0
      vagina 654.7
      vulva 654.8
    abruptio placentae 641.2
    acromion presentation 652.8
    affecting fetus or newborn 763.4
    anteversion, cervix or uterus 654.4
    atony, uterus, with hemorrhage 666.1
    bicornis or bicornuate uterus 654.0
    breech presentation 652.2
    brow presentation 652.4
    cephalopelvic disproportion (normally formed
      fetus) 653.4
    chin presentation 652.4
    cicatrix of cervix 654.6
    contracted pelvis (general) 653.1
      inlet 653.2
      outlet 653.3
    cord presentation or prolapse 663.0
    cystocele 654.4
    deformity (acquired) (congenital)
      pelvic organs or tissues NEC 654.9
      pelvis (bony) NEC 653.0
    displacement, uterus NEC 654.4
    disproportion NEC 653.9
    distress
      fetal 656.8
      maternal 669.0
    eclampsia 642.6
    face presentation 652.4
    failed
      forceps 660.7
      trial of labor NEC 660.6
      vacuum extraction 660.7
      ventouse 660.7
    fetal deformity 653.7
    fetal-maternal hemorrhage 656.0
    fetus, fetal
      distress 656.8
      prematurity 656.8

Delivery—*continued*
  fibroid (tumor) (uterus) 654.1
  footling 652.8
    with successful version 652.1
  hemorrhage (antepartum) (intrapartum) NEC
    641.9
  hydrocephalic fetus 653.6
  incarceration of uterus 654.3
  incoordinate uterine action 661.4
  inertia, uterus 661.2
    primary 661.0
    secondary 661.1
  lateroversion, uterus or cervix 654.4
  mal lie 652.9
  malposition
    fetus 652.9
      in multiple gestation 652.6
    pelvic organs or tissues NEC 654.9
    uterus NEC or cervix 654.4
  malpresentation NEC 652.9
    in multiple gestation 652.6
  maternal
    diabetes mellitus 648.0
    heart disease NEC 648.6
  meconium in liquor 656.8
    staining only 792.3
  oblique presentation 652.3
  oversize fetus 653.5
  pelvic tumor NEC 654.9
  placental insufficiency 656.5
  placenta previa 641.0
    with hemorrhage 641.1
  poor dilation, cervix 661.0
  pre-eclampsia 642.4
    severe 642.5
  previous
    cesarean delivery 654.2
    surgery (to)
      cervix 654.6
      gynecological NEC 654.9
      rectum 654.8
      uterus NEC 654.9
        from previous cesarean delivery 654.2
      vagina 654.7
  prolapse
    arm or hand 652.7
    uterus 654.4
  prolonged labor 662.1
  rectocele 654.4
  retroversion, uterus or cervix 654.3
  rigid
    cervix 654.6
    pelvic floor 654.4
    perineum 654.8
    vagina 654.7
    vulva 654.8
  sacculation, pregnant uterus 654.4
  scar(s)
    cervix 654.6
    cesarean delivery 654.2
    uterus NEC 654.9
      due to previous cesarean delivery 654.2
  Shirodkar suture in situ 654.5
  shoulder presentation 652.8
  stenosis or stricture, cervix 654.6
  transverse presentation or lie 652.3
  tumor, pelvic organs or tissues NEC 654.4
  umbilical cord presentation or prolapse 663.0
completely normal case—*see* category 650

Dementia—*continued*
  schizophrenic (*see also* Schizophrenia) 295.9
  senile 290.0
    with
      acute confusional state 290.3
      delirium 290.3
      delusional features 290.20
      depressive features 290.21
    depressed type 290.21
    exhaustion 290.0
    paranoid type 290.20
  simple type (acute) (*see also* Schizophrenia) 295.0
  simplex (acute) (*see also* Schizophrenia) 295.0
  syphilitic 094.1
  uremic—*see* Uremia
  vascular 290.40
    with
      delirium 290.41
      delusions 290.42
      depressed mood 290.43
Demerol dependence (*see also* Dependence) 304.0
Demineralization, ankle (*see also* Osteoporosis) 733.00
Demodex folliculorum (infestation) 133.8
de Morgan's spots (senile angiomas) 448.1
Demyelinating
  polyneuritis, chronic inflammatory 357.81
Demyelination, demyelinization
  central nervous system 341.9
    specified NEC 341.8
  corpus callosum (central) 341.8
  global 340
Dengue (fever) 061
  sandfly 061
  vaccination, prophylactic (against) V05.1
  virus hemorrhagic fever 065.4
Dens
  evaginatus 520.2
  in dente 520.2
  invaginatus 520.2
Density
  increased, bone (disseminated) (generalized) (spotted) 733.99
  lung (nodular) 518.89
Dental —*see also* condition
  examination only V72.2
Dentia praecox 520.6
Denticles (in pulp) 522.2
Dentigerous cyst 526.0
Dentin
  irregular (in pulp) 522.3
  opalescent 520.5
  secondary (in pulp) 522.3
  sensitive 521.89
Dentinogenesis imperfecta 520.5
Dentinoma (M9271/0) 213.1
  upper jaw (bone) 213.0
Dentition 520.7
  abnormal 520.6
  anomaly 520.6
  delayed 520.6
  difficult 520.7
  disorder of 520.6
  precocious 520.6
  retarded 520.6
Denture sore (mouth) 528.9

Dependence

> *Note—Use the following fifth-digit*
> *subclassification with category 304:*
>
> *0 unspecified*
> *1 continuous*
> *2 episodic*
> *3 in remission*

  with
    withdrawal symptoms
      alcohol 291.81
      drug 292.0
  14-hydroxy-dihydromorphinone 304.0
  absinthe 304.6
  acemorphan 304.0
  acetanilid(e) 304.6
  acetophenetidin 304.6
  acetorphine 304.0
  acetyldihydrocodeine 304.0
  acetyldihydrocodeinone 304.0
  Adalin 304.1
  Afghanistan black 304.3
  agrypnal 304.1
  alcohol, alcoholic (ethyl) (methyl) (wood) 303.9
    maternal, with suspected fetal damage
      affecting management of pregnancy 655.4
  allobarbitone 304.1
  allonal 304.1
  allylisopropylacetylurea 304.1
  alphaprodine (hydrochloride) 304.0
  Alurate 304.1
  Alvodine 304.0
  amethocaine 304.6
  amidone 304.0
  amidopyrine 304.6
  aminopyrine 304.6
  amobarbital 304.1
  amphetamine(s) (type) (drugs classifiable to 969.7) 304.4
  amylene hydrate 304.6
  amylobarbitone 304.1
  amylocaine 304.6
  Amytal (sodium) 304.1
  analgesic (drug) NEC 304.6
    synthetic with morphine-like effect 304.0
  anesthetic (agent) (drug) (gas) (general) (local) NEC 304.6
  Angel dust 304.6
  anileridine 304.0
  antipyrine 304.6
  anxiolytic 304.1
  aprobarbital 304.1
  aprobarbitone 304.1
  atropine 304.6
  Avertin (bromide) 304.6
  barbenyl 304.1
  barbital(s) 304.1
  barbitone 304.1
  barbiturate(s) (compounds) (drugs classifiable to 967.0) 304.1
  barbituric acid (and compounds) 304.1
  benzedrine 304.4
  benzylmorphine 304.0
  Beta-chlor 304.1
  bhang 304.3
  blue velvet 304.0
  Brevital 304.1
  bromal (hydrate) 304.1
  bromide(s) NEC 304.1
  bromine compounds NEC 304.1

Depletion
 carbohydrates 271.9
 complement factor 279.8
 extracellular fluid 276.52
 plasma 276.52
 potassium 276.8
  nephropathy 588.89
 salt or sodium 276.1
  causing heat exhaustion or prostration 992.4
  nephropathy 593.9
 volume 276.50
  extracellular fluid 276.52
  plasma 276.52

Deposit
 argentous, cornea 371.16
 bone, in Boeck's sarcoid 135
 calcareous, calcium—*see* Calcification
 cholesterol
  retina 362.82
  skin 709.3
  vitreous (humor) 379.22
 conjunctival 372.56
 cornea, corneal NEC 371.10
  argentous 371.16
  in
    cystinosis 270.0 *[371.15]*
    mucopolysaccharidosis 277.5 *[371.15]*
 crystalline, vitreous (humor) 379.22
 hemosiderin, in old scars of cornea 371.11
 metallic, in lens 366.45
 skin 709.3
 teeth, tooth (betel) (black) (green) (materia alba)
   (orange) (soft) (tobacco) 523.6
 urate, in kidney (*see also* Disease, renal) 593.9

Depraved appetite 307.52

Depression 311
 acute (*see also* Psychosis, affective) 296.2
  recurrent episode 296.3
  single episode 296.2
 agitated (*see also* Psychosis, affective) 296.2
  recurrent episode 296.3
  single episode 296.2
 anaclitic 309.21
 anxiety 300.4
 arches 734
  congenital 754.61
 autogenous (*see also* Psychosis, affective) 296.2
  recurrent episode 296.3
  single episode 296.2
 basal metabolic rate (BMR) 794.7
 bone marrow 289.9
 central nervous system 799.1
  newborn 779.2
 cerebral 331.9
  newborn 779.2
 cerebrovascular 437.8
  newborn 779.2
 chest wall 738.3
 endogenous (*see also* Psychosis, affective) 296.2
  recurrent episode 296.3
  single episode 296.2
 functional activity 780.99
 hysterical 300.11
 involutional, climacteric, or menopausal (*see
   also* Psychosis, affective) 296.2
  recurrent episode 296.3
  single episode 296.2
 manic (*see also* Psychosis, affective) 296.80
 medullary 348.8
  newborn 779.2
 mental 300.4

Depression—*continued*
 metatarsal heads—*see* Depression, arches
 metatarsus—*see* Depression, arches
 monopolar (*see also* Psychosis, affective) 296.2
  recurrent episode 296.3
  single episode 296.2
 nervous 300.4
 neurotic 300.4
 nose 738.0
 postpartum 648.4
 psychogenic 300.4
  reactive 298.0
 psychoneurotic 300.4
 psychotic (*see also* Psychosis, affective) 296.2
  reactive 298.0
  recurrent episode 296.3
  single episode 296.2
 reactive 300.4
  neurotic 300.4
  psychogenic 298.0
  psychoneurotic 300.4
  psychotic 298.0
 recurrent 296.3
 respiratory center 348.8
  newborn 770.89
 scapula 736.89
 senile 290.21
 situational (acute) (brief) 309.0
  prolonged 309.1
 skull 754.0
 sternum 738.3
 visual field 368.40

Depressive reaction —*see also* Reaction,
  depressive
 acute (transient) 309.0
  with anxiety 309.28
 prolonged 309.1
 situational (acute) 309.0
  prolonged 309.1

Deprivation
 cultural V62.4
 emotional V62.89
  affecting
    adult 995.82
    infant or child 995.51
 food 994.2
  specific substance NEC 269.8
 protein (familial) (kwashiorkor) 260
 sleep V69.4
 social V62.4
  affecting
    adult 995.82
    infant or child 995.51
 symptoms, syndrome
  alcohol 291.81
  drug 292.0
 vitamins (*see also* Deficiency, vitamin) 269.2
 water 994.3

de Quervain's
 disease (tendon sheath) 727.04
 thyroiditis (subacute granulomatous thyroiditis)
   245.1

Derangement
 ankle (internal) 718.97
  current injury (*see also* Dislocation, ankle)
    837.0
  recurrent 718.37
 cartilage (articular) NEC (*see also* Disorder,
   cartilage, articular) 718.0
  knee 717.9
    recurrent 718.36

Derangement—*continued*
  recurrent 718.3
  collateral ligament (knee) (medial) (tibial) 717.82
    current injury 844.1
      lateral (fibular) 844.0
    lateral (fibular) 717.81
      current injury 844.0
  cruciate ligament (knee) (posterior) 717.84
    anterior 717.83
      current injury 844.2
    current injury 844.2
  elbow (internal) 718.92
    current injury (*see also* Dislocation, elbow) 832.00
    recurrent 718.32
  gastrointestinal 536.9
  heart—*see* Disease, heart
  hip (joint) (internal) (old) 718.95
    current injury (*see also* Dislocation, hip) 835.00
    recurrent 718.35
  intervertebral disc—*see* Displacement, intervertebral disc
  joint (internal) 718.90
    ankle 718.97
    current injury—*see also* Dislocation, by site
      knee, meniscus or cartilage (*see also* Tear, meniscus) 836.2
    elbow 718.92
    foot 718.97
    hand 718.94
    hip 718.95
    knee 717.9
    multiple sites 718.99
    pelvic region 718.95
    recurrent 718.30
      ankle 718.37
      elbow 718.32
      foot 718.37
      hand 718.34
      hip 718.35
      knee 718.36
      multiple sites 718.39
      pelvic region 718.35
      shoulder (region) 718.31
      specified site NEC 718.38
      temporomandibular (old) 524.69
      wrist 718.33
    shoulder (region) 718.91
    specified site NEC 718.98
    spine NEC 724.9
    temporomandibular 524.69
    wrist 718.93
  knee (cartilage) (internal) 717.9
    current injury (*see also* Tear, meniscus) 836.2
    ligament 717.89
      capsular 717.85
      collateral—*see* Derangement, collateral ligament
      cruciate—*see* Derangement, cruciate ligament
      specified NEC 717.85
      recurrent 718.36
  low back NEC 724.9
  meniscus NEC (knee) 717.5
    current injury (*see also* Tear, meniscus) 836.2
    lateral 717.40
      anterior horn 717.42
      posterior horn 717.43
      specified NEC 717.49

Derangement—*continued*
    medial 717.3
      anterior horn 717.1
      posterior horn 717.2
    recurrent 718.3
    site other than knee—*see* Disorder, cartilage, articular
  mental (*see also* Psychosis) 298.9
  rotator cuff (recurrent) (tear) 726.10
    current 840.4
  sacroiliac (old) 724.6
    current—*see* Dislocation, sacroiliac
  semilunar cartilage (knee) 717.5
    current injury 836.2
      lateral 836.1
      medial 836.0
    recurrent 718.3
  shoulder (internal) 718.91
    current injury (*see also* Dislocation, shoulder) 831.00
    recurrent 718.31
  spine (recurrent) NEC 724.9
    current—*see* Dislocation, spine
  temporomandibular (internal) (joint) (old) 524.69
    current—*see* Dislocation, jaw
Dercum's disease or syndrome (adiposis dolorosa) 272.8
Derealization (neurotic) 300.6
Dermal —*see* condition
Dermaphytid —*see* Dermatophytosis
Dermatergosis —*see* Dermatitis
Dermatitis (allergic) (contact) (occupational) (venenata) 692.9
  ab igne 692.82
  acneiform 692.9
  actinic (due to sun) 692.70
    acute 692.72
    chronic NEC 692.74
    other than from sun NEC 692.82
  ambustionis
    due to
      burn or scald—*see* Burn, by site
      sunburn (*see also* Sunburn) 692.71
  amebic 006.6
  ammonia 691.0
  anaphylactoid NEC 692.9
  arsenical 692.4
  artefacta 698.4
    psychogenic 316 *[698.4]*
  asthmatic 691.8
  atopic (allergic) (intrinsic) 691.8
    psychogenic 316 *[691.8]*
  atrophicans 701.8
    diffusa 701.8
    maculosa 701.3
  berlock, berloque 692.72
  blastomycetic 116.0
  blister beetle 692.89
  Brucella NEC 023.9
  bullosa 694.9
    striata pratensis 692.6
  bullous 694.9
    mucosynechial, atrophic 694.60
      with ocular involvement 694.61
    seasonal 694.8
  calorica
    due to
      burn or scald—*see* Burn, by site
      cold 692.89
      sunburn (*see also* Sunburn) 692.71

Dermatitis—*continued*
  caterpillar 692.89
  cercarial 120.3
  combustionis
    due to
      burn or scald—*see* Burn, by site
      sunburn (*see also* Sunburn) 692.71
  congelationis 991.5
  contusiformis 695.2
  diabetic 250.8
  diaper 691.0
  diphtheritica 032.85
  due to
    acetone 692.2
    acids 692.4
    adhesive plaster 692.4
    alcohol (skin contact) (substances classifiable
      to 980.0-980.9) 692.4
      taken internally 693.8
    alkalis 692.4
    allergy NEC 692.9
    ammonia (household) (liquid) 692.4
    animal
      dander (cat) (dog) 692.84
      hair (cat) (dog) 692.84
    arnica 692.3
    arsenic 692.4
      taken internally 693.8
    blister beetle 692.89
    cantharides 692.3
    carbon disulphide 692.2
    caterpillar 692.89
    caustics 692.4
    cereal (ingested) 693.1
      contact with skin 692.5
    chemical(s) NEC 692.4
      internal 693.8
      irritant NEC 692.4
      taken internally 693.8
    chlorocompounds 692.2
    coffee (ingested) 693.1
      contact with skin 692.5
    cold weather 692.89
    cosmetics 692.81
    cyclohexanes 692.2
    dander, animal (cat) (dog) 692.84
    deodorant 692.81
    detergents 692.0
    dichromate 692.4
    drugs and medicinals (correct substance
      properly administered) (internal use) 693.0
      external (in contact with skin) 692.3
        wrong substance given or taken 976.9
          specified substance—*see* Table of drugs
            and chemicals
      wrong substance given or taken 977.9
        specified substance—*see* Table of drugs
          and chemicals
    dyes 692.89
      hair 692.89
    epidermophytosis—*see* Dermatophytosis
    esters 692.2
    external irritant NEC 692.9
      specified agent NEC 692.89
    eye shadow 692.81
    fish (ingested) 693.1
      contact with skin 692.5
    flour (ingested) 693.1
      contact with skin 692.5
    food (ingested) 693.1
      in contact with skin 692.5

Dermatitis—*continued*
    fruit (ingested) 693.1
      contact with skin 692.5
    fungicides 692.3
    furs 692.84
    glycols 692.2
    greases NEC 692.1
    hair, animal (cat) (dog) 692.84
    hair dyes 692.89
    hot
      objects and materials—*see* Burn, by site
      weather or places 692.89
    hydrocarbons 692.2
    infrared rays, except from sun 692.82
      solar NEC (*see also* Dermatitis, due to, sun)
        692.70
    ingested substance 693.9
      drugs and medicinals (*see also* Dermatitis,
        due to, drugs and medicinals) 693.0
      food 693.1
      specified substance NEC 693.8
    ingestion or injection of
      chemical 693.8
      drug (correct substance properly
        administered) 693.0
        wrong substance given or taken 977.9
          specified substance—*see* Table of drugs
            and chemicals
    insecticides 692.4
    internal agent 693.9
      drugs and medicinals (*see also* Dermatitis,
        due to, drugs and medicinals) 693.0
      food (ingested) 693.1
        in contact with skin 692.5
      specified agent NEC 693.8
    iodine 692.3
    iodoform 692.3
    irradiation 692.82
    jewelry 692.83
    keratolytics 692.3
    ketones 692.2
    lacquer tree (Rhus verniciflua) 692.6
    light (sun) NEC (*see also* Dermatitis, due to,
      sun) 692.70
      other 692.82
    low temperature 692.89
    mascara 692.81
    meat (ingested) 693.1
      contact with skin 692.5
    mercury, mercurials 692.3
    metals 692.83
    milk (ingested) 693.1
      contact with skin 692.5
    Neomycin 692.3
    nylon 692.4
    oils NEC 692.1
    paint solvent 692.2
    pediculocides 692.3
    petroleum products (substances classifiable to
      981) 692.4
    phenol 692.3
    photosensitiveness, photosensitivity (sun)
      692.72
      other light 692.82
    plants NEC 692.6
    plasters, medicated (any) 692.3
    plastic 692.4
    poison
      ivy (Rhus toxicodendron) 692.6
      oak (Rhus diversiloba) 692.6
      plant or vine 692.6

Dermatitis—*continued*
  perioral 695.3
  perstans 696.1
  photosensitivity (sun) 692.72
    other light 692.82
  pigmented purpuric lichenoid 709.1
  polymorpha dolorosa 694.0
  primary irritant 692.9
  pruriginosa 694.0
  pruritic NEC 692.9
  psoriasiform nodularis 696.2
  psychogenic 316
  purulent 686.00
  pustular contagious 051.2
  pyococcal 686.00
  pyocyaneus 686.09
  pyogenica 686.00
  radiation 692.82
  repens 696.1
  Ritter's (exfoliativa) 695.81
  Schamberg's (progressive pigmentary
      dermatosis) 709.09
  schistosome 120.3
  seasonal bullous 694.8
  seborrheic 690.10
    infantile 690.12
  sensitization NEC 692.9
  septic (*see also* Septicemia) 686.00
    gonococcal 098.89
  solar, solare NEC (*see also* Dermatitis, due to,
      sun) 692.70
  stasis 459.81
    due to
      postphlebitic syndrome 459.12
        with ulcer 459.13
      varicose veins—*see* Varicose
    ulcerated or with ulcer (varicose) 454.2
  sunburn (*see also* Sunburn) 692.71
  suppurative 686.00
  traumatic NEC 709.8
  trophoneurotica 694.0
  ultraviolet, except from sun 692.82
    due to sun NEC (*see also* Dermatitis, due to,
      sun) 692.70
  varicose 454.1
    with ulcer 454.2
  vegetans 686.8
  verrucosa 117.2
  xerotic 706.8
Dermatoarthritis, lipoid 272.8 *[713.0]*
Dermatochalasia, dermatochalasis 374.87
Dermatofibroma (lenticulare) (M8832/0)—*see
    also* Neoplasm, skin, benign
  protuberans (M8832/1)—*see* Neoplasm, skin,
    uncertain behavior
Dermatofibrosarcoma (protuberans) (M8832/3)
  see Neoplasm, skin, malignant
Dermatographia 708.3
Dermatolysis (congenital) (exfoliativa) 757.39
  acquired 701.8
  eyelids 374.34
  palpebrarum 374.34
  senile 701.8
Dermatomegaly NEC 701.8
Dermatomucomyositis 710.3
Dermatomycosis 111.9
  furfuracea 111.0
  specified type NEC 111.8
Dermatomyositis (acute) (chronic) 710.3
Dermatoneuritis of children 985.0
Dermatophiliasis 134.1
Dermatophytide —*see* Dermatophytosis

Dermatophytosis (Epidermophyton) (infection)
    (microsporum) (tinea) (Trichophyton) 110.9
  beard 110.0
  body 110.5
  deep seated 110.6
  fingernails 110.1
  foot 110.4
  groin 110.3
  hand 110.2
  nail 110.1
  perianal (area) 110.3
  scalp 110.0
  scrotal 110.8
  specified site NEC 110.8
  toenails 110.1
  vulva 110.8
Dermatopolyneuritis 985.0
Dermatorrhexis 756.83
  acquired 701.8
Dermatosclerosis (*see also* Scleroderma) 710.1
  localized 701.0
Dermatosis 709.9
  Andrews' 686.8
  atopic 691.8
  Bowen's (M8081/2)—*see* Neoplasm, skin, in situ
  bullous 694.9
    specified type NEC 694.8
  erythematosquamous 690.8
  exfoliativa 695.89
  factitial 698.4
  gonococcal 098.89
  herpetiformis 694.0
    juvenile 694.2
    senile 694.5
  hysterical 300.11
  linear IgA 694.8
  menstrual NEC 709.8
  neutrophilic, acute febrile 695.89
  occupational (*see also* Dermatitis) 692.9
  papulosa nigra 709.8
  pigmentary NEC 709.00
    progressive 709.09
    Schamberg's 709.09
    Siemens-Bloch 757.33
  progressive pigmentary 709.09
  psychogenic 316
  pustular subcorneal 694.1
  Schamberg's (progressive pigmentary) 709.09
  senile NEC 709.3
  Unna's (seborrheic dermatitis) 690.10
Dermographia 708.3
Dermographism 708.3
Dermoid (cyst) (M9084/0)—*see also* Neoplasm,
    by site, benign
  with malignant transformation (M9084/3) 183.0
Dermopathy
  infiltrative, with thyrotoxicosis 242.0
  senile NEC 709.3
Dermophytosis —*see* Dermatophytosis
Descemet's membrane —*see* condition
Descemetocele 371.72
Descending —*see* condition
Descensus uteri (complete) (incomplete) (partial)
    (without vaginal wall prolapse) 618.1
  with mention of vaginal wall prolapse—*see*
    Prolapse, uterovaginal
Desensitization to allergens V07.1
Desert
  rheumatism 114.0
  sore (*see also* Ulcer, skin) 707.9

Deviation—*continued*
  midline (jaw) (teeth) 524.29
    specified site NEC—*see* Malposition
  occlusal plane 524.76
  organ or site, congenital NEC—*see* Malposition,
      congenital
  septum (acquired) (nasal) 470
    congenital 754.0
  sexual 302.9
    bestiality 302.1
    coprophilia 302.89
    ego-dystonic
      homosexuality 302.0
      lesbianism 302.0
    erotomania 302.89
      Clérambault's 297.8
    exhibitionism (sexual) 302.4
    fetishism 302.81
      transvestic 302.3
    frotteurism 302.89
    homosexuality, ego-dystonic 302.0
      pedophilic 302.2
    lesbianism, ego-dystonic 302.0
    masochism 302.83
    narcissism 302.89
    necrophilia 302.89
    nymphomania 302.89
    pederosis 302.2
    pedophilia 302.2
    sadism 302.84
    sadomasochism 302.84
    satyriasis 302.89
    specified type NEC 302.89
    transvestic fetishism 302.3
    transvestism 302.3
    voyeurism 302.82
    zoophilia (erotica) 302.1
  teeth, midline 524.29
  trachea 519.19
  ureter (congenital) 753.4
Devic's disease 341.0
Device
  cerebral ventricle (communicating) in situ V45.2
  contraceptive—*see* Contraceptive, device
  drainage, cerebrospinal fluid V45.2
Devil's
  grip 074.1
  pinches (purpura simplex) 287.2
Devitalized tooth 522.9
Devonshire colic 984.9
  specified type of lead—*see* Table of drugs and
      chemicals
Dextraposition, aorta 747.21
  with ventricular septal defect, pulmonary
      stenosis or atresia, and hypertrophy of right
      ventricle 745.2
  in tetralogy of Fallot 745.2
Dextratransposition, aorta 745.11
Dextrinosis, limit (debrancher enzyme
    deficiency) 271.0
Dextrocardia (corrected) (false) (isolated)
    (secondary) (true) 746.87
  with
    complete transposition of viscera 759.3
    situs inversus 759.3
Dextroversion, kidney (left) 753.3
Dhobie itch 110.3

Diabetes, diabetic (brittle) (congenital) (familial)
    (mellitus) (poorly controlled) (severe) (slight)
    (without complication) 250.0

Note—Use the following fifth-digit
subclassification with category 250:

0 type II or unspecified type, not stated as
    uncontrolled
    Fifth-digit 0 is for use for type II patients,
    even if the patient requires insulin
1 type I [juvenile type], not stated as
    uncontrolled
2 type II or unspecified type, uncontrolled
    Fifth-digit 2 is for use for type II patients,
    even if the paiten requires insulin
3 type I [juvenile type], uncontrolled

---

  with
    coma (with ketoacidosis) 250.3
      hyperosmolar (nonketotic) 250.2
    complication NEC 250.9
      specified NEC 250.8
    gangrene 250.7 *[785.4]*
    hyperosmolarity 250.2
    ketosis, ketoacidosis 250.1
    osteomyelitis 250.8 *[731.8]*
    specified manifestations NEC 250.8
  acetonemia 250.1
  acidosis 250.1
  amyotrophy 250.6 *[358.1]*
  angiopathy, peripheral 250.7 *[443.81]*
  asymptomatic 790.29
  autonomic neuropathy (peripheral) 250.6 *[337.1]*
  bone change 250.8 *[731.8]*
  bronze, bronzed 275.0
  cataract 250.5 *[366.41]*
  chemical 790.29
    complicating pregnancy, childbirth, or
        puerperium 648.8
  coma (with ketoacidosis) 250.3
    hyperglycemic 250.3
    hyperosmolar (nonketotic) 250.2
    hypoglycemic 250.3
    insulin 250.3
  complicating pregnancy, childbirth, or
      puerperium (maternal) 648.0
    affecting fetus or newborn 775.0
  complication NEC 250.9
    specified NEC 250.8
  dorsal sclerosis 250.6 *[340]*
  dwarfism-obesity syndrome 258.1
  gangrene 250.7 *[785.4]*
  gastroparesis 250.6 *[536.3]*
  gestational 648.8
    complicating pregnancy, childbirth, or
        puerperium 648.8
  glaucoma 250.5 *[365.44]*
  glomerulosclerosis (intercapillary) 250.4 *[581.81]*
  glycogenosis, secondary 250.8 *[259.8]*
  hemochromatosis 275.0
  hyperosmolar coma 250.2
  hyperosmolarity 250.2
  hypertension-nephrosis syndrome 250.4 *[581.81]*
  hypoglycemia 250.8
  hypoglycemic shock 250.8
  insipidus 253.5

Diabetes, diabetic—*continued*
   nephrogenic 588.1
   pituitary 253.5
   vasopressin-resistant 588.1
  intercapillary glomerulosclerosis 250.4 *[581.81]*
  iritis 250.5 *[364.42]*
  ketosis, ketoacidosis 250.1
  Kimmelstiel (-Wilson) disease or syndrome
    (intercapillary glomerulosclerosis) 250.4
    [581.81]
  Lancereaux's (diabetes mellitus with marked
    emaciation) 250.8 *[261]*
  latent (chemical) 790.29
   complicating pregnancy, childbirth, or
    puerperium 648.8
  lipoidosis 250.8 *[272.7]*
  macular edema 250.5 *[362.07]*
  maternal
   with manifest disease in the infant 775.1
   affecting fetus or newborn 775.0
  microaneurysms, retinal 250.5 *[362.01]*
  mononeuropathy 250.6 *[355.9]*
  neonatal, transient 775.1
  nephropathy 250.4 *[583.81]*
  nephrosis (syndrome) 250.4 *[581.81]*
  neuralgia 250.6 *[357.2]*
  neuritis 250.6 *[357.2]*
  neurogenic arthropathy 250.6 *[713.5]*
  neuropathy 250.6 *[357.2]*
  nonclinical 790.29
  osteomyelitis 250.8 *[731.8]*
  peripheral autonomic neuropathy 250.6 *[337.1]*
  phosphate 275.3
  polyneuropathy 250.6 *[357.2]*
  renal (true) 271.4
  retinal
   edema 250.5 *[362.07]*
   hemorrhage 250.5 *[362.01]*
   microaneurysms 250.5 *[362.01]*
  retinitis 250.5 *[362.01]*
  retinopathy 250.5 *[362.01]*
   background 250.5 *[362.01]*
   nonproliferative 250.5 *[362.03]*
    mild 250.5 *[362.04]*
    moderate 250.5 *[362.05]*
    severe 250.5 *[362.06]*
   proliferative 250.5 *[362.02]*
  steroid induced
   correct substance properly administered 251.8
   overdose or wrong substance given or taken
    962.0
  stress 790.29
  subclinical 790.29
  subliminal 790.29
  sugar 250.0
  ulcer (skin) 250.8 *[707.9]*
   lower extremity 250.8 *[707.10]*
    ankle 250.8 *[707.13]*
    calf 250.8 *[707.12]*
    foot 250.8 *[707.15]*
    heel 250.8 *[707.14]*
    knee 250.8 *[707.19]*
    specified site NEC 250.8 *[707.19]*
    thigh 250.8 *[707.11]*
    toes 250.8 *[707.15]*
   specified site NEC 250.8 *[707.8]*
  xanthoma 250.8 *[272.2]*
Diacyclothrombopathia 287.1
Diagnosis deferred 799.9

Dialysis (intermittent) (treatment)
  anterior retinal (juvenile) (with detachment)
   361.04
  extracorporeal V56.0
  hemodialysis V56.0
   status only V45.1
  peritoneal V56.8
   status only V45.1
  renal V56.0
   status only V45.1
  specified type NEC V56.8
Diamond-Blackfan anemia or syndrome
  (congenital hypoplastic anemia) 284.01
Diamond-Gardener syndrome (autoerythrocyte
  sensitization) 287.2
Diaper rash 691.0
Diaphoresis (excessive) NEC (*see also*
  Hyperhidrosis) 780.8
Diaphragm —*see* condition
Diaphragmalgia 786.52
Diaphragmitis 519.4
Diaphyseal aclasis 756.4
Diaphysitis 733.99
Diarrhea, diarrheal (acute) (autumn) (bilious)
  (bloody) (catarrhal) (choleraic) (chronic)
  (gravis) (green) (infantile) (lienteric)
  (noninfectious) (presumed noninfectious)
  (putrefactive) (secondary) (sporadic)
  (summer) (symptomatic) (thermic) 787.91
  achlorhydric 536.0
  allergic 558.3
  amebic (*see also* Amebiasis) 006.9
   with abscess—*see* Abscess, amebic
   acute 006.0
   chronic 006.1
   nondysenteric 006.2
  bacillary—*see* Dysentery, bacillary
  bacterial NEC 008.5
  balantidial 007.0
  bile salt-induced 579.8
  cachectic NEC 787.91
  chilomastix 007.8
  choleriformis 001.1
  coccidial 007.2
  Cochin-China 579.1
   anguilluliasis 127.2
   psilosis 579.1
  Dientamoeba 007.8
  dietetic 787.91
  due to
   achylia gastrica 536.8
   Aerobacter aerogenes 008.2
   Bacillus coli—*see* Enteritis, E. coli
   bacteria NEC 008.5
   bile salts 579.8
   Capillaria
    hepatica 128.8
    philippinensis 127.5
   Clostridium perfringens (C) (F) 008.46
   Enterobacter aerogenes 008.2
   enterococci 008.49
   Escherichia coli—*see* Enteritis, E. coli
   Giardia lamblia 007.1
   Heterophyes heterophyes 121.6
   irritating foods 787.91
   Metagonimus yokogawai 121.5
   Necator americanus 126.1
   Paracolobactrum arizonae 008.1
   Paracolon bacillus NEC 008.47
    Arizona 008.1
   Proteus (bacillus) (mirabilis) (Morganii) 008.3

Diarrhea, diarrheal—*continued*
　Pseudomonas aeruginosa 008.42
　S. japonicum 120.2
　specified organism NEC 008.8
　　bacterial 008.49
　　viral NEC 008.69
　Staphylococcus 008.41
　Streptococcus 008.49
　　anaerobic 008.46
　Strongyloides stercoralis 127.2
　Trichuris trichiuria 127.3
　virus NEC (*see also* Enteritis, viral) 008.69
　dysenteric 009.2
　　due to specified organism NEC 008.8
　dyspeptic 787.91
　endemic 009.3
　epidemic 009.3
　fermentative 787.91
　flagellate 007.9
　Flexner's (ulcerative) 004.1
　functional 564.5
　　following gastrointestinal surgery 564.4
　　psychogenic 306.4
　giardial 007.1
　Giardia lamblia 007.1
　hill 579.1
　hyperperistalsis (nervous) 306.4
　infectious 009.2
　　presumed 009.3
　inflammatory 787.91
　　due to specified organism NEC 008.8
　malarial (*see also* Malaria) 084.6
　mite 133.8
　mycotic 117.9
　nervous 306.4
　neurogenic 564.5
　parenteral NEC 009.2
　postgastrectomy 564.4
　postvagotomy 564.4
　prostaglandin induced 579.8
　protozoal NEC 007.9
　psychogenic 306.4
　septic 009.2
　　due to specified organism NEC 008.8
　specified organism NEC 008.8
　　bacterial 008.49
　　viral NEC 008.69
　Staphylococcus 008.41
　Streptococcus 008.49
　　anaerobic 088.46
　toxic 558.2
　travelers' 009.2
　　due to specified organism NEC 008.8
　trichomonal 007.3
　tropical 579.1
　tuberculous 014.8
　ulcerative (chronic) (*see also* Colitis, ulcerative)
　　556.9
　viral (*see also* Enteritis, viral) 008.8
　zymotic NEC 009.2
Diastasis
　cranial bones 733.99
　　congenital 756.0
　joint (traumatic)—*see* Dislocation, by site
　muscle 728.84
　　congenital 756.89
　recti (abdomen) 728.84
　　complicating delivery 665.8
　　congenital 756.79
Diastema, teeth, tooth 524.30
Diastematomyelia 742.51

Diataxia, cerebral, infantile 343.0
Diathesis
　allergic V15.09
　bleeding (familial) 287.9
　cystine (familial) 270.0
　gouty 274.9
　hemorrhagic (familial) 287.9
　　newborn NEC 776.0
　oxalic 271.8
　scrofulous (*see also* Tuberculosis) 017.2
　spasmophilic (*see also* Tetany) 781.7
　ulcer 536.9
　uric acid 274.9
Diaz's disease or osteochondrosis 732.5
Dibothriocephaliasis 123.4
　larval 123.5
Dibothriocephalus (infection) (infestation)
　　(latus) 123.4
　larval 123.5
Dicephalus 759.4
Dichotomy, teeth 520.2
Dichromat, dichromata (congenital) 368.59
Dichromatopsia (congenital) 368.59
Dichuchwa 104.0
Dicroceliasis 121.8
Didelphys, didelphic (*see also* Double uterus)
　　752.2
Didymitis (*see also* Epididymitis) 604.90
Died —*see also* Death
　without
　medical attention (cause unknown) 798.9
　sign of disease 798.2
Dientamoeba diarrhea 007.8
Dietary
　inadequacy or deficiency 269.9
　surveillance and counseling V65.3
Dietl's crisis 593.4
Dieulafoy lesion (hemorrhagic)
　of
　　duodenum 537.84
　　esophagus 530.82
　　intestine 569.86
　　stomach 537.84
Dieulafoy's ulcer —*see* Ulcer, stomach
Difficult
　birth, affecting fetus or newborn 763.9
　delivery NEC 669.9
Difficulty
　feeding 783.3
　　adult 783.3
　　breast 676.8
　　child 783.3
　　elderly 783.3
　　infant 783.3
　newborn 779.3
　nonorganic (infant) NEC 307.59
　mechanical, gastroduodenal stoma 537.89
　reading 315.00
　specific, spelling 315.09
　swallowing (*see also* Dysphagia) 787.2
　walking 719.7
Diffuse —*see* condition
Diffused ganglion 727.42
DiGeorge's syndrome (thymic hypoplasia)
　　279.11
Digestive —*see* condition
Di Guglielmo's disease or syndrome (M9841/3)
　　207.0
Diktyoma (M9051/3)—*see* Neoplasm, by site,
　　malignant
Dilaceration, tooth 520.4

Dilatation
- anus 564.89
  - venule—*see* Hemorrhoids
- aorta (focal) (general) (*see also* Aneurysm, aorta) 441.9
  - congenital 747.29
  - infectional 093.0
  - ruptured 441.5
  - syphilitic 093.0
- appendix (cystic) 543.9
- artery 447.8
- bile duct (common) (cystic) (congenital) 751.69
  - acquired 576.8
- bladder (sphincter) 596.8
  - congenital 753.8
  - in pregnancy or childbirth 654.4
    - causing obstructed labor 660.2
      - affecting fetus or newborn 763.1
- blood vessel 459.89
- bronchus, bronchi 494.0
  - with acute exacerbation 494.1
- calyx (due to obstruction) 593.89
- capillaries 448.9
- cardiac (acute) (chronic) (*see also* Hypertrophy, cardiac) 429.3
  - congenital 746.89
    - valve NEC 746.89
      - pulmonary 746.09
  - hypertensive (*see also* Hypertension, heart) 402.90
- cavum septi pellucidi 742.4
- cecum 564.89
  - psychogenic 306.4
- cervix (uteri)—*see also* Incompetency, cervix
  - incomplete, poor, slow
    - affecting fetus or newborn 763.7
    - complicating delivery 661.0
      - affecting fetus or newborn 763.7
- colon 564.7
  - congenital 751.3
  - due to mechanical obstruction 560.89
  - psychogenic 306.4
- common bile duct (congenital) 751.69
  - acquired 576.8
    - with calculus, choledocholithiasis, or stones—*see* Choledocholithiasis
- cystic duct 751.69
  - acquired (any bile duct) 575.8
- duct, mammary 610.4
- duodenum 564.89
- esophagus 530.89
  - congenital 750.4
  - due to
    - achalasia 530.0
    - cardiospasm 530.0
- Eustachian tube, congenital 744.24
- fontanel 756.0
- gallbladder 575.8
  - congenital 751.69
- gastric 536.8
  - acute 536.1
  - psychogenic 306.4
- heart (acute) (chronic) (*see also* Hypertrophy, cardiac) 429.3
  - congenital 746.89
  - hypertensive (*see also* Hypertension, heart) 402.90
  - valve—*see also* Endocarditis
    - congenital 746.89
- ileum 564.89
  - psychogenic 306.4

Dilatation—*continued*
- inguinal rings—*see* Hernia, inguinal
- jejunum 564.89
  - psychogenic 306.4
- kidney (calyx) (collecting structures) (cystic) (parenchyma) (pelvis) 593.89
- lacrimal passages 375.69
- lymphatic vessel 457.1
- mammary duct 610.4
- Meckel's diverticulum (congenital) 751.0
- meningeal vessels, congenital 742.8
- myocardium (acute) (chronic) (*see also* Hypertrophy, cardiac) 429.3
- organ or site, congenital NEC—*see* Distortion
- pancreatic duct 577.8
- pelvis, kidney 593.89
- pericardium—*see* Pericarditis
- pharynx 478.29
- prostate 602.8
- pulmonary
  - artery (idiopathic) 417.8
    - congenital 747.3
  - valve, congenital 746.09
- pupil 379.43
- rectum 564.89
- renal 593.89
- saccule vestibularis, congenital 744.05
- salivary gland (duct) 527.8
- sphincter ani 564.89
- stomach 536.8
  - acute 536.1
  - psychogenic 306.4
- submaxillary duct 527.8
- trachea, congenital 748.3
- ureter (idiopathic) 593.89
  - congenital 753.20
  - due to obstruction 593.5
- urethra (acquired) 599.84
- vasomotor 443.9
- vein 459.89
- ventricular, ventricle (acute) (chronic) (*see also* Hypertrophy, cardiac) 429.3
  - cerebral, congenital 742.4
  - hypertensive (*see also* Hypertension, heart) 402.90
- venule 459.89
  - anus—*see* Hemorrhoids
- vesical orifice 596.8

Dilated, dilation —*see* Dilatation

Diminished
- hearing (acuity) (*see also* Deafness) 389.9
- pulse pressure 785.9
- vision NEC 369.9
- vital capacity 794.2

Diminuta taenia 123.6

Diminution, sense or sensation (cold) (heat) (tactile) (vibratory) (*see also* Disturbance, sensation) 782.0

Dimitri-Sturge-Weber disease (encephalocutaneous angiomatosis) 759.6

Dimple
- parasacral 685.1
  - with abscess 685.0
- pilonidal 685.1
  - with abscess 685.0
- postanal 685.1
  - with abscess 685.0

Dioctophyma renale (infection) (infestation) 128.8

Dipetalonemiasis 125.4

Diphallus 752.69

Diphtheria, diphtheritic (gangrenous)
    (hemorrhagic) 032.9
  carrier (suspected) of V02.4
  cutaneous 032.85
  cystitis 032.84
  faucial 032.0
  infection of wound 032.85
  inoculation (anti) (not sick) V03.5
  laryngeal 032.3
  myocarditis 032.82
  nasal anterior 032.2
  nasopharyngeal 032.1
  neurological complication 032.89
  peritonitis 032.83
  specified site NEC 032.89
Diphyllobothriasis (intestine) 123.4
  larval 123.5
Diplacusis 388.41
Diplegia (upper limbs) 344.2
  brain or cerebral 437.8
  congenital 343.0
  facial 351.0
    congenital 352.6
  infantile or congenital (cerebral) (spastic)
    (spinal) 343.0
  lower limbs 344.1
  syphilitic, congenital 090.49
Diplococcus, diplococcal —*see* condition
Diplomyelia 742.59
Diplopia 368.2
  refractive 368.15
Dipsomania (*see also* Alcoholism) 303.9
  with psychosis (*see also* Psychosis, alcoholic)
    291.9
Dipylidiasis 123.8
  intestine 123.8
Direction, teeth, abnormal 524.30
Dirt-eating child 307.52
Disability
  heart—*see* Disease, heart
  learning NEC 315.2
  special spelling 315.09
Disarticulation (*see also* Derangement, joint)
    718.9
  meaning
    amputation
      status—*see* Absence, by site
      traumatic —*see* Amputation, traumatic
    dislocation, traumatic or congenital—*see*
      Dislocation
Disaster, cerebrovascular (*see also* Disease,
    cerebrovascular, acute) 436
Discharge
  anal NEC 787.99
  breast (female) (male) 611.79
  conjunctiva 372.89
  continued locomotor idiopathic (*see also*
    Epilepsy) 345.5
  diencephalic autonomic idiopathic (*see also*
    Epilepsy) 345.5
  ear 388.60
    blood 388.69
    cerebrospinal fluid 388.61
  excessive urine 788.42
  eye 379.93
  nasal 478.19
  nipple 611.79
  patterned motor idiopathic (*see also* Epilepsy)
    345.5
  penile 788.7
  postnasal—*see* Sinusitis

Discharge—*continued*
  sinus, from mediastinum 510.0
  umbilicus 789.9
  urethral 788.7
    bloody 599.84
  vaginal 623.5
Discitis 722.90
  cervical, cervicothoracic 722.91
  lumbar, lumbosacral 722.93
  thoracic, thoracolumbar 722.92
Discogenic syndrome —*see* Displacement,
    intervertebral disc
Discoid
  kidney 753.3
  meniscus, congenital 717.5
  semilunar cartilage 717.5
Discoloration
  mouth 528.9
  nails 703.8
  teeth 521.7
    due to
      drugs 521.7
      metals (copper) (silver) 521.7
      pulpal bleeding 521.7
    during formation 520.8
    extrinsic 523.6
    intrinsic posteruptive 521.7
Discomfort
  chest 786.59
  visual 368.13
Discomycosis —*see* Actinomycosis
Discontinuity, ossicles, ossicular chain 385.23
Discrepancy
  centric occlusion
    maximum intercuspation 524.55
    of teeth 524.55
  leg length (acquired) 736.81
    congenital 755.30
  uterine size-date 649.6
Discrimination
  political V62.4
  racial V62.4
  religious V62.4
  sex V62.4
Disease, diseased —*see also* Syndrome
  Abrami's (acquired hemolytic jaundice) 283.9
  absorbent system 459.89
  accumulation—*see* Thesaurismosis
  acid-peptic 536.8
  Acosta's 993.2
  Adams-Stokes (-Morgagni) (syncope with heart
    block) 426.9
  Addison's (bronze) (primary adrenal
    insufficiency) 255.4
    anemia (pernicious) 281.0
    tuberculous (*see also* Tuberculosis) 017.6
  Addison-Gull—*see* Xanthoma
  adenoids (and tonsils) (chronic) 474.9
  adrenal (gland) (capsule) (cortex) 255.9
    hyperfunction 255.3
    hypofunction 255.4
    specified type NEC 255.8
  ainhum (dactylolysis spontanea) 136.0
  akamushi (scrub typhus) 081.2
  Akureyri (epidemic neuromyasthenia) 049.8
  Albarrán's (colibacilluria) 791.9
  Albers-Schönberg's (marble bones) 756.52
  Albert's 726.71
  Albright (-Martin) (-Bantam) 275.49
  Alibert's (mycosis fungoides) (M9700/3) 202.1
  Alibert-Bazin (M9700/3) 202.1

Disease, diseased—*continued*
  Bernhardt (-Roth) 355.1
  beryllium 503
  Besnier-Boeck (-Schaumann) (sarcoidosis) 135
  Best's 362.76
  Beurmann's (sporotrichosis) 117.1
  Bielschowsky (-Jansky) 330.1
  Biermer's (pernicious anemia) 281.0
  Biett's (discoid lupus erythematosus) 695.4
  bile duct (*see also* Disease, biliary) 576.9
  biliary (duct) (tract) 576.9
    with calculus, choledocholithiasis, or
      stones—*see* Choledocholithiasis
  Billroth's (meningocele) (*see also* Spina bifida)
    741.9
  Binswanger's 290.12
  Bird's (oxaluria) 271.8
  bird fanciers' 495.2
  black lung 500
  bladder 596.9
    specified NEC 596.8
  bleeder's 286.0
  Bloch-Sulzberger (incontinentia pigmenti)
    757.33
  Blocq's (astasia-abasia) 307.9
  blood (-forming organs) 289.9
    specified NEC 289.89
    vessel 459.9
  Bloodgood's 610.1
  Blount's (tibia vara) 732.4
  blue 746.9
  Bodechtel-Guttmann (subacute sclerosing
    panencephalitis) 046.2
  Boeck's (sarcoidosis) 135
  bone 733.90
    fibrocystic NEC 733.29
      jaw 526.2
    marrow 289.9
    Paget's (osteitis deformans) 731.0
    specified type NEC 733.99
    von Recklinghausen's (osteitis fibrosa cystica)
      252.01
  Bonfils'—*see* Disease, Hodgkin's
  Borna 062.9
  Bornholm (epidemic pleurodynia) 074.1
  Bostock's (*see also* Fever, hay) 477.9
  Bouchard's (myopathic dilatation of the
    stomach) 536.1
  Bouillaud's (rheumatic heart disease) 391.9
  Bourneville (-Brissaud) (tuberous sclerosis)
    759.5
  Bouveret (-Hoffmann) (paroxysmal tachycardia)
    427.2
  bowel 569.9
    functional 564.9
      psychogenic 306.4
  Bowen's (M8081/2)—*see* Neoplasm, skin, in
    situ
  Bozzolo's (multiple myeloma) (M9730/3) 203.0
  Bradley's (epidemic vomiting) 078.82
  Brailsford's 732.3
    radius, head 732.3
    tarsal, scaphoid 732.5
  Brailsford-Morquio (mucopolysaccharidosis IV)
    277.5
  brain 348.9
    Alzheimer's 331.0
      with dementia—*see* Alzheimer's, dementia
    arterial, artery 437.9
    arteriosclerotic 437.0
    congenital 742.9

Disease, diseased—*continued*
  degenerative—*see* Degeneration, brain
  inflammatory—*see also* Encephalitis
    late effect—*see* category 326
  organic 348.9
    arteriosclerotic 437.0
  parasitic NEC 123.9
  Pick's 331.11
    with dementia
      with behavioral disturbance 331.11
        [294.11]
      without behavioral disturbance 331.11
        [294.10]
  senile 331.2
  braziers' 985.8
  breast 611.9
    cystic (chronic) 610.1
    fibrocystic 610.1
    inflammatory 611.0
    Paget's (M8540/3) 174.0
    puerperal, postpartum NEC 676.3
    specified NEC 611.8
  Breda's (*see also* Yaws) 102.9
  Breisky's (kraurosis vulvae) 624.0
  Bretonneau's (diphtheritic malignant angina)
    032.0
  Bright's (*see also* Nephritis) 583.9
    arteriosclerotic (*see also* Hypertension,
      kidney) 403.90
  Brill's (recrudescent typhus) 081.1
    flea-borne 081.0
    louse-borne 081.1
  Brill-Symmers (follicular lymphoma)
    (M9690/3) 202.0
  Brill-Zinsser (recrudescent typhus) 081.1
  Brinton's (leather bottle stomach) (M8142/3)
    151.9
  Brion-Kayser (*see also* Fever, paratyphoid)
    002.9
  broad
    beta 272.2
    ligament, noninflammatory 620.9
      specified NEC 620.8
  Brocq's 691.8
    meaning
      atopic (diffuse) neurodermatitis 691.8
      dermatitis herpetiformis 694.0
      lichen simplex chronicus 698.3
      parapsoriasis 696.2
      prurigo 698.2
  Brocq-Duhring (dermatitis herpetiformis) 694.0
  Brodie's (joint) (*see also* Osteomyelitis) 730.1
  bronchi 519.19
  bronchopulmonary 519.19
  bronze (Addison's) 255.4
    tuberculous (*see also* Tuberculosis) 017.6
  Brown-Séquard 344.89
  Bruck's 733.99
  Bruck-de Lange (Amsterdam dwarf, mental
    retardation, and brachycephaly) 759.89
  Bruhl's (splenic anemia with fever) 285.8
  Bruton's (X-linked agammaglobulinemia)
    279.04
  buccal cavity 528.9
  Buchanan's (juvenile osteochondrosis, iliac
    crest) 732.1
  Buchman's (osteochondrosis juvenile) 732.1
  Budgerigar-fanciers' 495.2
  Büdinger-Ludloff-Läwen 717.89
  Buerger's (thromboangiitis obliterans) 443.1

Disease, diseased—*continued*
  Bürger-Grütz (essential familial hyperlipemia)
    272.3
  Burns' (lower ulna) 732.3
  bursa 727.9
  Bury's (erythema elevatum diutinum) 695.89
  Buschke's 710.1
  Busquet's (*see also* Osteomyelitis) 730.1
  Busse-Buschke (cryptococcosis) 117.5
  C$_2$ (*see also* Alcoholism) 303.9
  Caffey's (infantile cortical hyperostosis) 756.59
  caisson 993.3
  calculous 592.9
  California 114.0
  Calvé (-Perthes) (osteochondrosis, femoral
    capital) 732.1
  Camurati-Engelmann (diaphyseal sclerosis)
    756.59
  Canavan's 330.0
  capillaries 448.9
  Carapata 087.1
  cardiac-*see* Disease, heart
  cardiopulmonary, chronic 416.9
  cardiorenal (arteriosclerotic) (hepatic)
    (hypertensive) (vascular) (*see also*
    Hypertension, cardiorenal) 404.90
  cardiovascular (arteriosclerotic) 429.2
    congenital 746.9
    hypertensive (*see also* Hypertension, heart)
      402.90
      benign 402.10
      malignant 402.00
     renal (*see also* Hypertension, cardiorenal)
      404.90
    syphilitic (asymptomatic) 093.9
  carotid gland 259.8
  Carrión's (Bartonellosis) 088.0
  cartilage NEC 733.90
    specified NEC 733.99
  Castellani's 104.8
  cat-scratch 078.3
  Cavare's (familial periodic paralysis) 359.3
  Cazenave's (pemphigus) 694.4
  cecum 569.9
  celiac (adult) 579.0
    infantile 579.0
  cellular tissue NEC 709.9
  central core 359.0
  cerebellar, cerebellum—*see* Disease, brain
  cerebral (*see also* Disease, brain) 348.9
    arterial, artery 437.9
    degenerative—*see* Degeneration, brain
  cerebrospinal 349.9
  cerebrovascular NEC 437.9
    acute 436
      embolic—*see* Embolism, brain
      late effect—*see* Late effect(s) (of)
        cerebrovascular disease
      puerperal, postpartum, childbirth 674.0
      thrombotic—*see* Thrombosis, brain
    arteriosclerotic 437.0
    embolic—*see* Embolism, brain
    ischemic, generalized NEC 437.1
    late effect—*see* Late effect(s) (of)
      cerebrovascular disease
    occlusive 437.1
    puerperal, postpartum, childbirth 674.0
    specified type NEC 437.8
    thrombotic—*see* Thrombosis, brain
  ceroid storage 272.7

Disease, diseased—*continued*
  cervix (uteri)
    inflammatory 616.9
      specified NEC 616.89
    noninflammatory 622.9
      specified NEC 622.8
  Chabert's 022.9
  Chagas' (*see also* Trypanosomiasis, American)
    086.2
  Chandler's (osteochondritis dissecans, hip)
    732.7
  Charcot's (joint) 094.0 *[713.5]*
    spinal cord 094.0
  Charcot-Marie-Tooth 356.1
  Charlouis' (*see also* Yaws) 102.9
  Cheadle (-Möller) (-Barlow) (infantile scurvy)
    267
  Chédiak-Steinbrinck (-Higashi) (congenital
    gigantism of peroxidase granules) 288.2
  cheek, inner 528.9
  chest 519.9
  Chiari's (hepatic vein thrombosis) 453.0
  Chicago (North American blastomycosis) 116.0
  chignon (white piedra) 111.2
  chigoe, chigo (jigger) 134.1
  childhood granulomatous 288.1
  Chinese liver fluke 121.1
  chlamydial NEC 078.88
  cholecystic (*see also* Disease, gallbladder) 575.9
  choroid 363.9
    degenerative (*see also* Degeneration, choroid)
      363.40
    hereditary (*see also* Dystrophy, choroid)
      363.50
    specified type NEC 363.8
  Christian's (chronic histiocytosis X) 277.89
  Christian-Weber (nodular nonsuppurative
    panniculitis) 729.30
  Christmas 286.1
  ciliary body 364.9
  circulatory (system) NEC 459.9
    chronic, maternal, affecting fetus or newborn
      760.3
    specified NEC 459.89
    syphilitic 093.9
      congenital 090.5
  Civatte's (poikiloderma) 709.09
  climacteric 627.2
    male 608.89
  coagulation factor deficiency (congenital) (*see
    also* Defect, coagulation) 286.9
  Coats' 362.12
  coccidioidal pulmonary 114.5
    acute 114.0
    chronic 114.4
    primary 114.0
    residual 114.4
  Cockayne's (microcephaly and dwarfism)
    759.89
  Cogan's 370.52
  cold
    agglutinin 283.0
      or hemoglobinuria 283.0
        paroxysmal (cold) (nocturnal) 283.2
      hemagglutinin (chronic) 283.0
  collagen NEC 710.9
    nonvascular 710.9
    specified NEC 710.8
    vascular (allergic) (*see also* Angiitis,
      hypersensitivity) 446.20

Disease, diseased—*continued*
  colon 569.9
    functional 564.9
      congenital 751.3
    ischemic 557.0
  combined system (of spinal cord) 266.2 *[336.2]*
    with anemia (pernicious) 281.0 *[336.2]*
  compressed air 993.3
  Concato's (pericardial polyserositis) 423.2
    peritoneal 568.82
    pleural—*see* Pleurisy
  congenital NEC 799.89
  conjunctiva 372.9
    chlamydial 077.98
      specified NEC 077.8
    specified type NEC 372.89
    viral 077.99
      specified NEC 077.8
  connective tissue, diffuse (*see also* Disease,
    collagen) 710.9
  Conor and Bruch's (boutonneuse fever) 082.1
  Conradi (-Hünermann) 756.59
  Cooley's (erythroblastic anemia) 282.49
  Cooper's 610.1
  Corbus' 607.1
  cork-handlers' 495.3
  cornea (*see also* Keratopathy) 371.9
  coronary (*see also* Ischemia, heart) 414.9
    congenital 746.85
    ostial, syphilitic 093.20
      aortic 093.22
      mitral 093.21
      pulmonary 093.24
      tricuspid 093.23
  Corrigan's—*see* Insufficiency, aortic
  Cotugno's 724.3
  Coxsackie (virus) NEC 074.8
  cranial nerve NEC 352.9
  Creutzfeldt-Jakob (new variant) 046.1
    with dementia
      with behavioral disturbance 046.1 *[294.11]*
      without behavioral disturbance 046.1
        [294.10]
  Crigler-Najjar (congenital hyperbilirubinemia)
    277.4
  Crocq's (acrocyanosis) 443.89
  Crohn's (intestine) (*see also* Enteritis, regional)
    555.9
  Crouzon's (craniofacial dysostosis) 756.0
  Cruchet's (encephalitis lethargica) 049.8
  Cruveilhier's 335.21
  Cruz-Chagas (*see also* Trypanosomiasis,
    American) 086.2
  crystal deposition (*see also* Arthritis, due to,
    crystals) 712.9
  Csillag's (lichen sclerosus et atrophicus) 701.0
  Curschmann's 359.2
  Cushing's (pituitary basophilism) 255.0
  cystic
    breast (chronic) 610.1
    kidney, congenital (*see also* Cystic, disease,
      kidney) 753.10
    liver, congenital 751.62
    lung 518.89
      congenital 748.4
    pancreas 577.2
      congenital 751.7
    renal, congenital (*see also* Cystic, disease,
      kidney) 753.10
    semilunar cartilage 717.5
  cysticercus 123.1

Disease, diseased—*continued*
  cystine storage (with renal sclerosis) 270.0
  cytomegalic inclusion (generalized) 078.5
    with
      pneumonia 078.5 *[484.1]*
    congenital 771.1
  Daae (-Finsen) (epidemic pleurodynia) 074.1
  dancing 297.8
  Danielssen's (anesthetic leprosy) 030.1
  Darier's (congenital) (keratosis follicularis)
    757.39
    erythema annulare centrifugum 695.0
    vitamin A deficiency 264.8
  Darling's (histoplasmosis) (*see also*
    Histoplasmosis, American) 115.00
  Davies' 425.0
  de Beurmann-Gougerot (sporotrichosis) 117.1
  Débove's (splenomegaly) 789.2
  deer fly (*see also* Tularemia) 021.9
  deficiency 269.9
  degenerative—*see also* Degeneration
    disc—*see* Degeneration, intervertebral disc
  Degos' 447.8
  Déjérine (-Sottas) 356.0
  Deleage's 359.89
  demyelinating, demyelinizating (brain stem)
    (central nervous system) 341.9
    multiple sclerosis 340
    specified NEC 341.8
  de Quervain's (tendon sheath) 727.04
    thyroid (subacute granulomatous thyroiditis)
      245.1
  Dercum's (adiposis dolorosa) 272.8
  Deutschländer's—*see* Fracture, foot
  Devergie's (pityriasis rubra pilaris) 696.4
  Devic's 341.0
  diaphorase deficiency 289.7
  diaphragm 519.4
  diarrheal, infectious 009.2
  diatomaceous earth 502
  Diaz's (osteochondrosis astragalus) 732.5
  digestive system 569.9
  Di Guglielmo's (erythemic myelosis) (M9841/3)
    207.0
  Dimitri-Sturge-Weber (encephalocutaneous
    angiomatosis) 759.6
  disc, degenerative—*see* Degeneration,
    intervertebral disc
  discogenic (*see also* Disease, intervertebral disc)
    722.90
  diverticular—*see* Diverticula
  Down's (mongolism) 758.0
  Dubini's (electric chorea) 049.8
  Dubois' (thymus gland) 090.5
  Duchenne's 094.0
    locomotor ataxia 094.0
    muscular dystrophy 359.1
    paralysis 335.22
    pseudohypertrophy, muscles 359.1
  Duchenne-Griesinger 359.1
  ductless glands 259.9
  Duhring's (dermatitis herpetiformis) 694.0
  Dukes (-Filatov) 057.8
  duodenum NEC 537.9
    specified NEC 537.89
  Duplay's 726.2
  Dupré's (meningism) 781.6
  Dupuytren's (muscle contracture) 728.6
  Durand-Nicolas-Favre (climatic bubo) 099.1
  Duroziez's (congenital mitral stenosis) 746.5
  Dutton's (trypanosomiasis) 086.9

Disease, diseased—*continued*
    psychogenic 306.4
  Gaucher's (adult) (cerebroside lipidosis)
    (infantile) 272.7
  Gayet's (superior hemorrhagic
    polioencephalitis) 265.1
  Gee (-Herter) (-Heubner) (-Thaysen)
    (nontropical sprue) 579.0
  generalized neoplastic (M8000/6) 199.0
  genital organs NEC
    female 629.9
      specified NEC 629.89
    male 608.9
  Gerhardt's (erythromelalgia) 443.82
  Gerlier's (epidemic vertigo) 078.81
  Gibert's (pityriasis rosea) 696.3
  Gibney' s (perispondylitis) 720.9
  Gierke's (glycogenosis I) 271.0
  Gilbert's (familial nonhemolytic jaundice) 277.4
  Gilchrist's (North American blastomycosis)
    116.0
  Gilford (-Hutchinson) (progeria) 259.8
  Gilles de la Tourette's (motor-verbal tic) 307.23
  Giovannini's 117.9
  gland (lymph) 289.9
  Glanzmann's (hereditary hemorrhagic
    thrombasthenia) 287.1
  glassblowers' 527.1
  Glénard's (enteroptosis) 569.89
  Glisson's (*see also* Rickets) 268.0
  glomerular
    membranous, idiopathic 581.1
    minimal change 581.3
  glycogen storage (Andersen's) (Cori types 1-7)
    (Forbes') (McArdle-Schmid-Pearson)
    (Pompe's) (types I-VII) 271.0
    cardiac 271.0 *[425.7]*
    generalized 271.0
    glucose-6-phosphatase deficiency 271.0
    heart 271.0 *[425.7]*
    hepatorenal 271.0
    liver and kidneys 271.0
    myocardium 271.0 *[425.7]*
    von Gierke's (glycogenosis I) 271.0
  Goldflam-Erb 358.00
  Goldscheider's (epidermolysis bullosa) 757.39
  Goldstein's (familial hemorrhagic
    telangiectasia) 448.0
  gonococcal NEC 098.0
  Goodall's (epidemic vomiting) 078.82
  Gordon's (exudative enteropathy) 579.8
  Gougerot's (trisymptomatic) 709.1
  Gougerot-Carteaud (confluent reticulate
    papillomatosis) 701.8
  Gougerot-Hailey-Hailey (benign familial
    chronic pemphigus) 757.39
  graft-versus-host (bone marrow) 996.85
    due to organ transplant NEC—*see*
      Complications, transplant, organ
  grain-handlers' 495.8
  Grancher's (splenopneumonia)—*see* Pneumonia
  granulomatous (childhood) (chronic) 288.1
  graphite lung 503
  Graves' (exophthalmic goiter) 242.0
  Greenfield's 330.0
  green monkey 078.89
  Griesinger's (*see also* Ancylostomiasis) 126.9
  grinders' 502
  Grisel's 723.5
  Gruby's (tinea tonsurans) 110.0
  Guertin's (electric chorea) 049.8

Disease, diseased—*continued*
  Guillain-Barré 357.0
  Guinon's (motor-verbal tic) 307.23
  Gull's (thyroid atrophy with myxedema) 244.8
  Gull and Sutton's—*see* Hypertension, kidney
  gum NEC 523.9
  Günther's (congenital erythropoietic porphyria)
    277.1
  gynecological 629.9
    specified NEC 629.89
  H 270.0
  Haas' 732.3
  Habermann's (acute parapsoriasis varioliformis)
    696.2
  Haff 985.1
  Hageman (congenital factor XII deficiency) (*see*
    also Defect, congenital) 286.3
  Haglund's (osteochondrosis os tibiale externum)
    732.5
  Hagner's (hypertrophic pulmonary
    osteoarthropathy) 731.2
  Hailey-Hailey (benign familial chronic
    pemphigus) 757.39
  hair (follicles) NEC 704.9
    specified type NEC 704.8
  Hallervorden-Spatz 333.0
  Hallopeau's (lichen sclerosus et atrophicus)
    701.0
  Hamman's (spontaneous mediastinal
    emphysema) 518.1
  hand, foot, and mouth 074.3
  Hand-Schüller-Christian (chronic histiocytosis
    X) 277.89
  Hanot's—*see* Cirrhosis, biliary
  Hansen's (leprosy) 030.9
    benign form 030.1
    malignant form 030.0
  Harada's 363.22
  Harley's (intermittent hemoglobinuria) 283.2
  Hart's (pellagra-cerebellar ataxia renal
    aminoaciduria) 270.0
  Hartnup (pellagra-cerebellar ataxia-renal
    aminoaciduria) 270.0
  Hashimoto's (struma lymphomatosa) 245.2
  Hb—*see* Disease, hemoglobin
  heart (organic) 429.9
    with
      acute pulmonary edema (*see also* Failure,
        ventricular, left) 428.1
        hypertensive 402.91
          with renal failure 404.92
          benign 402.11
            with renal failure 404.12
          malignant 402.01
            with renal failure 404.02
      kidney disease—*see* Hypertension,
        cardiorenal
      rheumatic fever (conditions classifiable to
        390)
        active 391.9
          with chorea 392.0
        inactive or quiescent (with chorea) 398.90
    amyloid 277.39 *[425.7]*
    aortic (valve) (*see also* Endocarditis, aortic)
      424.1
    arteriosclerotic or sclerotic (minimal)
      (senile)—*see* Arteriosclerosis, coronary
    artery, arterial —*see* Arteriosclerosis,
      coronary
    atherosclerotic —*see* Arteriosclerosis,
      coronary

Disease, diseased—*continued*
    hereditary persistence, fetal (HPFH) ("Swiss
       variety") 282.7
    high fetal gene 282.7
    I thalassemia 282.49
    M 289.7
    S—*see also* Disease, sickle-cell, Hb-S
       thalassemia (without crisis) 282.41
         with
           crisis 282.42
           vaso-occlusive pain 282.42
    spherocytosis 282.7
    unstable, hemolytic 282.7
    Zurich (Hb-Zurich) 282.7
   hemolytic (fetus) (newborn) 773.2
    autoimmune (cold type) (warm type) 283.0
    due to or with
      incompatibility
        ABO (blood group) 773.1
        blood (group) (Duffy) (Kell) (Kidd)
          (Lewis) (M) (S) NEC 773.2
        Rh (blood group) (factor) 773.0
      Rh negative mother 773.0
    unstable hemoglobin 282.7
   hemorrhagic 287.9
    newborn 776.0
   Henoch (-Schönlein) (purpura nervosa) 287.0
   hepatic—*see* Disease, liver
   hepatolenticular 275.1
   heredodegenerative NEC
    brain 331.89
    spinal cord 336.8
   Hers' (glycogenosis VI) 271.0
   Herter (-Gee) (-Heubner) (nontropical sprue)
    579.0
   Herxheimer's (diffuse idiopathic cutaneous
    atrophy) 701.8
   Heubner's 094.89
   Heubner-Herter (nontropical sprue) 579.0
   high fetal gene or hemoglobin thalassemia
    282.49
   Hildenbrand's (typhus) 081.9
   hip (joint) NEC 719.95
    congenital 755.63
    suppurative 711.05
    tuberculous (*see also* Tuberculosis) 015.1
     [730.85]
   Hippel's (retinocerebral angiomatosis) 759.6
   Hirschfeld's (acute diabetes mellitus) (*see also*
    Diabetes) 250.0
   Hirschsprung's (congenital megacolon) 751.3
   His (-Werner) (trench fever) 083.1
   HIV 042
   Hodgkin's (M9650/3) 201.9

> *Note—Use the following fifth-digit*
> *subclassification with categories 201:*
>
> 0 *unspecified site*
> 1 *lymph nodes of head, face, and neck*
> 2 *intrathoracic lymph nodes*
> 3 *intra-abdominal lymph nodes*
> 4 *lymph nodes of axilla and upper limb*
> 5 *lymph nodes of inguinal region and*
>   *lower limb*
> 6 *intrapelvic lymph nodes*
> 7 *spleen*
> 8 *lymph nodes of multiple sites*

    lymphocytic
     depletion (M9653/3) 201.7
      diffuse fibrosis (M9654/3) 201.7

Disease, diseased—*continued*
    reticular type (M9655/3) 201.7
     predominance (M9651/3) 201.4
    lymphocytic-histiocytic predominance
     (M9651/3) 201.4
    mixed cellularity (M9652/3) 201.6
    nodular sclerosis (M9656/3) 201.5
     cellular phase (M9657/3) 201.5
   Hodgson's 441.9
    ruptured 441.5
   Hoffa (-Kastert) (liposynovitis prepatellaris)
    272.8
   Holla (*see also* Spherocytosis) 282.0
   homozygous-Hb-S 282.61
   hoof and mouth 078.4
   hookworm (*see also* Ancylostomiasis) 126.9
   Horton's (temporal arteritis) 446.5
   host-versus-graft (immune or nonimmune cause)
    996.80
    bone marrow 996.85
    heart 996.83
    intestines 996.87
    kidney 996.81
    liver 996.82
    lung 996.84
    pancreas 996.86
    specified NEC 996.89
   HPFH (hereditary persistence of fetal
    hemoglobin) ("Swiss variety") 282.7
   Huchard's (continued arterial hypertension)
    401.9
   Huguier's (uterine fibroma) 218.9
   human immunodeficiency (virus) 042
   hunger 251.1
   Hunt's
    dyssynergia cerebellaris myoclonica 334.2
    herpetic geniculate ganglionitis 053.11
   Huntington's 333.4
   Huppert's (multiple myeloma) (M9730/3) 203.0
   Hurler's (mucopolysaccharidosis I) 277.5
   Hutchinson's, meaning
    angioma serpiginosum 709.1
    cheiropompholyx 705.81
    prurigo estivalis 692.72
   Hutchinson-Boeck (sarcoidosis) 135
   Hutchinson-Gilford (progeria) 259.8
   hyaline (diffuse) (generalized) 728.9
    membrane (lung) (newborn) 769
   hydatid (*see also* Echinococcus) 122.9
   Hyde's (prurigo nodularis) 698.3
   hyperkinetic (*see also* Hyperkinesia) 314.9
    heart 429.82
   hypertensive (*see also* Hypertension) 401.9
   hypophysis 253.9
    hyperfunction 253.1
    hypofunction 253.2
   Iceland (epidemic neuromyasthenia) 049.8
   I cell 272.7
   ill-defined 799.89
   immunologic NEC 279.9
   immunoproliferative 203.8
   inclusion 078.5
    salivary gland 078.5
   infancy, early NEC 779.9
   infective NEC 136.9
   inguinal gland 289.9
   internal semilunar cartilage, cystic 717.5
   intervertebral disc 722.90
    with myelopathy 722.70
    cervical, cervicothoracic 722.91
     with myelopathy 722.71

Disease, diseased—*continued*
  lumbar, lumbosacral 722.93
    with myelopathy 722.73
  thoracic, thoracolumbar 722.92
    with myelopathy 722.72
  intestine 569.9
   functional 564.9
    congenital 751.3
    psychogenic 306.4
   lardaceous 277.39
   organic 569.9
   protozoal NEC 007.9
  iris 364.9
  iron
   metabolism 275.0
   storage 275.0
  Isambert's (*see also* Tuberculosis, larynx) 012.3
  Iselin's (osteochondrosis, fifth metatarsal) 732.5
  Island (scrub typhus) 081.2
  itai-itai 985.5
  Jadassohn's (maculopapular erythroderma)
    696.2
  Jadassohn-Pellizari's (anetoderma) 701.3
  Jakob-Creutzfeldt (new variant) 046.1
   with dementia
    with behavioral disturbance 046.1 *[294.11]*
    without behavioral disturbance 046.1
      [294.10]
  Jaksch (-Luzet) (pseudoleukemia infantum)
    285.8
  Janet's 300.89
  Jansky-Bielschowsky 330.1
  jaw NEC 526.9
   fibrocystic 526.2
  Jensen's 363.05
  Jeune's (asphyxiating thoracic dystrophy) 756.4
  jigger 134.1
  Johnson-Stevens (erythema multiforme
    exudativum) 695.1
  joint NEC 719.9
   ankle 719.97
   Charcot 094.0 *[713.5]*
   degenerative (*see also* Osteoarthrosis) 715.9
    multiple 715.09
    spine (*see also* Spondylosis) 721.90
   elbow 719.92
   foot 719.97
   hand 719.94
   hip 719.95
   hypertrophic (chronic) (degenerative) (*see also*
    Osteoarthrosis) 715.9
    spine (*see also* Spondylosis) 721.90
   knee 719.96
   Luschka 721.90
   multiple sites 719.99
   pelvic region 719.95
   sacroiliac 724.6
   shoulder (region) 719.91
   specified site NEC 719.98
   spine NEC 724.9
    pseudarthrosis following fusion 733.82
    sacroiliac 724.6
   wrist 719.93
  Jourdain's (acute gingivitis) 523.00
  Jüngling's (sarcoidosis) 135
  Kahler (-Bozzolo) (multiple myeloma)
    (M9730/3) 203.0
  Kalischer's 759.6
  Kaposi's 757.33
   lichen ruber 697.8
    acuminatus 696.4

Disease, diseased—*continued*
  moniliformis 697.8
  xeroderma pigmentosum 757.33
  Kaschin-Beck (endemic polyarthritis) 716.00
   ankle 716.07
   arm 716.02
    lower (and wrist) 716.03
    upper (and elbow) 716.02
   foot (and ankle) 716.07
   forearm (and wrist) 716.03
   hand 716.04
   leg 716.06
    lower 716.06
    upper 716.05
   multiple sites 716.09
   pelvic region (hip) (thigh) 716.05
   shoulder region 716.01
   specified site NEC 716.08
  Katayama 120.2
  Kawasaki 446.1
  Kedani (scrub typhus) 081.2
  kidney (functional) (pelvis) (*see also* Disease,
    renal) 593.9
   chronic 585.9
    requiring chronic dialysis 585.6
    stage
     I 585.1
     II (mild) 585.2
     III (moderate) 585.3
     IV (severe) 585.4
     V 585.5
   cystic (congenital) 753.10
    multiple 753.19
    single 753.11
    specified NEC 753.19
   fibrocystic (congenital) 753.19
   in gout 274.10
   polycystic (congenital) 753.12
    adult type (APKD) 753.13
    autosomal dominant 753.13
    autosomal recessive 753.14
    childhood type (CPKD) 753.14
    infantile type 753.14
  Kienböck's (carpal lunate) (wrist) 732.3
  Kimmelstiel (-Wilson) (intercapillary
    glomerulosclerosis) 250.4 *[581.81]*
  Kinnier Wilson's (hepatolenticular
    degeneration) 275.1
  kissing 075
  Kleb's (*see also* Nephritis) 583.9
  Klinger's 446.4
  Klippel's 723.8
  Klippel-Feil (brevicollis) 756.16
  knight's 911.1
  Köbner's (epidermolysis bullosa) 757.39
  Koenig-Wichmann (pemphigus) 694.4
  Köhler's
   first (osteoarthrosis juvenilis) 732.5
   second (Freiberg's infraction, metatarsal head)
    732.5
   patellar 732.4
   tarsal navicular (bone) (osteoarthrosis
    juvenilis) 732.5
  Köhler-Freiberg (infraction, metatarsal head)
    732.5
  Köhler-Mouchet (osteoarthrosis juvenilis) 732.5
  Köhler-Pellegrini-Stieda (calcification, knee
    joint) 726.62
  Kok 759.89
  König's (osteochondritis dissecans) 732.7

Disease, diseased—*continued*
  Korsakoff's (nonalcoholic) 294.0
    alcoholic 291.1
  Kostmann's (infantile genetic agranulocytosis)
    288.01
  Krabbe's 330.0
  Kraepelin-Morel (*see also* Schizophrenia) 295.9
  Kraft-Weber-Dimitri 759.6
  Kufs' 330.1
  Kugelberg-Welander 335.11
  Kuhnt-Junius 362.52
  Kümmell's (-Verneuil) (spondylitis) 721.7
  Kundrat's (lymphosarcoma) 200.1
  kuru 046.0
  Kussmaul (-Meier) (polyarteritis nodosa) 446.0
  Kyasanur Forest 065.2
  Kyrle's (hyperkeratosis follicularis in cutem
    penetrans) 701.1
  labia
    inflammatory 616.9
      specified NEC 616.89
    noninflammatory 624.9
      specified NEC 624.8
  labyrinth, ear 386.8
  lacrimal system (apparatus) (passages) 375.9
    gland 375.00
    specified NEC 375.89
  Lafora's 333.2
  Lagleyze-von Hippel (retinocerebral
    angiomatosis) 759.6
  Lancereaux-Mathieu (leptospiral jaundice)
    100.0
  Landry's 357.0
  Lane's 569.89
  lardaceous (any site) 277.39
  Larrey-Weil (leptospiral jaundice) 100.0
  Larsen (-Johansson) (juvenile osteopathia
    patellae) 732.4
  larynx 478.70
  Lasègue's (persecution mania) 297.9
  Leber's 377.16
  Lederer's (acquired infectious hemolytic
    anemia) 283.19
  Legg's (capital femoral osteochondrosis) 732.1
  Legg-Calvé-Perthes (capital femoral
    osteochondrosis) 732.1
  Legg-Calvé-Waldenström (femoral capital
    osteochondrosis) 732.1
  Legg-Perthes (femoral capital osteochondrosis)
    732.1
  Legionnaires' 482.84
  Leigh's 330.8
  Leiner's (exfoliative dermatitis) 695.89
  Leloir's (lupus erythematosus) 695.4
  Lenegre's 426.0
  lens (eye) 379.39
  Leriche's (osteoporosis, posttraumatic) 733.7
  Letterer-Siwe (acute histiocytosis X) (M9722/3)
    202.5
  Lev's (acquired complete heart block) 426.0
  Lewandowski's (*see also* Tuberculosis) 017.0
  Lewandowski-Lutz (epidermodysplasia
    verruciformis) 078.19
  Lewy body 331.82
    with dementia
      with behavioral disturbance 331.82 *[294.11]*
      without behavioral disturbance 331.82
        [294.10]
  Leyden's (periodic vomiting) 536.2
  Libman-Sacks (verrucous endocarditis) 710.0
    [424.91]

Disease, diseased—*continued*
  Lichtheim's (subacute combined sclerosis with
    pernicious anemia) 281.0 *[336.2]*
  ligament 728.9
  light chain 203.0
  Lightwood's (renal tubular acidosis) 588.89
  Lignac's (cystinosis) 270.0
  Lindau's (retinocerebral angiomatosis) 759.6
  Lindau-von Hippel (angiomatosis
    retinocerebellosa) 759.6
  lip NEC 528.5
  lipidosis 272.7
  lipoid storage NEC 272.7
  Lipschültz's 616.50
  Little's—*see* Palsy, cerebral
  liver 573.9
    alcoholic 571.3
      acute 571.1
      chronic 571.3
    chronic 571.9
      alcoholic 571.3
    cystic, congenital 751.62
    drug-induced 573.3
    due to
      chemicals 573.3
      fluorinated agents 573.3
      hypersensitivity drugs 573.3
      isoniazids 573.3
    fibrocystic (congenital) 751.62
    glycogen storage 271.0
    organic 573.9
    polycystic (congenital) 751.62
  Lobo's (keloid blastomycosis) 116.2
  Lobstein's (brittle bones and blue sclera) 756.61
  locomotor system 334.9
  Lorain's (pituitary dwarfism) 253.3
  Lou Gehrig's 335.20
  Lucas-Championnière (fibrinous bronchitis)
    466.0
  Ludwig's (submaxillary cellulitis) 528.3
  luetic—*see* Syphilis
  lumbosacral region 724.6
  lung NEC 518.89
    black 500
    congenital 748.60
    cystic 518.89
      congenital 748.4
    fibroid (chronic) (*see also* Fibrosis, lung) 515
    fluke 121.2
      Oriental 121.2
    in
      amyloidosis 277.39 *[517.8]*
      polymyositis 710.4 *[517.8]*
      sarcoidosis 135 *[517.8]*
      Sjögren's syndrome 710.2 *[517.8]*
      syphilis 095.1
      systemic lupus erythematosus 710.0 *[517.8]*
      systemic sclerosis 710.1 *[517.2]*
    interstitial (chronic) 515
      acute 136.3
    nonspecific, chronic 496
    obstructive (chronic) (COPD) 496
      with
        acute
          bronchitis 491.22
          exacerbation NEC 491.21
        alveolitis, allergic (*see also* Alveolitis,
          allergic) 495.9
        asthma (chronic) (obstructive) 493.2
        bronchiectasis 494.0
          with exacerbation (acute) 494.1

Disease, diseased—*continued*
　　bronchitis (chronic) 491.20
　　　　with
　　　　　　acute bronchitis 491.22
　　　　　　exacerbation (acute) 491.21
　　　　　　decompensated 491.21
　　　　　　　　with exacerbation 491.21
　　　　　　emphysema NEC 492.8
　　　　　diffuse (with fibrosis) 496
　　　polycystic 518.89
　　　　　asthma (chronic) (obstructive) 493.2
　　　　　congenital 748.4
　　　purulent (cavitary) 513.0
　　　restrictive 518.89
　　　rheumatoid 714.81
　　　　diffuse interstitial 714.81
　　　specified NEC 518.89
　　Lutembacher's (atrial septal defect with mitral
　　　　stenosis) 745.5
　　Lutz-Miescher (elastosis perforans serpiginosa)
　　　　701.1
　　Lutz-Splendore-de Almeida (Brazilian
　　　　blastomycosis) 116.1
　　Lyell's (toxic epidermal necrolysis) 695.1
　　　due to drug
　　　　correct substance properly administered
　　　　　　695.1
　　　　overdose or wrong substance given or taken
　　　　　　977.9
　　　　　specific drug—*see* Table of drugs and
　　　　　　chemicals
　　Lyme 088.81
　　lymphatic (gland) (system) 289.9
　　　channel (noninfective) 457.9
　　　vessel (noninfective) 457.9
　　　　specified NEC 457.8
　　lymphoproliferative (chronic) (M9970/1) 238.79
　　Machado-Joseph 334.8
　　Madelung's (lipomatosis) 272.8
　　Madura (actinomycotic) 039.9
　　　mycotic 117.4
　　Magitot's 526.4
　　Majocchi's (purpura annularis telangiectodes)
　　　　709.1
　　malarial (*see also* Malaria) 084.6
　　Malassez's (cystic) 608.89
　　Malibu 919.8
　　　infected 919.9
　　malignant (M8000/3)—*see also* Neoplasm, by
　　　　site, malignant
　　　previous, affecting management of pregnancy
　　　　V23.8
　　Manson's 120.1
　　maple bark 495.6
　　maple syrup (urine) 270.3
　　Marburg (virus) 078.89
　　Marchiafava (-Bignami) 341.8
　　Marfan's 090.49
　　　congenital syphilis 090.49
　　　meaning Marfan's syndrome 759.82
　　Marie-Bamberger (hypertrophic pulmonary
　　　　osteoarthropathy) (secondary) 731.2
　　　primary or idiopathic (acropachyderma)
　　　　757.39
　　　pulmonary (hypertrophic osteoarthropathy)
　　　　731.2
　　Marie-Strümpell (ankylosing spondylitis) 720.0
　　Marion's (bladder neck obstruction) 596.0
　　Marsh's (exophthalmic goiter) 242.0
　　Martin's 715.27

Disease, diseased—*continued*
　　mast cell 757.33
　　　systemic (M9741/3) 202.6
　　mastoid (*see also* Mastoiditis) 383.9
　　　process 385.9
　　maternal, unrelated to pregnancy NEC, affecting
　　　　fetus or newborn 760.9
　　Mathieu's (leptospiral jaundice) 100.0
　　Mauclaire's 732.3
　　Mauriac's (erythema nodosum syphiliticum)
　　　　091.3
　　Maxcy's 081.0
　　McArdle (-Schmid-Pearson) (glycogenosis V)
　　　　271.0
　　mediastinum NEC 519.3
　　Medin's (*see also* Poliomyelitis) 045.9
　　Mediterranean (with hemoglobinopathy) 282.49
　　medullary center (idiopathic) (respiratory) 348.8
　　Meige's (chronic hereditary edema) 757.0
　　Meleda 757.39
　　Ménétrier's (hypertrophic gastritis) 535.2
　　Ménière's (active) 386.00
　　　cochlear 386.02
　　　cochleovestibular 386.01
　　　inactive 386.04
　　　in remission 386.04
　　　vestibular 386.03
　　meningeal—*see* Meningitis
　　mental (*see also* Psychosis) 298.9
　　Merzbacher-Pelizaeus 330.0
　　mesenchymal 710.9
　　mesenteric embolic 557.0
　　metabolic NEC 277.9
　　metal polishers' 502
　　metastatic—*see* Metastasis
　　Mibelli's 757.39
　　microdrepanocytic 282.49
　　microvascular —*code to condition*
　　Miescher's 709.3
　　Mikulicz's (dryness of mouth, absent or
　　　　decreased lacrimation) 527.1
　　Milkman (-Looser) (osteomalacia with
　　　　pseudofractures) 268.2
　　Miller's (osteomalacia) 268.2
　　Mills' 335.29
　　Milroy's (chronic hereditary edema) 757.0
　　Minamata 985.0
　　Minor's 336.1
　　Minot's (hemorrhagic disease, newborn) 776.0
　　Minot-von Willebrand-Jürgens
　　　　(angiohemophilia) 286.4
　　Mitchell's (erythromelalgia) 443.82
　　mitral—*see* Endocarditis, mitral
　　Mljet (mal de Meleda) 757.39
　　Möbius', Moebius' 346.8
　　Moeller's 267
　　Möller (-Barlow) (infantile scurvy) 267
　　Mönckeberg's (*see also* arteriosclerosis,
　　　　extremities) 440.20
　　Mondor's (thrombophlebitis of breast) 451.89
　　Monge's 993.2
　　Morel-Kraepelin (*see also* Schizophrenia) 295.9
　　Morgagni's (syndrome) (hyperostosis frontalis
　　　　interna) 733.3
　　Morgagni-Adams-Stokes (syncope with heart
　　　　block) 426.9
　　Morquio (-Brailsford) (-Ullrich)
　　　　(mucopolysaccharidosis IV) 277.5
　　Morton's (with metatarsalgia) 355.6
　　Morvan's 336.0
　　motor neuron (bulbar) (mixed type) 335.20

Disease, diseased—*continued*
 Mouchet's (juvenile osteochondrosis, foot)
  732.5
 mouth 528.9
 Moyamoya 437.5
 Mucha's (acute parapsoriasis varioliformis)
  696.2
 mu-chain 273.2
 mucolipidosis (I) (II) (III) 272.7
 Münchmeyer's (exostosis luxurians) 728.11
 Murri's (intermittent hemoglobinuria) 283.2
 muscle 359.9
  inflammatory 728.9
  ocular 378.9
 musculoskeletal system 729.9
 mushroom workers' 495.5
 Myà's (congenital dilation, colon) 751.3
 mycotic 117.9
 myeloproliferative (chronic) (M9960/1) 238.79
 myocardium, myocardial (*see also*
   Degeneration, myocardial) 429.1
  hypertensive (*see also* Hypertension, heart)
   402.90
  primary (idiopathic) 425.4
 myoneural 358.9
 Naegeli's 287.1
 nail 703.9
  specified type NEC 703.8
 Nairobi sheep 066.1
 nasal 478.19
  cavity NEC 478.19
  sinus (chronic)—*see* Sinusitis
 navel (newborn) NEC 779.89
  delayed separation of umbilical cord 779.83
 nemaline body 359.0
 neoplastic, generalized (M8000/6) 199.0
 nerve—*see* Disorder, nerve
 nervous system (central) 349.9
  autonomic, peripheral (*see also* Neuropathy,
    peripheral, autonomic) 337.9
  congenital 742.9
  inflammatory—*see* Encephalitis
  parasympathetic (*see also* Neuropathy,
    peripheral, autonomic) 337.9
  peripheral NEC 355.9
  specified NEC 349.89
  sympathetic (*see also* Neuropathy, peripheral,
    autonomic) 337.9
  vegetative (*see also* Neuropathy, peripheral,
    autonomic) 337.9
 Nettleship's (urticaria pigmentosa) 757.33
 Neumann's (pemphigus vegetans) 694.4
 neurologic (central) NEC (*see also* Disease,
    nervous system) 349.9
  peripheral NEC 355.9
 neuromuscular system NEC 358.9
 Newcastle 077.8
 Nicolas (-Durand) -Favre (climatic bubo) 099.1
 Niemann-Pick (lipid histiocytosis) 272.7
 nipple 611.9
  Paget's (M8540/3) 174.0
 Nishimoto (-Takeuchi) 437.5
 nonarthropod-borne NEC 078.89
  central nervous system NEC 049.9
  enterovirus NEC 078.89
 non-autoimmune hemolytic NEC 283.10
 Nonne-Milroy-Meige (chronic hereditary
    edema) 757.0
 Norrie's (congenital progressive
    oculoacousticocerebral degeneration) 743.8
 nose 478.19

Disease, diseased—*continued*
 nucleus pulposus—*see* Disease, intervertebral
  disc
 nutritional 269.9
  maternal, affecting fetus or newborn 760.4
 oasthouse, urine 270.2
 obliterative vascular 447.1
 Odelberg's (juvenile osteochondrosis) 732.1
 Oguchi's (retina) 368.61
 Ohara's (*see also* Tularemia) 021.9
 Ollier's (chondrodysplasia) 756.4
 Opitz's (congestive splenomegaly) 289.51
 Oppenheim's 358.8
 Oppenheim-Urbach (necrobiosis lipoidica
    diabeticorum) 250.8 *[709.3]*
 optic nerve NEC 377.49
 orbit 376.9
  specified NEC 376.89
 Oriental liver fluke 121.1
 Oriental lung fluke 121.2
 Ormond's 593.4
 Osgood's tibia (tubercle) 732.4
 Osgood-Schlatter 732.4
 Osler (-Vaquez) (polycythemia vera) (M9950/1)
    238.4
 Osler-Rendu (familial hemorrhagic
    telangiectasia) 448.0
 osteofibrocystic 252.01
 Otto's 715.35
 outer ear 380.9
 ovary (noninflammatory) NEC 620.9
  cystic 620.2
  polycystic 256.4
  specified NEC 620.8
 Owren's (congenital) (*see also* Defect,
    coagulation) 286.3
 Paas' 756.59
 Paget's (osteitis deformans) 731.0
  with infiltrating duct carcinoma of the breast
    (M8541/3)—*see* Neoplasm, breast,
    malignant
  bone 731.0
   osteosarcoma in (M9184/3)—*see* Neoplasm,
    bone, malignant
  breast (M8540/3) 174.0
  extramammary (M8542/3)—*see also*
    Neoplasm, skin, malignant
   anus 154.3
    skin 173.5
  malignant (M8540/3)
   breast 174.0
   specified site NEC (M8542/3)—*see*
    Neoplasm, skin, malignant
   unspecified site 174.0
  mammary (M8540/3) 174.0
  nipple (M8540/3) 174.0
 palate (soft) 528.9
 Paltauf-Sternberg 201.9
 pancreas 577.9
  cystic 577.2
   congenital 751.7
  fibrocystic 277.00
 Panner's 732.3
  capitellum humeri 732.3
  head of humerus 732.3
  tarsal navicular (bone) (osteochondrosis)
    732.5
 panvalvular—*see* Endocarditis, mitral
 parametrium 629.9
 parasitic NEC 136.9
  cerebral NEC 123.9

Disease, diseased—*continued*
  polycystic (congenital) 759.89
    kidney or renal 753.12
      adult type (APKD) 753.13
      autosomal dominant 753.13
      autosomal recessive 753.14
      childhood type (CPKD) 753.14
      infantile type 753.14
    liver or hepatic 751.62
    lung or pulmonary 518.89
      congenital 748.4
    ovary, ovaries 256.4
    spleen 759.0
  Pompe's (glycogenosis II) 271.0
  Poncet's (tuberculous rheumatism) (*see also* Tuberculosis) 015.9
  Posada-Wernicke 114.9
  Potain's (pulmonary edema) 514
  Pott's (*see also* Tuberculosis) 015.0 *[730.88]*
    osteomyelitis 015.0 *[730.88]*
    paraplegia 015.0 *[730.88]*
    spinal curvature 015.0 *[737.43]*
    spondylitis 015.0 *[720.81]*
  Potter's 753.0
  Poulet's 714.2
  pregnancy NEC (*see also* Pregnancy) 646.9
  Preiser's (osteoporosis) 733.09
  Pringle's (tuberous sclerosis) 759.5
  Profichet's 729.9
  prostate 602.9
    specified type NEC 602.8
  protozoal NEC 136.8
    intestine, intestinal NEC 007.9
  pseudo-Hurler's (mucolipidosis III) 272.7
  psychiatric (*see also* Psychosis) 298.9
  psychotic (*see also* Psychosis) 298.9
  Puente's (simple glandular cheilitis) 528.5
  puerperal NEC (*see also* Puerperal) 674.9
  pulmonary—*see also* Disease, lung
    amyloid 277.39 *[517.8]*
    artery 417.9
    circulation, circulatory 417.9
      specified NEC 417.8
    diffuse obstructive (chronic) 496
      with
        acute bronchitis 491.22
        asthma (chronic) (obstructive) 493.2
        bronchitis (chronic) 491.20
          with exacerbation (acute) 491.21
        exacerbation NEC (acute) 491.21
    heart (chronic) 416.9
      specified NEC 416.8
    hypertensive (vascular) 416.0
      cardiovascular 416.0
    obstructive diffuse (chronic) 496
      decompensated 491.21
        with exacerbation 491.21
      with
        acute bronchitis 491.22
        asthma (chronic) (obstructive) 493.2
        bronchitis (chronic) 491.20
          with
            exacerbation (acute) 491.21
          acute 491.22
        exacerbation NEC (acute) 491.21
    valve (*see also* Endocarditis, pulmonary) 424.3
  pulp (dental) NEC 522.9
  pulseless 446.7
  Putnam's (subacute combined sclerosis with pernicious anemia) 281.0 *[336.2]*

Disease, diseased—*continued*
  Pyle (-Cohn) (craniometaphyseal dysplasia) 756.89
  pyramidal tract 333.90
  Quervain's
    tendon sheath 727.04
    thyroid (subacute granulomatous thyroiditis) 245.1
  Quincke's—*see* Edema, angioneurotic
  Quinquaud (acne decalvans) 704.09
  rag sorters' 022.1
  Raynaud's (Paroxysmal digital cyanosis) 443.0
  reactive airway—*see* Asthma
  Recklinghausen's (M9540/1) 237.71
    bone (osteitis fibrosa cystica) 252.01
  Recklinghausen-Applebaum (hemochromatosis) 275.0
  Reclus' (cystic) 610.1
  rectum NEC 569.49
  Refsum's (heredopathia atactica polyneuritiformis) 356.3
  Reichmann's (gastrosuccorrhea) 536.8
  Reimann's (periodic) 277.31
  Reiter's 099.3
  renal (functional) (pelvis) (*see also* Disease, kidney) 593.9
    with
      edema (*see also* Nephrosis) 581.9
      exudative nephritis 583.89
      lesion of interstitial nephritis 583.89
      stated generalized cause—*see* Nephritis
    acute 593.9
    basement membrane NEC 583.89
      with
        pulmonary hemorrhage (Goodpasture's syndrome) 446.21 *[583.81]*
    chronic (*see also* Disease, kidney, chronic) 585.9
    complicating pregnancy or puerperium NEC 646.2
      with hypertension—*see* Toxemia, of pregnancy
      affecting fetus or newborn 760.1
    cystic, congenital (*see also* Cystic, disease, kidney) 753.10
    diabetic 250.4 *[583.81]*
    due to
      amyloidosis 277.39 *[583.81]*
      diabetes mellitus 250.4 *[583.81]*
      systemic lupus erythematosis 710.0 *[583.81]*
    end-stage 585.6
    exudative 583.89
    fibrocystic (congenital) 753.19
    gonococcal 098.19 *[583.81]*
    gouty 274.10
    hypertensive (*see also* Hypertension, kidney) 403.90
    immune complex NEC 583.89
    interstitial (diffuse) (focal) 583.89
    lupus 710.0 *[583.81]*
    maternal, affecting fetus or newborn 760.1
      hypertensive 760.0
    phosphate-losing (tubular) 588.0
    polycystic (congenital) 753.12
      adult type (APKD) 753.13
      autosomal dominant 753.13
      autosomal recessive 753.14
      childhood type (CPKD) 753.14
      infantile type 753.14
    specified lesion or cause NEC (*see also* Glomerulonephritis) 583.89

Disease, diseased—*continued*
   subacute 581.9
   syphilitic 095.4
   tuberculous (*see also* Tuberculosis) 016.0
     [583.81]
   tubular (*see also* Nephrosis, tubular) 584.5
  Rendu-Olser-Weber (familial hemorrhagic
    telangiectasia) 448.0
  renovascular (arteriosclerotic) (*see also*
    Hypertension, kidney) 403.90
  respiratory (tract) 519.9
   acute or subacute (upper) NEC 465.9
    due to fumes or vapors 506.3
    multiple sites NEC 465.8
    noninfectious 478.9
    streptococcal 034.0
   chronic 519.9
    arising in the perinatal period 770.7
    due to fumes or vapors 506.4
   due to
    aspiration of liquids or solids 508.9
    external agents NEC 508.9
     specified NEC 508.8
    fumes or vapors 506.9
     acute or subacute NEC 506.3
     chronic 506.4
   fetus or newborn NEC 770.9
   obstructive 496
   specified type NEC 519.8
   upper (acute) (infectious) NEC 465.9
    multiple sites NEC 465.8
    noninfectious NEC 478.9
    streptococcal 034.0
  retina, retinal NEC 362.9
   Batten's or Batten-Mayou 330.1 *[362.71]*
   degeneration 362.89
   vascular lesion 362.17
  rheumatic (*see also* Arthritis) 716.8
   heart—*see* Disease, heart, rheumatic
  rheumatoid (heart)—*see* Arthritis, rheumatoid
  rickettsial NEC 083.9
   specified type NEC 083.8
  Riedel's (ligneous thyroiditis) 245.3
  Riga (-Fede) (cachectic aphthae) 529.0
  Riggs' (compound periodontitis) 523.40
  Ritter's 695.81
  Rivalta's (cervicofacial actinomycosis) 039.3
  Robles' (onchocerciasis) 125.3 *[360.13]*
  Roger's (congenital interventricular septal
    defect) 745.4
  Rokitansky's (*see also* Necrosis, liver) 570
  Romberg's 349.89
  Rosenthal's (factor XI deficiency) 286.2
  Rossbach's (hyperchlorhydria) 536.8
   psychogenic 306.4
  Roth (-Bernhardt) 355.1
  Runeberg's (progressive pernicious anemia)
    281.0
  Rust's (tuberculous spondylitis) (*see also*
    Tuberculosis) 015.0 *[720.81]*
  Rustitskii's (multiple myeloma) (M9730/3)
    203.0
  Ruysch's (Hirschsprung's disease) 751.3
  Sachs (-Tay) 330.1
  sacroiliac NEC 724.6
  salivary gland or duct NEC 527.9
   inclusion 078.5
    streptococcal 034.0
   virus 078.5
  Sander's (paranoia) 297.1
  Sandhoff's 330.1

Disease, diseased—*continued*
  sandworm 126.9
  Savill's (epidemic exfoliative dermatitis) 695.89
  Schamberg's (progressive pigmentary
    dermatosis) 709.09
  Schaumann's (sarcoidosis) 135
  Schenck's (sporotrichosis) 117.1
  Scheuermann's (osteochondrosis) 732.0
  Schilder (-Flatau) 341.1
  Schimmelbusch's 610.1
  Schlatter's tibia (tubercle) 732.4
  Schlatter-Osgood 732.4
  Schmorl's 722.30
   cervical 722.39
   lumbar, lumbosacral 722.32
   specified region NEC 722.39
   thoracic, thoracolumbar 722.31
  Scholz's 330.0
  Schönlein (-Henoch) (purpura rheumatica) 287.0
  Schottmüller's (*see also* Fever, paratyphoid)
    002.9
  Schüller-Christian (chronic histiocytosis X)
    277.89
  Schultz's (agranulocytosis) 288.09
  Schwalbe-Ziehen-Oppenheimer 333.6
  Schweninger-Buzzi (macular atrophy) 701.3
  sclera 379.19
  scrofulous (*see also* Tuberculosis) 017.2
  scrotum 608.9
  sebaceous glands NEC 706.9
  Secretan's (posttraumatic edema) 782.3
  semilunar cartilage, cystic 717.5
  seminal vesicle 608.9
  Senear-Usher (pemphigus erythematosus) 694.4
  serum NEC 999.5
  Sever's (osteochondrosis calcaneum) 732.5
  Sézary's (reticulosis) (M9701/3) 202.2
  Shaver's (bauxite pneumoconiosis) 503
  Sheehan's (postpartum pituitary necrosis) 253.2
  shimamushi (scrub typhus) 081.2
  shipyard 077.1
  sickle-cell 282.60
   with
    crisis 282.62
    Hb-S disease 282.61
    other abnormal hemoglobin (Hb-D) (Hb-E)
     (Hb-G) (Hb-J) (Hb-K) (Hb-O) (Hb-P)
     (high fetal gene) (without crisis) 282.68
    with crisis 282.69
   elliptocytosis 282.60
   Hb-C (without crisis) 282.63
    with
     crisis 282.64
     vaso-occlusive pain 282.64
   Hb-S 282.61
    with
     crisis 282.62
     Hb-C (without crisis) 282.63
      with
       crisis 282.64
       vaso-occlusive pain 282.64
     other abnormal hemoglobin (Hb-D) (Hb-E)
      (Hb-G) (Hb-J) (Hb-K) (Hb-O) (Hb-P)
      (high fetal gene) (without crisis) 282.68
     with crisis 282.69
   spherocytosis 282.60
   thalassemia (without crisis) 282.41
    with
     crisis 282.42
     vaso-occlusive pain 282.42
  Siegal-Cattan-Mamou (periodic) 277.31

Disease, diseased—*continued*
  silo fillers' 506.9
  Simian B 054.3
  Simmonds' (pituitary cachexia) 253.2
  Simons' (progressive lipodystrophy) 272.6
  Sinding-Larsen (juvenile osteopathia patellae)
    732.4
  sinus—*see also* Sinusitis
    brain 437.9
    specified NEC 478.19
  Sirkari's 085.0
  sixth 057.8
  Sjögren (-Gougerot) 710.2
    with lung involvement 710.2 *[517.8]*
  Skevas-Zerfus 989.5
  skin NEC 709.9
    due to metabolic disorder 277.9
    specified type NEC 709.8
  sleeping (*see also* Narcolepsy) 347.00
    meaning sleeping sickness (*see also*
      Trypanosomiasis) 086.5
  small vessel 443.9
  Smith-Strang (oasthouse urine) 270.2
  Sneddon-Wilkinson (subcorneal pustular
    dermatosis) 694.1
  South African creeping 133.8
  Spencer's (epidemic vomiting) 078.82
  Spielmeyer-Stock 330.1
  Spielmeyer-Vogt 330.1
  spine, spinal 733.90
    combined system (*see also* Degeneration,
      combined) 266.2 *[336.2]*
      with pernicious anemia 281.0 *[336.2]*
    cord NEC 336.9
      congenital 742.9
    demyelinating NEC 341.8
    joint (*see also* Disease, joint, spine) 724.9
    tuberculous 015.0 *[730.8]*
  spinocerebellar 334.9
    specified NEC 334.8
  spleen (organic) (postinfectional) 289.50
    amyloid 277.39
    lardaceous 277.39
    polycystic 759.0
    specified NEC 289.59
  sponge divers' 989.5
  Stanton's (melioidosis) 025
  Stargardt's 362.75
  Startle 759.89
  Steinert's 359.2
  Sternberg's—*see* Disease, Hodgkin's
  Stevens-Johnson (erythema multiforme
    exudativum) 695.1
  Sticker's (erythema infectiosum) 057.0
  Stieda's (calcification, knee joint) 726.62
  Still's (juvenile rheumatoid arthritis) 714.30
  Stiller's (asthenia) 780.79
  Stokes' (exophthalmic goiter) 242.0
  Stokes-Adams (syncope with heart block) 426.9
  Stokvis (-Talma) (enterogenous cyanosis) 289.7
  stomach NEC (organic) 537.9
    functional 536.9
      psychogenic 306.4
    lardaceous 277.39
  stonemasons' 502
  storage
    glycogen (*see also* Disease, glycogen storage)
      271.0
    lipid 272.7
    mucopolysaccharide 277.5

Disease, diseased—*continued*
  striatopallidal system 333.90
    specified NEC 333.89
  Strümpell-Marie (ankylosing spondylitis) 720.0
  Stuart's (congenital factor X deficiency) (*see
    also* Defect, coagulation) 286.3
  Stuart-Prower (congenital factor X deficiency)
    (*see also* Defect, coagulation) 286.3
  Sturge (-Weber) (-Dimitri) (encephalocutaneous
    angiomatosis) 759.6
  Stuttgart 100.89
  Sudeck's 733.7
  supporting structures of teeth NEC 525.9
  suprarenal (gland) (capsule) 255.9
    hyperfunction 255.3
    hypofunction 255.4
  Sutton's 709.09
  Sutton and Gull's—*see* Hypertension, kidney
  sweat glands NEC 705.9
    specified type NEC 705.89
  sweating 078.2
  Sweeley-Klionsky 272.4
  Swift (-Feer) 985.0
  swimming pool (bacillus) 031.1
  swineherd's 100.89
  Sylvest's (epidemic pleurodynia) 074.1
  Symmers (follicular lymphoma) (M9690/3)
    202.0
  sympathetic nervous system (*see also*
    Neuropathy, peripheral, autonomic) 337.9
  synovium 727.9
  syphilitic—*see* Syphilis
  systemic tissue mast cell (M9741/3) 202.6
  Taenzer's 757.4
  Takayasu's (pulseless) 446.7
  Talma's 728.85
  Tangier (familial high-density lipoprotein
    deficiency) 272.5
  Tarral-Besnier (pityriasis rubra pilaris) 696.4
  Tay-Sachs 330.1
  Taylor's 701.8
  tear duct 375.69
  teeth, tooth 525.9
    hard tissues 521.9
      specified NEC 521.89
    pulp NEC 522.9
  tendon 727.9
    inflammatory NEC 727.9
  terminal vessel 443.9
  testis 608.9
  Thaysen-Gee (nontropical sprue) 579.0
  Thomsen's 359.2
  Thomson's (congenital poikiloderma) 757.33
  Thornwaldt's, Tornwaldt's (pharyngeal bursitis)
    478.29
  throat 478.20
    septic 034.0
  thromboembolic (*see also* Embolism) 444.9
  thymus (gland) 254.9
    specified NEC 254.8
  thyroid (gland) NEC 246.9
    heart (*see also* Hyperthyroidism) 242.9
      [425.7]
    lardaceous 277.39
    specified NEC 246.8
  Tietze's 733.6
  Tommaselli's
    correct substance properly administered 599.7
    overdose or wrong substance given or taken
      961.4
  tongue 529.9

Disease, diseased—*continued*
  tonsils, tonsillar (and adenoids) (chronic) 474.9
    specified NEC 474.8
  tooth, teeth 525.9
    hard tissues 521.9
      specified NEC 521.89
    pulp NEC 522.9
  Tornwaldt's (pharyngeal bursitis) 478.29
  Tourette's 307.23
  trachea 519.19
  tricuspid—*see* Endocarditis, tricuspid
  triglyceride-storage, type I, II, III 272.7
  triple vessel (coronary arteries) —*see*
      Arteriosclerosis, coronary
  trisymptomatic, Gougerot's 709.1
  trophoblastic (*see also* Hydatidiform mole) 630
    previous, affecting management of pregnancy
        V23.1
  tsutsugamushi (scrub typhus) 081.2
  tube (fallopian), noninflammatory 620.9
    specified NEC 620.8
  tuberculous NEC (*see also* Tuberculosis) 011.9
  tubo-ovarian
    inflammatory (*see also* Salpingo-oophoritis)
        614.2
    noninflammatory 620.9
      specified NEC 620.8
  tubotympanic, chronic (with anterior perforation
      of ear drum) 382.1
  tympanum 385.9
  Uhl's 746.84
  umbilicus (newborn) NEC 779.89
    delayed separation 779.83
  Underwood's (sclerema neonatorum) 778.1
  undiagnosed 799.9
  Unna's (seborrheic dermatitis) 690.18
  unstable hemoglobin hemolytic 282.7
  Unverricht (-Lundborg) 333.2
  Urbach-Oppenheim (necrobiosis lipoidica
      diabeticorum) 250.8 *[709.3]*
  Urbach-Wiethe (lipoid proteinosis) 272.8
  ureter 593.9
  urethra 599.9
    specified type NEC 599.84
  urinary (tract) 599.9
    bladder 596.9
      specified NEC 596.8
    maternal, affecting fetus or newborn 760.1
  Usher-Senear (pemphigus erythematosus) 694.4
  uterus (organic) 621.9
    infective (*see also* Endometritis) 615.9
    inflammatory (*see also* Endometritis) 615.9
    noninflammatory 621.9
      specified type NEC 621.8
  uveal tract
    anterior 364.9
    posterior 363.9
  vagabonds' 132.1
  vagina, vaginal
    inflammatory 616.9
      specified NEC 616.89
    noninflammatory 623.9
      specified NEC 623.8
  Valsuani's (progressive pernicious anemia,
      puerperal) 648.2
    complicating pregnancy or puerperium 648.2
  valve, valvular—*see* Endocarditis
  van Bogaert-Nijssen (-Peiffer) 330.0
  van Creveld-von Gierke (glycogenosis I) 271.0
  van den Bergh's (enterogenous cyanosis) 289.7
  van Neck's (juvenile osteochondrosis) 732.1

Disease, diseased—*continued*
  Vaquez (-Osler) (polycythemia vera) (M9950/1)
      238.4
  vascular 459.9
    arteriosclerotic—*see* Arteriosclerosis
    hypertensive—*see* Hypertension
    obliterative 447.1
      peripheral 443.9
    occlusive 459.9
    peripheral (occlusive) 443.9
      in diabetes mellitus 250.7 *[443.81]*
      specified type NEC 443.89
  vas deferens 608.9
  vasomotor 443.9
  vasospastic 443.9
  vein 459.9
  venereal 099.9
    fifth 099.1
    sixth 099.1
    chlamydial NEC 099.50
      anus 099.52
      bladder 099.53
      cervix 099.53
      epididymis 099.54
      genitourinary NEC 099.55
        lower 099.53
        specified NEC 099.54
      pelvic inflammatory disease 099.54
      perihepatic 099.56
      peritoneum 099.56
      pharynx 099.51
      rectum 099.52
      specified site NEC 099.59
      testis 099.54
      vagina 099.53
      vulva 099.53
    complicating pregnancy, childbirth, or
        puerperium 647.2
    specified nature or type NEC 099.8
      chlamydial—*see* Disease, venereal,
          chlamydial
  Verneuil's (syphilitic bursitis) 095.7
  Verse's (calcinosis intervertebralis) 275.49
      [722.90]
  vertebra, vertebral NEC 733.90
    disc—*see* Disease, Intervertebral disc
  vibration NEC 994.9
  Vidal's (lichen simplex chronicus) 698.3
  Vincent's (trench mouth) 101
  Virchow's 733.99
  virus (filterable) NEC 078.89
    arbovirus NEC 066.9
    arthropod-borne NEC 066.9
    central nervous system NEC 049.9
      specified type NEC 049.8
    complicating pregnancy, childbirth, or
        puerperium 647.6
    contact (with) V01.79
      varicella V01.71
    exposure to V01.79
      varicella V01.71
    Marburg 078.89
    maternal
      with fetal damage affecting management of
          pregnancy 655.3
    nonarthropod-borne NEC 078.89
      central nervous system NEC 049.9
        specified NEC 049.8
    vaccination, prophylactic (against) V04.89
  vitreous 379.29
  vocal cords NEC 478.5

Note—"Closed" includes simple, complete, partial, uncomplicated, and unspecified dislocation. "Open" includes dislocation specified as infected or compound and dislocation with foreign body. "Chronic," "habitual," "old," or "recurrent" dislocations should be coded as indicated under the entry "Dislocation, recurrent"; and "pathological" as indicated under the entry "Dislocation, pathological." For late effect of dislocation see Late, effect, dislocation.

Dislocation—*continued*
　　open 839.9
　　Bell-Daly 723.8
　　breast bone (closed) 839.61
　　　open 839.71
　　capsule, joint—*see* Dislocation, by site
　　carpal (bone)—*see* Dislocation, wrist
　　carpometacarpal (joint) (closed) 833.04
　　　open 833.14
　　cartilage (joint)—*see also* Dislocation, by site
　　　knee—*see* Tear, meniscus
　　cervical, cervicodorsal, or cervicothoracic
　　　　(spine) (vertebra)—*see* Dislocation,
　　　　vertebra, cervical
　　chiropractic (*see also* Lesion, nonallopathic)
　　　739.9
　　chondrocostal—*see* Dislocation, costochondral
　　chronic—*see* Dislocation, recurrent
　　clavicle (closed) 831.04
　　　open 831.14
　　coccyx (closed) 839.41
　　　open 839.51
　　collar bone (closed) 831.04
　　　open 831.14
　　compound (open) NEC 839.9
　　congenital NEC 755.8
　　　hip (*see also* Dislocation, hip, congenital)
　　　　754.30
　　　lens 743.37
　　　rib 756.3
　　　sacroiliac 755.69
　　　spine NEC 756.19
　　　vertebra 756.19
　　coracoid (closed) 831.09
　　　open 831.19
　　costal cartilage (closed) 839.69
　　　open 839.79
　　costochondral (closed) 839.69
　　　open 839.79
　　cricoarytenoid articulation (closed) 839.69
　　　open 839.79
　　cricothyroid (cartilage) articulation (closed)
　　　839.69
　　　open 839.79
　　dorsal vertebrae (closed) 839.21
　　　open 839.31
　　ear ossicle 385.23
　　elbow (closed) 832.00
　　　anterior (closed) 832.01
　　　　open 832.11
　　　congenital 754.89
　　　divergent (closed) 832.09
　　　　open 832.19
　　　lateral (closed) 832.04
　　　　open 832.14
　　　medial (closed) 832.03
　　　　open 832.13
　　　open 832.10
　　　posterior (closed) 832.02
　　　　open 832.12
　　　recurrent 718.32
　　　specified type NEC 832.09
　　　　open 832.19
　　eye 360.81
　　　lateral 376.36
　　eyeball 360.81
　　　lateral 376.36
　　femur
　　　distal end (closed) 836.50
　　　　anterior 836.52
　　　　　open 836.62

Dislocation—*continued*
　　　lateral 836.53
　　　　open 836.63
　　　medial 836.54
　　　　open 836.64
　　　open 836.60
　　　posterior 836.51
　　　　open 836.61
　　　proximal end (closed) 835.00
　　　　anterior (pubic) 835.03
　　　　　open 835.13
　　　　obturator 835.02
　　　　　open 835.12
　　　　open 835.10
　　　　posterior 835.01
　　　　　open 835.11
　　fibula
　　　distal end (closed) 837.0
　　　　open 837.1
　　　proximal end (closed) 836.59
　　　　open 836.69
　　finger(s) (phalanx) (thumb) (closed) 834.00
　　　interphalangeal (joint) 834.02
　　　　open 834.12
　　　metacarpal (bone), distal end 834.01
　　　　open 834.11
　　　metacarpophalangeal (joint) 834.01
　　　　open 834.11
　　　open 834.10
　　　recurrent 718.34
　　foot (closed) 838.00
　　　open 838.10
　　　recurrent 718.37
　　forearm (closed) 839.8
　　　open 839.9
　　fracture—*see* Fracture, by site
　　glenoid (closed) 831.09
　　　open 831.19
　　habitual—*see* Dislocation, recurrent
　　hand (closed) 839.8
　　　open 839.9
　　hip (closed) 835.00
　　　anterior 835.03
　　　　obturator 835.02
　　　　　open 835.12
　　　　open 835.13
　　　congenital (unilateral) 754.30
　　　　with subluxation of other hip 754.35
　　　　bilateral 754.31
　　　developmental 718.75
　　　open 835.10
　　　posterior 835.01
　　　　open 835.11
　　　recurrent 718.35
　　humerus (closed) 831.00
　　　distal end (*see also* Dislocation, elbow) 832.00
　　　open 831.10
　　　proximal end (closed) 831.00
　　　　anterior (subclavicular) (subcoracoid)
　　　　　(subglenoid) (closed) 831.01
　　　　　open 831.11
　　　　inferior (closed) 831.03
　　　　　open 831.13
　　　　open 831.10
　　　　posterior (closed) 831.02
　　　　　open 831.12
　　implant—*see* Complications, mechanical
　　incus 385.23
　　infracoracoid (closed) 831.01
　　　open 831.11

Dislocation—*continued*
    congenital 756.19
      multiple sites 839.08
        open 839.18
      open 839.10
    congenital 756.19
    dorsal 839.21
      open 839.31
      recurrent 724.9
    lumbar, lumbosacral 839.20
      open 839.30
    non-traumatic —*see* Displacement,
      intervertebral disc
    open NEC 839.50
    recurrent 724.9
    specified region NEC 839.49
      open 839.59
    thoracic 839.21
      open 839.31
  wrist (carpal bone) (scaphoid) (semilunar)
    (closed) 833.00
    carpometacarpal (joint) 833.04
      open 833.14
    metacarpal bone, proximal end 833.05
      open 833.15
    midcarpal (joint) 833.03
      open 833.13
    open 833.10
    radiocarpal (joint) 833.02
      open 833.12
    radioulnar (joint) 833.01
      open 833.11
    recurrent 718.33
    specified site NEC 833.09
      open 833.19
  xiphoid cartilage (closed) 839.61
    open 839.71

Dislodgement
  artificial skin graft 996.55
  decellularized allodermis graft 996.55

Disobedience, hostile (covert) (overt) (*see also*
  Disturbance, conduct) 312.0

Disorder —*see also* Disease
  academic underachievement, childhood and
    adolescence 313.83
  accommodation 367.51
    drug-induced 367.89
    toxic 367.89
  adjustment (*see also* Reaction, adjustment)
    309.9
    with
      anxiety 309.24
      anxiety and depressed mood 309.28
      depressed mood 309.0
      disturbance of conduct 309.3
      disturbance of emotions and conduct 309.4
  adrenal (capsule) (cortex) (gland) 255.9
    specified type NEC 255.8
  adrenogenital 255.2
  affective (*see also* Psychosis, affective) 296.90
    atypical 296.81
  aggressive, unsocialized (*see also* Disturbance,
    conduct) 312.0
  alcohol, alcoholic (*see also* Alcohol) 291.9
  allergic—*see* Allergy
  amino acid (metabolic) (*see also* Disturbance,
    metabolism, amino acid) 270.9
    albinism 270.2
    alkaptonuria 270.2
    argininosuccinicaciduria 270.6
    beta-amino-isobutyricaciduria 277.2

Disorder—*continued*
  cystathioninuria 270.4
  cystinosis 270.0
  cystinuria 270.0
  glycinuria 270.0
  homocystinuria 270.4
  imidazole 270.5
  maple syrup (urine) disease 270.3
  neonatal, transitory 775.89
  oasthouse urine disease 270.2
  ochronosis 270.2
  phenylketonuria 270.1
  phenylpyruvic oligophrenia 270.1
  purine NEC 277.2
  pyrimidine NEC 277.2
  renal transport NEC 270.0
  specified type NEC 270.8
  transport NEC 270.0
    renal 270.0
  xanthinuria 277.2
  amnestic (*see also* Amnestic syndrome) 294.08
    alcohol-induced persisting 291.1
    drug-induced persisting 292.83
    in conditions classified elsewhere 294.0
  anaerobic glycolysis with anemia 282.3
  anxiety (*see also* Anxiety) 300.00
    due to or associated with physical condition
      293.84
  arteriole 447.9
    specified type NEC 447.8
  artery 447.9
    specified type NEC 447.8
  articulation—*see* Disorder, joint
  Asperger's 299.8
  attachment of infancy or early childhood 313.89
  attention deficit 314.00
    with hyperactivity 314.01
    predominantly
      combined hyperactive/inattentive 314.01
      hyperactive/impulsive 314.01
      inattentive 314.00
    residual type 314.8
  autistic 299.0
  autoimmune NEC 279.4
    hemolytic (cold type) (warm type) 283.0
    parathyroid 252.1
    thyroid 245.2
  avoidant, childhood or adolescence 313.21
  balance
    acid-base 276.9
      mixed (with hypercapnia) 276.4
    electrolyte 276.9
    fluid 276.9
  behavior NEC (*see also* Disturbance, conduct)
    312.9
    disruptive 312.9
  bilirubin excretion 277.4
  bipolar (affective) (alternating) 296.80

---

*Note—Use the following fifth-digit
subclassification with categories 296.0-296.6:*

0	*unspecified*
1	*mild*
2	*moderate*
3	*severe, without mention of psychotic behavior*
4	*severe, specified as with psychotic behavior*
5	*in partial or unspecified remission*
6	*in full remission*

Disorder—*continued*
  atypical 296.7
  currently
    depressed 296.5
    hypomanic 296.4
    manic 296.4
  mixed 296.6
  specified type NEC 296.89
  type I 296.7
    most recent episode (or current)
      depressed 296.5
      hypomanic 296.4
      manic 296.4
      mixed 296.6
      unspecified 296.7
    single manic episode 296.0
  type II (recurrent major depressive episodes with hypomania) 296.89
  bladder 596.9
    functional NEC 596.59
    specified NEC 596.8
  bone NEC 733.90
    specified NEC 733.99
  brachial plexus 353.0
  branched-chain amino-acid degradation 270.3
  breast 611.9
    puerperal, postpartum 676.3
    specified NEC 611.8
  Briquet's 300.81
  bursa 727.9
    shoulder region 726.10
  carbohydrate metabolism, congenital 271.9
  cardiac, functional 427.9
    postoperative 997.1
    psychogenic 306.2
  cardiovascular, psychogenic 306.2
  cartilage NEC 733.90
    articular 718.00
      ankle 718.07
      elbow 718.02
      foot 718.07
      hand 718.04
      hip 718.05
      knee 717.9
      multiple sites 718.09
      pelvic region 718.05
      shoulder region 718.01
      specified
        site NEC 718.08
        type NEC 733.99
      wrist 718.03
  catatonic—*see* Catatonia
  central auditory processing 315.32
  cervical region NEC 723.9
  cervical root (nerve) NEC 353.2
  character NEC (*see also* Disorder, personality) 301.9
  coagulation (factor) (*see also* Defect, coagulation) 286.9
    factor VIII (congenital) (functional) 286.0
    factor IX (congenital) (functional) 286.1
    neonatal, transitory 776.3
  coccyx 724.70
    specified NEC 724.79
  cognitive 294.9
  colon 569.9
    functional 564.9
      congenital 751.3
  communication 307.9
  conduct (*see also* Disturbance, conduct) 312.9
    adjustment reaction 309.3

Disorder—*continued*
  adolescent onset type 312.82
  childhood onset type 312.81
  compulsive 312.30
    specified type NEC 312.39
  hyperkinetic 314.2
  onset unspecified 312.89
  socialized (type) 312.20
    aggressive 312.23
    unaggressive 312.21
  specified NEC 312.89
  conduction, heart 426.9
    specified NEC 426.89
  conflict
    sexual orientation 302.0
  congenital
    glycosylation (CDG) 271.8
  convulsive (secondary) (*see also* Convulsions) 780.39
    due to injury at birth 767.0
    idiopathic 780.39
  coordination 781.3
  cornea NEC 371.89
    due to contact lens 371.82
  corticosteroid metabolism NEC 255.2
  cranial nerve—*see* Disorder, nerve, cranial
  cyclothymic 301.13
  degradation, branched-chain amino acid 270.3
  delusional 297.1
  dentition 520.6
  depersonalization 300.6
  depressive NEC 311
    atypical 296.82
    major (*see also* Psychosis, affective) 296.2
      recurrent episode 296.3
      single episode 296.2
  development, specific 315.9
    associated with hyperkinesia 314.1
    coordination 315.4
    language 315.31
    learning 315.2
      arithmetical 315.1
      reading 315.00
    mixed 315.5
    motor coordination 315.4
    specified type NEC 315.8
    speech 315.39
  diaphragm 519.4
  digestive 536.9
    fetus or newborn 777.9
      specified NEC 777.8
    psychogenic 306.4
  disintegrative, childhood 299.1
  dissociative 300.15
    identity 300.14
    nocturnal 307.47
  drug-related 292.9
  dysmorphic body 300.7
  dysthymic 300.4
  ear 388.9
    degenerative NEC 388.00
    external 380.9
      specified 380.89
    pinna 380.30
    specified type NEC 388.8
    vascular NEC 388.00
  eating NEC 307.50
  electrolyte NEC 276.9
    with
      abortion—*see* Abortion, by type, with metabolic disorder

Disorder—*continued*
  lactation 676.9
  language (developmental) (expressive) 315.31
    mixed receptive-expressive 315.32
  learning 315.9
  ligament 728.9
  ligamentous attachments, peripheral—*see also*
    Enthesopathy
    spine 720.1
  limb NEC 729.9
    psychogenic 306.0
  lipid
    metabolism, congenital 272.9
    storage 272.7
  lipoprotein deficiency (familial) 272.5
  low back NEC 724.9
    psychogenic 306.0
  lumbosacral
    plexus 353.1
    root (nerve) NEC 353.4
  lymphoproliferative (chronic) NEC (M9970/1)
    238.79
  major depressive (*see also* Psychosis, affective)
    296.2
    recurrent episode 296.3
    single episode 296.2
  male erectile 607.84
    nonorganic origin 302.72
  manic (*see also* Psychosis, affective) 296.0
    atypical 296.81
  mathematics 315.1
  meniscus NEC (*see also* Disorder, cartilage,
    articular) 718.0
  menopausal 627.9
    specified NEC 627.8
  menstrual 626.9
    psychogenic 306.52
    specified NEC 626.8
  mental (nonpsychotic) 300.9
    affecting management of pregnancy,
      childbirth, or puerperium 648.4
    drug-induced 292.9
      hallucinogen persistent perception 292.89
      specified type NEC 292.89
    due to or associated with
      alcoholism 291.9
      drug consumption NEC 292.9
        specified type NEC 292.89
      physical condition NEC 293.9
    induced by drug 292.9
      specified type NEC 292.89
    neurotic (*see also* Neurosis) 300.9
    of infancy, childhood or adolescence 313.9
    persistent
      other
        due to conditions classified elsewhere
          294.8
      unspecified
        due to conditions classified elsewhere
          294.9
    presenile 310.1
      psychotic NEC 290.10
    previous, affecting management of pregnancy
      V23.8
    psychoneurotic (*see also* Neurosis) 300.9
    psychotic (*see also* Psychosis) 298.9
      brief 298.8
      senile 290.20
    specific, following organic brain damage
      310.9

Disorder—*continued*
    cognitive or personality change of other type
      310.1
    frontal lobe syndrome 310.0
    postconcussional syndrome 310.2
    specified type NEC 310.8
  transient
    in conditions classified elsewhere 293.9
  metabolism NEC 277.9
    with
      abortion—*see* Abortion, by type, with
        metabolic disorder
      ectopic pregnancy (*see also* categories
        633.0-633.9) 639.4
      molar pregnancy (*see also* categories
        630-632) 639.4
    alkaptonuria 270.2
    amino acid (*see also* Disorder, amino acid)
      270.9
      specified type NEC 270.8
    ammonia 270.6
    arginine 270.6
    argininosuccinic acid 270.6
    basal 794.7
    bilirubin 277.4
    calcium 275.40
    carbohydrate 271.9
      specified type NEC 271.8
    cholesterol 272.9
    citrulline 270.6
    copper 275.1
    corticosteroid 255.2
    cystine storage 270.0
    cystinuria 270.0
    fat 272.9
    fatty acid oxidation 277.85
    following
      abortion 639.4
      ectopic or molar pregnancy 639.4
    fructosemia 271.2
    fructosuria 271.2
    fucosidosis 271.8
    due to conditions classified elsewhere
      294.8galactose-1-phosphate uridyl
      transferase 271.1
    glutamine 270.7
    glycine 270.7
    glycogen storage NEC 271.0
      hepatorenal 271.0
    hemochromatosis 275.0
    in labor and delivery 669.0
    iron 275.0
    lactose 271.3
    lipid 272.9
      specified type NEC 272.8
      storage 272.7
    lipoprotein—*see also* Hyperlipemia deficiency
      (familial) 272.5
    lysine 270.7
    magnesium 275.2
    mannosidosis 271.8
    mineral 275.9
      specified type NEC 275.8
    mitochondrial 277.87
    mucopolysaccharide 277.5
    nitrogen 270.9
    ornithine 270.6
    oxalosis 271.8
    pentosuria 271.8
    phenylketonuria 270.1
    phosphate 275.3

Disorder—*continued*
   phosphorus 275.3
   plasma protein 273.9
     specified type NEC 273.8
   porphyrin 277.1
   purine 277.2
   pyrimidine 277.2
   serine 270.7
   sodium 276.9
   specified type NEC 277.89
   steroid 255.2
   threonine 270.7
   urea cycle 270.6
   xylose 271.8
  micturition NEC 788.69
   psychogenic 306.53
  misery and unhappiness, of childhood and
     adolescence 313.1
  mitochondrial metabolism 277.87
  mitral valve 424.0
  mood (*see also* Disorder, bipolar) 296.90
   episodic 296.90
     specified NEC 296.99
   in conditions classified elsewhere 293.83
  motor tic 307.20
   chronic 307.22
   transient (childhood) 307.21
  movement NEC 333.90
   hysterical 300.11
   medication-induced 333.90
   periodic limb 327.51
   sleep related, unspecified 780.58
     other organic 327.59
   specified type NEC 333.99
   stereotypic 307.3
  mucopolysaccharide 277.5
  muscle 728.9
   psychogenic 306.0
   specified type NEC 728.3
  muscular attachments, peripheral—*see also*
     Enthesopathy
   spine 720.1
  musculoskeletal system NEC 729.9
   psychogenic 306.0
  myeloproliferative (chronic) NEC (M9960/1)
     238.79
  myoneural 358.9
   due to lead 358.2
   specified type NEC 358.8
   toxic 358.2
  myotonic 359.2
  neck region NEC 723.9
  nerve 349.9
   abducens NEC 378.54
   accessory 352.4
   acoustic 388.5
   auditory 388.5
   auriculotemporal 350.8
   axillary 353.0
   cerebral—*see* Disorder, nerve, cranial
   cranial 352.9
     first 352.0
     second 377.49
     third
       partial 378.51
       total 378.52
     fourth 378.53
     fifth 350.9
     sixth 378.54
     seventh NEC 351.9
     eighth 388.5

Disorder—*continued*
     ninth 352.2
     tenth 352.3
     eleventh 352.4
     twelfth 352.5
     multiple 352.6
   entrapment—*see* Neuropathy, entrapment
   facial 351.9
     specified NEC 351.8
   femoral 355.2
   glossopharyngeal NEC 352.2
   hypoglossal 352.5
   iliohypogastric 355.79
   ilioinguinal 355.79
   intercostal 353.8
   lateral
     cutaneous of thigh 355.1
     popliteal 355.3
   lower limb NEC 355.8
   medial, popliteal 355.4
   median NEC 354.1
   obturator 355.79
   oculomotor
     partial 378.51
     total 378.52
   olfactory 352.0
   optic 377.49
     hypoplasia 377.43
     ischemic 377.41
     nutritional 377.33
     toxic 377.34
   peroneal 355.3
   phrenic 354.8
   plantar 355.6
   pneumogastric 352.3
   posterior tibial 355.5
   radial 354.3
   recurrent laryngeal 352.3
   root 353.9
     specified NEC 353.8
   saphenous 355.79
   sciatic NEC 355.0
   specified NEC 355.9
     lower limb 355.79
     upper limb 354.8
   spinal 355.9
   sympathetic NEC 337.9
   trigeminal 350.9
     specified NEC 350.8
   trochlear 378.53
   ulnar 354.2
   upper limb NEC 354.9
   vagus 352.3
  nervous system NEC 349.9
   autonomic (peripheral) (*see also* Neuropathy,
     peripheral, autonomic) 337.9
   cranial 352.9
   parasympathetic (*see also* Neuropathy,
     peripheral, autonomic) 337.9
   specified type NEC 349.89
   sympathetic (*see also* Neuropathy, peripheral,
     autonomic) 337.9
   vegetative (*see also* Neuropathy, peripheral,
     autonomic) 337.9
  neurohypophysis NEC 253.6
  neurological NEC 781.99
   peripheral NEC 355.9
  neuromuscular NEC 358.9
   hereditary NEC 359.1
   specified NEC 358.8
   toxic 358.2

Disorder—*continued*
    free running type 327.34
    in conditions classified elsewhere 327.37
    irregular sleep-wake type 327.33
    jet lag type 327.35
    other 327.39
    shift work type 327.36
  drug induced 292.85
  initiation or maintenance (*see also* Insomnia) 780.52
    nonorganic origin (transient) 307.41
      persistent 307.42
  nonorganic origin 307.40
    specified type NEC 307.49
  organic specified type NEC 327.8
  periodic limb movement 327.51
  specified NEC 780.59
  wake
    cycle—*see* Disorder, sleep, circadian rhythm
    schedule—*see* Disorder, sleep, circadian rhythm
    with apnea—*see* Apnea, sleep
social, of childhood and adolescence 313.22
soft tissue 729.9
somatization 300.81
somatoform (atypical) (undifferentiated) 300.82
  severe 300.81
  specified type NEC 300.89
speech NEC 784.5
  nonorganic origin 307.9
spine NEC 724.9
  ligamentous or muscular attachments, peripheral 720.1
steroid metabolism NEC 255.2
stomach (functional) (*see also* Disorder, gastric) 536.9
  psychogenic 306.4
storage, iron 275.0
stress (*see also* Reaction, stress, acute) 308.3
  posttraumatic
    acute 309.81
    brief 309.81
    chronic 309.81
substitution 300.11
suspected—*see* Observation
synovium 727.9
temperature regulation, fetus or newborn 778.4
temporomandibular joint NEC 524.60
  sounds on opening or closing 524.64
  specified NEC 524.69
tendon 727.9
  shoulder region 726.10
thoracic root (nerve) NEC 353.3
thyrocalcitonin secretion 246.0
thyroid (gland) NEC 246.9
  specified type NEC 246.8
tic 307.20
  chronic (motor or vocal) 307.22
  motor-verbal 307.23
  organic origin 333.1
  transient (of childhood) 307.21
tooth NEC 525.9
  development NEC 520.9
    specified type NEC 520.8
  eruption 520.6
  specified type NEC 525.8
Tourette's 307.23
transport, carbohydrate 271.9
  specified type NEC 271.8
tubular, phosphate-losing 588.0
tympanic membrane 384.9

Disorder—*continued*
unaggressive, unsocialized (*see also* Disturbance, conduct) 312.1
undersocialized, unsocialized—*see also* Disturbance, conduct
  aggressive (type) 312.0
  unaggressive (type) 312.1
vision, visual NEC 368.9
  binocular NEC 368.30
  cortex 377.73
    associated with
      inflammatory disorders 377.73
      neoplasms 377.71
      vascular disorders 377.72
  pathway NEC 377.63
    associated with
      inflammatory disorders 377.63
      neoplasms 377.61
      vascular disorders 377.62
vocal tic
  chronic 307.22
wakefulness (*see also* Hypersomnia) 780.54
  nonorganic origin (transient) 307.43
    persistent 307.44
written expression 315.2
Disorganized globe 360.29
Displacement, displaced

> *Note—For acquired displacement of bones, cartilage, joints, tendons, due to injury, see also Dislocation. Displacements at ages under one year should be considered congenital, provided there is no indication the condition was acquired after birth.*

acquired traumatic of bond, cartilage, joint, tendon NEC (without fracture) (*see also* Dislocation) 839.8
  with fracture—*see* Fracture, by site
adrenal gland (congenital) 759.1
alveolus and teeth, vertical 524.75
appendix, retrocecal (congenital) 751.5
auricle (congenital) 744.29
bladder (acquired) 596.8
  congenital 753.8
brachial plexus (congenital) 742.8
brain stem, caudal 742.4
canaliculus lacrimalis 743.65
cardia, through esophageal hiatus 750.6
cerebellum, caudal 742.4
cervix —*see* Displacement, uterus
colon (congenital) 751.4
device, implant, or graft—*see* Complications, mechanical
epithelium
  columnar of cervix 622.10
  cuboidal, beyond limits of external os (uterus) 752.49
esophageal mucosa into cardia of stomach, congenital 750.4
esophagus (acquired) 530.89
  congenital 750.4
eyeball (acquired) (old) 376.36
  congenital 743.8
  current injury 871.3
  lateral 376.36
fallopian tube (acquired) 620.4
  congenital 752.19
  opening (congenital) 752.19
gallbladder (congenital) 751.69

Displacement, displaced—*continued*
  gastric mucosa 750.7
    into
      duodenum 750.7
      esophagus 750.7
      Meckel's diverticulum, congenital 750.7
  globe (acquired) (lateral) (old) 376.36
    current injury 871.3
  graft
    artificial skin graft 996.55
    decellularized allodermis graft 996.55
  heart (congenital) 746.87
    acquired 429.89
  hymen (congenital) (upward) 752.49
  internal prosthesis NEC—*see* Complications,
    mechanical
  intervertebral disc (with neuritis, radiculitis,
    sciatica, or other pain) 722.2
    with myelopathy 722.70
    cervical, cervicodorsal, cervicothoracic 722.0
      with myelopathy 722.71
      due to major trauma—*see* Dislocation,
        vertebra, cervical
    due to trauma—*see* Dislocation, vertebra
    lumbar, lumbosacral 722.10
      with myelopathy 722.73
      due to major trauma—*see* Dislocation,
        vertebra, lumbar
    thoracic, thoracolumbar 722.11
      with myelopathy 722.72
      due to major trauma—*see* Dislocation,
        vertebra, thoracic
  intrauterine device 996.32
  kidney (acquired) 593.0
    congenital 753.3
  lacrimal apparatus or duct (congenital) 743.65
  macula (congenital) 743.55
  Meckel's diverticulum (congenital) 751.0
  nail (congenital) 757.5
    acquired 703.8
  opening of Wharton's duct in mouth 750.26
  organ or site, congenital NEC—*see* Malposition,
    congenital
  ovary (acquired) 620.4
    congenital 752.0
    free in peritoneal cavity (congenital) 752.0
    into hernial sac 620.4
  oviduct (acquired) 620.4
    congenital 752.19
  parathyroid (gland) 252.8
  parotid gland (congenital) 750.26
  punctum lacrimale (congenital) 743.65
  sacroiliac (congenital) (joint) 755.69
    current injury—*see* Dislocation, sacroiliac
    old 724.6
  spine (congenital) 756.19
  spleen, congenital 759.0
  stomach (congenital) 750.7
    acquired 537.89
  subglenoid (closed) 831.01
  sublingual duct (congenital) 750.26
  teeth, tooth 524.30
    horizontal 524.33
    vertical 524.34
  tongue (congenital) (downward) 750.19
  trachea (congenital) 748.3
  ureter or ureteric opening or orifice (congenital)
    753.4
  uterine opening of oviducts or fallopian tubes
    752.19

Displacement, displaced—*continued*
  uterus, uterine (*see also* Malposition, uterus)
    621.6
    congenital 752.3
  ventricular septum 746.89
    with rudimentary ventricle 746.89
  xyphoid bone (process) 738.3
Disproportion 653.9
  affecting fetus or newborn 763.1
  caused by
    conjoined twins 653.7
    contraction, pelvis (general) 653.1
      inlet 653.2
      midpelvic 653.8
      midplane 653.8
      outlet 653.3
    fetal
      ascites 653.7
      hydrocephalus 653.6
      hydrops 653.7
      meningomyelocele 653.7
      sacral teratoma 653.7
      tumor 653.7
    hydrocephalic fetus 653.6
    pelvis, pelvic, abnormality (bony) NEC 653.0
    unusually large fetus 653.5
  causing obstructed labor 660.1
  cephalopelvic, normally formed fetus 653.4
    causing obstructed labor 660.1
  fetal NEC 653.5
    causing obstructed labor 660.1
  fetopelvic, normally formed fetus 653.4
    causing obstructed labor 660.1
  mixed maternal and fetal origin, normally
    formed fetus 653.4
  pelvis, pelvic (bony) NEC 653.1
    causing obstructed labor 660.1
  specified type NEC 653.8
Disruption
  cesarean wound 674.1
  family V61.0
  gastrointestinal anastomosis 997.4
  ligament(s)—*see also* Sprain
    knee
      current injury—*see* Dislocation, knee
      old 717.89
        capsular 717.85
        collateral (medial) 717.82
          lateral 717.81
        cruciate (posterior) 717.84
          anterior 717.83
        specified site NEC 717.85
  marital V61.10
    involving divorce or estrangement V61.0
  operation wound (external) 998.32
    internal 998.31
  organ transplant, anastomosis site—*see*
    Complications, transplant, organ, by site
  ossicles, ossicular chain 385.23
    traumatic—*see* Fracture, skull, base
  parenchyma
    liver (hepatic)—*see* Laceration, liver, major
    spleen—*see* Laceration, spleen, parenchyma,
      massive
  phase-shift, of 24 hour sleep wake cycle,
    unspecified 780.55
    nonorganic origin 307.45
  sleep wake cycle (24 hour), unspecified 780.55
    circadian rhythm 327.33
    nonorganic origin 307.45

Distortion—*continued*
  glottis 748.3
  gyri 742.4
  hand bone(s) 755.59
  heart (auricle) (ventricle) 746.89
    valve (cusp) 746.89
  hepatic duct 751.69
  humerus 755.59
  hymen 752.49
  ileum 751.5
  intestine (large) (small) 751.5
    with anomalous adhesions, fixation or
        malrotation 751.4
  jaw NEC 524.89
  jejunum 751.5
  kidney 753.3
  knee (joint) 755.64
  labium (majus) (minus) 752.49
  larynx 748.3
  leg 755.69
  lens 743.36
  liver 751.69
  lumbar spine 756.19
    with disproportion (fetopelvic) 653.0
      affecting fetus or newborn 763.1
      causing obstructed labor 660.1
  lumbosacral (joint) (region) 756.19
  lung (fissures) (lobe) 748.69
  nerve 742.8
  nose 748.1
  organ
    of Corti 744.05
    or site not listed—*see* Anomaly, specified type
        NEC
  ossicles, ear 744.04
  ovary 752.0
  oviduct 752.19
  pancreas 751.7
  parathyroid (gland) 759.2
  patella 755.64
  peripheral vascular system NEC 747.60
    gastrointestinal 747.61
    lower limb 747.64
    renal 747.62
    spinal 747.82
    upper limb 747.63
  pituitary (gland) 759.2
  radius 755.59
  rectum 751.5
  rib 756.3
  sacroiliac joint 755.69
  sacrum 756.19
  scapula 755.59
  shoulder girdle 755.59
  site not listed—*see* Anomaly, specified type
      NEC
  skull bone(s) 756.0
    with
      anencephalus 740.0
      encephalocele 742.0
      hydrocephalus 742.3
        with spina bifida (*see also* Spina bifida)
            741.0
      microcephalus 742.1
  spinal cord 742.59
  spine 756.19
  spleen 759.0
  sternum 756.3
  thorax (wall) 756.3
  thymus (gland) 759.2

Distortion—*continued*
  thyroid (gland) 759.2
    cartilage 748.3
  tibia 755.69
  toe(s) 755.66
  tongue 750.19
  trachea (cartilage) 748.3
  ulna 755.59
  ureter 753.4
    causing obstruction 753.20
  urethra 753.8
    causing obstruction 753.6
  uterus 752.3
  vagina 752.49
  vein (peripheral) NEC (*see also* Distortion,
      peripheral vascular system) 747.60
    great 747.49
    portal 747.49
    pulmonary 747.49
  vena cava (inferior) (superior) 747.49
  vertebra 756.19
  visual NEC 368.15
    shape or size 368.14
  vulva 752.49
  wrist (bones) (joint) 755.59
Distress
  abdomen 789.0
  colon 789.0
  emotional V40.9
  epigastric 789.0
  fetal (syndrome) 768.4
    affecting management of pregnancy or
        childbirth 656.8
    liveborn infant 768.4
      first noted
        before onset of labor 768.2
        during labor and delivery 768.3
      stillborn infant (death before onset of labor)
          768.0
        death during labor 768.1
  gastrointestinal (functional) 536.9
    psychogenic 306.4
  intestinal (functional) NEC 564.9
    psychogenic 306.4
  intrauterine (*see* Distress, fetal)
  leg 729.5
  maternal 669.0
  mental V40.9
  respiratory 786.09
    acute (adult) 518.82
    adult syndrome (following shock, surgery, or
        trauma) 518.5
      specified NEC 518.82
    fetus or newborn 770.89
    syndrome (idiopathic) (newborn) 769
  stomach 536.9
    psychogenic 306.4
Distribution vessel, atypical NEC 747.60
  coronary artery 746.85
  spinal 747.82
Districhiasis 704.2
Disturbance —*see also* Disease
  absorption NEC 579.9
    calcium 269.3
    carbohydrate 579.8
    fat 579.8
    protein 579.8
    specified type NEC 579.8
    vitamin (*see also* Deficiency, vitamin) 269.2
  acid-base equilibrium 276.9

Disturbance—*continued*
  activity and attention, simple, with hyperkinesis
      314.01
  amino acid (metabolic) (*see also* Disorder,
      amino acid) 270.9
    imidazole 270.5
    maple syrup (urine) disease 270.3
    transport 270.0
  assimilation, food 579.9
  attention, simple 314.00
    with hyperactivity 314.01
  auditory, nerve, except deafness 388.5
  behavior (*see also* Disturbance, conduct) 312.9
  blood clotting (hypoproteinemia) (mechanism)
      (*see also* Defect, coagulation) 286.9
  central nervous system NEC 349.9
  cerebral nerve NEC 352.9
  circulatory 459.9
  conduct 312.9

---

*Note—Use the following fifth-digit
subclassification with categories 312.0-312.2:*

0 *unspecified*
1 *mild*
2 *moderate*
3 *severe*

---

    adjustment reaction 309.3
    adolescent onset type 312.82
    childhood onset type 312.81
    compulsive 312.30
      intermittent explosive disorder 312.34
      isolated explosive disorder 312.35
      kleptomania 312.32
      pathological gambling 312.31
      pyromania 312.33
    hyperkinetic 314.2
    intermittent explosive 312.34
    isolated explosive 312.35
    memory (*see also* Amnesia) 780.99
    mixed with emotions 312.4
    socialized (type) 312.20
      aggressive 312.23
      unaggressive 312.21
    specified type NEC 312.89
    undersocialized, unsocialized
      aggressive (type) 312.0
      unaggressive (type) 312.1
  coordination 781.3
  cranial nerve NEC 352.9
  deep sensibility—*see* Disturbance, sensation
  digestive 536.9
    psychogenic 306.4
  electrolyte—*see* Imbalance, electrolyte
  emotions specific to childhood or adolescence
      313.9
    with
      academic underachievement 313.83
      anxiety and fearfulness 313.0
      elective mutism 313.23
      identity disorder 313.82
      jealousy 313.3
      misery and unhappiness 313.1
      oppositional defiant disorder 313.81
      overanxiousness 313.0
      sensitivity 313.21
      shyness 313.21
      social withdrawal 313.22
      withdrawal reaction 313.22
    involving relationship problems 313.3
    mixed 313.89

Disturbance—*continued*
  specified type NEC 313.89
  endocrine (gland) 259.9
    neonatal, transitory 775.9
      specified NEC 775.89
  equilibrium 780.4
  feeding (elderly) (infant) 783.3
    newborn 779.3
    nonorganic origin NEC 307.59
    psychogenic NEC 307.59
  fructose metabolism 271.2
  gait 781.2
    hysterical 300.11
  gastric (functional) 536.9
    motility 536.8
    psychogenic 306.4
    secretion 536.8
  gastrointestinal (functional) 536.9
    psychogenic 306.4
  habit, child 307.9
  hearing, except deafness 388.40
  heart, functional (conditions classifiable to 426,
      427, 428)
    due to presence of (cardiac) prosthesis 429.4
    postoperative (immediate) 997.1
      long-term effect of cardiac surgery 429.4
    psychogenic 306.2
  hormone 259.9
  innervation uterus, sympathetic,
      parasympathetic 621.8
  keratinization NEC
    gingiva 523.10
    lip 528.5
    oral (mucosa) (soft tissue) 528.79
      residual ridge mucosa
        excessive 528.72
        minimal 528.71
    tongue 528.79
  labyrinth, labyrinthine (vestibule) 386.9
  learning, specific NEC 315.2
  memory (*see also* Amnesia) 780.93
    mild, following organic brain damage 310.8
  mental (*see also* Disorder, mental) 300.9
    associated with diseases classified elsewhere
        316
  metabolism (acquired) (congenital) (*see also*
      Disorder, metabolism) 277.9
    with
      abortion—*see* Abortion, by type, with
          metabolic disorder
      ectopic pregnancy (*see also* categories
          633.0-633.9) 639.4
      molar pregnancy (*see also* categories
          630-632) 639.4
    amino acid (*see also* Disorder, amino acid)
        270.9
      aromatic NEC 270.2
      branched-chain 270.3
      specified type NEC 270.8
      straight-chain NEC 270.7
      sulfur-bearing 270.4
      transport 270.0
    ammonia 270.6
    arginine 270.6
    argininosuccinic acid 270.6
    carbohydrate NEC 271.9
    cholesterol 272.9
    citrulline 270.6
    cystathionine 270.4
    fat 272.9

Division—*continued*
  ligament (partial or complete) (current)—*see also* Sprain, by site
    with open wound—*see* Wound, open, by site
  muscle (partial or complete) (current)—*see also* Sprain, by site
    with open wound—*see* Wound, open, by site
  nerve—*see* Injury, nerve, by site
  penis glans 752.69
  spinal cord—*see* Injury, spinal, by site
  vein 459.9
    traumatic—*see* Injury, vascular, by site
Divorce V61.0
Dix-Hallpike neurolabyrinthitis 386.12
Dizziness 780.4
  hysterical 300.11
  psychogenic 306.9
Doan-Wiseman syndrome (primary splenic neutropenia) 289.53
Dog bite —*see* Wound, open, by site
Döhle-Heller aortitis 093.1
Döhle body-panmyelopathic syndrome 288.2
Dolichocephaly, dolichocephalus 754.0
Dolichocolon 751.5
Dolichostenomelia 759.82
Donohue's syndrome (leprechaunism) 259.8
Donor
  blood V59.01
    other blood components V59.09
    stem cells V59.02
    whole blood V59.01
  bone V59.2
    marrow V59.3
  cornea V59.5
  egg (oocyte) (ovum) V59.70
    age 35 and over V59.73
      anonymous recipient V59.73
      designated recipient V59.74
    under age 35 V59.71
      anonymous recipient V59.71
      designated recipient V59.72
  heart V59.8
  kidney V59.4
  liver V59.6
  lung V59.8
  lymphocyte V59.8
  organ V59.9
    specified NEC V59.8
  potential, examination of V70.8
  skin V59.1
  specified organ or tissue NEC V59.8
  sperm V59.8
  stem cells V59.02
  tissue V59.9
    specified type NEC V59.8
Donovanosis (granuloma venereum) 099.2
DOPS (diffuse obstructive pulmonary syndrome) 496
Double
  albumin 273.8
  aortic arch 747.21
  auditory canal 744.29
  auricle (heart) 746.82
  bladder 753.8
  external (cervical) os 752.49
  kidney with double pelvis (renal) 753.3
  larynx 748.3
  meatus urinarius 753.8
  organ or site NEC—*see* Accessory
  orifice
    heart valve NEC 746.89

Double—*continued*
    pulmonary 746.09
  outlet, right ventricle 745.11
  pelvis (renal) with double ureter 753.4
  penis 752.69
  tongue 750.13
  ureter (one or both sides) 753.4
    with double pelvis (renal) 753.4
  urethra 753.8
  urinary meatus 753.8
  uterus (any degree) 752.2
    with doubling of cervix and vagina 752.2
    in pregnancy or childbirth 654.0
      affecting fetus or newborn 763.89
  vagina 752.49
    with doubling of cervix and uterus 752.2
  vision 368.2
  vocal cords 748.3
  vulva 752.49
  whammy (syndrome) 360.81
Douglas' pouch, cul-de-sac —*see* condition
Down's disease or syndrome (mongolism) 758.0
Down-growth, epithelial (anterior chamber) 364.61
Dracontiasis 125.7
Dracunculiasis 125.7
Dracunculosis 125.7
Drainage
  abscess (spontaneous)—*see* Abscess
  anomalous pulmonary veins to hepatic veins or right atrium 747.41
  stump (amputation) (surgical) 997.62
  suprapubic, bladder 596.8
Dream state, hysterical 300.13
Drepanocytic anemia (*see also* Disease, sickle cell) 282.60
Dresbach's syndrome (elliptocytosis) 282.1
Dreschlera (infection) 118
  hawaiiensis 117.8
Dressler's syndrome (postmyocardial infarction) 411.0
Dribbling (post-void) 788.35
Drift, ulnar 736.09
Drinking (alcohol)—*see also* Alcoholism
  excessive, to excess NEC (*see also* Abuse, drugs, nondependent) 305.0
    bouts, periodic 305.0
    continual 303.9
    episodic 305.0
    habitual 303.9
    periodic 305.0
Drip, postnasal (chronic) 784.91
  due to
    allergic rhinitis —*see* Rhinitis, allergic
    common cold 460
    gastroesophageal reflux —*see* Reflux, gastroesophageal
    nasopharyngitis —*see* Nasopharyngitis
    other known condition —*code to condition*
    sinusitis —*see* Sinusitis
Drivers' license examination V70.3
Droop
  Cooper's 611.8
  facial 781.94
Drop
  finger 736.29
  foot 736.79
  hematocrit (precipitous) 790.01
  toe 735.8
  wrist 736.05

Dropped
  dead 798.1
  heart beats 426.6
Dropsy, dropsical (*see also* Edema) 782.3
  abdomen 789.5
  amnion (*see also* Hydramnios) 657
  brain—*see* Hydrocephalus
  cardiac (*see also* Failure, heart) 428.0
  cardiorenal (*see also* Hypertension, cardiorenal) 404.90
  chest 511.9
  fetus or newborn 778.0
    due to isoimmunization 773.3
  gangrenous (*see also* Gangrene) 785.4
  heart (*see also* Failure, heart) 428.0
  hepatic—*see* Cirrhosis, liver
  infantile—*see* Hydrops, fetalis
  kidney (*see also* Nephrosis) 581.9
  liver—*see* Cirrhosis, liver
  lung 514
  malarial (*see also* Malaria) 084.9
  neonatorum—*see* Hydrops, fetalis
  nephritic 581.9
  newborn—*see* Hydrops, fetalis
  nutritional 269.9
  ovary 620.8
  pericardium (*see also* Pericarditis) 423.9
  renal (*see also* Nephrosis) 581.9
  uremic—*see* Uremia
Drowned, drowning 994.1
  lung 518.5
Drowsiness 780.09
Drug —*see also* condition
  addiction (*see also* listing under Dependence) 304.9
  adverse effect NEC, correct substance properly administered 995.20
  allergy 995.27
  dependence (*see also* listing under Dependence) 304.9
  habit (*see also* listing under Dependence) 304.9
  hypersensitivity 995.27
  induced
    circadian rhythm sleep disorder 292.85
    hypersomnia 292.85
    insomnia 292.85
    mental disorder 292.9
      anxiety 292.89
      mood 292.84
      sexual 292.89
      sleep 292.85
      specified type 292.89
    parasomnia 292.85
    persisting
      amnestic disorder 292.83
      dementia 292.82
    psychotic disorder
      with
        delusions 292.11
        hallucinations 292.12
    sleep disorder 292.85
  intoxication 292.89
  overdose—*see* Table of drugs and chemicals
  poisoning—*see* Table of drugs and chemicals
  therapy (maintenance) status NEC
    chemotherapy, antineoplastic V58.11
    immunotherapy, antineoplastic V58.12
    long-term (current) use V58.69
      antibiotics V58.62
      anticoagulants V58.61

Drug—*continued*
    anti-inflammatories, non-steroidal (NSAID) V58.64
    antiplatelets V58.63
    antithrombotics V58.63
    aspirin V58.66
    insulin V58.67
    steroids V58.65
  wrong substance given or taken in error—*see* Table of drugs and chemicals
Drunkenness (*see also* Abuse, drugs, nondependent) 305.0
  acute in alcoholism (*see also* Alcoholism) 303.0
  chronic (*see also* Alcoholism) 303.9
  pathologic 291.4
  simple (acute) 305.0
    in alcoholism 303.0
  sleep 307.47
Drusen
  optic disc or papilla 377.21
  retina (colloid) (hyaloid degeneration) 362.57
    hereditary 362.77
Drusenfieber 075
Dry, dryness —*see also* condition
  eye 375.15
    syndrome 375.15
  larynx 478.79
  mouth 527.7
  nose 478.19
  skin syndrome 701.1
  socket (teeth) 526.5
  throat 478.29
DSAP (disseminated superficial actinic porokeratosis) 692.75
Duane's retraction syndrome 378.71
Duane-Stilling-Turk syndrome (ocular retraction syndrome) 378.71
Dubin-Johnson disease or syndrome 277.4
Dubini's disease (electric chorea) 049.8
Dubois' abscess or disease 090.5
Duchenne's
  disease 094.0
    locomotor ataxia 094.0
    muscular dystrophy 359.1
    pseudohypertrophy, muscles 359.1
  paralysis 335.22
  syndrome 335.22
Duchenne-Aran myelopathic muscular atrophy (nonprogressive) (progressive) 335.21
Duchenne-Griesinger disease 359.1
Ducrey's
  bacillus 099.0
  chancre 099.0
  disease (chancroid) 099.0
Duct, ductus —*see* condition
Duengero 061
Duhring's disease (dermatitis herpetiformis) 694.0
Dukes (-Filatov) disease 057.8
Dullness
  cardiac (decreased) (increased) 785.3
Dumb ague (*see also* Malaria) 084.6
Dumbness (*see also* Aphasia) 784.3
Dumdum fever 085.0
Dumping syndrome (postgastrectomy) 564.2
  nonsurgical 536.8
Duodenitis (nonspecific) (peptic) 535.60
  due to
    Strongyloides stercoralis 127.2
  with hemorrhage 535.61
Duodenocholangitis 575.8
Duodenum, duodenal —*see* condition

Duplay's disease, periarthritis, or syndrome 726.2

Duplex —*see also* Accessory
kidney 753.3
placenta—*see* Placenta, abnormal
uterus 752.2

Duplication —*see also* Accessory
anus 751.5
aortic arch 747.21
appendix 751.5
biliary duct (any) 751.69
bladder 753.8
cecum 751.5
  and appendix 751.5
clitoris 752.49
cystic duct 751.69
digestive organs 751.8
duodenum 751.5
esophagus 750.4
fallopian tube 752.19
frontonasal process 756.0
gallbladder 751.69
ileum 751.5
intestine (large) (small) 751.5
jejunum 751.5
kidney 753.3
liver 751.69
nose 748.1
pancreas 751.7
penis 752.69
respiratory organs NEC 748.9
salivary duct 750.22
spinal cord (incomplete) 742.51
stomach 750.7
ureter 753.4
vagina 752.49
vas deferens 752.89
vocal cords 748.3

Dupré's disease or syndrome (meningism) 781.6

Dupuytren's
contraction 728.6
disease (muscle contracture) 728.6
fracture (closed) 824.4
  ankle (closed) 824.4
    open 824.5
  fibula (closed) 824.4
    open 824.5
  open 824.5
  radius (closed) 813.42
    open 813.52
muscle contracture 728.6

Durand-Nicolas-Favre disease (climatic bubo) 099.1

Duroziez's disease (congenital mitral stenosis) 746.5

Dust
conjunctivitis 372.05
reticulation (occupational) 504

Dutton's
disease (trypanosomiasis) 086.9
relapsing fever (West African) 087.1

Dwarf, dwarfism 259.4
with infantilism (hypophyseal) 253.3
achondroplastic 756.4
Amsterdam 759.89
bird-headed 759.89
congenital 259.4
constitutional 259.4
hypophyseal 253.3
infantile 259.4
Levi type 253.3

Dwarf, dwarfism—*continued*
Lorain-Levi (pituitary) 253.3
Lorain type (pituitary) 253.3
metatropic 756.4
nephrotic-glycosuric, with hypophosphatemic rickets 270.0
nutritional 263.2
ovarian 758.6
pancreatic 577.8
pituitary 253.3
polydystrophic 277.5
primordial 253.3
psychosocial 259.4
renal 588.0
  with hypertension—*see* Hypertension, kidney
Russell's (uterine dwarfism and craniofacial dysostosis) 759.89

Dyke-Young anemia or syndrome (acquired macrocytic hemolytic anemia) (secondary) (symptomatic) 283.9

Dynia abnormality (*see also* Defect, coagulation) 286.9

Dysacousis 388.40

Dysadrenocortism 255.9
hyperfunction 255.3
hypofunction 255.4

Dysarthria 784.5

Dysautonomia (*see also* Neuropathy, peripheral, autonomic) 337.9
familial 742.8

Dysbarism 993.3

Dysbasia 719.7
angiosclerotica intermittens 443.9
  due to atherosclerosis 440.21
hysterical 300.11
lordotica (progressiva) 333.6
nonorganic origin 307.9
psychogenic 307.9

Dysbetalipoproteinemia (familial) 272.2

Dyscalculia 315.1

Dyschezia (*see also* Constipation) 564.00

Dyschondroplasia (with hemangiomata) 756.4
Voorhoeve's 756.4

Dyschondrosteosis 756.59

Dyschromia 709.00

Dyscollagenosis 710.9

Dyscoria 743.41

Dyscraniopyophalangy 759.89

Dyscrasia
blood 289.9
  with antepartum hemorrhage 641.3
  fetus or newborn NEC 776.9
  hemorrhage, subungual 287.8
  puerperal, postpartum 666.3
ovary 256.8
plasma cell 273.9
pluriglandular 258.9
polyglandular 258.9

Dysdiadochokinesia 781.3

Dysectasia, vesical neck 596.8

Dysendocrinism 259.9

Dysentery, dysenteric (bilious) (catarrhal) (diarrhea) (epidemic) (gangrenous) (hemorrhagic) (infectious) (sporadic) (tropical) (ulcerative) 009.0
abscess, liver (*see also* Abscess, amebic) 006.3
amebic (*see also* Amebiasis) 006.9
  with abscess—*see* Abscess, amebic
  acute 006.0
  carrier (suspected) of V02.2

Dysentery, dysenteric—*continued*
  chronic 006.1
  arthritis (*see also* Arthritis, due to, dysentery)
    009.0 *[711.3]*
    bacillary 004.9 *[711.3]*
  asylum 004.9
  bacillary 004.9
    arthritis 004.9 *[711.3]*
    Boyd 004.2
    Flexner 004.1
    Schmitz (-Stutzer) 004.0
    Shiga 004.0
    Shigella 004.9
      group A 004.0
      group B 004.1
      group C 004.2
      group D 004.3
      specified type NEC 004.8
    Sonne 004.3
    specified type NEC 004.8
  bacterium 004.9
  balantidial 007.0
  Balantidium coli 007.0
  Boyd's 004.2
  Chilomastix 007.8
  Chinese 004.9
  choleriform 001.1
  coccidial 007.2
  Dientamoeba fragilis 007.8
  due to specified organism NEC—*see* Enteritis,
    due to, by organism
  Embadomonas 007.8
  Endolimax nana—*see* Dysentery, amebic
  Entamoba, entamebic—*see* Dysentery, amebic
  Flexner's 004.1
  Flexner-Boyd 004.2
  giardial 007.1
  Giardia lamblia 007.1
  Hiss-Russell 004.1
  lamblia 007.1
  leishmanial 085.0
  malarial (*see also* Malaria) 084.6
  metazoal 127.9
  Monilia 112.89
  protozoal NEC 007.9
  Russell's 004.8
  salmonella 003.0
  schistosomal 120.1
  Schmitz (-Stutzer) 004.0
  Shiga 004.0
  Shigella NEC (*see also* Dysentery, bacillary)
    004.9
    boydii 004.2
    dysenteriae 004.0
      Schmitz 004.0
      Shiga 004.0
    flexneri 004.1
    Group A 004.0
    Group B 004.1
    Group C 004.2
    Group D 004.3
    Schmitz 004.0
    Shiga 004.0
    Sonnei 004.3
  Sonne 004.3
  strongyloidiasis 127.2
  trichomonal 007.3
  tuberculous (*see also* Tuberculosis) 014.8
  viral (*see also* Enteritis, viral) 008.8
Dysequilibrium 780.4
Dysesthesia 782.0
  hysterical 300.11

Dysfibrinogenemia (congenital) (*see also* Defect,
  coagulation) 286.3
Dysfunction
  adrenal (cortical) 255.9
    hyperfunction 255.3
    hypofunction 255.4
  associated with sleep stages or arousal from
    sleep 780.56
    nonorganic origin 307.47
  bladder NEC 596.59
  bleeding, uterus 626.8
  brain, minimal (*see also* Hyperkinesia) 314.9
  cerebral 348.30
  colon 564.9
    psychogenic 306.4
  colostomy or enterostomy 569.62
  cystic duct 575.8
  diastolic 429.9
    with heart failure—*see* Failure, heart
    due to
      cardiomyopathy—*see* Cardiomyopathy
      hypertension—*see* Hypertension, heart
  endocrine NEC 259.9
  endometrium 621.8
  enteric stoma 569.62
  enterostomy 569.62
  erectile 607.84
    nonorganic origin 302.72
  esophagostomy 530.87
  Eustachian tube 381.81
  gallbladder 575.8
  gastrointestinal 536.9
  gland, glandular NEC 259.9
  heart 427.9
    postoperative (immediate) 997.1
      long-term effect of cardiac surgery 429.4
  hemoglobin 289.89
  hepatic 573.9
  hepatocellular NEC 573.9
  hypophysis 253.9
    hyperfunction 253.1
    hypofunction 253.2
    posterior lobe 253.6
      hypofunction 253.5
  kidney (*see also* Disease, renal) 593.9
  labyrinthine 386.50
    specified NEC 386.58
  liver 573.9
    constitutional 277.4
  minimal brain (child) (*see also* Hyperkinesia)
    314.9
  ovary, ovarian 256.9
    hyperfunction 256.1
      estrogen 256.0
    hypofunction 256.39
      postablative 256.2
    postablative 256.2
    specified NEC 256.8
  papillary muscle 429.81
    with myocardial infarction 410.8
  parathyroid 252.8
    hyperfunction 252.00
    hypofunction 252.1
  pineal gland 259.8
  pituitary (gland) 253.9
    hyperfunction 253.1
    hypofunction 253.2
    posterior 253.6
      hypofunction 253.5
  placental—*see* Placenta, insufficiency
  platelets (blood) 287.1

Dysfunction—*continued*
  polyglandular 258.9
    specified NEC 258.8
  psychosexual 302.70
    with
      dyspareunia (functional) (psychogenic)
          302.76
      frigidity 302.72
      impotence 302.72
      inhibition
        orgasm
          female 302.73
          male 302.74
        sexual
          desire 302.71
          excitement 302.72
      premature ejaculation 302.75
      sexual aversion 302.79
      specified disorder NEC 302.79
      vaginismus 306.51
  pylorus 537.9
  rectum 564.9
    psychogenic 306.4
  segmental (*see also* Dysfunction, somatic) 739.9
  senile 797
  sexual 302.70
  sinoatrial node 427.81
  somatic 739.9
    abdomen 739.9
    acromioclavicular 739.7
    cervical 739.1
    cervicothoracic 739.1
    costochondral 739.8
    costovertebral 739.8
    extremities
      lower 739.6
      upper 739.7
    head 739.0
    hip 739.5
    umbar, lumbosacral 739.3
    occipitocervical 739.0
    pelvic 739.5
    pubic 739.5
    rib cage 739.8
    sacral 739.4
    sacrococcygeal 739.4
    sacroiliac 739.4
    specified site NEC 739.9
    sternochondral 739.8
    sternoclavicular 739.7
    temporomandibular 739.0
    thoracic, thoracolumbar 739.2
  stomach 536.9
    psychogenic 306.4
  suprarenal 255.9
    hyperfunction 255.3
    hypofunction 255.4
  symbolic NEC 784.60
    specified type NEC 784.69
  systolic 429.9
    with heart failure—*see* Failure, heart
  temporomandibular (joint)
      (joint-pain-syndrome) NEC 524.60
    sounds on opening or closing 524.64
    specified NEC 524.69
  testicular 257.9
    hyperfunction 257.0
    hypofunction 257.2
    specified type NEC 257.8
  thymus 254.9
  thyroid 246.9

Dysfunction—*continued*
  complicating pregnancy, childbirth, or
      puerperium 648.1
    hyperfunction—*see* Hyperthyroidism
    hypofunction—*see* Hypothyroidism
  uterus, complicating delivery 661.9
    affecting fetus or newborn 763.7
    hypertonic 661.4
    hypotonic 661.2
      primary 661.0
      secondary 661.1
  velopharyngeal (acquired) 528.9
    congenital 750.29
  ventricular 429.9
    with congestive heart failure (*see also* Failure,
        heart) 428.0
    due to
      cardiomyopathy—*see* Cardiomyopathy
      hypertension—*see* Hypertension, heart
    left, reversible following sudden emotional
        stress 429.83
  vesicourethral NEC 596.59
  vestibular 386.50
    specified type NEC 386.58
Dysgammaglobulinemia 279.06
Dysgenesis
  gonadal (due to chromosomal anomaly) 758.6
    pure 752.7
  kidney(s) 753.0
  ovarian 758.6
  renal 753.0
  reticular 279.2
  seminiferous tubules 758.6
  tidal platelet 287.31
Dysgerminoma (M9060/3)
  specified site—*see* Neoplasm, by site, malignant
  unspecified site
    female 183.0
    male 186.9
Dysgeusia 781.1
Dysgraphia 781.3
Dyshidrosis 705.81
Dysidrosis 705.81
Dysinsulinism 251.8
Dyskaryotic cervical smear 795.09
Dyskeratosis (*see also* Keratosis) 701.1
  bullosa hereditaria 757.39
  cervix 622.10
  congenital 757.39
  follicularis 757.39
    vitamin A deficiency 264.8
  gingiva 523.8
  oral soft tissue NEC 528.79
  tongue 528.79
  uterus NEC 621.8
Dyskinesia 781.3
  biliary 575.8
  esophagus 530.5
  hysterical 300.11
  intestinal 564.89
  neuroleptic-induced tardive 333.85
  nonorganic origin 307.9
  orofacial 333.82
    due to drugs 333.85
  psychogenic 307.9
  subacute, due to drugs 333.85
  tardive (oral) 333.85
Dyslalia 784.5
  developmental 315.39
Dyslexia 784.61
  developmental 315.02
  secondary to organic lesion 784.61

Dysplasia—*continued*
  neuroectodermal 759.6
  oculoauriculovertebral 756.0
  oculodentodigital 759.89
  olfactogenital 253.4
  osteo-onycho-arthro (hereditary) 756.89
  periosteum 733.99
  polyostotic fibrous 756.54
  progressive diaphyseal 756.59
  prostate 602.3
    intraepithelial neoplasia I [PIN I] 602.3
    intraepithelial neoplasia II [PIN II] 602.3
    intraepithelial neoplasia III [PIN III] 233.4
  renal 753.15
  renofacialis 753.0
  retinal NEC 743.56
  retrolental 362.21
  spinal cord 742.9
  thymic, with immunodeficiency 279.2
  vagina 623.0
  vocal cord 478.5
  vulva 624.8
    intraepithelial neoplasia I [VIN I] 624.0
    intraepithelial neoplasia II [VIN II] 624.0
    intraepithelial neoplasia III [VIN III] 233.3
    VIN I 624.0
    VIN II 624.0
    VIN III 233.3
Dyspnea (nocturnal) (paroxysmal) 786.09
  asthmatic (bronchial) (*see also* Asthma) 493.9
    with bronchitis (*see also* Asthma) 493.9
      chronic 493.2
    cardiac (*see also* Failure, ventricular, left) 428.1
  cardiac (*see also* Failure, ventricular, left) 428.1
  functional 300.11
  hyperventilation 786.01
  hysterical 300.11
  Monday morning 504
  newborn 770.89
  psychogenic 306.1
  uremic—*see* Uremia
Dyspraxia 781.3
  syndrome 315.4
Dysproteinemia 273.8
  transient with copper deficiency 281.4
Dysprothrombinemia (constitutional) (*see also*
    Defect, coagulation) 286.3
Dysreflexia, autonomic 337.3
Dysrhythmia
  cardiac 427.9
    postoperative (immediate) 997.1
      long-term effect of cardiac surgery 429.4
    specified type NEC 427.89
  cerebral or cortical 348.30
Dyssecretosis, mucoserous 710.2
**Dyssocial reaction without manifest psychiatric
    disorder**
  adolescent V71.02
  adult V71.01
  child V71.02
Dyssomnia NEC 780.56
  nonorganic origin 307.47
Dyssplenism 289.4
Dyssynergia
  biliary (*see also* Disease, biliary) 576.8
  cerebellaris myoclonica 334.2
  detrusor sphincter (bladder) 596.55
  ventricular 429.89
Dystasia, hereditary areflexic 334.3
Dysthymia 300.4
Dysthymic disorder 300.4
Dysthyroidism 246.9

Dystocia 660.9
  affecting fetus or newborn 763.1
  cervical 661.0
    affecting fetus or newborn 763.7
  contraction ring 661.4
    affecting fetus or newborn 763.7
  fetal 660.9
    abnormal size 653.5
    affecting fetus or newborn 763.1
    deformity 653.7
  maternal 660.9
    affecting fetus or newborn 763.1
  positional 660.0
    affecting fetus or newborn 763.1
  shoulder (girdle) 660.4
    affecting fetus or newborn 763.1
  uterine NEC 661.4
    affecting fetus or newborn 763.7
Dystonia
  acute
    due to drugs 333.72
    neuroleptic-induced acute 333.72
  deformans progressiva 333.6
  lenticularis 333.6
  musculorum deformans 333.6
  torsion (idiopathic) 333.6
    acquired 333.79
    fragments (of) 333.89
    genetic 333.6
    symptomatic 333.79
Dystonic
  movements 781.0
Dystopia kidney 753.3
Dystrophy, dystrophia 783.9
  adiposogenital 253.8
  asphyxiating thoracic 756.4
  Becker's type 359.1
  brevicollis 756.16
  Bruch's membrane 362.77
  cervical (sympathetic) NEC 337.0
  chondro-osseus with punctate epiphyseal
      dysplasia 756.59
  choroid (hereditary) 363.50
    central (areolar) (partial) 363.53
      total (gyrate) 363.54
    circinate 363.53
    circumpapillary (partial) 363.51
      total 363.52
    diffuse
      partial 363.56
      total 363.57
    generalized
      partial 363.56
      total 363.57
    gyrate
      central 363.54
      generalized 363.57
    helicoid 363.52
    peripapillary—*see* Dystrophy, choroid,
        circumpapillary
    serpiginous 363.54
  cornea (hereditary) 371.50
    anterior NEC 371.52
    Cogan's 371.52
    combined 371.57
    crystalline 371.56
    endothelial (Fuchs') 371.57
    epithelial 371.50
      juvenile 371.51
        microscopic cystic 371.52
    granular 371.53

E

Eagle-Barrett syndrome 756.71
Eales' disease (syndrome) 362.18
Ear —*see also* condition
  ache 388.70
    otogenic 388.71
    referred 388.72
  lop 744.29
  piercing V50.3
  swimmers' acute 380.12
  tank 380.12
  tropical 111.8 *[380.15]*
  wax 380.4
Earache 388.70
  otogenic 388.71
  referred 388.72
Early satiety 780.94
Eaton-Lambert syndrome (*see also* Neoplasm,
  by site, malignant) 199.1 *[358.1]*
Eberth's disease (typhoid fever) 002.0
Ebstein's
  anomaly or syndrome (downward displacement,
    tricuspid valve into right ventricle) 746.2
  disease (diabetes) 250.4 *[581.81]*
Eccentro-osteochondrodysplasia 277.5
Ecchondroma (M9210/0)—*see* Neoplasm, bone,
  benign
Ecchondrosis (M9210/1) 238.0
Ecchordosis physaliphora 756.0
Ecchymosis (multiple) 459.89
  conjunctiva 372.72
  eye (traumatic) 921.0
  eyelids (traumatic) 921.1
  newborn 772.6
  spontaneous 782.7
  traumatic—*see* Contusion
Echinococciasis —*see* Echinococcus
Echinococcosis —*see* Echinococcus
Echinococcus (infection) 122.9
  granulosus 122.4
    liver 122.0
    lung 122.1
    orbit 122.3 *[376.13]*
    specified site NEC 122.3
    thyroid 122.2
  liver NEC 122.8
    granulosus 122.0
    multilocularis 122.5
  lung NEC 122.9
    granulosus 122.1
    multilocularis 122.6
  multilocularis 122.7
    liver 122.5
    specified site NEC 122.6
  orbit 122.9 *[376.13]*
    granulosus 122.3 *[376.13]*
    multilocularis 122.6 *[376.13]*
  specified site NEC 122.9
    granulosus 122.3
    multilocularis 122.6 *[376.13]*
  thyroid NEC 122.9
    granulosus 122.2
    multilocularis 122.6
Echinorhynchiasis 127.7
Echinostomiasis 121.8
Echolalia 784.69
ECHO virus infection NEC 079.1

Eclampsia, eclamptic (coma) (convulsions)
  (delirium) 780.39
  female, child-bearing age NEC—*see* Eclampsia,
    pregnancy
  gravidarum—*see* Eclampsia, pregnancy
  male 780.39
  not associated with pregnancy or childbirth
    780.39
  pregnancy, childbirth or puerperium 642.6
    with pre-existing hypertension 642.7
    affecting fetus or newborn 760.0
  uremic 586
Eclipse blindness (total) 363.31
Economic circumstance affecting care V60.9
  specified type NEC V60.8
Economo's disease (encephalitis lethargica)
  049.8
Ectasia, ectasis
  aorta (*see also* Aneurysm, aorta) 441.9
    ruptured 441.5
  breast 610.4
  capillary 448.9
  cornea (marginal) (postinfectional) 371.71
  duct (mammary) 610.4
  kidney 593.89
  mammary duct (gland) 610.4
  papillary 448.9
  renal 593.89
  salivary gland (duct) 527.8
  scar, cornea 371.71
  sclera 379.11
Ecthyma 686.8
  contagiosum 051.2
  gangrenosum 686.09
  infectiosum 051.2
Ectocardia 746.87
Ectodermal dysplasia, congenital 757.31
Ectodermosis erosiva pluriorificialis 695.1
Ectopic, ectopia (congenital) 759.89
  abdominal viscera 751.8
    due to defect in anterior abdominal wall
      756.79
  ACTH syndrome 255.0
  adrenal gland 759.1
  anus 751.5
  auricular beats 427.61
  beats 427.60
  bladder 753.5
  bone and cartilage in lung 748.69
  brain 742.4
  breast tissue 757.6
  cardiac 746.87
  cerebral 742.4
  cordis 746.87
  endometrium 617.9
  gallbladder 751.69
  gastric mucosa 750.7
  gestation—*see* Pregnancy, ectopic
  heart 746.87
  hormone secretion NEC 259.3
  hyperparathyroidism 259.3
  kidney (crossed) (intrathoracic) (pelvis) 753.3
    in pregnancy or childbirth 654.4
      causing obstructed labor 660.2
  lens 743.37
  lentis 743.37
  mole—*see* Pregnancy, ectopic

Edema, edematous—*continued*
  due to external agent—*see* Condition,
    respiratory, acute, due to specified agent
  heart (*see also* Failure, heart) 428.0
    newborn 779.89
  heat 992.7
  hereditary (legs) 757.0
  inanition 262
  infectious 782.3
  intracranial 348.5
    due to injury at birth 767.8
  iris 364.8
  joint (*see also* Effusion, joint) 719.0
  larynx (*see also* Edema, glottis) 478.6
  legs 782.3
    due to venous obstruction 459.2
    hereditary 757.0
  localized 782.3
    due to venous obstruction 459.2
      lower extremity 459.2
  lower extremities—*see* Edema, legs
  lungs 514
    acute 518.4
      with heart disease or failure (*see also*
        Failure, ventricular, left) 428.1
        congestive 428.0
      chemical (due to fumes or vapors) 506.1
      due to
        external agent(s) NEC 508.9
          specified NEC 508.8
        fumes and vapors (chemical) (inhalation)
          506.1
        radiation 508.0
    chemical (acute) 506.1
      chronic 506.4
    chronic 514
      chemical (due to fumes or vapors) 506.4
      due to
        external agent(s) NEC 508.9
          specified NEC 508.8
        fumes or vapors (chemical) (inhalation)
          506.4
        radiation 508.1
    due to
      external agent 508.9
        specified NEC 508.8
      high altitude 993.2
      near drowning 994.1
    postoperative 518.4
    terminal 514
  lymphatic 457.1
    due to mastectomy operation 457.0
  macula 362.83
    cystoid 362.53
    diabetic 250.5 *[362.07]*
  malignant (*see also* Gangrene, gas) 040.0
  Milroy's 757.0
  nasopharynx 478.25
  neonatorum 778.5
  nutritional (newborn) 262
    with dyspigmentation, skin and hair 260
  optic disc or nerve—*see* Papilledema
  orbit 376.33
    circulatory 459.89
  palate (soft) (hard) 528.9
  pancreas 577.8
  penis 607.83
  periodic 995.1
    hereditary 277.6
  pharynx 478.25
  pitting 782.3

Edema, edematous—*continued*
  pulmonary—*see* Edema, lung
  Quincke's 995.1
    hereditary 277.6
  renal (*see also* Nephrosis) 581.9
  retina (localized) (macular) (peripheral) 362.83
    cystoid 362.53
    diabetic 250.5 *[362.07]*
  salt 276.0
  scrotum 608.86
  seminal vesicle 608.86
  spermatic cord 608.86
  spinal cord 336.1
  starvation 262
  stasis (*see also* Hypertension, venous) 459.30
  subconjunctival 372.73
  subglottic (*see also* Edema, glottis) 478.6
  supraglottic (*see also* Edema, glottis) 478.6
  testis 608.86
  toxic NEC 782.3
  traumatic NEC 782.3
  tunica vaginalis 608.86
  vas deferens 608.86
  vocal cord—*see* Edema, glottis
  vulva (acute) 624.8
Edentia (complete) (partial) (*see also* Absence,
  tooth) 520.0
  acquired (*see also* Edentulism) 525.40
    due to
      caries 525.13
      extraction 525.10
      periodontal disease 525.12
      specified NEC 525.19
      trauma 525.11
  causing malocclusion 524.30
  congenital (deficiency of tooth buds) 520.0
Edentulism 525.40
  complete 525.40
    class I 525.41
    class II 525.42
    class III 525.43
    class IV 525.44
  partial 525.50
    class I 525.51
    class II 525.52
    class III 525.53
    class IV 525.54
Edsall's disease 992.2
Educational handicap V62.3
Edwards' syndrome 758.2
Effect, adverse NEC
  abnormal gravitational (G) forces or states 994.9
  air pressure—*see* Effect, adverse, atmospheric
    pressure
  altitude (high)—*see* Effect, adverse, high
    altitude
  anesthetic
    in labor and delivery NEC 668.9
      affecting fetus or newborn 763.5
  antitoxin—*see* Complications, vaccination
  atmospheric pressure 993.9
    due to explosion 993.4
    high 993.3
    low—*see* Effect, adverse, high altitude
    specified effect NEC 993.8
  biological, correct substance properly
    administered (*see also* Effect, adverse, drug)
    995.20
  blood (derivatives) (serum) (transfusion)—*see*
    Complications, transfusion
  chemical substance NEC 989.9

Elevation—*continued*
  blood pressure (*see also* Hypertension) 401.9
    reading (incidental) (isolated) (nonspecific),
      no diagnosis of hypertension 796.2
  body temperature (of unknown origin) (*see also*
    Pyrexia) 780.6
  C-reactive protein (CRP) 790.95
  cancer antigen 125 [CA 125] 795.82
  carcinoembryonic antigen [CEA] 795.81
  conjugate, eye 378.81
  CRP (C-reactive protein) 790.95
  diaphragm, congenital 756.6
  glucose
    fasting 790.21
    tolerance test 790.22
  immunoglobulin level 795.79
  indolacetic acid 791.9
  lactic acid dehydrogenase (LDH) level 790.4
  leukocytes 288.60
  lipase 790.5
  lipoprotein a level 272.8
  liver function test (LFT) 790.6
    alkaline phosphatase 790.5
    aminotransferase 790.4
    bilirubin 782.4
    hepatic enzyme NEC 790.5
    lactate dehydrogenase 790.4
  lymphocytes 288.61
  prostate specific antigen (PSA) 790.93
  renin 790.99
    in hypertension (*see also* Hypertension,
      renovascular) 405.91
  Rh titer 999.7
  scapula, congenital 755.52
  sedimentation rate 790.1
  SGOT 790.4
  SGPT 790.4
  transaminase 790.4
  vanillylmandelic acid 791.9
  venous pressure 459.89
  VMA 791.9
  white blood cell count 288.60
    specified NEC 288.69
Elliptocytosis (congenital) (hereditary) 282.1
  Hb-C (disease) 282.7
  hemoglobin disease 282.7
  sickle-cell (disease) 282.60
    trait 282.5
Ellis-van Creveld disease or syndrome
  (chondroectodermal dysplasia) 756.55
Ellison-Zollinger syndrome (gastric
  hypersecretion with pancreatic islet cell
  tumor) 251.5
Elongation, elongated (congenital)—*see also*
  Distortion
  bone 756.9
  cervix (uteri) 752.49
    acquired 622.6
    hypertrophic 622.6
  colon 751.5
  common bile duct 751.69
  cystic duct 751.69
  frenulum, penis 752.69
  labia minora, acquired 624.8
  ligamentum patellae 756.89
  petiolus (epiglottidis) 748.3
  styloid bone (process) 733.99
  tooth, teeth 520.2
  uvula 750.26
    acquired 528.9
Elschnig bodies or pearls 366.51
El Tor cholera 001.1

Emaciation (due to malnutrition) 261
Emancipation disorder 309.22
Embadomoniasis 007.8
Embarrassment heart, cardiac —*see* Disease,
  heart
Embedded tooth, teeth 520.6
  root only 525.3
Embolic —*see* condition
Embolism 444.9
  with
    abortion—*see* Abortion, by type, with
      embolism
    ectopic pregnancy (*see also* categories
      633.0-633.9) 639.6
    molar pregnancy (*see also* categories 630-632)
      639.6
  air (any site) 958.0
    with
      abortion—*see* Abortion, by type, with
        embolism
      ectopic pregnancy (*see also* categories
        633.0-633.9) 639.6
      molar pregnancy (*see also* categories
        630-632) 639.6
    due to implanted device—*see* Complications,
      due to (presence of) any device, implant,
      or graft classified to 996.0-996.5 NEC
    following
      abortion 639.6
      ectopic or molar pregnancy 639.6
      infusion, perfusion, or transfusion 999.1
    in pregnancy, childbirth, or puerperium 673.0
    traumatic 958.0
  amniotic fluid (pulmonary) 673.1
    with
      abortion—*see* Abortion, by type, with
        embolism
      ectopic pregnancy (*see also* categories
        633.0-633.9) 639.6
      molar pregnancy (*see also* categories
        630-632) 639.6
    following
      abortion 639.6
      ectopic or molar pregnancy 639.6
  aorta, aortic 444.1
    abdominal 444.0
    bifurcation 444.0
    saddle 444.0
    thoracic 444.1
  artery 444.9
    auditory, internal 433.8
    basilar (*see also* Occlusion, artery, basilar)
      433.0
    bladder 444.89
    carotid (common) (internal) (*see also*
      Occlusion, artery, carotid) 433.1
    cerebellar (anterior inferior) (posterior
      inferior) (superior) 433.8
    cerebral (*see also* Embolism, brain) 434.1
    choroidal (anterior) 433.8
    communicating posterior 433.8
    coronary (*see also* Infarct, myocardium) 410.9
      without myocardial infarction 411.81
    extremity 444.22
      lower 444.22
      upper 444.21
    hypophyseal 433.8
    mesenteric (with gangrene) 557.0
    ophthalmic (*see also* Occlusion, retina) 362.30
    peripheral 444.22
    pontine 433.8

Embolism—*continued*
    ectopic pregnancy (*see also* categories
        633.0-633.9) 639.6
    molar pregnancy (*see also* categories
        630-632) 639.6
  following
    abortion 639.6
    ectopic or molar pregnancy 639.6
  iatrogenic 415.11
  in pregnancy, childbirth, or puerperium—*see*
    Embolism, obstetrical
  postoperative 415.11
  pyemic (multiple) 038.9
    with
      abortion—*see* Abortion, by type, with
        embolism
      ectopic pregnancy (*see also* categories
        633.0-633.9) 639.6
      molar pregnancy (*see also* categories
        630-632) 639.6
    Aerobacter aerogenes 038.49
    enteric gram-negative bacilli 038.40
    Enterobacter aerogenes 038.49
    Escherichia coli 038.42
    following
      abortion 639.6
      ectopic or molar pregnancy 639.6
    Hemophilus influenzae 038.41
    pneumococcal 038.2
    Proteus vulgaris 038.49
    Pseudomonas (aeruginosa) 038.43
    puerperal, postpartum, childbirth (any
      organism) 673.3
    Serratia 038.44
    specified organism NEC 038.8
    staphylococcal 038.10
      aureus 038.11
      specified organism NEC 038.19
    streptococcal 038.0
  renal (artery) 593.81
    vein 453.3
  retina, retinal (*see also* Occlusion, retina) 362.30
  saddle (aorta) 444.0
  septicemic—*see* Embolism, pyemic
  sinus—*see* Embolism, intracranial venous sinus
  soap
    with
      abortion—*see* Abortion, by type, with
        embolism
      ectopic pregnancy (*see also* categories
        633.0-633.9) 639.6
      molar pregnancy (*see also* categories
        630-632) 639.6
    following
      abortion 639.6
      ectopic or molar pregnancy 639.6
  spinal cord (nonpyogenic) 336.1
    in pregnancy or puerperium 671.5
    pyogenic origin 324.1
      late effect—*see* category 326
  spleen, splenic (artery) 444.89
  thrombus (thromboembolism) following
    infusion, perfusion, or transfusion 999.2
  upper extremity 444.21
  vein 453.9
    with inflammation or phlebitis—*see*
      Thrombophlebitis
    cerebral (*see also* Embolism, brain) 434.1
    coronary (*see also* Infarct, myocardium) 410.9
      without myocardial infarction 411.81
    hepatic 453.0

Embolism—*continued*
  lower extremity 453.8
    deep 453.40
      calf 453.42
      distal (lower leg) 453.42
      femoral 453.41
      iliac 453.41
      lower leg 453.42
      peroneal 453.42
      popliteal 453.41
      proximal (upper leg) 453.41
      thigh 453.41
      tibial 453.42
  mesenteric (with gangrene) 557.0
  portal 452
  pulmonary—*see* Embolism, pulmonary
  renal 453.3
  specified NEC 453.8
    with inflammation or phlebitis—*see*
      Thrombophlebitis
  vena cava (inferior) (superior) 453.2
  vessels of brain (*see also* Embolism, brain)
    434.1
Embolization —*see* Embolism
Embolus —*see* Embolism
Embryoma (M9080/1)—*see also* Neoplasm, by
  site, uncertain behavior
  benign (M9080/0)—*see* Neoplasm, by site,
    benign
  kidney (M8960/3) 189.0
  liver (M8970/3) 155.0
  malignant (M9080/3)—*see also* Neoplasm, by
    site, malignant
    kidney (M8960/3) 189.0
    liver (M8970/3) 155.0
    testis (M9070/3) 186.9
      undescended 186.0
  testis (M9070/3) 186.9
    undescended 186.0
Embryonic
  circulation 747.9
  heart 747.9
  vas deferens 752.89
Embryopathia NEC 759.9
Embryotomy, fetal 763.89
Embryotoxon 743.43
  interfering with vision 743.42
Emesis —*see also* Vomiting
  gravidarum—*see* Hyperemesis, gravidarum
Emissions, nocturnal (semen) 608.89
Emotional
  crisis—*see* Crisis, emotional
  disorder (*see also* Disorder, mental) 300.9
  instability (excessive) 301.3
  overlay—*see* Reaction, adjustment
  upset 300.9
Emotionality, pathological 301.3
Emotogenic disease (*see also* Disorder,
  psychogenic) 306.9
Emphysema (atrophic) (centriacinar)
  (centrilobular) (chronic) (diffuse) (essential)
  (hypertrophic) (interlobular) (lung)
  (obstructive) (panlobular) (paracicatricial)
  (paracinar) (postural) (pulmonary) (senile)
  (subpleural) (traction) (unilateral) (unilobular)
  (vesicular) 492.8
  with bronchitis
    chronic 491.20
      with
        acute bronchitis 491.22
        exacerbation (acute) 491.21

Emphysema—*continued*
  bullous (giant) 492.0
  cellular tissue 958.7
    surgical 998.81
  compensatory 518.2
  congenital 770.2
  conjunctiva 372.89
  connective tissue 958.7
    surgical 998.81
  due to fumes or vapors 506.4
  eye 376.89
  eyelid 374.85
    surgical 998.81
    traumatic 958.7
  fetus or newborn (interstitial) (mediastinal)
    (unilobular) 770.2
  heart 416.9
  interstitial 518.1
    congenital 770.2
    fetus or newborn 770.2
  laminated tissue 958.7
    surgical 998.81
  mediastinal 518.1
    fetus or newborn 770.2
  newborn (interstitial) (mediastinal) (unilobular)
    770.2
  obstructive diffuse with fibrosis 492.8
  orbit 376.89
  subcutaneous 958.7
    due to trauma 958.7
    nontraumatic 518.1
    surgical 998.81
  surgical 998.81
  thymus (gland) (congenital) 254.8
  traumatic 958.7
  tuberculous (*see also* Tuberculosis, pulmonary)
    011.9
Employment examination (certification) V70.5
Empty sella (turcica) syndrome 253.8
Empyema (chest) (diaphragmatic) (double)
    (encapsulated) (general) (interlobar) (lung)
    (medial) (necessitatis) (perforating chest wall)
    (pleura) (pneumococcal) (residual)
    (sacculated) (streptococcal)
    (supradiaphragmatic) 510.9
  with fistula 510.0
  accessory sinus (chronic) (*see also* Sinusitis)
    473.9
  acute 510.9
    with fistula 510.0
  antrum (chronic) (*see also* Sinusitis, maxillary)
    473.0
  brain (any part) (*see also* Abscess, brain) 324.0
  ethmoidal (sinus) (chronic) (*see also* Sinusitis,
    ethmoidal) 473.2
  extradural (*see also* Abscess, extradural) 324.9
  frontal (sinus) (chronic) (*see also* Sinusitis,
    frontal) 473.1
  gallbladder (*see also* Cholecystitis, acute) 575.0
  mastoid (process) (acute) (*see also* Mastoiditis,
    acute) 383.00
  maxilla, maxillary 526.4
    sinus (chronic) (*see also* Sinusitis, maxillary)
      473.0
  nasal sinus (chronic) (*see also* Sinusitis) 473.9
  sinus (accessory) (nasal) (*see also* Sinusitis)
    473.9
  sphenoidal (chronic) (sinus) (*see also* Sinusitis,
    sphenoidal) 473.3
  subarachnoid (*see also* Abscess, extradural)
    324.9

Empyema—*continued*
  subdural (*see also* Abscess, extradural) 324.9
  tuberculous (*see also* Tuberculosis, pleura)
    012.0
  ureter (*see also* Ureteritis) 593.89
  ventricular (*see also* Abscess, brain) 324.0
Enameloma 520.2
Encephalitis (bacterial) (chronic) (hemorrhagic)
    (idiopathic) (nonepidemic) (spurious)
    (subacute) 323.9
  acute—*see also* Encephalitis, viral
    disseminated (postinfectious) NEC 136.9
      [323.61]
      postimmunization or postvaccination 323.51
    inclusional 049.8
    inclusion body 049.8
    necrotizing 049.8
  arboviral, arbovirus NEC 064
  arthropod-borne (*see also* Encephalitis, viral,
    arthropod-borne) 064
  Australian X 062.4
  Bwamba fever 066.3
  California (virus) 062.5
  Central European 063.2
  Czechoslovakian 063.2
  Dawson's (inclusion body) 046.2
  diffuse sclerosing 046.2
  due to
    actinomycosis 039.8 *[323.41]*
    cat-scratch disease 078.3 *[323.01]*
    infection classified elsewhere 136.9 *[323.41]*
    infectious mononucleosis 075 *[323.01]*
    malaria (*see also* Malaria) 084.6 *[323.2]*
    Negishi virus 064
    ornithosis 073.7 *[323.01]*
    prophylactic inoculation against smallpox
      323.51
    rickettsiosis (*see also* Rickettsiosis) 083.9
      [323.1]
    rubella 056.01
    toxoplasmosis (acquired) 130.0
      congenital (active) 771.2 *[323.41]*
    typhus (fever) (*see also* Typhus) 081.9 *[323.1]*
    vaccination (smallpox) 323.51
  Eastern equine 062.2
  endemic 049.8
  epidemic 049.8
  equine (acute) (infectious) (viral) 062.9
    Eastern 062.2
    Venezuelan 066.2
    Western 062.1
  Far Eastern 063.0
  following vaccination or other immunization
    procedure 323.51
  herpes 054.3
  Ilheus (virus) 062.8
  inclusion body 046.2
  infectious (acute) (virus) NEC 049.8
  influenzal 487.8 *[323.41]*
    lethargic 049.8
  Japanese (B type) 062.0
  La Crosse 062.5
  Langat 063.8
  late effect—*see* Late, effect, encephalitis
  lead 984.9 *[323.71]*
  lethargic (acute) (infectious) (influenzal) 049.8
  lethargica 049.8
  louping ill 063.1
  lupus 710.0 *[323.81]*
  lymphatica 049.0
  Mengo 049.8

Encephalitis—*continued*
  meningococcal 036.1
  mumps 072.2
  Murray Valley 062.4
  myoclonic 049.8
  Negishi virus 064
  otitic NEC 382.4 *[323.41]*
  parasitic NEC 123.9 *[323.41]*
  periaxialis (concentrica) (diffusa) 341.1
  postchickenpox 052.0
  postexanthematous NEC 057.9 *[323.62]*
  postimmunization 323.51
  postinfectious NEC 136.9 *[323.62]*
  postmeasles 055.0
  posttraumatic 323.81
  postvaccinal (smallpox) 323.51
  postvaricella 052.0
  postviral NEC 079.99 *[323.62]*
    postexanthematous 057.9 *[323.62]*
      specified NEC 057.8 *[323.62]*
  Powassan 063.8
  progressive subcortical (Binswanger's) 290.12
  Rasmussen 323.81
  Rio Bravo 049.8
  rubella 056.01
  Russian
    autumnal 062.0
    spring-summer type (taiga) 063.0
  saturnine 984.9 *[323.71]*
  Semliki Forest 062.8
  serous 048
  slow-acting virus NEC 046.8
  specified cause NEC 323.81
  St. Louis type 062.3
  subacute sclerosing 046.2
  subcorticalis chronica 290.12
  summer 062.0
  suppurative 324.0
  syphilitic 094.81
    congenital 090.41
  tick-borne 063.9
  torula, torular 117.5 *[323.41]*
  toxic NEC 989.9 *[323.71]*
  toxoplasmic (acquired) 130.0
    congenital (active) 771.2 *[323.41]*
  trichinosis 124 *[323.41]*
  Trypanosomiasis (*see also* Trypanosomiasis) 086.9 *[323.2]*
  tuberculous (*see also* Tuberculosis) 013.6
  type B (Japanese) 062.0
  type C 062.3
  van Bogaert's 046.2
  Venezuelan 066.2
  Vienna type 049.8
  viral, virus 049.9
    arthropod-borne NEC 064
      mosquito-borne 062.9
        Australian X disease 062.4
        California virus 062.5
        Eastern equine 062.2
        Ilheus virus 062.8
        Japanese (B type) 062.0
        Murray Valley 062.4
        specified type NEC 062.8
        St. Louis 062.3
        type B 062.0
        type C 062.3
        Western equine 062.1
      tick-borne 063.9
        biundulant 063.2
        Central European 063.2

Encephalitis—*continued*
        Czechoslovakian 063.2
        diphasic meningoencephalitis 063.2
        Far Eastern 063.0
        Langat 063.8
        louping ill 063.1
        Powassan 063.8
        Russian spring-summer (taiga) 063.0
        specified type NEC 063.8
      vector unknown 064
    slow acting NEC 046.8
    specified type NEC 049.8
    vaccination, prophylactic (against) V05.0
  von Economo's 049.8
  Western equine 062.1
  West Nile type 066.41
Encephalocele 742.0
  orbit 376.81
Encephalocystocele 742.0
Encephalomalacia (brain) (cerebellar) (cerebral) (cerebrospinal) (*see also* Softening, brain) 434.9
  due to
    hemorrhage (*see also* Hemorrhage, brain) 431
    recurrent spasm of artery 435.9
  embolic (cerebral) (*see also* Embolism, brain) 434.1
  subcorticalis chronicus arteriosclerotica 290.12
  thrombotic (*see also* Thrombosis, brain) 434.0
Encephalomeningitis —*see* Meningoencephalitis
Encephalomeningocele 742.0
Encephalomeningomyelitis —*see* Meningoencephalitis
Encephalomeningopathy (*see also* Meningoencephalitis) 349.9
Encephalomyelitis (chronic) (granulomatous) (hemorrhagic necrotizing, acute) (myalgic, benign) (*see also* Encephalitis) 323.9
  abortive disseminated 049.8
  acute disseminated (ADEM) (postinfectious) 136.9 *[323.61]*
    infectious 136.9 *[323.61]*
    noninfectious 323.81
    postimmunization 323.51
  due to
    cat-scratch disease 078.3 *[323.01]*
    infectious mononucleosis 075 *[323.01]*
    ornithosis 073.7 *[323.01]*
    vaccination (any) 323.51
  equine (acute) (infectious) 062.9
    Eastern 062.2
    Venezuelan 066.2
    Western 062.1
  funicularis infectiosa 049.8
  late effect—*see* Late, effect, encephalitis
  Munch-Peterson's 049.8
  postchickenpox 052.0
  postimmunization 323.51
  postmeasles 055.0
  postvaccinal (smallpox) 323.51
  rubella 056.01
  specified cause NEC 323.81
  syphilitic 094.81
  West Nile 066.41
Encephalomyelocele 742.0
Encephalomyelomeningitis —*see* Meningoencephalitis
Encephalomyeloneuropathy 349.9
Encephalomyelopathy 349.9
  subacute necrotizing (infantile) 330.8
Encephalomyeloradiculitis (acute) 357.0

Encephalomyeloradiculoneuritis (acute) 357.0
Encephalomyeloradiculopathy 349.9
Encephalomyocarditis 074.23
Encephalopathia hyperbilirubinemica
   newborn 774.7
  due to isoimmunization (conditions classifiable
    to 773.0-773.2) 773.4
Encephalopathy (acute) 348.30
  alcoholic 291.2
  anoxic—*see* Damage, brain, anoxic
  arteriosclerotic 437.0
    late effect—*see* Late effect(s) (of)
      cerebrovascular disease
  bilirubin, newborn 774.7
    due to isoimmunization 773.4
  congenital 742.9
  demyelinating (callosal) 341.8
  due to
    birth injury (intracranial) 767.8
    dialysis 294.8
      transient 293.9
    hyperinsulinism—*see* Hyperinsulinism
    influenza (virus) 487.8
    lack of vitamin (*see also* Deficiency, vitamin)
      269.2
    nicotinic acid deficiency 291.2
    serum (nontherapeutic) (therapeutic) 999.5
    syphilis 094.81
    trauma (postconcussional) 310.2
      current (*see also* Concussion, brain) 850.9
        with skull fracture—*see* Fracture, skull, by
          site, with intracranial injury
    vaccination 323.51
  hepatic 572.2
  hyperbilirubinemic, newborn 774.7
    due to isoimmunization (conditions
      classifiable to 773.0-773.2) 773.4
  hypertensive 437.2
  hypoglycemic 251.2
  hypoxic—*see also* Damage, brain, anoxic
    ischemic (HIE) 768.7
  infantile cystic necrotizing (congenital) 341.8
  lead 984.9 *[323.71]*
  leukopolio 330.0
  metabolic (*see also* Delirium) 348.31
    toxic 349.82
  necrotizing
    hemorrhagic 323.61
    subacute 330.8
  other specified type NEC 348.39
  pellagrous 265.2
  portal-systemic 572.2
  postcontusional 310.2
  posttraumatic 310.2
  saturnine 984.9 *[323.71]*
  septic 348.31
  spongioform, subacute (viral) 046.1
  subacute
    necrotizing 330.8
    spongioform 046.1
    viral, spongioform 046.1
  subcortical progressive (Schilder) 341.1
    chronic (Binswanger's) 290.12
  toxic 349.82
    metabolic 349.82
  traumatic (postconcussional) 310.2
    current (*see also* Concussion, brain) 850.9
      with skull fracture—*see* Fracture, skull, by
        site, with intracranial injury
  vitamin B deficiency NEC 266.9
  Wernicke's (superior hemorrhagic
    polioencephalitis) 265.1

Enchephalorrhagia (*see also* Hemorrhage,
   brain) 432.9
  healed or old V12.59
  late effect—*see* Late effect(s) (of)
    cerebrovascular disease
Encephalosis, posttraumatic 310.2
Enchondroma (M9220/0)—*see also* Neoplasm,
   bone, benign
  multiple, congenital 756.4
Enchondromatosis (cartilaginous) (congenital)
   (multiple) 756.4
Enchondroses, multiple (cartilaginous)
   (congenital) 756.4
Encopresis (*see also* Incontinence, feces) 787.6
  nonorganic origin 307.7
Encounter for —*see also* Admission for
  administrative purpose only V68.9
    referral of patient without examination or
      treatment V68.81
    specified purpose NEC V68.89
  chemotherapy, antineoplastic V58.11
  end-of-life care V66.7
  hospice care V66.7
  immunotherapy, antineoplastic V58.12
  palliative care V66.7
  radiotherapy V58.0
  respirator (ventilator) dependence
    during
      mechanical failure V46.14
      power failure V46.12
    for weaning V46.13
  screening mammogram NEC V76.12
    for high-risk patient V76.11
  paternity testing V70.4
  terminal care V66.7
  weaning from respirator (ventilator) V46.13
Encystment —*see* Cyst
End-of-life care V66.7
Endamebiasis —*see* Amebiasis
Endamoeba —*see* Amebiasis
Endarteritis (bacterial, subacute) (infective)
   (septic) 447.6
  brain, cerebral or cerebrospinal 437.4
    late effect—*see* Late effect(s) (of)
      cerebrovascular disease
  coronary (artery) —*see* Arteriosclerosis,
    coronary
  deformans—*see* Arteriosclerosis
  embolic (*see also* Embolism) 444.9
  obliterans—*see also* Arteriosclerosis
    pulmonary 417.8
  pulmonary 417.8
  retina 362.18
  senile—*see* Arteriosclerosis
  syphilitic 093.89
    brain or cerebral 094.89
    congenital 090.5
    spinal 094.89
  tuberculous (*see also* Tuberculosis) 017.9
Endemic —*see* condition
Endocarditis (chronic) (indeterminate)
   (interstitial) (marantis) (nonbacterial
   thrombotic) (residual) (sclerotic) (sclerous)
   (senile) (valvular) 424.90
  with
    rheumatic fever (conditions classifiable to
      390)
      active—*see* Endocarditis, acute, rheumatic
      inactive or quiescent (with chorea) 397.9
  acute or subacute 421.9

Endocarditis—*continued*
rheumatic (aortic) (mitral) (pulmonary)
(tricuspid) 391.1
with chorea (acute) (rheumatic)
(Sydenham's) 392.0
aortic (heart) (nonrheumatic) (valve) 424.1
with
mitral (valve) disease 396.9
active or acute 391.1
with chorea (acute) (rheumatic)
(Sydenham's) 392.0
rheumatic fever (conditions classifiable to
390)
active—*see* Endocarditis, acute, rheumatic
inactive or quiescent (with chorea) 395.9
with mitral disease 396.9
acute or subacute 421.9
arteriosclerotic 424.1
congenital 746.89
hypertensive 424.1
rheumatic (chronic) (inactive) 395.9
with mitral (valve) disease 396.9
active or acute 391.1
with chorea (acute) (rheumatic)
(Sydenham's) 392.0
active or acute 391.1
with chorea (acute) (rheumatic)
(Sydenham's) 392.0
specified cause, except rheumatic 424.1
syphilitic 093.22
arteriosclerotic or due to arteriosclerosis 424.99
atypical verrucous (Libman-Sacks) 710.0
[424.91]
bacterial (acute) (any valve) (chronic) (subacute)
421.0
blastomycotic 116.0 *[421.1]*
candidal 112.81
congenital 425.3
constrictive 421.0
Coxsackie 074.22
due to
blastomycosis 116.0 *[421.1]*
candidiasis 112.81
Coxsackie (virus) 074.22
disseminated lupus erythematosus 710.0
[424.91]
histoplasmosis (*see also* Histoplasmosis) 115.94
hypertension (benign) 424.99
moniliasis 112.81
prosthetic cardiac valve 996.61
Q fever 083.0 *[421.1]*
serratia marcescens 421.0
typhoid (fever) 002.0 *[421.1]*
fetal 425.3
gonococcal 098.84
hypertensive 424.99
infectious or infective (acute) (any valve)
(chronic) (subacute) 421.0
lenta (acute) (any valve) (chronic) (subacute)
421.0
Libman-Sacks 710.0 *[424.91]*
Loeffler's (parietal fibroplastic) 421.0
malignant (acute) (any valve) (chronic)
(subacute) 421.0
meningococcal 036.42
mitral (chronic) (double) (fibroid) (heart)
(inactive) (valve) (with chorea) 394.9
with
aortic (valve) disease 396.9
active or acute 391.1

Endocarditis—*continued*
with chorea (acute) (rheumatic)
(Sydenham's) 392.0
rheumatic fever (conditions classifiable to
390)
active—*see* Endocarditis, acute, rheumatic
inactive or quiescent (with chorea) 394.9
with aortic valve disease 396.9
active or acute 391.1
bacterial 421.0
with chorea (acute) (rheumatic)
(Sydenham's) 392.0
arteriosclerotic 424.0
congenital 746.89
hypertensive 424.0
nonrheumatic 424.0
acute or subacute 421.9
syphilitic 093.21
monilial 112.81
mycotic (acute) (any valve) (chronic) (subacute)
421.0
pneumococcic (acute) (any valve) (chronic)
(subacute) 421.0
pulmonary (chronic) (heart) (valve) 424.3
with
rheumatic fever (conditions classifiable to
390)
active—*see* Endocarditis, acute, rheumatic
inactive or quiescent (with chorea) 397.1
acute or subacute 421.9
rheumatic 391.1
with chorea (acute) (rheumatic)
(Sydenham's) 392.0
arteriosclerotic or due to arteriosclerosis 424.3
congenital 746.09
hypertensive or due to hypertension (benign)
424.3
rheumatic (chronic) (inactive) (with chorea)
397.1
active or acute 391.1
with chorea (acute) (rheumatic)
(Sydenham's) 392.0
syphilitic 093.24
purulent (acute) (any valve) (chronic) (subacute)
421.0
rheumatic (chronic) (inactive) (with chorea)
397.9
active or acute (aortic) (mitral) (pulmonary)
(tricuspid) 391.1
with chorea (acute) (rheumatic)
(Sydenham's) 392.0
septic (acute) (any valve) (chronic) (subacute)
421.0
specified cause, except rheumatic 424.99
streptococcal (acute) (any valve) (chronic)
(subacute) 421.0
subacute—*see* Endocarditis, acute
suppurative (any valve) (acute) (chronic)
(subacute) 421.0
syphilitic NEC 093.20
toxic (*see also* Endocarditis, acute) 421.9
tricuspid (chronic) (heart) (inactive) (rheumatic)
(valve) (with chorea) 397.0
with
rheumatic fever (conditions classifiable to
390)
active—*see* Endocarditis, acute, rheumatic
inactive or quiescent (with chorea) 397.0
active or acute 391.1
with chorea (acute) (rheumatic)
(Sydenham's) 392.0

Endocarditis—*continued*
   arteriosclerotic 424.2
   congenital 746.89
   hypertensive 424.2
   nonrheumatic 424.2
     acute or subacute 421.9
   specified cause, except rheumatic 424.2
   syphilitic 093.23
   tuberculous (*see also* Tuberculosis) 017.9
     [424.91]
   typhoid 002.0 *[421.1]*
   ulcerative (acute) (any valve) (chronic)
     (subacute) 421.0
   vegetative (acute) (any valve) (chronic)
     (subacute) 421.0
   verrucous (acute) (any valve) (chronic)
     (subacute) NEC 710.0 *[424.91]*
     nonbacterial 710.0 *[424.91]*
     nonrheumatic 710.0 *[424.91]*
Endocardium, endocardial —*see also* condition
   cushion defect 745.60
     specified type NEC 745.69
Endocervicitis (*see also* Cervicitis) 616.0
  due to
    intrauterine (contraceptive) device 996.65
  gonorrheal (acute) 098.15
   chronic or duration of 2 months or over 098.35
  hyperplastic 616.0
  syphilitic 095.8
  trichomonal 131.09
  tuberculous (*see also* Tuberculosis) 016.7
Endocrine —*see* condition
Endocrinopathy, pluriglandular 258.9
Endodontitis 522.0
Endomastoiditis (*see also* Mastoiditis) 383.9
Endometrioma 617.9
Endometriosis 617.9
  appendix 617.5
  bladder 617.8
  bowel 617.5
  broad ligament 617.3
  cervix 617.0
  colon 617.5
  cul-de-sac (Douglas') 617.3
  exocervix 617.0
  fallopian tube 617.2
  female genital organ NEC 617.8
  gallbladder 617.8
  in scar of skin 617.6
  internal 617.0
  intestine 617.5
  lung 617.8
  myometrium 617.0
  ovary 617.1
  parametrium 617.3
  pelvic peritoneum 617.3
  peritoneal (pelvic) 617.3
  rectovaginal septum 617.4
  rectum 617.5
  round ligament 617.3
  skin 617.6
  specified site NEC 617.8
  stromal (M8931/1) 236.0
  umbilicus 617.8
  uterus 617.0
   internal 617.0
  vagina 617.4
  vulva 617.8

Endometritis (nonspecific) (purulent) (septic)
   (suppurative) 615.9
  with
   abortion—*see* Abortion, by type, with sepsis
   ectopic pregnancy (*see also* categories
     633.0-633.9) 639.0
   molar pregnancy (*see also* categories 630-632)
     639.0
  acute 615.0
  blennorrhagic 098.16
   acute 098.16
   chronic or duration of 2 months or over 098.36
  cervix, cervical (*see also* Cervicitis) 616.0
   hyperplastic 616.0
  chronic 615.1
  complicating pregnancy 646.6
   affecting fetus or newborn 760.8
  decidual 615.9
  following
   abortion 639.0
   ectopic or molar pregnancy 639.0
  gonorrheal (acute) 098.16
   chronic or duration of 2 months or over 098.36
  hyperplastic (*see also* Hyperplasia,
    endometrium) 621.30
   cervix 616.0
  polypoid—*see* Endometritis, hyperplastic
  puerperal, postpartum, childbirth 670
  senile (atrophic) 615.9
  subacute 615.0
  tuberculous (*see also* Tuberculosis) 016.7
Endometrium —*see* condition
Endomyocardiopathy, South African 425.2
Endomyocarditis —*see* Endocarditis
Endomyofibrosis 425.0
Endomyometritis (*see also* Endometritis) 615.9
Endopericarditis —*see* Endocarditis
Endoperineuritis —*see* Disorder, nerve
Endophlebitis (*see also* Phlebitis) 451.9
  leg 451.2
   deep (vessels) 451.19
   superficial (vessels) 451.0
  portal (vein) 572.1
  retina 362.18
  specified site NEC 451.89
  syphilitic 093.89
Endophthalmia (*see also* Endophthalmitis) 360.00
  gonorrheal 098.42
Endophthalmitis (globe) (infective) (metastatic)
   (purulent) (subacute) 360.00
  acute 360.01
  bleb associated 379.63
  chronic 360.03
  parasitic 360.13
  phacoanaphylactic 360.19
  specified type NEC 360.19
  sympathetic 360.11
Endosalpingioma (M9111/1) 236.2
Endosteitis —*see* Osteomyelitis
Endothelioma, bone (M9260/3)—*see* Neoplasm,
   bone, malignant
Endotheliosis 287.8
  hemorrhagic infectional 287.8
Endotoxemia —*code to condition*
Endotoxic shock 785.52
Endotrachelitis (*see also* Cervicitis) 616.0
Enema rash 692.89
Engel-von Recklinghausen disease or syndrome
   (osteitis fibrosa cystica) 252.01
Engelmann's disease (diaphyseal sclerosis)
   756.59

English disease (*see also* Rickets) 268.0
Engman's disease (infectious eczematoid dermatitis) 690.8
Engorgement
  breast 611.79
    newborn 778.7
    puerperal, postpartum 676.2
  liver 573.9
  lung 514
  pulmonary 514
  retina, venous 362.37
  stomach 536.8
  venous, retina 362.37
Enlargement, enlarged *—see also* Hypertrophy
  abdomen 789.3
  adenoids 474.12
    and tonsils 474.10
  alveolar process or ridge 525.8
  apertures of diaphragm (congenital) 756.6
  blind spot, visual field 368.42
  gingival 523.8
  heart, cardiac (*see also* Hypertrophy, cardiac) 429.3
  lacrimal gland, chronic 375.03
  liver (*see also* Hypertrophy, liver) 789.1
  lymph gland or node 785.6
  orbit 376.46
  organ or site, congenital NEC—*see* Anomaly, specified type NEC
  parathyroid (gland) 252.01
  pituitary fossa 793.0
  prostate (simple) (soft) 600.00
    with
      other lower urinary tract symptoms (LUTS) 600.01
      urinary
        obstruction 600.01
        retention 600.01
  sella turcica 793.0
  spleen (*see also* Splenomegaly) 789.2
    congenital 759.0
  thymus (congenital) (gland) 254.0
  thyroid (gland) (*see also* Goiter) 240.9
  tongue 529.8
  tonsils 474.11
    and adenoids 474.10
  uterus 621.2
Enophthalmos 376.50
  due to
    atrophy of orbital tissue 376.51
    surgery 376.52
    trauma 376.52
Enostosis 526.89
Entamebiasis *—see* Amebiasis
Entamebic *—see* Amebiasis
Entanglement, umbilical cord (s) 663.3
  with compression 663.2
  affecting fetus or newborn 762.5
  around neck with compression 663.1
  twins in monoamniotic sac 663.2
Enteralgia 789.0
Enteric *—see* condition
Enteritis (acute) (catarrhal) (choleraic) (chronic) (congestive) (diarrheal) (exudative) (follicular) (hemorrhagic) (infantile) (lienteric) (noninfectious) (perforative) (phlegmonous) (presumed noninfectious) (pseudomembranous) 558.9
  adaptive 564.9
  aertrycke infection 003.0
  allergic 558.3

Enteritis—*continued*
  amebic (*see also* Amebiasis) 006.9
    with abscess—*see* Abscess, amebic
    acute 006.0
      with abscess—*see* Abscess, amebic
      nondysenteric 006.2
    chronic 006.1
      with abscess—*see* Abscess, amebic
      nondysenteric 006.2
    nondysenteric 006.2
  anaerobic (cocci) (gram-negative) (gram-positive) (mixed) NEC 008.46
  bacillary NEC 004.9
  bacterial NEC 008.5
    specified NEC 008.49
  Bacteroides (fragilis) (melaninogeniscus) (oralis) 008.46
  Butyrivibrio (fibriosolvens) 008.46
  Campylobacter 008.43
  Candida 112.85
  Chilomastix 007.8
  choleriformis 001.1
  chronic 558.9
    ulcerative (*see also* Colitis, ulcerative) 556.9
  cicatrizing (chronic) 555.0
  Clostridium
    botulinum 005.1
    difficile 008.45
    haemolyticum 008.46
    novyi 008.46
    perfringens (C) (F) 008.46
    specified type NEC 008.46
  coccidial 007.2
  dietetic 558.9
  due to
    achylia gastrica 536.8
    adenovirus 008.62
    Aerobacter aerogenes 008.2
    anaerobes—*see* Enteritis, anaerobic 008.46
    Arizona (bacillus) 008.1
    astrovirus 008.66
    Bacillus coli—*see* Enteritis, E. coli 008.0
    bacteria NEC 008.5
      specified NEC 008.49
    Bacteroides 008.46
    Butyrivibrio (fibriosolvens) 008.46
    Calcivirus 008.65
    Campylobacter 008.43
    Clostridium—*see* Enteritis, Clostridium
    Cockle agent 008.64
    Coxsackie (virus) 008.67
    Ditchling agent 008.64
    ECHO virus 008.67
    Enterobacter aerogenes 008.2
    enterococci 008.49
    enterovirus NEC 008.67
    Escherichia coli—*see* Enteritis, E. coli
    Eubacterium 008.46
    Fusobacterium (nucleatum) 008.46
    gram-negative bacteria NEC 008.47
      anaerobic NEC 008.46
    Hawaii agent 008.63
    irritating foods 558.9
    Klebsiella aerogenes 008.47
    Marin County agent 008.66
    Montgomery County agent 008.63
    Norwalk-like agent 008.63
    Norwalk virus 008.63
    Otofuke agent 008.63
    Paracolobactrum arizonae 008.1

Epilepsia
  partialis continua (*see also* Epilepsy) 345.7
  procursiva (*see also* Epilepsy) 345.8
Epilepsy, epileptic (idiopathic) 345.9

> *Note—use the following fifth-digit*
> *subclassification with categories 345.0, 345.1,*
> *345.4-345.9*
>
> 0 *without mention of intractable epilepsy*
> 1 *with intractable epilepsy*

  abdominal 345.5
  absence (attack) 345.0
  akinetic 345.0
    psychomotor 345.4
  automatism 345.4
  autonomic diencephalic 345.5
  brain 345.9
  Bravais-Jacksonian 345.5
  cerebral 345.9
  climacteric 345.9
  clonic 345.1
  clouded state 345.9
  coma 345.3
  communicating 345.4
  complicating pregnancy, childbirth or the
    puerperium 649.4
  congenital 345.9
  convulsions 345.9
  cortical (focal) (motor) 345.5
  cursive (running) 345.8
  cysticercosis 123.1
  deterioration
    with behavioral disturbance 345.9 *[294.11]*
    without behavioral disturbance 345.9 *[294.10]*
  due to syphilis 094.89
  equivalent 345.5
  fit 345.9
  focal (motor) 345.5
  gelastic 345.8
  generalized 345.9
    convulsive 345.1
    flexion 345.1
    nonconvulsive 345.0
  grand mal (idiopathic) 345.1
  Jacksonian (motor) (sensory) 345.5
  Kojevnikoff's, Kojevnikov's, Kojewnikoff's
    345.7
  laryngeal 786.2
  limbic system 345.4
  localization related (focal) (partial) and epileptic
    syndromes
    with
      complex partial seizures 345.4
      simple partial seizures 345.5
  major (motor) 345.1
  minor 345.0
  mixed (type) 345.9
  motor partial 345.5
  musicogenic 345.1
  myoclonus, myoclonic 345.1
    progressive (familial) 333.2
  nonconvulsive, generalized 345.0
  parasitic NEC 123.9
  partial (focalized) 345.5
    with
      impairment of consciousness 345.4
      memory and ideational disturbances 345.4
    abdominal type 345.5
    motor type 345.5
    psychomotor type 345.4

Epilepsy, epileptic—*continued*
  psychosensory type 345.4
  secondarily generalized 345.4
  sensory type 345.5
  somatomotor type 345.5
  somatosensory type 345.5
  temporal lobe type 345.4
  visceral type 345.5
  visual type 345.5
  without impairment of consciousness 345.5
  peripheral 345.9
  petit mal 345.0
  photokinetic 345.8
  progressive myoclonic (familial) 333.2
  psychic equivalent 345.5
  psychomotor 345.4
  psychosensory 345.4
  reflex 345.1
  seizure 345.9
  senile 345.9
  sensory-induced 345.5
  sleep (*see also* Narcolepsy) 347.00
  somatomotor type 345.5
  somatosensory 345.5
  specified type NEC 345.8
  status (grand mal) 345.3
    focal motor 345.7
    petit mal 345.2
    psychomotor 345.7
    temporal lobe 345.7
  symptomatic 345.9
  temporal lobe 345.4
  tonic (-clonic) 345.1
  traumatic (injury unspecified) 907.0
    injury specified—*see* Late, effect (of)
      specified injury
  twilight 293.0
  uncinate (gyrus) 345.4
  Unverricht (-Lundborg) (familial myoclonic)
    333.2
  visceral 345.5
  visual 345.5
Epileptiform
  convulsions 780.39
  seizure 780.39
Epiloia 759.5
Epimenorrhea 626.2
Epipharyngitis (*see also* Nasopharyngitis) 460
Epiphora 375.20
  due to
    excess lacrimation 375.21
    insufficient drainage 375.22
Epiphyseal arrest 733.91
  femoral head 732.2
Epiphyseolysis, epiphysiolysis (*see also*
  Osteochondrosis) 732.9
Epiphysitis (*see also* Osteochondrosis) 732.9
  juvenile 732.6
  marginal (Scheuermann's) 732.0
  os calcis 732.5
  syphilitic (congenital) 090.0
  vertebral (Scheuermann's) 732.0
Epiplocele (*see also* Hernia) 553.9
Epiploitis (*see also* Peritonitis) 567.9
Epiplosarcomphalocele (*see also* Hernia,
  umbilicus) 553.1
Episcleritis 379.00
  gouty 274.89 *[379.09]*
  nodular 379.02
  periodica fugax 379.01
    angioneurotic—*see* Edema, angioneurotic

Episcleritis—*continued*
  specified NEC 379.09
  staphylococcal 379.00
  suppurative 379.00
  syphilitic 095.0
  tuberculous (*see also* Tuberculosis) 017.3
    [379.09]
Episode
  brain (*see also* Disease, cerebrovascular, acute)
    436
  cerebral (*see also* Disease, cerebrovascular,
    acute) 436
  depersonalization (in neurotic state) 300.6
  hyporesponsive 780.09
  psychotic (*see also* Psychosis) 298.9
    organic, transient 293.9
  schizophrenic (acute) NEC (*see also*
    Schizophrenia) 295.4
Epispadias
  female 753.8
  male 752.62
Episplenitis 289.59
Epistaxis (multiple) 784.7
  hereditary 448.0
  vicarious menstruation 625.8
Epithelioma (malignant) (M8011/3)—*see also*
  Neoplasm, by site, malignant
  adenoides cysticum (M8100/0)—*see* Neoplasm,
    skin, benign
  basal cell (M8090/3)—*see* Neoplasm, skin,
    malignant
  benign (M8011/0)—*see* Neoplasm, by site,
    benign
  Bowen's (M8081/2)—*see* Neoplasm, skin, in
    situ
  calcifying (benign) (Malherbe's)
    (M8110/0)—*see* Neoplasm, skin, benign
  external site—*see* Neoplasm, skin, malignant
  intraepidermal, Jadassohn (M8096/0)—*see*
    Neoplasm, skin, benign
  squamous cell (M8070/3)—*see* Neoplasm, by
    site, malignant
Epitheliopathy
  pigment, retina 363.15
  posterior multifocal placoid (acute) 363.15
Epithelium, epithelial —*see* condition
Epituberculosis (allergic) (with atelectasis) (*see*
  also Tuberculosis) 010.8
Eponychia 757.5
Epstein's
  nephrosis or syndrome (*see also* Nephrosis)
    581.9
  pearl (mouth) 528.4
Epstein-Barr infection (viral) 075
  chronic 780.79 *[139.8]*
Epulis (giant cell) (gingiva) 523.8
Equinia 024
Equinovarus (congenital) 754.51
  acquired 736.71
Equivalent
  convulsive (abdominal) (*see also* Epilepsy)
    345.5
  epileptic (psychic) (*see also* Epilepsy) 345.5
Erb's
  disease 359.1
  palsy, paralysis (birth) (brachial) (newborn) 767.6
    spinal (spastic) syphilitic 094.89
  pseudohypertrophic muscular dystrophy 359.1
Erb (-Duchenne) paralysis (birth injury)
  (newborn) 767.6
Erb-Goldflam disease or syndrome 358.00

Erdheim's syndrome (acromegalic
  macrospondylitis) 253.0
Erection, painful (persistent) 607.3
Ergosterol deficiency (vitamin D) 268.9
  with
    osteomalacia 268.2
    rickets (*see also* Rickets) 268.0
Ergotism (ergotized grain) 988.2
  from ergot used as drug (migraine therapy)
    correct substance properly administered 349.82
    overdose or wrong substance given or taken 975.0
Erichsen's disease (railway spine) 300.16
Erlacher-Blount syndrome (tibia vara) 732.4
Erosio interdigitalis blastomycetica 112.3
Erosion
  arteriosclerotic plaque—*see* Arteriosclerosis, by
    site
  artery NEC 447.2
    without rupture 447.8
  bone 733.99
  bronchus 519.19
  cartilage (joint) 733.99
  cervix (uteri) (acquired) (chronic) (congenital)
    622.0
    with mention of cervicitis 616.0
  cornea (recurrent) (*see also* Keratitis) 371.42
    traumatic 918.1
  dental (idiopathic) (occupational) 521.30
    extending into
      dentine 521.32
      pulp 521.33
    generalized 521.35
    limited to enamel 521.31
    localized 521.34
  duodenum, postpyloric—*see* Ulcer, duodenum
  esophagus 530.89
  gastric 535.4
  intestine 569.89
  lymphatic vessel 457.8
  pylorus, pyloric (ulcer) 535.4
  sclera 379.16
  spine, aneurysmal 094.89
  spleen 289.59
  stomach 535.4
  teeth (idiopathic) (occupational) (*see also* Erosion,
    dental) 521.30
    due to
      medicine 521.30
      persistent vomiting 521.30
  urethra 599.84
  uterus 621.8
  vertebra 733.99
Erotomania 302.89
  Clérambault's 297.8
Error
  in diet 269.9
  refractive 367.9
    astigmatism (*see also* Astigmatism) 367.20
    drug-induced 367.89
    hypermetropia 367.0
    hyperopia 367.0
    myopia 367.1
    presbyopia 367.4
    toxic 367.89
Eructation 787.3
  nervous 306.4
  psychogenic 306.4
Eruption
  creeping 126.9
  drug—*see* Dermatitis, due to, drug
  Hutchinson, summer 692.72

Eruption—*continued*
  Kaposi's varicelliform 054.0
  napkin (psoriasiform) 691.0
  polymorphous
    light (sun) 692.72
      other source 692.82
  psoriasiform, napkin 691.0
  recalcitrant pustular 694.8
  ringed 695.89
  skin (*see also* Dermatitis) 782.1
    creeping (meaning hookworm) 126.9
    due to
      chemical(s) NEC 692.4
        internal use 693.8
      drug—*see* Dermatitis, due to, drug
      prophylactic inoculation or vaccination
          against disease—*see* Dermatitis, due to,
          vaccine
      smallpox vaccination NEC—*see* Dermatitis,
          due to, vaccine
    erysipeloid 027.1
    feigned 698.4
    Hutchinson, summer 692.72
    Kaposi's, varicelliform 054.0
      vaccinia 999.0
    lichenoid, axilla 698.3
    polymorphous, due to light 692.72
    toxic NEC 695.0
    vesicular 709.8
  teeth, tooth
    accelerated 520.6
    delayed 520.6
    difficult 520.6
    disturbance of 520.6
    in abnormal sequence 520.6
    incomplete 520.6
    late 520.6
    natal 520.6
    neonatal 520.6
    obstructed 520.6
    partial 520.6
    persistent primary 520.6
    premature 520.6
    prenatal 520.6
  vesicular 709.8
Erysipelas (gangrenous) (infantile) (newborn)
    (phlegmonous) (suppurative) 035
  external ear 035 *[380.13]*
  puerperal, postpartum, childbirth 670
Erysipelatoid (Rosenbach's) 027.1
Erysipeloid (Rosenbach's) 027.1
Erythema, erythematous (generalized) 695.9
  ab igne—*see* Burn, by site, first degree
  annulare (centrifugum) (rheumaticum) 695.0
  arthriticum epidemicum 026.1
  brucellum (*see also* Brucellosis) 023.9
  bullosum 695.1
  caloricum—*see* Burn, by site, first degree
  chronicum migrans 088.81
    chronicum 088.81
  circinatum 695.1
  diaper 691.0
  due to
    chemical (contact) NEC 692.4
      internal 693.8
    drug (internal use) 693.0
      contact 692.3
  elevatum diutinum 695.89
  endemic 265.2
  epidemic, arthritic 026.1
  figuratum perstans 695.0

Erythema, erythematous—*continued*
  gluteal 691.0
  gyratum (perstans) (repens) 695.1
  heat—*see* Burn, by site, first degree
  ichthyosiforme congenitum 757.1
  induratum (primary) (scrofulosorum) (*see also*
      Tuberculosis) 017.1
    nontuberculous 695.2
  infantum febrile 057.8
  infectional NEC 695.9
  infectiosum 057.0
  inflammation NEC 695.9
  intertrigo 695.89
  iris 695.1
  lupus (discoid) (localized) (*see also* Lupus,
      erythematosus) 695.4
  marginatum 695.0
    rheumaticum—*see* Fever, rheumatic
  medicamentosum—*see* Dermatitis, due to, drug
  migrans 529.1
  multiforme 695.1
    bullosum 695.1
    conjunctiva 695.1
    exudativum (Hebra) 695.1
    pemphigoides 694.5
  napkin 691.0
  neonatorum 778.8
  nodosum 695.2
    tuberculous (*see also* Tuberculosis) 017.1
  nummular, nummulare 695.1
  palmar 695.0
  palmaris hereditarium 695.0
  pernio 991.5
  perstans solare 692.72
  rash, newborn 778.8
  scarlatiniform (exfoliative) (recurrent) 695.0
  simplex marginatum 057.8
  solare (*see also* Sunburn) 692.71
  streptogenes 696.5
  toxic, toxicum NEC 695.0
    newborn 778.8
  tuberculous (primary) (*see also* Tuberculosis)
      017.0
  venenatum 695.0
Erythematosus —*see* condition
Erythematous —*see* condition
Erythermalgia (primary) 443.82
Erythralgia 443.82
Erythrasma 039.0
Erythredema 985.0
  polyneuritica 985.0
  polyneuropathy 985.0
Erythremia (acute) (M9841/3) 207.0
  chronic (M9842/3) 207.1
  secondary 289.0
Erythroblastopenia (acquired) 284.8
  congenital 284.01
Erythroblastophthisis 284.01
Erythroblastosis (fetalis) (newborn) 773.2
  due to
    ABO
      antibodies 773.1
      incompatibility, maternal/fetal 773.1
      isoimmunization 773.1
    Rh
      antibodies 773.0
      incompatibility, maternal/fetal 773.0
      isoimmunization 773.0
Erythrocyanosis (crurum) 443.89
Erythrocythemia —*see* Erythremia
Erythrocytopenia 285.9

Erythrocytosis (megalosplenic)
  familial 289.6
  oval, hereditary (*see also* Elliptocytosis) 282.1
  secondary 289.0
  stress 289.0
Erythroderma (*see also* Erythema) 695.9
  desquamativa (in infants) 695.89
  exfoliative 695.89
  ichthyosiform, congenital 757.1
  infantum 695.89
  maculopapular 696.2
  neonatorum 778.8
  psoriaticum 696.1
  secondary 695.9
Erythrogenesis imperfecta 284.09
Erythroleukemia (M9840/3) 207.0
Erythromelalgia 443.82
Erythromelia 701.8
Erythropenia 285.9
Erythrophagocytosis 289.9
Erythrophobia 300.23
Erythroplakia
  oral mucosa 528.79
  tongue 528.79
Erythroplasia (Queyrat) (M8080/2)
  specified site—*see* Neoplasm, skin, in situ
  unspecified site 233.5
Erythropoiesis, idiopathic ineffective 285.0
Escaped beats, heart 427.60
  postoperative 997.1
Esoenteritis —*see* Enteritis
Esophagalgia 530.89
Esophagectasis 530.89
  due to cardiospasm 530.0
Esophagismus 530.5
Esophagitis (alkaline) (chemical) (chronic)
    (infectional) (necrotic) (postoperative) 530.10
  acute 530.12
  candidal 112.84
  reflux 530.11
  specified NEC 530.19
  tuberculous (*see also* Tuberculosis) 017.8
  ulcerative 530.19
Esophagocele 530.6
Esophagodynia 530.89
Esophagomalacia 530.89
Esophagoptosis 530.89
Esophagospasm 530.5
Esophagostenosis 530.3
Esophagostomiasis 127.7
Esophagostomy
  complication 530.87
    infection 530.86
    malfunctioning 530.87
    mechanical 530.87
Esophagotracheal —*see* condition
Esophagus —*see* condition
Esophoria 378.41
  convergence, excess 378.84
  divergence, insufficiency 378.85
Esotropia (nonaccommodative) 378.00
  accommodative 378.35
  alternating 378.05
    with
      A pattern 378.06
      specified noncomitancy NEC 378.08
      V pattern 378.07
      X pattern 378.08
      Y pattern 378.08
    intermittent 378.22

Esotropia—*continued*
  intermittent 378.20
    alternating 378.22
    monocular 378.21
  monocular 378.01
    with
      A pattern 378.02
      specified noncomitancy NEC 378.04
      V pattern 378.03
      X pattern 378.04
      Y pattern 378.04
    intermittent 378.21
Espundia 085.5
Essential —*see* condition
Esterapenia 289.89
Esthesioneuroblastoma (M9522/3) 160.0
Esthesioneurocytoma (M9521/3) 160.0
Esthesioneuroepithelioma (M9523/3) 160.0
Esthiomene 099.1
Estivo-autumnal
  fever 084.0
  malaria 084.0
Estrangement V61.0
Estriasis 134.0
Ethanolaminuria 270.8
Ethanolism (*see also* Alcoholism) 303.9
Ether dependence, dependency (*see also*
    Dependence) 304.6
Etherism (*see also* Dependence) 304.6
Ethmoid, ethmoidal —*see* condition
Ethmoiditis (chronic) (nonpurulent) (purulent)
    (*see also* Sinusitis, ethmoidal) 473.2
  influenzal 487.1
  Woakes' 471.1
Ethylism (*see also* Alcoholism) 303.9
Eulenburg's disease (congenital paramyotonia)
    359.2
Eunuchism 257.2
Eunuchoidism 257.2
  hypogonadotropic 257.2
European blastomycosis 117.5
Eustachian —*see* condition
Euthyroid sick syndrome 790.94
Euthyroidism 244.9
Evaluation
  fetal lung maturity 659.8
  for suspected condition (*see also* Observation) V71.9
    abuse V71.81
    exposure
      antrax V71.82
      biologic agent NEC V71.83
      SARS V71.83
    neglect V71.81
    newborn—*see* Observation, suspected,
      condition, newborn
    specified condition NEC V71.89
  mental health V70.2
    requested by authority V70.1
  nursing care V63.8
  social service V63.8
Evans' syndrome (thrombocytopenic purpura)
    287.32
Eventration
  colon into chest—*see* Hernia, diaphragm
  diaphragm (congenital) 756.6
Eversion
  bladder 596.8
  cervix (uteri) 622.0
    with mention of cervicitis 616.0
  foot NEC 736.79

Excess, excessive, excessively—*continued*
  D (dietary) 278.4
    administered as drug (chronic) (prolonged
      excessive intake) 278.4
      reaction to sudden overdose 963.5
  weight 278.02
    gain 783.1
      of pregnancy 646.1
    loss 783.21
Excitability, abnormal, under minor stress
  309.29
Excitation
  catatonic (*see also* Schizophrenia) 295.2
  psychogenic 298.1
  reactive (from emotional stress, psychological
    trauma) 298.1
Excitement
  manic (*see also* Psychosis, affective) 296.0
    recurrent episode 296.1
    single episode 296.0
  mental, reactive (from emotional stress,
    psychological trauma) 298.1
  state, reactive (from emotional stress,
    psychological trauma) 298.1
Excluded pupils 364.76
Excoriation (traumatic) (*see also* Injury,
  superficial, by site) 919.8
  neurotic 698.4
Excyclophoria 378.44
Excyclotropia 378.33
Exencephalus, exencephaly 742.0
Exercise
  breathing V57.0
  remedial NEC V57.1
  therapeutic NEC V57.1
Exfoliation, teeth due to systemic causes 525.0
Exfoliative —*see also* condition
  dermatitis 695.89
Exhaustion, exhaustive (physical NEC) 780.79
  battle (*see also* Reaction, stress, acute) 308.9
  cardiac (*see also* Failure, heart) 428.9
  delirium (*see also* Reaction, stress, acute) 308.9
  due to
    cold 991.8
    excessive exertion 994.5
    exposure 994.4
  fetus or newborn 779.89
  heart (*see also* Failure, heart) 428.9
  heat 992.5
    due to
      salt depletion 992.4
      water depletion 992.3
  manic (*see also* Psychosis, affective) 296.0
    recurrent episode 296.1
    single episode 296.0
  maternal, complicating delivery 669.8
    affecting fetus or newborn 763.89
  mental 300.5
  myocardium, myocardial (*see also* Failure,
    heart) 428.9
  nervous 300.5
  old age 797
  postinfectional NEC 780.79
  psychogenic 300.5
  psychosis (*see also* Reaction, stress, acute)
    308.9
  senile 797
    dementia 290.0
Exhibitionism (sexual) 302.4
Exomphalos 756.79

Exophoria 378.42
  convergence, insufficiency 378.83
  divergence, excess 378.85
Exophthalmic
  cachexia 242.0
  goiter 242.0
  ophthalmoplegia 242.0 *[376.22]*
Exophthalmos 376.30
  congenital 743.66
  constant 376.31
  endocrine NEC 259.9 *[376.22]*
  hyperthyroidism 242.0 *[376.21]*
  intermittent NEC 376.34
  malignant 242.0 *[376.21]*
  pulsating 376.35
    endocrine NEC 259.9 *[376.22]*
  thyrotoxic 242.0 *[376.21]*
Exostosis 726.91
  cartilaginous (M9210/0)—*see* Neoplasm, bone,
    benign
  congenital 756.4
  ear canal, external 380.81
  gonococcal 098.89
  hip 726.5
  intracranial 733.3
  jaw (bone) 526.81
  luxurians 728.11
  multiple (cancellous) (congenital) (hereditary)
    756.4
  nasal bones 726.91
  orbit, orbital 376.42
  osteocartilaginous (M9210/0)—*see* Neoplasm,
    bone, benign
  spine 721.8
    with spondylosis—*see* Spondylosis
  syphilitic 095.5
  wrist 726.4
Exotropia 378.10
  alternating 378.15
    with
      A pattern 378.16
      specified noncomitancy 378.18
      V pattern 378.17
      X pattern 378.18
      Y pattern 378.18
    intermittent 378.24
  intermittent 378.20
    alternating 378.24
    monocular 378.23
  monocular 378.11
    with
      A pattern 378.12
      specified noncomitancy NEC 378.14
      V pattern 378.13
      X pattern 378.14
      Y pattern 378.14
    intermittent 378.23
Explanation of
  investigation finding V65.4
  medication V65.4
Exposure 994.9
  cold 991.9
    specified effect NEC 991.8
  effects of 994.9
  exhaustion due to 994.4
  to
    AIDS virus V01.79
    antrax V01.81
    asbestos V15.84
    body fluids (hazardous) V15.85
    cholera V01.0

Exposure—*continued*
  communicable disease V01.9
    specified type NEC V01.89
  Escherichia coli (E. coli) V01.83
  German measles V01.4
  gonorrhea V01.6
  hazardous body fluids V15.85
  HIV V01.79
  human immunodeficiency virus V01.79
  lead V15.86
  meningococcus V01.84
  parasitic disease V01.89
  poliomyelitis V01.2
  potentially hazardous body fluids V15.85
  rabies V01.5
  rubella V01.4
  SARS-associated coronavirus V01.82
  smallpox V01.3
  syphilis V01.6
  tuberculosis V01.1
  varicella V01.71
  venereal disease V01.6
  viral disease NEC V01.79
    varicella V01.71
Exsanguination, fetal 772.0
Exstrophy
  abdominal content 751.8
  bladder (urinary) 753.5
Extensive —*see* condition
Extra —*see also* Accessory
  rib 756.3
    cervical 756.2
Extraction
  with hook 763.89
  breech NEC 669.6
    affecting fetus or newborn 763.0
  cataract postsurgical V45.61
  manual NEC 669.8
    affecting fetus or newborn 763.89
Extrasystole 427.60
  atrial 427.61
  postoperative 997.1
  ventricular 427.69
Extrauterine gestation or pregnancy —*see*
  Pregnancy, ectopic
Extravasation
  blood 459.0
    lower extremity 459.0
  chyle into mesentery 457.8
  pelvicalyceal 593.4
  pyelosinus 593.4
  urine 788.8
    from ureter 788.8
Extremity —*see* condition
Extrophy —*see* Exstrophy
Extroversion
  bladder 753.5
  uterus 618.1
    complicating delivery 665.2
      affecting fetus or newborn 763.89
    postpartal (old) 618.1
Extruded tooth 524.34
Extrusion
  alveolus and teeth 524.75
  breast implant (prosthetic) 996.54
  device, implant, or graft—*see* Complications,
    mechanical
  eye implant (ball) (globe) 996.59
  intervertebral disc—*see* Displacement,
    intervertebral disc
  lacrimal gland 375.43

Extrusion—*continued*
  mesh (reinforcing) 996.59
  ocular lens implant 996.53
  prosthetic device NEC—*see* Complications,
    mechanical
  vitreous 379.26
Exudate, pleura —*see* Effusion, pleura
Exudates, retina 362.82
Exudative —*see* condition
Eye, eyeball, eyelid—*see* condition
Eyestrain 368.13
Eyeworm disease of Africa 125.2

F

Faber's anemia or syndrome (achlorhydric anemia) 280.9

Fabry's disease (angiokeratoma corporis diffusum) 272.7

Face, facial —*see* condition

Facet of cornea 371.44

Faciocephalalgia, autonomic (*see also* Neuropathy, peripheral, autonomic) 337.9

Facioscapulohumeral myopathy 359.1

Factitious disorder, illness —*see* Illness, factitious

Factor
deficiency—*see* Deficiency, factor
psychic, associated with diseases classified elsewhere 316
risk—*see* Problem

Fahr-Volhard disease (malignant nephrosclerosis) 403.00

Failure, failed
adenohypophyseal 253.2
attempted abortion (legal) (*see also* Abortion, failed) 638.9
bone marrow (anemia) 284.9
acquired (secondary) 284.8
congenital 284.09
idiopathic 284.9
cardiac (*see also* Failure, heart) 428.9
newborn 779.89
cardiorenal (chronic) 428.9
hypertensive (*see also* Hypertension, cardiorenal) 404.93
cardiorespiratory 799.1
specified during or due to a procedure 997.1
long-term effect of cardiac surgery 429.4
cardiovascular (chronic) 428.9
cerebrovascular 437.8
cervical dilatation in labor 661.0
affecting fetus or newborn 763.7
circulation, circulatory 799.89
fetus or newborn 779.89
peripheral 785.50
compensation—*see* Disease, heart
congestive (*see also* Failure, heart) 428.0
coronary (*see also* Insufficiency, coronary) 411.89
dental restoration
marginal integrity 525.61
periodontal anatomical integrity 525.65
descent of head (at term) 652.5
affecting fetus or newborn 763.1
in labor 660.0
affecting fetus or newborn 763.1
device, implant, or graft—*see* Complications, mechanical
engagement of head NEC 652.5
in labor 660.0
extrarenal 788.9
fetal head to enter pelvic brim 652.5
affecting fetus or newborn 763.1
in labor 660.0
affecting fetus or newborn 763.1
forceps NEC 660.7
affecting fetus or newborn 763.1
fusion (joint) (spinal) 996.49
growth in childhood 783.43

Failure, failed—*continued*
heart (acute) (sudden) 428.9
with
abortion—*see* Abortion, by type, with specified complication NEC
acute pulmonary edema (*see also* Failure, ventricular, left) 428.1
with congestion (*see also* Failure, heart) 428.0
decompensation (*see also* Failure, heart) 428.0
dilation—*see* Disease, heart
ectopic pregnancy (*see also* categories 633.0-633.9) 639.8
molar pregnancy (*see also* categories 630-632) 639.8
arteriosclerotic 440.9
combined left-right sided 428.0
combined systolic and diastolic 428.40
acute 428.41
acute on chronic 428.43
chronic 428.42
compensated (*see also* Failure, heart) 428.0
complicating
abortion—*see* Abortion, by type, with specified complication NEC
delivery (cesarean) (instrumental) 669.4
ectopic pregnancy (*see also* categories 633.0-633.9) 639.8
molar pregnancy (*see also* categories 630-632) 639.8
obstetric anesthesia or sedation 668.1
surgery 997.1
congestive (compensated) (decompensated) (*see also* Failure, heart) 428.0
with rheumatic fever (conditions classifiable to 390)
active 391.8
inactive or quiescent (with chorea) 398.91
fetus or newborn 779.89
hypertensive (*see also* Hypertension, heart) 402.91
with renal disease (*see also* Hypertension, cardiorenal) 404.91
with renal failure 404.93
benign 402.11
malignant 402.01
rheumatic (chronic) (inactive) (with chorea) 398.91
active or acute 391.8
with chorea (Sydenham's) 392.0
decompensated (*see also* Failure, heart) 428.0
degenerative (*see also* Degeneration, myocardial) 429.1
diastolic 428.30
acute 428.31
acute or chronic 428.33
chronic 428.32
due to presence of (cardiac) prosthesis 429.4
fetus or newborn 779.89
following
abortion 639.8
cardiac surgery 429.4
ectopic or molar pregnancy 639.8
high output NEC 428.9

Fat *—continued*
  breast (aseptic) (segmental) 611.3
  mesentery 567.82
  omentum 567.82
  peritoneum 567.82
  pad 278.1
Fatal syncope 798.1
Fatigue 780.79
  auditory deafness (*see also* Deafness) 389.9
  chronic, syndrome 780.71
  combat (*see also* Reaction, stress, acute) 308.9
  during pregnancy 646.8
  general 780.79
    psychogenic 300.5
  heat (transient) 992.6
  muscle 729.89
  myocardium (*see also* Failure, heart) 428.9
  nervous 300.5
  neurosis 300.5
  operational 300.89
  postural 729.89
  posture 729.89
  psychogenic (general) 300.5
  senile 797
  syndrome NEC 300.5
    chronic 780.71
  undue 780.79
  voice 784.49
Fatness 278.02
Fatty *—see also* condition
  apron 278.1
  degeneration (diffuse) (general) NEC 272.8
    localized—*see* Degeneration, by site, fatty
    placenta—*see* Placenta, abnormal
  heart (enlarged) (*see also* Degeneration,
    myocardial) 429.1
  infiltration (diffuse) (general) (*see also*
    Degeneration, by site, fatty) 272.8
    heart (enlarged) (*see also* Degeneration,
      myocardial) 429.1
  liver 571.8
    alcoholic 571.0
  necrosis—*see* Degeneration, fatty
  phanerosis 272.8
Fauces *—see* condition
Fauchard's disease (periodontitis) 523.40
Faucitis 478.29
Faulty *—see also* condition
  position of teeth 524.30
Favism (anemia) 282.2
Favre-Racouchot disease (elastoidosis cutanea
  nodularis) 701.8
Favus 110.9
  beard 110.0
  capitis 110.0
  corporis 110.5
  eyelid 110.8
  foot 110.4
  hand 110.2
  scalp 110.0
  specified site NEC 110.8
Fear, fearfulness (complex) (reaction) 300.20
  child 313.0
  of
    animals 300.29
    closed spaces 300.29
    crowds 300.29
    eating in public 300.23
    heights 300.29
    open spaces 300.22
      with panic attacks 300.21

Fear, fearfulness—*continued*
  public speaking 300.23
  streets 300.22
    with panic attacks 300.21
  travel 300.22
    with panic attacks 300.21
  washing in public 300.23
  transient 308.0
Feared complaint unfounded V65.5
Febricula (continued) (simple) (*see also* Pyrexia)
  780.6
Febrile (*see also* Pyrexia) 780.6
  convulsion (simple) 780.31
    complex 780.32
  seizure (simple) 780.31
    atypical 780.32
    complex 780.32
    complicated 780.32
Febris (*see also* Fever) 780.6
  aestiva (*see also* Fever, hay) 477.9
  flava (*see also* Fever, yellow) 060.9
  melitensis 023.0
  pestis (*see also* Plague) 020.9
  puerperalis 672
  recurrens (*see also* Fever, relapsing) 087.9
    pediculo vestimenti 087.0
  rubra 034.1
  typhoidea 002.0
  typhosa 002.0
Fecal *—see* condition
Fecalith (impaction) 560.39
  with hernia—*see also* Hernia, by site, with
    obstruction
    gangrenous—*see* Hernia, by site, with
      gangrene
  appendix 543.9
  congenital 777.1
Fede's disease 529.0
Feeble-minded 317
Feeble rapid pulse due to shock following
  injury 958.4
Feeding
  faulty (elderly) (infant) 783.3
    newborn 779.3
  formula check V20.2
  improper (elderly) (infant) 783.3
    newborn 779.3
  problem (elderly) (infant) 783.3
    newborn 779.3
  nonorganic origin 307.59
Feer's disease 985.0
Feet *—see* condition
Feigned illness V65.2
Feil-Klippel syndrome (brevicollis) 756.16
Feinmesser's (hidrotic) ectodermal dysplasia
  757.31
Felix's disease (juvenile osteochondrosis, hip)
  732.1
Felon (any digit) (with lymphangitis) 681.01
  herpetic 054.6
Felty's syndrome (rheumatoid arthritis with
  splenomegaly and leukopenia) 714.1
Feminism in boys 302.6
Feminization, testicular 259.5
  with pseudohermaphroditism, male 259.5
Femoral hernia *—see* Hernia, femoral
Femora vara 736.32
Femur, femoral *—see* condition
Fenestrata placenta *—see* Placenta, abnormal

Fenestration, fenestrated —*see also* Imperfect, closure
  aorta-pulmonary 745.0
  aorticopulmonary 745.0
  aortopulmonary 745.0
  cusps, heart valve NEC 746.89
    pulmonary 746.09
  hymen 752.49
  pulmonic cusps 746.09
Fenwick's disease 537.89
Fermentation (gastric) (gastrointestinal) (stomach) 536.8
  intestine 564.89
    psychogenic 306.4
  psychogenic 306.4
Fernell's disease (aortic aneurysm) 441.9
Fertile eunuch syndrome 257.2
Fertility, meaning multiparity—*see* Multiparity
Fetal alcohol syndrome 760.71
Fetalis uterus 752.3
Fetid
  breath 784.99
  sweat 705.89
Fetishism 302.81
  transvestic 302.3
Fetomaternal hemorrhage
  affecting management of pregnancy 656.0
  fetus or newborn 772.0
Fetus, fetal —*see also* condition
  papyraceous 779.89
  type lung tissue 770.4
Fever 780.6
  with chills 780.6
    in malarial regions (*see also* Malaria) 084.6
  abortus NEC 023.9
  Aden 061
  African tick-borne 087.1
  American
    mountain tick 066.1
    spotted 082.0
  and ague (*see also* Malaria) 084.6
  aphthous 078.4
  arbovirus hemorrhagic 065.9
  Assam 085.0
  Australian A or Q 083.0
  Bangkok hemorrhagic 065.4
  biliary, Charcot's intermittent—*see* Choledocholithiasis
  bilious, hemoglobinuric 084.8
  blackwater 084.8
  blister 054.9
  Bonvale Dam 780.79
  boutonneuse 082.1
  brain 323.9
    late effect—*see* category 326
  breakbone 061
  Bullis 082.8
  Bunyamwera 066.3
  Burdwan 085.0
  Bwamba (encephalitis) 066.3
  Cameroon (*see also* Malaria) 084.6
  Canton 081.9
  catarrhal (acute) 460
    chronic 472.0
  cat-scratch 078.3
  cerebral 323.9
    late effect—*see* category 326
  cerebrospinal (meningococcal) (*see also* Meningitis, cerebrospinal) 036.0
  Chagres 084.0
  Chandipura 066.8

Fever—*continued*
  changuinola 066.0
  Charcot's (biliary) (hepatic) (intermittent)—*see* Choledocholithiasis
  Chikungunya (viral) 066.3
    hemorrhagic 065.4
  childbed 670
  Chitral 066.0
  Colombo (*see also* Fever, paratyphoid) 002.9
  Colorado tick (virus) 066.1
  congestive
    malarial (*see also* Malaria) 084.6
    remittent (*see also* Malaria) 084.6
  Congo virus 065.0
  continued 780.6
    malarial 084.0
  Corsican (*see also* Malaria) 084.6
  Crimean hemorrhagic 065.0
  Cyprus (*see also* Brucellosis) 023.9
  dandy 061
  deer fly (*see also* Tularemia) 021.9
  dehydration, newborn 778.4
  dengue (virus) 061
    hemorrhagic 065.4
  desert 114.0
  due to heat 992.0
  Dumdum 085.0
  enteric 002.0
  ephemeral (of unknown origin) (*see also* Pyrexia) 780.6
  epidemic, hemorrhagic of the Far East 065.0
  erysipelatous (*see also* Erysipelas) 035
  estivo-autumnal (malarial) 084.0
  etiocholanolone 277.31
  famine—*see also* Fever, relapsing
    meaning typhus—*see* Typhus
  Far Eastern hemorrhagic 065.0
  five day 083.1
  Fort Bragg 100.89
  gastroenteric 002.0
  gastromalarial (*see also* Malaria) 084.6
  Gibraltar (*see also* Brucellosis) 023.9
  glandular 075
  Guama (viral) 066.3
  Haverhill 026.1
  hay (allergic) (with rhinitis) 477.9
    with
      asthma (bronchial) (*see also* Asthma) 493.0
    due to
      dander, animal (cat) (dog) 477.2
      dust 477.8
      fowl 477.8
      hair, animal (cat) (dog) 477.2
      pollen, any plant or tree 477.0
      specified allergen other than pollen 477.8
  heat (effects) 992.0
  hematuric, bilious 084.8
  hemoglobinuric (malarial) 084.8
    bilious 084.8
  hemorrhagic (arthropod-borne) NEC 065.9
    with renal syndrome 078.6
    arenaviral 078.7
    Argentine 078.7
    Bangkok 065.4
    Bolivian 078.7
    Central Asian 065.0
    chikungunya 065.4
    Crimean 065.0
    dengue (virus) 065.4
    Ebola 065.8
    epidemic 078.6

Fever—*continued*
    endocarditis (aortic) (mitral) (pulmonary)
        (tricuspid) 391.1
      multiple sites 391.8
      myocarditis 391.2
      pancarditis, acute 391.8
      pericarditis 391.0
      specified type NEC 391.8
      valvulitis 391.1
    inactive or quiescent with cardiac hypertrophy
      398.99
      carditis 398.90
      endocarditis 397.9
        aortic (valve) 395.9
          with mitral (valve) disease 396.9
        mitral (valve) 394.9
          with aortic (valve) disease 396.9
        pulmonary (valve) 397.1
        tricuspid (valve) 397.0
      heart conditions (classifiable to 429.3, 429.6,
        429.9) 398.99
        failure (congestive) (conditions classifiable
          to 428.0, 428.9) 398.91
        left ventricular failure (conditions
          classifiable to 428.1) 398.91
        myocardial degeneration (conditions
          classifiable to 429.1) 398.0
        myocarditis (conditions classifiable to
          429.0) 398.0
        pancarditis 398.99
        pericarditis 393
  Rift Valley (viral) 066.3
  Rocky Mountain spotted 082.0
  rose 477.0
  Ross river (viral) 066.3
  Russian hemorrhagic 078.6
  sandfly 066.0
  San Joaquin (valley) 114.0
  São Paulo 082.0
  scarlet 034.1
  septic—*see* Septicemia
  seven-day 061
    Japan 100.89
    Queensland 100.89
  shin bone 083.1
  Singapore hemorrhagic 065.4
  solar 061
  sore 054.9
  South African tick-bite 087.1
  Southeast Asia hemorrhagic 065.4
  spinal—*see* Meningitis
  spirillary 026.0
  splenic (*see also* Anthrax) 022.9
  spotted (Rocky Mountain) 082.0
    American 082.0
    Brazilian 082.0
    Colombian 082.0
    meaning
      cerebrospinal meningitis 036.0
      typhus 082.9
  spring 309.23
  steroid
    correct substance properly administered 780.6
    overdose or wrong substance given or taken
      962.0
  streptobacillary 026.1
  subtertian 084.0
  Sumatran mite 081.2
  sun 061
  swamp 100.89
  sweating 078.2

Fever—*continued*
  swine 003.8
  sylvatic yellow 060.0
  Tahyna 062.5
  tertian—*see* Malaria, tertian
  Thailand hemorrhagic 065.4
  thermic 992.0
  three day 066.0
    with Coxsackie exanthem 074.8
  tick
    American mountain 066.1
    Colorado 066.1
    Kemerovo 066.1
    Mediterranean 082.1
    mountain 066.1
    nonexanthematous 066.1
    Quaranfil 066.1
  tick-bite NEC 066.1
  tick-borne NEC 066.1
    hemorrhagic NEC 065.3
  transitory of newborn 778.4
  trench 083.1
  tsutsugamushi 081.2
  typhogastric 002.0
  typhoid (abortive) (ambulant) (any site)
    (hemorrhagic) (infection) (intermittent)
    (malignant) (rheumatic) 002.0
  typhomalarial (*see also* Malaria) 084.6
  typhus—*see* Typhus
  undulant (*see also* Brucellosis) 023.9
  unknown origin (*see also* Pyrexia) 780.6
  uremic—*see* Uremia
  uveoparotid 135
  valley (Coccidioidomycosis) 114.0
  Venezuelan equine 066.2
  Volhynian 083.1
  Wesselsbron (viral) 066.3
  West
    African 084.8
    Nile (viral) 066.40
      with
        cranial nerve disorders 066.42
        encephalitis 066.41
        optic neuritis 066.42
        other complications 066.49
        other neurologic manifestations 066.42
        polyradiculitis 066.42
  Whitmore's 025
  Wolhynian 083.1
  worm 128.9
  Yaroslav hemorrhagic 078.6
  yellow 060.9
    jungle 060.0
    sylvatic 060.0
    urban 060.1
    vaccination, prophylactic (against) V04.4
  Zika (viral) 066.3
Fibrillation
  atrial (established) (paroxysmal) 427.31
  auricular (atrial) (established) 427.31
  cardiac (ventricular) 427.41
  coronary (*see also* Infarct, myocardium) 410.9
  heart (ventricular) 427.41
  muscular 728.9
  postoperative 997.1
  ventricular 427.41
Fibrin
  ball or bodies, pleural (sac) 511.0
  chamber, anterior (eye) (gelatinous exudate)
    364.04
Fibrinogenolysis (hemorrhagic)—*see*
  Fibrinolysis

Fibrinogenopenia (congenital) (hereditary) (*see also* Defect, coagulation) 286.3
  acquired 286.6
Fibrinolysis (acquired) (hemorrhagic) (pathologic) 286.6
  with
    abortion—*see* Abortion, by type, with hemorrhage, delayed or excessive
    ectopic pregnancy (*see also* categories 633.0-633.9) 639.1
    molar pregnancy (*see also* categories 630-632) 639.1
  antepartum or intrapartum 641.3
    affecting fetus or newborn 762.1
  following
    abortion 639.1
    ectopic or molar pregnancy 639.1
  newborn, transient 776.2
  postpartum 666.3
Fibrinopenia (hereditary) (*see also* Defect, coagulation) 286.3
  acquired 286.6
Fibrinopurulent —*see* condition
Fibrinous —*see* condition
Fibroadenoma (M9010/0)
  cellular intracanalicular (M9020/0) 217
  giant (intracanalicular) (M9020/0) 217
  intracanalicular (M9011/0)
    cellular (M9020/0) 217
    giant (M9020/0) 217
    specified site—*see* Neoplasm, by site, benign
    unspecified site 217
  juvenile (M9030/0) 217
  pericanalicular (M9012/0)
    specified site—*see* Neoplasm, by site, benign
    unspecified site 217
  phyllodes (M9020/0) 217
  prostate 600.20
    with
      other lower urinary tract symptoms (LUTS) 600.21
      urinary
        obstruction 600.21
        retention 600.21
  specified site—*see* Neoplasm, by site, benign
  unspecified site 217
Fibroadenosis, breast (chronic) (cystic) (diffuse) (periodic) (segmental) 610.2
Fibroangioma (M9160/0)—*see also* Neoplasm, by site, benign
  juvenile (M9160/0)
    specified site—*see* Neoplasm, by site, benign
    unspecified site 210.7
Fibrocellulitis progressiva ossificans 728.11
Fibrochondrosarcoma (M9220/3)—*see* Neoplasm, cartilage, malignant
Fibrocystic
  disease 277.00
    bone NEC 733.29
    breast 610.1
    jaw 526.2
    kidney (congenital) 753.19
    liver 751.62
    lung 518.89
      congenital 748.4
    pancreas 277.00
    kidney (congenital) 753.19
Fibrodysplasia ossificans multiplex (progressiva) 728.11
Fibroelastosis (cordis) (endocardial) (endomyocardial) 425.3

Fibroid (tumor) (M8890/0)—*see also* Neoplasm, connective tissue, benign
  disease, lung (chronic) (*see also* Fibrosis, lung) 515
  heart (disease) (*see also* Myocarditis) 429.0
  induration, lung (chronic) (*see also* Fibrosis, lung) 515
  in pregnancy or childbirth 654.1
    affecting fetus or newborn 763.89
    causing obstructed labor 660.2
      affecting fetus or newborn 763.1
  liver—*see* Cirrhosis, liver
  lung (*see also* Fibrosis, lung) 515
  pneumonia (chronic) (*see also* Fibrosis, lung) 515
  uterus (M8890/0) (*see also* Leiomyoma, uterus) 218.9
Fibrolipoma (M8851/0) (*see also* Lipoma, by site) 214.9
Fibroliposarcoma (M8850/3)—*see* Neoplasm, connective tissue, malignant
Fibroma (M8810/0)—*see also* Neoplasm, connective tissue, benign
  ameloblastic (M9330/0) 213.1
    upper jaw (bone) 213.0
  bone (nonossifying) 733.99
    ossifying (M9262/0)—*see* Neoplasm, bone, benign
  cementifying (M9274/0)—*see* Neoplasm, bone, benign
  chondromyxoid (M9241/0)—*see* Neoplasm, bone, benign
  desmoplastic (M8823/1)—*see* Neoplasm, connective tissue, uncertain behavior
  facial (M8813/0)—*see* Neoplasm, connective tissue, benign
  invasive (M8821/1)—*see* Neoplasm, connective tissue, uncertain behavior
  molle (M8851/0) (*see also* Lipoma, by site) 214.9
  myxoid (M8811/0)—*see* Neoplasm, connective tissue, benign
  nasopharynx, nasopharyngeal (juvenile) (M9160/0) 210.7
  nonosteogenic (nonossifying)—*see* Dysplasia, fibrous
  odontogenic (M9321/0) 213.1
    upper jaw (bone) 213.0
  ossifying (M9262/0)—*see* Neoplasm, bone, benign
  periosteal (M8812/0)—*see* Neoplasm, bone, benign
  prostate 600.20
    with
      other lower urinary tract symptoms (LUTS) 600.21
      urinary
        obstruction 600.21
        retention 600.21
  soft (M8851/0) (*see also* Lipoma, by site) 214.9
Fibromatosis 728.79
  abdominal (M8822/1)—*see* Neoplasm, connective tissue, uncertain behavior
  aggressive (M8821/1)—*see* Neoplasm, connective tissue, uncertain behavior
  congenital generalized (CGF) 759.89
  Dupuytren's 728.6
  gingival 523.8
  plantar fascia 728.71
  proliferative 728.79
  pseudosarcomatous (proliferative) (subcutaneous) 728.79

Fibromatosis—*continued*
  subcutaneous pseudosarcomatous (proliferative)
    728.79
Fibromyalgia 729.1
Fibromyoma (M8890/0)—*see also* Neoplasm,
  connective tissue, benign
  uterus (corpus) (*see also* Leiomyoma, uterus)
    218.9
    in pregnancy or childbirth 654.1
      affecting fetus or newborn 763.89
      causing obstructed labor 660.2
        affecting fetus or newborn 763.1
Fibromyositis (*see also* Myositis) 729.1
  scapulohumeral 726.2
Fibromyxolipoma (M8852/0) (*see also* Lipoma,
  by site) 214.9
Fibromyxoma (M8811/0)—*see* Neoplasm,
  connective tissue, benign
Fibromyxosarcoma (M8811/3)—*see* Neoplasm,
  connective tissue, malignant
Fibro-odontoma, ameloblastic (M9290/0) 213.1
  upper jaw (bone) 213.0
Fibro-osteoma (M9262/0)—*see* Neoplasm, bone,
  benign
Fibroplasia, retrolental 362.21
Fibropurulent —*see* condition
Fibrosarcoma (M8810/3)—*see also* Neoplasm,
  connective tissue, malignant
  ameloblastic (M9330/3) 170.1
    upper jaw (bone) 170.0
  congenital (M8814/3)—*see* Neoplasm,
    connective tissue, malignant
  fascial (M8813/3)—*see* Neoplasm, connective
    tissue, malignant
  infantile (M8814/3)—*see* Neoplasm, connective
    tissue, malignant
  odontogenic (M9330/3) 170.1
    upper jaw (bone) 170.0
  periosteal (M8812/3)—*see* Neoplasm, bone,
    malignant
Fibrosclerosis
  breast 610.3
  corpora cavernosa (penis) 607.89
  familial multifocal NEC 710.8
  multifocal (idiopathic) NEC 710.8
  penis (corpora cavernosa) 607.89
Fibrosis, fibrotic
  adrenal (gland) 255.8
  alveolar (diffuse) 516.3
  amnion 658.8
  anal papillae 569.49
  anus 569.49
  appendix, appendiceal, noninflammatory 543.9
  arteriocapillary—*see* Arteriosclerosis
  bauxite (of lung) 503
  biliary 576.8
    due to Clonorchis sinensis 121.1
  bladder 596.8
    interstitial 595.1
    localized submucosal 595.1
    panmural 595.1
  bone, diffuse 756.59
  breast 610.3
  capillary—*see also* Arteriosclerosis
    lung (chronic) (*see also* Fibrosis, lung) 515
  cardiac (*see also* Myocarditis) 429.0
  cervix 622.8
  chorion 658.8
  corpus cavernosum 607.89

Fibrosis, fibrotic—*continued*
  cystic (of pancreas) 277.00
    with
      manifestations
        gastrointestinal 277.03
        pulmonary 277.02
        specified NEC 277.09
      meconium ileus 277.01
      pulmonary exacerbation 277.02
  due to (presence of) any device, implant, or
    graft—*see* Complications, due to (presence
    of) any device, implant, or graft classified to
    996.0-996.5 NEC
  ejaculatory duct 608.89
  endocardium (*see also* Endocarditis) 424.90
  endomyocardial (African) 425.0
  epididymis 608.89
  eye muscle 378.62
  graphite (of lung) 503
  heart (*see also* Myocarditis) 429.0
  hepatic—*see also* Cirrhosis, liver
    due to Clonorchis sinensis 121.1
  hepatolienal—*see* Cirrhosis, liver
  hepatosplenic—*see* Cirrhosis, liver
  infrapatellar fat pad 729.31
  interstitial pulmonary, newborn 770.7
  intrascrotal 608.89
  kidney (*see also* Sclerosis, renal) 587
  liver—*see* Cirrhosis, liver
  lung (atrophic) (capillary) (chronic) (confluent)
    (massive) (perialveolar) (peribronchial) 515
    with
      anthracosilicosis (occupational) 500
      anthracosis (occupational) 500
      asbestosis (occupational) 501
      bagassosis (occupational) 495.1
      bauxite 503
      berylliosis (occupational) 503
      byssinosis (occupational) 504
      calcicosis (occupational) 502
      chalicosis (occupational) 502
      dust reticulation (occupational) 504
      farmers' lung 495.0
      gannister disease (occupational) 502
      graphite 503
      pneumonoconiosis (occupational) 505
      pneumosiderosis (occupational) 503
      siderosis (occupational) 503
      silicosis (occupational) 502
    tuberculosis (*see also* Tuberculosis) 011.4
    diffuse (idiopathic) (interstitial) 516.3
    due to
      bauxite 503
      fumes or vapors (chemical) (inhalation) 506.4
      graphite 503
    following radiation 508.1
    postinflammatory 515
    silicotic (massive) (occupational) 502
    tuberculous (*see also* Tuberculosis) 011.4
  lymphatic gland 289.3
  median bar 600.90
    with
      other lower urinary tract symptoms (LUTS)
        600.91
      urinary
        obstruction 600.91
        retention 600.91
  mediastinum (idiopathic) 519.3
  meninges 349.2
  muscle NEC 728.2
    iatrogenic (from injection) 999.9

Findings, abnormal, without diagnosis
　　(examination) (laboratory test) 796.4
　17-ketosteroids, elevated 791.9
　acetonuria 791.6
　acid phosphatase 790.5
　albumin-globulin ratio 790.99
　albuminuria 791.0
　alcohol in blood 790.3
　alkaline phosphatase 790.5
　amniotic fluid 792.3
　amylase 790.5
　anisocytosis 790.09
　antenatal screening 796.5
　anthrax positive 795.31
　antibody titers, elevated 795.79
　anticardiolipin antibody 795.79
　antigen-antibody reaction 795.79
　antiphospholipid antibody 795.79
　bacteriuria 791.9
　ballistocardiogram 794.39
　bicarbonate 276.9
　bile in urine 791.4
　bilirubin 277.4
　bleeding time (prolonged) 790.92
　blood culture, positive 790.7
　blood gas level 790.91
　blood sugar level 790.29
　　high 790.29
　　　fasting glucose 790.21
　　　glucose tolerance test 790.22
　　low 251.2
　C-reactive protein (CRP) 790.95
　calcium 275.40
　cancer antigen 125 [CA 125] 795.82
　carbonate 276.9
　carcinoembryonic antigen [CEA] 795.81
　casts, urine 791.7
　catecholamines 791.9
　cells, urine 791.7
　cerebrospinal fluid (color) (content) (pressure)
　　792.0
　cervical
　　high risk human papillomavirus (HPV) DNA
　　　test positive 795.05
　　low risk human papillomavirus (HPV) DNA
　　　test positive 795.09
　chloride 276.9
　cholesterol 272.9
　chromosome analysis 795.2
　chyluria 791.1
　circulation time 794.39
　cloudy dialysis effluent 792.5
　cloudy urine 791.9
　coagulation study 790.92
　cobalt, blood 790.6
　color of urine (unusual) NEC 791.9
　copper, blood 790.6
　crystals, urine 791.9
　culture, positive NEC 795.39
　　blood 790.7
　　HIV V08
　　human immunodeficiency virus V08
　　nose 795.39
　　skin lesion NEC 795.39
　　spinal fluid 792.0
　　sputum 795.39
　　stool 792.1
　　throat 795.39
　　urine 791.9
　　viral
　　　human immunodeficiency V08

Findings, abnormal —*continued*
　wound 795.39
　echocardiogram 793.2
　echoencephalogram 794.01
　echogram NEC—*see* Findings, abnormal,
　　structure
　electrocardiogram (ECG) (EKG) 794.31
　electroencephalogram (EEG) 794.02
　electrolyte level, urinary 791.9
　electromyogram (EMG) 794.17
　　ocular 794.14
　electro-oculogram (EOG) 794.12
　electroretinogram (ERG) 794.11
　enzymes, serum NEC 790.5
　fibrinogen titer coagulation study 790.92
　filling defect—*see* Filling defect
　function study NEC 794.9
　　auditory 794.15
　　bladder 794.9
　　brain 794.00
　　cardiac 794.30
　　endocrine NEC 794.6
　　　thyroid 794.5
　　kidney 794.4
　　liver 794.8
　　nervous system
　　　central 794.00
　　　peripheral 794.19
　　oculomotor 794.14
　　pancreas 794.9
　　placenta 794.9
　　pulmonary 794.2
　　retina 794.11
　　special senses 794.19
　　spleen 794.9
　　vestibular 794.16
　gallbladder, nonvisualization 793.3
　glucose 790.29
　　elevated
　　　fasting 790.21
　　　tolerance test 790.22
　glycosuria 791.5
　heart
　　shadow 793.2
　　sounds 785.3
　hematinuria 791.2
　hematocrit
　　drop (precipitous) 790.01
　　elevated 282.7
　　low 285.9
　hematologic NEC 790.99
　hematuria 599.7
　hemoglobin
　　elevated 282.7
　　low 285.9
　hemoglobinuria 791.2
　histological NEC 795.4
　hormones 259.9
　immunoglobulins, elevated 795.79
　indolacetic acid, elevated 791.9
　iron 790.6
　karyotype 795.2
　ketonuria 791.6
　lactic acid dehydrogenase (LDH) 790.4
　lead 790.6
　lipase 790.5
　lipids NEC 272.9
　lithium, blood 790.6
　liver function test 790.6
　lung field (coin lesion) (shadow) 793.1
　magnesium, blood 790.6

Findings, abnormal —*continued*
  lung 793.1
    musculoskeletal 793.7
    placenta 793.99
    retroperitoneum 793.6
    skin 793.99
    subcutaneous tissue NEC 793.99
  synovial fluid 792.9
  thermogram—*see* Finding, abnormal, structure
  throat culture, positive 795.39
  thyroid (function) 794.5
    metabolism (rate) 794.5
    scan 794.5
    uptake 794.5
  total proteins 790.99
  toxicology (drugs) (heavy metals) 796.0
  transaminase (level) 790.4
  triglycerides 272.9
  tuberculin skin test (without active tuberculosis)
    795.5
  tumor markers NEC 795.89
  ultrasound—*see also* Finding, abnormal,
    structure
    cardiogram 793.2
  uric acid, blood 790.6
  urine, urinary constituents 791.9
    acetone 791.6
    albumin 791.0
    bacteria 791.9
    bile 791.4
    blood 599.7
    casts or cells 791.7
    chyle 791.1
    culture, positive 791.9
    glucose 791.5
    hemoglobin 791.2
    ketone 791.6
    protein 791.0
    pus 791.9
    sugar 791.5
  vaginal fluid 792.9
  vanillylmandelic acid, elevated 791.9
  vectorcardiogram (VCG) 794.39
  ventriculogram (cerebral) 793.0
  VMA, elevated 791.9
  Wassermann reaction
    false positive 795.6
    positive 097.1
      follow-up of latent syphilis—*see* Syphilis,
        latent
      only finding—*see* Syphilis, latent
  white blood cell 288.9
    count 288.9
      elevated 288.60
      low 288.50
    differential 288.9
    morphology 288.9
  wound culture 795.39
  xerography 793.89
  zinc, blood 790.6
Finger —*see* condition
Fire, St. Anthony's (*see also* Erysipelas) 035
Fish
  hook stomach 537.89
  meal workers' lung 495.8
Fisher's syndrome 357.0
Fissure, fissured
  abdominal wall (congenital) 756.79
  anus, anal 565.0
    congenital 751.5
  buccal cavity 528.9

Fissure, fissured—*continued*
  clitoris (congenital) 752.49
  ear, lobule (congenital) 744.29
  epiglottis (congenital) 748.3
  larynx 478.79
    congenital 748.3
  lip 528.5
    congenital (*see also* Cleft, lip) 749.10
  nipple 611.2
    puerperal, postpartum 676.1
  palate (congenital) (*see also* Cleft, palate) 749.00
  postanal 565.0
  rectum 565.0
  skin 709.8
    streptococcal 686.9
  spine (congenital) (*see also* Spina bifida) 741.9
  sternum (congenital) 756.3
  tongue (acquired) 529.5
    congenital 750.13
Fistula (sinus) 686.9
  abdomen (wall) 569.81
    bladder 596.2
    intestine 569.81
    ureter 593.82
    uterus 619.2
  abdominorectal 569.81
  abdominosigmoidal 569.81
  abdominothoracic 510.0
  abdominouterine 619.2
    congenital 752.3
  abdominovesical 596.2
  accessory sinuses (*see also* Sinusitis) 473.9
  actinomycotic—*see* Actinomycosis
  alveolar
    antrum (*see also* Sinusitis, maxillary) 473.0
    process 522.7
  anorectal 565.1
  antrobuccal (*see also* Sinusitis, maxillary) 473.0
  antrum (*see also* Sinusitis, maxillary) 473.0
  anus, anal (infectional) (recurrent) 565.1
    congenital 751.5
    tuberculous (*see also* Tuberculosis) 014.8
  aortic sinus 747.29
  aortoduodenal 447.2
  appendix, appendicular 543.9
  arteriovenous (acquired) 447.0
    brain 437.3
      congenital 747.81
        ruptured (*see also* Hemorrhage,
          subarachnoid) 430
        ruptured (*see also* Hemorrhage,
          subarachnoid) 430
    cerebral 437.3
      congenital 747.81
    congenital (peripheral) 747.60
      brain—*see* Fistula, arteriovenous, brain,
        congenital
      coronary 746.85
      gastrointestinal 747.61
      lower limb 747.64
      pulmonary 747.3
      renal 747.62
      specified NEC 747.69
      upper limb 747.63
    coronary 414.19
      congenital 746.85
    heart 414.19
    pulmonary (vessels) 417.0
      congenital 747.3
    surgically created (for dialysis) V45.1
      complication NEC 996.73

Fistula—*continued*
    atherosclerosis —*see* Arteriosclerosis, extremities
    embolism 996.74
    infection or inflammation 996.62
    mechanical 996.1
    occlusion NEC 996.74
    thrombus 996.74
  traumatic—*see* Injury, blood vessel, by site
artery 447.2
aural 383.81
  congenital 744.49
auricle 383.81
  congenital 744.49
Bartholin's gland 619.8
bile duct (*see also* Fistula, biliary) 576.4
biliary (duct) (tract) 576.4
  congenital 751.69
bladder (neck) (sphincter) 596.2
  into seminal vesicle 596.2
bone 733.99
brain 348.8
  arteriovenous—*see* Fistula, arteriovenous, brain
branchial (cleft) 744.41
branchiogenous 744.41
breast 611.0
  puerperal, postpartum 675.1
bronchial 510.0
bronchocutaneous, bronchomediastinal, bronchopleural, bronchopleuromediastinal (infective) 510.0
  tuberculous (*see also* Tuberculosis) 011.3
bronchoesophageal 530.89
  congenital 750.3
buccal cavity (infective) 528.3
canal, ear 380.89
carotid-cavernous
  congenital 747.81
    with hemorrhage 430
    traumatic 900.82
    with hemorrhage (*see also* Hemorrhage, brain, traumatic) 853.0
    late effect 908.3
cecosigmoidal 569.81
cecum 569.81
cerebrospinal (fluid) 349.81
cervical, lateral (congenital) 744.41
cervicoaural (congenital) 744.49
cervicosigmoidal 619.1
cervicovesical 619.0
cervix 619.8
chest (wall) 510.0
cholecystocolic (*see also* Fistula, gallbladder) 575.5
cholecystocolonic (*see also* Fistula, gallbladder) 575.5
cholecystoduodenal (*see also* Fistula, gallbladder) 575.5
cholecystoenteric (*see also* Fistula, gallbladder) 575.5
cholecystogastric (*see also* Fistula, gallbladder) 575.5
cholecystointestinal (*see also* Fistula, gallbladder) 575.5
choledochoduodenal 576.4
cholocolic (*see also* Fistula, gallbladder) 575.5
coccyx 685.1
  with abscess 685.0
colon 569.81
colostomy 569.69

Fistula—*continued*
colovaginal (acquired) 619.1
common duct (bile duct) 576.4
congenital, NEC—*see* Anomaly, specified type NEC
cornea, causing hypotony 360.32
coronary, arteriovenous 414.19
  congenital 746.85
costal region 510.0
cul-de-sac, Douglas' 619.8
cutaneous 686.9
cystic duct (*see also* Fistula, gallbladder) 575.5
  congenital 751.69
dental 522.7
diaphragm 510.0
  bronchovisceral 510.0
  pleuroperitoneal 510.0
  pulmonoperitoneal 510.0
duodenum 537.4
ear (canal) (external) 380.89
enterocolic 569.81
enterocutaneous 569.81
enteroenteric 569.81
entero-uterine 619.1
  congenital 752.3
enterovaginal 619.1
  congenital 752.49
enterovesical 596.1
epididymis 608.89
  tuberculous (*see also* Tuberculosis) 016.4
esophagobronchial 530.89
  congenital 750.3
esophagocutaneous 530.89
esophagopleurocutaneous 530.89
esophagotracheal 530.84
  congenital 750.3
esophagus 530.89
  congenital 750.4
ethmoid (*see also* Sinusitis, ethmoidal) 473.2
eyeball (cornea) (sclera) 360.32
eyelid 373.11
fallopian tube (external) 619.2
fecal 569.81
  congenital 751.5
from periapical lesion 522.7
frontal sinus (*see also* Sinusitis, frontal) 473.1
gallbladder 575.5
  with calculus, cholelithiasis, stones (*see also* Cholelithiasis) 574.2
  congenital 751.69
gastric 537.4
gastrocolic 537.4
  congenital 750.7
  tuberculous (*see also* Tuberculosis) 014.8
gastroenterocolic 537.4
gastroesophageal 537.4
gastrojejunal 537.4
gastrojejunocolic 537.4
genital
  organs
    female 619.9
      specified site NEC 619.8
    male 608.89
  tract-skin (female) 619.2
hepatopleural 510.0
hepatopulmonary 510.0
horseshoe 565.1
ileorectal 569.81
ileosigmoidal 569.81
ileostomy 569.69
ileovesical 596.1

Fistula—*continued*
  ileum 569.81
  in ano 565.1
    tuberculous (*see also* Tuberculosis) 014.8
  inner ear (*see also* Fistula, labyrinth) 386.40
  intestine 569.81
  intestinocolonic (abdominal) 569.81
  intestinoureteral 593.82
  intestinouterine 619.1
  intestinovaginal 619.1
    congenital 752.49
  intestinovesical 596.1
  involving female genital tract 619.9
    digestive-genital 619.1
    genital tract-skin 619.2
    specified site NEC 619.8
    urinary-genital 619.0
  ischiorectal (fossa) 566
  jejunostomy 569.69
  jejunum 569.81
  joint 719.80
    ankle 719.87
    elbow 719.82
    foot 719.87
    hand 719.84
    hip 719.85
    knee 719.86
    multiple sites 719.89
    pelvic region 719.85
    shoulder (region) 719.81
    specified site NEC 719.88
    tuberculous—*see* Tuberculosis, joint
    wrist 719.83
  kidney 593.89
  labium (majus) (minus) 619.8
  labyrinth, labyrinthine NEC 386.40
    combined sites 386.48
    multiple sites 386.48
    oval window 386.42
    round window 386.41
  semicircular canal 386.43
  lacrimal, lachrymal (duct) (gland) (sac) 375.61
  lacrimonasal duct 375.61
  laryngotracheal 748.3
  larynx 478.79
  lip 528.5
    congenital 750.25
  lumbar, tuberculous (*see also* Tuberculosis)
    015.0 *[730.8]*
  lung 510.0
  lymphatic (node) (vessel) 457.8
  mamillary 611.0
  mammary (gland) 611.0
    puerperal, postpartum 675.1
  mastoid (process) (region) 383.1
  maxillary (*see also* Sinusitis, maxillary) 473.0
  mediastinal 510.0
  mediastinobronchial 510.0
  mediastinocutaneous 510.0
  middle ear 385.89
  mouth 528.3
  nasal 478.19
    sinus (*see also* Sinusitis) 473.9
  nasopharynx 478.29
  nipple—*see* Fistula, breast
  nose 478.19
  oral (cutaneous) 528.3
    maxillary (*see also* Sinusitis, maxillary) 473.0
    nasal (with cleft palate) (*see also* Cleft, palate)
      749.00
  orbit, orbital 376.10

Fistula—*continued*
  oro-antral (*see also* Sinusitis, maxillary) 473.0
  oval window (internal ear) 386.42
  oviduct (external) 619.2
  palate (hard) 526.89
    soft 528.9
  pancreatic 577.8
  pancreaticoduodenal 577.8
  parotid (gland) 527.4
    region 528.3
  pelvoabdominointestinal 569.81
  penis 607.89
  perianal 565.1
  pericardium (pleura) (sac) (*see also* Pericarditis)
    423.8
  pericecal 569.81
  perineal—*see* Fistula, perineum
  perineorectal 569.81
  perineosigmoidal 569.81
  perineo-urethroscrotal 608.89
  perineum, perineal (with urethral involvement)
    NEC 599.1
    tuberculous (*see also* Tuberculosis) 017.9
    ureter 593.82
  perirectal 565.1
    tuberculous (*see also* Tuberculosis) 014.8
  peritoneum (*see also* Peritonitis) 567.22
  periurethral 599.1
  pharyngo-esophageal 478.29
  pharynx 478.29
    branchial cleft (congenital) 744.41
  pilonidal (infected) (rectum) 685.1
    with abscess 685.0
  pleura, pleural, pleurocutaneous,
    pleuroperitoneal 510.0
    stomach 510.0
    tuberculous (*see also* Tuberculosis) 012.0
  pleuropericardial 423.8
  postauricular 383.81
  postoperative, persistent 998.6
  preauricular (congenital) 744.46
  prostate 602.8
  pulmonary 510.0
    arteriovenous 417.0
      congenital 747.3
    tuberculous (*see also* Tuberculosis,
      pulmonary) 011.9
  pulmonoperitoneal 510.0
  rectolabial 619.1
  rectosigmoid (intercommunicating) 569.81
  rectoureteral 593.82
  rectourethral 599.1
    congenital 753.8
  rectouterine 619.1
    congenital 752.3
  rectovaginal 619.1
    congenital 752.49
    old, postpartal 619.1
    tuberculous (*see also* Tuberculosis) 014.8
  rectovesical 596.1
    congenital 753.8
  rectovesicovaginal 619.1
  rectovulvar 619.1
    congenital 752.49
  rectum (to skin) 565.1
    tuberculous (*see also* Tuberculosis) 014.8
  renal 593.89
  retroauricular 383.81
  round window (internal ear) 386.41
  salivary duct or gland 527.4
    congenital 750.24

Fistula—*continued*
  sclera 360.32
  scrotum (urinary) 608.89
    tuberculous (*see also* Tuberculosis) 016.5
  semicircular canals (internal ear) 386.43
  sigmoid 569.81
    vesicoabdominal 596.1
  sigmoidovaginal 619.1
    congenital 752.49
  skin 686.9
    ureter 593.82
    vagina 619.2
  sphenoidal sinus (*see also* Sinusitis, sphenoidal)
      473.3
  splenocolic 289.59
  stercoral 569.81
  stomach 537.4
  sublingual gland 527.4
    congenital 750.24
  submaxillary
    gland 527.4
      congenital 750.24
    region 528.3
  thoracic 510.0
    duct 457.8
  thoracicoabdominal 510.0
  thoracicogastric 510.0
  thoracicointestinal 510.0
  thoracoabdominal 510.0
  thoracogastric 510.0
  thorax 510.0
  thyroglossal duct 759.2
  thyroid 246.8
  trachea (congenital) (external) (internal) 748.3
  tracheoesophageal 530.84
    congenital 750.3
    following tracheostomy 519.09
  traumatic
    arteriovenous (*see also* Injury, blood vessel,
        by site) 904.9
    brain—*see* Injury, intracranial
  tuberculous—*see* Tuberculosis, by site
  typhoid 002.0
  umbilical 759.89
  umbilico-urinary 753.8
  urachal, urachus 753.7
  ureter (persistent) 593.82
  ureteroabdominal 593.82
  ureterocervical 593.82
  ureterorectal 593.82
  ureterosigmoido-abdominal 593.82
  ureterovaginal 619.0
  ureterovesical 596.2
  urethra 599.1
    congenital 753.8
    tuberculous (*see also* Tuberculosis) 016.3
  urethroperineal 599.1
  urethroperineovesical 596.2
  urethrorectal 599.1
    congenital 753.8
  urethroscrotal 608.89
  urethrovaginal 619.0
  urethrovesical 596.2
  urethrovesicovaginal 619.0
  urinary (persistent) (recurrent) 599.1
  uteroabdominal (anterior wall) 619.2
    congenital 752.3
  uteroenteric 619.1
  uterofecal 619.1
  uterointestinal 619.1
    congenital 752.3

Fistula—*continued*
  uterorectal 619.1
    congenital 752.3
  uteroureteric 619.0
  uterovaginal 619.8
  uterovesical 619.0
    congenital 752.3
  uterus 619.8
  vagina (wall) 619.8
    postpartal, old 619.8
  vaginocutaneous (postpartal) 619.2
  vaginoileal (acquired) 619.1
  vaginoperineal 619.2
  vesical NEC 596.2
  vesicoabdominal 596.2
  vesicocervicovaginal 619.0
  vesicocolic 596.1
  vesicocutaneous 596.2
  vesicoenteric 596.1
  vesicointestinal 596.1
  vesicometrorectal 619.1
  vesicoperineal 596.2
  vesicorectal 596.1
    congenital 753.8
  vesicosigmoidal 596.1
  vesicosigmoidovaginal 619.1
  vesicoureteral 596.2
  vesicoureterovaginal 619.0
  vesicourethral 596.2
  vesicourethrorectal 596.1
  vesicouterine 619.0
    congenital 752.3
  vesicovaginal 619.0
  vulvorectal 619.1
    congenital 752.49
Fit 780.39
  apoplectic (*see also* Disease, cerebrovascular,
      acute) 436
    late effect—*see* Late effect(s) (of)
        cerebrovascular disease
  epileptic (*see also* Epilepsy) 345.9
  fainting 780.2
  hysterical 300.11
  newborn 779.0
Fitting (of)
  artificial
    arm (complete) (partial) V52.0
    breast V52.4
    eye(s) V52.2
    leg(s) (complete) (partial) V52.1
  brain neuropacemaker V53.02
  cardiac pacemaker V53.31
  carotid sinus pacemaker V53.39
  cerebral ventricle (communicating) shunt
      V53.01
  colostomy belt V53.5
  contact lenses V53.1
  cystostomy device V53.6
  defibrillator, automatic implantable V53.32
  dentures V52.3
  device, unspecified type V53.90
    abdominal V53.5
    cardiac
      defibrillator, automatic implantable V53.32
      pacemaker V53.31
      specified NEC V53.39
    cerebral ventricle (communicating) shunt
        V53.01
    insulin pump V53.91
    intrauterine contraceptive V25.1
    nervous system V53.09

Fitting—*continued*
  orthodontic V53.4
  orthoptic V53.1
  other device V53.99
  prosthetic V52.9
    breast V52.4
    dental V52.3
    eye V52.2
    specified type NEC V52.8
  special senses V53.09
  substitution
    auditory V53.09
    nervous system V53.09
    visual V53.09
  urinary V53.6
  diaphragm (contraceptive) V25.02
  glasses (reading) V53.1
  growth rod V54.02
  hearing aid V53.2
  ileostomy device V53.5
  intestinal appliance or device NEC V53.5
  intrauterine contraceptive device V25.1
  neuropacemaker (brain) (peripheral nerve)
    (spinal cord) V53.02
  orthodontic device V53.4
  orthopedic (device) V53.7
    brace V53.7
    cast V53.7
    corset V53.7
    shoes V53.7
  pacemaker (cardiac) V53.31
    brain V53.02
    carotid sinus V53.39
    peripheral nerve V53.02
    spinal cord V53.02
  prosthesis V52.9
    arm (complete) (partial) V52.0
    breast V52.4
    dental V52.3
    eye V52.2
    leg (complete) (partial) V52.1
    specified type NEC V52.8
  spectacles V53.1
  wheelchair V53.8
Fitz's syndrome (acute hemorrhagic pancreatitis)
  577.0
Fitz-Hugh and Curtis syndrome 098.86
  due to
    Chlamydia trachomatis 099.56
    Neisseria gonorrhoeae (gonococcal peritonitis)
      098.86
Fixation
  joint—*see* Ankylosis
  larynx 478.79
  pupil 364.76
  stapes 385.22
    deafness (*see also* Deafness, conductive)
      389.04
  uterus (acquired)—*see* Malposition, uterus
  vocal cord 478.5
Flaccid —*see* condition
  foot 736.79
  forearm 736.09
  palate, congenital 750.26
Flail
  chest 807.4
    newborn 767.3
  joint (paralytic) 718.80
    ankle 718.87
    elbow 718.82
    foot 718.87

Flail —*continued*
  hand 718.84
  hip 718.85
  knee 718.86
  multiple sites 718.89
  pelvic region 718.85
  shoulder (region) 718.81
  specified site NEC 718.88
  wrist 718.83
Flajani (-Basedow) syndrome or disease
  (exophthalmic goiter) 242.0
Flap, liver 572.8
Flare, anterior chamber (aqueous) (eye) 364.04
Flashback phenomena (drug) (hallucinogenic)
  292.89
Flat
  chamber (anterior) (eye) 360.34
  chest, congenital 754.89
  electroencephalogram (EEG) 348.8
  foot (acquired) (fixed type) (painful) (postural)
    (spastic) 734
    congenital 754.61
      rocker bottom 754.61
      vertical talus 754.61
    rachitic 268.1
    rocker bottom (congenital) 754.61
    vertical talus, congenital 754.61
  organ or site, congenital NEC—*see* Anomaly,
    specified type NEC
  pelvis 738.6
    with disproportion (fetopelvic) 653.2
      affecting fetus or newborn 763.1
      causing obstructed labor 660.1
        affecting fetus or newborn 763.1
    congenital 755.69
Flatau-Schilder disease 341.1
Flattening
  head, femur 736.39
  hip 736.39
  lip (congenital) 744.89
  nose (congenital) 754.0
    acquired 738.0
Flatulence 787.3
Flatus 787.3
  vaginalis 629.89
Flax dressers' disease 504
Flea bite —*see* Injury, superficial, by site
Fleischer (-Kayser) ring (corneal pigmentation)
  275.1 *[371.14]*
Fleischner's disease 732.3
Fleshy mole 631
Flexibilitas cerea (*see also* Catalepsy) 300.11
Flexion
  cervix —*see* Flexion, uterus
  contracture, joint (*see also* Contraction, joint)
    718.4
  deformity, joint (*see also* Contraction, joint) 736.9
    hip, congenital (*see also* Subluxation,
      congenital, hip) 754.32
  uterus (*see also* Malposition, uterus) 621.6
Flexner's
  bacillus 004.1
  diarrhea (ulcerative) 004.1
  dysentery 004.1
Flexner-Boyd dysentery 004.2
Flexure —*see* condition
Floater, vitreous 379.24
Floating
  cartilage (joint) (*see also* Disorder, cartilage,
    articular) 718.0
    knee 717.6

Foreign body

Note—For foreign body with open wound or other injury, see Wound, open, or the type of injury specified.

   accidentally left during a procedure 998.4
   anterior chamber (eye) 871.6
      magnetic 871.5
         retained or old 360.51
      retained or old 360.61
   ciliary body (eye) 871.6
      magnetic 871.5
         retained or old 360.52
      retained or old 360.62
   entering through orifice (current) (old)
      accessory sinus 932
      air passage (upper) 933.0
         lower 934.8
      alimentary canal 938
      alveolar process 935.0
      antrum (Highmore) 932
      anus 937
      appendix 936
      asphyxia due to (*see also* Asphyxia, food)
         933.1
      auditory canal 931
      auricle 931
      bladder 939.0
      bronchioles 934.8
      bronchus (main) 934.1
      buccal cavity 935.0
      canthus (inner) 930.1
      cecum 936
      cervix (canal) uterine 939.1
      coil, ileocecal 936
      colon 936
      conjunctiva 930.1
      conjunctival sac 930.1
      cornea 930.0
      digestive organ or tract NEC 938
      duodenum 936
      ear (external) 931
      esophagus 935.1
      eye (external) 930.9
         combined sites 930.8
         intraocular—*see* Foreign body, by site
         specified site NEC 930.8
      eyeball 930.8
         intraocular—*see* Foreign body, intraocular
      eyelid 930.1
         retained or old 374.86
      frontal sinus 932
      gastrointestinal tract 938
      genitourinary tract 939.9
      globe 930.8
         penetrating 871.6
            magnetic 871.5
               retained or old 360.50
            retained or old 360.60
      gum 935.0
      Highmore's antrum 932
      hypopharynx 933.0
      ileocecal coil 936
      ileum 936
      inspiration (of) 933.1
      intestine (large) (small) 936
      lacrimal apparatus, duct, gland, or sac 930.2

Foreign body—*continued*
   larynx 933.1
   lung 934.8
   maxillary sinus 932
   mouth 935.0
   nasal sinus 932
   nasopharynx 933.0
   nose (passage) 932
   nostril 932
   oral cavity 935.0
   palate 935.0
   penis 939.3
   pharynx 933.0
   pyriform sinus 933.0
   rectosigmoid 937
      junction 937
   rectum 937
   respiratory tract 934.9
      specified part NEC 934.8
   sclera 930.1
   sinus 932
      accessory 932
      frontal 932
      maxillary 932
      nasal 932
      pyriform 933.0
   small intestine 936
   stomach (hairball) 935.2
   suffocation by (*see also* Asphyxia, food) 933.1
   swallowed 938
      tongue 933.0
   tear ducts or glands 930.2
   throat 933.0
   tongue 935.0
      swallowed 933.0
   tonsil, tonsillar 933.0
      fossa 933.0
   trachea 934.0
   ureter 939.0
   urethra 939.0
   uterus (any part) 939.1
   vagina 939.2
   vulva 939.2
   wind pipe 934.0
 granuloma (old) 728.82
   bone 733.99
   in operative wound (inadvertently left) 998.4
      due to surgical material intentionally
         left—*see* Complications, due to
         (presence of) any device, implant, or
         graft classified to 996.0-996.5 NEC
   muscle 728.82
   skin 709.4
   soft tissue 709.1
   subcutaneous tissue 709.4
 in
   bone (residual) 733.99
   open wound—*see* Wound, open, by site
      complicated
   soft tissue (residual) 729.6
 inadvertently left in operation wound (causing
     adhesions, obstruction, or perforation) 998.4
 ingestion, ingested NEC 938
 inhalation or inspiration (*see also* Asphyxia,
     food) 933.1
 internal organ, not entering through an
     orifice—*see* Injury, internal, by site, with
     open wound
 intraocular (nonmagnetic) 871.6
   combined sites 871.6
      magnetic 871.5

Foreign body—*continued*
　　　retained or old 360.59
　　retained or old 360.69
　　magnetic 871.5
　　retained or old 360.50
　retained or old 360.60
　specified site NEC 871.6
　　magnetic 871.5
　　　retained or old 360.59
　　retained or old 360.69
　iris (nonmagnetic) 871.6
　　magnetic 871.5
　　　retained or old 360.52
　　retained or old 360.62
　lens (nonmagnetic) 871.6
　　magnetic 871.5
　　　retained or old 360.53
　　retained or old 360.63
　lid, eye 930.1
　ocular muscle 870.4
　　retained or old 376.6
　old or residual
　　bone 733.99
　　eyelid 374.86
　　middle ear 385.83
　　muscle 729.6
　　　ocular 376.6
　　retrobulbar 376.6
　　skin 729.6
　　　with granuloma 709.4
　　soft tissue 729.6
　　　with granuloma 709.4
　　subcutaneous tissue 729.6
　　　with granuloma 709.4
　operation wound, left accidentally 998.4
　orbit 870.4
　　retained or old 376.6
　posterior wall, eye 871.6
　　magnetic 871.5
　　　retained or old 360.55
　　retained or old 360.65
　respiratory tree 934.9
　　specified site NEC 934.8
　retained (old) (nonmagnetic) (in)
　　anterior chamber (eye) 360.61
　　　magnetic 360.51
　　ciliary body 360.62
　　　magnetic 360.52
　　eyelid 374.86
　　globe 360.60
　　　magnetic 360.50
　　intraocular 360.60
　　　magnetic 360.50
　　　specified site NEC 360.69
　　　　magnetic 360.59
　　iris 360.62
　　　magnetic 360.52
　　lens 360.63
　　　magnetic 360.53
　　muscle 729.6
　　orbit 376.6
　　posterior wall of globe 360.65
　　　magnetic 360.55
　　retina 360.65
　　　magnetic 360.55
　　retrobulbar 376.6
　　skin 729.6
　　　with granuloma 709.4
　　soft tissue 729.6
　　　with granuloma 709.4
　　subcutaneous tissue 729.6

Foreign body—*continued*
　　with granuloma 709.4
　　vitreous 360.64
　　　magnetic 360.54
　　retina 871.6
　　　magnetic 871.5
　　　　retained or old 360.55
　　　retained or old 360.65
　　superficial, without major open wound (*see also*
　　　Injury, superficial, by site) 919.6
　　swallowed NEC 938
　　vitreous (humor) 871.6
　　　magnetic 871.5
　　　　retained or old 360.54
　　　retained or old 360.64
Forking, aqueduct of Sylvius 742.3
　with spina bifida (*see also* Spina bifida) 741.0
Formation
　bone in scar tissue (skin) 709.3
　connective tissue in vitreous 379.25
　Elschnig pearls (postcataract extraction) 366.51
　hyaline in cornea 371.49
　sequestrum in bone (due to infection) (*see also*
　　Osteomyelitis) 730.1
　valve
　　colon, congenital 751.5
　　ureter (congenital) 753.29
Formication 782.0
Fort Bragg fever 100.89
Fossa —*see also* condition
　pyriform—*see* condition
Foster-Kennedy syndrome 377.04
Fothergill's
　disease, meaning scarlatina anginosa 034.1
　neuralgia (*see also* Neuralgia, trigeminal) 350.1
Foul breath 784.99
Found dead (cause unknown) 798.9
Foundling V20.0
Fournier's disease (idiopathic gangrene) 608.83
Fourth
　cranial nerve—*see* condition
　disease 057.8
　molar 520.1
Foville's syndrome 344.89
Fox's
　disease (apocrine miliaria) 705.82
　impetigo (contagiosa) 684
Fox-Fordyce disease (apocrine miliaria) 705.82

Fracture (abduction) (adduction) (avulsion) (compression) (crush) (dislocation) (oblique) (separation) (closed) 829.0

> *Note—For fracture of any of the following sites with fracture of other bones—see Fracture, multiple.*
>
> *"Closed" includes the following descriptions of fractures, with or without delayed healing, unless they are specified as open or compound:*
>
> > *comminuted*
> > *depressed*
> > *elevated*
> > *fissured*
> > *greenstick*
> > *impacted*
> > *linear*
> > *simple*
> > *slipped epiphysis*
> > *spiral*
> > *unspecified*
>
> *"Open" includes the following descriptions of fractures, with or without delayed healing:*
>
> > *compound*
> > *infected*
> > *missile*
> > *puncture*
> > *with foreign body*
>
> *For late effect of fracture, see Late, effect, fracture, by site.*

with
   internal injuries in same region (conditions classifiable to 860-869)—*see also* Injury, internal, by site
     pelvic region—*see* Fracture, pelvis
acetabulum (with visceral injury) (closed) 808.0
  open 808.1
acromion (process) (closed) 811.01
  open 811.11
alveolus (closed) 802.8
  open 802.9
ankle (malleolus) (closed) 824.8
  bimalleolar (Dupuytren's) (Pott's) 824.4
    open 824.5
  bone 825.21
    open 825.31
  lateral malleolus only (fibular) 824.2
    open 824.3
  medial malleolus only (tibial) 824.0
    open 824.1
  open 824.9
  pathologic 733.16
  talus 825.21
    open 825.31
  trimalleolar 824.6
    open 824.7
antrum—*see* Fracture, skull, base
arm (closed) 818.0
  and leg(s) (any bones) 828.0
    open 828.1
  both (any bones) (with rib(s)) (with sternum) 819.0
    open 819.1
  lower 813.80
    open 813.90
  open 818.1

Fracture—*continued*
  upper—*see* Fracture, humerus
astragalus (closed) 825.21
  open 825.31
atlas—*see* Fracture, vertebra, cervical, first
axis—*see* Fracture, vertebra, cervical, second
back—*see* Fracture, vertebra, by site
Barton's—*see* Fracture, radius, lower end
basal (skull)—*see* Fracture, skull, base
Bennett's (closed) 815.01
  open 815.11
bimalleolar (closed) 824.4
  open 824.5
bone (closed) NEC 829.0
  birth injury NEC 767.3
  open 829.1
  pathologic NEC (*see also* Fracture, pathologic) 733.10
  stress NEC (*see also* Fracture, stress) 733.95
boot top—*see* Fracture, fibula
boxers'—*see* Fracture, metacarpal bone(s)
breast bone—*see* Fracture, sternum
bucket handle (semilunar cartilage)—*see* Tear, meniscus
bursting—*see* Fracture, phalanx, hand, distal
calcaneus (closed) 825.0
  open 825.1
capitate (bone) (closed) 814.07
  open 814.17
capitellum (humerus) (closed) 812.49
  open 812.59
carpal bone(s) (wrist NEC) (closed) 814.00
  open 814.10
  specified site NEC 814.09
    open 814.19
cartilage, knee (semilunar)—*see* Tear, meniscus
cervical—*see* Fracture, vertebra, cervical
chauffeur's—*see* Fracture, ulna, lower end
chisel—*see* Fracture, radius, upper end
clavicle (interligamentous part) (closed) 810.00
  acromial end 810.03
    open 810.13
  due to birth trauma 767.2
  open 810.10
  shaft (middle third) 810.02
    open 810.12
  sternal end 810.01
    open 810.11
clayshovelers'—*see* Fracture, vertebra, cervical
coccyx—*see also* Fracture, vertebra, coccyx
  complicating delivery 665.6
collar bone—*see* Fracture, clavicle
Colles' (reversed) (closed) 813.41
  open 813.51
comminuted—*see* Fracture, by site
compression—*see also* Fracture, by site
  nontraumatic—*see* Fracture, pathologic
congenital 756.9
coracoid process (closed) 811.02
  open 811.12
coronoid process (ulna) (closed) 813.02
  mandible (closed) 802.23
    open 802.33
  open 813.12
corpus cavernosum penis 959.13
costochondral junction—*see* Fracture, rib
costosternal junction—*see* Fracture, rib
cranium—*see* Fracture, skull, by site
cricoid cartilage (closed) 807.5
  open 807.6
cuboid (ankle) (closed) 825.23

Fracture—*continued*
   open 825.33
  cuneiform
    foot (closed) 825.24
     open 825.34
    wrist (closed) 814.03
     open 814.13
  dental restorative material
    with loss of material 525.64
    without loss of material 525.63
  due to
    birth injury—*see* Birth injury, fracture
    gunshot—*see* Fracture, by site, open
    neoplasm—*see* Fracture, pathologic
    osteoporosis—*see* Fracture, pathologic
  Dupuytren's (ankle) (fibula) (closed) 824.4
    open 824.5
    radius 813.42
     open 813.52
  Duverney's—*see* Fracture, ilium
  elbow—*see also* Fracture, humerus, lower end
    olecranon (process) (closed) 813.01
     open 813.11
    supracondylar (closed) 812.41
     open 812.51
  ethmoid (bone) (sinus)—*see* Fracture, skull,
    base
  face bone(s) (closed) NEC 802.8
    with
     other bone(s)—*see also* Fracture, multiple,
      skull
     skull—*see also* Fracture, skull
      involving other bones—*see* Fracture,
       multiple, skull
    open 802.9
  fatigue—*see* Fracture, march
  femur, femoral (closed) 821.00
    cervicotrochanteric 820.03
     open 820.13
    condyles, epicondyles 821.21
     open 821.31
    distal end—*see* Fracture, femur, lower end
    epiphysis (separation)
     capital 820.01
      open 820.11
     head 820.01
      open 820.11
     lower 821.22
      open 821.32
     trochanteric 820.01
      open 820.11
     upper 820.01
      open 820.11
    head 820.09
     open 820.19
    lower end or extremity (distal end) (closed)
     821.20
     condyles, epicondyles 821.21
      open 821.31
     epiphysis (separation) 821.22
      open 821.32
     multiple sites 821.29
      open 821.39
     open 821.30
     specified site NEC 821.29
      open 821.39
     supracondylar 821.23
      open 821.33
     T-shaped 821.21
      open 821.31
    neck (closed) 820.8

Fracture—*continued*
    base (cervicotrochanteric) 820.03
     open 820.13
    extracapsular 820.20
     open 820.30
    intertrochanteric (section) 820.21
     open 820.31
    intracapsular 820.00
     open 820.10
    intratrochanteric 820.21
     open 821.31
    midcervical 820.02
     open 820.12
    open 820.9
    pathologic 733.14
     specified part NEC 733.15
    specified site NEC 820.09
     open 820.19
    transcervical 820.02
     open 820.12
    transtrochanteric 820.20
     open 820.30
   open 821.10
   pathologic 733.14
    specified part NEC 733.15
   peritrochanteric (section) 820.20
    open 820.30
   shaft (lower third) (middle third) (upper third)
    821.01
    open 821.11
   subcapital 820.09
    open 820.19
   subtrochanteric (region) (section) 820.22
    open 820.32
   supracondylar 821.23
    open 821.33
   transepiphyseal 820.01
    open 820.11
   trochanter (greater) (lesser) (*see also* Fracture,
    femur, neck, by site) 820.20
    open 820.30
   T-shaped, into knee joint 821.21
    open 821.31
   upper end 820.8
    open 820.9
  fibula (closed) 823.81
    with tibia 823.82
     open 823.92
    distal end 824.8
     open 824.9
    epiphysis
     lower 824.8
      open 824.9
     upper—*see* Fracture, fibula, upper end
    head—*see* Fracture, fibula, upper end
    involving ankle 824.2
     open 824.3
    lower end or extremity 824.8
     open 824.9
    malleolus (external) (lateral) 824.2
     open 824.3
    open NEC 823.91
    pathologic 733.16
    proximal end—*see* Fracture, fibula, upper end
    shaft 823.21
     with tibia 823.22
      open 823.32
     open 823.31
    stress 733.93
    torus 853.41
     with tibia 823.42

Fracture—*continued*
   upper end or extremity (epiphysis) (head)
      (proximal end) (styloid) 823.01
     with tibia 823.02
       open 823.12
      open 823.11
   finger(s), of one hand (closed) (*see also*
      Fracture, phalanx, hand) 816.00
     with
       metacarpal bone(s), of same hand 817.0
         open 817.1
       thumb of same hand 816.03
         open 816.13
      open 816.10
   foot, except toe(s) alone (closed) 825.20
     open 825.30
   forearm (closed) NEC 813.80
     lower end (distal end) (lower epiphysis)
       813.40
      open 813.50
     open 813.90
     shaft 813.20
      open 813.30
     upper end (proximal end) (upper epiphysis)
       813.00
      open 813.10
   fossa, anterior, middle, or posterior—*see*
      Fracture, skull, base
   frontal (bone)—*see also* Fracture, skull, vault
     sinus—*see* Fracture, skull base
   Galeazzi's—*see* Fracture, radius, lower end
   glenoid (cavity) (fossa) (scapula) (closed)
      811.03
     open 811.13
   Gosselin's—*see* Fracture, ankle
   greenstick—*see* Fracture, by site
   grenade-throwers'—*see* Fracture, humerus,
     shaft
   gutter—*see* Fracture, skull, vault
   hamate (closed) 814.08
     open 814.18
   hand, one (closed) 815.00
     carpals 814.00
      open 814.10
      specified site NEC 814.09
       open 814.19
     metacarpals 815.00
      open 815.10
     multiple, bones of one hand 817.0
      open 817.1
     open 815.10
     phalanges (*see also* Fracture, phalanx, hand)
       816.00
      open 816.10
   healing
     aftercare (*see also* Aftercare, fracture) V54.89
     change of cast V54.89
     complications—*see* condition
     convalescence V66.4
     removal of
      cast V54.89
      fixation device
       external V54.89
       internal V54.01
   heel bone (closed) 825.0
     open 825.1
   hip (closed) (*see also* Fracture, femur, neck)
      820.8
     open 820.9
     pathologic 733.14
   humerus (closed) 812.20

Fracture—*continued*
   anatomical neck 812.02
     open 812.12
   articular process (*see also* Fracture, humerus,
     condyle(s) 812.44
     open 812.54
   capitellum 812.49
     open 812.59
   condyle(s) 812.44
     lateral (external) 812.42
      open 812.52
     medial (internal epicondyle) 812.43
      open 812.53
     open 812.54
   distal end—*see* Fracture, humerus, lower end
   epiphysis
     lower (*see also* Fracture, humerus,
      condyle(s)) 812.44
      open 812.54
     upper 812.09
      open 812.19
   external condyle 812.42
     open 812.52
   great tuberosity 812.03
     open 812.13
   head 812.09
     open 812.19
   internal epicondyle 812.43
     open 812.53
   lesser tuberosity 812.09
     open 812.19
   lower end or extremity (distal end) (*see also*
     Fracture, humerus, by site) 812.40
     multiple sites NEC 812.49
      open 812.59
     open 812.50
     specified site NEC 812.49
      open 812.59
   neck 812.01
     open 812.11
   open 812.30
   pathologic 733.11
   proximal end—*see* Fracture, humerus, upper
     end
   shaft 812.21
     open 812.31
   supracondylar 812.41
     open 812.51
   surgical neck 812.01
     open 812.11
   trochlea 812.49
     open 812.59
   T-shaped 812.44
     open 812.54
   tuberosity—*see* Fracture, humerus, upper end
   upper end or extremity (proximal end) (*see
     also* Fracture, humerus, by site) 812.00
     open 812.10
     specified site NEC 812.09
      open 812.19
  hyoid bone (closed) 807.5
     open 807.6
  hyperextension—*see* Fracture, radius, lower end
  ilium (with visceral injury) (closed) 808.41
     open 808.51
  impaction, impacted—*see* Fracture, by site
  incus—*see* Fracture, skull, base
  innominate bone (with visceral injury) (closed)
     808.49
     open 808.59
  instep, of one foot (closed) 825.20

Fracture—*continued*
  multiple (closed) 829.0

> *Note—Multiple fractures of sites classifiable to*
> *the same three- or four-digit category are coded*
> *to that category, except for sites classifiable to*
> *810-818 or 820-827 in different limbs.*
>
> *Multiple fractures of sites classifiable to*
> *different fourth-digit subdivisions within the*
> *same three-digit category should be dealt with*
> *according to coding rules.*
>
> *Multiple fractures of sites classifiable to*
> *different three-digit categories (identifiable*
> *from the listing under "Fracture"), and of sites*
> *classifiable to 810-818 or 820-827 in different*
> *limbs should be coded according to the*
> *following list, which should be referred to in the*
> *following priority order: skull or face bones,*
> *pelvis or vertebral column, legs, arms.*

  arm (multiple bones in same arm except in
      hand alone) (sites classifiable to 810-817
      with sites classifiable to a different
      three-digit category in 810-817 in same
      arm) (closed) 818.0
    open 818.1
  arms, both or arm(s) with rib(s) or sternum
      (sites classifiable to 810-818 with sites
      classifiable to same range of categories in
      other limb or to 807) (closed) 819.0
    open 819.1
  bones of trunk NEC (closed) 809.0
    open 809.1
  hand, metacarpal bone(s) with phalanx or
      phalanges of same hand (sites classifiable
      to 815 with sites classifiable to 816 in
      same hand) (closed) 817.0
    open 817.1
  leg (multiple bones in same leg) (sites
      classifiable to 820-826 with sites
      classifiable to a different three-digit
      category in that range in same leg) (closed)
      827.0
    open 827.1
  legs, both or leg(s) with arm(s), rib(s), or
      sternum (sites classifiable to 820-
      827 with sites classifiable to same range of
      categories in other leg or to 807 or
      810-819) (closed) 828.0
    open 828.1
  open 829.1
  pelvis with other bones except skull or face
      bones (sites classifiable to 808 with sites
      classifiable to 805-807 or 810-829)
      (closed) 809.0
    open 809.1
  skull, specified or unspecified bones, or face
      bone(s) with any other bone(s) (sites
      classifiable to 800-803 with sites
      classifiable to 805-829) (closed) 804.0

Fracture—*continued*

> *Note—Use the following fifth-digit*
> *subclassification with categories 800, 801, 803,*
> *and 804:*
>
> *0 unspecified state of consciousness*
> *1 with no loss of consciousness*
> *2 with brief [less than one hour] loss of*
> *   consciousness*
> *3 with moderate [1-24 hours] loss of*
> *   consciousness*
> *4 with prolonged [more than 24 hours] loss of*
> *   consciousness and return to pre-existing*
> *   conscious level*
> *5 with prolonged [more than 24 hours] loss of*
> *   consciousness, without return to pre-existing*
> *   conscious level*
> *Use fifth-digit 5 to designate when a patient is*
> *unconcious and dies before regaining*
> *conciousness, regardless of the duration of the*
> *loss of conciousness*
> *6 with loss of consciousness of unspecified*
> *   duration*
> *9 with concussion, unspecified*

  with
    contusion, cerebral 804.1
    epidural hemorrhage 804.2
    extradural hemorrhage 804.2
    hemorrhage (intracranial) NEC 804.3
    intracranial injury NEC 804.4
    laceration, cerebral 804.1
    subarachnoid hemorrhage 804.2
    subdural hemorrhage 804.2
  open 804.5
    with
      contusion, cerebral 804.6
      epidural hemorrhage 804.7
      extradural hemorrhage 804.7
      hemorrhage (intracranial) NEC 804.8
      intracranial injury NEC 804.9
      laceration, cerebral 804.6
      subarachnoid hemorrhage 804.7
      subdural hemorrhage 804.7
  vertebral column with other bones, except
      skull or face bones (sites classifiable to
      805 or 806 with sites classifiable to
      807-808 or 810-829) (closed) 809.0
    open 809.1
nasal (bone(s)) (closed) 802.0
  open 802.1
  sinus—Fracture, skull, base
navicular
  carpal (wrist) (closed) 814.01
    open 814.11
  tarsal (ankle) (closed) 825.22
    open 825.32
neck—*see* Fracture, vertebra, cervical
neural arch—*see* Fracture, vertebra, by site
nonunion 733.82
nose, nasal (bone) (septum) (closed) 802.0
  open 802.1
occiput—*see* Fracture, skull, base
odontoid process—*see* Fracture, vertebra,
    cervical
olecranon (process) (ulna) (closed) 813.01
  open 813.11
open 829.1
orbit, orbital (bone) (region) (closed) 802.8
  floor (blow-out) 802.6
    open 802.7

> *Note—Use the following fifth-digit subclassification with categories 807.0-807.1:*
>
> *0 rib(s), unspecified*
> *1 one rib*
> *2 two ribs*
> *3 three ribs*
> *4 four ribs*
> *5 five ribs*
> *6 six ribs*
> *7 seven ribs*
> *8 eight or more ribs*
> *9 multiple ribs, unspecified*

Fracture—*continued*
    complicated 873.73
   sacrum—*see* Fracture, vertebra, sacrum
   scaphoid
     ankle (closed) 825.22
      open 825.32
     wrist (closed) 814.01
      open 814.11
   scapula (closed) 811.00
     acromial, acromion (process) 811.01
      open 811.11
     body 811.09
      open 811.19
     coracoid process 811.02
      open 811.12
     glenoid (cavity) (fossa) 811.03
      open 811.13
     neck 811.03
      open 811.13
     open 811.10
   semilunar
     bone, wrist (closed) 814.02
      open 814.12
     cartilage (interior) (knee)—*see* Tear, meniscus
   sesamoid bone—*see* Fracture, by site
   Shepherd's (closed) 825.21
     open 825.31
   shoulder—*see also* Fracture, humerus, upper
     end
     blade—*see* Fracture, scapula
   silverfork—*see* Fracture, radius, lower end
   sinus (ethmoid) (frontal) (maxillary) (nasal)
     (sphenoidal)—*see* Fracture, skull, base
     maxillary—*see* Fracture, maxilla
   Skillern's—*see* Fracture, radius, shaft
   skull (multiple NEC) (with face bones) (closed)
     803.0

Note—Use the following fifth-digit subclassification with categories 800, 801, 803, and 804:

0 unspecified state of consciousness
1 with no loss of consciousness
2 with brief [less than one hour] loss of consciousness
3 with moderate [1-24 hours] loss of consciousness
4 with prolonged [more than 24 hours] loss of consciousness and return to pre-existing conscious level
5 with prolonged [more than 24 hours] loss of consciousness, without return to pre-existing conscious level
Use fifth-digit 5 to designate when a patient is unconscious and dies before regaining consciousness, regardless of the duration of the loss of consciousness
6 with loss of consciousness of unspecified duration
9 with concussion, unspecified

---

     with
      contusion, cerebral 803.1
      epidural hemorrhage 803.2
      extradural hemorrhage 803.2
      hemorrhage (intracranial) NEC 803.3
      intracranial injury NEC 803.4
      laceration, cerebral 803.1
      other bones—*see* Fracture, multiple, skull
      subarachnoid hemorrhage 803.2

Fracture—*continued*
     subdural hemorrhage 803.2
   base (antrum) (ethmoid bone) (fossa) (internal
     ear) (nasal sinus) (occiput) (sphenoid)
     (temporal bone) (closed) 801.0
     with
      contusion, cerebral 801.1
      epidural hemorrhage 801.2
      extradural hemorrhage 801.2
      hemorrhage (intracranial) NEC 801.3
      intracranial injury NEC 801.4
      laceration, cerebral 801.1
      subarachnoid hemorrhage 801.2
      subdural hemorrhage 801.2
     open 801.5
      with
       contusion, cerebral 801.6
       epidural hemorrhage 801.7
       extradural hemorrhage 801.7
       hemorrhage (intracranial) NEC 801.8
       intracranial injury NEC 801.9
       laceration, cerebral 801.6
       subarachnoid hemorrhage 801.7
       subdural hemorrhage 801.7
   birth injury 767.3
   face bones—*see* Fracture, face bones
   open 803.5
     with
      contusion, cerebral 803.6
      epidural hemorrhage 803.7
      extradural hemorrhage 803.7
      hemorrhage (intracranial) NEC 803.8
      intracranial injury NEC 803.9
      laceration, cerebral 803.6
      subarachnoid hemorrhage 803.7
      subdural hemorrhage 803.7
   vault (frontal bone) (parietal bone) (vertex)
     (closed) 800.0
     with
      contusion, cerebral 800.1
      epidural hemorrhage 800.2
      extradural hemorrhage 800.2
      hemorrhage (intracranial) NEC 800.3
      intracranial injury NEC 800.4
      laceration, cerebral 800.1
      subarachnoid hemorrhage 800.2
      subdural hemorrhage 800.2
     open 800.5
      with
       contusion, cerebral 800.6
       epidural hemorrhage 800.7
       extradural hemorrhage 800.7
       hemorrhage (intracranial) NEC 800.8
       intracranial injury NEC 800.9
       laceration, cerebral 800.6
       subarachnoid hemorrhage 800.7
       subdural hemorrhage 800.7
  Smith's 813.41
   open 813.51
  sphenoid (bone) (sinus)—*see* Fracture, skull,
    base
  spine—*see also* Fracture, vertebra, by site
   due to birth trauma 767.4
  spinous process—*see* Fracture, vertebra, by site
  spontaneous—*see* Fracture, pathologic
  sprinters'—*see* Fracture, ilium
  stapes—*see* Fracture, skull, base
  stave—*see also* Fracture, metacarpus,
    metacarpal bone(s)
   spine—*see* Fracture, tibia, upper end
  sternum (closed) 807.2

Fracture—*continued*
  unciform (closed) 814.08
    open 814.18
  vertebra, vertebral (back) (body) (column)
    (neural arch) (pedicle) (spine) (spinous
    process) (transverse process) (closed) 805.8
    with
      hematomyelia—*see* Fracture, vertebra, by
        site, with spinal cord injury
      injury to
        cauda equina—*see* Fracture, vertebra,
          sacrum, with spinal cord injury
        nerve—*see* Fracture, vertebra, by site, with
          spinal cord injury
        paralysis—*see* Fracture, vertebra, by site,
          with spinal cord injury
        paraplegia—*see* Fracture, vertebra, by site,
          with spinal cord injury
        quadriplegia—*see* Fracture, vertebra, by site,
          with spinal cord injury
        spinal concussion—*see* Fracture, vertebra,
          by site, with spinal cord injury
      spinal cord injury (closed) NEC 806.8

Note—Use the following fifth-digit
subclassification with categories 806.0-806.3:

C_1-C_4 *or unspecified level and* D_1-D_6 (T_1-T_6) *or*
unspecified level with:

0 unspecified spinal cord injury
1 complete lesion of cord
2 anterior cord syndrome
3 central cord syndrome
4 specified injury NEC

C_5-C_7 *level and* D_7-D_{12} *level with:*

5 unspecified spinal cord injury
6 complete lesion of cord
7 anterior cord syndrome
8 central cord syndrome
9 specified injury NEC

---

      cervical 806.0
        open 806.1
      dorsal, dorsolumbar 806.2
        open 806.3
        open 806.9
      thoracic, thoracolumbar 806.2
        open 806.3
    atlanto-axial—*see* Fracture, vertebra, cervical
    cervical (hangman) (teardrop) (closed) 805.00
      with spinal cord injury—*see* Fracture,
        vertebra, with spinal cord injury, cervical
      first (atlas) 805.01
        open 805.11
      second (axis) 805.02
        open 805.12
      third 805.03
        open 805.13
      fourth 805.04
        open 805.14
      fifth 805.05
        open 805.15
      sixth 805.06
        open 805.16
      seventh 805.07
        open 805.17
      multiple sites 805.08
        open 805.18

Fracture—*continued*
  open 805.10
  coccyx (closed) 805.6
    with spinal cord injury (closed) 806.60
      cauda equina injury 806.62
        complete lesion 806.61
          open 806.71
        open 806.72
      open 806.70
      specified type NEC 806.69
        open 806.79
    open 805.7
  collapsed 733.13
  compression, not due to trauma 733.13
  dorsal (closed) 805.2
    with spinal cord injury—*see* Fracture,
      vertebra, with spinal cord injury, dorsal
    open 805.3
  dorsolumbar (closed) 805.2
    with spinal cord injury—*see* Fracture,
      vertebra, with spinal cord injury, dorsal
    open 805.3
  due to osteoporosis 733.13
  fetus or newborn 767.4
  lumbar (closed) 805.4
    with spinal cord injury (closed) 806.4
      open 806.5
    open 805.5
  nontraumatic 733.13
  open NEC 805.9
  pathologic 733.13
  sacrum (closed) 805.6
    with spinal cord injury 806.60
      cauda equina injury 806.62
        complete lesion 806.61
          open 806.71
        open 806.72
      open 806.70
      specified type NEC 806.69
        open 806.79
    open 805.7
  site unspecified (closed) 805.8
    with spinal cord injury (closed) 806.8
      open 806.9
    open 805.9
  stress (any site) 733.95
  thoracic (closed) 805.2
    with spinal cord injury—*see* Fracture,
      vertebra, with spinal cord injury,
      thoracic
    open 805.3
  vertex—*see* Fracture, skull, vault
  vomer (bone) 802.0
    open 802.1
  Wagstaffe's—*see* Fracture, ankle
  wrist (closed) 814.00
    open 814.10
    pathologic 733.12
  xiphoid (process)—*see* Fracture, sternum
  zygoma (zygomatic arch) (closed) 802.4
    open 802.5
Fragile X syndrome 759.83
Fragilitas
  crinium 704.2
  hair 704.2
  ossium 756.51
    with blue sclera 756.51
  unguium 703.8
    congenital 757.5

Furuncle 680.9
  abdominal wall 680.2
  ankle 680.6
  anus 680.5
  arm (any part, above wrist) 680.3
  auditory canal, external 680.0
  axilla 680.3
  back (any part) 680.2
  breast 680.2
  buttock 680.5
  chest wall 680.2
  corpus cavernosum 607.2
  ear (any part) 680.0
  eyelid 373.13
  face (any part, except eye) 680.0
  finger (any) 680.4
  flank 680.2
  foot (any part) 680.7
  forearm 680.3
  gluteal (region) 680.5
  groin 680.2
  hand (any part) 680.4
  head (any part, except face) 680.8
  heel 680.7
  hip 680.6
  kidney (*see also* Abscess, kidney) 590.2
  knee 680.6
  labium (majus) (minus) 616.4
  lacrimal
    gland (*see also* Dacryoadenitis) 375.00
    passages (duct) (sac) (*see also* Dacryocystitis)
      375.30
  leg, any part except foot 680.6
  malignant 022.0
  multiple sites 680.9
  neck 680.1
  nose (external) (septum) 680.0
  orbit 376.01
  partes posteriores 680.5
  pectoral region 680.2
  penis 607.2
  perineum 680.2
  pinna 680.0
  scalp (any part) 680.8
  scrotum 608.4
  seminal vesicle 608.0
  shoulder 680.3
  skin NEC 680.9
  specified site NEC 680.8
  spermatic cord 608.4
  temple (region) 680.0
  testis 604.90
  thigh 680.6
  thumb 680.4
  toe (any) 680.7
  trunk 680.2
  tunica vaginalis 608.4
  umbilicus 680.2
  upper arm 680.3
  vas deferens 608.4
  vulva 616.4
  wrist 680.4
Furunculosis (*see also* Furuncle) 680.9
  external auditory meatus 680.0 *[380.13]*
Fusarium (infection) 118
Fusion, fused (congenital)
  anal (with urogenital canal) 751.5
  aorta and pulmonary artery 745.0
  astragaloscaphoid 755.67
  atria 745.5
  atrium and ventricle 745.69

Fusion, fused—*continued*
  auditory canal 744.02
  auricles, heart 745.5
  binocular, with defective stereopsis 368.33
  bone 756.9
  cervical spine—*see* Fusion, spine
  choanal 748.0
  commissure, mitral valve 746.5
  cranial sutures, premature 756.0
  cusps, heart valve NEC 746.89
    mitral 746.5
    tricuspid 746.89
  ear ossicles 744.04
  fingers (*see also* Syndactylism, fingers) 755.11
  hymen 752.42
  hymeno-urethral 599.89
    causing obstructed labor 660.1
      affecting fetus or newborn 763.1
  joint (acquired)—*see also* Ankylosis
    congenital 755.8
  kidneys (incomplete) 753.3
  labium (majus) (minus) 752.49
  larynx and trachea 748.3
  limb 755.8
    lower 755.69
    upper 755.59
  lobe, lung 748.5
  lumbosacral (acquired) 724.6
    congenital 756.15
    surgical V45.4
  nares (anterior) (posterior) 748.0
  nose, nasal 748.0
  nostril(s) 748.0
  organ or site NEC—*see* Anomaly, specified
    type NEC
  ossicles 756.9
    auditory 744.04
  pulmonary valve segment 746.02
  pulmonic cusps 746.02
  ribs 756.3
  sacroiliac (acquired) (joint) 724.6
    congenital 755.69
    surgical V45.4
  skull, imperfect 756.0
  spine (acquired) 724.9
    arthrodesis status V45.4
    congenital (vertebra) 756.15
    postoperative status V45.4
  sublingual duct with submaxillary duct at
    opening in mouth 750.26
  talonavicular (bar) 755.67
  teeth, tooth 520.2
  testes 752.89
  toes (*see also* Syndactylism, toes) 755.13
  trachea and esophagus 750.3
  twins 759.4
  urethral-hymenal 599.89
  vagina 752.49
  valve cusps—*see* Fusion, cusps, heart valve
  ventricles, heart 745.4
  vertebra (arch)—*see* Fusion, spine
  vulva 752.49
Fusospirillosis (mouth) (tongue) (tonsil) 101
Fussy infant (baby) 780.91

G

Gafsa boil 085.1
Gain, weight (abnormal) (excessive) (see also
   Weight, gain) 783.1
Gaisböck's disease or syndrome (polycythemia
   hypertonica) 289.0
Gait
  abnormality 781.2
    hysterical 300.11
  ataxic 781.2
    hysterical 300.11
  disturbance 781.2
    hysterical 300.11
  paralytic 781.2
  scissor 781.2
  spastic 781.2
  staggering 781.2
    hysterical 300.11
Galactocele (breast) (infected) 611.5
  puerperal, postpartum 676.8
Galactophoritis 611.0
  puerperal, postpartum 675.2
Galactorrhea 676.6
  not associated with childbirth 611.6
Galactosemia (classic) (congenital) 271.1
Galactosuria 271.1
Galacturia 791.1
  bilharziasis 120.0
Galen's vein —*see* condition
Gallbladder —*see also* condition
  acute (*see also* Disease, gallbladder) 575.0
Gall duct —*see* condition
Gallop rhythm 427.89
Gallstone (cholemic) (colic) (impacted)—*see*
   also Cholelithiasis
  causing intestinal obstruction 560.31
Gambling, pathological 312.31
Gammaloidosis 277.39
Gammopathy 273.9
  macroglobulinemia 273.3
  monoclonal (benign) (essential) (idiopathic)
    (with lymphoplasmacytic dyscrasia) 273.1
Gamna's disease (siderotic splenomegaly)
   289.51
Gampsodactylia (congenital) 754.71
Gamstorp's disease (adynamia episodica
   hereditaria) 359.3
Gandy-Nanta disease (siderotic splenomegaly)
   289.51
**Gang activity without manifest psychiatric
   disorder** V71.09
  adolescent V71.02
  adult V71.01
  child V71.02
Gangliocytoma (M9490/0)—*see* Neoplasm,
   connective tissue, benign
Ganglioglioma (M9505/1)—*see* Neoplasm, by
   site, uncertain behavior
Ganglion 727.43
  joint 727.41
  of yaws (early) (late) 102.6
  periosteal (*see also* Periostitis) 730.3
  tendon sheath (compound) (diffuse) 727.42
  tuberculous (*see also* Tuberculosis) 015.9
Ganglioneuroblastoma (M9490/3)—*see*
   Neoplasm, connective tissue, malignant
Ganglioneuroma (M9490/0)—*see also*
   Neoplasm, connective tissue, benign

Ganglioneuroma—*continued*
  malignant (M9490/3)—*see* Neoplasm,
   connective tissue, malignant
Ganglioneuromatosis (M9491/0)—*see*
   Neoplasm, connective tissue, benign
Ganglionitis
  fifth nerve (*see also* Neuralgia, trigeminal)
    350.1
  gasserian 350.1
  geniculate 351.1
    herpetic 053.11
    newborn 767.5
  herpes zoster 053.11
  herpetic geniculate (Hunt's syndrome) 053.11
Gangliosidosis 330.1
Gangosa 102.5
Gangrene, gangrenous (anemia) (artery)
   (cellulitis) (dermatitis) (dry) (infective)
   (moist) (pemphigus) (septic) (skin) (stasis)
   (ulcer) 785.4
  with
   arteriosclerosis (native artery) 440.24
    bypass graft 440.30
     autologous vein 440.31
     nonautologous biological 440.32
   diabetes (mellitus) 250.7 *[785.4]*
  abdomen (wall) 785.4
  adenitis 683
  alveolar 526.5
  angina 462
   diphtheritic 032.0
  anus 569.49
  appendices epiploicae—*see* Gangrene,
    mesentery
  appendix—*see* Appendicitis, acute
  arteriosclerotic —*see* Arteriosclerosis, with,
    gangrene
  auricle 785.4
  Bacillus welchii (*see also* Gangrene, gas) 040.0
  bile duct (*see also* Cholangitis) 576.8
  bladder 595.89
  bowel—*see* Gangrene, intestine
  cecum—*see* Gangrene, intestine
  Clostridium perfringens or welchii (*see also*
    Gangrene, gas) 040.0
  colon—*see* Gangrene, intestine
  connective tissue 785.4
  cornea 371.40
  corpora cavernosa (infective) 607.2
   noninfective 607.89
  cutaneous, spreading 785.4
  decubital (*see also* Decubitus) 707.00 *[785.4]*
  diabetic (any site) 250.7 *[785.4]*
  dropsical 785.4
  emphysematous (*see also* Gangrene, gas) 040.0
  epidemic (ergotized grain) 988.2
  epididymis (infectional) (*see also* Epididymitis)
    604.99
  erysipelas (*see also* Erysipelas) 035
  extremity (lower) (upper) 785.4
  gallbladder or duct (*see also* Cholecystitis,
    acute) 575.0
  gas (bacillus) 040.0
   with
    abortion—*see* Abortion, by type, with sepsis
    ectopic pregnancy (*see also* categories
     633.0-633.9) 639.0

Gangrene, gangrenous—*continued*
    molar pregnancy (*see also* categories
       630-632) 639.0
  following
    abortion 639.0
    ectopic or molar pregnancy 639.0
  puerperal, postpartum, childbirth 670
  glossitis 529.0
  gum 523.8
  hernia—*see* Hernia, by site, with gangrene
  hospital noma 528.1
  intestine, intestinal (acute) (hemorrhagic)
    (massive) 557.0
    with
      hernia—*see* Hernia, by site, with gangrene
      mesenteric embolism or infarction 557.0
      obstruction (*see also* Obstruction, intestine)
        560.9
  laryngitis 464.00
    with obstruction 464.01
  liver 573.8
  lung 513.0
    spirochetal 104.8
  lymphangitis 457.2
  Meleney's (cutaneous) 686.09
  mesentery 557.0
    with
      embolism or infarction 557.0
      intestinal obstruction (*see also* Obstruction,
        intestine) 560.9
  mouth 528.1
  noma 528.1
  orchitis 604.90
  ovary (*see also* Salpingo-oophoritis) 614.2
  pancreas 577.0
  penis (infectional) 607.2
    noninfective 607.89
  perineum 785.4
  pharynx 462
    septic 034.0
  pneumonia 513.0
  Pott's 440.24
  presenile 443.1
  pulmonary 513.0
  pulp, tooth 522.1
  quinsy 475
  Raynaud's (symmetric gangrene) 443.0 *[785.4]*
  rectum 569.49
  retropharyngeal 478.24
  rupture—*see* Hernia, by site, with gangrene
  scrotum 608.4
    noninfective 608.83
  senile 440.24
  sore throat 462
  spermatic cord 608.4
    noninfective 608.89
  spine 785.4
  spirochetal NEC 104.8
  spreading cutaneous 785.4
  stomach 537.89
  stomatitis 528.1
  symmetrical 443.0 *[785.4]*
  testis (infectional) (*see also* Orchitis) 604.99
    noninfective 608.89
  throat 462
    diphtheritic 032.0
  thyroid (gland) 246.8
  tonsillitis (acute) 463
  tooth (pulp) 522.1
  tuberculous NEC (*see also* Tuberculosis) 011.9
  tunica vaginalis 608.4

Gangrene, gangrenous—*continued*
  noninfective 608.89
  umbilicus 785.4
  uterus (*see also* Endometritis) 615.9
  uvulitis 528.3
  vas deferens 608.4
    noninfective 608.89
  vulva (*see also* Vulvitis) 616.10
Gannister disease (occupational) 502
  with tuberculosis—*see* Tuberculosis, pulmonary
Ganser's syndrome, hysterical 300.16
Gardner-Diamond syndrome (autoerythrocyte
  sensitization) 287.2
Gargoylism 277.5
Garré's
  disease (*see also* Osteomyelitis) 730.1
  osteitis (sclerosing) (*see also* Osteomyelitis)
    730.1
  osteomyelitis (*see also* Osteomyelitis) 730.1
Garrod's pads, knuckle 728.79
Gartner's duct
  cyst 752.41
  persistent 752.41
Gas
  asphyxia, asphyxiation, inhalation, poisoning,
    suffocation NEC 987.9
    specified gas—*see* Table of drugs and
      chemicals
  bacillus gangrene or infection—*see* Gas,
    gangrene
  cyst, mesentery 568.89
  excessive 787.3
  gangrene 040.0
    with
      abortion—*see* Abortion, by type, with sepsis
      ectopic pregnancy (*see also* categories
        633.0-633.9) 639.0
      molar pregnancy (*see also* categories
        630-632) 639.0
    following
      abortion 639.0
      ectopic or molar pregnancy 639.0
    puerperal, postpartum, childbirth 670
  on stomach 787.3
  pains 787.3
Gastradenitis 535.0
Gastralgia 536.8
  psychogenic 307.89
Gastrectasis, gastrectasia 536.1
  psychogenic 306.4
Gastric —*see* condition
Gastrinoma (M8153/1)
  malignant (M8153/3)
    pancreas 157.4
    specified site NEC—*see* Neoplasm, by site,
      malignant
    unspecified site 157.4
    specified site—*see* Neoplasm, by site,
      uncertain behavior
  unspecified site 235.5
Gastritis 535.5

Note—Use the following fifth-digit
subclassification for category 535:

0 without mention of hemorrhage
1 with hemorrhage

---

  acute 535.0
  alcoholic 535.3
  allergic 535.4

Genu—*continued*
  introrsum (acquired) 736.41
    congenital 755.64
    late effects of rickets 268.1
    rachitic (old) 268.1
  recurvatum (acquired) 736.5
    congenital 754.40
      with dislocation of knee 754.41
    late effects of rickets 268.1
  valgum (acquired) (knock-knee) 736.41
    congenital 755.64
    late effects of rickets 268.1
  varum (acquired) (bowleg) 736.42
    congenital 755.64
    late effects of rickets 268.1
Geographic tongue 529.1
Geophagia 307.52
Geotrichosis 117.9
  intestine 117.9
  lung 117.9
  mouth 117.9
Gephyrophobia 300.29
Gerbode defect 745.4
Gerhardt's
  disease (erythromelalgia) 443.82
  syndrome (vocal cord paralysis) 478.30
Gerlier's disease (epidemic vertigo) 078.81
German measles 056.9
  exposure to V01.4
Germinoblastoma (diffuse) (M9614/3) 202.8
  follicular (M9692/3) 202.0
Germinoma (M9064/3)—*see* Neoplasm, by site,
  malignant
Gerontoxon 371.41
Gerstmann's syndrome (finger agnosia) 784.69
Gestation (period)—*see also* Pregnancy
  ectopic NEC (*see also* Pregnancy, ectopic) 633.90
    with intrauterine pregnancy 633.91
Gestational proteinuria 646.2
  with hypertension—*see* Toxemia, of pregnancy
Ghon tubercle primary infection (*see also*
  Tuberculosis) 010.0
Ghost
  teeth 520.4
  vessels, cornea 370.64
Ghoul hand 102.3
Gianotti Crosti syndrome 057.8
  due to known virus—*see* Infection, virus
  due to unknown virus 057.8
Giant
  cell
    epulis 523.8
    peripheral (gingiva) 523.8
    tumor, tendon sheath 727.02
  colon (congenital) 751.3
  esophagus (congenital) 750.4
  kidney 753.3
  urticaria 995.1
    hereditary 277.6
Giardia lamblia infestation 007.1
Giardiasis 007.1
Gibert's disease (pityriasis rosea) 696.3
Gibraltar fever —*see* Brucellosis
Giddiness 780.4
  hysterical 300.11
  psychogenic 306.9
Gierke's disease (glycogenosis I) 271.0
Gigantism (cerebral) (hypophyseal) (pituitary)
  253.0

Gilbert's disease or cholemia (familial
  nonhemolytic jaundice) 277.4
Gilchrist's disease (North American
  blastomycosis) 116.0
Gilford (-Hutchinson) disease or syndrome
  (progeria) 259.8
Gilles de la Tourette's disease (motor-verbal tic)
  307.23
Gillespie's syndrome (dysplasia
  oculodentodigitalis) 759.89
Gingivitis 523.10
  acute 523.00
    necrotizing 101
    non-plaque induced 523.01
    plaque induced 523.00
  catarrhal 523.00
  chronic 523.10
    non-plaque induced 523.11
  desquamative 523.10
  expulsiva 523.40
  hyperplastic 523.10
  marginal, simple 523.10
  necrotizing, acute 101
  non-plaque induced 523.11
  pellagrous 265.2
  plaque induced 523.10
  ulcerative 523.10
    acute necrotizing 101
  Vincent's 101
Gingivoglossitis 529.0
Gingivopericementitis 523.40
Gingivosis 523.10
Gingivostomatitis 523.10
  herpetic 054.2
Giovannini's disease 117.9
GISA (glycopeptide intermediate staphylococcus
  aureus) V09.8
Gland, glandular —*see* condition
Glanders 024
Glanzmann (-Naegeli) disease or thrombasthenia
  287.1
Glassblowers' disease 527.1
Glaucoma (capsular) (inflammatory)
  (noninflammatory) (primary) 365.9
  with increased episcleral venous pressure 365.82
  absolute 360.42
  acute 365.22
    narrow angle 365.22
    secondary 365.60
  angle closure 365.20
    acute 365.22
    chronic 365.23
    intermittent 365.21
    interval 365.21
    residual stage 365.24
    subacute 365.21
  border line 365.00
  chronic 365.11
    noncongestive 365.11
    open angle 365.11
    simple 365.11
  closed angle—*see* Glaucoma, angle closure
  congenital 743.20
    associated with other eye anomalies 743.22
    simple 743.21
  congestive—*see* Glaucoma, narrow angle
  corticosteroid-induced (glaucomatous stage)
    365.31
    residual stage 365.32
  hemorrhagic 365.60
  hypersecretion 365.81

Glaucoma—*continued*
  in or with
    aniridia 743.45 *[365.42]*
    Axenfeld's anomaly 743.44 *[365.41]*
    concussion of globe 921.3 *[365.65]*
    congenital syndromes NEC 759.89 *[365.44]*
    dislocation of lens
      anterior 379.33 *[365.59]*
      posterior 379.34 *[365.59]*
    disorder of lens NEC 365.59
    epithelial down-growth 364.61 *[365.64]*
    glaucomatocyclitic crisis 364.22 *[365.62]*
    hypermature cataract 366.18 *[365.51]*
    hyphema 364.41 *[365.63]*
    inflammation, ocular 365.62
    iridocyclitis 364.3 *[365.62]*
    iris
      anomalies NEC 743.46 *[365.42]*
      atrophy, essential 364.51 *[365.42]*
      bombé 364.74 *[365.61]*
      rubeosis 364.42 *[365.63]*
    microcornea 743.41 *[365.43]*
    neurofibromatosis 237.71 *[365.44]*
    ocular
      cysts NEC 365.64
      disorders NEC 365.60
      trauma 365.65
      tumors NEC 365.64
    postdislocation of lens
      anterior 379.33 *[365.59]*
      posterior 379.34 *[365.59]*
    pseudoexfoliation of capsule 366.11 *[365.52]*
    pupillary block or seclusion 364.74 *[365.61]*
    recession of chamber angle 364.77 *[365.65]*
    retinal vein occlusion 362.35 *[365.63]*
    Rieger's anomaly or syndrome 743.44
      [365.41]
    rubeosis of iris 364.42 *[365.63]*
    seclusion of pupil 364.74 *[365.61]*
    spherophakia 743.36 *[365.59]*
    Sturge-Weber (-Dimitri) syndrome 759.6
      [365.44]
    systemic syndrome NEC 365.44
    tumor of globe 365.64
    vascular disorders NEC 365.63
  infantile 365.14
    congenital 743.20
      associated with other eye anomalies 743.22
      simple 743.21
  juvenile 365.14
  low tension 365.12
  malignant 365.83
  narrow angle (primary) 365.20
    acute 365.22
    chronic 365.23
    intermittent 365.21
    interval 365.21
    residual stage 365.24
    subacute 365.21
  newborn 743.20
    associated with other eye anomalies 743.22
    simple 743.21
  noncongestive (chronic) 365.11
  nonobstructive (chronic) 365.11
  obstructive 365.60
    due to lens changes 365.59
  open angle 365.10
    with
      borderline intraocular pressure 365.01
      cupping of optic discs 365.01
  primary 365.11

Glaucoma—*continued*
  residual stage 365.15
  phacolytic 365.51
    with hypermature cataract 366.18 *[365.51]*
  pigmentary 365.13
  postinfectious 365.60
  pseudoexfoliation 365.52
    with pseudoexfoliation of capsule 366.11
      [365.52]
  secondary NEC 365.60
  simple (chronic) 365.11
  simplex 365.11
  steroid responders 365.03
  suspect 365.00
  syphilitic 095.8
  traumatic NEC 365.65
    newborn 767.8
  tuberculous (*see also* Tuberculosis) 017.3
    [365.62]
  wide angle (*see also* Glaucoma, open angle)
    365.10
Glaucomatous flecks (subcapsular) 366.31
Glazed tongue 529.4
Gleet 098.2
Glénard's disease or syndrome (enteroptosis)
  569.89
Glinski-Simmonds syndrome (pituitary
  cachexia) 253.2
Glioblastoma (multiforme) (M9440/3)
  with sarcomatous component (M9442/3)
    specified site—*see* Neoplasm, by site,
      malignant
    unspecified site 191.9
  giant cell (M9441/3)
    specified site—*see* Neoplasm, by site, malignant
    unspecified site 191.9
  specified site—*see* Neoplasm, by site, malignant
  unspecified site 191.9
Glioma (malignant) (M9380/3)
  astrocytic (M9400/3)
    specified site—*see* Neoplasm, by site,
      malignant
    unspecified site 191.9
  mixed (M9382/3)
    specified site—*see* Neoplasm, by site,
      malignant
    unspecified site 191.9
  nose 748.1
  specified site NEC—*see* Neoplasm, by site,
    malignant
  subependymal (M9383/1) 237.5
  unspecified site 191.9
Gliomatosis cerebri (M9381/3) 191.0
Glioneuroma (M9505/1)—*see* Neoplasm, by
  site, uncertain behavior
Gliosarcoma (M9380/3)
  specified site—*see* Neoplasm, by site, malignant
  unspecified site 191.9
Gliosis (cerebral) 349.89
  spinal 336.0
Glisson's
  cirrhosis—*see* Cirrhosis, portal
  disease (*see also* Rickets) 268.0
Glissonitis 573.3
Globinuria 791.2
Globus 306.4
  hystericus 300.11
Glomangioma (M8712/0) (*see also*
  Hemangioma) 228.00
Glomangiosarcoma (M8710/3)—*see* Neoplasm,
  connective tissue, malignant

Glomerular nephritis (*see also* Nephritis) 583.9
Glomerulitis (*see also* Nephritis) 583.9
Glomerulonephritis (*see also* Nephritis) 583.9
  with
    edema (*see also* Nephrosis) 581.9
    lesion of
      exudative nephritis 583.89
      interstitial nephritis (diffuse) (focal) 583.89
      necrotizing glomerulitis 583.4
        acute 580.4
      chronic 582.4
      renal necrosis 583.9
        cortical 583.6
        medullary 583.7
      specified pathology NEC 583.89
        acute 580.89
        chronic 582.89
    necrosis, renal 583.9
      cortical 583.6
      medullary (papillary) 583.7
    specified pathology or lesion NEC 583.89
  acute 580.9
    with
      exudative nephritis 580.89
      interstitial nephritis (diffuse) (focal) 580.89
      necrotizing glomerulitis 580.4
    extracapillary with epithelial crescents 580.4
    poststreptococcal 580.0
    proliferative (diffuse) 580.0
    rapidly progressive 580.4
    specified pathology NEC 580.89
  arteriolar (*see also* Hypertension, kidney) 403.90
  arteriosclerotic (*see also* Hypertension, kidney) 403.90
  ascending (*see also* Pyelitis) 590.80
  basement membrane NEC 583.89
    with
      pulmonary hemorrhage (Goodpasture's syndrome) 446.21 *[583.81]*
  chronic 582.9
    with
      exudative nephritis 582.89
      interstitial nephritis (diffuse) (focal) 582.89
      necrotizing glomerulitis 582.4
      specified pathology or lesion NEC 582.89
    endothelial 582.2
    extracapillary with epithelial crescents 582.4
    hypocomplementemic persistent 582.2
    lobular 582.2
    membranoproliferative 582.2
    membranous 582.1
      and proliferative (mixed) 582.2
      sclerosing 582.1
    mesangiocapillary 582.2
    mixed membranous and proliferative 582.2
    proliferative (diffuse) 582.0
    rapidly progressive 582.4
    sclerosing 582.1
  cirrhotic—*see* Sclerosis, renal
  desquamative—*see* Nephrosis
  due to or associated with
    amyloidosis 277.39 *[583.81]*
      with nephrotic syndrome 277.39 *[581.81]*
      chronic 277.39 *[582.81]*
    diabetes mellitus 250.4 *[583.81]*
      with nephrotic syndrome 250.4 *[581.81]*
    diphtheria 032.89 *[580.81]*
    gonococcal infection (acute) 098.19 *[583.81]*
      chronic or duration or 2 months or over 098.39 *[583.81]*

Glomerulonephritis—*continued*
  infectious hepatitis 070.9 *[580.81]*
  malaria (with nephrotic syndrome) 084.9 *[581.81]*
  mumps 072.79 *[580.81]*
  polyarteritis (nodosa) (with nephrotic syndrome) 446.0 *[581.81]*
  specified pathology NEC 583.89
    acute 580.89
    chronic 582.89
  streptotrichosis 039.8 *[583.81]*
  subacute bacterial endocarditis 421.0 *[580.81]*
  syphilis (late) 095.4
    congenital 090.5 *[583.81]*
    early 091.69 *[583.81]*
  systemic lupus erythematosus 710.0 *[583.81]*
    with nephrotic syndrome 710.0 *[581.81]*
    chronic 710.0 *[582.81]*
  tuberculosis (*see also* Tuberculosis) 016.0 *[583.81]*
  typhoid fever 002.0 *[580.81]*
  extracapillary with epithelial crescents 583.4
    acute 580.4
    chronic 582.4
  exudative 583.89
    acute 580.89
    chronic 582.89
  focal (*see also* Nephritis) 583.9
    embolic 580.4
  granular 582.89
  granulomatous 582.89
  hydremic (*see also* Nephrosis) 581.9
  hypocomplementemic persistent 583.2
    with nephrotic syndrome 581.2
    chronic 582.2
  immune complex NEC 583.89
  infective (*see also* Pyelitis) 590.80
  interstitial (diffuse) (focal) 583.89
    with nephrotic syndrome 581.89
    acute 580.89
    chronic 582.89
  latent or quiescent 582.9
  lobular 583.2
    with nephrotic syndrome 581.2
    chronic 582.2
  membranoproliferative 583.2
    with nephrotic syndrome 581.2
    chronic 582.2
  membranous 583.1
    with nephrotic syndrome 581.1
    and proliferative (mixed) 583.2
      with nephrotic syndrome 581.2
      chronic 582.2
    chronic 582.1
    sclerosing 582.1
      with nephrotic syndrome 581.1
  mesangiocapillary 583.2
    with nephrotic syndrome 581.2
    chronic 582.2
  minimal change 581.3
  mixed membranous and proliferative 583.2
    with nephrotic syndrome 581.2
    chronic 582.2
  necrotizing 583.4
    acute 580.4
    chronic 582.4
  nephrotic (*see also* Nephrosis) 581.9
  old—*see* Glomerulonephritis, chronic
  parenchymatous 581.89
  poststreptococcal 580.0
  proliferative (diffuse) 583.0

Goiter—*continued*
  pulsating (*see also* Goiter, toxic) 242.0
  simple 240.0
  toxic 242.0

> *Note—Use the following fifth-digit*
> *subclassification with category 242:*
>
> *0* *without mention of thyrotoxic crisis*
>   *or storm*
> *1* *with mention of thyrotoxic crisis or storm*

    adenomatous 242.3
      multinodular 242.2
      uninodular 242.1
     multinodular 242.2
     nodular 242.3
      multinodular 242.2
      uninodular 242.1
     uninodular 242.1
   uninodular (nontoxic) 241.0
    toxic or with hyperthyroidism (*see also* Goiter, toxic) 242.1
Goldberg (-Maxwell) (-Morris) syndrome (testicular feminization) 259.5
Goldblatt's
  hypertension 440.1
  kidney 440.1
Goldenhar's syndrome (oculoauriculovertebral dysplasia) 756.0
Goldflam-Erb disease or syndrome 358.00
Goldscheider's disease (epidermolysis bullosa) 757.39
Goldstein's disease (familial hemorrhagic telangiectasia) 448.0
Golfer's elbow 726.32
Goltz-Gorlin syndrome (dermal hypoplasia) 757.39
Gonadoblastoma (M9073/1)
  specified site—*see* Neoplasm, by site uncertain behavior
  unspecified site
    female 236.2
    male 236.4
Gonecystitis (*see also* Vesiculitis) 608.0
Gongylonemiasis 125.6
  mouth 125.6
Goniosynechiae 364.73
Gonococcemia 098.89
Gonococcus, gonococcal (disease) (infection) (*see also* condition) 098.0
  anus 098.7
  bursa 098.52
  chronic NEC 098.2
  complicating pregnancy, childbirth, or puerperium 647.1
    affecting fetus or newborn 760.2
  conjunctiva, conjunctivitis (neonatorum) 098.40
  dermatosis 098.89
  endocardium 098.84
  epididymo-orchitis 098.13
    chronic or duration of 2 months or over 098.33
  eye (newborn) 098.40
  fallopian tube (chronic) 098.37
    acute 098.17
  genitourinary (acute) (organ) (system) (tract) (*see also* Gonorrhea) 098.0
    lower 098.0
      chronic 098.2
    upper 098.10
      chronic 098.30

Gonococcus, gonococcal—*continued*
  heart NEC 098.85
  joint 098.50
  keratoderma 098.81
  keratosis (blennorrhagica) 098.81
  lymphatic (gland) (node) 098.89
  meninges 098.82
  orchitis (acute) 098.13
    chronic or duration of 2 months or over 098.33
  pelvis (acute) 098.19
    chronic or duration of 2 months or over 098.39
  pericarditis 098.83
  peritonitis 098.86
  pharyngitis 098.6
  pharynx 098.6
  proctitis 098.7
  pyosalpinx (chronic) 098.37
    acute 098.17
  rectum 098.7
  septicemia 098.89
  skin 098.89
  specified site NEC 098.89
  synovitis 098.51
  tendon sheath 098.51
  throat 098.6
  urethra (acute) 098.0
    chronic or duration of 2 months or over 098.2
  vulva (acute) 098.0
    chronic or duration of 2 months or over 098.2
Gonocytoma (M9073/1)
  specified site—*see* Neoplasm, by site, uncertain behavior
  unspecified site
    female 236.2
    male 236.4
Gonorrhea 098.0
  acute 098.0
  Bartholin's gland (acute) 098.0
    chronic or duration of 2 months or over 098.2
  bladder (acute) 098.11
    chronic or duration of 2 months or over 098.31
  carrier (suspected of) V02.7
  cervix (acute) 098.15
    chronic or duration of 2 months or over 098.35
  chronic 098.2
  complicating pregnancy, childbirth, or puerperium 647.1
    affecting fetus or newborn 760.2
  conjunctiva, conjunctivitis (neonatorum) 098.40
  contact V01.6
  Cowper's gland (acute) 098.0
    chronic or duration of 2 months or over 098.2
  duration of two months or over 098.2
  exposure to V01.6
  fallopian tube (chronic) 098.37
    acute 098.17
  genitourinary (acute) (organ) (system) (tract) 098.0
    chronic 098.2
    duration of two months or over 098.2
  kidney (acute) 098.19
    chronic or duration of 2 months or over 098.39
  ovary (acute) 098.19
    chronic or duration of 2 months or over 098.39
  pelvis (acute) 098.19
    chronic or duration of 2 months or over 098.39
  penis (acute) 098.0
    chronic or duration of 2 months or over 098.2
  prostate (acute) 098.12
    chronic or duration of 2 months or over 098.32
  seminal vesicle (acute) 098.14

Granuloma—*continued*
  subcutaneous tissue 709.4
  fungoides 202.1
  gangraenescens 446.3
  giant cell (central) (jaw) (reparative) 526.3
    gingiva 523.8
    peripheral (gingiva) 523.8
  gland (lymph) 289.3
  Hodgkin's (M9661/3) 201.1
  ileum 569.89
  infectious NEC 136.9
  inguinale (Donovan) 099.2
    venereal 099.2
  intestine 569.89
  iridocyclitis 364.10
  jaw (bone) 526.3
    reparative giant cell 526.3
  kidney (*see also* Infection, kidney) 590.9
  lacrimal sac 375.81
  larynx 478.79
  lethal midline 446.3
  lipid 277.89
  lipoid 277.89
  liver 572.8
  lung (infectious) (*see also* Fibrosis, lung) 515
    coccidioidal 114.4
    eosinophilic 277.89
  lymph gland 289.3
  Majocchi's 110.6
  malignant, face 446.3
  mandible 526.3
  mediastinum 519.3
  midline 446.3
  monilial 112.3
  muscle 728.82
    from residual foreign body 728.82
  nasal sinus (*see also* Sinusitis) 473.9
  operation wound 998.59
    foreign body 998.4
    stitch (external) 998.89
      internal organ 998.89
    talc 998.7
  oral mucosa, eosinophilic or pyogenic 528.9
  orbit, orbital 376.11
  paracoccidioidal 116.1
  penis, venereal 099.2
  periapical 522.6
  peritoneum 568.89
    due to ova of helminths NEC (*see also*
      Helminthiasis) 128.9
  postmastoidectomy cavity 383.33
  postoperative–*see* Granuloma, operation wound
  prostate 601.8
  pudendi (ulcerating) 099.2
  pudendorum (ulcerative) 099.2
  pulp, internal (tooth) 521.49
  pyogenic, pyogenicum (skin) 686.1
    maxillary alveolar ridge 522.6
    oral mucosa 528.9
  rectum 569.49
  reticulohistiocytic 277.89
  rubrum nasi 705.89
  sarcoid 135
  Schistosoma 120.9
  septic (skin) 686.1
  silica (skin) 709.4
  sinus (accessory) (infectional) (nasal) (*see also*
    Sinusitis) 473.9
  skin (pyogenicum) 686.1
    from foreign body or material 709.4
  sperm 608.89

Granuloma—*continued*
  spine
    syphilitic (epidural) 094.89
    tuberculous (*see also* Tuberculosis) 015.0
      [730.88]
  stitch (postoperative) 998.89
    internal wound 998.89
  suppurative (skin) 686.1
  suture (postoperative) 998.89
    internal wound 998.89
  swimming pool 031.1
  talc 728.82
    in operation wound 998.7
  telangiectaticum (skin) 686.1
  tracheostomy 519.09
  trichophyticum 110.6
  tropicum 102.4
  umbilicus 686.1
    newborn 771.4
  urethra 599.84
  uveitis 364.10
  vagina 099.2
  venereum 099.2
  vocal cords 478.5
  Wegener's (necrotizing respiratory
    granulomatosis) 446.4
Granulomatosis NEC 686.1
  disciformis chronica et progressiva 709.3
  infantiseptica 771.2
  lipoid 277.89
  lipophagic, intestinal 040.2
  miliary 027.0
  necrotizing, respiratory 446.4
  progressive, septic 288.1
  Wegener's (necrotizing respiratory) 446.4
Granulomatous tissue —*see* Granuloma
Granulosis rubra nasi 705.89
Graphite fibrosis (of lung) 503
Graphospasm 300.89
  organic 333.84
Grating scapula 733.99
Gravel (urinary) (*see also* Calculus) 592.9
Graves' disease (exophthalmic goiter) (*see also*
  Goiter, toxic) 242.0
Gravis —*see* condition
Grawitz's tumor (hypernephroma) (M8312/3)
  189.0
Grayness, hair (premature) 704.3
  congenital 757.4
Gray or grey syndrome (chloramphenicol)
  (newborn) 779.4
Greenfield's disease 330.0
Green sickness 280.9
Greenstick fracture —*see* Fracture, by site
Greig's syndrome (hypertelorism) 756.0
Griesinger's disease (*see also* Ancylostomiasis)
  126.9
Grinder's
  asthma 502
  lung 502
  phthisis (*see also* Tuberculosis) 011.4
Grinding, teeth 306.8
Grip
  Dabney's 074.1
  devil's 074.1
Grippe, grippal —*see also* Influenza
  Balkan 083.0
  intestinal 487.8
  summer 074.8
Grippy cold 487.1
Grisel's disease 723.5

Groin —*see* condition
Grooved
  nails (transverse) 703.8
  tongue 529.5
    congenital 750.13
Ground itch 126.9
Growing pains, children 781.99
Growth (fungoid) (neoplastic) (new)
    (M8000/1)—*see also* Neoplasm, by site,
    unspecified nature
  adenoid (vegetative) 474.12
  benign (M8000/0)—*see* Neoplasm, by site,
    benign
  fetal, poor 764.9
    affecting management of pregnancy 656.5
  malignant (M8000/3)—*see* Neoplasm, by site
    malignant
  rapid, childhood V21.0
  secondary (M8000/6)—*see* Neoplasm, by site,
    malignant, secondary
GRSA (glycopeptide resistant staphylococcus
    aureus) V09.8
Gruber's hernia —*see* Hernia, Gruber's
Gruby's disease (tinea tonsurans) 110.0
G-trisomy 758.0
Guama fever 066.3
Gubler (-Millard) paralysis or syndrome 344.89
Guérin-Stern syndrome (arthrogryposis
    multiplex congenita) 754.89
Guertin's disease (electric chorea) 049.8
Guillain-Barré disease or syndrome 357.0
Guinea worms (infection) (infestation) 125.7
Guinon's disease (motor-verbal tic) 307.23
Gull's disease (thyroid atrophy with myxedema)
    244.8
Gull and Sutton's disease —*see* Hypertension,
    kidney
Gum —*see* condition
Gumboil 522.7
Gumma (syphilitic) 095.9
  artery 093.89
    cerebral or spinal 094.89
  bone 095.5
    of yaws (late) 102.6
  brain 094.89
  cauda equina 094.89
  central nervous system NEC 094.9
  ciliary body 095.8 *[364.11]*
  congenital 090.5
    testis 090.5
  eyelid 095.8 *[373.5]*
  heart 093.89
  intracranial 094.89
  iris 095.8 *[364.11]*
  kidney 095.4
  larynx 095.8
  leptomeninges 094.2
  liver 095.3
  meninges 094.2
  myocardium 093.82
  nasopharynx 095.8
  neurosyphilitic 094.9
  nose 095.8
  orbit 095.8
  palate (soft) 095.8
  penis 095.8
  pericardium 093.81
  pharynx 095.8
  pituitary 095.8
  scrofulous (*see also* Tuberculosis) 017.0

Gumma—*continued*
  skin 095.8
  specified site NEC 095.8
  spinal cord 094.89
  tongue 095.8
  tonsil 095.8
  trachea 095.8
  tuberculous (*see also* Tuberculosis) 017.0
  ulcerative due to yaws 102.4
  ureter 095.8
  yaws 102.4
    bone 102.6
Gunn's syndrome (jaw-winking syndrome)
    742.8
Gunshot wound —*see also* Wound, open, by site
  fracture—*see* Fracture, by site, open
  internal organs (abdomen, chest, or pelvis)—*see*
    Injury, internal, by site, with open wound
  intracranial—*see* Laceration, brain, with open
    intracranial wound
Günther's disease or syndrome (congenital
    erythropoietic porphyria) 277.1
Gustatory hallucination 780.1
Gynandrism 752.7
Gynandroblastoma (M8632/1)
  specified site—*see* Neoplasm, by site, uncertain
    behavior
  unspecified site
    female 236.2
    male 236.4
Gynandromorphism 752.7
Gynatresia (congenital) 752.49
Gynecoid pelvis, male 738.6
Gynecological examination V72.31
  for contraceptive maintenance V25.40
Gynecomastia 611.1
Gynephobia 300.29
Gyrate scalp 757.39

H

Hay
  asthma (*see also* Asthma) 493.0
    fever (allergic) (with rhinitis) 477.9with
        asthma (bronchial) (*see also* Asthma) 493.0
    allergic, due to grass, pollen, ragweed, or tree
        477.0
    conjunctivitis 372.05
    due to
      dander, animal (cat) (dog) 477.2
      dust 477.8
      fowl 477.8
      hair, animal (cat) (dog) 477.2
      pollen 477.0
      specified allergen other than pollen 477.8
Hayem-Faber syndrome (achlorhydric anemia)
    280.9
Hayem-Widal syndrome (acquired hemolytic
    jaundice) 283.9
Haygarth's nodosities 715.04
Hazard-Crile tumor (M8350/3) 193
Hb (abnormal)
  disease—*see* Disease, hemoglobin
  trait—*see* Trait
H disease 270.0
Head —*see also* condition
  banging 307.3
Headache 784.0
  allergic 346.2
  cluster 346.2
  due to
    loss, spinal fluid 349.0
    lumbar puncture 349.0
    saddle block 349.0
  emotional 307.81
  histamine 346.2
  lumbar puncture 349.0
  menopausal 627.2
  migraine 346.9
  nonorganic origin 307.81
  postspinal 349.0
  psychogenic 307.81
  psychophysiologic 307.81
  sick 346.1
  spinal 349.0
    complicating labor and delivery 668.8
    postpartum 668.8
  spinal fluid loss 349.0
  tension 307.81
  vascular 784.0
    migraine type 346.9
  vasomotor 346.9
Health
  advice V65.4
  audit V70.0
  checkup V70.0
  education V65.4
  hazard (*see also* History of) V15.9
    falling V15.88
    specified cause NEC V15.89
  instruction V65.4
  services provided because (of)
    boarding school residence V60.6
    holiday relief for person providing home care
        V60.5
    inadequate
      housing V60.1
      resources V60.2
    lack of housing V60.0
    no care available in home V60.4
    person living alone V60.3
    poverty V60.3

Health—*continued*
  residence in institution V60.6
  specified cause NEC V60.8
  vacation relief for person providing home care
      V60.5
Healthy
  donor (*see also* Donor) V59.9
  infant or child
    accompanying sick mother V65.0
    receiving care V20.1
  person
    accompanying sick relative V65.0
    admitted for sterilization V25.2
    receiving prophylactic inoculation or
        vaccination (*see also* Vaccination,
        prophylactic) V05.9
Hearing examination V72.19
  following failed hearing screening V72.11
Heart —*see* condition
Heartburn 787.1
  psychogenic 306.4
Heat (effects) 992.9
  apoplexy 992.0
  burn—*see also* Burn, by site
    from sun (*see also* Sunburn) 692.71
  collapse 992.1
  cramps 992.2
  dermatitis or eczema 692.89
  edema 992.7
  erythema—*see* Burn, by site
  excessive 992.9
    specified effect NEC 992.8
  exhaustion 992.5
    anhydrotic 992.3
    due to
      salt (and water) depletion 992.4
      water depletion 992.3
  fatigue (transient) 992.6
  fever 992.0
  hyperpyrexia 992.0
  prickly 705.1
  prostration—*see* Heat, exhaustion
  pyrexia 992.0
  rash 705.1
  specified effect NEC 992.8
  stroke 992.0
  sunburn (*see also* Sunburn) 692.71
  syncope 992.1
Heavy-chain disease 273.2
Heavy-for-dates (fetus or infant) 766.1
  4500 grams or more 766.0
  exceptionally 766.0
Hebephrenia, hebephrenic (acute) (*see also*
    Schizophrenia) 295.1
  dementia (praecox) (*see also* Schizophrenia)
      295.1
  schizophrenia (*see also* Schizophrenia) 295.1
Heberden's
  disease or nodes 715.04
  syndrome (angina pectoris) 413.9
Hebra's disease
  dermatitis exfoliativa 695.89
  erythema multiforme exudativum 695.1
  pityriasis 695.89
    maculata et circinata 696.3
  rubra 695.89
    pilaris 696.4
  prurigo 698.2
Hebra, nose 040.1
Hedinger's syndrome (malignant carcinoid)
    259.2
Heel —*see* condition

Heerfordt's disease or syndrome (uveoparotitis) 135
Hegglin's anomaly or syndrome 288.2
Heidenhain's disease 290.10
  with dementia 290.10
Heilmeyer-Schöner disease (M9842/3) 207.1
Heine-Medin disease (*see also* Poliomyelitis) 045.9
Heinz-body anemia, congenital 282.7
Heller's disease or syndrome (infantile psychosis) (*see also* Psychosis, childhood) 299.1
H.E.L.L.P. 642.5
Helminthiasis (*see also* Infestation, by specific parasite) 128.9
  Ancylostoma (*see also* Ancylostoma) 126.9
  intestinal 127.9
    mixed types (types classifiable to more than one of the titles 120.0-127.7) 127.8
    specified type 127.7
  mixed types (intestinal) (types classifiable to more than one of the titles 120.0-127.7) 127.8
  Necator americanus 126.1
  specified type NEC 128.8
  Trichinella 124
Heloma 700
Hemangioblastoma (M9161/1)—*see also* Neoplasm, connective tissue, uncertain behavior
  malignant (M9161//3)—*see* Neoplasm, connective tissue, malignant
Hemangioblastomatosis, cerebelloretinal 759.6
Hemangioendothelioma (M9130/1)—*see also* Neoplasm, by site, uncertain behavior
  benign (M9130/0) 228.00
  bone (diffuse) (M9130/3)—*see* Neoplasm, bone, malignant
  malignant (M9130/3)—*see* Neoplasm, connective tissue, malignant
  nervous system (M9130/0) 228.09
Hemangioendotheliosarcoma (M9130/3)—*see* Neoplasm, connective tissue, malignant
Hemangiofibroma (M9160/0)—*see* Neoplasm, by site, benign
Hemangiolipoma (M8861/0)—*see* Lipoma
Hemangioma (M9120/0) 228.00
  arteriovenous (M9123/0)—*see* Hemangioma, by site
  brain 228.02
  capillary (M9131/0)—*see* Hemangioma, by site
  cavernous (M9121/0)—*see* Hemangioma, by site
  central nervous system NEC 228.09
  choroid 228.09
  heart 228.09
  infantile (M9131/0)—*see* Hemangioma, by site
  intra-abdominal structures 228.04
  intracranial structures 228.02
  intramuscular (M9132/0)—*see* Hemangioma, by site
  iris 228.09
  juvenile (M9131/0)—*see* Hemangioma, by site
  malignant (M9120/3)—*see* Neoplasm, connective tissue, malignant
  meninges 228.09
    brain 228.02
    spinal cord 228.09
  peritoneum 228.04
  placenta—*see* Placenta, abnormal
  plexiform (M9131/0)—*see* Hemangioma, by site

Hemangioma—*continued*
  racemose (M9123/0)—*see* Hemangioma, by site
  retina 228.03
  retroperitoneal tissue 228.04
  sclerosing (M8832/0)—*see* Neoplasm, skin, benign
  simplex (M9131/0)—*see* Hemangioma, by site
  skin and subcutaneous tissue 228.01
  specified site NEC 228.09
  spinal cord 228.09
  venous (M9122/0)—*see* Hemangioma, by site
  verrucous keratotic (M9142/0)—*see* Hemangioma, by site
Hemangiomatosis (systemic) 757.32
  involving single site—*see* Hemangioma
Hemangiopericytoma (M9150/1)—*see also* Neoplasm, connective tissue, uncertain behavior
  benign (M9150/0)—*see* Neoplasm, connective tissue, benign
  malignant (M9150/3)—*see* Neoplasm, connective tissue, malignant
Hemangiosarcoma (M9120/3)—*see* Neoplasm, connective tissue, malignant
Hemarthrosis (nontraumatic) 719.0
  ankle 719.17
  elbow 719.12
  foot 719.17
  hand 719.14
  hip 719.15
  knee 719.16
  multiple sites 719.19
  pelvic region 719.15
  shoulder (region) 719.11
  specified site NEC 719.18
  traumatic—*see* Sprain, by site
  wrist 719.13
Hematemesis 578.0
  with ulcer—*see* Ulcer, by site, with hemorrhage
  due to S. japonicum 120.2
  Goldstein's (familial hemorrhagic telangiectasia) 448.0
  newborn 772.4
    due to swallowed maternal blood 777.3
Hematidrosis 705.89
Hematinuria (*see also* Hemoglobinuria) 791.2
  malarial 084.8
  paroxysmal 283.2
Hematite miners' lung 503
Hematobilia 576.8
Hematocele (congenital) (diffuse) (idiopathic) 608.83
  broad ligament 620.7
  canal of Nuck 629.0
  cord, male 608.83
  fallopian tube 620.8
  female NEC 629.0
  ischiorectal 569.89
  male NEC 608.83
  ovary 629.0
  pelvis, pelvic
    female 629.0
      with ectopic pregnancy (*see also* Pregnancy, ectopic) 633.90
        with intrauterine pregnancy 633.91
    male 608.83
  periuterine 629.0
  retrouterine 629.0
  scrotum 608.83
  spermatic cord (diffuse) 608.83
  testis 608.84

Hematocele—*continued*
 traumatic—*see* Injury, internal, pelvis
 tunica vaginalis 608.83
 uterine ligament 629.0
 uterus 621.4
 vagina 623.6
 vulva 624.5
Hematocephalus 742.4
Hematochezia (*see also* Melena) 578.1
Hematochyluria (*see also* Infestation, filarial)
 125.9
Hematocolpos 626.8
Hematocornea 371.12
Hematogenous —*see* condition
Hematoma (skin surface intact) (traumatic)—*see*
 also Contusion

> *Note—Hematomas are coded according to
> origin and the nature and site of the hematoma
> or the accompanying injury. Hematomas of
> unspecified origin are coded as injuries of the
> sites involved, except:*
> *(a) hematomas of genital organs which are
> coded as diseases of the organ involved
> unless they complicate pregnancy or
> delivery*
> *(b) hematomas of the eye which are coded as
> diseases of the eye.*
>
> *For late effect of hematoma classifiable to
> 920-924 see Late, effect, contusion*

 with
  crush injury—*see* Crush
  fracture—*see* Fracture, by site
  injury of internal organs—*see also* Injury,
   internal, by site
   kidney—*see* Hematoma, kidney, traumatic
   liver—*see* Hematoma, liver, traumatic
   spleen—*see* Hematoma, spleen
  nerve injury—*see* Injury, nerve
  open wound—*see* Wound, open, by site
  skin surface intact—*see* Contusion
 abdomen (wall)—*see* Contusion, abdomen
 amnion 658.8
 aorta, dissecting 441.00
  abdominal 441.02
  thoracic 441.01
  thoracoabdominal 441.03
 arterial (complicating trauma) 904.9
  specified site—*see* Injury, blood vessel, by
   site
 auricle (ear) 380.31
 birth injury 767.8
  skull 767.19

Hematoma—*continued*
 brain (traumatic) 853.0

> *Note—Use the following fifth-digit
> subclassification with categories 851-854:*
>
> *0 unspecified state of consciousness*
> *1 with no loss of consciousness*
> *2 with brief [less than one hour] loss of
> consciousness*
> *3 with moderate [1-24 hours] loss of
> consciousness*
> *4 with prolonged [more than 24 hours] loss of
> consciousness and return to pre-existing
> conscious level*
> *5 with prolonged [more than 24 hours] loss of
> consciousness, without return to pre-existing
> conscious level*
> *Use fifth-digit 5 to designate when a patient is
> unconscious and dies before regaining
> consciousness, regardless of the duration of the
> loss of consciousness*
> *6 with loss of consciousness of unspecified
> duration*
> *9 with concussion, unspecified*

 with
  cerebral
   contusion—*see* Contusion, brain
   laceration—*see* Laceration, brain
   open intracranial wound 853.1
   skull fracture—*see* Fracture, skull, by site
  extradural or epidural 852.4
   with open intracranial wound 852.5
   fetus or newborn 767.0
   nontraumatic 432.0
  fetus or newborn NEC 767.0
  nontraumatic (*see also* Hemorrhage, brain)
   431
   epidural or extradural 432.0
   newborn NEC 772.8
   subarachnoid, arachnoid, or meningeal (*see
    also* Hemorrhage, subarachnoid) 430
   subdural (*see also* Hemorrhage, subdural)
    432.1
  subarachnoid, arachnoid, or meningeal 852.0
   with open intracranial wound 852.1
   fetus or newborn 772.2
   nontraumatic (*see also* Hemorrhage,
    subarachnoid) 430
  subdural 852.2
   with open intracranial wound 852.3
   fetus or newborn (localized) 767.0
   nontraumatic (*see also* Hemorrhage,
    subdural) 432.1
 breast (nontraumatic) 611.8
 broad ligament (nontraumatic) 620.7
  complicating delivery 665.7
  traumatic—*see* Injury, internal, broad
   ligament
 calcified NEC 959.9
 capitis 920
  due to birth injury 767.19
  newborn 767.19
 cerebral—*see* Hematoma, brain
 cesarean section wound 674.3
 chorion—*see* Placenta, abnormal
 complicating delivery (perineum) (vulva) 664.5
  pelvic 665.7
  vagina 665.7
 corpus
  cavernosum (nontraumatic) 607.82

Hematoma—*continued*
　luteum (nontraumatic) (ruptured) 620.1
　dura (mater)—*see* Hematoma, brain, subdural
　epididymis (nontraumatic) 608.83
　epidural (traumatic)—*see also* Hematoma,
　　brain, extradural
　spinal—*see* Injury, spinal, by site
　episiotomy 674.3
　external ear 380.31
　extradural—*see also* Hematoma, brain,
　　extradural
　　fetus or newborn 767.0
　　nontraumatic 432.0
　　　fetus or newborn 767.0
　fallopian tube 620.8
　genital organ (nontraumatic)
　　female NEC 629.89
　　male NEC 608.83
　　traumatic (external site) 922.4
　　　internal—*see* Injury, internal, genital organ
　graafian follicle (ruptured) 620.0
　internal organs (abdomen, chest, or pelvis)—*see*
　　also Injury, internal, by site
　　kidney—*see* Hematoma, kidney, traumatic
　　liver—*see* Hematoma, liver, traumatic
　　spleen—*see* Hematoma, spleen
　intracranial—*see* Hematoma, brain
　kidney, cystic 593.81
　　traumatic 866.01
　　　with open wound into cavity 866.11
　labia (nontraumatic) 624.5
　lingual (and other parts of neck, scalp, or face,
　　except eye) 920
　liver (subcapsular) 573.8
　　birth injury 767.8
　　fetus or newborn 767.8
　　traumatic NEC 864.01
　　　with
　　　　laceration—*see* Laceration, liver
　　　　open wound into cavity 864.11
　mediastinum—*see* Injury, internal, mediastinum
　meninges, meningeal (brain)—*see also*
　　Hematoma, brain, subarachnoid
　　spinal—*see* Injury, spinal, by site
　mesosalpinx (nontraumatic) 620.8
　　traumatic—*see* Injury, internal, pelvis
　muscle (traumatic)—*see* Contusion, by site
　nasal (septum) (and other part(s) of neck, scalp,
　　or face, except eye) 920
　obstetrical surgical wound 674.3
　orbit, orbital (nontraumatic) 376.32
　　traumatic 921.2
　ovary (corpus luteum) (nontraumatic) 620.1
　　traumatic—*see* Injury, internal, ovary
　pelvis (female) (nontraumatic) 629.89
　　complicating delivery 665.7
　　male 608.83
　　traumatic—*see also* Injury, internal, pelvis
　　　specified organ NEC (*see also* Injury,
　　　　internal, pelvis) 867.6
　penis (nontraumatic) 607.82
　pericranial (and neck, or face any part, except
　　eye) 920
　　due to injury at birth 767.19
　perineal wound (obstetrical) 674.3
　　complicating delivery 664.5
　perirenal, cystic 593.81
　pinna 380.31
　placenta—*see* Placenta, abnormal
　postoperative 998.12
　retroperitoneal (nontraumatic) 568.81

Hematoma—*continued*
　traumatic—*see* Injury, internal,
　　retroperitoneum
　retropubic, male 568.81
　scalp (and neck, or face any part, except eye)
　　920
　　fetus or newborn 767.19
　scrotum (nontraumatic) 608.83
　　traumatic 922.4
　seminal vesicle (nontraumatic) 608.83
　　traumatic—*see* Injury, internal, seminal
　　　vesicle
　spermatic cord—*see also* Injury, internal,
　　spermatic cord
　　nontraumatic 608.83
　spinal (cord) (meninges)—*see also* Injury,
　　spinal, by site
　　fetus or newborn 767.4
　　nontraumatic 336.1
　spleen 865.01
　　with
　　　laceration—*see* Laceration, spleen
　　　open wound into cavity 865.11
　sternocleidomastoid, birth injury 767.8
　sternomastoid, birth injury 767.8
　subarachnoid—*see also* Hematoma, brain,
　　subarachnoid
　　fetus or newborn 772.2
　　nontraumatic (*see also* Hemorrhage,
　　　subarachnoid) 430
　　newborn 772.2
　subdural—*see also* Hematoma, brain, subdural
　　fetus or newborn (localized) 767.0
　　nontraumatic (*see also* Hemorrhage, subdural)
　　　432.1
　subperiosteal (syndrome) 267
　　traumatic—*see* Hematoma, by site
　superficial, fetus or newborn 772.6
　syncytium—*see* Placenta, abnormal
　testis (nontraumatic) 608.83
　　birth injury 767.8
　　traumatic 922.4
　tunica vaginalis (nontraumatic) 608.83
　umbilical cord 663.6
　　affecting fetus or newborn 762.6
　uterine ligament (nontraumatic) 620.7
　　traumatic—*see* Injury, internal, pelvis
　uterus 621.4
　　traumatic—*see* Injury, internal, pelvis
　vagina (nontraumatic) (ruptured) 623.6
　　complicating delivery 665.7
　　traumatic 922.4
　vas deferens (nontraumatic) 608.83
　　traumatic—*see* Injury, internal, vas deferens
　vitreous 379.23
　vocal cord 920
　vulva (nontraumatic) 624.5
　　complicating delivery 664.5
　　fetus or newborn 767.8
　　traumatic 922.4
Hematometra 621.4
Hematomyelia 336.1
　with fracture of vertebra (*see also* Fracture,
　　vertebra, by site, with spinal cord injury)
　　806.8
　fetus or newborn 767.4
Hematomyelitis 323.9
　late effect—*see* category 326
Hematoperitoneum (*see also* Hemoperitoneum)
　568.81

Hemiplegia—*continued*
  viral encephalitis 139.0
  middle alternating NEC 344.89
  newborn NEC 767.0
  seizure (current episode) (*see also* Disease,
    cerebrovascular, acute) 436
  spastic 342.1
    congenital or infantile 343.1
  specified NEC 342.8
  thrombotic (current) (*see also* Thrombosis,
    brain) 434.0
    late effect—*see* late effect(s) (of)
      cerebrovascular disease
Hemisection, spinal cord —*see* Fracture,
  vertebra, by site, with spinal cord injury
Hemispasm 781.0
  facial 781.0
Hemispatial neglect 781.8
Hemisporosis 117.9
Hemitremor 781.0
Hemivertebra 756.14
Hemobilia 576.8
Hemocholecyst 575.8
Hemochromatosis (acquired) (diabetic)
  (hereditary) (liver) (myocardium) (primary
  idiopathic) (secondary) 275.0
  with refractory anemia 238.72
Hemodialysis V56.0
Hemoglobin —*see also* condition
  abnormal (disease)—*see* Disease, hemoglobin
  AS genotype 282.5
  fetal, hereditary persistence 282.7
  high-oxygen-affinity 289.0
  low NEC 285.9
  S (Hb-S), heterozygous 282.5
Hemoglobinemia 283.2
  due to blood transfusion NEC 999.8
    bone marrow 996.85
  paroxysmal 283.2
Hemoglobinopathy (mixed) (*see also* Disease,
  hemoglobin) 282.7
  with thalassemia 282.49
  sickle-cell 282.60
    with thalassemia (without crisis) 282.41
      with
        crisis 282.42
        vaso-occlusive pain 282.42
Hemoglobinuria, hemoglobinuric 791.2
  with anemia, hemolytic, acquired (chronic) NEC
    283.2
  cold (agglutinin) (paroxysmal) (with Raynaud's
    syndrome) 283.2
  due to
    exertion 283.2
    hemolysis (from external causes) NEC 283.2
  exercise 283.2
  fever (malaria) 084.8
  infantile 791.2
  intermittent 283.2
  malarial 084.8
  march 283.2
  nocturnal (paroxysmal) 283.2
  paroxysmal (cold) (nocturnal) 283.2
Hemolymphangioma (M9175/0) 228.1
Hemolysis
  fetal—*see* Jaundice, fetus or newborn
  intravascular (disseminated) NEC 286.6
    with
      abortion—*see* Abortion, by type, with
        hemorrhage, delayed or excessive

Hemolysis—*continued*
    ectopic pregnancy (*see also* categories
      633.0-633.9) 639.1
      hemorrhage of pregnancy 641.3
        affecting fetus or newborn 762.1
      molar pregnancy (*see also* categories
        630-632) 639.1
  acute 283.2
  following
    abortion 639.1
    ectopic or molar pregnancy 639.1
  neonatal—*see* Jaundice, fetus or newborn
  transfusion NEC 999.8
    bone marrow 996.85
Hemolytic —*see also* condition
  anemia—*see* Anemia, hemolytic
  uremic syndrome 283.11
Hemometra 621.4
Hemopericardium (with effusion) 423.0
  newborn 772.8
  traumatic (*see also* Hemothorax, traumatic)
    860.2
    with open wound into thorax 860.3
Hemoperitoneum 568.81
  infectional (*see also* Peritonitis) 567.29
  traumatic—*see* Injury, internal, peritoneum
Hemophagocytic syndrome 288.4
  infection-associated 288.4
Hemophilia (familial) (hereditary) 286.0
  A 286.0
    carrier (asymptomatic) V83.01
      symptomatic V83.02
  B (Leyden) 286.1
  C 286.2
  calcipriva (*see also* Fibrinolysis) 286.7
  classical 286.0
  nonfamilial 286.7
  secondary 286.5
  vascular 286.4
Hemophilus influenzae NEC 041.5
  arachnoiditis (basic) (brain) (spinal) 320.0
    late effect—*see* category 326
  bronchopneumonia 482.2
  cerebral ventriculitis 320.0
    late effect—*see* category 326
  cerebrospinal inflammation 320.0
    late effect—*see* category 326
  infection NEC 041.5
  leptomeningitis 320.0
    late effect—*see* category 326
  meningitis (cerebral) (cerebrospinal) (spinal)
    320.0
    late effect—*see* category 326
  meningomyelitis 320.0
    late effect—*see* category 326
  pachymeningitis (adhesive) (fibrous)
    (hemorrhagic) (hypertrophic) (spinal) 320.0
    late effect—*see* category 326
  pneumonia (broncho-) 482.2
Hemophthalmos 360.43
Hemopneumothorax (*see also* Hemothorax)
  511.8
  traumatic 860.4
    with open wound into thorax 860.5
Hemoptysis 786.3
  due to Paragonimus (westermani) 121.2
  newborn 770.3
  tuberculous (*see also* Tuberculosis, pulmonary)
    011.9

Hemorrhage, hemorrhagic (nontraumatic) 459.0
  abdomen 459.0
  accidental (antepartum) 641.2
    affecting fetus or newborn 762.1
  adenoid 474.8
  adrenal (capsule) (gland) (medulla) 255.4
    newborn 772.5
  after labor—*see* Hemorrhage, postpartum
  alveolar
    lung, newborn 770.3
    process 525.8
  alveolus 525.8
  amputation stump (surgical) 998.11
    secondary, delayed 997.69
  anemia (chronic) 280.0
    acute 285.1
  antepartum—*see* Hemorrhage, pregnancy
  anus (sphincter) 569.3
  apoplexy (stroke) 432.9
  arachnoid—*see* Hemorrhage, subarachnoid
  artery NEC 459.0
    brain (*see also* Hemorrhage, brain) 431
    middle meningeal—*see* Hemorrhage,
      subarachnoid
  basilar (ganglion) (*see also* Hemorrhage, brain)
    431
  bladder 596.8
  blood dyscrasia 289.9
  bowel 578.9
    newborn 772.4
  brain (miliary) (nontraumatic) 431
    with
      birth injury 767.0
    arachnoid—*see* Hemorrhage, subarachnoid
    due to
      birth injury 767.0
      rupture of aneurysm (congenital) (*see also*
        Hemorrhage, subarachnoid) 430
        mycotic 431
      syphilis 094.89
    epidural or extradural—*see* Hemorrhage,
      extradural
    fetus or newborn (anoxic) (hypoxic) (due to
      birth trauma) (nontraumatic) 767.0
      intraventricular 772.10
        grade I 772.11
        grade II 772.12
        grade III 772.13
        grade IV 772.14
    iatrogenic 997.02
    postoperative 997.02
    puerperal, postpartum, childbirth 674.0
    stem 431
    subarachnoid, arachnoid or meningeal—*see*
      Hemorrhage, subarachnoid
    subdural—*see* Hemorrhage, subdural

Hemorrhage, hemorrhagic—*continued*
  traumatic NEC 853.0

> *Note—Use the following fifth-digit*
> *subclassification with categories 851-854:*
>
> *0 unspecified state of consciousness*
> *1 with no loss of consciousness*
> *2 with brief [less than one hour] loss of*
> *consciousness*
> *3 with moderate [1-24 hours] loss of*
> *consciousness*
> *4 with prolonged [more than 24 hours] loss of*
> *consciousness and return to pre-existing*
> *conscious level*
> *5 with prolonged [more than 24 hours] loss of*
> *consciousness, without return to pre-existing*
> *conscious level*
> *Use fifth-digit 5 to designate when a patient is*
> *unconscious and dies before regaining*
> *consciousness, regardless of the duration of the*
> *loss of consciousness*
> *6 with loss of consciousness of unspecified*
> *duration*
> *9 with concussion, unspecified*

    with
      cerebral
        contusion—*see* Contusion, brain
        laceration—*see* Laceration, brain
      open intracranial wound 853.1
      skull fracture—*see* Fracture, skull, by site
    extradural or epidural 852.4
      with open intracranial wound 852.5
    subarachnoid 852.0
      with open intracranial wound 852.1
    subdural 852.2
      with open intracranial wound 852.3
  breast 611.79
  bronchial tube—*see* Hemorrhage, lung
  bronchopulmonary—*see* Hemorrhage, lung
  bronchus (cause unknown) (*see also*
    Hemorrhage, lung) 786.3
  bulbar (*see also* Hemorrhage, brain) 431
  bursa 727.89
  capillary 448.9
    primary 287.8
  capsular—*see* Hemorrhage, brain
  cardiovascular 429.89
  cecum 578.9
  cephalic (*see also* Hemorrhage, brain) 431
  cerebellar (*see also* Hemorrhage, brain) 431
  cerebellum (*see also* Hemorrhage, brain) 431
  cerebral (*see also* Hemorrhage, brain) 431
    fetus or newborn (anoxic) (traumatic) 767.0
  cerebromeningeal (*see also* Hemorrhage, brain)
    431
  cerebrospinal (*see also* Hemorrhage, brain) 431
  cerebrovascular accident—*see* Hemorrhage,
    brain
  cerebrum (*see also* Hemorrhage, brain) 431
  cervix (stump) (uteri) 622.8
  cesarean section wound 674.3
  chamber, anterior (eye) 364.41
  childbirth—*see* Hemorrhage, complicating,
    delivery
  choroid 363.61
    expulsive 363.62
  ciliary body 364.41
  cochlea 386.8
  colon—*see* Hemorrhage, intestine
  complicating

Hemorrhage, hemorrhagic—*continued*
  delivery 641.9
    affecting fetus or newborn 762.1
    associated with
      afibrinogenemia 641.3
        affecting fetus or newborn 763.89
      coagulation defect 641.3
        affecting fetus or newborn 763.89
      hyperfibrinolysis 641.3
        affecting fetus or newborn 763.89
      hypofibrinogenemia 641.3
        affecting fetus or newborn 763.89
    due to
      low-lying placenta 641.1
        affecting fetus or newborn 762.0
      placenta previa 641.1
        affecting fetus or newborn 762.0
      premature separation of placenta 641.2
        affecting fetus or newborn 762.1
      retained
        placenta 666.0
        secundines 666.2
      trauma 641.8
        affecting fetus or newborn 763.89
      uterine leiomyoma 641.8
        affecting fetus or newborn 763.89
    surgical procedure 998.11
  concealed NEC 459.0
  congenital 772.9
  conjunctiva 372.72
    newborn 772.8
  cord, newborn 772.0
    slipped ligature 772.3
    stump 772.3
  corpus luteum (ruptured) 620.1
  cortical (*see also* Hemorrhage, brain) 431
  cranial 432.9
  cutaneous 782.7
    newborn 772.6
  cyst, pancreas 577.2
  cystitis—*see* Cystitis
  delayed
    with
      abortion—*see* Abortion, by type, with
        hemorrhage, delayed or excessive
      ectopic pregnancy (*see also* categories
        633.0-633.9) 639.1
      molar pregnancy (*see also* categories
        630-632) 639.1
    following
      abortion 639.1
      ectopic or molar pregnancy 639.1
    postpartum 666.2
  diathesis (familial) 287.9
    newborn 776.0
  disease 287.9
    newborn 776.0
    specified type NEC 287.8
  disorder 287.9
    due to intrinsic circulating anticoagulants
      286.5
    specified type NEC 287.8
  due to
    any device, implant, or graft (presence of)
      classifiable to 996.0-996.5—*see*
      Complications, due to (presence of) any
      device, implant, or graft classified to
      996.0—996.5 NEC
    intrinsic circulating anticoagulant 286.5
  duodenum, duodenal 537.89
    ulcer—*see* Ulcer, duodenum, with hemorrhage

Hemorrhage, hemorrhagic—*continued*
  dura mater—*see* Hemorrhage, subdural
  endotracheal—*see* Hemorrhage, lung
  epicranial subaponeurotic (massive) 767.11
  epidural—*see* Hemorrhage, extradural
  episiotomy 674.3
  esophagus 530.82
    varix (*see also* Varix, esophagus, bleeding)
      456.0
  excessive
    with
      abortion—*see* Abortion, by type, with
        hemorrhage, delayed or excessive
      ectopic pregnancy (*see also* categories
        633.0-633.9) 639.1
      molar pregnancy (*see also* categories
        630-632) 639.1
    following
      abortion 639.1
      ectopic or molar pregnancy 639.1
  external 459.0
  extradural (traumatic)—*see also* Hemorrhage,
    brain, traumatic, extradural
    birth injury 767.0
    fetus or newborn (anoxic) (traumatic) 767.0
    nontraumatic 432.0
  eye 360.43
    chamber (anterior) (aqueous) 364.41
    fundus 362.81
  eyelid 374.81
  fallopian tube 620.8
  fetomaternal 772.0
    affecting management of pregnancy or
      puerperium 656.0
  fetus, fetal 772.0
    from
      cut end of co-twin's cord 772.0
      placenta 772.0
      ruptured cord 772.0
      vasa previa 772.0
    into
      co-twin 772.0
      mother's circulation 772.0
        affecting management of pregnancy or
        puerperium 656.0
  fever (*see also* Fever, hemorrhagic) 065.9
    with renal syndrome 078.6
    arthropod-borne NEC 065.9
    Bangkok 065.4
    Crimean 065.0
    dengue virus 065.4
    epidemic 078.6
    Junin virus 078.7
    Korean 078.6
    Machupo virus 078.7
    mite-borne 065.8
    mosquito-borne 065.4
    Philippine 065.4
    Russian (Yaroslav) 078.6
    Singapore 065.4
    southeast Asia 065.4
    Thailand 065.4
    tick-borne NEC 065.3
  fibrinogenolysis (*see also* Fibrinolysis) 286.6
  fibrinolytic (acquired) (*see also* Fibrinolysis)
    286.6
  fontanel 767.19
  from tracheostomy stoma 519.09
  fundus, eye 362.81
  funis
    affecting fetus or newborn 772.0

Hemorrhage, hemorrhagic—*continued*
  complicating delivery 663.8
  gastric (*see also* Hemorrhage, stomach) 578.9
  gastroenteric 578.9
    newborn 772.4
  gastrointestinal (tract) 578.9
    newborn 772.4
  genitourinary (tract) NEC 599.89
  gingiva 523.8
  globe 360.43
  gravidarum—*see* Hemorrhage, pregnancy
  gum 523.8
  heart 429.89
  hypopharyngeal (throat) 784.8
  intermenstrual 626.6
    irregular 626.6
    regular 626.5
  internal (organs) 459.0
    capsule (*see also* Hemorrhage, brain) 431
    ear 386.8
    newborn 772.8
  intestine 578.9
    congenital 772.4
    newborn 772.4
  into
    bladder wall 596.7
    bursa 727.89
    corpus luysii (*see also* Hemorrhage, brain) 431
  intra-abdominal 459.0
    during or following surgery 998.11
  intra-alveolar, newborn (lung) 770.3
  intracerebral (*see also* Hemorrhage, brain) 431
  intracranial NEC 432.9
    puerperal, postpartum, childbirth 674.0
    traumatic—*see* Hemorrhage, brain, traumatic
  intramedullary NEC 336.1
  intraocular 360.43
  intraoperative 998.11
  intrapartum—*see* Hemorrhage, complicating,
    delivery
  intrapelvic
    female 629.89
    male 459.0
  intraperitoneal 459.0
  intrapontine (*see also* Hemorrhage, brain) 431
  intrauterine 621.4
    complicating delivery—*see* Hemorrhage,
      complicating, delivery
    in pregnancy or childbirth—*see* Hemorrhage,
      pregnancy
    postpartum (*see also* Hemorrhage,
      postpartum) 666.1
  intraventricular (*see also* Hemorrhage, brain)
    431
    fetus or newborn (anoxic) (traumatic) 772.10
      grade I 772.11
      grade II 772.12
      grade III 772.13
      grade IV 772.14
  intravesical 596.7
  iris (postinfectional) (postinflammatory) (toxic)
    364.41
  joint (nontraumatic) 719.10
    ankle 719.17
    elbow 719.12
    foot 719.17
    forearm 719.13
    hand 719.14
    hip 719.15
    knee 719.16
    lower leg 719.16

Hemorrhage, hemorrhagic—*continued*
    multiple sites 719.19
    pelvic region 719.15
    shoulder (region) 719.11
    specified site NEC 719.18
    thigh 719.15
    upper arm 719.12
    wrist 719.13
  kidney 593.81
  knee (joint) 719.16
  labyrinth 386.8
  leg NEC 459.0
  lenticular striate artery (*see also* Hemorrhage,
    brain) 431
  ligature, vessel 998.11
  liver 573.8
  lower extremity NEC 459.0
  lung 786.3
    newborn 770.3
    tuberculous (*see also* Tuberculosis,
      pulmonary) 011.9
  malaria 084.8
  marginal sinus 641.2
  massive subaponeurotic, birth injury 767.11
  maternal, affecting fetus or newborn 762.1
  mediastinum 786.3
  medulla (*see also* Hemorrhage, brain) 431
  membrane (brain) (*see also* Hemorrhage,
    subarachnoid) 430
    spinal cord—*see* Hemorrhage, spinal cord
  meninges, meningeal (brain) (middle) (*see also*
    Hemorrhage, subarachnoid) 430
    spinal cord—*see* Hemorrhage, spinal cord
  mesentery 568.81
  metritis 626.8
  midbrain (*see also* Hemorrhage, brain) 431
  mole 631
  mouth 528.9
  mucous membrane NEC 459.0
    newborn 772.8
  muscle 728.89
  nail (subungual) 703.8
  nasal turbinate 784.7
    newborn 772.8
  nasopharynx 478.29
  navel, newborn 772.3
  newborn 772.9
    adrenal 772.5
    alveolar (lung) 770.3
    brain (anoxic) (hypoxic) (due to birth trauma)
      767.0
    cerebral (anoxic) (hypoxic) (due to birth
      trauma) 767.0
    conjunctiva 772.8
    cutaneous 772.6
    diathesis 776.0
    due to vitamin K deficiency 776.0
    epicranial subaponeurotic (massive) 767.11
    gastrointestinal 772.4
    internal (organs) 772.8
    intestines 772.4
    intra-alveolar (lung) 770.3
    intracranial (from any perinatal cause) 767.0
    intraventricular (from any perinatal cause)
      772.10
      grade I 772.11
      grade II 772.12
      grade III 772.13
      grade IV 772.14
    lung 770.3
    pulmonary (massive) 770.3

Hemorrhage, hemorrhagic—*continued*
  newborn 772.4
  ulcer—*see* Ulcer, stomach, with hemorrhage
  subaponeurotic, newborn 767.11
    massive (birth injury) 767.11
  subarachnoid (nontraumatic) 430
    fetus or newborn (anoxic) (traumatic) 772.2
    puerperal, postpartum, childbirth 674.0
    traumatic—*see* Hemorrhage, brain, traumatic,
      subarachnoid
  subconjunctival 372.72
    due to birth injury 772.8
    newborn 772.8
  subcortical (*see also* Hemorrhage, brain) 431
  subcutaneous 782.7
  subdiaphragmatic 459.0
  subdural (nontraumatic) 432.1
    due to birth injury 767.0
    fetus or newborn (anoxic) (hypoxic) (due to
      birth trauma) 767.0
    puerperal, postpartum, childbirth 674.0
    spinal 336.1
    traumatic—*see* Hemorrhage, brain, traumatic,
      subdural
  subgaleal 767.11
  subhyaloid 362.81
  subperiosteal 733.99
  subretinal 362.81
  subtentorial (*see also* Hemorrhage, subdural)
    432.1
  subungual 703.8
    due to blood dyscrasia 287.8
  suprarenal (capsule) (gland) 255.4
    fetus or newborn 772.5
  tentorium (traumatic)—*see also* Hemorrhage,
    brain, traumatic
    fetus or newborn 767.0
    nontraumatic—*see* Hemorrhage, subdural
  testis 608.83
  thigh 459.0
  third stage 666.0
  thorax—*see* Hemorrhage, lung
  throat 784.8
  thrombocythemia 238.71
  thymus (gland) 254.8
  thyroid (gland) 246.3
    cyst 246.3
  tongue 529.8
  tonsil 474.8
    postoperative 998.11
  tooth socket (postextraction) 998.11
  trachea—*see* Hemorrhage, lung
  traumatic—*see also* nature of injury
    brain—*see* Hemorrhage, brain, traumatic
    recurring or secondary (following initial
      hemorrhage at time of injury) 958.2
  tuberculous NEC (*see also* Tuberculosis,
    pulmonary) 011.9
  tunica vaginalis 608.83
  ulcer—*see* Ulcer, by site, with hemorrhage
  umbilicus, umbilical cord 772.0
    after birth, newborn 772.3
    complicating delivery 663.8
      affecting fetus or newborn 772.0
    slipped ligature 772.3
    stump 772.3
  unavoidable (due to placenta previa) 641.1
    affecting fetus or newborn 762.0
  upper extremity 459.0
  urethra (idiopathic) 599.84
  uterus, uterine (abnormal) 626.9

Hemorrhage, hemorrhagic—*continued*
  climacteric 627.0
  complicating delivery—*see* Hemorrhage,
    complicating, delivery
  due to
    intrauterine contraceptive device 996.76
      perforating uterus 996.32
  functional or dysfunctional 626.8
  in pregnancy—*see* Hemorrhage, pregnancy
  intermenstrual 626.6
    irregular 626.6
    regular 626.5
  postmenopausal 627.1
  postpartum (*see also* Hemorrhage,
    postpartum) 666.1
  prepubertal 626.8
  pubertal 626.3
  puerperal (immediate) 666.1
  vagina 623.8
  vasa previa 663.5
    affecting fetus or newborn 772.0
  vas deferens 608.83
  ventricular (*see also* Hemorrhage, brain) 431
  vesical 596.8
  viscera 459.0
    newborn 772.8
  vitreous (humor) (intraocular) 379.23
  vocal cord 478.5
  vulva 624.8
Hemorrhoids (anus) (rectum) (without
  complication) 455.6
  bleeding, prolapsed, strangulated, or ulcerated
    NEC 455.8
    external 455.5
    internal 455.2
  complicated NEC 455.8
  complicating pregnancy and puerperium 671.8
  external 455.3
    with complication NEC 455.5
    bleeding, prolapsed, strangulated, or ulcerated
      455.5
    thrombosed 455.4
  internal 455.0
    with complication NEC 455.2
    bleeding, prolapsed, strangulated, or ulcerated
      455.2
    thrombosed 455.1
  residual skin tag 455.9
  sentinel pile 455.9
  thrombosed NEC 455.7
    external 455.4
    internal 455.1
Hemosalpinx 620.8
Hemosiderosis 275.0
  dietary 275.0
  pulmonary (idiopathic) 275.0 *[516.1]*
  transfusion NEC 999.8
    bone marrow 996.85
Hemospermia 608.82
Hemothorax 511.8
  bacterial, nontuberculous 511.1
  newborn 772.8
  nontuberculous 511.8
    bacterial 511.1
  pneumococcal 511.1
  postoperative 998.11
  staphylococcal 511.1
  streptococcal 511.1
  traumatic 860.2
    with
      open wound into thorax 860.3

> *Note—Use the following fifth-digit
> subclassification with category 550:*
>
> *0 unilateral or unspecified (not specified as
>   recurrent)*
> *1 unilateral or unspecified, recurrent*
> *2 bilateral (not specified as recurrent)*
> *3 bilateral, recurrent*

Hernia, hernial—*continued*
  with
      gangrene (obstructed) 551.8
      obstruction 552.8
        and gangrene 551.8
    Richter's (parietal) 553.9
      with
        gangrene (obstructed) 551.9
        obstruction 552.9
          and gangrene 551.9
    Rieux's, Riex's (retrocecal) 553.8
      with
        gangrene (obstructed) 551.8
        obstruction 552.8
          and gangrene 551.8
    sciatic 553.8
      with
        gangrene (obstructed) 551.8
        obstruction 552.8
          and gangrene 551.8
    scrotum, scrotal—*see* Hernia, inguinal
    sliding (inguinal)—*see also* Hernia, inguinal
      hiatus—*see* Hernia, hiatal
    spigelian 553.29
      with
        gangrene (obstructed) 551.29
        obstruction 552.29
          and gangrene 551.29
    spinal (*see also* Spina bifida) 741.9
      with hydrocephalus 741.0
    strangulated (*see also* Hernia, by site, with
        obstruction) 552.9
      gangrenous (with obstruction) (*see also*
          Hernia, by site, with gangrene) 551.9
    supraumbilicus (linea alba)—*see* Hernia,
        epigastric
    tendon 727.9
    testis (nontraumatic) 550.9
      meaning
        scrotal hernia 550.9
        symptomatic late syphilis 095.8
    Treitz's (fossa) 553.8
      with
        gangrene (obstructed) 551.8
        obstruction 552.8
          and gangrene 551.8
    tunica
      albuginea 608.89
      vaginalis 752.89
    umbilicus, umbilical 553.1
      with
        gangrene (obstructed) 551.1
        obstruction 552.1
          and gangrene 551.1
    ureter 593.89
      with obstruction 593.4
    uterus 621.8
      pregnant 654.4
    vaginal (posterior) 618.6
    Velpeau's (femoral) (*see also* Hernia, femoral)
        553.00
    ventral 553.20
      with
        gangrene (obstructed) 551.20
        obstruction 552.20
          and gangrene 551.20
      recurrent 553.21
        with
          gangrene (obstructed) 551.21
          obstruction 552.21
            and gangrene 551.21

Hernia, hernial—*continued*
  vesical
      congenital (female) (male) 756.71
      female (*see also* Cystocele, female) 618.01
      male 596.8
    vitreous (into anterior chamber) 379.21
      traumatic 871.1
Herniation —*see also* Hernia
    brain (stem) 348.4
    cerebral 348.4
    gastric mucosa (into duodenal bulb) 537.89
    mediastinum 519.3
    nucleus pulposus—*see* Displacement,
        intervertebral disc
Herpangina 074.0
Herpes, herpetic 054.9
    auricularis (zoster) 053.71
      simplex 054.73
    blepharitis (zoster) 053.20
      simplex 054.41
    circinate 110.5
    circinatus 110.5
      bullous 694.5
    conjunctiva (simplex) 054.43
      zoster 053.21
    cornea (simplex) 054.43
      disciform (simplex) 054.43
      zoster 053.21
    encephalitis 054.3
    eye (zoster) 053.29
      simplex 054.40
    eyelid (zoster) 053.20
      simplex 054.41
    febrilis 054.9
    fever 054.9
    geniculate ganglionitis 053.11
    genital, genitalis 054.10
      specified site NEC 054.19
    gestationis 646.8
    gingivostomatitis 054.2
    iridocyclitis (simplex) 054.44
      zoster 053.22
    iris (any site) 695.1
    iritis (simplex) 054.44
    keratitis (simplex) 054.43
      dendritic 054.42
      disciform 054.43
      interstitial 054.43
        zoster 053.21
    keratoconjunctivitis (simplex) 054.43
      zoster 053.21
    labialis 054.9
      meningococcal 036.89
    lip 054.9
    meningitis (simplex) 054.72
      zoster 053.0
    ophthalmicus (zoster) 053.20
      simplex 054.40
    otitis externa (zoster) 053.71
      simplex 054.73
    penis 054.13
    perianal 054.10
    pharyngitis 054.79
    progenitalis 054.10
    scrotum 054.19
    septicemia 054.5
    simplex 054.9
      complicated 054.8
        ophthalmic 054.40
          specified NEC 054.49
        specified NEC 054.79

Herpes, herpetic—*continued*
  congenital 771.2
  external ear 054.73
  keratitis 054.43
    dendritic 054.42
  meningitis 054.72
  myelitis 054.74
  neuritis 054.79
  specified complication NEC 054.79
    ophthalmic 054.49
  visceral 054.71
 stomatitis 054.2
 tonsurans 110.0
  maculosus (of Hebra) 696.3
 visceral 054.71
 vulva 054.12
 vulvovaginitis 054.11
 whitlow 054.6
 zoster 053.9
  auricularis 053.71
  complicated 053.8
    specified NEC 053.79
  conjunctiva 053.21
  cornea 053.21
  ear 053.71
  eye 053.29
  geniculate 053.11
  keratitis 053.21
    interstitial 053.21
  myelitis 053.14
  neuritis 053.10
  ophthalmicus(a) 053.20
  oticus 053.71
  otitis externa 053.71
  specified complication NEC 053.79
  specified site NEC 053.9
 zosteriform, intermediate type 053.9
Herrick's
 anemia (hemoglobin S disease) 282.61
 syndrome (hemoglobin S disease) 282.61
Hers' disease (glycogenosis VI) 271.0
Herter's infantilism (nontropical sprue) 579.0
Herter (-Gee) disease or syndrome (nontropical
 sprue) 579.0
Herxheimer's disease (diffuse idiopathic
 cutaneous atrophy) 701.8
Herxheimer's reaction 995.0
Hesitancy, urinary 788.64
Hesselbach's hernia —*see* Hernia, Hesselbach's
Heterochromia (congenital) 743.46
 acquired 364.53
 cataract 366.33
 cyclitis 364.21
 hair 704.3
 iritis 364.21
 retained metallic foreign body 360.62
  magnetic 360.52
 uveitis 364.21
Heterophoria 378.40
 alternating 378.45
 vertical 378.43
Heterophyes, small intestine 121.6
Heterophyiasis 121.6
Heteropsia 368.8
Heterotopia, heterotopic —*see also*
 Malposition, congenital
 cerebralis 742.4
 pancreas, pancreatic 751.7
 spinalis 742.59

Heterotropia 378.30
 intermittent 378.20
  vertical 378.31
 vertical (constant) (intermittent) 378.31
Heubner's disease 094.89
Heubner-Herter disease or syndrome
 (nontropical sprue) 579.0
Hexadactylism 755.00
Heyd's syndrome (hepatorenal) 572.4
HGSIL (high grade squamous intrepithelial
 lesion) 795.04
Hibernoma (M8880/0)—*see* Lipoma
Hiccough 786.8
 epidemic 078.89
 psychogenic 306.1
Hiccup (*see also* Hiccough) 786.8
Hicks (-Braxton) contractures 644.1
Hidden penis 752.65
Hidradenitis (axillaris) (suppurative) 705.83
Hidradenoma (nodular) (M8400/0)—*see also*
 Neoplasm, skin, benign
 clear cell (M8402/0)—*see* Neoplasm, skin,
  benign
 papillary (M8405/0)—*see* Neoplasm, skin,
  benign
Hidrocystoma (M8404/0)—*see* Neoplasm, skin,
 benign
HIE (hypoxic-ischemic encephalopathy) 768.7
High
 A_2 anemia 282.49
 altitude effects 993.2
  anoxia 993.2
  on
   ears 993.0
   sinuses 993.1
  polycythemia 289.0
 arch
  foot 755.67
  palate 750.26
 artery (arterial) tension (*see also* Hypertension)
  401.9
  without diagnosis of hypertension 796.2
 basal metabolic rate (BMR) 794.7
 blood pressure (*see also* Hypertension) 401.9
  incidental reading (isolated) (nonspecific), no
   diagnosis of hypertension 796.2
 compliance bladder 596.4
 diaphragm (congenital) 756.6
 frequency deafness (congenital) (regional) 389.8
 head at term 652.5
 output failure (cardiac) (*see also* Failure, heart)
  428.9
 oxygen-affinity hemoglobin 289.0
 palate 750.26
 risk
  behavior —*see* Problem
  cervical, human papillomavirus (HPV) DNA
   test positive 795.05
  family situation V61.9
   specified circumstance NEC V61.8
  individual NEC V62.89
  infant NEC V20.1
  patient taking drugs (prescribed) V67.51
   nonprescribed (*see also* Abuse, drugs,
    nondependent) 305.9
  pregnancy V23.9
   inadequate prenatal care V23.7
   specified problem NEC V23.8
 temperature (of unknown origin) (*see also*
  Pyrexia) 780.6
 thoracic rib 756.3

Hildenbrand's disease (typhus) 081.9
Hilger's syndrome 337.0
Hill diarrhea 579.1
Hilliard's lupus (*see also* Tuberculosis) 017.0
Hilum —*see* condition
Hip —*see* condition
Hippel's disease (retinocerebral angiomatosis) 759.6
Hippus 379.49
Hirschfeld's disease (acute diabetes mellitus) (*see also* Diabetes) 250.0
Hirschsprung's disease or megacolon (congenital) 751.3
Hirsuties (*see also* Hypertrichosis) 704.1
Hirsutism (*see also* Hypertrichosis) 704.1
Hirudiniasis (external) (internal) 134.2
His-Werner disease (trench fever) 083.1
Hiss-Russell dysentery 004.1
Histamine cephalgia 346.2
Histidinemia 270.5
Histidinuria 270.5
Histiocytic syndromes 288.4
Histiocytoma (M8832/0)—*see also* Neoplasm, skin, benign
  fibrous (M8830/0)—*see also* Neoplasm, skin, benign
    atypical (M8830/1)—*see* Neoplasm, connective tissue, uncertain behavior
    malignant (M8830/0)—*see* Neoplasm, connective tissue, malignant
Histiocytosis (acute) (chronic) (subacute) 277.89
  acute differentiated progressive (M9722/3) 202.5
  cholesterol 277.89
  essential 277.89
  lipid, lipoid (essential) 272.7
  lipochrome (familial) 288.1
  malignant (M9720/3) 202.3
  X (chronic) 277.89
    acute (progressive) (M9722/3) 202.5
Histoplasmosis 115.90
  with
    endocarditis 115.94
    meningitis 115.91
    pericarditis 115.93
    pneumonia 115.95
    retinitis 115.92
    specified manifestation NEC 115.99
  African (due to Histoplasma duboisii) 115.10
    with
      endocarditis 115.14
      meningitis 115.11
      pericarditis 115.13
      pneumonia 115.15
      retinitis 115.12
      specified manifestation NEC 115.19
  American (due to Histoplasma capsulatum) 115.00
    with
      endocarditis 115.04
      meningitis 115.01
      pericarditis 115.03
      pneumonia 115.05
      retinitis 115.02
      specified manifestation NEC 115.09
  Darling's—*see* Histoplasmosis, American
  large form (*see also* Histoplasmosis, African) 115.10
  lung 115.05
  small form (*see also* Histoplasmosis, American) 115.00

History (personal) of
  abuse
    emotional V15.42
    neglect V15.42
    physical V15.41
    sexual V15.41
  affective psychosis V11.1
  alcoholism V11.3
    specified as drinking problem (*see also* Abuse, drugs, nondependent) 305.0
  allergy to
    analgesic agent NEC V14.6
    anesthetic NEC V14.4
    antibiotic agent NEC V14.1
      penicillin V14.0
    anti-infective agent NEC V14.3
    diathesis V15.09
    drug V14.9
      specified type NEC V14.8
    eggs V15.03
    food additives V15.05
    insect bite V15.06
    latex V15.07
    medicinal agents V14.9
      specified type NEC V14.8
    milk products V15.02
    narcotic agent NEC V14.5
    nuts V15.05
      peanuts V15.01
    penicillin V14.0
    radiographic dye V15.08
    seafood V15.04
    serum V14.7
    specified food NEC V15.05
    specified nonmedicinal agents NEC V15.09
    spider bite V15.06
    sulfa V14.2
    sulfonamides V14.2
    therapeutic agent NEC V15.09
    vaccine V14.7
  anemia V12.3
  arthritis V13.4
  benign neoplasm of brain V12.41
  blood disease V12.3
  calculi, urinary V13.01
  cardiovascular disease V12.50
    myocardial infarction 412
  child abuse V15.41
  cigarette smoking V15.82
  circulatory system disease V12.50
    myocardial infarction 412
  congenital malformation V13.69
  contraception V15.7
  diathesis, allergic V15.09
  digestive system disease V12.70
    peptic ulcer V12.71
    polyps, colonic V12.72
    specified NEC V12.79
  disease (of) V13.9
    blood V12.3
    blood-forming organs V12.3
    cardiovascular system V12.50
    circulatory system V12.50
    digestive system V12.70
      peptic ulcer V12.71
      polyps, colonic V12.72
      specified NEC V12.79
    infectious V12.00
      malaria V12.03
      poliomyelitis V12.02
      specified NEC V12.09

History—*continued*
    tuberculosis V12.01
  parasitic V12.00
    specified NEC V12.09
  respiratory system V12.60
    pneumonia V12.61
    specified NEC V12.69
  skin V13.3
  specified site NEC V13.8
  subcutaneous tissue V13.3
  trophoblastic V13.1
    affecting management of pregnancy V23.1
 disorder (of) V13.9
  endocrine V12.2
  genital system V13.29
  hematological V12.3
  immunity V12.2
  mental V11.9
    affective type V11.1
    manic-depressive V11.1
    neurosis V11.2
    schizophrenia V11.0
    specified type NEC V11.8
  metabolic V12.2
  musculoskeletal NEC V13.5
  nervous system V12.40
    specified type NEC V12.49
  obstetric V13.29
    affecting management of current pregnancy V23.49
      pre-term labor V13.21
  sense organs V12.40
    specified type NEC V12.49
  specified site NEC V13.8
  urinary system V13.00
    calculi V13.01
    infection V13.02
    nephrotic syndrome V13.03
    specified NEC V13.09
 drug use
  nonprescribed (*see also* Abuse, drugs, nondependent) 305.9
  patent (*see also* Abuse, drugs, nondependent) 305.9
 effect NEC of external cause V15.89
 embolism (pulmonary) V12.51
 emotional abuse V15.42
 encephalitis V12.42
 endocrine disorder V12.2
 extracorporeal membrane oxygenation (ECMO) V15.87
 falling V15.88
 family
  allergy V19.6
  anemia V18.2
  arteriosclerosis V17.4
  arthritis V17.7
  asthma V17.5
  blindness V19.0
  blood disorder NEC V18.3
  cardiovascular disease V17.4
  carrier, genetic disease V18.9
  cerebrovascular disease V17.1
  chronic respiratory condition NEC V17.6
  colonic polyps V18.51
  congenital anomalies V19.5
  consanguinity V19.7
  coronary artery disease V17.3
  cystic fibrosis V18.1
  deafness V19.2
  diabetes mellitus V18.0

History—*continued*
 digestive disorders V18.59
 disease or disorder (of)
  allergic V19.6
  blood NEC V18.3
  cardiovascular NEC V17.4
  cerebrovascular V17.1
  colonic polyps V18.51
  coronary artery V17.3
  digestive V18.59
  ear NEC V19.3
  endocrine V18.1
  eye NEC V19.1
  genitourinary NEC V18.7
  hypertensive V17.4
  infectious V18.8
  ischemic heart V17.3
  kidney V18.69
    polycystic V18.61
  mental V17.0
  metabolic V18.1
  musculoskeletal NEC V17.89
    osteoporosis V17.81
  neurological NEC V17.2
  parasitic V18.8
  psychiatric condition V17.0
  skin condition V19.4
 ear disorder NEC V19.3
 endocrine disease V18.1
 epilepsy V17.2
 eye disorder NEC V19.1
 genetic disease carrier V18.9
 genitourinary disease NEC V18.7
 glomerulonephritis V18.69
 gout V18.1
 hay fever V17.6
 hearing loss V19.2
 hematopoietic neoplasia V16.7
 Hodgkin's disease V16.7
 Huntington's chorea V17.2
 hydrocephalus V19.5
 hypertension V17.4
 hypospadias V13.61
 infectious disease V18.8
 ischemic heart disease V17.3
 kidney disease V18.69
  polycystic V18.61
 leukemia V16.6
 lymphatic malignant neoplasia NEC V16.7
 malignant neoplasm (of) NEC V16.9
  anorectal V16.0
  anus V16.0
  appendix V16.0
  bladder V16.59
  bone V16.8
  brain V16.8
  breast V16.3
    male V16.8
  bronchus V16.1
  cecum V16.0
  cervix V16.49
  colon V16.0
  duodenum V16.0
  esophagus V16.0
  eye V16.8
  gallbladder V16.0
  gastrointestinal tract V16.0
  genital organs V16.40
  hemopoietic NEC V16.7
  ileum V16.0
  ilium V16.8

Hollow foot (congenital) 754.71
  acquired 736.73
Holmes' syndrome (visual disorientation) 368.16
Holoprosencephaly 742.2
  due to
    trisomy 13 758.1
    trisomy 18 758.2
Holthouse's hernia —*see* Hernia, inguinal
Homesickness 309.89
Homocystinemia 270.4
Homocystinuria 270.4
Homologous serum jaundice (prophylactic)
    (therapeutic)—*see* Hepatitis, viral
Homosexuality —*omit code*
  ego-dystonic 302.0
  pedophilic 302.2
  problems with 302.0
Homozygous Hb-S disease 282.61
Honeycomb lung 518.89
  congenital 748.4
Hong Kong ear 117.3
HOOD (hereditary osteo-onychodysplasia) 756.89
Hooded
  clitoris 752.49
  penis 752.69
Hookworm (anemia) (disease) (infestation)—*see*
    Ancylostomiasis
Hoppe-Goldflam syndrome 358.00
Hordeolum (external) (eyelid) 373.11
  internal 373.12
Horn
  cutaneous 702.8
    cheek 702.8
    eyelid 702.8
    penis 702.8
  iliac 756.89
  nail 703.8
    congenital 757.5
  papillary 700
Horner's
  syndrome (*see also* Neuropathy, peripheral,
    autonomic) 337.9
    traumatic 954.0
  teeth 520.4
Horseshoe kidney (congenital) 753.3
Horton's
  disease (temporal arteritis) 446.5
  headache or neuralgia 346.2
Hospice care V66.7
Hospitalism (in children) NEC 309.83
Hourglass contraction, contracture
  bladder 596.8
  gallbladder 575.2
    congenital 751.69
  stomach 536.8
    congenital 750.7
    psychogenic 306.4
  uterus 661.4
    affecting fetus or newborn 763.7
Household circumstance affecting care V60.9
  specified type NEC V60.8
Housemaid's knee 727.2
Housing circumstance affecting care V60.9
  specified type NEC V60.8
Huchard's disease (continued arterial
    hypertension) 401.9
Hudson-Stähli lines 371.11
Huguier's disease (uterine fibroma) 218.9
Hum, venous —*omit code*

Human bite (open wound)—*see also* Wound,
    open, by site
  intact skin surface—*see* Contusion
Human immunodeficiency virus (disease)
    (illness) 042
  infection V08
    with symptoms, symptomatic 042
Human immunodeficiency virus-2 infection
    079.53
Human immunovirus (disease) (illness)
    (infection)—*see* Human immunodeficiency
    virus (disease) (illness) (infection)
Human papillomavirus 079.4
  cervical
    high risk, DNA test positive 795.05
    low risk, DNA test positive 795.09
Human T-cell lymphotrophic virus I infection
    079.51
Human T-cell lymphotrophic virus II infection
    079.52
Human T-cell lymphotropic virus-III (disease)
    (illness) (infection)—*see* Human
    immunodeficiency virus (disease) (illness)
    (infection)
HTLV-I infection 079.51
HTLV-II infection 079.52
HTLV-III (disease) (illness) (infection)—*see*
    Human immunodeficiency virus (disease)
    (illness) (infection)
HTLV-III/LAV
    (disease) (illness) (infection)—*see* Human
      immunodeficiency virus (disease) (illness)
      (infection)
Humpback (acquired) 737.9
  congenital 756.19
Hunchback (acquired) 737.9
  congenital 756.19
Hunger 994.2
  air, psychogenic 306.1
  disease 251.1
Hunner's ulcer (*see also* Cystitis) 595.1
Hunt's
  neuralgia 053.11
  syndrome (herpetic geniculate ganglionitis)
      053.11
    dyssynergia cerebellaris myoclonica 334.2
Hunter's glossitis 529.4
Hunter (-Hurler) syndrome
    (mucopolysaccharidosis II) 277.5
Hunterian chancre 091.0
Huntington's
  chorea 333.4
  disease 333.4
Huppert's disease (multiple myeloma)
    (M9730/3) 203.0
Hurler (-Hunter) disease or syndrome
    (mucopolysaccharidosis II) 277.5
Hürthle cell
  adenocarcinoma (M8290/3) 193
  adenoma (M8290/0) 226
  carcinoma (M8290/3) 193
  tumor (M8290/0) 226
Hutchinson's
  disease meaning
    angioma serpiginosum 709.1
    cheiropompholyx 705.81
    prurigo estivalis 692.72
    summer eruption, or summer prurigo 692.72
  incisors 090.5

Hydropericardium (*see also* Pericarditis) 423.9
Hydroperitoneum 789.5
Hydrophobia 071
Hydrophthalmos (*see also* Buphthalmia) 743.20
Hydropneumohemothorax (*see also* Hemothorax) 511.8
Hydropneumopericarditis (*see also* Pericarditis) 423.9
Hydropneumopericardium (*see also* Pericarditis) 423.9
Hydropneumothorax 511.8
  nontuberculous 511.8
    bacterial 511.1
  pneumococcal 511.1
  staphylococcal 511.1
  streptococcal 511.1
  traumatic 860.0
    with open wound into thorax 860.1
  tuberculous (*see also* Tuberculosis, pleural) 012.0
Hydrops 782.3
  abdominis 789.5
  amnii (complicating pregnancy) (*see also* Hydramnios) 657
  articulorum intermittens (*see also* Rheumatism, palindromic) 719.3
  cardiac (*see also* Failure, heart) 428.0
  congenital—*see* Hydrops, fetalis
  endolymphatic (*see also* Disease, Ménière's) 386.00
  fetal(is) or newborn 778.0
    due to isoimmunization 773.3
  not due to isoimmunization 778.0
  gallbladder 575.3
  idiopathic (fetus or newborn) 778.0
  joint (*see also* Effusion, joint) 719.0
  labyrinth (*see also* Disease, Ménière's) 386.00
  meningeal NEC 331.4
  nutritional 262
  pericardium—*see* Pericarditis
  pleura (*see also* Hydrothorax) 511.8
  renal (*see also* Nephrosis) 581.9
  spermatic cord (*see also* Hydrocele) 603.9
Hydropyonephrosis (*see also* Pyelitis) 590.80
  chronic 590.00
Hydrorachis 742.53
Hydrorrhea (nasal) 478.19
  gravidarum 658.1
  pregnancy 658.1
Hydrosadenitis 705.83
Hydrosalpinx (fallopian tube) (follicularis) 614.1
Hydrothorax (double) (pleural) 511.8
  chylous (nonfilarial) 457.8
    filaria (*see also* Infestation, filarial) 125.9
  nontuberculous 511.8
    bacterial 511.1
  pneumococcal 511.1
  staphylococcal 511.1
  streptococcal 511.1
  traumatic 862.29
    with open wound into thorax 862.39
  tuberculous (*see also* Tuberculosis, pleura) 012.0
Hydroureter 593.5
  congenital 753.22
Hydroureteronephrosis (*see also* Hydronephrosis) 591
Hydrourethra 599.84
Hydroxykynureninuria 270.2
Hydroxyprolinemia 270.8
Hydroxyprolinuria 270.8

Hygroma (congenital) (cystic) (M9173/0) 228.1
  prepatellar 727.3
  subdural—*see* Hematoma, subdural
Hymen —*see* condition
Hymenolepiasis (diminuta) (infection) (infestation) (nana) 123.6
Hymenolepis (diminuta) (infection) (infestation) (nana) 123.6
Hypalgesia (*see also* Disturbance, sensation) 782.0
Hyperabduction syndrome 447.8
Hyperacidity, gastric 536.8
  psychogenic 306.4
Hyperactive, hyperactivity
  basal cell, uterine cervix 622.10
  bladder 596.51
  bowel (syndrome) 564.9
    sounds 787.5
  cervix epithelial (basal) 622.10
  child 314.01
  colon 564.9
  gastrointestinal 536.8
    psychogenic 306.4
  intestine 564.9
  labyrinth (unilateral) 386.51
    with loss of labyrinthine reactivity 386.58
    bilateral 386.52
  nasal mucous membrane 478.19
  stomach 536.8
  thyroid (gland) (*see also* Thyrotoxicosis) 242.9
Hyperacusis 388.42
Hyperadrenalism (cortical) 255.3
  medullary 255.6
Hyperadrenocorticism 255.3
  congenital 255.2
  iatrogenic
    correct substance properly administered 255.3
    overdose or wrong substance given or taken 962.0
Hyperaffectivity 301.11
Hyperaldosteronism (atypical) (hyperplastic) (normoaldosteronal) (normotensive) (primary) 255.10
  secondary 255.14
Hyperalgesia (*see also* Disturbance, sensation) 782.0
Hyperalimentation 783.6
  carotene 278.3
  specified NEC 278.8
  vitamin A 278.2
  vitamin D 278.4
Hyperaminoaciduria 270.9
  arginine 270.6
  citrulline 270.6
  cystine 270.0
  glycine 270.0
  lysine 270.7
  ornithine 270.6
  renal (types I, II, III) 270.0
Hyperammonemia (congenital) 270.6
Hyperamnesia 780.99
Hyperamylasemia 790.5
Hyperaphia 782.0
Hyperazotemia 791.9
Hyperbetalipoproteinemia (acquired) (essential) (familial) (hereditary) (primary) (secondary) 272.0
  with prebetalipoproteinemia 272.2

Hypergonadism
 ovarian 256.1
 testicular (infantile) (primary) 257.0
Hyperheparinemia (*see also* Circulating
  anticoagulants) 286.5
Hyperhidrosis, hyperidrosis 705.21
 axilla 705.21
 face 705.21
 focal (localized) 705.21
  primary 705.21
   axilla 705.21
   face 705.21
   palms 705.21
   soles 705.21
  secondary 705.22
   axilla 705.22
   face 705.22
   palms 705.22
   soles 705.22
 generalized 780.8
 palms 705.21
 psychogenic 306.3
 secondary 780.8
 soles 705.21
Hyperhistidinemia 270.5
Hyperinsulinism (ectopic) (functional) (organic)
  NEC 251.1
 iatrogenic 251.0
 reactive 251.2
 spontaneous 251.2
 therapeutic misadventure (from administration
   of insulin) 962.3
Hyperiodemia 276.9
Hyperirritability (cerebral), in newborn 779.1
Hyperkalemia 276.7
Hyperkeratosis (*see also* Keratosis) 701.1
 cervix 622.2
 congenital 757.39
 cornea 371.89
 due to yaws (early) (late) (palmar or plantar)
   102.3
 eccentrica 757.39
 figurata centrifuga atrophica 757.39
 follicularis 757.39
  in cutem penetrans 701.1
 limbic (cornea) 371.89
 palmoplantaris climacterica 701.1
 pinta (carate) 103.1
 senile (with pruritus) 702.0
 tongue 528.79
 universalis congenita 757.1
 vagina 623.1
 vocal cord 478.5
 vulva 624.0
Hyperkinesia, hyperkinetic (disease) (reaction)
  (syndrome) 314.9
 with
  attention deficit —*see* Disorder, attention deficit
  conduct disorder 314.2
  developmental delay 314.1
  simple disturbance of activity and attention
    314.01
  specified manifestation NEC 314.8
 heart (disease) 429.82
 of childhood or adolescence NEC 314.9
Hyperlacrimation (*see also* Epiphora) 375.20
Hyperlipemia (*see also* Hyperlipidemia) 272.4
Hyperlipidemia 272.4
 carbohydrate-induced 272.1
 combined 272.4
 endogenous 272.1

Hyperlipidemia—*continued*
 exogenous 272.3
 fat-induced 272.3
 group
  A 272.0
  B 272.1
  C 272.2
  D 272.3
 mixed 272.2
 specified type NEC 272.4
Hyperlipidosis 272.7
 hereditary 272.7
Hyperlipoproteinemia (acquired) (essential)
  (familial) (hereditary) (primary) (secondary)
  272.4
 Fredrickson type
  I 272.3
  IIa 272.0
  IIb 272.2
  III 272.2
  IV 272.1
  V 272.3
 low-density-lipoid-type (LDL) 272.0
 very-low-density-lipoid-type [VLDL] 272.1
Hyperlucent lung, unilateral 492.8
Hyperluteinization 256.1
Hyperlysinemia 270.7
Hypermagnesemia 275.2
 neonatal 775.5
Hypermaturity (fetus or newborn)
 post-term infant 766.21
 prolonged gestation infant 766.22
Hypermenorrhea 626.2
Hypermetabolism 794.7
Hypermethioninemia 270.4
Hypermetropia (congenital) 367.0
Hypermobility
 cecum 564.9
 coccyx 724.71
 colon 564.9
  psychogenic 306.4
 ileum 564.89
 joint (acquired) 718.80
  ankle 718.87
  elbow 718.82
  foot 718.87
  hand 718.84
  hip 718.85
  knee 718.86
  multiple sites 718.89
  pelvic region 718.85
  shoulder (region) 718.81
  specified site NEC 718.88
  wrist 718.83
 kidney, congenital 753.3
 meniscus (knee) 717.5
 scapula 718.81
 stomach 536.8
  psychogenic 306.4
 syndrome 728.5
 testis, congenital— 752.52
 urethral 599.81
Hypermotility
 gastrointestinal 536.8
 intestine 564.9
  psychogenic 306.4
 stomach 536.8
Hypernasality 784.49
Hypernatremia 276.0
 with water depletion 276.0
Hypernephroma (M8312/3) 189.0

Hypersteatosis 706.3
Hyperstimulation, ovarian 256.1
Hypersuprarenalism 255.3
Hypersusceptibility —*see* Allergy
Hyper-TBG-nemia 246.8
Hypertelorism 756.0
  orbit, orbital 376.41

> *"H" listing resumes after*
> *Hypertension table...*

Hypertension, hypertensive

	Malignant	Benign	Unspecified
(arterial) (arteriolar) (crisis) (degeneration) (disease) (essential) (fluctuating) (idiopathic) (intermittent) (labile) (low renin) (orthostatic) (paroxysmal) (primary) (systemic) (uncontrolled) (vascular)	401.0	401.1	401.9
with			
chronic kidney disease			
stage I through stage IV, or unspecified	403.00	403.10	403.90
stage V or end stage renal disease	403.01	403.11	403.91
heart involvement (conditions classifiable to 429.0-429.3, 429.8, 429.9 due to hypertension) (*see also* Hypertension, heart)	402.00	402.10	402.90
with kidney involvement—*see* Hypertension, cardiorenal			
renal involvement (only conditions classifiable to 585, 586, 587) (excludes conditions classifiable to 584) (*see also* Hypertension, kidney).	403.00	403.10	403.90
with heart involvement—*see* Hypertension, cardiorenal			
failure (and sclerosis) (*see also* Hypertension, kidney)	403.01	403.11	403.91
sclerosis without failure (*see also* Hypertension, kidney)	403.00	403.10	403.90
accelerated (*see also* Hypertension, by type, malignant)	401.0	—	—
antepartum—*see* Hypertension complicating pregnancy, childbirth, or the puerperium			
cardiorenal (disease)	404.00	404.10	404.90
with			
chronic kidney disease			
stage I through stage IV, or unspecified	404.00	404.10	404.90
and heart failure	404.01	404.11	404.91
stage V or end stage renal disease	404.02	404.12	404.92
and heart failure	404.03	404.13	404.93
heart failure	404.01	404.11	404.91
and chronic kidney disease	404.02	404.12	404.92
stage I through stage IV or unspecified	404.02	404.12	404.92
stage V or end stage renal disease	404.03	404.13	404.93
cardiovascular disease (arteriosclerotic) (sclerotic)	402.00	402.10	402.90
with			
heart failure	402.01	402.11	402.91
renal involvement (conditions classifiable to 403) (*see also* Hypertension, cardiorenal)	404.00	404.10	404.90
cardiovascular renal (disease) (sclerosis) (*see also* Hypertension cardiorenal)	404.00	404.10	404.90
cerebrovascular disease NEC	437.2	437.2	437.2
complicating pregnancy, childbirth, or the puerperium	642.2	642.0	642.9
with			
albuminuria (and edema) (mild)	—	—	642.4
severe	—	—	642.5
chronic kidney disease	642.2	642.2	642.2
and heart disease	642.2	642.2	642.2
edema (mild)	—	—	642.4
severe	—	—	642.5
heart disease	642.2	642.2	642.2
and chronic kidney disease	642.2	642.2	642.2
renal disease	642.2	642.2	642.2
and heart disease	642.2	642.2	642.2
chronic	642.2	642.0	642.0
with pre-eclampsia or eclampsia	642.7	642.7	642.7
fetus or newborn	760.0	760.0	760.0
essential	—	642.0	642.0
with pre-eclampsia or eclampsia	—	642.7	642.7
fetus or newborn	760.0	760.0	760.0
fetus or newborn	760.0	760.0	760.0
gestational	—	—	642.3
pre-existing	642.2	642.0	642.0
with pre-eclampsia or eclampsia	642.7	642.7	642.7
fetus or newborn	760.0	760.0	760.0
secondary to renal disease	642.1	642.1	642.1
with pre-eclampsia or eclampsia	642.7	642.7	642.7
fetus or newborn	760.0	760.0	760.0
transient	—	—	642.3
due to			
aldosteronism, primary	405.09	405.19	405.99
brain tumor	405.09	405.19	405.99
bulbar poliomyelitis	405.09	405.19	405.99
calculus			
kidney	405.09	405.19	405.99
ureter	405.09	405.19	405.99
coarctation, aorta	405.09	405.19	405.99
Cushing's disease	405.09	405.19	405.99
glomerulosclerosis (*see also* Hypertension, kidney)	403.00	403.10	403.90

	Malignant	Benign	Unspecified
periarteritis nodosa	405.09	405.19	405.99
pheochromocytoma	405.09	405.19	405.99
polycystic kidney(s)	405.09	405.19	405.99
polycythemia	405.09	405.19	405.99
porphyria	405.09	405.19	405.99
pyelonephritis	405.09	405.19	405.99
renal (artery)			
aneurysm	405.01	405.11	405.91
anomaly	405.01	405.11	405.91
embolism	405.01	405.11	405.91
fibromuscular hyperplasia	405.01	405.11	405.91
occlusion	405.01	405.11	405.91
stenosis	405.01	405.11	405.91
thrombosis	405.01	405.11	405.91
encephalopathy	437.2	437.2	437.2
gestational (transient) NEC	—	—	642.3
Goldblatt's	440.1	440.1	440.1
heart (disease) (conditions classifiable to 429.0-429.3, 429.8, 429.9 due to hypertension)	402.00	402.10	402.90
with			
heart failure	402.01	402.11	402.91
hypertensive kidney disease (conditions classifiable to 403) (*see also* Hypertension, cardiorenal)	404.00	404.10	404.90
renal sclerosis (*see also* Hypertension, cardiorenal)	404.00	404.10	404.90
intracranial, benign	—	348.2	—
intraocular	—	—	365.04
kidney	403.00	403.10	403.90
with			
chronic kidney disease			
stage I through stage IV, or unspecified	403.00	403.10	403.90
stage V or end stage renal disease	403.01	403.11	403.91
heart involvement (conditions classifiable to 429.0-429.3, 429.8, 429.9 due to hypertension) (*see also* Hypertension cardiorenal)	404.00	404.10	404.90
hypertensive heart (disease) (conditions classifiable to 402) (*see also* Hypertension, cardiorenal)	404.00	404.10	404.90
lesser circulation	—	—	416.0
necrotizing	401.0	—	—
ocular	—	—	365.04
portal (due to chronic liver disease)	—	—	572.3
postoperative	—	—	997.91
psychogenic	—	—	306.2
puerperal, postpartum—*see* Hypertension, complicating pregnancy, childbirth, or the puerperium			
pulmonary (artery)	—	—	416.8
idiopathic	—	—	416.0
primary	—	—	416.0
of newborn	—	—	747.83
with cor pulmonale (chronic)	—	—	416.8
acute	—	—	415.0
secondary	—	—	416.8
renal (disease) (*see also* Hypertension, kidney)	403.00	403.10	403.90
renovascular NEC	405.01	405.11	405.91
secondary NEC	405.09	405.19	405.99
due to			
aldosteronism, primary	405.09	405.19	405.99
brain tumor	405.09	405.19	405.99
bulbar poliomyelitis	405.09	405.19	405.99
calculus			
kidney	405.09	405.19	405.99
ureter	405.09	405.19	405.99
coarctation, aorta	405.09	405.19	405.99
Cushing's disease	405.09	405.19	405.99
glomerulosclerosis (*see also* Hypertension, kidney)	403.00	403.10	403.90
periarteritis nodosa	405.09	405.19	405.99
pheochromocytoma	405.09	405.19	405.99
polycystic kidney(s)	405.09	405.19	405.99
polycythemia	405.09	405.19	405.99
porphyria	405.09	405.19	405.99
pyelonephritis	405.09	405.19	405.99
renal (artery)			
aneurysm	405.01	405.11	405.91
anomaly	405.01	405.11	405.91
embolism	405.01	405.11	405.91
fibromuscular hyperplasia	405.01	405.11	405.91
occlusion	405.01	405.11	405.91
stenosis	405.01	405.11	405.91
thrombosis	405.01	405.11	405.91
transient	—	—	796.2

	Malignant	Benign	Unspecified
of pregnancy	—	—	642.3
venous, chronic (asymptomatic) (idiopathic)	—	—	459.30
due to			
deep vein thrombosis (*see also* Syndrome, postphlebetic)	—	—	459.10
with			
complication, NEC	—	—	459.39
inflammation	—	—	459.32
with ulcer	—	—	459.33
ulcer	—	—	459.31
with inflammation	—	—	459.33

Hyperthecosis, ovary 256.8
Hyperthermia (of unknown origin) (*see also*
　　Pyrexia) 780.6
　malignant (due to anesthesia) 995.86
　newborn 778.4
Hyperthymergasia (*see also* Psychosis,
　　affective) 296.0
　reactive (from emotional stress, psychological
　　　trauma) 298.1
　recurrent episode 296.1
　single episode 296.0
Hyperthymism 254.8
Hyperthyroid (recurrent)—*see* Hyperthyroidism
Hyperthyroidism (latent) (preadult) (recurrent)
　　(without goiter) 242.9

---
*Note—Use the following fifth-digit
subclassification with category 242:*

0　*without mention of thyrotoxic crisis or storm*
1　*with mention of thyrotoxic crisis or storm*

---

　with
　　goiter (diffuse) 242.0
　　　adenomatous 242.3
　　　　multinodular 242.2
　　　　uninodular 242.1
　　　nodular 242.3
　　　　multinodular 242.2
　　　　uninodular 242.1
　　　thyroid nodule 242.1
　　complicating pregnancy, childbirth, or
　　　puerperium 648.1
　　neonatal (transient) 775.3
Hypertonia —Hypertonicity
Hypertonicity
　bladder 596.51
　fetus or newborn 779.89
　gastrointestinal (tract) 536.8
　infancy 779.89
　　due to electrolyte imbalance 779.89
　muscle 728.85
　stomach 536.8
　　psychogenic 306.4
　uterus, uterine (contractions) 661.4
　　affecting fetus or newborn 763.7
Hypertony —*see* Hypertonicity
Hypertransaminemia 790.4
Hypertrichosis 704.1
　congenital 757.4
　eyelid 374.54
　lanuginosa 757.4
　　acquired 704.1
Hypertriglyceridemia, essential 272.1
Hypertrophy, hypertrophic
　adenoids (infectional) 474.12
　　and tonsils (faucial) (infective) (lingual)
　　　(lymphoid) 474.10
　adrenal 255.8
　alveolar process or ridge 525.8
　anal papillae 569.49
　apocrine gland 705.82
　artery NEC 447.8
　　carotid 447.8
　　congenital (peripheral) NEC 747.60
　　gastrointestinal 747.61
　　lower limb 747.64
　　renal 747.62
　　specified NEC 747.69
　　spinal 747.82
　arthritis (chronic) (*see also* Osteoarthrosis) 715.9

Hypertrophy, hypertrophic—*continued*
　spine (*see also* Spondylosis) 721.90
　arytenoid 478.79
　asymmetrical (heart) 429.9
　auricular—*see* Hypertrophy, cardiac
　Bartholin's gland 624.8
　bile duct 576.8
　bladder (sphincter) (trigone) 596.8
　blind spot, visual field 368.42
　bone 733.99
　brain 348.8
　breast 611.1
　　cystic 610.1
　　fetus or newborn 778.7
　　fibrocystic 610.1
　　massive pubertal 611.1
　　puerperal, postpartum 676.3
　　senile (parenchymatous) 611.1
　cardiac (chronic) (idiopathic) 429.3
　　with
　　　rheumatic fever (conditions classifiable to
　　　　390)
　　　　active 391.8
　　　　　with chorea 392.0
　　　　inactive or quiescent (with chorea) 398.99
　　congenital NEC 746.89
　　fatty (*see also* Degeneration, myocardial)
　　　429.1
　　hypertensive (*see also* Hypertension, heart)
　　　402.90
　　rheumatic (with chorea) 398.99
　　　active or acute 391.8
　　　　with chorea 392.0
　　valve (*see also* Endocarditis) 424.90
　　　congenital NEC 746.89
　cartilage 733.99
　cecum 569.89
　cervix (uteri) 622.6
　　congenital 752.49
　　elongation 622.6
　clitoris (cirrhotic) 624.2
　　congenital 752.49
　colon 569.89
　　congenital 751.3
　conjunctiva, lymphoid 372.73
　cornea 371.89
　corpora cavernosa 607.89
　duodenum 537.89
　endometrium (uterus) (*see also* Hyperplasia,
　　endometrium) 621.30
　　cervix 622.6
　epididymis 608.89
　esophageal hiatus (congenital) 756.6
　　with hernia—*see* Hernia, diaphragm
　eyelid 374.30
　falx, skull 733.99
　fat pad 729.30
　　infrapatellar 729.31
　　knee 729.31
　　orbital 374.34
　　popliteal 729.31
　　prepatellar 729.31
　　retropatellar 729.31
　　specified site NEC 729.39
　foot (congenital) 755.67
　frenum, frenulum (tongue) 529.8
　　linguae 529.8
　　lip 528.5
　gallbladder or cystic duct 575.8
　gastric mucosa 535.2
　gingiva 523.8

Hypertrophy, hypertrophic—*continued*
  gland, glandular (general) NEC 785.6
  gum (mucous membrane) 523.8
  heart (idiopathic)—*see also* Hypertrophy,
    cardiac
    valve—*see also* Endocarditis
      congenital NEC 746.89
  hemifacial 754.0
  hepatic—*see* Hypertrophy, liver
  hiatus (esophageal) 756.6
  hilus gland 785.6
  hymen, congenital 752.49
  ileum 569.89
  infrapatellar fat pad 729.31
  intestine 569.89
  jejunum 569.89
  kidney (compensatory) 593.1
    congenital 753.3
  labial frenulum 528.5
  labium (majus) (minus) 624.3
  lacrimal gland, chronic 375.03
  ligament 728.9
    spinal 724.8
  linguae frenulum 529.8
  lingual tonsil (infectional) 474.11
  lip (frenum) 528.5
    congenital 744.81
  liver 789.1
    acute 573.8
    cirrhotic—*see* Cirrhosis, liver
    congenital 751.69
    fatty—*see* Fatty, liver
  lymph gland 785.6
    tuberculous—*see* Tuberculosis, lymph gland
  mammary gland—*see* Hypertrophy, breast
  maxillary frenulum 528.5
  Meckel's diverticulum (congenital) 751.0
  medial meniscus, acquired 717.3
  median bar 600.90
    with
      other lower urinary tract symptoms (LUTS)
        600.91
      urinary
        obstruction 600.91
        retention 600.91
  mediastinum 519.3
  meibomian gland 373.2
  meniscus, knee, congenital 755.64
  metatarsal head 733.99
  metatarsus 733.99
  mouth 528.9
  mucous membrane
    alveolar process 523.8
    nose 478.19
    turbinate (nasal) 478.0
  muscle 728.9
  muscular coat, artery NEC 447.8
    carotid 447.8
    renal 447.3
  myocardium (*see also* Hypertrophy, cardiac)
    429.3
    idiopathic 425.4
  myometrium 621.2
  nail 703.8
    congenital 757.5
  nasal 478.19
    alae 478.19
    bone 738.0
    cartilage 478.19
    mucous membrane (septum) 478.19
    sinus (*see also* Sinusitis) 473.9

Hypertrophy, hypertrophic—*continued*
  turbinate 478.0
  nasopharynx, lymphoid (infectional) (tissue)
    (wall) 478.29
  neck, uterus 622.6
  nipple 611.1
  normal aperture diaphragm (congenital) 756.6
  nose (*see also* Hypertrophy, nasal) 478.19
  orbit 376.46
  organ or site, congenital NEC—*see* Anomaly,
    specified type NEC
  osteoarthropathy (pulmonary) 731.2
  ovary 620.8
  palate (hard) 526.89
    soft 528.9
  pancreas (congenital) 751.7
  papillae
    anal 569.49
    tongue 529.3
  parathyroid (gland) 252.01
  parotid gland 527.1
  penis 607.89
  phallus 607.89
    female (clitoris) 624.2
  pharyngeal tonsil 474.12
  pharyngitis 472.1
  pharynx 478.29
    lymphoid (infectional) (tissue) (wall) 478.29
  pituitary (fossa) (gland) 253.8
  popliteal fat pad 729.31
  preauricular (lymph) gland (Hampstead) 785.6
  prepuce (congenital) 605
    female 624.2
  prostate (asymptomatic) (early) (recurrent)
    600.90
    with
      other lower urinary tract symptoms (LUTS)
        600.91
      urinary
        obstruction 600.91
        retention 600.91
    adenofibromatous 600.20
      with
        other lower urinary tract symptoms
          (LUTS) 600.21
        urinary
          obstruction 600.21
          retention 600.21
    benign 600.00
      with
        other lower urinary tract symptoms
          (LUTS) 600.01
        urinary
          obstruction 600.01
          retention 600.01
    congenital 752.89
  psuedoedematous hypodermal 757.0
  pseudomuscular 359.1
  pylorus (muscle) (sphincter) 537.0
    congenital 750.5
    infantile 750.5
  rectal sphincter 569.49
  rectum 569.49
  renal 593.1
  rhinitis (turbinate) 472.0
  salivary duct or gland 527.1
    congenital 750.26
  scaphoid (tarsal) 733.99
  scar 701.4
  scrotum 608.89
  sella turcica 253.8

Hypertrophy, hypertrophic—*continued*
  seminal vesicle 608.89
  sigmoid 569.89
  skin condition NEC 701.9
  spermatic cord 608.89
  spinal ligament 724.8
  spleen—*see* Splenomegaly
  spondylitis (spine) (*see also* Spondylosis) 721.90
  stomach 537.89
  subaortic stenosis (idiopathic) 425.1
  sublingual gland 527.1
    congenital 750.26
  submaxillary gland 527.1
  suprarenal (gland) 255.8
  tendon 727.9
  testis 608.89
    congenital 752.89
  thymic, thymus (congenital) (gland) 254.0
  thyroid (gland) (*see also* Goiter) 240.9
    primary 242.0
    secondary 242.2
  toe (congenital) 755.65
    acquired 735.8
  tongue 529.8
    congenital 750.15
    frenum 529.8
    papillae (foliate) 529.3
  tonsil (faucial) (infective) (lingual) (lymphoid)
      474.11
    and adenoids 474.10
    with
      adenoiditis 474.01
        tonsillitis 474.00
          and adenoiditis 474.02
  tunica vaginalis 608.89
  turbinate (mucous membrane) 478.0
  ureter 593.89
  urethra 599.84
  uterus 621.2
    puerperal, postpartum 674.8
  uvula 528.9
  vagina 623.8
  vas deferens 608.89
  vein 459.89
  ventricle, ventricular (heart) (left) (right)—*see
      also* Hypertrophy, cardiac
    congenital 746.89
    due to hypertension (left) (right) (*see also*
        Hypertension, heart) 402.90
      benign 402.10
      malignant 402.00
    right with ventricular septal defect, pulmonary
        stenosis or atresia, and dextraposition of
        aorta 745.2
  verumontanum 599.89
  vesical 596.8
  vocal cord 478.5
  vulva 624.3
    stasis (nonfilarial) 624.3
Hypertropia (intermittent) (periodic) 378.31
Hypertyrosinemia 270.2
Hyperuricemia 790.6
Hypervalinemia 270.3
Hyperventilation (tetany) 786.01
  hysterical 300.11
  psychogenic 306.1
  syndrome 306.1
Hyperviscidosis 277.00
Hyperviscosity (of serum) (syndrome) NEC
    273.3
  polycythemic 289.0
  sclerocythemic 282.8

Hypervitaminosis (dietary) NEC 278.8
  A (dietary) 278.2
  D (dietary) 278.4
  from excessive administration or use of vitamin
      preparations (chronic) 278.8
    reaction to sudden overdose 963.5
  vitamin A 278.2
    reaction to sudden overdose 963.5
  vitamin D 278.4
    reaction to sudden overdose 963.5
  vitamin K
    correct substance properly administered 278.8
    overdose or wrong substance given or taken
        964.3
Hypervolemia 276.6
Hypesthesia (*see also* Disturbance, sensation)
    782.0
  cornea 371.81
Hyphema (anterior chamber) (ciliary body) (iris)
    364.41
  traumatic 921.3
Hyphemia —*see* Hyphema
Hypoacidity, gastric 536.8
  psychogenic 306.4
Hypoactive labyrinth (function)—*see*
    Hypofunction, labyrinth
Hypoadrenalism 255.4
  tuberculous (*see also* Tuberculosis) 017.6
Hypoadrenocorticism 255.4
  pituitary 253.4
Hypoalbuminemia 273.8
Hypoaldosteronism 255.4
Hypoalphalipoproteinemia 272.5
Hypobarism 993.2
Hypobaropathy 993.2
Hypobetalipoproteinemia (familial) 272.5
Hypocalcemia 275.41
  cow's milk 775.4
  dietary 269.3
  neonatal 775.4
  phosphate-loading 775.4
Hypocalcification, teeth 520.4
Hypochloremia 276.9
Hypochlorhydria 536.8
  neurotic 306.4
  psychogenic 306.4
Hypocholesteremia 272.5
Hypochondria (reaction) 300.7
Hypochondriac 300.7
Hypochondriasis 300.7
Hypochromasia blood cells 280.9
Hypochromic anemia 280.9
  due to blood loss (chronic) 280.0
    acute 285.1
  microcytic 280.9
Hypocoagulability (*see also* Defect, coagulation)
    286.9
Hypocomplementemia 279.8
Hypocythemia (progressive) 284.9
Hypodontia (*see also* Anodontia) 520.0
Hypoeosinophilia 288.59
Hypoesthesia (*see also* Disturbance, sensation)
    782.0
  cornea 371.81
  tactile 782.0
Hypoestrinism 256.39
Hypoestrogenism 256.39
Hypoferremia 280.9
  due to blood loss (chronic) 280.0

I

Iatrogenic syndrome of excess cortisol 255.0
Iceland disease (epidemic neuromyasthenia)
　　049.8
Ichthyosis (congenita) 757.1
　acquired 701.1
　fetalis gravior 757.1
　follicularis 757.1
　hystrix 757.39
　lamellar 757.1
　lingual 528.6
　palmaris and plantaris 757.39
　simplex 757.1
　vera 757.1
　vulgaris 757.1
Ichthyotoxism 988.0
　bacterial (*see also* Poisoning, food) 005.9
Icteroanemia, hemolytic (acquired) 283.9
　congenital (*see also* Spherocytosis) 282.0
Icterus (*see also* Jaundice) 782.4
　catarrhal—*see* Icterus, infectious
　conjunctiva 782.4
　　newborn 774.6
　epidemic—*see* Icterus, infectious
　febrilis—*see* Icterus, infectious
　fetus or newborn—*see* Jaundice, fetus or newborn
　gravis (*see also* Necrosis, liver) 570
　　complicating pregnancy 646.7
　　　affecting fetus or newborn 760.8
　　fetus or newborn NEC 773.0
　　obstetrical 646.7
　　　affecting fetus or newborn 760.8
　hematogenous (acquired) 283.9
　hemolytic (acquired) 283.9
　　congenital (*see also* Spherocytosis) 282.0
　hemorrhagic (acute) 100.0
　　leptospiral 100.0
　　newborn 776.0
　　spirochetal 100.0
　infectious 070.1
　　with hepatic coma 070.0
　　leptospiral 100.0
　　spirochetal 100.0
　intermittens juvenilis 277.4
　malignant (*see also* Necrosis, liver) 570
　neonatorum (*see also* Jaundice, fetus or
　　newborn) 774.6
　pernicious (*see also* Necrosis, liver) 570
　spirochetal 100.0
Ictus solaris, solis 992.0
Ideation
　suicidal V62.84
Identity disorder 313.82
　dissociative 300.14
　gender role (child) 302.6
　　adult 302.85
　psychosexual (child) 302.6
　　adult 302.85
Idioglossia 307.9
Idiopathic —*see* condition
Idiosyncrasy (*see also* Allergy) 995.3
　drug, medicinal substance, and biological—*see*
　　Allergy, drug
Idiot, idiocy (congenital) 318.2
　amaurotic (Bielschowsky) (-Jansky) (family)
　　(infantile (late)) (juvenile (late))
　　(Vogt-Spielmeyer) 330.1
　microcephalic 742.1

Idiot, idiocy—*continued*
　Mongolian 758.0
　oxycephalic 756.0
Id reaction (due to bacteria) 692.89
IgE asthma 493.0
Ileitis (chronic) (*see also* Enteritis) 558.9
　infectious 009.0
　noninfectious 558.9
　regional (ulcerative) 555.0
　　with large intestine 555.2
　segmental 555.0
　　with large intestine 555.2
　terminal (ulcerative) 555.0
　　with large intestine 555.2
Ileocolitis (*see also* Enteritis) 558.9
　infectious 009.0
　regional 555.2
　ulcerative 556.1
Ileostomy status V44.2
　with complication 569.60
Ileotyphus 002.0
Ileum —*see* condition
Ileus (adynamic) (bowel) (colon) (inhibitory)
　　(intestine) (neurogenic) (paralytic) 560.1
　arteriomesenteric duodenal 537.2
　due to gallstone (in intestine) 560.31
　duodenal, chronic 537.2
　following gastrointestinal surgery 997.4
　gallstone 560.31
　mechanical (*see also* Obstruction, intestine) 560.9
　meconium 777.1
　　due to cystic fibrosis 277.01
　myxedema 564.89
　postoperative 997.4
　transitory, newborn 777.4
Iliac —*see* condition
Iliotibial band friction syndrome 728.89
Ill, louping 063.1
Illegitimacy V61.6
Illness —*see also* Disease
　factitious 300.19
　　with
　　　combined psychological and physical signs
　　　　and symptoms 300.19
　　　physical symptoms 300.19
　　　predominantly
　　　　physical signs and symptoms 300.19
　　　　psychological symptoms 300.16
　chronic (with physical symptoms) 301.51
　heart—*see* Disease, heart
　manic-depressive (*see also* Psychosis, affective)
　　296.80
　mental (*see also* Disorder, mental) 300.9
Imbalance 781.2
　autonomic (*see also* Neuropathy, peripheral,
　　autonomic) 337.9
　electrolyte 276.9
　　with
　　　abortion—*see* Abortion, by type, with
　　　　metabolic disorder
　　　ectopic pregnancy (*see also* categories
　　　　633.0-633.9) 639.4
　　　hyperemesis gravidarum (before 22
　　　　completed weeks gestation) 643.1
　　　molar pregnancy (*see also* categories
　　　　630-632) 639.4
　　following

Impaired, impairment—*continued*
mastication 524.9
mild cognitive, so stated 331.83
mobility
  ear ossicles NEC 385.22
  incostapedial joint 385.22
  malleus 385.21
myocardium, myocardial (*see also*
    Insufficiency, myocardial) 428.0
neuromusculoskeletal NEC V49.89
  back V48.3
  head V48.2
  limb V49.2
  neck V48.3
  spine V48.3
  trunk V48.3
rectal sphincter 787.99
renal (*see also* Disease, renal) 593.9
  disorder resulting from 588.9
    specified NEC 588.89
spine V48.3
vision NEC 369.9
  both eyes NEC 369.3
  moderate 369.74
    both eyes 369.25
      with impairment of lesser eye (specified
          as)
        blind, not further specified 369.15
        low vision, not further specified 369.23
        near-total 369.17
        profound 369.18
        severe 369.24
        total 369.16
    one eye 369.74
      with vision of other eye (specified as)
        near-normal 369.75
        normal 369.76
  near-total 369.64
    both eyes 369.04
      with impairment of lesser eye (specified
          as)
        blind, not further specified 369.02
        total 369.03
    one eye 369.64
      with vision of other eye (specified as)
        near-normal 369.65
        normal 369.66
    one eye 369.60
      with low vision of other eye 369.10
  profound 369.67
    both eyes 369.08
      with impairment of lesser eye (specified
          as)
        blind, not further specified 369.05
        near-total 369.07
        total 369.06
    one eye 369.67
      with vision of other eye (specified as)
        near-normal 369.68
        normal 369.69
  severe 369.71
    both eyes 369.22
      with impairment of lesser eye (specified
          as)
        blind, not further specified 369.11
        low vision, not further specified 369.21
        near-total 369.13
        profound 369.14
        total 369.12
    one eye 369.71
      with vision of other eye (specified as)

Impaired, impairment—*continued*
        near-normal 369.72
        normal 369.73
  total
    both eyes 369.01
    one eye 369.61
      with vision of other eye (specified as)
        near-normal 369.62
        normal 369.63
Impaludism —*see* Malaria
Impediment, speech NEC 784.5
  psychogenic 307.9
  secondary to organic lesion 784.5
Impending
  cerebrovascular accident or attack 435.9
  coronary syndrome 411.1
  delirium tremens 291.0
  myocardial infarction 411.1
Imperception, auditory (acquired) (congenital)
    389.9
Imperfect
  aeration, lung (newborn) 770.5
  closure (congenital)
    alimentary tract NEC 751.8
      lower 751.5
      upper 750.8
    atrioventricular ostium 745.69
    atrium (secundum) 745.5
      primum 745.61
    branchial cleft or sinus 744.41
    choroid 743.59
    cricoid cartilage 748.3
    cusps, heart valve NEC 746.89
      pulmonary 746.09
    ductus
      arteriosus 747.0
      Botalli 747.0
    ear drum 744.29
      causing impairment of hearing 744.03
    endocardial cushion 745.60
    epiglottis 748.3
    esophagus with communication to bronchus or
        trachea 750.3
    Eustachian valve 746.89
    eyelid 743.62
    face, facial (*see also* Cleft, lip) 749.10
    foramen
      Botalli 745.5
      ovale 745.5
    genitalia, genital organ(s) or system
      female 752.89
        external 752.49
        internal NEC 752.89
        uterus 752.3
      male 752.89
        penis 752.69
    glottis 748.3
    heart valve (cusps) NEC 746.89
    interatrial ostium or septum 745.5
    interauricular ostium or septum 745.5
    interventricular ostium or septum 745.4
    iris 743.46
    kidney 753.3
    larynx 748.3
    lens 743.36
    lip (*see also* Cleft, lip) 749.10
    nasal septum or sinus 748.1
    nose 748.1
    omphalomesenteric duct 751.0
    optic nerve entry 743.57

Incompetency, incompetence, incompetent
  annular
    aortic (valve) (*see also* Insufficiency, aortic)
        424.1
    mitral (valve)—(*see also* Insufficiency, mitral)
        424.0
    pulmonary valve (heart) (*see also*
        Endocarditis, pulmonary) 424.3
  aortic (valve) (*see also* Insufficiency, aortic)
      424.1
    syphilitic 093.22
  cardiac (orifice) 530.0
    valve—*see* Endocarditis
  cervix, cervical (os) 622.5
    in pregnancy 654.5
      affecting fetus or newborn 761.0
  esophagogastric (junction) (sphincter) 530.0
  heart valve, congenital 746.89
  mitral (valve)—*see* Insufficiency, mitral
  papillary muscle (heart) 429.81
  pelvic fundus
    pubocervical tissue 618.81
    rectovaginal tissue 618.82
  pulmonary valve (heart) (*see also* Endocarditis,
      pulmonary) 424.3
    congenital 746.09
  tricuspid (annular) (rheumatic) (valve) (*see also*
      Endocarditis, tricuspid) 397.0
  valvular—*see* Endocarditis
  vein, venous (saphenous) (varicose) (*see also*
      Varicose, vein) 454.9
  velopharyngeal (closure)
    acquired 528.9
    congenital 750.29
Incomplete —*see also* condition
  bladder emptying 788.21
  expansion lungs (newborn) 770.5
  gestation (liveborn)—*see* Immaturity
  rotation—*see* Malrotation
Incontinence 788.30
  without sensory awareness 788.34
  anal sphincter 787.6
  continuous leakage 788.37
  feces 787.6
    due to hysteria 300.11
    nonorganic origin 307.7
  hysterical 300.11
  mixed (male) (female) (urge and stress) 788.33
  overflow 788.38
  paradoxical 788.39
  rectal 787.6
  specified NEC 788.39
  stress (female) 625.6
    male NEC 788.32
  urethral sphincter 599.84
  urge 788.31
    and stress (male) (female) 788.33
  urine 788.30
    active 788.30
    male 788.30
      stress 788.32
        and urge 788.33
      neurogenic 788.39
      nonorganic origin 307.6
      stress (female) 625.6
        male NEC 788.32
      urge 788.31
        and stress 788.33
Incontinentia pigmenti 757.33
Incoordinate
  uterus (action) (contractions) 661.4
    affecting fetus or newborn 763.7

Incoordination
  esophageal-pharyngeal (newborn) 787.2
  muscular 781.3
  papillary muscle 429.81
Increase, increased
  abnormal, in development 783.9
  androgens (ovarian) 256.1
  anticoagulants (antithrombin) (anti-VIIIa)
      (anti-IXa) (anti-Xa) (anti-XIa) 286.5
    postpartum 666.3
  cold sense (*see also* Disturbance, sensation)
      782.0
  estrogen 256.0
  function
    adrenal (cortex) 255.3
      medulla 255.6
    pituitary (anterior) (gland) (lobe) 253.1
      posterior 253.6
  heat sense (*see also* Disturbance, sensation) 782.0
  intracranial pressure 781.99
    injury at birth 767.8
  light reflex of retina 362.13
  permeability, capillary 448.9
  pressure
    intracranial 781.99
      injury at birth 767.8
    intraocular 365.00
  pulsations 785.9
  pulse pressure 785.9
  sphericity, lens 743.36
  splenic activity 289.4
  venous pressure 459.89
    portal 572.3
Incrustation, cornea, lead or zinc 930.0
Incyclophoria 378.44
Incyclotropia 378.33
Indeterminate sex 752.7
India rubber skin 756.83
Indicanuria 270.2
Indigestion (bilious) (functional) 536.8
  acid 536.8
  catarrhal 536.8
  due to decomposed food NEC 005.9
  fat 579.8
  nervous 306.4
  psychogenic 306.4
Indirect —*see* condition
Indolent bubo NEC 099.8
Induced
  abortion—*see* Abortion, induced
  birth, affecting fetus or newborn 763.89
  delivery—*see* Delivery
  labor—*see* Delivery
Induration, indurated
  brain 348.8
  breast (fibrous) 611.79
    puerperal, postpartum 676.3
  broad ligament 620.8
  chancre 091.0
    anus 091.1
    congenital 090.0
    extragenital NEC 091.2
  corpora cavernosa (penis) (plastic) 607.89
  liver (chronic) 573.8
    acute 573.8
  lung (black) (brown) (chronic) (fibroid) (*see*
      also Fibrosis, lung) 515
    essential brown 275.0 *[516.1]*
  penile 607.89
  phlebitic—*see* Phlebitis
  skin 782.8
  stomach 537.89

Induratio penis plastica 607.89
Industrial —*see* condition
Inebriety (*see also* Abuse, drugs, nondependent)
305.0
Inefficiency
kidney (*see also* Disease, renal) 593.9
thyroid (acquired) (gland) 244.9
Inelasticity, skin 782.8
Inequality, leg (acquired) (length) 736.81
congenital 755.30
Inertia
bladder 596.4
neurogenic 596.54
with cauda equina syndrome 344.61
stomach 536.8
psychogenic 306.4
uterus, uterine 661.2
affecting fetus or newborn 763.7
primary 661.0
secondary 661.1
vesical 596.4
neurogenic 596.54
with cauda equina 344.61
Infant —*see also* condition
excessive crying of 780.92
fussy (baby) 780.91
held for adoption V68.89
newborn—*see* Newborn
post-term (gestation period over 40 completed
weeks to 42 completed weeks) 766.21
prolonged gestation of (period over 42
completed weeks) 766.22
syndrome of diabetic mother 775.0
"Infant Hercules" syndrome 255.2
Infantile —*see also* condition
genitalia, genitals 259.0
in pregnancy or childbirth NEC 654.4
affecting fetus or newborn 763.89
causing obstructed labor 660.2
affecting fetus or newborn 763.1
heart 746.9
kidney 753.3
lack of care 995.52
macula degeneration 362.75
melanodontia 521.05
os, uterus (*see also* Infantile, genitalia) 259.0
pelvis 738.6
with disproportion (fetopelvic) 653.1
affecting fetus or newborn 763.1
causing obstructed labor 660.1
affecting fetus or newborn 763.1
penis 259.0
testis 257.2
uterus (*see also* Infantile, genitalia) 259.0
vulva 752.49
Infantilism 259.9
with dwarfism (hypophyseal) 253.3
Brissaud's (infantile myxedema) 244.9
celiac 579.0
Herter's (nontropical sprue) 579.0
hypophyseal 253.3
hypothalamic (with obesity) 253.8
idiopathic 259.9
intestinal 579.0
pancreatic 577.8
pituitary 253.3
renal 588.0
sexual (with obesity) 259.0
Infants, healthy liveborn —*see* Newborn

Infarct, infarction
adrenal (capsule) (gland) 255.4
amnion 658.8
anterior (with contiguous portion of
intraventricular septum) NEC (*see also*
Infarct, myocardium) 410.1
appendices epiploicae 557.0
bowel 557.0
brain (stem) 434.91
embolic (*see also* Embolism, brain) 434.11
healed or old, without residuals V12.59
iatrogenic 997.02
postoperative 997.02
puerperal, postpartum, childbirth 674.0
thrombotic (*see also* Thrombosis, brain)
434.01
breast 611.8
Brewer's (kidney) 593.81
cardiac (*see also* Infarct, myocardium) 410.9
cerebellar (*see also* Infarct, brain) 434.91
embolic (*see also* Embolism, brain) 434.11
cerebral (*see also* Infarct, brain) 434.91
embolic (*see also* Embolism, brain) 434.11
thrombotic (*see also* Infarct, brain) 434.01
chorion 658.8
colon (acute) (agnogenic) (embolic)
(hemorrhagic) (nonocclusive)
(nonthrombotic) (occlusive) (segmental)
(thrombotic) (with gangrene) 557.0
coronary artery (*see also* Infarct, myocardium)
410.9
cortical 434.91
embolic (*see also* Embolism) 444.9
fallopian tube 620.8
gallbladder 575.8
heart (*see also* Infarct, myocardium) 410.9
hepatic 573.4
hypophysis (anterior lobe) 253.8
impending (myocardium) 411.1
intestine (acute) (agnogenic) (embolic)
(hemorrhagic) (nonocclusive)
(nonthrombotic) (occlusive) (thrombotic)
(with gangrene) 557.0
kidney 593.81
liver 573.4
lung (embolic) (thrombotic) 415.19
with
abortion—*see* Abortion, by type, with,
embolism
ectopic pregnancy (*see also* categories
633.0-633.9) 639.6
molar pregnancy (*see also* categories
630-632) 639.6
following
abortion 639.6
ectopic or molar pregnancy 639.6
iatrogenic 415.11
in pregnancy, childbirth, or puerperium—*see*
Embolism, obstetrical
postoperative 415.11
lymph node or vessel 457.8
medullary (brain)—*see* Infarct, brain
meibomian gland (eyelid) 374.85
mesentery, mesenteric (embolic) (thrombotic)
(with gangrene) 557.0
midbrain—*see* Infarct, brain
myocardium, myocardial (acute or with a stated
duration of 8 weeks or less) (with
hypertension) 410.9

Infarct, infarction—*continued*

> *Note—use the following fifth-digit*
> *subclassification with category 410*
>
> 0 *episode unspecified*
> 1 *initial episode*
> 2 *subsequent episode without recurrence*

with symptoms after 8 weeks from date of
    infarction 414.8
anterior (wall) (with contiguous portion of
    intraventricular septum) NEC 410.1
anteroapical (with contiguous portion of
    intraventricular septum) 410.1
anterolateral (wall) 410.0
anteroseptal (with contiguous portion of
    intraventricular septum) 410.1
apical-lateral 410.5
atrial 410.8
basal-lateral 410.5
chronic (with symptoms after 8 weeks from
    date of infarction) 414.8
diagnosed on ECG, but presenting no
    symptoms 412
diaphragmatic wall (with contiguous portion
    of intraventricular septum) 410.4
healed or old, currently presenting no
    symptoms 412
high lateral 410.5
impending 411.1
inferior (wall) (with contiguous portion of
    intraventricular septum) 410.4
inferolateral (wall) 410.2
inferoposterior wall 410.3
lateral wall 410.5
non-ST elevation (NSTEMI) 410.7
nontransmural 410.7
papillary muscle 410.8
past (diagnosed on ECG or other special
    investigation, but currently presenting no
    symptoms) 412
    with symptoms NEC 414.8
posterior (strictly) (true) (wall) 410.6
posterobasal 410.6
posteroinferior 410.3
posterolateral 410.5
previous, currently presenting no symptoms
    412
septal 410.8
specified site NEC 410.8
ST elevation (STEMI) 410.9
    anterior (wall) 410.1
    anterolateral (wall) 410.0
    inferior (wall) 410.4
    inferolateral (wall) 410.2
    inferoposterior (wall) 410.3
    lateral (wall) 410.5
    posterior (strictly) (true) (wall) 410.6
    specified site NEC 410.8
subendocardial 410.7
syphilitic 093.82
non-ST elevation myocardial infarction
    (NSTEMI) 410.7
nontransmural 410.7
omentum 557.0
ovary 620.8
pancreas 577.8
papillary muscle (*see also* Infarct, myocardium)
    410.8
parathyroid gland 252.8
pituitary (gland) 253.8

Infarct, infarction—*continued*
placenta (complicating pregnancy) 656.7
    affecting fetus or newborn 762.2
pontine—*see* Infarct, brain
posterior NEC (*see also* Infarct, myocardium)
    410.6
prostate 602.8
pulmonary (artery) (hemorrhagic) (vein) 415.19
    with
        abortion—*see* Abortion, by type, with
            embolism
        ectopic pregnancy (*see also* categories
            633.0-633.9) 639.6
        molar pregnancy (*see also* categories
            630-632) 639.6
    following
        abortion 639.6
        ectopic or molar pregnancy 639.6
    iatrogenic 415.11
    in pregnancy, childbirth, or puerperium—*see*
        Embolism, obstetrical
    postoperative 415.11
renal 593.81
    embolic or thrombotic 593.81
retina, retinal 362.84
    with occlusion—*see* Occlusion, retina
spinal (acute) (cord) (embolic) (nonembolic) 336.1
spleen 289.59
    embolic or thrombotic 444.89
subchorionic—*see* Infarct, placenta
subendocardial (*see also* Infarct, myocardium)
    410.7
suprarenal (capsule) (gland) 255.4
syncytium—*see* Infarct, placenta
testis 608.83
thrombotic (*see also* Thrombosis) 453.9
    artery, arterial—*see* Embolism
thyroid (gland) 246.3
ventricle (heart) (*see also* Infarct, myocardium)
    410.9
Infecting —*see* condition
Infection, infected, infective (opportunistic)
    136.9
with lymphangitis—*see* Lymphangitis
abortion—*see* Abortion, by type, with sepsis
abscess (skin)—*see* Abscess, by site
Absidia 117.7
Acanthocheilonema (perstans) 125.4
    streptocerca 125.6
accessory sinus (chronic) (*see also* Sinusitis)
    473.9
Achorion—*see* Dermatophytosis
Acremonium falciforme 117.4
acromioclavicular (joint) 711.91
actinobacillus
    lignieresii 027.8
    mallei 024
    muris 026.1
actinomadura—*see* Actinomycosis
Actinomyces (israelii)—*see also* Actinomycosis
    muris-ratti 026.1
Actinomycetales (actinomadura) (Actinomyces)
    (Nocardia) (Streptomyces)—*see*
    Actinomycosis
actinomycotic NEC (*see also* Actinomycosis)
    039.9
adenoid (chronic) 474.01
    acute 463
    and tonsil (chronic) 474.02
        acute or subacute 463
adenovirus NEC 079.0

Infection, infected, infective—*continued*
  suis 023.2
  Brugia (Wuchereria) malayi 125.1
  bursa—*see* Bursitis
  buttocks (skin) 686.9
  Candida (albicans) (tropicalis) (*see also*
    Candidiasis) 112.9
    congenital 771.7
  Candiru 136.8
  Capillaria
    hepatica 128.8
    philippinensis 127.5
  cartilage 733.99
  cat liver fluke 121.0
  cellulitis—*see* Cellulitis, by site
  Cephalosporum falciforme 117.4
  Cercomonas hominis (intestinal) 007.3
  cerebrospinal (*see also* Meningitis) 322.9
    late effect—*see* category 326
  cervical gland 683
  cervix (*see also* Cervicitis) 616.0
  cesarean section wound 674.3
  Chilomastix (intestinal) 007.8
  Chlamydia 079.98
    specified NEC 079.88
  Cholera (*see also* Cholera) 001.9
  chorionic plate 658.8
  Cladosporium
    bantianum 117.8
    carrionii 117.2
    mansoni 111.1
    trichoides 117.8
    wernecki 111.1
  Clonorchis (sinensis) (liver) 121.1
  Clostridium (haemolyticum) (novyi) NEC
    041.84
    botulinum 005.1
    histolyticum (*see also* Gangrene, gas) 040.0
    oedematiens (*see also* Gangrene, gas) 040.0
    perfringens 041.83
      due to food 005.2
    septicum (*see also* Gangrene, gas) 040.0
    sordelii (*see also* Gangrene, gas) 040.0
    welchii (*see also* Gangrene, gas) 040.0
      due to food 005.2
  Coccidioides (immitis) (*see also*
    Coccidioidomycosis) 114.9
  coccus NEC 041.89
  colon (*see also* Enteritis, due to, by organism) 009.0
    bacillus—*see* Infection, Escherichia coli
  colostomy or enterostomy 569.61
  common duct 576.1
  complicating pregnancy, childbirth, or
    puerperium NEC 647.9
    affecting fetus or newborn 760.2
  Condiobolus 117.7
  congenital NEC 771.89
    Candida albicans 771.7
    chronic 771.2
    Cytomegalovirus 771.1
    hepatitis, viral 771.2
    Herpes simplex 771.2
    listeriosis 771.2
    malaria 771.2
    poliomyelitis 771.2
    rubella 771.0
    toxoplasmosis 771.2
    tuberculosis 771.2
    urinary (tract) 771.82
    vaccinia 771.2

Infection, infected, infective—*continued*
  coronavirus 079.89
    SARS-associated 079.82
  corpus luteum (*see also* Salpingo-oophoritis)
    614.2
  Corynebacterium diphtheriae—*see* Diphtheria
  Coxsackie (*see also* Coxsackie) 079.2
    endocardium 074.22
    heart NEC 074.20
    in diseases classified elsewhere—*see* category 079
    meninges 047.0
    myocardium 074.23
    pericardium 074.21
    pharynx 074.0
    specified disease NEC 074.8
    unspecified nature or site 079.2
  Cryptococcus neoformans 117.5
  Cryptosporidia 007.4
  Cunninghamella 117.7
  cyst—*see* Cyst
  Cysticercus cellulosae 123.1
  cytomegalovirus 078.5
    congenital 771.1
  dental (pulpal origin) 522.4
  deuteromycetes 117.4
  Dicrocoelium dendriticum 121.8
  Dipetalonema (perstans) 125.4
    streptocerca 125.6
  diphtherial—*see* Diphtheria
  Diphyllobothrium (adult) (latum) (pacificum)
    123.4
    larval 123.5
  Diplogonoporus (grandis) 123.8
  Dipylidium (caninum) 123.8
  Dirofilaria 125.6
  dog tapeworm 123.8
  Dracunculus medinensis 125.7
  Dreschlera 118
    hawaiiensis 117.8
  Ducrey's bacillus (any site) 099.0
  due to or resulting from
    device, implant, or graft (any) (presence
      of)—*see* Complications, infection and
      inflammation, due to (presence of) any
      device, implant, or graft classified to
      996.0-996.5 NEC
    injection, inoculation, infusion, transfusion, or
      vaccination (prophylactic) (therapeutic)
      999.3
    injury NEC—*see* Wound, open, by site,
      complicated
    surgery 998.59
  duodenum 535.6
  ear—*see also* Otitis
    external (*see also* Otitis, externa) 380.10
    inner (*see also* Labyrinthitis) 386.30
    middle —*see* Otitis, media
  Eaton's agent NEC 041.81
  Eberthella typhosa 002.0
  Ebola 078.89
  echinococcosis 122.9
  Echinococcus (*see also* Echinococcus) 122.9
  Echinostoma 121.8
  ECHO virus 079.1
    in diseases classified elsewhere—*see* category
      079
    unspecified nature or site 079.1
  Ehrlichiosis 082.40
    chaffeensis 082.41
    specified type NEC 082.49
  Endamoeba—*see* Infection, ameba

Infection, infected, infective—*continued*
  endocardium (*see also* Endocarditis) 421.0
  endocervix (*see also* Cervicitis) 616.0
  Entamoeba—*see* Infection, ameba
  enteric (*see also* Enteritis, due to, by organism)
    009.0
  Enterobacter aerogenes NEC 041.85
  Enterobacter sakazakii 041.85
  Enterobius vermicularis 127.4
  enterococcus NEC 041.04
  enterovirus NEC 079.89
    central nervous system NEC 048
    enteritis 008.67
    meningitis 047.9
  Entomophthora 117.7
  Epidermophyton—*see* Dermatophytosis
  epidermophytosis—*see* Dermatophytosis
  episiotomy 674.3
  Epstein-Barr virus 075
    chronic 780.79 *[139.8]*
  erysipeloid 027.1
  Erysipelothrix (insidiosa) (rhusiopathiae) 027.1
  erythema infectiosum 057.0
  Escherichia coli NEC 041.4
    enteritis—*see* Enteritis, E. coli
    generalized 038.42
    intestinal—*see* Enteritis, E. coli
  esophagostomy 530.86
  ethmoidal (chronic) (sinus) (*see also* Sinusitis,
    ethmoidal) 473.2
  Eubacterium 041.84
  Eustachian tube (ear) 381.50
    acute 381.51
    chronic 381.52
  exanthema subitum 057.8
  external auditory canal (meatus) (*see also* Otitis,
    externa) 380.10
  eye NEC 360.00
  eyelid 373.9
    specified NEC 373.8
  fallopian tube (*see also* Salpingo-oophoritis)
    614.2
  fascia 728.89
  Fasciola
    gigantica 121.3
    hepatica 121.3
  Fasciolopsis (buski) 121.4
  fetus (intra-amniotic)—*see* Infection, congenital
  filarial—*see* Infestation, filarial
  finger (skin) 686.9
    abscess (with lymphangitis) 681.00
      pulp 681.01
    cellulitis (with lymphangitis) 681.00
    distal closed space (with lymphangitis) 681.00
    nail 681.02
      fungus 110.1
  fish tapeworm 123.4
    larval 123.5
  flagellate, intestinal 007.9
  fluke—*see* Infestation, fluke
  focal
    teeth (pulpal origin) 522.4
    tonsils 474.00
      and adenoids 474.02
  Fonsecaea
    compactum 117.2
    pedrosoi 117.2
  food (*see also* Poisoning, food) 005.9
  foot (skin) 686.9
    fungus 110.4
  Francisella tularensis (*see also* Tularemia) 021.9

Infection, infected, infective—*continued*
  frontal sinus (chronic) (*see also* Sinusitis,
    frontal) 473.1
  fungus NEC 117.9
    beard 110.0
    body 110.5
    dermatiacious NEC 117.8
    foot 110.4
    groin 110.3
    hand 110.2
    nail 110.1
    pathogenic to compromised host only 118
    perianal (area) 110.3
    scalp 110.0
    scrotum 110.8
    skin 111.9
      foot 110.4
      hand 110.2
    toenails 110.1
    trachea 117.9
  Fusarium 118
  Fusobacterium 041.84
  gallbladder (*see also* Cholecystitis, acute) 575.0
  Gardnerella vaginalis 041.89
  gas bacillus (*see also* Gas, gangrene) 040.0
  gastric (*see also* Gastritis) 535.5
  Gastrodiscoides hominis 121.8
  gastroenteric (*see also* Enteritis, due to, by
    organism) 009.0
  gastrointestinal (*see also* Enteritis, due to, by
    organism) 009.0
  gastrostomy 536.41
  generalized NEC (*see also* Septicemia) 038.9
  genital organ or tract NEC
    female 614.9
      with
        abortion—*see* Abortion, by type, with
          sepsis
        ectopic pregnancy (*see also* categories
          633.0-633.9) 639.0
        molar pregnancy (*see also* categories
          630-632) 639.0
      complicating pregnancy 646.6
        affecting fetus or newborn 760.8
      following
        abortion 639.0
        ectopic or molar pregnancy 639.0
      puerperal, postpartum, childbirth 670
        minor or localized 646.6
          affecting fetus or newborn 760.8
    male 608.4
  genitourinary tract NEC 599.0
  Ghon tubercle, primary (*see also* Tuberculosis)
    010.0
  Giardia lamblia 007.1
  gingival (chronic) 523.10
    acute 523.00
    Vincent's 101
  glanders 024
  Glenosporopsis amazonica 116.2
  Gnathostoma spinigerum 128.1
  Gongylonema 125.6
  gonococcal NEC (*see also* Gonococcus) 098.0
  gram-negative bacilli NEC 041.85
    anaerobic 041.84
  guinea worm 125.7
  gum (*see also* Infection, gingival) 523.10
  Hantavirus 079.81
  heart 429.89
  Helicobacter pylori (H. pylori) 041.86
  helminths NEC 128.9

Infection, infected, infective—*continued*
  intestinal 127.9
    mixed (types classifiable to more than one
      category in 120.0-127.7) 127.8
    specified type NEC 127.7
    specified type NEC 128.8
  Hemophilus influenzae NEC 041.5
    generalized 038.41
  Herpes (simplex) (*see also* Herpes, simplex)
    054.9
    congenital 771.2
    zoster (*see also* Herpes, zoster) 053.9
      eye NEC 053.29
  Heterophyes heterophyes 121.6
  Histoplasma (*see also* Histoplasmosis) 115.90
    capsulatum (*see also* Histoplasmosis,
      American) 115.00
    duboisii (*see also* Histoplasmosis, African)
      115.10
  HIV V08
    with symptoms, symptomatic 042
  hookworm (*see also* Ancylostomiasis) 126.9
  human immunodeficiency virus V08
    with symptoms, symptomatic 042
  human papillomavirus 079.4
  hydrocele 603.1
  hydronephrosis 591
  Hymenolepis 123.6
  hypopharynx 478.29
  inguinal glands 683
    due to soft chancre 099.0
  intestine, intestinal (*see also* Enteritis, due to, by
    organism) 009.0
  intrauterine (*see also* Endometritis) 615.9
    complicating delivery 646.6
  isospora belli or hominis 007.2
  Japanese B encephalitis 062.0
  jaw (bone) (acute) (chronic) (lower) (subacute)
    (upper) 526.4
  joint—*see* Arthritis, infectious or infective
  kidney (cortex) (hematogenous) 590.9
    with
      abortion—*see* Abortion, by type, with
        urinary tract infection
      calculus 592.0
      ectopic pregnancy (*see also* categories
        633.0-633.9) 639.8
      molar pregnancy (*see also* categories
        630-632) 639.8
    complicating pregnancy or puerperium 646.6
      affecting fetus or newborn 760.1
    following
      abortion 639.8
      ectopic or molar pregnancy 639.8
    pelvis and ureter 590.3
  Klebsiella pneumoniae NEC 041.3
  knee (skin) NEC 686.9
    joint—*see* Arthritis, infectious
  Koch's (*see also* Tuberculosis, pulmonary)
    011.9
  labia (majora) (minora) (*see also* Vulvitis)
    616.10
  lacrimal
    gland (*see also* Dacryoadenitis) 375.00
    passages (duct) (sac) (*see also* Dacryocystitis)
      375.30
  larynx NEC 478.79
  leg (skin) NEC 686.9
  Leishmania (*see also* Leishmaniasis) 085.9
    braziliensis 085.5
    donovani 085.0

Infection, infected, infective—*continued*
  Ethiopica 085.3
  furunculosa 085.1
  infantum 085.0
  mexicana 085.4
  tropica (minor) 085.1
    major 085.2
  Leptosphaeria senegalensis 117.4
  leptospira (*see also* Leptospirosis) 100.9
    Australis 100.89
    Bataviae 100.89
    pyrogenes 100.89
    specified type NEC 100.89
  leptospirochetal NEC (*see also* Leptospirosis)
    100.9
  Leptothrix—*see* Actinomycosis
  Listeria monocytogenes (listeriosis) 027.0
    congenital 771.2
  liver fluke—*see* Infestation, fluke, liver
  Loa loa 125.2
    eyelid 125.2 *[373.6]*
  Loboa loboi 116.2
  local, skin (staphylococcal) (streptococcal) NEC
    686.9
    abscess—*see* Abscess, by site
    cellulitis—*see* Cellulitis, by site
    ulcer (*see also* Ulcer, skin) 707.9
  Loefflerella
    mallei 024
    whitmori 025
  lung 518.89
    atypical Mycobacterium 031.0
      tuberculous (*see also* Tuberculosis,
        pulmonary) 011.9
    basilar 518.89
    chronic 518.89
    fungus NEC 117.9
    spirochetal 104.8
    virus—*see* Pneumonia, virus
  lymph gland (axillary) (cervical) (inguinal) 683
    mesenteric 289.2
  lymphoid tissue, base of tongue or posterior
    pharynx, NEC 474.00
  madurella
    grisea 117.4
    mycetomii 117.4
  major
    with
      abortion—*see* Abortion, by type, with sepsis
      ectopic pregnancy (*see also* categories
        633.0-633.9) 639.0
      molar pregnancy (*see also* categories
        630-632) 639.0
    following
      abortion 639.0
      ectopic or molar pregnancy 639.0
    puerperal, postpartum, childbirth 670
  malarial—*see* Malaria
  Malassezia furfur 111.0
  Malleomyces
    mallei 024
    pseudomallei 025
  mammary gland 611.0
    puerperal, postpartum 675.2
  Mansonella (ozzardi) 125.5
  mastoid (suppurative)—*see* Mastoiditis
  maxilla, maxillary 526.4
    sinus (chronic) (*see also* Sinusitis, maxillary)
      473.0
  mediastinum 519.2
  medina 125.7

Infection, infected, infective—*continued*
  meibomian
    cyst 373.12
    gland 373.12
  melioidosis 025
  meninges (*see also* Meningitis) 320.9
  meningococcal (*see also* condition) 036.9
    brain 036.1
    cerebrospinal 036.0
    endocardium 036.42
    generalized 036.2
    meninges 036.0
    meningococcemia 036.2
    specified site NEC 036.89
  mesenteric lymph nodes or glands NEC 289.2
  Metagonimus 121.5
  metatarsophalangeal 711.97
  microorganism resistant to drugs—*see*
    Resistance (to), drugs by microorganisms
  Microsporidia 136.8
  microsporum, microsporic—*see*
    Dermatophytosis
  Mima polymorpha NEC 041.85
  mixed flora NEC 041.89
  Monilia (*see also* Candidiasis) 112.9
    neonatal 771.7
  monkeypox 057.8
  Monosporium apiospermum 117.6
  mouth (focus) NEC 528.9
    parasitic 112.0
  Mucor 117.7
  muscle NEC 728.89
  mycelium NEC 117.9
  mycetoma
    actinomycotic NEC (*see also* Actinomycosis) 039.9
    mycotic NEC 117.4
  Mycobacterium, mycobacterial (*see also*
    Mycobacterium) 031.9
  mycoplasma NEC 041.81
  mycotic NEC 117.9
    pathogenic to compromised host only 118
    skin NEC 111.9
    systemic 117.9
  myocardium NEC 422.90
  nail (chronic) (with lymphangitis) 681.9
    finger 681.02
      fungus 110.1
    ingrowing 703.0
    toe 681.11
      fungus 110.1
  nasal sinus (chronic) (*see also* Sinusitis) 473.9
  nasopharynx (chronic) 478.29
    acute 460
  navel 686.9
    newborn 771.4
  Neisserian—*see* Gonococcus
  Neotestudina rosatii 117.4
  newborn, generalized 771.89
  nipple 611.0
    puerperal, postpartum 675.0
      with breast 675.9
        specified type NEC 675.8
  Nocardia—*see* Actinomycosis
  nose 478.19
  nostril 478.19
  obstetrical surgical wound 674.3
  Oesophagostomum (apiostomum) 127.7
  Oestrus ovis 134.0
  Oidium albicans (*see also* Candidiasis) 112.9
  Onchocerca (volvulus) 125.3
    eye 125.3 *[360.13]*

Infection, infected, infective—*continued*
  eyelid 125.3 *[373.6]*
  operation wound 998.59
  Opisthorchis (felineus) (tenuicollis) (viverrini)
    121.0
  orbit 376.00
    chronic 376.10
  ovary (*see also* Salpingo-oophoritis) 614.2
  Oxyuris vermicularis 127.4
  pancreas 577.0
  Paracoccidioides brasiliensis 116.1
  Paragonimus (westermani) 121.2
  parainfluenza virus 079.89
  parameningococcus NEC 036.9
    with meningitis 036.0
  parasitic NEC 136.9
  paratyphoid 002.9
    Type A 002.1
    Type B 002.2
    Type C 002.3
  paraurethral ducts 597.89
  parotid gland 527.2
  Pasteurella NEC 027.2
    multocida (cat-bite) (dog-bite) 027.2
    pestis (*see also* Plague) 020.9
    pseudotuberculosis 027.2
    septica (cat-bite) (dog-bite) 027.2
    tularensis (*see also* Tularemia) 021.9
  pelvic, female (*see also* Disease, pelvis,
    inflammatory) 614.9
  penis (glans) (retention) NEC 607.2
    herpetic 054.13
  Peptococcus 041.84
  Peptostreptococcus 041.84
  periapical (pulpal origin) 522.4
  peridental 523.30
  perineal wound (obstetrical) 674.3
  periodontal 523.31
  periorbital 376.00
    chronic 376.10
  perirectal 569.49
  perirenal (*see also* Infection, kidney) 590.9
  peritoneal (*see also* Peritonitis) 567.9
  periureteral 593.89
  periurethral 597.89
  Petriellidium boydii 117.6
  pharynx 478.29
    Coxsackie virus 074.0
    phlegmonous 462
    posterior, lymphoid 474.00
  Phialophora
    gougerotii 117.8
    jeanselmei 117.8
    verrucosa 117.2
  Piedraia hortai 111.3
  pinna, acute 380.11
  pinta 103.9
    intermediate 103.1
    late 103.2
    mixed 103.3
    primary 103.0
  pinworm 127.4
  pityrosporum furfur 111.0
  pleuropneumonia-like organisms NEC (PPLO)
    041.81
  pneumococcal NEC 041.2
    generalized (purulent) 038.2
  Pneumococcus NEC 041.2
  postoperative wound 998.59
  posttraumatic NEC 958.3
  postvaccinal 999.3

Infection, infected, infective—*continued*
  prepuce NEC 607.1
  Propionibacterium 041.84
  prostate (capsule) (*see also* Prostatitis) 601.9
  Proteus (mirabilis) (morganii) (vulgaris) NEC
    041.6
    enteritis 008.3
  protozoal NEC 136.8
    intestinal NEC 007.9
  Pseudomonas NEC 041.7
    mallei 024
    pneumonia 482.1
    pseudomallei 025
  psittacosis 073.9
  puerperal, postpartum (major) 670
    minor 646.6
  pulmonary—*see* Infection, lung
  purulent—*see* Abscess
  putrid, generalized—*see* Septicemia
  pyemic—*see* Septicemia
  Pyrenochaeta romeroi 117.4
  Q fever 083.0
  rabies 071
  rectum (sphincter) 569.49
  renal (*see also* Infection, kidney) 590.9
    pelvis and ureter 590.3
  resistant to drugs—*see* Resistance (to), drugs by
    microorganisms
  respiratory 519.8
    chronic 519.8
    influenzal (acute) (upper) 487.1
    lung 518.89
    rhinovirus 460
    syncytial virus 079.6
    upper (acute) (infectious) NEC 465.9
      with flu, grippe, or influenza 487.1
      influenzal 487.1
      multiple sites NEC 465.8
      streptococcal 034.0
      viral NEC 465.9
  respiratory syncytial virus (RSV) 079.6
  resulting from presence of shunt or other
    internal prosthetic device—*see*
    Complications, infection and inflammation,
    due to (presence of) any device, implant, or
    graft classified to 996.0-996.5 NEC
  retroperitoneal 567.39
  retrovirus 079.50
    human immunodeficiency virus type 2
      [HIV-2] 079.53
    human T-cell lymphotrophic virus type I
      [HTLV-I] 079.51
    human T-cell lymphotrophic virus type II
      [HTLV-II] 079.52
    specified NEC 079.59
  Rhinocladium 117.1
  Rhinosporidium (*see*beri) 117.0
  rhinovirus
    in diseases classified elsewhere—*see* category
      079
    unspecified nature or site 079.3
  Rhizopus 117.7
  rickettsial 083.9
  rickettsialpox 083.2
  rubella (*see also* Rubella) 056.9
    congenital 771.0
  Saccharomyces (*see also* Candidiasis) 112.9
  Saksenaea 117.7
  salivary duct or gland (any) 527.2

Infection, infected, infective—*continued*
  Salmonella (aertrycke) (callinarum)
    (choleraesuis) (enteritidis) (suipestifer)
    (typhimurium) 003.9
    with
      arthritis 003.23
      gastroenteritis 003.0
      localized infection 003.20
        specified type NEC 003.29
      meningitis 003.21
      osteomyelitis 003.24
      pneumonia 003.22
      septicemia 003.1
      specified manifestation NEC 003.8
    due to food (poisoning) (any serotype) (*see*
      also Poisoning, food, due to, Salmonella)
    hirschfeldii 002.3
    localized 003.20
      specified type NEC 003.29
    paratyphi 002.9
      A 002.1
      B 002.2
      C 002.3
    schottmuelleri 002.2
    specified type NEC 003.8
    typhi 002.0
    typhosa 002.0
  saprophytic 136.8
  Sarcocystis, lindemanni 136.5
  SARS-associated coronavirus 079.82
  scabies 133.0
  Schistosoma—*see* Infestation, Schistosoma
  Schmorl's bacillus 040.3
  scratch or other superficial injury—*see* Injury,
    superficial, by site
  scrotum (acute) NEC 608.4
  secondary, burn or open wound (dislocation)
    (fracture) 958.3
  seminal vesicle (*see also* Vesiculitis) 608.0
  septic
    generalized—*see* Septicemia
    localized, skin (*see also* Abscess) 682.9
  septicemic—*see* Septicemia
  seroma 998.51
  Serratia (marcescens) 041.85
    generalized 038.44
  sheep liver fluke 121.3
  Shigella 004.9
    boydii 004.2
    dysenteriae 004.0
    Flexneri 004.1
    group
      A 004.0
      B 004.1
      C 004.2
      D 004.3
    Schmitz (-Stutzer) 004.0
    Schmitzii 004.0
    Shiga 004.0
    Sonnei 004.3
    specified type NEC 004.8
  Sin Nombre virus 079.81
  sinus (*see also* Sinusitis) 473.9
    pilonidal 685.1
      with abscess 685.0
    skin NEC 686.9
  Skene's duct or gland (*see also* Urethritis) 597.89
  skin (local) (staphylococcal) (streptococcal)
    NEC 686.9
    abscess—*see* Abscess, by site
    cellulitis—*see* Cellulitis, by site

Infertility—*continued*
    adhesions, peritubal 614.6 *[628.2]*
    anomaly
      cervical mucus 628.4
      congenital
        cervix 628.4
        fallopian tube 628.2
        uterus 628.3
        vagina 628.4
    anovulation 628.0
    dysmucorrhea 628.4
    endometritis, tuberculous (*see also*
      Tuberculosis) 016.7 *[628.3]*
    Stein-Leventhal syndrome 256.4 *[628.0]*
    due to
      adiposogenital dystrophy 253.8 *[628.1]*
      anterior pituitary disorder NEC 253.4
        [628.1]
        hyperfunction 253.1 *[628.1]*
      cervical anomaly 628.4
      fallopian tube anomaly 628.2
      ovarian failure 256.39 *[628.0]*
      Stein-Leventhal syndrome 256.4 *[628.0]*
      uterine anomaly 628.3
      vaginal anomaly 628.4
    nonimplantation 628.3
    origin
      cervical 628.4
      pituitary-hypothalamus NEC 253.8 *[628.1]*
        anterior pituitary NEC 253.4 *[628.1]*
          hyperfunction NEC 253.1 *[628.1]*
        dwarfism 253.3 *[628.1]*
        panhypopituitarism 253.2 *[628.1]*
      specified NEC 628.8
      tubal (block) (occlusion) (stenosis) 628.2
        adhesions 614.6 *[628.2]*
      uterine 628.3
      vaginal 628.4
    previous, requiring supervision of pregnancy
      V23.0
  male 606.9
    absolute 606.0
    due to
      azoospermia 606.0
      drug therapy 606.8
      extratesticular cause NEC 606.8
      germinal cell
        aplasia 606.0
        desquamation 606.1
      hypospermatogenesis 606.1
      infection 606.8
      obstruction, afferent ducts 606.8
      oligospermia 606.1
      radiation 606.8
      spermatogenic arrest (complete) 606.0
        incomplete 606.1
      systemic disease 606.8

Infestation 134.9
  Acanthocheilonema (perstans) 125.4
    streptocerca 125.6
  Acariasis 133.9
    demodex folliculorum 133.8
    Sarcoptes scabiei 133.0
    trombiculae 133.8
  Agamofilaria streptocerca 125.6
  Ancylostoma, Ankylostoma 126.9
    americanum 126.1
    braziliense 126.2
    canium 126.8
    ceylanicum 126.3
    duodenale 126.0

Infestation—*continued*
  new world 126.1
  old world 126.0
  Angiostrongylus cantonensis 128.8
  anisakiasis 127.1
  Anisakis larva 127.1
  arthropod NEC 134.1
  Ascaris lumbricoides 127.0
  Bacillus fusiformis 101
  Balantidium coli 007.0
  beef tapeworm 123.2
  Bothriocephalus (latus) 123.4
    larval 123.5
  broad tapeworm 123.4
    larval 123.5
  Brugia malayi 125.1
  Candiru 136.8
  Capillaria
    hepatica 128.8
    philippinensis 127.5
  cat liver fluke 121.0
  Cercomonas hominis (intestinal) 007.3
  cestodes 123.9
    specified type NEC 123.8
  chigger 133.8
  chigoe 134.1
  Chilomastix 007.8
  Clonorchis (sinensis) (liver) 121.1
  coccidia 007.2
  complicating pregnancy, childbirth, or
    puerperium 647.9
    affecting fetus or newborn 760.8
  Cysticercus cellulosae 123.1
  Demodex folliculorum 133.8
  Dermatobia (hominis) 134.0
  Dibothriocephalus (latus) 123.4
    larval 123.5
  Dicrocoelium dendriticum 121.8
  Diphyllobothrium (adult) (intestinal) (latum)
    (pacificum) 123.4
    larval 123.5
  Diplogonoporus (grandis) 123.8
  Dipylidium (caninum) 123.8
  Distoma hepaticum 121.3
  dog tapeworm 123.8
  Dracunculus medinensis 125.7
  dragon worm 125.7
  dwarf tapeworm 123.6
  Echinococcus (*see also* Echinococcus) 122.9
  Echinostoma ilocanum 121.8
  Embadomonas 007.8
  Endamoeba (histolytica)—*see* Infection, ameba
  Entamoeba (histolytica)—*see* Infection, ameba
  Enterobius vermicularis 127.4
  Epidermophyton—*see* Dermatophytosis
  eyeworm 125.2
  Fasciola
    gigantica 121.3
    hepatica 121.3
  Fasciolopsis (buski) (small intestine) 121.4
  filarial 125.9
    due to
      Acanthocheilonema (perstans) 125.4
        streptocerca 125.6
      Brugia (Wuchereria) malayi 125.1
      Dracunculus medinensis 125.7
      guinea worms 125.7
      Mansonella (ozzardi) 125.5
      Onchocerca volvulus 125.3
        eye 125.3 *[360.13]*
        eyelid 125.3 *[373.6]*

Inflammation—*continued*
    spleen 289.59
  catarrhal (*see also* Catarrh) 460
    vagina 616.10
  cecum (*see also* Appendicitis) 541
  cerebral (*see also* Encephalitis) 323.9
    late effect—*see* category 326
    membrane—*see* Meningitis
  cerebrospinal (*see also* Meningitis) 322.9
    late effect—*see* category 326
    meningococcal 036.0
    tuberculous (*see also* Tuberculosis) 013.6
  cervix (uteri) (*see also* Cervicitis) 616.0
  chest 519.9
  choroid NEC (*see also* Choroiditis) 363.20
  cicatrix (tissue)—*see* Cicatrix
  colon (*see also* Enteritis) 558.9
    granulomatous 555.1
    newborn 558.9
  connective tissue (diffuse) NEC 728.9
  cornea (*see also* Keratitis) 370.9
    with ulcer (*see also* Ulcer, cornea) 370.00
  corpora cavernosa (penis) 607.2
  cranial nerve—*see* Disorder, nerve, cranial
  diarrhea—*see* Diarrhea
  disc (intervertebral) (space) 722.90
    cervical, cervicothoracic 722.91
    lumbar, lumbosacral 722.93
    thoracic, thoracolumbar 722.93
  Douglas' cul-de-sac or pouch (chronic) (*see also* Disease, pelvis, inflammatory) 614.4
    acute 614.3
  due to (presence of) any device, implant, or graft classifiable to 996.0-996.5—*see* Complications, infection and inflammation, due to (presence of) any device, implant, or graft classified to 996.0-996.5 NEC
  duodenum 535.6
  dura mater—*see* Meningitis
  ear—*see also* Otitis
    external (*see also* Otitis, externa) 380.10
    inner (*see also* Labyrinthitis) 386.30
    middle—*see* Otitis media
  esophagus 530.10
  ethmoidal (chronic) (sinus) (*see also* Sinusitis, ethmoidal) 473.2
  Eustachian tube (catarrhal) 381.50
    acute 381.51
    chronic 381.52
  extrarectal 569.49
  eye 379.99
  eyelid 373.9
    specified NEC 373.8
  fallopian tube (*see also* Salpingo-oophoritis) 614.2
  fascia 728.9
  fetal membranes (acute) 658.4
    affecting fetus or newborn 762.7
  follicular, pharynx 472.1
  frontal (chronic) (sinus) (*see also* Sinusitis, frontal) 473.1
  gallbladder (*see also* Cholecystitis, acute) 575.0
  gall duct (*see also* Cholecystitis) 575.10
  gastrointestinal (*see also* Enteritis) 558.9
  genital organ (diffuse) (internal)
    female 614.9
      with
        abortion—*see* Abortion, by type, with sepsis
        ectopic pregnancy (*see also* categories 633.0-633.9) 639.0

Inflammation—*continued*
    molar pregnancy (*see also* categories 630-632) 639.0
    complicating pregnancy, childbirth, or puerperium 646.6
    affecting fetus or newborn 760.8
    following
      abortion 639.0
      ectopic or molar pregnancy 639.0
    male 608.4
  gland (lymph) (*see also* Lymphadenitis) 289.3
  glottis (*see also* Laryngitis) 464.00
    with obstruction 464.01
  granular, pharynx 472.1
  gum 523.10
  heart (*see also* Carditis) 429.89
  hepatic duct 576.8
  hernial sac—*see* Hernia, by site
  ileum (*see also* Enteritis) 558.9
    terminal or regional 555.0
    with large intestine 555.2
  intervertebral disc 722.90
    cervical, cervicothoracic 722.91
    lumbar, lumbosacral 722.93
    thoracic, thoracolumbar 722.92
  intestine (*see also* Enteritis) 558.9
  jaw (acute) (bone) (chronic) (lower) (suppurative) (upper) 526.4
  jejunum—*see* Enteritis
  joint NEC (*see also* Arthritis) 716.9
    sacroiliac 720.2
  kidney (*see also* Nephritis) 583.9
  knee (joint) 716.66
    tuberculous (active) (*see also* Tuberculosis) 015.2
  labium (majus) (minus) (*see also* Vulvitis) 616.10
  lacrimal
    gland (*see also* Dacryoadenitis) 375.00
    passages (duct) (sac) (*see also* Dacryocystitis) 375.30
  larynx (*see also* Laryngitis) 464.00
    with obstruction 464.01
    diphtheritic 032.3
  leg NEC 686.9
  lip 528.5
  liver (capsule) (*see also* Hepatitis) 573.3
    acute 570
    chronic 571.40
    suppurative 572.0
  lung (acute) (*see also* Pneumonia) 486
    chronic (interstitial) 518.89
  lymphatic vessel (*see also* Lymphangitis) 457.2
  lymph node or gland (*see also* Lymphadenitis) 289.3
  mammary gland 611.0
    puerperal, postpartum 675.2
  maxilla, maxillary 526.4
    sinus (chronic) (*see also* Sinusitis, maxillary) 473.0
  membranes of brain or spinal cord—*see* Meningitis
  meninges—*see* Meningitis
  mouth 528.00
  muscle 728.9
  myocardium (*see also* Myocarditis) 429.0
  nasal sinus (chronic) (*see also* Sinusitis) 473.9
  nasopharynx—*see* Nasopharyngitis
  navel 686.9
    newborn NEC 771.4
  nerve NEC 729.2

Influenza, influenzal—*continued*
  catarrhal 487.1
  epidemic 487.1
  gastric 487.8
  intestinal 487.8
  laryngitis 487.1
  maternal affecting fetus or newborn 760.2
    manifest influenza in infant 771.2
  pharyngitis 487.1
  pneumonia (any form) 487.0
  respiratory (upper) 487.1
  stomach 487.8
  vaccination, prophylactic (against) V04.81
Influenza-like disease 487.1
Infraction, Freiberg's (metatarsal head) 732.5
Infraeruption, teeth 524.34
Infusion complication, misadventure or
    reaction —*see* Complication, infusion
Ingestion
  chemical—*see* Table of drugs and chemicals
  drug or medicinal substance
    overdose or wrong substance given or taken
      977.9
      specified drug—*see* Table of drugs and
        chemicals
  foreign body NEC (*see also* Foreign body) 938
Ingrowing
  hair 704.8
  nail (finger) (toe) (infected) 703.0
Inguinal —*see also* condition
  testis 752.51
Inhalation
  carbon monoxide 986
  flame
    mouth 947.0
    lung 947.1
  food or foreign body (*see also* Asphyxia, food or
    foreign body) 933.1
  gas, fumes, or vapor (noxious) 987.9
    specified agent—*see* Table of drugs and
      chemicals
  liquid or vomitus (*see also* Asphyxia, food or
    foreign body) 933.1
  lower respiratory tract NEC 934.9
  meconium (fetus or newborn) 770.11
    with respiratory symptoms 770.12
  mucus (*see also* Asphyxia, mucus) 933.1
  oil (causing suffocation) (*see also* Asphyxia,
    food or foreign body) 933.1
  pneumonia—*see* Pneumonia, aspiration
  smoke 987.9
  steam 987.9
  stomach contents or secretions (*see also*
    Asphyxia, food or foreign body) 933.1
  in labor and deliver 668.0
Inhibition, inhibited
  academic as adjustment reaction 309.23
  orgasm
    female 302.73
    male 302.74
  sexual
    desire 302.71
    excitement 302.72
  work as adjustment reaction 309.23
Inhibitor, systemic lupus erythematosus
  (presence of) 286.5
Iniencephalus, iniencephaly 740.2
Injected eye 372.74

Injury 959.9

> *Note*—*For abrasion, insect bite (nonvenomous),
> blister, or scratch, see Injury, superficial. For
> laceration, traumatic rupture, tear, or
> penetrating wound of internal organs, such as
> heart, lung, liver, kidney, pelvic organs, whether
> or not accompanied by open wound in the same
> region, see Injury, internal. For nerve injury,
> see Injury, nerve. For late effect of injuries
> classifiable to 850-854, 860-869, 900-919,
> 950-959, see Late, effect, injury, by type.*

  abdomen, abdominal (viscera)—*see also* Injury,
    internal, abdomen
    muscle or wall 959.12
  acoustic, resulting in deafness 951.5
  adenoid 959.09
  adrenal (gland)—*see* Injury, internal, adrenal
  alveolar (process) 959.09
  ankle (and foot) (and knee) (and leg, except
    thigh) 959.7
  anterior chamber, eye 921.3
  anus 959.19
  aorta (thoracic) 901.0
    abdominal 902.0
  appendix—*see* Injury, internal, appendix
  arm, upper (and shoulder) 959.2
  artery (complicating trauma) (*see also* Injury,
    blood vessel, by site) 904.9
    cerebral or meningeal (*see also* Hemorrhage,
      brain, traumatic, subarachnoid) 852.0
  auditory canal (external) (meatus) 959.09
  auricle, auris, ear 959.09
  axilla 959.2
  back 959.19
  bile duct—*see* Injury, internal, bile duct
  birth—*see also* Birth, injury
    canal NEC, complicating delivery 665.9
  bladder (sphincter)—*see* Injury, internal,
    bladder
  blast (air) (hydraulic) (immersion) (underwater)
    NEC 869.0
    with open wound into cavity NEC 869.1
    abdomen or thorax—*see* Injury, internal, by
      site
    brain—*see* Concussion, brain
    ear (acoustic nerve trauma) 951.5
      with perforation of tympanic
        membrane—*see* Wound, open, ear, drum
  blood vessel NEC 904.9
    abdomen 902.9
      multiple 902.87
      specified NEC 902.89
    aorta (thoracic) 901.0
      abdominal 902.0
    arm NEC 903.9
    axillary 903.00
      artery 903.01
      vein 903.02
    azygos vein 901.89
    basilic vein 903.1
    brachial (artery) (vein) 903.1
    bronchial 901.89
    carotid artery 900.00
      common 900.01
      external 900.02
      internal 900.03
    celiac artery 902.20
      specified branch NEC 902.24
    cephalic vein (arm) 903.1
    colica dextra 902.26

> *Note—For injury of internal organ(s) by foreign*
> *body entering through a natural orifice (e.g.,*
> *inhaled, ingested, or swallowed)—see Foreign*
> *body, entering through orifice.*
>
> *For internal injury of any of the following sites*
> *with internal injury of any other of the sites—*
> *see Injury, internal, multiple.*

Injury—*continued*

specified site, except pelvis—*see* Injury, internal, by site
open wound into cavity 869.1
abdomen, abdominal (viscera) NEC 868.00
with
fracture, pelvis—*see* Fracture, pelvis
open wound into cavity 868.10
specified site NEC 868.09
with open wound into cavity 868.19
adrenal (gland) 868.01
with open wound into cavity 868.11
aorta (thoracic) 901.0
abdominal 902.0
appendix 863.85
with open wound into cavity 863.95
bile duct 868.02
with open wound into cavity 868.12
bladder (sphincter) 867.0
with
abortion—*see* Abortion, by type, with, damage to pelvic organs
ectopic pregnancy (*see also* categories 633.0-633.9) 639.2
molar pregnancy (*see also* categories 630-632) 639.2
open wound into cavity 867.1
following
abortion 639.2
ectopic or molar pregnancy 639.2
obstetrical trauma 665.5
affecting fetus or newborn 763.89
blood vessel—*see* Injury, blood vessel, by site
broad ligament 867.6
with open wound into cavity 867.7
bronchus, bronchi 862.21
with open wound into cavity 862.31
cecum 863.89
with open wound into cavity 863.99
cervix (uteri) 867.4
with
abortion—*see* Abortion, by type, with, damage to pelvic organs
ectopic pregnancy (*see also* categories 633.0-633.9) 639.2
molar pregnancy (*see also* categories 630-632) 639.2
open wound into cavity 867.5
following
abortion 639.2
ectopic or molar pregnancy 639.2
obstetrical trauma 665.3
affecting fetus or newborn 763.89
chest (*see also* Injury, internal, intrathoracic organs) 862.8
with open wound into cavity 862.9
colon 863.40
with
open wound into cavity 863.50
rectum 863.46
with open wound into cavity 863.56
ascending (right) 863.41
with open wound into cavity 863.51
descending (left) 863.43
with open wound into cavity 863.53
multiple sites 863.46
with open wound into cavity 863.56
sigmoid 863.44
with open wound into cavity 863.54
specified site NEC 863.49
with open wound into cavity 863.59

Injury—*continued*

transverse 863.42
with open wound into cavity 863.52
common duct 868.02
with open wound into cavity 868.12
complicating delivery 665.9
affecting fetus or newborn 763.89
diaphragm 862.0
with open wound into cavity 862.1
duodenum 863.21
with open wound into cavity 863.31
esophagus (intrathoracic) 862.22
with open wound into cavity 862.32
cervical region 874.4
complicated 874.5
fallopian tube 867.6
with open wound into cavity 867.7
gallbladder 868.02
with open wound into cavity 868.12
gastrointestinal tract NEC 863.80
with open wound into cavity 863.90
genital organ NEC 867.6
with open wound into cavity 867.7
heart 861.00
with open wound into thorax 861.10
ileum 863.29
with open wound into cavity 863.39
intestine NEC 863.89
with open wound into cavity 863.99
large NEC 863.40
with open wound into cavity 863.50
small NEC 863.20
with open wound into cavity 863.30
intra-abdominal (organ) 868.00
with open wound into cavity 868.10
multiple sites 868.09
with open wound into cavity 868.19
specified site NEC 868.09
with open wound into cavity 868.19
intrathoracic organs (multiple) 862.8
with open wound into cavity 862.9
diaphragm (only)—*see* Injury, internal, diaphragm
heart (only)—*see* Injury, internal, heart
lung (only)—*see* Injury, internal, lung
specified site NEC 862.29
with open wound into cavity 862.39
intrauterine (*see also* Injury, internal, uterus) 867.4
with open wound into cavity 867.5
jejunum 863.29
with open wound into cavity 863.39
kidney (subcapsular) 866.00
with
disruption of parenchyma (complete) 866.03
with open wound into cavity 866.13
hematoma (without rupture of capsule) 866.01
with open wound into cavity 866.11
laceration 866.02
with open wound into cavity 866.12
open wound into cavity 866.10
liver 864.00
with
contusion 864.01
with open wound into cavity 864.11
hematoma 864.01
with open wound into cavity 864.11
laceration 864.05
with open wound into cavity 864.15

Injury—*continued*
    major (disruption of hepatic parenchyma) 864.04
      with open wound into cavity 864.14
    minor (capsule only) 864.02
      with open wound into cavity 864.12
    moderate (involving parenchyma) 864.03
      with open wound into cavity 864.13
      multiple 864.04
    stellate 864.04
      with open wound in cavity 864.14
  open wound into cavity 864.10
lung 861.20
  with open wound into thorax 861.30
  hemopneumothorax—*see* Hemopneumothorax, traumatic
  hemothorax—*see* Hemothorax, traumatic
  pneumohemothorax—*see* Pneumohemothorax, traumatic
  pneumothorax—*see* Pneumothorax, traumatic
  transfusion related, acute (TRALI) 518.7
mediastinum 862.29
  with open wound into cavity 862.39
mesentery 863.89
  with open wound into cavity 863.99
mesosalpinx 867.6
  with open wound into cavity 867.7
multiple 869.0

> *Note—Multiple internal injuries of sites classifiable to the same three- or four-digit category should be classified to that category. Multiple injuries classifiable to different fourth-digit subdivisions of 861 (heart and lung injuries) should be dealt with according to coding rules.*

  with open wound into cavity 869.1
  intra-abdominal organ (sites classifiable to 863-868)
    with
      intrathoracic organ(s) (sites classifiable to 861-862) 869.0
        with open wound into cavity 869.1
      other intra-abdominal organ(s) (sites classifiable to 863-868, except where classifiable to the same three-digit category) 868.09
        with open wound into cavity 868.19
  intrathoracic organ (sites classifiable to 861-862)
    with
      intra-abdominal organ(s) (sites classifiable to 863-868) 869.0
        with open wound into cavity 869.1
      other intrathoracic organ(s) (sites classifiable to 861-862, except where classifiable to the same three-digit category) 862.8
        with open wound into cavity 862.9
myocardium—*see* Injury, internal, heart
ovary 867.6
  with open wound into cavity 867.7
pancreas (multiple sites) 863.84
  with open wound into cavity 863.94
  body 863.82
    with open wound into cavity 863.92
  head 863.81
    with open wound into cavity 863.91
  tail 863.83
    with open wound into cavity 863.93

Injury—*continued*
pelvis, pelvic (organs) (viscera) 867.8
  with
    fracture, pelvis—*see* Fracture, pelvis
    open wound into cavity 867.9
  specified site NEC 867.6
    with open wound into cavity 867.7
peritoneum 868.03
  with open wound into cavity 868.13
pleura 862.29
  with open wound into cavity 862.39
prostate 867.6
with open wound into cavity 867.7
rectum 863.45
  with
    colon 863.46
      with open wound into cavity 863.56
    open wound into cavity 863.55
retroperitoneum 868.04
  with open wound into cavity 868.14
round ligament 867.6
  with open wound into cavity 867.7
seminal vesicle 867.6
  with open wound into cavity 867.7
spermatic cord 867.6
  with open wound into cavity 867.7
  scrotal—*see* Wound, open, spermatic cord
spleen 865.00
  with
    disruption of parenchyma (massive) 865.04
      with open wound into cavity 865.14
    hematoma (without rupture of capsule) 865.01
      with open wound into cavity 865.11
    open wound into cavity 865.10
    tear, capsular 865.02
      with open wound into cavity 865.12
      extending into parenchyma 865.03
        with open wound into cavity 865.13
stomach 863.0
  with open wound into cavity 863.1
suprarenal gland (multiple) 868.01
  with open wound into cavity 868.11
thorax, thoracic (cavity) (organs) (multiple) (*see also* Injury, internal, intrathoracic organs) 862.8
  with open wound into cavity 862.9
thymus (gland) 862.29
  with open wound into cavity 862.39
trachea (intrathoracic) 862.29
  with open wound into cavity 862.39
  cervical region (*see also* Wound, open, trachea) 874.02
ureter 867.2
  with open wound into cavity 867.3
urethra (sphincter) 867.0
  with
    abortion—*see* Abortion, by type, with, damage to pelvic organs
    ectopic pregnancy (*see also* categories 633.0-633.9) 639.2
    molar pregnancy (*see also* categories 630-632) 639.2
    open wound into cavity 867.1
  following
    abortion 639.2
    ectopic or molar pregnancy 639.2
  obstetrical trauma 665.5
    affecting fetus or newborn 763.89

Injury—*continued*
uterus 867.4
  with
    abortion—*see* Abortion, by type, with,
      damage to pelvic organs
    ectopic pregnancy (*see also* categories
      633.0-633.9) 639.2
    molar pregnancy (*see also* categories
      630-632) 639.2
    open wound into cavity 867.5
  following
    abortion 639.2
    ectopic or molar pregnancy 639.2
  obstetrical trauma NEC 665.5
    affecting fetus or newborn 763.89
vas deferens 867.6
  with open wound into cavity 867.7
vesical (sphincter) 867.0
  with open wound into cavity 867.1
viscera (abdominal) (*see also* Injury, internal,
    multiple) 868.00
  with
    fracture, pelvis—*see* Fracture, pelvis
    open wound into cavity 868.10
    thoracic NEC (*see also* Injury, internal,
      intrathoracic organs) 862.8
      with open wound into cavity 862.9
interscapular region 959.19
intervertebral disc 959.19
intestine—*see* Injury, internal, intestine
intra-abdominal (organs) NEC—*see* Injury,
    internal, intra-abdominal
intracranial 854.0

Note—Use the following fifth-digit
subclassification with categories 851-854:

0 unspecifidd state of consciousness
1 with no loss of consciousness
2 with brief [less than one hour] loss of
*   consciousness*
3 with moderate [1-24 hours] loss of
*   consciousness*
4 with prolonged [more than 24 hours] loss of
*   consciousness and return to pre-existing*
*   conscious level*
5 with prolonged [more than 24 hours] loss of
*   consciousness, without return to pre-existing*
*   conscious level*
Use fifth-digit 5 to designate when a patient is
unconscious and dies before regaining
consciousness, regardless of the duration of the
loss of consciousness
6 with loss of consciousness of unspecified
*   duration*
9 with concussion, unspecified

---

  with
    open intracranial wound 854.1
    skull fracture—*see* Fracture, skull, by site
  contusion 851.8
    with open intracranial wound 851.9
    brain stem 851.4
      with open intracranial wound 851.5
    cerebellum 851.4
      with open intracranial wound 851.5
    cortex (cerebral) 851.0
      with open intracranial wound 851.2
  hematoma—*see* Injury, intracranial,
      hemorrhage
  hemorrhage 853.0
    with

Injury—*continued*
    laceration—*see* Injury, intracranial,
      laceration
    open intracranial wound 853.1
  extradural 852.4
    with open intracranial wound 852.5
  subarachnoid 852.0
    with open intracranial wound 852.1
  subdural 852.2
    with open intracranial wound 852.3
  laceration 851.8
    with open intracranial wound 851.9
    brain stem 851.6
      with open intracranial wound 851.7
    cerebellum 851.6
      with open intracranial wound 851.7
    cortex (cerebral) 851.2
      with open intracranial wound 851.3
intraocular—*see* Injury, eyeball, penetrating
intrathoracic organs (multiple)—*see* Injury,
    internal, intrathoracic organs
intrauterine—*see* Injury, internal, intrauterine
iris 921.3
  penetrating—*see* Injury, eyeball, penetrating
jaw 959.09
jejunum—*see* Injury, internal, jejunum
joint NEC 959.9
  old or residual 718.80
    ankle 718.87
    elbow 718.82
    foot 718.87
    hand 718.84
    hip 718.85
    knee 718.86
    multiple sites 718.89
    pelvic region 718.85
    shoulder (region) 718.81
    specified site NEC 718.88
    wrist 718.83
kidney—*see* Injury, internal, kidney
knee (and ankle) (and foot) (and leg, except
    thigh) 959.7
labium (majus) (minus) 959.14
labyrinth, ear 959.09
lacrimal apparatus, gland, or sac 921.1
  laceration 870.8
larynx 959.09
late effect—*see* Late, effects (of), injury
leg except thigh (and ankle) (and foot) (and
    knee) 959.7
  upper or thigh 959.6
lens, eye 921.3
  penetrating—*see* Injury, eyeball, penetrating
lid, eye—*see* Injury, eyelid
lip 959.09
liver—*see* Injury, internal, liver
lobe, parietal—*see* Injury, intracranial
lumbar (region) 959.19
  plexus 953.5
lumbosacral (region) 959.19
  plexus 953.5
lung—*see* Injury, internal, lung
malar region 959.09
mastoid region 959.09
maternal, during pregnancy, affecting fetus or
    newborn 760.5
maxilla 959.09
mediastinum—*see* Injury, internal, mediastinum
membrane
  brain (*see also* Injury, intracranial) 854.0
  tympanic 959.09

Injury—*continued*
  meningeal artery—*see* Hemorrhage, brain,
    traumatic, subarachnoid
  meninges (cerebral)—*see* Injury, intracranial
  mesenteric
    artery—*see* Injury, blood vessel, mesenteric,
      artery
    plexus, inferior 954.1
    vein—*see* Injury, blood vessel, mesenteric,
      vein
  mesentery—*see* Injury, internal, mesentery
  mesosalpinx—*see* Injury, internal, mesosalpinx
  middle ear 959.09
  midthoracic region 959.11
  mouth 959.09
  multiple (sites not classifiable to the same
    four-digit category in 959.0-959.7) 959.8
    internal 869.0
      with open wound into cavity 869.1
  musculocutaneous nerve 955.4
  nail
    finger 959.5
    toe 959.7
  nasal (septum) (sinus) 959.09
  nasopharynx 959.09
  neck (and face) 959.09
  nerve 957.9
    abducens 951.3
    abducent 951.3
    accessory 951.6
    acoustic 951.5
    ankle and foot 956.9
    anterior crural, femoral 956.1
    arm (*see also* Injury, nerve, upper limb) 955.9
    auditory 951.5
    axillary 955.0
    brachial plexus 953.4
    cervical sympathetic 954.0
    cranial 951.9
      first or olfactory 951.8
      second or optic 950.0
      third or oculomotor 951.0
      fourth or trochlear 951.1
      fifth or trigeminal 951.2
      sixth or abducens 951.3
      seventh or facial 951.4
      eighth, acoustic, or auditory 951.5
      ninth or glossopharyngeal 951.8
      tenth, pneumogastric, or vagus 951.8
      eleventh or accessory 951.6
      twelfth or hypoglossal 951.7
      newborn 767.7
    cutaneous sensory
      lower limb 956.4
      upper limb 955.5
    digital (finger) 955.6
      toe 956.5
    facial 951.4
      newborn 767.5
    femoral 956.1
    finger 955.9
    foot and ankle 956.9
    forearm 955.9
    glossopharyngeal 951.8
    hand and wrist 955.9
    head and neck, superficial 957.0
    hypoglossal 951.7
    involving several parts of body 957.8
    leg (*see also* Injury, nerve, lower limb) 956.9
    lower limb 956.9
      multiple 956.8

Injury—*continued*
    specified site NEC 956.5
    lumbar plexus 953.5
    lumbosacral plexus 953.5
    median 955.1
      forearm 955.1
      wrist and hand 955.1
    multiple (in several parts of body) (sites not
      classifiable to the same three-digit
      category) 957.8
    musculocutaneous 955.4
    musculospiral 955.3
      upper arm 955.3
    oculomotor 951.0
    olfactory 951.8
    optic 950.0
    pelvic girdle 956.9
      multiple sites 956.8
      specified site NEC 956.5
    peripheral 957.9
      multiple (in several regions) (sites not
        classifiable to the same three-digit
        category) 957.8
      specified site NEC 957.1
    peroneal 956.3
      ankle and foot 956.3
      lower leg 956.3
    plantar 956.5
    plexus 957.9
      celiac 954.1
      mesenteric, inferior 954.1
      spinal 953.9
        brachial 953.4
        lumbosacral 953.5
        multiple sites 953.8
      sympathetic NEC 954.1
    pneumogastric 951.8
    radial 955.3
      wrist and hand 955.3
    sacral plexus 953.5
    sciatic 956.0
      thigh 956.0
    shoulder girdle 955.9
      multiple 955.8
      specified site NEC 955.7
    specified site NEC 957.1
    spinal 953.9
      plexus—*see* Injury, nerve, plexus, spinal
      root 953.9
        cervical 953.0
        dorsal 953.1
        lumbar 953.2
        multiple sites 953.8
        sacral 953.3
    splanchnic 954.1
    sympathetic NEC 954.1
      cervical 954.0
    thigh 956.9
    tibial 956.5
      ankle and foot 956.2
      lower leg 956.5
      posterior 956.2
    toe 956.9
    trigeminal 951.2
    trochlear 951.1
    trunk, excluding shoulder and pelvic girdles
      954.9
      specified site NEC 954.8
      sympathetic NEC 954.1
    ulnar 955.2
      forearm 955.2

Injury—*continued*
 wrist (and hand) 955.2
 upper limb 955.9
  multiple 955.8
  specified site NEC 955.7
  vagus 951.8
  wrist and hand 955.9
 nervous system, diffuse 957.8
 nose (septum) 959.09
 obstetrical NEC 665.9
  affecting fetus or newborn 763.89
 occipital (region) (scalp) 959.09
  lobe (*see also* Injury, intracranial) 854.0
 optic 950.9
  chiasm 950.1
  cortex 950.3
  nerve 950.0
  pathways 950.2
 orbit, orbital (region) 921.2
  penetrating 870.3
   with foreign body 870.4
 ovary—*see* Injury, internal, ovary
 paint-gun—*see* Wound, open, by site,
  complicated
 palate (soft) 959.09
 pancreas—*see* Injury, internal, pancreas
 parathyroid (gland) 959.09
 parietal (region) (scalp) 959.09
  lobe—*see* Injury, intracranial
 pelvic
  floor 959.19
   complicating delivery 664.1
    affecting fetus or newborn 763.89
  joint or ligament, complicating delivery 665.6
   affecting fetus or newborn 763.89
  organs—*see also* Injury, internal, pelvis
   with
    abortion—*see* Abortion, by type, with
     damage to pelvic organs
    ectopic pregnancy (*see also* categories
     633.0-633.9) 639.2
    molar pregnancy (*see also* categories
     633.0-633.9) 639.2
   following
    abortion 639.2
    ectopic or molar pregnancy 639.2
   obstetrical trauma 665.5
    affecting fetus or newborn 763.89
 pelvis 959.19
 penis 959.14
  fracture of corpus cavernosum 959.13
 perineum 959.14
 peritoneum—*see* Injury, internal, peritoneum
 periurethral tissue
  with
   abortion—*see* Abortion, by type, with
    damage to pelvic organs
   ectopic pregnancy (*see also* categories
    633.0-633.9) 639.2
   molar pregnancy (*see also* categories
    630-632) 639.2
  complicating delivery 665.5
   affecting fetus or newborn 763.89
  following
   abortion 639.2
   ectopic or molar pregnancy 639.2
 phalanges
  foot 959.7
  hand 959.5
 pharynx 959.09
 pleura—*see* Injury, internal, pleura

Injury—*continued*
 popliteal space 959.7
 post-cardiac surgery (syndrome) 429.4
 prepuce 959.14
 prostate—*see* Injury, internal, prostate
 pubic region 959.19
 pudenda 959.14
 radiation NEC 990
 radioactive substance or radium NEC 990
 rectovaginal septum 959.14
 rectum—*see* Injury, internal, rectum
 retina 921.3
  penetrating—*see* Injury, eyeball, penetrating
 retroperitoneal—*see* Injury, internal,
  retroperitoneum
 roentgen rays NEC 990
 round ligament—*see* Injury, internal, round
  ligament
 sacral (region) 959.19
  plexus 953.5
 sacroiliac ligament NEC 959.19
 sacrum 959.19
 salivary ducts or glands 959.09
 scalp 959.09
  due to birth trauma 767.19
  fetus or newborn 767.19
 scapular region 959.2
 sclera 921.3
  penetrating—*see* Injury, eyeball, penetrating
  superficial 918.2
 scrotum 959.14
 seminal vesicle—*see* Injury, internal, seminal
  vesicle
 shoulder (and upper arm) 959.2
 sinus
  cavernous (*see also* Injury, intracranial) 854.0
  nasal 959.09
 skeleton NEC, birth injury 767.3
 skin NEC 959.9
 skull—*see* Fracture, skull, by site
 soft tissue (of external sites) (severe)—*see*
  Wound, open, by site
 specified site NEC 959.8
 spermatic cord—*see* Injury, internal, spermatic
  cord
 spinal (cord) 952.9
  with fracture, vertebra—*see* Fracture, vertebra,
   by site, with spinal cord injury
  cervical (C_1-C_4) 952.00
   with
    anterior cord syndrome 952.02
    central cord syndrome 952.03
    complete lesion of cord 952.01
    incomplete lesion NEC 952.04
    posterior cord syndrome 952.04
   C_5-C_7 level 952.05
    with
     anterior cord syndrome 952.07
     central cord syndrome 952.08
     complete lesion of cord 952.06
     incomplete lesion NEC 952.09
     posterior cord syndrome 952.09
    specified type NEC 952.09
   specified type NEC 952.04
  dorsal (D_1-D_6) (T_1-T_6) (thoracic) 952.10
   with
    anterior cord syndrome 952.12
    central cord syndrome 952.13
    complete lesion of cord 952.11
    incomplete lesion NEC 952.14
    posterior cord syndrome 952.14

Injury—*continued*
    D_7-D_{12} level (T_7-T_{12}) 952.15
      with
        anterior cord syndrome 952.17
        central cord syndrome 952.18
        complete lesion of cord 952.16
        incomplete lesion NEC 952.19
        posterior cord syndrome 952.19
      specified type NEC 952.19
      specified type NEC 952.14
    lumbar 952.2
    multiple sites 952.8
    nerve (root) NEC—*see* Injury, nerve, spinal, root
    plexus 953.9
      brachial 953.4
      lumbosacral 953.5
      multiple sites 953.8
    sacral 952.3
    thoracic (*see also* Injury, spinal, dorsal) 952.10
  spleen—*see* Injury, internal, spleen
  stellate ganglion 954.1
  sternal region 959.11
  stomach—*see* Injury, internal, stomach
  subconjunctival 921.1
  subcutaneous 959.9
  subdural—*see* Injury, intracranial
  submaxillary region 959.09
  submental region 959.09
  subungual
    fingers 959.5
    toes 959.7
  superficial 919

> *Note—Use the following fourth-digit subdivisions with categories 910-919:*
>
> *.0 Abrasion or friction burn without mention of infection*
> *.1 Abrasion or friction burn, infected*
> *.2 Blister without mention of infection*
> *.3 Blister, infected*
> *.4 Insect bite, nonvenomous, without mention of infection*
> *.5 Insect bite, nonvenomous, infected*
> *.6 Superficial foreign body (splinter) without major open wound and without mention of infection*
> *.7 Superficial foreign body (splinter) without major open wound, infected*
> *.8 Other and unspecified superficial injury without mention of infection*
> *.9 Other and unspecified superficial injury, infected*
>
> *For late effects of superficial injury, see category 906.2.*

  abdomen, abdominal (muscle) (wall) (and other part(s) of trunk) 911
  ankle (and hip, knee, leg, or thigh) 916
  anus (and other part(s) of trunk) 911
  arm 913
    upper (and shoulder) 912
  auditory canal (external) (meatus) (and other part(s) of face, neck, or scalp, except eye) 910
  axilla (and upper arm) 912
  back (and other part(s) of trunk) 911
  breast (and other part(s) of trunk) 911

Injury—*continued*
  brow (and other part(s) of face, neck or scalp, except eye) 910
  buttock (and other part(s) of trunk) 911
  canthus, eye 918.0
  cheek(s) (and other part(s) of face, neck, or scalp, except eye) 910
  chest wall (and other part(s) of trunk) 911
  chin (and other part(s) of face, neck, or scalp, except eye) 910
  clitoris (and other part(s) of trunk) 911
  conjunctiva 918.2
  cornea 918.1
    due to contact lens 371.82
  costal region (and other part(s) of trunk) 911
  ear(s) (auricle) (canal) (drum) (external) (and other part(s) of face, neck, or scalp, except eye) 910
  elbow (and forearm) (and wrist) 913
  epididymis (and other part(s) of trunk) 911
  epigastric region (and other part(s) of trunk) 911
  epiglottis (and other part(s) of face, neck, or scalp, except eye) 910
  eye(s) (and adnexa) NEC 918.9
  eyelid(s) (and periocular area) 918.0
  face (any part(s), except eye) (and neck or scalp) 910
  finger(s) (nail) (any) 915
  flank (and other part(s) of trunk) 911
  foot (phalanges) (and toe(s)) 917
  forearm (and elbow) (and wrist) 913
  forehead (and other part(s) of face, neck, or scalp, except eye) 910
  globe (eye) 918.9
  groin (and other part(s) of trunk) 911
  gum(s) (and other part(s) of face, neck, or scalp, except eye) 910
  hand(s) (except fingers alone) 914
  head (and other part(s) of face, neck, or scalp, except eye) 910
  heel (and foot or toe) 917
  hip (and ankle, knee, leg, or thigh) 916
  iliac region (and other part(s) of trunk) 911
  interscapular region (and other part(s) of trunk) 911
  iris 918.9
  knee (and ankle, hip, leg, or thigh) 916
  labium (majus) (minus) (and other part(s) of trunk) 911
  lacrimal (apparatus) (gland) (sac) 918.0
  leg (lower) (upper) (and ankle, hip, knee, or thigh) 916
  lip(s) (and other part(s) of face, neck, or scalp, except eye) 910
  lower extremity (except foot) 916
  lumbar region (and other part(s) of trunk) 911
  malar region (and other part(s) of face, neck, or scalp, except eye) 910
  mastoid region (and other part(s) of face, neck, or scalp, except eye) 910
  midthoracic region (and other part(s) of trunk) 911
  mouth (and other part(s) of face, neck, or scalp, except eye) 910
  multiple sites (not classifiable to the same three-digit category) 919
  nasal (septum) (and other part(s) of face, neck, or scalp, except eye) 910
  neck (and face or scalp, any part(s), except eye) 910

Injury—*continued*
    nose (septum) (and other part(s) of face, neck, or scalp, except eye) 910
    occipital region (and other part(s) of face, neck, or scalp, except eye) 910
    orbital region 918.0
    palate (soft) (and other part(s) of face, neck, or scalp, except eye) 910
    parietal region (and other part(s) of face, neck, or scalp, except eye) 910
    penis (and other part(s) of trunk) 911
    perineum (and other part(s) of trunk) 911
    periocular area 918.0
    pharynx (and other part(s) of face, neck, or scalp, except eye) 910
    popliteal space (and ankle, hip, leg, or thigh) 916
    prepuce (and other part(s) of trunk) 911
    pubic region (and other part(s) of trunk) 911
    pudenda (and other part(s) of trunk) 911
    sacral region (and other part(s) of trunk) 911
    salivary (ducts) (glands) (and other part(s) of face, neck, or scalp, except eye) 910
    scalp (and other part(s) of face or neck, except eye) 910
    scapular region (and upper arm) 912
    sclera 918.2
    scrotum (and other part(s) of trunk) 911
    shoulder (and upper arm) 912
    skin NEC 919
    specified site(s) NEC 919
    sternal region (and other part(s) of trunk) 911
    subconjunctival 918.2
    subcutaneous NEC 919
    submaxillary region (and other part(s) of face, neck, or scalp, except eye) 910
    submental region (and other part(s) of face, neck, or scalp, except eye) 910
    supraclavicular fossa (and other part(s) of face, neck or scalp, except eye) 910
    supraorbital 918.0
    temple (and other part(s) of face, neck, or scalp, except eye) 910
    temporal region (and other part(s) of face, neck, or scalp, except eye) 910
    testis (and other part(s) of trunk) 911
    thigh (and ankle, hip, knee, or leg) 916
    thorax, thoracic (external) (and other part(s) of trunk) 911
    throat (and other part(s) of face, neck, or scalp, except eye) 910
    thumb(s) (nail) 915
    toe(s) (nail) (subungual) (and foot) 917
    tongue (and other part(s) of face, neck, or scalp, except eye) 910
    tooth, teeth (*see also* Abrasion, dental) 521.20
    trunk (any part(s)) 911
    tunica vaginalis (and other part(s) of trunk) 911
    tympanum, tympanic membrane (and other part(s) of face, neck, or scalp, except eye) 910
    upper extremity NEC 913
    uvula (and other part(s) of face, neck, or scalp, except eye) 910
    vagina (and other part(s) of trunk) 911
    vulva (and other part(s) of trunk) 911
    wrist (and elbow) (and forearm) 913
  supraclavicular fossa 959.19
  supraorbital 959.09

Injury—*continued*
  surgical complication (external or internal site) 998.2
  symphysis pubis 959.19
    complicating delivery 665.6
      affecting fetus or newborn 763.89
  temple 959.09
  temporal region 959.09
  testis 959.14
  thigh (and hip) 959.6
  thorax, thoracic (external) 959.11
    cavity—*see* Injury, internal, thorax
    internal—*see* Injury, internal, intrathoracic organs
  throat 959.09
  thumb(s) (nail) 959.5
  thymus—*see* Injury, internal, thymus
  thyroid (gland) 959.09
  toe (nail) (any) 959.7
  tongue 959.09
  tonsil 959.09
  tooth NEC 873.63
    complicated 873.73
  trachea—*see* Injury, internal, trachea
  trunk 959.19
  tunica vaginalis 959.14
  tympanum, tympanic membrane 959.09
  ultraviolet rays NEC 990
  ureter—*see* Injury, internal, ureter
  urethra (sphincter)—*see* Injury, internal, urethra
  uterus—*see* Injury, internal, uterus
  uvula 959.09
  vagina 959.14
  vascular—*see* Injury, blood vessel
  vas deferens—*see* Injury, internal, vas deferens
  vein (*see also* Injury, blood vessel, by site) 904.9
  vena cava
    inferior 902.10
    superior 901.2
  vesical (sphincter)—*see* Injury, internal, vesical
  viscera (abdominal)—*see* Injury, internal, viscera
    with fracture, pelvis—*see* Fracture, pelvis
  visual 950.9
    cortex 950.3
  vitreous (humor) 871.2
  vulva 959.14
  whiplash (cervical spine) 847.0
  wringer—*see* Crush, by site
  wrist (and elbow) (and forearm) 959.3
  x-ray NEC 990
Inoculation —*see also* Vaccination
  complication or reaction—*see* Complication, vaccination
Insanity, insane (*see also* Psychosis) 298.9
  adolescent (*see also* Schizophrenia) 295.9
  alternating (*see also* Psychosis, affective, circular) 296.7
  confusional 298.9
    acute 293.0
    subacute 293.1
  delusional 298.9
  paralysis, general 094.1
    progressive 094.1
  paresis, general 094.1
  senile 290.20
Insect
  bite—*see* Injury, superficial, by site
  venomous, poisoning by 989.5
Insemination, artificial V26.1

Insuloma —*see* Insulinoma
Insult
  brain 437.9
    acute 436
  cerebral 437.9
    acute 436
  cerebrovascular 437.9
    acute 436
  vascular NEC 437.9
    acute 436
Insurance examination (certification) V70.3
Intemperance (*see also* Alcoholism) 303.9
Interception of pregnancy (menstrual
  extraction) V25.3
Interference
  balancing side 524.56
  non-working side 524.56
Intermenstrual
  bleeding 626.6
    irregular 626.6
    regular 626.5
  hemorrhage 626.6
    irregular 626.6
    regular 626.5
  ain(s) 625.2
Intermittent— *see* condition
Internal —*see* condition
Interproximal wear 521.10
Interruption
  aortic arch 747.11
  bundle of His 426.50
  fallopian tube (for sterilization) V25.2
  phase-shift, sleep cycle 307.45
  repeated REM-sleep 307.48
  sleep
    due to perceived environmental disturbances
      307.48
    phase-shift, of 24-hour sleep-wake cycle
      307.45
    repeated REM-sleep type 307.48
  vas deferens (for sterilization) V25.2
Intersexuality 752.7
Interstitial —*see* condition
Intertrigo 695.89
  labialis 528.5
Intervertebral disc —*see* condition
Intestine, intestinal —*see also* condition
  flu 487.8
Intolerance
  carbohydrate NEC 579.8
  cardiovascular exercise, with pain (at rest) (with
    less than ordinary activity) (with ordinary
    activity) V47.2
  cold 780.99
  disaccharide (hereditary) 271.3
  drug
    correct substance properly administered 995.27
    wrong substance given or taken in error 977.9
      specified drug—*see* Table of drugs and
        chemicals
  effort 306.2
  fat NEC 579.8
  foods NEC 579.8
  fructose (hereditary) 271.2
  glucose (-galactose) (congenital) 271.3
  gluten 579.0
  lactose (hereditary) (infantile) 271.3
  lysine (congenital) 270.7
  milk NEC 579.8
  protein (familial) 270.7
  starch NEC 579.8
  sucrose (-isomaltose) (congenital) 271.3

Intoxicated NEC (*see also* Alcoholism) 305.0
Intoxication
  acid 276.2
  acute
    alcoholic 305.0
      with alcoholism 303.0
      hangover effects 305.0
    caffeine 305.9
    hallucinogenic (*see also* Abuse, drugs,
      nondependent) 305.3
  alcohol (acute) 305.0
    with alcoholism 303.0
    hangover effects 305.0
    idiosyncratic 291.4
    pathological 291.4
  alimentary canal 558.2
  ammonia (hepatic) 572.2
  caffeine 305.9
  chemical—*see also* Table of drugs and
    chemicals
    via placenta or breast milk 760.70
      alcohol 760.71
      anticonvulsants 760.77
      antifungals 760.74
      anti-infective agents 760.74
      antimetabolics 760.78
      cocaine 760.75
      "crack" 760.75
      hallucinogenic agents NEC 760.73
      medicinal agents NEC 760.79
      narcotics 760.72
      obstetric anesthetic or analgesic drug 763.5
      specified agent NEC 760.79
      suspected, affecting management of
        pregnancy 655.5
  cocaine, through placenta or breast milk 760.75
  delirium
    alcohol 291.0
    drug 292.81
  drug 292.89
    with delirium 292.81
    correct substance properly administered (*see
      also* Allergy, drug) 995.27
    newborn 779.4
    obstetric anesthetic or sedation 668.9
      affecting fetus or newborn 763.5
    overdose or wrong substance given or
      taken—*see* Table of drugs and chemicals
    pathologic 292.2
    specific to newborn 779.4
    via placenta or breast milk 760.70
      alcohol 760.71
      anticonvulsants 760.77
      antifungals 760.74
      anti-infective agents 760.74
      antimetabolics 760.78
      cocaine 760.75
      "crack" 760.75
      hallucinogenic agents 760.73
      medicinal agents NEC 760.79
      narcotics 760.72
      obstetric anesthetic or analgesic drug 763.5
      specified agent NEC 760.79
      suspected, affecting management of
        pregnancy 655.5
  enteric—*see* Intoxication, intestinal
  fetus or newborn, via placenta or breast milk
    760.70
    alcohol 760.71
    anticonvulsants 760.77
    antifungals 760.74

Irritation—*continued*
  meninges (traumatic) (*see also* Injury,
    intracranial) 854.0
    nontraumatic—*see* Meningitis
  myocardium 306.2
  nerve—*see* Disorder, nerve
  nervous 799.2
  nose 478.19
  penis 607.89
  perineum 709.9
  peripheral
    autonomic nervous system (*see also*
      Neuropathy, peripheral, autonomic) 337.9
    nerve—*see* Disorder, nerve
  peritoneum (*see also* Peritonitis) 567.9
  pharynx 478.29
  plantar nerve 355.6
  spinal (cord) (traumatic)—*see also* Injury,
    spinal, by site
    nerve—*see also* Disorder, nerve
      root NEC 724.9
      traumatic—*see* Injury, nerve, spinal
    nontraumatic—*see* Myelitis
  stomach 536.9
    psychogenic 306.4
  sympathetic nerve NEC (*see also* Neuropathy,
    peripheral, autonomic) 337.9
  ulnar nerve 354.2
  vagina 623.9
Isambert's disease 012.3
Ischemia, ischemic 459.9
  basilar artery (with transient neurologic deficit)
    435.0
  bone NEC 733.40
  bowel (transient) 557.9
    acute 557.0
    chronic 557.1
    due to mesenteric artery insufficiency 557.1
  brain—*see also* Ischemia, cerebral
    recurrent focal 435.9
  cardiac (*see also* Ischemia, heart) 414.9
  cardiomyopathy 414.8
  carotid artery (with transient neurologic deficit)
    435.8
  cerebral (chronic) (generalized) 437.1
    arteriosclerotic 437.0
    intermittent (with transient neurologic deficit)
      435.9
    newborn 779.2
    puerperal, postpartum, childbirth 674.0
    recurrent focal (with transient neurologic
      deficit) 435.9
    transient (with transient neurologic deficit)
      435.9
  colon 557.9
    acute 557.0
    chronic 557.1
    due to mesenteric artery insufficiency 557.1
  coronary (chronic) (*see also* Ischemia, heart)
    414.9
  heart (chronic or with a stated duration of over 8
    weeks) 414.9
    acute or with a stated duration of 8 weeks or
      less (*see also* Infarct, myocardium) 410.9
      without myocardial infarction 411.89
        with coronary (artery) occlusion 411.81
    subacute 411.89
  intestine (transient) 557.9
    acute 557.0
    chronic 557.1
    due to mesenteric artery insufficiency 557.1

Ischemia, ischemic—*continued*
  kidney 593.81
  labyrinth 386.50
  muscles, leg 728.89
  myocardium, myocardial (chronic or with a
    stated duration of over 8 weeks) 414.8
    acute (*see also* Infarct, myocardium) 410.9
      without myocardial infarction 411.89
        with coronary (artery) occlusion 411.81
  renal 593.81
  retina, retinal 362.84
  small bowel 557.9
    acute 557.0
    chronic 557.1
    due to mesenteric artery insufficiency 557.1
  spinal cord 336.1
  subendocardial (*see also* Insufficiency,
    coronary) 411.89
  vertebral artery (with transient neurologic
    deficit) 435.1
Ischialgia (*see also* Sciatica) 724.3
Ischiopagus 759.4
Ischium, ischial —*see* condition
Ischomenia 626.8
Ischuria 788.5
Iselin's disease or osteochondrosis 732.5
Islands of
  parotid tissue in
    lymph nodes 750.26
    neck structures 750.26
  submaxillary glands in
    fascia 750.26
    lymph nodes 750.26
    neck muscles 750.26
Islet cell tumor, pancreas (M8150/0) 211.7
Isoimmunization NEC (*see also* Incompatibility)
  656.2
  fetus or newborn 773.2
    ABO blood groups 773.1
    Rhesus (Rh) factor 773.0
Isolation V07.0
  social V62.4
Isosporosis 007.2
Issue
  medical certificate NEC V68.0
    cause of death V68.0
    fitness V68.0
    incapacity V68.0
  repeat prescription NEC V68.1
    appliance V68.1
    contraceptive V25.40
      device NEC V25.49
        intrauterine V25.42
        specified type NEC V25.49
      pill V25.41
    glasses V68.1
    medicinal substance V68.1
Itch (*see also* Pruritus) 698.9
  bakers' 692.89
  barbers' 110.0
  bricklayers' 692.89
  cheese 133.8
  clam diggers' 120.3
  coolie 126.9
  copra 133.8
  Cuban 050.1
  dew 126.9
  dhobie 110.3
  eye 379.99
  filarial (*see also* Infestation, filarial) 125.9
  grain 133.8

Itch —*continued*
  grocers' 133.8
  ground 126.9
  harvest 133.8
  jock 110.3
  Malabar 110.9
    beard 110.0
    foot 110.4
    scalp 110.0
  meaning scabies 133.0
  Norwegian 133.0
  perianal 698.0
  poultrymen's 133.8
  sarcoptic 133.0
  scrub 134.1
  seven year V61.10
    meaning scabies 133.0
  straw 133.8
  swimmers' 120.3
  washerwoman's 692.4
  water 120.3
  winter 698.8
Itsenko-Cushing syndrome (pituitary
  basophilism) 255.0
Ivemark's syndrome (asplenia with congenital
  heart disease) 759.0
Ivory bones 756.52
Ixodes 134.8
Ixodiasis 134.8

J

Jaccoud's nodular fibrositis, chronic (Jaccoud's syndrome) 714.4
Jackson's
membrane 751.4
paralysis or syndrome 344.89
veil 751.4
Jacksonian
epilepsy (*see also* Epilepsy) 345.5
seizures (focal) (*see also* Epilepsy) 345.5
Jacob's ulcer (M8090/3)—*see* Neoplasm, skin, malignant, by site
Jacquet's dermatitis (diaper dermatitis) 691.0
Jadassohn's
blue nevus (M8780/0)—*see* Neoplasm, skin, benign
disease (maculopapular erythroderma) 696.2
intraepidermal epithelioma (M8096/0)—*see* Neoplasm, skin, benign
Jadassohn-Lewandowski syndrome (pachyonychia congenita) 757.5
Jadassohn-Pellizari's disease (anetoderma) 701.3
Jadassohn-Tièche nevus (M8780/0)—*see* Neoplasm, skin, benign
Jaffe-Lichtenstein (-Uehlinger) syndrome 252.01
Jahnke's syndrome (encephalocutaneous angiomatosis) 759.6
Jakob-Creutzfeldt disease (syndrome) (new variant) 046.1
with dementia
with behavioral disturbance 046.1 *[294.11]*
without behavioral disturbance 046.1 *[294.10]*
Jaksch (-Luzet) disease or syndrome (pseudoleukemia infantum) 285.8
Jamaican
neuropathy 349.82
paraplegic tropical ataxic-spastic syndrome 349.82
Janet's disease (psychasthenia) 300.89
Janiceps 759.4
Jansky-Bielschowsky amaurotic familial idiocy 330.1
Japanese
B type encephalitis 062.0
river fever 081.2
seven-day fever 100.89
Jaundice (yellow) 782.4
acholuric (familial) (splenomegalic) (*see also* Spherocytosis) 282.0
acquired 283.9
breast milk 774.39
catarrhal (acute) 070.1
with hepatic coma 070.0
chronic 571.9
epidemic—*see* Jaundice, epidemic
cholestatic (benign) 782.4
chronic idiopathic 277.4
epidemic (catarrhal) 070.1
with hepatic coma 070.0
leptospiral 100.0
spirochetal 100.0
febrile (acute) 070.1
with hepatic coma 070.0
leptospiral 100.0
spirochetal 100.0
fetus or newborn 774.6
due to or associated with

Jaundice—*continued*
ABO
antibodies 773.1
incompatibility, maternal/fetal 773.1
isoimmunization 773.1
absence or deficiency of enzyme system for bilirubin conjugation (congenital) 774.39
blood group incompatibility NEC 773.2
breast milk inhibitors to conjugation 774.39
associated with preterm delivery 774.2
bruising 774.1
Crigler-Najjar syndrome 277.4 *[774.31]*
delayed conjugation 774.30
associated with preterm delivery 774.2
development 774.39
drugs or toxins transmitted from mother 774.1
G-6-PD deficiency 282.2 *[774.0]*
galactosemia 271.1 *[774.5]*
Gilbert's syndrome 277.4 *[774.31]*
hepatocellular damage 774.4
hereditary hemolytic anemia (*see also* Anemia, hemolytic) 282.9 *[774.0]*
hypothyroidism, congenital 243 *[774.31]*
incompatibility, maternal/fetal NEC 773.2
infection 774.1
inspissated bile syndrome 774.4
isoimmunization NEC 773.2
mucoviscidosis 277.01 *[774.5]*
obliteration of bile duct, congenital 751.61 *[774.5]*
polycythemia 774.1
preterm delivery 774.2
red cell defect 282.9 *[774.0]*
Rh
antibodies 773.0
incompatibility, maternal/fetal 773.0
isoimmunization 773.0
spherocytosis (congenital) 282.0 *[774.0]*
swallowed maternal blood 774.1
physiological NEC 774.6
from injection, inoculation, infusion, or transfusion (blood) (plasma) (serum) (other substance) (onset within 8 months after administration)—*see* Hepatitis, viral
Gilbert's (familial nonhemolytic) 277.4
hematogenous 283.9
hemolytic (acquired) 283.9
congenital (*see also* Spherocytosis) 282.0
hemorrhagic (acute) 100.0
leptospiral 100.0
newborn 776.0
spirochetal 100.0
hepatocellular 573.8
homologous (serum)—*see* Hepatitis, viral
idiopathic, chronic 277.4
infectious (acute) (subacute) 070.1
with hepatic coma 070.0
leptospiral 100.0
spirochetal 100.0
leptospiral 100.0
malignant (*see also* Necrosis, liver) 570
newborn (physiological) (*see also* Jaundice, fetus or newborn) 774.6
nonhemolytic, congenital familial (Gilbert's) 277.4
nuclear, newborn (*see also* Kernicterus of newborn) 774.7

Jaundice—*continued*
  obstructive NEC (*see also* Obstruction, biliary)
    576.8
  postimmunization—*see* Hepatitis, viral
  posttransfusion—*see* Hepatitis, viral
  regurgitation (*see also* Obstruction, biliary)
    576.8
  serum (homologous) (prophylactic)
    (therapeutic)—*see* Hepatitis, viral
  spirochetal (hemorrhagic) 100.0
  symptomatic 782.4
    newborn 774.6
Jaw —*see* condition
Jaw-blinking 374.43
  congenital 742.8
Jaw-winking phenomenon or syndrome 742.8
Jealousy
  alcoholic 291.5
  childhood 313.3
  sibling 313.3
Jejunitis (*see also* Enteritis) 558.9
Jejunostomy status V44.4
Jejunum, jejunal —*see* condition
Jensen's disease 363.05
Jericho boil 085.1
Jerks, myoclonic 333.2
Jervell-Lange-Nielsen syndrome 426.82
Jeune's disease or syndrome (asphyxiating
    thoracic dystrophy) 756.4
Jigger disease 134.1
Job's syndrome (chronic granulomatous disease)
    288.1
Jod-Basedow phenomenon 242.8
Johnson-Stevens disease (erythema multiforme
    exudativum) 695.1
Joint —*see also* condition
  Charcot's 094.0 *[713.5]*
  false 733.82
  flail—*see* Flail, joint
  mice—*see* Loose, body, joint, by site
  sinus to bone 730.9
  von Gies' 095.8
Jordan's anomaly or syndrome 288.2
Josephs-Diamond-Blackfan anemia (congenital
    hypoplastic) 284.01
Joubert syndrome 759.89
Jumpers' knee 727.2
Jungle yellow fever 060.0
Jüngling's disease (sarcoidosis) 135
Junin virus hemorrhagic fever 078.7
Juvenile —*see also* condition
  delinquent 312.9
    group (*see also* Disturbance, conduct) 312.2
    neurotic 312.4

K

Kabuki syndrome 759.89
Kahler (-Bozzolo) disease (multiple myeloma)
    (M9730/3) 203.0
Kakergasia 300.9
Kakke 265.0
Kala-azar (Indian) (infantile) (Mediterranean)
    (Sudanese) 085.0
Kalischer's syndrome (encephalocutaneous
    angiomatosis) 759.6
Kallmann's syndrome (hypogonadotropic
    hypogonadism with anosmia) 253.4
Kanner's syndrome (autism) (*see also*
    Psychosis, childhood) 299.0
Kaolinosis 502
Kaposi's
    disease 757.33
        lichen ruber 696.4
            acuminatus 696.4
            moniliformis 697.8
        xeroderma pigmentosum 757.33
    sarcoma (M9140/3) 176.9
        adipose tissue 176.1
        aponeurosis 176.1
        artery 176.1
        blood vessel 176.1
        bursa 176.1
        connective tissue 176.1
        external genitalia 176.8
        fascia 176.1
        fatty tissue 176.1
        fibrous tissue 176.1
        gastrointestinal tract NEC 176.3
        ligament 176.1
        lung 176.4
        lymph
            gland(s) 176.5
            node(s) 176.5
        lymphatic(s) NEC 176.1
        muscle (skeletal) 176.1
        oral cavity NEC 176.8
        palate 176.2
        scrotum 176.8
        skin 176.0
        soft tissue 176.1
        specified site NEC 176.8
        subcutaneous tissue 176.1
        synovia 176.1
        tendon (sheath) 176.1
        vein 176.1
        vessel 176.1
        viscera NEC 176.9
        vulva 176.8
    varicelliform eruption 054.0
    vaccinia 999.0
Kartagener's syndrome or triad (sinusitis,
    bronchiectasis, situs inversus) 759.3
Kasabach-Merritt syndrome (capillary
    hemangioma associated with
    thrombocytopenic purpura) 287.39
Kaschin-Beck disease (endemic
    polyarthritis)—*see* Disease, Kaschin-Beck
Kast's syndrome (dyschondroplasia with
    hemangiomas) 756.4
Katatonia (*see also* Schizophrenia) 295.2
Katayama disease or fever 120.2
Kathisophobia 781.0
Kawasaki disease 446.1

Kayser-Fleischer ring (cornea) (pseudosclerosis)
    275.1 *[371.14]*
Kaznelson's syndrome (congenital hypoplastic
    anemia) 284.01
Kearns-Sayre syndrome 277.87
Kedani fever 081.2
Kelis 701.4
Kelly (-Patterson) syndrome (sideropenic
    dysphagia) 280.8
Keloid, cheloid 701.4
    Addison's (morphea) 701.0
    cornea 371.00
    Hawkins' 701.4
    scar 701.4
Keloma 701.4
Kenya fever 082.1
Keratectasia 371.71
    congenital 743.41
Keratinization NEC
    alveolar ridge mucosa
        excessive 528.72
        minimal 528.71
Keratitis (nodular) (nonulcerative) (simple)
    (zonular) NEC 370.9
    with ulceration (*see also* Ulcer, cornea) 370.00
    actinic 370.24
    arborescens 054.42
    areolar 370.22
    bullosa 370.8
    deep—*see* Keratitis, interstitial
    dendritic(a) 054.42
    desiccation 370.34
    diffuse interstitial 370.52
    disciform(is) 054.43
        varicella 052.7 *[370.44]*
    epithelialis vernalis 372.13 *[370.32]*
    exposure 370.34
    filamentary 370.23
    gonococcal (congenital) (prenatal) 098.43
    herpes, herpetic (simplex) NEC 054.43
        zoster 053.21
    hypopyon 370.04
    in
        chickenpox 052.7 *[370.44]*
        exanthema (*see also* Exanthem) 057.9
            [370.44]
        paravaccinia (*see also* Paravaccinia) 051.9
            [370.44]
        smallpox (*see also* Smallpox) 050.9 *[370.44]*
        vernal conjunctivitis 372.13 *[370.32]*
    interstitial (nonsyphilitic) 370.50
        with ulcer (*see also* Ulcer, cornea) 370.00
        diffuse 370.52
        herpes, herpetic (simplex) 054.43
            zoster 053.21
        syphilitic (congenital) (hereditary) 090.3
        tuberculous (*see also* Tuberculosis) 017.3
            [370.59]
    lagophthalmic 370.34
    macular 370.22
    neuroparalytic 370.35
    neurotrophic 370.35
    nummular 370.22
    oyster-shuckers' 370.8
    parenchymatous—*see* Keratitis, interstitial
    petrificans 370.8
    phlyctenular 370.31

Keraunoparalysis 994.0
Kerion (celsi) 110.0
Kernicterus of newborn (not due to
      isoimmunization) 774.7
   due to isoimmunization (conditions classifiable
      to 773.0-773.2) 773.4
Ketoacidosis 276.2
   diabetic 250.1
Ketonuria 791.6
   branched-chain, intermittent 270.3
Ketosis 276.2
   diabetic 250.1
Kidney —*see* condition
Kienböck's
   disease 732.3
      adult 732.8
   osteochondrosis 732.3
Kimmelstiel (-Wilson) disease or syndrome
      (intercapillary glomerulosclerosis) 250.4
      [581.81]
Kink, kinking
   appendix 543.9
   artery 447.1
   cystic duct, congenital 751.61
   hair (acquired) 704.2
   ileum or intestine (*see also* Obstruction,
      intestine) 560.9
   Lane's (*see also* Obstruction, intestine) 560.9
   organ or site, congenital NEC—*see* Anomaly,
      specified type NEC, by site
   ureter (pelvic junction) 593.3
      congenital 753.20
   vein(s) 459.2
      caval 459.2
      peripheral 459.2
Kinnier Wilson's disease (hepatolenticular
      degeneration) 275.1
Kissing
   osteophytes 721.5
   spine 721.5
   vertebra 721.5
Klauder's syndrome (erythema multiforme
      exudativum) 695.1
Kleb's disease (*see also* Nephritis) 583.9
Klein-Waardenburg syndrome
      (ptosisepicanthus) 270.2
Kleine-Levin syndrome 327.13
Kleptomania 312.32
Klinefelter's syndrome 758.7
Klinger's disease 446.4
Klippel's disease 723.8
Klippel-Feil disease or syndrome (brevicollis)
      756.16
Klippel-Trenaunay syndrome 759.89
Klumpke (-Déjérine) palsy, paralysis (birth)
      (newborn) 767.6
Klüver-Bucy (-Terzian) syndrome 310.0
Knee —*see* condition
Knifegrinders' rot (*see also* Tuberculosis) 011.4
Knock-knee (acquired) 736.41
   congenital 755.64
Knot
   intestinal, syndrome (volvulus) 560.2
   umbilical cord (true) 663.2
      affecting fetus or newborn 762.5
Knots, surfer 919.8
   infected 919.9
Knotting (of)
   hair 704.2
   intestine 560.2
Knuckle pads (Garrod's) 728.79

Köbner's disease (epidermolysis bullosa) 757.39
Koch's
   infection (*see also* Tuberculosis, pulmonary)
      011.9
   relapsing fever 087.9
Koch-Weeks conjunctivitis 372.03
Koenig-Wichman disease (pemphigus) 694.4
Köhler's disease (osteochondrosis) 732.5
   first (osteochondrosis juvenilis) 732.5
   second (Freiburg's infarction, metatarsal head)
      732.5
   patellar 732.4
   tarsal navicular (bone) (osteoarthosis juvenilis)
      732.5
Köhler-Mouchet disease (osteoarthrosis
      juvenilis) 732.5
Köhler-Pellegrini-Stieda disease or syndrome
      (calcification, knee joint) 726.62
Koilonychia 703.8
   congenital 757.5
Kojevnikov's, Kojewnikoff's epilepsy (*see also*
      Epilepsy) 345.7
König's
   disease (osteochondritis dissecans) 732.7
   syndrome 564.89
Koniophthisis (*see also* Tuberculosis) 011.4
Koplik's spots 055.9
Kopp's asthma 254.8
Korean hemorrhagic fever 078.6
Korsakoff (-Wernicke) disease, psychosis, or
      syndrome (nonalcoholic) 294.0
   alcoholic 291.1
Korsakov's disease —*see* Korsakoff's disease
Korsakow's disease —*see* Korsakoff's disease
Kostmann's disease or syndrome (infantile
      genetic agranulocytosis) 288.01
Krabbe's
   disease (leukodystrophy) 330.0
   syndrome
      congenital muscle hypoplasia 756.89
      cutaneocerebral angioma 759.6
Kraepelin-Morel disease (*see also*
      Schizophrenia) 295.9
Kraft-Weber-Dimitri disease 759.6
Kraurosis
   ani 569.49
   penis 607.0
   vagina 623.8
   vulva 624.0
Kreotoxism 005.9
Krukenberg's
   spindle 371.13
   tumor (M8490/6) 198.6
Kufs' disease 330.1
Kugelberg-Welander disease 335.11
Kuhnt-Junius degeneration or disease 362.52
Kulchitsky's cell carcinoma (carcinoid tumor of
      intestine) 259.2
Kümmell's disease or spondylitis 721.7
Kundrat's disease (lymphosarcoma) 200.1
Kunekune —*see* Dermatophytosis
Kunkel syndrome (lupoid hepatitis) 571.49
Kupffer cell sarcoma (M9124/3) 155.0
Kuru 046.0
Kussmaul's
   coma (diabetic) 250.3
   disease (polyarteritis nodosa) 446.0
   respiration (air hunger) 786.09
Kwashiorkor (marasmus type) 260
Kyasanur Forest disease 065.2

Kyphoscoliosis, kyphoscoliotic (acquired) (*see also* Scoliosis) 737.30
  congenital 756.19
  due to radiation 737.33
  heart (disease) 416.1
  idiopathic 737.30
    infantile
      progressive 737.32
      resolving 737.31
  late effect of rickets 268.1 *[737.43]*
  specified NEC 737.39
  thoracogenic 737.34
  tuberculous (*see also* Tuberculosis) 015.0
    [737.43]
Kyphosis, kyphotic (acquired) (postural) 737.10
  adolescent postural 737.0
  congenital 756.19
  dorsalis juvenilis 732.0
  due to or associated with
    Charcot-Marie-Tooth disease 356.1 *[737.41]*
    mucopolysaccharidosis 277.5 *[737.41]*
    neurofibromatosis 237.71 *[737.41]*
    osteitis
      deformans 731.0 *[737.41]*
      fibrosa cystica 252.01 *[737.41]*
    osteoporosis (*see also* Osteoporosis) 733.0
      [737.41]
    poliomyelitis (*see also* Poliomyelitis) 138
      [737.41]
    radiation 737.11
    tuberculosis (*see also* Tuberculosis) 015.0
      [737.41]
  Kümmell's 721.7
  late effect of rickets 268.1 *[737.41]*
  Morquio-Brailsford type (spinal) 277.5 *[737.41]*
  pelvis 738.6
  postlaminectomy 737.12
  specified cause NEC 737.19
  syphilitic, congenital 090.5 *[737.41]*
  tuberculous (*see also* Tuberculosis) 015.0
    [737.41]
Kyrle's disease (hyperkeratosis follicularis in
  cutem penetrans) 701.1

L

Labia, labium —*see* condition
Labiated hymen 752.49
Labile
blood pressure 796.2
emotions, emotionality 301.3
vasomotor system 443.9
Labioglossal paralysis 335.22
Labium leporinum (*see also* Cleft, lip) 749.10
Labor (*see also* Delivery)
with complications—*see* Delivery, complicated
abnormal NEC 661.9
affecting fetus or newborn 763.7
arrested active phase 661.1
affecting fetus or newborn 763.7
desultory 661.2
affecting fetus or newborn 763.7
dyscoordinate 661.4
affecting fetus or newborn 763.7
early onset (22-36 weeks gestation) 644.2
failed
induction 659.1
mechanical 659.0
medical 659.1
surgical 659.0
trial (vaginal delivery) 660.6
false 644.1
forced or induced, affecting fetus or newborn
763.89
hypertonic 661.4
affecting fetus or newborn 763.7
hypotonic 661.2
affecting fetus or newborn 763.7
primary 661.0
affecting fetus or newborn 763.7
secondary 661.1
affecting fetus or newborn 763.7
incoordinate 661.4
affecting fetus or newborn 763.7
irregular 661.2
affecting fetus or newborn 763.7
long—*see* Labor, prolonged
missed (at or near term) 656.4
obstructed NEC 660.9
affecting fetus or newborn 763.1
due to female genital mutilation 660.8
specified cause NEC 660.8
affecting fetus or newborn 763.1
pains, spurious 644.1
precipitate 661.3
affecting fetus or newborn 763.6
premature 644.2
threatened 644.0
prolonged or protracted 662.1
affecting fetus or newborn 763.89
first stage 662.0
affecting fetus or newborn 763.89
second stage 662.2
affecting fetus or newborn 763.89
threatened NEC 644.1
undelivered 644.1
Labored breathing (*see also* Hyperventilation)
786.09

Labyrinthitis (inner ear) (destructive) (latent)
386.30
circumscribed 386.32
diffuse 386.31
focal 386.32
purulent 386.33
serous 386.31
suppurative 386.33
syphilitic 095.8
toxic 386.34
viral 386.35
Laceration —*see also* Wound, open, by site
accidental, complicating surgery 998.2
Achilles tendon 845.09
with open wound 892.2
anus (sphincter) 879.6
with
abortion—*see* Abortion, by type, with
damage to pelvic organs
ectopic pregnancy (*see also* categories
633.0-633.9) 639.2
molar pregnancy (*see also* categories
630-632) 639.2
complicated 879.7
complicating delivery 664.2
with laceration of anal or rectal mucosa
664.3
following
abortion 639.2
ectopic or molar pregnancy 639.2
nontraumatic, nonpuerperal 565.0
bladder (urinary)
with
abortion—*see* Abortion, by type, with
damage to pelvic organs
ectopic pregnancy (*see also* categories
633.0-633.9) 639.2
molar pregnancy (*see also* categories
630-632) 639.2
following
abortion 639.2
ectopic or molar pregnancy 639.2
obstetrical trauma 665.5
blood vessel—*see* Injury, blood vessel, by site
bowel
with
abortion—*see* Abortion, by type, with
damage to pelvic organs
ectopic pregnancy (*see also* categories
633.0-633.9) 639.2
molar pregnancy (*see also* categories
630-632) 639.2
following
abortion 639.2
ectopic or molar pregnancy 639.2
obstetrical trauma 665.5
brain (with hemorrhage) (cerebral) (membrane)
851.8

Laceration—*continued*

> *Note—Use the following fifth-digit*
> *subclassification with categories 851-854:*
>
> *0 unspecified state of consciousness*
> *1 with no loss of consciousness*
> *2 with brief [less than one hour] loss of*
> *consciousness*
> *3 with moderate [1-24 hours] loss of*
> *consciousness*
> *4 with prolonged [more than 24 hours] loss of*
> *consciousness and return to pre-existing*
> *conscious level*
> *5 with prolonged [more than 24 hours] loss of*
> *consciousness, without return to pre-existing*
> *conscious level*
> *Use fifth-digit 5 to designate when a patient is*
> *unconscious and dies before regaining*
> *consciousness, regardless of the duration of the*
> *loss of consciousness*
> *6 with loss of consciousness of unspecified*
> *duration*
> *9 with concussion, unspecified*

   with
     open intracranial wound 851.9
     skull fracture—*see* Fracture, skull, by site
   cerebellum 851.6
     with open intracranial wound 851.7
   cortex 851.2
     with open intracranial wound 851.3
   during birth 767.0
   stem 851.6
     with open intracranial wound 851.7
  broad ligament
   with
     abortion—*see* Abortion, by type, with
      damage to pelvic organs
     ectopic pregnancy (*see also* categories
      633.0-633.9) 639.2
     molar pregnancy (*see also* categories
      630-632) 639.2
   following
     abortion 639.2
     ectopic or molar pregnancy 639.2
   nontraumatic 620.6
   obstetrical trauma 665.6
   syndrome (nontraumatic) 620.6
  capsule, joint—*see* Sprain, by site
  cardiac—*see* Laceration, heart
  causing eversion of cervix uteri (old) 622.0
  central, complicating delivery 664.4
  cerebellum—*see* Laceration, brain, cerebellum
  cerebral—*see also* Laceration, brain
   during birth 767.0
  cervix (uteri)
   with
     abortion—*see* Abortion, by type, with
      damage to pelvic organs
     ectopic pregnancy (*see also* categories
      633.0-633.9) 639.2
     molar pregnancy (*see also* categories
      630-632) 639.2
   following
     abortion 639.2
     ectopic or molar pregnancy 639.2
   nonpuerperal, nontraumatic 622.3
   obstetrical trauma (current) 665.3
   old (postpartal) 622.3
   traumatic—*see* Injury, internal, cervix
  chordae heart 429.5

Laceration—*continued*
  complicated 879.9
  cornea—*see* Laceration, eyeball
   superficial 918.1
  cortex (cerebral)—*see* Laceration, brain, cortex
  esophagus 530.89
  eye(s)—*see* Laceration, ocular
  eyeball NEC 871.4
   with prolapse or exposure of intraocular tissue
    871.1
   penetrating—*see* Penetrating wound, eyeball
   specified as without prolapse of intraocular
    tissue 871.0
  eyelid NEC 870.8
   full thickness 870.1
    involving lacrimal passages 870.2
   skin (and periocular area) 870.0
    penetrating—*see* Penetrating wound, orbit
  fourchette
   with
     abortion—*see* Abortion, by type, with
      damage to pelvic organs
     ectopic pregnancy (*see also* categories
      633.0-633.9) 639.2
     molar pregnancy (*see also* categories
      630-632) 639.2
   complicating delivery 664.0
   following
    abortion 639.2
    ectopic or molar pregnancy 639.2
  heart (without penetration of heart chambers)
   861.02
   with
     open wound into thorax 861.12
     penetration of heart chambers 861.03
      with open wound into thorax 861.13
  hernial sac—*see* Hernia, by site
  internal organ (abdomen) (chest) (pelvis)
   NEC—*see* Injury, internal, by site
  kidney (parenchyma) 866.02
   with
     complete disruption of parenchyma (rupture)
      866.03
      with open wound into cavity 866.13
     open wound into cavity 866.12
  labia
   complicating delivery 664.0
  ligament—*see also* Sprain, by site
   with open wound—*see* Wound, open, by site
  liver 864.05
   with open wound into cavity 864.15
   major (disruption of hepatic parenchyma)
    864.04
    with open wound into cavity 864.14
   minor (capsule only) 864.02
    with open wound into cavity 864.12
   moderate (involving parenchyma without
    major disruption) 864.03
    with open wound into cavity 864.13
   multiple 864.04
    with open wound into cavity 864.14
   stellate 864.04
    with open wound into cavity 864.14
  lung 861.22
   with open wound into thorax 861.32
  meninges—*see* Laceration, brain
  meniscus (knee) (*see also* Tear, meniscus) 836.2
   old 717.5
   site other than knee—*see also* Sprain, by site
    old NEC (*see also* Disorder, cartilage,
     articular) 718.0

Laryngotracheitis—*continued*
  streptococcal 034.0
  stridulous 478.75
  syphilitic 095.8
    congenital 090.5
  tuberculous (*see also* Tuberculosis, larynx)
    012.3
  Vincent's 101
Laryngotracheobronchitis (*see also* Bronchitis)
  490
  acute 466.0
  chronic 491.8
  viral 466.0
Laryngotracheobronchopneumonitis —*see*
  Pneumonia, broncho-
Larynx, laryngeal —*see* condition
Lasègue's disease (persecution mania) 297.9
Lassa fever 078.89
Lassitude (*see also* Weakness) 780.79
Late —*see also* condition
  infant
    post-term (gestation period over 40
      completed weeks to 42 completed
      weeks) 766.21
    prolonged gestation (period over 42
      completed weeks) 766.22
Late effect(s) (of) —*see also* condition
  abscess
    intracranial or intraspinal (conditions
      classifiable to 324)–*see* category 326
  adverse effect of drug, medicinal or biological
    substance 909.5
  allergic reaction 909.9
  amputation
    postoperative (late) 997.60
    traumatic (injury classifiable to 885-887 and
      895-897) 905.9
  burn (injury classifiable to 948-949) 906.9
    extremities NEC (injury classifiable to 943 or
      945) 906.7
      hand or wrist (injury classifiable to 944)
        906.6
    eye (injury classifiable to 940) 906.5
    face, head, and neck (injury classifiable to
      941) 906.5
    specified site NEC (injury classifiable to 942
      and 946-947) 906.8
  cerebrovascular disease (conditions classifiable
    to 430-437) 438.9
    with
      alterations of sensations 438.6
      aphasia 438.11
      apraxia 438.81
      ataxia 438.84
      cognitive deficits 438.0
      disturbances of vision 438.7
      dysphagia 438.82
      dysphasia 438.12
      facial droop 438.83
      facial weakness 438.83
      hemiplegia/hemiparesis
        affecting
          dominant side 438.21
          nondominant side 438.22
          unspecified side 438.20
      monoplegia of lower limb
        affecting
          dominant side 438.41
          nondominant side 438.42
          unspecified side 438.40
      monoplegia of upper limb

Late effect(s) (of)—*continued*
    affecting
      dominant side 438.31
      nondominant side 438.32
      unspecified side 438.30
    paralytic syndrome NEC
      affecting
        bilateral 438.53
        dominant side 438.51
        nondominant side 438.52
        unspecified side 438.50
    speech and language deficit 438.10
      specified type NEC 438.19
    vertigo 438.85
    specified type NEC 438.89
  childbirth complication(s) 677
  complication(s) of
    childbirth 677
    delivery 677
    pregnancy 677
    puerperium 677
    surgical and medical care (conditions
      classifiable to 996-999) 909.3
    trauma (conditions classifiable to 958) 908.6
  contusion (injury classifiable to 920-924) 906.3
  crushing (injury classifiable to 925-929) 906.4
  delivery complication(s) 677
  dislocation (injury classifiable to 830-839) 905.6
  encephalitis or encephalomyelitis (conditions
    classifiable to 323)—*see* category 326
    in infectious diseases 139.8
      viral (conditions classifiable to 049.8, 049.9,
        062-064) 139.0
  external cause NEC (conditions classifiable to
    995) 909.9
    certain conditions classifiable to categories
      991-994 909.4
  foreign body in orifice (injury classifiable to
    930-939) 908.5
  fracture (multiple) (injury classifiable to
    828-829) 905.5
    extremity
      lower (injury classifiable to 821-827) 905.4
        neck of femur (injury classifiable to 820)
          905.3
      upper (injury classifiable to 810-819) 905.2
    face and skull (injury classifiable to 800-804)
      905.0
    skull and face (injury classifiable to 800-804)
      905.0
    spine and trunk (injury classifiable to 805 and
      807-809) 905.1
      with spinal cord lesion (injury classifiable to
        806) 907.2
  infection
    pyogenic, intracranial—*see* category 326
  infectious diseases (conditions classifiable to
    001-136) NEC 139.8
  injury (injury classifiable to 959) 908.9
    blood vessel 908.3
      abdomen and pelvis (injury classifiable to
        902) 908.4
      extremity (injury classifiable to 903-904)
        908.3
      head and neck (injury classifiable to 900)
        908.3
        intracranial (injury classifiable to 850-854)
          907.0
        with skull fracture 905.0
      thorax (injury classifiable to 901) 908.4

Late effect(s) (of)—*continued*
- internal organ NEC (injury classifiable to 867 and 869) 908.2
  - abdomen (injury classifiable to 863-866 and 868) 908.1
  - thorax (injury classifiable to 860-862) 908.0
- intracranial (injury classifiable to 850-854) 907.0
  - with skull fracture (injury classifiable to 800-801 and 803-804) 905.0
- nerve NEC (injury classifiable to 957) 907.9
  - cranial (injury classifiable to 950-951) 907.1
  - peripheral NEC (injury classifiable to 957) 907.9
    - lower limb and pelvic girdle (injury classifiable to 956) 907.5
    - upper limb and shoulder girdle (injury classifiable to 955) 907.4
  - roots and plexus(es), spinal (injury classifiable to 953) 907.3
  - trunk (injury classifiable to 954) 907.3
- pregnancy complication(s) 677
- puerperal complication(s) 677
- spinal
  - cord (injury classifiable to 806 and 952) 907.2
  - nerve root(s) and plexus(es) (injury classifiable to 953) 907.3
- superficial (injury classifiable to 910-919) 906.2
- tendon (tendon injury classifiable to 840-848, 880-884 with .2, and 890-894 with .2) 905.8
- meningitis
  - bacterial (conditions classifiable to 320)—*see* category 326
  - unspecified cause (conditions classifiable to 322)—*see* category 326
- myelitis (*see also* Late, effect(s) (of), encephalitis)—*see* category 326
- parasitic diseases (conditions classifiable to 001-136 NEC) 139.8
- phlebitis or thrombophlebitis of intracranial venous sinuses (conditions classifiable to 325)—*see* category 326
- poisoning due to drug, medicinal or biological substance (conditions classifiable to 960-979) 909.0
- poliomyelitis, acute (conditions classifiable to 045) 138
- radiation (conditions classifiable to 990) 909.2
- rickets 268.1
- sprain and strain without mention of tendon injury (injury classifiable to 840-848, except tendon injury) 905.7
  - tendon involvement 905.8
- toxic effect of
  - drug, medicinal or biological substance (conditions classifiable to 960-979) 909.0
  - nonmedical substance (conditions classifiable to 980-989) 909.1
- trachoma (conditions classifiable to 076) 139.1
- tuberculosis 137.0
  - bones and joints (conditions classifiable to 015) 137.3
  - central nervous system (conditions classifiable to 013) 137.1
  - genitourinary (conditions classifiable to 016) 137.2
  - pulmonary (conditions classifiable to 010-012) 137.0

Late effect(s) (of)—*continued*
- specified organs NEC (conditions classifiable to 014, 017-018) 137.4
- viral encephalitis (conditions classifiable to 049.8, 049.9, 062-064) 139.0
- wound, open
  - extremity (injury classifiable to 880-884 and 890-894, except .2) 906.1
    - tendon (injury classifiable to 880-884 with .2 and 890-894 with .2) 905.8
  - head, neck, and trunk (injury classifiable to 870-879) 906.0

Latent —*see* condition

Lateral —*see* condition

Laterocession —*see* Lateroversion

Lateroflexion —*see* Lateroversion

Lateroversion
- cervix—*see* Lateroversion, uterus
- uterus, uterine (cervix) (postinfectional) (postpartal, old) 621.6
  - congenital 752.3
  - in pregnancy or childbirth 654.4
    - affecting fetus or newborn 763.89

Lathyrism 988.2

Launois' syndrome (pituitary gigantism) 253.0

Launois-Bensaude's lipomatosis 272.8

Launois-Cléret syndrome (adiposogenital dystrophy) 253.8

Laurence-Moon-Biedl syndrome (obesity, polydactyly, and mental retardation) 759.89

LAV (disease) (illness) (infection)—*see* Human immunodeficiency virus (disease) (illness) (infection)

LAV/HTLV-III (disease) (illness) (infection)—*see* Human immunodeficiency virus (disease) (illness) (infection)

Lawford's syndrome (encephalocutaneous angiomatosis) 759.6

Lax, laxity —*see also* Relaxation
- ligament 728.4
- skin (acquired) 701.8
  - congenital 756.83

Laxative habit (*see also* Abuse, drugs, nondependent) 305.9

Lazy leukocyte syndrome 288.09

LCAD (long chain/very long chain acyl CoA dehydrogenase deficiency, VLCAD) 277.85

LCHAD (long chain 3-hydroxyacyl CoA dehydrogenase deficiency) 277.85

Lead —*see also* condition
- exposure to V15.86
- incrustation of cornea 371.15
- poisoning 984.9
  - specified type of lead—*see* Table of drugs and chemicals

Lead miner's lung 503

Leakage
- amniotic fluid 658.1
  - with delayed delivery 658.2
  - affecting fetus or newborn 761.1
- bile from drainage tube (T tube) 997.4
- blood (microscopic), fetal, into maternal circulation 656.0
  - affecting management of pregnancy or puerperium 656.0
- device, implant, or graft—*see* Complications, mechanical
- spinal fluid at lumbar puncture site 997.09
- urine, continuous 788.37

Leaky heart —*see* Endocarditis

Learning defect, specific NEC
    (strephosymbolia) 315.2
Leather bottle stomach (M8142/3) 151.9
Leber's
    congenital amaurosis 362.76
    optic atrophy (hereditary) 377.16
Lederer's anemia or disease (acquired
    infectious hemolytic anemia) 283.19
Lederer-Brill syndrome (acquired infectious
    hemolytic anemia) 283.19
Leeches (aquatic) (land) 134.2
Left-sided neglect 781.8
Leg —*see* condition
Legal investigation V62.5
Legg (-Calvé) -Perthes disease or syndrome
    (osteochondrosis, femoral capital) 732.1
Legionnaires' disease 482.84
Leigh's disease 330.8
Leiner's disease (exfoliative dermatitis) 695.89
Leiofibromyoma (M8890/0)—*see also*
    Leiomyoma
    uterus (cervix) (corpus) (*see also* Leiomyoma,
        uterus) 218.9
Leiomyoblastoma (M8891/1)—*see* Neoplasm,
    connective tissue, uncertain behavior
Leiomyofibroma (M8890/0)—*see also*
    Neoplasm, connective tissue, benign
    uterus (cervix) (corpus) (*see also* Leiomyoma,
        uterus) 218.9
Leiomyoma (M8890/0)—*see also* Neoplasm,
    connective tissue, benign
    bizarre (M8893/0)—*see* Neoplasm, connective
        tissue, benign
    cellular (M8892/1)—*see* Neoplasm, connective
        tissue, uncertain behavior
    epithelioid (M8891/1)—*see* Neoplasm,
        connective tissue, uncertain behavior
    prostate (polypoid) 600.20
        with
            other lower urinary tract symptoms (LUTS)
                600.21
            urinary
                obstruction 600.21
                retention 600.21
    uterus (cervix) (corpus) 218.9
        interstitial 218.1
        intramural 218.1
        submucous 218.0
        subperitoneal 218.2
        subserous 218.2
        vascular (M8894/0)—*see* Neoplasm,
            connective tissue, benign
Leiomyomatosis (intravascular) (M8890/1)—*see*
    Neoplasm, connective tissue, uncertain
    behavior
Leiomyosarcoma (M8890/3)—*see also*
    Neoplasm, connective tissue, malignant
    epithelioid (M8891/3)—*see* Neoplasm,
        connective tissue, malignant
Leishmaniasis 085.9
    American 085.5
        cutaneous 085.4
        mucocutaneous 085.5
    Asian desert 085.2
    Brazilian 085.5
    cutaneous 085.9
        acute necrotizing 085.2
        American 085.4
        Asian desert 085.2
        diffuse 085.3

Leishmaniasis—*continued*
    dry form 085.1
    Ethiopian 085.3
    eyelid 085.5 *[373.6]*
    late 085.1
    lepromatous 085.3
    recurrent 085.1
    rural 085.2
    ulcerating 085.1
    urban 085.1
    wet form 085.2
    zoonotic form 085.2
    dermal—*see also* Leishmaniasis, cutaneous
        post kala-azar 085.0
    eyelid 085.5 *[373.6]*
    infantile 085.0
    Mediterranean 085.0
    mucocutaneous (American) 085.5
    naso-oral 085.5
    nasopharyngeal 085.5
    Old World 085.1
    tegumentaria diffusa 085.4
    vaccination, prophylactic (against) V05.2
    visceral (Indian) 085.0
Leishmanoid, dermal —*see also* Leishmaniasis,
    cutaneous
    post kala-azar 085.0
Leloir's disease 695.4
Lemiere syndrome 451.89
Lenegre's disease 426.0
Lengthening, leg 736.81
Lennox-Gastaut syndrome 345.0
    with tonic seizures 345.1
Lennox's syndrome (*see also* Epilepsy) 345.0
Lens —*see* condition
Lenticonus (anterior) (posterior) (congenital)
    743.36
Lenticular degeneration, progressive 275.1
Lentiglobus (posterior) (congenital) 743.36
Lentigo (congenital) 709.09
    juvenile 709.09
    Maligna (M8742/2)—*see also* Neoplasm, skin,
        in situ
    melanoma (M8742/3)—*see* Melanoma
    senile 709.09
Leonine leprosy 030.0
Leontiasis
    ossium 733.3
    syphilitic 095.8
        congenital 090.5
Léopold-Lévi's syndrome (paroxysmal thyroid
    instability) 242.9
Lepore hemoglobin syndrome 282.49
Lepothrix 039.0
Lepra 030.9
    Willan's 696.1
Leprechaunism 259.8
Lepromatous leprosy 030.0
Leprosy 030.9
    anesthetic 030.1
    beriberi 030.1
    borderline (group B) (infiltrated) (neuritic) 030.3
    cornea (*see also* Leprosy, by type) 030.9
        [371.89]
    dimorphous (group B) (infiltrated)
        (lepromatous) (neuritic) (tuberculoid) 030.3
    eyelid 030.0 *[373.4]*
    indeterminate (group I) (macular) (neuritic)
        (uncharacteristic) 030.2
    leonine 030.0

Leprosy—*continued*
  lepromatous (diffuse) (infiltrated) (macular)
      (neuritic) (nodular) (type L) 030.0
  macular (early) (neuritic) (simple) 030.2
  maculoanesthetic 030.1
  mixed 030.0
  neuro 030.1
  nodular 030.0
  primary neuritic 030.3
  specified type or group NEC 030.8
  tubercular 030.1
  tuberculoid (macular) (maculoanesthetic)
      (major) (minor) (neuritic) (type T) 030.1
Leptocytosis, hereditary 282.49
Leptomeningitis (chronic) (circumscribed)
    (hemorrhagic) (nonsuppurative) (*see also*
    Meningitis) 322.9
  aseptic 047.9
    adenovirus 049.1
    Coxsackie virus 047.0
    ECHO virus 047.1
    enterovirus 047.9
    lymphocytic choriomeningitis 049.0
  epidemic 036.0
  late effect—*see* category 326
  meningococcal 036.0
  pneumococcal 320.1
  syphilitic 094.2
  tuberculous (*see also* Tuberculosis, meninges)
    013.0
Leptomeningopathy (*see also* Meningitis) 322.9
Leptospiral —*see* condition
Leptospirochetal —*see* condition
Leptospirosis 100.9
  autumnalis 100.89
  canicula 100.89
  grippotyphosa 100.89
  hebdomidis 100.89
  icterohemorrhagica 100.0
  nanukayami 100.89
  pomona 100.89
  Weil's disease 100.0
Leptothricosis —*see* Actinomycosis
Leptothrix infestation —*see* Actinomycosis
Leptotricosis —*see* Actinomycosis
Leptus dermatitis 133.8
Léri's pleonosteosis 756.89
Léri-Weill syndrome 756.59
Leriche syndrome (aortic bifurcation occlusion)
  444.0
Lermoyez's syndrome (*see also* Disease,
  Ménière's) 386.00
Lesbianism —*omit code*
  egodystonic 302.0
  problems with 302.0
Lesch-Nyhan syndrome (hypoxanthine-guanine-
  phosphoribosyltransferase deficiency) 277.2
Lesion(s)
  abducens nerve 378.54
  alveolar process 525.8
  anorectal 569.49
  aortic (valve)—*see* Endocarditis, aortic
  auditory nerve 388.5
  basal ganglion 333.90
  bile duct (*see also* Disease, biliary) 576.8
  bladder 596.9
  bone 733.90
  brachial plexus 353.0
  brain 348.8
    congenital 742.9

Lesion(s)—*continued*
  vascular (*see also* Lesion, cerebrovascular)
    437.9
    degenerative 437.1
    healed or old without residuals V12.59
    hypertensive 437.2
    late effect—*see* Late effect(s) (of)
      cerebrovascular disease
  buccal 528.9
  calcified—*see* Calcification
  canthus 373.9
  carate—*see* Pinta, lesions
  cardia 537.89
  cardiac—*see also* Disease, heart congenital 746.9
    valvular—*see* Endocarditis
  cauda equina 344.60
    with neurogenic bladder 344.61
  cecum 569.89
  cerebral—*see* Lesion, brain
  cerebrovascular (*see also* Disease,
    cerebrovascular NEC) 437.9
    degenerative 437.1
    healed or old without residuals V12.59
    hypertensive 437.2
    specified type NEC 437.8
  cervical root (nerve) NEC 353.2
  chiasmal 377.54
    associated with
      inflammatory disorders 377.54
      neoplasm NEC 377.52
      pituitary 377.51
      pituitary disorders 377.51
      vascular disorders 377.53
  chorda tympani 351.8
  coin, lung 793.1
  colon 569.89
  congenital—*see* Anomaly
  conjunctiva 372.9
  coronary artery (*see also* Ischemia, heart) 414.9
  cranial nerve 352.9
    first 352.0
    second 377.49
    third
      partial 378.51
      total 378.52
    fourth 378.53
    fifth 350.9
    sixth 378.54
    seventh 351.9
    eighth 388.5
    ninth 352.2
    tenth 352.3
    eleventh 352.4
    twelfth 352.5
  cystic—*see* Cyst
  degenerative—*see* Degeneration
  dermal (skin) 709.9
  Dieulafoy (hemorrhagic)
    of
      duodenum 537.84
      intestine 569.86
      stomach 537.84
  duodenum 537.89
    with obstruction 537.3
  eyelid 373.9
  gasserian ganglion 350.8
  gastric 537.89
  gastroduodenal 537.89
  gastrointestinal 569.89
  glossopharyngeal nerve 352.2
  heart (organic)—*see also* Disease, heart

Lesion(s)—*continued*
  traumatic NEC (*see also* nature and site of injury) 959.9
  tricuspid (valve)—*see* Endocarditis, tricuspid
  trigeminal nerve 350.9
  ulcerated or ulcerative—*see* Ulcer
  uterus NEC 621.9
  vagina 623.8
  vagus nerve 352.3
  valvular—*see* Endocarditis
  vascular 459.9
    affecting central nervous system (*see also* Lesion, cerebrovascular) 437.9
    following trauma (*see also* Injury, blood vessel, by site) 904.9
    retina 362.17
    traumatic—*see* Injury, blood vessel, by site
    umbilical cord 663.6
      affecting fetus or newborn 762.6
  visual
    cortex NEC (*see also* Disorder, visual, cortex) 377.73
    pathway NEC (*see also* Disorder, visual, pathway) 377.63
  warty—*see* Verruca
  white spot, on teeth 521.01
  x-ray NEC 990
Lethargic —*see* condition
Lethargy 780.79
Letterer-Siwe disease (acute histiocytosis X) (M9722/3) 202.5
Leucinosis 270.3
Leucocoria 360.44
Leucosarcoma (M9850/3) 207.8
Leukasmus 270.2
Leukemia, leukemic (congenital) (M9800/3) 208.9

> *Note—Use the following fifth-digit subclassification for categories 203-208:*
>
> *0 without mention of remission*
> *1 with remission*

  acute NEC (M9801/3) 208.0
  aleukemic NEC (M9804/3) 208.8
    granulocytic (M9864/3) 205.8
  basophilic (M9870/3) 205.1
  blast (cell) (M9801/3) 208.0
  blastic (M9801/3) 208.0
    granulocytic (M9861/3) 205.0
  chronic NEC (M9803/3) 208.1
  compound (M9810/3) 207.8
  eosinophilic (M9880/3) 205.1
  giant cell (M9910/3) 207.2
  granulocytic (M9860/3) 205.9
    acute (M9861/3) 205.0
    aleukemic (M9864/3) 205.8
    blastic (M9861/3) 205.0
    chronic (M9863/3) 205.1
    subacute (M9862/3) 205.2
    subleukemic (M9864/3) 205.8
  hairy cell (M9940/3) 202.4
  hemoblastic (M9801/3) 208.0
  histiocytic (M9890/3) 206.9
  lymphatic (M9820/3) 204.9
    acute (M9821/3) 204.0
    aleukemic (M9824/3) 204.8
    chronic (M9823/3) 204.1
    subacute (M9822/3) 204.2
    subleukemic (M9824/3) 204.8
  lymphoblastic (M9821/3) 204.0

Leukemia, leukemic—*continued*
  lymphocytic (M9820/3) 204.9
    acute (M9821/3) 204.0
    aleukemic (M9824/3) 204.8
    chronic (M9823/3) 204.1
    subacute (M9822/3) 204.2
    subleukemic (M9824/3) 204.8
  lymphogenous (M9820/3)—*see* Leukemia, lymphoid
  lymphoid (M9820/3) 204.9
    acute (M9821/3) 204.0
    aleukemic (M9824/3) 204.8
    blastic (M9821/3) 204.0
    chronic (M9823/3) 204.1
    subacute (M9822/3) 204.2
    subleukemic (M9824/3) 204.8
  lymphosarcoma cell (M9850/3) 207.8
  mast cell (M9900/3) 207.8
  megakaryocytic (M9910/3) 207.2
  megakaryocytoid (M9910/3) 207.2
  mixed (cell) (M9810/3) 207.8
  monoblastic (M9891/3) 206.0
  monocytic (Schilling-type) (M9890/3) 206.9
    acute (M9891/3) 206.0
    aleukemic (M9894/3) 206.8
    chronic (M9893/3) 206.1
    Naegeli-type (M9863/3) 205.1
    subacute (M9892/3) 206.2
    subleukemic (M9894/3) 206.8
  monocytoid (M9890/3) 206.9
    acute (M9891/3) 206.0
    aleukemic (M9894/3) 206.8
    chronic (M9893/3) 206.1
    myelogenous (M9863/3) 205.1
    subacute (M9892/3) 206.2
    subleukemic (M9894/3) 206.8
  monomyelocytic (M9860/3)—*see* Leukemia, myelomonocytic
  myeloblastic (M9861/3) 205.0
  myelocytic (M9863/3) 205.1
    acute (M9861/3) 205.0
  myelogenous (M9860/3) 205.9
    acute (M9861/3) 205.0
    aleukemic (M9864/3) 205.8
    chronic (M9863/3) 205.1
    monocytoid (M9863/3) 205.1
    subacute (M9862/3) 205.2
    subleukemic (M9864) 205.8
  myeloid (M9860/3) 205.9
    acute (M9861/3) 205.0
    aleukemic (M9864/3) 205.8
    chronic (M9863/3) 205.1
    subacute (M9862/3) 205.2
    subleukemic (M9864/3) 205.8
  myelomonocytic (M9860/3) 205.9
    acute (M9861/3) 205.0
    chronic (M9863/3) 205.1
  Naegeli-type monocytic (M9863/3) 205.1
  neutrophilic (M9865/3) 205.1
  plasma cell (M9830/3) 203.1
  plasmacytic (M9830/3) 203.1
  prolymphocytic (M9825/3)—*see* Leukemia, lymphoid
  promyelocytic, acute (M9866/3) 205.0
  Schilling-type monocytic (M9890/3)—*see* Leukemia, monocytic
  stem cell (M9801/3) 208.0
  subacute NEC (M9802/3) 208.2
  subleukemic NEC (M9804/3) 208.8
  thrombocytic (M9910/3) 207.2
  undifferentiated (M9801/3) 208.0

Leukemoid reaction (basophilic) (lymphocytic)
      (monocytic) (myelocytic) (neutrophilic)
      288.62
Leukoclastic vasculitis 446.29
Leukocoria 360.44
Leukocythemia —*see* Leukemia
Leukocytopenia 288.50
Leukocytosis 288.60
   basophilic 288.8
   eosinophilic 288.3
   lymphocytic 288.8
   monocytic 288.8
   neutrophilic 288.8
Leukoderma 709.09
   syphilitic 091.3
      late 095.8
Leukodermia (*see also* Leukoderma) 709.09
Leukodystrophy (cerebral) (globoid cell)
      (metachromatic) (progressive) (sudanophilic)
      330.0
Leukoedema, mouth or tongue 528.79
Leukoencephalitis
   acute hemorrhagic (postinfectious) NEC 136.9
      [323.61]
      postimmunization or postvaccinal 323.51
   subacute sclerosing 046.2
      van Bogaert's 046.2
   van Bogaert's (sclerosing) 046.2
Leukoencephalopathy (*see also* Encephalitis)
      323.9
   acute necrotizing hemorrhagic (postinfectious)
      136.9 *[323.61]*
      postimmunization or postvaccinal 323.51
   metachromatic 330.0
   multifocal (progressive) 046.3
   progressive multifocal 046.3
Leukoerythroblastosis 289.9
Leukoerythrosis 289.0
Leukokeratosis (*see also* Leukoplakia) 702.8
   mouth 528.6
   nicotina palati 528.79
   tongue 528.6
Leukokoria 360.44
Leukokoraurosis vulva, vulvae 624.0
Leukolymphosarcoma (M9850/3) 207.8
Leukoma (cornea) (interfering with central
      vision) 371.03
   adherent 371.04
Leukomalacia, periventricular 779.7
Leukomelanopathy, hereditary 288.2
Leukonychia (punctata) (striata) 703.8
   congenital 757.5
Leukopathia
   unguium 703.8
      congenital 757.5
Leukopenia 288.50
   basophilic 288.59
   cyclic 288.02
   eosinophilic 288.59
   familial 288.59
   malignant (see also Agranulocytosis) 288.09
   periodic 288.02
   transitory neonatal 776.7
Leukopenic —*see* condition
Leukoplakia 702.8
   anus 569.49
   bladder (postinfectional) 596.8
   buccal 528.6
   cervix (uteri) 622.2
   esophagus 530.83
   gingiva 528.6

Leukoplakia—*continued*
   kidney (pelvis) 593.89
   larynx 478.79
   lip 528.6
   mouth 528.6
   oral soft tissue (including tongue) (mucosa) 528.6
   palate 528.6
   pelvis (kidney) 593.89
   penis (infectional) 607.0
   rectum 569.49
   syphilitic 095.8
   tongue 528.6
   tonsil 478.29
   ureter (postinfectional) 593.89
   urethra (postinfectional) 599.84
   uterus 621.8
   vagina 623.1
   vesical 596.8
   vocal cords 478.5
   vulva 624.0
Leukopolioencephalopathy 330.0
Leukorrhea (vagina) 623.5
   due to trichomonas (vaginalis) 131.00
   trichomonal (Trichomonas vaginalis) 131.00
Leukosarcoma (M9850/3) 207.8
Leukosis (M9800/3)—*see* Leukemia
Lev's disease or syndrome (acquired complete
      heart block) 426.0
Levi's syndrome (pituitary dwarfism) 253.3
Levocardia (isolated) 746.87
   with situs inversus 759.3
Levulosuria 271.2
Lewandowski's disease (primary) (*see also*
      Tuberculosis) 017.0
Lewandowski-Lutz disease (epidermodysplasia
      verruciformis) 078.19
Lewy body dementia 331.82
Lewy body disease 331.82
Leyden's disease (periodic vomiting) 536.2
Leyden's-Möbius dystrophy 359.1
Leydig cell
   carcinoma (M8650/3)
      specified site—*see* Neoplasm, by site,
         malignant
      unspecified site
         female 183.0
         male 186.9
   tumor (M8650/1)
      benign (M8650/0)
         specified site—*see* Neoplasm, by site, benign
         unspecified site
            female 220
            male 222.0
      malignant (M8650/3)
         specified site—*see* Neoplasm, by site,
            malignant
         unspecified site
            female 183.0
            male 186.9
      specified site—*see* Neoplasm, by site, uncertain
         behavior
      unspecified site
         female 236.2
         male 236.4
Leydig-Sertoli cell tumor (M8631/0)
   specified site—*see* Neoplasm, by site, benign
   unspecified site
      female 220
      male 222.0
LGSIL (low grade squamous intraepithelial
      lesion) 795.03
Liar, pathologic 301.7

Libman-Sacks disease or syndrome 710.0
   [424.91]
Lice (infestation) 132.9
  body (pediculus corporis) 132.1
  crab 132.2
  head (pediculus capitis) 132.0
  mixed (classifiable to more than one of the
    categories 132.0-132.2) 132.3
  pubic (pediculus pubis) 132.2
Lichen 697.9
  albus 701.0
  annularis 695.89
  atrophicus 701.0
  corneus obtusus 698.3
  myxedematous 701.8
  nitidus 697.1
  pilaris 757.39
    acquired 701.1
  planopilaris 697.0
  planus (acute) (chronicus) (hypertrophic)
    (verrucous) 697.0
    morphoeicus 701.0
    sclerosus (et atrophicus) 701.0
  ruber 696.4
    acuminatus 696.4
    moniliformis 697.8
    obtusus corneus 698.3
    of Wilson 697.0
    planus 697.0
  sclerosus (et atrophicus) 701.0
  scrofulosus (primary) (*see also* Tuberculosis)
    017.0
  simplex (Vidal's) 698.3
    chronicus 698.3
    circumscriptus 698.3
  spinulosus 757.39
    mycotic 117.9
  striata 697.8
  urticatus 698.2
Lichenification 698.3
  nodular 698.3
Lichenoides tuberculosis (primary) (*see also*
  Tuberculosis) 017.0
Lichtheim's disease or syndrome (subacute
  combined sclerosis with pernicious anemia)
  281.0 *[336.2]*
Lien migrans 289.59
Lientery (*see also* Diarrhea) 787.91
  infectious 009.2
Life circumstance problem NEC V62.89
Li-Fraumeni cancer syndrome V84.01
Ligament —*see* condition
Light-for-dates (infant) 764.0
  with signs of fetal malnutrition 764.1
  affecting management of pregnancy 656.5
Light-headedness 780.4
Lightning (effects) (shock) (stroke) (struck by) 994.0
  burn—*see* Burn, by site
  foot 266.2
Lightwood's disease or syndrome (renal tubular
  acidosis) 588.89
Lignac's disease (cystinosis) 270.0
Lignac (-de Toni) (-Fanconi) (-Debré) syndrome
  (cystinosis) 270.0
Lignac (-Fanconi) syndrome (cystinosis) 270.0
Ligneous thyroiditis 245.3
Likoff's syndrome (angina in menopausal
  women) 413.9
Limb —*see* condition
Limitation of joint motion (*see also* Stiffness,
  joint) 719.5
  sacroiliac 724.6

Limit dextrinosis 271.0
Limited
  cardiac reserve—*see* Disease, heart
  duction, eye NEC 378.63
  mandibular range of motion 524.52
Lindau's disease (retinocerebral angiomatosis)
  759.6
Lindau (-von Hippel) disease (angiomatosis
  retinocerebellosa) 759.6
Linea corneae senilis 371.41
Lines
  Beau's (transverse furrows on fingernails) 703.8
  Harris' 733.91
  Hudson-Stähli 371.11
  Stähli's 371.11
Lingua
  geographical 529.1
  nigra (villosa) 529.3
  plicata 529.5
    congenital 750.13
  tylosis 528.6
Lingual (tongue)—*see also* condition
  thyroid 759.2
Linitis (gastric) 535.4
  plastica (M8142/3) 151.9
Lioderma essentialis (cum melanosis et
  telangiectasia) 757.33
Lip —*see also* condition
  biting 528.9
Lipalgia 272.8
Lipedema —*see* Edema
Lipemia (*see also* Hyperlipidemia) 272.4
  retina, retinalis 272.3
Lipidosis 272.7
  cephalin 272.7
  cerebral (infantile) (juvenile) (late) 330.1
  cerebroretinal 330.1 *[362.71]*
  cerebroside 272.7
  cerebrospinal 272.7
  chemically-induced 272.7
  cholesterol 272.7
  diabetic 250.8 *[272.7]*
  dystopic (hereditary) 272.7
  glycolipid 272.7
  hepatosplenomegalic 272.3
  hereditary, dystopic 272.7
  sulfatide 330.0
Lipoadenoma (M8324/0)—*see* Neoplasm, by
  site, benign
Lipoblastoma (M8881/0)—*see* Lipoma, by site
Lipoblastomatosis (M8881/0)—*see* Lipoma, by
  site
Lipochondrodystrophy 277.5
Lipochrome histiocytosis (familial) 288.1
Lipodystrophia progressiva 272.6
Lipodystrophy (progressive) 272.6
  insulin 272.6
  intestinal 040.2
  mesenteric 567.82
Lipofibroma (M8851/0)—*see* Lipoma, by site
Lipoglycoproteinosis 272.8
Lipogranuloma, sclerosing 709.8
Lipogranulomatosis (disseminated) 272.8
  kidney 272.8
Lipoid —*see* condition
  histiocytosis 272.7
    essential 272.7
  nephrosis (*see also* Nephrosis) 581.3
  proteinosis of Urbach 272.8
Lipoidemia (*see also* Hyperlipidemia) 272.4
Lipoidosis (*see also* Lipidosis) 272.7

Lymphangiomyomatosis (M9174/1)—*see*
    Neoplasm, connective tissue, uncertain
    behavior
Lymphangiosarcoma (M9170/3)—*see*
    Neoplasm, connective tissue, malignant
Lymphangitis 457.2
    with
        abortion—*see* Abortion, by type, with sepsis
        abscess—*see* Abscess, by site
        cellulitis—*see* Abscess, by site
        ectopic pregnancy (*see also* categories
            633.0-633.9) 639.0
        molar pregnancy (*see also* categories 630-632)
            639.0
    acute (with abscess or cellulitis) 682.9
        specified site—*see* Abscess, by site
    breast, puerperal, postpartum 675.2
    chancroidal 099.0
    chronic (any site) 457.2
    due to
        Brugia (Wuchereria) malayi 125.1
        Wuchereria bancrofti 125.0
    following
        abortion 639.0
        ectopic or molar pregnancy 639.0
    gangrenous 457.2
    penis
        acute 607.2
        gonococcal (acute) 098.0
            chronic or duration of 2 months or more
                098.2
    puerperal, postpartum, childbirth 670
    strumous, tuberculous (*see also* Tuberculosis)
        017.2
    subacute (any site) 457.2
    tuberculous—*see* Tuberculosis, lymph gland
Lymphatic (vessel)—*see* condition
Lymphatism 254.8
    scrofulous (*see also* Tuberculosis) 017.2
Lymphectasia 457.1
Lymphedema (*see also* Elephantiasis) 457.1
    acquired (chronic) 457.1
    chronic hereditary 757.0
    congenital 757.0
    idiopathic hereditary 757.0
    praecox 457.1
    secondary 457.1
    surgical NEC 997.99
        postmastectomy (syndrome) 457.0
Lymph-hemangioma (M9120/0)—*see*
    Hemangioma, by site
Lymphoblastic —*see* condition
Lymphoblastoma (diffuse) (M9630/3) 200.1
    giant follicular (M9690/3) 202.0
    macrofollicular (M9690/3) 202.0
Lymphoblastosis, acute benign 075
Lymphocele 457.8
Lymphocythemia 288.51
Lymphocytic —*see also* condition
    chorioencephalitis (acute) (serous) 049.0
    choriomeningitis (acute) (serous) 049.0
Lymphocytoma (diffuse) (malignant) (M9620/3)
    200.1
Lymphocytomatosis (M9620/3) 200.1
Lymphocytopenia 288.51
Lymphocytosis (symptomatic) 288.61
    infectious (acute) 078.89
Lymphoepithelioma (M8082/3)—*see* Neoplasm,
    by site, malignant

Lymphogranuloma (malignant) (M9650/3) 201.9
    inguinale 099.1
    venereal (any site) 099.1
        with stricture of rectum 099.1
    venereum 099.1
Lymphogranulomatosis (malignant) (M9650/3)
    201.9
    benign (Boeck's sarcoid) (Schaumann's) 135
    Hodgkin's (M9650/3) 201.9
Lymphohistiocytosis, familial hemophagocytic
    288.4
Lymphoid —*see* condition
Lympholeukoblastoma (M9850/3) 207.8
Lympholeukosarcoma (M9850/3) 207.8
Lymphoma (malignant) (M9590/3) 202.8

---

*Note—Use the following fifth-digit
subclassification with categories 200-202:*

0 *unspecifidd site*
1 *lymph nodes of head, face and neck*
2 *intrathoracic lymph nodes*
3 *intra-abdominal lymph nodes*
4 *lymph nodes of axilla and upper limb*
5 *lymph nodes of inguinal region and
   lower limb*
6 *intrapelvic lymph nodes*
7 *spleen*
8 *lymph nodes of multiple sites*

---

    wenign (M9580/0)—*see* Neoplasm, by site, benign
    Burkitt's type (lymphoblastic) (undifferentiated)
        (M9750/3) 200.2
    Castleman's (mediastinal lymph node hyperplasia)
        785.6
    centroblastic-centrocytic
        diffuse (M9614/3) 202.8
        follicular (M9692/3) 202.0
    centroblastic type (diffuse) (M9632/3) 202.8
        follicular (M9697/3) 202.0
    centrocytic (M9622/3) 202.8
    compound (M9613/3) 200.8
    convoluted cell type (lymphoblastic) (M9602/3)
        202.8
    diffuse NEC (M9590/3) 202.8
    follicular (giant) (M9690/3) 202.0
        center cell (diffuse) (M9615/3) 202.8
            cleaved (diffuse) (M9623/3) 202.8
                follicular (M9695/3) 202.0
            non-cleaved (diffuse) (M9633/3) 202.8
                follicular (M9698/3) 202.0
        centroblastic-centrocytic (M9692/3) 202.0
        centroblastic type (M9697/3) 202.0
        lymphocytic
            intermediate differentiation (M9694/3) 202.0
            poorly differentiated (M9696/3) 202.0
        mixed (cell type) (lymphocytic-histiocytic)
            (small cell and large cell) (M9691/3) 202.0
    germinocytic (M9622/3) 202.8
    giant, follicular or follicle (M9690/3) 202.0
    histiocytic (diffuse) (M9640/3) 200.0
        nodular (M9642/3) 200.0
        pleomorphic cell type (M9641/3) 200.0
    Hodgkin's (M9650/3) (*see also* Disease,
        Hodgkin's) 201.9
    immunoblastic (type) (M9612/3) 200.8
    large cell (M9640/3) 200.0
        nodular (M9642/3) 200.0
        pleomorphic cell type (M9641/3) 200.0
    lymphoblastic (diffuse) (M9630/3) 200.1
        Burkitt's type (M9750/3) 200.2
        convoluted cell type (M9602/3) 202.8

Lymphoma—*continued*
  lymphocytic (cell type) (diffuse) (M9620/3) 200.1
    with plasmacytoid differentiation, diffuse
      (M9611/3) 200.8
    intermediate differentiation (diffuse)
      (M9621/3) 200.1
     follicular (M9694/3) 202.0
     nodular (M9694/3) 202.0
    nodular (M9690/3) 202.0
    poorly differentiated (diffuse) (M9630/3) 200.1
     follicular (M9696/3) 202.0
     nodular (M9696/3) 202.0
    well differentiated (diffuse) (M9620/3) 200.1
     follicular (M9693/3) 202.0
     nodular (M9693/3) 202.0
  lymphocytic-histiocytic, mixed (diffuse)
    (M9613/3) 200.8
    follicular (M9691/3) 202.0
    nodular (M9691/3) 202.0
  lymphoplasmacytoid type (M9611/3) 200.8
  lymphosarcoma type (M9610/3) 200.1
  macrofollicular (M9690/3) 202.0
  mixed cell type (diffuse) (M9613/3) 200.8
    follicular (M9691/3) 202.0
    nodular (M9691/3) 202.0
  nodular (M9690/3) 202.0
    histiocytic (M9642/3) 200.0
    lymphocytic (M9690.3) 202.0
     intermediate differentiation (M9694/3) 202.0
     poorly differentiated (M9696/3) 202.0
    mixed (cell type) (lymphocytic-histiocytic)
     (small cell and large cell) (M9691/3) 202.0
  non-Hodgkin's type NEC (M9591/3) 202.8
  reticulum cell (type) (M9640/3) 200.0
  small cell and large cell, mixed (diffuse)
    (M9613/3) 200.8
    follicular (M9691/3) 202.0
    nodular (9691/3) 202.0
  stem cell (type) (M9601/3) 202.8
  T-cell 202.1
  undifferentiated (cell type) (non-Burkitt's)
    (M9600/3) 202.8
    Burkitt's type (M9750/3) 200.2
Lymphomatosis (M9590/3)—*see also*
  Lymphoma
  granulomatous 099.1
Lymphopathia
  venereum 099.1
  veneris 099.1
Lymphopenia 288.51
  familial 279.2
Lymphoreticulosis, benign (of inoculation)
  078.3
Lymphorrhea 457.8
Lymphosarcoma (M9610/3) 200.1
  diffuse (M9610/3) 200.1
    with plasmacytoid differentiation (M9611/3)
     200.8
    lymphoplasmacytic (M9611/3) 200.8
  follicular (giant) (M9690/3) 202.0
    lymphoblastic (M9696/3) 202.0
    lymphocytic, intermediate differentiation
     (M9694/3) 202.0
    mixed cell type (M9691/3) 202.0
  giant follicular (M9690/3) 202.0
  Hodgkin's (M9650/3) 201.9
  immunoblastic (M9612/3) 200.8
  lymphoblastic (diffuse) (M9630/3) 200.1
    follicular (M9696/3) 202.0
    nodular (M9696/3) 202.0
  lymphocytic (diffuse) (M9620/3) 200.1

Lymphosarcoma—*continued*
  intermediate differentiation (diffuse)
    (M9621/3) 200.1
    follicular (M9694/3) 202.0
    nodular (M9694/3) 202.0
  mixed cell type (diffuse) (M9613/3) 200.8
    follicular (M9691/3) 202.0
    nodular (M9691/3) 202.0
  nodular (M9690/3) 202.0
    lymphoblastic (M9696/3) 202.0
    lymphocytic, intermediate differentiation
     (M9694/3) 202.0
    mixed cell type (M9691/3) 202.0
  prolymphocytic (M9631/3) 200.1
  reticulum cell (M9640/3) 200.0
Lymphostasis 457.8
Lypemania (*see also* Melancholia) 296.2
Lyssa 071

M

Macacus ear 744.29
Maceration
  fetus (cause not stated) 779.9
  wet feet, tropical (syndrome) 991.4
Machado-Joseph disease 334.8
Machupo virus hemorrhagic fever 078.7
Macleod's syndrome (abnormal transradiancy,
    one lung) 492.8
Macrocephalia, macrocephaly 756.0
Macrocheilia (congenital) 744.81
Macrochilia (congenital) 744.81
Macrocolon (congenital) 751.3
Macrocornea 743.41
  associated with buphthalmos 743.22
Macrocytic —*see* condition
Macrocytosis 289.89
Macrodactylia, macrodactylism (fingers)
    (thumbs) 755.57
  toes 755.65
Macrodontia 520.2
Macroencephaly 742.4
Macrogenia 524.05
Macrogenitosomia (female) (male) (praecox)
    255.2
Macrogingivae 523.8
Macroglobulinemia (essential) (idiopathic)
    (monoclonal) (primary) (syndrome)
    (Waldenström's) 273.3
Macroglossia (congenital) 750.15
  acquired 529.8
Macrognathia, macrognathism (congenital)
    524.00
  mandibular 524.02
    alveolar 524.72
  maxillary 524.01
    alveolar 524.71
Macrogyria (congenital) 742.4
Macrohydrocephalus (*see also* Hydrocephalus)
    331.4
Macromastia (*see also* Hypertrophy, breast)
    611.1
Macrophage activation syndrome 288.4
Macropsia 368.14
Macrosigmoid 564.7
  congenital 751.3
Macrospondylitis, acromegalic 253.0
Macrostomia (congenital) 744.83
Macrotia (external ear) (congenital) 744.22
Macula
  cornea, corneal
    congenital 743.43
      interfering with vision 743.42
     interfering with central vision 371.03
     not interfering with central vision 371.02
    degeneration (*see also* Degeneration, macula)
      362.50
     hereditary (*see also* Dystrophy, retina) 362.70
    edema, cystoid 362.53
Maculae ceruleae 132.1
Macules and papules 709.8
Maculopathy, toxic 362.55
Madarosis 374.55
Madelung's
  deformity (radius) 755.54
  disease (lipomatosis) 272.8
  lipomatosis 272.8

Madness (*see also* Psychosis) 298.9
  myxedema (acute) 293.0
    subacute 293.1
Madura
  disease (actinomycotic) 039.9
    mycotic 117.4
  foot (actinomycotic) 039.4
    mycotic 117.4
Maduromycosis (actinomycotic) 039.9
  mycotic 117.4
Maffucci's syndrome (dyschondroplasia with
    hemangiomas) 756.4
Magenblase syndrome 306.4
Main en griffe (acquired) 736.06
  congenital 755.59
Maintenance
  chemotherapy regimen or treatment V58.11
  dialysis regimen or treatment
    extracorporeal (renal) V56.0
    peritoneal V56.8
    renal V56.0
  drug therapy or regimen
    chemotherapy, antineoplastic V58.11
    immunotherapy, antineoplastic V58.12
  external fixation NEC V54.89
  radiotherapy V58.0
  traction NEC V54.89
Majocchi's
  disease (purpura annularis telangiectodes) 709.1
  granuloma 110.6
Major —*see* condition
Mal
  cerebral (idiopathic) (*see also* Epilepsy) 345.9
  comital (*see also* Epilepsy) 345.9
  de los pintos (*see also* Pinta) 103.9
  de Meleda 757.39
  de mer 994.6
  lie—*see* Presentation, fetal
  perforant (*see also* Ulcer, lower extremity)
    707.15
Malabar itch 110.9
  beard 110.0
  foot 110.4
  scalp 110.0
Malabsorption 579.9
  calcium 579.8
  carbohydrate 579.8
  disaccharide 271.3
  drug-induced 579.8
  due to bacterial overgrowth 579.8
  fat 579.8
  folate, congenital 281.2
  galactose 271.1
  glucose-galactose (congenital) 271.3
  intestinal 579.9
  isomaltose 271.3
  lactose (hereditary) 271.3
  methionine 270.4
  monosaccharide 271.8
  postgastrectomy 579.3
  postsurgical 579.3
  protein 579.8
  sucrose (-isomaltose) (congenital) 271.3
  syndrome 579.9
    postgastrectomy 579.3
    postsurgical 579.3
Malacia, bone 268.2
  juvenile (*see also* Rickets) 268.0

Malformation—*continued*
  specified type NEC 748.8
  Rieger's 743.44
  sense organs NEC 742.9
    specified type NEC 742.8
  skin 757.9
    specified type NEC 757.8
  spinal cord 742.9
  teeth, tooth NEC 520.9
  tendon 756.9
  throat 750.9
  umbilical cord (complicating delivery) 663.9
    affecting fetus or newborn 762.6
  umbilicus 759.9
  urinary system NEC 753.9
    specified type NEC 753.8
Malfunction —*see also* Dysfunction
  arterial graft 996.1
  cardiac pacemaker 996.01
  catheter device—*see* Complications,
    mechanical, catheter
  colostomy 569.62
    valve 569.62
  cystostomy 997.5
  device, implant, or graft NEC—*see*
    Complications, mechanical
  enteric stoma 569.62
  enterostomy 569.62
  esophagostomy 530.87
  gastroenteric 536.8
  gastrostomy 536.42
  ileostomy
    valve 569.62
  nephrostomy 997.5
  pacemaker—*see* Complications, mechanical,
    pacemaker
  prosthetic device, internal—*see* Complications,
    mechanical
  tracheostomy 519.02
  valve
    colostomy 569.62
    ileostomy 569.62
  vascular graft or shunt 996.1
Malgaigne's fracture (closed) 808.43
  open 808.53
Malherbe's
  calcifying epithelioma (M8110/0)—*see*
    Neoplasm, skin, benign
  tumor (M8110/0)—*see* Neoplasm, skin, benign
Malibu disease 919.8
  infected 919.9
Malignancy (M8000/3)—*see* Neoplasm, by site,
  malignant
Malignant —*see* condition
Malingerer, malingering V65.2
Mallet, finger (acquired) 736.1
  congenital 755.59
  late effect of rickets 268.1
Malleus 024
Mallory's bodies 034.1
Mallory-Weiss syndrome 530.7
Malnutrition (calorie) 263.9
  complicating pregnancy 648.9
  degree
    first 263.1
    second 263.0
    third 262
    mild 263.1
    moderate 263.0
    severe 261
      protein-calorie 262

Malnutrition—*continued*
  fetus 764.2
    "light-for-dates" 764.1
  following gastrointestinal surgery 579.3
  intrauterine or fetal 764.2
    fetus or infant "light-for-dates" 764.1
  lack of care, or neglect (child) (infant) 995.52
    adult 995.84
  malignant 260
  mild 263.1
  moderate 263.0
  protein 260
  protein-calorie 263.9
    severe 262
    specified type NEC 263.8
  severe 261
    protein-calorie NEC 262
Malocclusion (teeth) 524.4
  angle's class I 524.21
  angle's class II 524.22
  angle's class III 524.23
  due to
    abnormal swallowing 524.59
    accessory teeth (causing crowding) 524.31
    dentofacial abnormality NEC 524.89
    impacted teeth (causing crowding) 520.6
    missing teeth 524.30
    mouth breathing 524.59
    sleep posture 524.59
    supernumerary teeth (causing crowding)
      524.31
    thumb sucking 524.59
    tongue, lip, or finger habits 524.59
  temporomandibular (joint) 524.69
Malposition
  cardiac apex (congenital) 746.87
  cervix—*see* Malposition, uterus
  congenital
    adrenal (gland) 759.1
    alimentary tract 751.8
      lower 751.5
      upper 750.8
    aorta 747.21
    appendix 751.5
    arterial trunk 747.29
    artery (peripheral) NEC (*see also* Malposition,
      congenital, peripheral vascular system)
      747.60
      coronary 746.85
      pulmonary 747.3
    auditory canal 744.29
      causing impairment of hearing 744.02
    auricle (ear) 744.29
      causing impairment of hearing 744.02
      cervical 744.43
    biliary duct or passage 751.69
    bladder (mucosa) 753.8
      exteriorized or extroverted 753.5
    brachial plexus 742.8
    brain tissue 742.4
    breast 757.6
    bronchus 748.3
    cardiac apex 746.87
    cecum 751.5
    clavicle 755.51
    colon 751.5
    digestive organ or tract NEC 751.8
      lower 751.5
      upper 750.8
    ear (auricle) (external) 744.29
      ossicles 744.04

Malposition—*continued*
  endocrine (gland) NEC 759.2
  epiglottis 748.3
  Eustachian tube 744.24
  eye 743.8
  facial features 744.89
  fallopian tube 752.19
  finger(s) 755.59
    supernumerary 755.01
  foot 755.67
  gallbladder 751.69
  gastrointestinal tract 751.8
  genitalia, genital organ(s) or tract
    female 752.89
      external 752.49
      internal NEC 752.89
    male 752.89
      penis 752.69
      scrotal transposition 752.81
  glottis 748.3
  hand 755.59
  heart 746.87
    dextrocardia 746.87
      with complete transposition of viscera
        759.3
  hepatic duct 751.69
  hip (joint) (*see also* Dislocation, hip,
    congenital) 754.30
  intestine (large) (small) 751.5
    with anomalous adhesions, fixation, or
      malrotation 751.4
  joint NEC 755.8
  kidney 753.3
  larynx 748.3
  limb 755.8
    lower 755.69
    upper 755.59
  liver 751.69
  lung (lobe) 748.69
  nail(s) 757.5
  nerve 742.8
  nervous system NEC 742.8
  nose, nasal (septum) 748.1
  organ or site NEC—*see* Anomaly, specified
    type NEC, by site
  ovary 752.0
  pancreas 751.7
  parathyroid (gland) 759.2
  patella 755.64
  peripheral vascular system 747.60
    gastrointestinal 747.61
    lower limb 747.64
    renal 747.62
    specified NEC 747.69
    spinal 747.82
    upper limb 747.63
  pituitary (gland) 759.2
  respiratory organ or system NEC 748.9
  rib (cage) 756.3
    supernumerary in cervical region 756.2
  scapula 755.59
  shoulder 755.59
  spinal cord 742.59
  spine 756.19
  spleen 759.0
  sternum 756.3
  stomach 750.7
  symphysis pubis 755.69
  testis (undescended) 752.51
  thymus (gland) 759.2
  thyroid (gland) (tissue) 759.2

Malposition—*continued*
  cartilage 748.3
  toe(s) 755.66
    supernumerary 755.02
  tongue 750.19
  trachea 748.3
  uterus 752.3
  vein(s) (peripheral) NEC (*see also*
      Malposition, congenital, peripheral
      vascular system) 747.60
    great 747.49
    portal 747.49
    pulmonary 747.49
  vena cava (inferior) (superior) 747.49
  device, implant, or graft—*see* Complications,
    mechanical
  fetus NEC (*see also* Presentation, fetal) 652.9
    with successful version 652.1
    affecting fetus or newborn 763.1
    before labor, affecting fetus or newborn 761.7
    causing obstructed labor 660.0
    in multiple gestation (one fetus or more) 652.6
      with locking 660.5
      causing obstructed labor 660.0
  gallbladder (*see also* Disease, gallbladder) 575.8
  gastrointestinal tract 569.89
    congenital 751.8
  heart (*see also* Malposition, congenital, heart)
    746.87
  intestine 569.89
    congenital 751.5
  pelvic organs or tissues
    in pregnancy or childbirth 654.4
      affecting fetus or newborn 763.89
      causing obstructed labor 660.2
        affecting fetus or newborn 763.1
  placenta—*see* Placenta, previa
  stomach 537.89
    congenital 750.7
  tooth, teeth 524.30
    with impaction 520.6
  uterus (acquired) (acute) (adherent) (any degree)
      (asymptomatic) (postinfectional) (postpartal,
      old) 621.6
    anteflexion or anteversion (*see also*
      Anteversion, uterus) 621.6
    congenital 752.3
    flexion 621.6
      lateral (*see also* Lateroversion, uterus) 621.6
    in pregnancy or childbirth 654.4
      affecting fetus or newborn 763.89
      causing obstructed labor 660.2
        affecting fetus or newborn 763.1
    inversion 621.6
    lateral (flexion) (version) (*see also*
      Lateroversion, uterus) 621.6
    lateroflexion (*see also* Lateroversion, uterus)
      621.6
    lateroversion (*see also* Lateroversion, uterus)
      621.6
    retroflexion or retroversion (*see also*
      Retroversion, uterus) 621.6
Malposture 729.9
Malpresentation, fetus (*see also* Presentation,
    fetal) 652.9
Malrotation
  cecum 751.4
  colon 751.4
  intestine 751.4
  kidney 753.3
Malta fever (*see also* Brucellosis) 023.9
Maltosuria 271.3

Maltreatment (of)
  adult 995.80
    emotional 995.82
    multiple forms 995.85
    neglect (nutritional) 995.84
    physical 995.81
    psychological 995.82
    sexual 995.83
  child 995.50
    emotional 995.51
    multiple forms 995.59
    neglect (nutritional) 995.52
    psychological 995.51
    physical 995.54
      shaken infant syndrome 995.55
    sexual 995.53
  spouse (*see also* Maltreatment, adult) 995.80
Malt workers' lung 495.4
Malum coxae senilis 715.25
Malunion, fracture 733.81
Mammillitis (*see also* Mastitis) 611.0
  puerperal, postpartum 675.2
Mammitis (*see also* Mastitis) 611.0
  puerperal, postpartum 675.2
Mammographic
  calcification 793.89
  calculus 793.89
  microcalcification 793.81
Mammoplasia 611.1
Management
  contraceptive V25.9
    specified type NEC V25.8
  procreative V26.9
    specified type NEC V26.8
Mangled NEC (*see also* nature and site of injury)
  959.9
Mania (monopolar) (*see also* Psychosis,
    affective) 296.0
  alcoholic (acute) (chronic) 291.9
  Bell's—*see* Mania, chronic
  chronic 296.0
    recurrent episode 296.1
    single episode 296.0
  compulsive 300.3
  delirious (acute) 296.0
    recurrent episode 296.1
    single episode 296.0
  epileptic (*see also* Epilepsy) 345.4
  hysterical 300.10
  inhibited 296.89
  puerperal (after delivery) 296.0
    recurrent episode 296.1
    single episode 296.0
  recurrent episode 296.1
  senile 290.8
  single episode 296.0
  stupor 296.89
  stuporous 296.89
  unproductive 296.89
Manic-depressive insanity, psychosis reaction,
    or syndrome (*see also* Psychosis, affective)
    296.80
  circular (alternating) 296.7
    currently
      depressed 296.5
      episode unspecified 296.7
      hypomanic, previously depressed 296.4
      manic 296.4
    mixed 296.6
  depressed (type), depressive 296.2
    atypical 296.82

Manic-depressive insanity—*continued*
    recurrent episode 296.3
    single episode 296.2
  hypomanic 296.0
    recurrent episode 296.1
    single episode 296.0
  manic 296.0
    atypical 296.81
    recurrent episode 296.1
    single episode 296.0
  mixed NEC 296.89
  perplexed 296.89
  stuporous 296.89
Manifestations, rheumatoid
  lungs 714.81
  pannus—*see* Arthritis, rheumatoid
  subcutaneous nodules—*see* Arthritis,
    rheumatoid
Mankowsky's syndrome (familial dysplastic
    osteopathy) 731.2
Mannoheptulosuria 271.8
Mannosidosis 271.8
Manson's
  disease (schistosomiasis) 120.1
  pyosis (pemphigus contagiosus) 684
  schistosomiasis 120.1
Mansonellosis 125.5
Manual —*see* condition
Maple bark disease 495.6
Maple bark-strippers' lung 495.6
Maple syrup (urine) disease or syndrome 270.3
Marable's syndrome (celiac artery compression)
    447.4
Marasmus 261
  brain 331.9
  due to malnutrition 261
  intestinal 569.89
  nutritional 261
  senile 797
  tuberculous NEC (*see also* Tuberculosis) 011.9
Marble
  bones 756.52
  skin 782.61
Marburg disease (virus) 078.89
March
  foot 733.94
  hemoglobinuria 283.2
Marchand multiple nodular hyperplasia (liver)
    571.5
Marchesani (-Weill) syndrome
    (brachymorphism and ectopia lentis) 759.89
Marchiafava (-Bignami) disease or syndrome
    341.8
Marchiafava-Micheli syndrome (paroxysmal
    nocturnal hemoglobinuria) 283.2
Marcus Gunn's syndrome (jaw-winking
    syndrome) 742.8
Marfan's
  congenital syphilis 090.49
  disease 090.49
  syndrome (arachnodactyly) 759.82
    meaning congenital syphilis 090.49
      with luxation of lens 090.49 *[379.32]*
Marginal
  implantation, placenta—*see* Placenta, previa
  placenta—*see* Placenta, previa
  sinus (hemorrhage) (rupture) 641.2
    affecting fetus or newborn 762.1
Marie's
  cerebellar ataxia 334.2
  syndrome (acromegaly) 253.0

Marie-Bamberger disease or syndrome
  (hypertrophic) (pulmonary) (secondary) 731.2
  idiopathic (acropachyderma) 757.39
  primary (acropachyderma) 757.39
**Marie-Charcot-Tooth neuropathic atrophy,
  muscle** 356.1
Marie-Strümpell arthritis or disease
  (ankylosing spondylitis) 720.0
Marihuana, marijuana
  abuse (*see also* Abuse, drugs, nondependent) 305.2
  dependence (*see also* Dependence) 304.3
Marion's disease (bladder neck obstruction)
  596.0
Marital conflict V61.10
Mark
  port wine 757.32
  raspberry 757.32
  strawberry 757.32
  stretch 701.3
  tattoo 709.09
Maroteaux-Lamy syndrome
  (mucopolysaccharidosis VI) 277.5
Marriage license examination V70.3
Marrow (bone)
  arrest 284.9
  megakaryocytic 287.30
  poor function 289.9
Marseilles fever 082.1
Marsh's disease (exophthalmic goiter) 242.0
Marshall's (hidrotic) ectodermal dysplasia
  757.31
Marsh fever (*see also* Malaria) 084.6
Martin's disease 715.27
Martin-Albright syndrome
  (pseudohypoparathyroidism) 275.49
Martorell-Fabre syndrome (pulseless disease)
  446.7
**Masculinization, female with adrenal
  hyperplasia** 255.2
Masculinovoblastoma (M8670/0) 220
Masochism 302.83
Masons' lung 502
Mass
  abdominal 789.3
  anus 787.99
  bone 733.90
  breast 611.72
  cheek 784.2
  chest 786.6
  cystic—*see* Cyst
  ear 388.8
  epigastric 789.3
  eye 379.92
  female genital organ 625.8
  gum 784.2
  head 784.2
  intracranial 784.2
  joint 719.60
    ankle 719.67
    elbow 719.62
    foot 719.67
    hand 719.64
    hip 719.65
    knee 719.66
    multiple sites 719.69
    pelvic region 719.65
    shoulder (region) 719.61
    specified site NEC 719.68
    wrist 719.63
  kidney (*see also* Disease, kidney) 593.9

Mass—*continued*
  lung 786.6
  lymph node 785.6
  malignant (M8000/3)—*see* Neoplasm, by site,
    malignant
  mediastinal 786.6
  mouth 784.2
  muscle (limb) 729.89
  neck 784.2
  nose or sinus 784.2
  palate 784.2
  pelvis, pelvic 789.3
  penis 607.89
  perineum 625.8
  rectum 787.99
  scrotum 608.89
  skin 782.2
  specified organ NEC—*see* Disease of specified
    organ or site
  splenic 789.2
  substernal 786.6
    thyroid (*see also* Goiter) 240.9
  superficial (localized) 782.2
  testes 608.89
  throat 784.2
  tongue 784.2
  umbilicus 789.3
  uterus 625.8
  vagina 625.8
  vulva 625.8
Massive —*see* condition
Mastalgia 611.71
  psychogenic 307.89
Mast cell
  disease 757.33
    systemic (M9741/3) 202.6
  leukemia (M9900/3) 207.8
  sarcoma (M9742/3) 202.6
  tumor (M9740/1) 238.5
    malignant (M9740/3) 202.6
Masters-Allen syndrome 620.6
Mastitis (acute) (adolescent) (diffuse)
  (interstitial) (lobular) (nonpuerperal)
  (nonsuppurative) (parenchymatous)
  (phlegmonous) (simple) (subacute)
  (suppurative) 611.0
  chronic (cystic) (fibrocystic) 610.1
  cystic 610.1
    Schimmelbusch's type 610.1
  fibrocystic 610.1
  infective 611.0
  lactational 675.2
  lymphangitis 611.0
  neonatal (noninfective) 778.7
    infective 771.5
  periductal 610.4
  plasma cell 610.4
  puerperal, postpartum, (interstitial)
    (nonpurulent) (parenchymatous) 675.2
    purulent 675.1
    stagnation 676.2
  puerperalis 675.2
  retromammary 611.0
    puerperal, postpartum 675.1
  submammary 611.0
    puerperal, postpartum 675.1
Mastocytoma (M9740/1) 238.5
  malignant (M9740/3) 202.6
Mastocytosis 757.33
  malignant (M9741/3) 202.6
  systemic (M9741/3) 202.6

Measles (black) (hemorrhagic) (suppressed) 055.9
  with
    encephalitis 055.0
    keratitis 055.71
    keratoconjunctivitis 055.71
    otitis media 055.2
    pneumonia 055.1
  complication 055.8
    specified type NEC 055.79
  encephalitis 055.0
  French 056.9
  German 056.9
  keratitis 055.71
  keratoconjunctivitis 055.71
  liberty 056.9
  otitis media 055.2
  pneumonia 055.1
  specified complications NEC 055.79
  vaccination, prophylactic (against) V04.2
Meatitis, urethral (*see also* Urethritis) 597.89
Meat poisoning —*see* Poisoning, food
Meatus, meatal —*see* condition
Meat-wrappers' asthma 506.9
Meckel's
  diverticulitis 751.0
  diverticulum (displaced) (hypertrophic) 751.0
Meconium
  aspiration 770.11
    with
      pneumonia 770.12
      pneumonitis 770.12
      respiratory symptoms 770.12
     below vocal cords 770.11
      with respiratory symptoms 770.12
    syndrome 770.12
  delayed passage in newborn 777.1
  ileus 777.1
    due to cystic fibrosis 277.01
  in liquor 792.3
    noted during delivery 656.8
  insufflation 770.11
    with respiratory symptoms 770.12
  obstruction
    fetus or newborn 777.1
      in mucoviscidosis 277.01
  passage of 792.3
    noted during delivery 763.84
  peritonitis 777.6
  plug syndrome (newborn) NEC 777.1
  staining 779.84
Median —*see also* condition
  arcuate ligament syndrome 447.4
  bar (prostate) 600.90
    with
      other lower urinary tract symptoms (LUTS) 600.91
      urinary
        obstruction 600.91
        retention 600.91
  vesical orifice 600.90
    with
      other lower urinary tract symptoms (LUTS) 600.91
      urinary
        obstruction 600.91
        retention 600.91
  rhomboid glossitis 529.2
Mediastinal shift 793.2

Mediastinitis (acute) (chronic) 519.2
  actinomycotic 039.8
  syphilitic 095.8
  tuberculous (*see also* Tuberculosis) 012.8
Mediastinopericarditis (*see also* Pericarditis) 423.9
  acute 420.90
  chronic 423.8
    rheumatic 393
  rheumatic, chronic 393
Mediastinum, mediastinal —*see* condition
Medical services provided for —*see* Health, services provided because (of)
Medicine poisoning (by overdose) (wrong substance given or taken in error) 977.9
  specified drug or substance—*see* Table of drugs and chemicals
Medin's disease (poliomyelitis) 045.9
Mediterranean
  anemia (with other hemoglobinopathy) 282.49
  disease or syndrome (hemipathic) 282.49
  fever (*see also* Brucellosis) 023.9
    familial 277.31
  kala-azar 085.0
  leishmaniasis 085.0
  tick fever 082.1
Medulla —*see* condition
Medullary
  cystic kidney 753.16
  sponge kidney 753.17
Medullated fibers
  optic (nerve) 743.57
  retina 362.85
Medulloblastoma (M9470/3)
  desmoplastic (M9471/3) 191.6
  specified site—*see* Neoplasm, by site, malignant
  unspecified site 191.6
Medulloepithelioma (M9501/3)—*see also* Neoplasm, by site, malignant
  teratoid (M9502/3)—*see* Neoplasm, by site, malignant
Medullomyoblastoma (M9472/3)
  specified site—*see* Neoplasm, by site, malignant
  unspecified site 191.6
Meekeren-Ehlers-Danlos syndrome 756.83
Megacaryocytic —*see* condition
Megacolon (acquired) (functional) (not Hirschsprung's disease) 564.7
  aganglionic 751.3
  congenital, congenitum 751.3
  Hirschsprung's (disease) 751.3
  psychogenic 306.4
  toxic (*see also* Colitis, ulcerative) 556.9
Megaduodenum 537.3
Megaesophagus (functional) 530.0
  congenital 750.4
Megakaryocytic —*see* condition
Megalencephaly 742.4
Megalerythema (epidermicum) (infectiosum) 057.0
Megalia, cutis et ossium 757.39
Megaloappendix 751.5
Megalocephalus, megalocephaly NEC 756.0
Megalocornea 743.41
  associated with buphthalmos 743.22
Megalocytic anemia 281.9
Megalodactylia (fingers) (thumbs) 755.57
  toes 755.65
Megaloduodenum 751.5
Megaloesophagus (functional) 530.0
  congenital 750.4
Megalogastria (congenital) 750.7

> *Note—Except where otherwise indicated, the
> morphological varieties of melanoma in the list
> below should be coded by site as for
> "Melanoma (malignant)." Internal sites should
> be coded to malignant neoplasm of those sites.*

Meninges, meningeal *—see* condition
Meningioma (M9530/0)*—see also* Neoplasm, meninges, benign
  angioblastic (M9535/0)*—see* Neoplasm, meninges, benign
  angiomatous (M9534/0)*—see* Neoplasm, meninges, benign
  endotheliomatous (M9531/0)*—see* Neoplasm, meninges, benign
  fibroblastic (M9532/0)*—see* Neoplasm, meninges, benign
  fibrous (M9532/0)*—see* Neoplasm, meninges, benign
  hemangioblastic (M9535/0)*—see* Neoplasm, meninges, benign
  hemangiopericytic (M9536/0)*—see* Neoplasm, meninges, benign
  malignant (M9530/3)*—see* Neoplasm, meninges, malignant
  meningiothelial (M9531/0)*—see* Neoplasm, meninges, benign
  meningotheliomatous (M9531/0)*—see* Neoplasm, meninges, benign
  mixed (M9537/0)*—see* Neoplasm, meninges, benign
  multiple (M9530/1) 237.6
  papillary (M9538/1) 237.6
  psammomatous (M9533/0)*—see* Neoplasm, meninges, benign
  syncytial (M9531/0)*—see* Neoplasm, meninges, benign
  transitional (M9537/0)*—see* Neoplasm, meninges, benign
Meningiomatosis (diffuse) (M9530/1) 237.6
Meningism (*see also* Meningismus) 781.6
Meningismus (infectional) (pneumococcal) 781.6
  due to serum or vaccine 997.09 *[321.8]*
  influenzal NEC 487.8
Meningitis (basal) (basic) (basilar) (brain) (cerebral) (cervical) (congestive) (diffuse) (hemorrhagic) (infantile) (membranous) (metastatic) (nonspecific) (pontine) (progressive) (simple) (spinal) (subacute) (sympathetica) (toxic) 322.9
  abacterial NEC (*see also* Meningitis, aseptic) 047.9
  actinomycotic 039.8 *[320.7]*
  adenoviral 049.1
  Aerobacter aerogenes 320.82
  anaerobes (cocci) (gram-negative) (gram-positive) (mixed) (NEC) 320.81
  arbovirus NEC 066.9 *[321.2]*
    specified type NEC 066.8 *[321.2]*
  aseptic (acute) NEC 047.9
    adenovirus 049.1
    Coxsackie virus 047.0
    due to
      adenovirus 049.1
      Coxsackie virus 047.0
      ECHO virus 047.1
      enterovirus 047.9
      mumps 072.1
      poliovirus (*see also* Poliomyelitis) 045.2 *[321.2]*
    ECHO virus 047.1
    herpes (simplex) virus 054.72
      zoster 053.0
    leptospiral 100.81
    lymphocytic choriomeningitis 049.0
    noninfective 322.0
  Bacillus pyocyaneus 320.89

Meningitis—*continued*
  bacterial NEC 320.9
    anaerobic 320.81
    gram-negative 320.82
      anaerobic 320.81
  Bacteroides (fragilis) (oralis) (melaninogenicus) 320.81
  cancerous (M8000/6) 198.4
  candidal 112.83
  carcinomatous (M8010/6) 198.4
  caseous (*see also* Tuberculosis, meninges) 013.0
  cerebrospinal (acute) (chronic) (diplococcal) (endemic) (epidemic) (fulminant) (infectious) (malignant) (meningococcal) (sporadic) 036.0
    carrier (suspected) of V02.59
  chronic NEC 322.2
  clear cerebrospinal fluid NEC 322.0
  Clostridium (haemolyticum) (novyi) NEC 320.81
  coccidioidomycosis 114.2
  Coxsackie virus 047.0
  cryptococcal 117.5 *[321.0]*
  diplococcal 036.0
    gram-negative 036.0
    gram-positive 320.1
  Diplococcus pneumoniae 320.1
  due to
    actinomycosis 039.8 *[320.7]*
    adenovirus 049.1
    coccidiomycosis 114.2
    enterovirus 047.9
      specified NEC 047.8
    histoplasmosis (*see also* Histoplasmosis) 115.91
    Listerosis 027.0 *[320.7]*
    Lyme disease 088.81 *[320.7]*
    moniliasis 112.83
    mumps 072.1
    neurosyphilis 094.2
    nonbacterial organisms NEC 321.8
    oidiomycosis 112.83
    poliovirus (*see also* Poliomyelitis) 045.2 *[321.2]*
    preventive immunization, inoculation, or vaccination 997.09 *[321.8]*
    sarcoidosis 135 *[321.4]*
    sporotrichosis 117.1 *[321.1]*
    syphilis 094.2
      acute 091.81
      congenital 090.42
      secondary 091.81
    trypanosomiasis (*see also* Trypanosomiasis) 086.9 *[321.3]*
    whooping cough 033.9 *[320.7]*
  E. coli 320.82
  ECHO virus 047.1
  endothelial-leukocytic, benign, recurrent 047.9
  Enterobacter aerogenes 320.82
  enteroviral 047.9
    specified type NEC 047.8
  enterovirus 047.9
    specified NEC 047.8
  eosinophilic 322.1
  epidemic NEC 036.0
  Escherichia coli (E. coli) 320.82
  Eubacterium 320.81
  fibrinopurulent NEC 320.9
    specified type NEC 320.89
  Friedländer (bacillus) 320.82
  fungal NEC 117.9 *[321.1]*
  Fusobacterium 320.81
  gonococcal 098.82

Meningitis—*continued*
  gram-negative bacteria NEC 320.82
    anaerobic 320.81
    cocci 036.0
      specified NEC 320.82
  gram-negative cocci NEC 036.0
    specified NEC 320.82
  gram-positive cocci NEC 320.9
  H. influenzae 320.0
  herpes (simplex) virus 054.72
    zoster 053.0
  infectious NEC 320.9
  influenzal 320.0
  Klebsiella pneumoniae 320.82
  late effect—*see* Late, effect, meningitis
  leptospiral (aseptic) 100.81
  Listerella (monocytogenes) 027.0 *[320.7]*
  Listeria monocytogenes 027.0 *[320.7]*
  lymphocytic (acute) (benign) (serous) 049.0
    choriomeningitis virus 049.0
  meningococcal (chronic) 036.0
  Mima polymorpha 320.82
  Mollaret's 047.9
  monilial 112.83
  mumps (virus) 072.1
  mycotic NEC 117.9 *[321.1]*—
  Neisseria 036.0
  neurosyphilis 094.2
  nonbacterial NEC (*see also* Meningitis, aseptic)
    047.9
  nonpyogenic NEC 322.0
  oidiomycosis 112.83
  ossificans 349.2
  Peptococcus 320.81
  Peptostreptococcus 320.81
  pneumococcal 320.1
  poliovirus (*see also* Poliomyelitis) 045.2 *[321.2]*
  Proprionibacterium 320.81
  Proteus morganii 320.82
  Pseudomonas (aeruginosa) (pyocyaneus) 320.82
  purulent NEC 320.9
    specified organism NEC 320.89
  pyogenic NEC 320.9
    specified organism NEC 320.89
  Salmonella 003.21
  septic NEC 320.9
    specified organism NEC 320.89
  serosa circumscripta NEC 322.0
  serous NEC (*see also* Meningitis, aseptic) 047.9
    lymphocytic 049.0
    syndrome 348.2
  Serratia (marcescens) 320.82
  specified organism NEC 320.89
  sporadic cerebrospinal 036.0
  sporotrichosis 117.1 *[321.1]*
  staphylococcal 320.3
  sterile 997.09
  streptococcal (acute) 320.2
  suppurative 320.9
    specified organism NEC 320.89
  syphilitic 094.2
    acute 091.81
    congenital 090.42
    secondary 091.81
  torula 117.5 *[321.0]*
  traumatic (complication of injury) 958.8
  Treponema (denticola) (macrodenticum) 320.81
  trypanosomiasis 086.1 *[321.3]*
  tuberculous (*see also* Tuberculosis, meninges)
    013.0
  typhoid 002.0 *[320.7]*

Meningitis—*continued*
  Veillonella 320.81
  Vibrio vulnificus 320.82
  viral, virus NEC (*see also* Meningitis, aseptic)
    047.9
  Wallgren's (*see also* Meningitis, aseptic) 047.9
Meningocele (congenital) (spinal) (*see also* Spina
    bifida) 741.9
  acquired (traumatic) 349.2
  cerebral 742.0
  cranial 742.0
Meningocerebritis —*see* Meningoencephalitis
Meningococcemia (acute) (chronic) 036.2
Meningococcus, meningococcal (*see also*
    condition) 036.9
  adrenalitis, hemorrhagic 036.3
  carditis 036.40
  carrier (suspected) of V02.59
  cerebrospinal fever 036.0
  encephalitis 036.1
  endocarditis 036.42
  exposure to V01.84
  infection NEC 036.9
  meningitis (cerebrospinal) 036.0
  myocarditis 036.43
  optic neuritis 036.81
  pericarditis 036.41
  septicemia (chronic) 036.2
Meningoencephalitis (*see also* Encephalitis)
    323.9
  acute NEC 048
  bacterial, purulent, pyogenic, or septic—*see*
    Meningitis
  chronic NEC 094.1
  diffuse NEC 094.1
  diphasic 063.2
  due to
    actinomycosis 039.8 *[320.7]*
    blastomycosis NEC (*see also* Blastomycosis)
      116.0 *[323.41]*
    free-living amebae 136.2
    Listeria monocytogenes 027.0 *[320.7]*
    Lyme disease 088.81 *[320.7]*
    mumps 072.2
    Naegleria (amebae) (gruberi) (organisms)
      136.2
    rubella 056.01
    sporotrichosis 117.1 *[321.1]*
    toxoplasmosis (acquired) 130.0
      congenital (active) 771.2 *[323.41]*
    Trypanosoma 086.1 *[323.2]*
  epidemic 036.0
  herpes 054.3
  herpetic 054.3
  H. influenzae 320.0
  infectious (acute) 048
  influenzal 320.0
  late effect—*see* category 326
  Listeria monocytogenes 027.0 *[320.7]*
  lymphocytic (serous) 049.0
  mumps 072.2
  parasitic NEC 123.9 *[323.41]*
  pneumococcal 320.1
  primary amebic 136.2
  rubella 056.01
  serous 048
    lymphocytic 049.0
  specific 094.2
  staphylococcal 320.3
  streptococcal 320.2
  syphilitic 094.2

Mental—*continued*
  insufficiency (congenital) (*see also* Retardation, mental) 319
  observation without need for further medical care NEC V71.09
  retardation (*see also* Retardation, mental) 319
  subnormality (*see also* Retardation, mental) 319
    mild 317
      moderate 318.0
      profound 318.2
      severe 318.1
  upset (*see also* Disorder, mental) 300.9
Meralgia paresthetica 355.1
Mercurial —*see* condition
Mercurialism NEC 985.0
Merergasia 300.9
Merkel cell tumor —*see* Neoplasm, by site, malignant
Merocele (*see also* Hernia, femoral) 553.00
Meromelia 755.4
  lower limb 755.30
    intercalary 755.32
      femur 755.34
        tibiofibular (complete) (incomplete) 755.33
      fibula 755.37
      metatarsal(s) 755.38
      tibia 755.36
      tibiofibular 755.35
    terminal (complete) (partial) (transverse) 755.31
    longitudinal 755.32
      metatarsal(s) 755.38
      phalange(s) 755.39
      tarsal(s) 755.38
    transverse 755.31
  upper limb 755.20
    intercalary 755.22
      carpal(s) 755.28
      humeral 755.24
        radioulnar (complete) (incomplete) 755.23
      metacarpal(s) 755.28
      phalange(s) 755.29
      radial 755.26
      radioulnar 755.25
      ulnar 755.27
    terminal (complete) (partial) (transverse) 755.21
    longitudinal 755.22
      carpal(s) 755.28
      metacarpal(s) 755.28
      phalange(s) 755.29
    transverse 755.21
Merosmia 781.1
MERRF syndrome (myoclonus with epilepsy and with ragged red fibers) 277.87
Merycism (*see also* Rumination)—*see also* Vomiting
  psychogenic 307.53
Merzbacher-Pelizaeus disease 330.0
Mesaortitis —*see* Aortitis
Mesarteritis —*see* Arteritis
Mesencephalitis (*see also* Encephalitis) 323.9
  late effect—*see* category 326
Mesenchymoma (M8990/1)—*see also* Neoplasm, connective tissue, uncertain behavior
  benign (M8990/0)—*see* Neoplasm, connective tissue, benign
  malignant (M8990/3)—*see* Neoplasm, connective tissue, malignant

Mesenteritis
  retractile 567.82
  sclerosing 567.82
Mesentery, mesenteric —*see* condition
Mesiodens, mesiodentes 520.1
  causing crowding 524.31
Mesio-occlusion 524.23
Mesocardia (with asplenia) 746.87
Mesocolon —*see* condition
Mesonephroma (malignant) (M9110/3)—*see also* Neoplasm, by site, malignant
  benign (M9110/0)—*see* Neoplasm, by site, benign
Mesophlebitis —*see* Phlebitis
Mesostromal dysgenesis 743.51
Mesothelioma (malignant) (M9050/3)—*see also* Neoplasm, by site, malignant
  benign (M9050/0)—*see* Neoplasm, by site, benign
  biphasic type (M9053/3)—*see also* Neoplasm, by site, malignant
    benign (M9053/0)—*see* Neoplasm, by site, benign
  epithelioid (M9052/3)—*see also* Neoplasm, by site, malignant
    benign (M9052/0)—*see* Neoplasm, by site, benign
  fibrous (M9051/3)—*see also* Neoplasm, by site, malignant
    benign (M9051/0)—*see* Neoplasm, by site, benign
Metabolic syndrome 277.7
Metabolism disorder 277.9
  specified type NEC 277.89
Metagonimiasis 121.5
Metagonimus infestation (small intestine) 121.5
Metal
  pigmentation (skin) 709.00
  polishers' disease 502
Metalliferous miners' lung 503
Metamorphopsia 368.14
Metaplasia
  bone, in skin 709.3
  breast 611.8
  cervix—*omit code*
  endometrium (squamous) 621.8
  esophagus 530.85
  intestinal, of gastric mucosa 537.89
  kidney (pelvis) (squamous) (*see also* Disease, renal) 593.89
  myelogenous 289.89
  myeloid 289.89
    agnogenic 238.76
    megakaryocytic 238.76
  spleen 289.59
  squamous cell
    amnion 658.8
    bladder 596.8
    cervix—*see* condition
    trachea 519.19
    tracheobronchial tree 519.19
    uterus 621.8
      cervix—*see* condition
Metastasis, metastatic
  abscess—*see* Abscess
  calcification 275.40
  cancer, neoplasm, or disease
    from specified site (M8000/3)—*see* Neoplasm, by site, malignant
    to specified site (M8000/6)—*see* Neoplasm, by site, secondary
  deposits (in) (M8000/6)—*see* Neoplasm, by site, secondary

Metastasis, metastatic—*continued*
  pneumonia 038.8 *[484.8]*
  spread (to) (M8000/6)—*see* Neoplasm, by site,
    secondary
Metatarsalgia 726.70
  anterior 355.6
  due to Freiberg's disease 732.5
  Morton's 355.6
Metatarsus, metatarsal —*see also* condition
  adductus varus (congenital) 754.53
  abductus valgus (congenital) 764.60
  primus varus 754.52
  valgus (adductus) (congenital) 754.60
  varus (abductus) (congenital) 754.53
    primus 754.52
Methemoglobinemia 289.7
  acquired (with sulfhemoglobinemia) 289.7
  congenital 289.7
  enzymatic 289.7
  Hb-M disease 289.7
  hereditary 289.7
  toxic 289.7
Methemoglobinuria (*see also* Hemoglobinuria)
  791.2
Methicillin-resistant staphylococcus aureus
  (MRSA) V09.0
Methioninemia 270.4
Metritis (catarrhal) (septic) (suppurative) (*see*
  also Endometritis) 615.9
  blennorrhagic 098.16
    chronic or duration of 2 months or over 098.36
  cervical (*see also* Cervicitis) 616.0
  gonococcal 098.16
    chronic or duration of 2 months or over 098.36
  hemorrhagic 626.8
  puerperal, postpartum, childbirth 670
  tuberculous (*see also* Tuberculosis) 016.7
Metropathia hemorrhagica 626.8
Metroperitonitis (*see also* Peritonitis, pelvic,
  female) 614.5
Metrorrhagia 626.6
  arising during pregnancy—*see* Hemorrhage,
    pregnancy
  postpartum NEC 666.2
  primary 626.6
  psychogenic 306.59
  puerperal 666.2
Metrorrhexis —*see* Rupture, uterus
Metrosalpingitis (*see also* Salpingo-oophoritis)
  614.2
Metrostaxis 626.6
Metrovaginitis (*see also* Endometritis) 615.9
  gonococcal (acute) 098.16
    chronic or duration of 2 months or over 098.36
Mexican fever —*see* Typhus, Mexican
Meyenburg-Altherr-Uehlinger syndrome
  733.99
Meyer-Schwickerath and Weyers syndrome
  (dysplasia oculodentodigitalis) 759.89
Meynert's amentia (nonalcoholic) 294.0
  alcoholic 291.1
Mibelli's disease 757.39
Mice, joint (*see also* Loose, body, joint) 718.1
  knee 717.6
Micheli-Rietti syndrome (thalassemia minor)
  282.49
Michotte's syndrome 721.5
Micrencephalon, micrencephaly 742.1
Microalbuminuria 791.0
Microaneurysm, retina 362.14
  diabetic 250.5 *[362.01]*

Microangiopathy 443.9
  diabetic (peripheral) 250.7 *[443.81]*
    retinal 250.5 *[362.01]*
  peripheral 443.9
    diabetic 250.7 *[443.81]*
  retinal 362.18
    diabetic 250.5 *[362.01]*
  thrombotic 446.6
    Moschcowitz's (thrombotic thrombocytopenic
     purpura) 446.6
Microcalcification, mammographic 793.81
Microcephalus, microcephalic, microcephaly
  742.1
  due to toxoplasmosis (congenital) 771.2
Microcheilia 744.82
Microcolon (congenital) 751.5
Microcornea (congenital) 743.41
Microcytic —*see* condition
Microdeletions NEC 758.33
Microdontia 520.2
Microdrepanocytosis (thalassemia-Hb-S
  disease) 282.49
Microembolism
  atherothrombotic—*see also* Atheroembolism
  retina 362.33
Microencephalon 742.1
Microfilaria streptocerca infestation 125.3
Microgastria (congenital) 750.7
Microgenia 524.06
Microgenitalia (congenital) 752.89
  penis 752.64
Microglioma (M9710/3)
  specified site—*see* Neoplasm, by site, malignant
  unspecified site 191.9
Microglossia (congenital) 750.16
Micrognathia, micrognathism (congenital) 524.00
  mandibular 524.04
    alveolar 524.74
  maxillary 524.03
    alveolar 524.73
Microgyria (congenital) 742.2
Microinfarct, heart (*see also* Insufficiency,
  coronary) 411.89
Microlithiasis, alveolar, pulmonary 516.2
Micromyelia (congenital) 742.59
Micropenis 752.64
Microphakia (congenital) 743.36
Microphthalmia (congenital) (*see also*
  Microphthalmos) 743.10
Microphthalmos (congenital) 743.10
  associated with eye and adnexal anomalies NEC
    743.12
  due to toxoplasmosis (congenital) 771.2
  isolated 743.11
  simple 743.11
  syndrome 759.89
Micropsia 368.14
Microsporidiosis 136.8
Microsporon furfur infestation 111.0
Microsporosis (*see also* Dermatophytosis) 110.9
  nigra 111.1
Microstomia (congenital) 744.84
Microthelia 757.6
Microthromboembolism —*see* Embolism
Microtia (congenital) (external ear) 744.23
Microtropia 378.34
Micturition
  disorder NEC 788.69
    psychogenic 306.53
  frequency 788.41

Mite (s)
  diarrhea 133.8
  grain (itch) 133.8
  hair follicle (itch) 133.8
  in sputum 133.8
**Mitochondrial encephalopathy, lactic acidosis
    and stroke-like episodes** (MELAS
    syndrome) 277.87
**Mitochondrial neurogastrointestinal
    encephalopathy syndrome (MNGIE)** 277.87
Mitral —*see* condition
Mittelschmerz 625.2
Mixed —*see* condition
Mljet disease (mal de Meleda) 757.39
Mobile, mobility
  cecum 751.4
  coccyx 733.99
  excessive—*see* Hypermobility
  gallbladder 751.69
  kidney 593.0
    congenital 753.3
  organ or site, congenital NEC—*see* Malposition,
      congenital
  spleen 289.59
Mobitz heart block (atrioventricular) 426.10
  type I (Wenckebach's) 426.13
  type II 426.12
Möbius'
  disease 346.8
  syndrome
    congenital oculofacial paralysis 352.6
    ophthalmoplegic migraine 346.8
Moeller (-Barlow) disease (infantile scurvy) 267
  glossitis 529.4
Mohr's syndrome (Types I and II) 759.89
Mola destruens (M9100/1) 236.1
Molarization, premolars 520.2
Molar pregnancy 631
  hydatidiform (delivered) (undelivered) 630
Mold (s) in vitreous 117.9
Molding, head (during birth)—*omit code*
Mole (pigmented) (M8720/0)—*see also*
    Neoplasm, skin, benign
  blood 631
  Breus' 631
  cancerous (M8720/3)—*see* Melanoma
  carneous 631
  destructive (M9100/1) 236.1
  ectopic—*see* Pregnancy, ectopic
  fleshy 631
  hemorrhagic 631
  hydatid, hydatidiform (benign) (complicating
      pregnancy) (delivered) (undelivered) (*see
      also* Hydatidiform mole) 630
    invasive (M9100/1) 236.1
    malignant (M9100/1) 236.1
    previous, affecting management of pregnancy
        V23.1
  invasive (hydatidiform) (M9100/1) 236.1
  malignant
    meaning
      malignant hydatidiform mole (M9100/1) 236.1
      melanoma (M8720/3)—*see* Melanoma
  nonpigmented (M8730/0)—*see* Neoplasm, skin,
      benign
  pregnancy NEC 631
  skin (M8720/0)—*see* Neoplasm, skin, benign
  tubal—*see* Pregnancy, tubal
  vesicular (*see also* Hydatidiform mole) 630
Molimen, molimina (menstrual) 625.4
Mollaret's meningitis 047.9

Mollities (cerebellar) (cerebral) 437.8
  ossium 268.2
Molluscum
  contagiosum 078.0
  epitheliale 078.0
  fibrosum (M8851/0)—*see* Lipoma, by site
  pendulum (M8851/0)—*see* Lipoma, by site
**Mönckeberg's arteriosclerosis, degeneration
    disease, or sclerosis** (*see also*
    Arteriosclerosis, extremities) 440.20
Monday fever 504
Monday morning dyspnea or asthma 504
Mondini's malformation (cochlea) 744.05
Mondor's disease (thrombophlebitis of breast)
    451.89
**Mongolian, mongolianism, mongolism
    mongoloid** 758.0
  spot 757.33
Monilethrix (congenital) 757.4
Monilia infestation —*see* Candidiasis
Moniliasis —*see also* Candidiasis
  neonatal 771.7
  vulvovaginitis 112.1
Monkeypox 057.8
Monoarthritis 716.60
  ankle 716.67
  arm 716.62
    lower (and wrist) 716.63
    upper (and elbow) 716.62
  foot (and ankle) 716.67
  forearm (and wrist) 716.63
  hand 716.64
  leg 716.66
    lower 716.66
    upper 716.65
  pelvic region (hip) (thigh) 716.65
  shoulder (region) 716.61
  specified site NEC 716.68
Monoblastic —*see* condition
Monochromatism (cone) (rod) 368.54
Monocytic —*see* condition
Monocytopenia 288.59
Monocytosis (symptomatic) 288.63
Monofixation syndrome 378.34
Monomania (*see also* Psychosis) 298.9
Mononeuritis 355.9
  cranial nerve—*see* Disorder, nerve, cranial
  femoral nerve 355.2
  lateral
    cutaneous nerve of thigh 355.1
    popliteal nerve 355.3
  lower limb 355.8
    specified nerve NEC 355.79
  medial popliteal nerve 355.4
  median nerve 354.1
  multiplex 354.5
  plantar nerve 355.6
  posterior tibial nerve 355.5
  radial nerve 354.3
  sciatic nerve 355.0
  ulnar nerve 354.2
  upper limb 354.9
    specified nerve NEC 354.8
  vestibular 388.5
Mononeuropathy (*see also* Mononeuritis) 355.9
  diabetic NEC 250.6 *[355.9]*
    lower limb 250.6 *[355.8]*
    upper limb 250.6 *[354.9]*
  iliohypogastric nerve 355.79
  ilioinguinal nerve 355.79

Mouse, joint (*see also* Loose, body, joint) 718.1
  knee 717.6
Mouth —*see* condition
Movable
  coccyx 724.71
  kidney (*see also* Disease, renal) 593.0
    congenital 753.3
  organ or site, congenital NEC—*see* Malposition,
    congenital
  spleen 289.59
Movement
  abnormal (dystonic) (involuntary) 781.0
  decreased fetal 655.7
  paradoxical facial 374.43
Moya Moya disease 437.5
Mozart's ear 744.29
MRSA (methicillin-resistant staphylococcus
  aureus) V09.0
Mucha's disease (acute parapsoriasis
  varioliformis) 696.2
Mucha-Haberman syndrome (acute
  parapsoriasis varioliformis) 696.2
Mu-chain disease 273.2
Mucinosis (cutaneous) (papular) 701.8
Mucocele
  appendix 543.9
  buccal cavity 528.9
  gallbladder (*see also* Disease, gallbladder) 575.3
  lacrimal sac 375.43
  orbit (eye) 376.81
  salivary gland (any) 527.6
  sinus (accessory) (nasal) 478.19
  turbinate (bone) (middle) (nasal) 478.19
  uterus 621.8
Mucocutaneous lymph node syndrome (acute)
  (febrile) (infantile) 446.1
Mucoenteritis 564.9
Mucolipidosis I, II, III 272.7
Mucopolysaccharidosis (types 1-6) 277.5
  cardiopathy 277.5 *[425.7]*
Mucormycosis (lung) 117.7
Mucositis —*see also* Inflammation, by site
  528.00
  cervix (ulcerative) 616.81
  due to
    antineoplastic therapy (ulcerative) 528.01
    other drugs (ulcerative) 528.02
    specified NEC 528.09
  gastrointestinal (ulcerative) 538
  nasal (ulcerative) 478.11
  necroticans agranulocytica (*see also*
    Agranulocytosis) 288.09
  ulcerative 528.00
  vagina (ulcerative) 616.81
  vulva (ulcerative) 616.81
Mucous —*see also* condition
  patches (syphilitic) 091.3
    congenital 090.0
Mucoviscidosis 277.00
  with meconium obstruction 277.01
Mucus
  asphyxia or suffocation (*see also* Asphyxia,
    mucus) 933.1
    newborn 770.18
  in stool 792.1
  plug (*see also* Asphyxia, mucus) 933.1
    aspiration, of newborn 770.17
    tracheobronchial 519.19
      newborn 770.18
Muguet 112.0
Mulberry molars 090.5

Mullerian mixed tumor (M8950/3)—*see*
  Neoplasm, by site, malignant
Multicystic kidney 753.19
Multilobed placenta —*see* Placenta, abnormal
Multinodular prostate 600.10
  with
    urinary
      obstruction 600.11
      retention 600.11
Multiparity V61.5
  affecting
    fetus or newborn 763.89
    management of
      labor and delivery 659.4
      pregnancy V23.3
  requiring contraceptive management (*see also*
    Contraception) V25.9
Multipartita placenta —*see* Placenta, abnormal
Multiple, multiplex —*see also* condition
  birth
    affecting fetus or newborn 761.5
    healthy liveborn—*see* Newborn, multiple
  digits (congenital) 755.00
    fingers 755.01
    toes 755.02
  organ or site NEC—*see* Accessory
  personality 300.14
  renal arteries 747.62
Mumps 072.9
  with complication 072.8
    specified type NEC 072.79
  encephalitis 072.2
  hepatitis 072.71
  meningitis (aseptic) 072.1
  meningoencephalitis 072.2
  oophoritis 072.79
  orchitis 072.0
  pancreatitis 072.3
  polyneuropathy 072.72
  vaccination, prophylactic (against) V04.6
Mumu (*see also* Infestation, filarial) 125.9
Münchausen syndrome 301.51
Münchmeyer's disease or syndrome (exostosis
  luxurians) 728.11
Mural —*see* condition
Murmur (cardiac) (heart) (nonorganic) (organic)
  785.2
  abdominal 787.5
  aortic (valve) (*see also* Endocarditis, aortic) 424.1
  benign—*omit code*
  cardiorespiratory 785.2
  diastolic—*see* condition
  Flint (*see also* Endocarditis, aortic) 424.1
  functional—*omit code*
  Graham Steell (pulmonic regurgitation) (*see also*
    Endocarditis, pulmonary) 424.3
  innocent—*omit code*
  insignificant—*omit code*
  midsystolic 785.2
  mitral (valve)—*see* stenosis, mitral
  physiologic—*see* condition
  presystolic, mitral—*see* Insufficiency, mitral
  pulmonic (valve) (*see also* Endocarditis,
    pulmonary) 424.3
  Still's (vibratory)—*omit code*
  systolic (valvular)—*see* condition
  tricuspid (valve)—*see* Endocarditis, tricuspid
  valvular—*see* condition
  vibratory—*omit code*
  undiagnosed 785.2
Murri's disease (intermittent hemoglobinuria)
  283.2
Muscae volitantes 379.24

Muscle, muscular —*see* condition
Musculoneuralgia 729.1
Mushrooming hip 718.95
Mushroom workers' (pickers') lung 495.5
Mutation
 factor V leiden 289.81
 prothrombin gene 289.81
Mutism (*see also* Aphasia) 784.3
 akinetic 784.3
 deaf (acquired) (congenital) 389.7
 hysterical 300.11
 selective (elective) 313.23
  adjustment reaction 309.83
Myà's disease (congenital dilation, colon) 751.3
Myalgia (intercostal) 729.1
 eosinophilia syndrome 710.5
 epidemic 074.1
  cervical 078.89
 psychogenic 307.89
 traumatic NEC 959.9
Myasthenia 358.00
 cordis—*see* Failure, heart
 gravis 358.00
  with exacerbation (acute) 358.01
  in crisis 358.01
  neonatal 775.2
  pseudoparalytica 358.00
 stomach 536.8
  psychogenic 306.4
 syndrome in
  botulism 005.1 *[358.1]*
  diabetes mellitus 250.6 *[358.1]*
  hypothyroidism (*see also* Hypothyroidism)
   244.9 *[358.1]*
  malignant neoplasm NEC 199.1 *[358.1]*
  pernicious anemia 281.0 *[358.1]*
  thyrotoxicosis (*see also* Thyrotoxicosis) 242.9
   [358.1]
Myasthenic 728.87
Mycelium infection NEC 117.9
Mycetismus 988.1
Mycetoma (actinomycotic) 039.9
 bone 039.8
  mycotic 117.4
 foot 039.4
  mycotic 117.4
 madurae 039.9
  mycotic 117.4
 maduromycotic 039.9
  mycotic 117.4
 mycotic 117.4
 nocardial 039.9
Mycobacteriosis —*see* Mycobacterium
Mycobacterium, mycobacterial (infection) 031.9
 acid-fast (bacilli) 031.9
 anonymous (*see also* Mycobacterium, atypical)
  031.9
 atypical (acid-fast bacilli) 031.9
  cutaneous 031.1
  pulmonary 031.0
   tuberculous (*see also* Tuberculosis,
    pulmonary) 011.9
  specified site NEC 031.8
 avium 031.0
  intracellulare complex bacteremia (MAC)
   031.2
 balnei 031.1
 Battey 031.0
 cutaneous 031.1
 disseminated 031.2
  avium-intracellulare complex (DMAC) 031.2

Mycobacterium, mycobacterial—*continued*
 fortuitum 031.0
 intracellulare (battey bacillus) 031.0
 kakerifu 031.8
 kansasii 031.0
 kasongo 031.8
 leprae—*see* Leprosy
 luciflavum 031.0
 marinum 031.1
 pulmonary 031.0
  tuberculous (*see also* Tuberculosis,
   pulmonary) 011.9
 scrofulaceum 031.1
 tuberculosis (human, bovine)—*see also*
  Tuberculosis
  avian type 031.0
 ulcerans 031.1
 xenopi 031.0
Mycosis, mycotic 117.9
 cutaneous NEC 111.9
 ear 111.8 *[380.15]*
 fungoides (M9700/3) 202.1
 mouth 112.0
 pharynx 117.9
 skin NEC 111.9
 stomatitis 112.0
 systemic NEC 117.9
 tonsil 117.9
 vagina, vaginitis 112.1
Mydriasis (persistent) (pupil) 379.43
Myelatelia 742.59
Myelinoclasis, perivascular, acute
  (postinfectious) NEC 136.9 *[323.61]*
 postimmunization or postvaccinal 323.51
Myelinosis, central pontine 341.8
Myelitis (ascending) (cerebellar) (childhood)
  (chronic) (descending) (diffuse)
  (disseminated) (pressure) (progressive) (spinal
  cord) (subacute) (*see also* Encephalitis) 323.9
 acute (transverse) 341.20
  idiopathic 341.22
  in conditions classified elsewhere 341.21
 due to
  infection classified elsewhere 136.9 *[323.42]*
  specified cause NEC 323.82
  vaccination (any) 323.52
  viral diseases classified elsewhere 323.02
 herpes simplex 054.74
 herpes zoster 053.14
 late effect—*see* category 326
 optic neuritis in 341.0
 postchickenpox 052.2
 postimmunization 323.52
 postinfectious 136.9 *[323.63]*
 postvaccinal 323.52
 postvaricella 052.2
 syphilitic (transverse) 094.89
 toxic 989.9 *[323.72]*
 transverse 323.82
  acute 341.20
   idiopathic 341.22
   in conditions classified elsewhere 341.21
  idiopathic 341.22
 tuberculous (*see also* Tuberculosis) 013.6
 virus 049.9
Myeloblastic —*see* condition
Myelocele (*see also* Spina bifida) 741.9
 with hydrocephalus 741.0
Myelocystocele (*see also* Spina bifida) 741.9
Myelocytic —*see* condition
Myelocytoma 205.1

Myocarditis—*continued*
    inactive or quiescent (with chorea) 398.0
  active (nonrheumatic) 422.90
    rheumatic 391.2
      with chorea (acute) (rheumatic)
        (Sydenham's) 392.0
  acute or subacute (interstitial) 422.90
    due to Streptococcus (beta-hemolytic) 391.2
    idiopathic 422.91
    rheumatic 391.2
      with chorea (acute) (rheumatic)
        (Sydenham's) 392.0
    specified type NEC 422.99
  aseptic of newborn 074.23
  bacterial (acute) 422.92
  chagasic 086.0
  chronic (interstitial) 429.0
  congenital 746.89
  constrictive 425.4
  Coxsackie (virus) 074.23
  diphtheritic 032.82
  due to or in
    Coxsackie (virus) 074.23
    diphtheria 032.82
    epidemic louse-borne typhus 080 *[422.0]*
    influenza 487.8 *[422.0]*
    Lyme disease 088.81 *[422.0]*
    scarlet fever 034.1 *[422.0]*
    toxoplasmosis (acquired) 130.3
    tuberculosis (*see also* Tuberculosis) 017.9
      [422.0]
    typhoid 002.0 *[422.0]*
    typhus NEC 081.9 *[422.0]*
  eosinophilic 422.91
  epidemic of newborn 074.23
  Fiedler's (acute) (isolated) (subacute) 422.91
  giant cell (acute) (subacute) 422.91
  gonococcal 098.85
  granulomatous (idiopathic) (isolated)
    (nonspecific) 422.91
  hypertensive (*see also* Hypertension, heart)
    402.90
  idiopathic 422.91
    granulomatous 422.91
  infective 422.92
  influenzal 487.8 *[422.0]*
  isolated (diffuse) (granulomatous) 422.91
  malignant 422.99
  meningococcal 036.43
  nonrheumatic, active 422.90
  parenchymatous 422.90
  pneumococcal (acute) (subacute) 422.92
  rheumatic (chronic) (inactive) (with chorea)
    398.0
    active or acute 391.2
      with chorea (acute) (rheumatic)
        (Sydenham's) 392.0
  septic 422.92
  specific (giant cell) (productive) 422.91
  staphylococcal (acute) (subacute) 422.92
  suppurative 422.92
  syphilitic (chronic) 093.82
  toxic 422.93
    rheumatic (*see also* Myocarditis, acute
      rheumatic) 391.2
  tuberculous (*see also* Tuberculosis) 017.9
    [422.0]
  typhoid 002.0 *[422.0]*
  valvular—*see* Endocarditis
  viral, except Coxsackie 422.91
    Coxsackie 074.23
    of newborn (Coxsackie) 074.23

Myocardium, myocardial —*see* condition
Myocardosis (*see also* Cardiomyopathy) 425.4
Myoclonia (essential) 333.2
  epileptica 333.2
  Friedrich's 333.2
  massive 333.2
Myoclonic
  epilepsy, familial (progressive) 333.2
  jerks 333.2
Myoclonus (familial essential) (multifocal)
  (simplex) 333.2
  with epilepsy and with ragged red fibers
    (MERRF syndrome) 277.87
  facial 351.8
  massive (infantile) 333.2
  pharyngeal 478.29
Myodiastasis 728.84
Myoendocarditis —*see also* Endocarditis
  acute or subacute 421.9
Myoepithelioma (M8982/0)—*see* Neoplasm, by
  site, benign
Myofascitis (acute) 729.1
  low back 724.2
Myofibroma (M8890/0)—*see also* Neoplasm,
  connective tissue, benign
  uterus (cervix) (corpus) (*see also* Leiomyoma)
    218.9
Myofibromatosis
  infantile 759.89
Myofibrosis 728.2
  heart (*see also* Myocarditis) 429.0
  humeroscapular region 726.2
  scapulohumeral 726.2
Myofibrositis (*see also* Myositis) 729.1
  scapulohumeral 726.2
Myogelosis (occupational) 728.89
Myoglobinuria 791.3
Myoglobulinuria, primary 791.3
Myokymia —*see also* Myoclonus
  facial 351.8
Myolipoma (M8860/0)
  specified site—*see* Neoplasm, connective tissue,
    benign
  unspecified site 223.0
Myoma (M8895/0)—*see also* Neoplasm,
  connective tissue, benign
  cervix (stump) (uterus) (*see also* Leiomyoma)
    218.9
  malignant (M8895/3)—*see* Neoplasm,
    connective tissue, malignant
  prostate 600.20
    with
      other lower urinary tract symptoms (LUTS)
        600.21
      urinary
        obstruction 600.21
        retention 600.21
  uterus (cervix) (corpus) (*see also* Leiomyoma)
    218.9
    in pregnancy or childbirth 654.1
      affecting fetus or newborn 763.89
      causing obstructed labor 660.2
        affecting fetus or newborn 763.1
Myomalacia 728.9
  cordis, heart (*see also* Degeneration,
    myocardial) 429.1
Myometritis (*see also* Endometritis) 615.9
Myometrium —*see* condition
Myonecrosis, clostridial 040.0

N

Naegeli's
  disease (hereditary hemorrhagic
     thrombasthenia) 287.1
  leukemia, monocytic (M9863/3) 205.1
  syndrome (incontinentia pigmenti) 757.33
Naffziger's syndrome 353.0
Naga sore (*see also* Ulcer, skin) 707.9
Nägele's pelvis 738.6
  with disproportion (fetopelvic) 653.0
    affecting fetus or newborn 763.1
    causing obstructed labor 660.1
     affecting fetus or newborn 763.1
Nager-de Reynier syndrome (dysostosis
   mandibularis) 756.0
Nail —*see also* condition
  biting 307.9
  patella syndrome (hereditary
    osteo-onychodysplasia) 756.89
Nanism, nanosomia (*see also* Dwarfism) 259.4
  hypophyseal 253.3
  pituitary 253.3
  renis, renalis 588.0
Nanukayami 100.89
Napkin rash 691.0
Narcissism 301.81
Narcolepsy 347.00
  with cataplexy 347.01
  in conditions classified elsewhere 347.10
    with cataplexy 347.11
Narcosis
  carbon dioxide (respiratory) 786.09
  due to drug
    correct substance properly administered
     780.09
    overdose or wrong substance given or taken
     977.9
     specified drug—*see* Table of drugs and
      chemicals
Narcotism (chronic) (*see also* listing under
   Dependence) 304.9
  acute
    correct substance properly administered
     349.82
    overdose or wrong substance given or taken
     967.8
     specified drug—*see* Table of drugs and
      chemicals
NARP syndrome (Neuropathy, ataxia and
   retinitis pigmentosa) 277.87
Narrow
  anterior chamber angle 365.02
  pelvis (inlet) (outlet)—*see* Contraction, pelvis
Narrowing
  artery NEC 447.1
    auditory, internal 433.8
    basilar 433.0
     with other precerebral artery 433.3
      bilateral 433.3
    carotid 433.1
     with other precerebral artery 433.3
      bilateral 433.3
    cerebellar 433.8
    choroidal 433.8
    communicating posterior 433.8
    coronary —*see also* Arteriosclerosis, coronary
     congenital 746.85
      due to syphilis 090.5

Narrowing—*continued*
    hypophyseal 433.8
    pontine 433.8
    precerebral NEC 433.9
     multiple or bilateral 433.3
     specified NEC 433.8
    vertebral 433.2
     with other precerebral artery 433.3
     bilateral 433.3
  auditory canal (external) (*see also* Stricture, ear
    canal, acquired) 380.50
  cerebral arteries 437.0
  cicatricial—*see* Cicatrix
  congenital—*see* Anomaly, congenital
  coronary artery—*see* Narrowing, artery,
    coronary
  ear, middle 385.22
  Eustachian tube (*see also* Obstruction,
    Eustachian tube) 381.60
  eyelid 374.46
    congenital 743.62
  intervertebral disc or space NEC—*see*
    Degeneration, intervertebral disc
  joint space, hip 719.85
  larynx 478.74
  lids 374.46
    congenital 743.62
  mesenteric artery (with gangrene) 557.0
  palate 524.89
  palpebral fissure 374.46
  retinal artery 362.13
  ureter 593.3
  urethra (*see also* Stricture, urethra) 598.9
Narrowness, abnormal, eyelid 743.62
Nasal —*see* condition
Nasolacrimal —*see* condition
Nasopharyngeal —*see also* condition
  bursa 478.29
  pituitary gland 759.2
  torticollis 723.5
Nasopharyngitis (acute) (infective) (subacute)
   460
  chronic 472.2
    due to external agent—*see* Condition,
     respiratory, chronic, due to
  due to external agent—*see* Condition,
    respiratory, due to
  septic 034.0
  streptococcal 034.0
  suppurative (chronic) 472.2
  ulcerative (chronic) 472.2
Nasopharynx, nasopharyngeal —*see* condition
Natal tooth, teeth 520.6
Nausea (*see also* Vomiting) 787.02
  epidemic 078.82
  gravidarum—*see* Hyperemesis, gravidarum
  marina 994.6
  with vomiting 787.01
Naval —*see* condition
Neapolitan fever (*see also* Brucellosis) 023.9
Nearsightedness 367.1
Near-syncope 780.2
Nebécourt's syndrome 253.3
Nebula, cornea (eye) 371.01
  congenital 743.43
    interfering with vision 743.42
Necator americanus infestation 126.1
Necatoriasis 126.1

Neck —*see* condition
Necrencephalus (*see also* Softening, brain) 437.8
Necrobacillosis 040.3
Necrobiosis 799.89
  brain or cerebral (*see also* Softening, brain)
    437.8
  lipoidica 709.3
    diabeticorum 250.8 *[709.3]*
Necrodermolysis 695.1
Necrolysis, toxic epidermal 695.1
  due to drug
    correct substance properly administered 695.1
    overdose or wrong substance given or taken
      977.9
      specified drug—*see* Table of drugs and
        chemicals
Necrophilia 302.89
Necrosis, necrotic
  adrenal (capsule) (gland) 255.8
  antrum, nasal sinus 478.19
  aorta (hyaline) (*see also* Aneurysm, aorta) 441.9
    cystic medial 441.00
      abdominal 441.02
      thoracic 441.01
      thoracoabdominal 441.03
    ruptured 441.5
  arteritis 446.0
  artery 447.5
  aseptic, bone 733.40
    femur (head) (neck) 733.42
      medial condyle 733.43
    humoral head 733.41
    medial femoral condyle 733.43
    specified site NEC 733.49
    talus 733.44
  avascular, bone NEC (*see also* Necrosis, aseptic,
    bone) 733.40
  bladder (aseptic) (sphincter) 596.8
  bone (*see also* Osteomyelitis) 730.1
    acute 730.0
    aseptic or avascular 733.40
      femur (head) (neck) 733.42
        medial condyle 733.43
      humoral head 733.41
      medial femoral condyle 733.43
      specified site NEC 733.49
      talus 733.44
    ethmoid 478.19
    ischemic 733.40
    jaw 526.4
    marrow 289.89
    Paget's (osteitis deformans) 731.0
    tuberculous—*see* Tuberculosis, bone
  brain (softening) (*see also* Softening, brain)
    437.8
  breast (aseptic) (fat) (segmental) 611.3
  bronchus, bronchi 519.19
  central nervous system NEC (*see also*
    Softening, brain) 437.8
  cerebellar (*see also* Softening, brain) 437.8
  cerebral (softening) (*see also* Softening, brain)
    437.8
  cerebrospinal (softening) (*see also* Softening,
    brain) 437.8
  cornea (*see also* Keratitis) 371.40
  cortical, kidney 583.6
  cystic medial (aorta) 441.00
    abdominal 441.02
    thoracic 441.01
    thoracoabdominal 441.03
  dental 521.09

Necrosis, necrotic— *continued*
  pulp 522.1
  due to swallowing corrosive substance—*see*
    Burn, by site
  ear (ossicle) 385.24
  esophagus 530.89
  ethmoid (bone) 478.19
  eyelid 374.50
  fat, fatty (generalized) (*see also* Degeneration,
    fatty) 272.8
    abdominal wall 567.82
    breast (aseptic) (segmental) 611.3
    intestine 569.89
    localized—*see* Degeneration, by site, fatty
    mesentery 567.82
    omentum 567.82
    pancreas 577.8
    peritoneum 567.82
    skin (subcutaneous) 709.3
      newborn 778.1
  femur (aseptic) (avascular) 733.42
    head 733.42
    medial condyle 733.43
    neck 733.42
  gallbladder (*see also* Cholecystitis, acute) 575.0
  gangrenous 785.4
  gastric 537.89
  glottis 478.79
  heart (myocardium)—*see* Infarct, myocardium
  hepatic (*see also* Necrosis, liver) 570
  hip (aseptic) (avascular) 733.42
  intestine (acute) (hemorrhagic) (massive) 557.0
  ischemic 785.4
  jaw 526.4
  kidney (bilateral) 583.9
    acute 584.9
    cortical 583.6
      acute 584.6
        with
          abortion—*see* Abortion, by type, with
            renal failure
          ectopic pregnancy (*see also* categories
            633.0-633.9) 639.3
          molar pregnancy (*see also* categories
            630-632) 639.3
        complicating pregnancy 646.2
          affecting fetus or newborn 760.1
        following labor and delivery 669.3
    medullary (papillary) (*see also* Pyelitis)
      590.80
      in
        acute renal failure 584.7
        nephritis, nephropathy 583.7
    papillary (*see also* Pyelitis) 590.80
      in
        acute renal failure 584.7
        nephritis, nephropathy 583.7
    tubular 584.5
      with
        abortion—*see* Abortion, by type, with
          renal failure
        ectopic pregnancy (*see also* categories
          633.0-633.9) 639.3
        molar pregnancy (*see also* categories
          630-632) 639.3
      complicating
        abortion 639.3
        ectopic or molar pregnancy 639.3
        pregnancy 646.2
          affecting fetus or newborn 760.1
      following labor and delivery 669.3

Necrosis, necrotic—*continued*
      traumatic 958.5
   larynx 478.79
   liver (acute) (congenital) (diffuse) (massive)
      (subacute) 570
    with
      abortion—*see* Abortion, by type, with
        specified complication NEC
      ectopic pregnancy (*see also* categories
        633.0-633.9) 639.8
      molar pregnancy (*see also* categories
        630-632) 639.8
    complicating pregnancy 646.7
      affecting fetus or newborn 760.8
    following
      abortion 639.8
      ectopic or molar pregnancy 639.8
    obstetrical 646.7
    postabortal 639.8
    puerperal, postpartum 674.8
    toxic 573.3
   lung 513.0
   lymphatic gland 683
   mammary gland 611.3
   mastoid (chronic) 383.1
   mesentery 557.0
    fat 567.82
   mitral valve—*see* Insufficiency, mitral
   myocardium, myocardial—*see* Infarct,
    myocardium
   nose (septum) 478.19
   omentum 557.0
    with mesenteric infarction 557.0
    fat 567.82
   orbit, orbital 376.10
   ossicles, ear (aseptic) 385.24
   ovary (*see also* Salpingo-oophoritis) 614.2
   pancreas (aseptic) (duct) (fat) 577.8
    acute 577.0
    infective 577.0
   papillary, kidney (*see also* Pyelitis) 590.80
   perineum 624.8
   peritoneum 557.0
    with mesenteric infarction 557.0
    fat 567.82
   pharynx 462
    in granulocytopenia 288.09
   phosphorus 983.9
   pituitary (gland) (postpartum) (Sheehan) 253.2
   placenta (*see also* Placenta, abnormal) 656.7
   pneumonia 513.0
   pulmonary 513.0
   pulp (dental) 522.1
   pylorus 537.89
   radiation—*see* Necrosis, by site
   radium—*see* Necrosis, by site
   renal—*see* Necrosis, kidney
   sclera 379.19
   scrotum 608.89
   skin or subcutaneous tissue 709.8
    due to burn—*see* Burn, by site
    gangrenous 785.4
   spine, spinal (column) 730.18
    acute 730.18
    cord 336.1
   spleen 289.59
   stomach 537.89
   stomatitis 528.1
   subcutaneous fat 709.3
    fetus or newborn 778.1
   subendocardial—*see* Infarct, myocardium

Necrosis, necrotic—*continued*
  suprarenal (capsule) (gland) 255.8
  teeth, tooth 521.09
  testis 608.89
  thymus (gland) 254.8
  tonsil 474.8
  trachea 519.19
  tuberculous NEC—*see* Tuberculosis
  tubular (acute) (anoxic) (toxic) 584.5
   due to a procedure 997.5
  umbilical cord, affecting fetus or newborn 762.6
  vagina 623.8
  vertebra (lumbar) 730.18
   acute 730.18
   tuberculous (*see also* Tuberculosis) 015.0
    [730.8]
  vesical (aseptic) (bladder) 596.8
  vulva 624.8
  x-ray—*see* Necrosis, by site
Necrospermia 606.0
Necrotizing angiitis 446.0
Negativism 301.7
Neglect (child) (newborn) NEC 995.52
  adult 995.84
  after or at birth 995.52
  hemispatial 781.8
  left-sided 781.8
  sensory 781.8
  visuospatial 781.8
Negri bodies 071
Neill-Dingwall syndrome (microcephaly and
  dwarfism) 759.89
Neisserian infection NEC—*see* Gonococcus
Nematodiasis NEC (*see also* Infestation,
  Nematode) 127.9
  ancylostoma (*see also* Ancylostomiasis) 126.9
Neoformans cryptococcus infection 117.5
Neonatal —*see also* condition
  adrenoleukodystrophy 277.86
  teeth, tooth 520.6
Neonatorum —*see* condition

      "N" listing resumes after
      "Neoplasm, neoplastic" table...

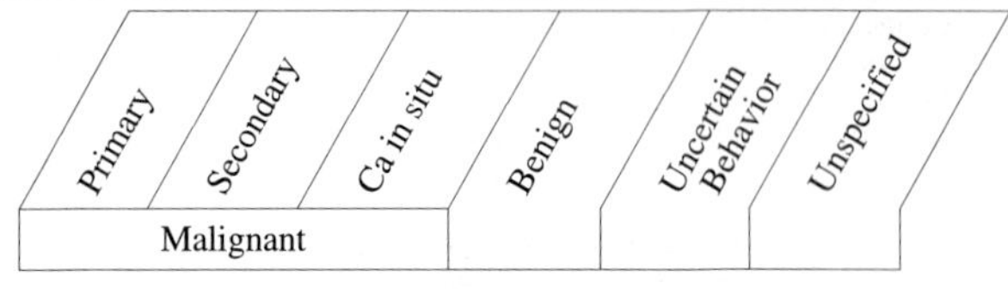

	Primary	Secondary	Ca in situ	Benign	Uncertain Behavior	Unspecified
Neoplasm, neoplastic	199.1	199.1	234.9	229.9	238.9	239.9

Note—1. The list below gives the code numbers for neoplasms by anatomical site. For each site there are six possible code numbers according to whether the neoplasm in question is malignant, benign, in situ, of uncertain behavior, or of unspecified nature. The description of the neoplasm will often indicate which of the six columns is appropriate; e.g., malignant melanoma of skin, benign fibroadenoma of breast, carcinoma in situ of cervix uteri.

Where such descriptors are not present, the remainder of the Index should be consulted where guidance is given to the appropriate column for each morphological (histological) variety listed; e.g., Mesonephroma—see Neoplasm, malignant; Embryoma—see also Neoplasm, uncertain behavior; Disease, Bowen's—see Neoplasm, skin, in situ. However, the guidance in the Index can be overridden if one of the descriptors mentioned above is present; e.g., malignant adenoma of colon is coded to 153.9 and not to 211.3 as the adjective "malignant" overrides the Index entry "Adenoma—see also Neoplasm, benign."

*Note—2. Sites marked with the sign * (e.g., face NEC*) should be classified to malignant neoplasm of skin of these sites if the variety of neoplasm is a squamous cell carcinoma or an epidermoid carcinoma and to benign neoplasm of skin of these sites if the variety of neoplasm is a papilloma (any type).*

	Primary	Secondary	Ca in situ	Benign	Uncertain Behavior	Unspecified
abdomen, abdominal	195.2	198.89	234.8	229.8	238.8	239.8
cavity	195.2	198.89	234.8	229.8	238.8	239.8
organ	195.2	198.89	234.8	229.8	238.8	239.8
viscera	195.2	198.89	234.8	229.8	238.8	239.8
wall	173.5	198.2	232.5	216.5	238.2	239.2
connective tissue	171.5	198.89	—	215.5	238.1	239.2
abdominopelvic	195.8	198.89	234.8	229.8	238.8	239.8
accessory sinus—*see* Neoplasm, sinus						
acoustic nerve	192.0	198.4	—	225.1	237.9	239.7
acromion (process)	170.4	198.5	—	213.4	238.0	239.2
adenoid (pharynx) (tissue)	147.1	198.89	230.0	210.7	235.1	239.0
adipose tissue (*see also* Neoplasm,						
connective tissue)	171.9	198.89	—	215.9	238.1	239.2
adnexa (uterine)	183.9	198.82	233.3	221.8	236.3	239.5
adrenal (cortex) (gland)						
(medulla)	194.0	198.7	234.8	227.0	237.2	239.7
ala nasi (external)	173.3	198.2	232.3	216.3	238.2	239.2
alimentary canal or						
tract NEC	159.9	197.8	230.9	211.9	235.5	239.0
alveolar	143.9	198.89	230.0	210.4	235.1	239.0
mucosa	143.9	198.89	230.0	210.4	235.1	239.0
lower	143.1	198.89	230.0	210.4	235.1	239.0
upper	143.0	198.89	230.0	210.4	235.1	239.0
ridge or process	170.1	198.5	—	213.1	238.0	239.2
carcinoma	143.9	—	—	—	—	—
lower	143.1	—	—	—	—	—
upper	143.0	—	—	—	—	—
lower	170.1	198.5	—	213.1	238.0	239.2
mucosa	143.9	198.89	230.0	210.4	235.1	239.0
lower	143.1	198.89	230.0	210.4	235.1	239.0
upper	143.0	198.89	230.0	210.4	235.1	239.0
upper	170.0	198.5	—	213.0	238.0	239.2
sulcus	145.1	198.89	230.0	210.4	235.1	239.0
alveolus	143.9	198.89	230.0	210.4	235.1	239.0
lower	143.1	198.89	230.0	210.4	235.1	239.0
upper	143.0	198.89	230.0	210.4	235.1	239.0
ampulla of Vater	156.2	197.8	230.8	211.5	235.3	239.0
ankle NEC*	195.5	198.89	232.7	229.8	238.8	239.8
anorectum, anorectal						
(junction)	154.8	197.5	230.7	211.4	235.2	239.0
antecubital fossa or space*	195.4	198.89	232.6	229.8	238.8	239.8
antrum (Highmore)						
(maxillary)	160.2	197.3	231.8	212.0	235.9	239.1

	Malignant					
	Primary	Secondary	Ca in situ	Benign	Uncertain Behavior	Unspecified
pyloric	151.2	197.8	230.2	211.1	235.2	239.0
tympanicum	160.1	197.3	231.8	212.0	235.9	239.1
anus, anal	154.3	197.5	230.6	211.4	235.5	239.0
canal	154.2	197.5	230.5	211.4	235.5	239.0
contiguous sites with rectosigmoid junction or rectum	154.8	—	—	—	—	—
margin	173.5	198.2	232.5	216.5	238.2	239.2
skin	173.5	198.2	232.5	216.5	238.2	239.2
sphincter	154.2	197.5	230.5	211.4	235.5	239.0
aorta (thoracic)	171.4	198.89	—	215.4	238.1	239.2
abdominal	171.5	198.89	—	215.5	238.1	239.2
aortic body	194.6	198.89	—	227.6	237.3	239.7
aponeurosis	171.9	198.89	—	215.9	238.1	239.2
palmar	171.2	198.89	—	215.2	238.1	239.2
plantar	171.3	198.89	—	215.3	238.1	239.2
appendix	153.5	197.5	230.3	211.3	235.2	239.0
arachnoid (cerebral)	192.1	198.4	—	225.2	237.6	239.7
spinal	192.3	198.4	—	225.4	237.6	239.7
areola (female)	174.0	198.81	233.0	217	238.3	239.3
male	175.0	198.81	233.0	217	238.3	239.3
arm NEC*	195.4	198.89	232.6	229.8	238.8	239.8
artery—*see* Neoplasm, connective tissue						
aryepiglottic fold	148.2	198.89	230.0	210.8	235.1	239.0
hypopharyngeal aspect	148.2	198.89	230.0	210.8	235.1	239.0
laryngeal aspect	161.1	197.3	231.0	212.1	235.6	239.1
marginal zone	148.2	198.89	230.0	210.8	235.1	239.0
arytenoid (cartilage)	161.3	197.3	231.0	212.1	235.6	239.1
fold—*see* Neoplasm, aryepiglottic						
atlas	170.2	198.5	—	213.2	238.0	239.2
atrium, cardiac	164.1	198.89	—	212.7	238.8	239.8
auditory						
canal (external) (skin)	173.2	198.2	232.2	216.2	238.2	239.2
internal	160.1	197.3	231.8	212.0	235.9	239.1
nerve	192.0	198.4	—	225.1	237.9	239.7
tube	160.1	197.3	231.8	212.0	235.9	239.1
opening	147.2	198.89	230.0	210.7	235.1	239.0
auricle, ear	173.2	198.2	232.2	216.2	238.2	239.2
cartilage	171.0	198.89	—	215.0	238.1	239.2
auricular canal (external)	173.2	198.2	232.2	216.2	238.2	239.2
internal	160.1	197.3	231.8	212.0	235.9	239.1
autonomic nerve or nervous system NEC	171.9	198.89	—	215.9	238.1	239.2
axilla, axillary	195.1	198.89	234.8	229.8	238.8	239.8
fold	173.5	198.2	232.5	216.5	238.2	239.2
back NEC*	195.8	198.89	232.5	229.8	238.8	239.8
Bartholin's gland	184.1	198.82	233.3	221.2	236.3	239.5
basal ganglia	191.0	198.3	—	225.0	237.5	239.6
basis pedunculi	191.7	198.3	—	225.0	237.5	239.6
bile or biliary (tract)	156.9	197.8	230.8	211.5	235.3	239.0
canaliculi (biliferi) (intrahepatic)	155.1	197.8	230.8	211.5	235.3	239.0
canals, interlobular	155.1	197.8	230.8	211.5	235.3	239.0
contiguous sites	156.8	—	—	—	—	—
duct or passage (common) (cyst) (extrahepatic)	156.1	197.8	230.8	211.5	235.3	239.0
contiguous sites with gallbladder	156.8	—	—	—	—	—
interlobular	155.1	197.8	230.8	211.5	235.3	239.0
intrahepatic	155.1	197.8	230.8	211.5	235.3	239.0
and extrahepatic	156.9	197.8	230.8	211.5	235.3	239.0
bladder (urinary)	188.9	198.1	233.7	223.3	236.7	239.4
contiguous sites	188.8	—	—	—	—	—
dome	188.1	198.1	233.7	223.3	236.7	239.4

	Malignant			Benign	Uncertain Behavior	Unspecified
	Primary	Secondary	Ca in situ			
neck	188.5	198.1	233.7	223.3	236.7	239.4
orifice	188.9	198.1	233.7	223.3	236.7	239.4
ureteric	188.6	198.1	233.7	223.3	236.7	239.4
urethral	188.5	198.1	233.7	223.3	236.7	239.4
sphincter	188.8	198.1	233.7	223.3	236.7	239.4
trigone	188.0	198.1	233.7	223.3	236.7	239.4
urachus	188.7	—	233.7	223.3	236.7	239.4
wall	188.9	198.1	233.7	223.3	236.7	239.4
anterior	188.3	198.1	233.7	223.3	236.7	239.4
lateral	188.2	198.1	233.7	223.3	236.7	239.4
posterior	188.4	198.1	233.7	223.3	236.7	239.4
blood vessel—*see* Neoplasm, connective tissue						
bone (periosteum)	170.9	198.5	—	213.9	238.0	239.2

Note—Carcinomas and adenocarcinomas, of any type other than intraosseous or odontogenic, of the sites listed under "Neoplasm, bone" should be considered as constituting metastatic spread from an unspecified primary site and coded to 198.5 for morbidity coding and to 199.1 for underlying cause of death coding.

	Malignant			Benign	Uncertain Behavior	Unspecified
	Primary	Secondary	Ca in situ			
acetabulum	170.6	198.5	—	213.6	238.0	239.2
acromion (process)	170.4	198.5	—	213.4	238.0	239.2
ankle	170.8	198.5	—	213.8	238.0	239.2
arm NEC	170.4	198.5	—	213.4	238.0	239.2
astragalus	170.8	198.5	—	213.8	238.0	239.2
atlas	170.2	198.5	—	213.2	238.0	239.2
axis	170.2	198.5	—	213.2	238.0	239.2
back NEC	170.2	198.5	—	213.2	238.0	239.2
calcaneus	170.8	198.5	—	213.8	238.0	239.2
calvarium	170.0	198.5	—	213.0	238.0	239.2
carpus (any)	170.5	198.5	—	213.5	238.0	239.2
cartilage NEC	170.9	198.5	—	213.9	238.0	239.2
clavicle	170.3	198.5	—	213.3	238.0	239.2
clivus	170.0	198.5	—	213.0	238.0	239.2
coccygeal vertebra	170.6	198.5	—	213.6	238.0	239.2
coccyx	170.6	198.5	—	213.6	238.0	239.2
costal cartilage	170.3	198.5	—	213.3	238.0	239.2
costovertebral joint	170.3	198.5	—	213.3	238.0	239.2
cranial	170.0	198.5	—	213.0	238.0	239.2
cuboid	170.8	198.5	—	213.8	238.0	239.2
cuneiform	170.9	198.5	—	213.9	238.0	239.2
ankle	170.8	198.5	—	213.8	238.0	239.2
wrist	170.5	198.5	—	213.5	238.0	239.2
digital	170.9	198.5	—	213.9	238.0	239.2
finger	170.5	198.5	—	213.5	238.0	239.2
toe	170.8	198.5	—	213.8	238.0	239.2
elbow	170.4	198.5	—	213.4	238.0	239.2
ethmoid (labyrinth)	170.0	198.5	—	213.0	238.0	239.2
face	170.0	198.5	—	213.0	238.0	239.2
lower jaw	170.1	198.5	—	213.1	238.0	239.2
femur (any part)	170.7	198.5	—	213.7	238.0	239.2
fibula (any part)	170.7	198.5	—	213.7	238.0	239.2
finger (any)	170.5	198.5	—	213.5	238.0	239.2
foot	170.8	198.5	—	213.8	238.0	239.2
forearm	170.4	198.5	—	213.4	238.0	239.2
frontal	170.0	198.5	—	213.0	238.0	239.2
hand	170.5	198.5	—	213.5	238.0	239.2
heel	170.8	198.5	—	213.8	238.0	239.2
hip	170.6	198.5	—	213.6	238.0	239.2
humerus (any part)	170.4	198.5	—	213.4	238.0	239.2
hyoid	170.0	198.5	—	213.0	238.0	239.2
ilium	170.6	198.5	—	213.6	238.0	239.2
innominate	170.6	198.5	—	213.6	238.0	239.2
intervertebral cartilage or disc	170.2	198.5	—	213.2	238.0	239.2

| | Malignant | | | | | |
	Primary	Secondary	Ca in situ	Benign	Uncertain Behavior	Unspecified
ischium	170.6	198.5	—	213.6	238.0	239.2
jaw (lower)	170.1	198.5	—	213.1	238.0	239.2
upper	170.0	198.5	—	213.0	238.0	239.2
knee	170.7	198.5	—	213.7	238.0	239.2
leg NEC	170.7	198.5	—	213.7	238.0	239.2
limb NEC	170.9	198.5	—	213.9	238.0	239.2
lower (long bones)	170.7	198.5	—	213.7	238.0	239.2
short bones	170.8	198.5	—	213.8	238.0	239.2
upper (long bones)	170.4	198.5	—	213.4	238.0	239.2
short bones	170.5	198.5	—	213.5	238.0	239.2
long	170.9	198.5	—	213.9	238.0	239.2
lower limbs NEC	170.7	198.5	—	213.7	238.0	239.2
upper limbs NEC	170.4	198.5	—	213.4	238.0	239.2
malar	170.0	198.5	—	213.0	238.0	239.2
mandible	170.1	198.5	—	213.1	238.0	239.2
marrow NEC	202.9	198.5	—	—	—	238.79
mastoid	170.0	198.5	—	213.0	238.0	239.2
maxilla, maxillary (superior)	170.0	198.5	—	213.0	238.0	239.2
inferior	170.1	198.5	—	213.1	238.0	239.2
metacarpus (any)	170.5	198.5	—	213.5	238.0	239.2
metatarsus (any)	170.8	198.5	—	213.8	238.0	239.2
navicular (ankle)	170.8	198.5	—	213.8	238.0	239.2
hand	170.5	198.5	—	213.5	238.0	239.2
nose, nasal	170.0	198.5	—	213.0	238.0	239.2
occipital	170.0	198.5	—	213.0	238.0	239.2
orbit	170.0	198.5	—	213.0	238.0	239.2
parietal	170.0	198.5	—	213.0	238.0	239.2
patella	170.8	198.5	—	213.8	238.0	239.2
pelvic	170.6	198.5	—	213.6	238.0	239.2
phalanges	170.9	198.5	—	213.9	238.0	239.2
foot	170.8	198.5	—	213.8	238.0	239.2
hand	170.5	198.5	—	213.5	238.0	239.2
pubic	170.6	198.5	—	213.6	238.0	239.2
radius (any part)	170.4	198.5	—	213.4	238.0	239.2
rib	170.3	198.5	—	213.3	238.0	239.2
sacral vertebra	170.6	198.5	—	213.6	238.0	239.2
sacrum	170.6	198.5	—	213.6	238.0	239.2
scaphoid (of hand)	170.5	198.5	—	213.5	238.0	239.2
of ankle	170.8	198.5	—	213.8	238.0	239.2
scapula (any part)	170.4	198.5	—	213.4	238.0	239.2
sella turcica	170.0	198.5	—	213.0	238.0	239.2
short	170.9	198.5	—	213.9	238.0	239.2
lower limb	170.8	198.5	—	213.8	238.0	239.2
upper limb	170.5	198.5	—	213.5	238.0	239.2
shoulder	170.4	198.5	—	213.4	238.0	239.2
skeleton, skeletal NEC	170.9	198.5	—	213.9	238.0	239.2
skull	170.0	198.5	—	213.0	238.0	239.2
sphenoid	170.0	198.5	—	213.0	238.0	239.2
spine, spinal (column)	170.2	198.5	—	213.2	238.0	239.2
coccyx	170.6	198.5	—	213.6	238.0	239.2
sacrum	170.6	198.5	—	213.6	238.0	239.2
sternum	170.3	198.5	—	213.3	238.0	239.2
tarsus (any)	170.8	198.5	—	213.8	238.0	239.2
temporal	170.0	198.5	—	213.0	238.0	239.2
thumb	170.5	198.5	—	213.5	238.0	239.2
tibia (any part)	170.7	198.5	—	213.7	238.0	239.2
toe (any)	170.8	198.5	—	213.8	238.0	239.2
trapezium	170.5	198.5	—	213.5	238.0	239.2
trapezoid	170.5	198.5	—	213.5	238.0	239.2
turbinate	170.0	198.5	—	213.0	238.0	239.2
ulna (any part)	170.4	198.5	—	213.4	238.0	239.2
unciform	170.5	198.5	—	213.5	238.0	239.2

	Malignant					
	Primary	Secondary	Ca in situ	Benign	Uncertain Behavior	Unspecified
vertebra (column)	170.2	198.5	—	213.2	238.0	239.2
coccyx	170.6	198.5	—	213.6	238.0	239.2
sacrum	170.6	198.5	—	213.6	238.0	239.2
vomer	170.0	198.5	—	213.0	238.0	239.2
wrist	170.5	198.5	—	213.5	238.0	239.2
xiphoid process	170.3	198.5	—	213.3	238.0	239.2
zygomatic	170.0	198.5	—	213.0	238.0	239.2
book-leaf (mouth)	145.8	198.89	230.0	210.4	235.1	239.0
bowel—*see* Neoplasm, intestine						
brachial plexus	171.2	198.89	—	215.2	238.1	239.2
brain NEC	191.9	198.3	—	225.0	237.5	239.6
basal ganglia	191.0	198.3	—	225.0	237.5	239.6
cerebellopontine angle	191.6	198.3	—	225.0	237.5	239.6
cerebellum NOS	191.6	198.3	—	225.0	237.5	239.6
cerebrum	191.0	198.3	—	225.0	237.5	239.6
choroid plexus	191.5	198.3	—	225.0	237.5	239.6
contiguous sites	191.8	—	—	—	—	—
corpus callosum	191.8	198.3	—	225.0	237.5	239.6
corpus striatum	191.0	198.3	—	225.0	237.5	239.6
cortex (cerebral)	191.0	198.3	—	225.0	237.5	239.6
frontal lobe	191.1	198.3	—	225.0	237.5	239.6
globus pallidus	191.0	198.3	—	225.0	237.5	239.6
hippocampus	191.2	198.3	—	225.0	237.5	239.6
hypothalamus	191.0	198.3	—	225.0	237.5	239.6
internal capsule	191.0	198.3	—	225.0	237.5	239.6
medulla oblongata	191.7	198.3	—	225.0	237.5	239.6
meninges	192.1	198.4	—	225.2	237.6	239.7
midbrain	191.7	198.3	—	225.0	237.5	239.6
occipital lobe	191.4	198.3	—	225.0	237.5	239.6
parietal lobe	191.3	198.3	—	225.0	237.5	239.6
peduncle	191.7	198.3	—	225.0	237.5	239.6
pons	191.7	198.3	—	225.0	237.5	239.6
stem	191.7	198.3	—	225.0	237.5	239.6
tapetum	191.8	198.3	—	225.0	237.5	239.6
temporal lobe	191.2	198.3	—	225.0	237.5	239.6
thalamus	191.0	198.3	—	225.0	237.5	239.6
uncus	191.2	198.3	—	225.0	237.5	239.6
ventricle (floor)	191.5	198.3	—	225.0	237.5	239.6
branchial (cleft) (vestiges)	146.8	198.89	230.0	210.6	235.1	239.0
breast (connective tissue) (female) (glandular tissue) (soft parts)	174.9	198.81	233.0	217	238.3	239.3
areola	174.0	198.81	233.0	217	238.3	239.3
male	175.0	198.81	233.0	217	238.3	239.3
axillary tail	174.6	198.81	233.0	217	238.3	239.3
central portion	174.1	198.81	233.0	217	238.3	239.3
contiguous sites	174.8	—	—	—	—	—
ectopic sites	174.8	198.81	233.0	217	238.3	239.3
inner	174.8	198.81	233.0	217	238.3	239.3
lower	174.8	198.81	233.0	217	238.3	239.3
lower-inner quadrant	174.3	198.81	233.0	217	238.3	239.3
lower-outer quadrant	174.5	198.81	233.0	217	238.3	239.3
male	175.9	198.81	233.0	217	238.3	239.3
areola	175.0	198.81	233.0	217	238.3	239.3
ectopic tissue	175.9	198.81	233.0	217	238.3	239.3
nipple	175.0	198.81	233.0	217	238.3	239.3
mastectomy site (skin)	173.5	198.2	—	—	—	—
specified as breast tissue	174.8	198.81	—	—	—	—
midline	174.8	198.81	233.0	217	238.3	239.3
nipple	174.0	198.81	233.0	217	238.3	239.3
male	175.0	198.81	233.0	217	238.3	239.3
outer	174.8	198.81	233.0	217	238.3	239.3
skin	173.5	198.2	232.5	216.5	238.2	239.2

	Malignant			Benign	Uncertain Behavior	Unspecified
	Primary	Secondary	Ca in situ			
tail (axillary)	174.6	198.81	233.0	217	238.3	239.3
upper	174.8	198.81	233.0	217	238.3	239.3
upper-inner quadrant	174.2	198.81	233.0	217	238.3	239.3
upper-outer quadrant	174.4	198.81	233.0	217	238.3	239.3
broad ligament	183.3	198.82	233.3	221.0	236.3	239.5
bronchiogenic, bronchogenic						
(lung)	162.9	197.0	231.2	212.3	235.7	239.1
bronchiole	162.9	197.0	231.2	212.3	235.7	239.1
bronchus	162.9	197.0	231.2	212.3	235.7	239.1
carina	162.2	197.0	231.2	212.3	235.7	239.1
contiguous sites with						
lung or trachea	162.8	—	—	—	—	—
lower lobe of lung	162.5	197.0	231.2	212.3	235.7	239.1
main	162.2	197.0	231.2	212.3	235.7	239.1
middle lobe of lung.	162.4	197.0	231.2	212.3	235.7	239.1
upper lobe of lung	162.3	197.0	231.2	212.3	235.7	239.1
brow	173.3	198.2	232.3	216.3	238.2	239.2
buccal (cavity)	145.9	198.89	230.0	210.4	235.1	239.0
commissure.	145.0	198.89	230.0	210.4	235.1	239.0
groove (lower) (upper)	145.1	198.89	230.0	210.4	235.1	239.0
mucosa	145.0	198.89	230.0	210.4	235.1	239.0
sulcus (lower) (upper)	145.1	198.89	230.0	210.4	235.1	239.0
bulbourethral gland.	189.3	198.1	233.9	223.81	236.99	239.5
bursa—*see* Neoplasm,						
connective tissue						
buttock NEC*	195.3	198.89	232.5	229.8	238.8	239.8
calf*	195.5	198.89	232.7	229.8	238.8	239.8
calvarium.	170.0	198.5	—	213.0	238.0	239.2
calyx, renal	189.1	198.0	233.9	223.1	236.91	239.5
canal						
anal	154.2	197.5	230.5	211.4	235.5	239.0
auditory (external)	173.2	198.2	232.2	216.2	238.2	239.2
auricular (external).	173.2	198.2	232.2	216.2	238.2	239.2
canaliculi, biliary (biliferi)						
(intrahepatic)	155.1	197.8	230.8	211.5	235.3	239.0
canthus (eye) (inner)						
(outer)	173.1	198.2	232.1	216.1	238.2	239.2
capillary—*see* Neoplasm,						
connective tissue						
caput coli	153.4	197.5	230.3	211.3	235.2	239.0
cardia (gastric)	151.0	197.8	230.2	211.1	235.2	239.0
cardiac orifice (stomach).	151.0	197.8	230.2	211.1	235.2	239.0
cardio-esophageal junction.	151.0	197.8	230.2	211.1	235.2	239.0
cardio-esophagus.	151.0	197.8	230.2	211.1	235.2	239.0
carina (bronchus).	162.2	197.0	231.2	212.3	235.7	239.1
carotid (artery)	171.0	198.89	—	215.0	238.1	239.2
body	194.5	198.89	—	227.5	237.3	239.7
carpus (any bone)	170.5	198.5	—	213.5	238.0	239.2
cartilage (articular) (joint) NEC—*see also*						
Neoplasm, bone	170.9	198.5	—	213.9	238.0	239.2
arytenoid	161.3	197.3	231.0	212.1	235.6	239.1
auricular	171.0	198.89	—	215.0	238.1	239.2
bronchi	162.2	197.3	—	212.3	235.7	239.1
connective tissue—*see* Neoplasm,						
connective tissue						
costal	170.3	198.5	—	213.3	238.0	239.2
cricoid	161.3	197.3	231.0	212.1	235.6	239.1
cuneiform.	161.3	197.3	231.0	212.1	235.6	239.1
ear (external)	171.0	198.89	—	215.0	238.1	239.2
ensiform	170.3	198.5	—	213.3	238.0	239.2
epiglottis	161.1	197.3	231.0	212.1	235.6	239.1
anterior surface.	146.4	198.89	230.0	210.6	235.1	239.0
eyelid.	171.0	198.89	—	215.0	238.1	239.2

	Malignant			Benign	Uncertain Behavior	Unspecified
	Primary	Secondary	Ca in situ			
intervertebral	170.2	198.5	—	213.2	238.0	239.2
larynx, laryngeal	161.3	197.3	231.0	212.1	235.6	239.1
nose, nasal	160.0	197.3	231.8	212.0	235.9	239.1
pinna	171.0	198.89	—	215.0	238.1	239.2
rib	170.3	198.5	—	213.3	238.0	239.2
semilunar (knee)	170.7	198.5	—	213.7	238.0	239.2
thyroid	161.3	197.3	231.0	212.1	235.6	239.1
trachea	162.0	197.3	231.1	212.2	235.7	239.1
cauda equina	192.2	198.3	—	225.3	237.5	239.7
cavity						
buccal	145.9	198.89	230.0	210.4	235.1	239.0
nasal	160.0	197.3	231.8	212.0	235.9	239.1
oral	145.9	198.89	230.0	210.4	235.1	239.0
peritoneal	158.9	197.6	—	211.8	235.4	239.0
tympanic	160.1	197.3	231.8	212.0	235.9	239.1
cecum	153.4	197.5	230.3	211.3	235.2	239.0
central						
nervous system—*see*						
Neoplasm, nervous system						
white matter	191.0	198.3	—	225.0	237.5	239.6
cerebellopontine (angle)	191.6	198.3	—	225.0	237.5	239.6
cerebellum, cerebellar	191.6	198.3	—	225.0	237.5	239.6
cerebrum, cerebral (cortex)						
(hemisphere)						
(white matter)	191.0	198.3	—	225.0	237.5	239.6
meninges	192.1	198.4	—	225.2	237.6	239.7
peduncle	191.7	198.3	—	225.0	237.5	239.6
ventricle (any)	191.5	198.3	—	225.0	237.5	239.6
cervical region	195.0	198.89	234.8	229.8	238.8	239.8
cervix (cervical) (uteri)						
(uterus)	180.9	198.82	233.1	219.0	236.0	239.5
canal	180.0	198.82	233.1	219.0	236.0	239.5
contiguous sites	180.8	—	—	—	—	—
endocervix (canal) (gland)	180.0	198.82	233.1	219.0	236.0	239.5
exocervix	180.1	198.82	233.1	219.0	236.0	239.5
external os	180.1	198.82	233.1	219.0	236.0	239.5
internal os	180.0	198.82	233.1	219.0	236.0	239.5
nabothian gland	180.0	198.82	233.1	219.0	236.0	239.5
squamocolumnar junction	180.8	198.82	233.1	219.0	236.0	239.5
stump	180.8	198.82	233.1	219.0	236.0	239.5
cheek	195.0	198.89	234.8	229.8	238.8	239.8
external	173.3	198.2	232.3	216.3	238.2	239.2
inner aspect	145.0	198.89	230.0	210.4	235.1	239.0
internal	145.0	198.89	230.0	210.4	235.1	239.0
mucosa	145.0	198.89	230.0	210.4	235.1	239.0
chest (wall) NEC	195.1	198.89	234.8	229.8	238.8	239.8
chiasma opticum	192.0	198.4	—	225.1	237.9	239.7
chin	173.3	198.2	232.3	216.3	238.2	239.2
choana	147.3	198.89	230.0	210.7	235.1	239.0
cholangiole	155.1	197.8	230.8	211.5	235.3	239.0
choledochal duct	156.1	197.8	230.8	211.5	235.3	239.0
choroid	190.6	198.4	234.0	224.6	238.8	239.8
plexus	191.5	198.3	—	225.0	237.5	239.6
ciliary body	190.0	198.4	234.0	224.0	238.8	239.8
clavicle	170.3	198.5	—	213.3	238.0	239.2
clitoris	184.3	198.82	233.3	221.2	236.3	239.5
clivus	170.0	198.5	—	213.0	238.0	239.2
cloacogenic zone	154.8	197.5	230.7	211.4	235.5	239.0
coccygeal						
body or glomus	194.6	198.89	—	227.6	237.3	239.7
vertebra	170.6	198.5	—	213.6	238.0	239.2
coccyx	170.6	198.5	—	213.6	238.0	239.2
colon—*see also* Neoplasm,						

	Malignant					
	Primary	Secondary	Ca in situ	Benign	Uncertain Behavior	Unspecified
intestine, large						
and rectum	154.0	197.5	230.4	211.4	235.2	239.0
column, spinal—*see* Neoplasm, spine						
columnella	173.3	198.2	232.3	216.3	238.2	239.2
commissure						
labial, lip	140.6	198.89	230.0	210.4	235.1	239.0
laryngeal	161.0	197.3	231.0	212.1	235.6	239.1
common (bile) duct	156.1	197.8	230.8	211.5	235.3	239.0
concha	173.2	198.2	232.2	216.2	238.2	239.2
nose	160.0	197.3	231.8	212.0	235.9	239.1
conjunctiva	190.3	198.4	234.0	224.3	238.8	239.8
connective tissue NEC	171.9	198.89	—	215.9	238.1	239.2

Note—For neoplasms of connective tissue (blood vessel, bursa, fasica, ligament, muscle, peripheral nerves, sympathetic and parasympathetic nerves, and ganglia, synovia, tendon, etc.) or of morphological types that indicate connective tissue, code according to the list under "Neoplasm, connective tissue;" for sites that do not appear in this list, code to neoplasm of that site; e.g.: liposarcoma, shoulder 171.2; leiomyosarcoma, stomach 151.9; neurofibroma, chest wall 215.4.

Morphological types that indicate connective tissue appear in their proper palce in the alphabetic index with the instruction "see Neoplasm, connective tissue..."

	Primary	Secondary	Ca in situ	Benign	Uncertain Behavior	Unspecified
abdomen	171.5	198.89	—	215.5	238.1	239.2
abdominal wall	171.5	198.89	—	215.5	238.1	239.2
ankle	171.3	198.89	—	215.3	238.1	239.2
antecubital fossa or space	171.2	198.89	—	215.2	238.1	239.2
arm	171.2	198.89	—	215.2	238.1	239.2
auricle (ear)	171.0	198.89	—	215.0	238.1	239.2
axilla	171.4	198.89	—	215.4	238.1	239.2
back	171.7	198.89	—	215.7	238.1	239.2
breast (female) (*see also*						
Neoplasm, breast)	174.9	198.81	233.0	217	238.3	239.3
male	175.9	198.81	233.0	217	238.3	239.3
buttock	171.6	198.89	—	215.6	238.1	239.2
calf	171.3	198.89	—	215.3	238.1	239.2
cervical region	171.0	198.89	—	215.0	238.1	239.2
cheek	171.0	198.89	—	215.0	238.1	239.2
chest (wall)	171.4	198.89	—	215.4	238.1	239.2
chin	171.0	198.89	—	215.0	238.1	239.2
contiguous sites	171.8	—	—	—	—	—
diaphragm	171.4	198.89	—	215.4	238.1	239.2
ear (external)	171.0	198.89	—	215.0	238.1	239.2
elbow	171.2	198.89	—	215.2	238.1	239.2
extrarectal	171.6	198.89	—	215.6	238.1	239.2
extremity	171.8	198.89	—	215.8	238.1	239.2
lower	171.3	198.89	—	215.3	238.1	239.2
upper	171.2	198.89	—	215.2	238.1	239.2
eyelid	171.0	198.89	—	215.0	238.1	239.2
face	171.0	198.89	—	215.0	238.1	239.2
finger	171.2	198.89	—	215.2	238.1	239.2
flank	171.7	198.89	—	215.7	238.1	239.2
foot	171.3	198.89	—	215.3	238.1	239.2
forearm	171.2	198.89	—	215.2	238.1	239.2
forehead	171.0	198.89	—	215.0	238.1	239.2
gastric	171.5	198.89	—	215.5	238.1	—
gastrointestinal	171.5	198.89	—	215.5	238.1	—
gluteal region	171.6	198.89	—	215.6	238.1	239.2
great vessels NEC	171.4	198.89	—	215.4	238.1	239.2
groin	171.6	198.89	—	215.6	238.1	239.2
hand	171.2	198.89	—	215.2	238.1	239.2
head	171.0	198.89	—	215.0	238.1	239.2
heel	171.3	198.89	—	215.3	238.1	239.2
hip	171.3	198.89	—	215.3	238.1	239.2
hypochondrium	171.5	198.89	—	215.5	238.1	239.2
iliopsoas muscle	171.6	198.89	—	215.5	238.1	239.2

	Malignant					
	Primary	Secondary	Ca in situ	Benign	Uncertain Behavior	Unspecified
infraclavicular region	171.4	198.89	—	215.4	238.1	239.2
inguinal (canal) (region)	171.6	198.89	—	215.6	238.1	239.2
intestine	171.5	198.89	—	215.5	238.1	—
intrathoracic	171.4	198.89	—	215.4	238.1	239.2
ischorectal fossa	171.6	198.89	—	215.6	238.1	239.2
jaw	143.9	198.89	230.0	210.4	235.1	239.0
knee	171.3	198.89	—	215.3	238.1	239.2
leg	171.3	198.89	—	215.3	238.1	239.2
limb NEC.	171.9	198.89	—	215.8	238.1	239.2
lower	171.3	198.89	—	215.3	238.1	239.2
upper	171.2	198.89	—	215.2	238.1	239.2
nates	171.6	198.89	—	215.6	238.1	239.2
neck	171.0	198.89	—	215.0	238.1	239.2
orbit	190.1	198.4	234.0	224.1	238.8	239.8
pararectal	171.6	198.89	—	215.6	238.1	239.2
para-urethral	171.6	198.89	—	215.6	238.1	239.2
paravaginal	171.6	198.89	—	215.6	238.1	239.2
pelvis (floor)	171.6	198.89	—	215.6	238.1	239.2
pelvo-abdominal	171.8	198.89	—	215.8	238.1	239.2
perineum	171.6	198.89	—	215.6	238.1	239.2
perirectal (tissue)	171.6	198.89	—	215.6	238.1	239.2
periurethral (tissue)	171.6	198.89	—	215.6	238.1	239.2
popliteal fossa or space	171.3	198.89	—	215.3	238.1	239.2
presacral	171.6	198.89	—	215.6	238.1	239.2
psoas muscle	171.5	198.89	—	215.5	238.1	239.2
pterygoid fossa	171.0	198.89	—	215.0	238.1	239.2
rectovaginal septum or wall	171.6	198.89	—	215.6	238.1	239.2
rectovesical	171.6	198.89	—	215.6	238.1	239.2
retroperitoneum	158.0	197.6	—	211.8	235.4	239.0
sacrococcygeal region	171.6	198.89	—	215.6	238.1	239.2
scalp	171.0	198.89	—	215.0	238.1	239.2
scapular region	171.4	198.89	—	215.4	238.1	239.2
shoulder	171.2	198.89	—	215.2	238.1	239.2
skin (dermis) NEC	173.9	198.2	232.9	216.9	238.2	239.2
stomach	171.5	198.89	—	215.5	238.1	—
submental	171.0	198.89	—	215.0	238.1	239.2
supraclavicular region	171.0	198.89	—	215.0	238.1	239.2
temple	171.0	198.89	—	215.0	238.1	239.2
temporal region	171.0	198.89	—	215.0	238.1	239.2
thigh	171.3	198.89	—	215.3	238.1	239.2
thoracic (duct) (wall)	171.4	198.89	—	215.4	238.1	239.2
thorax	171.4	198.89	—	215.4	238.1	239.2
thumb	171.2	198.89	—	215.2	238.1	239.2
toe	171.3	198.89	—	215.3	238.1	239.2
trunk	171.7	198.89	—	215.7	238.1	239.2
umbilicus	171.5	198.89	—	215.5	238.1	239.2
vesicorectal	171.6	198.89	—	215.6	238.1	239.2
wrist	171.2	198.89	—	215.2	238.1	239.2
conus medullaris	192.2	198.3	—	225.3	237.5	239.7
cord (true) (vocal)	161.0	197.3	231.0	212.1	235.6	239.1
false	161.1	197.3	231.0	212.1	235.6	239.1
spermatic	187.6	198.82	233.6	222.8	236.6	239.5
spinal (cervical) (lumbar) (thoracic)	192.2	198.3	—	225.3	237.5	239.7
cornea (limbus)	190.4	198.4	234.0	224.4	238.8	239.8
corpus						
albicans	183.0	198.6	233.3	220	236.2	239.5
callosum, brain	191.8	198.3	—	225.0	237.5	239.6
cavernosum	187.3	198.82	233.5	222.1	236.6	239.5
gastric	151.4	197.8	230.2	211.1	235.2	239.0
penis	187.3	198.82	233.5	222.1	236.6	239.5
striatum, cerebrum	191.0	198.3	—	225.0	237.5	239.6

	Malignant			Benign	Uncertain Behavior	Unspecified
	Primary	Secondary	Ca in situ			
uteri	182.0	198.82	233.2	219.1	236.0	239.5
isthmus	182.1	198.82	233.2	219.1	236.0	239.5
cortex						
adrenal	194.0	198.7	234.8	227.0	237.2	239.7
cerebral	191.0	198.3	—	225.0	237.5	239.6
costal cartilage	170.3	198.5	—	213.3	238.0	239.2
costovertebral joint	170.3	198.5	—	213.3	238.0	239.2
Cowper's gland	189.3	198.1	233.9	223.81	236.99	239.5
cranial (fossa, any)	191.9	198.3	—	225.0	237.5	239.6
meninges	192.1	198.4	—	225.2	237.6	239.7
nerve (any)	192.0	198.4	—	225.1	237.9	239.7
craniobuccal pouch	194.3	198.89	234.8	227.3	237.0	239.7
craniopharyngeal (duct)						
(pouch)	194.3	198.89	234.8	227.3	237.0	239.7
cricoid	148.0	198.89	230.0	210.8	235.1	239.0
cartilage	161.3	197.3	231.0	212.1	235.6	239.1
cricopharynx	148.0	198.89	230.0	210.8	235.1	239.0
crypt of Morgagni	154.8	197.5	230.7	211.4	235.2	239.0
crystalline lens	190.0	198.4	234.0	224.0	238.8	239.8
cul-de-sac (Douglas')	158.8	197.6	—	211.8	235.4	239.0
cuneiform cartilage	161.3	197.3	231.0	212.1	235.6	239.1
cutaneous—*see* Neoplasm, skin						
cutis—*see* Neoplasm, skin						
cystic (bile) duct (common)	156.1	197.8	230.8	211.5	235.3	239.0
dermis—*see* Neoplasm, skin						
diaphragm	171.4	198.89	—	215.4	238.1	239.2
digestive organs, system,						
tube, tract NEC	159.9	197.8	230.9	211.9	235.5	239.0
contiguous sites with						
peritoneum	159.8	—	—	—	—	—
disc, intervertebral	170.2	198.5	—	213.2	238.0	239.2
disease, generalized	199.0	199.0	234.9	229.9	238.9	199.0
disseminated	199.0	199.0	234.9	229.9	238.9	199.0
Douglas' cul-de-sac or pouch	158.8	197.6	—	211.8	235.4	239.0
duodenojejunal junction	152.8	197.4	230.7	211.2	235.2	239.0
duodenum	152.0	197.4	230.7	211.2	235.2	239.0
dura (cranial) (mater)	192.1	198.4	—	225.2	237.6	239.7
cerebral	192.1	198.4	—	225.2	237.6	239.7
spinal	192.3	198.4	—	225.4	237.6	239.7
ear (external)	173.2	198.2	232.2	216.2	238.2	239.2
auricle or auris	173.2	198.2	232.2	216.2	238.2	239.2
canal, external	173.2	198.2	232.2	216.2	238.2	239.2
cartilage	171.0	198.89	—	215.0	238.1	239.2
external meatus	173.2	198.2	232.2	216.2	238.2	239.2
inner	160.1	197.3	231.8	212.0	235.9	239.8
lobule	173.2	198.2	232.2	216.2	238.2	239.2
middle	160.1	197.3	231.8	212.0	235.9	239.8
contiguous sites with						
accessory sinuses						
or nasal cavities	160.8	—	—	—	—	—
skin	173.2	198.2	232.2	216.2	238.2	239.2
earlobe	173.2	198.2	232.2	216.2	238.2	239.2
ejaculatory duct	187.8	198.82	233.6	222.8	236.6	239.5
elbow NEC*	195.4	198.89	232.6	229.8	238.8	239.8
endocardium	164.1	198.89	—	212.7	238.8	239.8
endocervix (canal) (gland)	180.0	198.82	233.1	219.0	236.0	239.5
endocrine gland NEC	194.9	198.89	—	227.9	237.4	239.7
pluriglandular NEC	194.8	198.89	234.8	227.8	237.4	239.7
endometrium (gland)						
(stroma)	182.0	198.82	233.2	219.1	236.0	239.5
ensiform cartilage	170.3	198.5	—	213.3	238.0	239.2
enteric—*see* Neoplasm, intestine						
ependyma (brain)	191.5	198.3	—	225.0	237.5	239.6

| | Malignant | | | | | |
	Primary	Secondary	Ca in situ	Benign	Uncertain Behavior	Unspecified
epicardium	164.1	198.89	—	212.7	238.8	239.8
epididymis	187.5	198.82	233.6	222.3	236.6	239.5
epidural	192.9	198.4	—	225.9	237.9	239.7
epiglottis	161.1	197.3	231.0	212.1	235.6	239.1
anterior aspect or surface	146.4	198.89	230.0	210.6	235.1	239.0
cartilage	161.3	197.3	231.0	212.1	235.6	239.1
free border (margin)	146.4	198.89	230.0	210.6	235.1	239.0
junctional region	146.5	198.89	230.0	210.6	235.1	239.0
posterior (laryngeal) surface	161.1	197.3	231.0	212.1	235.6	239.1
suprahyoid portion	161.1	197.3	231.0	212.1	235.6	239.1
esophagogastric junction	151.0	197.8	230.2	211.1	235.2	239.0
esophagus	150.9	197.8	230.1	211.0	235.5	239.0
abdominal	150.2	197.8	230.1	211.0	235.5	239.0
cervical	150.0	197.8	230.1	211.0	235.5	239.0
contiguous sites	150.8	—	—	—	—	—
distal (third)	150.5	197.8	230.1	211.0	235.5	239.0
lower (third)	150.5	197.8	230.1	211.0	235.5	239.0
middle (third)	150.4	197.8	230.1	211.0	235.5	239.0
proximal (third)	150.3	197.8	230.1	211.0	235.5	239.0
specified part NEC	150.8	197.8	230.1	211.0	235.5	239.0
thoracic	150.1	197.8	230.1	211.0	235.5	239.0
upper (third)	150.3	197.8	230.1	211.0	235.5	239.0
ethmoid (sinus)	160.3	197.3	231.8	212.0	235.9	239.1
bone or labyrinth	170.0	198.5	—	213.0	238.0	239.2
Eustachian tube	160.1	197.3	231.8	212.0	235.9	239.1
exocervix	180.1	198.82	233.1	219.0	236.0	239.5
external						
meatus (ear)	173.2	198.2	232.2	216.2	238.2	239.2
os, cervix uteri	180.1	198.82	233.1	219.0	236.0	239.5
extradural	192.9	198.4	—	225.9	237.9	239.7
extrahepatic (bile) duct	156.1	197.8	230.8	211.5	235.3	239.0
contiguous sites with gallbladder	156.8	—	—	—	—	—
extraocular muscle	190.1	198.4	234.0	224.1	238.8	239.8
extrarectal	195.3	198.89	234.8	229.8	238.8	239.8
extremity*	195.8	198.89	232.8	229.8	238.8	239.8
lower*	195.5	198.89	232.7	229.8	238.8	239.8
upper*	195.4	198.89	232.6	229.8	238.8	239.8
eye NEC	190.9	198.4	234.0	224.9	238.8	239.8
contiguous sites	190.8	—	—	—	—	—
specified sites NEC	190.8	198.4	234.0	224.8	238.8	239.8
eyeball	190.0	198.4	234.0	224.0	238.8	239.8
eyebrow	173.3	198.2	232.3	216.3	238.2	239.2
eyelid (lower) (skin) (upper)	173.1	198.2	232.1	216.1	238.2	239.2
cartilage	171.0	198.89	—	215.0	238.1	239.2
face NEC*	195.0	198.89	232.3	229.8	238.8	239.8
fallopian tube (accessory)	183.2	198.82	233.3	221.0	236.3	239.5
falx (cerebelli) (cerebri)	192.1	198.4	—	225.2	237.6	239.7
fascia—*see also* Neoplasm, connective tissue						
palmar	171.2	198.89	—	215.2	238.1	239.2
plantar	171.3	198.89	—	215.3	238.1	239.2
fatty tissue—*see* Neoplasm, connective tissue						
fauces, faucial NEC	146.9	198.89	230.0	210.6	235.1	239.0
pillars	146.2	198.89	230.0	210.6	235.1	239.0
tonsil	146.0	198.89	230.0	210.5	235.1	239.0
femur (any part)	170.7	198.5	—	213.7	238.0	239.2
fetal membrane	181	198.82	233.2	219.8	236.1	239.5
fibrous tissue—*see* Neoplasm, connective tissue						
fibula (any part)	170.7	198.5	—	213.7	238.0	239.2
filum terminale	192.2	198.3	—	225.3	237.5	239.7
finger NEC*	195.4	198.89	232.6	229.8	238.8	239.8
flank NEC*	195.8	198.89	232.5	229.8	238.8	239.8

	Malignant					
	Primary	Secondary	Ca in situ	Benign	Uncertain Behavior	Unspecified
follicle, nabothian	180.0	198.82	233.1	219.0	236.0	239.5
foot NEC*	195.5	198.89	232.7	229.8	238.8	239.8
forearm NEC*	195.4	198.89	232.6	229.8	238.8	239.8
forehead (skin)	173.3	198.2	232.3	216.3	238.2	239.2
foreskin	187.1	198.82	233.5	222.1	236.6	239.5
fornix						
pharyngeal	147.3	198.89	230.0	210.7	235.1	239.0
vagina	184.0	198.82	233.3	221.1	236.3	239.5
fossa (of)						
anterior (cranial)	191.9	198.3	—	225.0	237.5	239.6
cranial	191.9	198.3	—	225.0	237.5	239.6
ischiorectal	195.3	198.89	234.8	229.8	238.8	239.8
middle (cranial)	191.9	198.3	—	225.0	237.5	239.6
pituitary	194.3	198.89	234.8	227.3	237.0	239.7
posterior (cranial)	191.9	198.3	—	225.0	237.5	239.6
pterygoid	171.0	198.89	—	215.0	238.1	239.2
pyriform	148.1	198.89	230.0	210.8	235.1	239.0
Rosenmüller	147.2	198.89	230.0	210.7	235.1	239.0
tonsillar	146.1	198.89	230.0	210.6	235.1	239.0
fourchette	184.4	198.82	233.3	221.2	236.3	239.5
frenulum						
labii—*see* Neoplasm, lip, internal						
linguae	141.3	198.89	230.0	210.1	235.1	239.0
frontal						
bone	170.0	198.5	—	213.0	238.0	239.2
lobe, brain	191.1	198.3	—	225.0	237.5	239.6
meninges	192.1	198.4	—	225.2	237.6	239.7
pole	191.1	198.3	—	225.0	237.5	239.6
sinus	160.4	197.3	231.8	212.0	235.9	239.1
fundus						
stomach	151.3	197.8	230.2	211.1	235.2	239.0
uterus	182.0	198.82	233.2	219.1	236.0	239.5
gall duct (extrahepatic)	156.1	197.8	230.8	211.5	235.3	239.0
intrahepatic	155.1	197.8	230.8	211.5	235.3	239.0
gallbladder	156.0	197.8	230.8	211.5	235.3	239.0
contiguous sites with extrahepatic bile ducts	156.8	—	—	—	—	—
ganglia (*see also* Neoplasm, connective tissue)	171.9	198.89	—	215.9	238.1	239.2
basal	191.0	198.3	—	225.0	237.5	239.6
ganglion (*see also* Neoplasm, connective tissue)	171.9	198.89	—	215.9	238.1	239.2
cranial nerve	192.0	198.4	—	225.1	237.9	239.7
Gartner's duct	184.0	198.82	233.3	221.1	236.3	239.5
gastric—*see* Neoplasm, stomach						
gastrocolic	159.8	197.8	230.9	211.9	235.5	239.0
gastroesophageal junction	151.0	197.8	230.2	211.1	235.2	239.0
gastrointestinal (tract) NEC	159.9	197.8	230.9	211.9	235.5	239.0
generalized	199.0	199.0	234.9	229.9	238.9	199.0
genital organ or tract						
female NEC	184.9	198.82	233.3	221.9	236.3	239.5
contiguous sites	184.8	—	—	—	—	—
specified site NEC	184.8	198.82	233.3	221.8	236.3	239.5
male NEC	187.9	198.82	233.6	222.9	236.6	239.5
contiguous sites	187.8	—	—	—	—	—
specified site NEC	187.8	198.82	233.6	222.8	236.6	239.5
genitourinary tract						
female	184.9	198.82	233.3	221.9	236.3	239.5
male	187.9	198.82	233.6	222.9	236.6	239.5
gingiva (alveolar) (marginal)	143.9	198.89	230.0	210.4	235.1	239.0
lower	143.1	198.89	230.0	210.4	235.1	239.0
mandibular	143.1	198.89	230.0	210.4	235.1	239.0
maxillary	143.0	198.89	230.0	210.4	235.1	239.0

	Malignant					
	Primary	Secondary	Ca in situ	Benign	Uncertain Behavior	Unspecified
upper	143.0	198.89	230.0	210.4	235.1	239.0
gland, glandular (lymphatic) (system)—*see also* Neoplasm, lymph gland						
endocrine NEC	194.9	198.89	—	227.9	237.4	239.7
salivary—*see* Neoplasm, salivary, gland						
glans penis	187.2	198.82	233.5	222.1	236.6	239.5
globus pallidus	191.0	198.3	—	225.0	237.5	239.6
glomus						
coccygeal	194.6	198.89	—	227.6	237.3	239.7
jugularis	194.6	198.89	—	227.6	237.3	239.7
glosso-epiglottic fold(s)	146.4	198.89	230.0	210.6	235.1	239.0
glossopalatine fold	146.2	198.89	230.0	210.6	235.1	239.0
glossopharyngeal sulcus	146.1	198.89	230.0	210.6	235.1	239.0
glottis	161.0	197.3	231.0	212.1	235.6	239.1
gluteal region*	195.3	198.89	232.5	229.8	238.8	239.8
great vessels NEC	171.4	198.89	—	215.4	238.1	239.2
groin NEC*	195.3	198.89	232.5	229.8	238.8	239.8
gum	143.9	198.89	230.0	210.4	235.1	239.0
contiguous sites	143.8	—	—	—	—	—
lower	143.1	198.89	230.0	210.4	235.1	239.0
upper	143.0	198.89	230.0	210.4	235.1	239.0
hand NEC*	195.4	198.89	232.6	229.8	238.8	239.8
head NEC*	195.0	198.89	232.4	229.8	238.8	239.8
heart	164.1	198.89	—	212.7	238.8	239.8
contiguous sites with mediastinum or thymus	164.8	—	—	—	—	—
heel NEC*	195.5	198.89	232.7	229.8	238.8	239.8
helix	173.2	198.2	232.2	216.2	238.2	239.2
hematopoietic, hemopoietic tissue NEC	202.8	198.89	—	—	—	238.79
hemisphere, cerebral	191.0	198.3	—	225.0	237.5	239.6
hemorrhoidal zone	154.2	197.5	230.5	211.4	235.5	239.0
hepatic	155.2	197.7	230.8	211.5	235.3	239.0
duct (bile)	156.1	197.8	230.8	211.5	235.3	239.0
flexure (colon)	153.0	197.5	230.3	211.3	235.2	239.0
primary	155.0	—	—	—	—	—
hilus of lung	162.2	197.0	231.2	212.3	235.7	239.1
hip NEC*	195.5	198.89	232.7	229.8	238.8	239.8
hippocampus, brain	191.2	198.3	—	225.0	237.5	239.6
humerus (any part)	170.4	198.5	—	213.4	238.0	239.2
hymen	184.0	198.82	233.3	221.1	236.3	239.5
hypopharynx, hypopharyngeal NEC	148.9	198.89	230.0	210.8	235.1	239.0
contiguous sites	148.8	—	—	—	—	—
postcricoid region	148.0	198.89	230.0	210.8	235.1	239.0
posterior wall	148.3	198.89	230.0	210.8	235.1	239.0
pyriform fossa (sinus)	148.1	198.89	230.0	210.8	235.1	239.0
specified site NEC	148.8	198.89	230.0	210.8	235.1	239.0
wall	148.9	198.89	230.0	210.8	235.1	239.0
posterior	148.3	198.89	230.0	210.8	235.1	239.0
hypophysis	194.3	198.89	234.8	227.3	237.0	239.7
hypothalamus	191.0	198.3	—	225.0	237.5	239.6
ileocecum, ileocecal (coil, junction, valve)	153.4	197.5	230.3	211.3	235.2	239.0
ileum	152.2	197.4	230.7	211.2	235.2	239.0
ilium	170.6	198.5	—	213.6	238.0	239.2
immunoproliferative NEC	203.8	—	—	—	—	—
infraclavicular (region)*	195.1	198.89	232.5	229.8	238.8	239.8
inguinal (region)*	195.3	198.89	232.5	229.8	238.8	239.8
insula	191.0	198.3	—	225.0	237.5	239.6

| | Malignant | | | | | |
	Primary	Secondary	Ca in situ	Benign	Uncertain Behavior	Unspecified
insular tissue (pancreas)	157.4	197.8	230.9	211.7	235.5	239.0
brain	191.0	198.3	—	225.0	237.5	239.6
interarytenoid fold	148.2	198.89	230.0	210.8	235.1	239.0
hypopharyngeal aspect	148.2	198.89	230.0	210.8	235.1	239.0
laryngeal aspect	161.1	197.3	231.0	212.1	235.6	239.1
marginal zone	148.2	198.89	230.0	210.8	235.1	239.0
interdental papillae	143.9	198.89	230.0	210.4	235.1	239.0
lower	143.1	198.89	230.0	210.4	235.1	239.0
upper	143.0	198.89	230.0	210.4	235.1	239.0
internal						
capsule	191.0	198.3	—	225.0	237.5	239.6
os (cervix)	180.0	198.82	233.1	219.0	236.0	239.5
intervertebral cartilage						
or disc	170.2	198.5	—	213.2	238.0	239.2
intestine, intestinal	159.0	197.8	230.7	211.9	235.2	239.0
large	153.9	197.5	230.3	211.3	235.2	239.0
appendix	153.5	197.5	230.3	211.3	235.2	239.0
caput coli	153.4	197.5	230.3	211.3	235.2	239.0
cecum	153.4	197.5	230.3	211.3	235.2	239.0
colon	153.9	197.5	230.3	211.3	235.2	239.0
and rectum	154.0	197.5	230.4	211.4	235.2	239.0
ascending	153.6	197.5	230.3	211.3	235.2	239.0
caput	153.4	197.5	230.3	211.3	235.2	239.0
contiguous sites	153.8	—	—	—	—	—
descending	153.2	197.5	230.3	211.3	235.2	239.0
distal	153.2	197.5	230.3	211.3	235.2	239.0
left	153.2	197.5	230.3	211.3	235.2	239.0
pelvic	153.3	197.5	230.3	211.3	235.2	239.0
right	153.6	197.5	230.3	211.3	235.2	239.0
sigmoid (flexure)	153.3	197.5	230.3	211.3	235.2	239.0
transverse	153.1	197.5	230.3	211.3	235.2	239.0
contiguous sites	153.8	—	—	—	—	—
hepatic flexure	153.0	197.5	230.3	211.3	235.2	239.0
ileocecum,ileocecal						
(coil, valve)	153.4	197.5	230.3	211.3	235.2	239.0
sigmoid flexure (lower)						
(upper)	153.3	197.5	230.3	211.3	235.2	239.0
splenic flexure	153.7	197.5	230.3	211.3	235.2	239.0
small	152.9	197.4	230.7	211.2	235.2	239.0
contiguous sites	152.8	—	—	—	—	—
duodenum	152.0	197.4	230.7	211.2	235.2	239.0
ileum	152.2	197.4	230.7	211.2	235.2	239.0
jejunum	152.1	197.4	230.7	211.2	235.2	239.0
tract NEC	159.0	197.8	230.7	211.9	235.2	239.0
intra-abdominal	195.2	198.89	234.8	229.8	238.8	239.8
intracranial NEC	191.9	198.3	—	225.0	237.5	239.6
intrahepatic (bile) duct	155.1	197.8	230.8	211.5	235.3	239.0
intraocular	190.0	198.4	234.0	224.0	238.8	239.8
intraorbital	190.1	198.4	234.0	224.1	238.8	239.8
intrasellar	194.3	198.89	234.8	227.3	237.0	239.7
intrathoracic (cavity)						
(organs NEC)	195.1	198.89	234.8	229.8	238.8	239.8
contiguous sites with respiratory						
organs	165.8	—	—	—	—	—
iris	190.0	198.4	234.0	224.0	238.8	239.8
ischiorectal (fossa)	195.3	198.89	234.8	229.8	238.8	239.8
ischium	170.6	198.5	—	213.6	238.0	239.2
island of Reil	191.0	198.3	—	225.0	237.5	239.6
islands or islets of Langerhans	157.4	197.8	230.9	211.7	235.5	239.0
isthmus uteri	182.1	198.82	233.2	219.1	236.0	239.5
jaw	195.0	198.89	234.8	229.8	238.8	239.8
bone	170.1	198.5	—	213.1	238.0	239.2
carcinoma	143.9	—	—	—	—	—

	Malignant			Benign	Uncertain Behavior	Unspecified
	Primary	Secondary	Ca in situ			
lower	143.1	—	—	—	—	—
upper	143.0	—	—	—	—	—
lower	170.1	198.5	—	213.1	238.0	239.2
upper	170.0	198.5	—	213.0	238.0	239.2
carcinoma (any type)						
(lower) (upper)	195.0	—	—	—	—	—
skin	173.3	198.2	232.3	216.3	238.2	239.2
soft tissues	143.9	198.89	230.0	210.4	235.1	239.0
lower	143.1	198.89	230.0	210.4	235.1	239.0
upper	143.0	198.89	230.0	210.4	235.1	239.0
jejunum	152.1	197.4	230.7	211.2	235.2	239.0
joint NEC (*see also*						
Neoplasm, bone)	170.9	198.5	—	213.9	238.0	239.2
acromioclavicular	170.4	198.5	—	213.4	238.0	239.2
bursa or synovial membrane—*see*						
Neoplasm, connective tissue						
costovertebral	170.3	198.5	—	213.3	238.0	239.2
sternocostal	170.3	198.5	—	213.3	238.0	239.2
temporomandibular	170.1	198.5	—	213.1	238.0	239.2
junction						
anorectal	154.8	197.5	230.7	211.4	235.5	239.0
cardioesophageal	151.0	197.8	230.2	211.1	235.2	239.0
esophagogastric	151.0	197.8	230.2	211.1	235.2	239.0
gastroesophageal	151.0	197.8	230.2	211.1	235.2	239.0
hard and soft palate	145.5	198.89	230.0	210.4	235.1	239.0
ileocecal	153.4	197.5	230.3	211.3	235.2	239.0
pelvirectal	154.0	197.5	230.4	211.4	235.2	239.0
pelviureteric	189.1	198.0	233.9	223.1	236.91	239.5
rectosigmoid	154.0	197.5	230.4	211.4	235.2	239.0
squamocolumnar, of cervix	180.8	198.82	233.1	219.0	236.0	239.5
kidney (parenchyma)	189.0	198.0	233.9	223.0	236.91	239.5
calyx	189.1	198.0	233.9	223.1	236.91	239.5
hilus	189.1	198.0	233.9	223.1	236.91	239.5
pelvis	189.1	198.0	233.9	223.1	236.91	239.5
knee NEC*	195.5	198.89	232.7	229.8	238.8	239.8
labia (skin)	184.4	198.82	233.3	221.2	236.3	239.5
majora	184.1	198.82	233.3	221.2	236.3	239.5
minora	184.2	198.82	233.3	221.2	236.3	239.5
labial—*see also* Neoplasm, lip						
sulcus (lower) (upper)	145.1	198.89	230.0	210.4	235.1	239.0
labium (skin)	184.4	198.82	233.3	221.2	236.3	239.5
majus	184.1	198.82	233.3	221.2	236.3	239.5
minus	184.2	198.82	233.3	221.2	236.3	239.5
lacrimal						
canaliculi	190.7	198.4	234.0	224.7	238.8	239.8
duct (nasal)	190.7	198.4	234.0	224.7	238.8	239.8
gland	190.2	198.4	234.0	224.2	238.8	239.8
punctum	190.7	198.4	234.0	224.7	238.8	239.8
sac	190.7	198.4	234.0	224.7	238.8	239.8
Langerhans, islands or islets	157.4	197.8	230.9	211.7	235.5	239.0
laryngopharynx	148.9	198.89	230.0	210.8	235.1	239.0
larynx, laryngeal NEC	161.9	197.3	231.0	212.1	235.6	239.1
aryepiglottic fold	161.1	197.3	231.0	212.1	235.6	239.1
cartilage (arytenoid)						
(cricoid) (cuneiform)						
(thyroid)	161.3	197.3	231.0	212.1	235.6	239.1
commissure (anterior)						
(posterior)	161.0	197.3	231.0	212.1	235.6	239.1
contiguous sites	161.8	—	—	—	—	—
extrinsic NEC	161.1	197.3	231.0	212.1	235.6	239.1
meaning hypopharynx	148.9	198.89	230.0	210.8	235.1	239.0
interarytenoid fold	161.1	197.3	231.0	212.1	235.6	239.1
intrinsic	161.0	197.3	231.0	212.1	235.6	239.1

| | Malignant | | | | | |
	Primary	Secondary	Ca in situ	Benign	Uncertain Behavior	Unspecified
ventricular band	161.1	197.3	231.0	212.1	235.6	239.1
leg NEC*	195.5	198.89	232.7	229.8	238.8	239.8
lens, crystalline	190.0	198.4	234.0	224.0	238.8	239.8
lid (lower) (upper)	173.1	198.2	232.1	216.1	238.2	239.2
ligament—*see also* Neoplasm, connective tissue						
broad	183.3	198.82	233.3	221.0	236.3	239.5
Mackenrodt's	183.8	198.82	233.3	221.8	236.3	239.5
non-uterine—*see* Neoplasm, connective tissue						
round	183.5	198.82	—	221.0	236.3	239.5
sacro-uterine	183.4	198.82	—	221.0	236.3	239.5
uterine	183.4	198.82	—	221.0	236.3	239.5
utero-ovarian	183.8	198.82	233.3	221.8	236.3	239.5
uterosacral	183.4	198.82	—	221.0	236.3	239.5
limb*	195.8	198.89	232.8	229.8	238.8	239.8
lower*	195.5	198.89	232.7	229.8	238.8	239.8
upper*	195.4	198.89	232.6	229.8	238.8	239.8
limbus of cornea	190.4	198.4	234.0	224.4	238.8	239.8
lingual NEC (*see also* Neoplasm, tongue)	141.9	198.89	230.0	210.1	235.1	239.0
lingula, lung	162.3	197.0	231.2	212.3	235.7	239.1
lip (external) (lipstick area) (vermillion border)	140.9	198.89	230.0	210.0	235.1	239.0
buccal aspect—*see* Neoplasm, lip, internal						
commissure	140.6	198.89	230.0	210.4	235.1	239.0
contiguous sites	140.8	—	—	—	—	—
with oral cavity or pharynx	149.8	—	—	—	—	—
frenulum—*see* Neoplasm, lip, internal						
inner aspect—*see* Neoplasm, lip, internal						
internal (buccal) (frenulum) (mucosa) (oral)	140.5	198.89	230.0	210.0	235.1	239.0
lower	140.4	198.89	230.0	210.0	235.1	239.0
upper	140.3	198.89	230.0	210.0	235.1	239.0
lower	140.1	198.89	230.0	210.0	235.1	239.0
internal (buccal) (frenulum) (mucosa) (oral)	140.4	198.89	230.0	210.0	235.1	239.0
mucosa—*see* Neoplasm, lip, internal						
oral aspect—*see* Neoplasm, lip, internal						
skin (commissure) (lower) (upper)	173.0	198.2	232.0	216.0	238.2	239.2
upper	140.0	198.89	230.0	210.0	235.1	239.0
internal (buccal) (frenulum) (mucosa) (oral)	140.3	198.89	230.0	210.0	235.1	239.0
liver	155.2	197.7	230.8	211.5	235.3	239.0
primary	155.0	—	—	—	—	—
lobe						
azygos	162.3	197.0	231.2	212.3	235.7	239.1
frontal	191.1	198.3	—	225.0	237.5	239.6
lower	162.5	197.0	231.2	212.3	235.7	239.1
middle	162.4	197.0	231.2	212.3	235.7	239.1
occipital	191.4	198.3	—	225.0	237.5	239.6
parietal	191.3	198.3	—	225.0	237.5	239.6
temporal	191.2	198.3	—	225.0	237.5	239.6
upper	162.3	197.0	231.2	212.3	235.7	239.1
lumbosacral plexus	171.6	198.4	—	215.6	238.1	239.2
lung	162.9	197.0	231.2	212.3	235.7	239.1
azygos lobe	162.3	197.0	231.2	212.3	235.7	239.1
carina	162.2	197.0	231.2	212.3	235.7	239.1
contiguous sites with bronchus or trachea	162.8	—	—	—	—	—
hilus	162.2	197.0	231.2	212.3	235.7	239.1

	Malignant					
	Primary	Secondary	Ca in situ	Benign	Uncertain Behavior	Unspecified
lingula	162.3	197.0	231.2	212.3	235.7	239.1
lobe NEC	162.9	197.0	231.2	212.3	235.7	239.1
lower lobe	162.5	197.0	231.2	212.3	235.7	239.1
main bronchus	162.2	197.0	231.2	212.3	235.7	239.1
middle lobe	162.4	197.0	231.2	212.3	235.7	239.1
upper lobe	162.3	197.0	231.2	212.3	235.7	239.1
lymph, lymphatic						
channel NEC (*see also* Neoplasm, connective tissue)	171.9	198.89	—	215.9	238.1	239.2
gland (secondary)	—	196.9	—	229.0	238.8	239.8
abdominal	—	196.2	—	229.0	238.8	239.8
aortic	—	196.2	—	229.0	238.8	239.8
arm	—	196.3	—	229.0	238.8	239.8
auricular (anterior) (posterior)	—	196.0	—	229.0	238.8	239.8
axilla, axillary	—	196.3	—	229.0	238.8	239.8
brachial	—	196.3	—	229.0	238.8	239.8
bronchial	—	196.1	—	229.0	238.8	239.8
bronchopulmonary	—	196.1	—	229.0	238.8	239.8
celiac	—	196.2	—	229.0	238.8	239.8
cervical	—	196.0	—	229.0	238.8	239.8
cervicofacial	—	196.0	—	229.0	238.8	239.8
Cloquet	—	196.5	—	229.0	238.8	239.8
colic	—	196.2	—	229.0	238.8	239.8
common duct	—	196.2	—	229.0	238.8	239.8
cubital	—	196.3	—	229.0	238.8	239.8
diaphragmatic	—	196.1	—	229.0	238.8	239.8
epigastric, inferior	—	196.6	—	229.0	238.8	239.8
epitrochlear	—	196.3	—	229.0	238.8	239.8
esophageal	—	196.1	—	229.0	238.8	239.8
face	—	196.0	—	229.0	238.8	239.8
femoral	—	196.5	—	229.0	238.8	239.8
gastric	—	196.2	—	229.0	238.8	239.8
groin	—	196.5	—	229.0	238.8	239.8
head	—	196.0	—	229.0	238.8	239.8
hepatic	—	196.2	—	229.0	238.8	239.8
hilar (pulmonary)	—	196.1	—	229.0	238.8	239.8
splenic	—	196.2	—	229.0	238.8	239.8
hypogastric	—	196.6	—	229.0	238.8	239.8
ileocolic	—	196.2	—	229.0	238.8	239.8
iliac	—	196.6	—	229.0	238.8	239.8
infraclavicular	—	196.3	—	229.0	238.8	239.8
inguina, inguinal	—	196.5	—	229.0	238.8	239.8
innominate	—	196.1	—	229.0	238.8	239.8
intercostal	—	196.1	—	229.0	238.8	239.8
intestinal	—	196.2	—	229.0	238.8	239.8
intrabdominal	—	196.2	—	229.0	238.8	239.8
intrapelvic	—	196.6	—	229.0	238.8	239.8
intrathoracic	—	196.1	—	229.0	238.8	239.9
jugular	—	196.0	—	229.0	238.8	239.8
leg	—	196.5	—	229.0	238.8	239.8
limb						
lower	—	196.5	—	229.0	238.8	239.8
upper	—	196.3	—	229.0	238.8	239.8
lower limb	—	196.5	—	229.0	238.8	238.9
lumbar	—	196.2	—	229.0	238.8	239.8
mandibular	—	196.0	—	229.0	238.8	239.8
mediastinal	—	196.1	—	229.0	238.8	239.8
mesenteric (inferior) (superior)	—	196.2	—	229.0	238.8	239.8
midcolic	—	196.2	—	229.0	238.8	239.8
multiple sites in categories 196.0-196.6	—	196.8	—	229.0	238.8	239.8

	Malignant			Benign	Uncertain Behavior	Unspecified
	Primary	Secondary	Ca in situ			
neck	—	196.0	—	229.0	238.8	239.8
obturator	—	196.6	—	229.0	238.8	239.8
occipital	—	196.0	—	229.0	238.8	239.8
pancreatic	—	196.2	—	229.0	238.8	239.8
para-aortic	—	196.2	—	229.0	238.8	239.8
paracervical	—	196.6	—	229.0	238.8	239.8
parametrial	—	196.6	—	229.0	238.8	239.8
parasternal	—	196.1	—	229.0	238.8	239.8
parotid	—	196.0	—	229.0	238.8	239.8
pectoral	—	196.3	—	229.0	238.8	239.8
pelvic	—	196.6	—	229.0	238.8	239.8
peri-aortic	—	196.2	—	229.0	238.8	239.8
peripancreatic	—	196.2	—	229.0	238.8	239.8
popliteal	—	196.5	—	229.0	238.8	239.8
porta hepatis	—	196.2	—	229.0	238.8	239.8
portal	—	196.2	—	229.0	238.8	239.8
preauricular	—	196.0	—	229.0	238.8	239.8
prelaryngeal	—	196.0	—	229.0	238.8	239.8
presymphysial	—	196.6	—	229.0	238.8	239.8
pretracheal	—	196.0	—	229.0	238.8	239.8
primary (any site) NEC	202.9	—	—	—	—	—
pulmonary (hiler)	—	196.1	—	229.0	238.8	239.8
pyloric	—	196.2	—	229.0	238.8	239.8
retroperitoneal	—	196.2	—	229.0	238.8	239.8
retropharyngeal	—	196.0	—	229.0	238.8	239.8
Rosenmüller's	—	196.5	—	229.0	238.8	239.8
sacral	—	196.6	—	229.0	238.8	239.8
scalene	—	196.0	—	229.0	238.8	239.8
site NEC	—	196.9	—	229.0	238.8	239.8
splenic (hilar)	—	196.2	—	229.0	238.8	239.8
subclavicular	—	196.3	—	229.0	238.8	239.8
subinguinal	—	196.5	—	229.0	238.8	239.8
sublingual	—	196.0	—	229.0	238.8	239.8
submandibular	—	196.0	—	229.0	238.8	239.8
submaxillary	—	196.0	—	229.0	238.8	239.8
submental	—	196.0	—	229.0	238.8	239.8
subscapular	—	196.3	—	229.0	238.8	239.8
supraclavicular	—	196.0	—	229.0	238.8	239.8
thoracic	—	196.1	—	229.0	238.8	239.8
tibial	—	196.5	—	229.0	238.8	239.8
tracheal	—	196.1	—	229.0	238.8	239.8
tracheobronchial	—	196.1	—	229.0	238.8	239.8
upper limb	—	196.3	—	229.0	238.8	239.8
Virchow's	—	196.0	—	229.0	238.8	239.8
node—*see also* Neoplasm, lymph gland						
primary NEC	202.9	—	—	—	—	—
vessel (*see also* Neoplasm, connective tissue)	171.9	198.89	—	215.9	238.1	239.2
Mackenrodt's ligament	183.8	198.82	233.3	221.8	236.3	239.5
malar	170.0	198.5	—	213.0	238.0	239.2
region—*see* Neoplasm, cheek						
mammary gland—*see* Neoplasm, breast						
mandible	170.1	198.5	—	213.1	238.0	239.2
alveolar						
mucosa	143.1	198.89	230.0	210.4	235.1	239.0
ridge or process	170.1	198.5	—	213.1	238.0	239.2
carcinoma	143.1	—	—	—	—	—
carcinoma	143.1	—	—	—	—	—
marrow (bone) NEC	202.9	198.5	—	—	—	238.79
mastectomy site (skin)	173.5	198.2	—	—	—	—
specified as breast tissue	174.8	198.81	—	—	—	—

	Malignant			Benign	Uncertain Behavior	Unspecified
	Primary	Secondary	Ca in situ			
mastoid (air cells) (antrum) (cavity)	160.1	197.3	231.8	212.0	235.9	239.1
bone or process	170.0	198.5	—	213.0	238.0	239.2
maxilla, maxillary (superior)	170.0	198.5	—	213.0	238.0	239.2
alveolar						
mucosa	143.0	198.89	230.0	210.4	235.1	239.0
ridge or process	170.0	198.5	—	213.0	238.0	239.2
carcinoma	143.0	—	—	—	—	—
antrum	160.2	197.3	231.8	212.0	235.9	239.1
carcinoma	143.0	—	—	—	—	—
inferior—*see* Neoplasm, mandible						
sinus	160.2	197.3	231.8	212.0	235.9	239.1
meatus						
external (ear)	173.2	198.2	232.2	216.2	238.2	239.2
Meckel's diverticulum	152.3	197.4	230.7	211.2	235.2	239.0
mediastinum, mediastinal	164.9	197.1	—	212.5	235.8	239.8
anterior	164.2	197.1	—	212.5	235.8	239.8
contiguous sites with heart and thymus	164.8	—	—	—	—	—
posterior	164.3	197.1	—	212.5	235.8	239.8
medulla						
adrenal	194.0	198.7	234.8	227.0	237.2	239.7
oblongata	191.7	198.3	—	225.0	237.5	239.6
meibomian gland	173.1	198.2	232.1	216.1	238.2	239.2
melanoma —*see* Melanoma						
meninges (brain) (cerebral) (cranial) (intracranial)	192.1	198.4	—	225.2	237.6	239.7
spinal (cord)	192.3	198.4	—	225.4	237.6	239.7
meniscus, knee joint (lateral) (medial)	170.7	198.5	—	213.7	238.0	239.2
mesentery, mesenteric	158.8	197.6	—	211.8	235.4	239.0
mesoappendix	158.8	197.6	—	211.8	235.4	239.0
mesocolon	158.8	197.6	—	211.8	235.4	239.0
mesopharynx—*see* Neoplasm, oropharynx						
mesosalpinx	183.3	198.82	233.3	221.0	236.3	239.5
mesovarium	183.3	198.82	233.3	221.0	236.3	239.5
metacarpus (any bone)	170.5	198.5	—	213.5	238.0	239.2
metastatic NEC—*see also* Neoplasm, by site, secondary	—	199.1	—	—	—	—
metatarsus (any bone)	170.8	198.5	—	213.8	238.0	239.2
midbrain	191.7	198.3	—	225.0	237.5	239.6
milk duct—*see* Neoplasm, breast						
mons						
pubis	184.4	198.82	233.3	221.2	236.3	239.5
veneris	184.4	198.82	233.3	221.2	236.3	239.5
motor tract	192.9	198.4	—	225.9	237.9	239.7
brain	191.9	198.3	—	225.0	237.5	239.6
spinal	192.2	198.3	—	225.3	237.5	239.7
mouth	145.9	198.89	230.0	210.4	235.1	239.0
contiguous sites	145.8	—	—	—	—	—
floor	144.9	198.89	230.0	210.3	235.1	239.0
anterior portion	144.0	198.89	230.0	210.3	235.1	239.0
contiguous sites	144.8	—	—	—	—	—
lateral portion	144.1	198.89	230.0	210.3	235.1	239.0
roof	145.5	198.89	230.0	210.4	235.1	239.0
specified part NEC	145.8	198.89	230.0	210.4	235.1	239.0
vestibule	145.1	198.89	230.0	210.4	235.1	239.0
mucosa						
alveolar (ridge or process)	143.9	198.89	230.0	210.4	235.1	239.0
lower	143.1	198.89	230.0	210.4	235.1	239.0
upper	143.0	198.89	230.0	210.4	235.1	239.0
buccal	145.0	198.89	230.0	210.4	235.1	239.0
cheek	145.0	198.89	230.0	210.4	235.1	239.0

	Malignant					
	Primary	Secondary	Ca in situ	Benign	Uncertain Behavior	Unspecified
lip—*see* Neoplasm, lip, internal						
nasal	160.0	197.3	231.8	212.0	235.9	239.1
oral	145.0	198.89	230.0	210.4	235.1	239.0
Müllerian duct						
female	184.8	198.82	233.3	221.8	236.3	239.5
male	187.8	198.82	233.6	222.8	236.6	239.5
multiple sites NEC	199.0	199.0	234.9	229.9	238.9	199.0
muscle—*see also* Neoplasm, connective tissue						
extraocular	190.1	198.4	234.0	224.1	238.8	239.8
myocardium	164.1	198.89	—	212.7	238.8	239.8
myometrium	182.0	198.82	233.2	219.1	236.0	239.5
myopericardium	164.1	198.89	—	212.7	238.8	239.8
nabothian gland (follicle)	180.0	198.82	233.1	219.0	236.0	239.5
nail	173.9	198.2	232.9	216.9	238.2	239.2
finger	173.6	198.2	232.6	216.6	238.2	239.2
toe	173.7	198.2	232.7	216.7	238.2	239.2
nares, naris (anterior) (posterior)	160.0	197.3	231.8	212.0	235.9	239.1
nasal—*see* Neoplasm, nose						
nasolabial groove	173.3	198.2	232.3	216.3	238.2	239.2
nasolacrimal duct	190.7	198.4	234.0	224.7	238.8	239.8
nasopharynx, nasopharyngeal	147.9	198.89	230.0	210.7	235.1	239.0
contiguous sites	147.8	—	—	—	—	—
floor	147.3	198.89	230.0	210.7	235.1	239.0
roof	147.0	198.89	230.0	210.7	235.1	239.0
specified site NEC	147.8	198.89	230.0	210.7	235.1	239.0
wall	147.9	198.89	230.0	210.7	235.1	239.0
anterior	147.3	198.89	230.0	210.7	235.1	239.0
lateral	147.2	198.89	230.0	210.7	235.1	239.0
posterior	147.1	198.89	230.0	210.7	235.1	239.0
superior	147.0	198.89	230.0	210.7	235.1	239.0
nates	173.5	198.2	232.5	216.5	238.2	239.2
neck NEC*	195.0	198.89	234.8	229.8	238.8	239.8
nerve (autonomic) (ganglion) (parasympathetic) (peripheral) (sympathetic)—*see also* Neoplasm, connective tissue						
abducens	192.0	198.4	—	225.1	237.9	239.7
accessory (spinal)	192.0	198.4	—	225.1	237.9	239.7
acoustic	192.0	198.4	—	225.1	237.9	239.7
auditory	192.0	198.4	—	225.1	237.9	239.7
brachial	171.2	198.89	—	215.2	238.1	239.2
cranial (any)	192.0	198.4	—	225.1	237.9	239.7
facial	192.0	198.4	—	225.1	237.9	239.7
femoral	171.3	198.89	—	215.3	238.1	239.2
glossopharyngeal	192.0	198.4	—	225.1	237.9	239.7
hypoglossal	192.0	198.4	—	225.1	237.9	239.7
intercostal	171.4	198.89	—	215.4	238.1	239.2
lumbar	171.7	198.89	—	215.7	238.1	239.2
median	171.2	198.89	—	215.2	238.1	239.2
obturator	171.3	198.89	—	215.3	238.1	239.2
oculomotor	192.0	198.4	—	225.1	237.9	239.7
olfactory	192.0	198.4	—	225.1	237.9	239.7
optic	192.0	198.4	—	225.1	237.9	239.7
peripheral NEC	171.9	198.89	—	215.9	238.1	239.2
radial	171.2	198.89	—	215.2	238.1	239.2
sacral	171.6	198.89	—	215.6	238.1	239.2
sciatic	171.3	198.89	—	215.3	238.1	239.2
spinal NEC	171.9	198.89	—	215.9	238.1	239.2
trigeminal	192.0	198.4	—	225.1	237.9	239.7
trochlear	192.0	198.4	—	225.1	237.9	239.7
ulnar	171.2	198.89	—	215.2	238.1	239.2

	Malignant			Benign	Uncertain Behavior	Unspecified
	Primary	Secondary	Ca in situ			
vagus	192.0	198.4	—	225.1	237.9	239.7
nervous system (central)						
NEC	192.9	198.4	—	225.9	237.9	239.7
autonomic NEC	171.9	198.89	—	215.9	238.1	239.2
brain—*see also* Neoplasm, brain						
membrane or meninges	192.1	198.4	—	225.2	237.6	239.7
contiguous sites	192.8	—	—	—	—	—
parasympathetic NEC	171.9	198.89	—	215.9	238.1	239.2
sympathetic NEC	171.9	198.89	—	215.9	238.1	239.2
nipple (female)	174.0	198.81	233.0	217	238.3	239.3
male	175.0	198.81	233.0	217	238.3	239.3
nose, nasal	195.0	198.89	234.8	229.8	238.8	239.8
ala (external)	173.3	198.2	232.3	216.3	238.2	239.2
bone	170.0	198.5	—	213.0	238.0	239.2
cartilage	160.0	197.3	231.8	212.0	235.9	239.1
cavity	160.0	197.3	231.8	212.0	235.9	239.1
contiguous sites with accessory						
sinuses or middle ear	160.8	—	—	—	—	—
choana	147.3	198.89	230.0	210.7	235.1	239.0
external (skin)	173.3	198.2	232.3	216.3	238.2	239.2
fossa	160.0	197.3	231.8	212.0	235.9	239.1
internal	160.0	197.3	231.8	212.0	235.9	239.1
mucosa	160.0	197.3	231.8	212.0	235.9	239.1
septum	160.0	197.3	231.8	212.0	235.9	239.1
posterior margin	147.3	198.89	230.0	210.7	235.1	239.0
sinus—*see* Neoplasm, sinus						
skin	173.3	198.2	232.3	216.3	238.2	239.2
turbinate (mucosa)	160.0	197.3	231.8	212.0	235.9	239.1
bone	170.0	198.5	—	213.0	238.0	239.2
vestibule	160.0	197.3	231.8	212.0	235.9	239.1
nostril	160.0	197.3	231.8	212.0	235.9	239.1
nucleus pulposus	170.2	198.5	—	213.2	238.0	239.2
occipital						
bone	170.0	198.5	—	213.0	238.0	239.2
lobe or pole, brain	191.4	198.3	—	225.0	237.5	239.6
odontogenic—*see* Neoplasm,						
jaw bone						
oesophagus—*see* Neoplasm,						
esophagus						
olfactory nerve or bulb	192.0	198.4	—	225.1	237.9	239.7
olive (brain)	191.7	198.3	—	225.0	237.5	239.6
omentum	158.8	197.6	—	211.8	235.4	239.0
operculum (brain)	191.0	198.3	—	225.0	237.5	239.6
optic nerve, chiasm, or tract	192.0	198.4	—	225.1	237.9	239.7
oral (cavity)	145.9	198.89	230.0	210.4	235.1	239.0
contiguous sites with lip						
or pharynx	149.8	—	—	—	—	—
ill-defined	149.9	198.89	230.0	210.4	235.1	239.0
mucosa	145.9	198.89	230.0	210.4	235.1	239.0
orbit	190.1	198.4	234.0	224.1	238.8	239.8
bone	170.0	198.5	—	213.0	238.0	239.2
eye	190.1	198.4	234.0	224.1	238.8	239.8
soft parts	190.1	198.4	234.0	224.1	238.8	239.8
organ of Zuckerkandl	194.6	198.89	—	227.6	237.3	239.7
oropharynx	146.9	198.89	230.0	210.6	235.1	239.0
branchial cleft (vestige)	146.8	198.89	230.0	210.6	235.1	239.0
contiguous sites	146.8	—	—	—	—	—
junctional region	146.5	198.89	230.0	210.6	235.1	239.0
lateral wall	146.6	198.89	230.0	210.6	235.1	239.0
pillars of fauces	146.2	198.89	230.0	210.6	235.1	239.0
posterior wall	146.7	198.89	230.0	210.6	235.1	239.0
specified part NEC	146.8	198.89	230.0	210.6	235.1	239.0
vallecula	146.3	198.89	230.0	210.6	235.1	239.0

| | Malignant | | | | | |
	Primary	Secondary	Ca in situ	Benign	Uncertain Behavior	Unspecified
os						
external	180.1	198.82	233.1	219.0	236.0	239.5
internal	180.0	198.82	233.1	219.0	236.0	239.5
ovary	183.0	198.6	233.3	220	236.2	239.5
oviduct	183.2	198.82	233.3	221.0	236.3	239.5
palate	145.5	198.89	230.0	210.4	235.1	239.0
hard	145.2	198.89	230.0	210.4	235.1	239.0
junction of hard and soft						
palate	145.5	198.89	230.0	210.4	235.1	239.0
soft	145.3	198.89	230.0	210.4	235.1	239.0
nasopharyngeal surface	147.3	198.89	230.0	210.7	235.1	239.0
posterior surface	147.3	198.89	230.0	210.7	235.1	239.0
superior surface	147.3	198.89	230.0	210.7	235.1	239.0
palatoglossal arch	146.2	198.89	230.0	210.6	235.1	239.0
palatopharyngeal arch	146.2	198.89	230.0	210.6	235.1	239.0
pallium	191.0	198.3	—	225.0	237.5	239.6
palpebra	173.1	198.2	232.1	216.1	238.2	239.2
pancreas	157.9	197.8	230.9	211.6	235.5	239.0
body	157.1	197.8	230.9	211.6	235.5	239.0
contiguous sites	157.8	—	—	—	—	—
duct (of Santorini) (of						
Wirsung)	157.3	197.8	230.9	211.6	235.5	239.0
ectopic tissue	157.8	197.8	230.9	211.6	235.5	239.0
head	157.0	197.8	230.9	211.6	235.5	239.0
islet cells	157.4	197.8	230.9	211.7	235.5	239.0
neck	157.8	197.8	230.9	211.6	235.5	239.0
tail	157.2	197.8	230.9	211.6	235.5	239.0
para-aortic body	194.6	198.89	—	227.6	237.3	239.7
paraganglion NEC	194.6	198.89	—	227.6	237.3	239.7
parametrium	183.4	198.82	—	221.0	236.3	239.5
paranephric	158.0	197.6	—	211.8	235.4	239.0
pararectal	195.3	198.89	—	229.8	238.8	239.8
parasagittal (region)	195.0	198.89	234.8	229.8	238.8	239.8
parasellar	192.9	198.4	—	225.9	237.9	239.7
parathyroid (gland)	194.1	198.89	234.8	227.1	237.4	239.7
paraurethral	195.3	198.89	—	229.8	238.8	239.8
gland	189.4	198.1	233.9	223.89	236.99	239.5
paravaginal	195.3	198.89	—	229.8	238.8	239.8
parenchyma, kidney	189.0	198.0	233.9	223.0	236.91	239.5
parietal						
bone	170.0	198.5	—	213.0	238.0	239.2
lobe, brain	191.3	198.3	—	225.0	237.5	239.6
paroophoron	183.3	198.82	233.3	221.0	236.3	239.5
parotid (duct) (gland)	142.0	198.89	230.0	210.2	235.0	239.0
parovarium	183.3	198.82	233.3	221.0	236.3	239.5
patella	170.8	198.5	—	213.8	238.0	239.2
peduncle, cerebral	191.7	198.3	—	225.0	237.5	239.6
pelvirectal junction	154.0	197.5	230.4	211.4	235.2	239.0
pelvis, pelvic	195.3	198.89	234.8	229.8	238.8	239.8
bone	170.6	198.5	—	213.6	238.0	239.2
floor	195.3	198.89	234.8	229.8	238.8	239.8
renal	189.1	198.0	233.9	223.1	236.91	239.5
viscera	195.3	198.89	234.8	229.8	238.8	239.8
wall	195.3	198.89	234.8	229.8	238.8	239.8
pelvo-abdominal	195.8	198.89	234.8	229.8	238.8	239.8
penis	187.4	198.82	233.5	222.1	236.6	239.5
body	187.3	198.82	233.5	222.1	236.6	239.5
corpus (cavernosum)	187.3	198.82	233.5	222.1	236.6	239.5
glans	187.2	198.82	233.5	222.1	236.6	239.5
skin NEC	187.4	198.82	233.5	222.1	236.6	239.5
periadrenal (tissue)	158.0	197.6	—	211.8	235.4	239.0
perianal (skin)	173.5	198.2	232.5	216.5	238.2	239.2
pericardium	164.1	198.89	—	212.7	238.8	239.8

	Malignant					
	Primary	Secondary	Ca in situ	Benign	Uncertain Behavior	Unspecified
perinephric	158.0	197.6	—	211.8	235.4	239.0
perineum	195.3	198.89	234.8	229.8	238.8	239.8
periodontal tissue NEC	143.9	198.89	230.0	210.4	235.1	239.0
periosteum—*see* Neoplasm, bone						
peripancreatic	158.0	197.6	—	211.8	235.4	239.0
peripheral nerve NEC	171.9	198.89	—	215.9	238.1	239.2
perirectal (tissue)	195.3	198.89	—	229.8	238.8	239.8
perirenal (tissue)	158.0	197.6	—	211.8	235.4	239.0
peritoneum, peritoneal						
(cavity)	158.9	197.6	—	211.8	235.4	239.0
contiguous sites	158.8	—	—	—	—	—
with digestive organs	159.8	—	—	—	—	—
parietal	158.8	197.6	—	211.8	235.4	239.0
pelvic	158.8	197.6	—	211.8	235.4	239.0
specified part NEC	158.8	197.6	—	211.8	235.4	239.0
peritonsillar (tissue)	195.0	198.89	234.8	229.8	238.8	239.8
periurethral tissue	195.3	198.89	—	229.8	238.8	239.8
phalanges	170.9	198.5	—	213.9	238.0	239.2
foot	170.8	198.5	—	213.8	238.0	239.2
hand	170.5	198.5	—	213.5	238.0	239.2
pharynx, pharyngeal	149.0	198.89	230.0	210.9	235.1	239.0
bursa	147.1	198.89	230.0	210.7	235.1	239.0
fornix	147.3	198.89	230.0	210.7	235.1	239.0
recess	147.2	198.89	230.0	210.7	235.1	239.0
region	149.0	198.89	230.0	210.9	235.1	239.0
tonsil	147.1	198.89	230.0	210.7	235.1	239.0
wall (lateral) (posterior)	149.0	198.89	230.0	210.9	235.1	239.0
pia mater (cerebral) (cranial)	192.1	198.4	—	225.2	237.6	239.7
spinal	192.3	198.4	—	225.4	237.6	239.7
pillars of fauces	146.2	198.89	230.0	210.6	235.1	239.0
pineal (body) (gland)	194.4	198.89	234.8	227.4	237.1	239.7
pinna (ear) NEC	173.2	198.2	232.2	216.2	238.2	239.2
cartilage	171.0	198.89	—	215.0	238.1	239.2
piriform fossa or sinus	148.1	198.89	230.0	210.8	235.1	239.0
pituitary (body) (fossa)						
(gland) (lobe)	194.3	198.89	234.8	227.3	237.0	239.7
placenta	181	198.82	233.2	219.8	236.1	239.5
pleura, pleural (cavity)	163.9	197.2	—	212.4	235.8	239.1
contiguous sites	163.8	—	—	—	—	—
parietal	163.0	197.2	—	212.4	235.8	239.1
visceral	163.1	197.2	—	212.4	235.8	239.1
plexus						
brachial	171.2	198.89	—	215.2	238.1	239.2
cervical	171.0	198.89	—	215.0	238.1	239.2
choroid	191.5	198.3	—	225.0	237.5	239.6
lumbosacral	171.6	198.89	—	215.6	238.1	239.2
sacral	171.6	198.89	—	215.6	238.1	239.2
pluri-endocrine	194.8	198.89	234.8	227.8	237.4	239.7
pole						
frontal	191.1	198.3	—	225.0	237.5	239.6
occipital	191.4	198.3	—	225.0	237.5	239.6
pons (varolii)	191.7	198.3	—	225.0	237.5	239.6
popliteal fossa or space*	195.5	198.89	234.8	229.8	238.8	239.8
postcricoid (region)	148.0	198.89	230.0	210.8	235.1	239.0
posterior fossa (cranial)	191.9	198.3	—	225.0	237.5	239.6
postnasal space	147.9	198.89	230.0	210.7	235.1	239.0
prepuce	187.1	198.82	233.5	222.1	236.6	239.5
prepylorus	151.1	197.8	230.2	211.1	235.2	239.0
presacral (region)	195.3	198.89	—	229.8	238.8	239.8
prostate (gland)	185	198.82	233.4	222.2	236.5	239.5
utricle	189.3	198.1	233.9	223.81	236.99	239.5
pterygoid fossa	171.0	198.89	—	215.0	238.1	239.2
pubic bone	170.6	198.5	—	213.6	238.0	239.2

	Malignant					
	Primary	Secondary	Ca in situ	Benign	Uncertain Behavior	Unspecified
pudenda, pudendum (female)	184.4	198.82	233.3	221.2	236.3	239.5
pulmonary	162.9	197.0	231.2	212.3	235.7	239.1
putamen	191.0	198.3	—	225.0	237.5	239.6
pyloric						
antrum	151.2	197.8	230.2	211.1	235.2	239.0
canal	151.1	197.8	230.2	211.1	235.2	239.0
pylorus	151.1	197.8	230.2	211.1	235.2	239.0
pyramid (brain)	191.7	198.3	—	225.0	237.5	239.6
pyriform fossa or sinus	148.1	198.89	230.0	210.8	235.1	239.0
radius (any part)	170.4	198.5	—	213.4	238.0	239.2
Rathke's pouch	194.3	198.89	234.8	227.3	237.0	239.7
rectosigmoid (colon)						
(junction)	154.0	197.5	230.4	211.4	235.2	239.0
contiguous sites with						
anus or rectum	154.8	—	—	—	—	—
rectouterine pouch	158.8	197.6	—	211.8	235.4	239.0
rectovaginal septum or wall	195.3	198.89	234.8	229.8	238.8	239.8
rectovesical septum	195.3	198.89	234.8	229.8	238.8	239.8
rectum (ampulla)	154.1	197.5	230.4	211.4	235.2	239.0
and colon	154.0	197.5	230.4	211.4	235.2	239.0
contiguous sites with anus or						
rectosigmoid junction	154.8	—	—	—	—	—
renal	189.0	198.0	233.9	223.0	236.91	239.5
calyx	189.1	198.0	233.9	223.1	236.91	239.5
hilus	189.1	198.0	233.9	223.1	236.91	239.5
parenchyma	189.0	198.0	233.9	223.0	236.91	239.5
pelvis	189.1	198.0	233.9	223.1	236.91	239.5
respiratory						
organs or system NEC	165.9	197.3	231.9	212.9	235.9	239.1
contiguous sites with						
intrathoracic organs	165.8	—	—	—	—	—
specified sites NEC	165.8	197.3	231.8	212.8	235.9	239.1
tract NEC	165.9	197.3	231.9	212.9	235.9	239.1
upper	165.0	197.3	231.9	212.9	235.9	239.1
retina	190.5	198.4	234.0	224.5	238.8	239.8
retrobulbar	190.1	198.4	—	224.1	238.8	239.8
retrocecal	158.0	197.6	—	211.8	235.4	239.0
retromolar (area) (triangle)						
(trigone)	145.6	198.89	230.0	210.4	235.1	239.0
retro-orbital	195.0	198.89	234.8	229.8	238.8	239.8
retroperitoneal (space)						
(tissue)	158.0	197.6	—	211.8	235.4	239.0
contiguous sites	158.8	—	—	—	—	—
retroperitoneum	158.0	197.6	—	211.8	235.4	239.0
contiguous sites	158.8	—	—	—	—	—
retropharyngeal	149.0	198.89	230.0	210.9	235.1	239.0
retrovesical (septum)	195.3	198.89	234.8	229.8	238.8	239.8
rhinencephalon	191.0	198.3	—	225.0	237.5	239.6
rib	170.3	198.5	—	213.3	238.0	239.2
Rosenmüller's fossa	147.2	198.89	230.0	210.7	235.1	239.0
round ligament	183.5	198.82	—	221.0	236.3	239.5
sacrococcyx, sacrococcygeal	170.6	198.5	—	213.6	238.0	239.2
region	195.3	198.89	234.8	229.8	238.8	239.8
sacrouterine ligament	183.4	198.82	—	221.0	236.3	239.5
sacrum, sacral (vertebra)	170.6	198.5	—	213.6	238.0	239.2
salivary gland or duct						
(major)	142.9	198.89	230.0	210.2	235.0	239.0
contiguous sites	142.8	—	—	—	—	—
minor NEC	145.9	198.89	230.0	210.4	235.1	239.0
parotid	142.0	198.89	230.0	210.2	235.0	239.0
pluriglandular	142.8	198.89	230.0	210.2	235.0	239.0
sublingual	142.2	198.89	230.0	210.2	235.0	239.0
submandibular	142.1	198.89	230.0	210.2	235.0	239.0

	Malignant			Benign	Uncertain Behavior	Unspecified
	Primary	Secondary	Ca in situ			
submaxillary	142.1	198.89	230.0	210.2	235.0	239.0
salpinx (uterine)	183.2	198.82	233.3	221.0	236.3	239.5
Santorini's duct	157.3	197.8	230.9	211.6	235.5	239.0
scalp	173.4	198.2	232.4	216.4	238.2	239.2
scapula (any part)	170.4	198.5	—	213.4	238.0	239.2
scapular region	195.1	198.89	234.8	229.8	238.8	239.8
scar NEC (*see also* Neoplasm, skin)	173.9	198.2	232.9	216.9	238.2	239.2
sciatic nerve	171.3	198.89	—	215.3	238.1	239.2
sclera	190.0	198.4	234.0	224.0	238.8	239.8
scrotum (skin)	187.7	198.82	233.6	222.4	236.6	239.5
sebaceous gland—*see* Neoplasm, skin						
sella turcica	194.3	198.89	234.8	227.3	237.0	239.7
bone	170.0	198.5	—	213.0	238.0	239.2
semilunar cartilage (knee)	170.7	198.5	—	213.7	238.0	239.2
seminal vesicle	187.8	198.82	233.6	222.8	236.6	239.5
septum						
nasal	160.0	197.3	231.8	212.0	235.9	239.1
posterior margin	147.3	198.89	230.0	210.7	235.1	239.0
rectovaginal	195.3	198.89	234.8	229.8	238.8	239.8
rectovesical	195.3	198.89	234.8	229.8	238.8	239.8
urethrovaginal	184.9	198.82	233.3	221.9	236.3	239.5
vesicovaginal	184.9	198.82	233.3	221.9	236.3	239.5
shoulder NEC*	195.4	198.89	232.6	229.8	238.8	239.8
sigmoid flexure (lower) (upper)	153.3	197.5	230.3	211.3	235.2	239.0
sinus (accessory)	160.9	197.3	231.8	212.0	235.9	239.1
bone (any)	170.0	198.5	—	213.0	238.0	239.2
contiguous sites with middle ear or nasal cavities	160.8	—	—	—	—	—
ethmoidal	160.3	197.3	231.8	212.0	235.9	239.1
frontal	160.4	197.3	231.8	212.0	235.9	239.1
maxillary	160.2	197.3	231.8	212.0	235.9	239.1
nasal, paranasal NEC	160.9	197.3	231.8	212.0	235.9	239.1
pyriform	148.1	198.89	230.0	210.8	235.1	239.0
sphenoidal	160.5	197.3	231.8	212.0	235.9	239.1
skeleton, skeletal NEC	170.9	198.5	—	213.9	238.0	239.2
Skene's gland	189.4	198.1	233.9	223.89	236.99	239.5
skin NEC	173.9	198.2	232.9	216.9	238.2	239.2
abdominal wall	173.5	198.2	232.5	216.5	238.2	239.2
ala nasi	173.3	198.2	232.3	216.3	238.2	239.2
ankle	173.7	198.2	232.7	216.7	238.2	239.2
antecubital space	173.6	198.2	232.6	216.6	238.2	239.2
anus	173.5	198.2	232.5	216.5	238.2	239.2
arm	173.6	198.2	232.6	216.6	238.2	239.2
auditory canal (external)	173.2	198.2	232.2	216.2	238.2	239.2
auricle (ear)	173.2	198.2	232.2	216.2	238.2	239.2
auricular canal (external)	173.2	198.2	232.2	216.2	238.2	239.2
axilla, axillary fold	173.5	198.2	232.5	216.5	238.2	239.2
back	173.5	198.2	232.5	216.5	238.2	239.2
breast	173.5	198.2	232.5	216.5	238.2	239.2
brow	173.3	198.2	232.3	216.3	238.2	239.2
buttock	173.5	198.2	232.5	216.5	238.2	239.2
calf	173.7	198.2	232.7	216.7	238.2	239.2
canthus (eye) (inner) (outer)	173.1	198.2	232.1	216.1	238.2	239.2
cervical region	173.4	198.2	232.4	216.4	238.2	239.2
cheek (external)	173.3	198.2	232.3	216.3	238.2	239.2
chest (wall)	173.5	198.2	232.5	216.5	238.2	239.2
chin	173.3	198.2	232.3	216.3	238.2	239.2
clavicular area	173.5	198.2	232.5	216.5	238.2	239.2
clitoris	184.3	198.82	233.3	221.2	236.3	239.5
columnella	173.3	198.2	232.3	216.3	238.2	239.2

	Malignant			Benign	Uncertain Behavior	Unspecified
	Primary	Secondary	Ca in situ			
concha	173.2	198.2	232.2	216.2	238.2	239.2
contiguous sites	173.8	—	—	—	—	—
ear (external)	173.2	198.2	232.2	216.2	238.2	239.2
elbow	173.6	198.2	232.6	216.6	238.2	239.2
eyebrow	173.3	198.2	232.3	216.3	238.2	239.2
eyelid	173.1	198.2	232.1	216.1	238.2	239.2
face NEC	173.3	198.2	232.3	216.3	238.2	239.2
female genital organs						
(external)	184.4	198.82	233.3	221.2	236.3	239.5
clitoris	184.3	198.82	233.3	221.2	236.3	239.5
labium NEC	184.4	198.82	233.3	221.2	236.3	239.5
majus	184.1	198.82	233.3	221.2	236.3	239.5
minus	184.2	198.82	233.3	221.2	236.3	239.5
pudendum	184.4	198.82	233.3	221.2	236.3	239.5
vulva	184.4	198.82	233.3	221.2	236.3	239.5
finger	173.6	198.2	232.6	216.6	238.2	239.2
flank	173.5	198.2	232.5	216.5	238.2	239.2
foot	173.7	198.2	232.7	216.7	238.2	239.2
forearm	173.6	198.2	232.6	216.6	238.2	239.2
forehead	173.3	198.2	232.3	216.3	238.2	239.2
glabella	173.3	198.2	232.3	216.3	238.2	239.2
gluteal region	173.5	198.2	232.5	216.5	238.2	239.2
groin	173.5	198.2	232.5	216.5	238.2	239.2
hand	173.6	198.2	232.6	216.6	238.2	239.2
head NEC	173.4	198.2	232.4	216.4	238.2	239.2
heel	173.7	198.2	232.7	216.7	238.2	239.2
helix	173.2	198.2	232.2	216.2	238.2	239.2
hip	173.7	198.2	232.7	216.7	238.2	239.2
infraclavicular region	173.5	198.2	232.5	216.5	238.2	239.2
inguinal region	173.5	198.2	232.5	216.5	238.2	239.2
jaw	173.3	198.2	232.3	216.3	238.2	239.2
knee	173.7	198.2	232.7	216.7	238.2	239.2
labia						
majora	184.1	198.82	233.3	221.2	236.3	239.5
minora	184.2	198.82	233.3	221.2	236.3	239.5
leg	173.7	198.2	232.7	216.7	238.2	239.2
lid (lower) (upper)	173.1	198.2	232.1	216.1	238.2	239.2
limb NEC	173.9	198.2	232.9	216.9	238.2	239.5
lower	173.7	198.2	232.7	216.7	238.2	239.2
upper	173.6	198.2	232.6	216.6	238.2	239.2
lip (lower) (upper)	173.0	198.2	232.0	216.0	238.2	239.2
male genital organs	187.9	198.82	233.6	222.9	236.6	239.5
penis	187.4	198.82	233.5	222.1	236.6	239.5
prepuce	187.1	198.82	233.5	222.1	236.6	239.5
scrotum	187.7	198.82	233.6	222.4	236.6	239.5
mastectomy site	173.5	198.2	—	—	—	—
specified as breast tissue	174.8	198.81	—	—	—	
meatus, acoustic (external)	173.2	198.2	232.2	216.2	238.2	239.2
melanoma —*see* Melanoma						
nates	173.5	198.2	232.5	216.5	238.2	239.2
neck	173.4	198.2	232.4	216.4	238.2	239.2
nose (external)	173.3	198.2	232.3	216.3	238.2	239.2
palm	173.6	198.2	232.6	216.6	238.2	239.2
palpebra	173.1	198.2	232.1	216.1	238.2	239.2
penis NEC	187.4	198.82	233.5	222.1	236.6	239.5
perianal	173.5	198.2	232.5	216.5	238.2	239.2
perineum	173.5	198.2	232.5	216.5	238.2	239.2
pinna	173.2	198.2	232.2	216.2	238.2	239.2
plantar	173.7	198.2	232.7	216.7	238.2	239.2
popliteal fossa or space	173.7	198.2	232.7	216.7	238.2	239.2
prepuce	187.1	198.82	233.5	222.1	236.6	239.5
pubes	173.5	198.2	232.5	216.5	238.2	239.2
sacrococcygeal region	173.5	198.2	232.5	216.5	238.2	239.2

	Malignant					
	Primary	Secondary	Ca in situ	Benign	Uncertain Behavior	Unspecified
scalp	173.4	198.2	232.4	216.4	238.2	239.2
scapular region	173.5	198.2	232.5	216.5	238.2	239.2
scrotum	187.7	198.82	233.6	222.4	236.6	239.5
shoulder	173.6	198.2	232.6	216.6	238.2	239.2
sole (foot)	173.7	198.2	232.7	216.7	238.2	239.2
specified sites NEC	173.8	198.2	232.8	216.8	232.8	239.2
submammary fold	173.5	198.2	232.5	216.5	238.2	239.2
supraclavicular region	173.4	198.2	232.4	216.4	238.2	239.2
temple	173.3	198.2	232.3	216.3	238.2	239.2
thigh	173.7	198.2	232.7	216.7	238.2	239.2
thoracic wall	173.5	198.2	232.5	216.5	238.2	239.2
thumb	173.6	198.2	232.6	216.6	238.2	239.2
toe	173.7	198.2	232.7	216.7	238.2	239.2
tragus	173.2	198.2	232.2	216.2	238.2	239.2
trunk	173.5	198.2	232.5	216.5	238.2	239.2
umbilicus	173.5	198.2	232.5	216.5	238.2	239.2
vulva	184.4	198.82	233.3	221.2	236.3	239.5
wrist	173.6	198.2	232.6	216.6	238.2	239.2
skull	170.0	198.5	—	213.0	238.0	239.2
soft parts or tissues—*see* Neoplasm, connective tissue						
specified site NEC	195.8	198.89	234.8	229.8	238.8	239.8
spermatic cord	187.6	198.82	233.6	222.8	236.6	239.5
sphenoid	160.5	197.3	231.8	212.0	235.9	239.1
bone	170.0	198.5	—	213.0	238.0	239.2
sinus	160.5	197.3	231.8	212.0	235.9	239.1
sphincter						
anal	154.2	197.5	230.5	211.4	235.5	239.0
of Oddi	156.1	197.8	230.8	211.5	235.3	239.0
spine, spinal (column)	170.2	198.5	—	213.2	238.0	239.2
bulb	191.7	198.3	—	225.0	237.5	239.6
coccyx	170.6	198.5	—	213.6	238.0	239.2
cord (cervical) (lumbar) (sacral) (thoracic)	192.2	198.3	—	225.3	237.5	239.7
dura mater	192.3	198.4	—	225.4	237.6	239.7
lumbosacral	170.2	198.5	—	213.2	238.0	239.2
membrane	192.3	198.4	—	225.4	237.6	239.7
meninges	192.3	198.4	—	225.4	237.6	239.7
nerve (root)	171.9	198.89	—	215.9	238.1	239.2
pia mater	192.3	198.4	—	225.4	237.6	239.7
root	171.9	198.89	—	215.9	238.1	239.2
sacrum	170.6	198.5	—	213.6	238.0	239.2
spleen, splenic NEC	159.1	197.8	230.9	211.9	235.5	239.0
flexure (colon)	153.7	197.5	230.3	211.3	235.2	239.0
stem, brain	191.7	198.3	—	225.0	237.5	239.6
Stensen's duct	142.0	198.89	230.0	210.2	235.0	239.0
sternum	170.3	198.5	—	213.3	238.0	239.2
stomach	151.9	197.8	230.2	211.1	235.2	239.0
antrum (pyloric)	151.2	197.8	230.2	211.1	235.2	239.0
body	151.4	197.8	230.2	211.1	235.2	239.0
cardia	151.0	197.8	230.2	211.1	235.2	239.0
cardiac orifice	151.0	197.8	230.2	211.1	235.2	239.0
contiguous sites	151.8	—	—	—	—	—
corpus	151.4	197.8	230.2	211.1	235.2	239.0
fundus	151.3	197.8	230.2	211.1	235.2	239.0
greater curvature NEC	151.6	197.8	230.2	211.1	235.2	239.0
lesser curvature NEC	151.5	197.8	230.2	211.1	235.2	239.0
prepylorus	151.1	197.8	230.2	211.1	235.2	239.0
pylorus	151.1	197.8	230.2	211.1	235.2	239.0
wall NEC	151.9	197.8	230.2	211.1	235.2	239.0
anterior NEC	151.8	197.8	230.2	211.1	235.2	239.0
posterior NEC	151.8	197.8	230.2	211.1	235.2	239.0
stroma, endometrial	182.0	198.82	233.2	219.1	236.0	239.5

| | Malignant | | | | | |
	Primary	Secondary	Ca in situ	Benign	Uncertain Behavior	Unspecified
stump, cervical	180.8	198.82	233.1	219.0	236.0	239.5
subcutaneous (nodule) (tissue) NEC—*see* Neoplasm, connective tissue						
subdural	192.1	198.4	—	225.2	237.6	239.7
subglottis, subglottic	161.2	197.3	231.0	212.1	235.6	239.1
sublingual	144.9	198.89	230.0	210.3	235.1	239.0
gland or duct	142.2	198.89	230.0	210.2	235.0	239.0
submandibular gland	142.1	198.89	230.0	210.2	235.0	239.0
submaxillary gland or duct	142.1	198.89	230.0	210.2	235.0	239.0
submental	195.0	198.89	234.8	229.8	238.8	239.8
subpleural	162.9	197.0	—	212.3	235.7	239.1
substernal	164.2	197.1	—	212.5	235.8	239.8
sudoriferous, sudoriparous gland, site unspecified	173.9	198.2	232.9	216.9	238.2	239.2
specified site—*see* Neoplasm, skin						
supraclavicular region	195.0	198.89	234.8	229.8	238.8	239.8
supraglottis	161.1	197.3	231.0	212.1	235.6	239.1
suprarenal (capsule) (cortex) (gland) (medulla)	194.0	198.7	234.8	227.0	237.2	239.7
suprasellar (region)	191.9	198.3	—	225.0	237.5	239.6
sweat gland (apocrine) (eccrine), site unspecified	173.9	198.2	232.9	216.9	238.2	239.2
specified site—*see* Neoplasm, skin						
sympathetic nerve or nervous system NEC	171.9	198.89	—	215.9	238.1	239.2
symphysis pubis	170.6	198.5	—	213.6	238.0	239.2
synovial membrane—*see* Neoplasm, connective tissue						
tapetum, brain	191.8	198.3	—	225.0	237.5	239.6
tarsus (any bone)	170.8	198.5	—	213.8	238.0	239.2
temple (skin)	173.3	198.2	232.3	216.3	238.2	239.2
temporal						
bone	170.0	198.5	—	213.0	238.0	239.2
lobe or pole	191.2	198.3	—	225.0	237.5	239.6
region	195.0	198.89	234.8	229.8	238.8	239.8
skin	173.3	198.2	232.3	216.3	238.2	239.2
tendon (sheath)—*see* Neoplasm, connective tissue						
tentorium (cerebelli)	192.1	198.4	—	225.2	237.6	239.7
testis, testes (descended) (scrotal)	186.9	198.82	233.6	222.0	236.4	239.5
ectopic	186.0	198.82	233.6	222.0	236.4	239.5
retained	186.0	198.82	233.6	222.0	236.4	239.5
undescended	186.0	198.82	233.6	222.0	236.4	239.5
thalamus	191.0	198.3	—	225.0	237.5	239.6
thigh NEC*	195.5	198.89	234.8	229.8	238.8	239.8
thorax, thoracic (cavity) (organs NEC)	195.1	198.89	234.8	229.8	238.8	239.8
duct	171.4	198.89	—	215.4	238.1	239.2
wall NEC	195.1	198.89	234.8	229.8	238.8	239.8
throat	149.0	198.89	230.0	210.9	235.1	239.0
thumb NEC*	195.4	198.89	232.6	229.8	238.8	239.8
thymus (gland)	164.0	198.89	—	212.6	235.8	239.8
contiguous sites with heart and mediastinum	164.8	—	—	—	—	—
thyroglossal duct	193	198.89	234.8	226	237.4	239.7
thyroid (gland)	193	198.89	234.8	226	237.4	239.7
cartilage	161.3	197.3	231.0	212.1	235.6	239.1
tibia (any part)	170.7	198.5	—	213.7	238.0	239.2
toe NEC*	195.5	198.89	232.7	229.8	238.8	239.8
tongue	141.9	198.89	230.0	210.1	235.1	239.0
anterior (two-thirds) NEC	141.4	198.89	230.0	210.1	235.1	239.0

	Malignant					
	Primary	Secondary	Ca in situ	Benign	Uncertain Behavior	Unspecified
dorsal surface	141.1	198.89	230.0	210.1	235.1	239.0
ventral surface	141.3	198.89	230.0	210.1	235.1	239.0
base (dorsal surface)	141.0	198.89	230.0	210.1	235.1	239.0
border (lateral)	141.2	198.89	230.0	210.1	235.1	239.0
contiguous sites	141.8	—	—	—	—	—
dorsal surface NEC	141.1	198.89	230.0	210.1	235.1	239.0
fixed part NEC	141.0	198.89	230.0	210.1	235.1	239.0
foramen cecum	141.1	198.89	230.0	210.1	235.1	239.0
frenulum linguae	141.3	198.89	230.0	210.1	235.1	239.0
junctional zone	141.5	198.89	230.0	210.1	235.1	239.0
margin (lateral)	141.2	198.89	230.0	210.1	235.1	239.0
midline NEC	141.1	198.89	230.0	210.1	235.1	239.0
mobile part NEC	141.4	198.89	230.0	210.1	235.1	239.0
posterior (third)	141.0	198.89	230.0	210.1	235.1	239.0
root	141.0	198.89	230.0	210.1	235.1	239.0
surface (dorsal)	141.1	198.89	230.0	210.1	235.1	239.0
base	141.0	198.89	230.0	210.1	235.1	239.0
ventral	141.3	198.89	230.0	210.1	235.1	239.0
tip	141.2	198.89	230.0	210.1	235.1	239.0
tonsil	141.6	198.89	230.0	210.1	235.1	239.0
tonsil	146.0	198.89	230.0	210.5	235.1	239.0
fauces, faucial	146.0	198.89	230.0	210.5	235.1	239.0
lingual	141.6	198.89	230.0	210.1	235.1	239.0
palatine	146.0	198.89	230.0	210.5	235.1	239.0
pharyngeal	147.1	198.89	230.0	210.7	235.1	239.0
pillar (anterior) (posterior)	146.2	198.89	230.0	210.6	235.1	239.0
tonsillar fossa	146.1	198.89	230.0	210.6	235.1	239.0
tooth socket NEC	143.9	198.89	230.0	210.4	235.1	239.0
trachea (cartilage) (mucosa)	162.0	197.3	231.1	212.2	235.7	239.1
contiguous sites with bronchus or lung	162.8	—	—	—	—	—
tracheobronchial	162.8	197.3	231.1	212.2	235.7	239.1
contiguous sites with lung	162.8	—	—	—	—	—
tragus	173.2	198.2	232.2	216.2	238.2	239.2
trunk NEC*	195.8	198.89	232.5	229.8	238.8	239.8
tubo-ovarian	183.8	198.82	233.3	221.8	236.3	239.5
tunica vaginalis	187.8	198.82	233.6	222.8	236.6	239.5
turbinate (bone)	170.0	198.5	—	213.0	238.0	239.2
nasal	160.0	197.3	231.8	212.0	235.9	239.1
tympanic cavity	160.1	197.3	231.8	212.0	235.9	239.1
ulna (any part)	170.4	198.5	—	213.4	238.0	239.2
umbilicus, umbilical	173.5	198.2	232.5	216.5	238.2	239.2
uncus, brain	191.2	198.3	—	225.0	237.5	239.6
unknown site or unspecified	199.1	199.1	234.9	229.9	238.9	239.9
urachus	188.7	198.1	233.7	223.3	236.7	239.4
ureter, ureteral	189.2	198.1	233.9	223.2	236.91	239.5
orifice (bladder)	188.6	198.1	233.7	223.3	236.7	239.4
ureter-bladder (junction)	188.6	198.1	233.7	223.3	236.7	239.4
urethra, urethral (gland)	189.3	198.1	233.9	223.81	236.99	239.5
orifice, internal	188.5	198.1	233.7	223.3	236.7	239.4
urethrovaginal (septum)	184.9	198.82	233.3	221.9	236.3	239.5
urinary organ or system NEC	189.9	198.1	233.9	223.9	236.99	239.5
bladder—*see* Neoplasm, bladder						
contiguous sites	189.8	—	—	—	—	—
specified sites NEC	189.8	198.1	233.9	223.89	236.99	239.5
utero-ovarian	183.8	198.82	233.3	221.8	236.3	239.5
ligament	183.3	198.82	—	221.0	236.3	239.5
uterosacral ligament	183.4	198.82	—	221.0	236.3	239.5
uterus, uteri, uterine	179	198.82	233.2	219.9	236.0	239.5
adnexa NEC	183.9	198.82	233.3	221.8	236.3	239.5
contiguous sites	183.8	—	—	—	—	—
body	182.0	198.82	233.2	219.1	236.0	239.5
contiguous sites	182.8	—	—	—	—	—

	Malignant					
	Primary	Secondary	Ca in situ	Benign	Uncertain Behavior	Unspecified
cervix	180.9	198.82	233.1	219.0	236.0	239.5
cornu	182.0	198.82	233.2	219.1	236.0	239.5
corpus	182.0	198.82	233.2	219.1	236.0	239.5
endocervix (canal) (gland)	180.0	198.82	233.1	219.0	236.0	239.5
endometrium	182.0	198.82	233.2	219.1	236.0	239.5
exocervix	180.1	198.82	233.1	219.0	236.0	239.5
external os	180.1	198.82	233.1	219.0	236.0	239.5
fundus	182.0	198.82	233.2	219.1	236.0	239.5
internal os	180.0	198.82	233.1	219.0	236.0	239.5
isthmus	182.1	198.82	233.2	219.1	236.0	239.5
ligament	183.4	198.82	—	221.0	236.3	239.5
broad	183.3	198.82	233.3	221.0	236.3	239.5
round	183.5	198.82	—	221.0	236.3	239.5
lower segment	182.1	198.82	233.2	219.1	236.0	239.5
myometrium	182.0	198.82	233.2	219.1	236.0	239.5
squamocolumnar junction	180.8	198.82	233.1	219.0	236.0	239.5
tube	183.2	198.82	233.3	221.0	236.3	239.5
utricle, prostatic	189.3	198.1	233.9	223.81	236.99	239.5
uveal tract	190.0	198.4	234.0	224.0	238.8	239.8
uvula	145.4	198.89	230.0	210.4	235.1	239.0
vagina, vaginal (fornix) (vault) (wall)	184.0	198.82	233.3	221.1	236.3	239.5
vaginovesical	184.9	198.82	233.3	221.9	236.3	239.5
septum	194.9	198.82	233.3	221.9	236.3	239.5
vallecula (epiglottis)	146.3	198.89	230.0	210.6	235.1	239.0
vascular—*see* Neoplasm, connective tissue						
vas deferens	187.6	198.82	233.6	222.8	236.6	239.5
Vater's ampulla	156.2	197.8	230.8	211.5	235.3	239.0
vein, venous—*see* Neoplasm, connective tissue						
vena cava (abdominal) (inferior)	171.5	198.89	—	215.5	238.1	239.2
superior	171.4	198.89	—	215.4	238.1	239.2
ventricle (cerebral) (floor) (fourth) (lateral) (third)	191.5	198.3	—	225.0	237.5	239.6
cardiac (left) (right)	164.1	198.89	—	212.7	238.8	239.8
ventricular band of larynx	161.1	197.3	231.0	212.1	235.6	239.1
ventriculus—*see* Neoplasm, stomach						
vermillion border—*see* Neoplasm, lip						
vermis, cerebellum	191.6	198.3	—	225.0	237.5	239.6
vertebra (column)	170.2	198.5	—	213.2	238.0	239.2
coccyx	170.6	198.5	—	213.6	238.0	239.2
sacrum	170.6	198.5	—	213.6	238.0	239.2
vesical—*see* Neoplasm, bladder						
vesicle, seminal	187.8	198.82	233.6	222.8	236.6	239.5
vesicocervical tissue	184.9	198.82	233.3	221.9	236.3	239.5
vesicorectal	195.3	198.89	234.8	229.8	238.8	239.8
vesicovaginal	184.9	198.82	233.3	221.9	236.3	239.5
septum	184.9	198.82	233.3	221.9	236.3	239.5
vessel (blood)—*see* Neoplasm, connective tissue						
vestibular gland, greater	184.1	198.82	233.3	221.2	236.3	239.5
vestibule						
mouth	145.1	198.89	230.0	210.4	235.1	239.0
nose	160.0	197.3	231.8	212.0	235.9	239.1
Virchow's gland	—	196.0	—	229.0	238.8	239.8
viscera NEC	195.8	198.89	234.8	229.8	238.8	239.8
vocal cords (true)	161.0	197.3	231.0	212.1	235.6	239.1
false	161.1	197.3	231.0	212.1	235.6	239.1
vomer	170.0	198.5	—	213.0	238.0	239.2

	Malignant					
	Primary	Secondary	Ca in situ	Benign	Uncertain Behavior	Unspecified
vulva	184.4	198.82	233.3	221.2	236.3	239.5
vulvovaginal gland	184.4	198.82	233.3	221.2	236.3	239.5
Waldeyer's ring	149.1	198.89	230.0	210.9	235.1	239.0
Wharton's duct	142.1	198.89	230.0	210.2	235.0	239.0
white matter (central) (cerebral)	191.0	198.3	—	225.0	237.5	239.6
windpipe	162.0	197.3	231.1	212.2	235.7	239.1
Wirsung's duct	157.3	197.8	230.9	211.6	235.5	239.0
wolffian (body) (duct)						
female	184.8	198.82	233.3	221.8	236.3	239.5
male	187.8	198.82	233.6	222.8	236.6	239.5
womb—*see* Neoplasm, uterus						
wrist NEC*	195.4	198.89	232.6	229.8	238.8	239.8
xiphoid process	170.3	198.5	—	213.3	238.0	239.2
Zuckerkandl's organ	194.6	198.89	—	227.6	237.3	239.7

Neovascularization
  choroid 362.16
  ciliary body 364.42
  cornea 370.60
    deep 370.63
    localized 370.61
  iris 364.42
  retina 362.16
  subretinal 362.16
Nephralgia 788.0
Nephritis, nephritic (albuminuric) (azotemic)
  (congenital) (degenerative) (diffuse)
  (disseminated) (epithelial) (familial) (focal)
  (granulomatous) (hemorrhagic) (infantile)
  (nonsuppurative, excretory) (uremic) 583.9
  with
    edema—*see* Nephrosis
    lesion of
      glomerulonephritis
        hypocomplementemic persistent 583.2
          with nephrotic syndrome 581.2
          chronic 582.2
        lobular 583.2
          with nephrotic syndrome 581.2
          chronic 582.2
        membranoproliferative 583.2
          with nephrotic syndrome 581.2
          chronic 582.2
        membranous 583.1
          with nephrotic syndrome 581.1
          chronic 582.1
        mesangiocapillary 583.2
          with nephrotic syndrome 581.2
          chronic 582.2
        mixed membranous and proliferative 583.2
          with nephrotic syndrome 581.2
          chronic 582.2
        proliferative (diffuse) 583.0
          with nephrotic syndrome 581.0
          acute 580.0
          chronic 582.0
        rapidly progressive 583.4
          acute 580.4
          chronic 582.4
      interstitial nephritis (diffuse) (focal) 583.89
        with nephrotic syndrome 581.89
        acute 580.89
        chronic 582.89
      necrotizing glomerulitis 583.4
        acute 580.4
        chronic 582.4
      renal necrosis 583.9
        cortical 583.6
        medullary 583.7
      specified pathology NEC 583.89
        with nephrotic syndrome 581.89
        acute 580.89
        chronic 582.89
    necrosis, renal 583.9
      cortical 583.6
      medullary (papillary) 583.7
    nephrotic syndrome (*see also* Nephrosis) 581.9
    papillary necrosis 583.7
    specified pathology NEC 583.89
  acute 580.9
    extracapillary with epithelial crescents 580.4
    hypertensive (*see also* Hypertension, kidney)
      403.90
    necrotizing 580.4
    poststreptococcal 580.0
    proliferative (diffuse) 580.0

Nephritis, nephritic—*continued*
    rapidly progressive 580.4
    specified pathology NEC 580.89
  amyloid 277.39 *[583.81]*
    chronic 277.39 *[582.81]*
  arteriolar (*see also* Hypertension, kidney)
    403.90
  arteriosclerotic (*see also* Hypertension, kidney)
    403.90
  ascending (*see also* Pyelitis) 590.80
  atrophic 582.9
  basement membrane NEC 583.89
    with
      pulmonary hemorrhage (Goodpasture's
        syndrome) 446.21 *[583.81]*
  calculous, calculus 592.0
  cardiac (*see also* Hypertension, kidney) 403.90
  cardiovascular (*see also* Hypertension, kidney)
    403.90
  chronic 582.9
    arteriosclerotic (*see also* Hypertension,
      kidney) 403.90
    hypertensive (*see also* Hypertension, kidney)
      403.90
  cirrhotic (*see also* Sclerosis, renal) 587
  complicating pregnancy, childbirth, or
    puerperium 646.2
    with hypertension 642.1
      affecting fetus or newborn 760.0
    affecting fetus or newborn 760.1
  croupous 580.9
  desquamative—*see* Nephrosis
  due to
    amyloidosis 277.39 *[583.81]*
      chronic 277.39 *[582.81]*
    arteriosclerosis (*see also* Hypertension,
      kidney) 403.90
    diabetes mellitus 250.4 *[583.81]*
      with nephrotic syndrome 250.4 *[581.81]*
    diphtheria 032.89 *[580.81]*
    gonococcal infection (acute) 098.19 *[583.81]*
      chronic or duration of 2 months or over
        098.39 *[583.81]*
    gout 274.10
    infectious hepatitis 070.9 *[580.81]*
    mumps 072.79 *[580.81]*
    specified kidney pathology NEC 583.89
      acute 580.89
      chronic 582.89
    streptotrichosis 039.8 *[583.81]*
    subacute bacterial endocarditis 421.0 *[580.81]*
    systemic lupus erythematosus 710.0 *[583.81]*
      chronic 710.0 *[582.81]*
    typhoid fever 002.0 *[580.81]*
  endothelial 582.2
  end stage (chronic) (terminal) NEC 585.6
  epimembranous 581.1
  exudative 583.89
    with nephrotic syndrome 581.89
    acute 580.89
    chronic 582.89
  gonococcal (acute) 098.19 *[583.81]*
    chronic or duration of 2 months or over 098.39
      [583.81]
  gouty 274.10
  hereditary (Alport's syndrome) 759.89
  hydremic—*see* Nephrosis
  hypertensive (*see also* Hypertension, kidney)
    403.90
  hypocomplementemic persistent 583.2
    with nephrotic syndrome 581.2

Nephritis, nephritic—*continued*
    chronic 582.2
    immune complex NEC 583.89
    infective (*see also* Pyelitis) 590.80
    interstitial (diffuse) (focal) 583.89
        with nephrotic syndrome 581.89
        acute 580.89
        chronic 582.89
    latent or quiescent—*see* Nephritis, chronic
    lead 984.9
        specified type of lead—*see* Table of drugs and chemicals
    lobular 583.2
        with nephrotic syndrome 581.2
        chronic 582.2
    lupus 710.0 *[583.81]*
        acute 710.0 *[580.81]*
        chronic 710.0 *[582.81]*
    membranoproliferative 583.2
        with nephrotic syndrome 581.2
        chronic 582.2
    membranous 583.1
        with nephrotic syndrome 581.1
        chronic 582.1
    mesangiocapillary 583.2
        with nephrotic syndrome 581.2
        chronic 582.2
    minimal change 581.3
    mixed membranous and proliferative 583.2
        with nephrotic syndrome 581.2
        chronic 582.2
    necrotic, necrotizing 583.4
        acute 580.4
        chronic 582.4
    nephrotic—*see* Nephrosis
    old—*see* Nephritis, chronic
    parenchymatous 581.89
    polycystic 753.12
        adult type (APKD) 753.13
        autosomal dominant 753.13
        autosomal recessive 753.14
        childhood type (CPKD) 753.14
        infantile type 753.14
    poststreptococcal 580.0
    pregnancy—*see* Nephritis, complicating pregnancy
    proliferative 583.0
        with nephrotic syndrome 581.0
        acute 580.0
        chronic 582.0
    purulent (*see also* Pyelitis) 590.80
    rapidly progressive 583.4
        acute 580.4
        chronic 582.4
    salt-losing or salt-wasting (*see also* Disease, renal) 593.9
    saturnine 984.9
        specified type of lead—*see* Table of drugs and chemicals
    septic (*see also* Pyelitis) 590.80
    specified pathology NEC 583.89
        acute 580.89
        chronic 582.89
    staphylococcal (*see also* Pyelitis) 590.80
    streptotrichosis 039.8 *[583.81]*
    subacute (*see also* Nephrosis) 581.9
    suppurative (*see also* Pyelitis) 590.80
    syphilitic (late) 095.4
        congenital 090.5 *[583.81]*
        early 091.69 *[583.81]*
    terminal (chronic) (end-stage) NEC 585.6

Nephritis, nephritic—*continued*
   toxic—*see* Nephritis, acute
   tubal, tubular—*see* Nephrosis, tubular
   tuberculous (*see also* Tuberculosis) 016.0 *[583.81]*
   type II (Ellis)—*see* Nephrosis
   vascular—*see* Hypertension, kidney
   war 580.9
Nephroblastoma (M8960/3) 189.0
   epithelial (M8961/3) 189.0
   mesenchymal (M8962/3) 189.0
Nephrocalcinosis 275.49
Nephrocystitis, pustular (*see also* Pyelitis) 590.80
Nephrolithiasis (congenital) (pelvis) (recurrent) 592.0
   uric acid 274.11
Nephroma (M8960/3) 189.0
   mesoblastic (M8960/1) 236.9
Nephronephritis (*see also* Nephrosis) 581.9
Nephronopthisis 753.16
Nephropathy (*see also* Nephritis) 583.9
   with
      exudative nephritis 583.89
      interstitial nephritis (diffuse) (focal) 583.89
      medullary necrosis 583.7
      necrosis 583.9
         cortical 583.6
         medullary or papillary 583.7
      papillary necrosis 583.7
      specified lesion or cause NEC 583.89
   analgesic 583.89
      with medullary necrosis, acute 584.7
   arteriolar (*see also* Hypertension, kidney) 403.90
   arteriosclerotic (*see also* Hypertension, kidney) 403.90
   complicating pregnancy 646.2
   diabetic 250.4 *[583.81]*
   gouty 274.10
      specified type NEC 274.19
   hereditary amyloid 277.31
   hypercalcemic 588.89
   hypertensive (*see also* Hypertension, kidney) 403.90
   hypokalemic (vacuolar) 588.89
   IgA 583.9
   obstructive 593.89
      congenital 753.20
   phenacetin 584.7
   phosphate-losing 588.0
   potassium depletion 588.89
   proliferative (*see also* Nephritis, proliferative) 583.0
   protein-losing 588.89
   salt-losing or salt-wasting (*see also* Disease, renal) 593.9
   sickle-cell (*see also* Disease, sickle-cell) 282.60 *[583.81]*
   toxic 584.5
   vasomotor 584.5
   water-losing 588.89
Nephroptosis (*see also* Disease, renal) 593.0
   congenital (displaced) 753.3
Nephropyosis (*see also* Abscess, kidney) 590.2
Nephrorrhagia 593.81
Nephrosclerosis (arteriolar) (arteriosclerotic) (chronic) (hyaline) (*see also* Hypertension, kidney) 403.90
   gouty 274.10
   hyperplastic (arteriolar) (*see also* Hypertension, kidney) 403.90
   senile (*see also* Sclerosis, renal) 587

Nephrosis, nephrotic (Epstein's) (syndrome) 581.9
  with
    lesion of
      focal glomerulosclerosis 581.1
      glomerulonephritis
        endothelial 581.2
        hypocomplementemic persistent 581.2
        lobular 581.2
        membranoproliferative 581.2
        membranous 581.1
        mesangiocapillary 581.2
        minimal change 581.3
        mixed membranous and proliferative 581.2
        proliferative 581.0
      segmental hyalinosis 581.1
      specified pathology NEC 581.89
  acute—*see* Nephrosis, tubular
  anoxic—*see* Nephrosis, tubular
  arteriosclerotic (*see also* Hypertension, kidney) 403.90
  chemical—*see* Nephrosis, tubular
  cholemic 572.4
  complicating pregnancy, childbirth, or puerperium—*see* Nephritis, complicating pregnancy
  diabetic 250.4 *[581.81]*
  hemoglobinuric—*see* Nephrosis, tubular
  in
    amyloidosis 277.39 *[581.81]*
    diabetes mellitus 250.4 *[581.81]*
    epidemic hemorrhagic fever 078.6
    malaria 084.9 *[581.81]*
    polyarteritis 446.0 *[581.81]*
    systemic lupus erythematosus 710.0 *[581.81]*
  ischemic—*see* Nephrosis, tubular
  lipoid 581.3
  lower nephron—*see* Nephrosis, tubular
  lupoid 710.0 *[581.81]*
  lupus 710.0 *[581.81]*
  malarial 084.9 *[581.81]*
  minimal change 581.3
  necrotizing—*see* Nephrosis, tubular
  osmotic (sucrose) 588.89
  polyarteritic 446.0 *[581.81]*
  radiation 581.9
  specified lesion or cause NEC 581.89
  syphilitic 095.4
  toxic—*see* Nephrosis, tubular
  tubular (acute) 584.5
    due to a procedure 997.5
    radiation 581.9
Nephrosonephritis hemorrhagic (endemic) 078.6
Nephrostomy status V44.6
  with complication 997.5
Nerve —*see* condition
Nerves 799.2
Nervous (*see also* condition) 799.2
  breakdown 300.9
  heart 306.2
  stomach 306.4
  tension 799.2
Nervousness 799.2
Nesidioblastoma (M8150/0)
  pancreas 211.7
  specified site NEC—*see* Neoplasm, by site, benign
  unspecified site 211.7
Netherton's syndrome (ichthyosiform erythroderma) 757.1

Nettle rash 708.8
Nettleship's disease (urticaria pigmentosa) 757.33
Neumann's disease (pemphigus vegetans) 694.4
Neuralgia, neuralgic (acute) (*see also* Neuritis) 729.2
  accessory (nerve) 352.4
  acoustic (nerve) 388.5
  ankle 355.8
  anterior crural 355.8
  anus 787.99
  arm 723.4
  auditory (nerve) 388.5
  axilla 353.0
  bladder 788.1
  brachial 723.4
  brain—*see* Disorder, nerve, cranial
  broad ligament 625.9
  cerebral—*see* Disorder, nerve, cranial
  ciliary 346.2
  cranial nerve—*see also* Disorder, nerve, cranial
    fifth or trigeminal (*see also* Neuralgia, trigeminal) 350.1
  ear 388.71
    middle 352.1
  facial 351.8
  finger 354.9
  flank 355.8
  foot 355.8
  forearm 354.9
  Fothergill's (*see also* Neuralgia, trigeminal) 350.1
    postherpetic 053.12
  glossopharyngeal (nerve) 352.1
  groin 355.8
  hand 354.9
  heel 355.8
  Horton's 346.2
  Hunt's 053.11
  hypoglossal (nerve) 352.5
  iliac region 355.8
  infraorbital (*see also* Neuralgia, trigeminal) 350.1
  inguinal 355.8
  intercostal (nerve) 353.8
    postherpetic 053.19
  jaw 352.1
  kidney 788.0
  knee 355.8
  loin 355.8
  malarial (*see also* Malaria) 084.6
  mastoid 385.89
  maxilla 352.1
  median thenar 354.1
  metatarsal 355.6
  middle ear 352.1
  migrainous 346.2
  Morton's 355.6
  nerve, cranial—*see* Disorder, nerve, cranial
  nose 352.0
  occipital 723.8
  olfactory (nerve) 352.0
  ophthalmic 377.30
    postherpetic 053.19
  optic (nerve) 377.30
  penis 607.9
  perineum 355.8
  pleura 511.0
  postherpetic NEC 053.19
    geniculate ganglion 053.11
    ophthalmic 053.19
    trifacial 053.12

Neuralgia, neuralgic—*continued*
   trigeminal 053.12
  pubic region 355.8
  radial (nerve) 723.4
  rectum 787.99
  sacroiliac joint 724.3
  sciatic (nerve) 724.3
  scrotum 608.9
  seminal vesicle 608.9
  shoulder 354.9
  Sluder's 337.0
  specified nerve NEC—*see* Disorder, nerve
  spermatic cord 608.9
  sphenopalatine (ganglion) 337.0
  subscapular (nerve) 723.4
  suprascapular (nerve) 723.4
  testis 608.89
  thenar (median) 354.1
  thigh 355.8
  tongue 352.5
  trifacial (nerve) (*see also* Neuralgia, trigeminal)
    350.1
  trigeminal (nerve) 350.1
   postherpetic 053.12
  tympanic plexus 388.71
  ulnar (nerve) 723.4
  vagus (nerve) 352.3
  wrist 354.9
  writers' 300.89
   organic 333.84
Neurapraxia —*see* Injury, nerve
Neurasthenia 300.5
  cardiac 306.2
  gastric 306.4
  heart 306.2
  postfebrile 780.79
  postviral 780.79
Neurilemmoma (M9560/0)—*see also* Neoplasm,
  connective tissue, benign
  acoustic (nerve) 225.1
  malignant (M9560/3)—*see also* Neoplasm,
   connective tissue, malignant
   acoustic (nerve) 192.0
Neurilemmosarcoma (M9560/3)—*see*
  Neoplasm, connective tissue, malignant
Neurilemoma —*see* Neurilemmoma
Neurinoma (M9560/0)—*see* Neurilemmoma
Neurinomatosis (M9560/1)—*see also* Neoplasm,
  connective tissue, uncertain behavior
  centralis 759.5
Neuritis (*see also* Neuralgia) 729.2
  abducens (nerve) 378.54
  accessory (nerve) 352.4
  acoustic (nerve) 388.5
   syphilitic 094.86
  alcoholic 357.5
   with psychosis 291.1
  amyloid, any site 277.39 *[357.4]*
  anterior crural 355.8
  arising during pregnancy 646.4
  arm 723.4
  ascending 355.2
  auditory (nerve) 388.5
  brachial (nerve) NEC 723.4
   due to displacement, intervertebral disc 722.0
  cervical 723.4
  chest (wall) 353.8
  costal region 353.8
  cranial nerve—*see also* Disorder, nerve, cranial
   first or olfactory 352.0
   second or optic 377.30

Neuritis—*continued*
  third or oculomotor 378.52
  fourth or trochlear 378.53
  fifth or trigeminal (*see also* Neuralgia,
   trigeminal) 350.1
  sixth or abducens 378.54
  seventh or facial 351.8
   newborn 767.5
  eighth or acoustic 388.5
  ninth or glossopharyngeal 352.1
  tenth or vagus 352.3
  eleventh or accessory 352.4
  twelfth or hypoglossal 352.5
  Déjérine-Sottas 356.0
  diabetic 250.6 *[357.2]*
  diphtheritic 032.89 *[357.4]*
  due to
   beriberi 265.0 *[357.4]*
   displacement, prolapse, protrusion, or rupture
    of intervertebral disc 722.2
    cervical 722.0
    lumbar, lumbosacral 722.10
    thoracic, thoracolumbar 722.11
   herniation, nucleus pulposus 722.2
    cervical 722.0
    lumbar, lumbosacral 722.10
    thoracic, thoracolumbar 722.11
  endemic 265.0 *[357.4]*
  facial (nerve) 351.8
   newborn 767.5
  general—*see* Polyneuropathy
  geniculate ganglion 351.1
   due to herpes 053.11
  glossopharyngeal (nerve) 352.1
  gouty 274.89 *[357.4]*
  hypoglossal (nerve) 352.5
  ilioinguinal (nerve) 355.8
  in diseases classified elsewhere—*see*
   Polyneuropathy, in
  infectious (multiple) 357.0
  intercostal (nerve) 353.8
  interstitial hypertrophic progressive NEC 356.9
  leg 355.8
  lumbosacral NEC 724.4
  median (nerve) 354.1
   thenar 354.1
  multiple (acute) (infective) 356.9
   endemic 265.0 *[357.4]*
  multiplex endemica 265.0 *[357.4]*
  nerve root (*see also* Radiculitis) 729.2
  oculomotor (nerve) 378.52
  olfactory (nerve) 352.0
  optic (nerve) 377.30
   in myelitis 341.0
   meningococcal 036.81
  pelvic 355.8
  peripheral (nerve)—*see also* Neuropathy,
   peripheral
   complicating pregnancy or puerperium 646.4
   specified nerve NEC—*see* Mononeuritis
  pneumogastric (nerve) 352.3
  postchickenpox 052.7
  postherpetic 053.19
  progressive hypertrophic interstitial NEC 356.9
  puerperal, postpartum 646.4
  radial (nerve) 723.4
  retrobulbar 377.32
   syphilitic 094.85
  rheumatic (chronic) 729.2
  sacral region 355.8
  sciatic (nerve) 724.3

Neuropathy, neuropathic—*continued*
    ilioinguinal nerve 355.79
    lateral cutaneous nerve of thigh 355.1
    median nerve 354.0
    obturator nerve 355.79
    peroneal nerve 355.3
    posterior tibial nerve 355.5
    saphenous nerve 355.79
    ulnar nerve 354.2
  facial nerve 351.9
  hereditary 356.9
    peripheral 356.0
    sensory (radicular) 356.2
  hypertrophic
    Charcot-Marie-Tooth 356.1
    Déjérine-Sottas 356.0
    interstitial 356.9
    Refsum 356.3
  intercostal nerve 354.8
  ischemic—*see* Disorder, nerve
  Jamaican (ginger) 357.7
  leg NEC 355.8
  lower extremity NEC 355.8
  lumbar plexus 353.1
  median nerve 354.1
  motor
    acute 357.82
  multiple (acute) (chronic) (*see also*
      Polyneuropathy) 356.9
  optic 377.39
    ischemic 377.41
    nutritional 377.33
    toxic 377.34
  peripheral (nerve) (*see also* Polyneuropathy)
      356.9
    arm NEC 354.9
    autonomic 337.9
      amyloid 277.39 *[337.1]*
      idiopathic 337.0
      in
        amyloidosis 277.39 *[337.1]*
        diabetes (mellitus) 250.6 *[337.1]*
        diseases classified elsewhere 337.1
        gout 274.89 *[337.1]*
        hyperthyroidism 242.9 *[337.1]*
    due to
      antitetanus serum 357.6
      arsenic 357.7
      drugs 357.6
      lead 357.7
      organophosphate compounds 357.7
      toxic agent NEC 357.7
    hereditary 356.0
    idiopathic 356.9
      progressive 356.4
      specified type NEC 356.8
    in diseases classified elsewhere—*see*
        Polyneuropathy, in
    leg NEC 355.8
    lower extremity NEC 355.8
    upper extremity NEC 354.9
  plantar nerves 355.6
  progressive hypertrophic interstitial 356.9
  radicular NEC 729.2
    brachial 723.4
    cervical NEC 723.4
    hereditary sensory 356.2
    lumbar 724.4
    lumbosacral 724.4
    thoracic NEC 724.4
  sacral plexus 353.1

Neuropathy, neuropathic—*continued*
  sciatic 355.0
  spinal nerve NEC 355.9
    root (*see also* Radiculitis) 729.2
  toxic 357.7
  trigeminal sensory 350.8
  ulnar nerve 354.2
  upper extremity NEC 354.9
  uremic 585.9 *[357.4]*
  vitamin B$_{12}$ 266.2 *[357.4]*
    with anemia (pernicious) 281.0 *[357.4]*
      due to dietary deficiency 281.1 *[357.4]*
Neurophthisis —*see also* Disorder, nerve
  peripheral 356.9
    diabetic 250.6 *[357.2]*
Neuropraxia —*see* Injury,nerve
Neuroretinitis 363.05
  syphilitic 094.85
Neurosarcoma 9M9540/3)—sde Neoplasm,
    connective tissue, malignant
Neurosclerosis —*see* Disorder, nerve
Neurosis, neurotic 300.9
  accident 300.16
  anancastic, anankastic 300.3
  anxiety (state) 300.00
    generalized 300.02
    panic type 300.01
  asthenic 300.5
  bladder 306.53
  cardiac (reflex) 306.2
  cardiovascular 306.2
  climacteric, unspecified type 627.2
  colon 306.4
  compensation 300.16
  compulsive, compulsion 300.3
  conversion 300.11
  craft 300.89
  cutaneous 306.3
  depersonalization 300.6
  depressive (reaction) (type) 300.4
  endocrine 306.6
  environmental 300.89
  fatigue 300.5
  functional (*see also* Disorder, psychosomatic)
      306.9
  gastric 306.4
  gastrointestinal 306.4
  genitourinary 306.50
  heart 306.2
  hypochondriacal 300.7
  hysterical 300.10
    conversion type 300.11
    dissociative type 300.15
  impulsive 300.3
  incoordination 306.0
    larynx 306.1
    vocal cord 306.1
  intestine 306.4
  larynx 306.1
    hysterical 300.11
    sensory 306.1
  menopause, unspecified type 627.2
  mixed NEC 300.89
  musculoskeletal 306.0
  obsessional 300.3
    phobia 300.3
  obsessive-compulsive 300.3
  occupational 300.89
  ocular 306.7
  oral 307.0
  organ (*see also* Disorder, psychosomatic) 306.9

Neurosis, neurotic—*continued*
pharynx 306.1
phobic 300.20
posttraumatic (acute) (situational) 309.81
chronic 309.81
psychasthenic (type) 300.89
railroad 300.16
rectum 306.4
respiratory 306.1
rumination 306.4
senile 300.89
sexual 302.70
situational 300.89
specified type NEC 300.89
state 300.9
with depersonalization episode 300.6
stomach 306.4
vasomotor 306.2
visceral 306.4
war 300.16
Neurospongioblastosis diffusa 759.5
Neurosyphilis (arrested) (early) (inactive) (late)
(latent) (recurrent) 094.9
with ataxia (cerebellar) (locomotor) (spastic)
(spinal) 094.0
acute meningitis 094.2
aneurysm 094.89
arachnoid (adhesive) 094.2
arteritis (any artery) 094.89
asymptomatic 094.3
congenital 090.40
dura (mater) 094.89
general paresis 094.1
gumma 094.9
hemorrhagic 094.9
juvenile (asymptomatic) (meningeal) 090.40
leptomeninges (aseptic) 094.2
meningeal 094.2
meninges (adhesive) 094.2
meningovascular (diffuse) 094.2
optic atrophy 094.84
parenchymatous (degenerative) 094.1
paresis (*see also* Paresis, general) 094.1
paretic (*see also* Paresis, general) 094.1
relapse 094.9
remission in (sustained) 094.9
serological 094.3
specified nature or site NEC 094.89
tabes (dorsalis) 094.0
juvenile 090.40
tabetic 094.0
juvenile 090.40
taboparesis 094.1
juvenile 090.40
thrombosis 094.89
vascular 094.89
Neurotic (*see also* Neurosis) 300.9
excoriation 698.4
psychogenic 306.3
Neurotmesis —*see* Injury, nerve, by site
Neurotoxemia —*see* Toxemia
Neutro-oclusion 524.21
Neutropenia, neutropenic (idiopathic)
(pernicious) (primary) 288.00
chronic 288.09
hypoplastic 288.09
congenital (nontransient) 288.01
cyclic 288.02
drug induced 288.03
due to infection 288.04
fever 288.00

Neutropenia, neutropenic— *continued*
genetic 288.01
immune 288.09
infantile 288.01
malignant 288.09
neonatal, transitory (isoimmune) (maternal
transfer) 776.7
periodic 288.02
splenic 289.53
splenomegaly 289.53
toxic 288.09
Neutrophilia, hereditary giant 288.2
Nevocarcinoma (M8720/3)—*see* Melanoma
Nevus (M8720/0)—*see also* Neoplasm, skin,
benign

*Note—Except where otherwise indicated, the
varieties of nevus in the list below that are
followed by a morphology code number (M——
-/0) should be coded by site as for "Neoplasm,
skin, benign."*

acanthotic 702.8
achromic (M8730/0)
amelanotic (M8730/0)
anemic, anemicus 709.09
angiomatous (M9120/0) (*see also* Hemangioma)
228.00
araneus 448.1
avasculosus 709.09
balloon cell (M8722/0)
bathing trunk (M8761/1) 238.2
blue (M8780/0)
cellular (M8790/0)
giant (M8790/0)
Jadassohn's (M8780/0)
malignant (M8780/3)—*see* Melanoma
capillary (M9131/0) (*see also* Hemangioma)
228.00
cavernous (M9121/0) (*see also* Hemangioma)
228.00
cellular (M8720/0)
blue (M8790/0)
comedonicus 757.33
compound (M8760/0)
conjunctiva (M8720/0) 224.3
dermal (M8750/0)
and epidermal (M8760/0)
epithelioid cell (and spindle cell) (M8770/0)
flammeus 757.32
osteohypertrophic 759.89
hairy (M8720/0)
halo (M8723/0)
hemangiomatous (M9120/0) (*see also*
Hemangioma) 228.00
intradermal (M8750/0)
intraepidermal (M8740/0)
involuting (M8724/0)
Jadassohn's (blue) (M8780/0)
junction, junctional (M8740/0)
malignant melanoma in (M8740/3)—*see*
Melanoma
juvenile (M8770/0)
lymphatic (M9170/0) 228.1
magnocellular (M8726/0)
specified site—*see* Neoplasm, by site, benign
unspecified site 224.0
malignant (M8720/3)—*see* Melanoma
meaning hemangioma (M9120/0) (*see also*
Hemangioma) 228.00
melanotic (pigmented) (M8720/0)
multiplex 759.5

Nevus—*continued*
  nonneoplastic 448.1
  nonpigmented (M8730/0)
  nonvascular (M8720/0)
  oral mucosa, white sponge 750.26
  osteohypertrophic, flammeus 759.89
  papillaris (M8720/0)
  papillomatosus (M8720/0)
  pigmented (M8720/0)
    giant (M8761/1)—*see also* Neoplasm, skin,
      uncertain behavior
      malignant melanoma in (M8761/3)—*see*
        Melanoma
    systematicus 757.33
  pilosus (M8720/0)
  port wine 757.32
  sanguineous 757.32
  sebaceous (senile) 702.8
  senile 448.1
  spider 448.1
  spindle cell (and epithelioid cell) (M8770/0)
  stellar 448.1
  strawberry 757.32
  syringocystadenomatous papilliferous
    (M8406/0)
  unius lateris 757.33
  Unna's 757.32
  vascular 757.32
  verrucous 757.33
  white sponge (oral mucosa) 750.26
Newborn (infant) (liveborn)
  affected by maternal abuse of drugs (gestational)
      (via placenta) (via breast milk) (*see also*
      Noxious, substances transmitted through
      placenta or breast milk (affecting fetus or
      newborn)) 760.70
  apnea 770.81
    obstructive 770.82
    specified NEC 770.82
  cardiomyopathy 425.4
    congenital 425.3
  convulsion 779.0
  electrolyte imbalance NEC (transitory) 775.5
  gestation
    24 completed weeks 765.22
    25-26 completed weeks 765.23
    27-28 completed weeks 765.24
    29-30 completed weeks 765.25
    31-32 completed weeks 765.26
    33-34 completed weeks 765.27
    35-36 completed weeks 765.28
    37 or more completed weeks 765.29
    less than 24 completed weeks 765.21
    unspecified completed weeks 765.20
  infection 771.89
    candida 771.7
    mastitis 771.5
    specified NEC 771.89
    urinary tract 771.82
  mastitis 771.5
  multiple NEC
    born in hospital (without mention of cesarean
        delivery or section) V37.00
      with cesarean delivery or section V37.01
    born outside hospital
      hospitalized V37.1
      not hospitalized V37.2
    mates all liveborn
      born in hospital (without mention of
          cesarean delivery or section) V34.00
        with cesarean delivery or section V34.01

Newborn—*continued*
    born outside hospital
      hospitalized V34.1
      not hospitalized V34.2
    mates all stillborn
      born in hospital (without mention of
          cesarean delivery or section) V35.00
        with cesarean delivery or section V35.01
      born outside hospital
        hospitalized V35.1
        not hospitalized V35.2
    mates liveborn and stillborn
      born in hospital (without mention of
          cesarean delivery or section) V36.00
        with cesarean delivery or section V36.01
      born outside hospital
        hospitalized V36.1
        not hospitalized V36.2
  omphalitis 771.4
  seizure 779.0
  sepsis 771.81
  single
    born in hospital (without mention of cesarean
        delivery or section) V30.00
      with cesarean delivery or section V30.01
    born outside hospital
      hospitalized V30.1
      not hospitalized V30.2
  specified condition NEC 779.89
  twin NEC
    born in hospital (without mention of cesarean
        delivery or section) V33.00
      with cesarean delivery or section V33.01
    born outside hospital
      hospitalized V33.1
      not hospitalized V33.2
    mate liveborn
      born in hospital V31.0
      born outside hospital
        hospitalized V31.1
        not hospitalized V31.2
    mate stillborn
      born in hospital V32.0
      born outside hospital
        hospitalized V32.1
        not hospitalized V32.2
  unspecified as to single or multiple birth
    born in hospital (without mention of cesarean
        delivery or section) V39.00
      with cesarean delivery or section V39.01
    born outside hospital
      hospitalized V39.1
      not hospitalized V39.2
Newcastle's conjunctivitis or disease 077.8
Nezelof's syndrome (pure alymphocytosis) 279.13
Niacin (amide) deficiency 265.2
Nicolas-Durand-Favre disease (climatic bubo)
  099.1
Nicolas-Favre disease (climatic bubo) 099.1
Nicotinic acid (amide) deficiency 265.2
Niemann-Pick disease (lipid histiocytosis)
  (splenomegaly) 272.7
Night
  blindness (*see also* Blindness, night) 368.60
    congenital 368.61
    vitamin A deficiency 264.5
  cramps 729.82
  sweats 780.8
  terrors, child 307.46
Nightmare 307.47
  REM-sleep type 307.47
Nipple —*see* condition

Nisbet's chancre 099.0
Nishimoto (-Takeuchi) disease 437.5
Nitritoid crisis or reaction —*see* Crisis, nitritoid
Nitrogen retention, extrarenal 788.9
Nitrosohemoglobinemia 289.89
Njovera 104.0
No
 diagnosis 799.9
 disease (found) V71.9
 room at the inn V65.0
Nocardiasis —*see* Nocardiosis
Nocardiosis 039.9
 with pneumonia 039.1
 lung 039.1
 specified type NEC 039.8
Nocturia 788.43
 psychogenic 306.53
Nocturnal —*see also* condition
 dyspnea (paroxysmal) 786.09
 emissions 608.89
 enuresis 788.36
  psychogenic 307.6
 frequency (micturition) 788.43
  psychogenic 306.53
Nodal rhythm disorder 427.89
Nodding of head 781.0
Node (s)—*see also* Nodule
 Heberden's 715.04
 larynx 478.79
 lymph—*see* condition
 milkers' 051.1
 Osler's 421.0
 rheumatic 729.89
 Schmorl's 722.30
  lumbar, lumbosacral 722.32
  specified region NEC 722.39
  thoracic, thoracolumbar 722.31
 singers' 478.5
 skin NEC 782.2
 tuberculous—*see* Tuberculosis, lymph gland
 vocal cords 478.5
Nodosities, Haygarth's 715.04
Nodule(s), nodular
 actinomycotic (*see also* Actinomycosis) 039.9
 arthritic—*see* Arthritis, nodosa
 cutaneous 782.2
 Haygarth's 715.04
 inflammatory—*see* Inflammation
 juxta-articular 102.7
  syphilitic 095.7
  yaws 102.7
 larynx 478.79
 lung, solitary 518.89
  emphysematous 492.8
 milkers' 051.1
 prostate 600.10
  with
   urinary
    obstruction 600.11
    retention 600.11
 rheumatic 729.89
 rheumatoid—*see* Arthritis rheumatoid
 scrotum (inflammatory) 608.4
 singers' 478.5
 skin NEC 782.2
 solitary, lung 518.89
  emphysematous 492.8
 subcutaneous 782.2

Nodule(s), nodular—*continued*
 thyroid (gland) (nontoxic) (uninodular) 241.0
  with
   hyperthyroidism 242.1
   thyrotoxicosis 242.1
  toxic or with hyperthyroidism 242.1
 vocal cords 478.5
Noma (gangrenous) (hospital) (infective) 528.1
 auricle (*see also* Gangrene) 785.4
 mouth 528.1
 pudendi (*see also* Vulvitis) 616.10
 vulvae (*see also* Vulvitis) 616.10
Nomadism V60.0
Non-adherence
 artificial skin graft 996.55
 decellularized allodermis graft 996.55
Non-autoimmune hemolytic anemia NEC 283.10
Nonclosure —*see also* Imperfect, closure
 ductus
  arteriosus 747.0
  Botalli 747.0
 Eustachian valve 746.89
 foramen
  Botalli 745.5
  ovale 745.5
Noncompliance with medical treatment V15.81
Nondescent (congenital)—*see also* Malposition,
  congenital
 cecum 751.4
 colon 751.4
 testis 752.51
Nondevelopment
 brain 742.1
  specified part 742.2
 heart 746.89
 organ or site, congenital NEC—*see* Hypoplasia
Nonengagement
 head NEC 652.5
  in labor 660.1
   affecting fetus or newborn 763.1
Nonexanthematous tick fever 066.1
Nonexpansion, lung (newborn) NEC 770.4
Nonfunctioning
 cystic duct (*see also* Disease, gallbladder) 575.8
 gallbladder (*see also* Disease, gallbladder) 575.8
 kidney (*see also* Disease, renal) 593.9
 labyrinth 386.58
Nonhealing
 stump (surgical) 997.60
 wound, surgical 998.83
Nonimplantation of ovum, causing infertility
  628.3
Noninsufflation, fallopian tube 628.2
Nonne-Milroy-Meige syndrome (chronic
  hereditary edema) 757.0
Nonovulation 628.0
Nonpatent fallopian tube 628.2
Nonpneumatization, lung NEC 770.4
Nonreflex bladder 596.54
  with cauda equina 344.61
Nonretention of food —*see also* Vomiting
Nonrotation —*see* Malrotation
Nonsecretion, urine (*see also* Anuria) 788.5
 newborn 753.3
Nonunion
 fracture 733.82
 organ or site, congenital NEC—*see* Imperfect,
  closure
 symphysis pubis, congenital 755.69
 top sacrum, congenital 756.19
Nonviability 765.0

Nonvisualization, gallbladder 793.3
Nonvitalized tooth 522.9
Non-working side interference 524.56
Normal
  delivery—*see* category 650
  menses V65.5
  state (feared complaint unfounded) V65.5
Normoblastosis 289.89
Normocytic anemia (infectional) 285.9
  due to blood loss (chronic) 280.0
    acute 285.1
Norrie's disease (congenital) (progressive
  oculoacousticocerebral degeneration) 743.8
North American blastomycosis 116.0
Norwegian itch 133.0
Nose, nasal —*see* condition
Nosebleed 784.7
Nosomania 298.9
Nosophobia 300.29
Nostalgia 309.89
Notch of iris 743.46
Notched lip, congenital (*see also* Cleft, lip) 749.10
Notching nose, congenital (tip) 748.1
Nothnagel's
  syndrome 378.52
  vasomotor acroparesthesia 443.89
Novy's relapsing fever (American) 087.1
Noxious
  foodstuffs, poisoning by
    fish 988.0
    fungi 988.1
    mushrooms 988.1
    plants (food) 988.2
    shellfish 988.0
    specified type NEC 988.8
    toadstool 988.1
  substances transmitted through placenta or
    breast milk (affecting fetus or newborn)
    760.70
    acetretin 760.78
    alcohol 760.71
    aminopterin 760.78
    antiandrogens 760.79
    anticonvulsant 760.77
    antifungal 760.74
    anti-infective agents 760.74
    antimetabolic 760.78
    atorvastatin 760.78
    carbamazepine 760.77
    cocaine 760.75
    "crack" 760.75
    diethylstilbestrol (DES) 760.76
    divalproex sodium 760.77
    endocrine disrupting chemicals 760.79
    estrogens 760.79
    etretinate 760.78
    fluconazole 760.74
    fluvastatin 760.78
    hallucinogenic agents NEC 760.73
    hormones 760.79
    lithium 760.79
    lovastatin 760.78
    medicinal agents NEC 760.79
    methotrexate 760.78
    misoprostil 760.79
    narcotics 760.72
    obstetric anesthetic or analgesic 763.5
    phenobarbital 760.77
    phenytoin 760.77
    pravastatin 760.78

Noxious—*continued*
    progestins 760.79
    retinoic acid 760.78
    simvastatin 760.78
    solvents 760.79
    specified agent NEC 760.79
    statins 760.78
    suspected, affecting management of pregnancy
      655.5
    tetracycline 760.74
    thalidomide 760.79
    trimethadione 760.77
    valproate 760.77
    valproic acid 760.77
    vitamin A 760.78
Nuchal hitch (arm) 652.8
Nucleus pulposus —*see* condition
Numbness 782.0
Nuns' knee 727.2
Nursemaid's
  elbow 832.0
  shoulder 831.0
Nutmeg liver 573.8
Nutrition, deficient or insufficient (particular
    kind of food) 269.9
  due to
    insufficient food 994.2
    lack of
      care (child) (infant) 995.52
        adult 995.84
      food 994.2
Nyctalopia (*see also* Blindness, night) 368.60
  vitamin A deficiency 264.5
Nycturia 788.43
  psychogenic 306.53
Nymphomania 302.89
Nystagmus 379.50
  associated with vestibular system disorders
    379.54
  benign paroxysmal positional 386.11
  central positional 386.2
  congenital 379.51
  deprivation 379.53
  dissociated 379.55
  latent 379.52
  miners' 300.89
  positional
    benign paroxysmal 386.11
    central 386.2
  specified NEC 379.56
  vestibular 379.54
  visual deprivation 379.53

O

Obstruction, obstructed—*continued*
  gastric outlet 537.0
  gastrointestinal (*see also* Obstruction, intestine)
    560.9
  glottis 478.79
  hepatic 573.8
    duct (*see also* Obstruction, biliary) 576.2
      congenital 751.61
  icterus (*see also* Obstruction, biliary) 576.8
    congenital 751.61
  ileocecal coil (*see also* Obstruction, intestine)
    560.9
  ileum (*see also* Obstruction, intestine) 560.9
  iliofemoral (artery) 444.81
  internal anastomosis—*see* Complications,
    mechanical, graft
  intestine (mechanical) (neurogenic)
    (paroxysmal) (postinfectional) (reflex) 560.9
    with
      adhesions (intestinal) (peritoneal) 560.81
      hernia—*see also* Hernia, by site, with
        obstruction
        gangrenous—*see* Hernia, by site, with
          gangrene
    adynamic (*see also* Ileus) 560.1
    by gallstone 560.31
    congenital or infantile (small) 751.1
      large 751.2
    due to
      Ascaris lumbricoides 127.0
      mural thickening 560.89
      procedure 997.4
        involving urinary tract 997.5
    impaction 560.39
    infantile—*see* Obstruction, intestine,
      congenital
    newborn
      due to
        fecaliths 777.1
        inspissated milk 777.2
        meconium (plug) 777.1
          in mucoviscidosis 277.01
        transitory 777.4
    specified cause NEC 560.89
    transitory, newborn 777.4
    volvulus 560.2
  intracardiac ball valve prosthesis 996.02
  jaundice (*see also* Obstruction, biliary) 576.8
    congenital 751.61
  jejunum (*see also* Obstruction, intestine) 560.9
  kidney 593.89
  labor 660.9
    affecting fetus or newborn 763.1
    by
      bony pelvis (conditions classifiable to
        653.0-653.9) 660.1
      deep transverse arrest 660.3
      impacted shoulder 660.4
      locked twins 660.5
      malposition (fetus) (conditions classifiable
        to 652.0-652.9) 660.0
        head during labor 660.3
      persistent occipitoposterior position 660.3
      soft tissue, pelvic (conditions classifiable to
        654.0-654.9) 660.2
  lacrimal
    canaliculi 375.53
    congenital 743.65
    punctum 375.52
    sac 375.54
  lacrimonasal duct 375.56

Obstruction, obstructed—*continued*
    congenital 743.65
    neonatal 375.55
  lacteal, with steatorrhea 579.2
  laryngitis (*see also* Laryngitis) 464.01
  larynx 478.79
    congenital 748.3
  liver 573.8
    cirrhotic (*see also* Cirrhosis, liver) 571.5
  lung 518.89
    with
      asthma—*see* Asthma
      bronchitis (chronic) 491.20
      emphysema NEC 492.8
    airway, chronic 496
    chronic NEC 496
      with
        asthma (chronic) (obstructive) 493.2
    disease, chronic 496
      with
        asthma (chronic) (obstructive) 493.2
    emphysematous 492.8
  lymphatic 457.1
  meconium
    fetus or newborn 777.1
      in mucoviscidosis 277.01
    newborn due to fecaliths 777.1
  mediastinum 519.3
  mitral (rheumatic)—*see* Stenosis, mitral
  nasal 478.19
    duct 375.56
      neonatal 375.55
    sinus—*see* Sinusitis
  nasolacrimal duct 375.56
    congenital 743.65
    neonatal 375.55
  nasopharynx 478.29
  nose 478.19
  organ or site, congenital NEC—*see* Atresia
  pancreatic duct 577.8
  parotid gland 527.8
  pelviureteral junction (*see also* Obstruction,
    ureter) 593.4
  pharynx 478.29
  portal (circulation) (vein) 452
  prostate 600.90
    with
      other lower urinary tract symptoms (LUTS)
        600.91
      urinary
        obstruction 600.91
        retention 600.91
    valve (urinary) 596.0
  pulmonary
    valve (heart) (*see also* Endocarditis,
      pulmonary) 424.3
    vein, isolated 747.49
  pyemic—*see* Septicemia
  pylorus (acquired) 537.0
    congenital 750.5
    infantile 750.5
  rectosigmoid (*see also* Obstruction, intestine)
    560.9
  rectum 569.49
  renal 593.89
  respiratory 519.8
    chronic 496
  retinal (artery) (vein) (central) (*see also*
    Occlusion, retina) 362.30
  salivary duct (any) 527.8
    with calculus 527.5

Obstruction, obstructed—*continued*
  sigmoid (*see also* Obstruction, intestine) 560.9
  sinus (accessory) (nasal) (*see also* Sinusitis)
      473.9
  Stensen's duct 527.8
  stomach 537.89
    acute 536.1
    congenital 750.7
  submaxillary gland 527.8
    with calculus 527.5
  thoracic duct 457.1
  thrombotic—*see* Thrombosis
  tooth eruption 520.6
  trachea 519.19
  tracheostomy airway 519.09
  tricuspid—*see* Endocarditis, tricuspid
  upper respiratory, congenital 748.8
  ureter (functional) 593.4
    congenital 753.20
    due to calculus 592.1
  ureteropelvic junction, congenital 753.21
  ureterovesical junction, congenital 753.22
  urethra 599.60
    congenital 753.6
  urinary (moderate) 599.60
    organ or tract (lower) 599.60
      due to
        benign prostatic hypertrophy (BPH)—*see*
            category 600
        specified NEC 599.69
          due to
            benign prostatic hypertrophy
                (BPH)—*see* category 600
      prostatic valve 596.0
      specified NEC 599.69
        due to
          benign prostatic hypertrophy (BPH)—*see*
              category 600
  uropathy 599.60
  uterus 621.8
  vagina 623.2
  valvular—*see* Endocarditis
  vascular graft or shunt 996.1
    atherosclerosis —*see* Arteriosclerosis,
        coronary
    embolism 996.74
    occlusion NEC 996.74
    thrombus 996.74
  vein, venous 459.2
    caval (inferior) (superior) 459.2
    thrombotic—*see* Thrombosis
  vena cava (inferior) (superior) 459.2
  ventricular shunt 996.2
  vesical 596.0
  vesicourethral orifice 596.0
  vessel NEC 459.9
Obturator —*see* condition
Occlusal
  plane deviation 524.76
  wear, teeth 521.10
Occlusion
  anus 569.49
    congenital 751.2
    infantile 751.2
  aortoiliac (chronic) 444.0
  aqueduct of Sylvius 331.4
    congenital 742.3
      with spina bifida (*see also* Spina bifida) 741.0
  arteries of extremities, lower 444.22
    without thrombus or embolus (*see also*
        Arteriosclerosis, extremities) 440.20

Occlusion—*continued*
  due to stricture or stenosis 447.1
  upper 444.21
    without thrombus or embolus (*see also*
        Arteriosclerosis, extremities) 440.20
    due to stricture or stenosis 447.1
  artery NEC (*see also* Embolism, artery) 444.9
    auditory, internal 433.8
    basilar 433.0
      with other precerebral artery 433.3
      bilateral 433.3
    brain or cerebral (*see also* Infarct, brain) 434.9
    carotid 433.1
      with other precerebral artery 433.3
      bilateral 433.3
    cerebellar (anterior inferior) (posterior
        inferior) (superior) 433.8
    cerebral (*see also* Infarct, brain) 434.9
    choroidal (anterior) 433.8
    communicating posterior 433.8
    coronary (thrombotic) (*see also* Infarct,
        myocardium) 410.9
      acute 410.9
        without myocardial infarction 411.81
      healed or old 412
    hypophyseal 433.8
    iliac 444.81
    mesenteric (embolic) (thrombotic) (with
        gangrene) 557.0
    pontine 433.8
    precerebral NEC 433.9
      late effect—*see* Late effect(s) (of)
          cerebrovascular disease
      multiple or bilateral 433.3
      puerperal, postpartum, childbirth 674.0
      specified NEC 433.8
    renal 593.81
    retinal—*see* Occlusion, retina, artery
    spinal 433.8
    vertebral 433.2
      with other precerebral artery 433.3
      bilateral 433.3
  basilar (artery)—*see* Occlusion, artery, basilar
  bile duct (any) (*see also* Obstruction, biliary)
      576.2
  bowel (*see also* Obstruction, intestine) 560.9
  brain (artery) (vascular) (*see also* Infarct, brain)
      434.9
  breast (duct) 611.8
  carotid (artery) (common) (internal)—*see*
      Occlusion, artery, carotid
  cerebellar (anterior inferior) (artery) (posterior
      inferior) (superior) 433.8
  cerebral (artery) (*see also* Infarct, brain) 434.9
  cerebrovascular (*see also* Infarct, brain) 434.9
    diffuse 437.0
  cervical canal (*see also* Stricture, cervix) 622.4
    by falciparum malaria 084.0
  cervix (uteri) (*see also* Stricture, cervix) 622.4
  choanal 748.0
  choroidal (artery) 433.8
  colon (*see also* Obstruction, intestine) 560.9
  communicating posterior artery 433.8
  coronary (artery) (thrombotic) (*see also* Infarct,
      myocardium) 410.9
    acute 410.9
      without myocardial infarction 411.81
    healed or old 412
    without myocardial infarction 411.81
  cystic duct (*see also* Obstruction, gallbladder)
      575.2

Occlusion—*continued*
congenital 751.69
disto
division I 524.22
division II 524.22
embolic—*see* Embolism
fallopian tube 628.2
congenital 752.19
gallbladder (*see also* Obstruction, gallbladder)
575.2
congenital 751.69
jaundice from 751.69 *[774.5]*
gingiva, traumatic 523.8
hymen 623.3
congenital 752.42
hypophyseal (artery) 433.8
iliac artery 444.81
intestine (*see also* Obstruction, intestine) 560.9
kidney 593.89
lacrimal apparatus—*see* Stenosis, lacrimal
lung 518.89
lymph or lymphatic channel 457.1
mammary duct 611.8
mesenteric artery (embolic) (thrombotic) (with
gangrene) 557.0
nose 478.1
congenital 748.0
organ or site, congenital NEC—*see* Atresia
oviduct 628.2
congenital 752.19
periodontal, traumatic 523.8
peripheral arteries (lower extremity) 444.22
without thrombus or embolus (*see also*
Arteriosclerosis, extremities) 440.20
due to stricture or stenosis 447.1
upper extremity 444.21
without thrombus or embolus (*see also*
Arteriosclerosis, extremities) 440.20
due to stricture or stenosis 447.1
pontine (artery) 433.8
posterior lingual, of mandibular teeth 524.29
precerebral artery—*see* Occlusion, artery,
precerebral NEC
puncta lacrimalia 375.52
pupil 364.74
pylorus (*see also* Stricture, pylorus) 537.0
renal artery 593.81
retina, retinal (vascular) 362.30
artery, arterial 362.30
branch 362.32
central (total) 362.31
partial 362.33
transient 362.34
tributary 362.32
vein 362.30
branch 362.36
central (total) 362.35
incipient 362.37
partial 362.37
tributary 362.36
spinal artery 433.8
stent
coronary 996.72
teeth (mandibular) (posterior lingual) 524.29
thoracic duct 457.1
tubal 628.2
ureter (complete) (partial) 593.4
congenital 753.29
urethra (*see also* Stricture, urethra) 598.9
congenital 753.6
uterus 621.8

Occlusion—*continued*
vagina 623.2
vascular NEC 459.9
vein—*see* Thrombosis
vena cava (inferior) (superior) 453.2
ventricle (brain) NEC 331.4
vertebral (artery)—*see* Occlusion, artery,
vertebral
vessel (blood) NEC 459.9
vulva 624.8
Occlusio pupillae 364.74
Occupational
problems NEC V62.2
therapy V57.21
Ochlophobia 300.29
Ochronosis (alkaptonuric) (congenital)
(endogenous) 270.2
with chloasma of eyelid 270.2
Ocular muscle —*see also* condition
myopathy 359.1
torticollis 781.93
Oculoauriculovertebral dysplasia 756.0
Oculogyric
crisis or disturbance 378.87
psychogenic 306.7
Oculomotor syndrome 378.81
Oddi's sphincter spasm 576.5
Odelberg's disease (juvenile osteochondrosis)
732.1
Odontalgia 525.9
Odontoameloblastoma (M9311/0) 213.1
upper jaw (bone) 213.0
Odontoclasia 521.05
Odontoclasis 873.63
complicated 873.73
Odontodysplasia, regional 520.4
Odontogenesis imperfecta 520.5
Odontoma (M9280/0) 213.1
ameloblastic (M9311/0) 213.1
upper jaw (bone) 213.0
calcified (M9280/0) 213.1
upper jaw (bone) 213.0
complex (M9282/0) 213.1
upper jaw (bone) 213.0
compound (M9281/0) 213.1
upper jaw (bone) 213.0
fibroameloblastic (M9290/0) 213.1
upper jaw (bone) 213.0
follicular 526.0
upper jaw (bone) 213.0
Odontomyelitis (closed) (open) 522.0
Odontonecrosis 521.09
Odontorrhagia 525.8
Odontosarcoma, ameloblastic (M9290/3) 170.1
upper jaw (bone) 170.0
Odynophagia 787.2
Oesophagostomiasis 127.7
Oesophagostomum infestation 127.7
Oestriasis 134.0
Ogilvie's syndrome (sympathicotonic colon
obstruction) 560.89
Oguchi's disease (retina) 368.61
Ohara's disease (*see also* Tularemia) 021.9
Oidiomycosis (*see also* Candidiasis) 112.9
Oidiomycotic meningitis 112.83
Oidium albicans infection (*see also* Candidiasis)
112.9
Old age 797
dementia (of) 290.0
Olfactory —*see* condition
Oligemia 285.9

Oligergasia (*see also* Retardation, mental) 319
Oligoamnios 658.0
  affecting fetus or newborn 761.2
Oligoastrocytoma, mixed (M9382/3)
  specified site—*see* Neoplasm, by site, malignant
  unspecified site 191.9
Oligocythemia 285.9
Oligodendroblastoma (M9460/3)
  specified site—*see* Neoplasm, by site, malignant
  unspecified site 191.9
Oligodendroglioma (M9450/3)
  anaplastic type (M9451/3)
    specified site—*see* Neoplasm, by site,
      malignant
    unspecified site 191.9
  specified site—*see* Neoplasm, by site, malignant
  unspecified site 191.9
Oligodendroma —*see* Oligodendroglioma
Oligodontia (*see also* Anodontia) 520.0
Oligoencephalon 742.1
Oligohydramnios 658.0
  affecting fetus or newborn 761.2
  due to premature rupture of membranes 658.1
    affecting fetus or newborn 761.2
Oligohydrosis 705.0
Oligomenorrhea 626.1
Oligophrenia (*see also* Retardation, mental) 319
  phenylpyruvic 270.1
Oligospermia 606.1
Oligotrichia 704.09
  congenita 757.4
Oliguria 788.5
  with
    abortion—*see* Abortion, by type, with renal
      failure
    ectopic pregnancy (*see also* categories
      633.0-633.9) 639.3
    molar pregnancy (*see also* categories 630-632)
      639.3
  complicating
    abortion 639.3
    ectopic or molar pregnancy 639.3
    pregnancy 646.2
      with hypertension—*see* Toxemia, of
        pregnancy
  due to a procedure 997.5
  following labor and delivery 669.3
  heart or cardiac—*see* Failure, heart
  puerperal, postpartum 669.3
  specified due to a procedure 997.5
Ollier's disease (chondrodysplasia) 756.4
Omentitis (*see also* Peritonitis) 567.9
Omentocele (*see also* Hernia, omental) 553.8
Omentum, omental —*see* condition
Omphalitis (congenital) (newborn) 771.4
  not of newborn 686.9
  tetanus 771.3
Omphalocele 756.79
Omphalomesenteric duct, persistent 751.0
Omphalorrhagia, newborn 772.3
Omsk hemorrhagic fever 065.1
Onanism 307.9
Onchocerciasis 125.3
  eye 125.3 *[360.13]*
Onchocercosis 125.3
Oncocytoma (M8290/0)—*see* Neoplasm, by site,
  benign
Ondine's curse 348.8
Oneirophrenia (*see also* Schizophrenia) 295.4
Onychauxis 703.8
  congenital 757.5

Onychia (with lymphangitis) 681.9
  dermatophytic 110.1
  finger 681.02
  toe 681.11
Onychitis (with lymphangitis) 681.9
  finger 681.02
  toe 681.11
Onychocryptosis 703.0
Onychodystrophy 703.8
  congenital 757.5
Onychogryphosis 703.8
Onychogryposis 703.8
Onycholysis 703.8
Onychomadesis 703.8
Onychomalacia 703.8
Onychomycosis 110.1
  finger 110.1
  toe 110.1
Onycho-osteodysplasia 756.89
Onychophagy 307.9
Onychoptosis 703.8
Onychorrhexis 703.8
  congenital 757.5
Onychoschizia 703.8
Onychotrophia (*see also* Atrophy, nail) 703.8
O'nyong-nyong fever 066.3
Onyxis (finger) (toe) 703.0
Onyxitis (with lymphangitis) 681.9
  finger 681.02
  toe 681.11
Oocyte (egg) (ovum)
  donor V59.70
    age 35 and over V59.73
      anonymous recipient V59.73
      designated recipient V59.74
    under age 35 V59.71
      anonymous recipient V59.71
      designated recipient V59.72
Oophoritis (cystic) (infectional) (interstitial) (*see
  also* Salpingo-oophoritis) 614.2
  complicating pregnancy 646.6
  fetal (acute) 752.0
  gonococcal (acute) 098.19
    chronic or duration of 2 months or over 098.39
  tuberculous (*see also* Tuberculosis) 016.6
Opacity, opacities
  cornea 371.00
    central 371.03
    congenital 743.43
      interfering with vision 743.42
    degenerative (*see also* Degeneration, cornea)
      371.40
    hereditary (*see also* Dystrophy, cornea) 371.50
    inflammatory (*see also* Keratitis) 370.9
    late effect of trachoma (healed) 139.1
    minor 371.01
    peripheral 371.02
  enamel (fluoride) (nonfluoride) (teeth) 520.3
  lens (*see also* Cataract) 366.9
  snowball 379.22
  vitreous (humor) 379.24
    congenital 743.51
Opalescent dentin (hereditary) 520.5
Open, opening
  abnormal, organ or site, congenital—*see*
    Imperfect, closure
  angle with
    borderline intraocular pressure 365.01
    cupping of discs 365.01
  bite (anterior) (posterior) 524.29

Open, opening—*continued*
  false—*see* Imperfect, closure
  margin on tooth restoration 525.61
  restoration margins 525.61
  wound—*see* Wound, open, by site
Operation
  causing mutilation of fetus 763.89
  destructive, on live fetus, to facilitate birth 763.89
  for delivery, fetus or newborn 763.89
  maternal, unrelated to current delivery, affecting
    fetus or newborn 760.6
Operational fatigue 300.89
Operative —*see* condition
Operculitis (chronic) 523.40
  acute 523.30
Operculum, retina 361.32
  with detachment 361.01
Ophiasis 704.01
Ophthalmia (*see also* Conjunctivitis) 372.30
  actinic rays 370.24
  allergic (acute) 372.05
    chronic 372.14
  blennorrhagic (neonatorum) 098.40
  catarrhal 372.03
  diphtheritic 032.81
  Egyptian 076.1
  electric, electrica 370.24
  gonococcal (neonatorum) 098.40
  metastatic 360.11
  migraine 346.8
  neonatorum, newborn 771.6
    gonococcal 098.40
  nodosa 360.14
  phlyctenular 370.31
    with ulcer (*see also* Ulcer, cornea) 370.00
  sympathetic 360.11
Ophthalmitis —*see* Ophthalmia
Ophthalmocele (congenital) 743.66
Ophthalmoneuromyelitis 341.0
**Ophthalmopathy, infiltrative with
  thyrotoxicosis** 242.0
Ophthalmoplegia (*see also* Strabismus) 378.9
  anterior internuclear 378.86
  ataxia-areflexia syndrome 357.0
  bilateral 378.9
  diabetic 250.5 *[378.86]*
  exophthalmic 242.0 *[376.22]*
  external 378.55
    progressive 378.72
    total 378.56
  interna(l) (complete) (total) 367.52
  internuclear 378.86
  migraine 346.8
  painful 378.55
  Parinaud's 378.81
  progressive external 378.72
  supranuclear, progressive 333.0
  total (external) 378.56
    internal 367.52
  unilateral 378.9
Opisthognathism 524.00
Opisthorchiasis (felineus) (tenuicollis)
  (viverrini) 121.0
Opisthotonos, opisthotonus 781.0
Opitz's disease (congestive splenomegaly)
  289.51
Opiumism (*see also* Dependence) 304.0
Oppenheim's disease 358.8
Oppenheim-Urbach disease or syndrome
  (necrobiosis lipoidica diabeticorum) 250.8
  [709.3]

Opsoclonia 379.59
Optic nerve —*see* condition
Orbit —*see* condition
Orchioblastoma (M9071/3) 186.9
Orchitis (nonspecific) (septic) 604.90
  with abscess 604.0
  blennorrhagic (acute) 098.13
    chronic or duration of 2 months or over 098.33
  diphtheritic 032.89 *[604.91]*
  filarial 125.9 *[604.91]*
  gangrenous 604.99
  gonococcal (acute) 098.13
    chronic or duration of 2 months or over 098.33
  mumps 072.0
  parotidea 072.0
  suppurative 604.99
  syphilitic 095.8 *[604.91]*
  tuberculous (*see also* Tuberculosis) 016.5 *[608.81]*
Orf 051.2
Organic —*see also* condition
  heart—*see* Disease, heart
  insufficiency 799.89
Oriental
  bilharziasis 120.2
  schistosomiasis 120.2
  sore 085.1
Orientation
  ego-dystonic sexual 302.0
Orifice —*see* condition
Origin, both great vessels from right ventricle
  745.11
Ormond's disease or syndrome 593.4
Ornithosis 073.9
  with
    complication 073.8
      specified NEC 073.7
    pneumonia 073.0
    pneumonitis (lobular) 073.0
Orodigitofacial dysostosis 759.89
Oropouche fever 066.3
Orotaciduria, oroticaciduria (congenital)
  (hereditary) (pyrimidine deficiency) 281.4
Oroya fever 088.0
Orthodontics V58.5
  adjustment V53.4
  aftercare V58.5
  fitting V53.4
Orthopnea 786.02
Orthoptic training V57.4
Os, uterus —*see* condition
Osgood-Schlatter
  disease 732.4
  osteochondrosis 732.4
Osler's
  disease (M9950/1) (polycythemia vera) 238.4
  nodes 421.0
Osler-Rendu disease (familial hemorrhagic
  telangiectasia) 448.0
Osler-Vaquez disease (M9950/1) (polycythemia
  vera) 238.4
Osler-Weber-Rendu syndrome (familial
  hemorrhagic telangiectasia) 448.0
Osmidrosis 705.89
Osseous —*see* condition
Ossification
  artery—*see* Arteriosclerosis
  auricle (ear) 380.39
  bronchus 519.19
  cardiac (*see also* Degeneration, myocardial) 429.1
  cartilage (senile) 733.99

> *Note—Use the following fifth-digit*
> *subclassification with category 715:*
>
> *0 site unspecified*
> *1 shoulder region*
> *2 upper arm*
> *3 forearm*
> *4 hand*
> *5 pelvic region and thigh*
> *6 lower leg*
> *7 ankle and foot*
> *8 other specified sites except spine*
> *9 multiple sites*

Osteochondrosis—*continued*
  coxae juvenilis 732.1
  deformans juvenilis (coxae) (hip) 732.1
    Scheuermann's 732.0
    spine 732.0
    tibia 732.4
    vertebra 732.0
  Diaz's (astragalus) 732.5
  dissecans (knee) (shoulder) 732.7
  femoral capital epiphysis 732.1
  femur (head) (juvenile) 732.1
  foot (juvenile) 732.5
  Freiberg's (disease) (second metatarsal) 732.5
  Haas' 732.3
  Haglund's (os tibiale externum) 732.5
  hand (juvenile) 732.3
  head of
    femur 732.1
    humerus (juvenile) 732.3
  hip (juvenile) 732.1
  humerus (juvenile) 732.3
  iliac crest (juvenile) 732.1
  ilium (juvenile) 732.1
  ischiopubic synchondrosis 732.1
  Iselin's (osteochondrosis fifth metatarsal) 732.5
  juvenile, juvenilis 732.6
    arm 732.3
    capital femoral epiphysis 732.1
    capitellum humeri 732.3
    capitular epiphysis 732.1
    carpal scaphoid 732.3
    clavicle, sternal epiphysis 732.6
    coxae 732.1
    deformans 732.1
    foot 732.5
    hand 732.3
    hip and pelvis 732.1
    lower extremity, except foot 732.4
    lunate, wrist 732.3
    medial cuneiform bone 732.5
    metatarsal (head) 732.5
    metatarsophalangeal 732.5
    navicular, ankle 732.5
    patella 732.4
    primary patellar center (of Köhler) 732.4
    specified site NEC 732.6
    spine 732.0
    tarsal scaphoid 732.5
    tibia (epiphysis) (tuberosity) 732.4
    upper extremity 732.3
    vertebra (body) (Calvé) 732.0
      epiphyseal plates (of Scheuermann) 732.0
  Kienböck's (disease) 732.3
  Köhler's (disease) (navicular, ankle) 732.5
    patellar 732.4
    tarsal navicular 732.5
  Legg-Calvé-Perthes (disease) 732.1
  lower extremity (juvenile) 732.4
  lunate bone 732.3
  Mauclaire's 732.3
  metacarpal heads (of Mauclaire) 732.3
  metatarsal (fifth) (head) (second) 732.5
  navicular, ankle 732.5
  os calcis 732.5
  Osgood-Schlatter 732.4
  os tibiale externum 732.5
  Panner's 732.3
  patella (juvenile) 732.4
  patellar center
    primary (of Köhler) 732.4
    secondary (of Sinding-Larsen) 732.4

Osteochondrosis—*continued*
  pelvis (juvenile) 732.1
  Pierson's 732.1
  radial head (juvenile) 732.3
  Scheuermann's 732.0
  Sever's (calcaneum) 732.5
  Sinding-Larsen (secondary patellar center) 732.4
  spine (juvenile) 732.0
    adult 732.8
  symphysis pubis (of Pierson) (juvenile) 732.1
  syphilitic (congenital) 090.0
  tarsal (navicular) (scaphoid) 732.5
  tibia (proximal) (tubercle) 732.4
  tuberculous—*see* Tuberculosis, bone
  ulna 732.3
  upper extremity (juvenile) 732.3
  van Neck's (juvenile osteochondrosis) 732.1
  vertebral (juvenile) 732.0
    adult 732.8
Osteoclastoma (M9250/1) 238.0
  malignant (M9250/3)—*see* Neoplasm, bone,
    malignant
Osteocopic pain 733.90
Osteodynia 733.90
Osteodystrophy
  azotemic 588.0
  chronica deformans hypertrophica 731.0
  congenital 756.50
    specified type NEC 756.59
  deformans 731.0
  fibrosa localisata 731.0
  parathyroid 252.01
  renal 588.0
Osteofibroma (M9262/0)—*see* Neoplasm, bone,
  benign
Osteofibrosarcoma (M9182/3)—*see* Neoplasm,
  bone, malignant
Osteogenesis imperfecta 756.51
Osteogenic —*see* condition
Osteoma (M9180/0)—*see also* Neoplasm, bone,
  benign
  osteoid (M9191/0)—*see also* Neoplasm, bone,
    benign
    giant (M9200/0)—*see* Neoplasm, bone, benign
Osteomalacia 268.2
  chronica deformans hypertrophica 731.0
  due to vitamin D deficiency 268.2
  infantile (*see also* Rickets) 268.0
  juvenile (*see also* Rickets) 268.0
  pelvis 268.2
  vitamin D-resistant 275.3
Osteomalacic bone 268.2
Osteomalacosis 268.2
Osteomyelitis (general) (infective) (localized)
    (neonatal) (purulent) (pyogenic) (septic)
    (staphylococcal) (streptococcal) (suppurative)
    (with periostitis) 730.2

> *Note—Use the following fifth-digit*
> *subclassification with category 730:*
>
> *0 site unspecified*
> *1 shoulder region*
> *2 upper arm*
> *3 forearm*
> *4 hand*
> *5 pelvic region and thigh*
> *6 lower leg*
> *7 ankle and foot*
> *8 other specified sites*
> *9 multiple sites*

Osteomyelitis—*continued*
  acute or subacute 730.0
  chronic or old 730.1
  due to or associated with
      diabetes mellitus 250.8 *[731.8]*
      tuberculosis (*see also* Tuberculosis, bone)
          015.9 *[730.8]*
          limb bones 015.5 *[730.8]*
          specified bones NEC 015.7 *[730.8]*
          spine 015.0 *[730.8]*
          typhoid 002.0 *[730.8]*
  Garré's 730.1
  jaw (acute) (chronic) (lower) (neonatal)
      (suppurative) (upper) 526.4
  nonsuppurating 730.1
  orbital 376.03
  petrous bone (*see also* Petrositis) 383.20
  Salmonella 003.24
  sclerosing, nonsuppurative 730.1
  sicca 730.1
  syphilitic 095.5
      congenital 090.0 *[730.8]*
  tuberculous—*see* Tuberculosis, bone
  typhoid 002.0 *[730.8]*
Osteomyelofibrosis 289.89
Osteomyelosclerosis 289.89
Osteonecrosis 733.40
  meaning osteomyelitis 730.1
Osteo-onycho-arthro dysplasia 756.89
Osteo-onychodysplasia, hereditary 756.89
Osteopathia
  condensans disseminata 756.53
  hyperostotica multiplex infantilis 756.59
  hypertrophica toxica 731.2
  striata 756.4
Osteopathy resulting from poliomyelitis (*see
      also* Poliomyelitis) 045.9 *[730.7]*
  familial dysplastic 731.2
Osteopecilia 756.53
Osteopenia 733.90
Osteoperiostitis (*see also* Osteomyelitis) 730.2
  ossificans toxica 731.2
  toxica ossificans 731.2
Osteopetrosis (familial) 756.52
Osteophyte —*see* Exostosis
Osteophytosis —*see* Exostosis
Osteopoikilosis 756.53
Osteoporosis (generalized) 733.00
  circumscripta 731.0
  disuse 733.03
  drug-induced 733.09
  idiopathic 733.02
  postmenopausal 733.01
  posttraumatic 733.7
  screening V82.81
  senile 733.01
  specified type NEC 733.09
Osteoporosis-osteomalacia syndrome 268.2
Osteopsathyrosis 756.51
Osteoradionecrosis, jaw 526.89
Osteosarcoma (M9180/3)—*see also* Neoplasm,
      bone, malignant
  chondroblastic (M9181/3)—*see* Neoplasm,
      bone, malignant
  fibroblastic (M9182/3)—*see* Neoplasm, bone,
      malignant
  in Paget's disease of bone (M9184/3)—*see*
      Neoplasm, bone, malignant
  juxtacortical (M9190/3)—*see* Neoplasm, bone,
      malignant

Osteosarcoma—*continued*
  parosteal (M9190/3)—*see* Neoplasm, bone,
      malignant
  telangiectatic (M9183/3)—*see* Neoplasm, bone,
      malignant
Osteosclerosis 756.52
  fragilis (generalisata) 756.52
Osteosclerotic anemia 289.89
Osteosis
  acromegaloid 757.39
  cutis 709.3
  parathyroid 252.01
  renal fibrocystic 588.0
Österreicher-Turner syndrome 756.89
Ostium
  atrioventriculare commune 745.69
  primum (arteriosum) (defect) (persistent) 745.61
  secundum (arteriosum) (defect) (patent)
      (persistent) 745.5
Ostrum-Furst syndrome 756.59
Otalgia 388.70
  otogenic 388.71
  referred 388.72
Othematoma 380.31
Otitic hydrocephalus 348.2
Otitis 382.9
  with effusion 381.4
      purulent 382.4
      secretory 381.4
      serous 381.4
      suppurative 382.4
  acute 382.9
  adhesive (*see also* Adhesions, middle ear)
      385.10
  chronic 382.9
      with effusion 381.3
      mucoid, mucous (simple) 381.20
      purulent 382.3
      secretory 381.3
      serous 381.10
      suppurative 382.3
  diffuse parasitic 136.8
  externa (acute) (diffuse) (hemorrhagica) 380.10
      actinic 380.22
      candidal 112.82
      chemical 380.22
      chronic 380.23
          mycotic—*see* Otitis, externa, mycotic
          specified type NEC 380.23
      circumscribed 380.10
      contact 380.22
      due to
          erysipelas 035 *[380.13]*
          impetigo 684 *[380.13]*
          seborrheic dermatitis 690.10 *[380.13]*
      eczematoid 380.22
      furuncular 680.0 *[380.13]*
      infective 380.10
          chronic 380.16
      malignant 380.14
      mycotic (chronic) 380.15
          due to
              aspergillosis 117.3 *[380.15]*
              moniliasis 112.82
              otomycosis 111.8 *[380.15]*
      reactive 380.22
      specified type NEC 380.22
      tropical 111.8 *[380.15]*
  insidiosa (*see also* Otosclerosis) 387.9
  interna (*see also* Labyrinthitis) 386.30

P

Pacemaker syndrome 429.4
Pachyderma, pachydermia 701.8
  laryngis 478.5
  laryngitis 478.79
  larynx (verrucosa) 478.79
Pachydermatitis 701.8
Pachydermatocele (congenital) 757.39
  acquired 701.8
Pachydermatosis 701.8
Pachydermoperiostitis
  secondary 731.2
Pachydermoperiostosis
  primary idiopathic 757.39
  secondary 731.2
Pachymeningitis (adhesive) (basal) (brain)
      (cerebral) (cervical) (chronic) (circumscribed)
      (external) (fibrous) (hemorrhagic)
      (hypertrophic) (internal) (purulent) (spinal)
      (suppurative) (*see also* Meningitis) 322.9
  gonococcal 098.82
Pachyonychia (congenital) 757.5
  acquired 703.8
Pachyperiosteodermia
  primary or idiopathic 757.39
  secondary 731.2
Pachyperiostosis
  primary or idiopathic 757.39
  secondary 731.2
Pacinian tumor (M9507/0)—*see* Neoplasm,
    skin, benign
Pads, knuckle or Garrod's 728.79
Paget's disease (osteitis deformans) 731.0
  with infiltrating duct carcinoma of the breast
      (M8541/3)—*see* Neoplasm, breast,
      malignant
  bone 731.0
    osteosarcoma in (M9184/3)—*see* Neoplasm,
        bone, malignant
  breast (M8540/3) 174.0
  extramammary (M8542/3)—*see also* Neoplasm,
      skin, malignant
    anus 154.3
      skin 173.5
  malignant (M8540/3)
    breast 174.0
    specified site NEC (M8542/3)—*see*
        Neoplasm, skin, malignant
    unspecified site 174.0
  mammary (M8540/3) 174.0
  necrosis of bone 731.0
  nipple (M8540/3) 174.0
  osteitis deformans 731.0
Paget-Schroetter syndrome (intermittent venous
    claudication) 453.8
Pain(s) 780.96
  abdominal 789.0
  acute 338.19
    due to trauma 338.11
    postoperative 338.18
      post-thoracotomy 338.12
  adnexa (uteri) 625.9
  alimentary, due to vascular insufficiency 557.9
  anginoid (*see also* Pain, precordial) 786.51
  anus 569.42
  arch 729.5
  arm 729.5
  axillary 729.5

Pain(s)—*continued*
  back (postural) 724.5
    low 724.2
    psychogenic 307.89
  bile duct 576.9
  bladder 788.9
  bone 733.90
  breast 611.71
    psychogenic 307.89
  broad ligament 625.9
  cancer associated 338.3
  cartilage NEC 733.90
  cecum 789.0
  cervicobrachial 723.3
  chest (central) 786.50
    atypical 786.59
    midsternal 786.51
    musculoskeletal 786.59
    noncardiac 786.59
    substernal 786.51
    wall (anterior) 786.52
  chronic 338.29
    associated with significant psychosocial
        dysfunction 338.4
    due to trauma 338.21
    postoperative 338.28
      post-thoracotomy 338.22
    syndrome 338.4
  coccyx 724.79
  colon 789.0
  common duct 576.9
  coronary—*see* Angina
  costochondral 786.52
  diaphragm 786.52
  due to (presence of) any device, implant, or graft
      classifiable to 996.0-996.5—*see*
      Complications, due to (presence of) any
      device, implant, or graft classified to
      996.0-996.5 NEC
  malignancy (primary) (secondary) 338.3
  ear (*see also* Otalgia) 388.70
  epigastric, epigastrium 789.0
  extremity (lower) (upper) 729.5
  eye 379.91
  face, facial 784.0
    atypical 350.2
    nerve 351.8
  false (labor) 644.1
  female genital organ NEC 625.9
    psychogenic 307.89
  finger 729.5
  flank 789.0
  foot 729.5
  gallbladder 575.9
  gas (intestinal) 787.3
  gastric 536.8
  generalized 780.96
  genital organ
    female 625.9
    male 608.9
    psychogenic 307.89
  groin 789.0
  growing 781.99
  hand 729.5
  head (*see also* Headache) 784.0
  heart (*see also* Pain, precordial) 786.51
  infraorbital (*see also* Neuralgia, trigeminal)
      350.1

Palatoplegia 528.9
Palatoschisis (*see also* Cleft, palate) 749.00
Palilalia 784.69
Palindromic arthritis (*see also* Rheumatism,
   palindromic) 719.3
Palliative care V66.7
Pallor 782.61
   temporal, optic disc 377.15
Palmar —*see also* condition
   fascia—*see* condition
Palpable
   cecum 569.89
   kidney 593.89
   liver 573.9
   lymph nodes 785.6
   ovary 620.8
   prostate 602.9
   spleen (*see also* Splenomegaly) 789.2
   uterus 625.8
Palpitation (heart) 785.1
   psychogenic 306.2
Palsy (*see also* Paralysis) 344.9
   atrophic diffuse 335.20
   Bell's 351.0
      newborn 767.5
   birth 767.7
   brachial plexus 353.0
      fetus or newborn 767.6
   brain—*see also* Palsy, cerebral
      noncongenital or noninfantile 344.89
         due to vascular lesion—*see* category 438
         late effect—*see* Late effect(s) (of)
            cerebrovascular disease
      syphilitic 094.89
         congenital 090.49
   bulbar (chronic) (progressive) 335.22
      pseudo NEC 335.23
      supranuclear NEC 344.89
   cerebral (congenital) (infantile) (spastic) 343.9
      athetoid 333.71
      diplegic 343.0
         mue to prevhous vascular lesion—*see*
            category 438
         late effect—*see* Late effect(s) (of)
            cerebrovascular disease
      hemiplegic 343.1
      monoplegic 343.3
      noncongenital or noninfantile 437.8
         mue to prevhous vascular lesion—*see*
            category 438
         late effect—*see* Late effect(s) (of)
            cerebrovascular disease
      paraplegic 343.0
      quadriplegic 343.2
      spastic, not congenital or infantile 344.89
      syphilitic 094.89
         congenital 090.49
      tetraplegic 343.2
   cranial nerve—*see also* Disorder, nerve, cranial
      multiple 352.6
   creeping 335.21
   divers' 993.3
   Erb's (birth injury) 767.6
   facial 351.0
      newborn 767.5
   glossopharyngeal 352.2
   Klumpke (-Déjérine) 767.6
   lead 984.9
      specified type of lead—*see* Table of drugs and
         chemicals
   median nerve (tardy) 354.0

Palsy—*continued*
   peroneal nerve (acute) (tardy) 355.3
   progressive supranuclear 333.0
   pseudobulbar NEC 335.23
   radial nerve (acute) 354.3
   seventh nerve 351.0
      newborn 767.5
   shaking (*see also* Parkinsonism) 332.0
   spastic (cerebral) (spinal) 343.9
      hemiplegic 343.1
   specified nerve NEC—*see* Disorder, nerve
   supranuclear NEC 356.8
      progressive 333.0
   ulnar nerve (tardy) 354.2
   wasting 335.21
Paltauf-Sternberg disease 201.9
Paludism —*see* Malaria
Panama fever 084.0
Panaris (with lymphangitis) 681.9
   finger 681.02
   toe 681.11
Panaritium (with lymphangitis) 681.9
   finger 681.02
   toe 681.11
Panarteritis (nodosa) 446.0
   brain or cerebral 437.4
Pancake heart 793.2
   with cor pulmonale (chronic) 416.9
Pancarditis (acute) (chronic) 429.89
   with
      rheumatic
         fever (active) (acute) (chronic) (subacute)
            391.8
            inactive or quiescent 398.99
     rheumatic, acute 391.8
      chronic or inactive 398.99
Pancoast's syndrome or tumor (carcinoma,
   pulmonary apex) (M8010/3) 162.3
Pancoast-Tobias syndrome (M8010/3)
   (carcinoma, pulmonary apex) 162.3
Pancolitis 556.6
Pancreas, pancreatic —*see* condition
Pancreatitis 577.0
   acute (edematous) (hemorrhagic) (recurrent) 577.0
   annular 577.0
   apoplectic 577.0
   calcereous 577.0
   chronic (infectious) 577.1
      recurrent 577.1
   cystic 577.2
   fibrous 577.8
   gangrenous 577.0
   hemorrhagic (acute) 577.0
   interstitial (chronic) 577.1
      acute 577.0
   malignant 577.0
   mumps 072.3
   painless 577.1
   recurrent 577.1
   relapsing 577.1
   subacute 577.0
   suppurative 577.0
   syphilitic 095.8
Pancreatolithiasis 577.8
Pancytolysis 289.9
Pancytopenia (acquired) 284.1
   with malformations 284.09
   congenital 284.09
Panencephalitis —*see also* Encephalitis
   subacute, sclerosing 046.2

Panhematopenia 284.8
  congenital 284.09
  constitutional 284.09
  splenic, primary 289.4
Panhemocytopenia 284.8
  congenital 284.09
  constitutional 284.09
Panhypogonadism 257.2
Panhypopituitarism 253.2
  prepubertal 253.3
Panic (attack) (state) 300.01
  reaction to exceptional stress (transient) 308.0
Panmyelopathy, familial constitutional 284.09
Panmyelophthisis 284.2
  acquired (secondary) 284.8
  congenital 284.2
  idiopathic 284.9
Panmyelosis (acute) (M9951/1) 238.79
Panner's disease 732.3
  capitellum humeri 732.3
  head of humerus 732.3
  tarsal navicular (bone) (osteochondrosis) 732.5
Panneuritis endemica 265.0 *[357.4]*
Panniculitis 729.30
  back 724.8
  knee 729.31
  mesenteric 567.82
  neck 723.6
  nodular, nonsuppurative 729.30
  sacral 724.8
  specified site NEC 729.39
Panniculus adiposus (abdominal) 278.1
Pannus (corneal) 370.62
  abdominal (symptomatic) 278.1
  allergic eczematous 370.62
  degenerativus 370.62
  keratic 370.62
  rheumatoid—*see* Arthritis, rheumatoid
  trachomatosus, trachomatous (active) 076.1
    [370.62]
    late effect 139.1
Panophthalmitis 360.02
Panotitis —*see* Otitis media
Pansinusitis (chronic) (hyperplastic)
  (nonpurulent) (purulent) 473.8
  acute 461.8
  due to fungus NEC 117.9
  tuberculous (*see also* Tuberculosis) 012.8
Panuveitis 360.12
  sympathetic 360.11
Panvalvular disease —*see* Endocarditis, mitral
Papageienkrankheit 073.9
Papanicolaou smear
  cervix (screening test) V76.2
    as part of gynecological examination V72.31
    for suspected malignant neoplasm V76.2
      no disease found V71.1
    inadequate sample 795.08
    nonspecific abnormal finding 795.00
      with
        atypical squamous cells—changes of
          undetermined significance
          cannot exclude high grade squamous
            intraepithelial lesion (ASC-H)
            795.02
          of undetermined significance (ASC-US)
            795.01
        cytologic evidence of malignancy 795.06
        high grade squamous intraepithelial lesion
          (HGSIL) 795.04

Papanicolaou smear—*continued*
    low grade squamous intraepithelial lesion
      (LGSIL) 795.03
    nonspecific finding NEC 795.09
    to confirm findings of recent normal smear
      following initial abnormal smear V72.32
    unsatisfactory 795.08
  other specified site—*see also* Screening,
    malignant neoplasm
    for suspected malignant neoplasm—*see also*
      Screening, malignant neoplasm
    no disease found V71.1
    nonspecific abnormal finding 795.1
  vagina V76.47
    following hysterectomy for malignant
      condition V67.01
Papilledema 377.00
  associated with
    decreased ocular pressure 377.02
    increased intracranial pressure 377.01
    retinal disorder 377.03
  choked disc 377.00
  infectional 377.00
Papillitis 377.31
  anus 569.49
  chronic lingual 529.4
  necrotizing, kidney 584.7
  optic 377.31
  rectum 569.49
  renal, necrotizing 584.7
  tongue 529.0
Papilloma (M8050/0)—*see also* Neoplasm, by
  site, benign

> *Note—Except where otherwise indicated, the*
> *morphological varieties of papilloma in the list*
> *below should be coded by site as for*
> *"Neoplasm, benign."*

  acuminatum (female) (male) 078.11
  bladder (urinary) (transitional cell) (M8120/1)
    236.7
    benign (M8120/0) 223.3
  choroid plexus (M9390/0) 225.0
    anaplastic type (M9390/3) 191.5
    malignant (M9390/3) 191.5
  ductal (M8503/0)
  dyskeratotic (M8052/0)
  epidermoid (M8052/0)
  hyperkeratotic (M8052/0)
  intracystic (M8504/0)
  intraductal (M8503/0)
  inverted (M8053/0)
  keratotic (M8052/0)
  parakeratotic (M8052/0)
  pinta (primary) 103.0
  renal pelvis (transitional cell) (M8120/1) 236.99
    benign (M8120/0) 223.1
  Schneiderian (M8121/0)
    specified site—*see* Neoplasm, by site, benign
    unspecified site 212.0
  serous surface (M8461/0)
    borderline malignancy (M8461/1)
      specified site—*see* Neoplasm, by site,
        uncertain behavior
      unspecified site 236.2
    specified site—*see* Neoplasm, by site, benign
    unspecified site 220
  squamous (cell) (M8052/0)
  transitional (cell) (M8120/0)
    bladder (urinary) (M8120/1) 236.7

Papilloma—*continued*
    inverted type (M8121/1)—*see* Neoplasm, by
        site, uncertain behavior
    renal pelvis (M8120/1) 236.91
    ureter (M8120/1) 236.91
    ureter (transitional cell) (M8120/1) 236.91
        benign (M8120/0) 223.2
    urothelial (M8120/1)—*see* Neoplasm, by site,
        uncertain behavior
    verrucous (M8051/0)
    villous (M8261/1)—*see* Neoplasm, by site,
        uncertain behavior
    yaws, plantar or palmar 102.1
Papillomata, multiple, of yaws 102.1
Papillomatosis (M8060/0)—*see also* Neoplasm,
    by site, benign
    confluent and reticulate 701.8
    cutaneous 701.8
    ductal, breast 610.1
    Gougerot-Carteaud (confluent reticulate) 701.8
    intraductal (diffuse) (M8505/0)—*see* Neoplasm,
        by site, benign
    subareolar duct (M8506/0) 217
Papillon-Léage and Psaume syndrome
    (orodigitofacial dysostosis) 759.89
Papule 709.8
    carate (primary) 103.0
    fibrous, of nose (M8724/0) 216.3
    pinta (primary) 103.0
Papulosis, malignant 447.8
Papyraceous fetus 779.89
    complicating pregnancy 646.0
Paracephalus 759.7
Parachute mitral valve 746.5
Paracoccidioidomycosis 116.1
    mucocutaneous-lymphangitic 116.1
    pulmonary 116.1
    visceral 116.1
Paracoccidiomycosis —*see*
    Paracoccidioidomycosis
Paracusis 388.40
Paradentosis 523.5
Paradoxical facial movements 374.43
Paraffinoma 999.9
Paraganglioma (M8680/1)
    adrenal (M8700/0) 227.0
        malignant (M8700/3) 194.0
    aortic body (M8691/1) 237.3
        malignant (M8691/3) 194.6
    carotid body (M8692/1) 237.3
        malignant (M8692/3) 194.5
    chromaffin (M8700/0)—*see also* Neoplasm, by
        site, benign
        malignant (M8700/3)—*see* Neoplasm, by site,
            malignant
    extra-adrenal (M8693/1)
        malignant (M8693/3)
            specified site—*see* Neoplasm, by site,
                malignant
            unspecified site 194.6
        specified site—*see* Neoplasm, by site,
            uncertain behavior
        unspecified site 237.3
    glomus jugulare (M8690/1) 237.3
        malignant (M8690/3) 194.6
    jugular (M8690/1) 237.3
        malignant (M8680/3)
            specified site—*see* Neoplasm, by site,
                malignant
            unspecified site 194.6

Paraganglioma—*continued*
    nonchromaffin (M8693/1)
        malignant (M8693/3)
            specified site—*see* Neoplasm, by site,
                malignant
            unspecified site 194.6
        specified site—*see* Neoplasm, by site,
            uncertain behavior
        unspecified site 237.3
    parasympathetic (M8682/1)
        specified site—*see* Neoplasm, by site,
            uncertain behavior
        unspecified site 237.3
    specified site—*see* Neoplasm, by site, uncertain
        behavior
    sympathetic (M8681/1)
        specified site—*see* Neoplasm, by site,
            uncertain behavior
        unspecified site 237.3
    unspecified site 237.3
Parageusia 781.1
    psychogenic 306.7
Paragonimiasis 121.2
Paragranuloma, Hodgkin's (M9660/3) 201.0
Parahemophilia (*see also* Defect, coagulation)
    286.3
Parakeratosis 690.8
    psoriasiformis 696.2
    variegata 696.2
Paralysis, paralytic (complete) (incomplete) 344.9
    with
        broken
            back—*see* Fracture, vertebra, by site, with
                spinal cord injury
            neck—*see* Fracture, vertebra, cervical, with
                spinal cord injury
        fracture, vertebra—*see* Fracture, vertebra, by
            site, with spinal cord injury
        syphilis 094.89
    abdomen and back muscles 355.9
    abdominal muscles 355.9
    abducens (nerve) 378.54
    abductor 355.9
        lower extremity 355.8
        upper extremity 354.9
    accessory nerve 352.4
    accommodation 367.51
        hysterical 300.11
    acoustic nerve 388.5
    agitans 332.0
        arteriosclerotic 332.0
    alternating 344.89
        oculomotor 344.89
    amyotrophic 335.20
    ankle 355.8
    anterior serratus 355.9
    anus (sphincter) 569.49
    apoplectic (current episode) (*see also* Disease,
        cerebrovascular, acute) 436
        late effect—*see* Late effect(s) (of)
            cerebrovascular disease
        category 438
    arm 344.40
        affecting
            dominant side 344.41
            nondominant side 344.42
        both 344.2
        due to old CVA—*see* Category 438
        hysterical 300.11
        late effect—*see* Late effect(s) (of)
            cerebrovascular disease

Paralysis, paralytic—*continued*
　psychogenic 306.0
　transient 781.4
　　traumatic NDC (*see also* Injury, nerve,
　　　upper limb) 955.9
　arteriosclerotic (current episode) 437.0
　　late effect—*see* Late effect(s) (of)
　　　cerebrovascular disease
　ascending (spinal), acute 357.0
　associated, nuclear 344.89
　asthenic bulbar 358.00
　ataxic NEC 334.9
　　general 094.1
　athetoid 333.71
　atrophic 356.9
　　infantile, acute (*see also* Poliomyelitis, with
　　　paralysis) 045.1
　　muscle NEC 355.9
　　progressive 335.21
　　spinal (acute) (*see also* Poliomyelitis, with
　　　paralysis) 045.1
　attack (*see also* Disease, cerebrovascular, acute)
　　436
　axillary 353.0
　Babinski-Nageotte's 344.89
　Bell's 351.0
　　newborn 767.5
　Benedikt's 344.89
　birth (injury) 767.7
　　brain 767.0
　　intracranial 767.0
　　spinal cord 767.4
　bladder (sphincter) 596.53
　　neurogenic 596.54
　　　with cauda equina syndrome 344.61
　　puerperal, postpartum, childbirth 665.5
　　sensory 596.54
　　　with cauda equina 344.61
　　spastic 596.54
　　　with cauda equina 344.61
　bowel, colon, or intestine (*see also* Ileus) 560.1
　brachial plexus 353.0
　　due to birth injury 767.6
　　newborn 767.6
　brain
　　congenital—*see* Palsy, cerebral
　　current episode 437.8
　　diplegia 344.2
　　due to previous vascular lesion—*see* category
　　　438
　　hemiplegia 342.9
　　　due to previous vascular lesion—*see*
　　　　category 438
　　　late effect—*see* Late effect(s) (of)
　　　　cerebrovascular disease
　　infantile—*see* Palsy, cerebral
　　late effect—*see* Late effect(s) (of)
　　　cerebrovascular disease
　　monoplegia—*see also* Monoplegia
　　　due to previous vascular lesion—*see*
　　　　category 438
　　　late effect—*see* Late effect(s) (of)
　　　　cerebrovascular disease
　　paraplegia 344.1
　　quadriplegia —*see* Quadriplegia
　　syphilitic, congenital 090.49
　　triplegia 344.89
　bronchi 519.19
　Brown-Séquard's 344.89
　bulbar (chronic) (progressive) 335.22
　　infantile (*see also* Poliomyelitis, bulbar) 045.0

Paralysis, paralytic—*continued*
　poliomyelitic (*see also* Poliomyelitis, bulbar)
　　045.0
　pseudo 335.23
　supranuclear 344.89
　bulbospinal 358.00
　cardiac (*see also* Failure, heart) 428.9
　cerebral
　　current episode 437.8
　　spastic, infantile—*see* Palsy, cerebral
　cerebrocerebellar 437.8
　　diplegic infantile 343.0
　cervical
　　plexus 353.2
　　sympathetic NEC 337.0
　Céstan-Chenais 344.89
　Charcot-Marie-Tooth type 356.1
　childhood—*see* Palsy, cerebral
　Clark's 343.9
　colon (*see also* Ileus) 560.1
　compressed air 993.3
　compression
　　arm NEC 354.9
　　cerebral—*see* Paralysis, brain
　　leg NEC 355.8
　　lower extremity NEC 355.8
　　upper extremity NEC 354.9
　congenital (cerebral) (spastic) (spinal)—*see*
　　Palsy, cerebral
　conjugate movement (of eye) 378.81
　　cortical (nuclear) (supranuclear) 378.81
　convergence 378.83
　cordis (*see also* Failure, heart) 428.9
　cortical (*see also* Paralysis, brain) 437.8
　cranial or cerebral nerve (*see also* Disorder,
　　nerve, cranial) 352.9
　creeping 335.21
　crossed leg 344.89
　crutch 953.4
　deglutition 784.99
　　hysterical 300.11
　dementia 094.1
　descending (spinal) NEC 335.9
　diaphragm (flaccid) 519.4
　　due to accidental section of phrenic nerve
　　　during procedure 998.2
　digestive organs NEC 564.89
　diplegic—*see* Diplegia
　divergence (nuclear) 378.85
　divers' 993.3
　Duchenne's 335.22
　due to intracranial or spinal birth injury—*see*
　　Palsy, cerebral
　embolic (current episode) (*see also* Embolism,
　　brain) 434.1
　　late effect —*see* Late effect(s) (of)
　　　cerebrovascular disease
　enteric (*see also* Ileus) 560.1
　　with hernia—*see* Hernia, by site, with
　　　obstruction
　Erb's syphilitic spastic spinal 094.89
　Erb (-Duchenne) (birth) (newborn) 767.6
　esophagus 530.89
　essential, infancy (*see also* Poliomyelitis) 045.9
　extremity
　　lower —*see* Paralysis, leg
　　spastic (hereditary) 343.3
　　　noncongenital or noninfantile 344.1
　　transient (cause unknown) 781.4
　　upper —*see* Paralysis, arm
　eye muscle (extrinsic) 378.55

Paralysis, paralytic—*continued*
  intrinsic 367.51
  facial (nerve) 351.0
    birth injury 767.5
    congenital 767.5
    following operation NEC 998.2
    newborn 767.5
  familial 359.3
    periodic 359.3
    spastic 334.1
  fauces 478.29
  finger NEC 354.9
  foot NEC 355.8
  gait 781.2
  gastric nerve 352.3
  gaze 378.81
  general 094.1
    ataxic 094.1
    insane 094.1
    juvenile 090.40
    progressive 094.1
    tabetic 094.1
  glossopharyngeal (nerve) 352.2
  glottis (*see also* Paralysis, vocal cord) 478.30
  gluteal 353.4
  Gubler (-Millard) 344.89
  hand 354.9
    hysterical 300.11
    psychogenic 306.0
  heart (*see also* Failure, heart) 428.9
  hemifacial, progressive 349.89
  hemiplegic—*see* Hemiplegia
  hyperkalemic periodic (familial) 359.3
  hypertensive (current episode) 437.8
  hypoglossal (nerve) 352.5
  hypokalemic periodic 359.3
  Hyrtl's sphincter (rectum) 569.49
  hysterical 300.11
  ileus (*see also* Ileus) 560.1
  infantile (*see also* Poliomyelitis) 045.9
    atrophic acute 045.1
    bulbar 045.0
    cerebral—*see* Palsy, cerebral
    paralytic 045.1
    progressive acute 045.9
    spastic—*see* Palsy, cerebral
    spinal 045.9
  infective (*see also* Poliomyelitis) 045.9
  inferior nuclear 344.9
  insane, general or progressive 094.1
  internuclear 378.86
  interosseous 355.9
  intestine (*see also* Ileus) 560.1
  intracranial (current episode) (*see also* Paralysis, brain) 437.8
    due to birth injury 767.0
  iris 379.49
    due to diphtheria (toxin) 032.81 *[379.49]*
  ischemic, Volkmann's (complicating trauma) 958.6
  isolated sleep, recurrent 327.43
  Jackson's 344.89
  jake 357.7
  Jamaica ginger (jake) 357.7
  juvenile general 090.40
  Klumpke (-Déjérine) (birth) (newborn) 767.6
  labioglossal (laryngeal) (pharyngeal) 335.22
  Landry's 357.0
  laryngeal nerve (recurrent) (superior) (*see also* Paralysis, vocal cord) 478.30
  larynx (*see also* Paralysis, vocal cord) 478.30

Paralysis, paralytic—*continued*
  due to diphtheria (toxin) 032.3
  late effect
    due to
      birth injury, brain or spinal (cord)—*see* Palsy, cerebral
      edema, brain or cerebral—*see* Paralysis, brain
      lesion
        cerebrovascular—*see* category 438
        late effect—*see* Late effect(s) (of) cerebrovascular disease
        spinal (cord)—*see* Paralysis, spinal
  lateral 335.24
  lead 984.9
    specified type of lead—*see* Table of drugs and chemicals
  left side—*see* Hemiplegia
  leg 344.30
    affecting
      dominant side 344.31
      nondominant side 344.32
    both (*see also* Paraplegia) 344.1
    crossed 344.89
    hysterical 300.11
    psychogenic 306.0
    transient or transitory 781.4
      traumatic NEC (*see also* Injury, nerve, lower limb) 956.9
  levator palpebrae superioris 374.31
  limb NEC 344.5
    all four—*see* Quadriplegia
    quadriplegia—*see* Quadriplegia
  lip 528.5
  Lissauer's 094.1
  local 355.9
  lower limb—*see also* Paralysis, leg
    both (*see also* Paraplegia) 344.1
  lung 518.89
    newborn 770.89
  median nerve 354.1
  medullary (tegmental) 344.89
  mesencephalic NEC 344.89
    tegmental 344.89
  middle alternating 344.89
  Millard-Gubler-Foville 344.89
  monoplegic—*see* Monoplegia
  motor NEC 344.9
    cerebral—*see* Paralysis, brain
    spinal—*see* Paralysis, spinal
  multiple
    cerebral—*see* Paralysis, brain
    spinal—*see* Paralysis, spinal
  muscle (flaccid) 359.9
    due to nerve lesion NEC 355.9
    eye (extrinsic) 378.55
      intrinsic 367.51
      oblique 378.51
    iris sphincter 364.8
    ischemic (complicating trauma) (Volkmann's) 958.6
    pseudohypertrophic 359.1
  muscular (atrophic) 359.9
    progressive 335.21
  musculocutaneous nerve 354.9
  musculospiral 354.9
  nerve—*see also* Disorder, nerve
    third or oculomotor (partial) 378.51
      total 378.52
    fourth or trochlear 378.53
    sixth or abducens 378.54

Paraplegia—*continued*
  cerebral (current episode) (*see also* Paralysis,
    brain) 437.8
  congenital or infantile (cerebral) (spastic)
    (spinal) 343.0
  cortical—*see* Paralysis, brain
  familial spastic 334.1
  functional (hysterical) 300.11
  hysterical 300.11
  infantile 343.0
  late effect 344.1
  Pott's (*see also* Tuberculosis) 015.0 *[730.88]*
  psychogenic 306.0
  spastic
    Erb's spinal 094.89
    hereditary 334.1
    not infantile or congenital 344.1
  spinal (cord)
    traumatic NEC—*see* Injury, spinal, by site
  syphilitic (spastic) 094.89
  traumatic NEC—*see* Injury, spinal, by site
Paraproteinemia 273.2
  benign (familial) 273.1
  monoclonal 273.1
  secondary to malignant or inflammatory disease
    273.1
Parapsoriasis 696.2
  en plaques 696.2
  guttata 696.2
  lichenoides chronica 696.2
  retiformis 696.2
  varioliformis (acuta) 696.2
Parascarlatina 057.8
Parasitic —*see also* condition
  disease NEC (*see also* Infestation, parasitic)
    136.9
    contact V01.89
    exposure to V01.89
    intestinal NEC 129
    skin NEC 134.9
  stomatitis 112.0
  sycosis 110.0
    beard 110.0
    scalp 110.0
  twin 759.4
Parasitism NEC 136.9
  intestinal NEC 129
  skin NEC 134.9
  specified—*see* Infestation
Parasitophobia 300.29
Parasomnia 307.47
  alcohol induced 291.82
  drug induced 292.85
  nonorganic origin 307.47
  organic 327.40
    in conditions classified elsewhere 327.44
    other 327.49
Paraspadias 752.69
Paraspasm facialis 351.8
Parathyroid gland —*see* condition
Parathyroiditis (autoimmune) 252.1
Parathyroprival tetany 252.1
Paratrachoma 077.0
Paratyphilitis (*see also* Appendicitis) 541
Paratyphoid (fever)—*see* Fever, paratyphoid
Paratyphus —*see* Fever, paratyphoid
Paraurethral duct 753.8
Para-urethritis 597.89
  gonococcal (acute) 098.0
    chronic or duration of 2 months or over 098.2

Paravaccinia NEC 051.9
  milkers' node 051.1
Paravaginitis (*see also* Vaginitis) 616.10
Parencephalitis (*see also* Encephalitis) 323.9
  late effect—*see* category 326
Parergasia 298.9
Paresis (*see also* Paralysis) 344.9
  accommodation 367.51
  bladder (spastic) (sphincter) (*see also* Paralysis,
    bladder) 596.53
    tabetic 094.0
  bowel, colon, or intestine (*see also* Ileus) 560.1
  brain or cerebral—*see* Paralysis, brain
  extrinsic muscle, eye 378.55
  general 094.1
    arrested 094.1
    brain 094.1
    cerebral 094.1
    insane 094.1
    juvenile 090.40
      remission 090.49
    progressive 094.1
    remission (sustained) 094.1
    tabetic 094.1
  heart (*see also* Failure, heart) 428.9
  infantile (*see also* Poliomyelitis) 045.9
  insane 094.1
  juvenile 090.40
  late effect—*see* Paralysis, late effect
  luetic (general) 094.1
  peripheral progressive 356.9
  pseudohypertrophic 359.1
  senile NEC 344.9
  stomach 536.3
  syphilitic (general) 094.1
    congenital 090.40
  transient, limb 781.4
  vesical (sphincter) NEC 596.53
Paresthesia (*see also* Disturbance, sensation)
  782.0
  Berger's (paresthesia of lower limb) 782.0
  Bernhardt 355.1
  Magnan's 782.0
Paretic —*see* condition
Parinaud's
  conjunctivitis 372.02
  oculoglandular syndrome 372.02
  ophthalmoplegia 378.81
  syndrome (paralysis of conjugate upward gaze)
    378.81
Parkes Weber and Dimitri syndrome
  (encephalocutaneous angiomatosis) 759.6
Parkinson's disease, syndrome, or tremor
  —*see Parkinsonism*
Parkinsonism (arteriosclerotic) (idiopathic)
  (primary) 332.0
  associated with orthostatic hypotension
    (idiopathic) (symptomatic) 333.0
  due to drugs 332.1
  neuroleptic-induced 332.1
  secondary 332.1
  syphilitic 094.82
Parodontitis 523.40
Parodontosis 523.5
Paronychia (with lymphangitis) 681.9
  candidal (chronic) 112.3
  chronic 681.9
    candidal 112.3
    finger 681.02
    toe 681.11
  finger 681.02

Perforation, perforative—*continued*
  broad ligament
    with
      abortion—*see* Abortion, by type, with
        damage to pelvic organs
      ectopic pregnancy (*see also* categories
        633.0-633.9) 639.2
      molar pregnancy (*see also* categories
        630-632) 639.2
    following
      abortion 639.2
      ectopic or molar pregnancy 639.2
    obstetrical trauma 665.6
  by
    device, implant, or graft—*see* Complications,
      mechanical
    foreign body left accidentally in operation
      wound 998.4
    instrument (any) during a procedure,
      accidental 998.2
  cecum 540.0
    with peritoneal abscess 540.1
  cervix (uteri)—*see also* Injury, internal, cervix
    with
      abortion—*see* Abortion, by type, with
        damage to pelvic organs
      ectopic pregnancy (*see also* categories
        633.0-633.9) 639.2
      molar pregnancy (*see also* categories
        630-632) 639.2
    following
      abortion 639.2
      ectopic or molar pregnancy 639.2
    obstetrical trauma 665.3
  colon 569.83
  common duct (bile) 576.3
  cornea (*see also* Ulcer, cornea) 370.00
    due to ulceration 370.06
  cystic duct 575.4
  diverticulum (*see also* Diverticula) 562.10
    small intestine 562.00
  duodenum, duodenal (ulcer)—*see* Ulcer,
    duodenum, with perforation
  ear drum—*see* Perforation, tympanum
  enteritis—*see* Enteritis
  esophagus 530.4
  ethmoidal sinus (*see also* Sinusitis, ethmoidal)
    473.2
  foreign body (external site)—*see also* Wound,
    open, by site, complicated
    internal site, by ingested object—*see* Foreign
      body
  frontal sinus (*see also* Sinusitis, frontal) 473.1
  gallbladder or duct (*see also* Disease,
    gallbladder) 575.4
  gastric (ulcer)—*see* Ulcer, stomach, with
    perforation
  heart valve—*see* Endocarditis
  ileum (*see also* Perforation, intestine) 569.83
  instrumental
    external—*see* Wound, open, by site
    pregnant uterus, complicating delivery 665.9
    surgical (accidental) (blood vessel) (nerve)
      (organ) 998.2
  intestine 569.83
    with
      abortion—*see* Abortion, by type, with
        damage to pelvic organs
      ectopic pregnancy (*see also* categories
        633.0-633.9) 639.2

Perforation, perforative—*continued*
    molar pregnancy (*see also* categories
      630-632) 639.2
    fetus or newborn 777.6
    obstetrical trauma 665.5
    ulcerative NEC 569.83
  jejunum, jejunal 569.83
    ulcer—*see* Ulcer, gastrojejunal, with
      perforation
  mastoid (antrum) (cell) 383.89
  maxillary sinus (*see also* Sinusitis, maxillary)
    473.0
  membrana tympani—*see* Perforation, tympanum
  nasal
    septum 478.19
      congenital 748.1
      syphilitic 095.8
    sinus (*see also* Sinusitis) 473.9
      congenital 748.1
  palate (hard) 526.89
    soft 528.9
      syphilitic 095.8
    syphilitic 095.8
  palatine vault 526.89
    syphilitic 095.8
      congenital 090.5
  pelvic
    floor
      with
        abortion—*see* Abortion, by type, with
          damage to pelvic organs
        ectopic pregnancy (*see also* categories
          633.0-633.9) 639.2
        molar pregnancy (*see also* categories
          630-632) 639.2
      obstetrical trauma 664.1
    organ
      with
        abortion—*see* Abortion, by type, with
          damage to pelvic organs
        ectopic pregnancy (*see also* categories
          633.0-633.9) 639.2
        molar pregnancy (*see also* categories
          630-632) 639.2
      following
        abortion 639.2
        ectopic or molar pregnancy 639.2
      obstetrical trauma 665.5
  perineum—*see* Laceration, perineum
  periurethral tissue
    with
      abortion—*see* Abortion, by type, with
        damage to pelvic organs
      ectopic pregnancy (*see also* categories
        630-632) 639.2
      molar pregnancy (*see also* categories
        630-632) 639.2
  pharynx 478.29
  pylorus, pyloric (ulcer)—*see* Ulcer, stomach,
    with perforation
  rectum 569.49
  root canal space 526.61
  sigmoid 569.83
  sinus (accessory) (chronic) (nasal) (*see also*
    Sinusitis) 473.9
  sphenoidal sinus (*see also* Sinusitis, sphenoidal)
    473.3
  stomach (due to ulcer)—*see* Ulcer, stomach,
    with perforation
  surgical (accidental) (by instrument) (blood
    vessel) (nerve) (organ) 998.2

Perforation, perforative—*continued*
  traumatic
    external—*see* Wound, open, by site
    eye (*see also* Penetrating wound, ocular) 871.7
    internal organ—*see* Injury, internal, by site
    tympanum (membrane) (persistent
        posttraumatic) (postinflammatory) 384.20
      with
        otitis media—*see* Otitis media
      attic 384.22
      central 384.21
      healed 384.81
      marginal NEC 384.23
      multiple 384.24
      pars flaccida 384.22
      total 384.25
      traumatic—*see* Wound, open, ear, drum
  typhoid, gastrointestinal 002.0
  ulcer—*see* Ulcer, by site, with perforation
  ureter 593.89
  urethra
    with
      abortion—*see* Abortion, by type, with
          damage to pelvic organs
      ectopic pregnancy (*see also* categories
          633.0-633.9) 639.2
      molar pregnancy (*see also* categories
          630-632) 639.2
    following
      abortion 639.2
      ectopic or molar pregnancy 639.2
    obstetrical trauma 665.5
  uterus—*see also* Injury, internal, uterus
    with
      abortion—*see* Abortion, by type, with
          damage to pelvic organs
      ectopic pregnancy (*see also* categories
          633.0-633.9) 639.2
      molar pregnancy (*see also* categories
          630-632) 639.2
    by intrauterine contraceptive device 996.32
    following
      abortion 639.2
      ectopic or molar pregnancy 639.2
    obstetrical trauma—*see* Injury, internal,
        uterus, obstetrical trauma
  uvula 528.9
    syphilitic 095.8
  vagina—*see* Laceration, vagina
  viscus NEC 799.89
    traumatic 868.00
      with open wound into cavity 868.10
Periadenitis mucosa necrotica recurrens 528.2
Periangiitis 446.0
Periantritis 535.4
Periappendicitis (acute) (*see also* Appendicitis)
  541
Periarteritis (disseminated) (infectious)
  (necrotizing) (nodosa) 446.0
Periarthritis (joint) 726.90
  Duplay's 726.2
  gonococcal 098.50
  humeroscapularis 726.2
  scapulohumeral 726.2
  shoulder 726.2
  wrist 726.4
Periarthrosis (angioneural)—*see* Periarthritis
Peribronchitis 491.9
  tuberculous (*see also* Tuberculosis) 011.3
Pericapsulitis, adhesive (shoulder) 726.0

Pericarditis (granular) (with decompensation)
  (with effusion) 423.9
  with
    rheumatic fever (conditions classifiable to
        390)
      active (*see also* Pericarditis, rheumatic)
        391.0
      inactive or quiescent 393
  actinomycotic 039.8 *[420.0]*
  acute (nonrheumatic) 420.90
    with chorea (acute) (rheumatic) (Sydenham's)
        392.0
    bacterial 420.99
    benign 420.91
    hemorrhagic 420.90
    idiopathic 420.91
    infective 420.90
    nonspecific 420.91
    rheumatic 391.0
      with chorea (acute) (rheumatic)
          (Sydenham's) 392.0
    sicca 420.90
    viral 420.91
  adhesive or adherent (external) (internal) 423.1
    acute—*see* Pericarditis, acute
    rheumatic (external) (internal) 393
  amebic 006.8 *[420.0]*
  bacterial (acute) (subacute) (with serous or
      seropurulent effusion) 420.99
  calcareous 423.2
  cholesterol (chronic) 423.8
    acute 420.90
  chronic (nonrheumatic) 423.8
    rheumatic 393
  constrictive 423.2
  Coxsackie 074.21
  due to
    actinomycosis 039.8 *[420.0]*
    amebiasis 006.8 *[420.0]*
    Coxsackie (virus) 074.21
    histoplasmosis (*see also* Histoplasmosis)
        115.93
    nocardiosis 039.8 *[420.0]*
    tuberculosis (*see also* Tuberculosis) 017.9
        [420.0]
  fibrinocaseous (*see also* Tuberculosis) 017.9
      [420.0]
  fibrinopurulent 420.99
  fibrinous—*see* Pericarditis, rheumatic
  fibropurulent 420.99
  fibrous 423.1
  gonococcal 098.83
  hemorrhagic 423.0
  idiopathic (acute) 420.91
  infective (acute) 420.90
  meningococcal 036.41
  neoplastic (chronic) 423.8
    acute 420.90
  nonspecific 420.91
  obliterans, obliterating 423.1
  plastic 423.1
  pneumococcal (acute) 420.99
  postinfarction 411.0
  purulent (acute) 420.99
  rheumatic (active) (acute) (with effusion) (with
      pneumonia) 391.0
    with chorea (acute) (rheumatic) (Sydenham's)
        392.0
    chronic or inactive (with chorea) 393
  septic (acute) 420.99
  serofibrinous—*see* Pericarditis, rheumatic

Pericarditis—*continued*
staphylococcal (acute) 420.99
streptococcal (acute) 420.99
suppurative (acute) 420.99
syphilitic 093.81
tuberculous (acute) (chronic) (*see also*
Tuberculosis) 017.9 *[420.0]*
uremic 585.9 *[420.0]*
viral (acute) 420.91
Pericardium, pericardial —*see* condition
Pericellulitis (*see also* Cellulitis) 682.9
Pericementitis 523.40
acute 523.30
chronic (suppurative) 523.40
Pericholecystitis (*see also* Cholecystitis) 575.10
Perichondritis
auricle 380.00
acute 380.01
chronic 380.02
bronchus 491.9
ear (external) 380.00
acute 380.01
chronic 380.02
larynx 478.71
syphilitic 095.8
typhoid 002.0 *[478.71]*
nose 478.19
pinna 380.00
acute 380.01
chronic 380.02
trachea 478.9
Periclasia 523.5
Pericolitis 569.89
Pericoronitis (chronic) 523.40
acute 523.30
Pericystitis (*see also* Cystitis) 595.9
Pericytoma (M9150/1)—*see also* Neoplasm,
connective tissue, uncertain behavior
benign (M9150/0)—*see* Neoplasm, connective
tissue, benign
malignant (M9150/3)—*see* Neoplasm,
connective tissue, malignant
Peridacryocystitis, acute 375.32
Peridiverticulitis (*see also* Diverticulitis) 562.11
Periduodenitis 535.6
Periendocarditis (*see also* Endocarditis) 424.90
acute or subacute 421.9
Periepididymitis (*see also* Epididymitis) 604.90
Perifolliculitis (abscedens) 704.8
capitis, abscedens et suffodiens 704.8
dissecting, scalp 704.8
scalp 704.8
superficial pustular 704.8
Perigastritis (acute) 535.0
Perigastrojejunitis (acute) 535.0
Perihepatitis (acute) 573.3
chlamydial 099.56
gonococcal 098.86
Peri-ileitis (subacute) 569.89
Perilabyrinthitis (acute)—*see* Labyrinthitis
Perimeningitis —*see* Meningitis
Perimetritis (*see also* Endometritis) 615.9
Perimetrosalpingitis (*see also*
Salpingo-oophoritis) 614.2
Perineocele 618.05
Perinephric —*see* condition
Perinephritic —*see* condition
Perinephritis (*see also* Infection, kidney) 590.9
purulent (*see also* Abscess, kidney) 590.2
Perineum, perineal —*see* condition
Perineuritis NEC 729.2

Periodic —*see also* condition
disease (familial) 277.31
edema 995.1
hereditary 277.6
fever 277.31
limb movement disorder 327.51
paralysis (familial) 359.3
peritonitis 277.31
polyserositis 277.31
somnolence (*see also* Narcolepsy) 347.00
Periodontal
cyst 522.8
pocket 523.8
Periodontitis (chronic) (complex) (compound)
(simplex) 523.40
acute 523.33
aggressive 523.30
generalized 523.32
localized 523.31
apical 522.6
acute (pulpal origin) 522.4
generalized 523.42
localized 523.41
Periodontoclasia 523.5
Periodontosis 523.5
Periods —*see also* Menstruation
heavy 626.2
irregular 626.4
Perionychia (with lymphangitis) 681.9
finger 681.02
toe 681.11
Perioophoritis (*see also* Salpingo-oophoritis)
614.2
Periorchitis (*see also* Orchitis) 604.90
Periosteum, periosteal —*see* condition
Periostitis (circumscribed) (diffuse) (infective)
730.3

> *Note—Use the following fifth-digit*
> *subclassification with category 730:*
> *0 site unspdcified*
> *1 shoulder region*
> *2 upper arm*
> *3 forearm*
> *4 hand*
> *5 pelvic region and thigh*
> *6 lower leg*
> *7 ankle and foot*
> *8 other specified sites*
> *9 multiple sites*

with osteomyelitis (*see also* Osteomyelitis) 730.2
acute or subacute 730.0
chronic or old 730.1
albuminosa, albuminosus 730.3
alveolar 526.5
alveolodental 526.5
dental 526.5
gonorrheal 098.89
hyperplastica, generalized 731.2
jaw (lower) (upper) 526.4
monomelic 733.99
orbital 376.02
syphilitic 095.5
congenital 090.0 *[730.8]*
secondary 091.61
tuberculous (*see also* Tuberculosis, bone) 015.9
[730.8]
yaws (early) (hypertrophic) (late) 102.6

Periostosis (*see also* Periostitis) 730.3
  with osteomyelitis (*see also* Osteomyelitis) 730.2
    acute or subacute 730.0
    chronic or old 730.1
  hyperplastic 756.59
Peripartum cardiomyopathy 674.5
Periphlebitis (*see also* Phlebitis) 451.9
  lower extremity 451.2
    deep (vessels) 451.19
    superficial (vessels) 451.0
  portal 572.1
  retina 362.18
  superficial (vessels) 451.0
  tuberculous (*see also* Tuberculosis) 017.9
    retina 017.3 *[362.18]*
Peripneumonia —*see* Pneumonia
Periproctitis 569.49
Periprostatitis (*see also* Prostatitis) 601.9
Perirectal —*see* condition
Perirenal —*see* condition
Perisalpingitis (*see also* Salpingo-oophoritis)
  614.2
Perisigmoiditis 569.89
Perisplenitis (infectional) 289.59
Perispondylitis —*see* Spondylitis
Peristalsis reversed or visible 787.4
Peritendinitis (*see also* Tenosynovitis) 726.90
  adhesive (shoulder) 726.0
Perithelioma (M9150/1)—*see* Pericytoma
Peritoneum, peritoneal —*see also* condition
  equilibration test V56.32
Peritonitis (acute) (adhesive) (fibrinous)
    (hemorrhagic) (idiopathic) (localized)
    (perforative) (primary) (with adhesions) (with
    effusion) 567.9
  with or following
    abortion—*see* Abortion, by type, with sepsis
    abscess 567.21
    appendicitis 540.0
      with peritoneal abscess 540.1
    ectopic pregnancy (*see also* categories
      633.0-633.9) 639.0
    molar pregnancy (*see also* categories 630-632)
      639.0
  aseptic 998.7
  bacterial 567.29
    spontaneous 567.23
  bile, biliary 567.81
  chemical 998.7
  chlamydial 099.56
  chronic proliferative 567.89
  congenital NEC 777.6
  diaphragmatic 567.22
  diffuse NEC 567.29
  diphtheritic 032.83
  disseminated NEC 567.29
  due to
    bile 567.81
    foreign
      body or object accidentally left during a
        procedure (instrument) (sponge) (swab)
        998.4
      substance accidentally left during a procedure
        (chemical) (powder) (talc) 998.7
    talc 998.7
    urine 567.89
  fibrinopurulent 567.29
  fibrinous 567.29
  fibrocaseous (*see also* Tuberculosis) 014.0
  fibropurulent 567.29
  general, generalized (acute) 567.21

Peritonitis—*continued*
  gonococcal 098.86
  in infective disease NEC 136.9 *[567.0]*
  meconium (newborn) 777.6
  pancreatic 577.8
  paroxysmal, benign 277.31
  pelvic
    female (acute) 614.5
      chronic NEC 614.7
        with adhesions 614.6
        puerperal, postpartum, childbirth 670
    male (acute) 567.21
  periodic (familial) 277.31
  phlegmonous 567.29
  pneumococcal 567.1
  postabortal 639.0
  proliferative, chronic 567.89
  puerperal, postpartum, childbirth 670
  purulent 567.29
  septic 567.29
  spontaneous bacterial 567.23
  staphylococcal 567.29
  streptococcal 567.29
  subdiaphragmatic 567.29
  subphrenic 567.29
  suppurative 567.29
  syphilitic 095.2
    congenital 090.0 *[567.0]*
  talc 998.7
  tuberculous (*see also* Tuberculosis) 014.0
  urine 567.89
Peritonsillar —*see* condition
Peritonsillitis 475
Perityphlitis (*see also* Appendicitis) 541
Periureteritis 593.89
Periurethral —*see* condition
Periurethritis (gangrenous) 597.89
Periuterine —*see* condition
Perivaginitis (*see also* Vaginitis) 616.10
Perivasculitis, retinal 362.18
Perivasitis (chronic) 608.4
Periventricular leukomalacia 779.7
Perivesiculitis (seminal) (*see also* Vesiculitis)
  608.0
Perlèche 686.8
  due to
    moniliasis 112.0
    riboflavin deficiency 266.0
Pernicious —*see* condition
Pernio, perniosis 991.5
Persecution
  delusion 297.9
  social V62.4
Perseveration (tonic) 784.69
Persistence, persistent (congenital) 759.89
  anal membrane 751.2
  arteria stapedia 744.04
  atrioventricular canal 745.69
  bloody ejaculate 792.2
  branchial cleft 744.41
  bulbus cordis in left ventricle 745.8
  canal of Cloquet 743.51
  capsule (opaque) 743.51
  cilioretinal artery or vein 743.51
  cloaca 751.5
  communication—*see* Fistula, congenital
  convolutions
    aortic arch 747.21
    fallopian tube 752.19
    oviduct 752.19

Persistence, persistent—*continued*
  uterine tube 752.19
  double aortic arch 747.21
  ductus
    arteriosus 747.0
    Botalli 747.0
  fetal
    circulation 747.83
    form of cervix (uteri) 752.49
    hemoglobin (hereditary) ("Swiss variety")
      282.7
    pulmonary hypertension 747.83
  foramen
    Botalli 745.5
    ovale 745.5
  Gartner's duct 752.41
  hemoglobin, fetal (hereditary) (HPFH) 282.7
  hyaloid
    artery (generally incomplete) 743.51
    system 743.51
  hymen (tag)
    in pregnancy or childbirth 654.8
      causing obstructed labor 660.2
  lanugo 757.4
  left
    posterior cardinal vein 747.49
    root with right arch of aorta 747.21
    superior vena cava 747.49
  Meckel's diverticulum 751.0
  mesonephric duct 752.89
    fallopian tube 752.11
  mucosal disease (middle ear) (with posterior or
    superior marginal perforation of ear drum)
    382.2
  nail(s), anomalous 757.5
  occiput, anterior or posterior 660.3
    fetus or newborn 763.1
  omphalomesenteric duct 751.0
  organ or site NEC—*see* Anomaly, specified
    type NEC
  ostium
    atrioventriculare commune 745.69
    primum 745.61
    secundum 745.5
  ovarian rests in fallopian tube 752.19
  pancreatic tissue in intestinal tract 751.5
  primary (deciduous)
    teeth 520.6
    vitreous hyperplasia 743.51
  pulmonary hypertension 747.83
  pupillary membrane 743.46
    iris 743.46
  Rhesus (Rh) titer 999.7
  right aortic arch 747.21
  sinus
    urogenitalis 752.89
    venosus with imperfect incorporation in right
      auricle 747.49
  thymus (gland) 254.8
    hyperplasia 254.0
  thyroglossal duct 759.2
  thyrolingual duct 759.2
  truncus arteriosus or communis 745.0
  tunica vasculosa lentis 743.39
  umbilical sinus 753.7
  urachus 753.7
  vegetative state 780.03
  vitelline duct 751.0
  wolffian duct 752.89

Person (with)
  admitted for clinical research, as participant or
    control subject V70.7
  awaiting admission to adequate facility
    elsewhere V63.2
    undergoing social agency investigation V63.8
  concern (normal) about sick person in family
    V61.49
  consulting on behalf of another V65.19
    pediatric pre-birth visit for expectant mother
      V65.11
  feared
    complaint in whom no diagnosis was made
      V65.5
    condition not demonstrated V65.5
  feigning illness V65.2
  healthy, accompanying sick person V65.0
  living (in)
    alone V60.3
    boarding school V60.6
    residence remote from hospital or medical
      care facility V63.0
    residential institution V60.6
    without
      adequate
        financial resources V60.2
        housing (heating) (space) V60.1
      housing (permanent) (temporary) V60.0
      material resources V60.2
      person able to render necessary care V60.4
      shelter V60.0
  medical services in home not available V63.1
  on waiting list V63.2
    undergoing social agency investigation V63.8
  sick or handicapped in family V61.49
  "worried well" V65.5
Personality
  affective 301.10
  aggressive 301.3
  amoral 301.7
  anancastic, anankastic 301.4
  antisocial 301.7
  asocial 301.7
  asthenic 301.6
  avoidant 301.82
  borderline 301.83
  change 310.1
  compulsive 301.4
  cycloid 301.13
  cyclothymic 301.13
  dependent 301.6
  depressive (chronic) 301.12
  disorder, disturbance NEC 301.9
    with
      antisocial disturbance 301.7
      pattern disturbance NEC 301.9
      sociopathic disturbance 301.7
      trait disturbance 301.9
  dual 300.14
  dyssocial 301.7
  eccentric 301.89
    "haltlose" type 301.89
  emotionally unstable 301.59
  epileptoid 301.3
  explosive 301.3
  fanatic 301.0
  histrionic 301.50
  hyperthymic 301.11
  hypomanic 301.11
  hypothymic 301.12
  hysterical 301.50

Personality—*continued*
  immature 301.89
  inadequate 301.6
  labile 301.59
  masochistic 301.89
  morally defective 301.7
  multiple 300.14
  narcissistic 301.81
  obsessional 301.4
  obsessive-compulsive 301.4
  overconscientious 301.4
  paranoid 301.0
  passive (-dependent) 301.6
  passive-aggressive 301.84
  pathologic NEC 301.9
  pattern defect or disturbance 301.9
  pseudosocial 301.7
  psychoinfantile 301.59
  psychoneurotic NEC 301.89
  psychopathic 301.9
    with
      amoral trend 301.7
      antisocial trend 301.7
      asocial trend 301.7
      pathologic sexuality (*see also* Deviation,
        sexual) 302.9
      mixed types 301.9
    schizoid 301.20
      introverted 301.21
      schizotypal 301.22
      with sexual deviation (*see also* Deviation,
        sexual) 302.9
      antisocial 301.7
      dyssocial 301.7
    type A 301.4
    unstable (emotional) 301.59
Perthes' disease (capital femoral
  osteochondrosis) 732.1
Pertussis (*see also* Whooping cough) 033.9
  vaccination, prophylactic (against) V03.6
Peruvian wart 088.0
Perversion, perverted
  appetite 307.52
    hysterical 300.11
  function
    pineal gland 259.8
    pituitary gland 253.9
      anterior lobe
        deficient 253.2
        excessive 253.1
      posterior lobe 253.6
    placenta—*see* Placenta, abnormal
  sense of smell or taste 781.1
    psychogenic 306.7
  sexual (*see also* Deviation, sexual) 302.9
Pervious, congenital —*see also* Imperfect,
  closure
  ductus arteriosus 747.0
Pes (congenital) (*see also* Talipes) 754.70
  abductus (congenital) 754.60
    acquired 736.79
  acquired NEC 736.79
    planus 734
  adductus (congenital) 754.79
    acquired 736.79
  cavus 754.71
    acquired 736.73
  planovalgus (congenital) 754.69
    acquired 736.79
  planus (acquired) (any degree) 734
    congenital 754.61

Pes —*continued*
  rachitic 268.1
  valgus (congenital) 754.61
    acquired 736.79
  varus (congenital) 754.50
    acquired 736.79
Pest (*see also* Plague) 020.9
Pestis (*see also* Plague) 020.9
  bubonica 020.0
  fulminans 020.0
  minor 020.8
  pneumonica—*see* Plague, pneumonic
Petechia, petechiae 782.7
  fetus or newborn 772.6
Petechial
  fever 036.0
  typhus 081.9
Petges-Cléjat or Petges-Clégat syndrome
  (poikilodermatomyositis) 710.3
Petit's
  disease (*see also* Hernia, lumbar) 553.8
Petit mal (idiopathic) (*see also* Epilepsy) 345.0
  status 345.2
Petrellidosis 117.6
Petrositis 383.20
  acute 383.21
  chronic 383.22
Peutz-Jeghers disease or syndrome 759.6
Peyronie's disease 607.85
Pfeiffer's disease 075
Phacentocele 379.32
  traumatic 921.3
Phacoanaphylaxis 360.19
Phacocele (old) 379.32
  traumatic 921.3
Phaehyphomycosis 117.8
Phagedena (dry) (moist) (*see also* Gangrene)
  785.4
  arteriosclerotic 440.24
  geometric 686.09
  penis 607.89
  senile 440.24
  sloughing 785.4
  tropical (*see also* Ulcer, skin) 707.9
  vulva 616.50
Phagedenic —*see also* condition
  abscess—*see also* Abscess
    chancroid 099.0
  bubo NEC 099.8
  chancre 099.0
  ulcer (tropical) (*see also* Ulcer, skin) 707.9
Phagomania 307.52
Phakoma 362.89
Phantom limb (syndrome) 353.6
Pharyngeal —*see also* condition
  arch remnant 744.41
  pouch syndrome 279.11
Pharyngitis (acute) (catarrhal) (gangrenous)
  (infective) (malignant) (membranous)
  (phlegmonous) (pneumococcal)
  (pseudomembranous) (simple)
  (staphylococcal) (subacute) (suppurative)
  (ulcerative) (viral) 462
  with influenza, flu, or grippe 487.1
  aphthous 074.0
  atrophic 472.1
  chlamydial 099.51
  chronic 472.1
  Coxsackie virus 074.0
  diphtheritic (membranous) 032.0

Pharyngitis—*continued*
  follicular 472.1
  fusospirochetal 101
  gonococcal 098.6
  granular (chronic) 472.1
  herpetic 054.79
  hypertrophic 472.1
  infectional, chronic 472.1
  influenzal 487.1
  lymphonodular, acute 074.8
  septic 034.0
  streptococcal 034.0
  tuberculous (*see also* Tuberculosis) 012.8
  vesicular 074.0
Pharyngoconjunctival fever 077.2
Pharyngoconjunctivitis, viral 077.2
Pharyngolaryngitis (acute) 465.0
  chronic 478.9
  septic 034.0
Pharyngoplegia 478.29
Pharyngotonsillitis 465.8
  tuberculous 012.8
Pharyngotracheitis (acute) 465.8
  chronic 478.9
Pharynx, pharyngeal —*see* condition
Phase of life problem NEC V62.89
Phenomenon
  Arthus' 995.21
  flashback (drug) 292.89
  jaw-winking 742.8
  Jod-Basedow 242.8
  L. E. cell 710.0
  lupus erythematosus cell 710.0
  Pelger-Huët (hereditary hyposegmentation) 288.2
  Raynaud's (paroxysmal digital cyanosis)
      (secondary) 443.0
  Reilly's (*see also* Neuropathy, peripheral,
      autonomic) 337.9
  vasomotor 780.2
  vasospastic 443.9
  vasovagal 780.2
  Wenckebach's, heart block (second degree) 426.13
Phenylketonuria (PKU) 270.1
Phenylpyruvicaciduria 270.1
Pheochromoblastoma (M8700/3)
  specified site—*see* Neoplasm, by site, malignant
  unspecified site 194.0
Pheochromocytoma (M8700/0)
  malignant (M8700/3)
    specified site—*see* Neoplasm, by site,
        malignant
    unspecified site 194.0
  specified site—*see* Neoplasm, by site, benign
  unspecified site 227.0
Phimosis (congenital) 605
  chancroidal 099.0
  due to infection 605
Phlebectasia (*see also* Varicose, vein) 454.9
  congenital NEC 747.60
  esophagus (*see also* Varix, esophagus) 456.1
    with hemorrhage (*see also* Varix, esophagus,
        bleeding) 456.0
Phlebitis (infective) (pyemic) (septic)
      (suppurative) 451.9
  antecubital vein 451.82
  arm NEC 451.84
    axillary vein 451.89
    basilic vein 451.82
    deep 451.83
    superficial 451.82

Phlebitis—*continued*
  basilic vein 451.82
  blue 451.19
  brachial vein 451.83
  breast, superficial 451.89
  cavernous (venous) sinus—*see* Phlebitis,
      intracranial sinus
  cephalic vein 451.82
  cerebral (venous) sinus—*see* Phlebitis,
      intracranial sinus
  chest wall, superficial 451.89
  complicating pregnancy or puerperium 671.9
    affecting fetus or newborn 760.3
  cranial (venous) sinus—*see* Phlebitis,
      intracranial sinus
  deep (vessels) 451.19
    femoral vein 451.11
    specified vessel NEC 451.19
  due to implanted device—*see* Complications,
      due to (presence of) any device, implant, or
      graft classified to 996.0-996.5 NEC
  during or resulting from a procedure 997.2
  femoral vein (deep) (superficial) 451.11
  femoropopliteal 451.19
  following infusion, perfusion, or transfusion
      999.2
  gouty 274.89 *[451.9]*
  hepatic veins 451.89
  iliac vein 451.81
  iliofemoral 451.11
  intracranial sinus (any) (venous) 325
    late effect—*see* category 326
    nonpyogenic 437.6
      in pregnancy or puerperium 671.5
  jugular vein 451.89
  lateral (venous) sinus—*see* Phlebitis,
      intracranial sinus
  leg 451.2
    deep (vessels) 451.19
      femoral vein 451.11
      specified vessel NEC 451.19
    superficial (vessels) 451.0
      femoral vein 451.11
  longitudinal sinus—*see* Phlebitis, intracranial
      sinus
  lower extremity 451.2
    deep (vessels) 451.19
      femoral vein 451.11
      specified vessel NEC 451.19
    superficial (vessels) 451.0
      femoral vein 451.11
  migrans, migrating (superficial) 453.1
  pelvic
    with
      abortion—*see* Abortion, by type, with sepsis
      ectopic pregnancy (*see also* categories
          633.0-633.9) 639.0
      molar pregnancy (*see also* categories
          630-632) 639.0
    following
      abortion 639.0
      ectopic or molar pregnancy 639.0
    puerperal, postpartum 671.4
  popliteal vein 451.19
  portal (vein) 572.1
  postoperative 997.2
  pregnancy 671.9
    deep 671.3
    specified type NEC 671.5
    superficial 671.2

Phlebitis—*continued*
  puerperal, postpartum, childbirth 671.9
    deep 671.4
      lower extremities 671.2
      pelvis 671.4
      specified site NEC 671.5
      superficial 671.2
  radial vein 451.83
  retina 362.18
  saphenous (great) (long) 451.0
    accessory or small 451.0
  sinus (meninges)—*see* Phlebitis, intracranial
    sinus
  specified site NEC 451.89
  subclavian vein 451.89
  syphilitic 093.89
  tibial vein 451.19
  ulcer, ulcerative 451.9
    leg 451.2
      deep (vessels) 451.19
        femoral vein 451.11
        specified vessel NEC 451.19
      superficial (vessels) 451.0
        femoral vein 451.11
    lower extremity 451.2
      deep (vessels) 451.19
        femoral vein 451.11
        specified vessel NEC 451.19
      superficial (vessels) 451.0
  ulnar vein 451.83
  umbilicus 451.89
  upper extremity—*see* Phlebitis, arm
  uterus (septic) (*see also* Endometritis) 615.9
  varicose (leg) (lower extremity) (*see also*
    Varicose, vein) 454.1
Phlebofibrosis 459.89
Phleboliths 459.89
Phlebosclerosis 459.89
Phlebothrombosis —*see* Thrombosis
Phlebotomus fever 066.0
Phlegm, choked on 933.1
Phlegmasia
  alba dolens (deep vessels) 451.19
    complicating pregnancy 671.3
    nonpuerperal 451.19
    puerperal, postpartum, childbirth 671.4
  cerulea dolens 451.19
Phlegmon (*see also* Abscess) 682.9
  erysipelatous (*see also* Erysipelas) 035
  iliac 682.2
    fossa 540.1
  throat 478.29
Phlegmonous —*see* condition
Phlyctenulosis (allergic) (keratoconjunctivitis)
  (nontuberculous) 370.31
  cornea 370.31
    with ulcer (*see also* Ulcer, cornea) 370.00
  tuberculous (*see also* Tuberculosis) 017.3
    [370.31]
Phobia, phobic (reaction) 300.20
  animal 300.29
  isolated NEC 300.29
  obsessional 300.3
  simple NEC 300.29
  social 300.23
  specified NEC 300.29
  state 300.20
Phocas' disease 610.1
Phocomelia 755.4
  lower limb 755.32
    complete 755.33

Phocomelia—*continued*
    distal 755.35
    proximal 755.34
  upper limb 755.22
    complete 755.23
    distal 755.25
    proximal 755.24
Phoria (*see also* Heterophoria) 378.40
Phosphate-losing tubular disorder 588.0
Phosphatemia 275.3
Phosphaturia 275.3
Photoallergic response 692.72
Photocoproporphyria 277.1
Photodermatitis (sun) 692.72
  light other than sun 692.82
Photokeratitis 370.24
Photo-ophthalmia 370.24
Photophobia 368.13
Photopsia 368.15
Photoretinitis 363.31
Photoretinopathy 363.31
Photosensitiveness (sun) 692.72
  light other than sun 692.82
Photosensitization (sun) skin 692.72
  light other than sun 692.82
Phototoxic response 692.72
Phrenitis 323.9
Phrynoderma 264.8
Phthiriasis (pubis) (any site) 132.2
  with any infestation classifiable to 132.0
    and 132.1 132.3
Phthirus infestation —*see* Phthiriasis
Phthisis (*see also* Tuberculosis) 011.9
  bulbi (infectional) 360.41
  colliers' 011.4
  cornea 371.05
  eyeball (due to infection) 360.41
  millstone makers' 011.4
  miners' 011.4
  potters' 011.4
  sandblasters' 011.4
  stonemasons' 011.4
Phycomycosis 117.7
Physalopteriasis 127.7
Physical therapy NEC V57.1
  breathing exercises V57.0
Physiological cup, optic papilla
  borderline, glaucoma suspect 365.00
  enlarged 377.14
  glaucomatous 377.14
Phytobezoar 938
  intestine 936
  stomach 935.2
Pian (*see also* Yaws) 102.9
Pianoma 102.1
Piarhemia, piarrhemia (*see also* Hyperlipemia)
  272.4
  bilharziasis 120.9
Pica 307.52
  hysterical 300.11
Pick's
  cerebral atrophy 331.11
    with dementia
      with behavioral disturbance 331.11 *[294.11]*
      without behavioral disturbance 331.11
        [294.10]
  disease
    brain 331.11
      dementia in

Pitting (edema) (*see also* Edema) 782.3
  lip 782.3
  nail 703.8
    congenital 757.5
Pituitary gland —*see* condition
Pituitary snuff-takers' disease 495.8
Pityriasis 696.5
  alba 696.5
  capitis 690.11
  circinata (et maculata) 696.3
  Hebra's (exfoliative dermatitis) 695.89
  lichenoides et varioliformis 696.2
  maculata (et circinata) 696.3
  nigra 111.1
  pilaris 757.39
    acquired 701.1
    Hebra's 696.4
  rosea 696.3
  rotunda 696.3
  rubra (Hebra) 695.89
    pilaris 696.4
  sicca 690.18
  simplex 690.18
  specified type NEC 696.5
  streptogenes 696.5
  versicolor 111.0
    scrotal 111.0
Placenta, placental
  ablatio 641.2
    affecting fetus or newborn 762.1
  abnormal, abnormality 656.7
    with hemorrhage 641.8
      affecting fetus or newborn 762.1
    affecting fetus or newborn 762.2
  abruptio 641.2
    affecting fetus or newborn 762.1
  accessory lobe—*see* Placenta, abnormal
  accreta (without hemorrhage) 667.0
    with hemorrhage 666.0
  adherent (without hemorrhage) 667.0
    with hemorrhage 666.0
  apoplexy—*see* Placenta, separation
  battledore—*see* Placenta, abnormal
  bilobate—*see* Placenta, abnormal
  bipartita—*see* Placenta, abnormal
  carneous mole 631
  centralis—*see* Placenta, previa
  circumvallata—*see* Placenta, abnormal
  cyst (amniotic)—*see* Placenta, abnormal
  deficiency—*see* Placenta insufficiency
  degeneration—*see* Placenta, insufficiency
  detachment (partial) (premature) (with
    hemorrhage) 641.2
    affecting fetus or newborn 762.1
  dimidiata—*see* Placenta, abnormal
  disease 656.7
    affecting fetus or newborn 762.2
  duplex—*see* Placenta, abnormal
  dysfunction—*see* Placenta, insufficiency
  fenestrata—*see* Placenta, abnormal
  fibrosis—*see* Placenta, abnormal
  fleshy mole 631
  hematoma—*see* Placenta, abnormal
  hemorrhage NEC—*see* Placenta, separation
  hormone disturbance or malfunction—*see*
    Placenta, abnormal
  hyperplasia—*see* Placenta, abnormal
  increta (without hemorrhage) 667.0
    with hemorrhage 666.0
  infarction 656.7
    affecting fetus or newborn 762.2

Placenta, placental—*continued*
  insertion, vicious—*see* Placenta, previa
  insufficiency
    affecting
      fetus or newborn 762.2
      management of pregnancy 656.5
  lateral—*see* Placenta, previa
  low implantation or insertion—*see* Placenta,
    previa
  low-lying—*see* Placenta, previa
  malformation—*see* Placenta, abnormal
  malposition—*see* Placenta, previa
  marginalis, marginata—*see* Placenta, previa
  marginal sinus (hemorrhage) (rupture) 641.2
    affecting fetus or newborn 762.1
  membranacea—*see* Placenta, abnormal
  multilobed—*see* Placenta, abnormal
  multipartita—*see* Placenta, abnormal
  necrosis—*see* Placenta, abnormal
  percreta (without hemorrhage) 667.0
    with hemorrhage 666.0
  polyp 674.4
  previa (central) (centralis) (complete) (lateral)
    (marginal) (marginalis) (partial) (partialis)
    (total) (with hemorrhage) 641.1
    affecting fetus or newborn 762.0
    noted
      before labor, without hemorrhage (with
        cesarean delivery) 641.0
      during pregnancy (without hemorrhage)
        641.0
    without hemorrhage (before labor and
      delivery) (during pregnancy) 641.0
  retention (with hemorrhage) 666.0
    fragments, complicating puerperium (delayed
      hemorrhage) 666.2
      without hemorrhage 667.1
    postpartum, puerperal 666.2
    without hemorrhage 667.0
  separation (normally implanted) (partial)
    (premature) (with hemorrhage) 641.2
    affecting fetus or newborn 762.1
  septuplex—*see* Placenta, abnormal
  small—*see* Placenta, insufficiency
  softening (premature)—*see* Placenta, abnormal
  spuria—*see* Placenta, abnormal
  succenturiata—*see* Placenta, abnormal
  syphilitic 095.8
  transfusion syndromes 762.3
  transmission of chemical substance—*see*
    Absorption, chemical, through placenta
  trapped (with hemorrhage) 666.0
    without hemorrhage 667.0
  trilobate—*see* Placenta, abnormal
  tripartita—*see* Placenta, abnormal
  triplex—*see* Placenta, abnormal
  varicose vessel—*see* Placenta, abnormal
  vicious insertion—*see* Placenta, previa
Placentitis
  affecting fetus or newborn 762.7
  complicating pregnancy 658.4
Plagiocephaly (skull) 754.0
Plague 020.9
  abortive 020.8
  ambulatory 020.8
  bubonic 020.0
  cellulocutaneous 020.1
  lymphatic gland 020.0
  pneumonic 020.5
    primary 020.3
    secondary 020.4

Pneumoblastoma (M8981/3)—*see* Neoplasm,
lung, malignant
Pneumocephalus 348.8
Pneumococcemia 038.2
Pneumococcus, pneumococcal —*see* condition
Pneumoconiosis (due to) (inhalation of) 505
  aluminum 503
  asbestos 501
  bagasse 495.1
  bauxite 503
  beryllium 503
  carbon electrode makers' 503
  coal
    miners' (simple) 500
    workers' (simple) 500
  cotton dust 504
  diatomite fibrosis 502
  dust NEC 504
    inorganic 503
    lime 502
    marble 502
    organic NEC 504
  fumes or vapors (from silo) 506.9
  graphite 503
  hard metal 503
  mica 502
  moldy hay 495.0
  rheumatoid 714.81
  silica NEC 502
    and carbon 500
  silicate NEC 502
  talc 502
Pneumocystis carinii pneumonia 136.3
Pneumocystis jiroveci pneumonia 136.3
Pneumocystosis 136.3
  with pneumonia 136.3
Pneumoenteritis 025
Pneumohemopericardium (*see also* Pericarditis)
  423.9
Pneumohemothorax (*see also* Hemothorax)
  511.8
  traumatic 860.4
  with open wound into thorax 860.5
Pneumohydropericardium (*see also*
  Pericarditis) 423.9
Pneumohydrothorax (*see also* Hydrothorax) 511.8
Pneumomediastinum 518.1
  congenital 770.2
  fetus or newborn 770.2
Pneumomycosis 117.9
Pneumonia (acute) (Alpenstich) (benign)
    (bilateral) (brain) (cerebral) (circumscribed)
    (congestive) (creeping) (delayed resolution)
    (double) (epidemic) (fever) (flash) (fulminant)
    (fungoid) (granulomatous) (hemorrhagic)
    (incipient) (infantile) (infectious) (infiltration)
    (insular) (intermittent) (latent) (lobe)
    (migratory) (newborn) (organized)
    (overwhelming) (primary) (progressive)
    (pseudolobar) (purulent) (resolved)
    (secondary) (senile) (septic) (suppurative)
    (terminal) (true) (unresolved) (vesicular) 486
  with influenza, flu, or grippe 487.0
  adenoviral 480.0
  adynamic 514
  alba 090.0
  allergic 518.3
  alveolar—*see* Pneumonia, lobar
  anaerobes 482.81
  anthrax 022.1 *[484.5]*

Pneumonia—*continued*
  apex, apical—*see* Pneumonia, lobar
  ascaris 127.0 *[484.8]*
  aspiration 507.0
    due to
      aspiration of microorganisms
        bacterial 482.9
          specified type NEC 482.89
        specified organism NEC 483.8
          bacterial NEC 482.89
        viral 480.9
          specified type NEC 480.8
      food (regurgitated) 507.0
      gastric secretions 507.0
      milk 507.0
      oils, essences 507.1
      solids, liquids NEC 507.8
      vomitus 507.0
  fetal 770.18
    due to
      blood 770.16
      clear amniotic fluid 770.14
      meconium 770.12
      postnatal stomach contents 770.86
  newborn 770.18
    due to
      blood 770.16
      clear amniotic fluid 770.14
      meconium 770.12
      postnatal stomach contents 770.86
  asthenic 514
  atypical (disseminated, focal) (primary) 486
    with influenza 487.0
  bacillus 482.9
    specified type NEC 482.89
  bacterial 482.9
    specified type NEC 482.89
  Bacteroides (fragilis) (oralis) (melaninogenicus)
    482.81
  basal, basic, basilar—*see* Pneumonia, lobar
  broncho-, bronchial (confluent) (croupous)
    (diffuse) (disseminated) (hemorrhagic)
    (involving lobes) (lobar) (terminal) 485
    with influenza 487.0
  allergic 518.3
  aspiration (*see also* Pneumonia, aspiration)
    507.0
  bacterial 482.9
    specified type NEC 482.89
  capillary 466.19
    with bronchospasm or obstruction 466.19
  chronic (*see also* Fibrosis, lung) 515
  congenital (infective) 770.0
  diplococcal 481
  Eaton's agent 483.0
  Escherichia coli (E. coli) 482.82
  Friedländer's bacillus 482.0
  Hemophilus influenzae 482.2
  hiberno-vernal 083.0 *[484.8]*
  hypostatic 514
  influenzal 487.0
  inhalation (*see also* Pneumonia, aspiration) 507.0
    due to fumes or vapors (chemical) 506.0
  Klebsiella 482.0
  lipid 507.1
    endogenous 516.8
  Mycoplasma (pneumoniae) 483.0
  ornithosis 073.0
  pleuropneumonia-like organisms (PPLO) 483.0
  pneumococcal 481
  Proteus 482.83

Poisoning—*continued*
    Streptococcus 005.8
    Vibrio parahaemolyticus 005.4
    Vibrio vulnificus 005.81
  noxious or naturally toxic 988.0
    berries 988.2
    fish 988.0
    mushroom 988.1
    plants NEC 988.2
  ice cream—*see* Poisoning, food
  ichthyotoxism (bacterial) 005.9
  kreotoxism, food 005.9
  malarial—*see* Malaria
  meat—*see* Poisoning, food
  mushroom (noxious) 988.1
  mussel—*see also* Poisoning, food
    noxious 988.0
  noxious foodstuffs (*see also* Poisoning, food,
    noxious) 988.9
    specified type NEC 988.8
  plants, noxious 988.2
  pork—*see also* Poisoning, food
    specified NEC 988.8
    Trichinosis 124
  ptomaine—*see* Poisoning, food
  putrefaction, food—*see* Poisoning, food
  radiation 508.0
  Salmonella (*see also* Infection, Salmonella) 003.9
  sausage—*see also* Poisoning, food
    Trichinosis 124
  saxitoxin 988.0
  shellfish—*see also* Poisoning, food
    noxious 988.0
  Staphylococcus, food 005.0
  toxic, from disease NEC 799.89
  truffles—*see* Poisoning, food
  uremic—*see* Uremia
  uric acid 274.9
**Poison ivy, oak, sumac or other plant
  dermatitis** 692.6
Poker spine 720.0
Policeman's disease 729.2
Polioencephalitis (acute) (bulbar) (*see also*
  Poliomyelitis, bulbar) 045.0
  inferior 335.22
  influenzal 487.8
  superior hemorrhagic (acute) (Wernicke's)
    265.1
  Wernicke's (superior hemorrhagic) 265.1
Polioencephalomyelitis (acute) (anterior)
  (bulbar) (*see also* Polioencephalitis) 045.0
Polioencephalopathy, superior hemorrhagic
  265.1
  with
    beriberi 265.0
    pellagra 265.2
Poliomeningoencephalitis —*see*
  Meningoencephalitis
Poliomyelitis (acute) (anterior) (epidemic) 045.9

---

*Note—Use the following fifth-digit
subclassification with category 045:*

*0 poliovirus, unspecified type
1 poliovirus, type I
2 poliovirus, type II
3 poliovirus, type III*

---

  with
    paralysis 045.1
      bulbar 045.0
  abortive 045.2

Poliomyelitis—*continued*
  ascending 045.9
    progressive 045.9
  bulbar 045.0
  cerebral 045.0
  chronic 335.21
  congenital 771.2
  contact V01.2
  deformities 138
  exposure to V01.2
  late effect 138
  nonepidemic 045.9
  nonparalytic 045.2
  old with deformity 138
  posterior, acute 053.19
  residual 138
  sequelae 138
  spinal, acute 045.9
  syphilitic (chronic) 094.89
  vaccination, prophylactic (against) V04.0
Poliosis (eyebrow) (eyelashes) 704.3
  circumscripta (congenital) 757.4
    acquired 704.3
  congenital 757.4
Pollakiuria 788.41
  psychogenic 306.53
Pollinosis 477.0
Pollitzer's disease (hidradenitis suppurativa)
  705.83
Polyadenitis (*see also* Adenitis) 289.3
  malignant 020.0
Polyalgia 729.9
Polyangiitis (essential) 446.0
Polyarteritis (nodosa) (renal) 446.0
Polyarthralgia 719.49
  psychogenic 306.0
Polyarthritis, polyarthropathy NEC 716.59
  due to or associated with other specified
    conditions—*see* Arthritis, due to or
    associated with
  endemic (*see also* Disease, Kaschin-Beck) 716.0
  inflammatory 714.9
    specified type NEC 714.89
  juvenile (chronic) 714.30
    acute 714.31
  migratory—*see* Fever, rheumatic
  rheumatic 714.0
    fever (acute)—*see* Fever, rheumatic
Polycarential syndrome of infancy 260
Polychondritis (atrophic) (chronic) (relapsing)
  733.99
Polycoria 743.46
Polycystic (congenital) (disease) 759.89
  degeneration, kidney—*see* Polycystic, kidney
  kidney (congenital) 753.12
    adult type (APKD) 753.13
    autosomal dominant 753.13
    autosomal recessive 753.14
    childhood type (CPKD) 753.14
    infantile type 753.14
  liver 751.62
  lung 518.89
    congenital 748.4
  ovary, ovaries 256.4
  spleen 759.0
Polycythemia (primary) (rubra) (vera) (M9950/1)
  238.4
  acquired 289.0
  benign 289.0
    familial 289.6

Polycythemia—*continued*
  due to
    donor twin 776.4
    fall in plasma volume 289.0
    high altitude 289.0
    maternal-fetal transfusion 776.4
    stress 289.0
  emotional 289.0
  erythropoietin 289.0
  familial (benign) 289.6
  Gaisböck's (hypertonica) 289.0
  high altitude 289.0
  hypertonica 289.0
  hypoxemic 289.0
  neonatorum 776.4
  nephrogenous 289.0
  relative 289.0
  secondary 289.0
  spurious 289.0
  stress 289.0
Polycytosis cryptogenica 289.0
Polydactylism, polydactyly 755.00
  fingers 755.01
  toes 755.02
Polydipsia 783.5
Polydystrophic oligophrenia 277.5
Polyembryoma (M9072/3)—*see* Neoplasm, by
    site, malignant
Polygalactia 676.6
Polyglandular
  deficiency 258.9
  dyscrasia 258.9
  dysfunction 258.9
  syndrome 258.8
Polyhydramnios (*see also* Hydramnios) 657
Polymastia 757.6
Polymenorrhea 626.2
Polymicrogyria 742.2
Polymyalgia 725
  arteritica 446.5
  rheumatica 725
Polymyositis (acute) (chronic) (hemorrhagic) 710.4
  with involvement of
    lung 710.4 *[517.8]*
    skin 710.3
  ossificans (generalisata) (progressiva) 728.19
  Wagner's (dermatomyositis) 710.3
Polyneuritis, polyneuritic (*see also*
    Polyneuropathy) 356.9
  alcoholic 357.5
    with psychosis 291.1
  cranialis 352.6
  demyelinating, chronic inflammatory 357.81
  diabetic 250.6 *[357.2]*
  due to lack of vitamin NEC 269.2 *[357.4]*
  endemic 265.0 *[357.4]*
  erythredema 985.0
  febrile 357.0
  hereditary ataxic 356.3
  idiopathic, acute 357.0
  infective (acute) 357.0
  nutritional 269.9 *[357.4]*
  postinfectious 357.0
Polyneuropathy (peripheral) 356.9
  alcoholic 357.5
  amyloid 277.39 *[357.4]*
  arsenical 357.7
  critical illness 357.82
  diabetic 250.6 *[357.2]*

Polyneuropathy—*continued*
  due to
    antitetanus serum 357.6
    arsenic 357.7
    drug or medicinal substance 357.6
      correct substance properly administered 357.6
      overdose or wrong substance given or taken
        977.9
        specified drug—*see* Table of drugs and
          chemicals
    lack of vitamin NEC 269.2 *[357.4]*
    lead 357.7
    organophosphate compounds 357.7
    pellagra 265.2 *[357.4]*
    porphyria 277.1 *[357.4]*
    serum 357.6
    toxic agent NEC 357.7
  hereditary 356.0
  idiopathic 356.9
    progressive 356.4
  in
    amyloidosis 277.39 *[357.4]*
    avitaminosis 269.2 *[357.4]*
      specified NEC 269.1 *[357.4]*
    beriberi 265.0 *[357.4]*
    collagen vascular disease NEC 710.9 *[357.1]*
    deficiency
      B-complex NEC 266.2 *[357.4]*
      vitamin B 266.9 *[357.4]*
      vitamin B₆ 266.1 *[357.4]*
    diabetes 250.6 *[357.2]*
    diphtheria (*see also* Diphtheria) 032.89 *[357.4]*
    disseminated lupus erythematosus 710.0 *[357.1]*
    herpes zoster 053.13
    hypoglycemia 251.2 *[357.4]*
    malignant neoplasm (M8000/3) NEC 199.1
      [357.3]
    mumps 072.72
    pellagra 265.2 *[357.4]*
    polyarteritis nodosa 446.0 *[357.1]*
    porphyria 277.1 *[357.4]*
    rheumatoid arthritis 714.0 *[357.1]*
    sarcoidosis 135 *[357.4]*
    uremia 585.9 *[357.4]*
  lead 357.7
  nutritional 269.9 *[357.4]*
    specified NEC 269.8 *[357.4]*
  postherpetic 053.13
  progressive 356.4
  sensory (hereditary) 356.2
Polyonychia 757.5
Polyopia 368.2
  refractive 368.15
Polyorchism, polyorchidism (three testes)
    752.89
Polyorrhymenitis (peritoneal) (*see also*
    Polyserositis) 568.82
  pericardial 423.2
Polyostotic fibrous dysplasia 756.54
Polyotia 744.1
Polyp, polypus

> *Note—Polyps of organs or sites that do not*
> *appear in the list below should be coded to the*
> *residual category for diseases of the organ or*
> *site concerned.*

  accessory sinus 471.8
  adenoid tissue 471.0
  adenomatous (M8210/0)—*see also* Neoplasm,
    by site, benign

Poor —*continued*
  sucking reflex (newborn) 796.1
  vision NEC 369.9
Poradenitis, nostras 099.1
Porencephaly (congenital) (development) (true) 742.4
  acquired 348.0
  nondevelopmental 348.0
  traumatic (post) 310.2
Porocephaliasis 134.1
Porokeratosis 757.39
  disseminated superficial actinic (DSAP) 692.75
Poroma, eccrine (M8402/0)—*see* Neoplasm, skin, benign
Porphyria (acute) (congenital) (constitutional) (erythropoietic) (familial) (hepatica) (idiopathic) (idiosyncratic) (intermittent) (latent) (mixed hepatic) (photosensitive) (South African genetic) (Swedish) 277.1
  acquired 277.1
  cutaneatarda
    hereditaria 277.1
    symptomatica 277.1
  due to drugs
    correct substance properly administered 277.1
    overdose or wrong substance given or taken 977.9
      specified drug—*see* Table of drugs and chemicals
  secondary 277.1
  toxic NEC 277.1
  variegata 277.1
Porphyrinuria (acquired) (congenital) (secondary) 277.1
Porphyruria (acquired) (congenital) 277.1
Portal —*see* condition
Port wine nevus or mark 757.32
Posadas-Wernicke disease 114.9
Position
  fetus, abnormal (*see also* Presentation, fetal) 652.9
  teeth, faulty (*see also* Anomaly, position tooth) 524.30
Positive
  culture (nonspecific) 795.39
    AIDS virus V08
    blood 790.7
    HIV V08
    human immunodeficiency virus V08
    nose 795.39
    skin lesion NEC 795.39
    spinal fluid 792.0
    sputum 795.39
    stool 792.1
    throat 795.39
    urine 791.9
    wound 795.39
  findings, anthrax 795.31
  HIV V08
  human immunodeficiency virus (HIV) V08
  PPD 795.5
  serology
    AIDS virus V08
      inconclusive 795.71
    HIV V08
      inconclusive 795.71
    human immunodeficiency virus V08
      inconclusive 795.71
    syphilis 097.1
      with signs or symptoms—*see* Syphilis, by site and stage
      false 795.6

Positive—*continued*
  skin test 795.7
    tuberculin (without active tuberculosis) 795.5
  VDRL 097.1
    with signs or symptoms—*see* Syphilis, by site and stage
    false 795.6
  Wassermann reaction 097.1
    false 795.6
Postcardiotomy syndrome 429.4
Postcaval ureter 753.4
Postcholecystectomy syndrome 576.0
Postclimacteric bleeding 627.1
Postcommissurotomy syndrome 429.4
Postconcussional syndrome 310.2
Postcontusional syndrome 310.2
Postcricoid region —*see* condition
Post-dates (pregnancy) —*see* Pregnancy
Postencephalitic —*see also* condition syndrome 310.8
Posterior —*see* condition
Posterolateral sclerosis (spinal cord)—*see* Degeneration, combined
Postexanthematous —*see* condition
Postfebrile —*see* condition
Postgastrectomy dumping syndrome 564.2
Posthemiplegic chorea 344.89
Posthemorrhagic anemia (chronic) 280.0
  acute 285.1
  newborn 776.5
Posthepatitis syndrome 780.79
Postherpetic neuralgia (intercostal) (syndrome) (zoster) 053.19
  geniculate ganglion 053.11
  ophthalmica 053.19
  trigeminal 053.12
Posthitis 607.1
Postimmunization complication or reaction —*see Complications, vaccination*
Postinfectious —*see* condition
Postinfluenzal syndrome 780.79
Postlaminectomy syndrome 722.80
  cervical, cervicothoracic 722.81
  kyphosis 737.12
  lumbar, lumbosacral 722.83
  thoracic, thoracolumbar 722.82
Postleukotomy syndrome 310.0
Postlobectomy syndrome 310.0
Postmastectomy lymphedema (syndrome) 457.0
Postmaturity, postmature (fetus or newborn) (gestation period over 42 completed weeks) 766.22
  affecting management of pregnancy
    post-term pregnancy 645.1
    prolonged pregnancy 645.2
  syndrome 766.22
Postmeasles —*see also* condition
  complication 055.8
    specified NEC 055.79
Postmenopausal
  endometrium (atrophic) 627.8
    suppurative (*see also* Endometritis) 615.9
  hormone replacement therapy V07.4
  status (age related) (natural) V49.81
Postnasal drip 784.91
Postnatal —*see* condition
Postoperative —*see also* condition
  confusion state 293.9
  psychosis 293.9
  status NEC (*see also* Status (post)) V45.89
Postpancreatectomy hyperglycemia 251.3

Postpartum —*see also* condition
  anemia 648.2
  cardiomyopathy 674.5
  observation
    immediately after delivery V24.0
    routine follow-up V24.2
Postperfusion syndrome NEC 999.8
  bone marrow 996.85
Postpoliomyelitic —*see* condition
Postsurgery status NEC (*see also* Status (post) V45.89
Post-term (pregnancy) 645.1
  infant (gestation period over 40 completed weeks to 42 completed weeks) 766.21
Posttraumatic —*see* condition
Posttraumatic brain syndrome, nonpsychotic 310.2
Post-Traumatic Stress Disorder (PTSD) 309.81
Post-typhoid abscess 002.0
Postures, hysterical 300.11
Postvaccinal reaction or complication —*see* Complications, vaccination
Postvagotomy syndrome 564.2
Postvalvulotomy syndrome 429.4
Postvasectomy sperm count V25.8
Potain's disease (pulmonary edema) 514
Potain's syndrome (gastrectasis with dyspepsia) 536.1
Pott's
  curvature (spinal) (*see also* Tuberculosis) 015.0 *[737.43]*
  disease or paraplegia (*see also* Tuberculosis) 015.0 *[730.88]*
  fracture (closed) 824.4
    open 824.5
  gangrene 440.24
  osteomyelitis (*see also* Tuberculosis) 015.0 *[730.88]*
  spinal curvature (*see also* Tuberculosis) 015.0 *[737.43]*
  tumor, puffy (*see also* Osteomyelitis) 730.2
Potter's
  asthma 502
  disease 753.0
  facies 754.0
  lung 502
  syndrome (with renal agenesis) 753.0
Pouch
  bronchus 748.3
  Douglas'—*see* condition
  esophagus, esophageal (congenital) 750.4
    acquired 530.6
  gastric 537.1
  Hartmann's (abnormal sacculation of gallbladder neck) 575.8
    of intestine V44.3
      attention to V55.3
  pharynx, pharyngeal (congenital) 750.27
Poulet's disease 714.2
Poultrymen's itch 133.8
Poverty V60.2
Prader-Labhart-Willi-Fanconi syndrome (hypogenital dystrophy with diabetic tendency) 759.81
Prader-Willi syndrome (hypogenital dystrophy with diabetic tendency) 759.81
Preachers' voice 784.49
Pre-AIDS —*see* Human immunodeficiency virus (disease) (illness) (infection)
Preauricular appendage 744.1

Prebetalipoproteinemia (acquired) (essential) (familial) (hereditary) (primary) (secondary) 272.1
  with chylomicronemia 272.3
Precipitate labor 661.3
  affecting fetus or newborn 763.6
Preclimacteric bleeding 627.0
  menorrhagia 627.0
Precocious
  adrenarche 259.1
  menarche 259.1
  menstruation 626.8
  pubarche 259.1
  puberty NEC 259.1
  sexual development NEC 259.1
  thelarche 259.1
Precocity, sexual (constitutional) (cryptogenic) (female) (idiopathic) (male) NEC 259.1
  with adrenal hyperplasia 255.2
Precordial pain 786.51
  psychogenic 307.89
Predeciduous teeth 520.2
Prediabetes, prediabetic 790.29
  complicating pregnancy, childbirth, or puerperium 648.8
  fetus or newborn 775.89
Predislocation status of hip, at birth (*see also* Subluxation, congenital, hip) 754.32
Pre-eclampsia (mild) 642.4
  with pre-existing hypertension 642.7
  affecting fetus or newborn 760.0
  severe 642.5
  superimposed on pre-existing hypertensive disease 642.7
Preeruptive color change, teeth, tooth 520.8
Preexcitation 426.7
  atrioventricular conduction 426.7
  ventricular 426.7
Preglaucoma 365.00
Pregnancy (single) (uterine) (without sickness) V22.2

> *Note—Use the following fifth-digit subclassification with categories 640-648, 651-676:*
>
> *0 unspecified as to episode of care*
> *1 delivered, with or without mention of antepartum condition*
> *2 delivered, with mention of postpartum complication*
> *3 antepartum condition or complication*
> *4 postpartum condition or complication*

  abdominal (ectopic) 633.00
    affecting fetus or newborn 761.4
    with intrauterine pregnancy 633.01
  abnormal NEC 646.9
  ampullar—*see* Pregnancy, tubal
  broad ligament—*see* Pregnancy, cornual
  cervical—*see* Pregnancy, cornual
  combined (extrauterine and intrauterine)—*see* Pregnancy, cornual
  complicated (by) 646.9
    abnormal, abnormality NEC 646.9
      cervix 654.6
      cord (umbilical) 663.9
      glucose tolerance (conditions classifiable to 790.21-790.29) 648.8
      pelvic organs or tissues NEC 654.9
      pelvis (bony) 653.0

Pregnancy—*continued*
    perineum or vulva 654.8
    placenta, placental (vessel) 656.7
    position
      cervix 654.4
      placenta 641.1
        without hemorrhage 641.0
      uterus 654.4
    size, fetus 653.5
    uterus (congenital) 654.0
   abscess or cellulitis
    bladder 646.6
    genitourinary tract (conditions classifiable to
       590, 595, 597, 599.0, 614.0-614.5,
       614.7-614.9, 615) 646.6
    kidney 646.6
    urinary tract NEC 646.6
   adhesion, pelvic peritoneal 648.9
   air embolism 673.0
   albuminuria 646.2
    with hypertension—*see* Toxemia, of
      pregnancy
   amnionitis 658.4
   amniotic fluid embolism 673.1
   anemia (conditions classifiable to 280-285)
     648.2
   appendicitis 648.9
   atrophy, yellow (acute) (liver) (subacute)
     646.7
   bacilluria, asymptomatic 646.5
   bacteriuria, asymptomatic 646.5
   bariatric surgery status 649.2
   bicornis or bicornuate uterus 654.0
   biliary problems 646.8
   bone and joint disorders (conditions
     classifiable to 720-724 or conditions
     affecting lower limbs classifiable to
     711-719, 725-738) 648.7
   breech presentation 652.2
    with successful version 652.1
   cardiovascular disease (conditions classifiable
     to 390-398, 410-429) 648.6
    congenital (conditions classifiable to
      745-747) 648.5
   cerebrovascular disorders conditions
     (classifiable to 430-434, 436-437) 674.0
   cervicitis (conditions classifiable to 616.0)
     646.6
   chloasma (gravidarum) 646.8
   cholelithiasis 646.8
   chorea (gravidarum)—*see* Eclampsia,
     pregnancy
   coagulation defect 649.3
   contraction, pelvis (general) 653.1
    inlet 653.2
    outlet 653.3
   convulsions (eclamptic) (uremic) 642.6
    with pre-existing hypertension 642.7
   current disease or condition (nonobstetric)
    abnormal glucose tolerance 648.8
    anemia 648.2
    bone and joint (lower limb) 648.7
    cardiovascular 648.6
     congenital 648.5
    cerebrovascular 674.0
    diabetic 648.0
    drug dependence 648.3
    female genital mutilation 648.9
    genital organ or tract 646.6
    gonorrheal 647.1

Pregnancy—*continued*
    hypertensive 642.2
      chronic kidney 642.2
      renal 642.1
    infectious 647.9
      specified type NEC 647.8
    liver 646.7
    malarial 647.4
    nutritional deficiency 648.9
    parasitic NEC 647.8
    periodontal disease 648.9
    renal 646.2
      hypertensive 642.1
    rubella 647.5
    specified condition NEC 648.9
    syphilitic 647.0
    thyroid 648.1
    tuberculous 647.3
    urinary 646.6
    venereal 647.2
    viral NEC 647.6
   cystitis 646.6
   cystocele 654.4
   death of fetus (near term) 656.4
    early pregnancy (before 22 completed weeks
      gestation) 632
   deciduitis 646.6
   decreased fetal movements 655.7
   diabetes (mellitus) (conditions classifiable to
     250) 648.0
   disorders of liver 646.7
   displacement, uterus NEC 654.4
   disproportion—*see* Disproportion
   double uterus 654.0
   drug dependence (conditions classifiable to
     304) 648.3
   dysplasia, cervix 654.6
   early onset of delivery (spontaneous) 644.2
   eclampsia, eclamptic (coma) (convulsions)
     (delirium) (nephritis) (uremia) 642.6
    with pre-existing hypertension 642.7
   edema 646.1
    with hypertension—*see* Toxemia, of
      pregnancy
   effusion, amniotic fluid 658.1
    delayed delivery following 658.2
   embolism
    air 673.0
    amniotic fluid 673.1
    blood-clot 673.2
    cerebral 674.0
    pulmonary NEC 673.2
    pyemic 673.3
    septic 673.3
   emesis (gravidarum)—*see* Pregnancy,
     complicated, vomiting
   endometritis (conditions classifiable to
     615.0-615.9) 646.6
    decidual 646.6
   epilepsy 649.4
   excessive weight gain NEC 646.1
   face presentation 652.4
   failure, fetal head to enter pelvic brim 652.5
   false labor (pains) 644.1
   fatigue 646.8
   fatty metamorphosis of liver 646.7
   female genital mutilation 648.9
   fetal
    death (near term) 656.4
     early (before 22 completed weeks
      gestation) 632

Pregnancy—*continued*
  deformity 653.7
  distress 656.8
    reduction of multiple fetuses reduced to
      single fetus 651.7
  fibroid (tumor) (uterus) 654.1
  footling presentation 652.8
  with successful version 652.1
  gallbladder disease 646.8
  gastric banding status 649.2
  gastric bypass status for obesity 649.2
  goiter 648.1
  gonococcal infection (conditions classifiable
    to 098) 647.1
  gonorrhea (conditions classifiable to 098)
    647.1
  hemorrhage 641.9
    accidental 641.2
    before 22 completed weeks gestation NEC
      640.9
    cerebrovascular 674.0
    due to
      afibrinogenemia or other coagulation
        defect (conditions classifiable to
        286.0-286.9) 641.3
      leiomyoma, uterine 641.8
      marginal sinus (rupture) 641.2
      premature separation, placenta 641.2
      trauma 641.8
    early (before 22 completed weeks gestation)
      640.9
    threatened abortion 640.0
    unavoidable 641.1
  hepatitis (acute) (malignant) (subacute) 646.7
  viral 647.6
  herniation of uterus 654.4
  high head at term 652.5
  hydatidiform mole (delivered) (undelivered)
    630
  hydramnios 657
  hydrocephalic fetus 653.6
  hydrops amnii 657
  hydrorrhea 658.1
  hyperemesis (gravidarum)—*see* Hyperemesis,
    gravidarum
  hypertension—*see* Hypertension, complicating
    pregnancy
  hypertensive heart and chronic kidney disease
    642.2
  hypertensive
    chronic kidney disease 642.2
    heart and chronic kidney disease 642.2
    heart and renal disease 642.2
    heart disease 642.2
    renal disease 642.2
  hyperthyroidism 648.1
  hypothyroidism 648.1
  hysteralgia 646.8
  icterus gravis 646.7
  incarceration, uterus 654.3
  incompetent cervix (os) 654.5
  infection 647.9
    amniotic fluid 658.4
    bladder 646.6
    genital organ (conditions classifiable to
      614.0-614.5, 614.7-614.9, 615) 646.6
    kidney (conditions classifiable to
      590.0-590.9) 646.6
    urinary (tract) 646.6
      asymptomatic 646.5
  infective and parasitic diseases NEC 647.8

Pregnancy—*continued*
  inflammation
    bladder 646.6
    genital organ (conditions classifiable to
      614.0-614.5, 614.7-614.9, 615) 646.6
    urinary tract NEC 646.6
  injury 648.9
    obstetrical NEC 665.9
  insufficient weight gain 646.8
  intrauterine fetal death (near term) NEC 656.4
    early (before 22 completed weeks'
      gestation) 632
  malaria (conditions classifiable to 084) 647.4
  malformation, uterus (congenital) 654.0
  malnutrition (conditions classifiable to
    260-269) 648.9
  malposition
    fetus—*see* Pregnancy, complicated,
      malpresentation
    uterus or cervix 654.4
  malpresentation 652.9
    with successful version 652.1
    in multiple gestation 652.6
    specified type NEC 652.8
  marginal sinus hemorrhage or rupture 641.2
  maternal obesity syndrome 646.1
  menstruation 640.8
  mental disorders (conditions classifiable to
    290-303, 305.0, 305.2-305.9, 306-316,
    317-319) 648.4
  mentum presentation 652.4
  missed
    abortion 632
    delivery (at or near term) 656.4
    labor (at or near term) 656.4
  necrosis
    genital organ or tract (conditions classifiable
      to 614.0-614.5, 614.7-614.9, 615) 646.6
    liver (conditions classifiable to 570) 646.7
    renal, cortical 646.2
  nephritis or nephrosis (conditions classifiable
    to 580-589) 646.2
    with hypertension 642.1
  nephropathy NEC 646.2
  neuritis (peripheral) 646.4
  nutritional deficiency (conditions classifiable
    to 260-269) 648.9
  obesity 649.1
    surgery status 649.2
  oblique lie or presentation 652.3
    with successful version 652.1
  obstetrical trauma NEC 665.9
  oligohydramnios NEC 658.0
  onset of contractions before 37 weeks 644.0
  oversize fetus 653.5
  papyraceous fetus 646.0
  patent cervix 654.5
  pelvic inflammatory disease (conditions
    classifiable to 614.0-614.5, 614.7-614.9,
    615) 646.6
  pelvic peritoneal adhesion 648.9
  placenta, placental
    abnormality 656.7
    abruptio or ablatio 641.2
    detachment 641.2
    disease 656.7
    infarct 656.7
    low implantation 641.1
      without hemorrhage 641.0
    malformation 656.7
    malposition 641.1

Prolapse, prolapsed—*continued*
congenital 752.3
in pregnancy or childbirth 654.4
affecting fetus or newborn 763.1
causing obstructed labor 660.2
affecting fetus or newborn 763.1
postpartal (old) 618.1
uveal 871.1
vagina (anterior) (posterior) (vault) (wall)
(without uterine prolapse) 618.00
with uterine prolapse 618.4
complete 618.3
incomplete 618.2
paravaginal 618.02
posthysterectomy 618.5
specified NEC 618.09
vitreous (humor) 379.26
traumatic 871.1
womb—*see* Prolapse, uterus
Prolapsus, female 618.9
Proliferative —*see* condition
Prolinemia 270.8
Prolinuria 270.8
Prolonged, prolongation
bleeding time (*see also* Defect, coagulation)
790.92
"idiopathic" (in von Willebrand's disease)
286.4
coagulation time (*see also* Defect, coagulation)
790.92
gestation syndrome 766.22
labor 662.1
affecting fetus or newborn 763.89
first stage 662.0
second stage 662.2
PR interval 426.11
pregnancy 645.2
prothrombin time (*see also* Defect, coagulation)
790.92
QT interval 794.31
syndrome 426.82
rupture of membranes (24 hours or more prior to
onset of labor) 658.2
uterine contractions in labor 661.4
affecting fetus or newborn 763.7
Prominauris 744.29
Prominence
auricle (ear) (congenital) 744.29
acquired 380.32
ischial spine or sacral promontory
with disproportion (fetopelvic) 653.3
affecting fetus or newborn 763.1
causing obstructed labor 660.1
affecting fetus or newborn 763.1
nose (congenital) 748.1
acquired 738.0
Pronation
ankle 736.79
foot 736.79
congenital 755.67
Prophylactic
administration of
antibiotics V07.39
antitoxin, any V07.2
antivenin V07.2
chemotherapeutic agent NEC V07.39
fluoride V07.31
diphtheria antitoxin V07.2
gamma globulin V07.2
immune sera (gamma globulin) V07.2
RhoGAM V07.2

Prophylactic—*continued*
tetanus antitoxin V07.2
chemotherapy NEC V07.39
fluoride V07.31
hormone replacement (postmenopausal) V07.4
immunotherapy V07.2
measure V07.9
specified type NEC V07.8
postmenopausal hormone replacement V07.4
sterilization V25.2
Proptosis (ocular) (*see also* Exophthalmos)
376.30
thyroid 242.0
Propulsion
eyeball 360.81
Prosecution, anxiety concerning V62.5
Prostate, prostatic —*see* condition
Prostatism 600.90
with
other lower urinary tract symptoms (LUTS)
600.91
urinary
obstruction 600.91
retention 600.91
Prostatitis (congestive) (suppurative) 601.9
acute 601.0
cavitary 601.8
chlamydial 099.54
chronic 601.1
diverticular 601.8
due to Trichomonas (vaginalis) 131.03
fibrous 600.90
with
other lower urinary tract symptoms (LUTS)
600.91
urinary
obstruction 600.91
retention 600.91
gonococcal (acute) 098.12
chronic or duration of 2 months or over 098.32
granulomatous 601.8
hypertrophic 600.00
with
other lower urinary tract symptoms (LUTS)
600.01
urinary
obstruction 600.01
retention 600.01
specified type NEC 601.8
subacute 601.1
trichomonal 131.03
tuberculous (*see also* Tuberculosis) 016.5
[601.4]
Prostatocystitis 601.3
Prostatorrhea 602.8
Prostatoseminovesiculitis, trichomonal 131.03
Prostration 780.79
heat 992.5
anhydrotic 992.3
due to
salt (and water) depletion 992.4
water depletion 992.3
nervous 300.5
newborn 779.89
senile 797
Protanomaly 368.51
Protanopia (anomalous trichromat) (complete)
(incomplete) 368.51
Protein
deficiency 260
malnutrition 260
sickness (prophylactic) (therapeutic) 999.5

Pseudomyxoma peritonei (M8480/6) 197.6
Pseudoneuritis optic (nerve) 377.24
   papilla 377.24
      congenital 743.57
Pseudoneuroma —*see* Injury, nerve, by site
Pseudo-obstruction
   intestine (chronic) (idiopathic) (intermittent
      secondary) (primary) 564.89
     acute 560.89
Pseudopapilledema 377.24
Pseudoparalysis
   arm or leg 781.4
   atonic, congenital 358.8
Pseudopelade 704.09
Pseudophakia V43.1
Pseudopolycythemia 289.0
Pseudopolyposis, colon 556.4
Pseudoporencephaly 348.0
Pseudopseudohypoparathyroidism 275.49
Pseudopsychosis 300.16
Pseudopterygium 372.52
Pseudoptosis (eyelid) 374.34
Pseudorabies 078.89
Pseudoretinitis, pigmentosa 362.65
Pseudorickets 588.0
   senile (Pozzi's) 731.0
Pseudorubella 057.8
Pseudoscarlatina 057.8
Pseudosclerema 778.1
Pseudosclerosis (brain)
   Jakob's 046.1
   of Westphal (-Strümpell) (hepatolenticular
      degeneration) 275.1
   spastic 046.1
     with dementia
       with behavioral disturbance 046.1 *[294.11]*
       without behavioral disturbance 046.1 *[294.10]*
Pseudoseizure 780.39
   non-psychiatric 780.39
   psychiatric 300.11
Pseudotabes 799.89
   diabetic 250.6 *[337.1]*
Pseudotetanus (*see also* Convulsions) 780.39
Pseudotetany 781.7
   hysterical 300.11
Pseudothalassemia 285.0
Pseudotrichinosis 710.3
Pseudotruncus arteriosus 747.29
Pseudotuberculosis, pasteurella (infection) 027.2
Pseudotumor
   cerebri 348.2
   orbit (inflammatory) 376.11
Pseudo-Turner's syndrome 759.89
Pseudoxanthoma elasticum 757.39
Psilosis (sprue) (tropical) 579.1
   Monilia 112.89
   nontropical 579.0
   not sprue 704.00
Psittacosis 073.9
Psoitis 728.89
Psora NEC 696.1
Psoriasis 696.1
   any type, except arthropathic 696.1
   arthritic, arthropathic 696.0
   buccal 528.6
   flexural 696.1
   follicularis 696.1
   guttate 696.1
   inverse 696.1
   mouth 528.6

Psoriasis—*continued*
   nummularis 696.1
   psychogenic 316 *[696.1]*
   punctata 696.1
   pustular 696.1
   rupioides 696.1
   vulgaris 696.1
Psorospermiasis 136.4
Psorospermosis 136.4
   follicularis (vegetans) 757.39
Psychalgia 307.80
Psychasthenia 300.89
   compulsive 300.3
   mixed compulsive states 300.3
   obsession 300.3
Psychiatric disorder or problem NEC 300.9
Psychogenic —*see also* condition
   factors associated with physical conditions 316
Psychoneurosis, psychoneurotic (*see also*
    Neurosis) 300.9
   anxiety (state) 300.00
   climacteric 627.2
   compensation 300.16
   compulsion 300.3
   conversion hysteria 300.11
   depersonalization 300.6
   depressive type 300.4
   dissociative hysteria 300.15
   hypochondriacal 300.7
   hysteria 300.10
     conversion type 300.11
     dissociative type 300.15
   mixed NEC 300.89
   neurasthenic 300.5
   obsessional 300.3
   obsessive-compulsive 300.3
   occupational 300.89
   personality NEC 301.89
   phobia 300.20
   senile NEC 300.89
Psychopathic —*see also* condition
   constitution, posttraumatic 310.2
     with psychosis 293.9
   personality 301.9
     amoral trends 301.7
     antisocial trends 301.7
     asocial trends 301.7
     mixed types 301.7
   state 301.9
Psychopathy, sexual (*see also* Deviation, sexual)
    302.9
Psychophysiologic, psychophysiological
    condition—*see* Reaction, psychophysiologic
Psychose passionelle 297.8
Psychosexual identity disorder 302.6
   adult-life 302.85
   childhood 302.6
Psychosis 298.9
   acute hysterical 298.1
   affecting management of pregnancy, childbirth,
     or puerperium 648.4
   affective (*see also* Disorder, mood) 296.90
     drug induced 292.84
     due to or associated with physical condition
      293.83

Psychosis—*continued*

---
*Note—Use the following fifth-digit
subclassification with categories 296.0-296.6:*

0   *unspecified*
1   *mild*
2   *moderate*
3   *severe, without mention of psychotic
     behavior*
4   *severe, specified as with psychotic behavior*
5   *in partial or unspecified remission*
6   *in full remission*

---

   involutional 296.2
     recurrent episode 296.3
     single episode 296.2
   manic-depressive 296.80
     circular (alternating) 296.7
      currently depressed 296.5
      currently manic 296.4
     depressed type 296.2
      atypical 296.82
      recurrent episode 296.3
      single episode 296.2
     manic 296.0
      atypical 296.81
      recurrent episode 296.1
      single episode 296.0
     mixed type NEC 296.89
     specified type NEC 296.89
   senile 290.21
   specified type NEC 296.99
  alcoholic 291.9
   with
     anxiety 291.89
     delirium tremens 291.0
     delusions 291.5
     dementia 291.2
     hallucinosis 291.3
     jealousy 291.5
     mood disturbance 291.89
     paranoia 291.5
     persisting amnesia 291.1
     sexual dysfunction 291.89
     sleep disturbance 291.89
   amnestic confabulatory 291.1
   delirium tremens 291.0
   hallucinosis 291.3
   Korsakoff's, Korsakov's, Korsakow's 291.1
   paranoid type 291.5
   pathological intoxication 291.4
   polyneuritic 291.1
   specified type NEC 291.89
  alternating (*see also* Psychosis,
     manic-depressive, circular) 296.7
  anergastic (*see also* Psychosis, organic) 294.9
  arteriosclerotic 290.40
   with
     acute confusional state 290.41
     delirium 290.41
     delusions 290.42
     depressed mood 290.43
    depressed type 290.43
    paranoid type 290.42
    simple type 290.40
    uncomplicated 290.40
  atypical 298.9
   depressive 296.82
   manic 296.81
  borderline (schizophrenia) (*see also*
    Schizophrenia) 295.5

Psychosis—*continued*
  of childhood (*see also* Psychosis, childhood)
    299.8
   prepubertal 299.8
  brief reactive 298.8
  childhood, with origin specific to 299.9

---
*Note—Use the following fifth-digit
subclassification with category 299:*

0   *current or active state*
1   *residual state*

---

   atypical 299.8
   specified type NEC 299.8
  circular (*see also* Psychosis, manic-depressive,
    circular) 296.7
  climacteric (*see also* Psychosis, involutional)
    298.8
  confusional 298.9
   acute 293.0
   reactive 298.2
   subacute 293.1
  depressive (*see also* Psychosis, affective) 296.2
   atypical 296.82
   involutional 296.2
    recurrent episode 296.3
    single episode 296.2
   psychogenic 298.0
   reactive (emotional stress) (psychological
    trauma) 298.0
   recurrent episode 296.3
    with hypomania (bipolar II) 296.89
   single episode 296.2
  disintegrative, childhood (*see also* Psychosis,
    childhood) 299.1
  drug 292.9
   with
    affective syndrome 292.84
    amnestic syndrome 292.83
    anxiety 292.89
    delirium 292.81
     withdrawal 292.0
    delusions 292.11
    dementia 292.82
    depressive state 292.84
    hallucinations 292.12
    hallucinosis 292.12
    mood disorder 292.84
    mood disturbance 292.84
    organic personality syndrome NEC 292.89
    sexual dysfunction 292.89
    sleep disturbance 292.89
    withdrawal syndrome (and delirium) 292.0
   affective syndrome 292.84
   delusions 292.11
   hallucinatory state 292.12
   hallucinosis 292.12
   paranoid state 292.11
   specified type NEC 292.89
   withdrawal syndrome (and delirium) 292.0
  due to or associated with physical condition (*see
    also* Psychosis, organic) 293.9
  epileptic NEC 294.8
  excitation (psychogenic) (reactive) 298.1
  exhaustive (*see also* Reaction, stress, acute)
    308.9
  hypomanic (*see also* Psychosis, affective) 296.0
   recurrent episode 296.1
   single episode 296.0
  hysterical 298.8
   acute 298.1

Puerperal—*continued*
    liver (acute) (subacute) (conditions classifiable
        to 570) 674.8
      ovary 670
      renal cortex 669.3
    nephritis or nephrosis (conditions classifiable to
        580-589) 646.2
      with hypertension 642.1
    nutritional deficiency (conditions classifiable to
        260-269) 648.9
    occlusion, precerebral artery 674.0
    oliguria 669.3
    oophoritis 670
    ovaritis 670
    paralysis
      bladder (sphincter) 665.5
      cerebral 674.0
    paralytic stroke 674.0
    parametritis 670
    paravaginitis 646.6
    pelviperitonitis 670
    perimetritis 670
    perimetrosalpingitis 670
    perinephritis 646.6
    perioophoritis 670
    periphlebitis—*see* Puerperal, phlebitis
    perisalpingitis 670
    peritoneal infection 670
    peritonitis (pelvic) 670
    perivaginitis 646.6
    phlebitis 671.9
      deep 671.4
      intracranial sinus (venous) 671.5
      pelvic 671.4
      specified site NEC 671.5
      superficial 671.2
    phlegmasia alba dolens 671.4
    placental polyp 674.4
    pneumonia, embolic—*see* Puerperal, embolism
    prediabetes 648.8
    pre-eclampsia (mild) 642.4
      with pre-existing hypertension 642.7
      severe 642.5
    psychosis, unspecified (*see also* Psychosis,
      puerperal) 293.89
    pyelitis 646.6
    pyelocystitis 646.6
    pyelohydronephrosis 646.6
    pyelonephritis 646.6
    pyelonephrosis 646.6
    pyemia 670
    pyocystitis 646.6
    pyohemia 670
    pyometra 670
    pyonephritis 646.6
    pyonephrosis 646.6
    pyo-oophoritis 670
    pyosalpingitis 670
    pyosalpinx 670
    pyrexia (of unknown origin) 672
    renal
      disease NEC 646.2
      failure, acute 669.3
    retention
      decidua (fragments) (with delayed
        hemorrhage) 666.2
        without hemorrhage 667.1
      placenta (fragments) (with delayed
        hemorrhage) 666.2
        without hemorrhage 667.1

Puerperal—*continued*
    secundines (fragments) (with delayed
      hemorrhage) 666.2
      without hemorrhage 667.1
    retracted nipple 676.0
    rubella (conditions classifiable to 056) 647.5
    salpingitis 670
    salpingo-oophoritis 670
    salpingo-ovaritis 670
    salpingoperitonitis 670
    sapremia 670
    secondary perineal tear 674.2
    sepsis (pelvic) 670
    septicemia 670
    subinvolution (uterus) 674.8
    sudden death (cause unknown) 674.9
    suppuration—*see* Puerperal, abscess
    syphilis (conditions classifiable to 090-097)
      647.0
    tetanus 670
    thelitis 675.0
    thrombocytopenia 666.3
    thrombophlebitis (superficial) 671.2
      deep 671.4
      pelvic 671.4
      specified site NEC 671.5
    thrombosis (venous)—*see* Thrombosis,
      puerperal
    thyroid dysfunction (conditions classifiable to
      240-246) 648.1
    toxemia (*see also* Toxemia, of pregnancy) 642.4
      eclamptic 642.6
        with pre-existing hypertension 642.7
      pre-eclamptic (mild) 642.4
        with
          convulsions 642.6
          pre-existing hypertension 642.7
        severe 642.5
    tuberculosis (conditions classifiable to 010-018)
      647.3
    uremia 669.3
    vaginitis (conditions classifiable to 616.1) 646.6
    varicose veins (legs) 671.0
      vulva or perineum 671.1
    vulvitis (conditions classifiable to 616.1) 646.6
    vulvovaginitis (conditions classifiable to 616.1)
      646.6
    white leg 671.4
Pulled muscle —*see* Sprain, by site
Pulmolithiasis 518.89
Pulmonary —*see* condition
Pulmonitis (unknown etiology) 486
Pulpitis (acute) (anachoretic) (chronic)
    (hyperplastic) (putrescent) (suppurative)
    (ulcerative) 522.0
Pulpless tooth 522.9
Pulse
    alternating 427.89
      psychogenic 306.2
    bigeminal 427.89
    fast 785.0
    feeble, rapid, due to shock following injury
      958.4
    rapid 785.0
    slow 427.89
    strong 785.9
    trigeminal 427.89
    water-hammer (*see also* Insufficiency, aortic)
      424.1
    weak 785.9
Pulseless disease 446.7

Q

Q fever 083.0
  with pneumonia 083.0 *[484.8]*
Quadricuspid aortic valve 746.89
Quadrilateral fever 083.0
Quadriparesis —*see* Quadriplegia
  meaning muscle weakness 728.87
Quadriplegia 344.00
  with fracture, vertebra (process)—*see* Fracture,
      vertebra, cervical, with spinal cord injury
  brain (current episode) 437.8
  cerebral (current episode) 437.8
  C1-C4
    complete 344.01
    incomplete 344.02
  C5-C7
    complete 344.03
    incomplete 344.04
  congenital or infantile (cerebral) (spastic)
      (spinal) 343.2
  cortical 437.8
  embolic (current episode) (*see also* Embolism,
      brain) 434.1
  infantile (cerebral) (spastic) (spinal) 343.2
  newborn NEC 767.0
  specified NEC 344.09
  thrombotic (current episode) (*see also*
      Thrombosis, brain) 434.0
  traumatic—*see* Injury, spinal, cervical
Quadruplet
  affected by maternal complications of pregnancy
      761.5
  healthy liveborn—*see* Newborn, multiple
  pregnancy (complicating delivery) NEC 651.8
    with fetal loss and retention of one or more
        fetus(es) 651.5
    following (elective) fetal reduction 651.7
Quarrelsomeness 301.3
Quartan
  fever 084.2
  malaria (fever) 084.2
Queensland fever 083.0
  coastal 083.0
  seven-day 100.89
Quervain's disease 727.04
  thyroid (subacute granulomatous thyroiditis)
      245.1
Queyrat's erythroplasia (M8080/2)
  specified site—*see* Neoplasm, skin, in situ
  unspecified site 233.5
Quincke's disease or edema —*see* Edema,
  angioneurotic
Quinquaud's disease (acne decalvans) 704.09
Quinsy (gangrenous) 475
Quintan fever 083.1
Quintuplet
  affected by maternal complications of pregnancy
      761.5
  healthy liveborn—*see* Newborn, multiple
  pregnancy (complicating delivery) NEC 651.2
    with fetal loss and retention of one or more
        fetus(es) 651.6
    following (elective) fetal reduction 651.7
Quotidian
  fever 084.0
  malaria (fever) 084.0

R

Rabbia 071
Rabbit fever (*see also* Tularemia) 021.9
Rabies 071
  contact V01.5
  exposure to V01.5
  inoculation V04.5
    reaction—*see* Complications, vaccination
  vaccination, prophylactic (against) V04.5
Rachischisis (*see also* Spina bifida) 741.9
Rachitic —*see also* condition
  deformities of spine 268.1
  pelvis 268.1
    with disproportion (fetopelvic) 653.2
      affecting fetus or newborn 763.1
      causing obstructed labor 660.1
        affecting fetus or newborn 763.1
Rachitis, rachitism —*see also* Rickets
  acute 268.0
  fetalis 756.4
  renalis 588.0
  tarda 268.0
Racket nail 757.5
Radial nerve —*see* condition
Radiation effects or sickness —*see also* Effect,
    adverse, radiation
  cataract 366.46
  dermatitis 692.82
    sunburn (*see also* Sunburn) 692.71
Radiculitis (pressure) (vertebrogenic) 729.2
  accessory nerve 723.4
  anterior crural 724.4
  arm 723.4
  brachial 723.4
  cervical NEC 723.4
  due to displacement of intervertebral disc—*see*
      Neuritis, due to, displacement intervertebral
      disc
  leg 724.4
  lumbar NEC 724.4
  lumbosacral 724.4
  rheumatic 729.2
  syphilitic 094.89
  thoracic (with visceral pain) 724.4
Radiculomyelitis 357.0
  toxic, due to
    Clostridium tetani 037
    Corynebacterium diphtheriae 032.89
Radiculopathy (*see also* Radiculitis) 729.2
Radioactive substances, adverse effect —*see*
    Effect, adverse, radioactive substance
Radiodermal burns (acute) (chronic)
    (occupational)—*see* Burn, by site
Radiodermatitis 692.82
Radionecrosis —*see* Effect, adverse, radiation
Radiotherapy session V58.0
Radium, adverse effect —*see* Effect, adverse,
    radioactive substance
Raeder-Harbitz syndrome (pulseless disease) 446.7
Rage (*see also* Disturbance, conduct) 312.0
  meaning rabies 071
Rag sorters' disease 022.1
Raillietiniasis 123.8
Railroad neurosis 300.16
Railway spine 300.16
Raised —*see* Elevation
Raiva 071
Rake teeth, tooth 524.39
Rales 786.7

Ramifying renal pelvis 753.3
Ramsay Hunt syndrome (herpetic geniculate ganglionitis) 053.11
meaning dyssynergia cerebellaris myoclonica 334.2
Ranke's primary infiltration (*see also* Tuberculosis) 010.0
Ranula 527.6
congenital 750.26
Rape
adult 995.83
alleged, observation or examination V71.5
child 995.53
Rapid
feeble pulse, due to shock, following injury 958.4
heart (beat) 785.0
psychogenic 306.2
respiration 786.06
psychogenic 306.1
second stage (delivery) 661.3
affecting fetus or newborn 763.6
time-zone change syndrome 327.35
Rarefaction, bone 733.99
Rash 782.1
canker 034.1
diaper 691.0
drug (internal use) 693.0
contact 692.3
ECHO 9 virus 078.89
enema 692.89
food (*see also* Allergy, food) 693.1
heat 705.1
napkin 691.0
nettle 708.8
pustular 782.1
rose 782.1
epidemic 056.9
of infants 057.8
scarlet 034.1
serum (prophylactic) (therapeutic) 999.5
toxic 782.1
wandering tongue 529.1
Rasmussen's aneurysm (*see also* Tuberculosis) 011.2
Rat-bite fever 026.9
due to Streptobacillus moniliformis 026.1
spirochetal (morsus muris) 026.0
Rathke's pouch tumor (M9350/1) 237.0
Raymond (-Céstan) syndrome 433.8
Raynaud's
disease or syndrome (paroxysmal digital cyanosis) 443.0
gangrene (symmetric) 443.0 *[785.4]*
phenomenon (paroxysmal digital cyanosis) (secondary) 443.0
RDS 769
Reaction
acute situational maladjustment (*see also* Reaction, adjustment) 309.9
adaptation (*see also* Reaction, adjustment) 309.9
adjustment 309.9
with
anxious mood 309.24
with depressed mood 309.28
conduct disturbance 309.3
combined with disturbance of emotions 309.4
depressed mood 309.0
brief 309.0
with anxious mood 309.28

Reaction—*continued*
prolonged 309.1
elective mutism 309.83
mixed emotions and conduct 309.4
mutism, elective 309.83
physical symptoms 309.82
predominant disturbance (of)
conduct 309.3
emotions NEC 309.29
mixed 309.28
mixed, emotions and conduct 309.4
specified type NEC 309.89
specific academic or work inhibition 309.23
withdrawal 309.83
depressive 309.0
with conduct disturbance 309.4
brief 309.0
prolonged 309.1
specified type NEC 309.89
adverse food NEC 995.7
affective (*see also* Psychosis, affective) 296.90
specified type NEC 296.99
aggressive 301.3
unsocialized (*see also* Disturbance, conduct) 312.0
allergic (*see also* Allergy) 995.3
drug, medicinal substance, and biological—*see* Allergy, drug
food—*see* Allergy, food
serum 999.5
anaphylactic—*see* Shock, anaphylactic
anesthesia—*see* Anesthesia, complication
anger 312.0
antisocial 301.7
antitoxin (prophylactic) (therapeutic)—*see* Complications, vaccination
anxiety 300.00
Arthus 995.21
asthenic 300.5
compulsive 300.3
conversion (anesthetic) (autonomic) (hyperkinetic) (mixed paralytic) (paresthetic) 300.11
deoxyribonuclease (DNA) (DNase) hypersensitivity NEC 287.2
depressive 300.4
acute 309.0
affective (*see also* Psychosis, affective) 296.2
recurrent episode 296.3
single episode 296.2
brief 309.0
manic (*see also* Psychosis, affective) 296.80
neurotic 300.4
psychoneurotic 300.4
psychotic 298.0
dissociative 300.15
drug NEC (*see also* Table of Drugs and Chemicals) 995.20
allergic—*see also* Allergy, drug 995.27
correct substance properly administered 995.20
obstetric anesthetic or analgesic NEC 668.9
affecting fetus or newborn 763.5
specified drug—*see* Table of drugs and chemicals
overdose or poisoning 977.9
specified drug—*see* Table of drugs and chemicals
specific to newborn 779.4
transmitted via placenta or breast milk—*see* Absorption, drug, through placenta
withdrawal NEC 292.0

Reaction—*continued*
 infant of dependent mother 779.5
 wrong substance given or taken in error 977.9
  specified drug—*see* Table of drugs and
   chemicals
dyssocial 301.7
dystonic, acute, due to drugs 333.72
erysipeloid 027.1
fear 300.20
 child 313.0
fluid loss, cerebrospinal 349.0
food—*see also* Allergy, food
 adverse NEC 995.7
 anaphylactic shock—*see* Anaphylactic shock,
  due to food
foreign
 body NEC 728.82
  in operative wound (inadvertently left) 998.4
   due to surgical material intentionally
    left—*see* Complications, due to
    (presence of) any device, implant, or
    graft classified to 996.0-996.5 NEC
  substance accidentally left during a procedure
   (chemical) (powder) (talc) 998.7
   body or object (instrument) (sponge) (swab)
    998.4
graft-versus-host (GVH) 996.85
grief (acute) (brief) 309.0
 prolonged 309.1
gross stress (*see also* Reaction, stress, acute)
 308.9
group delinquent (*see also* Disturbance,
 conduct) 312.2
Herxheimer's 995.0
hyperkinetic (*see also* Hyperkinesia) 314.9
hypochondriacal 300.7
hypoglycemic, due to insulin 251.0
 therapeutic misadventure 962.3
hypomanic (*see also* Psychosis, affective) 296.0
 recurrent episode 296.1
 single episode 296.0
hysterical 300.10
 conversion type 300.11
 dissociative 300.15
id (bacterial cause) 692.89
immaturity NEC 301.89
 aggressive 301.3
 emotional instability 301.59
immunization—*see* Complications, vaccination
incompatibility
 blood group (ABO) (infusion) (transfusion)
  999.6
 Rh (factor) (infusion) (transfusion) 999.7
inflammatory—*see* Infection
infusion—*see* Complications, infusion
inoculation (immune serum)—*see*
 Complications, vaccination
insulin 995.23
involutional
 paranoid 297.2
 psychotic (*see also* Psychosis, affective,
  depressive) 296.2
leukemoid (basophilic) (lymphocytic)
 (monocytic) (myelocytic) (neutrophilic)
 288.62
LSD (*see also* Abuse, drugs, nondependent)
 305.3
lumbar puncture 349.0
manic-depressive (*see also* Psychosis, affective)
 296.80
 depressed 296.2

Reaction—*continued*
 recurrent episode 296.3
 single episode 296.2
 hypomanic 296.0
neurasthenic 300.5
neurogenic (*see also* Neurosis) 300.9
neurotic NEC 300.9
neurotic-depressive 300.4
nitritoid—*see* Crisis, nitritoid
obsessive-compulsive 300.3
organic 293.9
 acute 293.0
 subacute 293.1
overanxious, child or adolescent 313.0
paranoid (chronic) 297.9
 acute 298.3
 climacteric 297.2
 involutional 297.2
 menopausal 297.2
 senile 290.20
 simple 297.0
passive
 aggressive 301.84
 dependency 301.6
personality (*see also* Disorder, personality)
 301.9
phobic 300.20
postradiation—*see* Effect, adverse, radiation
psychogenic NEC 300.9
psychoneurotic (*see also* Neurosis) 300.9
 anxiety 300.00
 compulsive 300.3
 conversion 300.11
 depersonalization 300.6
 depressive 300.4
 dissociative 300.15
 hypochondriacal 300.7
 hysterical 300.10
  conversion type 300.11
  dissociative type 300.15
 neurasthenic 300.5
 obsessive 300.3
 obsessive-compulsive 300.3
 phobic 300.20
 tension state 300.9
psychophysiologic NEC (*see also* Disorder,
 psychosomatic) 306.9
 cardiovascular 306.2
 digestive 306.4
 endocrine 306.6
 gastrointestinal 306.4
 genitourinary 306.50
 heart 306.2
 hemic 306.8
 intestinal (large) (small) 306.4
 laryngeal 306.1
 lymphatic 306.8
 musculoskeletal 306.0
 pharyngeal 306.1
 respiratory 306.1
 skin 306.3
 special sense organs 306.7
psychosomatic (*see also* Disorder,
 psychosomatic) 306.9
psychotic (*see also* Psychosis) 298.9
 depressive 298.0
 due to or associated with physical condition
  (*see also* Psychosis, organic) 293.9
 involutional (*see also* Psychosis, affective)
  296.2
  recurrent episode 296.3

Reflex—*continued*
vasoconstriction 443.9
Reflux
vasovagal 780.2
esophageal 530.81
esophagitis 530.11
gastroesophageal 530.81
mitral—*see* Insufficiency, mitral
ureteral —*see* Reflux, vesicoureteral
vesicoureteral 593.70
with
reflux nephropathy 593.73
bilateral 593.72
unilateral 593.71
Reformed gallbladder 576.0
Reforming, artificial openings (*see also*
Attention to, artificial, opening) V55.9
Refractive error (*see also* Error, refractive) 367.9
Refsum's disease or syndrome (heredopathia
atactica polyneuritiformis) 356.3
Refusal of
food 307.59
hysterical 300.11
treatment because of, due to
patient's decision NEC V64.2
reason of conscience or religion V62.6
Regaud
tumor (M8082/3)—*see* Neoplasm, nasopharynx,
malignant
type carcinoma (M8082/3)—*see* Neoplasm,
nasopharynx, malignant
Regional —*see* condition
Regulation feeding (elderly) (infant) 783.3
newborn 779.3
Regurgitated
food, choked on 933.1
stomach contents, choked on 933.1
Regurgitation
aortic (valve) (*see also* Insufficiency, aortic)
424.1
congenital 746.4
syphilitic 093.22
food—*see also* Vomiting
with reswallowing—*see* Rumination
newborn 779.3
gastric contents—*see* Vomiting
heart—*see* Endocarditis
mitral (valve)—*see also* Insufficiency, mitral
congenital 746.6
myocardial—*see* Endocarditis
pulmonary (heart) (valve) (*see also*
Endocarditis, pulmonary) 424.3
stomach—*see* Vomiting
tricuspid—*see* Endocarditis, tricuspid
valve, valvular—*see* Endocarditis
vesicoureteral —*see* Reflux, vesicoureteral
Rehabilitation V57.9
multiple types V57.89
occupational V57.21
specified type NEC V57.89
speech V57.3
vocational V57.22
Reichmann's disease or syndrome
(gastrosuccorrhea) 536.8
Reifenstein's syndrome (hereditary familial
hypogonadism, male) 259.5
Reilly's syndrome or phenomenon (*see also*
Neuropathy, peripheral, autonomic) 337.9
Reimann's periodic disease 277.31
Reinsertion, contraceptive device V25.42
Reiter's disease, syndrome, or urethritis 099.3
[711.1]

Rejection
food, hysterical 300.11
transplant 996.80
bone marrow 996.85
corneal 996.51
organ (immune or nonimmune cause) 996.80
bone marrow 996.85
heart 996.83
intestines 996.87
kidney 996.81
liver 996.82
lung 996.84
pancreas 996.86
specified NEC 996.89
skin 996.52
artificial 996.55
decellularized allodermis 996.55
Relapsing fever 087.9
Carter's (Asiatic) 087.0
Dutton's (West African) 087.1
Koch's 087.9
louse-borne (epidemic) 087.0
Novy's (American) 087.1
Obermeyer's (European) 087.0
Spirillum 087.9
tick-borne (endemic) 087.1
Relaxation
anus (sphincter) 569.49
due to hysteria 300.11
arch (foot) 734
congenital 754.61
back ligaments 728.4
bladder (sphincter) 596.59
cardio-esophageal 530.89
cervix (*see also* Incompetency, cervix) 622.5
diaphragm 519.4
inguinal rings—*see* Hernia, inguinal
joint (capsule) (ligament) (paralytic) (*see also*
Derangement, joint) 718.90
congenital 755.8
lumbosacral joint 724.6
pelvic floor 618.89
pelvis 618.89
perineum 618.89
posture 729.9
rectum (sphincter) 569.49
sacroiliac (joint) 724.6
scrotum 608.89
urethra (sphincter) 599.84
uterus (outlet) 618.89
vagina (outlet) 618.89
vesical 596.59
Remains
canal of Cloquet 743.51
capsule (opaque) 743.51
Remittent fever (malarial) 084.6
Remnant
canal of Cloquet 743.51
capsule (opaque) 743.51
cervix, cervical stump (acquired) (postoperative)
622.8
cystic duct, postcholecystectomy 576.0
fingernail 703.8
congenital 757.5
meniscus, knee 717.5
thyroglossal duct 759.2
tonsil 474.8
infected 474.00
urachus 753.7
Remote effect of cancer —*see* Condition

Removal (of)
catheter (urinary) (indwelling) V53.6
from artificial opening—*see* Attention to,
artificial, opening
non-vascular V58.82
vascular V58.81
cerebral ventricle (communicating) shunt V53.01
device—*see also* Fitting (of)
contraceptive V25.42
fixation
external V54.89
internal V54.01
traction V54.89
drains V58.49
dressing
wound V58.30
nonsurgical V58.30
surgical V58.31
ileostomy V55.2
Kirschner wire V54.89
non-vascular catheter V58.82
pin V54.01
plaster cast V54.89
plate (fracture) V54.01
rod V54.01
screw V54.01
splint, external V54.89
subdermal implantable contraceptive V25.43
staples V58.32
sutures V58.32
traction device, external V54.89
vascular catheter V58.81
wound packing V58.30
nonsurgical V58.30
surgical V58.31
Ren
arcuatus 753.3
mobile, mobilis (*see also* Disease, renal) 593.0
congenital 753.3
unguliformis 753.3
Renal —*see also* condition
glomerulohyalinosis-diabetic syndrome 250.4
[581.81]
Rendu-Osler-Weber disease or syndrome
(familial hemorrhagic telangiectasia) 448.0
Reninoma (M8361/1) 236.91
Rénon-Delille syndrome 253.8
Repair
pelvic floor, previous, in pregnancy or childbirth
654.4
affecting fetus or newborn 763.89
scarred tissue V51
Replacement by artificial or mechanical device
or prosthesis of (*see also* Fitting (of))
artificial skin V43.83
bladder V43.5
blood vessel V43.4
breast V43.82
eye globe V43.0
heart
with
assist device V43.21
fully implantable artificial heart V43.22
valve V43.3
intestine V43.89
joint V43.60
ankle 43.66
elbow V43.62
finger V43.69
hip (partial) (total) V43.64
knee V43.65

Replacement—*continued*
shoulder V43.61
specified NEC V43.69
wrist V43.63
kidney V43.89
larynx V43.81
lens V43.1
limb(s) V43.7
liver V43.89
lung V43.89
organ NEC V43.89
pancreas V43.89
skin (artificial) V43.83
tissue NEC V43.89
Reprogramming
cardiac pacemaker V53.31
Request for expert evidence V68.2
Reserve, decreased or low
cardiac—*see* Disease, heart
kidney (*see also* Disease, renal) 593.9
Residual —*see also* condition
bladder 596.8
foreign body—*see* Retention, foreign body
state, schizophrenic (*see also* Schizophrenia)
295.6
urine 788.69
Resistance, resistant (to)

---

*Note—Use the following subclassification for
categories V09.5, V09.7, V09.8, V09.9.:*

*0 without mention of resistance to multiple
drugs*
1 with resistance to multiple drugs

V09.5   quinolones and fluoroquinolones
V09.7   antimycobacterial agents
V09.8   specified drugs NEC
V09.9   unspecified drugs

9 multiple sites

---

activated protein C 289.81
drugs by microorganisms V09.90
Amikacin V09.4
aminoglycosides V09.4
Amodiaquine V09.5
Amoxicillin V09.0
Ampicillin V09.0
antimycobacterial agents V09.7
Azithromycin V09.2
Azlocillin V09.0
Aztreonam V09.1
B-lactam antibiotics V09.1
Bacampicillin V09.0
Bacitracin V09.8
Benznidazole V09.8
Capreomycin V09.7
Carbenicillin V09.0
Cefaclor V09.1
Cefadroxil V09.1
Cefamandole V09.1
Cefatetan V09.1
Cefazolin V09.1
Cefixime V09.1
Cefonicid V09.1
Cefoperazone V09.1
Ceforanide V09.1
Cefotaxime V09.1
Cefoxitin V09.1
Ceftazidine V09.1
Ceftizoxime V09.1

Resistance, resistant (to)—*continued*
   Ceftriaxone V09.1
   Cefuroxime V09.1
   Cephalexin V09.1
   Cephaloglycin V09.1
   Cephaloridine V09.1
   cephalosporins V09.1
   Cephalothin V09.1
   Cephapirin V09.1
   Cephradine V09.1
   Chloramphenicol V09.8
   Chloraquine V09.5
   Chlorguanide V09.8
   Chlorproguanil V09.8
   Chlortetracycline V09.3
   Cinoxacin V09.5
   Ciprofloxacin V09.5
   Clarithromycin V09.2
   Clindamycin V09.8
   Clioquinol V09.5
   Clofazimine V09.7
   Cloxacillin V09.0
   Cyclacillin V09.0
   Cycloserine V09.7
   Dapsone [DZ] V09.7
   Demeclocycline V09.3
   Dicloxacillin V09.0
   Doxycycline V09.3
   Enoxacin V09.5
   Erythromycin V09.2
   Ethambutol [EMB] V09.7
   Ethionamide [ETA] V09.7
   fluoroquinolones NEC V09.5
   Gentamicin V09.4
   Halofantrine V09.8
   Imipenem V09.1
   Iodoquinol V09.5
   Isoniazid [INH] V09.7
   Kanamycin V09.4
   macrolides V09.2
   Mafenide V09.6
   MDRO (multiple drug resistant organisms)
      NOS V09.91
   Mefloquine V09.8
   Melassoprol V09.8
   Methacillin V09.0
   Methacycline V09.3
   Methenamine V09.8
   Methicillin V09.0
   Metronidazole V09.8
   Mezlocillin V09.0
   Minocycline V09.3
   multiple drug resistant organisms NOS V09.91
   Nafcillin V09.0
   Nalidixic Acid V09.5
   Natamycin V09.2
   Neomycin V09.4
   Netilmicin V09.4
   Nimorazole V09.8
   Nitrofurantoin V09.8
   Nitrofurtimox V09.8
   Norfloxacin V09.5
   Nystatin V09.2
   Ofloxacin V09.5
   Oleandomycin V09.2
   Oxacillin V09.0
   Oxytetracycline V09.3
   Para-amino salicylic acid [PAS] V09.7
   Paromomycin V09.4
   Penicillin (G)(V)(VK) V09.0
   penicillins V09.0

Resistance, resistant (to)—*continued*
   Pentamidine V09.8
   Piperacillin V09.0
   Primaquine V09.5
   Proguanil V09.8
   Pyrazinamide [PZA] V09.7
   Pyrimethamine/Sulfalene V09.8
   Pyrimethamine/Sulfodoxine V09.8
   Quinacrine V09.5
   Quinidine V09.8
   Quinine V09.8
   quinolones V09.5
   Rifabutin V09.7
   Rifampin [RIF] V09.7
   Rifamycin V09.7
   Rolitetracycline V09.3
   specified drugs NEC V09.8
   Spectinomycin V09.8
   Spiramycin V09.2
   Streptomycin [SM] V09.4
   Sulfacetamide V09.6
   Sulfacytine V90.6
   Sulfadiazine V09.6
   Sulfadoxine V09.6
   Sulfamethoxazole V09.6
   Sulfapyridine V09.6
   Sulfasalizine V09.6
   Sulfasoxazole V09.6
   sulfonamides V09.6
   Sulfoxone V09.7
   Tetracycline V09.3
   tetracyclines V09.3
   Thiamphenicol V09.8
   Ticarcillin V09.0
   Tinidazole V09.8
   Tobramycin V09.4
   Triamphenicol V09.8
   Trimethoprim V09.8
   Vancomycin V09.8
  insulin 277.7
  thyroid hormone 246.8
Resorption
  biliary 576.8
    purulent or putrid (*see also* Cholecystitis)
      576.8
  dental (roots) 521.40
   alveoli 525.8
   pathological
     external 521.42
     internal 521.41
     specified NEC 521.49
  septic—*see* Septicemia
  teeth (roots) 521.40
   pathological
     external 521.42
     internal 521.41
     specified NEC 521.49
Respiration
  asymmetrical 786.09
  bronchial 786.09
  Cheyne-Stokes (periodic respiration) 786.04
  decreased, due to shock following injury 958.4
  disorder of 786.00
   psychogenic 306.1
   specified NEC 786.09
  failure 518.81
   acute 518.81
   acute and chronic 518.84
   chronic 518.83
   newborn 770.84
  insufficiency 786.09

Retrocession —*see* Retroversion
Retrodisplacement —*see* Retroversion
Retroflection, retroflexion —*see* Retroversion
Retrognathia, retrognathism (mandibular)
(maxillary) 524.06
Retrograde
ejaculation 608.87
menstruation 626.8
Retroiliac ureter 753.4
Retroperineal —*see* condition
Retroperitoneal —*see* condition
Retroperitonitis 567.39
Retropharyngeal —*see* condition
Retroplacental —*see* condition
Retroposition —*see* Retroversion
Retrosternal thyroid (congenital) 759.2
Retroversion, retroverted
cervix *see* Retroversion, uterus
female NEC (*see also* Retroversion, uterus) 621.6
iris 364.70
testis (congenital) 752.51
uterus, uterine (acquired) (acute) (adherent) (any
degree) (asymptomatic) (cervix)
(postinfectional) (postpartal, old) 621.6
congenital 752.3
in pregnancy or childbirth 654.3
affecting fetus or newborn 763.89
causing obstructed labor 660.2
affecting fetus or newborn 763.1
Retrusion, premaxilla (developmental) 524.04
Rett's syndrome 330.8
Reverse, reversed
peristalsis 787.4
Reye's syndrome 331.81
Reye-Sheehan syndrome (postpartum pituitary
necrosis) 253.2
Rh (factor)
hemolytic disease 773.0
incompatibility, immunization, or sensitization
affecting management of pregnancy 656.1
fetus or newborn 773.0
transfusion reaction 999.7
negative mother, affecting fetus or newborn
773.0
titer elevated 999.7
transfusion reaction 999.7
Rhabdomyolysis (idiopathic) 728.88
Rhabdomyoma (M8900/0)—*see also* Neoplasm,
connective tissue, benign
adult (M8904/0)—*see* Neoplasm, connective
tissue, benign
fetal (M8903/0)—*see* Neoplasm, connective
tissue, benign
glycogenic (M8904/0)—*see* Neoplasm,
connective tissue, benign
Rhabdomyosarcoma (M8900/3)—*see also*
Neoplasm connective tissue, malignant
alveolar (M8920/3)—*see* Neoplasm, connective
tissue, malignant
embryonal (M8910/3)—*see* Neoplasm,
connective tissue malignant
mixed type (M8902/3)—*see* Neoplasm,
connective tissue, malignant
pleomorphic (M8901/3)—*see* Neoplasm,
connective tissue, malignant
Rhabdosarcoma (M8900/3)—*see*
Rhabdomyosarcoma
Rhesus (factor) (Rh) incompatibility—*see* Rh,
incompatibility
Rheumaticosis —*see* Rheumatism

Rheumatism, rheumatic (acute NEC) 729.0
adherent pericardium 393
arthritis
acute or subacute—*see* Fever, rheumatic
chronic 714.0
spine 720.0
articular (chronic) NEC (*see also* Arthritis)
716.9
acute or subacute—*see* Fever, rheumatic
back 724.9
blennorrhagic 098.59
carditis—*see* Disease, heart, rheumatic
cerebral—*see* Fever, rheumatic
chorea (acute)—*see* Chorea, rheumatic
chronic NEC 729.0
coronary arteritis 391.9
chronic 398.99
degeneration, myocardium (*see also*
Degeneration, myocardium, with rheumatic
fever) 398.0
desert 114.0
febrile—*see* Fever, rheumatic
fever—*see* Fever, rheumatic
gonococcal 098.59
gout 274.0
heart
disease (*see also* Disease, heart, rheumatic)
398.90
failure (chronic) (congestive) (inactive) 398.91
hemopericardium—*see* Rheumatic, pericarditis
hydropericardium—*see* Rheumatic, pericarditis
inflammatory (acute) (chronic) (subacute)—*see*
Fever, rheumatic
intercostal 729.0
meaning Tietze's disease 733.6
joint (chronic) NEC (*see also* Arthritis) 716.9
acute—*see* Fever, rheumatic
mediastinopericarditis—*see* Rheumatic,
pericarditis
muscular 729.0
myocardial degeneration (*see also*
Degeneration, myocardium, with rheumatic
fever) 398.0
myocarditis (chronic) (inactive) (with chorea)
398.0
active or acute 391.2
with chorea (acute) (rheumatic)
(Sydenham's) 392.0
myositis 729.1
neck 724.9
neuralgic 729.0
neuritis (acute) (chronic) 729.2
neuromuscular 729.0
nodose—*see* Arthritis, nodosa
nonarticular 729.0
palindromic 719.30
ankle 719.37
elbow 719.32
foot 719.37
hand 719.34
hip 719.35
knee 719.36
multiple sites 719.39
pelvic region 719.35
shoulder (region) 719.31
specified site NEC 719.38
wrist 719.33
pancarditis, acute 391.8
with chorea (acute) (rheumatic) (Sydenham's)
392.0
chronic or inactive 398.99

Rheumatism, rheumatic—*continued*
  pericarditis (active) (acute) (with effusion) (with pneumonia) 391.0
    with chorea (acute) (rheumatic) (Sydenham's) 392.0
    chronic or inactive 393
  pericardium—*see* Rheumatic, pericarditis
  pleuropericarditis—*see* Rheumatic, pericarditis
  pneumonia 390 *[517.1]*
  pneumonitis 390 *[517.1]*
  pneumopericarditis—*see* Rheumatic, pericarditis
  polyarthritis
    acute or subacute—*see* Fever, rheumatic
    chronic 714.0
  polyarticular NEC (*see also* Arthritis) 716.9
  psychogenic 306.0
  radiculitis 729.2
  sciatic 724.3
  septic—*see* Fever, rheumatic
  spine 724.9
  subacute NEC 729.0
  torticollis 723.5
  tuberculous NEC (*see also* Tuberculosis) 015.9
  typhoid fever 002.0
Rheumatoid —*see also* condition
  lungs 714.81
Rhinitis (atrophic) (catarrhal) (chronic) (croupous) (fibrinous) (hyperplastic) (hypertrophic) (membranous) (purulent) (suppurative) (ulcerative) 472.0
  with
    hay fever (*see also* Fever, hay) 477.9
      with asthma (bronchial) 493.0
    sore throat—*see* Nasopharyngitis
  acute 460
  allergic (nonseasonal) (seasonal) (*see also* Fever, hay) 477.9
    due to food 477.1
    with asthma (*see also* Asthma) 493.0
  granulomatous 472.0
  infective 460
  obstructive 472.0
  pneumococcal 460
  syphilitic 095.8
    congenital 090.0
  tuberculous (*see also* Tuberculosis) 012.8
  vasomotor (*see also* Fever, hay) 477.9
Rhinoantritis (chronic) 473.0
  acute 461.0
Rhinodacryolith 375.57
Rhinolalia (aperta) (clausa) (open) 784.49
Rhinolith 478.19
  nasal sinus (*see also* Sinusitis) 473.9
Rhinomegaly 478.19
Rhinopharyngitis (acute) (subacute) (*see also* Nasopharyngitis) 460
  chronic 472.2
  destructive ulcerating 102.5
  mutilans 102.5
Rhinophyma 695.3
Rhinorrhea 478.19
  cerebrospinal (fluid) 349.81
  paroxysmal (*see also* Fever, hay) 477.9
  spasmodic (*see also* Fever, hay) 477.9
Rhinosalpingitis 381.50
  acute 381.51
  chronic 381.52
Rhinoscleroma 040.1
Rhinosporidiosis 117.0
Rhinovirus infection 079.3

Rhizomelic chrondrodysplasia punctata 277.86
Rhizomelique, pseudopolyarthritic 446.5
Rhoads and Bomford anemia (refractory) 238.72
Rhus
  diversiloba dermatitis 692.6
  radicans dermatitis 692.6
  toxicodendron dermatitis 692.6
  venenata dermatitis 692.6
  verniciflua dermatitis 692.6
Rhythm
  atrioventricular nodal 427.89
  disorder 427.9
    coronary sinus 427.89
    ectopic 427.89
    nodal 427.89
  escape 427.89
  heart, abnormal 427.9
    fetus or newborn—*see* Abnormal, heart rate
  idioventricular 426.89
    accelerated 427.89
  nodal 427.89
  sleep, inversion 327.39
    nonorganic origin 307.45
Rhytidosis facialis 701.8
Rib —*see also* condition
  cervical 756.2
Riboflavin deficiency 266.0
Rice bodies (*see also* Loose, body, joint) 718.1
  knee 717.6
Richter's hernia —*see* Hernia, Richter's
Ricinism 988.2
Rickets (active) (acute) (adolescent) (adult) (chest wall) (congenital) (current) (infantile) (intestinal) 268.0
  celiac 579.0
  fetal 756.4
  hemorrhagic 267
  hypophosphatemic with nephrotic-glycosuric dwarfism 270.0
  kidney 588.0
  late effect 268.1
  renal 588.0
  scurvy 267
  vitamin D-resistant 275.3
Rickettsial disease 083.9
  specified type NEC 083.8
Rickettsialpox 083.2
Rickettsiosis NEC 083.9
  specified type NEC 083.8
  tick-borne 082.9
    specified type NEC 082.8
  vesicular 083.2
Ricord's chancre 091.0
Riddoch's syndrome (visual disorientation) 368.16
Rider's
  bone 733.99
  chancre 091.0
Ridge, alveolus —*see also* condition
  edentulous
    atrophy 525.20
      mandible 525.20
        minimal 525.21
        moderate 525.22
        severe 525.23
      maxilla 525.20
        minimal 525.24
        moderate 525.25
        severe 525.26
    flabby 525.20
Ridged ear 744.29

Rupture, ruptured—*continued*
  nontraumatic 593.89
  lacrimal apparatus (traumatic) 870.2
  lens (traumatic) 366.20
  ligament—*see also* Sprain, by site
    with open wound—*see* Wound, open, by site
    old (*see also* Disorder, cartilage, articular)
      718.0
  liver (traumatic) 864.04
    with open wound into cavity 864.14
    due to birth injury 767.8
    nontraumatic 573.8
  lymphatic (node) (vessel) 457.8
  marginal sinus (placental) (with hemorrhage)
    641.2
    affecting fetus or newborn 762.1
  meaning hernia—*see* Hernia
  membrana tympani (*see also* Perforation,
    tympanum) 384.20
    with otitis media—*see* Otitis media
    traumatic—*see* Wound, open, ear
  membranes (spontaneous)
    artificial
      delayed delivery following 658.3
        affecting fetus or newborn 761.1
        fetus or newborn 761.1
    delayed delivery following 658.2
      affecting fetus or newborn 761.1
    premature (less than 24 hours prior to onset of
      labor) 658.1
      affecting fetus or newborn 761.1
      delayed delivery following 658.2
        affecting fetus or newborn 761.1
  meningeal artery (*see also* Hemorrhage,
    subarachnoid) 430
    late effect—*see* Late effect(s) (of)
      cerebrovascular disease
  meniscus (knee)—*see also* Tear, meniscus
    old (*see also* Derangement, meniscus) 717.5
      site other than knee—*see* Disorder, cartilage,
        articular
    site other than knee—*see* Sprain, by site
  mesentery 568.89
    traumatic—*see* Injury, internal, mesentery
  mitral—*see* Insufficiency, mitral
  muscle (traumatic) NEC—*see also* Sprain, by
    site
    with open wound—*see* Wound, open, by site
    nontraumatic 728.83
  musculotendinous cuff (nontraumatic)
    (shoulder) 840.4
  mycotic aneurysm, causing cerebral hemorrhage
    (*see also* Hemorrhage, subarachnoid) 430
    late effect—*see* Late effect(s) (of)
      cerebrovascular disease
  myocardium, myocardial (*see also* Infarct,
    myocardium) 410.9
    traumatic 861.03
      with open wound into thorax 861.13
  nontraumatic (meaning hernia) (*see also* Hernia,
    by site) 553.9
  obstructed (*see also* Hernia, by site, with
    obstruction) 552.9
    gangrenous (*see also* Hernia, by site, with
      gangrene) 551.9
  operation wound 998.32
    internal 998.31
  ovary, ovarian 620.8
    corpus luteum 620.1
    follicle (graafian) 620.0
  oviduct 620.8

Rupture, ruptured—*continued*
  due to pregnancy—*see* Pregnancy, tubal
  pancreas 577.8
    traumatic—*see* Injury, internal, pancreas
  papillary muscle (ventricular) 429.6
  pelvic
    floor, complicating delivery 664.1
    organ NEC—*see* Injury, pelvic, organs
  penis (traumatic)—*see* Wound, open, penis
  perineum 624.8
    during delivery (*see also* Laceration,
      perineum, complicating delivery) 664.4
  pharynx (nontraumatic) (spontaneous) 478.29
  pregnant uterus (before onset of labor) 665.0
  prostate (traumatic)—*see* Injury, internal,
    prostate
  pulmonary
    artery 417.8
    valve (heart) (*see also* Endocarditis,
      pulmonary) 424.3
    vein 417.8
    vessel 417.8
  pupil, sphincter 364.75
  pus tube (*see also* Salpingo-oophoritis) 614.2
  pyosalpinx (*see also* Salpingo-oophoritis) 614.2
  rectum 569.49
    traumatic—*see* Injury, internal, rectum
  retina, retinal (traumatic) (without detachment)
    361.30
    with detachment (*see also* Detachment, retina,
      with retinal defect) 361.00
  rotator cuff (capsule) (traumatic) 840.4
    nontraumatic, complete 727.61
  sclera 871.0
  semilunar cartilage, knee (*see also* Tear,
    meniscus) 836.2
    old (*see also* Derangement, meniscus) 717.5
  septum (cardiac) 410.8
  sigmoid 569.89
    traumatic—*see* Injury, internal, colon, sigmoid
  sinus of Valsalva 747.29
  spinal cord—*see also* Injury, spinal, by site
    due to injury at birth 767.4
    fetus or newborn 767.4
    syphilitic 094.89
    traumatic—*see also* Injury, spinal, by site
      with fracture—*see* Fracture, vertebra, by
        site, with spinal cord injury
  spleen 289.59
    congenital 767.8
    due to injury at birth 767.8
    malarial 084.9
    nontraumatic 289.59
    spontaneous 289.59
    traumatic 865.04
      with open wound into cavity 865.14
  splenic vein 459.0
  stomach 537.89
    due to injury at birth 767.8
    traumatic—*see* Injury, internal, stomach
    ulcer—*see* Ulcer, stomach, with perforation
  synovium 727.50
    specified site NEC 727.59
  tendon (traumatic)—*see also* Sprain, by site
    with open wound—*see* Wound, open, by site
    Achilles 845.09
      nontraumatic 727.67
    ankle 845.09
      nontraumatic 727.68
    biceps (long bead) 840.8
      nontraumatic 727.62

S

Saber
 shin 090.5
 tibia 090.5
Sac, lacrimal —*see* condition
Saccharomyces infection (*see also* Candidiasis)
 112.9
Saccharopinuria 270.7
Saccular —*see* condition
Sacculation
 aorta (nonsyphilitic) (*see also* Aneurysm, aorta)
  441.9
  ruptured 441.5
  syphilitic 093.0
 bladder 596.3
 colon 569.89
 intralaryngeal (congenital) (ventricular) 748.3
 larynx (congenital) (ventricular) 748.3
 organ or site, congenital—*see* Distortion
 pregnant uterus, complicating delivery 654.4
  affecting fetus or newborn 763.1
   causing obstructed labor 660.2
    affecting fetus or newborn 763.1
 rectosigmoid 569.89
 sigmoid 569.89
 ureter 593.89
 urethra 599.2
 vesical 596.3
Sachs (-Tay) disease (amaurotic familial idiocy)
 330.1
Sacks-Libman disease 710.0 *[424.91]*
Sacralgia 724.6
Sacralization
 fifth lumbar vertebra 756.15
 incomplete (vertebra) 756.15
Sacrodynia 724.6
Sacroiliac joint —*see* condition
Sacroiliitis NEC 720.2
Sacrum —*see* condition
Saddle
 back 737.8
 embolus, aorta 444.0
 nose 738.0
  congenital 754.0
  due to syphilis 090.5
Sadism (sexual) 302.84
Saemisch's ulcer 370.04
Saenger's syndrome 379.46
Sago spleen 277.39
Sailors' skin 692.74
Saint
 Anthony's fire (*see also* Erysipelas) 035
 Guy's dance—*see* Chorea
 Louis-type encephalitis 062.3
 triad (*see also* Hernia, diaphragm) 553.3
 Vitus' dance—*see* Chorea
Salicylism
 correct substance properly administered 535.4
 overdose or wrong substance given or taken 965.1
Salivary duct or gland —*see also* condition
 virus disease 078.5
Salivation (excessive) (*see also* Ptyalism) 527.7
Salmonella (aertrycke) (choleraesuis) (enteritidis)
 (gallinarum) (suipestifer) (typhimurium) (*see
 also* Infection, Salmonella) 003.9
 arthritis 003.23
 carrier (suspected) of V02.3

Salmonella—*continued*
 meningitis 003.21
 osteomyelitis 003.24
 pneumonia 003.22
 septicemia 003.1
 typhosa 002.0
  carrier (suspected) of V02.1
Salmonellosis 003.0
 with pneumonia 003.22
Salpingitis (catarrhal) (fallopian tube) (nodular)
 (pseudofollicular) (purulent) (septic) (*see also*
 Salpingo-oophoritis) 614.2
 ear 381.50
  acute 381.51
  chronic 381.52
 Eustachian (tube) 381.50
  acute 381.51
  chronic 381.52
 follicularis 614.1
 gonococcal (chronic) 098.37
  acute 098.17
 interstitial, chronic 614.1
 isthmica nodosa 614.1
 old—*see* Salpingo-oophoritis, chronic
 puerperal, postpartum, childbirth 670
 specific (chronic) 098.37
  acute 098.17
 tuberculous (acute) (chronic) (*see also*
  Tuberculosis) 016.6
 venereal (chronic) 098.37
  acute 098.17
Salpingocele 620.4
Salpingo-oophoritis (catarrhal) (purulent)
 (ruptured) (septic) (suppurative) 614.2
 acute 614.0
  with
   abortion—*see* Abortion, by type, with sepsis
   ectopic pregnancy (*see also* categories
    633.0-633.9) 639.0
   molar pregnancy (*see also* categories
    630-632) 639.0
  following
   abortion 639.0
   ectopic or molar pregnancy 639.0
  gonococcal 098.17
  puerperal, postpartum, childbirth 670
  tuberculous (*see also* Tuberculosis) 016.6
 chronic 614.1
  gonococcal 098.37
  tuberculous (*see also* Tuberculosis) 016.6
 complicating pregnancy 646.6
  affecting fetus or newborn 760.8
 gonococcal (chronic) 098.37
  acute 098.17
 old—*see* Salpingo-oophoritis, chronic
 puerperal 670
 specific—*see* Salpingo-oophoritis, gonococcal
 subacute (*see also* Salpingo-oophoritis, acute)
  614.0
 tuberculous (acute) (chronic) (*see also*
  Tuberculosis) 016.6
 venereal—*see* Salpingo-oophoritis, gonococcal
Salpingo-ovaritis (*see also* Salpingo-oophoritis)
 614.2
Salpingoperitonitis (*see also*
 Salpingo-oophoritis) 614.2

Salt-losing
  nephritis (*see also* Disease, renal) 593.9
  syndrome (*see also* Disease, renal) 593.9
Salt-rheum (*see also* Eczema) 692.9
Salzmann's nodular dystrophy 371.46
Sampson's cyst or tumor 617.1
Sandblasters'
  asthma 502
  lung 502
Sander's disease (paranoia) 297.1
Sandfly fever 066.0
Sandhoff's disease 330.1
Sanfilippo's syndrome (mucopolysaccharidosis
  III) 277.5
Sanger-Brown's ataxia 334.2
San Joaquin Valley fever 114.0
São Paulo fever or typhus 082.0
Saponification, mesenteric 567.89
Sapremia —*see* Septicemia
Sarcocele (benign)
  syphilitic 095.8
    congenital 090.5
Sarcoepiplocele (*see also* Hernia) 553.9
Sarcoepiplomphalocele (*see also* Hernia,
  umbilicus) 553.1
Sarcoid (any site) 135
  with lung involvement 135 *[517.8]*
  Boeck's 135
  Darier-Roussy 135
  Spiegler-Fendt 686.8
Sarcoidosis 135
  cardiac 135 *[425.8]*
  lung 135 *[517.8]*
Sarcoma (M8800/3)—*see also* Neoplasm,
  connective tissue, malignant
  alveolar soft part (M9581/3)—*see* Neoplasm,
    connective tissue, malignant
  ameloblastic (M9330/3) 170.1
    upper jaw (bone) 170.0
  botryoid (M8910/3)—*see* Neoplasm, connective
    tissue, malignant
  botryoides (M8910/3)—*see* Neoplasm,
    connective tissue, malignant
  cerebellar (M9480/3) 191.6
    circumscribed (arachnoidal) (M9471/3) 191.6
  circumscribed (arachnoidal) cerebellar
    (M9471/3) 191.6
  clear cell, of tendons and aponeuroses
    (M9044/3)—*see* Neoplasm, connective
    tissue, malignant
  embryonal (M8991/3)—*see* Neoplasm,
    connective tissue, malignant
  endometrial (stromal) (M8930/3) 182.0
    isthmus 182.1
  endothelial (M9130/3)—*see also* Neoplasm,
    connective tissue, malignant
    bone (M9260/3)—*see* Neoplasm, bone,
      malignant
  epithelioid cell (M8804/3)—*see* Neoplasm,
    connective tissue, malignant
  Ewing's (M9260/3)—*see* Neoplasm, bone,
    malignant
  follicular dendritic cell 202.9
  germinoblastic (diffuse) (M9632/3) 202.8
    follicular (M9697/3) 202.0
  giant cell (M8802/3)—*see also* Neoplasm,
    connective tissue, malignant
    bone (M9250/3)—*see* Neoplasm, bone,
      malignant

Sarcoma—*continued*
  glomoid (M8710/3)—*see* Neoplasm, connective
    tissue, malignant
  granulocytic (M9930/3) 205.3
  hemangioendothelial (M9130/3)—*see*
    Neoplasm, connective tissue, malignant
  hemorrhagic, multiple (M9140/3)—*see*
    Kaposi's, sarcoma
  Hodgkin's (M9662/3) 201.2
  immunoblastic (M9612/3) 200.8
  interdigitating dendritic cell 202.9
  Kaposi's (M9140/3)—*see* Kaposi's, sarcoma
  Kupffer cell (M9124/3) 155.0
  Langerhans cell 202.9
  leptomeningeal (M9530/3)—*see* Neoplasm,
    meninges, malignant
  lymphangioendothelial (M9170/3)—*see*
    Neoplasm, connective tissue, malignant
  lymphoblastic (M9630/3) 200.1
  lymphocytic (M9620/3) 200.1
  mast cell (M9740/3) 202.6
  melanotic (M8720/3)—*see* Melanoma
  meningeal (M9530/3)—*see* Neoplasm,
    meninges, malignant
  meningothelial (M9530/3)—*see* Neoplasm,
    meninges, malignant
  mesenchymal (M8800/3)—*see also* Neoplasm,
    connective tissue, malignant
    mixed (M8990/3)—*see* Neoplasm, connective
      tissue, malignant
  mesothelial (M9050/3)—*see* Neoplasm, by site,
    malignant
  monstrocellular (M9481/3)
    specified site—*see* Neoplasm, by site, malignant
    unspecified site 191.9
  myeloid (M9930/3) 205.3
  neurogenic (M9540/3)—*see* Neoplasm,
    connective tissue, malignant
  odontogenic (M9270/3) 170.1
    upper jaw (bone) 170.0
  osteoblastic (M9180/3)—*see* Neoplasm, bone,
    malignant
  osteogenic (M9180/3)—*see also* Neoplasm,
    bone, malignant
    juxtacortical (M9190/3)—*see* Neoplasm,
      bone, malignant
    periosteal (M9190/3)—*see* Neoplasm, bone,
      malignant
  periosteal (M8812/3)—*see also* Neoplasm,
    bone, malignant
    osteogenic (M9190/3)—*see* Neoplasm, bone,
      malignant
  plasma cell (M9731/3) 203.8
  pleomorphic cell (M8802/3)—*see* Neoplasm,
    connective tissue, malignant
  reticuloendothelial (M9720/3) 202.3
  reticulum cell (M9640/3) 200.0
    nodular (M9642/3) 200.0
    pleomorphic cell type (M9641/3) 200.0
  round cell (M8803/3)—*see* Neoplasm,
    connective tissue, malignant
  small cell (M8803/3)—*see* Neoplasm,
    connective tissue, malignant
  spindle cell (M8801/3)—*see* Neoplasm,
    connective tissue, malignant
  stromal (endometrial) (M8930/3) 182.0
    isthmus 182.1
  synovial (M9040/3)—*see also* Neoplasm,
    connective tissue, malignant
    biphasic type (M9043/3)—*see* Neoplasm,
      connective tissue, malignant

Sarcoma—*continued*
   epithelioid cell type (M9042/3)—*see*
      Neoplasm, connective tissue, malignant
   spindle cell type (M9041/3)—*see* Neoplasm,
      connective tissue, malignant
Sarcomatosis
  meningeal (M9539/3)—*see* Neoplasm,
    meninges, malignant
  specified site NEC (M8800/3)—*see* Neoplasm,
    connective tissue, malignant
  unspecified site (M8800/6) 171.9
Sarcosinemia 270.8
Sarcosporidiosis 136.5
Satiety, early 780.94
Saturnine —*see* condition
Saturnism 984.9
  specified type of lead—*see* Table of drugs and
    chemicals
Satyriasis 302.89
Sauriasis —*see* Ichthyosis
Sauriderma 757.39
Sauriosis —*see* Ichthyosis
Savill's disease (epidemic exfoliative dermatitis)
    695.89
SBE (subacute bacterial endocarditis) 421.0
Scabies (any site) 133.0
Scabs 782.8
Scaglietti-Dagnini syndrome (acromegalic
    macrospondylitis) 253.0
Scald, scalded —*see also* Burn, by site
  skin syndrome 695.1
Scalenus anticus (anterior) syndrome 353.0
Scales 782.8
Scalp —*see* condition
Scaphocephaly 756.0
Scaphoiditis, tarsal 732.5
Scapulalgia 733.90
Scapulohumeral myopathy 359.1
Scar, scarring (*see also* Cicatrix) 709.2
  adherent 709.2
  atrophic 709.2
  cervix
    in pregnancy or childbirth 654.6
      affecting fetus or newborn 763.89
      causing obstructed labor 660.2
        affecting fetus or newborn 763.1
  cheloid 701.4
  chorioretinal 363.30
    disseminated 363.35
    macular 363.32
    peripheral 363.34
    posterior pole NEC 363.33
  choroid (*see also* Scar, chorioretinal) 363.30
  compression, pericardial 423.9
  congenital 757.39
  conjunctiva 372.64
  cornea 371.00
    xerophthalmic 264.6
  due to previous cesarean delivery, complicating
    pregnancy or childbirth 654.2
    affecting fetus or newborn 763.89
  duodenal (bulb) (cap) 537.3
  hypertrophic 701.4
  keloid 701.4
  labia 624.4
  lung (base) 518.89
  macula 363.32
    disseminated 363.35
    peripheral 363.34
  muscle 728.89

Scar, scarring—*continued*
  myocardium, myocardial 412
  painful 709.2
  papillary muscle 429.81
  posterior pole NEC 363.33
    macular—*see* Scar, macula
  postnecrotic (hepatic) (liver) 571.9
  psychic V15.49
  retina (*see also* Scar, chorioretinal) 363.30
  trachea 478.9
  uterus 621.8
    in pregnancy or childbirth NEC 654.9
      affecting fetus or newborn 763.89
      due to previous cesarean delivery 654.2
  vulva 624.4
Scarabiasis 134.1
Scarlatina 034.1
  anginosa 034.1
  maligna 034.1
  myocarditis, acute 034.1 *[422.0]*
    old (*see also* Myocarditis) 429.0
  otitis media 034.1 *[382.02]*
  ulcerosa 034.1
Scarlatinella 057.8
Scarlet fever (albuminuria) (angina)
    (convulsions) (lesions of lid) (rash) 034.1
Schamberg's disease, dermatitis, or dermatosis
    (progressive pigmentary dermatosis) 709.09
Schatzki's ring (esophagus) (lower) (congenital)
    750.3
  acquired 530.3
Schaufenster krankheit 413.9
Schaumann's
  benign lymphogranulomatosis 135
  disease (sarcoidosis) 135
  syndrome (sarcoidosis) 135
Scheie's syndrome (mucopolysaccharidosis IS)
    277.5
Schenck's disease (sporotrichosis) 117.1
Scheuermann's disease or osteochondrosis
    732.0
Scheuthauer-Marie-Sainton syndrome
    (cleidocranialis dysostosis) 755.59
Schilder (-Flatau) disease 341.1
Schilling-type monocytic leukemia (M9890/3)
    206.9
**Schimmelbusch's disease, cystic mastitis, or hy-
    perplasia** 610.1
Schirmer's syndrome (encephalocutaneous
    angiomatosis) 759.6
Schistocelia 756.79
Schistoglossia 750.13
Schistosoma infestation —*see* Infestation,
    Schistosoma
Schistosomiasis 120.9
  Asiatic 120.2
  bladder 120.0
  chestermani 120.8
  colon 120.1
  cutaneous 120.3
  due to
    S. hematobium 120.0
    S. japonicum 120.2
    S. mansoni 120.1
    S. mattheii 120.8
  eastern 120.2
  genitourinary tract 120.0
  intestinal 120.1
  lung 120.2
  Manson's (intestinal) 120.1

> *Note—Use the following fifth-digit*
> *subclassification with category 295:*
>
> *0 unspecified*
> *1 subchronic*
> *2 chronic*
> *3 subchronic with acute exacerbation*
> *4 chronic with acute exacerbation*
> *5 in remission*

Sclerosis, sclerotic—*continued*
  lobar, atrophic (of brain) 331.0
    with dementia
      with behavioral disturbance 331.0 *[294.11]*
      without behavioral disturbance 331.0 *[294.10]*
  lung (*see also* Fibrosis, lung) 515
  mastoid 383.1
  mitral—*see* Endocarditis, mitral
  Mönckeberg's (medial) (*see also*
    Arteriosclerosis, extremities) 440.20
  multiple (brain stem) (cerebral) (generalized)
    (spinal cord) 340
  myocardium, myocardial —*see*
    Arteriosclerosis, coronary
  nuclear (senile), eye 366.16
  ovary 620.8
  pancreas 577.8
  penis 607.89
  peripheral arteries NEC (*see also*
    Arteriosclerosis, extremities) 440.20
  plaques 340
  pluriglandular 258.8
  polyglandular 258.8
  posterior (spinal cord) (syphilitic) 094.0
  posterolateral (spinal cord)—*see* Degeneration,
    combined
  prepuce 607.89
  primary lateral 335.24
  progressive systemic 710.1
  pulmonary (*see also* Fibrosis, lung) 515
    artery 416.0
    valve (heart) (*see also* Endocarditis,
      pulmonary) 424.3
  renal 587
    with
      cystine storage disease 270.0
      hypertension (*see also* Hypertension,
        kidney) 403.90
      hypertensive heart disease (conditions
        classifiable to 402) (*see also*
        Hypertension, cardiorenal) 404.90
      arteriolar (hyaline) (*see also* Hypertension,
        kidney) 403.90
      hyperplastic (*see also* Hypertension, kidney)
        403.90
  retina (senile) (vascular) 362.17
  rheumatic
    aortic valve 395.9
    mitral valve 394.9
  Schilder's 341.1
  senile—*see* Arteriosclerosis
  spinal (cord) (general) (progressive) (transverse)
    336.8
    ascending 357.0
    combined—*see also* Degeneration, combined
      multiple 340
      syphilitic 094.89
    disseminated 340
    dorsolateral—*see* Degeneration, combined
    hereditary (Friedreich's) (mixed form) 334.0
    lateral (amyotrophic) 335.24
    multiple 340
    posterior (syphilitic) 094.0
  stomach 537.89
  subendocardial, congenital 425.3
  systemic (progressive) 710.1
    with lung involvement 710.1 *[517.2]*
  tricuspid (heart) (valve)—*see* Endocarditis,
    tricuspid
  tuberous (brain) 759.5

Sclerosis, sclerotic—*continued*
  tympanic membrane (*see also*
    Tympanosclerosis) 385.00
  valve, valvular (heart)—*see* Endocarditis
  vascular—*see* Arteriosclerosis
  vein 459.89
Sclerotenonitis 379.07
Sclerotitis (*see also* Scleritis) 379.00
  syphilitic 095.0
  tuberculous (*see also* Tuberculosis) 017.3
    [379.09]
Scoliosis (acquired) (postural) 737.30
  congenital 754.2
  due to or associated with
    Charcot-Marie-Tooth disease 356.1 *[737.43]*
    mucopolysaccharidosis 277.5 *[737.43]*
    neurofibromatosis 237.71 *[737.43]*
    osteitis
      deformans 731.0 *[737.43]*
      fibrosa cystica 252.01 *[737.43]*
    osteoporosis (*see also* Osteoporosis) 733.00
      [737.43]
    poliomyelitis 138 *[737.43]*
    radiation 737.33
    tuberculosis (*see also* Tuberculosis) 015.0
      [737.43]
  idiopathic 737.30
    infantile
      progressive 737.32
      resolving 737.31
  paralytic 737.39
  rachitic 268.1
  sciatic 724.3
  specified NEC 737.39
  thoracogenic 737.34
  tuberculous (*see also* Tuberculosis) 015.0
    [737.43]
Scoliotic pelvis 738.6
  with disproportion (fetopelvic) 653.0
    affecting fetus or newborn 763.1
    causing obstructed labor 660.1
      affecting fetus or newborn 763.1
Scorbutus, scorbutic 267
  anemia 281.8
Scotoma (ring) 368.44
  arcuate 368.43
  Bjerrum 368.43
  blind spot area 368.42
  central 368.41
  centrocecal 368.41
  paracecal 368.42
  paracentral 368.41
  scintillating 368.12
  Seidel 368.43
Scratch —*see* Injury, superficial, by site
Screening (for) V82.9
  alcoholism V79.1
  anemia, deficiency NEC V78.1
    iron V78.0
  anomaly, congenital V82.89
  antenatal, of mother V28.9
    alphafetoprotein levels, raised V28.1
    based on amniocentesis V28.2
      chromosomal anomalies V28.0
      raised alphafetoprotein levels V28.1
    fetal growth retardation using ultrasonics
      V28.4
    isoimmunization V28.5
    malformations using ultrasonics V28.3
    raised alphafetoprotein levels V28.1
    specified condition NEC V28.8

Seckel's syndrome 759.89
Seclusion pupil 364.74
Seclusiveness, child 313.22
Secondary —*see also* condition
    neoplasm—*see* Neoplasm, by site, malignant,
        secondary
Secretan's disease or syndrome (posttraumatic
    edema) 782.3
Secretion
    antidiuretic hormone, inappropriate (syndrome)
        253.6
    catecholamine, by pheochromocytoma 255.6
    hormone
        antidiuretic, inappropriate (syndrome) 253.6
        by
            carcinoid tumor 259.2
            pheochromocytoma 255.6
        ectopic NEC 259.3
    urinary
        excessive 788.42
        suppression 788.5
Section
    cesarean
        affecting fetus or newborn 763.4
        post mortem, affecting fetus or newborn 761.6
        previous, in pregnancy or childbirth 654.2
            affecting fetus or newborn 763.89
    nerve, traumatic—*see* Injury, nerve, by site
Seeligmann's syndrome (ichthyosis congenita)
    757.1
Segmentation, incomplete (congenital)—*see*
        also Fusion
    bone NEC 756.9
    lumbosacral (joint) 756.15
    vertebra 756.15
        lumbosacral 756.15
Seizure 780.39
    akinetic (idiopathic) (*see also* Epilepsy) 345.0
        psychomotor 345.4
    apoplexy, apoplectic (*see also* Disease,
        cerebrovascular, acute) 436
    atonic (*see also* Epilepsy) 345.0
    autonomic 300.11
    brain or cerebral (*see also* Disease,
        cerebrovascular, acute) 436
    convulsive (*see also* Convulsions) 780.39
    cortical (focal) (motor) (*see also* Epilepsy) 345.5
    epilepsy, epileptic (cryptogenic) (*see also*
        Epilepsy) 345.9
    epileptiform, epileptoid 780.39
        focal (*see also* Epilepsy) 345.5
    febrile (simple) 780.31
        atypical 780.32
        complex 780.32
        complicated 780.32
        with status epilepticus 345.3
    heart—*see* Disease, heart
    hysterical 300.11
    Jacksonian (focal) (*see also* Epilepsy) 345.5
        motor type 345.5
        sensory type 345.5
    newborn 779.0
    paralysis (*see also* Disease, cerebrovascular,
        acute) 436
    recurrent 345.9
        epileptic—*see* Epilepsy
    repetitive 780.39
        epileptic—*see* Epilepsy
    salaam (*see also* Epilepsy) 345.6
    uncinate (*see also* Epilepsy) 345.4
Self-mutilation 300.9
Semicoma 780.09

Semiconsciousness 780.09
Seminal
    vesicle—*see* condition
    vesiculitis (*see also* Vesiculitis) 608.0
Seminoma (M9061/3)
    anaplastic type (M9062/3)
        specified site—*see* Neoplasm, by site,
            malignant
        unspecified site 186.9
    specified site—*see* Neoplasm, by site, malignant
    spermatocytic (M9063/3)
        specified site—*see* Neoplasm, by site,
            malignant
        unspecified site 186.9
    unspecified site 186.9
Semliki Forest encephalitis 062.8
Senear-Usher disease or syndrome (pemphigus
    erythematosus) 694.4
Senecio jacobae dermatitis 692.6
Senectus 797
Senescence 797
Senile (*see also* condition) 797
    cervix (atrophic) 622.8
    degenerative atrophy, skin 701.3
    endometrium (atrophic) 621.8
    fallopian tube (atrophic) 620.3
    heart (failure) 797
    lung 492.8
    ovary (atrophic) 620.3
    syndrome 259.8
    vagina, vaginitis (atrophic) 627.3
    wart 702.0
Senility 797
    with
        acute confusional state 290.3
        delirium 290.3
        mental changes 290.9
        psychosis NEC (*see also* Psychosis, senile)
            290.20
    premature (syndrome) 259.8
Sensation
    burning (*see also* Disturbance, sensation) 782.0
        tongue 529.6
    choking 784.99
    loss of (*see also* Disturbance, sensation) 782.0
    prickling (*see also* Disturbance, sensation) 782.0
    tingling (*see also* Disturbance, sensation) 782.0
Sense loss (touch) (*see also* Disturbance,
    sensation) 782.0
    smell 781.1
    taste 781.1
Sensibility disturbance NEC (cortical) (deep)
    (vibratory) (*see also* Disturbance, sensation)
    782.0
Sensitive dentine 521.89
Sensitiver Beziehungswahn 297.8
Sensitivity, sensitization —*see also* Allergy
    autoerythrocyte 287.2
    carotid sinus 337.0
    child (excessive) 313.21
    cold, autoimmune 283.0
    methemoglobin 289.7
    suxamethonium 289.89
    tuberculin, without clinical or radiological
        symptoms 795.5
Sensory
    extinction 781.8
    neglect 781.8
Separation
    acromioclavicular—see Dislocation, shoulder
    anxiety, abnormal 309.21

Separation—*continued*
 apophysis, traumatic—*see* Fracture, by site
 choroid 363.70
  hemorrhagic 363.72
  serous 363.71
 costochondral (simple) (traumatic)—*see*
   Dislocation, costochondral
 delayed
  umbilical cord 779.83
 epiphysis, epiphyseal
  nontraumatic 732.9
   upper femoral 732.2
  traumatic—*see* Fracture, by site
 fracture—*see* Fracture, by site
 infundibulum cardiac from right ventricle by a
   partition 746.83
 joint (current) (traumatic)—*see* Dislocation, by
   site
 placenta (normally implanted)—*see* Placenta,
   separation
 pubic bone, obstetrical trauma 665.6
 retina, retinal (*see also* Detachment, retina)
   361.9
  layers 362.40
   sensory (*see also* Retinoschisis) 361.10
  pigment epithelium (exudative) 362.42
   hemorrhagic 362.43
 sternoclavicular (traumatic)—*see* Dislocation,
   sternoclavicular
 symphysis pubis, obstetrical trauma 665.6
 tracheal ring, incomplete (congenital) 748.3
Sepsis (generalized) 995.91
 with
  abortion—*see* Abortion, by type, with sepsis
  acute organ dysfunction 995.92
  ectopic pregnancy (*see also* categories
    633.0-633.9) 639.0
  molar pregnancy (*see also* categories 630-632)
    639.0
  multiple organ dysfunction (MOD) 995.92
 buccal 528.3
 complicating labor 659.3
 dental (pulpal origin) 522.4
 female genital organ NEC 614.9
 fetus (intrauterine) 771.81
 following
  abortion 639.0
  ectopic or molar pregnancy 639.0
  infusion, perfusion, or transfusion 999.3
 Friedländer's 038.49
 intraocular 360.00
 localized
  in operation wound 998.59
  skin (*see also* Abscess) 682.9
 malleus 024
 newborn (organism unspecified) NEC 771.81
 oral 528.3
 puerperal, postpartum, childbirth (pelvic) 670
 resulting from infusion, injection, transfusion, or
   vaccination 999.3
 severe 995.92
 skin, localized (*see also* Abscess) 682.9
 umbilical (newborn) (organism unspecified)
   771.89
  tetanus 771.3
 urinary 599.0
  meaning sepsis 995.91
  meaning urinary tract infection 599.0
Septate —*see also* Septum

Septic —*see also* condition
 adenoids 474.01
  and tonsils 474.02
 arm (with lymphangitis) 682.3
 embolus—*see* Embolism
 finger (with lymphangitis) 681.00
 foot (with lymphangitis) 682.7
 gallbladder (*see also* Cholecystitis) 575.8
 hand (with lymphangitis) 682.4
 joint (*see also* Arthritis, septic) 711.0
 kidney (*see also* Infection, kidney) 590.9
 leg (with lymphangitis) 682.6
 mouth 528.3
 nail 681.9
  finger 681.02
  toe 681.11
 shock (endotoxic) 785.52
 sore (*see also* Abscess) 682.9
  throat 034.0
   milk-borne 034.0
   streptococcal 034.0
 spleen (acute) 289.59
 teeth (pulpal origin) 522.4
 throat 034.0
 thrombus—*see* Thrombosis
 toe (with lymphangitis) 681.10
 tonsils 474.00
  and adenoids 474.02
 umbilical cord (newborn) (organism
   unspecified) 771.89
 uterus (*see also* Endometritis) 615.9
Septicemia, septicemic (generalized)
   (suppurative) 038.9
 with
  abortion—*see* Abortion, by type, with sepsis
  ectopic pregnancy (*see also* categories
    633.0-633.9) 639.0
  molar pregnancy (*see also* categories 630-632)
    639.0
 Aerobacter aerogenes 038.49
 anaerobic 038.3
 anthrax 022.3
 Bacillus coli 038.42
 Bacteroides 038.3
 Clostridium 038.3
 complicating labor 659.3
 cryptogenic 038.9
 enteric gram-negative bacilli 038.40
 Enterobacter aerogenes 038.49
 Erysipelothrix (insidiosa) (rhusiopathiae) 027.1
 Escherichia coli 038.42
 following
  abortion 639.0
  ectopic or molar pregnancy 639.0
  infusion, injection, transfusion, or vaccination
    999.3
 Friedländer's (bacillus) 038.49
 gangrenous 038.9
 gonococcal 098.89
 gram-negative (organism) 038.40
  anaerobic 038.3
 Hemophilus influenzae 038.41
 herpes (simplex) 054.5
 herpetic 054.5
 Listeria monocytogenes 027.0
 meningeal—*see* Meningitis
 meningococcal (chronic) (fulminating) 036.2
 navel, newborn (organism unspecified) 771.89
 newborn (organism unspecified) 771.81
 plague 020.2
 pneumococcal 038.2

Septicemia, septicemic—*continued*
  postabortal 639.0
  postoperative 998.59
  Proteus vulgaris 038.49
  Pseudomonas (aeruginosa) 038.43
  puerperal, postpartum 670
  Salmonella (aertrycke) (callinarum)
      (choleraesuis) (enteritidis) (suipestifer) 003.1
  Serratia 038.44
  Shigella (*see also* Dysentery, bacillary) 004.9
  specified organism NEC 038.8
  staphylococcal 038.10
    aureus 038.11
    specified organism NEC 038.19
  streptococcal (anaerobic) 038.0
  suipestifer 003.1
  umbilicus, newborn (organism unspecified)
      771.89
  viral 079.99
  Yersinia enterocolitica 038.49
Septum, septate (congenital)—*see also*
      Anomaly, specified type NEC
  anal 751.2
  aqueduct of Sylvius 742.3
    with spina bifida (*see also* Spina bifida) 741.0
  hymen 752.49
  uterus (*see also* Double, uterus) 752.2
  vagina 752.49
    in pregnancy or childbirth 654.7
      affecting fetus or newborn 763.89
      causing obstructed labor 660.2
        affecting fetus or newborn 763.1
Sequestration
  lung (congenital) (extralobar) (intralobar) 748.5
  orbit 376.10
  pulmonary artery (congenital) 747.3
  splenic 289.52
Sequestrum
  bone (*see also* Osteomyelitis) 730.1
    jaw 526.4
  dental 525.8
  jaw bone 526.4
  sinus (accessory) (nasal) (*see also* Sinusitis)
      473.9
    maxillary 473.0
Sequoiosis asthma 495.8
Serology for syphilis
  doubtful
    with signs or symptoms—*see* Syphilis, by site
      and stage
    follow-up of latent syphilis—*see* Syphilis,
      latent
  false positive 795.6
  negative, with signs or symptoms—*see* Syphilis,
      by site and stage
  positive 097.1
    with signs or symptoms—*see* Syphilis, by site
      and stage
    false 795.6
    follow-up of latent syphilis—*see* Syphilis,
      latent
    only finding—*see* Syphilis, latent
  reactivated 097.1
Seroma (postoperative) (non-infected) 998.13
  infected 998.51
Seropurulent —*see* condition
Serositis, multiple 569.89
  pericardial 423.2
  peritoneal 568.82
  pleural—*see* Pleurisy
Serotonin syndrome 333.99
Serous —*see* condition

Sertoli cell
  adenoma (M8640/0)
    specified site—*see* Neoplasm, by site, benign
    unspecified site
      female 220
      male 222.0
  carcinoma (M8640/3)
    specified site—*see* Neoplasm, by site,
      malignant
    unspecified site 186.9
  syndrome (germinal aplasia) 606.0
  tumor (M8640/0)
    with lipid storage (M8641/0)
      specified site—*see* Neoplasm, by site,
        benign
      unspecified site
        female 220
        male 222.0
    specified site—*see* Neoplasm, by site, benign
    unspecified site
      female 220
      male 222.0
Sertoli-Leydig cell tumor (M8631/0)
  specified site—*see* Neoplasm, by site, benign
  unspecified site
    female 220
    male 222.0
Serum
  allergy, allergic reaction 999.5
    shock 999.4
  arthritis 999.5 *[713.6]*
  complication or reaction NEC 999.5
  disease NEC 999.5
  hepatitis 070.3
  intoxication 999.5
  jaundice (homologous) *see* Hepatitis, viral
  neuritis 999.5
  poisoning NEC 999.5
  rash NEC 999.5
  reaction NEC 999.5
  sickness NEC 999.5
Sesamoiditis 733.99
Seven-day fever 061
  of
    Japan 100.89
    Queensland 100.89
Sever's disease or osteochondrosis (calcaneum)
    732.5
Sex chromosome mosaics 758.81
Sextuplet
  affected by maternal complications of pregnancy
      761.5
  healthy liveborn—*see* Newborn, multiple
  pregnancy (complicating delivery) NEC 651.8
    with fetal loss and retention of one or more
        fetus(es) 651.6
    following (elective) fetal reduction 651.7
Sexual
  anesthesia 302.72
  deviation (*see also* Deviation, sexual) 302.9
  disorder (*see also* Deviation, sexual) 302.9
  frigidity (female) 302.72
  function, disorder of (psychogenic) 302.70
    specified type NEC 302.79
  immaturity (female) (male) 259.0
  impotence 607.84
    organic origin NEC 607.84
    psychogenic 302.72
  precocity (constitutional) (cryptogenic) (female)
      (idiopathic) (male) NEC 259.1
    with adrenal hyperplasia 255.2
  sadism 302.84

Sexuality, pathological (*see also* Deviation,
    sexual) 302.9
Sézary's disease , reticulosis, or syndrome
    (M9701/3) 202.2
Shadow, lung 793.1
Shaken infant syndrome 995.55
Shaking
    head (tremor) 781.0
    palsy or paralysis (*see also* Parkinsonism) 332.0
Shallowness, acetabulum 736.39
Shaver's disease or syndrome (bauxite
    pneumoconiosis) 503
Shearing
    artificial skin graft 996.55
    decellularized allodermis graft 996.55
Sheath (tendon)—*see* condition
Shedding
    nail 703.8
    teeth, premature, primary (deciduous) 520.6
Sheehan's disease or syndrome (postpartum
    pituitary necrosis) 253.2
Shelf, rectal 569.49
Shell
    shock (current) (*see also* Reaction, stress, acute)
        308.9
        lasting state 300.16
    teeth 520.5
Shield kidney 753.3
Shift, mediastinal 793.2
Shifting
    pacemaker 427.89
    sleep-work schedule (affecting sleep) 327.36
Shiga's
    bacillus 004.0
    dysentery 004.0
Shigella (dysentery) (*see also* Dysentery,
    bacillary) 004.9
    carrier (suspected) of V02.3
Shigellosis (*see also* Dysentery, bacillary) 004.9
Shingles (*see also* Herpes, zoster) 053.9
    eye NEC 053.29
Shin splints 844.9
Shipyard eye or disease 077.1
Shirodkar suture, in pregnancy 654.5
Shock 785.50
    with
        abortion—*see* Abortion, by type, with shock
        ectopic pregnancy (*see also* categories
            633.0-633.9) 639.5
        molar pregnancy (*see also* categories 630-632)
            639.5
    allergic—*see* Shock, anaphylactic
    anaclitic 309.21
    anaphylactic 995.0
        chemical—*see* Table of drugs and chemicals
        correct medicinal substance properly
            administered 995.0
        drug or medicinal substance
            correct substance properly administered
                995.0
            overdose or wrong substance given or taken
                977.9
            specified drug—*see* Table of drugs and
                chemicals
        food—*see* Anaphylactic shock, due to, food
        following sting(s) 989.5
        immunization 999.4
        serum 999.4
    anaphylactoid—*see* Shock, anaphylactic
    anesthetic

Shock—*continued*
    correct substance properly administered 995.4
    overdose or wrong substance given 968.4
        specified anesthetic—*see* Table of drugs and
            chemicals
    birth, fetus or newborn NEC 779.89
    cardiogenic 785.51
    chemical substance—*see* Table of drugs and
        chemicals
    circulatory 785.59
    complicating
        abortion—*see* Abortion, by type, with shock
        ectopic pregnancy (*see also* categories
            633.0-633.9) 639.5
        labor and delivery 669.1
        molar pregnancy (*see also* categories 630-632)
            639.5
    culture 309.29
    due to
        drug 995.0
            correct substance properly administered
                995.0
            overdose or wrong substance given or taken
                977.9
            specified drug—*see* Table of drugs and
                chemicals
        food—*see* Anaphylactic shock, due to, food
    during labor and delivery 669.1
    electric 994.8
    endotoxic 785.52
        due to surgical procedure 998.0
    following
        abortion 639.5
        ectopic or molar pregnancy 639.5
        injury (immediate) (delayed) 958.4
        labor and delivery 669.1
    gram-negative 785.52
    hematogenic 785.59
    hemorrhagic
        due to
            disease 785.59
            surgery (intraoperative) (postoperative)
                998.0
            trauma 958.4
    hypovolemic NEC 785.59
        surgical 998.0
        traumatic 958.4
    insulin 251.0
        therapeutic misadventure 962.3
    kidney 584.5
        traumatic (following crushing) 958.5
    lightning 994.0
    lung 518.5
    nervous (*see also* Reaction, stress, acute) 308.9
    obstetric 669.1
        with
            abortion—*see* Abortion, by type, with shock
            ectopic pregnancy (*see also* categories
                633.0-633.9) 639.5
            molar pregnancy (*see also* categories
                630-632) 639.5
        following
            abortion 639.5
            ectopic or molar pregnancy 639.5
    paralysis, paralytic (*see also* Disease,
        cerebrovascular, acute) 436
        late effect—*see* Late effect(s) (of)
            cerebrovascular disease
    pleural (surgical) 998.0
        due to trauma 958.4
    postoperative 998.0

Shock—*continued*
  with
    abortion—*see* Abortion, by type, with shock
    ectopic pregnancy (*see also* categories
      633.0-633.9) 639.5
    molar pregnancy (*see also* categories
      630-632) 639.5
    following
      abortion 639.5
      ectopic or molar pregnancy 639.5
  psychic (*see also* Reaction, stress, acute) 308.9
    past history (of) V15.49
  psychogenic (*see also* Reaction, stress, acute)
    308.9
  septic 785.52
    with
      abortion—*see* Abortion, by type, with shock
      ectopic pregnancy (*see also* categories
        633.0-633.9) 639.5
      molar pregnancy (*see also* categories
        630-632) 639.5
    due to
      surgical procedure 998.0
      transfusion NEC 999.8
        bone marrow 996.85
    following
      abortion 639.5
      ectopic or molar pregnancy 639.5
      surgical procedure 998.0
      transfusion NEC 999.8
        bone marrow 996.85
  spinal—*see also* Injury, spinal, by site
    with spinal bone injury—*see* Fracture,
      vertebra, by site, with spinal cord injury
  surgical 998.0
  therapeutic misadventure NEC (*see also*
    Complications) 998.89
  thyroxin 962.7
  toxic 040.82
  transfusion—*see* Complications, transfusion
  traumatic (immediate) (delayed) 958.4
Shoemakers' chest 738.3
Short, shortening, shortness
  Achilles tendon (acquired) 727.81
  arm 736.89
    congenital 755.20
  back 737.9
  bowel syndrome 579.3
  breath 786.05
  chain acyl CoA dehydrogenase deficiency
    (SCAD) 277.85
  common bile duct, congenital 751.69
  cord (umbilical) 663.4
    affecting fetus or newborn 762.6
  cystic duct, congenital 751.69
  esophagus (congenital) 750.4
  femur (acquired) 736.81
    congenital 755.34
  frenulum linguae 750.0
  frenum, lingual 750.0
  hamstrings 727.81
  hip (acquired) 736.39
    congenital 755.63
  leg (acquired) 736.81
    congenital 755.30
  metatarsus (congenital) 754.79
    acquired 736.79
  organ or site, congenital NEC—*see* Distortion
  palate (congenital) 750.26
  P-R interval syndrome 426.81
  radius (acquired) 736.09

Short, shortening, shortness—*continued*
  congenital 755.26
  round ligament 629.89
  sleeper 307.49
  stature, constitutional (hereditary) 783.43
  tendon 727.81
    Achilles (acquired) 727.81
      congenital 754.79
    congenital 756.89
  thigh (acquired) 736.81
    congenital 755.34
  tibialis anticus 727.81
  umbilical cord 663.4
    affecting fetus or newborn 762.6
  urethra 599.84
  uvula (congenital) 750.26
  vagina 623.8
Shortsightedness 367.1
Shoshin (acute fulminating beriberi) 265.0
Shoulder —*see* condition
Shovel-shaped incisors 520.2
Shower, thromboembolic —*see* Embolism
Shunt (status)
  aortocoronary bypass V45.81
  arterial-venous (dialysis) V45.1
  arteriovenous, pulmonary (acquired) 417.0
    congenital 747.3
    traumatic (complication) 901.40
  cerebral ventricle (communicating) in situ V45.2
  coronary artery bypass V45.81
  surgical, prosthetic, with complications—*see*
    Complications, shunt
  vascular NEC V45.89
Shutdown
  renal 586
    with
      abortion—*see* Abortion, by type, with renal
        failure
      ectopic pregnancy (*see also* categories
        633.0-633.9) 639.3
      molar pregnancy (*see also* categories
        630-632) 639.3
    complicating
      abortion 639.3
      ectopic or molar pregnancy 639.3
    following labor and delivery 669.3
Shwachman's syndrome 288.02
Shy-Drager syndrome (orthostatic hypotension
  with multisystem degeneration) 333.0
Sialadenitis (any gland) (chronic) (suppurative)
  527.2
  epidemic—*see* Mumps
Sialadenosis, periodic 527.2
Sialaporia 527.7
Sialectasia 527.8
Sialitis 527.2
Sialoadenitis (*see also* Sialadenitis) 527.2
Sialoangitis 527.2
Sialodochitis (fibrinosa) 527.2
Sialodocholithiasis 527.5
Sialolithiasis 527.5
Sialorrhea (*see also* Ptyalism) 527.7
  periodic 527.2
Sialosis 527.8
  rheumatic 710.2
Siamese twin 759.4
Sicard's syndrome 352.6
Sicca syndrome (keratoconjunctivitis) 710.2
Sick 799.9
  cilia syndrome 759.89
  or handicapped person in family V61.49

Sickle-cell
  anemia (*see also* Disease, sickle-cell) 282.60
  disease (*see also* Disease, sickle-cell) 282.60
  hemoglobin
    C disease (without crisis) 282.63
      with
        crisis 282.64
        vaso-occlusive pain 282.64
    D disease (without crisis) 282.68
      with crisis 282.69
    E disease (without crisis) 282.68
      with crisis 282.69
    thalassemia (without crisis) 282.41
      with
        crisis 282.42
        vaso-occlusive pain 282.42
  trait 282.5
Sicklemia (*see also* Disease, sickle-cell) 282.60
  trait 282.5
Sickness
  air (travel) 994.6
  airplane 994.6
  alpine 993.2
  altitude 993.2
  Andes 993.2
  aviators' 993.2
  balloon 993.2
  car 994.6
  compressed air 993.3
  decompression 993.3
  green 280.9
  harvest 100.89
  milk 988.8
  morning 643.0
  motion 994.6
  mountain 993.2
    acute 289.0
  protein (*see also* Complications, vaccination) 999.5
  radiation NEC 990
  roundabout (motion) 994.6
  sea 994.6
  serum NEC 999.5
  sleeping (African) 086.5
    by Trypanosoma 086.5
      gambiense 086.3
      rhodesiense 086.4
    Gambian 086.3
    late effect 139.8
    Rhodesian 086.4
  sweating 078.2
  swing (motion) 994.6
  train (railway) (travel) 994.6
  travel (any vehicle) 994.6
Sick sinus syndrome 427.81
Sideropenia (*see also* Anemia, iron deficiency) 280.9
Siderosis (lung) (occupational) 503
  cornea 371.15
  eye (bulbi) (vitreous) 360.23
  lens 360.23
Siegal-Cattan-Mamou disease (periodic) 277.31
Siemens' syndrome
  ectodermal dysplasia 757.31
  keratosis follicularis spinulosa (decalvans) 757.39
Sighing respiration 786.7
Sigmoid
  flexure—*see* condition
  kidney 753.3
Sigmoiditis —*see* Enteritis
Silfverskiöld's syndrome 756.50

Silicosis, sillicotic (complicated) (occupational) (simple) 502
  fibrosis, lung (confluent) (massive) (occupational) 502
  non-nodular 503
  pulmonum 502
Silicotuberculosis (*see also* Tuberculosis) 011.4
Silo fillers' disease 506.9
Silver's syndrome (congenital hemihypertrophy and short stature) 759.89
Silver wire arteries, retina 362.13
Silvestroni-Bianco syndrome (thalassemia minima) 282.49
Simian crease 757.2
Simmonds' cachexia or disease (pituitary cachexia) 253.2
Simons' disease or syndrome (progressive lipodystrophy) 272.6
Simple, simplex —*see* condition
Sinding-Larsen disease (juvenile osteopathia patellae) 732.4
Singapore hemorrhagic fever 065.4
Singers' node or nodule 478.5
Single
  atrium 745.69
  coronary artery 746.85
  umbilical artery 747.5
  ventricle 745.3
Singultus 786.8
  epidemicus 078.89
Sinus —*see also* Fistula
  abdominal 569.81
  arrest 426.6
  arrhythmia 427.89
  bradycardia 427.89
    chronic 427.81
  branchial cleft (external) (internal) 744.41
  coccygeal (infected) 685.1
    with abscess 685.0
  dental 522.7
  dermal (congenital) 685.1
    with abscess 685.0
  draining—*see* Fistula
  infected, skin NEC 686.9
  marginal, ruptured or bleeding 641.2
    affecting fetus or newborn 762.1
  pause 426.6
  pericranii 742.0
  pilonidal (infected) (rectum) 685.1
    with abscess 685.0
  preauricular 744.46
  rectovaginal 619.1
  sacrococcygeal (dermoid) (infected) 685.1
    with abscess 685.0
  skin
    infected NEC 686.9
    noninfected—*see* Ulcer, skin
  tachycardia 427.89
  tarsi syndrome 726.79
  testis 608.89
  tract (postinfectional)—*see* Fistula
  urachus 753.7
Sinuses, Rokitansky-Aschoff (*see also* Disease, gallbladder) 575.8
Sinusitis (accessory) (nasal) (hyperplastic) (nonpurulent) (purulent) (chronic) 473.9
  with influenza, flu, or grippe 487.1
  acute 461.9
    ethmoidal 461.2
    frontal 461.1

Small, smallness—*continued*
infant, term 764.0
with malnutrition 764.1
affecting management of pregnancy 656.5
introitus, vagina 623.3
kidney, unknown cause 589.9
bilateral 589.1
unilateral 589.0
ovary 620.8
pelvis
with disproportion (fetopelvic) 653.1
affecting fetus or newborn 763.1
causing obstructed labor 660.1
affecting fetus or newborn 763.1
placenta—*see* Placenta, insufficiency
uterus 621.8
white kidney 582.9
Small-for-dates (*see also* Light-for-dates) 764.0
affecting management of pregnancy 656.5
Smallpox 050.9
contact V01.3
exposure to V01.3
hemorrhagic (pustular) 050.0
malignant 050.0
modified 050.2
vaccination
complications—*see* Complications,
vaccination
prophylactic (against) V04.1
Smith's fracture (separation) (closed) 813.41
open 813.51
Smith-Lemli-Opitz syndrome
(cerebrohepatorenal syndrome) 759.89
Smith-Magenis syndrome 758.33
Smith-Strang disease (oasthouse urine) 270.2
Smokers'
bronchitis 491.0
cough 491.0
syndrome (*see also* Abuse, drugs,
nondependent) 305.1
throat 472.1
tongue 528.6
Smoking complicating pregnancy, childbirth, or
the puerperium 649.0
Smothering spells 786.09
Snaggle teeth, tooth 524.39
Snapping
finger 727.05
hip 719.65
jaw 524.69
temporomandibular joint sounds on opening or
closing 524.64
knee 717.9
thumb 727.05
Sneddon-Wilkinson disease or syndrome
(subcorneal pustular dermatosis) 694.1
Sneezing 784.99
intractable 478.19
Sniffing
cocaine (*see also* Dependence) 304.2
ether (*see also* Dependence) 304.6
glue (airplane) (*see also* Dependence) 304.6
Snoring 786.09
Snow blindness 370.24
Snuffles (nonsyphilitic) 460
syphilitic (infant) 090.0
Social migrant V60.0
Sodoku 026.0
Soemmering's ring 366.51

Soft —*see also* condition
enlarged prostate 600.00
with
other lower urinary tract symptoms (LUTS)
600.01
urinary
obstruction 600.01
retention 600.01
nails 703.8
Softening
bone 268.2
brain (necrotic) (progressive) 434.9
arteriosclerotic 437.0
congenital 742.4
embolic (*see also* Embolism, brain) 434.1
hemorrhagic (*see also* Hemorrhage, brain) 431
occlusive 434.9
thrombotic (*see also* Thrombosis, brain) 434.0
cartilage 733.92
cerebellar—*see* Softening, brain
cerebral—*see* Softening, brain
cerebrospinal—*see* Softening, brain
myocardial, heart (*see also* Degeneration,
myocardial) 429.1
nails 703.8
spinal cord 336.8
stomach 537.89
Solar fever 061
Soldier's
heart 306.2
patches 423.1
Solitary
cyst
bone 733.21
kidney 593.2
kidney (congenital) 753.0
tubercle, brain (*see also* Tuberculosis, brain) 013.2
ulcer, bladder 596.8
Somatization reaction, somatic reaction (*see*
also Disorder, psychosomatic) 306.9
disorder 300.81
Somatoform disorder 300.82
atypical 300.82
severe 300.81
undifferentiated 300.82
Somnambulism 307.46
hysterical 300.13
Somnolence 780.09
nonorganic origin 307.43
periodic 349.89
Sonne dysentery 004.3
Soor 112.0
Sore
Delhi 085.1
desert (*see also* Ulcer, skin) 707.9
eye 379.99
Lahore 085.1
mouth 528.9
canker 528.2
due to dentures 528.9
muscle 729.1
Naga (*see also* Ulcer, skin) 707.9
oriental 085.1
pressure (*see also* Decubitus) 707.00
with gangrene (*see also* Decubitus) 707.00
[785.4]
skin NEC 709.9
soft 099.0
throat 462
with influenza, flu, or grippe 487.1
acute 462

Sore —*continued*
  chronic 472.1
  clergyman's 784.49
  coxsackie (virus) 074.0
  diphtheritic 032.0
  epidemic 034.0
  gangrenous 462
  herpetic 054.79
  influenzal 487.1
  malignant 462
  purulent 462
  putrid 462
  septic 034.0
  streptococcal (ulcerative) 034.0
  ulcerated 462
  viral NEC 462
    Coxsackie 074.0
  tropical (*see also* Ulcer, skin) 707.9
  veldt (*see also* Ulcer, skin) 707.9
Sotos' syndrome (cerebral gigantism) 253.0
Sounds
  friction, pleural 786.7
  succussion, chest 786.7
  temporomandibular joint
    on opening or closing 524.64
South African cardiomyopathy syndrome
  425.2
South American
  blastomycosis 116.1
  trypanosomiasis—*see* Trypanosomiasis
Southeast Asian hemorrhagic fever 065.4
Spacing, teeth, abnormal 524.30
  excessive 524.32
Spade-like hand (congenital) 754.89
Spading nail 703.8
  congenital 757.5
Spanemia 285.9
Spanish collar 605
Sparganosis 123.5
Spasm, spastic, spasticity (*see also* condition)
  781.0
  accommodation 367.53
  ampulla of Vater (*see also* Disease, gallbladder)
    576.8
  anus, ani (sphincter) (reflex) 564.6
    psychogenic 306.4
  artery NEC 443.9
    basilar 435.0
    carotid 435.8
    cerebral 435.9
      specified artery NEC 435.8
    retinal (*see also* Occlusion, retinal, artery)
      362.30
    vertebral 435.1
    vertebrobasilar 435.3
  Bell's 351.0
  bladder (sphincter, external or internal) 596.8
  bowel 564.9
    psychogenic 306.4
  bronchus, bronchiole 519.11
  cardia 530.0
  cardiac—*see* Angina
  carpopedal (*see also* Tetany) 781.7
  cecum 564.9
    psychogenic 306.4
  cerebral (arteries) (vascular) 435.9
    specified artery NEC 435.8
  cerebrovascular 435.9
  cervix, complicating delivery 661.4
    affecting fetus or newborn 763.7
  ciliary body (of accommodation) 367.53

Spasm, spastic, spasticity— *continued*
  colon 564.1
    psychogenic 306.4
  common duct (*see also* Disease, biliary) 576.8
  compulsive 307.22
  conjugate 378.82
  convergence 378.84
  coronary (artery)—*see* Angina
  diaphragm (reflex) 786.8
    psychogenic 306.1
  duodenum, duodenal (bulb) 564.89
  esophagus (diffuse) 530.5
    psychogenic 306.4
  facial 351.8
  fallopian tube 620.8
  gait 781.2
  gastrointestinal (tract) 536.8
    psychogenic 306.4
  glottis 478.75
    hysterical 300.11
    psychogenic 306.1
      specified as conversion reaction 300.11
    reflex through recurrent laryngeal nerve
      478.75
  habit 307.20
    chronic 307.22
    transient (of childhood) 307.21
  heart—*see* Angina
  hourglass—*see* Contraction, hourglass
  hysterical 300.11
  infantile (*see also* Epilepsy) 345.6
  internal oblique, eye 378.51
  intestinal 564.9
    psychogenic 306.4
  larynx, laryngeal 478.75
    hysterical 300.11
    psychogenic 306.1
      specified as conversion reaction 300.11
  levator palpebrae superioris 333.81
  lightning (*see also* Epilepsy) 345.6
  mobile 781.0
  muscle 728.85
    back 724.8
    psychogenic 306.0
  nerve, trigeminal 350.1
  nervous 306.0
  nodding 307.3
    infantile (*see also* Epilepsy) 345.6
  occupational 300.89
  oculogyric 378.87
  ophthalmic artery 362.30
  orbicularis 781.0
  perineal 625.8
  peroneo-extensor (*see also* Flat, foot) 734
  pharynx (reflex) 478.29
    hysterical 300.11
    psychogenic 306.1
      specified as conversion reaction 300.11
  pregnant uterus, complicating delivery 661.4
  psychogenic 306.0
  pylorus 537.81
    adult hypertrophic 537.0
    congenital or infantile 750.5
    psychogenic 306.4
  rectum (sphincter) 564.6
    psychogenic 306.4
  retinal artery NEC (*see also* Occlusion, retina,
    artery) 362.30
  sacroiliac 724.6
  salaam (infantile) (*see also* Epilepsy) 345.6
  saltatory 781.0

Spasm, spastic, spasticity—*continued*
  sigmoid 564.9
    psychogenic 306.4
  sphincter of Oddi (*see also* Disease, gallbladder)
    576.5
  stomach 536.8
    neurotic 306.4
  throat 478.29
    hysterical 300.11
    psychogenic 306.1
      specified as conversion reaction 300.11
  tic 307.20
    chronic 307.22
    transient (of childhood) 307.21
  tongue 529.8
  torsion 333.6
  trigeminal nerve 350.1
    postherpetic 053.12
  ureter 593.89
  urethra (sphincter) 599.84
  uterus 625.8
    complicating labor 661.4
      affecting fetus or newborn 763.7
  vagina 625.1
    psychogenic 306.51
  vascular NEC 443.9
  vasomotor NEC 443.9
  vein NEC 459.89
  vesical (sphincter, external or internal) 596.8
  viscera 789.0
Spasmodic —*see* condition
Spasmophilia (*see also* Tetany) 781.7
Spasmus nutans 307.3
Spastic —*see also* Spasm
  child 343.9
Spasticity —*see also* Spasm
  cerebral, child 343.9
Speakers' throat 784.49
Specific, specified —*see* condition
Speech
  defect, disorder, disturbance, impediment NEC
    784.5
    psychogenic 307.9
  therapy V57.3
Spells 780.39
  breath-holding 786.9
Spencer's disease (epidemic vomiting) 078.82
Spens' syndrome (syncope with heart block)
  426.9
Spermatic cord —*see* condition
Spermatocele 608.1
  congenital 752.89
Spermatocystitis 608.4
Spermatocytoma (M9063/3)
  specified site—*see* Neoplasm, by site, malignant
  unspecified site 186.9
Spermatorrhea 608.89
Sperm counts
  fertility testing V26.21
  following sterilization reversal V26.22
  postvasectomy V25.8
Sphacelus (*see also* Gangrene) 785.4
Sphenoidal —*see* condition
Sphenoiditis (chronic) (*see also* Sinusitis,
  sphenoidal) 473.3
Sphenopalatine ganglion neuralgia 337.0
Sphericity, increased, lens 743.36
Spherocytosis (congenital) (familial) (hereditary)
  282.0
  hemoglobin disease 287.7
  sickle-cell (disease) 282.60

Spherophakia 743.36
Sphincter —*see* condition
Sphincteritis, sphincter of Oddi (*see also*
  Cholecystitis) 576.8
Sphingolipidosis 272.7
Sphingolipodystrophy 272.7
Sphingomyelinosis 272.7
Spicule tooth 520.2
Spider
  finger 755.59
  nevus 448.1
  vascular 448.1
Spiegler-Fendt sarcoid 686.8
Spielmeyer-Stock disease 330.1
Spielmeyer-Vogt disease 330.1
Spina bifida (aperta) 741.9

Note—Use the following fifth-digit
subclassification with category 741:

0 unspecified region
1 cervical region
2 dorsal [thoracic] region
3 lumbar region

---

  with hydrocephalus 741.0
  fetal (suspected), affecting management of
    pregnancy 655.0
  occulta 756.17
Spindle, Krukenberg's 371.13
Spine, spinal —*see* condition
Spiradenoma (eccrine) (M8403/0)—*see*
  Neoplasm, skin, benign
Spirillosis NEC (*see also* Fever, relapsing) 087.9
Spirillum minus 026.0
Spirillum obermeieri infection 087.0
Spirochetal —*see* condition
Spirochetosis 104.9
  arthritic, arthritica 104.9 *[711.8]*
  bronchopulmonary 104.8
  icterohemorrhagica 100.0
  lung 104.8
Spitting blood (*see also* Hemoptysis) 786.3
Splanchnomegaly 569.89
Splanchnoptosis 569.89
Spleen, splenic —*see also* condition
  agenesis 759.0
  flexure syndrome 569.89
  neutropenia syndrome 289.53
  sequestration syndrome 289.52
Splenectasis (*see also* Splenomegaly) 789.2
Splenitis (interstitial) (malignant) (nonspecific)
  289.59
  malarial (*see also* Malaria) 084.6
  tuberculous (*see also* Tuberculosis) 017.7
Splenocele 289.59
Splenomegalia —*see* Splenomegaly
Splenomegalic —*see* condition
Splenomegaly 789.2
  Bengal 789.2
  cirrhotic 289.51
  congenital 759.0
  congestive, chronic 289.51
  cryptogenic 789.2
  Egyptian 120.1
  Gaucher's (cerebroside lipidosis) 272.7
  idiopathic 789.2
  malarial (*see also* Malaria) 084.6
  neutropenic 289.53
  Niemann-Pick (lipid histiocytosis) 272.7
  siderotic 289.51

Splenomegaly—*continued*
  syphilitic 095.8
    congenital 090.0
  tropical (Bengal) (idiopathic) 789.2
Splenopathy 289.50
Splenopneumonia —*see* Pneumonia
Splenoptosis 289.59
Splinter —*see* Injury, superficial, by site
Split, splitting
  heart sounds 427.89
  lip, congenital (*see also* Cleft, lip) 749.10
  nails 703.8
  urinary stream 788.61
Spoiled child reaction (*see also* Disturbance,
    conduct) 312.1
Spondylarthritis (*see also* Spondylosis) 721.90
Spondylarthrosis (*see also* Spondylosis) 721.90
Spondylitis 720.9
  ankylopoietica 720.0
  ankylosing (chronic) 720.0
  atrophic 720.9
    ligamentous 720.9
  chronic (traumatic) (*see also* Spondylosis)
    721.90
  deformans (chronic) (*see also* Spondylosis)
    721.90
  gonococcal 098.53
  gouty 274.0
  hypertrophic (*see also* Spondylosis) 721.90
  infectious NEC 720.9
  juvenile (adolescent) 720.0
  Kümmell's 721.7
  Marie-Strümpell (ankylosing) 720.0
  muscularis 720.9
  ossificans ligamentosa 721.6
  osteoarthritica (*see also* Spondylosis) 721.90
  posttraumatic 721.7
  proliferative 720.0
  rheumatoid 720.0
  rhizomelica 720.0
  sacroiliac NEC 720.2
  senescent (*see also* Spondylosis) 721.90
  senile (*see also* Spondylosis) 721.90
  static (*see also* Spondylosis) 721.90
  traumatic (chronic) (*see also* Spondylosis)
    721.90
  tuberculous (*see also* Tuberculosis) 015.0
    [720.81]
  typhosa 002.0 *[720.81]*
Spondyloarthrosis (*see also* Spondylosis) 721.90
Spondylolisthesis (congenital) (lumbosacral)
    756.12
  with disproportion (fetopelvic) 653.3
    affecting fetus or newborn 763.1
    causing obstructed labor 660.1
      affecting fetus or newborn 763.1
  acquired 738.4
  degenerative 738.4
  traumatic 738.4
    acute (lumbar)—*see* Fracture, vertebra,
      lumbar
    site other than lumbosacral—*see* Fracture,
      vertebra, by site
Spondylolysis (congenital) 756.11
  acquired 738.4
  cervical 756.19
  lumbosacral region 756.11
    with disproportion (fetopelvic) 653.3
      affecting fetus or newborn 763.1
      causing obstructed labor 660.1
        affecting fetus or newborn 763.1

Spondylopathy
  inflammatory 720.9
    specified type NEC 720.89
  traumatic 721.7
Spondylose rhizomelique 720.0
Spondylosis 721.90
  with
    disproportion 653.3
      affecting fetus or newborn 763.1
      causing obstructed labor 660.1
        affecting fetus or newborn 763.1
    myelopathy NEC 721.91
  cervical, cervicodorsal 721.0
    with myelopathy 721.1
  inflammatory 720.9
  lumbar, lumbosacral 721.3
    with myelopathy 721.42
  sacral 721.3
    with myelopathy 721.42
  thoracic 721.2
    with myelopathy 721.41
  traumatic 721.7
Sponge
  divers' disease 989.5
  inadvertently left in operation wound 998.4
  kidney (medullary) 753.17
Spongioblastoma (M9422/3)
  multiforme (M9440/3)
    specified site—*see* Neoplasm, by site,
      malignant
    unspecified site 191.9
  polare (M9423/3)
    specified site—*see* Neoplasm, by site,
      malignant
    unspecified site 191.9
  primitive polar (M9443/3)
    specified site—*see* Neoplasm, by site,
      malignant
    unspecified site 191.9
  specified site—*see* Neoplasm, by site, malignant
  unspecified site 191.9
Spongiocytoma (M9400/3)
  specified site—*see* Neoplasm, by site, malignant
  unspecified site 191.9
Spongioneuroblastoma (M9504/3)—*see*
  Neoplasm, by site, malignant
Spontaneous —*see also* condition
  fracture—*see* Fracture, pathologic
Spoon nail 703.8
  congenital 757.5
Sporadic —*see* condition
Sporotrichosis (bones) (cutaneous)
    (disseminated) (epidermal) (lymphatic)
    (lymphocutaneous) (mucous membranes)
    (pulmonary) (skeletal) (visceral) 117.1
Sporotrichum schenckii infection 117.1
Spots, spotting
  atrophic (skin) 701.3
  Bitôt's (in the young child) 264.1
  café au lait 709.09
  cayenne pepper 448.1
  complicating pregnancy 649.5
  cotton wool (retina) 362.83
  de Morgan's (senile angiomas) 448.1
  Fúchs' black (myopic) 360.21
  intermenstrual
    irregular 626.6
    regular 626.5
  interpalpebral 372.53
  Koplik's 055.9
  liver 709.09

Spots, spotting—*continued*
  Mongolian (pigmented) 757.33
  of pregnancy 641.9
  purpuric 782.7
  ruby 448.1
Spotted fever —*see* Fever, spotted
Sprain, strain (joint) (ligament) (muscle)
      (tendon) 848.9
  abdominal wall (muscle) 848.8
  Achilles tendon 845.09
  acromioclavicular 840.0
  ankle 845.00
    and foot 845.00
  anterior longitudinal, cervical 847.0
  arm 840.9
    upper 840.9
      and shoulder 840.9
  astragalus 845.00
  atlanto-axial 847.0
  atlanto-occipital 847.0
  atlas 847.0
  axis 847.0
  back (*see also* Sprain, spine) 847.9
  breast bone 848.40
  broad ligament—*see* Injury, internal, broad
      ligament
  calcaneofibular 845.02
  carpal 842.01
  carpometacarpal 842.11
  cartilage
    costal, without mention of injury to sternum
        848.3
      involving sternum 848.42
    ear 848.8
    knee 844.9
      with current tear (*see also* Tear, meniscus)
          836.2
    semilunar (knee) 844.8
      with current tear (*see also* Tear, meniscus)
          836.2
    septal, nose 848.0
    thyroid region 848.2
    xiphoid 848.49
  cervical, cervicodorsal, cervicothoracic 847.0
  chondrocostal, without mention of injury to
      sternum 848.3
    involving sternum 848.42
  chondrosternal 848.42
  chronic (joint)—*see* Derangement, joint
  clavicle 840.9
  coccyx 847.4
  collar bone 840.9
  collateral, knee (medial) (tibial) 844.1
    lateral (fibular) 844.0
    recurrent or old 717.89
      lateral 717.81
      medial 717.82
  coracoacromial 840.8
  coracoclavicular 840.1
  coracohumeral 840.2
  coracoid (process) 840.9
  coronary, knee 844.8
  costal cartilage, without mention of injury to
      sternum 848.3
    involving sternum 848.42
  cricoarytenoid articulation 848.2
  cricothyroid articulation 848.2
  cruciate
    knee 844.2
    old 717.89
      anterior 717.83

Sprain, strain—*continued*
      posterior 717.84
  deltoid
    ankle 845.01
    shoulder 840.8
  dorsal (spine) 847.1
  ear cartilage 848.8
  elbow 841.9
    and forearm 841.9
    specified site NEC 841.8
  femur (proximal end) 843.9
    distal end 844.9
  fibula (proximal end) 844.9
    distal end 845.00
  fibulocalcaneal 845.02
  finger(s) 842.10
  foot 845.10
    and ankle 845.00
  forearm 841.9
    and elbow 841.9
    specified site NEC 841.8
  glenoid (shoulder) (*see also* SLAP lesion) 840.8
  hand 842.10
  hip 843.9
    and thigh 843.9
  humerus (proximal end) 840.9
    distal end 841.9
  iliofemoral 843.0
  infraspinatus 840.3
  innominate
    acetabulum 843.9
    pubic junction 848.5
    sacral junction 846.1
  internal
    collateral, ankle 845.01
    semilunar cartilage 844.8
      with current tear (*see also* Tear, meniscus)
          836.2
      old 717.5
  interphalangeal
    finger 842.13
    toe 845.13
  ischiocapsular 843.1
  jaw (cartilage) (meniscus) 848.1
    old 524.69
  knee 844.9
    and leg 844.9
    old 717.5
      collateral
        lateral 717.81
        medial 717.82
      cruciate
        anterior 717.83
        posterior 717.84
  late effect—*see* Late, effects (of), sprain
  lateral collateral, knee 844.0
    old 717.81
  leg 844.9
    and knee 844.9
  ligamentum teres femoris 843.8
  low back 846.9
  lumbar (spine) 847.2
  lumbosacral 846.0
    chronic or old 724.6
  mandible 848.1
    old 524.69
  maxilla 848.1
  medial collateral, knee 844.1
    old 717.82
  meniscus
    jaw 848.1

Squamous —*see also* condition
  cell metaplasia
    bladder 596.8
    cervix—*see* condition
  epithelium in
    cervical canal (congenital) 752.49
    uterine mucosa (congenital) 752.3
  metaplasia
    bladder 596.8
    cervix—*see* condition
Squashed nose 738.0
  congenital 754.0
Squeeze, divers' 993.3
Squint (*see also* Strabismus) 378.9
  accommodative (*see also* Esotropia) 378.00
  concomitant (*see also* Heterotropia) 378.30
Stab —*see also* Wound, open, by site
  internal organs—*see* Injury, internal, by site,
      with open wound
Staggering gait 781.2
  hysterical 300.11
Staghorn calculus 592.0
Stähl's
  ear 744.29
  pigment line (cornea) 371.11
Stähli's pigment lines (cornea) 371.11
Stain, staining
  meconium 779.84
  port wine 757.32
  tooth, teeth (hard tissues) 521.7
    due to
      accretions 523.6
      deposits (betel) (black) (green) (materia
          alba) (orange) (tobacco) 523.6
      metals (copper) (silver) 521.7
      nicotine 523.6
      pulpal bleeding 521.7
      tobacco 523.6
Stammering 307.0
Standstill
  atrial 426.6
  auricular 426.6
  cardiac (*see also* Arrest, cardiac) 427.5
  sinoatrial 426.6
  sinus 426.6
  ventricular (*see also* Arrest, cardiac) 427.5
Stannosis 503
Stanton's disease (melioidosis) 025
Staphylitis (acute) (catarrhal) (chronic)
    (gangrenous) (membranous) (suppurative)
    (ulcerative) 528.3
Staphylococcemia 038.10
  aureus 038.11
  specified organism NEC 038.19
Staphylococcus, staphylococcal —*see* condition
Staphyloderma (skin) 686.00
Staphyloma 379.11
  anterior, localized 379.14
  ciliary 379.11
  cornea 371.73
  equatorial 379.13
  posterior 379.12
  posticum 379.12
  ring 379.15
  sclera NEC 379.11
Starch eating 307.52
Stargardt's disease 362.75
Starvation (inanition) (due to lack of food) 994.2
  edema 262
  voluntary NEC 307.1

Stasis
  bile (duct) (*see also* Disease, biliary) 576.8
  bronchus (*see also* Bronchitis) 490
  cardiac (*see also* Failure, heart) 428.0
  cecum 564.89
  colon 564.89
  dermatitis (*see also* Varix, with stasis
      dermatitis) 454.1
  duodenal 536.8
  eczema (*see also* Varix, with stasis dermatitis)
      454.1
  edema (*see also* Hypertension, venous) 459.30
  foot 991.4
  gastric 536.3
  ileocecal coil 564.89
  ileum 564.89
  intestinal 564.89
  jejunum 564.89
  kidney 586
  liver 571.9
    cirrhotic—*see* Cirrhosis, liver
  lymphatic 457.8
  pneumonia 514
  portal 571.9
  pulmonary 514
  rectal 564.89
  renal 586
    tubular 584.5
  stomach 536.3
  ulcer
    with varicose veins 454.0
    without varicose veins 459.81
  urine NEC (*see also* Retention, urine) 788.20
  venous 459.81
State
  affective and paranoid, mixed, organic psychotic
      294.8
  agitated 307.9
    acute reaction to stress 308.2
  anxiety (neurotic) (*see also* Anxiety) 300.00
    specified type NEC 300.09
  apprehension (*see also* Anxiety) 300.00
    specified type NEC 300.09
  climacteric, female 627.2
    following induced menopause 627.4
  clouded
    epileptic (*see also* Epilepsy) 345.9
    paroxysmal (idiopathic) (*see also* Epilepsy)
        345.9
  compulsive (mixed) (with obsession) 300.3
  confusional 298.9
    acute 293.0
      with
        arteriosclerotic dementia 290.41
        presenile brain disease 290.11
        senility 290.3
      alcoholic 291.0
      drug-induced 292.81
    epileptic 293.0
    postoperative 293.9
    reactive (emotional stress) (psychological
        trauma) 298.2
    subacute 293.1
  constitutional psychopathic 301.9
  convulsive (*see also* Convulsions) 780.39
  depressive NEC 311
    induced by drug 292.84
    neurotic 300.4
  dissociative 300.15
  hallucinatory 780.1
    induced by drug 292.12

State—*continued*
  hypercoagulable (primary) 289.81
    secondary 289.82
  hyperdynamic beta-adrenergic circulatory
    429.82
  locked-in 344.81
  menopausal 627.2
    artificial 627.4
    following induced menopause 627.4
  neurotic NEC 300.9
    with depersonalization episode 300.6
  obsessional 300.3
  oneiroid (*see also* Schizophrenia) 295.4
  panic 300.01
  paranoid 297.9
    alcohol-induced 291.5
    arteriosclerotic 290.42
    climacteric 297.2
    drug-induced 292.11
    in
      presenile brain disease 290.12
      senile brain disease 290.20
    involutional 297.2
    menopausal 297.2
    senile 290.20
    simple 297.0
  postleukotomy 310.0
  pregnant (*see also* Pregnancy) V22.2
  psychogenic, twilight 298.2
  psychotic, organic (*see also* Psychosis, organic)
    294.9
    mixed paranoid and affective 294.8
    senile or presenile NEC 290.9
    transient NEC 293.9
      with
        anxiety 293.84
        delusions 293.81
        depression 293.83
        hallucinations 293.82
  residual schizophrenic (*see also* Schizophrenia)
    295.6
  tension (*see also* Anxiety) 300.9
  transient organic psychotic 293.9
    anxiety type 293.84
    depressive type 293.83
    hallucinatory type 293.83
    paranoid type 293.81
    specified type NEC 293.89
  twilight
    epileptic 293.0
    psychogenic 298.2
  vegetative (persistent) 780.03
Status (post)
  absence
    epileptic (*see also* Epilepsy) 345.2
    of organ, acquired (postsurgical)—*see*
      Absence, by site, acquired
  anastomosis of intestine (for bypass) V45.3
  angioplasty, percutaneous transluminal coronary
    V45.82
  anginosus 413.9
  ankle prosthesis V43.66
  aortocoronary bypass or shunt V45.81
  arthrodesis V45.4
  artificially induced condition NEC V45.89
  artificial opening (of) V44.9
    gastrointestinal tract NEC V44.4
    specified site NEC V44.8
    urinary tract NEC V44.6
    vagina V44.7
  aspirator V46.0

Status—*continued*
  asthmaticus (*see also* Asthma) 493.9
  awaiting organ transplant V49.83
  bariatric surgery V45.86
    complicating pregnancy, childbirth, or the
      puerperium 649.2
  bed confinement V49.84
  breast implant removal V45.83
  cardiac
    device (in situ) V45.00
      defibrillator, automatic implantable V45.02
      pacemaker V45.01
        fitting or adjustment V53.3
      carotid sinus V45.09
        fitting or adjustment V53.3
  carotid sinus stimulator V45.09
  cataract extraction V45.61
  chemotherapy V66.2
    current V58.69
  circumcision, female 629.20
  clitorectomy (female genital mutilation type I)
    629.21
    with excision of labia minora (female genital
      mutilation type II) 629.22
  colostomy V44.3
  contraceptive device V45.59
    intrauterine V45.51
    subdermal V45.52
  convulsivus idiopathicus (*see also* Epilepsy)
    345.3
  coronary artery bypass or shunt V45.81
  cutting
    female genital 629.20
      specified NEC 629.29
      type I 629.21
      type II 629.22
      type III 629.23
      type IV 629.29
  cystostomy V44.50
    appendico-vesicostomy V44.52
    cutaneous-vesicostomy V44.51
    specified type NEC V44.59
  defibrillator, automatic implantable cardiac
    V45.02
  dental crowns V45.84
  dental fillings V45.84
  dental restoration V45.84
  dental sealant V49.82
  dialysis (hemo) (peritoneal) V45.1
  donor V59.9
  drug therapy or regimen V67.59
    high-risk medication NEC V67.51
  elbow prosthesis V43.62
  enterostomy V44.4
  epileptic, epilepticus (absence) (grand mal) (*see*
    also Epilepsy) 345.3
    focal motor 345.7
    partial 345.7
    petit mal 345.2
    psychomotor 345.7
    temporal lobe 345.7
  estrogen receptor
    negative [ER-] V86.1
    positive [ER+] V86.0
  eye (adnexa) surgery V45.69
  female genital
    cutting 629.20
      specified NEC 629.29
      type I 629.21
      type II 629.22
      type III 629.23

Status—*continued*
   liver V42.7
   lung V42.6
   organ V42.9
     specified site NEC V42.89
   pancreas V42.83
   peripheral stem cells V42.82
   skin V42.3
   stem cells, peripheral V42.82
   tissue V42.9
     specified type NEC V42.89
   vessel, blood V42.89
  tubal ligation V26.51
  ureterostomy V44.6
  urethrostomy V44.6
  vagina, artificial V44.7
  vasectomy V26.52
  vascular shunt NEC V45.89
   aortocoronary (bypass) V45.81
  ventilator (respirator) V46.11
   encounter
    during
     mechanical failure V46.14
     power failure V46.12
    for weaning V46.13
  wrist prosthesis V43.63
Stave fracture —*see* Fracture, metacarpus,
  metacarpal bone(s)
Steal
  subclavian artery 435.2
  vertebral artery 435.1
Stealing, solitary, child problem (*see also*
  Disturbance, conduct) 312.1
Steam burn —*see* Burn, by site
Steatocystoma multiplex 706.2
Steatoma (infected) 706.2
  eyelid (cystic) 374.84
   infected 373.13
Steatorrhea (chronic) 579.8
  with lacteal obstruction 579.2
  idiopathic 579.0
   adult 579.0
   infantile 579.0
  pancreatic 579.4
  primary 579.0
  secondary 579.8
  specified cause NEC 579.8
  tropical 579.1
Steatosis 272.8
  heart (*see also* Degeneration, myocardial) 429.1
  kidney 593.89
  liver 571.8
Steele-Richardson (-Olszewski) Syndrome
  333.0
Stein's syndrome (polycystic ovary) 256.4
Stein-Leventhal syndrome (polycystic ovary)
  256.4
Steinbrocker's syndrome (*see also* Neuropathy,
  peripheral, autonomic) 337.9
Steinert's disease 359.2
STEMI (ST elevation myocardial infarction) (*see*
  also Infarct, myocardium, ST elevation) 410.9
Stenocardia (*see also* Angina) 413.9
Stenocephaly 756.0
Stenosis (cicatricial)—*see also* Stricture
  ampulla of Vater 576.2
   with calculus, cholelithiasis, or stones—*see*
    Choledocholithiasis
  anus, anal (canal) (sphincter) 569.2
   congenital 751.2
  aorta (ascending) 747.22

Stenosis—*continued*
  arch 747.10
  arteriosclerotic 440.0
  calcified 440.0
  aortic (valve) 424.1
   with
    mitral (valve)
     insufficiency or incompetence 396.2
     stenosis or obstruction 396.0
   atypical 396.0
   congenital 746.3
   rheumatic 395.0
    with
     insufficiency, incompetency or
      regurgitation 395.2
      with mitral (valve) disease 396.8
     mitral (valve)
      disease (stenosis) 396.0
      insufficiency or incompetence 396.2
      stenosis or obstruction 396.0
   specified cause, except rheumatic 424.1
   syphilitic 093.22
  aqueduct of Sylvius (congenital) 742.3
   with spina bifida (*see also* Spina bifida) 741.0
   acquired 331.4
  artery NEC 447.1
   basilar—*see* Narrowing, artery, basilar
   carotid (common) (internal)—*see* Narrowing,
    artery, carotid
   celiac 447.4
   cerebral 437.0
    due to
     embolism (*see also* Embolism, brain)
      434.1
     thrombus (*see also* Thrombosis, brain)
      434.0
   precerebral—*see* Narrowing, artery,
    precerebral
   pulmonary (congenital) 747.3
    acquired 417.8
   renal 440.1
   vertebral—*see* Narrowing, artery, vertebral
  bile duct or biliary passage (*see also*
   Obstruction, biliary) 576.2
   congenital 751.61
  bladder neck (acquired) 596.0
   congenital 753.6
  brain 348.8
  bronchus 519.19
   syphilitic 095.8
  cardia (stomach) 537.89
   congenital 750.7
  cardiovascular (*see also* Disease,
   cardiovascular) 429.2
  carotid artery—*see* Narrowing, artery, carotid
  cervix, cervical (canal) 622.4
   congenital 752.49
   in pregnancy or childbirth 654.6
    affecting fetus or newborn 763.89
    causing obstructed labor 660.2
     affecting fetus or newborn 763.1
  colon (*see also* Obstruction, intestine) 560.9
   congenital 751.2
  colostomy 569.62
  common bile duct (*see also* Obstruction, biliary)
   576.2
   congenital 751.61
  coronary (artery) —*see* Arteriosclerosis,
   coronary
  cystic duct (*see also* Obstruction, gallbladder)
   575.2

Stenosis—*continued*
congenital 751.61
due to (presence of) any device, implant, or graft
classifiable to 996.0-996.5—*see*
Complications, due to (presence of) any
device, implant, or graft classified to
996.0-996.5 NEC
duodenum 537.3
congenital 751.1
ejaculatory duct NEC 608.89
endocervical os—*see* Stenosis, cervix
enterostomy 569.62
esophagostomy 530.87
esophagus 530.3
congenital 750.3
syphilitic 095.8
congenital 090.5
external ear canal 380.50
secondary to
inflammation 380.53
surgery 380.52
trauma 380.51
gallbladder (*see also* Obstruction, gallbladder)
575.2
glottis 478.74
heart valve (acquired)—*see also* Endocarditis
congenital NEC 746.89
aortic 746.3
mitral 746.5
pulmonary 746.02
tricuspid 746.1
hepatic duct (*see also* Obstruction, biliary) 576.2
hymen 623.3
hypertrophic subaortic (idiopathic) 425.1
infundibulum cardiac 746.83
intestine (*see also* Obstruction, intestine) 560.9
congenital (small) 751.1
large 751.2
lacrimal
canaliculi 375.53
duct 375.56
congenital 743.65
punctum 375.52
congenital 743.65
sac 375.54
congenital 743.65
lacrimonasal duct 375.56
congenital 743.65
neonatal 375.55
larynx 478.74
congenital 748.3
syphilitic 095.8
congenital 090.5
mitral (valve) (chronic) (inactive) 394.0
with
aortic (valve)
disease (insufficiency) 396.1
insufficiency or incompetence 396.1
stenosis or obstruction 396.0
incompetency, insufficiency or regurgitation
394.2
with aortic valve disease 396.8
active or acute 391.1
with chorea (acute) (rheumatic)
(Sydenham's) 392.0
congenital 746.5
specified cause, except rheumatic 424.0
syphilitic 093.21
myocardium, myocardial (*see also*
Degeneration, myocardial) 429.1
hypertrophic subaortic (idiopathic) 425.1

Stenosis—*continued*
nares (anterior) (posterior) 478.19
congenital 748.0
nasal duct 375.56
congenital 743.65
nasolacrimal duct 375.56
congenital 743.65
neonatal 375.55
organ or site, congenital NEC—*see* Atresia
papilla of Vater 576.2
with calculus, cholelithiasis, or stones—*see*
Choledocholithiasis
pulmonary (artery) (congenital) 747.3
with ventricular septal defect, dextraposition
of aorta and hypertrophy of right ventricle
745.2
acquired 417.8
infundibular 746.83
in tetralogy of Fallot 745.2
subvalvular 746.83
valve (*see also* Endocarditis, pulmonary)
424.3
congenital 746.02
vein 747.49
acquired 417.8
vessel NEC 417.8
pulmonic (congenital) 746.02
infundibular 746.83
subvalvular 746.83
pylorus (hypertrophic) 537.0
adult 537.0
congenital 750.5
infantile 750.5
rectum (sphincter) (*see also* Stricture, rectum)
569.2
renal artery 440.1
salivary duct (any) 527.8
sphincter of Oddi (*see also* Obstruction, biliary)
576.2
spinal 724.00
cervical 723.0
lumbar, lumbosacral 724.02
nerve (root) NEC 724.9
specified region NEC 724.09
thoracic, thoracolumbar 724.01
stomach, hourglass 537.6
subaortic 746.81
hypertrophic (idiopathic) 425.1
supra (valvular)-aortic 747.22
trachea 519.19
congenital 748.3
syphilitic 095.8
tuberculous (*see also* Tuberculosis) 012.8
tracheostomy 519.02
tricuspid (valve) (*see also* Endocarditis,
tricuspid) 397.0
congenital 746.1
nonrheumatic 424.2
tubal 628.2
ureter (*see also* Stricture, ureter) 593.3
congenital 753.29
urethra (*see also* Stricture, urethra) 598.9
vagina 623.2
congenital 752.49
in pregnancy or childbirth 654.7
affecting fetus or newborn 763.89
causing obstructed labor 660.2
affecting fetus or newborn 763.1
valve (cardiac) (heart) (*see also* Endocarditis)
424.90
congenital NEC 746.89

Strangury 788.1
Strawberry
  gallbladder (*see also* Disease, gallbladder) 575.6
  mark 757.32
  tongue (red) (white) 529.3
Straw itch 133.8
Streak, ovarian 752.0
Strephosymbolia 315.01
  secondary to organic lesion 784.69
Streptobacillary fever 026.1
Streptobacillus moniliformis 026.1
Streptococcemia 038.0
Streptococcicosis —*see* Infection, streptococcal
Streptococcus, streptococcal —*see* condition
Streptoderma 686.00
Streptomycosis —*see* Actinomycosis
Streptothricosis —*see* Actinomycosis
Streptothrix —*see* Actinomycosis
Streptotrichosis —*see* Actinomycosis
Stress
  fracture—*see* Fracture, stress
  polycythemia 289.0
  reaction (gross) (*see also* Reaction, stress, acute)
    308.9
Stretching, nerve —*see* Injury, nerve, by site
Striae (albicantes) (atrophicae) (cutis distensae)
    (distensae) 701.3
Striations of nails 703.8
Stricture (*see also* Stenosis) 799.89
  ampulla of Vater 576.2
    with calculus, cholelithiasis, or stones—*see*
        Choledocholithiasis
  anus (sphincter) 569.2
    congenital 751.2
    infantile 751.2
  aorta (ascending) 747.22
    arch 747.10
    arteriosclerotic 440.0
    calcified 440.0
  aortic (valve) (*see also* Stenosis, aortic) 424.1
    congenital 746.3
  aqueduct of Sylvius (congenital) 742.3
    with spina bifida (*see also* Spina bifida) 741.0
    acquired 331.4
  artery 447.1
    basilar—*see* Narrowing, artery, basilar
    carotid (common) (internal)—*see* Narrowing,
        artery, carotid
    celiac 447.4
    cerebral 437.0
      congenital 747.81
      due to
        embolism (*see also* Embolism, brain) 434.1
        thrombus (*see also* Thrombosis, brain)
            434.0
    congenital (peripheral) 747.60
      cerebral 747.81
      coronary 746.85
      gastrointestinal 747.61
      lower limb 747.64
      renal 747.62
      retinal 743.58
      specified NEC 747.69
      spinal 747.82
      umbilical 747.5
      upper limb 747.63
    coronary —*see* Arteriosclerosis, coronary
      congenital 746.85
    precerebral—*see* Narrowing, artery,
        precerebral NEC

Stricture—*continued*
  pulmonary (congenital) 747.3
    acquired 417.8
    renal 440.1
    vertebral—*see* Narrowing, artery, vertebral
  auditory canal (congenital) (external) 744.02
    acquired (*see also* Stricture, ear canal,
        acquired) 380.50
  bile duct or passage (any) (postoperative) (*see
    also* Obstruction, biliary) 576.2
    congenital 751.61
  bladder 596.8
    congenital 753.6
    neck 596.0
      congenital 753.6
  bowel (*see also* Obstruction, intestine) 560.9
  brain 348.8
  bronchus 519.19
    syphilitic 095.8
  cardia (stomach) 537.89
    congenital 750.7
  cardiac—*see also* Disease, heart
    orifice (stomach) 537.89
  cardiovascular (*see also* Disease,
    cardiovascular) 429.2
  carotid artery—*see* Narrowing, artery, carotid
  cecum (*see also* Obstruction, intestine) 560.9
  cervix, cervical (canal) 622.4
    congenital 752.49
    in pregnancy or childbirth 654.6
      affecting fetus or newborn 763.89
      causing obstructed labor 660.2
        affecting fetus or newborn 763.1
  colon (*see also* Obstruction, intestine) 560.9
    congenital 751.2
  colostomy 569.62
  common bile duct (*see also* Obstruction, biliary)
    576.2
    congenital 751.61
  coronary (artery) —*see* Arteriosclerosis,
    coronary
    congenital 746.85
  cystic duct (*see also* Obstruction, gallbladder)
    575.2
    congenital 751.61
  cystostomy 997.5
  digestive organs NEC, congenital 751.8
  duodenum 537.3
    congenital 751.1
  ear canal (external) (congenital) 744.02
    acquired 380.50
      secondary to
        inflammation 380.53
        surgery 380.52
        trauma 380.51
  ejaculatory duct 608.85
  enterostomy 569.62
  esophagostomy 530.87
  esophagus (corrosive) (peptic) 530.3
    congenital 750.3
    syphilitic 095.8
      congenital 090.5
  Eustachian tube (*see also* Obstruction,
    Eustachian tube) 381.60
    congenital 744.24
  fallopian tube 628.2
    gonococcal (chronic) 098.37
      acute 098.17
    tuberculous (*see also* Tuberculosis) 016.6
  gallbladder (*see also* Obstruction, gallbladder)
    575.2

Stricture—*continued*
    congenital 751.69
    glottis 478.74
    heart—*see also* Disease, heart
      congenital NEC 746.89
      valve—*see also* Endocarditis
        congenital NEC 746.89
          aortic 746.3
          mitral 746.5
          pulmonary 746.02
          tricuspid 746.1
    hepatic duct (*see also* Obstruction, biliary) 576.2
    hourglass, of stomach 537.6
    hymen 623.3
    hypopharynx 478.29
    intestine (*see also* Obstruction, intestine) 560.9
      congenital (small) 751.1
        large 751.2
      ischemic 557.1
    lacrimal
      canaliculi 375.53
        congenital 743.65
      punctum 375.52
        congenital 743.65
      sac 375.54
        congenital 743.65
    lacrimonasal duct 375.56
      congenital 743.65
      neonatal 375.55
    larynx 478.79
      congenital 748.3
      syphilitic 095.8
        congenital 090.5
    lung 518.89
    meatus
      ear (congenital) 744.02
        acquired (*see also* Stricture, ear canal,
          acquired) 380.50
      osseous (congenital) (ear) 744.03
        acquired (*see also* Stricture, ear canal,
          acquired) 380.50
      urinarius (*see also* Stricture, urethra) 598.9
        congenital 753.6
    mitral (valve) (*see also* Stenosis, mitral) 394.0
      congenital 746.5
      specified cause, except rheumatic 424.0
    myocardium, myocardial (*see also*
      Degeneration, myocardial) 429.1
      hypertrophic subaortic (idiopathic) 425.1
    nares (anterior) (posterior) 478.19
      congenital 748.0
    nasal duct 375.56
      congenital 743.65
      neonatal 375.55
    nasolacrimal duct 375.56
      congenital 743.65
      neonatal 375.55
    nasopharynx 478.29
      syphilitic 095.8
    nephrostomy 997.5
    nose 478.19
      congenital 748.0
    nostril (anterior) (posterior) 478.19
      congenital 748.0
    organ or site, congenital NEC—*see* Atresia
    osseous meatus (congenital) (ear) 744.03
      acquired (*see also* Stricture, ear canal,
        acquired) 380.50
    os uteri (*see also* Stricture, cervix) 622.4
    oviduct—*see* Stricture, fallopian tube
    pelviureteric junction 593.3

Stricture—*continued*
  pharynx (dilation) 478.29
  prostate 602.8
  pulmonary, pulmonic
    artery (congenital) 747.3
      acquired 417.8
      noncongenital 417.8
    infundibulum (congenital) 746.83
    valve (*see also* Endocarditis, pulmonary)
      424.3
      congenital 746.02
    vein (congenital) 747.49
      acquired 417.8
    vessel NEC 417.8
  punctum lacrimale 375.52
    congenital 743.65
  pylorus (hypertrophic) 537.0
    adult 537.0
    congenital 750.5
    infantile 750.5
  rectosigmoid 569.89
  rectum (sphincter) 569.2
    congenital 751.2
    due to
      chemical burn 947.3
      irradiation 569.2
      lymphogranuloma venereum 099.1
    gonococcal 098.7
    inflammatory 099.1
    syphilitic 095.8
    tuberculous (*see also* Tuberculosis) 014.8
  renal artery 440.1
  salivary duct or gland (any) 527.8
  sigmoid (flexure) (*see also* Obstruction,
    intestine) 560.9
  spermatic cord 608.85
  stoma (following) (of)
    colostomy 569.62
    cystostomy 997.5
    enterostomy 569.62
    esophagostomy 530.87
    gastrostomy 536.42
    ileostomy 569.62
    nephrostomy 997.5
    tracheostomy 519.02
    ureterostomy 997.5
  stomach 537.89
    congenital 750.7
    hourglass 537.6
  subaortic 746.81
    hypertrophic (acquired) (idiopathic) 425.1
  subglottic 478.74
  syphilitic NEC 095.8
  tendon (sheath) 727.81
  trachea 519.19
    congenital 748.3
    syphilitic 095.8
    tuberculous (*see also* Tuberculosis) 012.8
  tracheostomy 519.02
  tricuspid (valve) (*see also* Endocarditis,
    tricuspid) 397.0
    congenital 746.1
    nonrheumatic 424.2
  tunica vaginalis 608.85
  ureter (postoperative) 593.3
    congenital 753.29
    tuberculous (*see also* Tuberculosis) 016.2
  ureteropelvic junction 593.3
    congenital 753.21
  ureterovesical orifice 593.3
    congenital 753.22

Stricture—*continued*
  urethra (anterior) (meatal) (organic) (posterior) (spasmodic) 598.9
    associated with schistosomiasis (*see also* Schistosomiasis) 120.9 *[598.01]*
    congenital (valvular) 753.6
    due to
      infection 598.00
        syphilis 095.8 *[598.01]*
      trauma 598.1
    gonococcal 098.2 *[598.01]*
    gonorrheal 098.2 *[598.01]*
    infective 598.00
    late effect of injury 598.1
    postcatheterization 598.2
    postobstetric 598.1
    postoperative 598.2
    specified cause NEC 598.8
    syphilitic 095.8 *[598.01]*
    traumatic 598.1
    valvular, congenital 753.6
  urinary meatus (*see also* Stricture, urethra) 598.9
    congenital 753.6
  uterus, uterine 621.5
    os (external) (internal)—see Stricture, cervix
  vagina (outlet) 623.2
    congenital 752.49
  valve (cardiac) (heart) (*see also* Endocarditis) 424.90
    congenital (cardiac) (heart) NEC 746.89
      aortic 746.3
      mitral 746.5
      pulmonary 746.02
      tricuspid 746.1
      urethra 753.6
  valvular (*see also* Endocarditis) 424.90
  vascular graft or shunt 996.1
    atherosclerosis —*see* Arteriosclerosis, extremities
    embolism 996.74
    occlusion NEC 996.74
    thrombus 996.74
  vas deferens 608.85
    congenital 752.89
  vein 459.2
  vena cava (inferior) (superior) NEC 459.2
    congenital 747.49
  ventricular shunt 996.2
  vesicourethral orifice 596.0
    congenital 753.6
  vulva (acquired) 624.8
Stridor 786.1
  congenital (larynx) 748.3
Stridulous —*see* condition
Strippling of nails 703.8
Stroke 434.91
  apoplectic (*see also* Disease, cerebrovascular, acute) 436
  brain—*see* Infarct, brain
  embolic 434.11
  epileptic—*see* Epilepsy
  healed or old V12.59
  heart—*see* Disease, heart
  heat 992.0
  hemorrhagic—*see* Hemorrhage, brain
  iatrogenic 997.02
  in evolution 435.9
  ischemic 434.91
  late effect—*see* Late effect(s) (of) cerebrovascular disease

Stroke—*continued*
  lightning 994.0
  paralytic—*see* Infarct, brain
  postoperative 997.02
  progressive 435.9
  thrombotic 434.01
Stromatosis, endometrial (M8931/1) 236.0
Strong pulse 785.9
Strongyloides stercoralis infestation 127.2
Strongyloidiasis 127.2
Strongyloidosis 127.2
Strongylus (gibsoni) infestation 127.7
Strophulus (newborn) 779.89
  pruriginosus 698.2
Struck by lightning 994.0
Struma (*see also* Goiter) 240.9
  fibrosa 245.3
  Hashimoto (struma lymphomatosa) 245.2
  lymphomatosa 245.2
  nodosa (simplex) 241.9
    endemic 241.9
    multinodular 241.1
    sporadic 241.9
    toxic or with hyperthyroidism 242.3
      multinodular 242.2
      uninodular 242.1
    toxicosa 242.3
      multinodular 242.2
      uninodular 242.1
    uninodular 241.0
  ovarii (M9090/0) 220
    and carcinoid (M9091/1) 236.2
    malignant (M9090/3) 183.0
  Riedel's (ligneous thyroiditis) 245.3
  scrofulous (*see also* Tuberculosis) 017.2
  tuberculous (*see also* Tuberculosis) 017.2
    abscess 017.2
    adenitis 017.2
    lymphangitis 017.2
    ulcer 017.2
Strumipriva cachexia (*see also* Hypothyroidism) 244.9
Strümpell-Marie disease or spine (ankylosing spondylitis) 720.0
Strümpell-Westphal pseudosclerosis (hepatolenticular degeneration) 275.1
Stuart's disease (congenital factor X deficiency) (*see also* Defect, coagulation) 286.3
Stuart-Prower factor deficiency (congenital factor X deficiency) (*see also* Defect, coagulation) 286.3
Students' elbow 727.2
Stuffy nose 478.19
Stump —*see also* Amputation
  cervix, cervical (healed) 622.8
Stupor 780.09
  catatonic (*see also* Schizophrenia) 295.2
  circular (*see also* Psychosis, manic-depressive, circular) 296.7
  manic 296.89
  manic-depressive (*see also* Psychosis, affective) 296.89
  mental (anergic) (delusional) 298.9
  psychogenic 298.8
  reaction to exceptional stress (transient) 308.2
  traumatic NEC—*see also* Injury, intracranial
    with spinal (cord)
      lesion—*see* Injury, spinal, by site
      shock—*see* Injury, spinal, by site
Sturge (-Weber) (-Dimitri) disease or syndrome (encephalocutaneous angiomatosis) 759.6

Sunstroke 992.0

Superfecundation 651.9
  with fetal loss and retention of one or more
      fetus(es) 651.6
  following (elective) fetal reduction 651.7

Superfetation 651.9
  with fetal loss and retention of one or more
      fetus(es) 651.6
  following (elective) fetal reduction 651.7

Supernumerary (congenital)
  aortic cusps 746.89
  auditory ossicles 744.04
  bone 756.9
  breast 757.6
  carpal bones 755.56
  cusps, heart valve NEC 746.89
    mitral 746.5
    pulmonary 746.09
  digit(s) 755.00
    finger 755.01
    toe 755.02
  ear (lobule) 744.1
  fallopian tube 752.19
  finger 755.01
  hymen 752.49
  kidney 753.3
  lacrimal glands 743.64
  lacrimonasal duct 743.65
  lobule (ear) 744.1
  mitral cusps 746.5
  muscle 756.82
  nipples 757.6
  organ or site NEC—*see* Accessory
  ossicles, auditory 744.04
  ovary 752.0
  oviduct 752.19
  pulmonic cusps 746.09
  rib 756.3
    cervical or first 756.2
      syndrome 756.2
  roots (of teeth) 520.2
  spinal vertebra 756.19
  spleen 759.0
  tarsal bones 755.67
  teeth 520.1
    causing crowding 524.31
  testis 752.89
  thumb 755.01
  toe 755.02
  uterus 752.2
  vagina 752.49
  vertebra 756.19

Supervision (of)
  contraceptive method previously prescribed V25.40
    intrauterine device V25.42
    oral contraceptive (pill) V25.41
    specified type NEC V25.49
    subdermal implantable contraceptive V25.43
  dietary (for) V65.3
    allergy (food) V65.3
    colitis V65.3
    diabetes mellitus V65.3
    food allergy intolerance V65.3
    gastritis V65.3
    hypercholesterolemia V65.3
    hypoglycemia V65.3
    intolerance (food) V65.3
    obesity V65.3
    specified NEC V65.3
  lactation V24.1
  pregnancy—*see* Pregnancy, supervision of

Supplemental teeth 520.1
  causing crowding 524.31

Suppression
  binocular vision 368.31
  lactation 676.5
  menstruation 626.8
  ovarian secretion 256.39
  renal 586
  urinary secretion 788.5
  urine 788.5

Suppuration, suppurative —*see also* condition
  accessory sinus (chronic) (*see also* Sinusitis)
    473.9
  adrenal gland 255.8
  antrum (chronic) (*see also* Sinusitis, maxillary)
    473.0
  bladder (*see also* Cystitis) 595.89
  bowel 569.89
  brain 324.0
    late effect 326
  breast 611.0
    puerperal, postpartum 675.1
  dental periosteum 526.5
  diffuse (skin) 686.00
  ear (middle) (*see also* Otitis media) 382.4
    external (*see also* Otitis, externa) 380.10
    internal 386.33
  ethmoidal (sinus) (chronic) (*see also* Sinusitis,
    ethmoidal) 473.2
  fallopian tube (*see also* Salpingo-oophoritis)
    614.2
  frontal (sinus) (chronic) (*see also* Sinusitis,
    frontal) 473.1
  gallbladder (*see also* Cholecystitis, acute) 575.0
  gum 523.30
  hernial sac—*see* Hernia, by site
  intestine 569.89
  joint (*see also* Arthritis, suppurative) 711.0
  labyrinthine 386.33
  lung 513.0
  mammary gland 611.0
    puerperal, postpartum 675.1
  maxilla, maxillary 526.4
    sinus (chronic) (*see also* Sinusitis, maxillary)
      473.0
  muscle 728.0
  nasal sinus (chronic) (*see also* Sinusitis) 473.9
  pancreas 577.0
  parotid gland 527.2
  pelvis, pelvic
    female (*see also* Disease, pelvis,
      inflammatory) 614.4
      acute 614.3
    male (*see also* Peritonitis) 567.21
  pericranial (*see also* Osteomyelitis) 730.2
  salivary duct or gland (any) 527.2
  sinus (nasal) (*see also* Sinusitis) 473.9
  sphenoidal (sinus) (chronic) (*see also* Sinusitis,
    sphenoidal) 473.3
  thymus (gland) 254.1
  thyroid (gland) 245.0
  tonsil 474.8
  uterus (*see also* Endometritis) 615.9
  vagina 616.10
  wound—*see also* Wound, open, by site,
    complicated
    dislocation—*see* Dislocation, by site,
      compound
    fracture—*see* Fracture, by site, open
    scratch or other superficial injury—*see* Injury,
      superficial, by site

Swelling—*continued*
  mediastinal 786.6
  mouth 784.2
  muscle (limb) 729.81
  neck 784.2
  nose or sinus 784.2
  palate 784.2
  pelvis 789.3
  penis 607.83
  perineum 625.8
  rectum 787.99
  scrotum 608.86
  skin 782.2
  splenic (*see also* Splenomegaly) 789.2
  substernal 786.6
  superficial, localized (skin) 782.2
  testicle 608.86
  throat 784.2
  toe 729.81
  tongue 784.2
  tubular (*see also* Disease, renal) 593.9
  umbilicus 789.3
  uterus 625.8
  vagina 625.8
  vulva 625.8
  wandering, due to Gnathostoma (spinigerum) 128.1
  white—*see* Tuberculosis, arthritis
Swift's disease 985.0
Swimmers'
  ear (acute) 380.12
  itch 120.3
Swimming in the head 780.4
Swollen —*see also* Swelling
  glands 785.6
Swyer-James syndrome (unilateral hyperlucent lung) 492.8
Swyer's syndrome (XY pure gonadal dysgenesis) 752.7
Sycosis 704.8
  barbae (not parasitic) 704.8
  contagiosa 110.0
  lupoid 704.8
  mycotic 110.0
  parasitic 110.0
  vulgaris 704.8
Sydenham's chorea —*see* Chorea, Sydenham's
Sylvatic yellow fever 060.0
Sylvest's disease (epidemic pleurodynia) 074.1
Symblepharon 372.63
  congenital 743.62
Symonds' syndrome 348.2
Sympathetic —*see* condition
Sympatheticotonia (*see also* Neuropathy, peripheral, autonomic) 337.9
Sympathicoblastoma (M9500/3)
  specified site—*see* Neoplasm, by site, malignant
  unspecified site 194.0
Sympathicogonioma (M9500/3)—*see* Sympathicoblastoma
Sympathoblastoma (M9500/3)—*see* Sympathicoblastoma
Sympathogonioma (M9500/3)—*see* Sympathicoblastoma
Symphalangy (*see also* Syndactylism) 755.10
Symptoms, specified (general) NEC 780.99
  abdomen NEC 789.9
  bone NEC 733.90
  breast NEC 611.79
  cardiac NEC 785.9

Symptoms, specified—*continued*
  cardiovascular NEC 785.9
  chest NEC 786.9
  development NEC 783.9
  digestive system NEC 787.99
  eye NEC 379.99
  gastrointestinal tract NEC 787.99
  genital organs NEC
    female 625.9
    male 608.9
  head and neck NEC 784.99
  heart NEC 785.9
  joint NEC 719.60
    ankle 719.67
    elbow 719.62
    foot 719.67
    hand 719.64
    hip 719.65
    knee 719.66
    multiple sites 719.69
    pelvic region 719.65
    shoulder (region) 719.61
    specified site NEC 719.68
    wrist 719.63
  larynx NEC 784.99
  limbs NEC 729.89
  lymphatic system NEC 785.9
  menopausal 627.2
  metabolism NEC 783.9
  mouth NEC 528.9
  muscle NEC 728.9
  musculoskeletal NEC 781.99
    limbs NEC 729.89
  nervous system NEC 781.99
  neurotic NEC 300.9
  nutrition, metabolism, and development NEC 783.9
  pelvis NEC 789.9
    female 625.9
  peritoneum NEC 789.9
  respiratory system NEC 786.9
  skin and integument NEC 782.9
  subcutaneous tissue NEC 782.9
  throat NEC 784.99
  tonsil NEC 784.99
  urinary system NEC 788.9
  vascular NEC 785.9
Sympus 759.89
Synarthrosis 719.80
  ankle 719.87
  elbow 719.82
  foot 719.87
  hand 719.84
  hip 719.85
  knee 719.86
  multiple sites 719.89
  pelvic region 719.85
  shoulder (region) 719.81
  specified site NEC 719.88
  wrist 719.83
Syncephalus 759.4
Synchondrosis 756.9
  abnormal (congenital) 756.9
  ischiopubic (van Neck's) 732.1
Synchysis (senile) (vitreous humor) 379.21
  scintillans 379.22
Syncope (near) (pre-) 780.2
  anginosa 413.9
  bradycardia 427.89
  cardiac 780.2
  carotid sinus 337.0
  complicating delivery 669.2

Syndrome—*continued*
  Cockayne-Weber (epidermolysis bullosa) 757.39
  Coffin-Lowry 759.89
  Cogan's (nonsyphilitic interstitial keratitis) 370.52
  cold injury (newborn) 778.2
  Collet (-Sicard) 352.6
  combined immunity deficiency 279.2
  compartment(al) (anterior) (deep) (posterior) 958.8
    nontraumatic
      abdomen 729.73
      arm 729.71
      buttock 729.72
      fingers 729.71
      foot 729.72
      forearm 729.71
      hand 729.71
      hip 729.72
      leg 729.72
      lower extremity 729.72
      shoulder 729.71
      specified site NEC 729.79
      thigh 729.72
      toes 729.72
      upper extremity 729.71
      wrist 729.71
    traumatic 958.90
      abdomen 958.93
      arm 958.91
      buttock 958.92
      fingers 958.91
      foot 958.92
      forearm 958.91
      hand 958.91
      hip 958.92
      leg 958.92
      lower extremity 958.92
      shoulder 958.91
      specified site NEC 958.99
      thigh 958.92
      tibial 958.92
      toes 958.92
      upper extremity 958.91
      wrist 958.91
  compression 958.5
    cauda equina 344.60
      with neurogenic bladder 344.61
  concussion 310.2
  congenital
    affecting more than one system 759.7
      specified type NEC 759.89
    congenital central alveolar hypoventilation 327.25
    facial diplegia 352.6
    muscular hypertrophy-cerebral 759.89
  congestion-fibrosis (pelvic) 625.5
  conjunctivourethrosynovial 099.3
  Conn (-Louis) (primary aldosteronism) 255.12
  Conradi (-Hünermann) (chondrodysplasia calcificans congenita) 756.59
  conus medullaris 336.8
  Cooke-Apert-Gallais (adrenogenital) 255.2
  Cornelia de Lange's (Amsterdam dwarf, mental retardation, and brachycephaly) 759.8
  coronary insufficiency or intermediate 411.1
  cor pulmonale 416.9
  corticosexual 255.2
  Costen's (complex) 524.60
  costochondral junction 733.6
  costoclavicular 353.0

Syndrome—*continued*
  costovertebral 253.0
  Cotard's (paranoia) 297.1
  Cowden 759.6
  craniovertebral 723.2
  Creutzfeldt-Jakob (new variant) 046.1
    with dementia
      with behavioral disturbance 046.1 *[294.11]*
      without behavioral disturbance 046.1 *[294.10]*
  crib death 798.0
  cricopharyngeal 787.2
  cri-du-chat 758.31
  Crigler-Najjar (congenital hyperbilirubinemia) 277.4
  crocodile tears 351.8
  Cronkhite-Canada 211.3
  croup 464.4
  CRST (cutaneous systemic sclerosis) 710.1
  crush 958.5
  crushed lung (*see also* Injury, internal, lung) 861.20
  Cruveilhier-Baumgarten (cirrhosis of liver) 571.5
  cubital tunnel 354.2
  Cuiffini-Pancoast (M8010/3) (carcinoma, pulmonary apex) 162.3
  Curschmann (-Batten) (-Steinert) 359.2
  Cushing's (iatrogenic) (idiopathic) (pituitary basophilism) (pituitary-dependent) 255.0
    overdose or wrong substance given or taken 962.0
  Cyriax's (slipping rib) 733.99
  cystic duct stump 576.0
  Da Costa's (neurocirculatory asthenia) 306.2
  Dameshek's (erythroblastic anemia) 282.49
  Dana-Putnam (subacute combined sclerosis with pernicious anemia) 281.0 *[336.2]*
  Danbolt (-Closs) (acrodermatitis enteropathica) 686.8
  Dandy-Walker (atresia, foramen of Magendie) 742.3
    with spina bifida (*see also* Spina bifida) 741.0
  Danlos' 756.83
  Davies-Colley (slipping rib) 733.99
  dead fetus 641.3
  defeminization 255.2
  defibrination (*see also* Fibrinolysis) 286.6
  Degos' 447.8
  Deiters' nucleus 386.19
  Déjérine-Roussy 338.0
  Déjérine-Thomas 333.0
  de Lange's (Amsterdam dwarf, mental retardation, and brachycephaly) (Cornelia) 759.89
  Del Castillo's (germinal aplasia) 606.0
  deletion chromosomes 758.39
  delusional
    induced by drug 292.11
  dementia-aphonia, of childhood (*see also* Psychosis, childhood) 299.1
  demyelinating NEC 341.9
  denial visual hallucination 307.9
  depersonalization 300.6
  Dercum's (adiposis dolorosa) 272.8
  de Toni-Fanconi (-Debré) (cystinosis) 270.0
  diabetes-dwarfism-obesity (juvenile) 258.1
  diabetes mellitus-hypertension-nephrosis 250.4 *[581.81]*
  diabetes mellitus in newborn infant 775.1
  diabetes-nephrosis 250.4 *[581.81]*

Syndrome—*continued*
  diabetic amyotrophy 250.6 *[358.1]*
  Diamond-Blackfan (congenital hypoplastic
    anemia) 284.01
  Diamond-Gardener (autoerythrocyte
    sensitization) 287.2
  DIC (diffuse or disseminated intravascular
    coagulopathy) (*see also* Fibrinolysis) 286.6
  diencephalohypophyseal NEC 253.8
  diffuse cervicobrachial 723.3
  diffuse obstructive pulmonary 496
  DiGeorge's (thymic hypoplasia) 279.11
  Dighton's 756.51
  Di Guglielmo's (erythremic myelosis)
    (M9841/3) 207.0
  disequilibrium 276.9
  disseminated platelet thrombosis 446.6
  Ditthomska 307.81
  Doan-Wiseman (primary splenic neutropenia)
    289.53
  Döhle body-panmyelopathic 288.2
  Donohue's (leprechaunism) 259.8
  dorsolateral medullary (*see also* Disease,
    cerebrovascular, acute) 436
  double athetosis 333.71
  double whammy 360.81
  Down's (mongolism) 758.0
  Dresbach's (elliptocytosis) 282.1
  Dressler's (postmyocardial infarction) 411.0
    hemoglobinuria 283.2
    postcardiotomy 429.4
  drug withdrawal, infant, of dependent mother
    779.5
  dry skin 701.1
    eye 375.15
  DSAP (disseminated superficial actinic
    porokeratosis) 692.75
  Duane's (retraction) 378.71
  Duane-Stilling-Türk (ocular retraction
    syndrome) 378.71
  Dubin-Johnson (constitutional
    hyperbilirubinemia) 277.4
  Dubin-Sprinz (constitutional
    hyperbilirubinemia) 277.4
  Duchenne's 335.22
  due to abnormality
    autosomal NEC (*see also* Abnormal,
      autosomes NEC) 758.5
      13 758.1
      18 758.2
      21 or 22 758.0
      D_1 758.1
      E_3 758.2
      G 758.0
    chromosomal 758.89
      sex 758.81
  dumping 564.2
    nonsurgical 536.8
  Duplay's 726.2
  Dupré's (meningism) 781.6
  Dyke-Young (acquired macrocytic hemolytic
    anemia) 283.9
  dyspraxia 315.4
  dystocia, dystrophia 654.9
  Eagle-Barrett 756.71
  Eales' 362.18
  Eaton-Lambert (*see also* Neoplasm, by site,
    malignant) 199.1 *[358.1]*
  Ebstein's (downward displacement, tricuspid
    valve into right ventricle) 746.2
  ectopic ACTH secretion 255.0

Syndrome—*continued*
  eczema-thrombocytopenia 279.12
  Eddowes' (brittle bones and blue sclera) 756.51
  Edwards' 758.2
  efferent loop 537.89
  effort (aviators') (psychogenic) 306.2
  Ehlers-Danlos 756.83
  Eisenmenger's (ventricular septal defect) 745.4
  Ekbom's (restless legs) 333.94
  Ekman's (brittle bones and blue sclera) 756.51
  electric feet 266.2
  Elephant man 237.71
  Ellison-Zollinger (gastric hypersecretion with
    pancreatic islet cell tumor) 251.5
  Ellis-van Creveld (chondroectodermal
    dysplasia) 756.55
  embryonic fixation 270.2
  empty sella (turcica) 253.8
  endocrine-hypertensive 255.3
  Engel-von Recklinghausen (osteitis fibrosa
    cystica) 252.01
  enteroarticular 099.3
  entrapment—*see* Neuropathy, entrapment
  eosinophilia myalgia 710.5
  epidemic vomiting 078.82
  Epstein's—*see* Nephrosis
  Erb (-Oppenheim) -Goldflam 358.00
  Erdheim's (acromegalic macrospondylitis)
    253.0
  Erlacher-Blount (tibia vara) 732.4
  erythrocyte fragmentation 283.19
  euthyroid sick 790.94
  Evans' (thrombocytopenic purpura) 287.32
  excess cortisol, iatrogenic 255.0
  exhaustion 300.5
  extrapyramidal 333.90
  eyelid-malar-mandible 756.0
  eye retraction 378.71
  Faber's (achlorhydric anemia) 280.9
  Fabry (-Anderson) (angiokeratoma corporis
    diffusum) 272.7
  facet 724.8
  Fallot's 745.2
  falx (*see also* Hemorrhage, brain) 431
  familial eczema-thrombocytopenia 279.12
  Fanconi's (anemia) (congenital pancytopenia)
    284.09
  Fanconi (-de Toni) (-Debré) (cystinosis) 270.0
  Farber (-Uzman) (disseminated
    lipogranulomatosis) 272.8
  fatigue NEC 300.5
    chronic 780.71
  faulty bowel habit (idiopathic megacolon) 564.7
  FDH (focal dermal hypoplasia) 757.39
  fecal reservoir 560.39
  Feil-Klippel (brevicollis) 756.16
  Felty's (rheumatoid arthritis with splenomegaly
    and leukopenia) 714.1
  fertile eunuch 257.2
  fetal alcohol 760.71
    late effect 760.71
  fibrillation-flutter 427.32
  fibrositis (periarticular) 729.0
  Fiedler's (acute isolated myocarditis) 422.91
  Fiessinger-Leroy (-Reiter) 099.3
  Fiessinger-Rendu (erythema multiforme
    exudativum) 695.1
  first arch 756.0
  fish odor 270.8
  Fisher's 357.0
  Fitz's (acute hemorrhagic pancreatitis) 577.0

Syndrome—*continued*
  Fitz-Hugh and Curtis 098.86
    due to
      Chlamydia trachomatis 099.56
      Neisseria gonorrhoeae (gonococcal
        peritonitis) 098.86
  Flajani (-Basedow) (exophthalmic goiter) 242.0
  floppy
    infant 781.99
    valve (mitral) 424.0
  flush 259.2
  Foix-Alajouanine 336.1
  Fong's (hereditary osteo-onychodysplasia)
    756.89
  foramen magnum 348.4
  Forbes-Albright (nonpuerperal amenorrhea and
    lactation associated with pituitary tumor)
    253.1
  Foster-Kennedy 377.04
  Foville's (peduncular) 344.89
  Fragile X 759.83
  Franceschetti's (mandibulofacial dysostosis)
    756.0
  Fraser's 759.89
  Freeman-Sheldon 759.89
  Frey's (auriculotemporal) 705.22
  Friderichsen-Waterhouse 036.3
  Friedrich-Erb-Arnold (acropachyderma) 757.39
  Fröhlich's (adiposogenital dystrophy) 253.8
  Froin's 336.8
  Frommel-Chiari 676.6
  frontal lobe 310.0
  Fuller Albright's (osteitis fibrosa disseminata)
    756.59
  Fukuhara 277.87
  functional
    bowel 564.9
    prepubertal castrate 752.89
  Gaisböck's (polycythemia hypertonica) 289.0
  ganglion (basal, brain) 333.90
    geniculi 351.1
  Ganser's, hysterical 300.16
  Gardner-Diamond (autoerythrocyte
    sensitization) 287.2
  gastroesophageal junction 530.0
  gastroesophageal laceration-hemorrhage 530.7
  gastrojejunal loop obstruction 537.89
  Gayet-Wernicke's (superior hemorrhagic
    polioencephalitis) 265.1
  Gee-Herter-Heubner (nontropical sprue) 579.0
  Gélineau's (*see also* Narcolepsy) 347.00
  genito-anorectal 099.1
  Gerhardt's (vocal cord paralysis) 478.30
  Gerstmann's (finger agnosia) 784.69
  Giannotti Crosti 057.8
    due to known virus—*see* Infection, virus
    due to unknown virus 057.8
  Gilbert's 277.4
  Gilford (-Hutchinson) (progeria) 259.8
  Gilles de la Tourette's 307.23
  Gillespie's (dysplasia oculodentodigitalis)
    759.89
  Glénard's (enteroptosis) 569.89
  Glinski-Simmonds (pituitary cachexia) 253.2
  glucuronyl transferase 277.4
  glue ear 381.20
  Goldberg (-Maxwell) (-Morris) (testicular
    feminization) 259.5
  Goldenhar's (oculoauriculovertebral dysplasia)
    756.0
  Goldflam-Erb 358.00

Syndrome—*continued*
  Goltz-Gorlin (dermal hypoplasia) 757.39
  Good's 279.06
  Goodpasture's (pneumorenal) 446.21
  Gopalan's (burning feet) 266.2
  Gorlin-Chaudhry-Moss 759.89
  Gougerot (-Houwer) -Sjögren
    (keratoconjunctivitis sicca) 710.2
  Gougerot-Blum (pigmented purpuric lichenoid
    dermatitis) 709.1
  Gougerot-Carteaud (confluent reticulate
    papillomatosis) 701.8
  Gouley's (constrictive pericarditis) 423.2
  Gowers' (vasovagal attack) 780.2
  Gowers-Paton-Kennedy 377.04
  Gradenigo's 383.02
  Gray or grey (chloramphenicol) (newborn)
    779.4
  Greig's (hypertelorism) 756.0
  Gubler-Millard 344.89
  Guérin-Stern (arthrogryposis multiplex
    congenita) 754.89
  Guillain-Barré (-Strohl) 357.0
  Gunn's (jaw-winking syndrome) 742.8
  Günther's (congenital erythropoietic porphyria)
    277.1
  gustatory sweating 350.8
  H_3O 759.81
  Hadfield-Clarke (pancreatic infantilism) 577.8
  Haglund-Läwen-Fründ 717.89
  hairless women 257.8
  hair tourniquet—*see also* Injury, superficial, by
    site
    finger 915.8
      infected 915.9
    penis 911.8
      infected 911.9
    toe 917.8
      infected 917.9
  Hallermann-Streiff 756.0
  Hallervorden-Spatz 333.0
  Hamman's (spontaneous mediastinal
    emphysema) 518.1
  Hamman-Rich (diffuse interstitial pulmonary
    fibrosis) 516.3
  Hand-Schüller-Christian (chronic histiocytosis
    X) 277.89
  hand-foot 282.61
  Hanot-Chauffard (-Troisier) (bronze diabetes)
    275.0
  Harada's 363.22
  Hare's (M8010/3) (carcinoma, pulmonary apex)
    162.3
  Harkavy's 446.0
  harlequin color change 779.89
  Harris' (organic hyperinsulinism) 251.1
  Hart's (pellagra-cerebellar ataxia-renal
    aminoaciduria) 270.0
  Hayem-Faber (achlorhydric anemia) 280.9
  Hayem-Widal (acquired hemolytic jaundice)
    283.9
  Heberden's (angina pectoris) 413.9
  Hedinger's (malignant carcinoid) 259.2
  Hegglin's 288.2
  Heller's (infantile psychosis) (*see also*
    Psychosis, childhood) 299.1
  H.E.L.L.P. 642.5
  hemolytic-uremic (adult) (child) 283.11
  hemophagocytic 288.4
    infection-associated 288.4

Syndrome—*continued*

Hench-Rosenberg (palindromic arthritis) (*see also* Rheumatism, palindromic) 719.3
Henoch-Schönlein (allergic purpura) 287.0
hepatic flexure 569.89
hepatorenal 572.4
  due to a procedure 997.4
  following delivery 674.8
hepatourologic 572.4
Herrick's (hemoglobin S disease) 282.61
Herter (-Gee) (nontropical sprue) 579.0
Heubner-Herter (nontropical sprue) 579.0
Heyd's (hepatorenal) 572.4
HHHO 759.81
high grade myelodysplastic 238.73
  with 5q deletion 238.73
Hilger's 337.0
histiocytic 288.4
Hoffa (-Kastert) (liposynovitis prepatellaris) 272.8
Hoffmann's 244.9 *[359.5]*
Hoffmann-Bouveret (paroxysmal tachycardia) 427.2
Hoffmann-Werdnig 335.0
Holländer-Simons (progressive lipodystrophy) 272.6
Holmes' (visual disorientation) 368.16
Holmes-Adie 379.46
Hoppe-Goldflam 358.00
Yorner's (sde also Neuropathy, peripheral, autonomic) 337.9
  traumatic—*see* Injury, nerve, cervical sympathetic
hospital addiction 301.51
Hunt's (herpetic geniculate ganglionitis) 053.11
  dyssynergia cerebellaris myoclonica 334.2
Hunter (-Hurler) (mucopolysaccharidosis II) 277.5
hunterian glossitis 529.4
Hurler (-Hunter) (mucopolysaccharidosis II) 277.5
Hutchinson's incisors or teeth 090.5
Hutchinson-Boeck (sarcoidosis) 135
Hutchinson-Gilford (progeria) 259.8
hydralazine
  correct substance properly administered 695.4
  overdose or wrong substance given or taken 972.6
hydraulic concussion (abdomen) (*see also* Injury, internal, abdomen) 868.00
hyperabduction 447.8
hyperactive bowel 564.9
hyperaldosteronism with hypokalemic alkalosis (Bartter's) 255.13
hypercalcemic 275.42
hypercoagulation NEC 289.89
hypereosinophilic (idiopathic) 288.3
hyperkalemic 276.7
hyperkinetic—*see also* Hyperkinesia
  heart 429.82
hyperlipemia-hemolytic anemia-icterus 571.1
hypermobility 728.5
hypernatremia 276.0
hyperosmolarity 276.0
hypersomnia-bulimia 349.89
hypersplenic 289.4
hypersympathetic (*see also* Neuropathy, peripheral, autonomic) 337.9
hypertransfusion, newborn 776.4
hyperventilation, psychogenic 306.1
hyperviscosity (of serum) NEC 273.3
  polycythemic 289.0

Syndrome—*continued*

sclerothymic 282.8
hypoglycemic (familial) (neonatal) 251.2
  functional 251.1
hypokalemic 276.8
hypophyseal 253.8
hypophyseothalamic 253.8
hypopituitarism 253.2
hypoplastic left heart 746.7
hypopotassemia 276.8
hyposmolality 276.1
hypotension, maternal 669.2
hypotonia-hypomentia-hypogonadism-obesity 759.81
ICF (intravascular coagulation-fibrinolysis) (*see also* Fibrinolysis) 286.6
idiopathic cardiorespiratory distress, newborn 769
idiopathic nephrotic (infantile) 581.9
Imerslund (-Gräsbeck) (anemia due to familial selective vitamin B_{12} malabsorption) 281.1
immobility (paraplegic) 728.3
immunity deficiency, combined 279.2
impending coronary 411.1
impingement
  shoulder 726.2
  vertebral bodies 724.4
inappropriate secretion of antidiuretic hormone (ADH) 253.6
incomplete
  mandibulofacial 756.0
infant
  death, sudden (SIDS) 798.0
  Hercules 255.2
  of diabetic mother 775.0
  shaken 995.55
infantilism 253.3
inferior vena cava 459.2
influenza-like 487.1
inspissated bile, newborn 774.4
insufficient sleep 307.44
intermediate coronary (artery) 411.1
internal carotid artery (*see also* Occlusion, artery, carotid) 433.1
interspinous ligament 724.8
intestinal
  carcinoid 259.2
  gas 787.3
  knot 560.2
intravascular
  coagulation-fibrinolysis (ICF) (*see also* Fibrinolysis) 286.6
  coagulopathy (*see also* Fibrinolysis) 286.6
inverted Marfan's 759.89
IRDS (idiopathic respiratory distress, newborn) 769
irritable
  bowel 564.1
  heart 306.2
  weakness 300.5
ischemic bowel (transient) 557.9
  chronic 557.1
  due to mesenteric artery insufficiency 557.1
Itsenko-Cushing (pituitary basophilism) 255.0
IVC (intravascular coagulopathy) (*see also* Fibrinolysis) 286.6
Ivemark's (asplenia with congenital heart disease) 759.0
Jaccoud's 714.4
Jackson's 344.89

Syndrome—*continued*
  Jadassohn-Lewandowski (pachyonychia
      congenita) 757.5
  Jaffe-Lichtenstein (-Uehlinger) 252.01
  Jahnke's (encephalocutaneous angiomatosis)
      759.6
  Jakob-Creutzfeldt (new variant) 046.1
    with dementia
        with behavioral disturbance 046.1 *[294.11]*
        without behavioral disturbance 046.1
            [294.10]
  Jaksch's (pseudoleukemia infantum) 285.8
  Jaksch-Hayem (-Luzet) (pseudoleukemia
      infantum) 285.8
  jaw-winking 742.8
  jejunal 564.2
  Jervell-Lange-Nielsen 426.82
  jet lag 327.35
  Jeune's (asphyxiating thoracic dystrophy of
      newborn) 756.4
  Job's (chronic granulomatous disease) 288.1
  Jordan's 288.2
  Joseph-Diamond-Blackfan (congenital
      hypoplastic anemia) 284.01
  Joubert 759.89
  jugular foramen 352.6
  Kabuki 759.89
  Kahler's (multiple myeloma) (M9730/3) 203.0
  Kalischer's (encephalocutaneous angiomatosis)
      759.6
  Kallmann's (hypogonadotropic hypogonadism
      with anosmia) 253.4
  Kanner's (autism) (*see also* Psychosis,
      childhood) 299.0
  Kartagener's (sinusitis, bronchiectasis, situs
      inversus) 759.3
  Kasabach-Merritt (capillary hemangioma
      associated with thrombocytopenic purpura)
      287.39
  Kast's (dyschondroplasia with hemangiomas)
      756.4
  Kaznelson's (congenital hypoplastic anemia)
      284.01
  Kearns-Sayre 277.87
  Kelly's (sideropenic dysphagia) 280.8
  Kimmelstiel-Wilson (intercapillary
      glomerulosclerosis) 250.4 *[581.81]*
  Klauder's (erythema multiforme exudativum)
      695.1
  Klein-Waardenburg (ptosis-epicanthus) 270.2
  Kleine-Levin 327.13
  Klinefelter's 758.7
  Klippel-Feil (brevicollis) 756.16
  Klippel-Trenaunay 759.89
  Klumpke (-Déjérine) (injury to brachial plexus
      at birth) 767.6
  Klüver-Bucy (-Terzian) 310.0
  Köhler-Pellegrini-Stieda (calcification, knee
      joint) 726.62
  König's 564.89
  Korsakoff's (nonalcoholic) 294.0
      alcoholic 291.1
  Korsakoff (-Wernicke) (nonalcoholic) 294.0
      alcoholic 291.1
  Kostmann's (infantile genetic agranulocytosis)
      288.01
  Krabbe's
    congenital muscle hypoplasia 756.89
    cutaneocerebral angioma 759.6
  Kunkel (lupoid hepatitis) 571.49
  labyrinthine 386.50

Syndrome—*continued*
  laceration, broad ligament 620.6
  Langdon Down (mongolism) 758.0
  Larsen's (flattened facies and multiple
      congenital dislocations) 755.8
  lateral
    cutaneous nerve of thigh 355.1
        medullary (*see also* Disease, cerebrovascular
            acute) 436
  Launois' (pituitary gigantism) 253.0
  Launois-Cléret (adiposogenital dystrophy) 253.8
  Laurence-Moon (-Bardet) -Biedl (obesity,
      polydactyly, and mental retardation) 759.8
  Lawford's (encephalocutaneous angiomatosis)
      759.6
  lazy
    leukocyte 288.09
    posture 728.3
  Lederer-Brill (acquired infectious hemolytic
      anemia) 283.19
  Legg-Calvé-Perthes (osteochondrosis capital
      femoral) 732.1
  Lemiere 451.89
  Lennox's (*see also* Epilepsy) 345.0
  Lennox-Gastaut syndrome 345.0
    with tonic seizures 345.1
  lenticular 275.1
  Léopold-Lévi's (paroxysmal thyroid instability)
      242.9
  Lepore hemoglobin 282.49
  Léri-Weill 756.59
  Leriche's (aortic bifurcation occlusion) 444.0
  Lermoyez's (*see also* Disease, Ménière's)
      386.00
  Lesch-Nyhan (hypoxanthine-guanine-
      phosphoribosyltransferase deficiency) 277.2
  Lev's (acquired complete heart block) 426.0
  Levi's (pituitary dwarfism) 253.3
  Lévy-Roussy 334.3
  Lichtheim's (subacute combined sclerosis with
      pernicious anemia) 281.0 *[336.2]*
  Li-Fraumeni V84.01
  Lightwood's (renal tubular acidosis) 588.89
  Lignac (-de Toni) (-Fanconi) (-Debré)
      (cystinosis) 270.0
  Likoff's (angina in menopausal women) 413.9
  liver-kidney 572.4
  Lloyd's 258.1
  lobotomy 310.0
  Löffler's (eosinophilic pneumonitis) 518.3
  Löfgren's (sarcoidosis) 135
  long arm 18 or 21 deletion 758.39
  Looser (-Debray) -Milkman (osteomalacia with
      pseudofractures) 268.2
  Lorain-Levi (pituitary dwarfism) 253.3
  Louis-Bar (ataxia-telangiectasia) 334.8
  low
    atmospheric pressure 993.2
    back 724.2
        psychogenic 306.0
    output (cardiac) (*see also* Failure, heart) 428.9
  Lowe's (oculocerebrorenal dystrophy) 270.8
  Lowe-Terrey-MacLachlan (oculocerebrorenal
      dystrophy) 270.8
  lower radicular, newborn 767.4
  Lown (-Ganong)-Levine (short P-R interval,
      normal QRS complex, and supraventricular
      tachycardia) 426.81
  Lucey-Driscoll (jaundice due to delayed
      conjugation) 774.30
  Luetscher's (dehydration) 276.51

Syndrome—*continued*
- lumbar vertebral 724.4
- Lutembacher's (atrial septal defect with mitral stenosis) 745.5
- Lyell's (toxic epidermal necrolysis) 695.1
  - due to drug
    - correct substance properly administered 695.1
    - overdose or wrong substance given or taken 977.9
      - specified drug—*see* Table of drugs and chemicals
- MacLeod's 492.8
- macrogenitosomia praecox 259.8
- macroglobulinemia 273.3
- macrophage activation 288.4
- Maffucci's (dyschondroplasia with hemangiomas) 756.4
- Magenblase 306.4
- magnesium-deficiency 781.7
- Mal de Debarquement 780.4
- malabsorption 579.9
  - postsurgical 579.3
  - spinal fluid 331.3
- malignant carcinoid 259.2
- Mallory-Weiss 530.7
- mandibulofacial dysostosis 756.0
- manic-depressive (*see also* Psychosis, affective) 296.80
- Mankowsky's (familial dysplastic osteopathy) 731.2
- maple syrup (urine) 270.3
- Marable's (celiac artery compression) 447.4
- Marchesani (-Weill) (brachymorphism and ectopia lentis) 759.89
- Marchiafava-Bignami 341.8
- Marchiafava-Micheli (paroxysmal nocturnal hemoglobinuria) 283.2
- Marcus Gunn's (jaw-winking syndrome) 742.8
- Marfan's (arachnodactyly) 759.82
  - meaning congenital syphilis 090.49
    - with luxation of lens 090.49 *[379.32]*
- Marie's (acromegaly) 253.0
  - primary or idiopathic (acropachyderma) 757.39
  - secondary (hypertrophic pulmonary osteoarthropathy) 731.2
- Markus-Adie 379.46
- Maroteaux-Lamy (mucopolysaccharidosis VI) 277.5
- Martin's 715.27
- Martin-Albright (pseudohypoparathyroidism) 275.49
- Martorell-Fabré (pulseless disease) 446.7
- massive aspiration of newborn 770.18
- Masters-Allen 620.6
- mastocytosis 757.33
- maternal hypotension 669.2
- maternal obesity 646.1
- May (-Hegglin) 288.2
- McArdle (-Schmid) (-Pearson) (glycogenosis V) 271.0
- McCune-Albright (osteitis fibrosa disseminata) 756.59
- McQuarrie's (idiopathic familial hypoglycemia) 251.2
- meconium
  - aspiration 770.12
  - plug (newborn) NEC 777.1
- median arcuate ligament 447.4
- mediastinal fibrosis 519.3

Syndrome—*continued*
- Meekeren-Ehlers-Danlos 756.83
- Meige (blepharospasm-oromandibular dystonia) 333.82
- -Milroy (chronic hereditary edema) 757.0
- MELAS (mitochondrial encephalopathy, lactic acidosis and stroke-like episodes) 277.87
- Melkersson (-Rosenthal) 351.8
- Mende's (ptosis-epicanthus) 270.2
- Mendelson's (resulting from a procedure) 997.3
  - during labor 668.0
  - obstetric 668.0
- Ménétrier's (hypertrophic gastritis) 535.2
- Ménière's (*see also* Disease, Ménière's) 386.00
- meningo-eruptive 047.1
- Menkes' 759.89
  - glutamic acid 759.89
  - maple syrup (urine) disease 270.3
- menopause 627.2
  - postartificial 627.4
- menstruation 625.4
- MERRF (myoclonus with epilepsy and with ragged red fibers) 277.87
- mesenteric
  - artery, superior 557.1
  - vascular insufficiency (with gangrene) 557.1
- metabolic 277.7
- metastatic carcinoid 259.2
- Meyenburg-Altherr-Uehlinger 733.99
- Meyer-Schwickerath and Weyers (dysplasia oculodentodigitalis) 759.89
- Micheli-Rietti (thalassemia minor) 282.49
- Michotte's 721.5
- micrognathia-glossoptosis 756.0
- microphthalmos (congenital) 759.89
- midbrain 348.8
- middle
  - lobe (lung) (right) 518.0
  - radicular 353.0
- Miescher's
  - familial acanthosis nigricans 701.2
  - granulomatosis disciformis 709.3
- Mieten's 759.89
- migraine 346.0
- Mikity-Wilson (pulmonary dysmaturity) 770.7
- Mikulicz's (dryness of mouth, absent or decreased lacrimation) 527.1
- milk alkali (milk drinkers') 275.42
- Milkman (-Looser) (osteomalacia with pseudofractures) 268.2
- Millard-Gubler 344.89
- Miller-Dieker 758.33
- Miller Fisher's 357.0
- Milles' (encephalocutaneous angiomatosis) 759.6
- Minkowski-Chauffard (*see also* Spherocytosis) 282.0
- Mirizzi's (hepatic duct stenosis) 576.2
  - with calculus, cholelithiasis, or stones—*see* Choledocholithiasis
- mitochondrial neurogastrointestinal encephalopathy (MNGIE) 277.87
- mitral
  - click (-murmur) 785.2
  - valve prolapse 424.0
- MNGIE (mitochondrial neurogastrointestinal encephalopathy) 277.87
- Möbius'
  - congenital oculofacial paralysis 352.6
  - ophthalmoplegic migraine 346.8
- Mohr's (Types I and II) 759.89

Syndrome—*continued*
  monofixation 378.34
  Moore's (*see also* Epilepsy) 345.5
  Morel-Moore (hyperostosis frontalis interna)
      733.3
  Morel-Morgagni (hyperostosis frontalis interna)
      733.3
  Morgagni (-Stewart-Morel) (hyperostosis
      frontalis interna) 733.3
  Morgagni-Adams-Stokes (syncope with heart
      block) 426.9
  Morquio (-Brailsford) (-Ullrich)
      (mucopolysaccharidosis IV) 277.5
  Morris (testicular feminization) 259.5
  Morton's (foot) (metatarsalgia) (metatarsal
      neuralgia) (neuralgia) (neuroma) (toe) 355.6
  Moschcowitz (-Singer-Symmers) (thrombotic
      thrombocytopenic purpura) 446.6
  Mounier-Kuhn 748.3
    with
      acute exacerbation 494.1
      bronchiectasis 494.0
        with (acute) exacerbation 494.1
      acquired 519.19
        with bronchiectasis 494.0
          with (acute) exacerbation 494.1
  Mucha-Haberman (acute parapsoriasis
      varioliformis) 696.2
  mucocutaneous lymph node (acute) (febrile)
      (infantile) (MCLS) 446.1
  multiple
    deficiency 260
    operations 301.51
  Munchausen's 301.51
  Münchmeyer's (exostosis luxurians) 728.11
  Murchison-Sanderson—*see* Disease, Hodgkin's
  myasthenic—*see* Myasthenia, syndrome
  myelodysplastic 238.75
    with 5q deletion 238.74
    high grade with 5q deletion 238.73
  myeloproliferative (chronic) (M9960/1) 238.79
  myofascial pain NEC 729.1
  Naffziger's 353.0
  Nager-de Reynier (dysostosis mandibularis)
      756.0
  nail-patella (hereditary osteo-onychodysplasia)
      756.89
  NARP (neuropathy, ataxia and retinitis
      pigmentosa) 277.87
  Nebécourt's 253.3
  Neill-Dingwall (microencephaly and dwarfism)
      759.89
  nephrotic (*see also* Nephrosis) 581.9
    diabetic 250.4 *[581.81]*
  Netherton's (ichthyosiform erythroderma) 757.1
  neurocutaneous 759.6
  neuroleptic malignant 333.92
  Nezelof's (pure alymphocytosis) 279.13
  Niemann-Pick (lipid histiocytosis) 272.7
  Nonne-Milroy-Meige (chronic hereditary
      edema) 757.0
  nonsense 300.16
  Noonan's 759.89
  Nothnagel's
    ophthalmoplegia-cerebellar ataxia 378.52
    vasomotor acroparesthesia 443.89
  nucleus ambiguous-hypoglossal 352.6
  OAV (oculoauriculovertebral dysplasia) 756.0
  obsessional 300.3
  oculocutaneous 364.24
  oculomotor 378.81

Syndrome—*continued*
  oculourethroarticular 099.3
  Ogilvie's (sympathicotonic colon obstruction)
      560.89
  ophthalmoplegia-cerebellar ataxia 378.52
  Oppenheim-Urbach (necrobiosis lipoidica
      diabeticorum) 250.8 *[709.3]*
  oral-facial-digital 759.89
  organic
    affective NEC 293.83
      drug-induced 292.84
    anxiety 293.84
    delusional 293.81
      alcohol-induced 291.5
      drug-induced 292.11
      due to or associated with
        arteriosclerosis 290.42
          presenile brain disease 290.12
          senility 290.20
    depressive 293.83
      drug-induced 292.84
      due to or associated with
        arteriosclerosis 290.43
          presenile brain disease 290.13
          senile brain disease 290.21
    hallucinosis 293.82
      drug-induced 292.84
  organic affective 293.83
    induced by drug 292.84
  organic personality 310.1
    induced by drug 292.89
  Ormond's 593.4
  orodigitofacial 759.89
  orthostatic hypotensive-dysautonomic-
      dyskinetic 333.0
  Osler-Weber-Rendu (familial hemorrhagic
      telangiectasia) 448.0
  osteodermopathic hyperostosis 757.39
  osteoporosis-osteomalacia 268.2
  Österreicher-Turner (hereditary
      osteo-onychodysplasia) 756.89
  Ostrum-Furst 756.59
  otolith 386.19
  otopalatodigital 759.89
  outlet (thoracic) 353.0
  ovarian remnant 620.8
  ovarian vein 593.4
  Owren's (*see also* Defect, coagulation) 286.3
  OX 758.6
  pacemaker 429.4
  Paget-Schroetter (intermittent venous
      claudication) 453.8
  pain —*see also* Pain
    central 338.0
    chronic 338.4
    myelopathic 338.0
    thalamic (hypersthetic) 338.0
  painful
    apicocostal vertebral (M8010/3) 162.3
    arc 726.19
    bruising 287.2
    feet 266.2
  Pancoast's (carcinoma, pulmonary apex)
      (M8010/3) 162.3
  panhypopituitary (postpartum) 253.2
  papillary muscle 429.81
    with myocardial infarction 410.8
  Papillon-Léage and Psaume (orodigitofacial
      dysostosis) 759.89
  parabiotic (transfusion)
    donor (twin) 772.0

Syndrome—*continued*
   recipient (twin) 776.4
  paralysis agitans 332.0
  paralytic 344.9
   specified type NEC 344.89
  Paraneoplastic —*see* condition
  Parinaud's (paralysis of conjugate upward gaze)
    378.81
   oculoglandular 372.02
  Parkes Weber and Dimitri (encephalocutaneous
    angiomatosis) 759.6
  Parkinson's (*see* also Parkinsonism) 332.0
  parkinsonian (*see* also Parkinsonism) 332.0
  Parry's (exophthalmic goiter) 242.0
  Parry-Romberg 349.89
  Parsonage-Aldren-Turner 353.5
  Parsonage-Turner 353.5
  Patau's (trisomy D_1) 758.1
  patellofemoral 719.46
  Paterson (-Brown) (-Kelly) (sideropenic
    dysphagia) 280.8
  Payr's (splenic flexure syndrome) 569.89
  pectoral girdle 447.8
  pectoralis minor 447.8
  Pelger-Huët (hereditary hyposegmentation)
    288.2
  pellagra-cerebellar ataxia-renal aminoaciduria
    270.0
  Pellegrini-Stieda 726.62
  pellagroid 265.2
  Pellizzi's (pineal) 259.8
  pelvic congestion (-fibrosis) 625.5
  Pendred's (familial goiter with deaf-mutism)
    243
  Penfield's (*see also* Epilepsy) 345.5
  Penta X 758.81
  peptic ulcer—*see* Ulcer, peptic 533.9
  perabduction 447.8
  periodic 277.31
  periurethral fibrosis 593.4
  persistent fetal circulation 747.83
  Petges-Cléjat (poikilodermatomyositis) 710.3
  Peutz-Jeghers 759.6
  Pfeiffer (acrocephalosyndactyly) 755.55
  phantom limb 353.6
  pharyngeal pouch 279.11
  Pick's (pericardial pseudocirrhosis of liver)
    423.2
   heart 423.2
   liver 423.2
  Pick-Herxheimer (diffuse idiopathic cutaneous
    atrophy) 701.8
  Pickwickian (cardiopulmonary obesity) 278.8
  PIE (pulmonary infiltration with eosinophilia)
    518.3
  Pierre Marie-Bamberger (hypertrophic
    pulmonary osteoarthropathy) 731.2
  Pierre Mauriac's (diabetes-dwarfism-obesity)
    258.1
  Pierre Robin 756.0
  pigment dispersion, iris 364.53
  pineal 259.8
  pink puffer 492.8
  pituitary 253.0
  placental
   dysfunction 762.2
   insufficiency 762.2
   transfusion 762.3
  plantar fascia 728.71
  plica knee 727.83
  Plummer-Vinson (sideropenic dysphagia) 280.8

Syndrome—*continued*
  pluricarential of infancy 260
  plurideficiency of infancy 260
  pluriglandular (compensatory) 258.8
  polycarential of infancy 260
  polyglandular 258.8
  polysplenia 759.0
  pontine 433.8
  popliteal
   artery entrapment 447.8
   web 756.89
  postartificial menopause 627.4
  postcardiac injury
   postcardiotomy 429.4
   postmyocardial infarction 411.0
  postcardiotomy 429.4
  postcholecystectomy 576.0
  postcommissurotomy 429.4
  postconcussional 310.2
  postcontusional 310.2
  postencephalitic 310.8
  posterior
   cervical sympathetic 723.2
   fossa compression 348.4
   inferior cerebellar artery (*see also* Disease,
    cerebrovascular, acute) 436
   reversible encephalopathy (PRES) 348.39
  postgastrectomy (dumping) 564.2
  post-gastric surgery 564.2
  posthepatitis 780.79
  postherpetic (neuralgia) (zoster) 053.19
   geniculate ganglion 053.11
   ophthalmica 053.19
  postimmunization—*see* Complications,
    vaccination
  postinfarction 411.0
  postinfluenza (asthenia) 780.79
  postirradiation 990
  postlaminectomy 722.80
   cervical, cervicothoracic 722.81
   lumbar, lumbosacral 722.83
   thoracic, thoracolumbar 722.82
  postleukotomy 310.0
  postlobotomy 310.0
  postmastectomy lymphedema 457.0
  postmature (of newborn) 766.22
  postmyocardial infarction 411.0
  postoperative NEC 998.9
   blind loop 579.2
  postpartum panhypopituitary 253.2
  postperfusion NEC 999.8
   bone marrow 996.85
  postpericardiotomy 429.4
  postphlebitic (asymptomatic) 459.10
   with
    complications NEC 459.19
    inflammation 459.12
     and ulcer 459.13
    stasis dermatitis 459.12
     with ulcer 459.13
    ulcer 459.11
     with inflammation 459.13
  postpolio (myelitis) 138
  postvagotomy 564.2
  postvalvulotomy 429.4
  postviral (asthenia) NEC 780.79
  Potain's (gastrectasis with dyspepsia) 536.1
  potassium intoxication 276.7
  Potter's 753.0
  Prader (-Labhart) -Willi (-Fanconi) 759.81
  preinfarction 411.1

Syndrome—*continued*
  preleukemic 238.75
  premature senility 259.8
  premenstrual 625.4
  premenstrual tension 625.4
  pre ulcer 536.9
  Prinzmetal-Massumi (anterior chest wall
      syndrome) 786.52
  Profichet's 729.9
  progeria 259.8
  progressive pallidal degeneration 333.0
  prolonged gestation 766.22
  Proteus (dermal hypoplasia) 757.39
  prune belly 756.71
  prurigo-asthma 691.8
  pseudocarpal tunnel (sublimis) 354.0
  pseudohermaphroditism-virilism-hirsutism
      255.2
  pseudoparalytica 358.00
  pseudo-Turner's 759.89
  psycho-organic 293.9
    acute 293.0
    anxiety type 293.84
    depressive type 293.83
    hallucinatory type 293.82
    nonpsychotic severity 310.1
      specified focal (partial) NEC 310.8
    paranoid type 293.81
    specified type NEC 293.89
    subacute 293.1
  pterygolymphangiectasia 758.6
  ptosis-epicanthus 270.2
  pulmonary
    arteriosclerosis 416.0
    hypoperfusion (idiopathic) 769
    renal (hemorrhagic) 446.21
  pulseless 446.7
  Putnam-Dana (subacute combined sclerosis with
      pernicious anemia) 281.0 *[336.2]*
  pyloroduodenal 537.89
  pyramidopallidonigral 332.0
  pyriformis 355.0
  QT interval prolongation 426.82
  radicular NEC 729.2
    lower limbs 724.4
    upper limbs 723.4
      newborn 767.4
  Raeder-Harbitz (pulseless disease) 446.7
  Ramsay Hunt's
    dyssynergia cerebellaris myoclonica 334.2
    herpetic geniculate ganglionitis 053.11
  rapid time-zone change 327.35
  Raymond (-Céstan) 433.8
  Raynaud's (paroxysmal digital cyanosis) 443.0
  RDS (respiratory distress syndrome, newborn)
      769
  Refsum's (heredopathia atactica
      polyneuritiformis) 356.3
  Reichmann's (gastrosuccorrhea) 536.8
  Reifenstein's (hereditary familial
      hypogonadism, male) 259.5
  Reilly's (*see also* Neuropathy, peripheral,
      autonomic) 337.9
  Reiter's 099.3
  renal glomerulohyalinosis-diabetic 250.4
      [581.81]
  Rendu-Osler-Weber (familial hemorrhagic
      telangiectasia) 448.0
  renofacial (congenital biliary fibroangiomatosis)
      753.0
  Rénon-Delille 253.8

Syndrome—*continued*
  respiratory distress (idiopathic) (newborn) 769
    adult (following shock, surgery, or trauma)
        518.5
      specified NEC 518.82
    type II 770.6
  restless legs (RLS) 333.94
  retinoblastoma (familial) 190.5
  retraction (Duane's) 378.71
  retroperitoneal fibrosis 593.4
  retroviral seroconversion (acute) V08
  Rett's 330.8
  Reye's 331.81
  Reye-Sheehan (postpartum pituitary necrosis)
      253.2
  Riddoch's (visual disorientation) 368.16
  Ridley's (*see also* Failure, ventricular, left)
      428.1
  Rieger's (mesodermal dysgenesis, anterior
      ocular segment) 743.44
  Rietti-Greppi-Micheli (thalassemia minor)
      282.49
  right ventricular obstruction—*see* Failure heart
  Riley-Day (familial dysautonomia) 742.8
  Robin's 756.0
  Rokitansky-Kuster-Hauser (congenital absence,
      vagina) 752.49
  Romano-Ward (prolonged QT interval
      syndrome) 426.82
  Romberg's 349.89
  Rosen-Castleman-Liebow (pulmonary
      proteinosis) 516.0
  rotator cuff, shoulder 726.10
  Roth's 355.1
  Rothmund's (congenital poikiloderma) 757.33
  Rotor's (idiopathic hyperbilirubinemia) 277.4
  Roussy-Lévy 334.3
  Roy (-Jutras) (acropachyderma) 757.39
  rubella (congenital) 771.0
  Rubinstein-Taybi's (brachydactylia, short
      stature, and mental retardation) 759.89
  Rud's (mental deficiency, epilepsy, and
      infantilism) 759.89
  Ruiter-Pompen (-Wyers) (angiokeratoma
      corporis diffusum) 272.7
  Runge's (postmaturity) 766.22
  Russell (-Silver) (congenital hemihypertrophy
      and short stature) 759.89
  Rytand-Lipsitch (complete atrioventricular
      block) 426.0
  sacralization-scoliosis-sciatica 756.15
  sacroiliac 724.6
  Saenger's 379.46
  salt
    depletion (*see also* Disease, renal) 593.9
      due to heat NEC 992.8
        causing heat exhaustion or prostration
            992.4
    low (*see also* Disease, renal) 593.9
  salt-losing (*see also* Disease, renal) 593.9
  Sanfilippo's (mucopolysaccharidosis III) 277.5
  Scaglietti-Dagnini (acromegalic
      macrospondylitis) 253.0
  scalded skin 695.1
  scalenus anticus (anterior) 353.0
  scapulocostal 354.8
  scapuloperoneal 359.1
  scapulovertebral 723.4
  Schaumann's (sarcoidosis) 135
  Scheie's (mucopolysaccharidosis IS) 277.5

Syndrome—*continued*
　Scheuthauer-Marie-Sainton (cleidocranialis
　　dysostosis) 755.59
　Schirmer's (encephalocutaneous angiomatosis)
　　759.6
　schizophrenic, of childhood NEC (*see also*
　　Psychosis, childhood) 299.9
　Schmidt's
　　sphallo-pharyngo-laryngeal hemiplegia 352.6
　　thyroid-adrenocortical insufficiency 258.1
　　vagoaccessory 352.6
　Schneider's 047.9
　Schnitzler 273.1
　Scholte's (malignant carcinoid) 259.2
　Scholz (-Bielschowsky-Henneberg) 330.0
　Schroeder's (endocrine-hypertensive) 255.3
　Schüller-Christian (chronic histiocytosis X)
　　277.89
　Schultz's (agranulocytosis) 288.09
　Schwartz (-Jampel) 756.89
　Schwartz-Bartter (inappropriate secretion of
　　antidiuretic hormone) 253.6
　Scimitar (anomalous venous drainage, right lung
　　to inferior vena cave) 747.49
　sclerocystic ovary 256.4
　sea-blue histiocyte 272.7
　Seabright-Bantam (pseudohypoparathyroidism)
　　275.49
　Seckel's 759.89
　Secretan's (posttraumatic edema) 782.3
　secretoinhibitor (keratoconjunctivitis sicca)
　　710.2
　Seeligmann's (ichthyosis congenita) 757.1
　Senear-Usher (pemphigus erythematosus) 694.4
　senilism 259.8
　seroconversion, retroviral (acute) V08
　serotonin 333.99
　serous meningitis 348.2
　Sertoli cell (germinal aplasia) 606.0
　sex chromosome mosaic 758.81
　Sézary's (reticulosis) (M9701/3) 202.2
　shaken infant 995.55
　Shaver's (bauxite pneumoconiosis) 503
　Sheehan's (postpartum pituitary necrosis) 253.2
　shock (traumatic) 958.4
　　kidney 584.5
　　　following crush injury 958.5
　　lung 518.5
　　neurogenic 308.9
　　psychic 308.9
　short
　　bowel 579.3
　　P-R interval 426.81
　shoulder-arm (*see also* Neuropathy, peripheral,
　　autonomic) 337.9
　shoulder-girdle 723.4
　shoulder-hand (*see also* Neuropathy, peripheral,
　　autonomic) 337.9
　Shwachman's 288.02
　Shy-Drager (orthostatic hypotension with
　　multisystem degeneration) 333.0
　Sicard's 352.6
　sicca (keratoconjunctivitis) 710.2
　sick
　　cell 276.1
　　cilia 759.89
　　sinus 427.81
　sideropenic 280.8
　Siemens'
　　ectodermal dysplasia 757.31

Syndrome—*continued*
　keratosis follicularis spinulosa (decalvans)
　　757.39
　Silfverskiöld's (osteochondrodystrophy,
　　extremities) 756.50
　Silver's (congenital hemihypertrophy and short
　　stature) 759.89
　Silvestroni-Bianco (thalassemia minima) 282.49
　Simons' (progressive lipodystrophy) 272.6
　sinus tarsi 726.79
　sinusitis-bronchiectasis-situs inversus 759.3
　Sipple's (medullary thyroid
　　carcinoma-pheochromocytoma) 193
　Sjögren (-Gougerot) (keratoconjunctivitis sicca)
　　710.2
　　with lung involvement 710.2 *[517.8]*
　Sjögren-Larsson (ichthyosis congenita) 757.1
　Slocumb's 255.3
　Sluder's 337.0
　Smith-Lemli-Opitz (cerebrohepatorenal
　　syndrome) 759.89
　Smith-Magenis 758.33
　smokers' 305.1
　Sneddon-Wilkinson (subcorneal pustular
　　dermatosis) 694.1
　Sotos' (cerebral gigantism) 253.0
　South African cardiomyopathy 425.2
　spasmodic
　　upward movement, eyes(s) 378.82
　　winking 307.20
　Spens' (syncope with heart block) 426.9
　spherophakia-brachymorphia 759.89
　spinal cord injury—*see also* Injury, spinal, by
　　site
　　with fracture, vertebra—*see* Fracture, vertebra,
　　　by site, with spinal cord injury
　　cervical—*see* Injury, spinal, cervical
　　fluid malabsorption (acquired) 331.3
　splenic
　　agenesis 759.0
　　flexure 569.89
　　neutropenia 289.53
　　sequestration 289.52
　Spurway's (brittle bones and blue sclera) 756.51
　staphylococcal scalded skin 695.1
　Stein's (polycystic ovary) 256.4
　Stein-Leventhal (polycystic ovary) 256.4
　Steinbrocker's (*see also* Neuropathy, peripheral,
　　autonomic) 337.9
　Stevens-Johnson (erythema multiforme
　　exudativum) 695.1
　Stewart-Morel (hyperostosis frontalis interna)
　　733.3
　Stickler 759.89
　stiff-baby 759.89
　stiff-man 333.91
　Still's (juvenile rheumatoid arthritis) 714.30
　Still-Felty (rheumatoid arthritis with
　　splenomegaly and leukopenia) 714.1
　Stilling-Türk-Duane (ocular retraction
　　syndrome) 378.71
　Stojano's (subcostal) 098.86
　Stokes (-Adams) (syncope with heart block)
　　426.9
　Stokvis-Talma (enterogenous cyanosis) 289.7
　stone heart (*see also* Failure, ventricular, left)
　　428.1
　straight-back 756.19
　stroke (*see also* Disease, cerebrovascular, acute)
　　436
　　little 435.9

Syndrome—*continued*
  Sturge-Kalischer-Weber (encephalotrigeminal angiomatosis) 759.6
  Sturge-Weber (-Dimitri) (encephalocutaneous angiomatosis) 759.6
  subclavian-carotid obstruction (chronic) 446.7
  subclavian steal 435.2
  subcoracoid-pectoralis minor 447.8
  subcostal 098.86
    nerve compression 354.8
  subperiosteal hematoma 267
  subphrenic interposition 751.4
  sudden infant death (SIDS) 798.0
  Sudeck's 733.7
  Sudeck-Leriche 733.7
  superior
    cerebellar artery (*see also* Disease, cerebrovascular, acute) 436
    mesenteric artery 557.1
    pulmonary sulcus (tumor) (M8010/3) 162.3
    vena cava 459.2
  suprarenal cortical 255.3
  supraspinatus 726.10
  swallowed blood 777.3
  sweat retention 705.1
  Sweet's (acute febrile neutrophilic dermatosis) 695.89
  Swyer-James (unilateral hyperlucent lung) 492.8
  Swyer's (XY pure gonadal dysgenesis) 752.7
  Symonds' 348.2
  sympathetic
    cervical paralysis 337.0
    pelvic 625.5
  syndactylic oxycephaly 755.55
  syphilitic-cardiovascular 093.89
  systemic
    fibrosclerosing 710.8
    inflammatory response (SIRS) 995.90
      due to
        infectious process 995.91
          with acute organ dysfunction 995.92
        non-infectious process 995.93
          with acute organ dysfunction 995.94
  systolic click (-murmur) 785.2
  Tabagism 305.1
  tachycardia-bradycardia 427.81
  Takayasu (-Onishi) (pulseless disease) 446.7
  Takotsubo 429.83
  Tapia's 352.6
  tarsal tunnel 355.5
  Taussig-Bing (transposition, aorta and overriding pulmonary artery) 745.11
  Taybi's (otopalatodigital) 759.89
  Taylor's 625.5
  teething 520.7
  tegmental 344.89
  telangiectasis-pigmentation-cataract 757.33
  temporal 383.02
    lobectomy behavior 310.0
  temporomandibular joint-pain-dysfunction [TMJ] NEC 524.60
    specified NEC 524.69
  Terry's 362.21
  testicular feminization 259.5
  testis, nonvirilizing 257.8
  tethered (spinal) cord 742.59
  thalamic 338.0
  Thibierge-Weissenbach (cutaneous systemic sclerosis) 710.1
  Thiele 724.6
  thoracic outlet (compression) 353.0

Syndrome—*continued*
  thoracogenous rheumatic (hypertrophic pulmonary osteoarthropathy) 731.2
  Thorn's (*see also* Disease, renal) 593.9
  Thorson-Biörck (malignant carcinoid) 259.2
  thrombopenia-hemangioma 287.39
  thyroid-adrenocortical insufficiency 258.1
  Tietze's 733.6
  time-zone (rapid) 327.35
  Tobias' (carcinoma, pulmonary apex) (M8010/3) 162.3
  toilet seat 926.0
  Tolosa-Hunt 378.55
  Toni-Fanconi (cystinosis) 270.0
  Touraine's (hereditary osteo-onychodysplasia) 756.89
  Touraine-Solente-Golé (acropachyderma) 757.39
  toxic
    oil 710.5
    shock 040.82
  transfusion
    fetal-maternal 772.0
    twin
      donor (infant) 772.0
      recipient (infant) 776.4
  transient left ventricular apical ballooning 429.83
  Treacher Collins' (incomplete mandibulofacial dysostosis) 756.0
  trigeminal plate 259.8
  triple X female 758.81
  trisomy NEC 758.5
    13 or D$_1$ 758.1
    16-18 or E 758.2
    18 or E$_3$ 758.2
    20 758.5
    21 or G (mongolism) 758.0
    22 or G (mongolism) 758.0
    G 758.0
  Troisier-Hanot-Chauffard (bronze diabetes) 275.0
  tropical wet feet 991.4
  Trousseau's (thrombophlebitis migrans visceral cancer) 453.1
  Türk's (ocular retraction syndrome) 378.71
  Turner's 758.6
  Turner-Varny 758.6
  twin-to-twin transfusion 762.3
    recipient twin 776.4
  Uehlinger's (acropachyderma) 757.39
  Ullrich (-Bonnevie) (-Turner) 758.6
  Ullrich-Feichtiger 759.89
  underwater blast injury (abdominal) (*see also* Injury, internal, abdomen) 868.00
  universal joint, cervix 620.6
  Unverricht (-Lundborg) 333.2
  Unverricht-Wagner (dermatomyositis) 710.3
  upward gaze 378.81
  Urbach-Oppenheim (necrobiosis lipoidica diabeticorum) 250.8 *[709.3]*
  Urbach-Wiethe (lipoid proteinosis) 272.8
  uremia, chronic 585.9
  urethral 597.81
  urethro-oculoarticular 099.3
  urethro-oculosynovial 099.3
  urohepatic 572.4
  uveocutaneous 364.24
  uveomeningeal, uveomeningitis 363.22
  vagohypoglossal 352.6
  vagovagal 780.2

Synechia—*continued*
  intrauterine (traumatic) 621.5
  posterior 364.71
  vulvae, congenital 752.49
Synesthesia (*see also* Disturbance, sensation)
  782.0
Synodontia 520.2
Synophthalmus 759.89
Synorchidism 752.89
Synorchism 752.89
Synostosis (congenital) 756.59
  astragaloscaphoid 755.67
  radioulnar 755.53
  talonavicular (bar) 755.67
  tarsal 755.67
Synovial —*see* condition
Synovioma (M9040/3)—*see also* Neoplasm,
    connective tissue, malignant
  benign (M9040/3)—*see* Neoplasm, connective
    tissue, benign
Synoviosarcoma (M9040/3)—*see* Neoplasm,
    connective tissue, malignant
Synovitis 727.00
  chronic crepitant, wrist 727.2
  due to crystals—*see* Arthritis, due to crystals
  gonococcal 098.51
  gouty 274.0
  syphilitic 095.7
    congenital 090.0
  traumatic, current—*see* Sprain, by site
  tuberculous—*see* Tuberculosis, synovitis
  villonodular 719.20
    ankle 719.27
    elbow 719.22
    foot 719.27
    hand 719.24
    hip 719.25
    knee 719.26
    multiple sites 719.29
    pelvic region 719.25
    shoulder (region) 719.21
    specified site NEC 719.28
    wrist 719.23
Syphilide 091.3
  congenital 090.0
  newborn 090.0
  tubercular 095.8
    congenital 090.0
Syphilis, syphilitic (acquired) 097.9
  with lung involvement 095.1
  abdomen (late) 095.2
  acoustic nerve 094.86
  adenopathy (secondary) 091.4
  adrenal (gland) 095.8
    with cortical hypofunction 095.8
  age under 2 years NEC (*see also* Syphilis,
      congenital) 090.9
    acquired 097.9
  alopecia (secondary) 091.82
  anemia 095.8
  aneurysm (artery) (ruptured) 093.89
    aorta 093.0
    central nervous system 094.89
    congenital 090.5
  anus 095.8
    primary 091.1
    secondary 091.3
  aorta, aortic (arch) (abdominal) (insufficiency)
      (pulmonary) (regurgitation) (stenosis)
      (thoracic) 093.89
    aneurysm 093.0

Syphilis, syphilitic—*continued*
  arachnoid (adhesive) 094.2
  artery 093.89
    cerebral 094.89
    spinal 094.89
  arthropathy (neurogenic) (tabetic) 094.0 *[713.5]*
  asymptomatic—*see* Syphilis, latent
  ataxia, locomotor (progressive) 094.0
  atrophoderma maculatum 091.3
  auricular fibrillation 093.89
  Bell's palsy 094.89
  bladder 095.8
  bone 095.5
    secondary 091.61
  brain 094.89
  breast 095.8
  bronchus 095.8
  bubo 091.0
  bulbar palsy 094.89
  bursa (late) 095.7
  cardiac decompensation 093.89
  cardiovascular (early) (late) (primary)
      (secondary) (tertiary) 093.9
    specified type and site NEC 093.89
  causing death under 2 years of age (*see also*
      Syphilis, congenital) 090.9
    stated to be acquired NEC 097.9
  central nervous system (any site) (early) (late)
      (latent) (primary) (recurrent) (relapse)
      (secondary) (tertiary) 094.9
    with
      ataxia 094.0
      paralysis, general 094.1
        juvenile 090.40
      paresis (general) 094.1
        juvenile 090.40
      tabes (dorsalis) 094.0
        juvenile 090.40
      taboparesis 094.1
        juvenile 090.40
    aneurysm (ruptured) 094.87
    congenital 090.40
    juvenile 090.40
    remission in (sustained) 094.9
    serology doubtful, negative, or positive 094.9
    specified nature or site NEC 094.89
    vascular 094.89
  cerebral 094.89
    meningovascular 094.2
    nerves 094.89
    sclerosis 094.89
    thrombosis 094.89
  cerebrospinal 094.89
    tabetic 094.0
  cerebrovascular 094.89
  cervix 095.8
  chancre (multiple) 091.0
    extragenital 091.2
    Rollet's 091.0
  Charcot's joint 094.0 *[713.5]*
  choked disc 094.89 *[377.00]*
  chorioretinitis 091.51
    congenital 090.0 *[363.13]*
    late 094.83
  choroiditis 091.51
    congenital 090.0 *[363.13]*
    late 094.83
    prenatal 090.0 *[363.13]*
  choroidoretinitis (secondary) 091.51
    congenital 090.0 *[363.13]*
    late 094.83

Syphilis, syphilitic—*continued*
  secondary 091.61
  peripheral nerve 095.8
  petrous bone (late) 095.5
  pharynx 095.8
    secondary 091.3
  pituitary (gland) 095.8
  placenta 095.8
  pleura (late) 095.8
  pneumonia, white 090.0
  pontine (lesion) 094.89
  portal vein 093.89
  primary NEC 091.2
    anal 091.1
    and secondary (*see also* Syphilis, secondary)
      091.9
    cardiovascular 093.9
    central nervous system 094.9
    extragenital chancre NEC 091.2
    fingers 091.2
    genital 091.0
    lip 091.2
    specified site NEC 091.2
    tonsils 091.2
  prostate 095.8
  psychosis (intracranial gumma) 094.89
  ptosis (eyelid) 094.89
  pulmonary (late) 095.1
    artery 093.89
  pulmonum 095.1
  pyelonephritis 095.4
  recently acquired, symptomatic NEC 091.89
  rectum 095.8
  respiratory tract 095.8
  retina
    late 094.83
    neurorecidive 094.83
  retrobulbar neuritis 094.85
  salpingitis 095.8
  sclera (late) 095.0
  sclerosis
    cerebral 094.89
    coronary 093.89
    multiple 094.89
    subacute 094.89
  scotoma (central) 095.8
  scrotum 095.8
  secondary (and primary) 091.9
    adenopathy 091.4
    anus 091.3
    bone 091.61
    cardiovascular 093.9
    central nervous system 094.9
    chorioretinitis, choroiditis 091.51
    hepatitis 091.62
    liver 091.62
    lymphadenitis 091.4
    meningitis, acute 091.81
    mouth 091.3
    mucous membranes 091.3
    periosteum 091.61
    periostitis 091.61
    pharynx 091.3
    relapse (treated) (untreated) 091.7
    skin 091.3
    specified form NEC 091.89
    tonsil 091.3
    ulcer 091.3
    viscera 091.69
    vulva 091.3
  seminal vesicle (late) 095.8

Syphilis, syphilitic—*continued*
  seronegative
    with signs or symptoms—*see* Syphilis, by site
      and stage
  seropositive
    with signs or symptoms—*see* Syphilis, by site
      and stage
    follow-up of latent syphilis—*see* Syphilis,
      latent
    only finding—*see* Syphilis, latent
  seventh nerve (paralysis) 094.89
  sinus 095.8
  sinusitis 095.8
  skeletal system 095.5
  skin (early) (secondary) (with ulceration) 091.3
    late or tertiary 095.8
  small intestine 095.8
  spastic spinal paralysis 094.0
  spermatic cord (late) 095.8
  spinal (cord) 094.89
    with
      paresis 094.1
      tabes 094.0
  spleen 095.8
  splenomegaly 095.8
  spondylitis 095.5
  staphyloma 095.8
  stigmata (congenital) 090.5
  stomach 095.8
  synovium (late) 095.7
  tabes dorsalis (early) (late) 094.0
    juvenile 090.40
  tabetic type 094.0
    juvenile 090.40
  taboparesis 094.1
    juvenile 090.40
  tachycardia 093.89
  tendon (late) 095.7
  tertiary 097.0
    with symptoms 095.8
    cardiovascular 093.9
    central nervous system 094.9
    multiple NEC 095.8
    specified site NEC 095.8
  testis 095.8
  thorax 095.8
  throat 095.8
  thymus (gland) 095.8
  thyroid (late) 095.8
  tongue 095.8
  tonsil (lingual) 095.8
    primary 091.2
    secondary 091.3
  trachea 095.8
  tricuspid valve 093.23
  tumor, brain 094.89
  tunica vaginalis (late) 095.8
  ulcer (any site) (early) (secondary) 091.3
    late 095.9
    perforating 095.9
      foot 094.0
  urethra (stricture) 095.8
  urogenital 095.8
  uterus 095.8
  uveal tract (secondary) 091.50
    late 095.8 *[363.13]*
  uveitis (secondary) 091.50
    late 095.8 *[363.13]*
  uvula (late) 095.8
    perforated 095.8
  vagina 091.0

Syphilis, syphilitic—*continued*
  late 095.8
 valvulitis NEC 093.20
 vascular 093.89
   brain or cerebral 094.89
 vein 093.89
   cerebral 094.89
 ventriculi 095.8
 vesicae urinariae 095.8
 viscera (abdominal) 095.2
   secondary 091.69
 vitreous (hemorrhage) (opacities) 095.8
 vulva 091.0
   late 095.8
   secondary 091.3
Syphiloma 095.9
 cardiovascular system 093.9
 central nervous system 094.9
 circulatory system 093.9
 congenital 090.5
Syphilophobia 300.29
Syringadenoma (M8400/0)—*see also* Neoplasm,
   skin, benign
 papillary (M8406/0)—*see* Neoplasm, skin,
   benign
Syringobulbia 336.0
Syringocarcinoma (M8400/3)—*see* Neoplasm,
   skin, malignant
Syringocystadenoma (M8400/0)—*see also*
   Neoplasm, skin, benign
 papillary (M8406/0)—*see* Neoplasm, skin,
   benign
Syringocystoma (M8407/0)—*see* Neoplasm,
   skin, benign
Syringoma (M8407/0)—*see also* Neoplasm, skin,
   benign
 chondroid (M8940/0)—*see* Neoplasm, by site,
   benign
Syringomyelia 336.0
Syringomyelitis 323.9
 late effect—*see* category 326
Syringomyelocele (*see also* Spina bifida) 741.9
Syringopontia 336.0
System, systemic —*see also* condition
 disease, combined—*see* Degeneration,
   combined
 fibrosclerosing syndrome 710.8
 inflammatory response syndrome (SIRS) 995.90
   due to
     infectious process 995.91
       with acute organ dysfunction 995.92
     non-infectious process 995.93
       with acute organ dysfunction 995.94
 lupus erythematosus 710.0
   inhibitor 286.5

T

Tab —*see* Tag
Tabacism 989.8
Tabacosis 989.8
Tabardillo 080
  flea-borne 081.0
  louse-borne 080
Tabes, tabetic
  with
    central nervous system syphilis 094.0
    Charcot's joint 094.0 *[713.5]*
    cord bladder 094.0
    crisis, viscera (any) 094.0
    paralysis, general 094.1
    paresis (general) 094.1
    perforating ulcer 094.0
  arthropathy 094.0 *[713.5]*
  bladder 094.0
  bone 094.0
  cerebrospinal 094.0
  congenital 090.40
  conjugal 094.0
  dorsalis 094.0
    neurosyphilis 094.0
  early 094.0
  juvenile 090.40
  latent 094.0
  mesenterica (*see also* Tuberculosis) 014.8
  paralysis insane, general 094.1
  peripheral (nonsyphilitic) 799.89
  spasmodic 094.0
    not dorsal or dorsalis 343.9
  syphilis (cerebrospinal) 094.0
Taboparalysis 094.1
Taboparesis (remission) 094.1
  with
    Charcot's joint 094.1 *[713.5]*
    cord bladder 094.1
    perforating ulcer 094.1
  juvenile 090.40
Tache noir 923.20
Tachyalimentation 579.3
Tachyarrhythmia, tachyrhythmia —*see also*
    Tachycardia
  paroxysmal with sinus bradycardia 427.81
Tachycardia 785.0
  atrial 427.89
  auricular 427.89
  AV nodal re-entry (re-entrant) 427.89
  newborn 779.82
  nodal 427.89
    nonparoxysmal atrioventricular 426.89
    nonparoxysmal atrioventricular (nodal) 426.89
  paroxysmal 427.2
    with sinus bradycardia 427.81
    atrial (PAT) 427.0
      psychogenic 316 *[427.0]*
    atrioventricular (AV) 427.0
      psychogenic 316 *[427.0]*
    essential 427.2
    junctional 427.0
    nodal 427.0
    psychogenic 316 *[427.2]*
      atrial 316 *[427.0]*
      supraventricular 316 *[427.0]*
      ventricular 316 *[427.1]*
    supraventricular 427.0
      psychogenic 316 *[427.0]*
    ventricular 427.1

Tachycardia—*continued*
    psychogenic 316 *[427.1]*
  postoperative 997.1
  psychogenic 306.2
  sick sinus 427.81
  sinoauricular 427.89
  sinus 427.89
  supraventricular 427.89
  ventricular (paroxysmal) 427.1
    psychogenic 316 *[427.1]*
Tachygastria 536.8
Tachypnea 786.06
  hysterical 300.11
  newborn (idiopathic) (transitory) 770.6
  psychogenic 306.1
  transitory, of newborn 770.6
Taenia (infection) (infestation) (*see also*
    Infestation, taenia) 123.3
  diminuta 123.6
  echinococcal infestation (*see also*
    Echinococcus) 122.9
  nana 123.6
  saginata infestation 123.2
  solium (intestinal form) 123.0
    larval form 123.1
Taeniasis (intestine) (*see also* Infestation, Taenia)
    123.3
  saginata 123.2
  solium 123.0
Taenzer's disease 757.4
Tag (hypertrophied skin) (infected) 701.9
  adenoid 474.8
  anus 455.9
  endocardial (*see also* Endocarditis) 424.90
  hemorrhoidal 455.9
  hymen 623.8
  perineal 624.8
  preauricular 744.1
  rectum 455.9
  sentinel 455.9
  skin 701.9
    accessory 757.39
    anus 455.9
    congenital 757.39
    preauricular 744.1
    rectum 455.9
  tonsil 474.8
  urethra, urethral 599.84
  vulva 624.8
Tahyna fever 062.5
Takayasu (-Onishi) disease or syndrome
    (pulseless disease) 446.7
Takotsubo syndrome 429.83
Talc granuloma 728.82
  in operation wound 998.7
Talcosis 502
Talipes (congenital) 754.70
  acquired NEC 736.79
    planus 734
  asymmetric 754.79
    acquired 736.79
  calcaneovalgus 754.62
    acquired 736.76
  calcaneovarus 754.59
    acquired 736.76
  calcaneus 754.79
    acquired 736.76

Tear, torn—*continued*
    anterior horn 836.1
      old 717.42
    bucket handle 836.1
      old 717.41
    old 717.40
    posterior horn 836.1
      old 717.43
    specified site NEC 836.1
      old 717.49
  medial 836.0
    anterior horn 836.0
      old 717.1
    bucket handle 836.0
      old 717.0
    old 717.3
    posterior horn 836.0
      old 717.2
  old NEC 717.5
  site other than knee—*see* Sprain, by site
  muscle—*see also* Sprain, by site
  with open wound—*see* Wound, open by site
  pelvic
    floor, complicating delivery 664.1
    organ NEC
      with
        abortion—*see* Abortion, by type, with
          damage to pelvic organs
        ectopic pregnancy (*see also* categories
          633.0-633.9) 639.2
        molar pregnancy (*see also* categories
          630-632) 639.2
      following
        abortion 639.2
        ectopic or molar pregnancy 639.2
      obstetrical trauma 665.5
  perineum—*see also* Laceration, perineum
    obstetrical trauma 665.5
  periurethral tissue
    with
      abortion—*see* Abortion, by type, with
        damage to pelvic organs
      ectopic pregnancy (*see also* categories
        633.0-633.9) 639.2
      molar pregnancy (*see also* categories
        630-632) 639.2
    following
      abortion 639.2
      ectopic or molar pregnancy 639.2
    obstetrical trauma 665.5
  rectovaginal septum—*see* Laceration,
    rectovaginal septum
  retina, retinal (recent) (with detachment) 361.00
    without detachment 361.30
    dialysis (juvenile) (with detachment) 361.04
    giant (with detachment) 361.03
    horseshoe (without detachment) 361.32
    multiple (with detachment) 361.02
      without detachment 361.33
    old
      delimited (partial) 361.06
      partial 361.06
      total or subtotal 361.07
    partial (without detachment)
      giant 361.03
      multiple defects 361.02
      old (delimited) 361.06
      single defect 361.01
    round hole (without detachment) 361.31
    single defect (with detachment) 361.01
    total or subtotal (recent) 361.05

Tear, torn—*continued*
    old 361.07
  rotator cuff (traumatic) 840.4
    current injury 840.4
    degenerative 726.10
    nontraumatic 727.61
  semilunar cartilage, knee (*see also* Tear,
    meniscus) 836.2
    old 717.5
  tendon—*see also* Sprain, by site
    with open wound—*see* Wound, open by site
  tentorial, at birth 767.0
  umbilical cord
    affecting fetus or newborn 772.0
    complicating delivery 663.8
  urethra
    with
      abortion—*see* Abortion, by type, with
        damage to pelvic organs
      ectopic pregnancy (*see also* categories
        633.0-633.9) 639.2
      molar pregnancy (*see also* categories
        630-632) 639.2
    following
      abortion 639.2
      ectopic or molar pregnancy 639.2
    obstetrical trauma 665.5
  uterus—*see* Injury, internal, uterus
  vagina—*see* Laceration, vagina
  vessel, from catheter 998.2
  vulva, complicating delivery 664.0
Tear stone 375.57
Teeth, tooth —*see also* condition
  grinding 306.8
  prenatal 520.6
Teething 520.7
  syndrome 520.7
Tegmental syndrome 344.89
Telangiectasia, telangiectasis (verrucous) 448.9
  ataxic (cerebellar) 334.8
  familial 448.0
  hemorrhagic, hereditary (congenital) (senile)
    448.0
  hereditary hemorrhagic 448.0
  retina 362.15
  spider 448.1
Telecanthus (congenital) 743.63
Telescoped bowel or intestine (*see also*
  Intussusception) 560.0
Teletherapy, adverse effect NEC 990
Telogen effluvium 704.02
Temperature
  body, high (of unknown origin) (*see also*
    Pyrexia) 780.6
  cold, trauma from 991.9
    newborn 778.2
    specified effect NEC 991.8
  high
    body (of unknown origin) (*see also* Pyrexia)
      780.6
    trauma from—*see* Heat
Temper tantrum (childhood) (*see also*
  Disturbance, conduct) 312.1
Temple —*see* condition
Temporal —*see also* condition
  lobe syndrome 310.0
Temporomandibular joint-pain-dysfunction
  syndrome 524.60
Temporosphenoidal —*see* condition

Tendency
  bleeding (*see also* Defect, coagulation) 286.9
  homosexual, ego-dystonic 302.0
  paranoid 301.0
  suicide 300.9
Tenderness
  abdominal (generalized) (localized) 789.6
  rebound 789.6
  skin 782.0
Tendinitis, tendonitis (*see also* Tenosynovitis)
    726.90
  Achilles 726.71
  adhesive 726.90
    shoulder 726.0
  calcific 727.82
    shoulder 726.11
  gluteal 726.5
  patellar 726.64
  peroneal 726.79
  pes anserinus 726.61
  psoas 726.5
  tibialis (anterior) (posterior) 726.72
  trochanteric 726.5
Tendon —*see* condition
Tendosynovitis —*see* Tenosynovitis
Tendovaginitis —*see* Tenosynovitis
Tenesmus 787.99
  rectal 787.99
  vesical 788.9
Tenia —*see* Taenia
Teniasis —*see* Taeniasis
Tennis elbow 726.32
Tenonitis —*see also* Tenosynovitis
  eye (capsule) 376.04
Tenontosynovitis —*see* Tenosynovitis
Tenontothecitis —*see* Tenosynovitis
Tenophyte 727.9
Tenosynovitis 727.00
  adhesive 726.90
    shoulder 726.0
  ankle 727.06
  bicipital (calcifying) 726.12
  buttock 727.09
  due to crystals—*see* Arthritis, due to crystals
  elbow 727.09
  finger 727.05
  foot 727.06
  gonococcal 098.51
  hand 727.05
  hip 727.09
  knee 727.09
  radial styloid 727.04
  shoulder 726.10
    adhesive 726.0
  spine 720.1
  supraspinatus 726.10
  toe 727.06
  tuberculous—*see* Tuberculosis, tenosynovitis
  wrist 727.05
Tenovaginitis —*see* Tenosynovitis
Tension
  arterial, high (*see also* Hypertension) 401.9
    without diagnosis of hypertension 796.2
  headache 307.81
  intraocular (elevated) 365.00
  nervous 799.2
  ocular (elevated) 365.00
  pneumothorax 512.0
    iatrogenic 512.1
    postoperative 512.1
    spontaneous 512.0

Tension—*continued*
  premenstrual 625.4
  state 300.9
Tentorium —*see* condition
Teratencephalus 759.89
Teratism 759.7
Teratoblastoma (malignant) (M9080/3)—*see*
    Neoplasm, by site, malignant
Teratocarcinoma (M9081/3)—*see also*
    Neoplasm, by site, malignant
  liver 155.0
Teratoma (solid) (M9080/1)—*see also*
    Neoplasm, by site, uncertain behavior
  adult (cystic) (M9080/0)—*see* Neoplasm, by
    site, benign
  and embryonal carcinoma, mixed
      (M9081/3)—*see* Neoplasm, by site,
      malignant
  benign (M9080/0)—*see* Neoplasm, by site,
    benign
  combined with choriocarcinoma
      (M9101/3)—*see* Neoplasm, by site,
      malignant
  cystic (adult) (M9080/0)—*see* Neoplasm, by
    site, benign
  differentiated type (M9080/0)—*see* Neoplasm,
    by site, benign
  embryonal (M9080/3)—*see also* Neoplasm, by
    site, malignant
    liver 155.0
  fetal
    sacral, causing fetopelvic disproportion 653.7
  immature (M9080/3)—*see* Neoplasm, by site,
    malignant
  liver (M9080/3) 155.0
    adult, benign, cystic, differentiated type or
      mature (M9080/0) 211.5
  malignant (M9080/3)—*see also* Neoplasm, by
    site, malignant
    anaplastic type (M9082/3)—*see* Neoplasm, by
      site, malignant
    intermediate type (M9083/3)—*see* Neoplasm,
      by site, malignant
    liver (M9080/3) 155.0
    trophoblastic (M9102/3)
      specified site—*see* Neoplasm, by site,
        malignant
      unspecified site 186.9
    undifferentiated type (M9082/3)—*see*
      Neoplasm, by site, malignant
  mature (M9080/0)—*see* Neoplasm, by site,
    benign
  ovary (M9080/0) 220
    embryonal, immature, or malignant (M9080/3)
      183.0
  suprasellar (M9080/3)—*see* Neoplasm, by site,
    malignant
  testis (M9080/3) 186.9
    adult, benign, cystic, differentiated type or
      mature (M9080/0) 222.0
  undescended 186.0
Terminal care V66.7
Termination
  anomalous—*see also* Malposition, congenital
    portal vein 747.49
    right pulmonary vein 747.42
  pregnancy (legal) (therapeutic) (*see* Abortion,
      legal) 635.9
    fetus NEC 779.6
    illegal (*see also* Abortion, illegal) 636.9
Ternidens diminutus infestation 127.7
Terrors, night (child) 307.46

Terry's syndrome 362.21
Tertiary —*see* condition
Tessellated fundus, retina (tigroid) 362.89
Test(s)
  adequacy
    hemodialysis V56.31
    peritoneal dialysis V56.32
  AIDS virus V72.6
  allergen V72.7
  bacterial disease NEC (*see also* Screening, by
    name of disease) V74.9
  basal metabolic rate V72.6
  blood-alcohol V70.4
  blood-drug V70.4
    for therapeutic drug monitoring V58.83
  blood typing V72.86
    Rh typing V72.86
  developmental, infant or child V20.2
  Dick V74.8
  fertility V26.21
  genetic
    female V26.32
    for genetic disease carrier status
      female V26.31
      male V26.34
    male V26.39
  hearing V72.19
    following failed hearing screening V72.11
  HIV V72.6
  human immunodeficiency virus V72.6
  Kveim V82.89
  laboratory V72.6
    for medicolegal reason V70.4
  male partner of habitual aborter V26.35
  Mantoux (for tuberculosis) V74.1
  mycotic organism V75.4
  parasitic agent NEC V75.8
  paternity V70.4
  peritoneal equilibration V56.32
  pregnancy
    negative result V72.41
    positive result V72.42
      first pregnancy V72.42
    unconfirmed V72.40
  preoperative V72.84
    cardiovascular V72.81
    respiratory V72.82
    specified NEC V72.83
  procreative management NEC V26.29
    genetic disease carrier status
      female V26.31
      male V26.34
  Rh typing V72.86
  sarcoidosis V82.89
  Schick V74.3
  Schultz-Charlton V74.8
  skin, diagnostic
    allergy V72.7
    bacterial agent NEC (*see also* Screening, by
      name of disease) V74.9
    Dick V74.8
    hypersensitivity V72.7
    Kveim V82.89
    Mantoux V74.1
    mycotic organism V75.4
    parasitic agent NEC V75.8
    sarcoidosis V82.89
    Schick V74.3
    Schultz-Charlton V74.8
    tuberculin V74.1
  specified type NEC V72.85

Test(s)—*continued*
  tuberculin V74.1
  vision V72.0
  Wassermann
    positive (*see also* Serology for syphilis,
      positive) 097.1
    false 795.6
Testicle, testicular, testis —*see also* condition
  feminization (syndrome) 259.5
Tetanus, tetanic (cephalic) (convulsions) 037
  with
    abortion—*see* Abortion, by type, with sepsis
    ectopic pregnancy (*see also* categories
      633.0-633.9) 639.0
    molar pregnancy (*see* categories 630-632) 639.0
  following
    abortion 639.0
    ectopic or molar pregnancy 639.0
  inoculation V03.7
    reaction (due to serum)—*see* Complications,
      vaccination
  neonatorum 771.3
  puerperal, postpartum, childbirth 670
Tetany, tetanic 781.7
  alkalosis 276.3
  associated with rickets 268.0
  convulsions 781.7
    hysterical 300.11
  functional (hysterical) 300.11
  hyperkinetic 781.7
    hysterical 300.11
  hyperpnea 786.01
    hysterical 300.11
    psychogenic 306.1
  hyperventilation 786.01
    hysterical 300.11
    psychogenic 306.1
  hypocalcemic, neonatal 775.4
  hysterical 300.11
  neonatal 775.4
  parathyroid (gland) 252.1
  parathyroprival 252.1
  postoperative 252.1
  postthyroidectomy 252.1
  pseudotetany 781.7
    hysterical 300.11
  psychogenic 306.1
    specified as conversion reaction 300.11
Tetralogy of Fallot 745.2
Tetraplegia —*see* Quadriplegia
Thailand hemorrhagic fever 065.4
Thalassanemia 282.49
Thalassemia (alpha) (beta) (disease) (Hb-C)
  (Hb-D) (Hb-E) (Hb-H) (Hb-I) (high fetal
  gene) (high fetal hemoglobin) (intermedia)
  (major) (minima) (minor) (mixed) (trait) (with
  other hemoglobinopathy) 282.49
  Hb-S (without crisis) 282.41
  with
    crisis 282.42
    vaso-occlusive pain 282.42
  sickle-cell (without crisis) 282.41
  with
    crisis 282.42
    vaso-occlusive pain 282.42
Thalassemic variants 282.49
Thaysen-Gee disease (nontropical sprue) 579.0
Thecoma (M8600/0) 220
  malignant (M8600/3) 183.0
Thelarche, precocious 259.1
Thelitis 611.0
  puerperal, postpartum 675.0

Thrombosis, thrombotic—*continued*
    without myocardial infarction 411.81
    extremities 444.22
      lower 444.22
      upper 444.21
    femoral 444.22
    hepatic 444.89
    hypophyseal 433.8
    meningeal, anterior or posterior 433.8
    mesenteric (with gangrene) 557.0
    ophthalmic (*see also* Occlusion, retina) 362.30
    pontine 433.8
    popliteal 444.22
    precerebral—*see* Occlusion, artery,
      precerebral NEC
    pulmonary 415.19
      iatrogenic 415.11
      postoperative 415.11
    renal 593.81
    retinal (*see also* Occlusion, retina) 362.30
    specified site NEC 444.89
    spinal, anterior or posterior 433.8
    traumatic (complication) (early) (*see also*
      Injury, blood vessel, by site) 904.9
    vertebral (*see also* Occlusion, artery,
      vertebral) 433.2
    with other precerebral artery 433.3
  atrial (endocardial) 424.90
    due to syphilis 093.89
    without endocarditis 429.89
  auricular (*see also* Infarct, myocardium) 410.9
  axillary (vein) 453.8
  basilar (artery) (*see also* Occlusion, artery,
    basilar) 433.0
  bland NEC 453.9
  brain (artery) (stem) 434.0
    due to syphilis 094.89
    iatrogenic 997.02
    late effect—*see* Late effect(s) (of)
      cerebrovascular disease
    postoperative 997.02
    puerperal, postpartum, childbirth 674.0
    sinus (*see also* Thrombosis, intracranial
      venous sinus) 325
  capillary 448.9
    arteriolar, generalized 446.6
  cardiac (*see also* Infarct, myocardium) 410.9
    due to syphilis 093.89
    healed or specified as old 412
    valve—*see* Endocarditis
  carotid (artery) (common) (internal) (*see also*
    Occlusion, artery, carotid) 433.1
    with other precerebral artery 433.3
  cavernous sinus (venous)—*see* Thrombosis,
    intracranial venous sinus
  cerebellar artery (anterior inferior) (posterior
    inferior) (superior) 433.8
    late effect—*see* Late effect(s) (of)
      cerebrovascular disease
  cerebral (arteries) (*see also* Thrombosis, brain)
    434.0
    late effect—*see* Late effect(s) (of)
      cerebrovascular disease
  coronary (artery) (*see also* Infarct, myocardium)
    410.9
    due to syphilis 093.89
    healed or specified as old 412
    without myocardial infarction 411.81
  corpus cavernosum 607.82
  cortical (*see also* Thrombosis, brain) 434.0

Thrombosis, thrombotic—*continued*
  due to (presence of) any device, implant, or graft
    classifiable to 996.0-996.5—*see*
    Complications, due to (presence of) any
    device, implant, or graft classified to
    996.0-996.5 NEC
  effort 453.8
  endocardial—*see* Infarct, myocardium
  eye (*see also* Occlusion, retina) 362.30
  femoral (vein) 453.8
    with inflammation or phlebitis 451.11
    artery 444.22
    deep 453.41
  genital organ, male 608.83
  heart (chamber) (*see also* Infarct, myocardium)
    410.9
  hepatic (vein) 453.0
    artery 444.89
    infectional or septic 572.1
  iliac (vein) 453.8
    with inflammation or phlebitis 451.81
    artery (common) (external) (internal) 444.81
  inflammation, vein—*see* Thrombophlebitis
  internal carotid artery (*see also* Occlusion,
    artery, carotid) 433.1
    with other precerebral artery 433.3
  intestine (with gangrene) 557.0
  intracranial (*see also* Thrombosis, brain) 434.0
    venous sinus (any) 325
      nonpyogenic origin 437.6
        in pregnancy or puerperium 671.5
  intramural (*see also* Infarct, myocardium) 410.9
    without
      cardiac condition 429.89
      coronary artery disease 429.89
      myocardial infarction 429.89
    healed or specified as old 412
  jugular (bulb) 453.8
  kidney 593.81
    artery 593.81
  lateral sinus (venous)—*see* Thrombosis,
    intracranial venous sinus
  leg 453.8
    with inflammation or phlebitis—*see*
      Thrombophlebitis
    deep (vessels) 453.40
      lower (distal) 453.42
      upper (proximal) 453.41
    superficial (vessels) 453.8
  liver (venous) 453.0
    artery 444.89
    infectional or septic 572.1
    portal vein 452
  longitudinal sinus (venous)—*see* Thrombosis,
    intracranial venous sinus
  lower extremity 453.8
    deep vessels 453.40
      calf 453.42
      distal (lower leg) 453.42
      femoral 453.41
      iliac 453.41
      lower leg 453.42
      peroneal 453.42
      popliteal 453.41
      proximal (upper leg) 453.41
      thigh 453.41
      tibial 453.42
  lung 415.19
    iatrogenic 415.11
    postoperative 415.11
  marantic, dural sinus 437.6

Thrombosis, thrombotic—*continued*
  meninges (brain) (*see also* Thrombosis, brain)
    434.0
  mesenteric (artery) (with gangrene) 557.0
    vein (inferior) (superior) 557.0
  mitral—*see* Insufficiency, mitral
  mural (heart chamber) (*see also* Infarct,
    myocardium) 410.9
    without
      cardiac condition 429.89
      coronary artery disease 429.89
      myocardial infarction 429.89
    due to syphilis 093.89
    following myocardial infarction 429.79
    healed or specified as old 412
  omentum (with gangrene) 557.0
  ophthalmic (artery) (*see also* Occlusion, retina)
    362.30
  pampiniform plexus (male) 608.83
    female 620.8
  parietal (*see also* Infarct, myocardium) 410.9
  penis, penile 607.82
  peripheral arteries 444.22
    lower 444.22
    upper 444.21
  platelet 446.6
  portal 452
    due to syphilis 093.89
    infectional or septic 572.1
  precerebral artery—*see also* Occlusion, artery,
    precerebral NEC
  pregnancy 671.9
    deep (vein) 671.3
    superficial (vein) 671.2
  puerperal, postpartum, childbirth 671.9
    brain (artery) 674.0
      venous 671.5
    cardiac 674.8
    cerebral (artery) 674.0
      venous 671.5
    deep (vein) 671.4
    intracranial sinus (nonpyogenic) (venous)
      671.5
    pelvic 671.4
    pulmonary (artery) 673.2
    specified site NEC 671.5
    superficial 671.2
  pulmonary (artery) (vein) 415.19
    iatrogenic 415.11
    postoperative 415.11
  radial vein 451.83
  renal (artery) 593.81
    vein 453.3
  resulting from presence of shunt or other
    internal prosthetic device—*see*
    Complications, due to (presence of) any
    device, implant, or graft classified to
    996.0-996.5 NEC
  retina, retinal (artery) 362.30
    arterial branch 362.32
    central 362.31
    partial 362.33
    vein
      central 362.35
      tributary (branch) 362.36
  scrotum 608.83
  seminal vesicle 608.83
  sigmoid (venous) sinus (*see* Thrombosis,
    intracranial venous sinus) 325
  silent NEC 453.9

Thrombosis, thrombotic—*continued*
  sinus, intracranial (venous) (any) (*see also*
    Thrombosis, intracranial venous sinus) 325
  softening, brain (*see also* Thrombosis, brain)
    434.0
  specified site NEC 453.8
  spermatic cord 608.83
  spinal cord 336.1
    due to syphilis 094.89
    in pregnancy or puerperium 671.5
    pyogenic origin 324.1
      late effect—*see* category 326
  spleen, splenic 289.59
    artery 444.89
  testis 608.83
  traumatic (complication) (early) (*see also* Injury,
    blood vessel, by site) 904.9
  tricuspid—*see* Endocarditis, tricuspid
  tumor—*see* Neoplasm, by site
  tunica vaginalis 608.83
  umbilical cord (vessels) 663.6
    affecting fetus or newborn 762.6
  vas deferens 608.83
  vein
    deep 453.40
    lower extremity—*see* Thrombosis, lower
      extremity
  vena cava (inferior) (superior) 453.2
Thrombus —*see* Thrombosis
Thrush 112.0
  newborn 771.7
Thumb —*see also* condition
  gamekeeper's 842.12
  sucking (child problem) 307.9
Thygeson's superficial punctate keratitis
  370.21
Thymergasia (*see also* Psychosis, affective)
  296.80
Thymitis 254.8
Thymoma (benign) (M8580/0) 212.6
  malignant (M8580/3) 164.0
Thymus, thymic (gland)—*see* condition
Thyrocele (*see also* Goiter) 240.9
Thyroglossal —*see also* condition
  cyst 759.2
  duct, persistent 759.2
Thyroid (body) (gland)—*see also* condition
  hormone resistance 246.8
  lingual 759.2
Thyroiditis 245.9
  acute (pyogenic) (suppurative) 245.0
    nonsuppurative 245.0
  autoimmune 245.2
  chronic (nonspecific) (sclerosing) 245.8
    fibrous 245.3
    lymphadenoid 245.2
    lymphocytic 245.2
    lymphoid 245.2
  complicating pregnancy, childbirth, or
    puerperium 648.1
  de Quervain's (subacute granulomatous) 245.1
  fibrous (chronic) 245.3
  giant (cell) (follicular) 245.1
  granulomatous (de Quervain's) (subacute) 245.1
  Hashimoto's (struma lymphomatosa) 245.2
  iatrogenic 245.4
  invasive (fibrous) 245.3
  ligneous 245.3
  lymphocytic (chronic) 245.2
  lymphoid 245.2
  lymphomatous 245.2

Thyroiditis—*continued*
  pseudotuberculous 245.1
  pyogenic 245.0
  radiation 245.4
  Riedel's (ligneous) 245.3
  subacute 245.1
  suppurative 245.0
  tuberculous (*see also* Tuberculosis) 017.5
  viral 245.1
  woody 245.3
Thyrolingual duct, persistent 759.2
Thyromegaly 240.9
Thyrotoxic
  crisis or storm (*see also* Thyrotoxicosis) 242.9
  heart failure (*see also* Thyrotoxicosis) 242.9
    [425.7]
Thyrotoxicosis 242.9

> *Note—Use the following fifth-digit*
> *subclassification with category 242:*
>
> 0 *without mention of thyrotoxic crisis or storm*
> 1 *with mention of thyrotoxic crisis or storm*

  with
    goiter (diffuse) 242.0
      adenomatous 242.3
        multinodular 242.2
        uninodular 242.1
      nodular 242.3
        multinodular 242.2
        uninodular 242.1
    infiltrative
      dermopathy 242.0
      ophthalmopathy 242.0
    thyroid acropachy 242.0
  complicating pregnancy, childbirth, or
    puerperium 648.1
  due to
    ectopic thyroid nodule 242.4
    ingestion of (excessive) thyroid material 242.8
    specified cause NEC 242.8
  factitia 242.8
  heart 242.9 [425.7]
  neonatal (transient) 775.3
TIA (transient ischemic attack) 435.9
  with transient neurologic deficit 435.9
  late effect—*see* Late effect(s) (of)
    cerebrovascular disease
Tibia vara 732.4
Tic 307.20
  breathing 307.20
  child problem 307.21
  compulsive 307.22
  convulsive 307.20
  degenerative (generalized) (localized) 333.3
    facial 351.8
  douloureux (*see also* Neuralgia, trigeminal)
    350.1
    atypical 350.2
  habit 307.20
    chronic (motor or vocal) 307.22
    transient (of childhood) 307.21
  lid 307.20
    transient (of childhood) 307.21
  motor-verbal 307.23
  occupational 300.89
  orbicularis 307.20
    transient (of childhood) 307.21
  organic origin 333.3
  postchoreic—*see* Chorea
  psychogenic 307.20

Tic —*continued*
  compulsive 307.22
  salaam 781.0
  spasm 307.20
    chronic (motor or vocal) 307.22
    transient (of childhood) 307.21
Tick (-borne) fever NEC 066.1
  American mountain 066.1
  Colorado 066.1
  hemorrhagic NEC 065.3
    Crimean 065.0
    Kyasanur Forest 065.2
    Omsk 065.1
  mountain 066.1
  nonexanthematous 066.1
Tick-bite fever NEC 066.1
  African 087.1
  Colorado (virus) 066.1
  Rocky Mountain 082.0
Tick paralysis 989.5
Tics and spasms, compulsive 307.22
Tietze's disease or syndrome 733.6
Tight, tightness
  anus 564.89
  chest 786.59
  fascia (lata) 728.9
  foreskin (congenital) 605
  hymen 623.3
  introitus (acquired) (congenital) 623.3
  rectal sphincter 564.89
  tendon 727.81
    Achilles (heel) 727.81
  urethral sphincter 598.9
Tilting vertebra 737.9
Timidity, child 313.21
Tinea (intersecta) (tarsi) 110.9
  amiantacea 110.0
  asbestina 110.0
  barbae 110.0
  beard 110.0
  black dot 110.0
  blanca 111.2
  capitis 110.0
  corporis 110.5
  cruris 110.3
  decalvans 704.09
  flava 111.0
  foot 110.4
  furfuracea 111.0
  imbricata (Tokelau) 110.5
  lepothrix 039.0
  manuum 110.2
  microsporic (*see also* Dermatophytosis) 110.9
  nigra 111.1
  nodosa 111.2
  pedis 110.4
  scalp 110.0
  specified site NEC 110.8
  sycosis 110.0
  tonsurans 110.0
  trichophytic (*see also* Dermatophytosis) 110.9
  unguium 110.1
  versicolor 111.0
Tingling sensation (*see also* Disturbance,
    sensation) 782.0
Tin-miners' lung 503
Tinnitus (aurium) 388.30
  audible 388.32
  objective 388.32
  subjective 388.31
Tipped, teeth 524.33

Tipping
pelvis 738.6
with disproportion (fetopelvic) 653.0
affecting fetus or newborn 763.1
causing obstructed labor 660.1
affecting fetus or newborn 763.1
teeth 524.33
Tiredness 780.79
Tissue —*see* condition
Tobacco
abuse (affecting health) NEC (*see also* Abuse,
drugs, nondependent) 305.1
heart 989.8
use disorder complicating pregnancy, childbirth,
or the puerperium 649.0
Tobias' syndrome (carcinoma, pulmonary apex)
(M8010/3) 162.3
Tocopherol deficiency 269.1
Todd's
cirrhosis—*see* Cirrhosis, biliary
paralysis (postepileptic transitory paralysis)
344.89
Toe —*see* condition
Toilet, artificial opening (*see also* Attention to,
artificial, opening) V55.9
Tokelau ringworm 110.5
Tollwut 071
Tolosa-Hunt syndrome 378.55
Tommaselli's disease
correct substance properly administered 599.7
overdose or wrong substance given or taken 961.4
Tongue —*see also* condition
worms 134.1
Tongue tie 750.0
Toni-Fanconi syndrome (cystinosis) 270.0
Tonic pupil 379.46
Tonsil —*see* condition
Tonsillitis (acute) (catarrhal) (croupous)
(follicular) (gangrenous) (infective) (lacunar)
(lingual) (malignant) (membranous)
(phlegmonous) (pneumococcal)
(pseudomembranous) (purulent) (septic)
(staphylococcal) (subacute) (suppurative)
(toxic) (ulcerative) (vesicular) (viral) 463
with influenza, flu, or grippe 487.1
chronic 474.00
diphtheritic (membranous) 032.0
hypertrophic 474.00
influenzal 487.1
parenchymatous 475
streptococcal 034.0
tuberculous (*see also* Tuberculosis) 012.8
Vincent's 101
Tonsillopharyngitis 465.8
Tooth, teeth —*see* condition
Toothache 525.9
Topagnosis 782.0
Tophi (gouty) 274.0
ear 274.81
heart 274.82
specified site NEC 274.82
Torn —*see* Tear, torn
Tornwaldt's bursitis (disease) (pharyngeal
bursitis) 478.29
cyst 478.26
Torpid liver 573.9

Torsion
accessory tube 620.5
adnexa (female) 620.5
aorta (congenital) 747.29
acquired 447.1
appendix
epididymis 608.24
testis 608.23
bile duct 576.8
with calculus, choledocholithiasis or
stones—*see* Choledocholithiasis
congenital 751.69
bowel, colon, or intestine 560.2
cervix (*see* Malposition, uterus)
duodenum 537.3
dystonia—*see* Dystonia, torsion
epididymis 608.24
appendix 608.24
fallopian tube 620.5
gallbladder (*see also* Disease, gallbladder) 575.8
congenital 751.69
gastric 537.89
hydatid of Morgagni (female) 620.5
kidney (pedicle) 593.89
Meckel's diverticulum (congenital) 751.0
mesentery 560.2
omentum 560.2
organ or site, congenital NEC—*see* Anomaly,
specified type NEC
ovary (pedicle) 620.5
congenital 752.0
oviduct 620.5
penis 607.89
congenital 752.69
renal 593.89
spasm—*see* Dystonia, torsion
spermatic cord 608.22
extravaginal 608.21
intravaginal 608.22
spleen 289.59
testicle, testis 608.20
appendix 608.23
tibia 736.89
umbilical cord—*see* Compression, umbilical
cord
uterus (*see also* Malposition, uterus) 621.6
Torticollis (intermittent) (spastic) 723.5
congenital 754.1
sternomastoid 754.1
due to birth injury 767.8
hysterical 300.11
ocular 781.93
psychogenic 306.0
specified as conversion reaction 300.11
rheumatic 723.5
rheumatoid 714.0
spasmodic 333.83
traumatic, current NEC 847.0
Tortuous
artery 447.1
fallopian tube 752.19
organ or site, congenital NEC—*see* Distortion
renal vessel, congenital 747.62
retina vessel (congenital) 743.58
acquired 362.17
ureter 593.4
urethra 599.84
vein—*see* Varicose, vein
Torula, torular (infection) 117.5
histolytica 117.5
lung 117.5
Torulosis 117.5

Torus
  fracture
    fibula 823.41
      with tibia 823.42
    radius 813.45
    tibia 823.40
      with fibula 823.42
  mandibularis 526.81
  palatinus 526.81
Touch, vitreous 997.99
Touraine's syndrome (hereditary
  osteo-onychodysplasia) 756.89
Touraine-Solente-Golé syndrome
  (acropachyderma) 757.39
Tourette's disease (motor-verbal tic) 307.23
Tower skull 756.0
  with exophthalmos 756.0
Toxemia 799.89
  with
    abortion—*see* Abortion, by type, with toxemia
  bacterial—*see* Septicemia
  biliary (*see also* Disease, biliary) 576.8
  burn—*see* Burn, by site
  congenital NEC 779.89
  eclamptic 642.6
    with pre-existing hypertension 642.7
  erysipelatous (*see also* Erysipelas) 035
  fatigue 799.89
  fetus or newborn NEC 779.89
  food (*see also* Poisoning, food) 005.9
  gastric 537.89
  gastrointestinal 558.2
  intestinal 558.2
  kidney (*see also* Disease, renal) 593.9
  lung 518.89
  malarial NEC (*see also* Malaria) 084.6
  maternal (of pregnancy), affecting fetus or
    newborn 760.0
  myocardial—*see* Myocarditis, toxic
  of pregnancy (mild) (pre-eclamptic) 642.4
    with
      convulsions 642.6
      pre-existing hypertension 642.7
    affecting fetus or newborn 760.0
    severe 642.5
  pre-eclamptic—*see* Toxemia, of pregnancy
  puerperal, postpartum—*see* Toxemia, of
    pregnancy
  pulmonary 518.89
  renal (*see also* Disease, renal) 593.9
  septic (*see also* Septicemia) 038.9
  small intestine 558.2
  staphylococcal 038.10
    aureus 038.11
    due to food 005.0
    specified organism NEC 038.19
  stasis 799.89
  stomach 537.89
  uremic (*see also* Uremia) 586
  urinary 586
Toxemica cerebropathia psychica
  (nonalcoholic) 294.0
  alcoholic 291.1
Toxic (poisoning)—*see also* condition
  from drug or poison—*see* Table of drugs and
    chemicals
  oil syndrome 710.5
  shock syndrome 040.82
  thyroid (gland) (*see also* Thyrotoxicosis) 242.9
Toxicemia —*see* Toxemia

Toxicity
  dilantin
    asymptomatic 796.0
    symptomatic—*see* Table of Drugs and Chemicals
  drug
    asymptomatic 796.0
    symptomatic—*see* Table of Drugs and Chemicals
  fava bean 282.2
  from drug or poison
    asymptomatic 796.0
    symptomatic—*see* Table of Drugs and
      Chemicals
Toxicosis (*see also* Toxemia) 799.89
  capillary, hemorrhagic 287.0
Toxinfection 799.89
  gastrointestinal 558.2
Toxocariasis 128.0
Toxoplasma infection, generalized 130.9
Toxoplasmosis (acquired) 130.9
  with pneumonia 130.4
  congenital, active 771.2
  disseminated (multisystemic) 130.8
  maternal
    with suspected damage to fetus affecting
      management of pregnancy 655.4
    affecting fetus or newborn 760.2
      manifest toxoplasmosis in fetus or newborn
        771.2
  multiple sites 130.8
  multisystemic disseminated 130.8
  specified site NEC 130.7
Trabeculation, bladder 596.8
Trachea —*see* condition
Tracheitis (acute)(catarrhal)(infantile)
  (membranous) (plastic) (pneumococcal)
  (septic) (suppurative) (viral) 464.10
  with
    bronchitis 490
      acute or subacute 466.0
      chronic 491.8
      tuberculosis—*see* Tuberculosis, pulmonary
    laryngitis (acute) 464.20
      with obstruction 464.21
      chronic 476.1
      tuberculous (*see also* Tuberculosis, larynx)
        012.3
    obstruction 464.11
  chronic 491.8
    with
      bronchitis (chronic) 491.8
      laryngitis (chronic) 476.1
    due to external agent—*see* Condition,
      respiratory, chronic, due to
  diphtheritic (membranous) 032.3
    due to external agent—*see* Inflammation,
      respiratory, upper, due to
  edematous 464.11
  influenzal 487.1
  streptococcal 034.0
  syphilitic 095.8
  tuberculous (*see also* Tuberculosis) 012.8
Trachelitis (nonvenereal) (*see also* Cervicitis) 616.0
  trichomonal 131.09
Tracheobronchial —*see* condition
Tracheobronchitis (*see also* Bronchitis) 490
  acute or subacute 466.0
    with bronchospasm or obstruction 466.0
  chronic 491.8
  influenzal 487.1
  senile 491.8

Tracheobronchomegaly (congenital) 748.3
  with bronchiectasis 494.0
    with (acute) exacerbation 494.1
  acquired 519.19
    with bronchiectasis 494.0
      with (acute) exacerbation 494.1
Tracheobronchopneumonitis —*see* Pneumonia,
    broncho
Tracheocele (external) (internal) 519.19
  congenital 748.3
Tracheomalacia 519.19
  congenital 748.3
Tracheopharyngitis (acute) 465.8
  chronic 478.9
    due to external agent—*see* Condition,
        respiratory, chronic, due to
    due to external agent—*see* Inflammation,
        respiratory, upper, due to
Tracheostenosis 519.19
  congenital 748.3
Tracheostomy
  attention to V55.0
  complication 519.00
    granuloma 519.09
    hemorrhage 519.09
    infection 519.01
    malfunctioning 519.02
    obstruction 519.09
    sepsis 519.01
  status V44.0
  stenosis 519.02
Trachoma, trachomatous 076.9
  active (stage) 076.1
  contraction of conjunctiva 076.1
  dubium 076.0
  healed or late effect 139.1
  initial (stage) 076.0
  Türck's (chronic catarrhal laryngitis) 476.0
Trachyphonia 784.49
Training
  insulin pump V65.46
  orthoptic V57.4
  orthotic V57.81
Train sickness 994.6
Trait
  hemoglobin
    abnormal NEC 282.7
      with thalassemia 282.49
    C (*see also* Disease, hemoglobin, C) 282.7
      with elliptocytosis 282.7
    S (Hb-S) 282.5
  Lepore 282.49
    with other abnormal hemoglobin NEC 282.49
  paranoid 301.0
  sickle-cell 282.5
    with
      elliptocytosis 282.5
      spherocytosis 282.5
Traits, paranoid 301.0
Tramp V60.0
Trance 780.09
  hysterical 300.13
Transaminasemia 790.4
Transfusion, blood
  donor V59.01
    stem cells V59.02
  incompatible 999.6
  reaction or complication—*see* Complications,
      transfusion
  related acute lung injury (TRALI) 518.7

Transfusion, blood—*continued*
  syndrome
    fetomaternal 772.0
    twin-to-twin
      blood loss (donor twin) 772.0
      recipient twin 776.4
  without reported diagnosis V58.2
Transient —*see also* condition
  alteration of awareness 780.02
  blindness 368.12
  deafness (ischemic) 388.02
  global amnesia 437.7
  person (homeless) NEC V60.0
Transitional, lumbosacral joint of vertebra
    756.19
Translocation
  autosomes NEC 758.5
    13-15 758.1
    16-18 758.2
    21 or 22 758.0
    balanced in normal individual 758.4
    D_1 758.1
    E_3 758.2
    G 758.0
  balanced autosomal in normal individual 758.4
  chromosomes NEC 758.89
  Down's syndrome 758.0
Translucency, iris 364.53
Transmission of chemical substances through
    the placenta
  (affecting fetus or newborn) 760.70
  alcohol 760.71
  anticonvulsants 760.77
  antifungals 760.74
  anti-infective agents 760.74
  antimetabolics 760.78
  cocaine 760.75
  "crack" 760.75
  diethylstilbestrol [DES] 760.76
  hallucinogenic agents 760.73
  medicinal agents NEC 760.79
  narcotics 760.72
  obstetric anesthetic or analgesic drug 763.5
  specified agent NEC 760.79
  suspected, affecting management of pregnancy
      655.5
Transplant(ed)
  bone V42.4
    marrow V42.81
  complication—*see also* Complications, due to
      (presence of) any device, implant, or graft
      classified to 996.0-996.5 NEC
    bone marrow 996.85
    corneal graft NEC 996.79
      infection or inflammation 996.69
      reaction 996.51
      rejection 996.51
    organ (failure) (immune or nonimmune cause)
        (infection) (rejection) 996.80
      bone marrow 996.85
      heart 996.83
      intestines 996.87
      kidney 996.81
      liver 996.82
      lung 996.84
      pancreas 996.86
      specified NEC 996.89
    skin NEC 996.79
      infection or inflammation 996.69
      rejection 996.52
        artificial 996.55

Trichocephalosis 127.3
Trichocephalus infestation 127.3
Trichoclasis 704.2
Trichoepithelioma (M8100/0)—*see also*
    Neoplasm, skin, benign
  breast 217
    genital organ NEC—*see* Neoplasm, by site,
      benign
    malignant (M8100/3)—*see* Neoplasm, skin,
      malignant
Trichofolliculoma (M8101/0)—*see* Neoplasm,
    skin, benign
Tricholemmoma (M8102/0)—*see* Neoplasm,
    skin, benign
Trichomatosis 704.2
Trichomoniasis 131.9
  bladder 131.09
  cervix 131.09
  intestinal 007.3
  prostate 131.03
  seminal vesicle 131.09
  specified site NEC 131.8
  urethra 131.02
  urogenitalis 131.00
  vagina 131.01
  vulva 131.01
  vulvovaginal 131.01
Trichomycosis 039.0
  axillaris 039.0
  nodosa 111.2
  nodularis 111.2
  rubra 039.0
Trichonocardiosis (axillaris) (palmellina) 039.0
Trichonodosis 704.2
Trichophytid, trichophyton infection (*see also*
    Dermatophytosis) 110.9
Trichophytide —*see* Dermatophytosis
Trichophytobezoar 938
  intestine 936
  stomach 935.2
Trichophytosis —*see* Dermatophytosis
Trichoptilosis 704.2
Trichorrhexis (nodosa) 704.2
Trichosporosis nodosa 111.2
Trichostasis spinulosa (congenital) 757.4
Trichostrongyliasis (small intestine) 127.6
Trichostrongylosis 127.6
Trichostrongylus (instabilis) infection 127.6
Trichotillomania 312.39
Trichromat, anomalous (congenital) 368.59
Trichromatopsia, anomalous (congenital)
    368.59
Trichuriasis 127.3
Trichuris trichiuria (any site) (infection)
    (infestation) 127.3
Tricuspid (valve)—*see* condition
Trifid —*see also* Accessory
  kidney (pelvis) 753.3
  tongue 750.13
Trigeminal neuralgia (*see also* Neuralgia,
    trigeminal) 350.1
Trigeminoencephaloangiomatosis 759.6
Trigeminy 427.89
  postoperative 997.1
Trigger finger (acquired) 727.03
  congenital 756.89
Trigonitis (bladder) (chronic)
    (pseudomembranous) 595.3
  tuberculous (*see also* Tuberculosis) 016.1
Trigonocephaly 756.0
Trihexosidosis 272.7

Trilobate placenta —*see* Placenta, abnormal
Trilocular heart 745.8
Trimethylaminuria 270.8
Tripartita placenta —*see* Placenta, abnormal
Triple —*see also* Accessory
  kidneys 753.3
  uteri 752.2
  X female 758.81
Triplegia 344.89
  congenital or infantile 343.8
Triplet
  affected by maternal complications of pregnancy
      761.5
  healthy liveborn—*see* Newborn, multiple
  pregnancy (complicating delivery) NEC 651.1
      with fetal loss and retention of one or more
          fetus(es) 651.4
      following (elective) fetal reduction 651.7
Triplex placenta —*see* Placenta, abnormal
Triplication —*see* Accessory
Trismus 781.0
  neonatorum 771.3
  newborn 771.3
Trisomy (syndrome) NEC 758.5
  13 (partial) 758.1
  16-18 758.2
  18 (partial) 758.2
  21 (partial) 758.0
  22 758.0
  autosomes NEC 758.5
  D_1 758.1
  E_3 758.2
  G (group) 758.0
  group D_1 758.1
  group E 758.2
  group G 758.0
Tritanomaly 368.53
Tritanopia 368.53
Troisier-Hanot-Chauffard syndrome (bronze
    diabetes) 275.0
Trombidiosis 133.8
Trophedema (hereditary) 757.0
  congenital 757.0
Trophoblastic disease (*see also* Hydatidiform
    mole) 630
  previous, affecting management of pregnancy
      V23.1
Tropholymphedema 757.0
Trophoneurosis NEC 356.9
  arm NEC 354.9
  disseminated 710.1
  facial 349.89
  leg NEC 355.8
  lower extremity NEC 355.8
  upper extremity NEC 354.9
Tropical —*see also* condition
  maceration feet (syndrome) 991.4
  wet foot (syndrome) 991.4
Trouble —*see also* Disease
  bowel 569.9
  heart—*see* Disease, heart
  intestine 569.9
  kidney (*see also* Disease, renal) 593.9
  nervous 799.2
  sinus (*see also* Sinusitis) 473.9
Trousseau's syndrome (thrombophlebitis
    migrans) 453.1
Truancy, childhood —*see also* Disturbance,
    conduct
  socialized 312.2
  undersocialized, unsocialized 312.1

Truncus
  arteriosus (persistent) 745.0
  common 745.0
  communis 745.0
Trunk —*see* condition
Trychophytide —*see* Dermatophytosis
Trypanosoma infestation —*see*
    Trypanosomiasis
Trypanosomiasis 086.9
  with meningoencephalitis 086.9 *[323.2]*
  African 086.5
    due to Trypanosoma 086.5
      gambiense 086.3
      rhodesiense 086.4
  American 086.2
    with
      heart involvement 086.0
      other organ involvement 086.1
    without mention of organ involvement 086.2
  Brazilian—*see* Trypanosomiasis, American
  Chagas'—*see* Trypanosomiasis, American
  due to Trypanosoma
    cruzi—*see* Trypanosomiasis, American
    gambiense 086.3
    rhodesiense 086.4
  gambiensis, Gambian 086.3
  North American—*see* Trypanosomiasis,
    American
  rhodesiensis, Rhodesian 086.4
  South American—*see* Trypanosomiasis,
    American
T-shaped incisors 520.2
Tsutsugamushi fever 081.2
Tube, tubal, tubular —*see also* condition
  ligation, admission for V25.2
Tubercle —*see also* Tuberculosis
  brain, solitary 013.2
  Darwin's 744.29
  epithelioid noncaseating 135
  Ghon, primary infection 010.0
Tuberculid, tuberculide (indurating) (lichenoid)
    (miliary) (papulonecrotic) (primary) (skin)
    (subcutaneous) (*see also* Tuberculosis) 017.0
Tuberculoma —*see also* Tuberculosis
  brain (any part) 013.2
  meninges (cerebral) (spinal) 013.1
  spinal cord 013.4

Tuberculosis, tubercular, tuberculous
    (calcification) (calcified) (caseous)
    (chromogenic acid-fast bacilli) (congenital)
    (degeneration) (disease) (fibrocaseous)
    (fistula) (gangrene) (interstitial) (isolated
    circumscribed lesions) (necrosis)
    (parenchymatous) (ulcerative) 011.9

Note—Use the following fifth-digit
subclassification with categories 010-018:

0 *unspecified*
1 *bacteriological or histological examination*
   not done
2 *bacteriological or histological examination*
   unknown (at present)
3 *tubercle bacilli found (in sputum) by*
   microscopy
4 *tubercle bacilli not found (in sputum) by*
   microscopy, but found by bacterial culture
5 *tubercle bacilli not found by bacteriological*
   examination, but tuberculosis confirmed
   histologically
6 *tubercle bacilli not found by bacteriological or*
   histological examination, but tuberculosis
   confirmed by other methods [inoculation of
   animals]

For tuberculous conditions specified as late
effects or sequelae, see category 137.

---

  abdomen 014.8
    lymph gland 014.8
  abscess 011.9
    arm 017.9
    bone (*see also* Osteomyelitis, due to,
        tuberculosis) 015.9 *[730.8]*
      hip 015.1 *[730.85]*
      knee 015.2 *[730.86]*
      sacrum 015.0 *[730.88]*
      specified site NEC 015.7 *[730.88]*
      spinal 015.0 *[730.88]*
      vertebra 015.0 *[730.88]*
    brain 013.3
    breast 017.9
    Cowper's gland 016.5
    dura (mater) 013.8
      brain 013.3
      spinal cord 013.5
    epidural 013.8
      brain 013.3
      spinal cord 013.5
    frontal sinus—*see* Tuberculosis, sinus
    genital organs NEC 016.9
      female 016.7
      male 016.5
    genitourinary NEC 016.9
    gland (lymphatic)—*see* Tuberculosis, lymph
        gland
    hip 015.1
    iliopsoas 015.0 *[730.88]*
    intestine 014.8
    ischiorectal 014.8
    joint 015.9
      hip 015.1
      knee 015.2
      specified joint NEC 015.8
      vertebral 015.0 *[730.88]*
    kidney 016.0 *[590.81]*
    knee 015.2
    lumbar 015.0 *[730.88]*
    lung 011.2

Tuberculosis, tubercular—*continued*
    affecting fetus or newborn 760.2
    congenital 771.2
    conjunctiva 017.3 *[370.31]*
    connective tissue 017.9
      bone—*see* Tuberculosis, bone
    contact V01.1
    converter (tuberculin skin test) (without disease)
      795.5
    cornea (ulcer) 017.3 *[370.31]*
    Cowper's gland 016.5
    coxae 015.1 *[730.85]*
    coxalgia 015.1 *[730.85]*
    cul-de-sac of Douglas 014.8
    curvature, spine 015.0 *[737.40]*
    cutis (colliquativa) (primary) 017.0
    cyst, ovary 016.6
    cystitis 016.1
    dacryocystitis 017.3 *[375.32]*
    dactylitis 015.5
    diarrhea 014.8
    diffuse (*see also* Tuberculosis, miliary) 018.9
      lung—*see* Tuberculosis, pulmonary
      meninges 013.0
    digestive tract 014.8
    disseminated (*see also* Tuberculosis, miliary)
      018.9
      meninges 013.0
    duodenum 014.8
    dura (mater) 013.9
      abscess 013.8
        cerebral 013.3
        spinal 013.5
    dysentery 014.8
    ear (inner) (middle) 017.4
      bone 015.6
      external (primary) 017.0
      skin (primary) 017.0
    elbow 015.8
    emphysema—*see* Tuberculosis, pulmonary
    empyema 012.0
    encephalitis 013.6
    endarteritis 017.9
    endocarditis (any valve) 017.9 *[424.91]*
    endocardium (any valve) 017.9 *[424.91]*
    endocrine glands NEC 017.9
    endometrium 016.7
    enteric, enterica 014.8
    enteritis 014.8
    enterocolitis 014.8
    epididymis 016.4
    epididymitis 016.4
    epidural abscess 013.8
      brain 013.3
      spinal cord 013.5
    epiglottis 012.3
    episcleritis 017.3 *[379.00]*
    erythema (induratum) (nodosum) (primary)
      017.1
    esophagus 017.8
    Eustachian tube 017.4
    exposure to V01.1
    exudative 012.0
      primary, progressive 010.1
    eye 017.3
      glaucoma 017.3 *[365.62]*
    eyelid (primary) 017.0
      lupus 017.0 *[373.4]*
    fallopian tube 016.6
    fascia 017.9
    fauces 012.8

Tuberculosis, tubercular—*continued*
    finger 017.9
    first infection 010.0
    fistula, perirectal 014.8
    Florida 011.6
    foot 017.9
    funnel pelvis 137.3
    gallbladder 017.9
    galloping (*see also* Tuberculosis, pulmonary)
      011.9
    ganglionic 015.9
    gastritis 017.9
    gastrocolic fistula 014.8
    gastroenteritis 014.8
    gastrointestinal tract 014.8
    general, generalized 018.9
      acute 018.0
      chronic 018.8
    genital organs NEC 016.9
      female 016.7
      male 016.5
    genitourinary NEC 016.9
    genu 015.2
    glandulae suprarenalis 017.6
    glandular, general 017.2
    glottis 012.3
    grinders' 011.4
    groin 017.2
    gum 017.9
    hand 017.9
    heart 017.9 *[425.8]*
    hematogenous—*see* Tuberculosis, miliary
    hemoptysis (*see also* Tuberculosis, pulmonary)
      011.9
    hemorrhage NEC (*see also* Tuberculosis,
      pulmonary) 011.9
    hemothorax 012.0
    hepatitis 017.9
    hilar lymph nodes 012.1
      primary, progressive 010.8
    hip (disease) (joint) 015.1
      bone 015.1 *[730.85]*
    hydrocephalus 013.8
    hydropneumothorax 012.0
    hydrothorax 012.0
    hypoadrenalism 017.6
    hypopharynx 012.8
    ileocecal (hyperplastic) 014.8
    ileocolitis 014.8
    ileum 014.8
    iliac spine (superior) 015.0 *[730.88]*
    incipient NEC (*see also* Tuberculosis,
      pulmonary) 011.9
    indurativa (primary) 017.1
    infantile 010.0
    infection NEC 011.9
      without clinical manifestation 010.0
    infraclavicular gland 017.2
    inguinal gland 017.2
    inguinalis 017.2
    intestine (any part) 014.8
    iris 017.3 *[364.11]*
    iritis 017.3 *[364.11]*
    ischiorectal 014.8
    jaw 015.7 *[730.88]*
    jejunum 014.8
    joint 015.9
      hip 015.1
      knee 015.2
      specified site NEC 015.8
      vertebral 015.0 *[730.88]*

Tuberculosis, tubercular—*continued*
  phthisis NEC (*see also* Tuberculosis,
     pulmonary) 011.9
  pituitary gland 017.9
  placenta 016.7
  pleura, pleural, pleurisy, pleuritis (fibrinous)
     (obliterative) (purulent) (simple plastic)
     (with effusion) 012.0
    primary, progressive 010.1
  pneumonia, pneumonic 011.6
  pneumothorax 011.7
  polyserositis 018.9
    acute 018.0
    chronic 018.8
  potters' 011.4
  prepuce 016.5
  primary 010.9
    complex 010.0
    complicated 010.8
      with pleurisy or effusion 010.1
    progressive 010.8
      with pleurisy or effusion 010.1
    skin 017.0
  proctitis 014.8
  prostate 016.5 *[601.4]*
  prostatitis 016.5 *[601.4]*
  pulmonaris (*see also* Tuberculosis, pulmonary)
     011.9
  pulmonary (artery) (incipient) (malignant)
     (multiple round foci) (pernicious)
     (reinfection stage) 011.9
    cavitated or with cavitation 011.2
      primary, progressive 010.8
    childhood type or first infection 010.0
    chromogenic acid-fast bacilli 795.39
    fibrosis or fibrotic 011.4
    infiltrative 011.0
      primary, progressive 010.9
    nodular 011.1
    specified NEC 011.8
    sputum positive only 795.39
    status following surgical collapse of lung NEC
     011.9
  pyelitis 016.0 *[590.81]*
  pyelonephritis 016.0 *[590.81]*
  pyemia—*see* Tuberculosis, miliary
  pyonephrosis 016.0
  pyopneumothorax 012.0
  pyothorax 012.0
  rectum (with abscess) 014.8
    fistula 014.8
  reinfection stage (*see also* Tuberculosis,
     pulmonary) 011.9
  renal 016.0
  renis 016.0
  reproductive organ 016.7
  respiratory NEC (*see also* Tuberculosis,
     pulmonary) 011.9
    specified site NEC 012.8
  retina 017.3 *[363.13]*
  retroperitoneal (lymph gland or node) 014.8
    gland 014.8
  retropharyngeal abscess 012.8
  rheumatism 015.9
  rhinitis 012.8
  sacroiliac (joint) 015.8
  sacrum 015.0 *[730.88]*
  salivary gland 017.9
  salpingitis (acute) (chronic) 016.6
  sandblasters' 011.4
  sclera 017.3 *[379.09]*

Tuberculosis, tubercular—*continued*
  scoliosis 015.0 *[737.43]*
  scrofulous 017.2
  scrotum 016.5
  seminal tract or vesicle 016.5 *[608.81]*
  senile NEC (*see also* Tuberculosis, pulmonary)
     011.9
  septic NEC (*see also* Tuberculosis, miliary)
     018.9
  shoulder 015.8
    blade 015.7 *[730.8]*
  sigmoid 014.8
  sinus (accessory) (nasal) 012.8
    bone 015.7 *[730.88]*
    epididymis 016.4
  skeletal NEC (*see also* Osteomyelitis, due to
     tuberculosis) 015.9 *[730.8]*
  skin (any site) (primary) 017.0
  small intestine 014.8
  soft palate 017.9
  spermatic cord 016.5
  spinal
    column 015.0 *[730.88]*
    cord 013.4
    disease 015.0 *[730.88]*
    medulla 013.4
    membrane 013.0
    meninges 013.0
  spine 015.0 *[730.88]*
  spleen 017.7
  splenitis 017.7
  spondylitis 015.0 *[720.81]*
  spontaneous pneumothorax—*see* Tuberculosis,
     pulmonary
  sternoclavicular joint 015.8
  stomach 017.9
  stonemasons' 011.4
  struma 017.2
  subcutaneous tissue (cellular) (primary) 017.0
  subcutis (primary) 017.0
  subdeltoid bursa 017.9
  submaxillary 017.9
    region 017.9
  supraclavicular gland 017.2
  suprarenal (capsule) (gland) 017.6
  swelling, joint (*see also* Tuberculosis, joint)
     015.9
  symphysis pubis 015.7 *[730.88]*
  synovitis 015.9 *[727.01]*
    hip 015.1 *[727.01]*
    knee 015.2 *[727.01]*
    specified site NEC 015.8 *[727.01]*
    spine or vertebra 015.0 *[727.01]*
  systemic—*see* Tuberculosis, miliary
  tarsitis (eyelid) 017.0 *[373.4]*
    ankle (bone) 015.5 *[730.87]*
  tendon (sheath)—*see* Tuberculosis,
     tenosynovitis
  tenosynovitis 015.9 *[727.01]*
    hip 015.1 *[727.01]*
    knee 015.2 *[727.01]*
    specified site NEC 015.8 *[727.01]*
    spine or vertebra 015.0 *[727.01]*
  testis 016.5 *[608.81]*
  throat 012.8
  thymus gland 017.9
  thyroid gland 017.5
  toe 017.9
  tongue 017.9
  tonsil (lingual) 012.8
  tonsillitis 012.8

Tuberculosis, tubercular—*continued*
  trachea, tracheal 012.8
    gland 012.1
      primary, progressive 010.8
    isolated 012.2
  tracheobronchial 011.3
    glandular 012.1
      primary, progressive 010.8
    isolated 012.2
    lymph gland or node 012.1
      primary, progressive 010.8
  tubal 016.6
  tunica vaginalis 016.5
  typhlitis 014.8
  ulcer (primary) (skin) 017.0
    bowel or intestine 014.8
    specified site NEC—*see* Tuberculosis, by site
  unspecified site—*see* Tuberculosis, pulmonary
  ureter 016.2
  urethra, urethral 016.3
  urinary organ or tract 016.3
    kidney 016.0
  uterus 016.7
  uveal tract 017.3 *[363.13]*
  uvula 017.9
  vaccination, prophylactic (against) V03.2
  vagina 016.7
  vas deferens 016.5
  vein 017.9
  verruca (primary) 017.0
  verrucosa (cutis) (primary) 017.0
  vertebra (column) 015.0 *[730.88]*
  vesiculitis 016.5 *[608.81]*
  viscera NEC 014.8
  vulva 016.7 *[616.51]*
  wrist (joint) 015.8
    bone 015.5 *[730.83]*
Tuberculum
  auriculae 744.29
  occlusal 520.2
  paramolare 520.2
Tuberosity
  jaw, excessive 524.07
  maxillary, entire 524.07
Tuberous sclerosis (brain) 759.5
Tubo-ovarian —*see* condition
Tuboplasty, after previous sterilization V26.0
Tubotympanitis 381.10
Tularemia 021.9
  with
    conjunctivitis 021.3
    pneumonia 021.2
  bronchopneumonic 021.2
  conjunctivitis 021.3
  cryptogenic 021.1
  disseminated 021.8
  enteric 021.1
  generalized 021.8
  glandular 021.8
  intestinal 021.1
  oculoglandular 021.3
  ophthalmic 021.3
  pneumonia 021.2
  pulmonary 021.2
  specified NEC 021.8
  typhoidal 021.1
  ulceroglandular 021.0
  vaccination, prophylactic (against) V03.4
Tularensis conjunctivitis 021.3
Tumefaction —*see also* Swelling
  liver (*see also* Hypertrophy, liver) 789.1

Tumor (M8000/1)—*see also* Neoplasm, by site,
  unspecified nature
  Abrikossov's (M9580/0)—*see also* Neoplasm,
    connective tissue, benign
    malignant (M9580/3)—*see* Neoplasm,
      connective tissue, malignant
  acinar cell (M8550/1)—*see* Neoplasm, by site,
    uncertain behavior
  acinic cell (M8550/1)—*see* Neoplasm, by site,
    uncertain behavior
  adenomatoid (M9054/0)—*see also* Neoplasm,
    by site, benign
    odontogenic (M9300/0) 213.1
      upper jaw (bone) 213.0
  adnexal (skin) (M8390/0)—*see* Neoplasm, skin,
    benign
  adrenal
    cortical (benign) (M8370/0) 227.0
      malignant (M8370/3) 194.0
    rest (M8671/0)—*see* Neoplasm, by site,
      benign
  alpha cell (M8152/0)
    malignant (M8152/3)
      pancreas 157.4
      specified site NEC—*see* Neoplasm, by site,
        malignant
      unspecified site 157.4
    pancreas 211.7
    specified site NEC—*see* Neoplasm, by site,
      benign
    unspecified site 211.7
  aneurysmal (*see also* Aneurysm) 442.9
  aortic body (M8691/1) 237.3
    malignant (M8691/3) 194.6
  argentaffin (M8241/1)—*see* Neoplasm, by site,
    uncertain behavior
  basal cell (M8090/1)—*see also* Neoplasm, skin,
    uncertain behavior
  benign (M8000/0)—*see* Neoplasm, by site,
    benign
  beta cell (M8151/0)
    malignant (M8151/3)
      pancreas 157.4
      specified site—*see* Neoplasm, by site,
        malignant
      unspecified site 157.4
    pancreas 211.7
    specified site NEC—*see* Neoplasm, by site,
      benign
    unspecified site 211.7
  blood—*see* Hematoma
  brenner (M9000/0) 220
    borderline malignancy (M9000/1) 236.2
    malignant (M9000/3) 183.0
    proliferating (M9000/1) 236.2
  Brooke's (M8100/0)—*see* Neoplasm, skin,
    benign
  brown fat (M8880/0)—*see* Lipoma, by site
  Burkitt's (M9750/3) 200.2
  calcifying epithelial odontogenic (M9340/0)
    213.1
    upper jaw (bone) 213.0
  carcinoid (M8240/1)—*see* Carcinoid
  carotid body (M8692/1) 237.3
    malignant (M8692/3) 194.5
  Castleman's (mediastinal lymph node
    hyperplasia) 785.6
  cells (M8001/1)—*see also* Neoplasm, by site,
    unspecified nature
    benign (M8001/0)—*see* Neoplasm, by site,
      benign

Tumor—*continued*

  malignant (M8000/3)—*see also* Neoplasm, by site, malignant

    fusiform cell (type) (M8004/3)—*see* Neoplasm, by site, malignant

    giant cell (type) (M8003/3)—*see* Neoplasm, by site, malignant

    mixed NEC (M8940/3)—*see* Neoplasm, by site, malignant

    small cell (type) (M8002/3)—*see* Neoplasm, by site, malignant

    spindle cell (type) (M8004/3)—*see* Neoplasm, by site, malignant

  mast cell (M9740/1) 238.5

    malignant (M9740/3) 202.6

  melanotic, neuroectodermal (M9363/0)—*see* Neoplasm, by site, benign

  Merkel cell—*see* Neoplasm, by site, malignant

  mesenchymal

    malignant (M8800/3)—*see* Neoplasm, connective tissue, malignant

    mixed (M8990/1)—*see* Neoplasm, connective tissue, uncertain behavior

  mesodermal, mixed (M8951/3)—*see also* Neoplasm, by site, malignant

    liver 155.0

  mesonephric (M9110/1)—*see also* Neoplasm, by site, uncertain behavior

    malignant (M9110/3)—*see* Neoplasm, by site, malignant

  metastatic

    from specified site (M8000/3)—*see* Neoplasm, by site, malignant

    to specified site (M8000/6)—*see* Neoplasm, by site, malignant, secondary

  mixed NEC (M8940/0)—*see also* Neoplasm, by site, benign

    malignant (M8940/3)—*see* Neoplasm, by site, malignant

  mucocarcinoid, malignant (M8243/3)—*see* Neoplasm, by site, malignant

  mucoepidermoid (M8430/1)—*see* Neoplasm, by site, uncertain behavior

  Mullerian, mixed (M8950/3)—*see* Neoplasm, by site, malignant

  myoepithelial (M8982/0)—*see* Neoplasm, by site, benign

  neurogenic olfactory (M9520/3) 160.0

  nonencapsulated sclerosing (M8350/3) 193

  odontogenic (M9270/1) 238.0

    adenomatoid (M9300/0) 213.1

      upper jaw (bone) 213.0

    benign (M9270/0) 213.1

      upper jaw (bone) 213.0

    calcifying epithelial (M9340/0) 213.1

      upper jaw (bone) 213.0

    malignant (M9270/3) 170.1

      upper jaw (bone) 170.0

    squamous (M9312/0) 213.1

      upper jaw (bone) 213.0

  ovarian stromal (M8590/1) 236.2

  ovary

    in pregnancy or childbirth 654.4

      affecting fetus or newborn 763.89

      causing obstructed labor 660.2

        affecting fetus or newborn 763.1

  pacinian (M9507/0)—*see* Neoplasm, skin, benign

  Pancoast's (M8010/3) 162.3

  papillary—*see* Papilloma

  pelvic, in pregnancy or childbirth 654.9

Tumor—*continued*

    affecting fetus or newborn 763.89

    causing obstructed labor 660.2

      affecting fetus or newborn 763.1

  phantom 300.11

  plasma cell (M9731/1) 238.6

    benign (M9731/0)—*see* Neoplasm, by site, benign

    malignant (M9731/3) 203.8

  polyvesicular vitelline (M9071/3)

    specified site—*see* Neoplasm, by site, malignant

    unspecified site

      female 183.0

      male 186.9

  Pott's puffy (*see also* Osteomyelitis) 730.2

  Rathke's pouch (M9350/1) 237.0

  regaud's (M8082/3)—*see* Neoplasm, nasopharynx, malignant

  rete cell (M8140/0) 222.0

  retinal anlage (M9363/0)—*see* Neoplasm, by site, benign

  Rokitansky's 620.2

  salivary gland type, mixed (M8940/0)—*see also* Neoplasm, by site, benign

    malignant (M8940/3)—*see* Neoplasm, by site, malignant

  Sampson's 617.1

  Schloffer's (*see also* Peritonitis) 567.29

  Schmincke (M8082/3)—*see* Neoplasm, nasopharynx, malignant

  sebaceous (*see also* Cyst, sebaceous) 706.2

  secondary (M8000/6)—*see* Neoplasm, by site, secondary

  Sertoli cell (M8640/0)

    with lipid storage (M8641/0)

      specified site—*see* Neoplasm, by site, benign

      unspecified site

        female 220

        male 222.0

    specified site—*see* Neoplasm, by site, benign

    unspecified site

      female 220

      male 222.0

  Sertoli-Leydig cell (M8631/0)

    specified site—*see* Neoplasm, by site, benign

    unspecified site

      female 220

      male 222.0

  sex cord (-stromal) (M8590/1)—*see* Neoplasm, by site, uncertain behavior

  skin appendage (M8390/0)—*see* Neoplasm, skin, benign

  soft tissue

    benign (M8800/0)—*see* Neoplasm, connective tissue, benign

    malignant (M8800/3)—*see* Neoplasm, connective tissue, malignant

  sternomastoid 754.1

  stromal

    abdomen

      benign 215.5

      malignant 171.5

      uncertain behavior 238.1

    digestive system 238.1

      benign 215.5

      malignant 171.5

      uncertain behavior 238.1

    gastric 238.1

      benign 215.5

Tumor—*continued*
   malignant 171.5
   uncertain behavior 238.1
  gastrointestinal 238.1
   benign 215.5
   malignant 171.5
   uncertain behavior 238.1
  intestine (small) (large) 238.1
   benign 215.5
   malignant 171.5
   uncertain behavior 238.1
  stomach 238.1
   benign 215.5
   malignant 171.5
   uncertain behavior 238.1
  superior sulcus (lung) (pulmonary) (syndrome) (M8010/3) 162.3
  suprasulcus (M8010/3) 162.3
  sweat gland (M8400/1)—*see also* Neoplasm, skin, uncertain behavior
   benign (M8400/0)—*see* Neoplasm, skin, benign
   malignant (M8400/3)—*see* Neoplasm, skin, malignant
  syphilitic brain 094.89
   congenital 090.49
  testicular stromal (M8590/1) 236.4
  theca cell (M8600/0) 220
  theca cell-granulosa cell (M8621/1) 236.2
  theca-lutein (M8610/0) 220
  turban (M8200/0) 216.4
  uterus
   in pregnancy or childbirth 654.1
    affecting fetus or newborn 763.89
    causing obstructed labor 660.2
     affecting fetus or newborn 763.1
  vagina
   in pregnancy or childbirth 654.7
    affecting fetus or newborn 763.89
    causing obstructed labor 660.2
     affecting fetus or newborn 763.1
  varicose (*see also* Varicose, vein) 454.9
  von Recklinghausen's (M9540/1) 237.71
  vulva
   in pregnancy or childbirth 654.8
    affecting fetus or newborn 763.89
    causing obstructed labor 660.2
     affecting fetus or newborn 763.1
  Warthin's (salivary gland) (M8561/0) 210.2
  white—*see also* Tuberculosis, arthritis
  White-Darier 757.39
  Wilms' (nephroblastoma) (M8960/3) 189.0
  yolk sac (M9071/3)
   specified site—*see* Neoplasm, by site, malignant
   unspecified site
    female 183.0
    male 186.9
Tumorlet (M8040/1)—*see* Neoplasm, by site, uncertain behavior
Tungiasis 134.1
Tunica vasculosa lentis 743.39
Tunnel vision 368.45
Turban tumor (M8200/0) 216.4
Türck's trachoma (chronic catarrhal laryngitis) 476.0
Türk's syndrome (ocular retraction syndrome) 378.71
Turner's
  hypoplasia (tooth) 520.4
  syndrome 758.6
  tooth 520.4

Turner-Kieser syndrome (hereditary osteo-onychodysplasia) 756.89
Turner-Varny syndrome 758.6
Turricephaly 756.0
Tussis convulsiva (*see also* Whooping cough) 033.9
Twin
  affected by maternal complications of pregnancy 761.5
  conjoined 759.4
  healthy liveborn—*see* Newborn, twin
  pregnancy (complicating delivery) NEC 651.0
   with fetal loss and retention of one fetus 651.3
   following (elective) fetal reduction 651.7
Twinning, teeth 520.2
Twist, twisted
  bowel, colon, or intestine 560.2
  hair (congenital) 757.4
  mesentery 560.2
  omentum 560.2
  organ or site, congenital NEC—*see* Anomaly, specified type NEC
  ovarian pedicle 620.5
   congenital 752.0
  umbilical cord—*see* Compression, umbilical cord
Twitch 781.0
Tylosis 700
  buccalis 528.6
  gingiva 523.8
  linguae 528.6
  palmaris et plantaris 757.39
Tympanism 787.3
Tympanites (abdominal) (intestine) 787.3
Tympanitis —*see* Myringitis
Tympanosclerosis 385.00
  involving
   combined sites NEC 385.09
    with tympanic membrane 385.03
   tympanic membrane 385.01
    with ossicles 385.02
     and middle ear 385.03
Tympanum —*see* condition
Tympany
  abdomen 787.3
  chest 786.7
Typhlitis (*see also* Appendicitis) 541
Typhoenteritis 002.0
Typhogastric fever 002.0
Typhoid (abortive) (ambulant) (any site) (fever) (hemorrhagic) (infection) (intermittent) (malignant) (rheumatic) 002.0
  with pneumonia 002.0 *[484.8]*
  abdominal 002.0
  carrier (suspected) of V02.1
  cholecystitis (current) 002.0
  clinical (Widal and blood test negative) 002.0
  endocarditis 002.0 *[421.1]*
  inoculation reaction—*see* Complications, vaccination
  meningitis 002.0 *[320.7]*
  mesenteric lymph nodes 002.0
  myocarditis 002.0 *[422.0]*
  osteomyelitis (*see also* Osteomyelitis, due to, typhoid) 002.0 *[730.8]*
  perichondritis, larynx 002.0 *[478.71]*
  pneumonia 002.0 *[484.8]*
  spine 002.0 *[720.81]*
  ulcer (perforating) 002.0
  vaccination, prophylactic (against) V03.1
  Widal negative 002.0

Typhomalaria (fever) (*see also* Malaria) 084.6
Typhomania 002.0
Typhoperitonitis 002.0
Typhus (fever) 081.9
  abdominal, abdominalis 002.0
  African tick 082.1
  amarillic (*see also* Fever, Yellow) 060.9
  brain 081.9
  cerebral 081.9
  classical 080
  endemic (flea-borne) 081.0
  epidemic (louse-borne) 080
  exanthematic NEC 080
  exanthematicus SAI 080
    brillii SAI 081.1
    Mexicanus SAI 081.0
    pediculo vestimenti causa 080
    typhus murinus 081.0
  flea-borne 081.0
  Indian tick 082.1
  Kenya tick 082.1
  louse-borne 080
  Mexican 081.0
    flea-borne 081.0
    louse-borne 080
    tabardillo 080
  mite-borne 081.2
  murine 081.0
  North Asian tick-borne 082.2
  petechial 081.9
  Queensland tick 082.3
  rat 081.0
  recrudescent 081.1
  recurrent (*see also* Fever, relapsing) 087.9
  São Paulo 082.0
  scrub (China) (India) (Malaya) (New Guinea)
    081.2
  shop (of Malaya) 081.0
  Siberian tick 082.2
  tick-borne NEC 082.9
  tropical 081.2
  vaccination, prophylactic (against) V05.8
Tyrosinemia 270.2
  neonatal 775.89
Tyrosinosis (Medes) (Sakai) 270.2
Tyrosinuria 270.2
Tyrosyluria 270.2

U

Uehlinger's syndrome (acropachyderma) 757.39
Uhl's anomaly or disease (hypoplasia of
   myocardium, right ventricle) 746.84
**Ulcer, ulcerated, ulcerating, ulceration, ulcer-
   ative** 707.9
  with gangrene 707.9 *[785.4]*
  abdomen (wall) (*see also* Ulcer, skin) 707.8
  ala, nose 478.19
  alveolar process 526.5
  amebic (intestine) 006.9
    skin 006.6
  anastomotic—*see* Ulcer, gastrojejunal
  anorectal 569.41
  antral—*see* Ulcer, stomach
  anus (sphincter) (solitary) 569.41
    varicose—*see* Varicose, ulcer, anus
  aorta —*see* Aneurysm
  aphthous (oral) (recurrent) 528.2
    genital organ(s)
      female 616.89
      male 60.89
      mouth 528.2
  arm (*see also* Ulcer, skin) 707.8
  arteriosclerotic plaque—*see* Arteriosclerosis, by
    site
  artery NEC 447.2
    without rupture 447.8
  atrophic NEC—*see* Ulcer, skin
  Barrett's (chronic peptic ulcer of esophagus)
    530.85
  bile duct 576.8
  bladder (solitary) (sphincter) 596.8
    bilharzial (*see also* Schistosomiasis) 120.9
      [595.4]
    submucosal (*see also* Cystitis) 595.1
    tuberculous (*see also* Tuberculosis) 016.1
  bleeding NEC—*see* Ulcer, peptic, with
    hemorrhage
  bone 730.9
  bowel (*see also* Ulcer, intestine) 569.82
  breast 611.0
  bronchitis 491.8
  bronchus 519.19
  buccal (cavity) (traumatic) 528.9
  burn (acute)—*see* Ulcer, duodenum
  Buruli 031.1
  buttock (*see also* Ulcer, skin) 707.8
    decubitus (*see also* Ulcer, decubitus) 707.00
  cancerous (M8000/3)—*see* Neoplasm, by site,
    malignant
  cardia—*see* Ulcer, stomach
  cardio-esophageal (peptic) 530.20
    with bleeding 530.21
  cecum (*see also* Ulcer, intestine) 569.82
  cervix (uteri) (trophic) 622.0
    with mention of cervicitis 616.0
  chancroidal 099.0
  chest (wall) (*see also* Ulcer, skin) 707.8
  Chiclero 085.4
  chin (pyogenic) (*see also* Ulcer, skin) 707.8
  chronic (cause unknown)—*see also* Ulcer, skin
    penis 607.89
  Cochin-China 085.1
  colitis —*see* Colitis, ulcerative
  colon (*see also* Ulcer, intestine) 569.82
  conjunctiva (acute) (postinfectional) 372.00

Ulcer, ulcerated, ulcerating—*continued*
  cornea (infectional) 370.00
    with perforation 370.06
    annular 370.02
    catarrhal 370.01
    central 370.03
    dendritic 054.42
    marginal 370.01
    mycotic 370.05
    phlyctenular, tuberculous (*see also*
      Tuberculosis) 017.3 *[370.31]*
    ring 370.02
    rodent 370.07
    serpent, serpiginous 370.04
    superficial marginal 370.01
    tuberculous (*see also* Tuberculosis) 017.3
      [370.31]
  corpus cavernosum (chronic) 607.89
  crural—*see* Ulcer, lower extremity
  Curling's—*see* Ulcer, duodenum
  Cushing's—*see* Ulcer, peptic
  cystitis (interstitial) 595.1
  decubitus (unspecified site) 707.00
    with gangrene 707.00 *[785.4]*
    ankle 707.06
    back
      lower 707.03
      upper 707.02
    buttock 707.05
    elbow 707.01
    head 707.09
    heel 707.07
    hip 707.04
    other site 707.09
    sacrum 707.03
    shoulder blades 707.02
  dendritic 054.42
  diabetes, diabetic (mellitus) 250.8 *[707.9]*
    lower limb 250.8 *[707.10]*
      ankle 250.8 *[707.13]*
      calf 250.8 *[707.12]*
      foot 250.8 *[707.15]*
      heel 250.8 *[707.14]*
      knee 250.8 *[707.19]*
      specified site NEC 250.8 *[707.19]*
      thigh 250.8 *[707.11]*
      toes 250.8 *[707.15]*
    specified site NEC 250.8 *[707.8]*
  Dieulafoy—*see* Lesion, Dieulafoy
  due to
    infection NEC—*see* Ulcer, skin
    radiation, radium—*see* Ulcer, by site
    trophic disturbance (any region)—*see* Ulcer,
      skin
    x-ray—*see* Ulcer, by site
  duodenum, duodenal (eroded) (peptic) 532.9

> *Note—Use the following fifth-digit*
> *subclassification with categories 531-534:*
>
> *0 without mention of obstruction*
> *1 with obstruction*

    with
      hemorrhage (chronic) 532.4
        and perforation 532.6
      perforation (chronic) 532.5
        and hemorrhage 532.6

Ulcer, ulcerated, ulcerating—*continued*
  acute 532.3
    with
      hemorrhage 532.0
        and perforation 532.2
      perforation 532.1
        and hemorrhage 532.2
    bleeding (recurrent)—*see* Ulcer, duodenum,
      with hemorrhage
  chronic 532.7
    with
      hemorrhage 532.4
        and perforation 532.6
      perforation 532.5
        and hemorrhage 532.6
    penetrating—*see* Ulcer, duodenum, with
      perforation
    perforating—*see* Ulcer, duodenum, with
      perforation
  dysenteric NEC 009.0
  elusive 595.1
  endocarditis (any valve) (acute) (chronic)
    (subacute) 421.0
  enteritis —*see* Colitis, ulcerative
  enterocolitis 556.0
  epiglottis 478.79
  esophagus (peptic) 530.20
    with bleeding 530.21
    due to ingestion
      aspirin 530.20
      chemicals 530.20
      medicinal agents 530.20
    fungal 530.20
    infectional 530.20
    varicose (*see also* Varix, esophagus) 456.1
      bleeding (*see also* Varix, esophagus,
        bleeding) 456.0
  eye NEC 360.00
    dendritic 054.42
  eyelid (region) 373.01
  face (*see also* Ulcer, skin) 707.8
  fauces 478.29
  Fenwick (-Hunner) (solitary) (*see also* Cystitis)
    595.1
  fistulous NEC—*see* Ulcer, skin
  foot (indolent) (*see also* Ulcer, lower extremity)
    707.15
    perforating 707.15
      leprous 030.1
      syphilitic 094.0
    trophic 707.15
    varicose 454.0
      inflamed or infected 454.2
  frambesial, initial or primary 102.0
  gallbladder or duct 575.8
  gall duct 576.8
  gangrenous (*see also* Gangrene) 785.4
  gastric—*see* Ulcer, stomach
  gastrocolic—*see* Ulcer, gastrojejunal
  gastroduodenal—*see* Ulcer, peptic
  gastroesophageal—*see* Ulcer, stomach
  gastrohepatic—*see* Ulcer, stomach
  gastrointestinal—*see* Ulcer, gastrojejunal
  gastrojejunal (eroded) (peptic) 534.9

> *Note—Use the following fifth-digit*
> *subclassification with categories 531-534:*
>
> *0 without mention of obstruction*
> *1 with obstruction*

Ulcer, ulcerated, ulcerating—*continued*
  with
    hemorrhage (chronic) 534.4
      and perforation 534.6
    perforation 534.5
      and hemorrhage 534.6
  acute 534.3
    with
      hemorrhage 534.0
        and perforation 534.2
      perforation 534.1
        and hemorrhage 534.2
    bleeding (recurrent)—*see* Ulcer, gastrojejunal,
      with hemorrhage
  chronic 534.7
    with
      hemorrhage 534.4
        and perforation 534.6
      perforation 534.5
        and hemorrhage 534.6
    penetrating—*see* Ulcer, gastrojejunal, with
      perforation
    perforating—*see* Ulcer, gastrojejunal, with
      perforation
  gastrojejunocolic—*see* Ulcer, gastrojejunal
  genital organ
    female 629.89
    male 608.89
  gingiva 523.8
  gingivitis 523.10
  glottis 478.79
  granuloma of pudenda 099.2
  groin (*see also* Ulcer, skin) 707.8
  gum 523.8
  gumma, due to yaws 102.4
  hand (*see also* Ulcer, skin) 707.8
  hard palate 528.9
  heel (*see also* Ulcer, lower extremity) 707.14
    decubitus (*see also* Ulcer, decubitus) 707.07
  hemorrhoids 455.8
    external 455.5
    internal 455.2
  hip (*see also* Ulcer, skin) 707.8
    decubitus (*see also* Ulcer, decubitus) 707.04
  Hunner's 595.1
  hypopharynx 478.29
  hypopyon (chronic) (subacute) 370.04
  hypostaticum—*see* Ulcer, varicose
  ileocolitis 556.1
  ileum (*see also* Ulcer, intestine) 569.82
  intestine, intestinal 569.82
    with perforation 569.83
    amebic 006.9
    duodenal—*see* Ulcer, duodenum
    granulocytopenic (with hemorrhage) 288.09
    marginal 569.82
    perforating 569.83
    small, primary 569.82
    stercoraceous 569.82
    stercoral 569.82
    tuberculous (*see also* Tuberculosis) 014.8
    typhoid (fever) 002.0
    varicose 456.8
  ischemic 707.9
    lower extremity (*see also* Ulcer, lower
      extremity) 707.10
    ankle 707.13
    calf 707.12
    foot 707.15
    heel 707.14
    knee 707.19

Ulcer, ulcerated, ulcerating—*continued*
    specified site NEC 707.19
      thigh 707.11
      toes 707.15
  jejunum, jejunal—*see* Ulcer, gastrojejunal
  keratitis (*see also* Ulcer, cornea) 370.00
  knee—*see* Ulcer, lower extremity
  labium (majus) (minus) 616.50
  laryngitis (*see also* Laryngitis) 464.00
    with obstruction 464.01
  larynx (aphthous) (contact) 478.79
    diphtheritic 032.3
  leg—*see* Ulcer, lower extremity
  lip 528.5
  Lipschütz's 616.50
  lower extremity (atrophic) (chronic)
     (neurogenic) (perforating) (pyogenic)
     (trophic) (tropical) 707.10
    with gangrene (*see also* Ulcer, lower
      extremity) 707.10 *[785.4]*
     arteriosclerotic 440.24
    ankle 707.13
    arteriosclerotic 440.23
     with gangrene 440.24
    calf 707.12
    decubitus 707.00
     with gangrene 707.00 *[785.4]*
     ankle 707.06
     buttock 707.05
     heel 707.07
     hip 707.04
    foot 707.15
    heel 707.14
    knee 707.19
    specified site NEC 707.19
    thigh 707.11
    toes 707.15
    varicose 454.0
     inflamed or infected 454.2
  luetic—*see* Ulcer, syphilitic
  lung 518.89
    tuberculous (*see also* Tuberculosis) 011.2
  malignant (M8000/3)—*see* Neoplasm, by site,
    malignant
  marginal NEC—*see* Ulcer, gastrojejunal
  meatus (urinarius) 597.89
  Meckel's diverticulum 751.0
  Meleney's (chronic undermining) 686.09
  Mooren's (cornea) 370.07
  mouth (traumatic) 528.9
  mycobacterial (skin) 031.1
  nasopharynx 478.29
  navel cord (newborn) 771.4
  neck (*see also* Ulcer, skin) 707.8
    uterus 622.0
  neurogenic NEC—*see* Ulcer, skin
  nose, nasal (infectional) (passage) 478.19
    septum 478.19
     varicose 456.8
    skin—*see* Ulcer, skin
    spirochetal NEC 104.8
  oral mucosa (traumatic) 528.9
  palate (soft) 528.9
  penetrating NEC—*see* Ulcer, peptic, with
    perforation
  penis (chronic) 607.89
  peptic (site unspecified) 533.9

Ulcer, ulcerated, ulcerating—*continued*

> *Note—Use the following fifth-digit*
> *subclassification with categories 531-534:*
>
> *0 without mention of obstruction*
> *1 with obstruction*

  with
    hemorrhage 533.4
     and perforation 533.6
    perforation (chronic) 533.5
     and hemorrhage 533.6
  acute 533.3
    with
     hemorrhage 533.0
      and perforation 533.2
     perforation 533.1
      and hemorrhage 533.2
  bleeding (recurrent)—*see* Ulcer, peptic, with
    hemorrhage
  chronic 533.7
    with
     hemorrhage 533.4
      and perforation 533.6
     perforation 533.5
      and hemorrhage 533.6
  penetrating—*see* Ulcer, peptic, with
    perforation
  perforating NEC (*see also* Ulcer, peptic, with
    perforation) 533.5
    skin 707.9
  perineum (*see also* Ulcer, skin) 707.8
  peritonsillar 474.8
  phagedenic (tropical) NEC—*see* Ulcer, skin
  pharynx 478.29
  phlebitis—*see* Phlebitis
  plaster (*see also* Ulcer, decubitus) 707.00
  popliteal space—*see* Ulcer, lower extremity
  postpyloric—*see* Ulcer, duodenum
  prepuce 607.89
  prepyloric—*see* Ulcer, stomach
  pressure (*see also* Ulcer, decubitus) 707.00
  primary of intestine 569.82
    with perforation 569.83
  proctitis 556.2
    with ulcerative sigmoiditis 556.3
  prostate 601.8
  pseudopeptic—*see* Ulcer, peptic
  pyloric—*see* Ulcer, stomach
  rectosigmoid 569.82
    with perforation 569.83
  rectum (sphincter) (solitary) 569.41
    stercoraceous, stercoral 569.41
    varicose—*see* Varicose, ulcer, anus
  retina (*see also* Chorioretinitis) 363.20
  rodent (M8090/3)—*see also* Neoplasm, skin,
    malignant
    cornea 370.07
  round—*see* Ulcer, stomach
  sacrum (region) (*see also* Ulcer, skin) 707.8
  Saemisch's 370.04
  scalp (*see also* Ulcer, skin) 707.8
  sclera 379.09
  scrofulous (*see also* Tuberculosis) 017.2
  scrotum 608.89
    tuberculous (*see also* Tuberculosis) 016.5
    varicose 456.4
  seminal vesicle 608.89
  sigmoid 569.82
    with perforation 569.83

Ulcer, ulcerated, ulcerating—*continued*
  skin (atrophic) (chronic) (neurogenic)
    (non-healing) (perforating) (pyogenic)
    (trophic) 707.9
    with gangrene 707.9 *[785.4]*
    amebic 006.6
    decubitus (*see also* Ulcer, decubitus) 707.00
      with gangrene 707.00 *[785.4]*
    in granulocytopenia 288.09
    lower extremity (*see also* Ulcer, lower
      extremity) 707.10
      with gangrene 707.10 *[785.4]*
        arteriosclerotic 440.24
      ankle 707.13
      arteriosclerotic 440.23
        with gangrene 440.24
      calf 707.12
      foot 707.15
      heel 707.14
      knee 707.19
      specified site NEC 707.19
      thigh 707.11
      toes 707.15
    mycobacterial 031.1
    syphilitic (early) (secondary) 091.3
    tuberculous (primary) (*see also* Tuberculosis)
      017.0
    varicose—*see* Ulcer, varicose
  sloughing NEC—*see* Ulcer, skin
  soft palate 528.9
  solitary, anus or rectum (sphincter) 569.41
  sore throat 462
    streptococcal 034.0
  spermatic cord 608.89
  spine (tuberculous) 015.0 *[730.88]*
  stasis (leg) (venous) 454.0
    with varicose veins 454.0
    inflamed or infected 454.2
    without varicose veins 459.81
  stercoral, stercoraceous 569.82
    with perforation 569.83
    anus or rectum 569.41
  stoma, stomal—*see* Ulcer, gastrojejunal
  stomach (eroded) (peptic) (round) 531.9

> *Note—Use the following fifth-digit*
> *subclassification with categories 531-534:*
>
> *0 without mention of obstruction*
> *1 with obstruction*

    with
      hemorrhage 531.4
        and perforation 531.6
      perforation (chronic) 531.5
        and hemorrhage 531.6
    acute 531.3
      with
        hemorrhage 531.0
          and perforation 531.2
        perforation 531.1
          and hemorrhage 531.2
    bleeding (recurrent)—*see* Ulcer, stomach,
      with hemorrhage
    chronic 531.7
      with
        hemorrhage 531.4
          and perforation 531.6
        perforation 531.5
          and hemorrhage 531.6
    penetrating—*see* Ulcer, stomach, with
      perforation

Ulcer, ulcerated, ulcerating—*continued*
    perforating—*see* Ulcer, stomach, with
      perforation
  stomatitis 528.00
  stress—*see* Ulcer, peptic
  strumous (tuberculous) (*see also* Tuberculosis)
    017.2
  submental (*see also* Ulcer, skin) 707.8
  submucosal, bladder 595.1
  syphilitic (any site) (early) (secondary) 091.3
    late 095.9
    perforating 095.9
      foot 094.0
  testis 608.89
  thigh—*see* Ulcer, lower extremity
  throat 478.29
    diphtheritic 032.0
  toe—*see* Ulcer, lower extremity
  tongue (traumatic) 529.0
  tonsil 474.8
    diphtheritic 032.0
  trachea 519.19
  trophic—*see* Ulcer, skin
  tropical NEC (*see also* Ulcer, skin) 707.9
  tuberculous—*see* Tuberculosis, ulcer
  tunica vaginalis 608.89
  turbinate 730.9
  typhoid (fever) 002.0
    perforating 002.0
  umbilicus (newborn) 771.4
  unspecified site NEC—*see* Ulcer, skin
  urethra (meatus) (*see also* Urethritis) 597.89
  uterus 621.8
    cervix 622.0
      with mention of cervicitis 616.0
    neck 622.0
      with mention of cervicitis 616.0
  vagina 616.89
  valve, heart 421.0
  varicose (lower extremity, any part) 454.0
    anus—*see* Varicose, ulcer, anus
    broad ligament 456.5
    esophagus (*see also* Varix, esophagus) 456.1
      bleeding (*see also* Varix, esophagus,
        bleeding) 456.0
    inflamed or infected 454.2
    nasal septum 456.8
    perineum 456.6
    rectum—*see* Varicose, ulcer, anus
    scrotum 456.4
    specified site NEC 456.8
    sublingual 456.3
    vulva 456.6
  vas deferens 608.89
  vesical (*see also* Ulcer, bladder) 596.8
  vulva (acute) (infectional) 616.50
    Behçet's syndrome 136.1 *[616.51]*
    herpetic 054.12
    tuberculous 016.7 *[616.51]*
  vulvobuccal, recurring 616.50
  x-ray—*see* Ulcer, by site
  yaws 102.4
Ulcerosa scarlatina 034.1
Ulcus —*see also* Ulcer
  cutis tuberculosum (*see also* Tuberculosis)
    017.0
  duodeni—*see* Ulcer, duodenum
  durum 091.0
    extragenital 091.2
  gastrojejunale—*see* Ulcer, gastrojejunal
  hypostaticum—*see* Ulcer, varicose

Uremia, uremic (absorption) (amaurosis)
  (amblyopia) (aphasia) (apoplexy) (coma)
  (delirium) (dementia) (dropsy) (dyspnea)
  (fever) (intoxication) (mania) (paralysis)
  (poisoning) (toxemia) (vomiting) 586
  with
    abortion—*see* Abortion, by type, with renal
      failure
    ectopic pregnancy (*see also* categories
      633.0-633.9) 639.3
    hypertension (*see also* Hypertension, kidney)
      403.91
    molar pregnancy (*see also* categories 630-632)
      639.3
  chronic 585.9
  complicating
    abortion 639.3
    ectopic or molar pregnancy 639.3
    hypertension (*see also* Hypertension, kidney)
      403.91
    labor and delivery 669.3
  congenital 779.89
  extrarenal 788.9
  hypertensive (chronic) (*see also* Hypertension,
    kidney) 403.91
  maternal NEC, affecting fetus or newborn 760.1
  neuropathy 585.9 *[357.4]*
  pericarditis 585.9 *[420.0]*
  prerenal 788.9
  pyelitic (*see also* Pyelitis) 590.80
Ureter, ureteral —*see* condition
Ureteralgia 788.0
Ureterectasis 593.89
Ureteritis 593.89
  cystica 590.3
  due to calculus 592.1
  gonococcal (acute) 098.19
    chronic or duration of 2 months or over 098.39
  nonspecific 593.89
Ureterocele (acquired) 593.89
  congenital 753.23
Ureterolith 592.1
Ureterolithiasis 592.1
Ureterostomy status V44.6
  with complication 997.5
Urethra, urethral —*see* condition
Urethralgia 788.9
Urethritis (abacterial) (acute) (allergic) (anterior)
  (chronic) (nonvenereal) (posterior) (recurrent)
  (simple) (subacute) (ulcerative)
  (undifferentiated) 597.80
  diplococcal (acute) 098.0
    chronic or duration of 2 months or over 098.2
  due to Trichomonas (vaginalis) 131.02
  gonococcal (acute) 098.0
    chronic or duration of 2 months or over 098.2
  nongonococcal (sexually transmitted) 099.40
    Chlamydia trachomatis 099.41
    Reiter's 099.3
    specified organism NEC 099.49
  nonspecific (sexually transmitted) (*see also*
    Urethritis, nongonococcal) 099.40
  not sexually transmitted 597.80
  Reiter's 099.3
  trichomonal or due to Trichomonas (vaginalis)
    131.02
  tuberculous (*see also* Tuberculosis) 016.3
  venereal NEC (*see also* Urethritis,
    nongonococcal) 099.40

Urethrocele
  female 618.03
    with uterine prolapse 618.4
      complete 618.3
      incomplete 618.2
  male 599.5
Urethrolithiasis 594.2
Urethro-oculoarticular syndrome 099.3
Urethro-oculosynovial syndrome 099.3
Urethrorectal —*see* condition
Urethrorrhagia 599.84
Urethrorrhea 788.7
Urethrostomy status V44.6
  with complication 997.5
Urethrotrigonitis 595.3
Urethrovaginal —*see* condition
Urhidrosis, uridrosis 705.89
Uric acid
  diathesis 274.9
  in blood 790.6
Uricacidemia 790.6
Uricemia 790.6
Uricosuria 791.9
Urination
  frequent 788.41
  painful 788.1
  urgency 788.63
Urine, urinary —*see also* condition
  abnormality NEC 788.69
  blood in (*see also* Hematuria) 599.7
  discharge, excessive 788.42
  enuresis 788.30
    nonorganic origin 307.6
  extravasation 788.8
  frequency 788.41
  hesitancy 788.64
  incontinence 788.30
    active 788.30
    female 788.30
      stress 625.6
        and urge 788.33
    male 788.30
      stress 788.32
        and urge 788.33
    mixed (stress and urge) 788.33
    neurogenic 788.39
    nonorganic origin 307.6
    overflow 788.38
    stress (female) 625.6
      male NEC 788.32
  intermittent stream 788.61
  pus in 791.9
  retention or stasis NEC 788.20
    bladder, incomplete emptying 788.21
    psychogenic 306.53
    specified NEC 788.29
  secretion
    deficient 788.5
    excessive 788.42
    frequency 788.41
  strain 788.65
  stream
    intermittent 788.61
    slowing 788.62
    splitting 788.61
    weak 788.62
  urgency 788.63
Urinemia —*see* Uremia

V

Vaccination
complication or reaction—*see* Complications, vaccination
not carried out V64.00
  because of
    acute illness V64.01
    allergy to vaccine or component V64.04
    caregiver refusal V64.05
    chronic illness V64.02
    immune compromised state V64.03
    patient had disease being vaccinated against V64.08
    patient refusal V64.06
    reason NEC V64.09
    religious reasons V64.07
prophylactic (against) V05.9
  arthropod-borne viral
    disease NEC V05.1
    encephalitis V05.0
  chickenpox V05.4
  cholera (alone) V03.0
    with typhoid-paratyphoid (cholera + TAB) V06.0
  common cold V04.7
  diphtheria (alone) V03.5
    with
      poliomyelitis (DTP + polio) V06.3
      tetanus V06.5
        pertussis combined [DTP] [DTaP] V06.1
        typhoid-paratyphoid (DTP + TAB) V06.2
  disease (single) NEC V05.9
    bacterial NEC V03.9
      specified type NEC V03.89
    combinations NEC V06.9
      specified type NEC V06.8
    specified type NEC V05.8
  encephalitis, viral, arthropod-borne V05.0
  Hemophilus influenzae, type B [Hib] V03.81
  hepatitis, viral V05.3
  influenza V04.81
    with
      Streptococcus pneumoniae [pneumococcus] V06.6
  leishmaniasis V05.2
  measles (alone) V04.2
    with mumps-rubella (MMR) V06.4
  mumps (alone) V04.6
    with measles and rubella (MMR) V06.4
  pertussis alone V03.6
  plague V03.3
  poliomyelitis V04.0
    with diphtheria-tetanus-pertussis (DTP + polio) V06.3
  rabies V04.5
  respiratory syncytial virus (RSV) V04.82
  rubella (alone) V04.3
    with measles and mumps (MMR) V06.4
  smallpox V04.1
  Streptococcus pneumoniae [pneumococcus] V03.82
    with
      influenza V06.6
  tetanus toxoid (alone) V03.7
    with diphtheria [Td] [DT] V06.5
      with
        pertussis [DTP] [DTaP] V06.1
          with poliomyelitis (DTP + polio) V06.3

Vaccination—*continued*
tuberculosis (BCG) V03.2
tularemia V03.4
typhoid-paratyphoid (TAB) (alone) V03.1
  with diphtheria-tetanus-pertussis (TAB + DTP) V06.2
varicella V05.4
viral
  disease NEC V04.89
  encephalitis, arthropod-borne V05.0
  hepatitis V05.3
yellow fever V04.4
Vaccinia (generalized) 999.0
congenital 771.2
conjunctiva 999.3
eyelids 999.0 *[373.5]*
localized 999.3
nose 999.3
not from vaccination 051.0
  eyelid 051.0 *[373.5]*
sine vaccinatione 051.0
without vaccination 051.0
Vacuum
extraction of fetus or newborn 763.3
in sinus (accessory) (nasal) (*see also* Sinusitis) 473.9
Vagabond V60.0
Vagabondage V60.0
Vagabonds' disease 132.1
Vagina, vaginal —*see* condition
Vaginalitis (tunica) 608.4
Vaginismus (reflex) 625.1
functional 306.51
hysterical 300.11
psychogenic 306.51
Vaginitis (acute) (chronic) (circumscribed) (diffuse) (emphysematous) (Hemophilus vaginalis) (nonspecific) (nonvenereal) (ulcerative) 616.10
with
  abortion—*see* Abortion, by type, with sepsis
  ectopic pregnancy (*see also* categories 633.0-633.9) 639.0
  molar pregnancy (*see also* categories 630-632) 639.0
adhesive, congenital 752.49
atrophic, postmenopausal 627.3
bacterial 616.10
blennorrhagic (acute) 098.0
  chronic or duration of 2 months or over 098.2
candidal 112.1
chlamydial 099.53
complicating pregnancy or puerperium 646.6
  affecting fetus or newborn 760.8
congenital (adhesive) 752.49
due to
  C. albicans 112.1
  Trichomonas (vaginalis) 131.01
following
  abortion 639.0
  ectopic or molar pregnancy 639.0
gonococcal (acute) 098.0
  chronic or duration of 2 months or over 098.2
granuloma 099.2
Monilia 112.1
mycotic 112.1
pinworm 127.4 *[616.11]*

Vasospasm 443.9
  cerebral (artery) 435.9
    with transient neurologic deficit 435.9
  coronary 413.1
  nerve
    arm NEC 354.9
    autonomic 337.9
    brachial plexus 353.0
    cervical plexus 353.2
    leg NEC 355.8
    lower extremity NEC 355.8
    peripheral NEC 355.9
    spinal NEC 355.9
    sympathetic 337.9
    upper extremity NEC 354.9
  peripheral NEC 443.9
  retina (artery) (*see also* Occlusion, retinal,
    artery) 362.30
Vasospastic —*see* condition
Vasovagal attack (paroxysmal) 780.2
  psychogenic 306.2
Vater's ampulla —*see* condition
VATER syndrome 759.89
Vegetation, vegetative
  adenoid (nasal fossa) 474.2
  consciousness (persistent) 780.03
  endocarditis (acute) (any valve) (chronic)
    (subacute) 421.0
  heart (mycotic) (valve) 421.0
  state (persistent) 780.03
Veil
  Jackson's 751.4
  over face (causing asphyxia) 768.9
Vein, venous —*see* condition
Veldt sore (*see also* Ulcer, skin) 707.9
Velo-cardio-facial syndrome 758.32
Velpeau's hernia —*see* Hernia, femoral
Venereal
  balanitis NEC 099.8
  bubo 099.1
  disease 099.9
    specified nature or type NEC 099.8
  granuloma inguinale 099.2
  lymphogranuloma (Durand-Nicolas-Favre), any
    site 099.1
  salpingitis 098.37
  urethritis (*see also* Urethritis, nongonococcal)
    099.40
  vaginitis NEC 099.8
  warts 078.19
Vengefulness, in child (*see also* Disturbance,
  conduct) 312.0
Venofibrosis 459.89
Venom, venomous
  bite or sting (animal or insect) 989.5
  poisoning 989.5
Venous —*see* condition
Ventouse delivery NEC 669.5
  affecting fetus or newborn 763.3
Ventral —*see* condition
Ventricle, ventricular —*see also* condition
  escape 427.69
  standstill (*see also* Arrest, cardiac) 427.5
Ventriculitis, cerebral (*see also* Meningitis)
  322.9
Ventriculostomy status V45.2
Verbiest's syndrome (claudicatio intermittens
  spinalis) 435.1
Vernet's syndrome 352.6
Verneuil's disease (syphilitic bursitis) 095.7

Verruca (filiformis) 078.10
  acuminata (any site) 078.11
  necrogenica (primary) (*see also* Tuberculosis)
    017.0
  peruana 088.0
  peruviana 088.0
  plana (juvenilis) 078.19
  plantaris 078.19
  seborrheica 702.19
    inflamed 702.11
  senilis 702.0
  tuberculosa (primary) (*see also* Tuberculosis)
    017.0
  venereal 078.19
  viral NEC 078.10
Verrucosities (*see also* Verruca) 078.10
Verrucous endocarditis (acute) (any valve)
  (chronic) (subacute) 710.0 *[424.91]*
  nonbacterial 710.0 *[424.91]*
Verruga
  peruana 088.0
  peruviana 088.0
Verse's disease (calcinosis intervertebralis)
  275.49 *[722.90]*
Version
  before labor, affecting fetus or newborn 761.7
  cephalic (correcting previous malposition) 652.1
    affecting fetus or newborn 763.1
  cervix (*see* Version, uterus)
  uterus (postinfectional) (postpartal, old) (*see*
    also Malposition, uterus) 621.6
    forward—*see* Anteversion, uterus
    lateral—*see* Lateroversion, uterus
Vertebra, vertebral —*see* condition
Vertigo 780.4
  auditory 386.19
  aural 386.19
  benign paroxysmal positional 386.11
  central origin 386.2
  cerebral 386.2
  Dix and Hallpike (epidemic) 386.12
  endemic paralytic 078.81
  epidemic 078.81
    Dix and Hallpike 386.12
    Gerlier's 078.81
    Pedersen's 386.12
    vestibular neuronitis 386.12
  epileptic—*see* Epilepsy
  Gerlier's (epidemic) 078.81
  hysterical 300.11
  labyrinthine 386.10
  laryngeal 786.2
  malignant positional 386.2
  Ménière's (*see also* Disease, Ménière's) 386.00
  menopausal 627.2
  otogenic 386.19
  paralytic 078.81
  paroxysmal positional, benign 386.11
  Pedersen's (epidemic) 386.12
  peripheral 386.10
    specified type NEC 386.19
  positional
    benign paroxysmal 386.11
    malignant 386.2
Verumontanitis (chronic) (*see also* Urethritis)
  597.89
Vesania (*see also* Psychosis) 298.9
Vesical —*see* condition
Vesicle
  cutaneous 709.8
  seminal—*see* condition
  skin 709.8

W

Waardenburg's syndrome 756.89
  meaning ptosis-epicanthus 270.2
Waardenburg-Klein syndrome
  (ptosis-epicanthus) 270.2
Wagner's disease (colloid milium) 709.3
Wagner (-Unverricht) syndrome
  (dermatomyositis) 710.3
Waiting list, person on V63.2
  undergoing social agency investigation V63.8
Wakefulness disorder (*see also* Hypersomnia)
  780.54
  nonorganic origin 307.43
Waldenström's
  disease (osteochondrosis, capital femoral) 732.1
  hepatitis (lupoid hepatitis) 571.49
  hypergammaglobulinemia 273.0
  macroglobulinemia 273.3
  purpura, hypergammaglobulinemic 273.0
  syndrome (macroglobulinemia) 273.3
Waldenström-Kjellberg syndrome (sideropenic
  dysphagia) 280.8
Walking
  difficulty 719.7
    psychogenic 307.9
  sleep 307.46
    hysterical 300.13
Wall, abdominal —*see* condition
Wallenberg's syndrome (posterior inferior
  cerebellar artery) (*see also* Disease,
  cerebrovascular, acute) 436
Wallgren's
  disease (obstruction of splenic vein with
    collateral circulation) 459.89
  meningitis (*see also* Meningitis, aseptic) 047.9
Wandering
  acetabulum 736.39
  gallbladder 751.69
  kidney, congenital 753.3
  organ or site, congenital NEC—*see* Malposition,
    congenital
  pacemaker (atrial) (heart) 427.89
  spleen 289.59
Wardrop's disease (with lymphangitis) 681.9
  finger 681.02
  toe 681.11
War neurosis 300.16
Wart (common) (digitate) (filiform) (infectious)
    (juvenile) (plantar) (viral) 078.10
  external genital organs (venereal) 078.19
  fig 078.19
  Hassall-Henle's (of cornea) 371.41
  Henle's (of cornea) 371.41
  juvenile 078.19
  moist 078.10
  Peruvian 088.0
  plantar 078.19
  prosector (*see also* Tuberculosis) 017.0
  seborrheic 702.19
    inflamed 702.11
  senile 702.0
  specified NEC 078.19
  syphilitic 091.3
  tuberculous (*see also* Tuberculosis) 017.0
  venereal (female) (male) 078.19
Warthin's tumor (salivary gland) (M8561/0)
  210.2

Washerwoman's itch 692.4
Wassilieff's disease (leptospiral jaundice) 100.0
Wasting
  disease 799.4
    due to malnutrition 261
  extreme (due to malnutrition) 261
  muscular NEC 728.2
  palsy, paralysis 335.21
  pelvic muscle 618.83
Water
  clefts 366.12
  deprivation of 994.3
  in joint (*see also* Effusion, joint) 719.0
  intoxication 276.6
  itch 120.3
  lack of 994.3
  loading 276.6
  on
    brain—*see* Hydrocephalus
    chest 511.8
  poisoning 276.6
Waterbrash 787.1
Water-hammer pulse (*see also* Insufficiency,
  aortic) 424.1
Waterhouse (-Friderichsen) disease or syndrome
  036.3
Water-losing nephritis 588.89
Wax in ear 380.4
Waxy
  degeneration, any site 277.39
  disease 277.39
  kidney 277.39 *[583.81]*
  liver (large) 277.39
  spleen 277.39
Weak, weakness (generalized) 780.79
  arches (acquired) 734
    congenital 754.61
  bladder sphincter 596.59
  congenital 779.89
  eye muscle—*see* Strabismus
  facial 781.94
  foot (double)—*see* Weak, arches
  heart, cardiac (*see also* Failure, heart) 428.9
    congenital 746.9
  mind 317
  muscle (generalized) 728.87
  myocardium (*see also* Failure, heart) 428.9
  newborn 779.89
  pelvic fundus
    pubocervical tissue 618.81
    rectovaginal tissue 618.82
  pulse 785.9
  senile 797
  valvular—*see* Endocarditis
Wear, worn, tooth, teeth (approximal) (hard
    tissues) (interproximal) (occlusal)—*see also*
    Attrition, teeth 521.10
Weather, weathered
  effects of
    cold NEC 991.9
      specified effect NEC 991.8
    hot (*see also* Heat) 992.9
  skin 692.74
Web, webbed (congenital)—*see also* Anomaly,
    specified type NEC
  canthus 743.63
  digits (*see also* Syndactylism) 755.10

Web, webbed—*continued*
  duodenal 751.5
  esophagus 750.3
  fingers (*see also* Syndactylism, fingers) 755.11
  larynx (glottic) (subglottic) 748.2
  neck (pterygium colli) 744.5
  Paterson-Kelly (sideropenic dysphagia) 280.8
  popliteal syndrome 756.89
  toes (*see also* Syndactylism, toes) 755.13
Weber's paralysis or syndrome 344.89
Weber-Christian disease or syndrome (nodular
  nonsuppurative panniculitis) 729.30
Weber-Cockayne syndrome (epidermolysis
  bullosa) 757.39
Weber-Dimitri syndrome 759.6
Weber-Gubler syndrome 344.89
Weber-Leyden syndrome 344.89
Weber-Osler syndrome (familial hemorrhagic
  telangiectasia) 448.0
Wedge-shaped or wedging vertebra (*see also*
  Osteoporosis) 733.00
Wegener's granulomatosis or syndrome 446.4
Wegner's disease (syphilitic osteochondritis)
  090.0
Weight
  gain (abnormal) (excessive) 783.1
    during pregnancy 646.1
      insufficient 646.8
  less than 1000 grams at birth 765.0
  loss (cause unknown) 783.21
Weightlessness 994.9
Weil's disease (leptospiral jaundice) 100.00
Weill-Marchesani syndrome (brachymorphism
  and ectopia lentis) 759.89
Weingarten's syndrome (tropical eosinophilia)
  518.3
Weir Mitchell's disease (erythromelalgia)
  443.82
Weiss-Baker syndrome (carotid sinus syncope)
  337.0
Weissenbach-Thibierge syndrome (cutaneous
  systemic sclerosis) 710.1
Wen (*see also* Cyst, sebaceous) 706.2
Wenckebach's phenomenon, heart block
  (second degree) 426.13
Werdnig-Hoffmann syndrome (muscular
  atrophy) 335.0
Werlhof's disease (*see also* Purpura,
  thrombocytopenic) 287.39
Werlhof-Wichmann syndrome (*see also*
  Purpura, thrombocytopenic) 287.39
Wermer's syndrome or disease (polyendocrine
  adenomatosis) 258.0
Werner's disease or syndrome (progeria
  adultorum) 259.8
Werner-His disease (trench fever) 083.1
Werner-Schultz disease (agranulocytosis)
  288.09
**Wernicke's encephalopathy, disease or
  syndrome** (superior hemorrhagic
  polioencephalitis) 265.1
Wernicke-Korsakoff syndrome or psychosis
  (nonalcoholic) 294.0
  alcoholic 291.1
Wernicke-Posadas disease (*see also*
  Coccidioidomycosis) 114.9
Wesselsbron fever 066.3
West African fever 084.8

West Nile
  encephalitis 066.41
  encephalomyelitis 066.41
  fever 066.40
    with
      cranial nerve disorders 066.42
      encephalitis 066.41
      optic neuritis 066.42
      other complications 066.49
      other neurologic manifestations 066.42
      polyradiculitis 066.42
  virus 066.40
Westphal-Strümpell syndrome
  (hepatolenticular degeneration) 275.1
Wet
  brain (alcoholic) (*see also* Alcoholism) 303.9
  feet, tropical (syndrome) (maceration) 991.4
  lung (syndrome)
    adult 518.5
    newborn 770.6
Wharton's duct —*see* condition
Wheal 709.8
Wheezing 786.07
Whiplash injury or syndrome 847.0
Whipple's disease or syndrome (intestinal
  lipodystrophy) 040.2
Whipworm 127.3
"Whistling face" syndrome (craniocarpotarsal
  dystrophy) 759.89
White —*see also* condition
  kidney
    large—*see* Nephrosis
    small 582.9
  leg, puerperal, postpartum, childbirth 671.4
    nonpuerperal 451.19
  mouth 112.0
  patches of mouth 528.6
  sponge nevus of oral mucosa 750.26
  spot lesions, teeth 521.01
White's disease (congenital) (keratosis
  follicularis) 757.39
Whitehead 706.2
Whitlow (with lymphangitis) 681.01
  herpetic 054.6
Whitmore's disease or fever (melioidosis) 025
Whooping cough 033.9
  with pneumonia 033.9 *[484.3]*
  due to
    Bordetella
      bronchoseptica 033.8
        with pneumonia 033.8 *[484.3]*
      parapertussis 033.1
        with pneumonia 033.1 *[484.3]*
      pertussis 033.0
        with pneumonia 033.0 *[484.3]*
    specified organism NEC 033.8
      with pneumonia 033.8 *[484.3]*
  vaccination, prophylactic (against) V03.6
Wichmann's asthma (laryngismus stridulus)
  478.75
Widal (-Abrami) syndrome (acquired hemolytic
  jaundice) 283.9
Widening aorta (*see also* Aneurysm, aorta)
  441.9
  ruptured 441.5
Wilkie's disease or syndrome 557.1
Wilkinson-Sneddon disease or syndrome
  (subcorneal pustular dermatosis) 694.1
Willan's lepra 696.1
Willan-Plumbe syndrome (psoriasis) 696.1

Willebrand (-Jürgens) syndrome or
  thrombopathy (angiohemophilia) 286.4
Willi-Prader syndrome (hypogenital dystrophy
  with diabetic tendency) 759.81
Willis' disease (diabetes mellitus) (*see also*
  Diabetes) 250.0
Wilms' tumor or neoplasm (nephroblastoma)
  (M8960/3) 189.0
Wilson's
  disease or syndrome (hepatolenticular
    degeneration) 275.1
  hepatolenticular degeneration 275.1
  lichen ruber 697.0
Wilson-Brocq disease (dermatitis exfoliativa)
  695.89
Wilson-Mikity syndrome 770.7
Window —*see also* Imperfect, closure
  aorticopulmonary 745.0
Winged scapula 736.89
Winter —*see also* condition
  vomiting disease 078.82
Wise's disease 696.2
Wiskott-Aldrich syndrome
  (eczema-thrombocytopenia) 279.12
Withdrawal symptoms, syndrome
  alcohol 291.81
    delirium (acute) 291.0
      chronic 291.1
      newborn 760.71
  drug or narcotic 292.0
  newborn, infant of dependent mother 779.5
  steroid NEC
    correct substance properly administered 255.4
    overdose or wrong substance given or taken
      962.0
Withdrawing reaction, child or adolescent
  313.22
Witts' anemia (achlorhydric anemia) 280.9
Witzelsucht 301.9
Woakes' syndrome (ethmoiditis) 471.1
Wohlfart-Kugelberg-Welander disease 335.11
Woillez's disease (acute idiopathic pulmonary
  congestion) 518.5
Wolff-Parkinson-White syndrome (anomalous
  atrioventricular excitation) 426.7
Wolhynian fever 083.1
Wolman's disease (primary familial
  xanthomatosis) 272.7
Wood asthma 495.8
Woolly, wooly hair (congenital) (nevus) 757.4
Wool-sorters' disease 022.1
Word
  blindness (congenital) (developmental) 315.01
    secondary to organic lesion 784.61
  deafness (secondary to organic lesion) 784.69
    developmental 315.31
Worm (s) (colic) (fever) (infection) (infestation)
  (*see also* Infestation) 128.9
  guinea 125.7
  in intestine NEC 127.9
Worm-eaten soles 102.3
Worn out (*see also* Exhaustion) 780.79
"Worried well" V65.5
Wound, open (by cutting or piercing instrument)
  (by firearms) (cut) (dissection) (incised)
  (laceration) (penetration) (perforating)
  (puncture) (with initial hemorrhage, not
  internal) 879.8

Wound, open—*continued*

> *Note—For fracture with open wound, see
> Fracture. For laceration, traumatic rupture,
> tear or penetrating wound of internal organs,
> such as heart, lung, liver, kidney, pelvic organs,
> etc., whether or not accompanied by open
> wound or fracture in the same region, see
> Injury, internal. For contused wound, see
> Contusion. For crush injury, see Crush. For
> abrasion, insect bite (nonvenomous), blister, or
> scratch, see Injury, superficial.*
>
> *Complicated includes wounds with:*
>   *delayed healing*
>   *delayed treatment*
>   *foreign body*
>   *primary infection*
>
> *For late effect of open wound, see Late, effect,
> wound, open, by site.*

  abdomen, abdominal (external) (muscle) 879.2
    complicated 879.3
    wall (anterior) 879.2
      complicated 879.3
      lateral 879.4
        complicated 879.5
  alveolar (process) 873.62
    complicated 873.72
  ankle 891.0
    with tendon involvement 891.2
    complicated 891.1
  anterior chamber, eye (*see also* Wound, open,
    intraocular) 871.9
  anus 879.6
    complicated 879.7
  arm 884.0
    with tendon involvement 884.2
    complicated 884.1
    forearm 881.00
      with tendon involvement 881.20
      complicated 881.10
    multiple sites—*see* Wound, open, multiple,
      upper limb
    upper 880.03
      with tendon involvement 880.23
      complicated 880.13
      multiple sites (with axillary or shoulder
        regions) 880.09
        with tendon involvement 880.29
        complicated 880.19
  artery—*see* Injury, blood vessel, by site
  auditory
    canal (external) (meatus) 872.02
      complicated 872.12
    ossicles (incus) (malleus) (stapes) 872.62
      complicated 872.72
  auricle, ear 872.01
    complicated 872.11
  axilla 880.02
    with tendon involvement 880.22
    complicated 880.12
      with tendon involvement 880.29
    involving other sites of upper arm 880.09
      complicated 880.19
  back 876.0
    complicated 876.1
  bladder—*see* Injury, internal, bladder
  blood vessel—*see* Injury, blood vessel, by site
  brain—*see* Injury, intracranial, with open
    intracranial wound

Wound, open—*continued*
  high-velocity (grease gun)—*see* Wound, open,
    complicated, by site
  hip 890.0
    with tendon involvement 890.2
    complicated 890.1
  hymen 878.6
    complicated 878.7
  hypochondrium 879.4
    complicated 879.5
  hypogastric region 879.2
    complicated 879.3
  iliac (region) 879.4
    complicated 879.5
  incidental to
    dislocation—*see* Dislocation, open, by site
    fracture—*see* Fracture, open, by site
    intracranial injury—*see* Injury, intracranial,
      with open intracranial wound
    nerve injury—*see* Injury, nerve, by site
  inguinal region 879.4
    complicated 879.5
  instep 892.0
    with tendon involvement 892.2
    complicated 892.1
  interscapular region 876.0
    complicated 876.1
  intracranial—*see* Injury, intracranial, with open
    intracranial wound
  intraocular 871.9
    with
      partial loss (of intraocular tissue) 871.2
      prolapse or exposure (of intraocular tissue)
        871.1
    laceration (*see also* Laceration, eyeball) 871.4
    penetrating 871.7
      with foreign body (nonmagnetic) 871.6
        magnetic 871.5
    without prolapse (of intraocular tissue) 871.0
  iris (*see also* Wound, open, eyeball) 871.9
  jaw (fracture not involved) 873.44
    with fracture—*see* Fracture, jaw
    complicated 873.54
  knee 891.0
    with tendon involvement 891.2
    complicated 891.1
  labium (majus) (minus) 878.4
    complicated 878.5
  lacrimal apparatus, gland, or sac 870.8
    with laceration of eyelid 870.2
  larynx 874.01
    with trachea 874.00
      complicated 874.10
    complicated 874.11
  leg (multiple) 891.0
    with tendon involvement 891.2
    complicated 891.1
    lower 891.0
      with tendon involvement 891.2
      complicated 891.1
    thigh 890.0
      with tendon involvement 890.2
      complicated 890.1
    upper 890.0
      with tendon involvement 890.2
      complicated 890.1
  lens (eye) (alone) (*see also* Cataract, traumatic)
    366.20
    with involvement of other eye structures—*see*
      Wound, open, eyeball

Wound, open—*continued*
  limb
    lower (multiple) NEC 894.0
      with tendon involvement 894.2
      complicated 894.1
    upper (multiple) NEC 884.0
      with tendon involvement 884.2
      complicated 884.1
  lip 873.43
    complicated 873.53
  loin 876.0
    complicated 876.1
  lumbar region 876.0
    complicated 876.1
  malar region 873.41
    complicated 873.51
  mastoid region 873.49
    complicated 873.59
  mediastinum—*see* Injury, internal, mediastinum
  midthoracic region 875.0
    complicated 875.1
  mouth 873.60
    complicated 873.70
    floor 873.64
      complicated 873.74
    multiple sites 873.69
      complicated 873.79
    specified site NEC 873.69
      complicated 873.79
  multiple, unspecified site(s) 879.8

> *Note—Multiple open wounds of sites
> classifiable to the same four-digit category
> should be classified to that category unless they
> are in different limbs.*
>
> *Multiple open wounds of sites classifiable to
> different four-digit categories, or to different
> limbs, should be coded separately.*

    complicated 879.9
    lower limb(s) (one or both) (sites classifiable
      to more than one three-digit category in
      890 to 893) 894.0
      with tendon involvement 894.2
      complicated 894.1
    upper limb(s) (one or both) (sites classifiable
      to more than one three-digit category in
      880 to 883) 884.0
      with tendon involvement 884.2
      complicated 884.1
  muscle—*see* Sprain, by site
  nail
    finger(s) 883.0
      complicated 883.1
    thumb 883.0
      complicated 883.1
    toe(s) 893.0
      complicated 893.1
  nape (neck) 874.8
    complicated 874.9
    specified part NEC 874.8
      complicated 874.9
  nasal—*see also* Wound, open, nose
    cavity 873.22
      complicated 873.32
    septum 873.21
      complicated 873.31
    sinuses 873.23
      complicated 873.33
  nasopharynx 873.22

Wound, open—*continued*
  complicated 893.1
 tongue 873.64
  complicated 873.74
 tonsil—*see* Wound, open, neck
 trachea (cervical region) 874.02
  with larynx 874.00
   complicated 874.10
  complicated 874.12
  intrathoracic—*see* Injury, internal, trachea
 trunk (multiple) NEC 879.6
  complicated 879.7
  specified site NEC 879.6
   complicated 879.7
 tunica vaginalis 878.2
  complicated 878.3
 tympanic membrane 872.61
  complicated 872.71
 tympanum 872.61
  complicated 872.71
 umbilical region 879.2
  complicated 879.3
 ureter—*see* Injury, internal, ureter
 urethra—*see* Injury, internal, urethra
 uterus—*see* Injury, internal, uterus
 uvula 873.69
  complicated 873.79
 vagina 878.6
  complicated 878.7
 vas deferens—*see* Injury, internal, vas deferens
 vitreous (humor) 871.2
 vulva 878.4
  complicated 878.5
 wrist 881.02
  with tendon involvement 881.22
  complicated 881.12
Wright's syndrome (hyperabduction) 447.8
 pneumonia 390 *[517.1]*
Wringer injury —*see* Crush injury, by site
Wrinkling of skin 701.8
Wrist —*see also* condition
 drop (acquired) 736.05
Wrong drug (given in error) NEC 977.9
 specified drug or substance—*see* Table of drugs
   and chemicals
Wry neck —*see also* Torticollis
 congenital 754.1
Wuchereria infestation 125.0
 bancrofti 125.0
 Brugia malayi 125.1
 malayi 125.1
Wuchereriasis 125.0
Wuchereriosis 125.0
Wuchernde struma langhans (M8332/3) 193

X

Xanthelasma 272.2
  eyelid 272.2 *[374.51]*
  palpebrarum 272.2 *[374.51]*
Xanthelasmatosis (essential) 272.2
Xanthelasmoidea 757.33
Xanthine stones 277.2
Xanthinuria 277.2
Xanthofibroma (M8831/0)—*see* Neoplasm,
  connective tissue, benign
Xanthoma(s), xanthomatosis 272.2
  with
    hyperlipoproteinemia
      type I 272.3
      type III 272.2
      type IV 272.1
      type V 272.3
  bone 272.7
  craniohypophyseal 277.89
  cutaneotendinous 272.7
  diabeticorum 250.8 *[272.2]*
  disseminatum 272.7
  eruptive 272.2
  eyelid 272.2 *[374.51]*
  familial 272.7
  hereditary 272.7
  hypercholesterinemic 272.0
  hypercholesterolemic 272.0
  hyperlipemic 272.4
  hyperlipidemic 272.4
  infantile 272.7
  joint 272.7
  juvenile 272.7
  multiple 272.7
  multiplex 272.7
  primary familial 272.7
  tendon (sheath) 272.7
  tuberosum 272.2
  tuberous 272.2
  tubo-eruptive 272.2
Xanthosis 709.09
  surgical 998.81
Xenophobia 300.29
Xeroderma (congenital) 757.39
  acquired 701.1
    eyelid 373.33
  eyelid 373.33
  pigmentosum 757.33
  vitamin A deficiency 264.8
Xerophthalmia 372.53
  vitamin A deficiency 264.7
Xerosis
  conjunctiva 372.53
    with Bitôt's spot 372.53
      vitamin A deficiency 264.1
    vitamin A deficiency 264.0
  cornea 371.40
    with corneal ulceration 370.00
      vitamin A deficiency 264.3
    vitamin A deficiency 264.2
  cutis 706.8
  skin 706.8
Xerostomia 527.7
Xiphodynia 733.90
Xiphoidalgia 733.90
Xiphoiditis 733.99
Xiphopagus 759.4
XO syndrome 758.6

X-ray
  effects, adverse, NEC 990
  of chest
    for suspected tuberculosis V71.2
    routine V72.5
XXX syndrome 758.81
XXXXY syndrome 758.81
XXY syndrome 758.7
Xyloketosuria 271.8
Xylosuria 271.8
Xylulosuria 271.8
XYY syndrome 758.81

Y

Yawning 786.09
  psychogenic 306.1
Yaws 102.9
  bone or joint lesions 102.6
  butter 102.1
  chancre 102.0
  cutaneous, less than five years after infection
      102.2
  early (cutaneous) (macular) (maculopapular)
      (micropapular) (papular) 102.2
    frambeside 102.2
    skin lesions NEC 102.2
  eyelid 102.9 *[373.4]*
  ganglion 102.6
  gangosis, gangosa 102.5
  gumma, gummata 102.4
    bone 102.6
  gummatous
    frambeside 102.4
    osteitis 102.6
    periostitis 102.6
  hydrarthrosis 102.6
  hyperkeratosis (early) (late) (palmar) (plantar)
      102.3
  initial lesions 102.0
  joint lesions 102.6
  juxta-articular nodules 102.7
  late nodular (ulcerated) 102.4
  latent (without clinical manifestations) (with
      positive serology) 102.8
  mother 102.0
  mucosal 102.7
  multiple papillomata 102.1
  nodular, late (ulcerated) 102.4
  osteitis 102.6
  papilloma, papillomata (palmar) (plantar) 102.1
  periostitis (hypertrophic) 102.6
  ulcers 102.4
  wet crab 102.1
Yeast infection (*see also* Candidiasis) 112.9
Yellow
  atrophy (liver) 570
    chronic 571.8
    resulting from administration of blood,
        plasma, serum, or other biological
        substance (within 8 months of
        administration)—*see* Hepatitis, viral
  fever—*see* Fever, yellow
  jack (*see also* Fever, yellow) 060.9
  jaundice (*see also* Jaundice) 782.4
Yersinia septica 027.8

Z

Zagari's disease (xerostomia) 527.7
Zahorsky's disease (exanthema subitum) 057.8
  syndrome (herpangina) 074.0
Zellweger syndrome 277.86
Zenker's diverticulum (esophagus) 530.6
Ziehen-Oppenheim disease 333.6
Zieve's syndrome (jaundice, hyperlipemia, and
    hemolytic anemia) 571.1
Zika fever 066.3
Zollinger-Ellison syndrome (gastric
    hypersecretion with pancreatic islet cell
    tumor) 251.5
Zona (*see also* Herpes, zoster) 053.9
Zoophilia (erotica) 302.1
Zoophobia 300.29
Zoster (herpes) (*see also* Herpes, zoster) 053.9
Zuelzer (-Ogden) anemia or syndrome
    (nutritional megaloblastic anemia) 281.2
Zygodactyly (*see also* Syndactylism) 755.10
Zygomycosis 117.7
Zymotic —*see* condition

SECTION 2

ALPHABETIC INDEX TO POISONING AND EXTERNAL CAUSES OF ADVERSE EFFECTS OF DRUGS AND OTHER CHEMICAL SUBSTANCES

TABLE OF DRUGS AND CHEMICALS

This table contains a classification of drugs and other chemical substances to identify poisoning states and external causes of adverse effects.

Each of the listed substances in the table is assigned a code according to the poisoning classification (960–989). These codes are used when there is a statement of poisoning, overdose, wrong substance given or taken, or intoxication.

The table also contains a listing of external causes of adverse effects. An adverse effect is a pathologic manifestation due to ingestion or exposure to drugs or other chemical substances (e.g., dermatitis, hypersensitivity reaction, aspirin gastritis). The adverse effect is to be identified by the appropriate code found in Section 1, Index to Diseases and Injuries. An external cause code can then be used to identify the circumstances involved. The table headings pertaining to external causes are defined below:

> **Accidental poisoning (E850–E869)**—accidental overdose of drug, wrong substance given or taken, drug taken inadvertently, accidents in the usage of drugs and biologicals in medical and surgical procedures, and to show external causes of poisonings classifiable to 980–989.

> **Therapeutic use (E930–E949)**—a correct substance properly administered in therapeutic or prophylactic dosage as the external cause of adverse effects.

> **Suicide attempt (E950–E952)**—instances in which self–inflicted injuries or poisonings are involved.

> **Assault (E961–E962)**—injury or poisoning inflicted by another person with the intent to injure or kill.

> **Undetermined (E980–E982)**—to be used when the intent of the poisoning or injury cannot be determined whether it was intentional or accidental.

The American Hospital Formulary Service list numbers are included in the table to help classify new drugs not identified in the table by name. The AHFS list numbers are keyed to the continually revised American Hospital Formulary Service (AHFS).* These listings are found in the table under the main term **Drug**.

Excluded from the table are radium and other radioactive substances. The classification of adverse effects and complications pertaining to these substances will be found in Section 1, Index to Diseases and Injuries, and Section 3, Index to External Causes of Injuries.

Although certain substances are indexed with one or more subentries, the majority are listed according to one use or state. It is recognized that many substances may be used in various ways, in medicine and in industry, and may cause adverse effects whatever the state of the agent (solid, liquid, or fumes arising from a liquid). In cases in which the reported data indicates a use or state not in the table, or which is clearly different from the one listed, an attempt should be made to classify the substance in the form which most nearly expresses the reported facts.

*American Hospital Formulary Service, 2 vol. (Washington, DC: American Society of Hospital Pharmacists, 1959)

Substance	Poisoning	Accident	Therapeutic Use	Suicide Attempt	Assault	Undetermined
		External Cause (E-Code)				
1–propanol	980.3	E860.4	—	E950.9	E962.1	E980.9
2–propanol	980.2	E860.3	—	E950.9	E962.1	E980.9
2, 4–D (dichlorophenoxyacetic acid)	989.4	E863.5	—	E950.6	E962.1	E980.7
2, 4–toluene diisocyanate	983.0	E864.0	—	E950.7	E962.1	E980.6
2, 4, 5–T (trichlorophenoxyacetic acid)	989.2	E863.5	—	E950.6	E962.1	E980.7
14–hydroxydihydromorphinone	965.09	E850.2	E935.2	E950.0	E962.0	E980.0
ABOB	961.7	E857	E931.7	E950.4	E962.0	E980.4
Abrus (seed)	988.2	E865.3	—	E950.9	E962.1	E980.9
Absinthe	980.0	E860.1	—	E950.9	E962.1	E980.9
beverage	980.0	E860.0	—	E950.9	E962.1	E980.9
Acenocoumarin, acenocoumarol	964.2	E858.2	E934.2	E950.4	E962.0	E980.4
Acepromazine	969.1	E853.0	E939.1	E950.3	E962.0	E980.3
Acetal	982.8	E862.4	—	E950.9	E962.1	E980.9
Acetaldehyde (vapor)	987.8	E869.8	—	E952.8	E962.2	E982.8
liquid	989.89	E866.8	—	E950.9	E962.1	E980.9
Acetaminophen	965.4	E850.4	E935.4	E950.0	E962.0	E980.0
Acetaminosalol	965.1	E850.3	E935.3	E950.0	E962.0	E980.0
Acetanilid(e)	965.4	E850.4	E935.4	E950.0	E962.0	E980.0
Acetarsol, acetarsone	961.1	E857	E931.1	E950.4	E962.0	E980.4
Acetazolamide	974.2	E858.5	E944.2	E950.4	E962.0	E980.4
Acetic						
acid	983.1	E864.1	—	E950.7	E962.1	E980.6
with sodium acetate (ointment)	976.3	E858.7	E946.3	E950.4	E962.0	E980.4
irrigating solution	974.5	E858.5	E944.5	E950.4	E962.0	E980.4
lotion	976.2	E858.7	E946.2	E950.4	E962.0	E980.4
anhydride	983.1	E864.1	—	E950.7	E962.1	E980.6
ether (vapor)	982.8	E862.4	—	E950.9	E962.1	E980.9
Acetohexamide	962.3	E858.0	E932.3	E950.4	E962.0	E980.4
Acetomenaphthone	964.3	E858.2	E934.3	E950.4	E962.0	E980.4
Acetomorphine	965.01	E850.0	E935.0	E950.0	E962.0	E980.0
Acetone (oils) (vapor)	982.8	E862.4	—	E950.9	E962.1	E980.9
Acetophenazine (maleate)	969.1	E853.0	E939.1	E950.3	E962.0	E980.3
Acetophenetidin	965.4	E850.4	E935.4	E950.0	E962.0	E980.0
Acetophenone	982.0	E862.4	—	E950.9	E962.1	E980.9
Acetorphine	965.09	E850.2	E935.2	E950.0	E962.0	E980.0
Acetosulfone (sodium)	961.8	E857	E931.8	E950.4	E962.0	E980.4
Acetrizoate (sodium)	977.8	E858.8	E947.8	E950.4	E962.0	E980.4
Acetylcarbromal	967.3	E852.2	E937.3	E950.2	E962.0	E980.2
Acetylcholine (chloride)	971.0	E855.3	E941.0	E950.4	E962.0	E980.4
Acetylcysteine	975.5	E858.6	E945.5	E950.4	E962.0	E980.4
Acetyldigitoxin	972.1	E858.3	E942.1	E950.4	E962.0	E980.4
Acetyldihydrocodeine	965.09	E850.2	E935.2	E950.0	E962.0	E980.0
Acetyldihydrocodeinone	965.09	E850.2	E935.2	E950.0	E962.0	E980.0
Acetylene (gas) (industrial)	987.1	E868.1	—	E951.8	E962.2	E981.8
incomplete combustion of — *see* Carbon monoxide, fuel, utility						
tetrachloride (vapor)	982.3	E862.4	—	E950.9	E962.1	E980.9
Acetyliodosalicylic acid	965.1	E850.3	E935.3	E950.0	E962.0	E980.0
Acetylphenylhydrazine	965.8	E850.8	E935.8	E950.0	E962.0	E980.0
Acetylsalicylic acid	965.1	E850.3	E935.3	E950.0	E962.0	E980.0
Achromycin	960.4	E856	E930.4	E950.4	E962.0	E980.4
ophthalmic preparation	976.5	E858.7	E946.5	E950.4	E962.0	E980.4
topical NEC	976.0	E858.7	E946.0	E950.4	E962.0	E980.4
Acidifying agents	963.2	E858.1	E933.2	E950.4	E962.0	E980.4
Acids (corrosive) NEC	983.1	E864.1	—	E950.7	E962.1	E980.6
Aconite (wild)	988.2	E865.4	—	E950.9	E962.1	E980.9
Aconitine (liniment)	976.8	E858.7	E946.8	E950.4	E962.0	E980.4
Aconitum ferox	988.2	E865.4	—	E950.9	E962.1	E980.9
Acridine	983.0	E864.0	—	E950.7	E962.1	E980.6
vapor	987.8	E869.8	—	E952.8	E962.2	E982.8

Substance	Poisoning	External Cause (E-Code)				
		Accident	Therapeutic Use	Suicide Attempt	Assault	Undetermined
Acriflavine	961.9	E857	E931.9	E950.4	E962.0	E980.4
Acrisorcin	976.0	E858.7	E946.0	E950.4	E962.0	E980.4
Acrolein (gas)	987.8	E869.8	—	E952.8	E962.2	E982.8
liquid	989.89	E866.8	—	E950.9	E962.1	E980.9
Actaea spicata	988.2	E865.4	—	E950.9	E962.1	E980.9
Acterol	961.5	E857	E931.5	E950.4	E962.0	E980.4
ACTH	962.4	E858.0	E932.4	E950.4	E962.0	E980.4
Acthar	962.4	E858.0	E932.4	E950.4	E962.0	E980.4
Actinomycin (C) (D)	960.7	E856	E930.7	E950.4	E962.0	E980.4
Adalin (acetyl)	967.3	E852.2	E937.3	E950.2	E962.0	E980.2
Adenosine (phosphate)	977.8	E858.8	E947.8	E950.4	E962.0	E980.4
Adhesives	989.89	E866.6	—	E950.9	E962.1	E980.9
ADH	962.5	E858.0	E932.5	E950.4	E962.0	E980.4
Adicillin	960.0	E856	E930.0	E950.4	E962.0	E980.4
Adiphenine	975.1	E855.6	E945.1	E950.4	E962.0	E980.4
Adjunct, pharmaceutical	977.4	E858.8	E947.4	E950.4	E962.0	E980.4
Adrenal (extract, cortex or medulla) (glucocorticoids) (hormones) (mineralocorticoids)	962.0	E858.0	E932.0	E950.4	E962.0	E980.4
ENT agent	976.6	E858.7	E946.6	E950.4	E962.0	E980.4
ophthalmic preparation	976.5	E858.7	E946.5	E950.4	E962.0	E980.4
topical NEC	976.0	E858.7	E946.0	E950.4	E962.0	E980.4
Adrenalin	971.2	E855.5	E941.2	E950.4	E962.0	E980.4
Adrenergic blocking agents	971.3	E855.6	E941.3	E950.4	E962.0	E980.4
Adrenergics	971.2	E855.5	E941.2	E950.4	E962.0	E980.4
Adrenochrome (derivatives)	972.8	E858.3	E942.8	E950.4	E962.0	E980.4
Adrenocorticotropic hormone	962.4	E858.0	E932.4	E950.4	E962.0	E980.4
Adrenocorticotropin	962.4	E858.0	E932.4	E950.4	E962.0	E980.4
Adriamycin	960.7	E856	E930.7	E950.4	E962.0	E980.4
Aerosol spray — *see* Sprays						
Aerosporin	960.8	E856	E930.8	E950.4	E962.0	E980.4
ENT agent	976.6	E858.7	E946.6	E950.4	E962.0	E980.4
ophthalmic preparation	976.5	E858.7	E946.5	E950.4	E962.0	E980.4
topical NEC	976.0	E858.7	E946.0	E950.4	E962.0	E980.4
Aethusa cynapium	988.2	E865.4	—	E950.9	E962.1	E980.9
Afghanistan black	969.6	E854.1	E939.6	E950.3	E962.0	E980.3
Aflatoxin	989.7	E865.9	—	E950.9	E962.1	E980.9
African boxwood	988.2	E865.4	—	E950.9	E962.1	E980.9
Agar (–agar)	973.3	E858.4	E943.3	E950.4	E962.0	E980.4
Agricultural agent NEC	989.89	E863.9	—	E950.6	E962.1	E980.7
Agrypnal	967.0	E851	E937.0	E950.1	E962.0	E980.1
Air contaminant(s), source or type not specified	987.9	E869.9	—	E952.9	E962.2	E982.9
specified type — *see* specific substance						
Akee	988.2	E865.4	—	E950.9	E962.1	E980.9
Akrinol	976.0	E858.7	E946.0	E950.4	E962.0	E980.4
Alantolactone	961.6	E857	E931.6	E950.4	E962.0	E980.4
Albamycin	960.8	E856	E930.8	E950.4	E962.0	E980.4
Albumin (normal human serum)	964.7	E858.2	E934.7	E950.4	E962.0	E980.4
Albuterol	975.7	E858.6	E945.7	E950.4	E962.0	E980.4
Alcohol	980.9	E860.9	—	E950.9	E962.1	E980.9
absolute	980.0	E860.1	—	E950.9	E962.1	E980.9
beverage	980.0	E860.0	E947.8	E950.9	E962.1	E980.9
amyl	980.3	E860.4	—	E950.9	E962.1	E980.9
antifreeze	980.1	E860.2	—	E950.9	E962.1	E980.9
butyl	980.3	E860.4	—	E950.9	E962.1	E980.9
dehydrated	980.0	E860.1	—	E950.9	E862.1	E980.9
beverage	980.0	E860.0	E947.8	E950.9	E962.1	E980.9
denatured	980.0	E860.1	—	E950.9	E962.1	E980.9
deterrents	977.3	E858.8	E947.3	E950.4	E962.0	E980.4
diagnostic (gastric function)	977.8	E858.8	E947.8	E950.4	E962.0	E980.4

Substance	Poisoning	Accident	Therapeutic Use	Suicide Attempt	Assault	Undetermined
			External Cause (E-Code)			
ethy l	980.0	E860.1	—	E950.9	E962.1	E980.9
beverage	980.0	E860.0	E947.8	E950.9	E962.1	E980.9
grain	980.0	E860.1	—	E950.9	E962.1	E980.9
beverage	980.0	E860.0	E947.8	E950.9	E962.1	E980.9
industrial	980.9	E860.9	—	E950.9	E962.1	E980.9
isopropyl	980.2	E860.3	—	E950.9	E962.1	E980.9
methyl	980.1	E860.2	—	E950.9	E962.1	E980.9
preparation for consumption	980.0	E860.0	E947.8	E950.9	E962.1	E980.9
propyl	980.3	E860.4	—	E950.9	E962.1	E980.9
secondary	980.2	E860.3	—	E950.9	E962.1	E980.9
radiator	980.1	E860.2	—	E950.9	E962.1	E980.9
rubbing	980.2	E860.3	—	E950.9	E962.1	E980.9
specified type NEC	980.8	E860.8	—	E950.9	E962.1	E980.9
surgical	980.9	E860.9	—	E950.9	E962.1	E980.9
vapor (from any type of alcohol)	987.8	E869.8	—	E952.8	E962.2	E982.8
wood	980.1	E860.2	—	E950.9	E962.1	E980.9
Alcuronium chloride	975.2	E858.6	E945.2	E950.4	E962.0	E980.4
Aldactone	974.4	E858.5	E944.4	E950.4	E962.0	E980.4
Aldicarb	989.3	E863.2	—	E950.6	E962.1	E980.7
Aldomet	972.6	E858.3	E942.6	E950.4	E962.0	E980.4
Aldosterone	962.0	E858.0	E932.0	E950.4	E962.0	E980.4
Aldrin (dust)	989.2	E863.0	—	E950.6	E962.1	E980.7
Algeldrate	973.0	E858.4	E943.0	E950.4	E962.0	E980.4
Alidase	963.4	E858.1	E933.4	E950.4	E962.0	E980.4
Aliphatic thiocyanates	989.0	E866.8	—	E950.9	E962.1	E980.9
Alkaline antiseptic solution (aromatic)	976.6	E858.7	E946.6	E950.4	E962.0	E980.4
Alkalinizing agents (medicinal)	963.3	E858.1	E933.3	E950.4	E962.0	E980.4
Alkalis, caustic	983.2	E864.2	—	E950.7	E962.1	E980.6
Alkalizing agents (medicinal)	963.3	E858.1	E933.3	E950.4	E962.0	E980.4
Alka–seltzer	965.1	E850.3	E935.3	E950.0	E962.0	E980.0
Alkavervir	972.6	E858.3	E942.6	E950.4	E962.0	E980.4
Allegron	969.0	E854.0	E939.0	E950.3	E962.0	E980.3
Alleve *see* Naproxen						
Allobarbital, allobarbitone	967.0	E851	E937.0	E950.1	E962.0	E980.1
Allopurinol	974.7	E858.5	E944.7	E950.4	E962.0	E980.4
Allylestrenol	962.2	E858.0	E932.2	E950.4	E962.0	E980.4
Allylisopropylacetylurea	967.8	E852.8	E937.8	E950.2	E962.0	E980.2
Allylisopropylmalonylurea	967.0	E851	E937.0	E950.1	E962.0	E980.1
Allyltribromide	967.3	E852.2	E937.3	E950.2	E962.0	E980.2
Aloe, aloes, aloin	973.1	E858.4	E943.1	E950.4	E962.0	E980.4
Alosetron	973.8	E858.4	E943.8	E950.4	E962.0	E980.4
Aloxidone	966.0	E855.0	E936.0	E950.4	E962.0	E980.4
Aloxiprin	965.1	E850.3	E935.3	E950.0	E962.0	E980.0
Alpha amylase	963.4	E858.1	E933.4	E950.4	E962.0	E980.4
Alphaprodine (hydrochloride)	965.09	E850.2	E935.2	E950.0	E962.0	E980.0
Alpha tocopherol	963.5	E858.1	E933.5	E950.4	E962.0	E980.4
Alseroxylon	972.6	E858.3	E942.6	E950.4	E962.0	E980.4
Alum (ammonium) (potassium)	983.2	E864.2	—	E950.7	E962.1	E980.6
medicinal (astringent) NEC	976.2	E858.7	E946.2	E950.4	E962.0	E980.4
Aluminium, aluminum (gel) (hydroxide)	973.0	E858.4	E943.0	E950.4	E962.0	E980.4
acetate solution	976.2	E858.7	E946.2	E950.4	E962.0	E980.4
aspirin	965.1	E850.3	E935.3	E950.0	E962.0	E980.0
carbonate	973.0	E858.4	E943.0	E950.4	E962.0	E980.4
glycinate	973.0	E858.4	E943.0	E950.4	E962.0	E980.4
nicotinate	972.2	E858.3	E942.2	E950.4	E962.0	E980.4
ointment (surgical) (topical)	976.3	E858.7	E946.3	E950.4	E962.0	E980.4
phosphate	973.0	E858.4	E943.0	E950.4	E962.0	E980.4
subacetate	976.2	E858.7	E946.2	E950.4	E962.0	E980.4
topical NEC	976.3	E858.7	E946.3	E950.4	E962.0	E980.4
Alurate	967.0	E851	E937.0	E950.1	E962.0	E980.1

Substance	Poisoning	Accident	Therapeutic Use	Suicide Attempt	Assault	Undetermined
		External Cause (E-Code)				
Alverine (citrate)	975.1	E858.6	E945.1	E950.4	E962.0	E980.4
Alvodine	965.09	E850.2	E935.2	E950.0	E962.0	E980.0
Amanita phalloides	988.1	E865.5	—	E950.9	E962.1	E980.9
Amantadine (hydrochloride)	966.4	E855.0	E936.4	E950.4	E962.0	E980.4
Ambazone	961.9	E857	E931.9	E950.4	E962.0	E980.4
Ambenonium	971.0	E855.3	E941.0	E950.4	E962.0	E980.4
Ambutonium bromide	971.1	E855.4	E941.1	E950.4	E962.0	E980.4
Ametazole	977.8	E858.8	E947.8	E950.4	E962.0	E980.4
Amethocaine (infiltration) (topical)	968.5	E855.2	E938.5	E950.4	E962.0	E980.4
nerve block (peripheral) (plexus)	968.6	E855.2	E938.6	E950.4	E962.0	E980.4
spinal	968.7	E855.2	E938.7	E950.4	E962.0	E980.4
Amethopterin	963.1	E858.1	E933.1	E950.4	E962.0	E980.4
Amfepramone	977.0	E858.8	E947.0	E950.4	E962.0	E980.4
Amidon	965.02	E850.1	E935.1	E950.0	E962.0	E980.0
Amidopyrine	965.5	E850.5	E935.5	E950.0	E962.0	E980.0
Aminacrine	976.0	E858.7	E946.0	E950.4	E962.0	E980.4
Aminitrozole	961.5	E857	E931.5	E950.4	E962.0	E980.4
Aminoacetic acid	974.5	E858.5	E944.5	E950.4	E962.0	E980.4
Amino acids	974.5	E858.5	E944.5	E950.4	E962.0	E980.4
Aminocaproic acid	964.4	E858.2	E934.4	E950.4	E962.0	E980.4
Aminoethylisothiourium	963.8	E858.1	E933.8	E950.4	E962.0	E980.4
Aminoglutethimide	966.3	E855.0	E936.3	E950.4	E962.0	E980.4
Aminometradine	974.3	E858.5	E944.3	E950.4	E962.0	E980.4
Aminopentamide	971.1	E855.4	E941.1	E950.4	E962.0	E980.4
Aminophenazone	965.5	E850.5	E935.5	E950.0	E962.0	E980.0
Aminophenol	983.0	E864.0	—	E950.7	E962.1	E980.6
Aminophenylpyridone	969.5	E853.8	E939.5	E950.3	E962.0	E980.3
Aminophyllin	975.7	E858.6	E945.7	E950.4	E962.0	E980.4
Aminopterin	963.1	E858.1	E933.1	E950.4	E962.0	E980.4
Aminopyrine	965.5	E850.5	E935.5	E950.0	E962.0	E980.0
Aminosalicylic acid	961.8	E857	E931.8	E950.4	E962.0	E980.4
Amiphenazole	970.1	E854.3	E940.1	E950.4	E962.0	E980.4
Amiquinsin	972.6	E858.3	E942.6	E950.4	E962.0	E980.4
Amisometradine	974.3	E858.5	E944.3	E950.4	E962.0	E980.4
Amitriptyline	969.0	E854.0	E939.0	E950.3	E962.0	E980.3
Ammonia (fumes) (gas) (vapor)	987.8	E869.8	—	E952.8	E962.2	E982.8
liquid (household) NEC	983.2	E861.4	—	E950.7	E961.1	E980.6
spirit, aromatic	970.8	E854.3	E940.8	E950.4	E962.0	E980.4
Ammoniated mercury	976.0	E858.7	E946.0	E950.4	E962.0	E980.4
Ammonium						
carbonate	983.2	E864.2	—	E950.7	E961.1	E980.6
chloride (acidifying agent)	963.2	E858.1	E933.2	E950.4	E962.0	E980.4
expectorant	975.5	E858.6	E945.5	E950.4	E962.0	E980.4
compounds (household) NEC	983.2	E861.4	—	E950.7	E961.1	E980.6
fumes (any usage)	987.8	E869.8	—	E952.8	E962.2	E982.8
industrial	983.2	E864.2	—	E950.7	E961.1	E980.6
ichthyosulfonate	976.4	E858.7	E946.4	E950.4	E962.0	E980.4
mandelate	961.9	E857	E931.9	E950.4	E962.0	E980.4
Amobarbital	967.0	E851	E937.0	E950.1	E962.0	E980.1
Amodiaquin(e)	961.4	E857	E931.4	E950.4	E962.0	E980.4
Amopyroquin(e)	961.4	E857	E931.4	E950.4	E962.0	E980.4
Amphenidone	969.5	E853.8	E939.5	E950.3	E962.0	E980.3
Amphetamine	969.7	E854.2	E939.7	E950.3	E962.0	E980.3
Amphomycin	960.8	E856	E930.8	E950.4	E962.0	E980.4
Amphotericin B	960.1	E856	E930.1	E950.4	E962.0	E980.4
topical	976.0	E858.7	E946.0	E950.4	E962.0	E980.4
Ampicillin	960.0	E856	E930.0	E950.4	E962.0	E980.4
Amprotropine	971.1	E855.4	E941.1	E950.4	E962.0	E980.4
Amygdalin	977.8	E858.8	E947.8	E950.4	E962.0	E980.4
Amyl						
acetate (vapor)	982.8	E862.4	—	E950.9	E962.1	E980.9

Substance	Poisoning	Accident	Therapeutic Use	Suicide Attempt	Assault	Undetermined
			External Cause (E-Code)			
alcohol	980.3	E860.4	—	E950.9	E962.1	E980.9
nitrite (medicinal)	972.4	E858.3	E942.4	E950.4	E962.0	E980.4
Amylase (alpha)	963.4	E858.1	E933.4	E950.4	E962.0	E980.4
Amylene hydrate	980.8	E860.8	—	E950.9	E962.1	E980.9
Amylobarbitone	967.0	E851	E937.0	E950.1	E962.0	E980.1
Amylocaine	968.9	E855.2	E938.9	E950.4	E962.0	E980.4
infiltration (subcutaneous)	968.5	E855.2	E938.5	E950.4	E962.0	E980.4
nerve block (peripheral) (plexus)	968.6	E855.2	E938.6	E950.4	E962.0	E980.4
spinal	968.7	E855.2	E938.7	E950.4	E962.0	E980.4
topical (surface)	968.5	E855.2	E938.5	E950.4	E962.0	E980.4
Amytal (sodium)	967.0	E851	E937.0	E950.1	E962.0	E980.1
Analeptics	970.0	E854.3	E940.0	E950.4	E962.0	E980.4
Analgesics	965.9	E850.9	E935.9	E950.0	E962.0	E980.0
aromatic NEC	965.4	E850.4	E935.4	E950.0	E962.0	E980.0
non–narcotic NEC	965.7	E850.7	E935.7	E950.0	E962.0	E980.0
specified NEC	965.8	E850.8	E935.8	E950.0	E962.0	E980.0
Anamirta cocculus	988.2	E865.3	—	E950.9	E962.1	E980.9
Ancillin	960.0	E856	E930.0	E950.4	E962.0	E980.4
Androgens (anabolic congeners)	962.1	E858.0	E932.1	E950.4	E962.0	E980.4
Androstalone	962.1	E858.0	E932.1	E950.4	E962.0	E980.4
Androsterone	962.1	E858.0	E932.1	E950.4	E962.0	E980.4
Anemone pulsatilla	988.2	E865.4	—	E950.9	E962.1	E980.9
Anesthesia, anesthetic (general) NEC	968.4	E855.1	E938.4	E950.4	E962.0	E980.4
block (nerve) (plexus)	968.6	E855.2	E938.6	E950.4	E962.0	E980.4
gaseous NEC	968.2	E855.1	E938.2	E950.4	E962.0	E980.4
halogenated hydrocarbon derivatives NEC	968.2	E855.1	E938.2	E950.4	E962.0	E980.4
infiltration (intradermal) (subcutaneous) (submucosal)	968.5	E855.2	E938.5	E950.4	E962.0	E980.4
intravenous	968.3	E855.1	E938.3	E950.4	E962.0	E980.4
local NEC	968.9	E855.2	E938.9	E950.4	E962.0	E980.4
nerve blocking (peripheral) (plexus)	968.6	E855.2	E938.6	E950.4	E962.0	E980.4
rectal NEC	968.3	E855.1	E938.3	E950.4	E962.0	E980.4
spinal	968.7	E855.2	E938.7	E950.4	E962.0	E980.4
surface	968.5	E855.2	E938.5	E950.4	E962.0	E980.4
topical	968.5	E855.2	E938.5	E950.4	E962.0	E980.4
Aneurine	963.5	E858.1	E933.5	E950.4	E962.0	E980.4
Angio–Conray	977.8	E858.8	E947.8	E950.4	E962.0	E980.4
Anginine see Glyceryl trinitrate						
Angiotensin	971.2	E855.5	E941.2	E950.4	E962.0	E980.4
Anhydrohydroxyprogesterone	962.2	E858.0	E932.2	E950.4	E962.0	E980.4
Anhydron	974.3	E858.5	E944.3	E950.4	E962.0	E980.4
Anileridine	965.09	E850.2	E935.2	E950.0	E962.0	E980.0
Aniline (dye) (liquid)	983.0	E864.0	—	E950.7	E962.1	E980.6
analgesic	965.4	E850.4	E935.4	E950.0	E962.0	E980.0
derivatives, therapeutic NEC	965.4	E850.4	E935.4	E950.0	E962.0	E980.0
vapor	987.8	E869.8	—	E952.8	E962.2	E982.8
Anisindione	964.2	E858.2	E934.2	E950.4	E962.0	E980.4
Anisotropine	971.1	E855.4	E941.1	E950.4	E962.0	E980.4
Anorexic agents	977.0	E858.8	E947.0	E950.4	E962.0	E980.4
Ant (bite) (sting)	989.5	E905.5	—	E950.9	E962.1	E980.9
Antabuse	977.3	E858.8	E947.3	E950.4	E962.0	E980.4
Antacids	973.0	E858.4	E943.0	E950.4	E962.0	E980.4
Antazoline	963.0	E858.1	E933.0	E950.4	E962.0	E980.4
Anthelmintics	961.6	E857	E931.6	E950.4	E962.0	E980.4
Anthralin	976.4	E858.7	E946.4	E950.4	E962.0	E980.4
Anthramycin	960.7	E856	E930.7	E950.4	E962.0	E980.4
Antiadrenergics	971.3	E855.6	E941.3	E950.4	E962.0	E980.4
Antiallergic agents	963.0	E858.1	E933.0	E950.4	E962.0	E980.4
Antianemic agents NEC	964.1	E858.2	E934.1	E950.4	E962.0	E980.4

Substance	Poisoning	Accident	Therapeutic Use	Suicide Attempt	Assault	Undetermined
			External Cause (E-Code)			
Antiaris toxicaria	988.2	E865.4	—	E950.9	E962.1	E980.9
Antiarteriosclerotic agents	972.2	E858.3	E942.2	E950.4	E962.0	E980.4
Antiasthmatics	975.7	E858.6	E945.7	E950.4	E962.0	E980.4
Antibiotics	960.9	E856	E930.9	E950.4	E962.0	E980.4
antifungal	960.1	E856	E930.1	E950.4	E962.0	E980.4
antimycobacterial	960.6	E856	E930.6	E950.4	E962.0	E980.4
antineoplastic	960.7	E856	E930.7	E950.4	E962.0	E980.4
cephalosporin (group)	960.5	E856	E930.5	E950.4	E962.0	E980.4
chloramphenicol (group)	960.2	E856	E930.2	E950.4	E962.0	E980.4
macrolides	960.3	E856	E930.3	E950.4	E962.0	E980.4
specified NEC	960.8	E856	E930.8	E950.4	E962.0	E980.4
tetracycline (group)	960.4	E856	E930.4	E950.4	E962.0	E980.4
Anticancer agents NEC	963.1	E858.1	E933.1	E950.4	E962.0	E980.4
antibiotics	960.7	E856	E930.7	E950.4	E962.0	E980.4
Anticholinergics	971.1	E855.4	E941.1	E950.4	E962.0	E980.4
Anticholinesterase (organophosphorus) (reversible)	971.0	E855.3	E941.0	E950.4	E962.0	E980.4
Anticoagulants	964.2	E858.2	E934.2	E950.4	E962.0	E980.4
antagonists	964.5	E858.2	E934.5	E950.4	E962.0	E980.4
Anti–common cold agents NEC	975.6	E858.6	E945.6	E950.4	E962.0	E980.4
Anticonvulsants NEC	966.3	E855.0	E936.3	E950.4	E962.0	E980.4
Antidepressants	969.0	E854.0	E939.0	E950.3	E962.0	E980.3
Antidiabetic agents	962.3	E858.0	E932.3	E950.4	E962.0	E980.4
Antidiarrheal agents	973.5	E858.4	E943.5	E950.4	E962.0	E980.4
Antidiuretic hormone	962.5	E858.0	E932.5	E950.4	E962.0	E980.4
Antidotes NEC	977.2	E858.8	E947.2	E950.4	E962.0	E980.4
Antiemetic agents	963.0	E858.1	E933.0	E950.4	E962.0	E980.4
Antiepilepsy agent NEC	966.3	E855.0	E936.3	E950.4	E962.0	E980.4
Antifertility pills	962.2	E858.0	E932.2	E950.4	E962.0	E980.4
Antiflatulents	973.8	E858.4	E943.8	E950.4	E962.0	E980.4
Antifreeze	989.89	E866.8	—	E950.9	E962.1	E980.9
alcohol	980.1	E860.2	—	E950.9	E962.1	E980.9
ethylene glycol	982.8	E862.4	—	E950.9	E962.1	E980.9
Antifungals (nonmedicinal) (sprays)	989.4	E863.6	—	E950.6	E962.1	E980.7
medicinal NEC	961.9	E857	E931.9	E950.4	E962.0	E980.4
antibiotic	960.1	E856	E930.1	E950.4	E962.0	E980.4
topical	976.0	E858.7	E946.0	E950.4	E962.0	E980.4
Antigastric secretion agents	973.0	E858.4	E943.0	E950.4	E962.0	E980.4
Antihelmintics	961.6	E857	E931.6	E950.4	E962.0	E980.4
Antihemophilic factor (human)	964.7	E858.2	E934.7	E950.4	E962.0	E980.4
Antihistamine	963.0	E858.1	E933.0	E950.4	E962.0	E980.4
Antihypertensive agents NEC	972.6	E858.3	E942.6	E950.4	E962.0	E980.4
Anti–infectives NEC	961.9	E857	E931.9	E950.4	E962.0	E980.4
antibiotics	960.9	E856	E930.9	E950.4	E962.0	E980.4
specified NEC	960.8	E856	E930.8	E950.4	E962.0	E980.4
antihelmintic	961.6	E857	E931.6	E950.4	E962.0	E980.4
antimalarial	961.4	E857	E931.4	E950.4	E962.0	E980.4
antimycobacterial NEC	961.8	E857	E931.8	E950.4	E962.0	E980.4
antibiotics	960.6	E856	E930.6	E950.4	E962.0	E980.4
antiprotozoal NEC	961.5	E857	E931.5	E950.4	E962.0	E980.4
blood	961.4	E857	E931.4	E950.4	E962.0	E980.4
antiviral	961.7	E857	E931.7	E950.4	E962.0	E980.4
arsenical	961.1	E857	E931.1	E950.4	E962.0	E980.4
ENT agents	976.6	E858.7	E946.6	E950.4	E962.0	E980.4
heavy metals NEC	961.2	E857	E931.2	E950.4	E962.0	E980.4
local	976.0	E858.7	E946.0	E950.4	E962.0	E980.4
ophthalmic preparation	976.5	E858.7	E946.5	E950.4	E962.0	E980.4
topical NEC	976.0	E858.7	E946.0	E950.4	E962.0	E980.4
Anti–inflammatory agents (topical)	976.0	E858.7	E946.0	E950.4	E962.0	E980.4
Antiknock (tetraethyl lead)	984.1	E862.1	—	E950.9	E962.1	E980.9
Antilipemics	972.2	E858.3	E942.2	E950.4	E962.0	E980.4

Substance	Poisoning	Accident	Therapeutic Use	Suicide Attempt	Assault	Undetermined
			External Cause (E-Code)			
Antimalarials	961.4	E857	E931.4	E950.4	E962.0	E980.4
Antimony (compounds) (vapor) NEC	985.4	E866.2	—	E950.9	E962.1	E980.9
anti–infectives	961.2	E857	E931.2	E950.4	E962.0	E980.4
pesticides (vapor)	985.4	E863.4	—	E950.6	E962.2	E980.7
potassium tartrate	961.2	E857	E931.2	E950.4	E962.0	E980.4
tartrated	961.2	E857	E931.2	E950.4	E962.0	E980.4
Antimuscarinic agents	971.1	E855.4	E941.1	E950.4	E962.0	E980.4
Antimycobacterials NEC	961.8	E857	E931.8	E950.4	E962.0	E980.4
antibiotics	960.6	E856	E930.6	E950.4	E962.0	E980.4
Antineoplastic agents	963.1	E858.1	E933.1	E950.4	E962.0	E980.4
antibiotics	960.7	E856	E930.7	E950.4	E962.0	E980.4
Anti–Parkinsonism agents	966.4	E855.0	E936.4	E950.4	E962.0	E980.4
Antiphlogistics	965.69	E850.6	E935.6	E950.0	E962.0	E980.0
Antiprotozoals NEC	961.5	E857	E931.5	E950.4	E962.0	E980.4
blood	961.4	E857	E931.4	E950.4	E962.0	E980.4
Antipruritics (local)	976.1	E858.7	E946.1	E950.4	E962.0	E980.4
Antipsychotic agents NEC	969.3	E853.8	E939.3	E950.3	E962.0	E980.3
Antipyretics	965.9	E850.9	E935.9	E950.0	E962.0	E980.0
specified NEC	965.8	E850.8	E935.8	E950.0	E962.0	E980.0
Antipyrine	965.5	E850.5	E935.5	E950.0	E962.0	E980.0
Antirabies serum (equine)	979.9	E858.8	E949.9	E950.4	E962.0	E980.4
Antirheumatics	965.69	E850.6	E935.6	E950.0	E962.0	E980.0
Antiseborrheics	976.4	E858.7	E946.4	E950.4	E962.0	E980.4
Antiseptics (external) (medicinal)	976.0	E858.7	E946.0	E950.4	E962.0	E980.4
Antistine	963.0	E858.1	E933.0	E950.4	E962.0	E980.4
Antithyroid agents	962.8	E858.0	E932.8	E950.4	E962.0	E980.4
Antitoxin, any	979.9	E858.8	E949.9	E950.4	E962.0	E980.4
Antituberculars	961.8	E857	E931.8	E950.4	E962.0	E980.4
antibiotics	960.6	E856	E930.6	E950.4	E962.0	E980.4
Antitussives	975.4	E858.6	E945.5	E950.4	E962.0	E980.4
Antivaricose agents (sclerosing)	972.7	E858.3	E942.7	E950.4	E962.0	E980.4
Antivenin (crotaline) (spider–bite)	979.9	E858.8	E949.9	E950.4	E962.0	E980.4
Antivert	963.0	E858.1	E933.0	E950.4	E962.0	E980.4
Antivirals NEC	961.7	E857	E931.7	E950.4	E962.0	E980.4
Ant poisons — *see* Pesticides						
Antrol	989.4	E863.4	—	E950.6	E962.1	E980.7
fungicide	989.4	E863.6	—	E950.6	E962.1	E980.7
Apomorphine hydrochloride (emetic)	973.6	E858.4	E943.6	E950.4	E962.0	E980.4
Appetite depressants, central	977.0	E858.8	E947.0	E950.4	E962.0	E980.4
Apresoline	972.6	E858.3	E942.6	E950.4	E962.0	E980.4
Aprobarbital, aprobarbitone	967.0	E851	E937.0	E950.1	E962.0	E980.1
Apronalide	967.8	E852.8	E937.8	E950.2	E962.0	E980.2
Aqua fortis	983.1	E864.1	—	E950.7	E962.1	E980.6
Arachis oil (topical)	976.3	E858.7	E946.3	E950.4	E962.0	E980.4
cathartic	973.2	E858.4	E943.2	E950.4	E962.0	E980.4
Aralen	961.4	E857	E931.4	E950.4	E962.0	E980.4
Arginine salts	974.5	E858.5	E944.5	E950.4	E962.0	E980.4
Argyrol	976.0	E858.7	E946.0	E950.4	E962.0	E980.4
ENT agent	976.6	E858.7	E946.6	E950.4	E962.0	E980.4
ophthalmic preparation	976.5	E858.7	E946.5	E950.4	E962.0	E980.4
Aristocort	962.0	E858.0	E932.0	E950.4	E962.0	E980.4
ENT agent	976.6	E858.7	E946.6	E950.4	E962.0	E980.4
ophthalmic preparation	976.5	E858.7	E946.5	E950.4	E962.0	E980.4
topical NEC	976.0	E858.7	E946.0	E950.4	E962.0	E980.4
Aromatics, corrosive	983.0	E864.0	—	E950.7	E962.1	E980.6
disinfectants	983.0	E861.4	—	E950.7	E962.1	E980.6
Arsenate of lead (insecticide)	985.1	E863.4	—	E950.8	E962.1	E980.8
herbicide	985.1	E863.5	—	E950.8	E962.1	E980.8
Arsenic, arsenicals (compounds) (dust) (fumes) (vapor) NEC	985.1	E866.3	—	E950.8	E962.1	E980.8

Substance	Poisoning	Accident	Therapeutic Use	Suicide Attempt	Assault	Undetermined
			External Cause (E-Code)			
anti–infectives	961.1	E857	E931.1	E950.4	E962.0	E980.4
pesticide (dust) (fumes)	985.1	E863.4	—	E950.8	E962.1	E980.8
Arsine (gas)	985.1	E866.3	—	E950.8	E962.1	E980.8
Arsphenamine (silver)	961.1	E857	E931.1	E950.4	E962.0	E980.4
Arsthinol	961.1	E857	E931.1	E950.4	E962.0	E980.4
Artane	971.1	E855.4	E941.1	E950.4	E962.0	E980.4
Arthropod (venomous) NEC	989.5	E905.5	—	E950.9	E962.1	E980.9
Asbestos	989.81	E866.8	—	E950.9	E962.1	E980.9
Ascaridole	961.6	E857	E931.6	E950.4	E962.0	E980.4
Ascorbic acid	963.5	E858.1	E933.5	E950.4	E962.0	E980.4
Asiaticoside	976.0	E858.7	E946.0	E950.4	E962.0	E980.4
Aspidium (oleoresin)	961.6	E857	E931.6	E950.4	E962.0	E980.4
Aspirin	965.1	E850.3	E935.3	E950.0	E962.0	E980.0
Astringents (local)	976.2	E858.7	E946.2	E950.4	E962.0	E980.4
Atabrine	961.3	E857	E931.3	E950.4	E962.0	E980.4
Ataractics	969.5	E853.8	E939.5	E950.3	E962.0	E980.3
Atonia drug, intestinal	973.3	E858.4	E943.3	E950.4	E962.0	E980.4
Atophan	974.7	E858.5	E944.7	E950.4	E962.0	E980.4
Atropine	971.1	E855.4	E941.1	E950.4	E962.0	E980.4
Attapulgite	973.5	E858.4	E943.5	E950.4	E962.0	E980.4
Attenuvax	979.4	E858.8	E949.4	E950.4	E962.0	E980.4
Aureomycin	960.4	E856	E930.4	E950.4	E962.0	E980.4
ophthalmic preparation	976.5	E858.7	E946.5	E950.4	E962.0	E980.4
topical NEC	976.0	E858.7	E946.0	E950.4	E962.0	E980.4
Aurothioglucose	965.69	E850.6	E935.6	E950.0	E962.0	E980.0
Aurothioglycanide	965.69	E850.6	E935.6	E950.0	E962.0	E980.0
Aurothiomalate	965.69	E850.6	E935.6	E950.0	E962.0	E980.0
Automobile fuel	981	E862.1	—	E950.9	E962.1	E980.9
Autonomic nervous system agents NEC	971.9	E855.9	E941.9	E950.4	E962.0	E980.4
Avlosulfon	961.8	E857	E931.8	E950.4	E962.0	E980.4
Avomine	967.8	E852.8	E937.8	E950.2	E962.0	E980.2
Azacyclonol	969.5	E853.8	E939.5	E950.3	E962.0	E980.3
Azapetine	971.3	E855.6	E941.3	E950.4	E962.0	E980.4
Azaribine	963.1	E858.1	E933.1	E950.4	E962.0	E980.4
Azaserine	960.7	E856	E930.7	E950.4	E962.0	E980.4
Azathioprine	963.1	E858.1	E933.1	E950.4	E962.0	E980.4
Azosulfamide	961.0	E857	E931.0	E950.4	E962.0	E980.4
Azulfidine	961.0	E857	E931.0	E950.4	E962.0	E980.4
Azuresin	977.8	E858.8	E947.8	E950.4	E962.0	E980.4
Bacimycin	976.0	E858.7	E946.0	E950.4	E962.0	E980.4
ophthalmic preparation	976.5	E858.7	E946.5	E950.4	E962.0	E980.4
Bacitracin	960.8	E856	E930.8	E950.4	E962.0	E980.4
ENT agent	976.6	E858.7	E946.6	E950.4	E962.0	E980.4
ophthalmic preparation	976.5	E858.7	E946.5	E950.4	E962.0	E980.4
topical NEC	976.0	E858.7	E946.0	E950.4	E962.0	E980.4
Baking soda	963.3	E858.1	E933.3	E950.4	E962.0	E980.4
BAL	963.8	E858.1	E933.8	E950.4	E962.0	E980.4
Bamethan (sulfate)	972.5	E858.3	E942.5	E950.4	E962.0	E980.4
Bamipine	963.0	E858.1	E933.0	E950.4	E962.0	E980.4
Baneberry	988.2	E865.4	—	E950.9	E962.1	E980.9
Banewort	988.2	E865.4	—	E950.9	E962.1	E980.9
Barbenyl	967.0	E851	E937.0	E950.1	E962.0	E980.1
Barbital, barbitone	967.0	E851	E937.0	E950.1	E962.0	E980.1
Barbiturates, barbituric acid	967.0	E851	E937.0	E950.1	E962.0	E980.1
anesthetic (intravenous)	968.3	E855.1	E938.3	E950.4	E962.0	E980.4
Barium (carbonate) (chloride) (sulfate)	985.8	E866.4	—	E950.9	E962.1	E980.9
diagnostic agent	977.8	E858.8	E947.8	E950.4	E962.0	E980.4
pesticide	985.8	E863.4	—	E950.6	E962.1	E980.7
rodenticide	985.8	E863.7	—	E950.6	E962.1	E980.7
Barrier cream	976.3	E858.7	E946.3	E950.4	E962.0	E980.4
Battery acid or fluid	983.1	E864.1	—	E950.7	E962.1	E980.6

Substance	Poisoning	Accident	Therapeutic Use	Suicide Attempt	Assault	Undetermined
			External Cause (E-Code)			
Bay rum	980.8	E860.8	—	E950.9	E962.1	E980.9
BCG vaccine	978.0	E858.8	E948.0	E950.4	E962.0	E980.4
Bearsfoot	988.2	E865.4	—	E950.9	E962.1	E980.9
Beclamide	966.3	E855.0	E936.3	E950.4	E962.0	E980.4
Bee (sting) (venom)	989.5	E905.3	—	E950.9	E962.1	E980.9
Belladonna (alkaloids)	971.1	E855.4	E941.1	E950.4	E962.0	E980.4
Bemegride	970.0	E854.3	E940.0	E950.4	E962.0	E980.4
Benactyzine	969.8	E855.8	E939.8	E950.3	E962.0	E980.3
Benadryl	963.0	E858.1	E933.0	E950.4	E962.0	E980.4
Bendrofluazide	974.3	E858.5	E944.3	E950.4	E962.0	E980.4
Bendroflumethiazide	974.3	E858.5	E944.3	E950.4	E962.0	E980.4
Benemid	974.7	E858.5	E944.7	E950.4	E962.0	E980.4
Benethamine penicillin G	960.0	E856	E930.0	E950.4	E962.0	E980.4
Benisone	976.0	E858.7	E946.0	E950.4	E962.0	E980.4
Benoquin	976.8	E858.7	E946.8	E950.4	E962.0	E980.4
Benoxinate	968.5	E855.2	E938.5	E950.4	E962.0	E980.4
Bentonite	976.3	E858.7	E946.3	E950.4	E962.0	E980.4
Benzalkonium (chloride)	976.0	E858.7	E946.0	E950.4	E962.0	E980.4
ophthalmic preparation	976.5	E858.7	E946.5	E950.4	E962.0	E980.4
Benzamidosalicylate (calcium)	961.8	E857	E931.8	E950.4	E962.0	E980.4
Benzathine penicillin	960.0	E856	E930.0	E950.4	E962.0	E980.4
Benzcarbimine	963.1	E858.1	E933.1	E950.4	E962.0	E980.4
Benzedrex	971.2	E855.5	E941.2	E950.4	E962.0	E980.4
Benzedrine (amphetamine)	969.7	E854.2	E939.7	E950.3	E962.0	E980.3
Benzene (acetyl) (dimethyl) (methyl) (solvent) (vapor)	982.0	E862.4	—	E950.9	E962.1	E980.9
hexachloride (gamma) (insecticide) (vapor)	989.2	E863.0	—	E950.6	E962.1	E980.7
Benzethonium	976.0	E858.7	E946.0	E950.4	E962.0	E980.4
Benzhexol (chloride)	966.4	E855.0	E936.4	E950.4	E962.0	E980.4
Benzilonium	971.1	E855.4	E941.1	E950.4	E962.0	E980.4
Benzin(e) — *see* Ligroin						
Benziodarone	972.4	E858.3	E942.4	E950.4	E962.0	E980.4
Benzocaine	968.5	E855.2	E938.5	E950.4	E962.0	E980.4
Benzodiapin	969.4	E853.2	E939.4	E950.3	E962.0	E980.3
Benzodiazepines (tranquilizers) NEC	969.4	E853.2	E939.4	E950.3	E962.0	E980.3
Benzoic acid (with salicylic acid) (anti–infective)	976.0	E858.7	E946.0	E950.4	E962.0	E980.4
Benzoin	976.3	E858.7	E946.3	E950.4	E962.0	E980.4
Benzol (vapor)	982.0	E862.4	—	E950.9	E962.1	E980.9
Benzomorphan	965.09	E850.2	E935.2	E950.0	E962.0	E980.0
Benzonatate	975.4	E858.6	E945.4	E950.4	E962.0	E980.4
Benzothiadiazides	974.3	E858.5	E944.3	E950.4	E962.0	E980.4
Benzoylpas	961.8	E857	E931.8	E950.4	E962.0	E980.4
Benzperidol	969.5	E853.8	E939.5	E950.3	E962.0	E980.3
Benzphetamine	977.0	E858.8	E947.0	E950.4	E962.0	E980.4
Benzpyrinium	971.0	E855.3	E941.0	E950.4	E962.0	E980.4
Benzquinamide	963.0	E858.1	E933.0	E950.4	E962.0	E980.4
Benzthiazide	974.3	E858.5	E944.3	E950.4	E962.0	E980.4
Benztropine	971.1	E855.4	E941.1	E950.4	E962.0	E980.4
Benzyl						
acetate	982.8	E862.4	—	E950.9	E962.1	E980.9
benzoate (anti–infective)	976.0	E858.7	E946.0	E950.4	E962.0	E980.4
morphine	965.09	E850.2	E935.2	E950.0	E962.0	E980.0
penicillin	960.0	E856	E930.0	E950.4	E962.0	E980.4
Bephenium hydroxynapthoate	961.6	E857	E931.6	E950.4	E962.0	E980.4
Bergamot oil	989.89	E866.8	—	E950.9	E962.1	E980.9
Berries, poisonous	988.2	E865.3	—	E950.9	E962.1	E980.9
Beryllium (compounds) (fumes)	985.3	E866.4	—	E950.9	E962.1	E980.9
Beta–carotene	976.3	E858.7	E946.3	E950.4	E962.0	E980.4

Substance	Poisoning	External Cause (E-Code)				
		Accident	Therapeutic Use	Suicide Attempt	Assault	Undetermined
Beta–Chlor	967.1	E852.0	E937.1	E950.2	E962.0	E980.2
Betamethasone	962.0	E858.0	E932.0	E950.4	E962.0	E980.4
topical	976.0	E858.7	E946.0	E950.4	E962.0	E980.4
Betazole	977.8	E858.8	E947.8	E950.4	E962.0	E980.4
Bethanechol	971.0	E855.3	E941.0	E950.4	E962.0	E980.4
Bethanidine	972.6	E858.3	E942.6	E950.4	E962.0	E980.4
Betula oil	976.3	E858.7	E946.3	E950.4	E962.0	E980.4
Bhang	969.6	E854.1	E939.6	E950.3	E962.0	E980.3
Bialamicol	961.5	E857	E931.5	E950.4	E962.0	E980.4
Bichloride of mercury — *see* Mercury, chloride						
Bichromates (calcium) (crystals) (potassium) (sodium)	983.9	E864.3	—	E950.7	E962.1	E980.6
fumes	987.8	E869.8	—	E952.8	E962.2	E982.8
Biguanide derivatives, oral	962.3	E858.0	E932.3	E950.4	E962.0	E980.4
Biligrafin	977.8	E858.8	E947.8	E950.4	E962.0	E980.4
Bilopaque	977.8	E858.8	E947.8	E950.4	E962.0	E980.4
Bioflavonoids	972.8	E858.3	E942.8	E950.4	E962.0	E980.4
Biological substance NEC	979.9	E858.8	E949.9	E950.4	E962.0	E980.4
Biperiden	966.4	E855.0	E936.4	E950.4	E962.0	E980.4
Bisacodyl	973.1	E858.4	E943.1	E950.4	E962.0	E980.4
Bishydroxycoumarin	964.2	E858.2	E934.2	E950.4	E962.0	E980.4
Bismarsen	961.1	E857	E931.1	E950.4	E962.0	E980.4
Bismuth (compounds) NEC	985.8	E866.4	—	E950.9	E962.1	E980.9
anti–infectives	961.2	E857	E931.2	E950.4	E962.0	E980.4
subcarbonate	973.5	E858.4	E943.5	E950.4	E962.0	E980.4
sulfarsphenamine	961.1	E857	E931.1	E950.4	E962.0	E980.4
Bithionol	961.6	E857	E931.6	E950.4	E962.0	E980.4
Bitter almond oil	989.0	E866.8	—	E950.9	E962.1	E980.9
Bittersweet	988.2	E865.4	—	E950.9	E962.1	E980.9
Black						
flag	989.4	E863.4	—	E950.6	E962.1	E980.7
henbane	988.2	E865.4	—	E950.9	E962.1	E980.9
leaf (40)	989.4	E863.4	—	E950.6	E962.1	E980.7
widow spider (bite)	989.5	E905.1	—	E950.9	E962.1	E980.9
antivenin	979.9	E858.8	E949.9	E950.4	E962.0	E980.4
Blast furnace gas (carbon monoxide from)	986	E868.8	—	E952.1	E962.2	E982.1
Bleach NEC	983.9	E864.3	—	E950.7	E962.1	E980.6
Bleaching solutions	983.9	E864.3	—	E950.7	E962.1	E980.6
Bleomycin (sulfate)	960.7	E856	E930.7	E950.4	E962.0	E980.4
Blockain	968.9	E855.2	E938.9	E950.4	E962.0	E980.4
infiltration (subcutaneous)	968.5	E855.2	E938.5	E950.4	E962.0	E980.4
nerve block (peripheral) (plexus)	968.6	E855.2	E938.6	E950.4	E962.0	E980.4
topical (surface)	968.5	E855.2	E938.5	E950.4	E962.0	E980.4
Blood (derivatives) (natural) (plasma) (whole)	964.7	E858.2	E934.7	E950.4	E962.0	E980.4
affecting agent	964.9	E858.2	E934.9	E950.4	E962.0	E980.4
specified NEC	964.8	E858.2	E934.8	E950.4	E962.0	E980.4
substitute (macromolecular)	964.8	E858.2	E934.8	E950.4	E962.0	E980.4
Blue velvet	965.09	E850.2	E935.2	E950.0	E962.0	E980.0
Bone meal	989.89	E866.5	—	E950.9	E962.1	E980.9
Bonine	963.0	E858.1	E933.0	E950.4	E962.0	E980.4
Boracic acid	976.0	E858.7	E946.0	E950.4	E962.0	E980.4
ENT agent	976.6	E858.7	E946.6	E950.4	E962.0	E980.4
ophthalmic preparation	976.5	E858.7	E946.5	E950.4	E962.0	E980.4
Borate (cleanser) (sodium)	989.6	E861.3	—	E950.9	E962.1	E980.9
Borax (cleanser)	989.6	E861.3	—	E950.9	E962.1	E980.9
Boric acid	976.0	E858.7	E946.0	E950.4	E962.0	E980.4
ENT agent	976.6	E858.7	E946.6	E950.4	E962.0	E980.4
ophthalmic preparation	976.5	E858.7	E946.5	E950.4	E962.0	E980.4
Boron hydride NEC	989.89	E866.8	—	E950.9	E962.1	E980.9

Substance	Poisoning	External Cause (E-Code)				
		Accident	Therapeutic Use	Suicide Attempt	Assault	Undetermined
fumes or gas	987.8	E869.8	—	E952.8	E962.2	E982.8
Botox	975.3	E858.6	E945.3	E950.4	E962.0	E980.4
Brake fluid vapor	987.8	E869.8	—	E952.8	E962.2	E982.8
Brass (compounds) (fumes)	985.8	E866.4	—	E950.9	E962.1	E980.9
Brasso	981	E861.3	—	E950.9	E962.1	E980.9
Bretylium (tosylate)	972.6	E858.3	E942.6	E950.4	E962.0	E980.4
Brevital (sodium)	968.3	E855.1	E938.3	E950.4	E962.0	E980.4
British antilewisite	963.8	E858.1	E933.8	E950.4	E962.0	E980.4
Bromal (hydrate)	967.3	E852.2	E937.3	E950.2	E962.0	E980.2
Bromelains	963.4	E858.1	E933.4	E950.4	E962.0	E980.4
Bromides NEC	967.3	E852.2	E937.3	E950.2	E962.0	E980.2
Bromine (vapor)	987.8	E869.8	—	E952.8	E962.2	E982.8
compounds (medicinal)	967.3	E852.2	E937.3	E950.2	E962.0	E980.2
Bromisovalum	967.3	E852.2	E937.3	E950.2	E962.0	E980.2
Bromobenzyl cyanide	987.5	E869.3	—	E952.8	E962.2	E982.8
Bromodiphenhydramine	963.0	E858.1	E933.0	E950.4	E962.0	E980.4
Bromoform	967.3	E852.2	E937.3	E950.2	E962.0	E980.2
Bromophenol blue reagent	977.8	E858.8	E947.8	E950.4	E962.0	E980.4
Bromosalicylhydroxamic acid	961.8	E857	E931.8	E950.4	E962.0	E980.4
Bromo–seltzer	965.4	E850.4	E935.4	E950.0	E962.0	E980.0
Brompheniramine	963.0	E858.1	E933.0	E950.4	E962.0	E980.4
Bromural	967.3	E852.2	E937.3	E950.2	E962.0	E980.2
Brown spider (bite) (venom)	989.5	E905.1	—	E950.9	E962.1	E980.9
Brucia	988.2	E865.3	—	E950.9	E962.1	E980.9
Brucine	989.1	E863.7	—	E950.6	E962.1	E980.7
Brunswick green — *see* Copper						
Bruten — *see* Ibuprofen						
Bryonia (alba) (dioica)	988.2	E865.4	—	E950.9	E962.1	E980.9
Buclizine	969.5	E853.8	E939.5	E950.3	E962.0	E980.3
Bufferin	965.1	E850.3	E935.3	E950.0	E962.0	E980.0
Bufotenine	969.6	E854.1	E939.6	E950.3	E962.0	E980.3
Buphenine	971.2	E855.5	E941.2	E950.4	E962.0	E980.4
Bupivacaine	968.9	E855.2	E938.9	E950.4	E962.0	E980.4
infiltration (subcutaneous)	968.5	E855.2	E938.5	E950.4	E962.0	E980.4
nerve block (peripheral) (plexus)	968.6	E855.2	E938.6	E950.4	E962.0	E980.4
Busulfan	963.1	E858.1	E933.1	E950.4	E962.0	E980.4
Butabarbital (sodium)	967.0	E851	E937.0	E950.1	E962.0	E980.1
Butabarbitone	967.0	E851	E937.0	E950.1	E962.0	E980.1
Butabarpal	967.0	E851	E937.0	E950.1	E962.0	E980.1
Butacaine	968.5	E855.2	E938.5	E950.4	E962.0	E980.4
Butallylonal	967.0	E851	E937.0	E950.1	E962.0	E980.1
Butane (distributed in mobile container)	987.0	E868.0	—	E951.1	E962.2	E981.1
distributed through pipes	987.0	E867	—	E951.0	E962.2	E981.0
incomplete combustion of — *see* Carbon monoxide, butane						
Butanol	980.3	E860.4	—	E950.9	E962.1	E980.9
Butanone	982.8	E862.4	—	E950.9	E962.1	E980.9
Butaperazine	969.1	E853.0	E939.1	E950.3	E962.0	E980.3
Butazolidin	965.5	E850.5	E935.5	E950.0	E962.0	E980.0
Butethal	967.0	E851	E937.0	E950.1	E962.0	E980.1
Butethamate	971.1	E855.4	E941.1	E950.4	E962.0	E980.4
Buthalitone (sodium)	968.3	E855.1	E938.3	E950.4	E962.0	E980.4
Butisol (sodium)	967.0	E851	E937.0	E950.1	E962.0	E980.1
Butobarbital, butobarbitone	967.0	E851	E937.0	E950.1	E962.0	E980.1
Butriptyline	969.0	E854.0	E939.0	E950.3	E962.0	E980.3
Buttercups	988.2	E865.4	—	E950.9	E962.1	E980.9
Butter of antimony — *see* Antimony						
Butyl						
acetate (secondary)	982.8	E862.4	—	E950.9	E962.1	E980.9
alcohol	980.3	E860.4	—	E950.9	E962.1	E980.9

Substance	Poisoning	Accident	Therapeutic Use	Suicide Attempt	Assault	Undetermined
			External Cause (E-Code)			
carbinol	980.8	E860.8	—	E950.9	E962.1	E980.9
carbitol	982.8	E862.4	—	E950.9	E962.1	E980.9
cellosolve	982.8	E862.4	—	E950.9	E962.1	E980.9
chloral (hydrate)	967.1	E852.0	E937.1	E950.2	E962.0	E980.2
formate	982.8	E862.4	—	E950.9	E962.1	E980.9
scopolammonium bromide	971.1	E855.4	E941.1	E950.4	E962.0	E980.4
Butyn	968.5	E855.2	E938.5	E950.4	E962.0	E980.4
Butyrophenone (–based tranquilizers)	969.2	E853.1	E939.2	E950.3	E962.0	E980.3
Cacodyl, cacodylic acid — *see* Arsenic						
Cactinomycin	960.7	E856	E930.7	E950.4	E962.0	E980.4
Cade oil	976.4	E858.7	E946.4	E950.4	E962.0	E980.4
Cadmium (chloride) (compounds) (dust) (fumes) (oxide)	985.5	E866.4	—	E950.9	E962.1	E980.9
sulfide (medicinal) NEC	976.4	E858.7	E946.4	E950.4	E962.0	E980.4
Caffeine	969.7	E854.2	E939.7	E950.3	E962.0	E980.3
Calabar bean	988.2	E865.4	—	E950.9	E962.1	E980.9
Caladium seguinium	988.2	E865.4	—	E950.9	E962.1	E980.9
Calamine (liniment) (lotion)	976.3	E858.7	E946.3	E950.4	E962.0	E980.4
Calciferol	963.5	E858.1	E933.5	E950.4	E962.0	E980.4
Calcium (salts) NEC	974.5	E858.5	E944.5	E950.4	E962.0	E980.4
acetylsalicylate	965.1	E850.3	E935.3	E950.0	E962.0	E980.0
benzamidosalicylate	961.8	E857	E931.8	E950.4	E962.0	E980.4
carbaspirin	965.1	E850.3	E935.3	E950.0	E962.0	E980.0
carbamide (citrated)	977.3	E858.8	E947.3	E950.4	E962.0	E980.4
carbonate (antacid)	973.0	E858.4	E943.0	E950.4	E962.0	E980.4
cyanide (citrated)	977.3	E858.8	E947.3	E950.4	E962.0	E980.4
dioctyl sulfosuccinate	973.2	E858.4	E943.2	E950.4	E962.0	E980.4
disodium edathamil	963.8	E858.1	E933.8	E950.4	E962.0	E980.4
disodium edetate	963.8	E858.1	E933.8	E950.4	E962.0	E980.4
EDTA	963.8	E858.1	E933.8	E950.4	E962.0	E980.4
hydrate, hydroxide	983.2	E864.2	—	E950.7	E962.1	E980.6
mandelate	961.9	E857	E931.9	E950.4	E962.0	E980.4
oxide	983.2	E864.2	—	E950.7	E962.1	E980.6
Calomel — *see* Mercury, chloride						
Caloric agents NEC	974.5	E858.5	E944.5	E950.4	E962.0	E980.4
Calusterone	963.1	E858.1	E933.1	E950.4	E962.0	E980.4
Camoquin	961.4	E857	E931.4	E950.4	E962.0	E980.4
Camphor (oil)	976.1	E858.7	E946.1	E950.4	E962.0	E980.4
Candeptin	976.0	E858.7	E946.0	E950.4	E962.0	E980.4
Candicidin	976.0	E858.7	E946.0	E950.4	E962.0	E980.4
Cannabinols	969.6	E854.1	E939.6	E950.3	E962.0	E980.3
Cannabis (derivatives) (indica) (sativa)	969.6	E854.1	E939.6	E950.3	E962.0	E980.3
Canned heat	980.1	E860.2	—	E950.9	E962.1	E980.9
Cantharides, cantharidin, cantharis	976.8	E858.7	E946.8	E950.4	E962.0	E980.4
Capillary agents	972.8	E858.3	E942.8	E950.4	E962.0	E980.4
Capreomycin	960.6	E856	E930.6	E950.4	E962.0	E980.4
Captodiame, captodiamine	969.5	E853.8	E939.5	E950.3	E962.0	E980.3
Caramiphen (hydrochloride)	971.1	E855.4	E941.1	E950.4	E962.0	E980.4
Carbachol	971.0	E855.3	E941.0	E950.4	E962.0	E980.4
Carbacrylamine resins	974.5	E858.5	E944.5	E950.4	E962.0	E980.4
Carbamate (sedative)	967.8	E852.8	E937.8	E950.2	E962.0	E980.2
herbicide	989.3	E863.5	—	E950.6	E962.1	E980.7
insecticide	989.3	E863.2	—	E950.6	E962.1	E980.7
Carbamazepine	966.3	E855.0	E936.3	E950.4	E962.0	E980.4
Carbamic esters	967.8	E852.8	E937.8	E950.2	E962.0	E980.2
Carbamide	974.4	E858.5	E944.4	E950.4	E962.0	E980.4
topical	976.8	E858.7	E946.8	E950.4	E962.0	E980.4
Carbamylcholine chloride	971.0	E855.3	E941.0	E950.4	E962.0	E980.4
Carbarsone	961.1	E857	E931.1	E950.4	E962.0	E980.4
Carbaryl	989.3	E863.2	—	E950.6	E962.1	E980.7
Carbaspirin	965.1	E850.3	E935.3	E950.0	E962.0	E980.0

Substance	Poisoning	External Cause (E-Code)				
		Accident	Therapeutic Use	Suicide Attempt	Assault	Undetermined
Carbazochrome	972.8	E858.3	E942.8	E950.4	E962.0	E980.4
Carbenicillin	960.0	E856	E930.0	E950.4	E962.0	E980.4
Carbenoxolone	973.8	E858.4	E943.8	E950.4	E962.0	E980.4
Carbetapentane	975.4	E858.6	E945.4	E950.4	E962.0	E980.4
Carbimazole	962.8	E858.0	E932.8	E950.4	E962.0	E980.4
Carbinol	980.1	E860.2	—	E950.9	E962.1	E980.9
Carbinoxamine	963.0	E858.1	E933.0	E950.4	E962.0	E980.4
Carbitol	982.8	E862.4	—	E950.9	E962.1	E980.9
Carbocaine	968.9	E855.2	E938.9	E950.4	E962.0	E980.4
infiltration (subcutaneous)	968.5	E855.2	E938.5	E950.4	E962.0	E980.4
nerve block (peripheral) (plexus)	968.6	E855.2	E938.6	E950.4	E962.0	E980.4
topical (surface)	968.5	E855.2	E938.5	E950.4	E962.0	E980.4
Carbol–fuchsin solution	976.0	E858.7	E946.0	E950.4	E962.0	E980.4
Carbolic acid (*see also* Phenol)	983.0	E864.0	—	E950.7	E962.1	E980.6
Carbomycin	960.8	E856	E930.8	E950.4	E962.0	E980.4
Carbon						
bisulfide (liquid) (vapor)	982.2	E862.4	—	E950.9	E962.1	E980.9
dioxide (gas)	987.8	E869.8	—	E952.8	E962.2	E982.8
disulfide (liquid) (vapor)	982.2	E862.4	—	E950.9	E962.1	E980.9
monoxide (from incomplete combustion of) (in) NEC	986	E868.9	—	E952.1	E962.2	E982.1
blast furnace gas	986	E868.8	—	E952.1	E962.2	E982.1
butane (distributed in mobile container)	986	E868.0	—	E951.1	E962.2	E981.1
distributed through pipes	986	E867	—	E951.0	E962.2	E981.0
charcoal fumes	986	E868.3	—	E952.1	E962.2	E982.1
coal						
gas (piped)	986	E867	—	E951.0	E962.2	E981.0
solid (in domestic stoves, fireplaces)	986	E868.3	—	E952.1	E962.2	E982.1
coke (in domestic stoves, fireplaces)	986	E868.3	—	E952.1	E962.2	E982.1
exhaust gas (motor) not in transit	986	E868.2	—	E952.0	E962.2	E982.0
combustion engine, any not in watercraft	986	E868.2	—	E952.0	E962.2	E982.0
farm tractor, not in transit	986	E868.2	—	E952.0	E962.2	E982.0
gas engine	986	E868.2	—	E952.0	E962.2	E982.0
motor pump	986	E868.2	—	E952.0	E962.2	E982.0
motor vehicle, not in transit	986	E868.2	—	E952.0	E962.2	E982.0
fuel (in domestic use)	986	E868.3	—	E952.1	E962.2	E982.1
gas (piped)	986	E867	—	E951.0	E962.2	E981.0
in mobile container	986	E868.0	—	E951.1	E962.2	E981.1
utility	986	E868.1	—	E951.8	E962.2	E981.1
in mobile container	986	E868.0	—	E951.1	E962.2	E981.1
piped (natural)	986	E867	—	E951.0	E962.2	E981.0
illuminating gas	986	E868.1	—	E951.8	E962.2	E981.8
industrial fuels or gases, any	986	E868.8	—	E952.1	E962.2	E982.1
kerosene (in domestic stoves, fireplaces)	986	E868.3	—	E952.1	E962.2	E982.1
kiln gas or vapor	986	E868.8	—	E952.1	E962.2	E982.1
motor exhaust gas, not in transit	986	E868.2	—	E952.0	E962.2	E982.0
piped gas (manufactured) (natural)	986	E867	—	E951.0	E962.2	E981.0
producer gas	986	E868.8	—	E952.1	E962.2	E982.1
propane (distributed in mobile container)	986	E868.0	—	E951.1	E962.2	E981.1
distributed through pipes	986	E867	—	E951.0	E962.2	E981.0
specified source NEC	986	E868.8	—	E952.1	E962.2	E982.1
stove gas	986	E868.1	—	E951.8	E962.2	E981.8
piped	986	E867	—	E951.0	E962.2	E981.0
utility gas	986	E868.1	—	E951.8	E962.2	E981.8
piped	986	E867	—	E951.0	E962.2	E981.0

Substance	Poisoning	Accident	Therapeutic Use	Suicide Attempt	Assault	Undetermined
			External Cause (E-Code)			
water gas	986	E868.1	—	E951.8	E962.2	E981.8
wood (in domestic stoves, fireplaces)	986	E868.3	—	E952.1	E962.2	E982.1
tetrachloride (vapor) NEC	987.8	E869.8	—	E952.8	E962.2	E982.8
liquid (cleansing agent) NEC	982.1	E861.3	—	E950.9	E962.1	E980.9
solvent	982.1	E862.4	—	E950.9	E962.1	E980.9
Carbonic acid (gas)	987.8	E869.8	—	E952.8	E962.2	E982.8
anhydrase inhibitors	974.2	E858.5	E944.2	E950.4	E962.0	E980.4
Carbowax	976.3	E858.7	E946.3	E950.4	E962.0	E980.4
Carbrital	967.0	E851	E937.0	E950.1	E962.0	E980.1
Carbromal (derivatives)	967.3	E852.2	E937.3	E950.2	E962.0	E980.2
Cardiac						
depressants	972.0	E858.3	E942.0	E950.4	E962.0	E980.4
rhythm regulators	972.0	E858.3	E942.0	E950.4	E962.0	E980.4
Cardiografin	977.8	E858.8	E947.8	E950.4	E962.0	E980.4
Cardio–green	977.8	E858.8	E947.8	E950.4	E962.0	E980.4
Cardiotonic glycosides	972.1	E858.3	E942.1	E950.4	E962.0	E980.4
Cardiovascular agents NEC	972.9	E858.3	E942.9	E950.4	E962.0	E980.4
Cardrase	974.2	E858.5	E944.2	E950.4	E962.0	E980.4
Carfusin	976.0	E858.7	E946.0	E950.4	E962.0	E980.4
Carisoprodol	968.0	E855.1	E938.0	E950.4	E962.0	E980.4
Carmustine	963.1	E858.1	E933.1	E950.4	E962.0	E980.4
Carotene	963.5	E858.1	E933.5	E950.4	E962.0	E980.4
Carphenazine (maleate)	969.1	E853.0	E939.1	E950.3	E962.0	E980.3
Carter's Little Pills	973.1	E858.4	E943.1	E950.4	E962.0	E980.4
Cascara (sagrada)	973.1	E858.4	E943.1	E950.4	E962.0	E980.4
Cassava	988.2	E865.4	—	E950.9	E962.1	E980.9
Castellani's paint	976.0	E858.7	E946.0	E950.4	E962.0	E980.4
Castor						
bean	988.2	E865.3	—	E950.9	E962.1	E980.9
oil	973.1	E858.4	E943.1	E950.4	E962.0	E980.4
Caterpillar (sting)	989.5	E905.5	—	E950.9	E962.1	E980.9
Catha (edulis)	970.8	E854.3	E940.8	E950.4	E962.0	E980.4
Cathartics NEC	973.3	E858.4	E943.3	E950.4	E962.0	E980.4
contact	973.1	E858.4	E943.1	E950.4	E962.0	E980.4
emollient	973.2	E858.4	E943.2	E950.4	E962.0	E980.4
intestinal irritants	973.1	E858.4	E943.1	E950.4	E962.0	E980.4
saline	973.3	E858.4	E943.3	E950.4	E962.0	E980.4
Cathomycin	960.8	E856	E930.8	E950.4	E962.0	E980.4
Caustic(s)	983.9	E864.4	—	E950.7	E962.1	E980.6
alkali	983.2	E864.2	—	E950.7	E962.1	E980.6
hydroxide	983.2	E864.2	—	E950.7	E962.1	E980.6
potash	983.2	E864.2	—	E950.7	E962.1	E980.6
soda	983.2	E864.2	—	E950.7	E962.1	E980.6
specified NEC	983.9	E864.3	—	E950.7	E962.1	E980.6
Ceepryn	976.0	E858.7	E946.0	E950.4	E962.0	E980.4
ENT agent	976.6	E858.7	E946.6	E950.4	E962.0	E980.4
lozenges	976.6	E858.7	E946.6	E950.4	E962.0	E980.4
Celestone	962.0	E858.0	E932.0	E950.4	E962.0	E980.4
topical	976.0	E858.7	E946.0	E950.4	E962.0	E980.4
Cellosolve	982.8	E862.4	—	E950.9	E962.1	E980.9
Cell stimulants and proliferants	976.8	E858.7	E946.8	E950.4	E962.0	E980.4
Cellulose derivatives, cathartic	973.3	E858.4	E943.3	E950.4	E962.0	E980.4
nitrates (topical)	976.3	E858.7	E946.3	E950.4	E962.0	E980.4
Centipede (bite)	989.5	E905.4	—	E950.9	E962.1	E980.9
Central nervous system						
depressants	968.4	E855.1	E938.4	E950.4	E962.0	E980.4
anesthetic (general) NEC	968.4	E855.1	E938.4	E950.4	E962.0	E980.4
gases NEC	968.2	E855.1	E938.2	E950.4	E962.0	E980.4
intravenous	968.3	E855.1	E938.3	E950.4	E962.0	E980.4
barbiturates	967.0	E851	E937.0	E950.1	E962.0	E980.1
bromides	967.3	E852.2	E937.3	E950.2	E962.0	E980.2

Substance	Poisoning	Accident	Therapeutic Use	Suicide Attempt	Assault	Undetermined
			External Cause (E-Code)			
cannabis sativa	969.6	E854.1	E939.6	E950.3	E962.0	E980.3
chloral hydrate	967.1	E852.0	E937.1	E950.2	E962.0	E980.2
hallucinogenics	969.6	E854.1	E939.6	E950.3	E962.0	E980.3
hypnotics	967.9	E852.9	E937.9	E950.2	E962.0	E980.2
specified NEC	967.8	E852.8	E937.8	E950.2	E962.0	E980.2
muscle relaxants	968.0	E855.1	E938.0	E950.4	E962.0	E980.4
paraldehyde	967.2	E852.1	E937.2	E950.2	E962.0	E980.2
sedatives	967.9	E852.9	E937.9	E950.2	E962.0	E980.2
mixed NEC	967.6	E852.5	E937.6	E950.2	E962.0	E980.2
specified NEC	967.8	E852.8	E937.8	E950.2	E962.0	E980.2
muscle–tone depressants	968.0	E855.1	E938.0	E950.4	E962.0	E980.4
stimulants	970.9	E854.3	E940.9	E950.4	E962.0	E980.4
amphetamines	969.7	E854.2	E939.7	E950.3	E962.0	E980.3
analeptics	970.0	E854.3	E940.0	E950.4	E962.0	E980.4
antidepressants	969.0	E854.0	E939.0	E950.3	E962.0	E980.3
opiate antagonists	970.1	E854.3	E940.0	E950.4	E962.0	E980.4
specified NEC	970.8	E854.3	E940.8	E950.4	E962.0	E980.4
Cephalexin	960.5	E856	E930.5	E950.4	E962.0	E980.4
Cephaloglycin	960.5	E856	E930.5	E950.4	E962.0	E980.4
Cephaloridine	960.5	E856	E930.5	E950.4	E962.0	E980.4
Cephalosporins NEC	960.5	E856	E930.5	E950.4	E962.0	E980.4
N (adicillin)	960.0	E856	E930.0	E950.4	E962.0	E980.4
Cephalothin (sodium)	960.5	E856	E930.5	E950.4	E962.0	E980.4
Cerbera (odallam)	988.2	E865.4	—	E950.9	E962.1	E980.9
Cerberin	972.1	E858.3	E942.1	E950.4	E962.0	E980.4
Cerebral stimulants	970.9	E854.3	E940.9	E950.4	E962.0	E980.4
psychotherapeutic	969.7	E854.2	E939.7	E950.3	E962.0	E980.3
specified NEC	970.8	E854.3	E940.8	E950.4	E962.0	E980.4
Cetalkonium (chloride)	976.0	E858.7	E946.0	E950.4	E962.0	E980.4
Cetoxime	963.0	E858.1	E933.0	E950.4	E962.0	E980.4
Cetrimide	976.2	E858.7	E946.2	E950.4	E962.0	E980.4
Cetylpyridinium	976.0	E858.7	E946.0	E950.4	E962.0	E980.4
ENT agent	976.6	E858.7	E946.6	E950.4	E962.0	E980.4
lozenges	976.6	E858.7	E946.6	E950.4	E962.0	E980.4
Cevadilla — *see* Sabadilla						
Cevitamic acid	963.5	E858.1	E933.5	E950.4	E962.0	E980.4
Chalk, precipitated	973.0	E858.4	E943.0	E950.4	E962.0	E980.4
Charcoal						
fumes (carbon monoxide)	986	E868.3	—	E952.1	E962.2	E982.1
industrial	986	E868.8	—	E952.1	E962.2	E982.1
medicinal (activated)	973.0	E858.4	E943.0	E950.4	E962.0	E980.4
Chelating agents NEC	977.2	E858.8	E947.2	E950.4	E962.0	E980.4
Chelidonium majus	988.2	E865.4	—	E950.9	E962.1	E980.9
Chemical substance	989.9	E866.9	—	E950.9	E962.1	E980.9
specified NEC	989.89	E866.8	—	E950.9	E962.1	E980.9
Chemotherapy, antineoplastic	963.1	E858.1	E933.1	E950.4	E962.0	E980.4
Chenopodium (oil)	961.6	E857	E931.6	E950.4	E962.0	E980.4
Cherry laurel	988.2	E865.4	—	E950.9	E962.1	E980.9
Chiniofon	961.3	E857	E931.3	E950.4	E962.0	E980.4
Chlophedianol	975.4	E858.6	E945.4	E950.4	E962.0	E980.4
Chloral (betaine) (formamide) (hydrate)	967.1	E852.0	E937.1	E950.2	E962.0	E980.2
Chloralamide	967.1	E852.0	E937.1	E950.2	E962.0	E980.2
Chlorambucil	963.1	E858.1	E933.1	E950.4	E962.0	E980.4
Chloramphenicol	960.2	E856	E930.2	E950.4	E962.0	E980.4
ENT agent	976.6	E858.7	E946.6	E950.4	E962.0	E980.4
ophthalmic preparation	976.5	E858.7	E946.5	E950.4	E962.0	E980.4
topical NEC	976.0	E858.7	E946.0	E950.4	E962.0	E980.4
Chlorate(s) (potassium) (sodium) NEC	983.9	E864.3	—	E950.7	E962.1	E980.6
herbicides	989.4	E863.5	—	E950.6	E962.1	E980.7
Chlorcyclizine	963.0	E858.1	E933.0	E950.4	E962.0	E980.4

Substance	Poisoning	Accident	Therapeutic Use	Suicide Attempt	Assault	Undetermined
			External Cause (E-Code)			
Chlordan(e) (dust)	989.2	E863.0	—	E950.6	E962.1	E980.7
Chlordantoin	976.0	E858.7	E946.0	E950.4	E962.0	E980.4
Chlordiazepoxide	969.4	E853.2	E939.4	E950.3	E962.0	E980.3
Chloresium	976.8	E858.7	E946.8	E950.4	E962.0	E980.4
Chlorethiazol	967.1	E852.0	E937.1	E950.2	E962.0	E980.2
Chlorethyl — *see* Ethyl, chloride						
Chloretone	967.1	E852.0	E937.1	E950.2	E962.0	E980.2
Chlorex	982.3	E862.4	—	E950.9	E962.1	E980.9
Chlorhexadol	967.1	E852.0	E937.1	E950.2	E962.0	E980.2
Chlorhexidine (hydrochloride)	976.0	E858.7	E946.0	E950.4	E962.0	E980.4
Chlorhydroxyquinolin	976.0	E858.7	E946.0	E950.4	E962.0	E980.4
Chloride of lime (bleach)	983.9	E864.3	—	E950.7	E962.1	E980.6
Chlorinated						
camphene	989.2	E863.0	—	E950.6	E962.1	E980.7
diphenyl	989.89	E866.8	—	E950.9	E962.1	E980.9
hydrocarbons NEC	989.2	E863.0	—	E950.6	E962.1	E980.7
solvent	982.3	E862.4	—	E950.9	E962.1	E980.9
lime (bleach)	983.9	E864.3	—	E950.7	E962.1	E980.6
naphthalene — *see* Naphthalene						
pesticides NEC	989.2	E863.0	—	E950.6	E962.1	E980.7
soda — *see* Sodium, hypochlorite						
Chlorine (fumes) (gas)	987.6	E869.8	—	E952.8	E962.2	E982.8
bleach	983.9	E864.3	—	E950.7	E962.1	E980.6
compounds NEC	983.9	E864.3	—	E950.7	E962.1	E980.6
disinfectant	983.9	E861.4	—	E950.7	E962.1	E980.6
releasing agents NEC	983.9	E864.3	—	E950.7	E962.1	E980.6
Chlorisondamine	972.3	E858.3	E942.3	E950.4	E962.0	E980.4
Chlormadinone	962.2	E858.0	E932.2	E950.4	E962.0	E980.4
Chlormerodrin	974.0	E858.5	E944.0	E950.4	E962.0	E980.4
Chlormethiazole	967.1	E852.0	E937.1	E950.2	E962.0	E980.2
Chlormethylenecycline	960.4	E856	E930.4	E950.4	E962.0	E980.4
Chlormezanone	969.5	E853.8	E939.5	E950.3	E962.0	E980.3
Chloroacetophenone	987.5	E869.3	—	E952.8	E962.2	E982.8
Chloroaniline	983.0	E864.0	—	E950.7	E962.1	E980.6
Chlorobenzene, chlorobenzol	982.0	E862.4	—	E950.9	E962.1	E980.9
Chlorobutanol	967.1	E852.0	E937.1	E950.2	E962.0	E980.2
Chlorodinitrobenzene	983.0	E864.0	—	E950.7	E962.1	E980.6
dust or vapor	987.8	E869.8	—	E952.8	E962.2	E982.8
Chloroethane — *see* Ethyl, chloride						
Chloroform (fumes) (vapor)	987.8	E869.8	—	E952.8	E962.2	E982.8
anesthetic (gas)	968.2	E855.1	E938.2	E950.4	E962.0	E980.4
liquid NEC	968.4	E855.1	E938.4	E950.4	E962.0	E980.4
solvent	982.3	E862.4	—	E950.9	E962.1	E980.9
Chloroguanide	961.4	E857	E931.4	E950.4	E962.0	E980.4
Chloromycetin	960.2	E856	E930.2	E950.4	E962.0	E980.4
ENT agent	976.6	E858.7	E946.6	E950.4	E962.0	E980.4
ophthalmic preparation	976.5	E858.7	E946.5	E950.4	E962.0	E980.4
otic solution	976.6	E858.7	E946.6	E950.4	E962.0	E980.4
topical NEC	976.0	E858.7	E946.0	E950.4	E962.0	E980.4
Chloronitrobenzene	983.0	E864.0	—	E950.7	E962.1	E980.6
dust or vapor	987.8	E869.8	—	E952.8	E962.2	E982.8
Chlorophenol	983.0	E864.0	—	E950.7	E962.1	E980.6
Chlorophenothane	989.2	E863.0	—	E950.6	E962.1	E980.7
Chlorophyll (derivatives)	976.8	E858.7	E946.8	E950.4	E962.0	E980.4
Chloropicrin (fumes)	987.8	E869.8	—	E952.8	E962.2	E982.8
fumigant	989.4	E863.8	—	E950.6	E962.1	E980.7
fungicide	989.4	E863.6	—	E950.6	E962.1	E980.7
pesticide (fumes)	989.4	E863.4	—	E950.6	E962.1	E980.7
Chloroprocaine	968.9	E855.2	E938.9	E950.4	E962.0	E980.4
infiltration (subcutaneous)	968.5	E855.2	E938.5	E950.4	E962.0	E980.4
nerve block (peripheral) (plexus)	968.6	E855.2	E938.6	E950.4	E962.0	E980.4

Substance	Poisoning	Accident	Therapeutic Use	Suicide Attempt	Assault	Undetermined
		External Cause (E-Code)				
Chloroptic	976.5	E858.7	E946.5	E950.4	E962.0	E980.4
Chloropurine	963.1	E858.1	E933.1	E950.4	E962.0	E980.4
Chloroquine (hydrochloride) (phosphate)	961.4	E857	E931.4	E950.4	E962.0	E980.4
Chlorothen	963.0	E858.1	E933.0	E950.4	E962.0	E980.4
Chlorothiazide	974.3	E858.5	E944.3	E950.4	E962.0	E980.4
Chlorotrianisene	962.2	E858.0	E932.2	E950.4	E962.0	E980.4
Chlorovinyldichloroarsine	985.1	E866.3	—	E950.8	E962.1	E980.8
Chloroxylenol	976.0	E858.7	E946.0	E950.4	E962.0	E980.4
Chlorphenesin (carbamate)	968.0	E855.1	E938.0	E950.4	E962.0	E980.4
topical (antifungal)	976.0	E858.7	E946.0	E950.4	E962.0	E980.4
Chlorpheniramine	963.0	E858.1	E933.0	E950.4	E962.0	E980.4
Chlorophenoxamine	966.4	E855.0	E936.4	E950.4	E962.0	E980.4
Chlorophentermine	977.0	E858.8	E947.0	E950.4	E962.0	E980.4
Chlorproguanil	961.4	E857	E931.4	E950.4	E962.0	E980.4
Chlorpromazine	969.1	E853.0	E939.1	E950.3	E962.0	E980.3
Chlorpropamide	962.3	E858.0	E932.3	E950.4	E962.0	E980.4
Chlorprothixene	969.3	E853.8	E939.3	E950.3	E962.0	E980.3
Chlorquinaldol	976.0	E858.7	E946.0	E950.4	E962.0	E980.4
Chlortetracycline	960.4	E856	E930.4	E950.4	E962.0	E980.4
Chlorthalidone	974.4	E858.5	E944.4	E950.4	E962.0	E980.4
Chlortrianisene	962.2	E858.0	E932.2	E950.4	E962.0	E980.4
Chlor–Trimeton	963.0	E858.1	E933.0	E950.4	E962.0	E980.4
Chlorzoxazone	968.0	E855.1	E938.0	E950.4	E962.0	E980.4
Choke damp	987.8	E869.8	—	E952.8	E962.2	E982.8
Cholebrine	977.8	E858.8	E947.8	E950.4	E962.0	E980.4
Cholera vaccine	978.2	E858.8	E948.2	E950.4	E962.0	E980.4
Cholesterol–lowering agents	972.2	E858.3	E942.2	E950.4	E962.0	E980.4
Cholestyramine (resin)	972.2	E858.3	E942.2	E950.4	E962.0	E980.4
Cholic acid	973.4	E858.4	E943.4	E950.4	E962.0	E980.4
Choline						
dihydrogen citrate	977.1	E858.8	E947.1	E950.4	E962.0	E980.4
salicylate	965.1	E850.3	E935.3	E950.0	E962.0	E980.0
theophyllinate	974.1	E858.5	E944.1	E950.4	E962.0	E980.4
Cholinergics	971.0	E855.3	E941.0	E950.4	E962.0	E980.4
Cholografin	977.8	E858.8	E947.8	E950.4	E962.0	E980.4
Chorionic gonadotropin	962.4	E858.0	E932.4	E950.4	E962.0	E980.4
Chromates	983.9	E864.3	—	E950.7	E962.1	E980.6
dust or mist	987.8	E869.8	—	E952.8	E962.2	E982.8
lead	984.0	E866.0	—	E950.9	E962.1	E980.9
paint	984.0	E861.5	—	E950.9	E962.1	E980.9
Chromic acid	983.9	E864.3	—	E950.7	E962.1	E980.6
dust or mist	987.8	E869.8	—	E952.8	E962.2	E982.8
Chromium	985.6	E866.4	—	E950.9	E962.1	E980.9
compounds — *see* Chromates						
Chromonar	972.4	E858.3	E942.4	E950.4	E962.0	E980.4
Chromyl chloride	983.9	E864.3	—	E950.7	E962.1	E980.6
Chrysarobin (ointment)	976.4	E858.7	E946.4	E950.4	E962.0	E980.4
Chrysazin	973.1	E858.4	E943.1	E950.4	E962.0	E980.4
Chymar	963.4	E858.1	E933.4	E950.4	E962.0	E980.4
ophthalmic preparation	976.5	E858.7	E946.5	E950.4	E962.0	E980.4
Chymotrypsin	963.4	E858.1	E933.4	E950.4	E962.0	E980.4
ophthalmic preparation	976.5	E858.7	E946.5	E950.4	E962.0	E980.4
Cicuta maculata or virosa	988.2	E865.4	—	E950.9	E962.1	E980.9
Cigarette lighter fluid	981	E862.1	—	E950.9	E962.1	E980.9
Cinchocaine (spinal)	968.7	E855.2	E938.7	E950.4	E962.0	E980.4
topical (surface)	968.5	E855.2	E938.5	E950.4	E962.0	E980.4
Cinchona	961.4	E857	E931.4	E950.4	E962.0	E980.4
Cinchonine alkaloids	961.4	E857	E931.4	E950.4	E962.0	E980.4
Cinchophen	974.7	E858.5	E944.7	E950.4	E962.0	E980.4
Cinnarizine	963.0	E858.1	E933.0	E950.4	E962.0	E980.4

Substance	Poisoning	Accident	Therapeutic Use	Suicide Attempt	Assault	Undetermined
			External Cause (E-Code)			
Citanest	968.9	E855.2	E938.9	E950.4	E962.0	E980.4
infiltration (subcutaneous)	968.5	E855.2	E938.5	E950.4	E962.0	E980.4
nerve block (peripheral) (plexus)	968.6	E855.2	E938.6	E950.4	E962.0	E980.4
Citric acid	989.89	E866.8	—	E950.9	E962.1	E980.9
Citrovorum factor	964.1	E858.2	E934.1	E950.4	E962.0	E980.4
Claviceps purpurea	988.2	E865.4	—	E950.9	E962.1	E980.9
Cleaner, cleansing agent NEC	989.89	E861.3	—	E950.9	E962.1	E980.9
of paint or varnish	982.8	E862.9	—	E950.9	E962.1	E980.9
Clematis vitalba	988.2	E865.4	—	E950.9	E962.1	E980.9
Clemizole	963.0	E858.1	E933.0	E950.4	E962.0	E980.4
penicillin	960.0	E856	E930.0	E950.4	E962.0	E980.4
Clidinium	971.1	E855.4	E941.1	E950.4	E962.0	E980.4
Clindamycin	960.8	E856	E930.8	E950.4	E962.0	E980.4
Cliradon	965.09	E850.2	E935.2	E950.0	E962.0	E980.0
Clocortolone	962.0	E858.0	E932.0	E950.4	E962.0	E980.4
Clofedanol	975.4	E858.6	E945.4	E950.4	E962.0	E980.4
Clofibrate	972.2	E858.3	E942.2	E950.4	E962.0	E980.4
Clomethiazole	967.1	E852.0	E937.1	E950.2	E962.0	E980.2
Clomiphene	977.8	E858.8	E947.8	E950.4	E962.0	E980.4
Clonazepam	969.4	E853.2	E939.4	E950.3	E962.0	E980.3
Clonidine	972.6	E858.3	E942.6	E950.4	E962.0	E980.4
Clopamide	974.3	E858.5	E944.3	E950.4	E962.0	E980.4
Clorazepate	969.4	E853.2	E939.4	E950.3	E962.0	E980.3
Clorexolone	974.4	E858.5	E944.4	E950.4	E962.0	E980.4
Clorox (bleach)	983.9	E864.3	—	E950.7	E962.1	E980.6
Clortermine	977.0	E858.8	E947.0	E950.4	E962.0	E980.4
Clotrimazole	976.0	E858.7	E946.0	E950.4	E962.0	E980.4
Cloxacillin	960.0	E856	E930.0	E950.4	E962.0	E980.4
Coagulants NEC	964.5	E858.2	E934.5	E950.4	E962.0	E980.4
Coal (carbon monoxide from) — *see also* Carbon, monoxide, coal						
oil — *see* Kerosene						
tar NEC	983.0	E864.0	—	E950.7	E962.1	E980.6
fumes	987.8	E869.8	—	E952.8	E962.2	E982.8
medicinal (ointment)	976.4	E858.7	E946.4	E950.4	E962.0	E980.4
analgesics NEC	965.5	E850.5	E935.5	E950.0	E962.0	E980.0
naphtha (solvent)	981	E862.0	—	E950.9	E962.1	E980.9
Cobalt (fumes) (industrial)	985.8	E866.4	—	E950.9	E962.1	E980.9
Cobra (venom)	989.5	E905.0	—	E950.9	E962.1	E980.9
Coca (leaf)	970.8	E854.3	E940.8	E950.4	E962.0	E980.4
Cocaine (hydrochloride) (salt)	970.8	E854.3	E940.8	E950.4	E962.0	E980.4
topical anesthetic	968.5	E855.2	E938.5	E950.4	E962.0	E980.4
Coccidioidin	977.8	E858.8	E947.8	E950.4	E962.0	E980.4
Cocculus indicus	988.2	E865.3	—	E950.9	E962.1	E980.9
Cochineal	989.89	E866.8	—	E950.9	E962.1	E980.9
medicinal products	977.4	E858.8	E947.4	E950.4	E962.0	E980.4
Codeine	965.09	E850.2	E935.2	E950.0	E962.0	E980.0
Coffee	989.89	E866.8	—	E950.9	E962.1	E980.9
Cogentin	971.1	E855.4	E941.1	E950.4	E962.0	E980.4
Coke fumes or gas (carbon monoxide)	986	E868.3	—	E952.1	E962.2	E982.1
industrial use	986	E868.8	—	E952.1	E962.2	E982.1
Colace	973.2	E858.4	E943.2	E950.4	E962.0	E980.4
Colchicine	974.7	E858.5	E944.7	E950.4	E962.0	E980.4
Colchicum	988.2	E865.3	—	E950.9	E962.1	E980.9
Cold cream	976.3	E858.7	E946.3	E950.4	E962.0	E980.4
Colestipol	972.2	E858.3	E942.2	E950.4	E962.0	E980.4
Colistimethate	960.8	E856	E930.8	E950.4	E962.0	E980.4
Colistin	960.8	E856	E930.8	E950.4	E962.0	E980.4
Collagen	977.8	E866.8	E947.8	E950.9	E962.1	E980.9
Collagenase	976.8	E858.7	E946.8	E950.4	E962.0	E980.4
Collodion (flexible)	976.3	E858.7	E946.3	E950.4	E962.0	E980.4

Substance	Poisoning	Accident	Therapeutic Use	Suicide Attempt	Assault	Undetermined
			External Cause (E-Code)			
Colocynth	973.1	E858.4	E943.1	E950.4	E962.0	E980.4
Coloring matter — *see* Dye(s)						
Combustion gas — *see* Carbon, monoxide						
Compazine	969.1	E853.0	E939.1	E950.3	E962.0	E980.3
Compound						
42 (warfarin)	989.4	E863.7	—	E950.6	E962.1	E980.7
269 (endrin)	989.2	E863.0	—	E950.6	E962.1	E980.7
497 (dieldrin)	989.2	E863.0	—	E950.6	E962.1	E980.7
1080 (sodium fluoroacetate)	989.4	E863.7	—	E950.6	E962.1	E980.7
3422 (parathion)	989.3	E863.1	—	E950.6	E962.1	E980.7
3911 (phorate)	989.3	E863.1	—	E950.6	E962.1	E980.7
3956 (toxaphene)	989.2	E863.0	—	E950.6	E962.1	E980.7
4049 (malathion)	989.3	E863.1	—	E950.6	E962.1	E980.7
4124 (dicapthon)	989.4	E863.4	—	E950.6	E962.1	E980.7
E (cortisone)	962.0	E858.0	E932.0	E950.4	E962.0	E980.4
F (hydrocortisone)	962.0	E858.0	E932.0	E950.4	E962.0	E980.4
Congo red	977.8	E858.8	E947.8	E950.4	E962.0	E980.4
Coniine, conine	965.7	E850.7	E935.7	E950.0	E962.0	E980.0
Conium (maculatum)	988.2	E865.4	—	E950.9	E962.1	E980.9
Conjugated estrogens (equine)	962.2	E858.0	E932.2	E950.4	E962.0	E980.4
Contac	975.6	E858.6	E945.6	E950.4	E962.0	E980.4
Contact lens solution	976.5	E858.7	E946.5	E950.4	E962.0	E980.4
Contraceptives (oral)	962.2	E858.0	E932.2	E950.4	E962.0	E980.4
vaginal	976.8	E858.7	E946.8	E950.4	E962.0	E980.4
Contrast media (roentgenographic)	977.8	E858.8	E947.8	E950.4	E962.0	E980.4
Convallaria majalis	988.2	E865.4	—	E950.9	E962.1	E980.9
Copper (dust) (fumes) (salts) NEC	985.8	E866.4	—	E950.9	E962.1	E980.9
arsenate, arsenite	985.1	E866.3	—	E950.8	E962.1	E980.8
insecticide	985.1	E863.4	—	E950.8	E962.1	E980.8
emetic	973.6	E858.4	E943.6	E950.4	E962.0	E980.4
fungicide	985.8	E863.6	—	E950.6	E962.1	E980.7
insecticide	985.8	E863.4	—	E950.6	E962.1	E980.7
oleate	976.0	E858.7	E946.0	E950.4	E962.0	E980.4
sulfate	983.9	E864.3	—	E950.7	E962.1	E980.6
fungicide	983.9	E863.6	—	E950.7	E962.1	E980.6
cupric	973.6	E858.4	E943.6	E950.4	E962.0	E980.4
cuprous	983.9	E864.3	—	E950.7	E962.1	E980.6
Copperhead snake (bite) (venom)	989.5	E905.0	—	E950.9	E962.1	E980.9
Coral (sting)	989.5	E905.6	—	E950.9	E962.1	E980.9
snake (bite) (venom)	989.5	E905.0	—	E950.9	E962.1	E980.9
Cordran	976.0	E858.7	E946.0	E950.4	E962.0	E980.4
Corn cures	976.4	E858.7	E946.4	E950.4	E962.0	E980.4
Cornhusker's lotion	976.3	E858.7	E946.3	E950.4	E962.0	E980.4
Corn starch	976.3	E858.7	E946.3	E950.4	E962.0	E980.4
Corrosive	983.9	E864.4	—	E950.7	E962.1	E980.6
acids NEC	983.1	E864.1	—	E950.7	E962.1	E980.6
aromatics	983.0	E864.0	—	E950.7	E962.1	E980.6
disinfectant	983.0	E861.4	—	E950.7	E962.1	E980.6
fumes NEC	987.9	E869.9	—	E952.9	E962.2	E982.9
specified NEC	983.9	E864.3	—	E950.7	E962.1	E980.6
sublimate — *see* Mercury, chloride						
Cortate	962.0	E858.0	E932.0	E950.4	E962.0	E980.4
Cort–Dome	962.0	E858.0	E932.0	E950.4	E962.0	E980.4
ENT agent	976.6	E858.7	E946.6	E950.4	E962.0	E980.4
ophthalmic preparation	976.5	E858.7	E946.5	E950.4	E962.0	E980.4
topical NEC	976.0	E858.7	E946.0	E950.4	E962.0	E980.4
Cortef	962.0	E858.0	E932.0	E950.4	E962.0	E980.4
ENT agent	976.6	E858.7	E946.6	E950.4	E962.0	E980.4
ophthalmic preparation	976.5	E858.7	E946.5	E950.4	E962.0	E980.4
topical NEC	976.0	E858.7	E946.0	E950.4	E962.0	E980.4

Substance	Poisoning	Accident	Therapeutic Use	Suicide Attempt	Assault	Undetermined
			External Cause (E-Code)			
Corticosteroids (fluorinated)	962.0	E858.0	E932.0	E950.4	E962.0	E980.4
ENT agent	976.6	E858.7	E946.6	E950.4	E962.0	E980.4
ophthalmic preparation	976.5	E858.7	E946.5	E950.4	E962.0	E980.4
topical NEC	976.0	E858.7	E946.0	E950.4	E962.0	E980.4
Corticotropin	962.4	E858.0	E932.4	E950.4	E962.0	E980.4
Cortisol	962.0	E858.0	E932.0	E950.4	E962.0	E980.4
ENT agent	976.6	E858.7	E946.6	E950.4	E962.0	E980.4
ophthalmic preparation	976.5	E858.7	E946.5	E950.4	E962.0	E980.4
topical NEC	976.0	E858.7	E946.0	E950.4	E962.0	E980.4
Cortisone derivatives (acetate)	962.0	E858.0	E932.0	E950.4	E962.0	E980.4
ENT agent	976.6	E858.7	E946.6	E950.4	E962.0	E980.4
ophthalmic preparation	976.5	E858.7	E946.5	E950.4	E962.0	E980.4
topical NEC	976.0	E858.7	E946.0	E950.4	E962.0	E980.4
Cortogen	962.0	E858.0	E932.0	E950.4	E962.0	E980.4
ENT agent	976.6	E858.7	E946.6	E950.4	E962.0	E980.4
ophthalmic preparation	976.5	E858.7	E946.5	E950.4	E962.0	E980.4
Cortone	962.0	E858.0	E932.0	E950.4	E962.0	E980.4
ENT agent	976.6	E858.7	E946.6	E950.4	E962.0	E980.4
ophthalmic preparation	976.5	E858.7	E946.5	E950.4	E962.0	E980.4
Cortril	962.0	E858.0	E932.0	E950.4	E962.0	E980.4
ENT agent	976.6	E858.7	E946.6	E950.4	E962.0	E980.4
ophthalmic preparation	976.5	E858.7	E946.5	E950.4	E962.0	E980.4
topical NEC	976.0	E858.7	E946.0	E950.4	E962.0	E980.4
Cosmetics	989.89	E866.7	—	E950.9	E962.1	E980.9
Cosyntropin	977.8	E858.8	E947.8	E950.4	E962.0	E980.4
Cotarnine	964.5	E858.2	E934.5	E950.4	E962.0	E980.4
Cottonseed oil	976.3	E858.7	E946.3	E950.4	E962.0	E980.4
Cough mixtures (antitussives)	975.4	E858.6	E945.4	E950.4	E962.0	E980.4
containing opiates	965.09	E850.2	E935.2	E950.0	E962.0	E980.0
expectorants	975.5	E858.6	E945.5	E950.4	E962.0	E980.4
Coumadin	964.2	E858.2	E934.2	E950.4	E962.0	E980.4
rodenticide	989.4	E863.7	—	E950.6	E962.1	E980.7
Coumarin	964.2	E858.2	E934.2	E950.4	E962.0	E980.4
Coumetarol	964.2	E858.2	E934.2	E950.4	E962.0	E980.4
Cowbane	988.2	E865.4	—	E950.9	E962.1	E980.9
Cozyme	963.5	E858.1	E933.5	E950.4	E962.0	E980.4
Crack	970.8	E854.3	E940.8	E950.4	E962.0	E980.4
Creolin	983.0	E864.0	—	E950.7	E962.1	E980.6
disinfectant	983.0	E861.4	—	E950.7	E962.1	E980.6
Creosol (compound)	983.0	E864.0	—	E950.7	E962.1	E980.6
Creosote (beechwood) (coal tar)	983.0	E864.0	—	E950.7	E962.1	E980.6
medicinal (expectorant)	975.5	E858.6	E945.5	E950.4	E962.0	E980.4
syrup	975.5	E858.6	E945.5	E950.4	E962.0	E980.4
Cresol	983.0	E864.0	—	E950.7	E962.1	E980.6
disinfectant	983.0	E861.4	—	E950.7	E962.1	E980.6
Cresylic acid	983.0	E864.0	—	E950.7	E962.1	E980.6
Cropropamide	965.7	E850.7	E935.7	E950.0	E962.0	E980.0
with crotethamide	970.0	E854.3	E940.0	E950.4	E962.0	E980.4
Crotamiton	976.0	E858.7	E946.0	E950.4	E962.0	E980.4
Crotethamide	965.7	E850.7	E935.7	E950.0	E962.0	E980.0
with cropropamide	970.0	E854.3	E940.0	E950.4	E962.0	E980.4
Croton (oil)	973.1	E858.4	E943.1	E950.4	E962.0	E980.4
chloral	967.1	E852.0	E937.1	E950.2	E962.0	E980.2
Crude oil	981	E862.1	—	E950.9	E962.1	E980.9
Cryogenine	965.8	E850.8	E935.8	E950.0	E962.0	E980.0
Cryolite (pesticide)	989.4	E863.4	—	E950.6	E962.1	E980.7
Cryptenamine	972.6	E858.3	E942.6	E950.4	E962.0	E980.4
Crystal violet	976.0	E858.7	E946.0	E950.4	E962.0	E980.4
Cuckoopint	988.2	E865.4	—	E950.9	E962.1	E980.9
Cumetharol	964.2	E858.2	E934.2	E950.4	E962.0	E980.4
Cupric sulfate	973.6	E858.4	E943.6	E950.4	E962.0	E980.4

Substance	Poisoning	Accident	Therapeutic Use	Suicide Attempt	Assault	Undetermined
		External Cause (E-Code)				
Cuprous sulfate	983.9	E864.3	—	E950.7	E962.1	E980.6
Curare, curarine	975.2	E858.6	E945.2	E950.4	E962.0	E980.4
Cyanic acid — *see* Cyanide(s)						
Cyanide(s) (compounds) (hydrogen) (potassium) (sodium) NEC	989.0	E866.8	—	E950.9	E962.1	E980.9
dust or gas (inhalation) NEC	987.7	E869.8	—	E952.8	E962.2	E982.8
fumigant	989.0	E863.8	—	E950.6	E962.1	E980.7
mercuric — *see* Mercury						
pesticide (dust) (fumes)	989.0	E863.4	—	E950.6	E962.1	E980.7
Cyanocobalamin	964.1	E858.2	E934.1	E950.4	E962.0	E980.4
Cyanogen (chloride) (gas) NEC	987.8	E869.8	—	E952.8	E962.2	E982.8
Cyclaine	968.5	E855.2	E938.5	E950.4	E962.0	E980.4
Cyclamen europaeum	988.2	E865.4	—	E950.9	E962.1	E980.9
Cyclandelate	972.5	E858.3	E942.5	E950.4	E962.0	E980.4
Cyclazocine	965.09	E850.2	E935.2	E950.0	E962.0	E980.0
Cyclizine	963.0	E858.1	E933.0	E950.4	E962.0	E980.4
Cyclobarbital, cyclobarbitone	967.0	E851	E937.0	E950.1	E962.0	E980.1
Cycloguanil	961.4	E857	E931.4	E950.4	E962.0	E980.4
Cyclohexane	982.0	E862.4	—	E950.9	E962.1	E980.9
Cyclohexanol	980.8	E860.8	—	E950.9	E962.1	E980.9
Cyclohexanone	982.8	E862.4	—	E950.9	E962.1	E980.9
Cyclomethycaine	968.5	E855.2	E938.5	E950.4	E962.0	E980.4
Cyclopentamine	971.2	E855.5	E941.2	E950.4	E962.0	E980.4
Cyclopenthiazide	974.3	E858.5	E944.3	E950.4	E962.0	E980.4
Cyclopentolate	971.1	E855.4	E941.1	E950.4	E962.0	E980.4
Cyclophosphamide	963.1	E858.1	E933.1	E950.4	E962.0	E980.4
Cyclopropane	968.2	E855.1	E938.2	E950.4	E962.0	E980.4
Cycloserine	960.6	E856	E930.6	E950.4	E962.0	E980.4
Cyclothiazide	974.3	E858.5	E944.3	E950.4	E962.0	E980.4
Cycrimine	966.4	E855.0	E936.4	E950.4	E962.0	E980.4
Cymarin	972.1	E858.3	E942.1	E950.4	E962.0	E980.4
Cyproheptadine	963.0	E858.1	E933.0	E950.4	E962.0	E980.4
Cyprolidol	969.0	E854.0	E939.0	E950.3	E962.0	E980.3
Cytarabine	963.1	E858.1	E933.1	E950.4	E962.0	E980.4
Cytisus						
laburnum	988.2	E865.4	—	E950.9	E962.1	E980.9
scoparius	988.2	E865.4	—	E950.9	E962.1	E980.9
Cytomel	962.7	E858.0	E932.7	E950.4	E962.0	E980.4
Cytosine (antineoplastic)	963.1	E858.1	E933.1	E950.4	E962.0	E980.4
Cytoxan	963.1	E858.1	E933.1	E950.4	E962.0	E980.4
Dacarbazine	963.1	E858.1	E933.1	E950.4	E962.0	E980.4
Dactinomycin	960.7	E856	E930.7	E950.4	E962.0	E980.4
DADPS	961.8	E857	E931.8	E950.4	E962.0	E980.4
Dakin's solution (external)	976.0	E858.7	E946.0	E950.4	E962.0	E980.4
Dalmane	969.4	E853.2	E939.4	E950.3	E962.0	E980.3
DAM	977.2	E858.8	E947.2	E950.4	E962.0	E980.4
Danilone	964.2	E858.2	E934.2	E950.4	E962.0	E980.4
Danthron	973.1	E858.4	E943.1	E950.4	E962.0	E980.4
Dantrolene	975.2	E858.6	E945.2	E950.4	E962.0	E980.4
Daphne (gnidium) (mezereum)	988.2	E865.4	—	E950.9	E962.1	E980.9
berry	988.2	E865.3	—	E950.9	E962.1	E980.9
Dapsone	961.8	E857	E931.8	E950.4	E962.0	E980.4
Daraprim	961.4	E857	E931.4	E950.4	E962.0	E980.4
Darnel	988.2	E865.3	—	E950.9	E962.1	E980.9
Darvon	965.8	E850.8	E935.8	E950.0	E962.0	E980.0
Daunorubicin	960.7	E856	E930.7	E950.4	E962.0	E980.4
DBI	962.3	E858.0	E932.3	E950.4	E962.0	E980.4
D–Con (rodenticide)	989.4	E863.7	—	E950.6	E962.1	E980.7
DDS	961.8	E857	E931.8	E950.4	E962.0	E980.4
DDT	989.2	E863.0	—	E950.6	E962.1	E980.7

Substance	Poisoning	Accident	Therapeutic Use	Suicide Attempt	Assault	Undetermined
			External Cause (E-Code)			
Deadly nightshade	988.2	E865.4	—	E950.9	E962.1	E980.9
berry	988.2	E865.3	—	E950.9	E962.1	E980.9
Deanol	969.7	E854.2	E939.7	E950.3	E962.0	E980.3
Debrisoquine	972.6	E858.3	E942.6	E950.4	E962.0	E980.4
Decaborane	989.89	E866.8	—	E950.9	E962.1	E980.9
fumes	987.8	E869.8	—	E952.8	E962.2	E982.8
Decadron	962.0	E858.0	E932.0	E950.4	E962.0	E980.4
ENT agent	976.6	E858.7	E946.6	E950.4	E962.0	E980.4
ophthalmic preparation	976.5	E858.7	E946.5	E950.4	E962.0	E980.4
topical NEC	976.0	E858.7	E946.0	E950.4	E962.0	E980.4
Decahydronaphthalene	982.0	E862.4	—	E950.9	E962.1	E980.9
Decalin	982.0	E862.4	—	E950.9	E962.1	E980.9
Decamethonium	975.2	E858.6	E945.2	E950.4	E962.0	E980.4
Decholin	973.4	E858.4	E943.4	E950.4	E962.0	E980.4
sodium (diagnostic)	977.8	E858.8	E947.8	E950.4	E962.0	E980.4
Declomycin	960.4	E856	E930.4	E950.4	E962.0	E980.4
Deferoxamine	963.8	E858.1	E933.8	E950.4	E962.0	E980.4
Dehydrocholic acid	973.4	E858.4	E943.4	E950.4	E962.0	E980.4
DeKalin	982.0	E862.4	—	E950.9	E962.1	E980.9
Delalutin	962.2	E858.0	E932.2	E950.4	E962.0	E980.4
Delphinium	988.2	E865.3	—	E950.9	E962.1	E980.9
Deltasone	962.0	E858.0	E932.0	E950.4	E962.0	E980.4
Deltra	962.0	E858.0	E932.0	E950.4	E962.0	E980.4
Delvinal	967.0	E851	E937.0	E950.1	E962.0	E980.1
Demecarium (bromide)	971.0	E855.3	E941.0	E950.4	E962.0	E980.4
Demeclocycline	960.4	E856	E930.4	E950.4	E962.0	E980.4
Demecolcine	963.1	E858.1	E933.1	E950.4	E962.0	E980.4
Demelanizing agents	976.8	E858.7	E946.8	E950.4	E962.0	E980.4
Demerol	965.09	E850.2	E935.2	E950.0	E962.0	E980.0
Demethylchlortetracycline	960.4	E856	E930.4	E950.4	E962.0	E980.4
Demethyltetracycline	960.4	E856	E930.4	E950.4	E962.0	E980.4
Demeton	989.3	E863.1	—	E950.6	E962.1	E980.7
Demulcents	976.3	E858.7	E946.3	E950.4	E962.0	E980.4
Demulen	962.2	E858.0	E932.2	E950.4	E962.0	E980.4
Denatured alcohol	980.0	E860.1	—	E950.9	E962.1	E980.9
Dendrid	976.5	E858.7	E946.5	E950.4	E962.0	E980.4
Dental agents, topical	976.7	E858.7	E946.7	E950.4	E962.0	E980.4
Deodorant spray (feminine hygiene)	976.8	E858.7	E946.8	E950.4	E962.0	E980.4
Deoxyribonuclease	963.4	E858.1	E933.4	E950.4	E962.0	E980.4
Depressants						
appetite, central	977.0	E858.8	E947.0	E950.4	E962.0	E980.4
cardiac	972.0	E858.3	E942.0	E950.4	E962.0	E980.4
central nervous system (anesthetic)	968.4	E855.1	E938.4	E950.4	E962.0	E980.4
psychotherapeutic	969.5	E853.9	E939.5	E950.3	E962.0	E980.3
Dequalinium	976.0	E858.7	E946.0	E950.4	E962.0	E980.4
Dermolate	976.2	E858.7	E946.2	E950.4	E962.0	E980.4
DES	962.2	E858.0	E932.2	E950.4	E962.0	E980.4
Desenex	976.0	E858.7	E946.0	E950.4	E962.0	E980.4
Deserpidine	972.6	E858.3	E942.6	E950.4	E962.0	E980.4
Desipramine	969.0	E854.0	E939.0	E950.3	E962.0	E980.3
Deslanoside	972.1	E858.3	E942.1	E950.4	E962.0	E980.4
Desocodeine	965.09	E850.2	E935.2	E950.0	E962.0	E980.0
Desomorphine	965.09	E850.2	E935.2	E950.0	E962.0	E980.0
Desonide	976.0	E858.7	E946.0	E950.4	E962.0	E980.4
Desoxycorticosterone derivatives	962.0	E858.0	E932.0	E950.4	E962.0	E980.4
Desoxyephedrine	969.7	E854.2	E939.7	E950.3	E962.0	E980.3
DET	969.6	E854.1	E939.6	E950.3	E962.0	E980.3
Detergents (ingested) (synthetic)	989.6	E861.0	—	E950.9	E962.1	E980.9
external medication	976.2	E858.7	E946.2	E950.4	E962.0	E980.4
Deterrent, alcohol	977.3	E858.8	E947.3	E950.4	E962.0	E980.4
Detrothyronine	962.7	E858.0	E932.7	E950.4	E962.0	E980.4

Substance	Poisoning	Accident	Therapeutic Use	Suicide Attempt	Assault	Undetermined
		External Cause (E-Code)				
Dettol (external medication)	976.0	E858.7	E946.0	E950.4	E962.0	E980.4
Dexamethasone	962.0	E858.0	E932.0	E950.4	E962.0	E980.4
ENT agent	976.6	E858.7	E946.6	E950.4	E962.0	E980.4
ophthalmic preparation	976.5	E858.7	E946.5	E950.4	E962.0	E980.4
topical NEC	976.0	E858.7	E946.0	E950.4	E962.0	E980.4
Dexamphetamine	969.7	E854.2	E939.7	E950.3	E962.0	E980.3
Dexedrine	969.7	E854.2	E939.7	E950.3	E962.0	E980.3
Dexpanthenol	963.5	E858.1	E933.5	E950.4	E962.0	E980.4
Dextran	964.8	E858.2	E934.8	E950.4	E962.0	E980.4
Dextriferron	964.0	E858.2	E934.0	E950.4	E962.0	E980.4
Dextroamphetamine	969.7	E854.2	E939.7	E950.3	E962.0	E980.3
Dextro calcium pantothenate	963.5	E858.1	E933.5	E950.4	E962.0	E980.4
Dextromethorphan	975.4	E858.6	E945.4	E950.4	E962.0	E980.4
Dextromoramide	965.09	E850.2	E935.2	E950.0	E962.0	E980.0
Dextro pantothenyl alcohol	963.5	E858.1	E933.5	E950.4	E962.0	E980.4
topical	976.8	E858.7	E946.8	E950.4	E962.0	E980.4
Dextropropoxyphene (hydrochloride)	965.8	E850.8	E935.8	E950.0	E962.0	E980.0
Dextrorphan	965.09	E850.2	E935.2	E950.0	E962.0	E980.0
Dextrose NEC	974.5	E858.5	E944.5	E950.4	E962.0	E980.4
Dextrothyroxin	962.7	E858.0	E932.7	E950.4	E962.0	E980.4
DFP	971.0	E855.3	E941.0	E950.4	E962.0	E980.4
DHE–45	972.9	E858.3	E942.9	E950.4	E962.0	E980.4
Diabinese	962.3	E858.0	E932.3	E950.4	E962.0	E980.4
Diacetyl monoxime	977.2	E858.8	E947.2	E950.4	E962.0	E980.4
Diacetylmorphine	965.01	E850.0	E935.0	E950.0	E962.0	E980.0
Diagnostic agents	977.8	E858.8	E947.8	E950.4	E962.0	E980.4
Dial (soap)	976.2	E858.7	E946.2	E950.4	E962.0	E980.4
sedative	967.0	E851	E937.0	E950.1	E962.0	E980.1
Diallylbarbituric acid	967.0	E851	E937.0	E950.1	E962.0	E980.1
Diaminodiphenylsulfone	961.8	E857	E931.8	E950.4	E962.0	E980.4
Diamorphine	965.01	E850.0	E935.0	E950.0	E962.0	E980.0
Diamox	974.2	E858.5	E944.2	E950.4	E962.0	E980.4
Diamthazole	976.0	E858.7	E946.0	E950.4	E962.0	E980.4
Diaphenylsulfone	961.8	E857	E931.8	E950.4	E962.0	E980.4
Diasone (sodium)	961.8	E857	E931.8	E950.4	E962.0	E980.4
Diazepam	969.4	E853.2	E939.4	E950.3	E962.0	E980.3
Diazinon	989.3	E863.1	—	E950.6	E962.1	E980.7
Diazomethane (gas)	987.8	E869.8	—	E952.8	E962.2	E982.8
Diazoxide	972.5	E858.3	E942.5	E950.4	E962.0	E980.4
Dibenamine	971.3	E855.6	E941.3	E950.4	E962.0	E980.4
Dibenzheptropine	963.0	E858.1	E933.0	E950.4	E962.0	E980.4
Dibenzyline	971.3	E855.6	E941.3	E950.4	E962.0	E980.4
Diborane (gas)	987.8	E869.8	—	E952.8	E962.2	E982.8
Dibromomannitol	963.1	E858.1	E933.1	E950.4	E962.0	E980.4
Dibucaine (spinal)	968.7	E855.2	E938.7	E950.4	E962.0	E980.4
topical (surface)	968.5	E855.2	E938.5	E950.4	E962.0	E980.4
Dibunate sodium	975.4	E858.6	E945.4	E950.4	E962.0	E980.4
Dibutoline	971.1	E855.4	E941.1	E950.4	E962.0	E980.4
Dicapthon	989.4	E863.4	—	E950.6	E962.1	E980.7
Dichloralphenazone	967.1	E852.0	E937.1	E950.2	E962.0	E980.2
Dichlorodifluoromethane	987.4	E869.2	—	E952.8	E962.2	E982.8
Dichloroethane	982.3	E862.4	—	E950.9	E962.1	E980.9
Dichloroethylene	982.3	E862.4	—	E950.9	E962.1	E980.9
Dichloroethyl sulfide	987.8	E869.8	—	E952.8	E962.2	E982.8
Dichlorohydrin	982.3	E862.4	—	E950.9	E962.1	E980.9
Dichloromethane (solvent) (vapor)	982.3	E862.4	—	E950.9	E962.1	E980.9
Dichlorophen(e)	961.6	E857	E931.6	E950.4	E962.0	E980.4
Dichlorphenamide	974.2	E858.5	E944.2	E950.4	E962.0	E980.4
Dichlorvos	989.3	E863.1	—	E950.6	E962.1	E980.7
Diclofenac sodium	965.69	E850.6	E935.6	E950.0	E962.0	E980.0

Substance	Poisoning	Accident	Therapeutic Use	Suicide Attempt	Assault	Undetermined
		External Cause (E-Code)				
Dicoumarin, dicumarol	964.2	E858.2	E934.2	E950.4	E962.0	E980.4
Dicyanogen (gas)	987.8	E869.8	—	E952.8	E962.2	E982.8
Dicyclomine	971.1	E855.4	E941.1	E950.4	E962.0	E980.4
Dieldrin (vapor)	989.2	E863.0	—	E950.6	E962.1	E980.7
Dienestrol	962.2	E858.0	E932.2	E950.4	E962.0	E980.4
Dietetics	977.0	E858.8	E947.0	E950.4	E962.0	E980.4
Diethazine	966.4	E855.0	E936.4	E950.4	E962.0	E980.4
Diethyl						
barbituric acid	967.0	E851	E937.0	E950.1	E962.0	E980.1
carbamazine	961.6	E857	E931.6	E950.4	E962.0	E980.4
carbinol	980.8	E860.8	—	E950.9	E962.1	E980.9
carbonate	982.8	E862.4	—	E950.9	E962.1	E980.9
ether (vapor) — *see* Ether(s)						
propion	977.0	E858.8	E947.0	E950.4	E962.0	E980.4
stilbestrol	962.2	E858.0	E932.2	E950.4	E962.0	E980.4
Diethylene						
dioxide	982.8	E862.4	—	E950.9	E962.1	E980.9
glycol (monoacetate) (monoethyl ether)	982.8	E862.4	—	E950.9	E962.1	E980.9
Diethylsulfone–diethylmethane	967.8	E852.8	E937.8	E950.2	E962.0	E980.2
Difencloxazine	965.09	E850.2	E935.2	E950.0	E962.0	E980.0
Diffusin	963.4	E858.1	E933.4	E950.4	E962.0	E980.4
Diflos	971.0	E855.3	E941.0	E950.4	E962.0	E980.4
Digestants	973.4	E858.4	E943.4	E950.4	E962.0	E980.4
Digitalin(e)	972.1	E858.3	E942.1	E950.4	E962.0	E980.4
Digitalis glycosides	972.1	E858.3	E942.1	E950.4	E962.0	E980.4
Digitoxin	972.1	E858.3	E942.1	E950.4	E962.0	E980.4
Digoxin	972.1	E858.3	E942.1	E950.4	E962.0	E980.4
Dihydrocodeine	965.09	E850.2	E935.2	E950.0	E962.0	E980.0
Dihydrocodeinone	965.09	E850.2	E935.2	E950.0	E962.0	E980.0
Dihydroergocristine	972.9	E858.3	E942.9	E950.4	E962.0	E980.4
Dihydroergotamine	972.9	E858.3	E942.9	E950.4	E962.0	E980.4
Dihydroergotoxine	972.9	E858.3	E942.9	E950.4	E962.0	E980.4
Dihydrohydroxycodeinone	965.09	E850.2	E935.2	E950.0	E962.0	E980.0
Dihydrohydroxymorphinone	965.09	E850.2	E935.2	E950.0	E962.0	E980.0
Dihydroisocodeine	965.09	E850.2	E935.2	E950.0	E962.0	E980.0
Dihydromorphine	965.09	E850.2	E935.2	E950.0	E962.0	E980.0
Dihydromorphinone	965.09	E850.2	E935.2	E950.0	E962.0	E980.0
Dihydrostreptomycin	960.6	E856	E930.6	E950.4	E962.0	E980.4
Dihydrotachysterol	962.6	E858.0	E932.6	E950.4	E962.0	E980.4
Dihydroxyanthraquinone	973.1	E858.4	E943.1	E950.4	E962.0	E980.4
Dihydroxycodeinone	965.09	E850.2	E935.2	E950.0	E962.0	E980.0
Diiodohydroxyquin	961.3	E857	E931.3	E950.4	E962.0	E980.4
topical	976.0	E858.7	E946.0	E950.4	E962.0	E980.4
Diiodohydroxyquinoline	961.3	E857	E931.3	E950.4	E962.0	E980.4
Dilantin	966.1	E855.0	E936.1	E950.4	E962.0	E980.4
Dilaudid	965.09	E850.2	E935.2	E950.0	E962.0	E980.0
Diloxanide	961.5	E857	E931.5	E950.4	E962.0	E980.4
Dimefline	970.0	E854.3	E940.0	E950.4	E962.0	E980.4
Dimenhydrinate	963.0	E858.1	E933.0	E950.4	E962.0	E980.4
Dimercaprol	963.8	E858.1	E933.8	E950.4	E962.0	E980.4
Dimercaptopropanol	963.8	E858.1	E933.8	E950.4	E962.0	E980.4
Dimetane	963.0	E858.1	E933.0	E950.4	E962.0	E980.4
Dimethicone	976.3	E858.7	E946.3	E950.4	E962.0	E980.4
Dimethindene	963.0	E858.1	E933.0	E950.4	E962.0	E980.4
Dimethisoquin	968.5	E855.2	E938.5	E950.4	E962.0	E980.4
Dimethisterone	962.2	E858.0	E932.2	E950.4	E962.0	E980.4
Dimethoxanate	975.4	E858.6	E945.4	E950.4	E962.0	E980.4
Dimethyl						
arsine, arsinic acid — *see* Arsenic						
carbinol	980.2	E860.3	—	E950.9	E962.1	E980.9
diguanide	962.3	E858.0	E932.3	E950.4	E962.0	E980.4

Substance	Poisoning	Accident	Therapeutic Use	Suicide Attempt	Assault	Undetermined
		External Cause (E-Code)				
ketone	982.8	E862.4	—	E950.9	E962.1	E980.9
vapor	987.8	E869.8	—	E952.8	E962.2	E982.8
meperidine	965.09	E850.2	E935.2	E950.0	E962.0	E980.0
parathion	989.3	E863.1	—	E950.6	E962.1	E980.7
polysiloxane	973.8	E858.4	E943.8	E950.4	E962.0	E980.4
sulfate (fumes)	987.8	E869.8	—	E952.8	E962.2	E982.8
liquid	983.9	E864.3	—	E950.7	E962.1	E980.6
sulfoxide NEC	982.8	E862.4	—	E950.9	E962.1	E980.9
medicinal	976.4	E858.7	E946.4	E950.4	E962.0	E980.4
triptamine	969.6	E854.1	E939.6	E950.3	E962.0	E980.3
tubocurarine	975.2	E858.6	E945.2	E950.4	E962.0	E980.4
Dindevan	964.2	E858.2	E934.2	E950.4	E962.0	E980.4
Dinitro (–ortho–) cresol (herbicide) (spray)	989.4	E863.5	—	E950.6	E962.1	E980.7
insecticide	989.4	E863.4	—	E950.6	E962.1	E980.7
Dinitrobenzene	983.0	E864.0	—	E950.7	E962.1	E980.6
vapor	987.8	E869.8	—	E952.8	E962.2	E982.8
Dinitro–orthocresol (herbicide)	989.4	E863.5	—	E950.6	E962.1	E980.7
insecticide	989.4	E863.4	—	E950.6	E962.1	E980.7
Dinitrophenol (herbicide) (spray)	989.4	E863.5	—	E950.6	E962.1	E980.7
insecticide	989.4	E863.4	—	E950.6	E962.1	E980.7
Dinoprost	975.0	E858.6	E945.0	E950.4	E962.0	E980.4
Dioctyl sulfosuccinate (calcium) (sodium)	973.2	E858.4	E943.2	E950.4	E962.0	E980.4
Diodoquin	961.3	E857	E931.3	E950.4	E962.0	E980.4
Dione derivatives NEC	966.3	E855.0	E936.3	E950.4	E962.0	E980.4
Dionin	965.09	E850.2	E935.2	E950.0	E962.0	E980.0
Dioxane	982.8	E862.4	—	E950.9	E962.1	E980.9
Dioxin — *see* herbicide						
Dioxyline	972.5	E858.3	E942.5	E950.4	E962.0	E980.4
Dipentene	982.8	E862.4	—	E950.9	E962.1	E980.9
Diphemanil	971.1	E855.4	E941.1	E950.4	E962.0	E980.4
Diphenadione	964.2	E858.2	E934.2	E950.4	E962.0	E980.4
Diphenhydramine	963.0	E858.1	E933.0	E950.4	E962.0	E980.4
Diphenidol	963.0	E858.1	E933.0	E950.4	E962.0	E980.4
Diphenoxylate	973.5	E858.4	E943.5	E950.4	E962.0	E980.4
Diphenylchloroarsine	985.1	E866.3	—	E950.8	E962.1	E980.8
Diphenylhydantoin (sodium)	966.1	E855.0	E936.1	E950.4	E962.0	E980.4
Diphenylpyraline	963.0	E858.1	E933.0	E950.4	E962.0	E980.4
Diphtheria						
antitoxin	979.9	E858.8	E949.9	E950.4	E962.0	E980.4
toxoid	978.5	E858.8	E948.5	E950.4	E962.0	E980.4
with tetanus toxoid	978.9	E858.8	E948.9	E950.4	E962.0	E980.4
with pertussis component	978.6	E858.8	E948.6	E950.4	E962.0	E980.4
vaccine	978.5	E858.8	E948.5	E950.4	E962.0	E980.4
Dipipanone	965.09	E850.2	E935.2	E950.0	E962.0	E980.0
Diplovax	979.5	E858.8	E949.5	E950.4	E962.0	E980.4
Diprophylline	975.1	E858.6	E945.1	E950.4	E962.0	E980.4
Dipyridamole	972.4	E858.3	E942.4	E950.4	E962.0	E980.4
Dipyrone	965.5	E850.5	E935.5	E950.0	E962.0	E980.0
Diquat	989.4	E863.5	—	E950.6	E962.1	E980.7
Disinfectant NEC	983.9	E861.4	—	E950.7	E962.1	E980.6
alkaline	983.2	E861.4	—	E950.7	E962.1	E980.6
aromatic	983.0	E861.4	—	E950.7	E962.1	E980.6
Disipal	966.4	E855.0	E936.4	E950.4	E962.0	E980.4
Disodium edetate	963.8	E858.1	E933.8	E950.4	E962.0	E980.4
Disulfamide	974.4	E858.5	E944.4	E950.4	E962.0	E980.4
Disulfanilamide	961.0	E857	E931.0	E950.4	E962.0	E980.4
Disulfiram	977.3	E858.8	E947.3	E950.4	E962.0	E980.4
Dithiazanine	961.6	E857	E931.6	E950.4	E962.0	E980.4
Dithioglycerol	963.8	E858.1	E933.8	E950.4	E962.0	E980.4
Dithranol	976.4	E858.7	E946.4	E950.4	E962.0	E980.4

Substance	Poisoning	Accident	Therapeutic Use	Suicide Attempt	Assault	Undetermined
		External Cause (E-Code)				
Diucardin	974.3	E858.5	E944.3	E950.4	E962.0	E980.4
Diupres	974.3	E858.5	E944.3	E950.4	E962.0	E980.4
Diuretics NEC	974.4	E858.5	E944.4	E950.4	E962.0	E980.4
carbonic acid anhydrase inhibitors	974.2	E858.5	E944.2	E950.4	E962.0	E980.4
mercurial	974.0	E858.5	E944.0	E950.4	E962.0	E980.4
osmotic	974.4	E858.5	E944.4	E950.4	E962.0	E980.4
purine derivatives	974.1	E858.5	E944.1	E950.4	E962.0	E980.4
saluretic	974.3	E858.5	E944.3	E950.4	E962.0	E980.4
Diuril	974.3	E858.5	E944.3	E950.4	E962.0	E980.4
Divinyl ether	968.2	E855.1	E938.2	E950.4	E962.0	E980.4
D–lysergic acid diethylamide	969.6	E854.1	E939.6	E950.3	E962.0	E980.3
DMCT	960.4	E856	E930.4	E950.4	E962.0	E980.4
DMSO	982.8	E862.4	—	E950.9	E962.1	E980.9
DMT	969.6	E854.1	E939.6	E950.3	E962.0	E980.3
DNOC	989.4	E863.5	—	E950.6	E962.1	E980.7
DOCA	962.0	E858.0	E932.0	E950.4	E962.0	E980.4
Dolophine	965.02	E850.1	E935.1	E950.0	E962.0	E980.0
Doloxene	965.8	E850.8	E935.8	E950.0	E962.0	E980.0
DOM	969.6	E854.1	E939.6	E950.3	E962.0	E980.3
Domestic gas — *see* Gas, utility						
Domiphen (bromide) (lozenges)	976.6	E858.7	E946.6	E950.4	E962.0	E980.4
Dopa (levo)	966.4	E855.0	E936.4	E950.4	E962.0	E980.4
Dopamine	971.2	E855.5	E941.2	E950.4	E962.0	E980.4
Doriden	967.5	E852.4	E937.5	E950.2	E962.0	E980.2
Dormiral	967.0	E851	E937.0	E950.1	E962.0	E980.1
Dormison	967.8	E852.8	E937.8	E950.2	E962.0	E980.2
Dornase	963.4	E858.1	E933.4	E950.4	E962.0	E980.4
Dorsacaine	968.5	E855.2	E938.5	E950.4	E962.0	E980.4
Dothiepin hydrochloride	969.0	E854.0	E939.0	E950.3	E962.0	E980.3
Doxapram	970.0	E854.3	E940.0	E950.4	E962.0	E980.4
Doxepin	969.0	E854.0	E939.0	E950.3	E962.0	E980.3
Doxorubicin	960.7	E856	E930.7	E950.4	E962.0	E980.4
Doxycycline	960.4	E856	E930.4	E950.4	E962.0	E980.4
Doxylamine	963.0	E858.1	E933.0	E950.4	E962.0	E980.4
Dramamine	963.0	E858.1	E933.0	E950.4	E962.0	E980.4
Drano (drain cleaner)	983.2	E864.2	—	E950.7	E962.1	E980.6
Dromoran	965.09	E850.2	E935.2	E950.0	E962.0	E980.0
Dromostanolone	962.1	E858.0	E932.1	E950.4	E962.0	E980.4
Droperidol	969.2	E853.1	E939.2	E950.3	E962.0	E980.3
Drotrecogin alfa	964.2	E858.2	E934.2	E950.4	E962.0	E980.4
Drug	977.9	E858.9	E947.9	E950.5	E962.0	E980.5
specified NEC	977.8	E858.8	E947.8	E950.4	E962.0	E980.4
AHFS List						
4:00 antihistamine drugs	963.0	E858.1	E933.0	E950.4	E962.0	E980.4
8:04 amebacides	961.5	E857	E931.5	E950.4	E962.0	E980.4
arsenical anti–infectives	961.1	E857	E931.1	E950.4	E962.0	E980.4
quinoline derivatives	961.3	E857	E931.3	E950.4	E962.0	E980.4
8:08 anthelmintics	961.6	E857	E931.6	E950.4	E962.0	E980.4
quinoline derivatives	961.3	E857	E931.3	E950.4	E962.0	E980.4
8:12.04 antifungal antibiotics	960.1	E856	E930.1	E950.4	E962.0	E980.4
8:12.06 cephalosporins	960.5	E856	E930.5	E950.4	E962.0	E980.4
8:12.08 chloramphenicol	960.2	E856	E930.2	E950.4	E962.0	E980.4
8:12.12 erythromycins	960.3	E856	E930.3	E950.4	E962.0	E980.4
8:12.16 penicillins	960.0	E856	E930.0	E950.4	E962.0	E980.4
8:12.20 streptomycins	960.6	E856	E930.6	E950.4	E962.0	E980.4
8:12.24 tetracyclines	960.4	E856	E930.4	E950.4	E962.0	E980.4
8:12.28 other antibiotics	960.8	E856	E930.8	E950.4	E962.0	E980.4
antimycobacterial	960.6	E856	E930.6	E950.4	E962.0	E980.4
macrolides	960.3	E856	E930.3	E950.4	E962.0	E980.4
8:16 antituberculars	961.8	E857	E931.8	E950.4	E962.0	E980.4
antibiotics	960.6	E856	E930.6	E950.4	E962.0	E980.4

Substance	Poisoning	Accident	Therapeutic Use	Suicide Attempt	Assault	Undetermined
		External Cause (E-Code)				
8:18 antivirals	961.7	E857	E931.7	E950.4	E962.0	E980.4
8:20 plasmodicides (antimalarials)	961.4	E857	E931.4	E950.4	E962.0	E980.4
8:24 sulfonamides	961.0	E857	E931.0	E950.4	E962.0	E980.4
8:26 sulfones	961.8	E857	E931.8	E950.4	E962.0	E980.4
8:28 treponemicides	961.2	E857	E931.2	E950.4	E962.0	E980.4
8:32 trichomonacides	961.5	E857	E931.5	E950.4	E962.0	E980.4
quinoline derivatives	961.3	E857	E931.3	E950.4	E962.0	E980.4
nitrofuran derivatives	961.9	E857	E931.9	E950.4	E962.0	E980.4
8:36 urinary germicides	961.9	E857	E931.9	E950.4	E962.0	E980.4
quinoline derivatives	961.3	E857	E931.3	E950.4	E962.0	E980.4
8:40 other anti–infectives	961.9	E857	E931.9	E950.4	E962.0	E980.4
10:00 antineoplastic agents	963.1	E858.1	E933.1	E950.4	E962.0	E980.4
antibiotics	960.7	E856	E930.7	E950.4	E962.0	E980.4
progestogens	962.2	E858.0	E932.2	E950.4	E962.0	E980.4
12:04 parasympathomimetic (cholinergic) agents	971.0	E855.3	E941.0	E950.4	E962.0	E980.4
12:08 parasympatholytic (cholinergic –blocking) agents	971.1	E855.4	E941.1	E950.4	E962.0	E980.4
12:12 Sympathomimetic (adrenergic) agents	971.2	E855.5	E941.2	E950.4	E962.0	E980.4
12:16 sympatholytic (adrenergic– blocking) agents	971.3	E855.6	E941.3	E950.4	E962.0	E980.4
12:20 skeletal muscle relaxants central nervous system muscle-tone depressants	968.0	E855.1	E938.0	E950.4	E962.0	E980.4
myoneural blocking agents	975.2	E858.6	E945.2	E950.4	E962.0	E980.4
16:00 blood derivatives	964.7	E858.2	E934.7	E950.4	E962.0	E980.4
20:04 antianemia drugs	964.1	E858.2	E934.1	E950.4	E962.0	E980.4
20:04.04 iron preparations	964.0	E858.2	E934.0	E950.4	E962.0	E980.4
20:04.08 liver and stomach preparations	964.1	E858.2	E934.1	E950.4	E962.0	E980.4
20:12.04 anticoagulants	964.2	E858.2	E934.2	E950.4	E962.0	E980.4
20:12.08 antiheparin agents	964.5	E858.2	E934.5	E950.4	E962.0	E980.4
20:12.12 coagulants	964.5	E858.2	E934.5	E950.4	E962.0	E980.4
20:12.16 hemostatics NEC	964.5	E858.2	E934.5	E950.4	E962.0	E980.4
capillary active drugs	972.8	E858.3	E942.8	E950.4	E962.0	E980.4
24:04 cardiac drugs	972.9	E858.3	E942.9	E950.4	E962.0	E980.4
cardiotonic agents	972.1	E858.3	E942.1	E950.4	E962.0	E980.4
rhythm regulators	972.0	E858.3	E942.0	E950.4	E962.0	E980.4
24:06 antilipemic agents	972.2	E858.3	E942.2	E950.4	E962.0	E980.4
thyroid derivatives	962.7	E858.0	E932.7	E950.4	E962.0	E980.4
24:08 hypotensive agents	972.6	E858.3	E942.6	E950.4	E962.0	E980.4
adrenergic blocking agents	971.3	E855.6	E941.3	E950.4	E962.0	E980.4
ganglion blocking agents	972.3	E858.3	E942.3	E950.4	E962.0	E980.4
vasodilators	972.5	E858.3	E942.5	E950.4	E962.0	E980.4
24:12 vasodilating agents NEC	972.5	E858.3	E942.5	E950.4	E962.0	E980.4
coronary	972.4	E858.3	E942.4	E950.4	E962.0	E980.4
nicotinic acid derivatives	972.2	E858.3	E942.2	E950.4	E962.0	E980.4
24:16 sclerosing agents	972.7	E858.3	E942.7	E950.4	E962.0	E980.4
28:04 general anesthetics	968.4	E855.1	E938.4	E950.4	E962.0	E980.4
gaseous anesthetics	968.2	E855.1	E938.2	E950.4	E962.0	E980.4
halothane	968.1	E855.1	E938.1	E950.4	E962.0	E980.4
intravenous anesthetics	968.3	E855.1	E938.3	E950.4	E962.0	E980.4
28:08 analgesics and antipyretics	965.9	E850.9	E935.9	E950.0	E962.0	E980.0
antirheumatics	965.69	E850.6	E935.6	E950.0	E962.0	E980.0
aromatic analgesics	965.4	E850.4	E935.4	E950.0	E962.0	E980.0
non–narcotic NEC	965.7	E850.7	E935.7	E950.0	E962.0	E980.0
opium alkaloids	965.00	E850.2	E935.2	E950.0	E962.0	E980.0
heroin	965.01	E850.0	E935.0	E950.0	E962.0	E980.0
methadone	965.02	E850.1	E935.1	E950.0	E962.0	E980.0
specified type NEC	965.09	E850.2	E935.2	E950.0	E962.0	E980.0

Substance	Poisoning	Accident	Therapeutic Use	Suicide Attempt	Assault	Undetermined
			External Cause (E-Code)			
pyrazole derivatives	965.5	E850.5	E935.5	E950.0	E962.0	E980.0
salicylates	965.1	E850.3	E935.3	E950.0	E962.0	E980.0
specified NEC	965.8	E850.8	E935.8	E950.0	E962.0	E980.0
28:10 narcotic antagonists	970.1	E854.3	E940.1	E950.4	E962.0	E980.4
28:12 anticonvulsants	966.3	E855.0	E936.3	E950.4	E962.0	E980.4
barbiturates	967.0	E851	E937.0	E950.1	E962.0	E980.1
benzodiazepine–based tranquilizers	969.4	E853.2	E939.4	E950.3	E962.0	E980.3
bromides	967.3	E852.2	E937.3	E950.2	E962.0	E980.2
hydantoin derivatives	966.1	E855.0	E936.1	E950.4	E962.0	E980.4
oxazolidine (derivatives)	966.0	E855.0	E936.0	E950.4	E962.0	E980.4
succinimides	966.2	E855.0	E936.2	E950.4	E962.0	E980.4
28:16.04 antidepressants	969.0	E854.0	E939.0	E950.3	E962.0	E980.3
28:16.08 tranquilizers	969.5	E853.9	E939.5	E950.3	E962.0	E980.3
benzodiazepine–based	969.4	E853.2	E939.4	E950.3	E962.0	E980.3
butyrophenone–based	969.2	E853.1	E939.2	E950.3	E962.0	E980.3
major NEC	969.3	E853.8	E939.3	E950.3	E962.0	E980.3
phenothiazine–based	969.1	E853.0	E939.1	E950.3	E962.0	E980.3
28:16.12 other psychotherapeutic agents	969.8	E855.8	E939.8	E950.3	E962.0	E980.3
28:20 respiratory and cerebral stimulants	970.9	E854.3	E940.9	E950.4	E962.0	E980.4
analeptics	970.0	E854.3	E940.0	E950.4	E962.0	E980.4
anorexigenic agents	977.0	E858.8	E947.0	E950.4	E962.0	E980.4
psychostimulants	969.7	E854.2	E939.7	E950.3	E962.0	E980.3
specified NEC	970.8	E854.3	E940.8	E950.4	E962.0	E980.4
28:24 sedatives and hypnotics	967.9	E852.9	E937.9	E950.2	E962.0	E980.2
barbiturates	967.0	E851	E937.0	E950.1	E962.0	E980.1
benzodiazepine–based tranquilizers	969.4	E853.2	E939.4	E950.3	E962.0	E980.3
chloral hydrate (group)	967.1	E852.0	E937.1	E950.2	E962.0	E980.2
glutethamide group	967.5	E852.4	E937.5	E950.2	E962.0	E980.2
intravenous anesthetics	968.3	E855.1	E938.3	E950.4	E962.0	E980.4
methaqualone (compounds)	967.4	E852.3	E937.4	E950.2	E962.0	E980.2
paraldehyde	967.2	E852.1	E937.2	E950.2	E962.0	E980.2
phenothiazine–based tranquilizers	969.1	E853.0	E939.1	E950.3	E962.0	E980.3
specified NEC	967.8	E852.8	E937.8	E950.2	E962.0	E980.2
thiobarbiturates	968.3	E855.1	E938.3	E950.4	E962.0	E980.4
tranquilizer NEC	969.5	E853.9	E939.5	E950.3	E962.0	E980.3
36:04 to 36:88 diagnostic agents	977.8	E858.8	E947.8	E950.4	E962.0	E980.4
40:00 electrolyte, caloric, and water balance agents NEC	974.5	E858.5	E944.5	E950.4	E962.0	E980.4
40:04 acidifying agents	963.2	E858.1	E933.2	E950.4	E962.0	E980.4
40:08 alkalinizing agents	963.3	E858.1	E933.3	E950.4	E962.0	E980.4
40:10 ammonia detoxicants	974.5	E858.5	E944.5	E950.4	E962.0	E980.4
40:12 replacement solutions	974.5	E858.5	E944.5	E950.4	E962.0	E980.4
plasma expanders	964.8	E858.2	E934.8	E950.4	E962.0	E980.4
40:16 sodium–removing resins	974.5	E858.5	E944.5	E950.4	E962.0	E980.4
40:18 potassium–removing resins	974.5	E858.5	E944.5	E950.4	E962.0	E980.4
40:20 caloric agents	974.5	E858.5	E944.5	E950.4	E962.0	E980.4
40:24 salt and sugar substitutes	974.5	E858.5	E944.5	E950.4	E962.0	E980.4
40:28 diuretics NEC	974.4	E858.5	E944.4	E950.4	E962.0	E980.4
carbonic acid anhydrase inhibitors	974.2	E858.5	E944.2	E950.4	E962.0	E980.4
mercurials	974.0	E858.5	E944.0	E950.4	E962.0	E980.4
purine derivatives	974.1	E858.5	E944.1	E950.4	E962.0	E980.4
saluretics	974.3	E858.5	E944.3	E950.4	E962.0	E980.4
thiazides	974.3	E858.5	E944.3	E950.4	E962.1	E980.4
40:36 irrigating solutions	974.5	E858.5	E944.5	E950.4	E962.0	E980.4
40:40 uricosuric agents	974.7	E858.5	E944.7	E950.4	E962.0	E980.4
44:00 enzymes	963.4	E858.1	E933.4	E950.4	E962.0	E980.4
fibrinolysis–affecting agents	964.4	E858.2	E934.4	E950.4	E962.0	E980.4
gastric agents	973.4	E858.4	E943.4	E950.4	E962.0	E980.4
48:00 expectorants and cough preparations antihistamine agents	963.0	E858.1	E933.0	E950.4	E962.0	E980.4

Substance	Poisoning	External Cause (E-Code)				
		Accident	Therapeutic Use	Suicide Attempt	Assault	Undetermined
antitussives	975.4	E858.6	E945.4	E950.4	E962.0	E980.4
codeine derivatives	965.09	E850.2	E935.2	E950.0	E962.0	E980.0
expectorants	975.5	E858.6	E945.5	E950.4	E962.0	E980.4
narcotic agents NEC	965.09	E850.2	E935.2	E950.0	E962.0	E980.0
52:04 anti–infectives (EENT)						
ENT agent	976.6	E858.7	E946.6	E950.4	E962.0	E980.4
ophthalmic preparation	976.5	E858.7	E946.5	E950.4	E962.0	E980.4
52:04.04 antibiotics (EENT)						
ENT agent	976.6	E858.7	E946.6	E950.4	E962.0	E980.4
ophthalmic preparation	976.5	E858.7	E946.5	E950.4	E962.0	E980.4
52:04.06 antivirals (EENT)						
ENT agent	976.6	E858.7	E946.6	E950.4	E962.0	E980.4
ophthalmic preparation	976.5	E858.7	E946.5	E950.4	E962.0	E980.4
52:04.08 sulfonamides (EENT)						
ENT agent	976.6	E858.7	E946.6	E950.4	E962.0	E980.4
ophthalmic preparation	976.5	E858.7	E946.5	E950.4	E962.0	E980.4
52:04.12 miscellaneous anti–infectives (EENT)						
ENT agent	976.6	E858.7	E946.6	E950.4	E962.0	E980.4
ophthalmic preparation	976.5	E858.7	E946.5	E950.4	E962.0	E980.4
52:08 anti–inflammatory agents (EENT)						
ENT agent	976.6	E858.7	E946.6	E950.4	E962.0	E980.4
ophthalmic preparation	976.5	E858.7	E946.5	E950.4	E962.0	E980.4
52:10 carbonic anhydrase inhibitors	974.2	E858.5	E944.2	E950.4	E962.0	E980.4
52:12 contact lens solutions	976.5	E858.7	E946.5	E950.4	E962.0	E980.4
52:16 local anesthetics (EENT)	968.5	E855.2	E938.5	E950.4	E962.0	E980.4
52:20 miotics	971.0	E855.3	E941.0	E950.4	E962.0	E980.4
52:24 mydriatics						
adrenergics	971.2	E855.5	E941.2	E950.4	E962.0	E980.4
anticholinergics	971.1	E855.4	E941.1	E950.4	E962.0	E980.4
antimuscarinics	971.1	E855.4	E941.1	E950.4	E962.0	E980.4
parasympatholytics	971.1	E855.4	E941.1	E950.4	E962.0	E980.4
spasmolytics	971.1	E855.4	E941.1	E950.4	E962.0	E980.4
sympathomimetics	971.2	E855.5	E941.2	E950.4	E962.0	E980.4
52:28 mouth washes and gargles	976.6	E858.7	E946.6	E950.4	E962.0	E980.4
52:32 vasoconstrictors (EENT)	971.2	E855.5	E941.2	E950.4	E962.0	E980.4
52:36 unclassified agents (EENT)						
ENT agent	976.6	E858.7	E946.6	E950.4	E962.0	E980.4
ophthalmic preparation	976.5	E858.7	E946.5	E950.4	E962.0	E980.4
56:04 antacids and adsorbents	973.0	E858.4	E943.0	E950.4	E962.0	E980.4
56:08 antidiarrhea agents	973.5	E858.4	E943.5	E950.4	E962.0	E980.4
56:10 antiflatulents	973.8	E858.4	E943.8	E950.4	E962.0	E980.4
56:12 cathartics NEC	973.3	E858.4	E943.3	E950.4	E962.0	E980.4
emollients	973.2	E858.4	E943.2	E950.4	E962.0	E980.4
irritants	973.1	E858.4	E943.1	E950.4	E962.0	E980.4
56:16 digestants	973.4	E858.4	E943.4	E950.4	E962.0	E980.4
56:20 emetics and antiemetics						
antiemetics	963.0	E858.1	E933.0	E950.4	E962.0	E980.4
emetics	973.6	E858.4	E943.6	E950.4	E962.0	E980.4
56:24 lipotropic agents	977.1	E858.8	E947.1	E950.4	E962.0	E980.4
56:40 miscellaneous G.I. drugs	973.8	E858.4	E943.8	E950.4	E962.0	E980.4
60:00 gold compounds	965.69	E850.6	E935.6	E950.0	E962.0	E980.0
64:00 heavy metal antagonists	963.8	E858.1	E933.8	E950.4	E962.0	E980.4
68:04 adrenals	962.0	E858.0	E932.0	E950.4	E962.0	E980.4
68:08 androgens	962.1	E858.0	E932.1	E950.4	E962.0	E980.4
68:12 contraceptives, oral	962.2	E858.0	E932.2	E950.4	E962.0	E980.4
68:16 estrogens	962.2	E858.0	E932.2	E950.4	E962.0	E980.4
68:18 gonadotropins	962.4	E858.0	E932.4	E950.4	E962.0	E980.4
68:20 insulins and antidiabetic agents	962.3	E858.0	E932.3	E950.4	E962.0	E980.4
68:20.08 insulins	962.3	E858.0	E932.3	E950.4	E962.0	E980.4
68:24 parathyroid	962.6	E858.0	E932.6	E950.4	E962.0	E980.4

Substance	Poisoning	Accident	Therapeutic Use	Suicide Attempt	Assault	Undetermined
		External Cause (E-Code)				
68:28 pituitary (posterior)	962.5	E858.0	E932.5	E950.4	E962.0	E980.4
anterior	962.4	E858.0	E932.4	E950.4	E962.0	E980.4
68:32 progestogens	962.2	E858.0	E932.2	E950.4	E962.0	E980.4
68:34 other corpus luteum hormones NEC	962.2	E858.0	E932.2	E950.4	E962.0	E980.4
68:36 thyroid and antithyroid antithyroid	962.8	E858.0	E932.8	E950.4	E962.0	E980.4
thyroid (derivatives)	962.7	E858.0	E932.7	E950.4	E962.0	E980.4
72:00 local anesthetics NEC	968.9	E855.2	E938.9	E950.4	E962.0	E980.4
topical (surface)	968.5	E855.2	E938.5	E950.4	E962.0	E980.4
infiltration (intradermal) (subcutaneous) (submucosal)	968.5	E855.2	E938.5	E950.4	E962.0	E980.4
nerve blocking (peripheral) (plexus) (regional)	968.6	E855.2	E938.6	E950.4	E962.0	E980.4
spinal	968.7	E855.2	E938.7	E950.4	E962.0	E980.4
76:00 oxytocics	975.0	E858.6	E945.0	E950.4	E962.0	E980.4
78:00 radioactive agents	990	—	—	—	—	—
80:04 serums NEC	979.9	E858.8	E949.9	E950.4	E962.0	E980.4
immune gamma globulin (human)	964.6	E858.2	E934.6	E950.4	E962.0	E980.4
80:08 toxoids NEC	978.8	E858.8	E948.8	E950.4	E962.0	E980.4
diphtheria	978.5	E858.8	E948.5	E950.4	E962.0	E980.4
and tetanus	978.9	E858.8	E948.9	E950.4	E962.0	E980.4
with pertussis component	978.6	E858.8	E948.6	E950.4	E962.0	E980.4
tetanus	978.4	E858.8	E948.4	E950.4	E962.0	E980.4
and diphtheria	978.9	E858.8	E948.9	E950.4	E962.0	E980.4
with pertussis component	978.6	E858.8	E948.6	E950.4	E962.0	E980.4
80:12 vaccines	979.9	E858.8	E949.9	E950.4	E962.0	E980.4
bacterial NEC	978.8	E858.8	E948.8	E950.4	E962.0	E980.4
with other bacterial components	978.9	E858.8	E948.9	E950.4	E962.0	E980.4
pertussis component	978.6	E858.8	E948.6	E950.4	E962.0	E980.4
viral and rickettsial components	979.7	E858.8	E949.7	E950.4	E962.0	E980.4
rickettsial NEC	979.6	E858.8	E949.6	E950.4	E962.0	E980.4
with bacterial component	979.7	E858.8	E949.7	E950.4	E962.0	E980.4
pertussis component	978.6	E858.8	E948.6	E950.4	E962.0	E980.4
viral component	979.7	E858.8	E949.7	E950.4	E962.0	E980.4
viral NEC	979.6	E858.8	E949.6	E950.4	E962.0	E980.4
with bacterial component	979.7	E858.8	E949.7	E950.4	E962.0	E980.4
pertussis component	978.6	E858.8	E948.6	E950.4	E962.0	E980.4
rickettsial component	979.7	E858.8	E949.7	E950.4	E962.0	E980.4
84:04.04 antibiotics (skin and mucous membrane)	976.0	E858.7	E946.0	E950.4	E962.0	E980.4
84:04.08 fungicides (skin and mucous membrane)	976.0	E858.7	E946.0	E950.4	E962.0	E980.4
84:04.12 scabicides and pediculicides (skin and mucous membrane)	976.0	E858.7	E946.0	E950.4	E962.0	E980.4
84:04.16 miscellaneous local anti–infectives (skin and mucous membrane)	976.0	E858.7	E946.0	E950.4	E962.0	E980.4
84:06 anti–inflammatory agents (skin and mucous membrane)	976.0	E858.7	E946.0	E950.4	E962.0	E980.4
84:08 antipruritics and local anesthetics antipruritics	976.1	E858.7	E946.1	E950.4	E962.0	E980.4
local anesthetics	968.5	E855.2	E938.5	E950.4	E962.0	E980.4
84:12 astringents	976.2	E858.7	E946.2	E950.4	E962.0	E980.4
84:16 cell stimulants and proliferants	976.8	E858.7	E946.8	E950.4	E962.0	E980.4
84:20 detergents	976.2	E858.7	E946.2	E950.4	E962.0	E980.4

Substance	Poisoning	Accident	Therapeutic Use	Suicide Attempt	Assault	Undetermined
			External Cause (E-Code)			
84:24 emollients, demulcents, and protectants	976.3	E858.7	E946.3	E950.4	E962.0	E980.4
84:28 keratolytic agents	976.4	E858.7	E946.4	E950.4	E962.0	E980.4
84:32 keratoplastic agents	976.4	E858.7	E946.4	E950.4	E962.0	E980.4
84:36 miscellaneous agents (skin and mucous membrane)	976.8	E858.7	E946.8	E950.4	E962.0	E980.4
86:00 spasmolytic agents	975.1	E858.6	E945.1	E950.4	E962.0	E980.4
antiasthmatics	975.7	E858.6	E945.7	E950.4	E962.0	E980.4
papaverine	972.5	E858.3	E942.5	E950.4	E962.0	E980.4
theophylline	974.1	E858.5	E944.1	E950.4	E962.0	E980.4
88:04 vitamin A	963.5	E858.1	E933.5	E950.4	E962.0	E980.4
88:08 vitamin B complex	963.5	E858.1	E933.5	E950.4	E962.0	E980.4
hematopoietic vitamin	964.1	E858.2	E934.1	E950.4	E962.0	E980.4
nicotinic acid derivatives	972.2	E858.3	E942.2	E950.4	E962.0	E980.4
88:12 vitamin C	963.5	E858.1	E933.5	E950.4	E962.0	E980.4
88:16 vitamin D	963.5	E858.1	E933.5	E950.4	E962.0	E980.4
88:20 vitamin E	963.5	E858.1	E933.5	E950.4	E962.0	E980.4
88:24 vitamin K activity	964.3	E858.2	E934.3	E950.4	E962.0	E980.4
88:28 multivitamin preparations	963.5	E858.1	E933.5	E950.4	E962.0	E980.4
92:00 unclassified therapeutic agents	977.8	E858.8	E947.8	E950.4	E962.0	E980.4
Duboisine	971.1	E855.4	E941.1	E950.4	E962.0	E980.4
Dulcolax	973.1	E858.4	E943.1	E950.4	E962.0	E980.4
Duponol (C) (EP)	976.2	E858.7	E946.2	E950.4	E962.0	E980.4
Durabolin	962.1	E858.0	E932.1	E950.4	E962.0	E980.4
Dyclone	968.5	E855.2	E938.5	E950.4	E962.0	E980.4
Dyclonine	968.5	E855.2	E938.5	E950.4	E962.0	E980.4
Dydrogesterone	962.2	E858.0	E932.2	E950.4	E962.0	E980.4
Dyes NEC	989.89	E866.8	—	E950.9	E962.1	E980.9
diagnostic agents	977.8	E858.8	E947.8	E950.4	E962.0	E980.4
pharmaceutical NEC	977.4	E858.8	E947.4	E950.4	E962.0	E980.4
Dyfols	971.0	E855.3	E941.0	E950.4	E962.0	E980.4
Dymelor	962.3	E858.0	E932.3	E950.4	E962.0	E980.4
Dynamite	989.89	E866.8	—	E950.9	E962.1	E980.9
fumes	987.8	E869.8	—	E952.8	E962.2	E982.8
Dyphylline	975.1	E858.6	E945.1	E950.4	E962.0	E980.4
Ear preparations	976.6	E858.7	E946.6	E950.4	E962.0	E980.4
Echothiopate, ecothiopate	971.0	E855.3	E941.0	E950.4	E962.0	E980.4
Ecstasy	969.7	E854.2	E939.7	E950.3	E962.0	E980.3
Ectylurea	967.8	E852.8	E937.8	E950.2	E962.0	E980.2
Edathamil disodium	963.8	E858.1	E933.8	E950.4	E962.0	E980.4
Edecrin	974.4	E858.5	E944.4	E950.4	E962.0	E980.4
Edetate, disodium (calcium)	963.8	E858.1	E933.8	E950.4	E962.0	E980.4
Edrophonium	971.0	E855.3	E941.0	E950.4	E962.0	E980.4
Elase	976.8	E858.7	E946.8	E950.4	E962.0	E980.4
Elaterium	973.1	E858.4	E943.1	E950.4	E962.0	E980.4
Elder	988.2	E865.4	—	E950.9	E962.1	E980.9
berry (unripe)	988.2	E865.3	—	E950.9	E962.1	E980.9
Electrolytes NEC	974.5	E858.5	E944.5	E950.4	E962.0	E980.4
Electrolytic agent NEC	974.5	E858.5	E944.5	E950.4	E962.0	E980.4
Embramine	963.0	E858.1	E933.0	E950.4	E962.0	E980.4
Emetics	973.6	E858.4	E943.6	E950.4	E962.0	E980.4
Emetine (hydrochloride)	961.5	E857	E931.5	E950.4	E962.0	E980.4
Emollients	976.3	E858.7	E946.3	E950.4	E962.0	E980.4
Emylcamate	969.5	E853.8	E939.5	E950.3	E962.0	E980.3
Encyprate	969.0	E854.0	E939.0	E950.3	E962.0	E980.3
Endocaine	968.5	E855.2	E938.5	E950.4	E962.0	E980.4
Endrin	989.2	E863.0	—	E950.6	E962.1	E980.7
Enflurane	968.2	E855.1	E938.2	E950.4	E962.0	E980.4
Enovid	962.2	E858.0	E932.2	E950.4	E962.0	E980.4
ENT preparations (anti–infectives)	976.6	E858.7	E946.6	E950.4	E962.0	E980.4

Substance	Poisoning	Accident	Therapeutic Use	Suicide Attempt	Assault	Undetermined
			External Cause (E-Code)			
Enzodase	963.4	E858.1	E933.4	E950.4	E962.0	E980.4
Enzymes NEC	963.4	E858.1	E933.4	E950.4	E962.0	E980.4
Epanutin	966.1	E855.0	E936.1	E950.4	E962.0	E980.4
Ephedra (tincture)	971.2	E855.5	E941.2	E950.4	E962.0	E980.4
Ephedrine	971.2	E855.5	E941.2	E950.4	E962.0	E980.4
Epiestriol	962.2	E858.0	E932.2	E950.4	E962.0	E980.4
Epilim — *see* Sodium valproate						
Epinephrine	971.2	E855.5	E941.2	E950.4	E962.0	E980.4
Epsom salt	973.3	E858.4	E943.3	E950.4	E962.0	E980.4
Equanil	969.5	E853.8	E939.5	E950.3	E962.0	E980.3
Equisetum (diuretic)	974.4	E858.5	E944.4	E950.4	E962.0	E980.4
Ergometrine	975.0	E858.6	E945.0	E950.4	E962.0	E980.4
Ergonovine	975.0	E858.6	E945.0	E950.4	E962.0	E980.4
Ergot NEC	988.2	E865.4	—	E950.9	E962.1	E980.9
medicinal (alkaloids)	975.0	E858.6	E945.0	E950.4	E962.0	E980.4
Ergotamine (tartrate) (for migraine) NEC	972.9	E858.3	E942.9	E950.4	E962.0	E980.4
Ergotrate	975.0	E858.6	E945.0	E950.4	E962.0	E980.4
Erythrityl tetranitrate	972.4	E858.3	E942.4	E950.4	E962.0	E980.4
Erythrol tetranitrate	972.4	E858.3	E942.4	E950.4	E962.0	E980.4
Erythromycin	960.3	E856	E930.3	E950.4	E962.0	E980.4
ophthalmic preparation	976.5	E858.7	E946.5	E950.4	E962.0	E980.4
topical NEC	976.0	E858.7	E946.0	E950.4	E962.0	E980.4
Eserine	971.0	E855.3	E941.0	E950.4	E962.0	E980.4
Eskabarb	967.0	E851	E937.0	E950.1	E962.0	E980.1
Eskalith	969.8	E855.8	E939.8	E950.3	E962.0	E980.3
Estradiol (cypionate) (dipropionate) (valerate)	962.2	E858.0	E932.2	E950.4	E962.0	E980.4
Estriol	962.2	E858.0	E932.2	E950.4	E962.0	E980.4
Estrogens (with progestogens)	962.2	E858.0	E932.2	E950.4	E962.0	E980.4
Estrone	962.2	E858.0	E932.2	E950.4	E962.0	E980.4
Etafedrine	971.2	E855.5	E941.2	E950.4	E962.0	E980.4
Ethacrynate sodium	974.4	E858.5	E944.4	E950.4	E962.0	E980.4
Ethacrynic acid	974.4	E858.5	E944.4	E950.4	E962.0	E980.4
Ethambutol	961.8	E857	E931.8	E950.4	E962.0	E980.4
Ethamide	974.2	E858.5	E944.2	E950.4	E962.0	E980.4
Ethamivan	970.0	E854.3	E940.0	E950.4	E962.0	E980.4
Ethamsylate	964.5	E858.2	E934.5	E950.4	E962.0	E980.4
Ethanol	980.0	E860.1	—	E950.9	E962.1	E980.9
beverage	980.0	E860.0	—	E950.9	E962.1	E980.9
Ethchlorvynol	967.8	E852.8	E937.8	E950.2	E962.0	E980.2
Ethebenecid	974.7	E858.5	E944.7	E950.4	E962.0	E980.4
Ether(s) (diethyl) (ethyl) (vapor)	987.8	E869.8	—	E952.8	E962.2	E982.8
anesthetic	968.2	E855.1	E938.2	E950.4	E962.0	E980.4
petroleum — *see* Ligroin						
solvent	982.8	E862.4	—	E950.9	E962.1	E980.9
Ethidine chloride (vapor)	987.8	E869.8	—	E952.8	E962.2	E982.8
liquid (solvent)	982.3	E862.4	—	E950.9	E962.1	E980.9
Ethinamate	967.8	E852.8	E937.8	E950.2	E962.0	E980.2
Ethinylestradiol	962.2	E858.0	E932.2	E950.4	E962.0	E980.4
Ethionamide	961.8	E857	E931.8	E950.4	E962.0	E980.4
Ethisterone	962.2	E858.0	E932.2	E950.4	E962.0	E980.4
Ethobral	967.0	E851	E937.0	E950.1	E962.0	E980.1
Ethocaine (infiltration) (topical)	968.5	E855.2	E938.5	E950.4	E962.0	E980.4
nerve block (peripheral) (plexus)	968.6	E855.2	E938.6	E950.4	E962.0	E980.4
spinal	968.7	E855.2	E938.7	E950.4	E962.0	E980.4
Ethoheptazine (citrate)	965.7	E850.7	E935.7	E950.0	E962.0	E980.0
Ethopropazine	966.4	E855.0	E936.4	E950.4	E962.0	E980.4
Ethosuximide	966.2	E855.0	E936.2	E950.4	E962.0	E980.4
Ethotoin	966.1	E855.0	E936.1	E950.4	E962.0	E980.4
Ethoxazene	961.9	E857	E931.9	E950.4	E962.0	E980.4
Ethoxzolamide	974.2	E858.5	E944.2	E950.4	E962.0	E980.4

Substance	Poisoning	Accident	Therapeutic Use	Suicide Attempt	Assault	Undetermined
			External Cause (E-Code)			
Ethyl						
acetate (vapor)	982.8	E862.4	—	E950.9	E962.1	E980.9
alcohol	980.0	E860.1	—	E950.9	E962.1	E980.9
beverage	980.0	E860.0	—	E950.9	E962.1	E980.9
aldehyde (vapor)	987.8	E869.8	—	E952.8	E962.2	E982.8
liquid	989.89	E866.8	—	E950.9	E962.1	E980.9
aminobenzoate	968.5	E855.2	E938.5	E950.4	E962.0	E980.4
biscoumacetate	964.2	E858.2	E934.2	E950.4	E962.0	E980.4
bromide (anesthetic)	968.2	E855.1	E938.2	E950.4	E962.0	E980.4
carbamate (antineoplastic)	963.1	E858.1	E933.1	E950.4	E962.0	E980.4
carbinol	980.3	E860.4	—	E950.9	E962.1	E980.9
chaulmoograte	961.8	E857	E931.8	E950.4	E962.0	E980.4
chloride (vapor)	987.8	E869.8	—	E952.8	E962.2	E982.8
anesthetic (local)	968.5	E855.2	E938.5	E950.4	E962.0	E980.4
inhaled	968.2	E855.1	E938.2	E950.4	E962.0	E980.4
solvent	982.3	E862.4	—	E950.9	E962.1	E980.9
estranol	962.1	E858.0	E932.1	E950.4	E962.0	E980.4
ether — *see* Ether(s)						
formate (solvent) NEC	982.8	E862.4	—	E950.9	E962.1	E980.9
iodoacetate	987.5	E869.3	—	E952.8	E962.2	E982.8
lactate (solvent) NEC	982.8	E862.4	—	E950.9	E962.1	E980.9
methylcarbinol	980.8	E860.8	—	E950.9	E962.1	E980.9
morphine	965.09	E850.2	E935.2	E950.0	E962.0	E980.0
Ethylene (gas)	987.1	E869.8	—	E952.8	E962.2	E982.8
anesthetic (general)	968.2	E855.1	E938.2	E950.4	E962.0	E980.4
chlorohydrin (vapor)	982.3	E862.4	—	E950.9	E962.1	E980.9
dichloride (vapor)	982.3	E862.4	—	E950.9	E962.1	E980.9
glycol(s) (any) (vapor)	982.8	E862.4	—	E950.9	E962.1	E980.9
Ethylidene						
chloride NEC	982.3	E862.4	—	E950.9	E962.1	E980.9
diethyl ether	982.8	E862.4	—	E950.9	E962.1	E980.9
Ethynodiol	962.2	E858.0	E932.2	E950.4	E962.0	E980.4
Etidocaine	968.9	E855.2	E938.9	E950.4	E962.0	E980.4
infiltration (subcutaneous)	968.5	E855.2	E938.5	E950.4	E962.0	E980.4
nerve (peripheral) (plexus)	968.6	E855.2	E938.6	E950.4	E962.0	E980.4
Etilfen	967.0	E851	E937.0	E950.1	E962.0	E980.1
Etomide	965.7	E850.7	E935.7	E950.0	E962.0	E980.0
Etorphine	965.09	E850.2	E935.2	E950.0	E962.0	E980.0
Etoval	967.0	E851	E937.0	E950.1	E962.0	E980.1
Etryptamine	969.0	E854.0	E939.0	E950.3	E962.0	E980.3
Eucaine	968.5	E855.2	E938.5	E950.4	E962.0	E980.4
Eucalyptus (oil) NEC	975.5	E858.6	E945.5	E950.4	E962.0	E980.4
Eucatropine	971.1	E855.4	E941.1	E950.4	E962.0	E980.4
Eucodal	965.09	E850.2	E935.2	E950.0	E962.0	E980.0
Euneryl	967.0	E851	E937.0	E950.1	E962.0	E980.1
Euphthalmine	971.1	E855.4	E941.1	E950.4	E962.0	E980.4
Eurax	976.0	E858.7	E946.0	E950.4	E962.0	E980.4
Euresol	976.4	E858.7	E946.4	E950.4	E962.0	E980.4
Euthroid	962.7	E858.0	E932.7	E950.4	E962.0	E980.4
Evans blue	977.8	E858.8	E947.8	E950.4	E962.0	E980.4
Evipal	967.0	E851	E937.0	E950.1	E962.0	E980.1
sodium	968.3	E855.1	E938.3	E950.4	E962.0	E980.4
Evipan	967.0	E851	E937.0	E950.1	E962.0	E980.1
sodium	968.3	E855.1	E938.3	E950.4	E962.0	E980.4
Exalgin	965.4	E850.4	E935.4	E950.0	E962.0	E980.0
Excipients, pharmaceutical	977.4	E858.8	E947.4	E950.4	E962.0	E980.4
Exhaust gas — *see* Carbon, monoxide						
Ex–Lax (phenolphthalein)	973.1	E858.4	E943.1	E950.4	E962.0	E980.4
Expectorants	975.5	E858.6	E945.5	E950.4	E962.0	E980.4

Substance	Poisoning	Accident	Therapeutic Use	Suicide Attempt	Assault	Undetermined
			External Cause (E-Code)			
External medications (skin) (mucous membrane)	976.9	E858.7	E946.9	E950.4	E962.0	E980.4
dental agent	976.7	E858.7	E946.7	E950.4	E962.0	E980.4
ENT agent	976.6	E858.7	E946.6	E950.4	E962.0	E980.4
ophthalmic preparation	976.5	E858.7	E946.5	E950.4	E962.0	E980.4
specified NEC	976.8	E858.7	E946.8	E950.4	E962.0	E980.4
Eye agents (anti–infective)	976.5	E858.7	E946.5	E950.4	E962.0	E980.4
Factor IX complex (human)	964.5	E858.2	E934.5	E950.4	E962.0	E980.4
Fecal softeners	973.2	E858.4	E943.2	E950.4	E962.0	E980.4
Fenbutrazate	977.0	E858.8	E947.0	E950.4	E962.0	E980.4
Fencamfamin	970.8	E854.3	E940.8	E950.4	E962.0	E980.4
Fenfluramine	977.0	E858.8	E947.0	E950.4	E962.0	E980.4
Fenoprofen	965.61	E850.6	E935.6	E950.0	E962.0	E980.0
Fentanyl	965.09	E850.2	E935.2	E950.0	E962.0	E980.0
Fentazin	969.1	E853.0	E939.1	E950.3	E962.0	E980.3
Fenticlor, fentichlor	976.0	E858.7	E946.0	E950.4	E962.0	E980.4
Fer de lance (bite) (venom)	989.5	E905.0	—	E950.9	E962.1	E980.9
Ferric — *see* Iron						
Ferrocholinate	964.0	E858.2	E934.0	E950.4	E962.0	E980.4
Ferrous fumerate, gluconate, lactate, salt NEC, sulfate (medicinal)	964.0	E858.2	E934.0	E950.4	E962.0	E980.4
Ferrum — *see* Iron						
Fertilizers NEC	989.89	E866.5	—	E950.9	E962.1	E980.4
with herbicide mixture	989.4	E863.5	—	E950.6	E962.1	E980.7
Fibrinogen (human)	964.7	E858.2	E934.7	E950.4	E962.0	E980.4
Fibrinolysin	964.4	E858.2	E934.4	E950.4	E962.0	E980.4
Fibrinolysis–affecting agents	964.4	E858.2	E934.4	E950.4	E962.0	E980.4
Filix mas	961.6	E857	E931.6	E950.4	E962.0	E980.4
Fiorinal	965.1	E850.3	E935.3	E950.0	E962.0	E980.0
Fire damp	987.1	E869.8	—	E952.8	E962.2	E982.8
Fish, nonbacterial or noxious	988.0	E865.2	—	E950.9	E962.1	E980.9
shell	988.0	E865.1	—	E950.9	E962.1	E980.9
Flagyl	961.5	E857	E931.5	E950.4	E962.0	E980.4
Flavoxate	975.1	E858.6	E945.1	E950.4	E962.0	E980.4
Flaxedil	975.2	E858.6	E945.2	E950.4	E962.0	E980.4
Flaxseed (medicinal)	976.3	E858.7	E946.3	E950.4	E962.0	E980.4
Florantyrone	973.4	E858.4	E943.4	E950.4	E962.0	E980.4
Floraquin	961.3	E857	E931.3	E950.4	E962.0	E980.4
Florinef	962.0	E858.0	E932.0	E950.4	E962.0	E980.4
ENT agent	976.6	E858.7	E946.6	E950.4	E962.0	E980.4
ophthalmic preparation	976.5	E858.7	E946.5	E950.4	E962.0	E980.4
topical NEC	976.0	E858.7	E946.0	E950.4	E962.0	E980.4
Flowers of sulfur	976.4	E858.7	E946.4	E950.4	E962.0	E980.4
Floxuridine	963.1	E858.1	E933.1	E950.4	E962.0	E980.4
Flucytosine	961.9	E857	E931.9	E950.4	E962.0	E980.4
Fludrocortisone	962.0	E858.0	E932.0	E950.4	E962.0	E980.4
ENT agent	976.6	E858.7	E946.6	E950.4	E962.0	E980.4
ophthalmic preparation	976.5	E858.7	E946.5	E950.4	E962.0	E980.4
topical NEC	976.0	E858.7	E946.0	E950.4	E962.0	E980.4
Flumethasone	976.0	E858.7	E946.0	E950.4	E962.0	E980.4
Flumethiazide	974.3	E858.5	E944.3	E950.4	E962.0	E980.4
Flumidin	961.7	E857	E931.7	E950.4	E962.0	E980.4
Flunitrazepam	969.4	E853.2	E939.4	E950.3	E962.0	E980.3
Fluocinolone	976.0	E858.7	E946.0	E950.4	E962.0	E980.4
Fluocortolone	962.0	E858.0	E932.0	E950.4	E962.0	E980.4
Fluohydrocortisone	962.0	E858.0	E932.0	E950.4	E962.0	E980.4
ENT agent	976.6	E858.7	E946.6	E950.4	E962.0	E980.4
ophthalmic preparation	976.5	E858.7	E946.5	E950.4	E962.0	E980.4
topical NEC	976.0	E858.7	E946.0	E950.4	E962.0	E980.4
Fluonid	976.0	E858.7	E946.0	E950.4	E962.0	E980.4
Fluopromazine	969.1	E853.0	E939.1	E950.3	E962.0	E980.3

Substance	Poisoning	Accident	Therapeutic Use	Suicide Attempt	Assault	Undetermined
		External Cause (E-Code)				
Fluoracetate	989.4	E863.7	—	E950.6	E962.1	E980.7
Fluorescein (sodium)	977.8	E858.8	E947.8	E950.4	E962.0	E980.4
Fluoride(s) (pesticides) (sodium) NEC	989.4	E863.4	—	E950.6	E962.1	E980.7
hydrogen — *see* Hydrofluoric acid						
medicinal	976.7	E858.7	E946.7	E950.4	E962.0	E980.4
not pesticide NEC	983.9	E864.4	—	E950.7	E962.1	E980.6
stannous	976.7	E858.7	E946.7	E950.4	E962.0	E980.4
Fluorinated corticosteroids	962.0	E858.0	E932.0	E950.4	E962.0	E980.4
Fluorine (compounds) (gas)	987.8	E869.8	—	E952.8	E962.2	E982.8
salt — *see* Fluoride(s)						
Fluoristan	976.7	E858.7	E946.7	E950.4	E962.0	E980.4
Fluoroacetate	989.4	E863.7	—	E950.6	E962.1	E980.7
Fluorodeoxyuridine	963.1	E858.1	E933.1	E950.4	E962.0	E980.4
Fluorometholone (topical) NEC	976.0	E858.7	E946.0	E950.4	E962.0	E980.4
ophthalmic preparation	976.5	E858.7	E946.5	E950.4	E962.0	E980.4
Fluorouracil	963.1	E858.1	E933.1	E950.4	E962.0	E980.4
Fluothane	968.1	E855.1	E938.1	E950.4	E962.0	E980.4
Fluoxetine hydrochloride	969.0	E854.0	E939.0	E950.3	E962.0	E980.3
Fluoxymesterone	962.1	E858.0	E932.1	E950.4	E962.0	E980.4
Fluphenazine	969.1	E853.0	E939.1	E950.3	E962.0	E980.3
Fluprednisolone	962.0	E858.0	E932.0	E950.4	E962.0	E980.4
Flurandrenolide	976.0	E858.7	E946.0	E950.4	E962.0	E980.4
Flurazepam (hydrochloride)	969.4	E853.2	E939.4	E950.3	E962.0	E980.3
Flurbiprofen	965.61	E850.6	E935.6	E950.0	E962.0	E980.0
Flurobate	976.0	E858.7	E946.0	E950.4	E962.0	E980.4
Flurothyl	969.8	E855.8	E939.8	E950.3	E962.0	E980.3
Fluroxene	968.2	E855.1	E938.2	E950.4	E962.0	E980.4
Folacin	964.1	E858.2	E934.1	E950.4	E962.0	E980.4
Folic acid	964.1	E858.2	E934.1	E950.4	E962.0	E980.4
Follicle stimulating hormone	962.4	E858.0	E932.4	E950.4	E962.0	E980.4
Food, foodstuffs, nonbacterial or noxious	988.9	E865.9	—	E950.9	E962.1	E980.9
berries, seeds	988.2	E865.3	—	E950.9	E962.1	E980.9
fish	988.0	E865.2	—	E950.9	E962.1	E980.9
mushrooms	988.1	E865.5	—	E950.9	E962.1	E980.9
plants	988.2	E865.9	—	E950.9	E962.1	E980.9
specified type NEC	988.2	E865.4	—	E950.9	E962.1	E980.9
shellfish	988.0	E865.1	—	E950.9	E962.1	E980.9
specified NEC	988.8	E865.8	—	E950.9	E962.1	E980.9
Fool's parsley	988.2	E865.4	—	E950.9	E962.1	E980.9
Formaldehyde (solution)	989.89	E861.4	—	E950.9	E962.1	E980.9
fungicide	989.4	E863.6	—	E950.6	E962.1	E980.7
gas or vapor	987.8	E869.8	—	E952.8	E962.2	E982.8
Formalin	989.89	E861.4	—	E950.9	E962.1	E980.9
fungicide	989.4	E863.6	—	E950.6	E962.1	E980.7
vapor	987.8	E869.8	—	E952.8	E962.2	E982.8
Formic acid	983.1	E864.1	—	E950.7	E962.1	E980.6
vapor	987.8	E869.8	—	E952.8	E962.2	E982.8
Fowler's solution	985.1	E866.3	—	E950.8	E962.1	E980.8
Foxglove	988.2	E865.4	—	E950.9	E962.1	E980.9
Fox green	977.8	E858.8	E947.8	E950.4	E962.0	E980.4
Framycetin	960.8	E856	E930.8	E950.4	E962.0	E980.4
Frangula (extract)	973.1	E858.4	E943.1	E950.4	E962.0	E980.4
Frei antigen	977.8	E858.8	E947.8	E950.4	E962.0	E980.4
Freons	987.4	E869.2	—	E952.8	E962.2	E982.8
Fructose	974.5	E858.5	E944.5	E950.4	E962.0	E980.4
Frusemide	974.4	E858.5	E944.4	E950.4	E962.0	E980.4
FSH	962.4	E858.0	E932.4	E950.4	E962.0	E980.4
Fuel						
automobile	981	E862.1	—	E950.9	E962.1	E980.9
exhaust gas, not in transit	986	E868.2	—	E952.0	E962.2	E982.0

Substance	Poisoning	Accident	Therapeutic Use	Suicide Attempt	Assault	Undetermined
			External Cause (E-Code)			
vapor NEC	987.1	E869.8	—	E952.8	E962.2	E982.8
gas (domestic use) — *see also* Carbon, monoxide, fuel						
utility	987.1	E868.1	—	E951.8	E962.2	E981.8
incomplete combustion of — *see* Carbon, monoxide, fuel, utility						
in mobile container	987.0	E868.0	—	E951.1	E962.2	E981.1
piped (natural)	987.1	E867	—	E951.0	E962.2	E981.0
industrial, incomplete combustion	986	E868.3	—	E952.1	E962.2	E982.1
Fugillin	960.8	E856	E930.8	E950.4	E962.0	E980.4
Fulminate of mercury	985.0	E866.1	—	E950.9	E962.1	E980.9
Fulvicin	960.1	E856	E930.1	E950.4	E962.0	E980.4
Fumadil	960.8	E856	E930.8	E950.4	E962.0	E980.4
Fumagillin	960.8	E856	E930.8	E950.4	E962.0	E980.4
Fumes (from)	987.9	E869.9	—	E952.9	E962.2	E982.9
carbon monoxide — *see* Carbon, monoxide						
charcoal (domestic use)	986	E868.3	—	E952.1	E962.2	E982.1
chloroform — *see* Chloroform						
coke (in domestic stoves, fireplaces)	986	E868.3	—	E952.1	E962.2	E982.1
corrosive NEC	987.8	E869.8	—	E952.8	E962.2	E982.8
ether — *see* Ether(s)						
freons	987.4	E869.2	—	E952.8	E962.2	E982.8
hydrocarbons	987.1	E869.8	—	E952.8	E962.2	E982.8
petroleum (liquefied)	987.0	E868.0	—	E951.1	E962.2	E981.1
distributed through pipes (pure or mixed with air)	987.0	E867	—	E951.0	E962.2	E981.0
lead — *see* Lead						
metals — *see* specified metal						
nitrogen dioxide	987.2	E869.0	—	E952.8	E962.2	E982.8
pesticides — *see* Pesticides						
petroleum (liquefied)	987.0	E868.0	—	E951.1	E962.2	E981.1
distributed through pipes (pure or mixed with air)	987.0	E867	—	E951.0	E962.2	E981.0
polyester	987.8	E869.8	—	E952.8	E962.2	E982.8
specified source, other (*see also* substance specified)	987.8	E869.8	—	E952.8	E962.2	E982.8
sulfur dioxide	987.3	E869.1	—	E952.8	E962.2	E982.8
Fumigants	989.4	E863.8	—	E950.6	E962.1	E980.7
Fungi, noxious, used as food	988.1	E865.5	—	E950.9	E962.1	E980.9
Fungicides (*see also* Antifungals)	989.4	E863.6	—	E950.6	E962.1	E980.7
Fungizone	960.1	E856	E930.1	E950.4	E962.0	E980.4
topical	976.0	E858.7	E946.0	E950.4	E962.0	E980.4
Furacin	976.0	E858.7	E946.0	E950.4	E962.0	E980.4
Furadantin	961.9	E857	E931.9	E950.4	E962.0	E980.4
Furazolidone	961.9	E857	E931.9	E950.4	E962.0	E980.4
Furnace (coal burning) (domestic), gas from	986	E868.3	—	E952.1	E962.2	E982.1
industrial	986	E868.8	—	E952.1	E962.2	E982.1
Furniture polish	989.89	E861.2	—	E950.9	E962.1	E980.9
Furosemide	974.4	E858.5	E944.4	E950.4	E962.0	E980.4
Furoxone	961.9	E857	E931.9	E950.4	E962.0	E980.4
Fusel oil (amyl) (butyl) (propyl)	980.3	E860.4	—	E950.9	E962.1	E980.9
Fusidic acid	960.8	E856	E930.8	E950.4	E962.0	E980.4
Gallamine	975.2	E858.6	E945.2	E950.4	E962.0	E980.4
Gallotannic acid	976.2	E858.7	E946.2	E950.4	E962.0	E980.4
Gamboge	973.1	E858.4	E943.1	E950.4	E962.0	E980.4
Gamimune	964.6	E858.2	E934.6	E950.4	E962.0	E980.4
Gamma–benzene hexachloride (vapor)	989.2	E863.0	—	E950.6	E962.1	E980.7
Gamma globulin	964.6	E858.2	E934.6	E950.4	E962.0	E980.4
Gamma Hydroxy Butyrate (GHB)	968.4	E855.1	E938.4	E950.4	E962.0	E980.4
Gamulin	964.6	E858.2	E934.6	E950.4	E962.0	E980.4

Substance	Poisoning	Accident	Therapeutic Use	Suicide Attempt	Assault	Undetermined
		External Cause (E-Code)				
Ganglionic blocking agents	972.3	E858.3	E942.3	E950.4	E962.0	E980.4
Ganja	969.6	E854.1	E939.6	E950.3	E962.0	E980.3
Garamycin	960.8	E856	E930.8	E950.4	E962.0	E980.4
ophthalmic preparation	976.5	E858.7	E946.5	E950.4	E962.0	E980.4
topical NEC	976.0	E858.7	E946.0	E950.4	E962.0	E980.4
Gardenal	967.0	E851	E937.0	E950.1	E962.0	E980.1
Gardepanyl	967.0	E851	E937.0	E950.1	E962.0	E980.1
Gas	987.9	E869.9	—	E952.9	E962.2	E982.9
acetylene	987.1	E868.1	—	E951.8	E962.2	E981.8
incomplete combustion of — *see* Carbon, monoxide, fuel, utility						
air contaminants, source or type not specified	987.9	E869.9	—	E952.9	E962.2	E982.9
anesthetic (general) NEC	968.2	E855.1	E938.2	E950.4	E962.0	E980.4
blast furnace	986	E868.8	—	E952.1	E962.2	E982.1
butane — *see* Butane						
carbon monoxide — *see* Carbon, monoxide						
chlorine	987.6	E869.8	—	E952.8	E962.2	E982.8
coal — *see* Carbon, monoxide, coal						
cyanide	987.7	E869.8	—	E952.8	E962.2	E982.8
dicyanogen	987.8	E869.8	—	E952.8	E962.2	E982.8
domestic — *see* Gas, utility						
exhaust — *see* Carbon, monoxide, exhaust gas						
from wood– or coal–burning stove or fireplace	986	E868.3	—	E952.1	E962.2	E982.1
fuel (domestic use) — *see also* Carbon, monoxide, fuel						
industrial use	986	E868.8	—	E952.1	E962.2	E982.1
utility	987.1	E868.1	—	E951.8	E962.2	E981.8
incomplete combustion of — *see* Carbon, monoxide, fuel, utility						
in mobile container	987.0	E868.0	—	E951.1	E962.2	E981.1
piped (natural)	987.1	E867	—	E951.0	E962.2	E981.0
garage	986	E868.2	—	E952.0	E962.2	E982.0
hydrocarbon NEC	987.1	E869.8	—	E952.8	E962.2	E982.8
incomplete combustion of — *see* Carbon, monoxide, fuel, utility						
liquefied (mobile container)	987.0	E868.0	—	E951.1	E962.2	E981.1
piped	987.0	E867	—	E951.0	E962.2	E981.0
hydrocyanic acid	987.7	E869.8	—	E952.8	E962.2	E982.8
illuminating — *see* Gas, utility						
incomplete combustion, any — *see* Carbon, monoxide						
kiln	986	E868.8	—	E952.1	E962.2	E982.1
lacrimogenic	987.5	E869.3	—	E952.8	E962.2	E982.8
marsh	987.1	E869.8	—	E952.8	E962.2	E982.8
motor exhaust, not in transit	986	E868.8	—	E952.1	E962.2	E982.1
mustard — *see* Mustard, gas						
natural	987.1	E867	—	E951.0	E962.2	E981.0
nerve (war)	987.9	E869.9	—	E952.9	E962.2	E982.9
oils	981	E862.1	—	E950.9	E961.1	E980.9
petroleum (liquefied) (distributed in mobile containers)	987.0	E868.0	—	E951.1	E962.2	E981.1
piped (pure or mixed with air)	987.0	E867	—	E951.1	E962.2	E981.1
piped (manufactured) (natural) NEC	987.1	E867	—	E951.0	E962.2	E981.0
producer	986	E868.8	—	E952.1	E962.2	E982.1
propane — *see* Propane						
refrigerant (freon)	987.4	E869.2	—	E952.8	E962.2	E982.8
not freon	987.9	E869.9	—	E952.9	E962.2	E982.9
sewer	987.8	E869.8	—	E952.8	E962.2	E982.8

Substance	Poisoning	External Cause (E-Code)				
		Accident	Therapeutic Use	Suicide Attempt	Assault	Undetermined
specified source NEC (*see also* substance specified)	987.8	E869.8	—	E952.8	E962.2	E982.8
stove — *see* Gas, utility						
tear	987.5	E869.3	—	E952.8	E962.2	E982.8
utility (for cooking, heating, or lighting) (piped) NEC	987.1	E868.1	—	E951.8	E962.2	E981.8
incomplete combustion of — *see* Carbon, monoxide, fuel, utility						
in mobile container	987.0	E868.0	—	E951.1	E962.2	E981.1
piped (natural)	987.1	E867	—	E951.0	E962.2	E981.0
water	987.1	E868.1	—	E951.8	E962.2	E981.8
incomplete combustion of — *see* Carbon, monoxide, fuel, utility						
Gaseous substance — *see* Gas						
Gasoline, gasolene	981	E862.1	—	E950.9	E962.1	E980.9
vapor	987.1	E869.8	—	E952.8	E962.2	E982.8
Gastric enzymes	973.4	E858.4	E943.4	E950.4	E962.0	E980.4
Gastrografin	977.8	E858.8	E947.8	E950.4	E962.0	E980.4
Gastrointestinal agents	973.9	E858.4	E943.9	E950.4	E962.0	E980.4
specified NEC	973.8	E858.4	E943.8	E950.4	E962.0	E980.4
Gaultheria procumbens	988.2	E865.4	—	E950.9	E962.1	E980.9
Gelatin (intravenous)	964.8	E858.2	E934.8	E950.4	E962.0	E980.4
absorbable (sponge)	964.5	E858.2	E934.5	E950.4	E962.0	E980.4
Gelfilm	976.8	E858.7	E946.8	E950.4	E962.0	E980.4
Gelfoam	964.5	E858.2	E934.5	E950.4	E962.0	E980.4
Gelsemine	970.8	E854.3	E940.8	E950.4	E962.0	E980.4
Gelsemium (sempervirens)	988.2	E865.4	—	E950.9	E962.1	E980.9
Gemonil	967.0	E851	E937.0	E950.1	E962.0	E980.1
Gentamicin	960.8	E856	E930.8	E950.4	E962.0	E980.4
ophthalmic preparation	976.5	E858.7	E946.5	E950.4	E962.0	E980.4
topical NEC	976.0	E858.7	E946.0	E950.4	E962.0	E980.4
Gentian violet	976.0	E858.7	E946.0	E950.4	E962.0	E980.4
Gexane	976.0	E858.7	E946.0	E950.4	E962.0	E980.4
Gila monster (venom)	989.5	E905.0	—	E950.9	E962.1	E980.9
Ginger, Jamaica	989.89	E866.8	—	E950.9	E962.1	E980.9
Gitalin	972.1	E858.3	E942.1	E950.4	E962.0	E980.4
Gitoxin	972.1	E858.3	E942.1	E950.4	E962.0	E980.4
Glandular extract (medicinal) NEC	977.9	E858.9	E947.9	E950.5	E962.0	E980.5
Glaucarubin	961.5	E857	E931.5	E950.4	E962.0	E980.4
Globin zinc insulin	962.3	E858.0	E932.3	E950.4	E962.0	E980.4
Glucagon	962.3	E858.0	E932.3	E950.4	E962.0	E980.4
Glucochloral	967.1	E852.0	E937.1	E950.2	E962.0	E980.2
Glucocorticoids	962.0	E858.0	E932.0	E950.4	E962.0	E980.4
Glucose	974.5	E858.5	E944.5	E950.4	E962.0	E980.4
oxidase reagent	977.8	E858.8	E947.8	E950.4	E962.0	E980.4
Glucosulfone sodium	961.8	E857	E931.8	E950.4	E962.0	E980.4
Glue(s)	989.89	E866.6	—	E950.9	E962.1	E980.9
Glutamic acid (hydrochloride)	973.4	E858.4	E943.4	E950.4	E962.0	E980.4
Glutaraldehyde	989.89	E861.4	—	E950.9	E962.1	E980.9
Glutathione	963.8	E858.1	E933.8	E950.4	E962.0	E980.4
Glutethimide (group)	967.5	E852.4	E937.5	E950.2	E962.0	E980.2
Glycerin (lotion)	976.3	E858.7	E946.3	E950.4	E962.0	E980.4
Glycerol (topical)	976.3	E858.7	E946.3	E950.4	E962.0	E980.4
Glyceryl						
guaiacolate	975.5	E858.6	E945.5	E950.4	E962.0	E980.4
triacetate (topical)	976.0	E858.7	E946.0	E950.4	E962.0	E980.4
trinitrate	972.4	E858.3	E942.4	E950.4	E962.0	E980.4
Glycine	974.5	E858.5	E944.5	E950.4	E962.0	E980.4
Glycobiarsol	961.1	E857	E931.1	E950.4	E962.0	E980.4
Glycols (ether)	982.8	E862.4	—	E950.9	E962.1	E980.9
Glycopyrrolate	971.1	E855.4	E941.1	E950.4	E962.0	E980.4

Substance	Poisoning	Accident	Therapeutic Use	Suicide Attempt	Assault	Undetermined
			External Cause (E-Code)			
Glymidine	962.3	E858.0	E932.3	E950.4	E962.0	E980.4
Gold (compounds) (salts)	965.69	E850.6	E935.6	E950.0	E962.0	E980.0
Golden sulfide of antimony	985.4	E866.2	—	E950.9	E962.1	E980.9
Goldylocks	988.2	E865.4	—	E950.9	E962.1	E980.9
Gonadal tissue extract	962.9	E858.0	E932.9	E950.4	E962.0	E980.4
female	962.2	E858.0	E932.2	E950.4	E962.0	E980.4
male	962.1	E858.0	E932.1	E950.4	E962.0	E980.4
Gonadotropin	962.4	E858.0	E932.4	E950.4	E962.0	E980.4
Grain alcohol	980.0	E860.1	—	E950.9	E962.1	E980.9
beverage	980.0	E860.0	—	E950.9	E962.1	E980.9
Gramicidin	960.8	E856	E930.8	E950.4	E962.0	E980.4
Gratiola officinalis	988.2	E865.4	—	E950.9	E962.1	E980.9
Grease	989.89	E866.8	—	E950.9	E962.1	E980.9
Green hellebore	988.2	E865.4	—	E950.9	E962.1	E980.9
Green soap	976.2	E858.7	E946.2	E950.4	E962.0	E980.4
Grifulvin	960.1	E856	E930.1	E950.4	E962.0	E980.4
Griseofulvin	960.1	E856	E930.1	E950.4	E962.0	E980.4
Growth hormone	962.4	E858.0	E932.4	E950.4	E962.0	E980.4
Guaiacol	975.5	E858.6	E945.5	E950.4	E962.0	E980.4
Guaiac reagent	977.8	E858.8	E947.8	E950.4	E962.0	E980.4
Guaifenesin	975.5	E858.6	E945.5	E950.4	E962.0	E980.4
Guaiphenesin	975.5	E858.6	E945.5	E950.4	E962.0	E980.4
Guanatol	961.4	E857	E931.4	E950.4	E962.0	E980.4
Guanethidine	972.6	E858.3	E942.6	E950.4	E962.0	E980.4
Guano	989.89	E866.5	—	E950.9	E962.1	E980.9
Guanochlor	972.6	E858.3	E942.6	E950.4	E962.0	E980.4
Guanoctine	972.6	E858.3	E942.6	E950.4	E962.0	E980.4
Guanoxan	972.6	E858.3	E942.6	E950.4	E962.0	E980.4
Hair treatment agent NEC	976.4	E858.7	E946.4	E950.4	E962.0	E980.4
Halcinonide	976.0	E858.7	E946.0	E950.4	E962.0	E980.4
Halethazole	976.0	E858.7	E946.0	E950.4	E962.0	E980.4
Hallucinogens	969.6	E854.1	E939.6	E950.3	E962.0	E980.3
Haloperidol	969.2	E853.1	E939.2	E950.3	E962.0	E980.3
Haloprogin	976.0	E858.7	E946.0	E950.4	E962.0	E980.4
Halotex	976.0	E858.7	E946.0	E950.4	E962.0	E980.4
Halothane	968.1	E855.1	E938.1	E950.4	E962.0	E980.4
Halquinols	976.0	E858.7	E946.0	E950.4	E962.0	E980.4
Harmonyl	972.6	E858.3	E942.6	E950.4	E962.0	E980.4
Hartmann's solution	974.5	E858.5	E944.5	E950.4	E962.0	E980.4
Hashish	969.6	E854.1	E939.6	E950.3	E962.0	E980.3
Hawaiian wood rose seeds	969.6	E854.1	E939.6	E950.3	E962.0	E980.3
Headache cures, drugs, powders NEC	977.9	E858.9	E947.9	E950.5	E962.0	E980.9
Heavenly Blue (morning glory)	969.6	E854.1	E939.6	E950.3	E962.0	E980.3
Heavy metal						
antagonists	963.8	E858.1	E933.8	E950.4	E962.0	E980.4
anti–infectives	961.2	E857	E931.2	E950.4	E962.0	E980.4
Hedaquinium	976.0	E858.7	E946.0	E950.4	E962.0	E980.4
Hedge hyssop	988.2	E865.4	—	E950.9	E962.1	E980.9
Heet	976.8	E858.7	E946.8	E950.4	E962.0	E980.4
Helenin	961.6	E857	E931.6	E950.4	E962.0	E980.4
Hellebore (black) (green) (white)	988.2	E865.4	—	E950.9	E962.1	E980.9
Hemlock	988.2	E865.4	—	E950.9	E962.1	E980.9
Hemostatics	964.5	E858.2	E934.5	E950.4	E962.0	E980.4
capillary active drugs	972.8	E858.3	E942.8	E950.4	E962.0	E980.4
Henbane	988.2	E865.4	—	E950.9	E962.1	E980.9
Heparin (sodium)	964.2	E858.2	E934.2	E950.4	E962.0	E980.4
Heptabarbital, heptabarbitone	967.0	E851	E937.0	E950.1	E962.0	E980.1
Heptachlor	989.2	E863.0	—	E950.6	E962.1	E980.7
Heptalgin	965.09	E850.2	E935.2	E950.0	E962.0	E980.0
Herbicides	989.4	E863.5	—	E950.6	E962.1	E980.7

Substance	Poisoning	Accident	Therapeutic Use	Suicide Attempt	Assault	Undetermined
			External Cause (E-Code)			
Heroin	965.01	E850.0	E935.0	E950.0	E962.0	E980.0
Herplex	976.5	E858.7	E946.5	E950.4	E962.0	E980.4
HES	964.8	E858.2	E934.8	E950.4	E962.0	E980.4
Hetastarch	964.8	E858.2	E934.8	E950.4	E962.0	E980.4
Hexachlorocyclohexane	989.2	E863.0	—	E950.6	E962.1	E980.7
Hexachlorophene	976.2	E858.7	E946.2	E950.4	E962.0	E980.4
Hexadimethrine (bromide)	964.5	E858.2	E934.5	E950.4	E962.0	E980.4
Hexafluorenium	975.2	E858.6	E945.2	E950.4	E962.0	E980.4
Hexa–germ	976.2	E858.7	E946.2	E950.4	E962.0	E980.4
Hexahydrophenol	980.8	E860.8	—	E950.9	E962.1	E980.9
Hexalin	980.8	E860.8	—	E950.9	E962.1	E980.9
Hexamethonium	972.3	E858.3	E942.3	E950.4	E962.0	E980.4
Hexamethyleneamine	961.9	E857	E931.9	E950.4	E962.0	E980.4
Hexamine	961.9	E857	E931.9	E950.4	E962.0	E980.4
Hexanone	982.8	E862.4	—	E950.9	E962.1	E980.9
Hexapropymate	967.8	E852.8	E937.8	E950.2	E962.0	E980.2
Hexestrol	962.2	E858.0	E932.2	E950.4	E962.0	E980.4
Hexethal (sodium)	967.0	E851	E937.0	E950.1	E962.0	E980.1
Hexetidine	976.0	E858.7	E946.0	E950.4	E962.0	E980.4
Hexobarbital, hexobarbitone	967.0	E851	E937.0	E950.1	E962.0	E980.1
sodium (anesthetic)	968.3	E855.1	E938.3	E950.4	E962.0	E980.4
soluble	968.3	E855.1	E938.3	E950.4	E962.0	E980.4
Hexocyclium	971.1	E855.4	E941.1	E950.4	E962.0	E980.4
Hexoestrol	962.2	E858.0	E932.2	E950.4	E962.0	E980.4
Hexone	982.8	E862.4	—	E950.9	E962.1	E980.9
Hexylcaine	968.5	E855.2	E938.5	E950.4	E962.0	E980.4
Hexylresorcinol	961.6	E857	E931.6	E950.4	E962.0	E980.4
Hinkle's pills	973.1	E858.4	E943.1	E950.4	E962.0	E980.4
Histalog	977.8	E858.8	E947.8	E950.4	E962.0	E980.4
Histamine (phosphate)	972.5	E858.3	E942.5	E950.4	E962.0	E980.4
Histoplasmin	977.8	E858.8	E947.8	E950.4	E962.0	E980.4
Holly berries	988.2	E865.3	—	E950.9	E962.1	E980.9
Homatropine	971.1	E855.4	E941.1	E950.4	E962.0	E980.4
Homo–tet	964.6	E858.2	E934.6	E950.4	E962.0	E980.4
Hormones (synthetic substitute) NEC	962.9	E858.0	E932.9	E950.4	E962.0	E980.4
adrenal cortical steroids	962.0	E858.0	E932.0	E950.4	E962.0	E980.4
antidiabetic agents	962.3	E858.0	E932.3	E950.4	E962.0	E980.4
follicle stimulating	962.4	E858.0	E932.4	E950.4	E962.0	E980.4
gonadotropic	962.4	E858.0	E932.4	E950.4	E962.0	E980.4
growth	962.4	E858.0	E932.4	E950.4	E962.0	E980.4
ovarian (substitutes)	962.2	E858.0	E932.2	E950.4	E962.0	E980.4
parathyroid (derivatives)	962.6	E858.0	E932.6	E950.4	E962.0	E980.4
pituitary (posterior)	962.5	E858.0	E932.5	E950.4	E962.0	E980.4
anterior	962.4	E858.0	E932.4	E950.4	E962.0	E980.4
thyroid (derivative)	962.7	E858.0	E932.7	E950.4	E962.0	E980.4
Hornet (sting)	989.5	E905.3	—	E950.9	E962.1	E980.9
Horticulture agent NEC	989.4	E863.9	—	E950.6	E962.1	E980.7
Hyaluronidase	963.4	E858.1	E933.4	E950.4	E962.0	E980.4
Hyazyme	963.4	E858.1	E933.4	E950.4	E962.0	E980.4
Hycodan	965.09	E850.2	E935.2	E950.0	E962.0	E980.0
Hydantoin derivatives	966.1	E855.0	E936.1	E950.4	E962.0	E980.4
Hydeltra	962.0	E858.0	E932.0	E950.4	E962.0	E980.4
Hydergine	971.3	E855.6	E941.3	E950.4	E962.0	E980.4
Hydrabamine penicillin	960.0	E856	E930.0	E950.4	E962.0	E980.4
Hydralazine, hydrallazine	972.6	E858.3	E942.6	E950.4	E962.0	E980.4
Hydrargaphen	976.0	E858.7	E946.0	E950.4	E962.0	E980.4
Hydrazine	983.9	E864.3	—	E950.7	E962.1	E980.6
Hydriodic acid	975.5	E858.6	E945.5	E950.4	E962.0	E980.4
Hydrocarbon gas	987.1	E869.8	—	E952.8	E962.2	E982.8
incomplete combustion of — *see* Carbon, monoxide, fuel, utility						

Substance	Poisoning	Accident	Therapeutic Use	Suicide Attempt	Assault	Undetermined
			External Cause (E-Code)			
liquefied (mobile container)	987.0	E868.0	—	E951.1	E962.2	E981.1
piped (natural)	987.0	E867	—	E951.0	E962.2	E981.0
Hydrochloric acid (liquid)	983.1	E864.1	—	E950.7	E962.1	E980.6
medicinal	973.4	E858.4	E943.4	E950.4	E962.0	E980.4
vapor	987.8	E869.8	—	E952.8	E962.2	E982.8
Hydrochlorothiazide	974.3	E858.5	E944.3	E950.4	E962.0	E980.4
Hydrocodone	965.09	E850.2	E935.2	E950.0	E962.0	E980.0
Hydrocortisone	962.0	E858.0	E932.0	E950.4	E962.0	E980.4
ENT agent	976.6	E858.7	E946.6	E950.4	E962.0	E980.4
ophthalmic preparation	976.5	E858.7	E946.5	E950.4	E962.0	E980.4
topical NEC	976.0	E858.7	E946.0	E950.4	E962.0	E980.4
Hydrocortone	962.0	E858.0	E932.0	E950.4	E962.0	E980.4
ENT agent	976.6	E858.7	E946.6	E950.4	E962.0	E980.4
ophthalmic preparation	976.5	E858.7	E946.5	E950.4	E962.0	E980.4
topical NEC	976.0	E858.7	E946.0	E950.4	E962.0	E980.4
Hydrocyanic acid — *see* Cyanide(s)						
Hydroflumethiazide	974.3	E858.5	E944.3	E950.4	E962.0	E980.4
Hydrofluoric acid (liquid)	983.1	E864.1	—	E950.7	E962.1	E980.6
vapor	987.8	E869.8	—	E952.8	E962.2	E982.8
Hydrogen	987.8	E869.8	—	E952.8	E962.2	E982.8
arsenide	985.1	E866.3	—	E950.8	E961.1	E980.8
arseniureted	985.1	E866.3	—	E950.8	E961.1	E980.8
cyanide (salts)	989.0	E866.8	—	E950.9	E962.1	E980.9
gas	987.7	E869.8	—	E952.8	E962.2	E982.8
fluoride (liquid)	983.1	E864.1	—	E950.7	E962.1	E980.6
vapor	987.8	E869.8	—	E952.8	E962.2	E982.8
peroxide (solution)	976.6	E858.7	E946.6	E950.4	E962.0	E980.4
phosphureted	987.8	E869.8	—	E952.8	E962.2	E982.8
sulfide (gas)	987.8	E869.8	—	E952.8	E962.2	E982.8
arseniureted	985.1	E866.3	—	E950.8	E961.1	E980.8
sulfureted	987.8	E869.8	—	E952.8	E962.2	E982.8
Hydromorphinol	965.09	E850.2	E935.2	E950.0	E962.0	E980.0
Hydromorphinone	965.09	E850.2	E935.2	E950.0	E962.0	E980.0
Hydromorphone	965.09	E850.2	E935.2	E950.0	E962.0	E980.0
Hydromox	974.3	E858.5	E944.3	E950.4	E962.0	E980.4
Hydrophilic lotion	976.3	E858.7	E946.3	E950.4	E962.0	E980.4
Hydroquinone	983.0	E864.0	—	E950.7	E962.1	E980.6
vapor	987.8	E869.8	—	E952.8	E962.2	E982.8
Hydrosulfuric acid (gas)	987.8	E869.8	—	E952.8	E962.2	E982.8
Hydrous wool fat (lotion)	976.3	E858.7	E946.3	E950.4	E962.0	E980.4
Hydroxide, caustic	983.2	E864.2	—	E950.7	E962.1	E980.6
Hydroxocobalamin	964.1	E858.2	E934.1	E950.4	E962.0	E980.4
Hydroxyamphetamine	971.2	E855.5	E941.2	E950.4	E962.0	E980.4
Hydroxychloroquine	961.4	E857	E931.4	E950.4	E962.0	E980.4
Hydroxydihydrocodeinone	965.09	E850.2	E935.2	E950.0	E962.0	E980.0
Hydroxyethyl starch	964.8	E858.2	E934.8	E950.4	E962.0	E980.4
Hydroxyphenamate	969.5	E853.8	E939.5	E950.3	E962.0	E980.3
Hydroxyphenylbutazone	965.5	E850.5	E935.5	E950.0	E962.0	E980.0
Hydroxyprogesterone	962.2	E858.0	E932.2	E950.4	E962.0	E980.4
Hydroxyquinoline derivatives	961.3	E857	E931.3	E950.4	E962.0	E980.4
Hydroxystilbamidine	961.5	E857	E931.5	E950.4	E962.0	E980.4
Hydroxyurea	963.1	E858.1	E933.1	E950.4	E962.0	E980.4
Hydroxyzine	969.5	E853.8	E939.5	E950.3	E962.0	E980.3
Hyoscine (hydrobromide)	971.1	E855.4	E941.1	E950.4	E962.0	E980.4
Hyoscyamine	971.1	E855.4	E941.1	E950.4	E962.0	E980.4
Hyoscyamus (albus) (niger)	988.2	E865.4	—	E950.9	E962.1	E980.9
Hypaque	977.8	E858.8	E947.8	E950.4	E962.0	E980.4
Hypertussis	964.6	E858.2	E934.6	E950.4	E962.0	E980.4
Hypnotics NEC	967.9	E852.9	E937.9	E950.2	E962.0	E980.2
Hypochlorites — *see* Sodium, hypochlorite						

Substance	Poisoning	Accident	Therapeutic Use	Suicide Attempt	Assault	Undetermined
			External Cause (E-Code)			
Hypotensive agents NEC.	972.6	E858.3	E942.6	E950.4	E962.0	E980.4
Ibufenac	965.69	E850.6	E935.6	E950.0	E962.0	E980.0
ibuprofen	965.61	E850.6	E935.6	E950.0	E962.0	E980.0
ICG	977.8	E858.8	E947.8	E950.4	E962.0	E980.4
Ichthammol	976.4	E858.7	E946.4	E950.4	E962.0	E980.4
Ichthyol.	976.4	E858.7	E946.4	E950.4	E962.0	E980.4
Idoxuridine	976.5	E858.7	E946.5	E950.4	E962.0	E980.4
IDU	976.5	E858.7	E946.5	E950.4	E962.0	E980.4
Iletin	962.3	E858.0	E932.3	E950.4	E962.0	E980.4
Ilex	988.2	E865.4	—	E950.9	E962.1	E980.9
Illuminating gas — *see* Gas, utility						
Ilopan	963.5	E858.1	E933.5	E950.4	E962.0	E980.4
Ilotycin.	960.3	E856	E930.3	E950.4	E962.0	E980.4
ophthalmic preparation.	976.5	E858.7	E946.5	E950.4	E962.0	E980.4
topical NEC	976.0	E858.7	E946.0	E950.4	E962.0	E980.4
Imipramine	969.0	E854.0	E939.0	E950.3	E962.0	E980.3
Immu–G	964.6	E858.2	E934.6	E950.4	E962.0	E980.4
Immuglobin	964.6	E858.2	E934.6	E950.4	E962.0	E980.4
Immune serum globulin	964.6	E858.2	E934.6	E950.4	E962.0	E980.4
Immunosuppressive agents	963.1	E858.1	E933.1	E950.4	E962.0	E980.4
Immu–tetanus	964.6	E858.2	E934.6	E950.4	E962.0	E980.4
Indandione (derivatives)	964.2	E858.2	E934.2	E950.4	E962.0	E980.4
Inderal	972.0	E858.3	E942.0	E950.4	E962.0	E980.4
Indian						
hemp	969.6	E854.1	E939.6	E950.3	E962.0	E980.3
tobacco	988.2	E865.4	—	E950.9	E962.1	E980.9
Indigo carmine.	977.8	E858.8	E947.8	E950.4	E962.0	E980.4
Indocin.	965.69	E850.6	E935.6	E950.0	E962.0	E980.0
Indocyanine green	977.8	E858.8	E947.8	E950.4	E962.0	E980.4
Indomethacin	965.69	E850.6	E935.6	E950.0	E962.0	E980.0
Industrial						
alcohol	980.9	E860.9	—	E950.9	E962.1	E980.9
fumes	987.8	E869.8	—	E952.8	E962.2	E982.8
solvents (fumes) (vapors).	982.8	E862.9	—	E950.9	E962.1	E980.9
Influenza vaccine.	979.6	E858.8	E949.6	E950.4	E962.0	E982.8
Ingested substances NEC	989.9	E866.9	—	E950.9	E962.1	E980.9
INH (isoniazid)	961.8	E857	E931.8	E950.4	E962.0	E980.4
Inhalation, gas (noxious) — *see* Gas						
Ink.	989.89	E866.8	—	E950.9	E962.1	E980.9
Innovar	967.6	E852.5	E937.6	E950.2	E962.0	E980.2
Inositol niacinate	972.2	E858.3	E942.2	E950.4	E962.0	E980.4
Inproquone	963.1	E858.1	E933.1	E950.4	E962.0	E980.4
Insect (sting), venomous	989.5	E905.5	—	E950.9	E962.1	E980.9
Insecticides (*see also* Pesticides)	989.4	E863.4	—	E950.6	E962.1	E980.7
chlorinated.	989.2	E863.0	—	E950.6	E962.1	E980.7
mixtures.	989.4	E863.3	—	E950.6	E962.1	E980.7
organochlorine (compounds)	989.2	E863.0	—	E950.6	E962.1	E980.7
organophosphorus (compounds)	989.3	E863.1	—	E950.6	E962.1	E980.7
Insular tissue extract	962.3	E858.0	E932.3	E950.4	E962.0	E980.4
Insulin (amorphous) (globin) (isophane) (Lente) (NPH) (protamine) (Semilente) (Ultralente) (zinc)	962.3	E858.0	E932.3	E950.4	E962.0	E980.4
Intranarcon	968.3	E855.1	E938.3	E950.4	E962.0	E980.4
Inulin.	977.8	E858.8	E947.8	E950.4	E962.0	E980.4
Invert sugar	974.5	E858.5	E944.5	E950.4	E962.0	E980.4
Inza—*see* Naproxen						
Iodide NEC (*see also* Iodine).	976.0	E858.7	E946.0	E950.4	E962.0	E980.4
mercury (ointment)	976.0	E858.7	E946.0	E950.4	E962.0	E980.4
methylate	976.0	E858.7	E946.0	E950.4	E962.0	E980.4
potassium (expectorant) NEC	975.5	E858.6	E945.5	E950.4	E962.0	E980.4
Iodinated glycerol	975.5	E858.6	E945.5	E950.4	E962.0	E980.4

Substance	Poisoning	Accident	Therapeutic Use	Suicide Attempt	Assault	Undetermined
		External Cause (E-Code)				
Iodine (antiseptic, external) (tincture)						
NEC	976.0	E858.7	E946.0	E950.4	E962.0	E980.4
diagnostic	977.8	E858.8	E947.8	E950.4	E962.0	E980.4
for thyroid conditions (antithyroid)	962.8	E858.0	E932.8	E950.4	E962.0	E980.4
vapor	987.8	E869.8	—	E952.8	E962.2	E982.8
Iodized oil	977.8	E858.8	E947.8	E950.4	E962.0	E980.4
Iodobismitol	961.2	E857	E931.2	E950.4	E962.0	E980.4
Iodochlorhydroxyquin	961.3	E857	E931.3	E950.4	E962.0	E980.4
topical	976.0	E858.7	E946.0	E950.4	E962.0	E980.4
Iodoform	976.0	E858.7	E946.0	E950.4	E962.0	E980.4
Iodopanoic acid	977.8	E858.8	E947.8	E950.4	E962.0	E980.4
Iodophthalein	977.8	E858.8	E947.8	E950.4	E962.0	E980.4
Ion exchange resins	974.5	E858.5	E944.5	E950.4	E962.0	E980.4
Iopanoic acid	977.8	E858.8	E947.8	E950.4	E962.0	E980.4
Iophendylate	977.8	E858.8	E947.8	E950.4	E962.0	E980.4
Iothiouracil	962.8	E858.0	E932.8	E950.4	E962.0	E980.4
Ipecac	973.6	E858.4	E943.6	E950.4	E962.0	E980.4
Ipecacuanha	973.6	E858.4	E943.6	E950.4	E962.0	E980.4
Ipodate	977.8	E858.8	E947.8	E950.4	E962.0	E980.4
Ipral	967.0	E851	E937.0	E950.1	E962.0	E980.1
Ipratropium	975.1	E858.6	E945.1	E950.4	E962.0	E980.4
Iproniazid	969.0	E854.0	E939.0	E950.3	E962.0	E980.3
Iron (compounds) (medicinal)						
(preparations)	964.0	E858.2	E934.0	E950.4	E962.0	E980.4
dextran	964.0	E858.2	E934.0	E950.4	E962.0	E980.4
nonmedicinal (dust) (fumes) NEC	985.8	E866.4	—	E950.9	E962.1	E980.9
Irritant drug	977.9	E858.9	E947.9	E950.5	E962.0	E980.5
Ismelin	972.6	E858.3	E942.6	E950.4	E962.0	E980.4
Isoamyl nitrite	972.4	E858.3	E942.4	E950.4	E962.0	E980.4
Isobutyl acetate	982.8	E862.4	—	E950.9	E962.1	E980.9
Isocarboxazid	969.0	E854.0	E939.0	E950.3	E962.0	E980.3
Isoephedrine	971.2	E855.5	E941.2	E950.4	E962.0	E980.4
Isoetharine	971.2	E855.5	E941.2	E950.4	E962.0	E980.4
Isofluorophate	971.0	E855.3	E941.0	E950.4	E962.0	E980.4
Isoniazid (INH)	961.8	E857	E931.8	E950.4	E962.0	E980.4
Isopentaquine	961.4	E857	E931.4	E950.4	E962.0	E980.4
Isophane insulin	962.3	E858.0	E932.3	E950.4	E962.0	E980.4
Isopregnenone	962.2	E858.0	E932.2	E950.4	E962.0	E980.4
Isoprenaline	971.2	E855.5	E941.2	E950.4	E962.0	E980.4
Isopropamide	971.1	E855.4	E941.1	E950.4	E962.0	E980.4
Isopropanol	980.2	E860.3	—	E950.9	E962.1	E980.9
topical (germicide)	976.0	E858.7	E946.0	E950.4	E962.0	E980.4
Isopropyl						
acetate	982.8	E862.4	—	E950.9	E962.1	E980.9
alcohol	980.2	E860.3	—	E950.9	E962.1	E980.9
topical (germicide)	976.0	E858.7	E946.0	E950.4	E962.0	E980.4
ether	982.8	E862.4	—	E950.9	E962.1	E980.9
Isoproterenol	971.2	E855.5	E941.2	E950.4	E962.0	E980.4
Isosorbide dinitrate	972.4	E858.3	E942.4	E950.4	E962.0	E980.4
Isothipendyl	963.0	E858.1	E933.0	E950.4	E962.0	E980.4
Isoxazolyl penicillin	960.0	E856	E930.0	E950.4	E962.0	E980.4
Isoxsuprine hydrochloride	972.5	E858.3	E942.5	E950.4	E962.0	E980.4
I–thyroxine sodium	962.7	E858.0	E932.7	E950.4	E962.0	E980.4
Jaborandi (pilocarpus) (extract)	971.0	E855.3	E941.0	E950.4	E962.0	E980.4
Jalap	973.1	E858.4	E943.1	E950.4	E962.0	E980.4
Jamaica						
dogwood (bark)	965.7	E850.7	E935.7	E950.0	E962.0	E980.0
ginger	989.89	E866.8	—	E950.9	E962.1	E980.9
Jatropha	988.2	E865.4	—	E950.9	E962.1	E980.9
curcas	988.2	E865.3	—	E950.9	E962.1	E980.9

Substance	Poisoning	Accident	Therapeutic Use	Suicide Attempt	Assault	Undetermined
		External Cause (E-Code)				
Jectofer	964.0	E858.2	E934.0	E950.4	E962.0	E980.4
Jellyfish (sting)	989.5	E905.6	—	E950.9	E962.1	E980.9
Jequirity (bean)	988.2	E865.3	—	E950.9	E962.1	E980.9
Jimson weed	988.2	E865.4	—	E950.9	E962.1	E980.9
seeds	988.2	E865.3	—	E950.9	E962.1	E980.9
Juniper tar (oil) (ointment)	976.4	E858.7	E946.4	E950.4	E962.0	E980.4
Kallikrein	972.5	E858.3	E942.5	E950.4	E962.0	E980.4
Kanamycin	960.6	E856	E930.6	E950.4	E962.0	E980.4
Kantrex	960.6	E856	E930.6	E950.4	E962.0	E980.4
Kaolin	973.5	E858.4	E943.5	E950.4	E962.0	E980.4
Karaya (gum)	973.3	E858.4	E943.3	E950.4	E962.0	E980.4
Kemithal	968.3	E855.1	E938.3	E950.4	E962.0	E980.4
Kenacort	962.0	E858.0	E932.0	E950.4	E962.0	E980.4
Keratolytics	976.4	E858.7	E946.4	E950.4	E962.0	E980.4
Keratoplastics	976.4	E858.7	E946.4	E950.4	E962.0	E980.4
Kerosene, kerosine (fuel) (solvent) NEC	981	E862.1	—	E950.9	E962.1	E980.9
insecticide	981	E863.4	—	E950.6	E962.1	E980.7
vapor	987.1	E869.8	—	E952.8	E962.2	E982.8
Ketamine	968.3	E855.1	E938.3	E950.4	E962.0	E980.4
Ketobemidone	965.09	E850.2	E935.2	E950.0	E962.0	E980.0
Ketols	982.8	E862.4	—	E950.9	E962.1	E980.9
Ketone oils	982.8	E862.4	—	E950.9	E962.1	E980.9
Ketoprofen	965.61	E850.6	E935.6	E950.0	E962.0	E980.0
Kiln gas or vapor (carbon monoxide)	986	E868.8	—	E952.1	E962.2	E982.1
Konsyl	973.3	E858.4	E943.3	E950.4	E962.0	E980.4
Kosam seed	988.2	E865.3	—	E950.9	E962.1	E980.9
Krait (venom)	989.5	E905.0	—	E950.9	E962.1	E980.9
Kwell (insecticide)	989.2	E863.0	—	E950.6	E962.1	E980.7
anti–infective (topical)	976.0	E858.7	E946.0	E950.4	E962.0	E980.4
Laburnum (flowers) (seeds)	988.2	E865.3	—	E950.9	E962.1	E980.9
leaves	988.2	E865.4	—	E950.9	E962.1	E980.9
Lacquers	989.89	E861.6	—	E950.9	E962.1	E980.9
Lacrimogenic gas	987.5	E869.3	—	E952.8	E962.2	E982.8
Lactic acid	983.1	E864.1	—	E950.7	E962.1	E980.6
Lactobacillus acidophilus	973.5	E858.4	E943.5	E950.4	E962.0	E980.4
Lactoflavin	963.5	E858.1	E933.5	E950.4	E962.0	E980.4
Lactuca (virosa) (extract)	967.8	E852.8	E937.8	E950.2	E962.0	E980.2
Lactucarium	967.8	E852.8	E937.8	E950.2	E962.0	E980.2
Laevulose	974.5	E858.5	E944.5	E950.4	E962.0	E980.4
Lanatoside(C)	972.1	E858.3	E942.1	E950.4	E962.0	E980.4
Lanolin (lotion)	976.3	E858.7	E946.3	E950.4	E962.0	E980.4
Largactil	969.1	E853.0	E939.1	E950.3	E962.0	E980.3
Larkspur	988.2	E865.3	—	E950.9	E962.1	E980.9
Laroxyl	969.0	E854.0	E939.0	E950.3	E962.0	E980.3
Lasix	974.4	E858.5	E944.4	E950.4	E962.0	E980.4
Latex	989.82	E866.8	—	E950.9	E962.1	E980.9
Lathyrus (seed)	988.2	E865.3	—	E950.9	E962.1	E980.9
Laudanum	965.09	E850.2	E935.2	E950.0	E962.0	E980.0
Laudexium	975.2	E858.6	E945.2	E950.4	E962.0	E980.4
Laurel, black or cherry	988.2	E865.4	—	E950.9	E962.1	E980.9
Laurolinium	976.0	E858.7	E946.0	E950.4	E962.0	E980.4
Lauryl sulfoacetate	976.2	E858.7	E946.2	E950.4	E962.0	E980.4
Laxatives NEC	973.3	E858.4	E943.3	E950.4	E962.0	E980.4
emollient	973.2	E858.4	E943.2	E950.4	E962.0	E980.4
L–dopa	966.4	E855.0	E936.4	E950.4	E962.0	E980.4
L Tryptophan—*see* amino acid						
Lead (dust) (fumes) (vapor) NEC	984.9	E866.0	—	E950.9	E962.1	E980.9
acetate (dust)	984.1	E866.0	—	E950.9	E962.1	E980.9
anti–infectives	961.2	E857	E931.2	E950.4	E962.0	E980.4
antiknock compound (tetraethyl)	984.1	E862.1	—	E950.9	E962.1	E980.9

Substance	Poisoning	External Cause (E-Code)				
		Accident	Therapeutic Use	Suicide Attempt	Assault	Undetermined
arsenate, arsenite (dust) (insecticide) (vapor)	985.1	E863.4	—	E950.8	E962.1	E980.8
herbicide	985.1	E863.5	—	E950.8	E962.1	E980.8
carbonate	984.0	E866.0	—	E950.9	E962.1	E980.9
paint	984.0	E861.5	—	E950.9	E962.1	E980.9
chromate	984.0	E866.0	—	E950.9	E962.1	E980.9
paint	984.0	E861.5	—	E950.9	E962.1	E980.9
dioxide	984.0	E866.0	—	E950.9	E962.1	E980.9
inorganic (compound)	984.0	E866.0	—	E950.9	E962.1	E980.9
paint	984.0	E861.5	—	E950.9	E962.1	E980.9
iodine	984.0	E866.0	—	E950.9	E962.1	E980.9
pigment (paint)	984.0	E861.5	—	E950.9	E962.1	E980.9
monoxide (dust)	984.0	E866.0	—	E950.9	E962.1	E980.9
paint	984.0	E861.5	—	E950.9	E962.1	E980.9
organic	984.1	E866.0	—	E950.9	E962.1	E980.9
oxide	984.0	E866.0	—	E950.9	E962.1	E980.9
paint	984.0	E861.5	—	E950.9	E962.1	E980.9
paint	984.0	E861.5	—	E950.9	E962.1	E980.9
salts	984.0	E866.0	—	E950.9	E962.1	E980.9
specified compound NEC	984.8	E866.0	—	E950.9	E962.1	E980.9
tetra–ethyl	984.1	E862.1	—	E950.9	E962.1	E980.9
Lebanese red	969.6	E854.1	E939.6	E950.3	E962.0	E980.3
Lente Iletin (insulin)	962.3	E858.0	E932.3	E950.4	E962.0	E980.4
Leptazol	970.0	E854.3	E940.0	E950.4	E962.0	E980.4
Leritine	965.09	E850.2	E935.2	E950.0	E962.0	E980.0
Letter	962.7	E858.0	E932.7	E950.4	E962.0	E980.4
Lettuce opium	967.8	E852.8	E937.8	E950.2	E962.0	E980.2
Leucovorin (factor)	964.1	E858.2	E934.1	E950.4	E962.0	E980.4
Leukeran	963.1	E858.1	E933.1	E950.4	E962.0	E980.4
Levalbuterol	975.7	E858.6	E945.7	E950.4	E962.0	E980.4
Levallorphan	970.1	E854.3	E940.1	E950.4	E962.0	E980.4
Levanil	967.8	E852.8	E937.8	E950.2	E962.0	E980.2
Levarterenol	971.2	E855.5	E941.2	E950.4	E962.0	E980.4
Levodopa	966.4	E855.0	E936.4	E950.4	E962.0	E980.4
Levo–dromoran	965.09	E850.2	E935.2	E950.0	E962.0	E980.0
Levoid	962.7	E858.0	E932.7	E950.4	E962.0	E980.4
Levo–iso–methadone	965.02	E850.1	E935.1	E950.0	E962.0	E980.0
Levomepromazine	967.8	E852.8	E937.8	E950.2	E962.0	E980.2
Levoprome	967.8	E852.8	E937.8	E950.2	E962.0	E980.2
Levopropoxyphene	975.4	E858.6	E945.4	E950.4	E962.0	E980.4
Levorphan, levophanol	965.09	E850.2	E935.2	E950.0	E962.0	E980.0
Levothyroxine (sodium)	962.7	E858.0	E932.7	E950.4	E962.0	E980.4
Levsin	971.1	E855.4	E941.1	E950.4	E962.0	E980.4
Levulose	974.5	E858.5	E944.5	E950.4	E962.0	E980.4
Lewisite (gas)	985.1	E866.3	—	E950.8	E962.1	E980.8
Librium	969.4	E853.2	E939.4	E950.3	E962.0	E980.3
Lidex	976.0	E858.7	E946.0	E950.4	E962.0	E980.4
Lidocaine (infiltration) (topical)	968.5	E855.2	E938.5	E950.4	E962.0	E980.4
nerve block (peripheral) (plexus)	968.6	E855.2	E938.6	E950.4	E962.0	E980.4
spinal	968.7	E855.2	E938.7	E950.4	E962.0	E980.4
Lighter fluid	981	E862.1	—	E950.9	E962.1	E980.9
Lignocaine (infiltration) (topical)	968.5	E855.2	E938.5	E950.4	E962.0	E980.4
nerve block (peripheral) (plexus)	968.6	E855.2	E938.6	E950.4	E962.0	E980.4
spinal	968.7	E855.2	E938.7	E950.4	E962.0	E980.4
Ligroin(e) (solvent)	981	E862.0	—	E950.9	E962.1	E980.9
vapor	987.1	E869.8	—	E952.8	E962.2	E982.8
Ligustrum vulgare	988.2	E865.3	—	E950.9	E962.1	E980.9
Lily of the valley	988.2	E865.4	—	E950.9	E962.1	E980.9
Lime (chloride)	983.2	E864.2	—	E950.7	E962.1	E980.6
solution, sulferated	976.4	E858.7	E946.4	E950.4	E962.0	E980.4

Substance	Poisoning	Accident	Therapeutic Use	Suicide Attempt	Assault	Undetermined
		External Cause (E-Code)				
Limonene	982.8	E862.4	—	E950.9	E962.1	E980.9
Lincomycin	960.8	E856	E930.8	E950.4	E962.0	E980.4
Lindane (insecticide) (vapor)	989.2	E863.0	—	E950.6	E962.1	E980.7
anti–infective (topical)	976.0	E858.7	E946.0	E950.4	E962.0	E980.4
Liniments NEC	976.9	E858.7	E946.9	E950.4	E962.0	E980.4
Linoleic acid	972.2	E858.3	E942.2	E950.4	E962.0	E980.4
Liothyronine	962.7	E858.0	E932.7	E950.4	E962.0	E980.4
Liotrix	962.7	E858.0	E932.7	E950.4	E962.0	E980.4
Lipancreatin	973.4	E858.4	E943.4	E950.4	E962.0	E980.4
Lipo–Lutin	962.2	E858.0	E932.2	E950.4	E962.0	E980.4
Lipotropic agents	977.1	E858.8	E947.1	E950.4	E962.0	E980.4
Liquefied petroleum gases	987.0	E868.0	—	E951.1	E962.2	E981.1
piped (pure or mixed with air)	987.0	E867	—	E951.0	E962.2	E981.0
Liquid petrolatum	973.2	E858.4	E943.2	E950.4	E962.0	E980.4
substance	989.9	E866.9	—	E950.9	E962.1	E980.9
specified NEC	989.89	E866.8	—	E950.9	E962.1	E980.9
Lirugen	979.4	E858.8	E949.4	E950.4	E962.0	E980.4
Lithane	969.8	E855.8	E939.8	E950.3	E962.0	E980.3
Lithium	985.8	E866.4	—	E950.9	E962.1	E980.9
carbonate	969.8	E855.8	E939.8	E950.3	E962.0	E980.3
Lithonate	969.8	E855.8	E939.8	E950.3	E962.0	E980.3
Liver (extract) (injection) (preparations)	964.1	E858.2	E934.1	E950.4	E962.0	E980.4
Lizard (bite) (venom)	989.5	E905.0	—	E950.9	E962.1	E980.9
LMD	964.8	E858.2	E934.8	E950.4	E962.0	E980.4
Lobelia	988.2	E865.4	—	E950.9	E962.1	E980.9
Lobeline	970.0	E854.3	E940.0	E950.4	E962.0	E980.4
Locorten	976.0	E858.7	E946.0	E950.4	E962.0	E980.4
Lolium temulentum	988.2	E865.3	—	E950.9	E962.1	E980.9
Lomotil	973.5	E858.4	E943.5	E950.4	E962.0	E980.4
Lomustine	963.1	E858.1	E933.1	E950.4	E962.0	E980.4
Lophophora williamsii	969.6	E854.1	E939.6	E950.3	E962.0	E980.3
Lorazepam	969.4	E853.2	E939.4	E950.3	E962.0	E980.3
Lotions NEC	976.9	E858.7	E946.9	E950.4	E962.0	E980.4
Lotronex	973.8	E858.4	E943.8	E950.4	E962.0	E980.4
Lotusate	967.0	E851	E937.0	E950.1	E962.0	E980.1
Lowila	976.2	E858.7	E946.2	E950.4	E962.0	E980.4
Loxapine	969.3	E853.8	E939.3	E950.3	E962.0	E980.3
Lozenges (throat)	976.6	E858.7	E946.6	E950.4	E962.0	E980.4
LSD (25)	969.6	E854.1	E939.6	E950.3	E962.0	E980.3
Lubricating oil NEC	981	E862.2	—	E950.9	E962.1	E980.9
Lucanthone	961.6	E857	E931.6	E950.4	E962.0	E980.4
Luminal	967.0	E851	E937.0	E950.1	E962.0	E980.1
Lung irritant (gas) NEC	987.9	E869.9	—	E952.9	E962.2	E982.9
Lutocylol	962.2	E858.0	E932.2	E950.4	E962.0	E980.4
Lutromone	962.2	E858.0	E932.2	E950.4	E962.0	E980.4
Lututrin	975.0	E858.6	E945.0	E950.4	E962.0	E980.4
Lye (concentrated)	983.2	E864.2	—	E950.7	E962.1	E980.6
Lygranum (skin test)	977.8	E858.8	E947.8	E950.4	E962.0	E980.4
Lymecycline	960.4	E856	E930.4	E950.4	E962.0	E980.4
Lymphogranuloma venereum antigen	977.8	E858.8	E947.8	E950.4	E962.0	E980.4
Lynestrenol	962.2	E858.0	E932.2	E950.4	E962.0	E980.4
Lyovac Sodium Edecrin	974.4	E858.5	E944.4	E950.4	E962.0	E980.4
Lypressin	962.5	E858.0	E932.5	E950.4	E962.0	E980.4
Lysergic acid (amide) (diethylamide)	969.6	E854.1	E939.6	E950.3	E962.0	E980.3
Lysergide	969.6	E854.1	E939.6	E950.3	E962.0	E980.3
Lysine vasopressin	962.5	E858.0	E932.5	E950.4	E962.0	E980.4
Lysol	983.0	E864.0	—	E950.7	E962.1	E980.6
Lytta (vitatta)	976.8	E858.7	E946.8	E950.4	E962.0	E980.4
Mace	987.5	E869.3	—	E952.8	E962.2	E982.8
Macrolides (antibiotics)	960.3	E856	E930.3	E950.4	E962.0	E980.4
Mafenide	976.0	E858.7	E946.0	E950.4	E962.0	E980.4

Substance	Poisoning	Accident	Therapeutic Use	Suicide Attempt	Assault	Undetermined
			External Cause (E-Code)			
Magaldrate	973.0	E858.4	E943.0	E950.4	E962.0	E980.4
Magic mushroom	969.6	E854.1	E939.6	E950.3	E962.0	E980.3
Magnamycin	960.8	E856	E930.8	E950.4	E962.0	E980.4
Magnesia magma	973.0	E858.4	E943.0	E950.4	E962.0	E980.4
Magnesium (compounds) (fumes) NEC	985.8	E866.4	—	E950.9	E962.1	E980.9
antacid	973.0	E858.4	E943.0	E950.4	E962.0	E980.4
carbonate	973.0	E858.4	E943.0	E950.4	E962.0	E980.4
cathartic	973.3	E858.4	E943.3	E950.4	E962.0	E980.4
citrate	973.3	E858.4	E943.3	E950.4	E962.0	E980.4
hydroxide	973.0	E858.4	E943.0	E950.4	E962.0	E980.4
oxide	973.0	E858.4	E943.0	E950.4	E962.0	E980.4
sulfate (oral)	973.3	E858.4	E943.3	E950.4	E962.0	E980.4
intravenous	966.3	E855.0	E936.3	E950.4	E962.0	E980.4
trisilicate	973.0	E858.4	E943.0	E950.4	E962.0	E980.4
Malathion (insecticide)	989.3	E863.1	—	E950.6	E962.1	E980.7
Male fern (oleoresin)	961.6	E857	E931.6	E950.4	E962.0	E980.4
Mandelic acid	961.9	E857	E931.9	E950.4	E962.0	E980.4
Manganese compounds (fumes) NEC	985.2	E866.4	—	E950.9	E962.1	E980.9
Mannitol (diuretic) (medicinal) NEC	974.4	E858.5	E944.4	E950.4	E962.0	E980.4
hexanitrate	972.4	E858.3	E942.4	E950.4	E962.0	E980.4
mustard	963.1	E858.1	E933.1	E950.4	E962.0	E980.4
Mannomustine	963.1	E858.1	E933.1	E950.4	E962.0	E980.4
MAO inhibitors	969.0	E854.0	E939.0	E950.3	E962.0	E980.3
Mapharsen	961.1	E857	E931.1	E950.4	E962.0	E980.4
Marcaine	968.9	E855.2	E938.9	E950.4	E962.0	E980.4
infiltration (subcutaneous)	968.5	E855.2	E938.5	E950.4	E962.0	E980.4
nerve block (peripheral) (plexus)	968.6	E855.2	E938.6	E950.4	E962.0	E980.4
Marezine	963.0	E858.1	E933.0	E950.4	E962.0	E980.4
Marihuana, marijuana (derivatives)	969.6	E854.1	E939.6	E950.3	E962.0	E980.3
Marine animals or plants (sting)	989.5	E905.6	—	E950.9	E962.1	E980.9
Marplan	969.0	E854.0	E939.0	E950.3	E962.0	E980.3
Marsh gas	987.1	E869.8	—	E952.8	E962.2	E982.8
Marsilid	969.0	E854.0	E939.0	E950.3	E962.0	E980.3
Matulane	963.1	E858.1	E933.1	E950.4	E962.0	E980.4
Mazindol	977.0	E858.8	E947.0	E950.4	E962.0	E980.4
MDMA	969.7	E854.2	E939.7	E950.3	E962.0	E980.3
Meadow saffron	988.2	E865.3	—	E950.9	E962.1	E980.9
Measles vaccine	979.4	E858.8	E949.4	E950.4	E962.0	E980.4
Meat, noxious or nonbacterial	988.8	E865.0	—	E950.9	E962.1	E980.9
Mebanazine	969.0	E854.0	E939.0	E950.3	E962.0	E980.3
Mebaral	967.0	E851	E937.0	E950.1	E962.0	E980.1
Mebendazole	961.6	E857	E931.6	E950.4	E962.0	E980.4
Mebeverine	975.1	E858.6	E945.1	E950.4	E962.0	E980.4
Mebhydroline	963.0	E858.1	E933.0	E950.4	E962.0	E980.4
Mebrophenhydramine	963.0	E858.1	E933.0	E950.4	E962.0	E980.4
Mebutamate	969.5	E853.8	E939.5	E950.3	E962.0	E980.3
Mecamylamine (chloride)	972.3	E858.3	E942.3	E950.4	E962.0	E980.4
Mechlorethamine hydrochloride	963.1	E858.1	E933.1	E950.4	E962.0	E980.4
Meclizene (hydrochloride)	963.0	E858.1	E933.0	E950.4	E962.0	E980.4
Meclofenoxate	970.0	E854.3	E940.0	E950.4	E962.0	E980.4
Meclozine (hydrochloride)	963.0	E858.1	E933.0	E950.4	E962.0	E980.4
Medazepam	969.4	E853.2	E939.4	E950.3	E962.0	E980.3
Medicine, medicinal substance	977.9	E858.9	E947.9	E950.5	E962.0	E980.5
specified NEC	977.8	E858.8	E947.8	E950.4	E962.0	E980.4
Medinal	967.0	E851	E937.0	E950.1	E962.0	E980.1
Medomin	967.0	E851	E937.0	E950.1	E962.0	E980.1
Medroxyprogesterone	962.2	E858.0	E932.2	E950.4	E962.0	E980.4
Medrysone	976.5	E858.7	E946.5	E950.4	E962.0	E980.4
Mefenamic acid	965.7	E850.7	E935.7	E950.0	E962.0	E980.0
Megahallucinogen	969.6	E854.1	E939.6	E950.3	E962.0	E980.3

Substance	Poisoning	Accident	Therapeutic Use	Suicide Attempt	Assault	Undetermined
			External Cause (E-Code)			
Megestrol	962.2	E858.0	E932.2	E950.4	E962.0	E980.4
Meglumine	977.8	E858.8	E947.8	E950.4	E962.0	E980.4
Meladinin	976.3	E858.7	E946.3	E950.4	E962.0	E980.4
Melanizing agents	976.3	E858.7	E946.3	E950.4	E962.0	E980.4
Melarsoprol	961.1	E857	E931.1	E950.4	E962.0	E980.4
Melia azedarach	988.2	E865.3	—	E950.9	E962.1	E980.9
Mellaril	969.1	E853.0	E939.1	E950.3	E962.0	E980.3
Meloxine	976.3	E858.7	E946.3	E950.4	E962.0	E980.4
Melphalan	963.1	E858.1	E933.1	E950.4	E962.0	E980.4
Menadiol sodium diphosphate	964.3	E858.2	E934.3	E950.4	E962.0	E980.4
Menadione (sodium bisulfate)	964.3	E858.2	E934.3	E950.4	E962.0	E980.4
Menaphthone	964.3	E858.2	E934.3	E950.4	E962.0	E980.4
Meningococcal vaccine	978.8	E858.8	E948.8	E950.4	E962.0	E980.4
Menningovax–C	978.8	E858.8	E948.8	E950.4	E962.0	E980.4
Menotropins	962.4	E858.0	E932.4	E950.4	E962.0	E980.4
Menthol NEC	976.1	E858.7	E946.1	E950.4	E962.0	E980.4
Mepacrine	961.3	E857	E931.3	E950.4	E962.0	E980.4
Meparfynol	967.8	E852.8	E937.8	E950.2	E962.0	E980.2
Mepazine	969.1	E853.0	E939.1	E950.3	E962.0	E980.3
Mepenzolate	971.1	E855.4	E941.1	E950.4	E962.0	E980.4
Meperidine	965.09	E850.2	E935.2	E950.0	E962.0	E980.0
Mephenamin(e)	966.4	E855.0	E936.4	E950.4	E962.0	E980.4
Mephenesin (carbamate)	968.0	E855.1	E938.0	E950.4	E962.0	E980.4
Mephenoxalone	969.5	E853.8	E939.5	E950.3	E962.0	E980.3
Mephentermine	971.2	E855.5	E941.2	E950.4	E962.0	E980.4
Mephenytoin	966.1	E855.0	E936.1	E950.4	E962.0	E980.4
Mephobarbital	967.0	E851	E937.0	E950.1	E962.0	E980.1
Mepiperphenidol	971.1	E855.4	E941.1	E950.4	E962.0	E980.4
Mepivacaine	968.9	E855.2	E938.9	E950.4	E962.0	E980.4
infiltration (subcutaneous)	968.5	E855.2	E938.5	E950.4	E962.0	E980.4
nerve block (peripheral) (plexus)	968.6	E855.2	E938.6	E950.4	E962.0	E980.4
topical (surface)	968.5	E855.2	E938.5	E950.4	E962.0	E980.4
Meprednisone	962.0	E858.0	E932.0	E950.4	E962.0	E980.4
Meprobam	969.5	E853.8	E939.5	E950.3	E962.0	E980.3
Meprobamate	969.5	E853.8	E939.5	E950.3	E962.0	E980.3
Mepyramine (maleate)	963.0	E858.1	E933.0	E950.4	E962.0	E980.4
Meralluride	974.0	E858.5	E944.0	E950.4	E962.0	E980.4
Merbaphen	974.0	E858.5	E944.0	E950.4	E962.0	E980.4
Merbromin	976.0	E858.7	E946.0	E950.4	E962.0	E980.4
Mercaptomerin	974.0	E858.5	E944.0	E950.4	E962.0	E980.4
Mercaptopurine	963.1	E858.1	E933.1	E950.4	E962.0	E980.4
Mercumatilin	974.0	E858.5	E944.0	E950.4	E962.0	E980.4
Mercuramide	974.0	E858.5	E944.0	E950.4	E962.0	E980.4
Mercuranin	976.0	E858.7	E946.0	E950.4	E962.0	E980.4
Mercurochrome	976.0	E858.7	E946.0	E950.4	E962.0	E980.4
Mercury, mercuric, mercurous (compounds) (cyanide) (fumes) (nonmedicinal) (vapor) NEC	985.0	E866.1	—	E950.9	E962.1	E980.9
ammoniated	976.0	E858.7	E946.0	E950.4	E962.0	E980.4
anti–infective	961.2	E857	E931.2	E950.4	E962.0	E980.4
topical	976.0	E858.7	E946.0	E950.4	E962.0	E980.4
chloride (antiseptic) NEC	976.0	E858.7	E946.0	E950.4	E962.0	E980.4
fungicide	985.0	E863.6	—	E950.6	E962.1	E980.7
diuretic compounds	974.0	E858.5	E944.0	E950.4	E962.0	E980.4
fungicide	985.0	E863.6	—	E950.6	E962.1	E980.7
organic (fungicide)	985.0	E863.6	—	E950.6	E962.1	E980.7
Merethoxylline	974.0	E858.5	E944.0	E950.4	E962.0	E980.4
Mersalyl	974.0	E858.5	E944.0	E950.4	E962.0	E980.4
Merthiolate (topical)	976.0	E858.7	E946.0	E950.4	E962.0	E980.4
ophthalmic preparation	976.5	E858.7	E946.5	E950.4	E962.0	E980.4
Meruvax	979.4	E858.8	E949.4	E950.4	E962.0	E980.4

Substance	Poisoning	Accident	Therapeutic Use	Suicide Attempt	Assault	Undetermined
			External Cause (E-Code)			
Mescal buttons	969.6	E854.1	E939.6	E950.3	E962.0	E980.3
Mescaline (salts)	969.6	E854.1	E939.6	E950.3	E962.0	E980.3
Mesoridazine besylate	969.1	E853.0	E939.1	E950.3	E962.0	E980.3
Mestanolone	962.1	E858.0	E932.1	E950.4	E962.0	E980.4
Mestranol	962.2	E858.0	E932.2	E950.4	E962.0	E980.4
Metacresylacetate	976.0	E858.7	E946.0	E950.4	E962.0	E980.4
Metaldehyde (snail killer) NEC	989.4	E863.4	—	E950.6	E962.1	E980.7
Metals (heavy) (nonmedicinal) NEC	985.9	E866.4	—	E950.9	E962.1	E980.9
dust, fumes, or vapor NEC	985.9	E866.4	—	E950.9	E962.1	E980.9
light NEC	985.9	E866.4	—	E950.9	E962.1	E980.9
dust, fumes, or vapor NEC	985.9	E866.4	—	E950.9	E962.1	E980.9
pesticides (dust) (vapor)	985.9	E863.4	—	E950.6	E962.1	E980.7
Metamucil	973.3	E858.4	E943.3	E950.4	E962.0	E980.4
Metaphen	976.0	E858.7	E946.0	E950.4	E962.0	E980.4
Metaproterenol	975.1	E858.6	E945.1	E950.4	E962.0	E980.4
Metaraminol	972.8	E858.3	E942.8	E950.4	E962.0	E980.4
Metaxalone	968.0	E855.1	E938.0	E950.4	E962.0	E980.4
Metformin	962.3	E858.0	E932.3	E950.4	E962.0	E980.4
Methacycline	960.4	E856	E930.4	E950.4	E962.0	E980.4
Methadone	965.02	E850.1	E935.1	E950.0	E962.0	E980.0
Methallenestril	962.2	E858.0	E932.2	E950.4	E962.0	E980.4
Methamphetamine	969.7	E854.2	E939.7	E950.3	E962.0	E980.3
Methandienone	962.1	E858.0	E932.1	E950.4	E962.0	E980.4
Methandriol	962.1	E858.0	E932.1	E950.4	E962.0	E980.4
Methandrostenolone	962.1	E858.0	E932.1	E950.4	E962.0	E980.4
Methane gas	987.1	E869.8	—	E952.8	E962.2	E982.8
Methanol	980.1	E860.2	—	E950.9	E962.1	E980.9
vapor	987.8	E869.8	—	E952.8	E962.2	E982.8
Methantheline	971.1	E855.4	E941.1	E950.4	E962.0	E980.4
Methaphenilene	963.0	E858.1	E933.0	E950.4	E962.0	E980.4
Methapyrilene	963.0	E858.1	E933.0	E950.4	E962.0	E980.4
Methaqualone (compounds)	967.4	E852.3	E937.4	E950.2	E962.0	E980.2
Metharbital, metharbitone	967.0	E851	E937.0	E950.1	E962.0	E980.1
Methazolamide	974.2	E858.5	E944.2	E950.4	E962.0	E980.4
Methdilazine	963.0	E858.1	E933.0	E950.4	E962.0	E980.4
Methedrine	969.7	E854.2	E939.7	E950.3	E962.0	E980.3
Methenamine (mandelate)	961.9	E857	E931.9	E950.4	E962.0	E980.4
Methenolone	962.1	E858.0	E932.1	E950.4	E962.0	E980.4
Methergine	975.0	E858.6	E945.0	E950.4	E962.0	E980.4
Methiacil	962.8	E858.0	E932.8	E950.4	E962.0	E980.4
Methicillin (sodium)	960.0	E856	E930.0	E950.4	E962.0	E980.4
Methimazole	962.8	E858.0	E932.8	E950.4	E962.0	E980.4
Methionine	977.1	E858.8	E947.1	E950.4	E962.0	E980.4
Methisazone	961.7	E857	E931.7	E950.4	E962.0	E980.4
Methitural	967.0	E851	E937.0	E950.1	E962.0	E980.1
Methixene	971.1	E855.4	E941.1	E950.4	E962.0	E980.4
Methobarbital, methobarbitone	967.0	E851	E937.0	E950.1	E962.0	E980.1
Methocarbamol	968.0	E855.1	E938.0	E950.4	E962.0	E980.4
Methohexital, methohexitone (sodium)	968.3	E855.1	E938.3	E950.4	E962.0	E980.4
Methoin	966.1	E855.0	E936.1	E950.4	E962.0	E980.4
Methopholine	965.7	E850.7	E935.7	E950.0	E962.0	E980.0
Methorate	975.4	E858.6	E945.4	E950.4	E962.0	E980.4
Methoserpidine	972.6	E858.3	E942.6	E950.4	E962.0	E980.4
Methotrexate	963.1	E858.1	E933.1	E950.4	E962.0	E980.4
Methotrimeprazine	967.8	E852.8	E937.8	E950.2	E962.0	E980.2
Methoxa–Dome	976.3	E858.7	E946.3	E950.4	E962.0	E980.4
Methoxamine	971.2	E855.5	E941.2	E950.4	E962.0	E980.4
Methoxsalen	976.3	E858.7	E946.3	E950.4	E962.0	E980.4
Methoxybenzyl penicillin	960.0	E856	E930.0	E950.4	E962.0	E980.4
Methoxychlor	989.2	E863.0	—	E950.6	E962.1	E980.7

Substance	Poisoning	Accident	Therapeutic Use	Suicide Attempt	Assault	Undetermined
		External Cause (E-Code)				
Methoxyflurane	968.2	E855.1	E938.2	E950.4	E962.0	E980.4
Methoxyphenamine	971.2	E855.5	E941.2	E950.4	E962.0	E980.4
Methoxypromazine	969.1	E853.0	E939.1	E950.3	E962.0	E980.3
Methoxypsoralen	976.3	E858.7	E946.3	E950.4	E962.0	E980.4
Methscopolamine (bromide)	971.1	E855.4	E941.1	E950.4	E962.0	E980.4
Methsuximide	966.2	E855.0	E936.2	E950.4	E962.0	E980.4
Methyclothiazide	974.3	E858.5	E944.3	E950.4	E962.0	E980.4
Methyl						
acetate	982.8	E862.4	—	E950.9	E962.1	E980.9
acetone	982.8	E862.4	—	E950.9	E962.1	E980.9
alcohol	980.1	E860.2	—	E950.9	E962.1	E980.9
amphetamine	969.7	E854.2	E939.7	E950.3	E962.0	E980.3
androstanolone	962.1	E858.0	E932.1	E950.4	E962.0	E980.4
atropine	971.1	E855.4	E941.1	E950.4	E962.0	E980.4
benzene	982.0	E862.4	—	E950.9	E962.1	E980.9
bromide (gas)	987.8	E869.8	—	E952.8	E962.2	E982.8
fumigant	987.8	E863.8	—	E950.6	E962.2	E980.7
butanol	980.8	E860.8	—	E950.9	E962.1	E980.9
carbinol	980.1	E860.2	—	E950.9	E962.1	E980.9
cellosolve	982.8	E862.4	—	E950.9	E962.1	E980.9
cellulose	973.3	E858.4	E943.3	E950.4	E962.0	E980.4
chloride (gas)	987.8	E869.8	—	E952.8	E962.2	E982.8
cyclohexane	982.8	E862.4	—	E950.9	E962.1	E980.9
cyclohexanone	982.8	E862.4	—	E950.9	E962.1	E980.9
dihydromorphinone	965.09	E850.2	E935.2	E950.0	E962.0	E980.0
ergometrine	975.0	E858.6	E945.0	E950.4	E962.0	E980.4
ergonovine	975.0	E858.6	E945.0	E950.4	E962.0	E980.4
ethyl ketone	982.8	E862.4	—	E950.9	E962.1	E980.9
hydrazine	983.9	E864.3	—	E950.7	E962.1	E980.6
isobutyl ketone	982.8	E862.4	—	E950.9	E962.1	E980.9
morphine NEC	965.09	E850.2	E935.2	E950.0	E962.0	E980.0
parafynol	967.8	E852.8	E937.8	E950.2	E962.0	E980.2
parathion	989.3	E863.1	—	E950.6	E962.1	E980.7
pentynol NEC	967.8	E852.8	E937.8	E950.2	E962.0	E980.2
peridol	969.2	E853.1	E939.2	E950.3	E962.0	E980.3
phenidate	969.7	E854.2	E939.7	E950.3	E962.0	E980.3
prednisolone	962.0	E858.0	E932.0	E950.4	E962.0	E980.4
ENT agent	976.6	E858.7	E946.6	E950.4	E962.0	E980.4
ophthalmic preparation	976.5	E858.7	E946.5	E950.4	E962.0	E980.4
topical NEC	976.0	E858.7	E946.0	E950.4	E962.0	E980.4
propylcarbinol	980.8	E860.8	—	E950.9	E962.1	E980.9
rosaniline NEC	976.0	E858.7	E946.0	E950.4	E962.0	E980.4
salicylate NEC	976.3	E858.7	E946.3	E950.4	E962.0	E980.4
sulfate (fumes)	987.8	E869.8	—	E952.8	E962.2	E982.8
liquid	983.9	E864.3	—	E950.7	E962.1	E980.6
sulfonal	967.8	E852.8	E937.8	E950.2	E962.0	E980.2
testosterone	962.1	E858.0	E932.1	E950.4	E962.0	E980.4
thiouracil	962.8	E858.0	E932.8	E950.4	E962.0	E980.4
Methylated spirit	980.0	E860.1	—	E950.9	E962.1	E980.9
Methyldopa	972.6	E858.3	E942.6	E950.4	E962.0	E980.4
Methylene						
blue	961.9	E857	E931.9	E950.4	E962.0	E980.4
chloride or dichloride (solvent) NEC	982.3	E862.4	—	E950.9	E962.1	E980.9
Methylhexabital	967.0	E851	E937.0	E950.1	E962.0	E980.1
Methylparaben (ophthalmic)	976.5	E858.7	E946.5	E950.4	E962.0	E980.4
Methyprylon	967.5	E852.4	E937.5	E950.2	E962.0	E980.2
Methysergide	971.3	E855.6	E941.3	E950.4	E962.0	E980.4
Metoclopramide	963.0	E858.1	E933.0	E950.4	E962.0	E980.4
Metofoline	965.7	E850.7	E935.7	E950.0	E962.0	E980.0
Metopon	965.09	E850.2	E935.2	E950.0	E962.0	E980.0
Metronidazole	961.5	E857	E931.5	E950.4	E962.0	E980.4

Substance	Poisoning	Accident	Therapeutic Use	Suicide Attempt	Assault	Undetermined
			External Cause (E-Code)			
Metycaine	968.9	E855.2	E938.9	E950.4	E962.0	E980.4
infiltration (subcutaneous)	968.5	E855.2	E938.5	E950.4	E962.0	E980.4
nerve block (peripheral) (plexus)	968.6	E855.2	E938.6	E950.4	E962.0	E980.4
topical (surface)	968.5	E855.2	E938.5	E950.4	E962.0	E980.4
Metyrapone	977.8	E858.8	E947.8	E950.4	E962.0	E980.4
Mevinphos	989.3	E863.1	—	E950.6	E962.1	E980.7
Mezereon (berries)	988.2	E865.3	—	E950.9	E962.1	E980.9
Micatin	976.0	E858.7	E946.0	E950.4	E962.0	E980.4
Miconazole	976.0	E858.7	E946.0	E950.4	E962.0	E980.4
Midol	965.1	E850.3	E935.3	E950.0	E962.0	E980.0
Mifepristone	962.9	E858.0	E932.9	E950.4	E962.0	E980.4
Milk of magnesia	973.0	E858.4	E943.0	E950.4	E962.0	E980.4
Millipede (tropical) (venomous)	989.5	E905.4	—	E950.9	E962.1	E980.9
Miltown	969.5	E853.8	E939.5	E950.3	E962.0	E980.3
Mineral						
oil (medicinal)	973.2	E858.4	E943.2	E950.4	E962.0	E980.4
nonmedicinal	981	E862.1	—	E950.9	E962.1	E980.9
topical	976.3	E858.7	E946.3	E950.4	E962.0	E980.4
salts NEC	974.6	E858.5	E944.6	E950.4	E962.0	E980.4
spirits	981	E862.0	—	E950.9	E962.1	E980.9
Minocycline	960.4	E856	E930.4	E950.4	E962.0	E980.4
Mithramycin (antineoplastic)	960.7	E856	E930.7	E950.4	E962.0	E980.4
Mitobronitol	963.1	E858.1	E933.1	E950.4	E962.0	E980.4
Mitomycin (antineoplastic)	960.7	E856	E930.7	E950.4	E962.0	E980.4
Mitotane	963.1	E858.1	E933.1	E950.4	E962.0	E980.4
Moderil	972.6	E858.3	E942.6	E950.4	E962.0	E980.4
Mogadon—*see* Nitrazepam						
Molindone	969.3	E853.8	E939.3	E950.3	E962.0	E980.3
Monistat	976.0	E858.7	E946.0	E950.4	E962.0	E980.4
Monkshood	988.2	E865.4	—	E950.9	E962.1	E980.9
Monoamine oxidase inhibitors	969.0	E854.0	E939.0	E950.3	E962.0	E980.3
Monochlorobenzene	982.0	E862.4	—	E950.9	E962.1	E980.9
Monosodium glutamate	989.89	E866.8	—	E950.9	E962.1	E980.9
Monoxide, carbon — *see* Carbon, monoxide						
Moperone	969.2	E853.1	E939.2	E950.3	E962.0	E980.3
Morning glory seeds	969.6	E854.1	E939.6	E950.3	E962.0	E980.3
Moroxydine (hydrochloride)	961.7	E857	E931.7	E950.4	E962.0	E980.4
Morphazinamide	961.8	E857	E931.8	E950.4	E962.0	E980.4
Morphinans	965.09	E850.2	E935.2	E950.0	E962.0	E980.0
Morphine NEC	965.09	E850.2	E935.2	E950.0	E962.0	E980.0
antagonists	970.1	E854.3	E940.1	E950.4	E962.0	E980.4
Morpholinylethylmorphine	965.09	E850.2	E935.2	E950.0	E962.0	E980.0
Morrhuate sodium	972.7	E858.3	E942.7	E950.4	E962.0	E980.4
Moth balls (*see also* Pesticides)	989.4	E863.4	—	E950.6	E962.1	E980.7
naphthalene	983.0	E863.4	—	E950.7	E962.1	E980.6
Motor exhaust gas — *see* Carbon, monoxide, exhaust gas						
Mouth wash	976.6	E858.7	E946.6	E950.4	E962.0	E980.4
Mucolytic agent	975.5	E858.6	E945.5	E950.4	E962.0	E980.4
Mucomyst	975.5	E858.6	E945.5	E950.4	E962.0	E980.4
Mucous membrane agents (external)	976.9	E858.7	E946.9	E950.4	E962.0	E980.4
specified NEC	976.8	E858.7	E946.8	E950.4	E962.0	E980.4
Mumps						
immune globulin (human)	964.6	E858.2	E934.6	E950.4	E962.0	E980.4
skin test antigen	977.8	E858.8	E947.8	E950.4	E962.0	E980.4
vaccine	979.6	E858.8	E949.6	E950.4	E962.0	E980.4
Mumpsvax	979.6	E858.8	E949.6	E950.4	E962.0	E980.4
Muriatic acid — *see* Hydrochloric acid						
Muscarine	971.0	E855.3	E941.0	E950.4	E962.0	E980.4
Muscle affecting agents NEC	975.3	E858.6	E945.3	E950.4	E962.0	E980.4

Substance	Poisoning	Accident	Therapeutic Use	Suicide Attempt	Assault	Undetermined
		External Cause (E-Code)				
oxytocic	975.0	E858.6	E945.0	E950.4	E962.0	E980.4
relaxants	975.3	E858.6	E945.3	E950.4	E962.0	E980.4
central nervous system	968.0	E855.1	E938.0	E950.4	E962.0	E980.4
skeletal	975.2	E858.6	E945.2	E950.4	E962.0	E980.4
smooth	975.1	E858.6	E945.1	E950.4	E962.0	E980.4
Mushrooms, noxious	988.1	E865.5	—	E950.9	E962.1	E980.9
Mussel, noxious	988.0	E865.1	—	E950.9	E962.1	E980.9
Mustard (emetic)	973.6	E858.4	E943.6	E950.4	E962.0	E980.4
gas	987.8	E869.8	—	E952.8	E962.2	E982.8
nitrogen	963.1	E858.1	E933.1	E950.4	E962.0	E980.4
Mustine	963.1	E858.1	E933.1	E950.4	E962.0	E980.4
M–vac	979.4	E858.8	E949.4	E950.4	E962.0	E980.4
Mycifradin	960.8	E856	E930.8	E950.4	E962.0	E980.4
topical	976.0	E858.7	E946.0	E950.4	E962.0	E980.4
Mycitracin	960.8	E856	E930.8	E950.4	E962.0	E980.4
ophthalmic preparation	976.5	E858.7	E946.5	E950.4	E962.0	E980.4
Mycostatin	960.1	E856	E930.1	E950.4	E962.0	E980.4
topical	976.0	E858.7	E946.0	E950.4	E962.0	E980.4
Mydriacyl	971.1	E855.4	E941.1	E950.4	E962.0	E980.4
Myelobromal	963.1	E858.1	E933.1	E950.4	E962.0	E980.4
Myleran	963.1	E858.1	E933.1	E950.4	E962.0	E980.4
Myochrysin(e)	965.69	E850.6	E935.6	E950.0	E962.0	E980.0
Myoneural blocking agents	975.2	E858.6	E945.2	E950.4	E962.0	E980.4
Myristica fragrans	988.2	E865.3	—	E950.9	E962.1	E980.9
Myristicin	988.2	E865.3	—	E950.9	E962.1	E980.9
Mysoline	966.3	E855.0	E936.3	E950.4	E962.0	E980.4
Nafcillin (sodium)	960.0	E856	E930.0	E950.4	E962.0	E980.4
Nail polish remover	982.8	E862.4	—	E950.9	E962.1	E980.9
Nalidixic acid	961.9	E857	E931.9	E950.4	E962.0	E980.4
Nalorphine	970.1	E854.3	E940.1	E950.4	E962.0	E980.4
Naloxone	970.1	E854.3	E940.1	E950.4	E962.0	E980.4
Nandrolone (decanoate) (phenproprioate)	962.1	E858.0	E932.1	E950.4	E962.0	E980.4
Naphazoline	971.2	E855.5	E941.2	E950.4	E962.0	E980.4
Naphtha (painter's) (petroleum)	981	E862.0	—	E950.9	E962.1	E980.9
solvent	981	E862.0	—	E950.9	E962.1	E980.9
vapor	987.1	E869.8	—	E952.8	E962.2	E982.8
Naphthalene (chlorinated)	983.0	E864.0	—	E950.7	E962.1	E980.6
insecticide or moth repellent	983.0	E863.4	—	E950.7	E962.1	E980.6
vapor	987.8	E869.8	—	E952.8	E962.2	E982.8
Naphthol	983.0	E864.0	—	E950.7	E962.1	E980.6
Naphthylamine	983.0	E864.0	—	E950.7	E962.1	E980.6
Naprosyn—*see* Naproxen						
Naproxen	965.61	E850.6	E935.6	E950.0	E962.0	E980.0
Narcotic (drug)	967.9	E852.9	E937.9	E950.2	E962.0	E980.2
analgesic NEC	965.8	E850.8	E935.8	E950.0	E962.0	E980.0
antagonist	970.1	E854.3	E940.1	E950.4	E962.0	E980.4
specified NEC	967.8	E852.8	E937.8	E950.2	E962.0	E980.2
Narcotine	975.4	E858.6	E945.4	E950.4	E962.0	E980.4
Nardil	969.0	E854.0	E939.0	E950.3	E962.0	E980.3
Natrium cyanide — *see* Cyanide(s)						
Natural						
blood (product)	964.7	E858.2	E934.7	E950.4	E962.0	E980.4
gas (piped)	987.1	E867	—	E951.0	E962.2	E981.0
incomplete combustion	986	E867	—	E951.0	E962.2	E981.0
Nealbarbital, nealbarbitone	967.0	E851	E937.0	E950.1	E962.0	E980.1
Nectadon	975.4	E858.6	E945.4	E950.4	E962.0	E980.4
Nematocyst (sting)	989.5	E905.6	—	E950.9	E962.1	E980.9
Nembutal	967.0	E851	E937.0	E950.1	E962.0	E980.1
Neoarsphenamine	961.1	E857	E931.1	E950.4	E962.0	E980.4
Neocinchophen	974.7	E858.5	E944.7	E950.4	E962.0	E980.4
Neomycin	960.8	E856	E930.8	E950.4	E962.0	E980.4

Substance	Poisoning	Accident	Therapeutic Use	Suicide Attempt	Assault	Undetermined
		External Cause (E-Code)				
ENT agent	976.6	E858.7	E946.6	E950.4	E962.0	E980.4
ophthalmic preparation	976.5	E858.7	E946.5	E950.4	E962.0	E980.4
topical NEC	976.0	E858.7	E946.0	E950.4	E962.0	E980.4
Neonal	967.0	E851	E937.0	E950.1	E962.0	E980.1
Neoprontosil	961.0	E857	E931.0	E950.4	E962.0	E980.4
Neosalvarsan	961.1	E857	E931.1	E950.4	E962.0	E980.4
Neosilversalvarsan	961.1	E857	E931.1	E950.4	E962.0	E980.4
Neosporin	960.8	E856	E930.8	E950.4	E962.0	E980.4
ENT agent	976.6	E858.7	E946.6	E950.4	E962.0	E980.4
ophthalmic preparation	976.5	E858.7	E946.5	E950.4	E962.0	E980.4
topical NEC	976.0	E858.7	E946.0	E950.4	E962.0	E980.4
Neostigmine	971.0	E855.3	E941.0	E950.4	E962.0	E980.4
Neraval	967.0	E851	E937.0	E950.1	E962.0	E980.1
Neravan	967.0	E851	E937.0	E950.1	E962.0	E980.1
Nerium oleander	988.2	E865.4	—	E950.9	E962.1	E980.9
Nerve gases (war)	987.9	E869.9	—	E952.9	E962.2	E982.9
Nesacaine	968.9	E855.2	E938.9	E950.4	E962.0	E980.4
infiltration (subcutaneous)	968.5	E855.2	E938.5	E950.4	E962.0	E980.4
nerve block (peripheral) (plexus)	968.6	E855.2	E938.6	E950.4	E962.0	E980.4
Neurobarb	967.0	E851	E937.0	E950.1	E962.0	E980.1
Neuroleptics NEC	969.3	E853.8	E939.3	E950.3	E962.0	E980.3
Neuroprotective agent	977.8	E858.8	E947.8	E950.4	E962.0	E980.4
Neutral spirits	980.0	E860.1	—	E950.9	E962.1	E980.9
beverage	980.0	E860.0	—	E950.9	E962.1	E980.9
Niacin, niacinamide	972.2	E858.3	E942.2	E950.4	E962.0	E980.4
Nialamide	969.0	E854.0	E939.0	E950.3	E962.0	E980.3
Nickle (carbonyl) (compounds) (fumes) (tetracarbonyl) (vapor)	985.8	E866.4	—	E950.9	E962.1	E980.9
Niclosamide	961.6	E857	E931.6	E950.4	E962.0	E980.4
Nicomorphine	965.09	E850.2	E935.2	E950.0	E962.0	E980.0
Nicotinamide	972.2	E858.3	E942.2	E950.4	E962.0	E980.4
Nicotine (insecticide) (spray) (sulfate) NEC	989.4	E863.4	—	E950.6	E962.1	E980.7
not insecticide	989.89	E866.8	—	E950.9	E962.1	E980.9
Nicotinic acid (derivatives)	972.2	E858.3	E942.2	E950.4	E962.0	E980.4
Nicotinyl alcohol	972.2	E858.3	E942.2	E950.4	E962.0	E980.4
Nicoumalone	964.2	E858.2	E934.2	E950.4	E962.0	E980.4
Nifenazone	965.5	E850.5	E935.5	E950.0	E962.0	E980.0
Nifuraldezone	961.9	E857	E931.9	E950.4	E962.0	E980.4
Nightshade (deadly)	988.2	E865.4	—	E950.9	E962.1	E980.9
Nikethamide	970.0	E854.3	E940.0	E950.4	E962.0	E980.4
Nilstat	960.1	E856	E930.1	E950.4	E962.0	E980.4
topical	976.0	E858.7	E946.0	E950.4	E962.0	E980.4
Nimodipine	977.8	E858.8	E947.8	E950.4	E962.0	E980.4
Niridazole	961.6	E857	E931.6	E950.4	E962.0	E980.4
Nisentil	965.09	E850.2	E935.2	E950.0	E962.0	E980.0
Nitrates	972.4	E858.3	E942.4	E950.4	E962.0	E980.4
Nitrazepam	969.4	E853.2	E939.4	E950.3	E962.0	E980.3
Nitric						
acid (liquid)	983.1	E864.1	—	E950.7	E962.1	E980.6
vapor	987.8	E869.8	—	E952.8	E962.2	E982.8
oxide (gas)	987.2	E869.0	—	E952.8	E962.2	E982.8
Nitrite, amyl (medicinal) (vapor)	972.4	E858.3	E942.4	E950.4	E962.0	E980.4
Nitroaniline	983.0	E864.0	—	E950.7	E962.1	E980.6
vapor	987.8	E869.8	—	E952.8	E962.2	E982.8
Nitrobenzene, nitrobenzol	983.0	E864.0	—	E950.7	E962.1	E980.6
vapor	987.8	E869.8	—	E952.8	E962.2	E982.8
Nitrocellulose	976.3	E858.7	E946.3	E950.4	E962.0	E980.4
Nitrofuran derivatives	961.9	E857	E931.9	E950.4	E962.0	E980.4
Nitrofurantoin	961.9	E857	E931.9	E950.4	E962.0	E980.4
Nitrofurazone	976.0	E858.7	E946.0	E950.4	E962.0	E980.4

Substance	Poisoning	Accident	Therapeutic Use	Suicide Attempt	Assault	Undetermined
			External Cause (E-Code)			
Nitrogen (dioxide) (gas) (oxide)	987.2	E869.0	—	E952.8	E962.2	E982.8
mustard (antineoplastic)	963.1	E858.1	E933.1	E950.4	E962.0	E980.4
Nitroglycerin, nitroglycerol (medicinal)	972.4	E858.3	E942.4	E950.4	E962.0	E980.4
nonmedicinal	989.89	E866.8	—	E950.9	E962.1	E980.9
fumes	987.8	E869.8	—	E952.8	E962.2	E982.8
Nitrohydrochloric acid	983.1	E864.1	—	E950.7	E962.1	E980.6
Nitromersol	976.0	E858.7	E946.0	E950.4	E962.0	E980.4
Nitronaphthalene	983.0	E864.0	—	E950.7	E962.2	E980.6
Nitrophenol	983.0	E864.0	—	E950.7	E962.2	E980.6
Nitrothiazol	961.6	E857	E931.6	E950.4	E962.0	E980.4
Nitrotoluene, nitrotoluol	983.0	E864.0	—	E950.7	E962.1	E980.6
vapor	987.8	E869.8	—	E952.8	E962.2	E982.8
Nitrous	968.2	E855.1	E938.2	E950.4	E962.0	E980.4
acid (liquid)	983.1	E864.1	—	E950.7	E962.1	E980.6
fumes	987.2	E869.0	—	E952.8	E962.2	E982.8
oxide (anesthetic) NEC	968.2	E855.1	E938.2	E950.4	E962.0	E980.4
Nitrozone	976.0	E858.7	E946.0	E950.4	E962.0	E980.4
Noctec	967.1	E852.0	E937.1	E950.2	E962.0	E980.2
Noludar	967.5	E852.4	E937.5	E950.2	E962.0	E980.2
Noptil	967.0	E851	E937.0	E950.1	E962.0	E980.1
Noradrenalin	971.2	E855.5	E941.2	E950.4	E962.0	E980.4
Noramidopyrine	965.5	E850.5	E935.5	E950.0	E962.0	E980.0
Norepinephrine	971.2	E855.5	E941.2	E950.4	E962.0	E980.4
Norethandrolone	962.1	E858.0	E932.1	E950.4	E962.0	E980.4
Norethindrone	962.2	E858.0	E932.2	E950.4	E962.0	E980.4
Norethisterone	962.2	E858.0	E932.2	E950.4	E962.0	E980.4
Norethynodrel	962.2	E858.0	E932.2	E950.4	E962.0	E980.4
Norlestrin	962.2	E858.0	E932.2	E950.4	E962.0	E980.4
Norlutin	962.2	E858.0	E932.2	E950.4	E962.0	E980.4
Normison—*see* Benzodiazepines						
Normorphine	965.09	E850.2	E935.2	E950.0	E962.0	E980.0
Nortriptyline	969.0	E854.0	E939.0	E950.3	E962.0	E980.3
Noscapine	975.4	E858.6	E945.4	E950.4	E962.0	E980.4
Nose preparations	976.6	E858.7	E946.6	E950.4	E962.0	E980.4
Novobiocin	960.8	E856	E930.8	E950.4	E962.0	E980.4
Novocain (infiltration) (topical)	968.5	E855.2	E938.5	E950.4	E962.0	E980.4
nerve block (peripheral) (plexus)	968.6	E855.2	E938.6	E950.4	E962.0	E980.4
spinal	968.7	E855.2	E938.7	E950.4	E962.0	E980.4
Noxythiolin	961.9	E857	E931.9	E950.4	E962.0	E980.4
NPH Iletin (insulin)	962.3	E858.0	E932.3	E950.4	E962.0	E980.4
Numorphan	965.09	E850.2	E935.2	E950.0	E962.0	E980.0
Nunol	967.0	E851	E937.0	E950.1	E962.0	E980.1
Nupercaine (spinal anesthetic)	968.7	E855.2	E938.7	E950.4	E962.0	E980.4
topical (surface)	968.5	E855.2	E938.5	E950.4	E962.0	E980.4
Nutmeg oil (liniment)	976.3	E858.7	E946.3	E950.4	E962.0	E980.4
Nux vomica	989.1	E863.7	—	E950.6	E962.1	E980.7
Nydrazid	961.8	E857	E931.8	E950.4	E962.0	E980.4
Nylidrin	971.2	E855.5	E941.2	E950.4	E962.0	E980.4
Nystatin	960.1	E856	E930.1	E950.4	E962.0	E980.4
topical	976.0	E858.7	E946.0	E950.4	E962.0	E980.4
Nytol	963.0	E858.1	E933.0	E950.4	E962.0	E980.4
Oblivion	967.8	E852.8	E937.8	E950.2	E962.0	E980.2
Octyl nitrite	972.4	E858.3	E942.4	E950.4	E962.0	E980.4
Oestradiol (cypionate) (dipropionate) (valerate)	962.2	E858.0	E932.2	E950.4	E962.0	E980.4
Oestriol	962.2	E858.0	E932.2	E950.4	E962.0	E980.4
Oestrone	962.2	E858.0	E932.2	E950.4	E962.0	E980.4
Oil (of) NEC	989.89	E866.8	—	E950.9	E962.1	E980.9
bitter almond	989.0	E866.8	—	E950.9	E962.1	E980.9
camphor	976.1	E858.7	E946.1	E950.4	E962.0	E980.4
colors	989.89	E861.6	—	E950.9	E962.1	E980.9

Substance	Poisoning	Accident	Therapeutic Use	Suicide Attempt	Assault	Undetermined
			External Cause (E-Code)			
fumes	987.8	E869.8	—	E952.8	E962.2	E982.8
lubricating	981	E862.2	—	E950.9	E962.1	E980.9
specified source, other — *see* substance specified						
vitriol (liquid)	983.1	E864.1	—	E950.7	E962.1	E980.6
fumes	987.8	E869.8	—	E952.8	E962.2	E982.8
wintergreen (bitter) NEC	976.3	E858.7	E946.3	E950.4	E962.0	E980.4
Ointments NEC	976.9	E858.7	E946.9	E950.4	E962.0	E980.4
Oleander	988.2	E865.4	—	E950.9	E962.1	E980.9
Oleandomycin	960.3	E856	E930.3	E950.4	E962.0	E980.4
Oleovitamin A	963.5	E858.1	E933.5	E950.4	E962.0	E980.4
Oleum ricini	973.1	E858.4	E943.1	E950.4	E962.0	E980.4
Olive oil (medicinal) NEC	973.2	E858.4	E943.2	E950.4	E962.0	E980.4
OMPA	989.3	E863.1	—	E950.6	E962.1	E980.7
Oncovin	963.1	E858.1	E933.1	E950.4	E962.0	E980.4
Ophthaine	968.5	E855.2	E938.5	E950.4	E962.0	E980.4
Ophthetic	968.5	E855.2	E938.5	E950.4	E962.0	E980.4
Opiates, opioids, opium NEC	965.00	E850.2	E935.2	E950.0	E962.0	E980.0
antagonists	970.1	E854.3	E940.1	E950.4	E962.0	E980.4
Oracon	962.2	E858.0	E932.2	E950.4	E962.0	E980.4
Oragrafin	977.8	E858.8	E947.8	E950.4	E962.0	E980.4
Oral contraceptives	962.2	E858.0	E932.2	E950.4	E962.0	E980.4
Orciprenaline	975.1	E858.6	E945.1	E950.4	E962.0	E980.4
Organidin	975.5	E858.6	E945.5	E950.4	E962.0	E980.4
Organophosphates	989.3	E863.1	—	E950.6	E962.1	E980.7
Orimune	979.5	E858.8	E949.5	E950.4	E962.0	E980.4
Orinase	962.3	E858.0	E932.3	E950.4	E962.0	E980.4
Orphenadrine	966.4	E855.0	E936.4	E950.4	E962.0	E980.4
Ortal (sodium)	967.0	E851	E937.0	E950.1	E962.0	E980.1
Orthoboric acid	976.0	E858.7	E946.0	E950.4	E962.0	E980.4
ENT agent	976.6	E858.7	E946.6	E950.4	E962.0	E980.4
ophthalmic preparation	976.5	E858.7	E946.5	E950.4	E962.0	E980.4
Orthocaine	968.5	E855.2	E938.5	E950.4	E962.0	E980.4
Ortho–Novum	962.2	E858.0	E932.2	E950.4	E962.0	E980.4
Orthotolidine (reagent)	977.8	E858.8	E947.8	E950.4	E962.0	E980.4
Osmic acid (liquid)	983.1	E864.1	—	E950.7	E962.1	E980.6
fumes	987.8	E869.8	—	E952.8	E962.2	E982.8
Osmotic diuretics	974.4	E858.5	E944.4	E950.4	E962.0	E980.4
Ouabain	972.1	E858.3	E942.1	E950.4	E962.0	E980.4
Ovarian hormones (synthetic substitutes)	962.2	E858.0	E932.2	E950.4	E962.0	E980.4
Ovral	962.2	E858.0	E932.2	E950.4	E962.0	E980.4
Ovulation suppressants	962.2	E858.0	E932.2	E950.4	E962.0	E980.4
Ovulen	962.2	E858.0	E932.2	E950.4	E962.0	E980.4
Oxacillin (sodium)	960.0	E856	E930.0	E950.4	E962.0	E980.4
Oxalic acid	983.1	E864.1	—	E950.7	E962.1	E980.6
Oxanamide	969.5	E853.8	E939.5	E950.3	E962.0	E980.3
Oxandrolone	962.1	E858.0	E932.1	E950.4	E962.0	E980.4
Oxaprozin	965.61	E850.6	E935.6	E950.0	E962.0	E980.0
Oxazepam	969.4	E853.2	E939.4	E950.3	E962.0	E980.3
Oxazolidine derivatives	966.0	E855.0	E936.0	E950.4	E962.0	E980.4
Ox bile extract	973.4	E858.4	E943.4	E950.4	E962.0	E980.4
Oxedrine	971.2	E855.5	E941.2	E950.4	E962.0	E980.4
Oxeladin	975.4	E858.6	E945.4	E950.4	E962.0	E980.4
Oxethazaine NEC	968.5	E855.2	E938.5	E950.4	E962.0	E980.4
Oxidizing agents NEC	983.9	E864.3	—	E950.7	E962.1	E980.6
Oxolinic acid	961.3	E857	E931.3	E950.4	E962.0	E980.4
Oxophenarsine	961.1	E857	E931.1	E950.4	E962.0	E980.4
Oxsoralen	976.3	E858.7	E946.3	E950.4	E962.0	E980.4
Oxtriphylline	975.7	E858.6	E945.7	E950.4	E962.0	E980.4
Oxybuprocaine	968.5	E855.2	E938.5	E950.4	E962.0	E980.4

Substance	Poisoning	Accident	Therapeutic Use	Suicide Attempt	Assault	Undetermined
			External Cause (E-Code)			
Oxybutynin	975.1	E858.6	E945.1	E950.4	E962.0	E980.4
Oxycodone	965.09	E850.2	E935.2	E950.0	E962.0	E980.0
Oxygen	987.8	E869.8	—	E952.8	E962.2	E982.8
Oxylone	976.0	E858.7	E946.0	E950.4	E962.0	E980.4
ophthalmic preparation	976.5	E858.7	E946.5	E950.4	E962.0	E980.4
Oxymesterone	962.1	E858.0	E932.1	E950.4	E962.0	E980.4
Oxymetazoline	971.2	E855.5	E941.2	E950.4	E962.0	E980.4
Oxymetholone	962.1	E858.0	E932.1	E950.4	E962.0	E980.4
Oxymorphone	965.09	E850.2	E935.2	E950.0	E962.0	E980.0
Oxypertine	969.0	E854.0	E939.0	E950.3	E962.0	E980.3
Oxyphenbutazone	965.5	E850.5	E935.5	E950.0	E962.0	E980.0
Oxyphencyclimine	971.1	E855.4	E941.1	E950.4	E962.0	E980.4
Oxyphenisatin	973.1	E858.4	E943.1	E950.4	E962.0	E980.4
Oxyphenonium	971.1	E855.4	E941.1	E950.4	E962.0	E980.4
Oxyquinoline	961.3	E857	E931.3	E950.4	E962.0	E980.4
Oxytetracycline	960.4	E856	E930.4	E950.4	E962.0	E980.4
Oxytocics	975.0	E858.6	E945.0	E950.4	E962.0	E980.4
Oxytocin	975.0	E858.6	E945.0	E950.4	E962.0	E980.4
Ozone	987.8	E869.8	—	E952.8	E962.2	E982.8
PABA	976.3	E858.7	E946.3	E950.4	E962.0	E980.4
Packed red cells	964.7	E858.2	E934.7	E950.4	E962.0	E980.4
Paint NEC	989.89	E861.6	—	E950.9	E962.1	E980.9
cleaner	982.8	E862.9	—	E950.9	E962.1	E980.9
fumes NEC	987.8	E869.8	—	E952.8	E962.1	E982.8
lead (fumes)	984.0	E861.5	—	E950.9	E962.1	E980.9
solvent NEC	982.8	E862.9	—	E950.9	E962.1	E980.9
stripper	982.8	E862.9	—	E950.9	E962.1	E980.9
Palfium	965.09	E850.2	E935.2	E950.0	E962.0	E980.0
Palivizumab	979.9	E858.8	E949.6	E950.4	E962.0	E980.4
Paludrine	961.4	E857	E931.4	E950.4	E962.0	E980.4
PAM	977.2	E855.8	E947.2	E950.4	E962.0	E980.4
Pamaquine (naphthoate)	961.4	E857	E931.4	E950.4	E962.0	E980.4
Pamprin	965.1	E850.3	E935.3	E950.0	E962.0	E980.0
Panadol	965.4	E850.4	E935.4	E950.0	E962.0	E980.0
Pancreatic dornase (mucolytic)	963.4	E858.1	E933.4	E950.4	E962.0	E980.4
Pancreatin	973.4	E858.4	E943.4	E950.4	E962.0	E980.4
Pancrelipase	973.4	E858.4	E943.4	E950.4	E962.0	E980.4
Pangamic acid	963.5	E858.1	E933.5	E950.4	E962.0	E980.4
Panthenol	963.5	E858.1	E933.5	E950.4	E962.0	E980.4
topical	976.8	E858.7	E946.8	E950.4	E962.0	E980.4
Pantopaque	977.8	E858.8	E947.8	E950.4	E962.0	E980.4
Pantopon	965.00	E850.2	E935.2	E950.0	E962.0	E980.0
Pantothenic acid	963.5	E858.1	E933.5	E950.4	E962.0	E980.4
Panwarfin	964.2	E858.2	E934.2	E950.4	E962.0	E980.4
Papain	973.4	E858.4	E943.4	E950.4	E962.0	E980.4
Papaverine	972.5	E858.3	E942.5	E950.4	E962.0	E980.4
Para–aminobenzoic acid	976.3	E858.7	E946.3	E950.4	E962.0	E980.4
Para–aminophenol derivatives	965.4	E850.4	E935.4	E950.0	E962.0	E980.0
Para–aminosalicylic acid (derivatives)	961.8	E857	E931.8	E950.4	E962.0	E980.4
Paracetaldehyde (medicinal)	967.2	E852.1	E937.2	E950.2	E962.0	E980.2
Paracetamol	965.4	E850.4	E935.4	E950.0	E962.0	E980.0
Paracodin	965.09	E850.2	E935.2	E950.0	E962.0	E980.0
Paradione	966.0	E855.0	E936.0	E950.4	E962.0	E980.4
Paraffin(s) (wax)	981	E862.3	—	E950.9	E962.1	E980.9
liquid (medicinal)	973.2	E858.4	E943.2	E950.4	E962.0	E980.4
nonmedicinal (oil)	981	E962.1	—	E950.9	E962.1	E980.9
Paraldehyde (medicinal)	967.2	E852.1	E937.2	E950.2	E962.0	E980.2
Paramethadione	966.0	E855.0	E936.0	E950.4	E962.0	E980.4
Paramethasone	962.0	E858.0	E932.0	E950.4	E962.0	E980.4
Paraquat	989.4	E863.5	—	E950.6	E962.1	E980.7
Parasympatholytics	971.1	E855.4	E941.1	E950.4	E962.0	E980.4

Substance	Poisoning	Accident	Therapeutic Use	Suicide Attempt	Assault	Undetermined
			External Cause (E-Code)			
Parasympathomimetics	971.0	E855.3	E941.0	E950.4	E962.0	E980.4
Parathion	989.3	E863.1	—	E950.6	E962.1	E980.7
Parathormone	962.6	E858.0	E932.6	E950.4	E962.0	E980.4
Parathyroid (derivatives)	962.6	E858.0	E932.6	E950.4	E962.0	E980.4
Paratyphoid vaccine	978.1	E858.8	E948.1	E950.4	E962.0	E980.4
Paredrine	971.2	E855.5	E941.2	E950.4	E962.0	E980.4
Paregoric	965.00	E850.2	E935.2	E950.0	E962.0	E980.0
Pargyline	972.3	E858.3	E942.3	E950.4	E962.0	E980.4
Paris green	985.1	E866.3	—	E950.8	E962.1	E980.8
insecticide	985.1	E863.4	—	E950.8	E962.1	E980.8
Parnate	969.0	E854.0	E939.0	E950.3	E962.0	E980.3
Paromomycin	960.8	E856	E930.8	E950.4	E962.0	E980.4
Paroxypropione	963.1	E858.1	E933.1	E950.4	E962.0	E980.4
Parzone	965.09	E850.2	E935.2	E950.0	E962.0	E980.0
PAS	961.8	E857	E931.8	E950.4	E962.0	E980.4
PCBs	981	E862.3	—	E950.9	E962.1	E980.9
PCP (pentachlorophenol)	989.4	E863.6	—	E950.6	E962.1	E980.7
herbicide	989.4	E863.5	—	E950.6	E962.1	E980.7
insecticide	989.4	E863.4	—	E950.6	E962.1	E980.7
phencyclidine	968.3	E855.1	E938.3	E950.4	E962.0	E980.4
Peach kernel oil (emulsion)	973.2	E858.4	E943.2	E950.4	E962.0	E980.4
Peanut oil (emulsion) NEC	973.2	E858.4	E943.2	E950.4	E962.0	E980.4
topical	976.3	E858.7	E946.3	E950.4	E962.0	E980.4
Pearly Gates (morning glory seeds)	969.6	E854.1	E939.6	E950.3	E962.0	E980.3
Pecazine	969.1	E853.0	E939.1	E950.3	E962.0	E980.3
Pecilocin	960.1	E856	E930.1	E950.4	E962.0	E980.4
Pectin (with kaolin) NEC	973.5	E858.4	E943.5	E950.4	E962.0	E980.4
Pelletierine tannate	961.6	E857	E931.6	E950.4	E962.0	E980.4
Pemoline	969.7	E854.2	E939.7	E950.3	E962.0	E980.3
Pempidine	972.3	E858.3	E942.3	E950.4	E962.0	E980.4
Penamecillin	960.0	E856	E930.0	E950.4	E962.0	E980.4
Penethamate hydriodide	960.0	E856	E930.0	E950.4	E962.0	E980.4
Penicillamine	963.8	E858.1	E933.8	E950.4	E962.0	E980.4
Penicillin (any type)	960.0	E856	E930.0	E950.4	E962.0	E980.4
Penicillinase	963.4	E858.1	E933.4	E950.4	E962.0	E980.4
Pentachlorophenol (fungicide)	989.4	E863.6	—	E950.6	E962.1	E980.7
herbicide	989.4	E863.5	—	E950.6	E962.1	E980.7
insecticide	989.4	E863.4	—	E950.6	E962.1	E980.7
Pentaerythritol	972.4	E858.3	E942.4	E950.4	E962.0	E980.4
chloral	967.1	E852.0	E937.1	E950.2	E962.0	E980.2
tetranitrate NEC	972.4	E858.3	E942.4	E950.4	E962.0	E980.4
Pentagastrin	977.8	E858.8	E947.8	E950.4	E962.0	E980.4
Pentalin	982.3	E862.4	—	E950.9	E962.1	E980.9
Pentamethonium (bromide)	972.3	E858.3	E942.3	E950.4	E962.0	E980.4
Pentamidine	961.5	E857	E931.5	E950.4	E962.0	E980.4
Pentanol	980.8	E860.8	—	E950.9	E962.1	E980.9
Pentaquine	961.4	E857	E931.4	E950.4	E962.0	E980.4
Pentazocine	965.8	E850.8	E935.8	E950.0	E962.0	E980.0
Penthienate	971.1	E855.4	E941.1	E950.4	E962.0	E980.4
Pentobarbital, pentobarbitone (sodium)	967.0	E851	E937.0	E950.1	E962.0	E980.1
Pentolinium (tartrate)	972.3	E858.3	E942.3	E950.4	E962.0	E980.4
Pentothal	968.3	E855.1	E938.3	E950.4	E962.0	E980.4
Pentylenetetrazol	970.0	E854.3	E940.0	E950.4	E962.0	E980.4
Pentylsalicylamide	961.8	E857	E931.8	E950.4	E962.0	E980.4
Pepsin	973.4	E858.4	E943.4	E950.4	E962.0	E980.4
Peptavlon	977.8	E858.8	E947.8	E950.4	E962.0	E980.4
Percaine (spinal)	968.7	E855.2	E938.7	E950.4	E962.0	E980.4
topical (surface)	968.5	E855.2	E938.5	E950.4	E962.0	E980.4
Perchloroethylene (vapor)	982.3	E862.4	—	E950.9	E962.1	E980.9
medicinal	961.6	E857	E931.6	E950.4	E962.0	E980.4

Substance	Poisoning	Accident	Therapeutic Use	Suicide Attempt	Assault	Undetermined
		External Cause (E-Code)				
Percodan	965.09	E850.2	E935.2	E950.0	E962.0	E980.0
Percogesic	965.09	E850.2	E935.2	E950.0	E962.0	E980.0
Percorten	962.0	E858.0	E932.0	E950.4	E962.0	E980.4
Pergonal	962.4	E858.0	E932.4	E950.4	E962.0	E980.4
Perhexiline	972.4	E858.3	E942.4	E950.4	E962.0	E980.4
Periactin	963.0	E858.1	E933.0	E950.4	E962.0	E980.4
Periclor	967.1	E852.0	E937.1	E950.2	E962.0	E980.2
Pericyazine	969.1	E853.0	E939.1	E950.3	E962.0	E980.3
Peritrate	972.4	E858.3	E942.4	E950.4	E962.0	E980.4
Permanganates NEC	983.9	E864.3	—	E950.7	E962.1	E980.6
potassium (topical)	976.0	E858.7	E946.0	E950.4	E962.0	E980.4
Pernocton	967.0	E851	E937.0	E950.1	E962.0	E980.1
Pernoston	967.0	E851	E937.0	E950.1	E962.0	E980.1
Peronin(e)	965.09	E850.2	E935.2	E950.0	E962.0	E980.0
Perphenazine	969.1	E853.0	E939.1	E950.3	E962.0	E980.3
Pertofrane	969.0	E854	E939.0	E950.3	E962.0	E980.3
Pertussis						
immune serum (human)	964.6	E858.2	E934.6	E950.4	E962.0	E980.4
vaccine (with diphtheria toxoid) (with						
tetanus toxoid)	978.6	E858.8	E948.6	E950.4	E962.0	E980.4
Peruvian balsam	976.8	E858.7	E946.8	E950.4	E962.0	E980.4
Pesticides (dust) (fumes) (vapor)	989.4	E863.4	—	E950.6	E962.1	E980.7
arsenic	985.1	E863.4	—	E950.8	E962.1	E980.8
chlorinated	989.2	E863.0	—	E950.6	E962.1	E980.7
cyanide	989.0	E863.4	—	E950.6	E962.1	E980.7
kerosene	981	E863.4	—	E950.6	E962.1	E980.7
mixture (of compounds)	989.4	E863.3	—	E950.6	E962.1	E980.7
naphthalene	983.0	E863.4	—	E950.7	E962.1	E980.6
organochlorine (compounds)	989.2	E863.0	—	E950.6	E962.1	E980.7
petroleum (distillate) (products)						
NEC	981	E863.4	—	E950.6	E962.1	E980.7
specified ingredient NEC	989.4	E863.4	—	E950.6	E962.1	E980.7
strychnine	989.1	E863.4	—	E950.6	E962.1	E980.7
thallium	985.8	E863.7	—	E950.6	E962.1	E980.7
Pethidine (hydrochloride)	965.09	E850.2	E935.2	E950.0	E962.0	E980.0
Petrichloral	967.1	E852.0	E937.1	E950.2	E962.0	E980.2
Petrol	981	E862.1	—	E950.9	E962.1	E980.9
vapor	987.1	E869.8	—	E952.8	E962.2	E982.8
Petrolatum (jelly) (ointment)	976.3	E858.7	E946.3	E950.4	E962.0	E980.4
hydrophilic	976.3	E858.7	E946.3	E950.4	E962.0	E980.4
liquid	973.2	E858.4	E943.2	E950.4	E962.0	E980.4
topical	976.3	E858.7	E946.3	E950.4	E962.0	E980.4
nonmedicinal	981	E862.1	—	E950.9	E962.1	E980.9
Petroleum (cleaners) (fuels) (products)						
NEC	981	E862.1	—	E950.9	E962.1	E980.9
benzin(e) — *see* Ligroin						
ether — *see* Ligroin						
jelly — *see* Petrolatum						
naphtha — *see* Ligroin						
pesticide	981	E863.4	—	E950.6	E962.1	E980.7
solids	981	E862.3	—	E950.9	E962.1	E980.9
solvents	981	E862.0	—	E950.9	E962.1	E980.9
vapor	987.1	E869.8	—	E952.8	E962.2	E982.8
Peyote	969.6	E854.1	E939.6	E950.3	E962.0	E980.3
Phanodorm, phanodorm	967.0	E851	E937.0	E950.1	E962.0	E980.1
Phanquinone, phanquone	961.5	E857	E931.5	E950.4	E962.0	E980.4
Pharmaceutical excipient or adjunct	977.4	E858.8	E947.4	E950.4	E962.0	E980.4
Phenacemide	966.3	E855.0	E936.3	E950.4	E962.0	E980.4
Phenacetin	965.4	E850.4	E935.4	E950.0	E962.0	E980.0
Phenadoxone	965.09	E850.2	E935.2	E950.0	E962.0	E980.0
Phenaglycodol	969.5	E853.8	E939.5	E950.3	E962.0	E980.3

Substance	Poisoning	External Cause (E-Code)				
		Accident	Therapeutic Use	Suicide Attempt	Assault	Undetermined
Phenantoin	966.1	E855.0	E936.1	E950.4	E962.0	E980.4
Phenaphthazine reagent	977.8	E858.8	E947.8	E950.4	E962.0	E980.4
Phenazocine	965.09	E850.2	E935.2	E950.0	E962.0	E980.0
Phenazone	965.5	E850.5	E935.5	E950.0	E962.0	E980.0
Phenazopyridine	976.1	E858.7	E946.1	E950.4	E962.0	E980.4
Phenbenicillin	960.0	E856	E930.0	E950.4	E962.0	E980.4
Phenbutrazate	977.0	E858.8	E947.0	E950.4	E962.0	E980.4
Phencyclidine	968.3	E855.1	E938.3	E950.4	E962.0	E980.4
Phendimetrazine	977.0	E858.8	E947.0	E950.4	E962.0	E980.4
Phenelzine	969.0	E854.0	E939.0	E950.3	E962.0	E980.3
Phenergan	967.8	E852.8	E937.8	E950.2	E962.0	E980.2
Phenethicillin (potassium)	960.0	E856	E930.0	E950.4	E962.0	E980.4
Phenetsal	965.1	E850.3	E935.3	E950.0	E962.0	E980.0
Pheneturide	966.3	E855.0	E936.3	E950.4	E962.0	E980.4
Phenformin	962.3	E858.0	E932.3	E950.4	E962.0	E980.4
Phenglutarimide	971.1	E855.4	E941.1	E950.4	E962.0	E980.4
Phenicarbazide	965.8	E850.8	E935.8	E950.0	E962.0	E980.0
Phenindamine (tartrate)	963.0	E858.1	E933.0	E950.4	E962.0	E980.4
Phenindione	964.2	E858.2	E934.2	E950.4	E962.0	E980.4
Pheniprazine	969.0	E854.0	E939.0	E950.3	E962.0	E980.3
Pheniramine (maleate)	963.0	E858.1	E933.0	E950.4	E962.0	E980.4
Phenmetrazine	977.0	E858.8	E947.0	E950.4	E962.0	E980.4
Phenobal	967.0	E851	E937.0	E950.1	E962.0	E980.1
Phenobarbital	967.0	E851	E937.0	E950.1	E962.0	E980.1
Phenobarbitone	967.0	E851	E937.0	E950.1	E962.0	E980.1
Phenoctide	976.0	E858.7	E946.0	E950.4	E962.0	E980.4
Phenol (derivatives) NEC	983.0	E864.0	—	E950.7	E962.1	E980.6
disinfectant	983.0	E864.0	—	E950.7	E962.1	E980.6
pesticide	989.4	E863.4	—	E950.6	E962.1	E980.7
red	977.8	E858.8	E947.8	E950.4	E962.0	E980.4
Phenolphthalein	973.1	E858.4	E943.1	E950.4	E962.0	E980.4
Phenolsulfonphthalein	977.8	E858.8	E947.8	E950.4	E962.0	E980.4
Phenomorphan	965.09	E850.2	E935.2	E950.0	E962.0	E980.0
Phenonyl	967.0	E851	E937.0	E950.1	E962.0	E980.1
Phenoperidine	965.09	E850.2	E935.2	E950.0	E962.0	E980.0
Phenoquin	974.7	E858.5	E944.7	E950.4	E962.0	E980.4
Phenothiazines (tranquilizers) NEC	969.1	E853.0	E939.1	E950.3	E962.0	E980.3
insecticide	989.3	E863.4	—	E950.6	E962.1	E980.7
Phenoxybenzamine	971.3	E855.6	E941.3	E950.4	E962.0	E980.4
Phenoxymethyl penicillin	960.0	E856	E930.0	E950.4	E962.0	E980.4
Phenprocoumon	964.2	E858.2	E934.2	E950.4	E962.0	E980.4
Phensuximide	966.2	E855.0	E936.2	E950.4	E962.0	E980.4
Phentermine	977.0	E858.8	E947.0	E950.4	E962.0	E980.4
Phentolamine	971.3	E855.6	E941.3	E950.4	E962.0	E980.4
Phenyl						
butazone	965.5	E850.5	E935.5	E950.0	E962.0	E980.0
enediamine	983.0	E864.0	—	E950.7	E962.1	E980.6
hydrazine	983.0	E864.0	—	E950.7	E962.1	E980.6
antineoplastic	963.1	E858.1	E933.1	E950.4	E962.0	E980.4
mercuric compounds — *see* Mercury						
salicylate	976.3	E858.7	E946.3	E950.4	E962.0	E980.4
Phenylephrin	971.2	E855.5	E941.2	E950.4	E962.0	E980.4
Phenylethybiguanide	962.3	E858.0	E932.3	E950.4	E962.0	E980.4
Phenylpropanolamine	971.2	E855.5	E941.2	E950.4	E962.0	E980.4
Phenylsulfthion	989.3	E863.1	—	E950.6	E962.1	E980.7
Phenyramidol, phenyramidon	965.7	E850.7	E935.7	E950.0	E962.0	E980.0
Phenytoin	966.1	E855.0	E936.1	E950.4	E962.0	E980.4
pHisoHex	976.2	E858.7	E946.2	E950.4	E962.0	E980.4
Pholcodine	965.09	E850.2	E935.2	E950.0	E962.0	E980.0
Phorate	989.3	E863.1	—	E950.6	E962.1	E980.7

Substance	Poisoning	Accident	Therapeutic Use	Suicide Attempt	Assault	Undetermined
		External Cause (E-Code)				
Phosdrin	989.3	E863.1	—	E950.6	E962.1	E980.7
Phosgene (gas)	987.8	E869.8	—	E952.8	E962.2	E982.8
Phosphate (tricresyl)	989.89	E866.8	—	E950.9	E962.1	E980.9
organic	989.3	E863.1	—	E950.6	E962.1	E980.7
solvent	982.8	E862.4	—	E950.9	E926.1	E980.9
Phosphine	987.8	E869.8	—	E952.8	E962.2	E982.8
fumigant	987.8	E863.8	—	E950.6	E962.2	E980.7
Phospholine	971.0	E855.3	E941.0	E950.4	E962.0	E980.4
Phosphoric acid	983.1	E864.1	—	E950.7	E962.1	E980.6
Phosphorus (compounds) NEC	983.9	E864.3	—	E950.7	E962.1	E980.6
rodenticide	983.9	E863.7	—	E950.7	E962.1	E980.6
Phthalimidogluarimide	967.8	E852.8	E937.8	E950.2	E962.0	E980.2
Phthalylsulfathiazole	961.0	E857	E931.0	E950.4	E962.0	E980.4
Phylloquinone	964.3	E858.2	E934.3	E950.4	E962.0	E980.4
Physeptone	965.02	E850.1	E935.1	E950.0	E962.0	E980.0
Physostigma venenosum	988.2	E865.4	—	E950.9	E962.1	E980.9
Physostigmine	971.0	E855.3	E941.0	E950.4	E962.0	E980.4
Phytolacca decandra	988.2	E865.4	—	E950.9	E962.1	E980.9
Phytomenadione	964.3	E858.2	E934.3	E950.4	E962.0	E980.4
Phytonadione	964.3	E858.2	E934.3	E950.4	E962.0	E980.4
Picric (acid)	983.0	E864.0	—	E950.7	E962.1	E980.6
Picrotoxin	970.0	E854.3	E940.0	E950.4	E962.0	E980.4
Pilocarpine	971.0	E855.3	E941.0	E950.4	E962.0	E980.4
Pilocarpus (jaborandi) extract	971.0	E855.3	E941.0	E950.4	E962.0	E980.4
Pimaricin	960.1	E856	E930.1	E950.4	E962.0	E980.4
Piminodine	965.09	E850.2	E935.2	E950.0	E962.0	E980.0
Pine oil, pinesol (disinfectant)	983.9	E861.4	—	E950.7	E962.1	E980.6
Pinkroot	961.6	E857	E931.6	E950.4	E962.0	E980.4
Pipadone	965.09	E850.2	E935.2	E950.0	E962.0	E980.0
Pipamazine	963.0	E858.1	E933.0	E950.4	E962.0	E980.4
Pipazethate	975.4	E858.6	E945.4	E950.4	E962.0	E980.4
Pipenzolate	971.1	E855.4	E941.1	E950.4	E962.0	E980.4
Piperacetazine	969.1	E853.0	E939.1	E950.3	E962.0	E980.3
Piperazine NEC	961.6	E857	E931.6	E950.4	E962.0	E980.4
estrone sulfate	962.2	E858.0	E932.2	E950.4	E962.0	E980.4
Piper cubeba	988.2	E865.4	—	E950.9	E962.1	E980.9
Piperidione	975.4	E858.6	E945.4	E950.4	E962.0	E980.4
Piperidolate	971.1	E855.4	E941.1	E950.4	E962.0	E980.4
Piperocaine	968.9	E855.2	E938.9	E950.4	E962.0	E980.4
infiltration (subcutaneous)	968.5	E855.2	E938.5	E950.4	E962.0	E980.4
nerve block (peripheral) (plexus)	968.6	E855.2	E938.6	E950.4	E962.0	E980.4
topical (surface)	968.5	E855.2	E938.5	E950.4	E962.0	E980.4
Pipobroman	963.1	E858.1	E933.1	E950.4	E962.0	E980.4
Pipradrol	970.8	E854.3	E940.8	E950.4	E962.0	E980.4
Piscidia (bark) (erythrina)	965.7	E850.7	E935.7	E950.0	E962.0	E980.0
Pitch	983.0	E864.0	—	E950.7	E962.1	E980.6
Pitkin's solution	968.7	E855.2	E938.7	E950.4	E962.0	E980.4
Pitocin	975.0	E858.6	E945.0	E950.4	E962.0	E980.4
Pitressin (tannate)	962.5	E858.0	E932.5	E950.4	E962.0	E980.4
Pituitary extracts (posterior)	962.5	E858.0	E932.5	E950.4	E962.0	E980.4
anterior	962.4	E858.0	E932.4	E950.4	E962.0	E980.4
Pituitrin	962.5	E858.0	E932.5	E950.4	E962.0	E980.4
Placental extract	962.9	E858.0	E932.9	E950.4	E962.0	E980.4
Placidyl	967.8	E852.8	E937.8	E950.2	E962.0	E980.2
Plague vaccine	978.3	E858.8	E948.3	E950.4	E962.0	E980.4
Plant foods or fertilizers NEC	989.89	E866.5	—	E950.9	E962.1	E980.9
mixed with herbicides	989.4	E863.5	—	E950.6	E962.1	E980.7
Plants, noxious, used as food	988.2	E865.9	—	E950.9	E962.1	E980.9
berries and seeds	988.2	E865.3	—	E950.9	E962.1	E980.9
specified type NEC	988.2	E865.4	—	E950.9	E962.1	E980.9
Plasma (blood)	964.7	E858.2	E934.7	E950.4	E962.0	E980.4

Substance	Poisoning	Accident	Therapeutic Use	Suicide Attempt	Assault	Undetermined
			External Cause (E-Code)			
expanders	964.8	E858.2	E934.8	E950.4	E962.0	E980.4
Plasmanate	964.7	E858.2	E934.7	E950.4	E962.0	E980.4
Plegicil	969.1	E853.0	E939.1	E950.3	E962.0	E980.3
Podophyllin	976.4	E858.7	E946.4	E950.4	E962.0	E980.4
Podophyllum resin	976.4	E858.7	E946.4	E950.4	E962.0	E980.4
Poison NEC	989.9	E866.9	—	E950.9	E962.1	E980.9
Poisonous berries	988.2	E865.3	—	E950.9	E962.1	E980.9
Pokeweed (any part)	988.2	E865.4	—	E950.9	E962.1	E980.9
Poldine	971.1	E855.4	E941.1	E950.4	E962.0	E980.4
Poliomyelitis vaccine	979.5	E858.8	E949.5	E950.4	E962.0	E980.4
Poliovirus vaccine	979.5	E858.8	E949.5	E950.4	E962.0	E980.4
Polish (car) (floor) (furniture) (metal) (silver)	989.89	E861.2	—	E950.9	E962.1	E980.9
abrasive	989.89	E861.3	—	E950.9	E962.1	E980.9
porcelain	989.89	E861.3	—	E950.9	E962.1	E980.9
Poloxalkol	973.2	E858.4	E943.2	E950.4	E962.0	E980.4
Polyaminostyrene resins	974.5	E858.5	E944.5	E950.4	E962.0	E980.4
Polychlorinated biphenyl—*see* PCBs						
Polycycline	960.4	E856	E930.4	E950.4	E962.0	E980.4
Polyester resin hardener	982.8	E862.4	—	E950.9	E962.1	E980.9
fumes	987.8	E869.8	—	E952.8	E962.2	E982.8
Polyestradiol (phosphate)	962.2	E858.0	E932.2	E950.4	E962.0	E980.4
Polyethanolamine alkyl sulfate	976.2	E858.7	E946.2	E950.4	E962.0	E980.4
Polyethylene glycol	976.3	E858.7	E946.3	E950.4	E962.0	E980.4
Polyferose	964.0	E858.2	E934.0	E950.4	E962.0	E980.4
Polymyxin B	960.8	E856	E930.8	E950.4	E962.0	E980.4
ENT agent	976.6	E858.7	E946.6	E950.4	E962.0	E980.4
ophthalmic preparation	976.5	E858.7	E946.5	E950.4	E962.0	E980.4
topical NEC	976.0	E858.7	E946.0	E950.4	E962.0	E980.4
Polynoxylin(e)	976.0	E858.7	E946.0	E950.4	E962.0	E980.4
Polyoxymethyleneurea	976.0	E858.7	E946.0	E950.4	E962.0	E980.4
Polytetrafluoroethylene (inhaled)	987.8	E869.8	—	E952.8	E962.2	E982.8
Polythiazide	974.3	E858.5	E944.3	E950.4	E962.0	E980.4
Polyvinylpyrrolidone	964.8	E858.2	E934.8	E950.4	E962.0	E980.4
Pontocaine (hydrochloride) (infiltration) (topical)	968.5	E855.2	E938.5	E950.4	E962.0	E980.4
nerve block (peripheral) (plexus)	968.6	E855.2	E938.6	E950.4	E962.0	E980.4
spinal	968.7	E855.2	E938.7	E950.4	E962.0	E980.4
Pot	969.6	E854.1	E939.6	E950.3	E962.0	E980.3
Potash (caustic)	983.2	E864.2	—	E950.7	E962.1	E980.6
Potassic saline injection (lactated)	974.5	E858.5	E944.5	E950.4	E962.0	E980.4
Potassium (salts) NEC	974.5	E858.5	E944.5	E950.4	E962.0	E980.4
aminosalicylate	961.8	E857	E931.8	E950.4	E962.0	E980.4
arsenite (solution)	985.1	E866.3	—	E950.8	E962.1	E980.8
bichromate	983.9	E864.3	—	E950.7	E962.1	E980.6
bisulfate	983.9	E864.3	—	E950.7	E962.1	E980.6
bromide (medicinal) NEC	967.3	E852.2	E937.3	E950.2	E962.0	E980.2
carbonate	983.2	E864.2	—	E950.7	E962.1	E980.6
chlorate NEC	983.9	E864.3	—	E950.7	E962.1	E980.6
cyanide — *see* Cyanide						
hydroxide	983.2	E864.2	—	E950.7	E962.1	E980.6
iodide (expectorant) NEC	975.5	E858.6	E945.5	E950.4	E962.0	E980.4
nitrate	989.89	E866.8	—	E950.9	E962.1	E980.9
oxalate	983.9	E864.3	—	E950.7	E962.1	E980.6
perchlorate NEC	977.8	E858.8	E947.8	E950.4	E962.0	E980.4
antithyroid	962.8	E858.0	E932.8	E950.4	E962.0	E980.4
permanganate	976.0	E858.7	E946.0	E950.4	E962.0	E980.4
nonmedicinal	983.9	E864.3	—	E950.7	E962.1	E980.6
Povidone–iodine (anti–infective) NEC	976.0	E858.7	E946.0	E950.4	E962.0	E980.4
Practolol	972.0	E858.3	E942.0	E950.4	E962.0	E980.4

Substance	Poisoning	Accident	Therapeutic Use	Suicide Attempt	Assault	Undetermined
		External Cause (E-Code)				
Pralidoxime (chloride)	977.2	E858.8	E947.2	E950.4	E962.0	E980.4
Pramoxine	968.5	E855.2	E938.5	E950.4	E962.0	E980.4
Prazosin	972.6	E858.3	E942.6	E950.4	E962.0	E980.4
Prednisolone	962.0	E858.0	E932.0	E950.4	E962.0	E980.4
ENT agent	976.6	E858.7	E946.6	E950.4	E962.0	E980.4
ophthalmic preparation	976.5	E858.7	E946.5	E950.4	E962.0	E980.4
topical NEC	976.0	E858.7	E946.0	E950.4	E962.0	E980.4
Prednisone	962.0	E858.0	E932.0	E950.4	E962.0	E980.4
Pregnanediol	962.2	E858.0	E932.2	E950.4	E962.0	E980.4
Pregneninolone	962.2	E858.0	E932.2	E950.4	E962.0	E980.4
Preludin	977.0	E858.8	E947.0	E950.4	E962.0	E980.4
Premarin	962.2	E858.0	E932.2	E950.4	E962.0	E980.4
Prenylamine	972.4	E858.3	E942.4	E950.4	E962.0	E980.4
Preparation H	976.8	E858.7	E946.8	E950.4	E962.0	E980.4
Preservatives	989.89	E866.8	—	E950.9	E962.1	E980.9
Pride of China	988.2	E865.3	—	E950.9	E962.1	E980.9
Prilocaine	968.9	E855.2	E938.9	E950.4	E962.0	E980.4
infiltration (subcutaneous)	968.5	E855.2	E938.5	E950.4	E962.0	E980.4
nerve block (peripheral) (plexus)	968.6	E855.2	E938.6	E950.4	E962.0	E980.4
Primaquine	961.4	E857	E931.4	E950.4	E962.0	E980.4
Primidone	966.3	E855.0	E936.3	E950.4	E962.0	E980.4
Primula (veris)	988.2	E865.4	—	E950.9	E962.1	E980.9
Prinadol	965.09	E850.2	E935.2	E950.0	E962.0	E980.0
Priscol, Priscoline	971.3	E855.6	E941.3	E950.4	E962.0	E980.4
Privet	988.2	E865.4	—	E950.9	E962.1	E980.9
Privine	971.2	E855.5	E941.2	E950.4	E962.0	E980.4
Pro–Banthine	971.1	E855.4	E941.1	E950.4	E962.0	E980.4
Probarbital	967.0	E851	E937.0	E950.1	E962.0	E980.1
Probenecid	974.7	E858.5	E944.7	E950.4	E962.0	E980.4
Procainamide (hydrochloride)	972.0	E858.3	E942.0	E950.4	E962.0	E980.4
Procaine (hydrochloride) (infiltration) (topical)	968.5	E855.2	E938.5	E950.4	E962.0	E980.4
nerve block (peripheral) (plexus)	968.6	E855.2	E938.6	E950.4	E962.0	E980.4
penicillin G	960.0	E856	E930.0	E950.4	E962.0	E980.4
spinal	968.7	E855.2	E938.7	E950.4	E962.0	E980.4
Procalmidol	969.5	E853.8	E939.5	E950.3	E962.0	E980.3
Procarbazine	963.1	E858.1	E933.1	E950.4	E962.0	E980.4
Prochlorperazine	969.1	E853.0	E939.1	E950.3	E962.0	E980.3
Procyclidine	966.4	E855.0	E936.4	E950.4	E962.0	E980.4
Producer gas	986	E868.8	—	E952.1	E962.2	E982.1
Profenamine	966.4	E855.0	E936.4	E950.4	E962.0	E980.4
Profenil	975.1	E858.6	E945.1	E950.4	E962.0	E980.4
Progesterones	962.2	E858.0	E932.2	E950.4	E962.0	E980.4
Progestin	962.2	E858.0	E932.2	E950.4	E962.0	E980.4
Progestogens (with estrogens)	962.2	E858.0	E932.2	E950.4	E962.0	E980.4
Progestone	962.2	E858.0	E932.2	E950.4	E962.0	E980.4
Proguanil	961.4	E857	E931.4	E950.4	E962.0	E980.4
Prolactin	962.4	E858.0	E932.4	E950.4	E962.0	E980.4
Proloid	962.7	E858.0	E932.7	E950.4	E962.0	E980.4
Proluton	962.2	E858.0	E932.2	E950.4	E962.0	E980.4
Promacetin	961.8	E857	E931.8	E950.4	E962.0	E980.4
Promazine	969.1	E853.0	E939.1	E950.3	E962.0	E980.3
Promedol	965.09	E850.2	E935.2	E950.0	E962.0	E980.0
Promethazine	967.8	E852.8	E937.8	E950.2	E962.0	E980.2
Promin	961.8	E857	E931.8	E950.4	E962.0	E980.4
Pronestyl (hydrochloride)	972.0	E858.3	E942.0	E950.4	E962.0	E980.4
Pronetalol, pronethalol	972.0	E858.3	E942.0	E950.4	E962.0	E980.4
Prontosil	961.0	E857	E931.0	E950.4	E962.0	E980.4
Propamidine isethionate	961.5	E857	E931.5	E950.4	E962.0	E980.4
Propanal (medicinal)	967.8	E852.8	E937.8	E950.2	E962.0	E980.2

Substance	Poisoning	Accident	Therapeutic Use	Suicide Attempt	Assault	Undetermined
		External Cause (E-Code)				
Propane (gas) (distributed in mobile container)	987.0	E868.0	—	E951.1	E962.2	E981.1
distributed through pipes	987.0	E867	—	E951.0	E962.2	E981.0
incomplete combustion of – *see* Carbon monoxide, Propane						
Propanidid	968.3	E855.1	E938.3	E950.4	E962.0	E980.4
Propanol	980.3	E860.4	—	E950.9	E962.1	E980.9
Propantheline	971.1	E855.4	E941.1	E950.4	E962.0	E980.4
Proparacaine	968.5	E855.2	E938.5	E950.4	E962.0	E980.4
Propatyl nitrate	972.4	E858.3	E942.4	E950.4	E962.0	E980.4
Propicillin	960.0	E856	E930.0	E950.4	E962.0	E980.4
Propiolactone (vapor)	987.8	E869.8	—	E952.8	E962.2	E982.8
Propiomazine	967.8	E852.8	E937.8	E950.2	E962.0	E980.2
Propionaldehyde (medicinal)	967.8	E852.8	E937.8	E950.2	E962.0	E980.2
Propionate compound	976.0	E858.7	E946.0	E950.4	E962.0	E980.4
Propion gel	976.0	E858.7	E946.0	E950.4	E962.0	E980.4
Propitocaine	968.9	E855.2	E938.9	E950.4	E962.0	E980.4
infiltration (subcutaneous)	968.5	E855.2	E938.5	E950.4	E962.0	E980.4
nerve block (peripheral) (plexus)	968.6	E855.2	E938.6	E950.4	E962.0	E980.4
Propoxur	989.3	E863.2	—	E950.6	E962.1	E980.7
Propoxycaine	968.9	E855.2	E938.9	E950.4	E962.0	E980.4
infiltration (subcutaneous)	968.5	E855.2	E938.5	E950.4	E962.0	E980.4
nerve block (peripheral) (plexus)	968.6	E855.2	E938.6	E950.4	E962.0	E980.4
topical (surface)	968.5	E855.2	E938.5	E950.4	E962.0	E980.4
Propoxyphene (hydrochloride)	965.8	E850.8	E935.8	E950.0	E962.0	E980.0
Propranolol	972.0	E858.3	E942.0	E950.4	E962.0	E980.4
Propyl						
alcohol	980.3	E860.4	—	E950.9	E962.1	E980.9
carbinol	980.3	E860.4	—	E950.9	E962.1	E980.9
hexadrine	971.2	E855.5	E941.2	E950.4	E962.0	E980.4
iodone	977.8	E858.8	E947.8	E950.4	E962.0	E980.4
thiouracil	962.8	E858.0	E932.8	E950.4	E962.0	E980.4
Propylene	987.1	E869.8	—	E952.8	E962.2	E982.8
Propylparaben (ophthalmic)	976.5	E858.7	E946.5	E950.4	E962.0	E980.4
Proscillaridin	972.1	E858.3	E942.1	E950.4	E962.0	E980.4
Prostaglandins	975.0	E858.6	E945.0	E950.4	E962.0	E980.4
Prostigmin	971.0	E855.3	E941.0	E950.4	E962.0	E980.4
Protamine (sulfate)	964.5	E858.2	E934.5	E950.4	E962.0	E980.4
zinc insulin	962.3	E858.0	E932.3	E950.4	E962.0	E980.4
Protectants (topical)	976.3	E858.7	E946.3	E950.4	E962.0	E980.4
Protein hydrolysate	974.5	E858.5	E944.5	E950.4	E962.0	E980.4
Prothiaden—*see* Dothiepin hydrochloride						
Prothionamide	961.8	E857	E931.8	E950.4	E962.0	E980.4
Prothipendyl	969.5	E853.8	E939.5	E950.3	E962.0	E980.3
Protokylol	971.2	E855.5	E941.2	E950.4	E962.0	E980.4
Protopam	977.2	E858.8	E947.2	E950.4	E962.0	E980.4
Protoveratrine(s) (A) (B)	972.6	E858.3	E942.6	E950.4	E962.0	E980.4
Protriptyline	969.0	E854.0	E939.0	E950.3	E962.0	E980.3
Provera	962.2	E858.0	E932.2	E950.4	E962.0	E980.4
Provitamin A	963.5	E858.1	E933.5	E950.4	E962.0	E980.4
Proxymetacaine	968.5	E855.2	E938.5	E950.4	E962.0	E980.4
Proxyphylline	975.1	E858.6	E945.1	E950.4	E962.0	E980.4
Prozac—*see* Fluoxetine hydrochloride						
Prunus						
laurocerasus	988.2	E865.4	—	E950.9	E962.1	E980.9
virginiana	988.2	E865.4	—	E950.9	E962.1	E980.9
Prussic acid	989.0	E866.8	—	E950.9	E962.1	E980.9
vapor	987.7	E869.8	—	E952.8	E962.2	E982.8
Pseudoephedrine	971.2	E855.5	E941.2	E950.4	E962.0	E980.4
Psilocin	969.6	E854.1	E939.6	E950.3	E962.0	E980.3

Substance	Poisoning	Accident	Therapeutic Use	Suicide Attempt	Assault	Undetermined
			External Cause (E-Code)			
Psilocybin	969.6	E854.1	E939.6	E950.3	E962.0	E980.3
PSP	977.8	E858.8	E947.8	E950.4	E962.0	E980.4
Psychedelic agents	969.6	E854.1	E939.6	E950.3	E962.0	E980.3
Psychodysleptics	969.6	E854.1	E939.6	E950.3	E962.0	E980.3
Psychostimulants	969.7	E854.2	E939.7	E950.3	E962.0	E980.3
Psychotherapeutic agents	969.9	E855.9	E939.9	E950.3	E962.0	E980.3
antidepressants	969.0	E854.0	E939.0	E950.3	E962.0	E980.3
specified NEC	969.8	E855.8	E939.8	E950.3	E962.0	E980.3
tranquilizers NEC	969.5	E853.9	E939.5	E950.3	E962.0	E980.3
Psychotomimetic agents	969.6	E854.1	E939.6	E950.3	E962.0	E980.3
Psychotropic agents	969.9	E854.8	E939.9	E950.3	E962.0	E980.3
specified NEC	969.8	E854.8	E939.8	E950.3	E962.0	E980.3
Psyllium	973.3	E858.4	E943.3	E950.4	E962.0	E980.4
Pteroylglutamic acid	964.1	E858.2	E934.1	E950.4	E962.0	E980.4
Pteroyltriglutamate	963.1	E858.1	E933.1	E950.4	E962.0	E980.4
PTFE	987.8	E869.8	—	E952.8	E962.2	E982.8
Pulsatilla	988.2	E865.4	—	E950.9	E962.1	E980.9
Purex (bleach)	983.9	E864.3	—	E950.7	E962.1	E980.6
Purine diuretics	974.1	E858.5	E944.1	E950.4	E962.0	E980.4
Purinethol	963.1	E858.1	E933.1	E950.4	E962.0	E980.4
PVP	964.8	E858.2	E934.8	E950.4	E962.0	E980.4
Pyrabital	965.7	E850.7	E935.7	E950.0	E962.0	E980.0
Pyramidon	965.5	E850.5	E935.5	E950.0	E962.0	E980.0
Pyrantel (pamoate)	961.6	E857	E931.6	E950.4	E962.0	E980.4
Pyrathiazine	963.0	E858.1	E933.0	E950.4	E962.0	E980.4
Pyrazinamide	961.8	E857	E931.8	E950.4	E962.0	E980.4
Pyrazinoic acid (amide)	961.8	E857	E931.8	E950.4	E962.0	E980.4
Pyrazole (derivatives)	965.5	E850.5	E935.5	E950.0	E962.0	E980.0
Pyrazolone (analgesics)	965.5	E850.5	E935.5	E950.0	E962.0	E980.0
Pyrethrins, pyrethrum	989.4	E863.4	—	E950.6	E962.1	E980.7
Pyribenzamine	963.0	E858.1	E933.0	E950.4	E962.0	E980.4
Pyridine (liquid) (vapor)	982.0	E862.4	—	E950.9	E962.1	E980.9
aldoxime chloride	977.2	E858.8	E947.2	E950.4	E962.0	E980.4
Pyridium	976.1	E858.7	E946.1	E950.4	E962.0	E980.4
Pyridostigmine	971.0	E855.3	E941.0	E950.4	E962.0	E980.4
Pyridoxine	963.5	E858.1	E933.5	E950.4	E962.0	E980.4
Pyrilamine	963.0	E858.1	E933.0	E950.4	E962.0	E980.4
Pyrimethamine	961.4	E857	E931.4	E950.4	E962.0	E980.4
Pyrogallic acid	983.0	E864.0	—	E950.7	E962.1	E980.6
Pyroxylin	976.3	E858.7	E946.3	E950.4	E962.0	E980.4
Pyrrobutamine	963.0	E858.1	E933.0	E950.4	E962.0	E980.4
Pyrrocaine	968.5	E855.2	E938.5	E950.4	E962.0	E980.4
Pyrvinium (pamoate)	961.6	E857	E931.6	E950.4	E962.0	E980.4
PZI	962.3	E858.0	E932.3	E950.4	E962.0	E980.4
Quaalude	967.4	E852.3	E937.4	E950.2	E962.0	E980.2
Quaternary ammonium derivatives	971.1	E855.4	E941.1	E950.4	E962.0	E980.4
Quicklime	983.2	E864.2	—	E950.7	E962.1	E980.6
Quinacrine	961.3	E857	E931.3	E950.4	E962.0	E980.4
Quinaglute	972.0	E858.3	E942.0	E950.4	E962.0	E980.4
Quinalbarbitone	967.0	E851	E937.0	E950.1	E962.0	E980.1
Quinestradiol	962.2	E858.0	E932.2	E950.4	E962.0	E980.4
Quinethazone	974.3	E858.5	E944.3	E950.4	E962.0	E980.4
Quinidine (gluconate) (polygalacturonate) (salts) (sulfate)	972.0	E858.3	E942.0	E950.4	E962.0	E980.4
Quinine	961.4	E857	E931.4	E950.4	E962.0	E980.4
Quiniobine	961.3	E857	E931.3	E950.4	E962.0	E980.4
Quinolines	961.3	E857	E931.3	E950.4	E962.0	E980.4
Quotane	968.5	E855.2	E938.5	E950.4	E962.0	E980.4
Rabies						
immune globulin (human)	964.6	E858.2	E934.6	E950.4	E962.0	E980.4
vaccine	979.1	E858.8	E949.1	E950.4	E962.0	E980.4

Substance	Poisoning	Accident	Therapeutic Use	Suicide Attempt	Assault	Undetermined
		External Cause (E-Code)				
Racemoramide	965.09	E850.2	E935.2	E950.0	E962.0	E980.0
Racemorphan	965.09	E850.2	E935.2	E950.0	E962.0	E980.0
Radiator alcohol	980.1	E860.2	—	E950.9	E962.1	E980.9
Radio–opaque (drugs) (materials)	977.8	E858.8	E947.8	E950.4	E962.0	E980.4
Ranunculus	988.2	E865.4	—	E950.9	E962.1	E980.9
Rat poison	989.4	E863.7	—	E950.6	E962.1	E980.7
Rattlesnake (venom)	989.5	E905.0	—	E950.9	E962.1	E980.9
Raudixin	972.6	E858.3	E942.6	E950.4	E962.0	E980.4
Rautensin	972.6	E858.3	E942.6	E950.4	E962.0	E980.4
Rautina	972.6	E858.3	E942.6	E950.4	E962.0	E980.4
Rautotal	972.6	E858.3	E942.6	E950.4	E962.0	E980.4
Rauwiloid	972.6	E858.3	E942.6	E950.4	E962.0	E980.4
Rauwoldin	972.6	E858.3	E942.6	E950.4	E962.0	E980.4
Rauwolfia (alkaloids)	972.6	E858.3	E942.6	E950.4	E962.0	E980.4
Realgar	985.1	E866.3	—	E950.8	E962.1	E980.8
Red cells, packed	964.7	E858.2	E934.7	E950.4	E962.0	E980.4
Reducing agents, industrial NEC	983.9	E864.3	—	E950.7	E962.1	E980.6
Refrigerant gas (freon)	987.4	E869.2	—	E952.8	E962.2	E982.8
not freon	987.9	E869.9	—	E952.9	E962.2	E982.9
Regroton	974.4	E858.5	E944.4	E950.4	E962.0	E980.4
Rela	968.0	E855.1	E938.0	E950.4	E962.0	E980.4
Relaxants, skeletal muscle (autonomic)	975.2	E858.6	E945.2	E950.4	E962.0	E980.4
central nervous system	968.0	E855.1	E938.0	E950.4	E962.0	E980.4
Renese	974.3	E858.5	E944.3	E950.4	E962.0	E980.4
Renografin	977.8	E858.8	E947.8	E950.4	E962.0	E980.4
Replacement solutions	974.5	E858.5	E944.5	E950.4	E962.0	E980.4
Rescinnamine	972.6	E858.3	E942.6	E950.4	E962.0	E980.4
Reserpine	972.6	E858.3	E942.6	E950.4	E962.0	E980.4
Resorcin, resorcinol	976.4	E858.7	E946.4	E950.4	E962.0	E980.4
Respaire	975.5	E858.6	E945.5	E950.4	E962.0	E980.4
Respiratory agents NEC	975.8	E858.6	E945.8	E950.4	E962.0	E980.4
Retinoic acid	976.8	E858.7	E946.8	E950.4	E962.0	E980.4
Retinol	963.5	E858.1	E933.5	E950.4	E962.0	E980.4
Rh_0 (D) immune globulin (human)	964.6	E858.2	E934.6	E950.4	E962.0	E980.4
Rhodine	965.1	E850.3	E935.3	E950.0	E962.0	E980.0
RhoGAM	964.6	E858.2	E934.6	E950.4	E962.0	E980.4
Riboflavin	963.5	E858.1	E933.5	E950.4	E962.0	E980.4
Ricin	989.89	E866.8	—	E950.9	E962.1	E980.9
Ricinus communis	988.2	E865.3	—	E950.9	E962.1	E980.9
Rickettsial vaccine NEC	979.6	E858.8	E949.6	E950.4	E962.0	E980.4
with viral and bacterial vaccine	979.7	E858.8	E949.7	E950.4	E962.0	E980.4
Rifampin	960.6	E856	E930.6	E950.4	E962.0	E980.4
Rimifon	961.8	E857	E931.8	E950.4	E962.0	E980.4
Ringer's injection (lactated)	974.5	E858.5	E944.5	E950.4	E962.0	E980.4
Ristocetin	960.8	E856	E930.8	E950.4	E962.0	E980.4
Ritalin	969.7	E854.2	E939.7	E950.3	E962.0	E980.3
Roach killers — *see* Pesticides						
Rocky Mountain spotted fever vaccine	979.6	E858.8	E949.6	E950.4	E962.0	E980.4
Rodenticides	989.4	E863.7	—	E950.6	E962.1	E980.7
Rohypnol	969.4	E853.2	E939.4	E950.3	E962.0	E980.3
Rolaids	973.0	E858.4	E943.0	E950.4	E962.0	E980.4
Rolitetracycline	960.4	E856	E930.4	E950.4	E962.0	E980.4
Romilar	975.4	E858.6	E945.4	E950.4	E962.0	E980.4
Rose water ointment	976.3	E858.7	E946.3	E950.4	E962.0	E980.4
Rotenone	989.4	E863.7	—	E950.6	E962.1	E980.7
Rotoxamine	963.0	E858.1	E933.0	E950.4	E962.0	E980.4
Rough–on–rats	989.4	E863.7	—	E950.6	E962.1	E980.7
Rubbing alcohol	980.2	E860.3	—	E950.9	E962.1	E980.9
Rubella virus vaccine	979.4	E858.8	E949.4	E950.4	E962.0	E980.4
Rubelogen	979.4	E858.8	E949.4	E950.4	E962.0	E980.4

Substance	Poisoning	Accident	Therapeutic Use	Suicide Attempt	Assault	Undetermined
		External Cause (E-Code)				
Rubeovax	979.4	E858.8	E949.4	E950.4	E962.0	E980.4
Rubidomycin	960.7	E856	E930.7	E950.4	E962.0	E980.4
Rue	988.2	E965.4	—	E950.9	E962.1	E980.9
RU486	962.9	E858.0	E932.9	E950.4	E962.0	E980.4
Ruta	988.2	E865.4	—	E950.9	E962.1	E980.9
Sabadilla (medicinal)	976.0	E858.7	E946.0	E950.4	E962.0	E980.4
pesticide	989.4	E863.4	—	E950.6	E962.1	E980.7
Sabin oral vaccine	979.5	E858.8	E949.5	E950.4	E962.0	E980.4
Saccharated iron oxide	964.0	E858.2	E934.0	E950.4	E962.0	E980.4
Saccharin	974.5	E858.5	E944.5	E950.4	E962.0	E980.4
Safflower oil	972.2	E858.3	E942.2	E950.4	E962.0	E980.4
Salbutamol sulfate	975.7	E858.6	E945.7	E950.4	E962.0	E980.4
Salicylamide	965.1	E850.3	E935.3	E950.0	E962.0	E980.0
Salicylate(s)	965.1	E850.3	E935.3	E950.0	E962.0	E980.0
methyl	976.3	E858.7	E946.3	E950.4	E962.0	E980.4
theobromine calcium	974.1	E858.5	E944.1	E950.4	E962.0	E980.4
Salicylazosulfapyridine	961.0	E857	E931.0	E950.4	E962.0	E980.4
Salicylhydroxamic acid	976.0	E858.7	E946.0	E950.4	E962.0	E980.4
Salicylic acid (keratolytic) NEC	976.4	E858.7	E946.4	E950.4	E962.0	E980.4
congeners	965.1	E850.3	E935.3	E950.0	E962.0	E980.0
salts	965.1	E850.3	E935.3	E950.0	E962.0	E980.0
Saliniazid	961.8	E857	E931.8	E950.4	E962.0	E980.4
Salol	976.3	E858.7	E946.3	E950.4	E962.0	E980.4
Salt (substitute) NEC	974.5	E858.5	E944.5	E950.4	E962.0	E980.4
Saluretics	974.3	E858.5	E944.3	E950.4	E962.0	E980.4
Saluron	974.3	E858.5	E944.3	E950.4	E962.0	E980.4
Salvarsan 606 (neosilver) (silver)	961.1	E857	E931.1	E950.4	E962.0	E980.4
Sambucus canadensis	988.2	E865.4	—	E950.9	E962.1	E980.9
berry	988.2	E865.3	—	E950.9	E962.1	E980.9
Sandril	972.6	E858.3	E942.6	E950.4	E962.0	E980.4
Sanguinaria canadensis	988.2	E865.4	—	E950.9	E962.1	E980.9
Saniflush (cleaner)	983.9	E861.3	—	E950.7	E962.1	E980.6
Santonin	961.6	E857	E931.6	E950.4	E962.0	E980.4
Santyl	976.8	E858.7	E946.8	E950.4	E962.0	E980.4
Sarkomycin	960.7	E856	E930.7	E950.4	E962.0	E980.4
Saroten	969.0	E854.0	E939.0	E950.3	E962.0	E980.3
Saturnine – *see* Lead						
Savin (oil)	976.4	E858.7	E946.4	E950.4	E962.0	E980.4
Scammony	973.1	E858.4	E943.1	E950.4	E962.0	E980.4
Scarlet red	976.8	E858.7	E946.8	E950.4	E962.0	E980.4
Scheele's green	985.1	E866.3	—	E950.8	E962.1	E980.8
insecticide	985.1	E863.4	—	E950.8	E962.1	E980.8
Schradan	989.3	E863.1	—	E950.6	E962.1	E980.7
Schweinfurt (h) green	985.1	E866.3	—	E950.8	E962.1	E980.8
insecticide	985.1	E863.4	—	E950.8	E962.1	E980.8
Scilla — *see* Squill						
Sclerosing agents	972.7	E858.3	E942.7	E950.4	E962.0	E980.4
Scopolamine	971.1	E855.4	E941.1	E950.4	E962.0	E980.4
Scouring powder	989.89	E861.3	—	E950.9	E962.1	E980.9
Sea						
anemone (sting)	989.5	E905.6	—	E950.9	E962.1	E980.9
cucumber (sting)	989.5	E905.6	—	E950.9	E962.1	E980.9
snake (bite) (venom)	989.5	E905.0	—	E950.9	E962.1	E980.9
urchin spine (puncture)	989.5	E905.6	—	E950.9	E962.1	E980.9
Secbutabarbital	967.0	E851	E937.0	E950.1	E962.0	E980.1
Secbutabaritone	967.0	E851	E937.0	E950.1	E962.0	E980.1
Secobarbital	967.0	E851	E937.0	E950.1	E962.0	E980.1
Seconal	967.0	E851	E937.0	E950.1	E962.0	E980.1
Secretin	977.8	E858.8	E947.8	E950.4	E962.0	E980.4
Sedatives, nonbarbiturate	967.9	E852.9	E937.9	E950.2	E962.0	E980.2
specified NEC	967.8	E852.8	E937.8	E950.2	E962.0	E980.2

Substance	Poisoning	Accident	Therapeutic Use	Suicide Attempt	Assault	Undetermined
		External Cause (E-Code)				
Sedormid	967.8	E852.8	E937.8	E950.2	E962.0	E980.2
Seed (plant)	988.2	E865.3	—	E950.9	E962.1	E980.9
disinfectant or dressing	989.89	E866.5	—	E950.9	E962.1	E980.9
Selenium (fumes) NEC	985.8	E866.4	—	E950.9	E962.1	E980.9
disulfide or sulfide	976.4	E858.7	E946.4	E950.4	E962.0	E980.4
Selsun	976.4	E858.7	E946.4	E950.4	E962.0	E980.4
Senna	973.1	E858.4	E943.1	E950.4	E962.0	E980.4
Septisol	976.2	E858.7	E946.2	E950.4	E962.0	E980.4
Serax	969.4	E853.2	E939.4	E950.3	E962.0	E980.3
Serenesil	967.8	E852.8	E937.8	E950.2	E962.0	E980.2
Serenium (hydrochloride)	961.9	E857	E931.9	E950.4	E962.0	E980.4
Serepax—*see* Oxazepam						
Sernyl	968.3	E855.1	E938.3	E950.4	E962.0	E980.4
Serotonin	977.8	E858.8	E947.8	E950.4	E962.0	E980.4
Serpasil	972.6	E858.3	E942.6	E950.4	E962.0	E980.4
Sewer gas	987.8	E869.8	—	E952.8	E962.2	E982.8
Shampoo	989.6	E861.0	—	E950.9	E962.1	E980.9
Shellfish, nonbacterial or noxious	988.0	E865.1	—	E950.9	E962.1	E980.9
Silicones NEC	989.83	E866.8	E947.8	E950.9	E962.1	E980.9
Silvadene	976.0	E858.7	E946.0	E950.4	E962.0	E980.4
Silver (compound) (medicinal) NEC	976.0	E858.7	E946.0	E950.4	E962.0	E980.4
anti–infectives	976.0	E858.7	E946.0	E950.4	E962.0	E980.4
arsphenamine	961.1	E857	E931.1	E950.4	E962.0	E980.4
nitrate	976.0	E858.7	E946.0	E950.4	E962.0	E980.4
ophthalmic preparation	976.5	E858.7	E946.5	E950.4	E962.0	E980.4
toughened (keratolytic)	976.4	E858.7	E946.4	E950.4	E962.0	E980.4
nonmedicinal (dust)	985.8	E866.4	—	E950.9	E962.1	E980.9
protein (mild) (strong)	976.0	E858.7	E946.0	E950.4	E962.0	E980.4
salvarsan	961.1	E857	E931.1	E950.4	E962.0	E980.4
Simethicone	973.8	E858.4	E943.8	E950.4	E962.0	E980.4
Sinequan	969.0	E854.0	E939.0	E950.3	E962.0	E980.3
Singoserp	972.6	E858.3	E942.6	E950.4	E962.0	E980.4
Sintrom	964.2	E858.2	E934.2	E950.4	E962.0	E980.4
Sitosterols	972.2	E858.3	E942.2	E950.4	E962.0	E980.4
Skeletal muscle relaxants	975.2	E858.6	E945.2	E950.4	E962.0	E980.4
Skin						
agents (external)	976.9	E858.7	E946.9	E950.4	E962.0	E980.4
specified NEC	976.8	E858.7	E946.8	E950.4	E962.0	E980.4
test antigen	977.8	E858.8	E947.8	E950.4	E962.0	E980.4
Sleep–eze	963.0	E858.1	E933.0	E950.4	E962.0	E980.4
Sleeping draught (drug) (pill) (tablet)	967.9	E852.9	E937.9	E950.2	E962.0	E980.2
Smallpox vaccine	979.0	E858.8	E949.0	E950.4	E962.0	E980.4
Smelter fumes NEC	985.9	E866.4	—	E950.9	E962.1	E980.9
Smog	987.3	E869.1	—	E952.8	E962.2	E982.8
Smoke NEC	987.9	E869.9	—	E952.9	E962.2	E982.9
Smooth muscle relaxant	975.1	E858.6	E945.1	E950.4	E962.0	E980.4
Snail killer	989.4	E863.4	—	E950.6	E962.1	E980.7
Snake (bite) (venom)	989.5	E905.0	—	E950.9	E962.1	E980.9
Snuff	989.89	E866.8	—	E950.9	E962.1	E980.9
Soap (powder) (product)	989.6	E861.1	—	E950.9	E962.1	E980.9
medicinal, soft	976.2	E858.7	E946.2	E950.4	E962.0	E980.4
Soda (caustic)	983.2	E864.2	—	E950.7	E962.1	E980.6
bicarb	963.3	E858.1	E933.3	E950.4	E962.0	E980.4
chlorinated — Sodium, hypochlorite						
Sodium						
acetosulfone	961.8	E857	E931.8	E950.4	E962.0	E980.4
acetrizoate	977.8	E858.8	E947.8	E950.4	E962.0	E980.4
amytal	967.0	E851	E937.0	E950.1	E962.0	E980.1
arsenate — see Arsenic						
bicarbonate	963.3	E858.1	E933.3	E950.4	E962.0	E980.4

Substance	Poisoning	Accident	Therapeutic Use	Suicide Attempt	Assault	Undetermined
			External Cause (E-Code)			
bichromate	983.9	E864.3	—	E950.7	E962.1	E980.6
biphosphate	963.2	E858.1	E933.2	E950.4	E962.0	E980.4
bisulfate	983.9	E864.3	—	E950.7	E962.1	E980.6
borate (cleanser)	989.6	E861.3	—	E950.9	E962.1	E980.9
bromide NEC	967.3	E852.2	E937.3	E950.2	E962.0	E980.2
cacodylate (nonmedicinal) NEC	978.8	E858.8	E948.8	E950.4	E962.0	E980.4
anti–infective	961.1	E857	E931.1	E950.4	E962.0	E980.4
herbicide	989.4	E863.5	—	E950.6	E962.1	E980.7
calcium edetate	963.8	E858.1	E933.8	E950.4	E962.0	E980.4
carbonate NEC	983.2	E864.2	—	E950.7	E962.1	E980.6
chlorate NEC	983.9	E864.3	—	E950.7	E962.1	E980.6
herbicide	983.9	E863.5	—	E950.7	E962.1	E980.6
chloride NEC	974.5	E858.5	E944.5	E950.4	E962.0	E980.4
chromate	983.9	E864.3	—	E950.7	E962.1	E980.6
citrate	963.3	E858.1	E933.3	E950.4	E962.0	E980.4
cyanide — see Cyanide(s)						
cyclamate	974.5	E858.5	E944.5	E950.4	E962.0	E980.4
diatrizoate	977.8	E858.8	E947.8	E950.4	E962.0	E980.4
dibunate	975.4	E858.6	E945.4	E950.4	E962.0	E980.4
dioctyl sulfosuccinate	973.2	E858.4	E943.2	E950.4	E962.0	E980.4
edetate	963.8	E858.1	E933.8	E950.4	E962.0	E980.4
ethacrynate	974.4	E858.5	E944.4	E950.4	E962.0	E980.4
fluoracetate (dust) (rodenticide)	989.4	E863.7	—	E950.6	E962.1	E980.7
fluoride — see Fluoride(s)						
free salt	974.5	E858.5	E944.5	E950.4	E962.0	E980.4
glucosulfone	961.8	E857	E931.8	E950.4	E962.0	E980.4
hydroxide	983.2	E864.2	—	E950.7	E962.1	E980.6
hypochlorite (bleach) NEC	983.9	E864.3	—	E950.7	E962.1	E980.6
disinfectant	983.9	E861.4	—	E950.7	E962.1	E980.6
medicinal (anti–infective) (external)	976.0	E858.7	E946.0	E950.4	E962.0	E980.4
vapor	987.8	E869.8	—	E952.8	E962.2	E982.8
hyposulfite	976.0	E858.7	E946.0	E950.4	E962.0	E980.4
indigotindisulfonate	977.8	E858.8	E947.8	E950.4	E962.0	E980.4
iodide	977.8	E858.8	E947.8	E950.4	E962.0	E980.4
iothalamate	977.8	E858.8	E947.8	E950.4	E962.0	E980.4
iron edetate	964.0	E858.2	E934.0	E950.4	E962.0	E980.4
lactate	963.3	E858.1	E933.3	E950.4	E962.0	E980.4
lauryl sulfate	976.2	E858.7	E946.2	E950.4	E962.0	E980.4
L–triiodothyronine	962.7	E858.0	E932.7	E950.4	E962.0	E980.4
metrizoate	977.8	E858.8	E947.8	E950.4	E962.0	E980.4
monofluoracetate (dust) (rodenticide)	989.4	E863.7	—	E950.6	E962.1	E980.7
morrhuate	972.7	E858.3	E942.7	E950.4	E962.0	E980.4
nafcillin	960.0	E856	E930.0	E950.4	E962.0	E980.4
nitrate (oxidizing agent)	983.9	E864.3	—	E950.7	E962.1	E980.6
nitrite (medicinal)	972.4	E858.3	E942.4	E950.4	E962.0	E980.4
nitroferricyanide	972.6	E858.3	E942.6	E950.4	E962.0	E980.4
nitroprusside	972.6	E858.3	E942.6	E950.4	E962.0	E980.4
para–aminohippurate	977.8	E858.8	E947.8	E950.4	E962.0	E980.4
perborate (non-medicinal) NEC	989.89	E866.8	—	E950.9	E962.1	E980.9
medicinal	976.6	E858.7	E946.6	E950.4	E962.0	E980.4
soap	989.6	E861.1	—	E950.9	E962.1	E980.9
percarbonate — *see* Sodium, perborate						
phosphate	973.3	E858.4	E943.3	E950.4	E962.0	E980.4
polystyrene sulfonate	974.5	E858.5	E944.5	E950.4	E962.0	E980.4
propionate	976.0	E858.7	E946.0	E950.4	E962.0	E980.4
psylliate	972.7	E858.3	E942.7	E950.4	E962.0	E980.4
removing resins	974.5	E858.5	E944.5	E950.4	E962.0	E980.4
salicylate	965.1	E850.3	E935.3	E950.0	E962.0	E980.0
sulfate	973.3	E858.4	E943.3	E950.4	E962.0	E980.4
sulfoxone	961.8	E857	E931.8	E950.4	E962.0	E980.4
tetradecyl sulfate	972.7	E858.3	E942.7	E950.4	E962.0	E980.4

Substance	Poisoning	Accident	Therapeutic Use	Suicide Attempt	Assault	Undetermined
		External Cause (E-Code)				
thiopental	968.3	E855.1	E938.3	E950.4	E962.0	E980.4
thiosalicylate	965.1	E850.3	E935.3	E950.0	E962.0	E980.0
thiosulfate	976.0	E858.7	E946.0	E950.4	E962.0	E980.4
tolbutamide	977.8	E858.8	E947.8	E950.4	E962.0	E980.4
tyropanoate	977.8	E858.8	E947.8	E950.4	E962.0	E980.4
valproate	966.3	E855.0	E936.3	E950.4	E962.0	E980.4
Solanine	977.8	E858.8	E947.8	E950.4	E962.0	E980.4
Solanum dulcamara	988.2	E865.4	—	E950.9	E962.1	E980.9
Solapsone	961.8	E857	E931.8	E950.4	E962.0	E980.4
Solasulfone	961.8	E857	E931.8	E950.4	E962.0	E980.4
Soldering fluid	983.1	E864.1	—	E950.7	E962.1	E980.6
Solid substance	989.9	E866.9	—	E950.9	E962.1	E980.9
specified NEC	989.9	E866.8	—	E950.9	E962.1	E980.9
Solvents, industrial	982.8	E862.9	—	E950.9	E962.1	E980.9
naphtha	981	E862.0	—	E950.9	E962.1	E980.9
petroleum	981	E862.0	—	E950.9	E962.1	E980.9
specified NEC	982.8	E862.4	—	E950.9	E962.1	E980.9
Soma	968.0	E855.1	E938.0	E950.4	E962.0	E980.4
Somatotropin	962.4	E858.0	E932.4	E950.4	E962.0	E980.4
Sominex	963.0	E858.1	E933.0	E950.4	E962.0	E980.4
Somnos	967.1	E852.0	E937.1	E950.2	E962.0	E980.2
Somonal	967.0	E851	E937.0	E950.1	E962.0	E980.1
Soneryl	967.0	E851	E937.0	E950.1	E962.0	E980.1
Soothing syrup	977.9	E858.9	E947.9	E950.5	E962.0	E980.5
Sopor	967.4	E852.3	E937.4	E950.2	E962.0	E980.2
Soporific drug	967.9	E852.9	E937.9	E950.2	E962.0	E980.2
specified type NEC	967.8	E852.8	E937.8	E950.2	E962.0	E980.2
Sorbitol NEC	977.4	E858.8	E947.4	E950.4	E962.0	E980.4
Sotradecol	972.7	E858.3	E942.7	E950.4	E962.0	E980.4
Spacoline	975.1	E858.6	E945.1	E950.4	E962.0	E980.4
Spanish fly	976.8	E858.7	E946.8	E950.4	E962.0	E980.4
Sparine	969.1	E853.0	E939.1	E950.3	E962.0	E980.3
Sparteine	975.0	E858.6	E945.0	E950.4	E962.0	E980.4
Spasmolytics	975.1	E858.6	E945.1	E950.4	E962.0	E980.4
anticholinergics	971.1	E855.4	E941.1	E950.4	E962.0	E980.4
Spectinomycin	960.8	E856	E930.8	E950.4	E962.0	E980.4
Speed	969.7	E854.2	E939.7	E950.3	E962.0	E980.3
Spermicides	976.8	E858.7	E946.8	E950.4	E962.0	E980.4
Spider (bite) (venom)	989.5	E905.1	—	E950.9	E962.1	E980.9
antivenin	979.9	E858.8	E949.9	E950.4	E962.0	E980.4
Spigelia (root)	961.6	E857	E931.6	E950.4	E962.0	E980.4
Spiperone	969.2	E853.1	E939.2	E950.3	E962.0	E980.3
Spiramycin	960.3	E856	E930.3	E950.4	E962.0	E980.4
Spirilene	969.5	E853.8	E939.5	E950.3	E962.0	E980.3
Spirit(s) (neutral) NEC	980.0	E860.1	—	E950.9	E962.1	E980.9
beverage	980.0	E860.0	—	E950.9	E962.1	E980.9
industrial	980.9	E860.9	—	E950.9	E962.1	E980.9
mineral	981	E862.0	—	E950.9	E962.1	E980.9
of salt — *see* Hydrochloric acid						
surgical	980.9	E860.9	—	E950.9	E962.1	E980.9
Spironolactone	974.4	E858.5	E944.4	E950.4	E962.0	E980.4
Sponge, absorbable (gelatin)	964.5	E858.2	E934.5	E950.4	E962.0	E980.4
Sporostacin	976.0	E858.7	E946.0	E950.4	E962.0	E980.4
Sprays (aerosol)	989.89	E866.8	—	E950.9	E962.1	E980.9
cosmetic	989.89	E866.7	—	E950.9	E962.1	E980.9
medicinal NEC	977.9	E858.9	E947.9	E950.5	E962.0	E980.5
pesticides — *see* Pesticides						
specified content — *see* substance specified						
Spurge flax	988.2	E865.4	—	E950.9	E962.1	E980.9

Substance	Poisoning	Accident	Therapeutic Use	Suicide Attempt	Assault	Undetermined
			External Cause (E-Code)			
Spurges	988.2	E865.4	—	E950.9	E962.1	E980.9
Squill (expectorant) NEC	975.5	E858.6	E945.5	E950.4	E962.0	E980.4
rat poison	989.4	E863.7	—	E950.6	E962.1	E980.7
Squirting cucumber (cathartic)	973.1	E858.4	E943.1	E950.4	E962.0	E980.4
Stains	989.89	E866.8	—	E950.9	E962.1	E980.9
Stannous — *see also* Tin						
fluoride	976.7	E858.7	E946.7	E950.4	E962.0	E980.4
Stanolone	962.1	E858.0	E932.1	E950.4	E962.0	E980.4
Stanozolol	962.1	E853.0	E932.1	E950.4	E962.0	E980.4
Staphisagria or stavesacre (pediculicide)	976.0	E858.7	E946.0	E950.4	E962.0	E980.4
Stelazine	969.1	E853.0	E939.1	E950.3	E962.0	E980.3
Stemetil	969.1	E853.0	E939.1	E950.3	E962.0	E980.3
Sterculia (cathartic) (gum)	973.3	E858.4	E943.3	E950.4	E962.0	E980.4
Sternutator gas	987.8	E869.8	—	E952.8	E962.2	E982.8
Steroids NEC	962.0	E858.0	E932.0	E950.4	E962.0	E980.4
ENT agent	976.6	E858.7	E946.6	E950.4	E962.0	E980.4
ophthalmic preparation	976.5	E858.7	E946.5	E950.4	E962.0	E980.4
topical NEC	976.0	E858.7	E946.0	E950.4	E962.0	E980.4
Stibine	985.8	E866.4	—	E950.9	E962.1	E980.9
Stibophen	961.2	E857	E931.2	E950.4	E962.0	E980.4
Stilbamide, stilbamidine	961.5	E857	E931.5	E950.4	E962.0	E980.4
Stilbestrol	962.2	E858.0	E932.2	E950.4	E962.0	E980.4
Stimulants (central nervous system)	970.9	E854.3	E940.9	E950.4	E962.0	E980.4
analeptics	970.0	E854.3	E940.0	E950.4	E962.0	E980.4
opiate antagonist	970.1	E854.3	E940.1	E950.4	E962.0	E980.4
psychotherapeutic NEC	969.0	E854.0	E939.0	E950.3	E962.0	E980.3
specified NEC	970.8	E854.3	E940.8	E950.4	E962.0	E980.4
Storage batteries (acid) (cells)	983.1	E864.1	—	E950.7	E962.1	E980.6
Stovaine	968.9	E855.2	E938.9	E950.4	E962.0	E980.4
infiltration (subcutaneous)	968.5	E855.2	E938.5	E950.4	E962.0	E980.4
nerve block (peripheral) (plexus)	968.6	E855.2	E938.6	E950.5	E962.0	E980.4
spinal	968.7	E855.2	E938.7	E950.4	E962.0	E980.4
topical (surface)	968.5	E855.2	E938.5	E950.4	E962.0	E980.4
Stovarsal	961.1	E857	E931.1	E950.4	E962.0	E980.4
Stove gas — *see* Gas, utility						
Stoxil	976.5	E858.7	E946.5	E950.4	E962.0	E980.4
STP	969.6	E854.1	E939.6	E950.3	E962.0	E980.3
Stramonium (medicinal) NEC	971.1	E855.4	E941.1	E950.4	E962.0	E980.4
natural state	988.2	E865.4	—	E950.9	E962.1	E980.9
Streptodornase	964.4	E858.2	E934.4	E950.4	E962.0	E980.4
Streptoduocin	960.6	E856	E930.6	E950.4	E962.0	E980.4
Streptokinase	964.4	E858.2	E934.4	E950.4	E962.0	E980.4
Streptomycin	960.6	E856	E930.6	E950.4	E962.0	E980.4
Streptozocin	960.7	E856	E930.7	E950.4	E962.0	E980.4
Stripper (paint) (solvent)	982.8	E862.9	—	E950.9	E962.1	E980.9
Strobane	989.2	E863.0	—	E950.6	E962.1	E980.7
Strophanthin	972.1	E858.3	E942.1	E950.4	E962.0	E980.4
Strophanthus hispidus or kombe	988.2	E865.4	—	E950.9	E962.1	E980.9
Strychnine (rodenticide) (salts)	989.1	E863.7	—	E950.6	E962.1	E980.7
medicinal NEC	970.8	E854.3	E940.8	E950.4	E962.0	E980.4
Strychnos (ignatii) — *see* Strychnine						
Styramate	968.0	E855.1	E938.0	E950.4	E962.0	E980.4
Styrene	983.0	E864.0	—	E950.7	E962.1	E980.6
Succinimide (anticonvulsant)	966.2	E855.0	E936.2	E950.4	E962.0	E980.4
mercuric — *see* Mercury						
Succinylcholine	975.2	E858.6	E945.2	E950.4	E962.0	E980.4
Succinylsulfathiazole	961.0	E857	E931.0	E950.4	E962.0	E980.4
Sucrose	974.5	E858.5	E944.5	E950.4	E962.0	E980.4
Sulfacetamide	961.0	E857	E931.0	E950.4	E962.0	E980.4
ophthalmic preparation	976.5	E858.7	E946.5	E950.4	E962.0	E980.4
Sulfachlorpyridazine	961.0	E857	E931.0	E950.4	E962.0	E980.4

Substance	Poisoning	Accident	Therapeutic Use	Suicide Attempt	Assault	Undetermined
		External Cause (E-Code)				
Sulfacytine	961.0	E857	E931.0	E950.4	E962.0	E980.4
Sulfadiazine	961.0	E857	E931.0	E950.4	E962.0	E980.4
silver (topical)	976.0	E858.7	E946.0	E950.4	E962.0	E980.4
Sulfadimethoxine	961.0	E857	E931.0	E950.4	E962.0	E980.4
Sulfadimidine	961.0	E857	E931.0	E950.4	E962.0	E980.4
Sulfaethidole	961.0	E857	E931.0	E950.4	E962.0	E980.4
Sulfafurazole	961.0	E857	E931.0	E950.4	E962.0	E980.4
Sulfaguanidine	961.0	E857	E931.0	E950.4	E962.0	E980.4
Sulfamerazine	961.0	E857	E931.0	E950.4	E962.0	E980.4
Sulfameter	961.0	E857	E931.0	E950.4	E962.0	E980.4
Sulfamethizole	961.0	E857	E931.0	E950.4	E962.0	E980.4
Sulfamethoxazole	961.0	E857	E931.0	E950.4	E962.0	E980.4
Sulfamethoxydiazine	961.0	E857	E931.0	E950.4	E962.0	E980.4
Sulfamethoxypyridazine	961.0	E857	E931.0	E950.4	E962.0	E980.4
Sulfamethylthiazole	961.0	E857	E931.0	E950.4	E962.0	E980.4
Sulfamylon	976.0	E858.7	E946.0	E950.4	E962.0	E980.4
Sulfan blue (diagnostic dye)	977.8	E858.8	E947.8	E950.4	E962.0	E980.4
Sulfanilamide	961.0	E857	E931.0	E950.4	E962.0	E980.4
Sulfanilylguanidine	961.0	E857	E931.0	E950.4	E962.0	E980.4
Sulfaphenazole	961.0	E857	E931.0	E950.4	E962.0	E980.4
Sulfaphenylthiazole	961.0	E857	E931.0	E950.4	E962.0	E980.4
Sulfaproxyline	961.0	E857	E931.0	E950.4	E962.0	E980.4
Sulfapyridine	961.0	E857	E931.0	E950.4	E962.0	E980.4
Sulfapyrimidine	961.0	E857	E931.0	E950.4	E962.0	E980.4
Sulfarsphenamine	961.1	E857	E931.1	E950.4	E962.0	E980.4
Sulfasalazine	961.0	E857	E931.0	E950.4	E962.0	E980.4
Sulfasomizole	961.0	E857	E931.0	E950.4	E962.0	E980.4
Sulfasuxidine	961.0	E857	E931.0	E950.4	E962.0	E980.4
Sulfinpyrazone	974.7	E858.5	E944.7	E950.4	E962.0	E980.4
Sulfisoxazole	961.0	E857	E931.0	E950.4	E962.0	E980.4
ophthalmic preparation	976.5	E858.7	E946.5	E950.4	E962.0	E980.4
Sulfomyxin	960.8	E856	E930.8	E950.4	E962.0	E980.4
Sulfonal	967.8	E852.8	E937.8	E950.2	E962.0	E980.2
Sulfonamides (mixtures)	961.0	E857	E931.0	E950.4	E962.0	E980.4
Sulfones	961.8	E857	E931.8	E950.4	E962.0	E980.4
Sulfonethylmethane	967.8	E852.8	E937.8	E950.2	E962.0	E980.2
Sulfonmethane	967.8	E852.8	E937.8	E950.2	E962.0	E980.2
Sulfonphthal, sulfonphthol	977.8	E858.8	E947.8	E950.4	E962.0	E980.4
Sulfonylurea derivatives, oral	962.3	E858.0	E932.3	E950.4	E962.0	E980.4
Sulfoxone	961.8	E857	E931.8	E950.4	E962.0	E980.4
Sulfur, sulfureted, sulfuric, sulfurous, sulfuryl (compounds) NEC	989.89	E866.8	—	E950.9	E962.1	E980.9
acid	983.1	E864.1	—	E950.7	E962.1	E980.6
dioxide	987.3	E869.1	—	E952.8	E962.2	E982.8
ether — *see* Ether(s)						
hydrogen	987.8	E869.8	—	E952.8	E962.2	E982.8
medicinal (keratolytic) (ointment) NEC	976.4	E858.7	E946.4	E950.4	E962.0	E980.4
pesticide (vapor)	989.4	E863.4	—	E950.6	E962.1	E980.7
vapor NEC	987.8	E869.8	—	E952.8	E962.2	E982.8
Sulkowitch's reagent	977.8	E858.8	E947.8	E950.4	E962.0	E980.4
Sulph — *see also* Sulf–						
Sulphadione	961.8	E857	E931.8	E950.4	E962.0	E980.4
Sulthiame, sultiame	966.3	E855.0	E936.3	E950.4	E962.0	E980.4
Superinone	975.5	E858.6	E945.5	E950.4	E962.0	E980.4
Suramin	961.5	E857	E931.5	E950.4	E962.0	E980.4
Surfacaine	968.5	E855.2	E938.5	E950.4	E962.0	E980.4
Surital	968.3	E855.1	E938.3	E950.4	E962.0	E980.4
Sutilains	976.8	E858.7	E946.8	E950.4	E962.0	E980.4
Suxamethonium (bromide) (chloride) (iodide)	975.2	E858.6	E945.2	E950.4	E962.0	E980.4

Substance	Poisoning	Accident	Therapeutic Use	Suicide Attempt	Assault	Undetermined
			External Cause (E-Code)			
Suxethonium (bromide)	975.2	E858.6	E945.2	E950.4	E962.0	E980.4
Sweet oil (birch)	976.3	E858.7	E946.3	E950.4	E962.0	E980.4
Sym–dichloroethyl ether	982.3	E862.4	—	E950.9	E962.1	E980.9
Sympatholytics	971.3	E855.6	E941.3	E950.4	E962.0	E980.4
Sympathomimetics	971.2	E855.5	E941.2	E950.4	E962.0	E980.4
Synagis	979.6	E858.8	E949.6	E950.4	E962.0	E980.4
Synalar	976.0	E858.7	E946.0	E950.4	E962.0	E980.4
Synthroid	962.7	E858.0	E932.7	E950.4	E962.0	E980.4
Syntocinon	975.0	E858.6	E945.0	E950.4	E962.0	E950.4
Syrosingopine	972.6	E858.3	E942.6	E950.4	E962.0	E980.4
Systemic agents (primarily)	963.9	E858.1	E933.9	E950.4	E962.0	E980.4
specified NEC	963.8	E858.1	E933.8	E950.4	E962.0	E980.4
Tablets (*see also* specified substance)	977.9	E858.9	E947.9	E950.5	E962.0	E980.5
Tace	962.2	E858.0	E932.2	E950.4	E962.0	E980.4
Tacrine	971.0	E855.3	E941.0	E950.4	E962.0	E980.4
Talbutal	967.0	E851	E937.0	E950.1	E962.0	E980.1
Talc	976.3	E858.7	E946.3	E950.4	E962.0	E980.4
Talcum	976.3	E858.7	E946.3	E950.4	E962.0	E980.4
Tandearil, tanderil	965.5	E850.5	E935.5	E950.0	E962.0	E980.0
Tannic acid	983.1	E864.1	—	E950.7	E962.1	E980.6
medicinal (astringent)	976.2	E858.7	E946.2	E950.4	E962.0	E980.4
Tannin — *see* Tannic acid						
Tansy	988.2	E865.4	—	E950.9	E962.1	E980.9
TAO	960.3	E856	E930.3	E950.4	E962.0	E980.4
Tapazole	962.8	E858.0	E932.8	E950.4	E962.0	E980.4
Tar NEC	983.0	E864.0	—	E950.7	E962.1	E980.6
camphor — *see* Naphthalene						
fumes	987.8	E869.8	—	E952.8	E962.2	E982.8
Taractan	969.3	E853.8	E939.3	E950.3	E962.0	E980.3
Tarantula (venomous)	989.5	E905.1	—	E950.9	E962.1	E980.9
Tartar emetic (anti–infective)	961.2	E857	E931.2	E950.4	E962.0	E980.4
Tartaric acid	983.1	E864.1	—	E950.7	E962.1	E980.6
Tartrated antimony (anti–infective)	961.2	E857	E931.2	E950.4	E962.0	E980.4
TCA — *see* Trichloroacetic acid						
TDI	983.0	E864.0	—	E950.7	E962.1	E980.6
vapor	987.8	E869.8	—	E952.8	E962.2	E982.8
Tear gas	987.5	E869.3	—	E952.8	E962.2	E982.8
Teclothiazide	974.3	E858.5	E944.3	E950.4	E962.0	E980.4
Tegretol	966.3	E855.0	E936.3	E950.4	E962.0	E980.4
Telepaque	977.8	E858.8	E947.8	E950.4	E962.0	E980.4
Tellurium	985.8	E866.4	—	E950.9	E962.1	E980.9
fumes	985.8	E866.4	—	E950.9	E962.1	E980.9
TEM	963.1	E858.1	E933.1	E950.4	E962.0	E980.4
Temazepan—*see* Benzodiazepines						
TEPA	963.1	E858.1	E933.1	E950.4	E962.0	E980.4
TEPP	989.3	E863.1	—	E950.6	E962.1	E980.7
Terbutaline	971.2	E855.5	E941.2	E950.4	E962.0	E980.4
Teroxalene	961.6	E857	E931.6	E950.4	E962.0	E980.4
Terpin hydrate	975.5	E858.6	E945.5	E950.4	E962.0	E980.4
Terramycin	960.4	E856	E930.4	E950.4	E962.0	E980.4
Tessalon	975.4	E858.6	E945.4	E950.4	E962.0	E980.4
Testosterone	962.1	E858.0	E932.1	E950.4	E962.0	E980.4
Tetanus (vaccine)	978.4	E858.8	E948.4	E950.4	E962.0	E980.4
antitoxin	979.9	E858.8	E949.9	E950.4	E962.0	E980.4
immune globulin (human)	964.6	E858.2	E934.6	E950.4	E962.0	E980.4
toxoid	978.4	E858.8	E948.4	E950.4	E962.0	E980.4
with diphtheria toxoid	978.9	E858.8	E948.9	E950.4	E962.0	E980.4
with pertussis	978.6	E858.8	E948.6	E950.4	E962.0	E980.4
Tetrabenazine	969.5	E853.8	E939.5	E950.3	E962.0	E980.3
Tetracaine (infiltration) (topical)	968.5	E855.2	E938.5	E950.4	E962.0	E980.4
nerve block (peripheral) (plexus)	968.6	E855.2	E938.6	E950.4	E962.0	E980.4

Substance	Poisoning	Accident	Therapeutic Use	Suicide Attempt	Assault	Undetermined
		External Cause (E-Code)				
spinal	968.7	E855.2	E938.7	E950.4	E962.0	E980.4
Tetrachlorethylene—*see* Tetrachloroethylene						
Tetrachlormethiazide	974.3	E858.5	E944.3	E950.4	E962.0	E980.4
Tetrachloroethane (liquid) (vapor)	982.3	E862.4	—	E950.9	E962.1	E980.9
paint or varnish	982.3	E861.6	—	E950.9	E962.1	E980.9
Tetrachloroethylene (liquid) (vapor)	982.3	E862.4	—	E950.9	E962.1	E980.9
medicinal	961.6	E857	E931.6	E950.4	E962.0	E980.4
Tetrachloromethane — *see* Carbon, tetrachloride						
Tetracycline	960.4	E856	E930.4	E950.4	E962.0	E980.4
ophthalmic preparation	976.5	E858.7	E946.5	E950.4	E962.0	E980.4
topical NEC	976.0	E858.7	E946.0	E950.4	E962.0	E980.4
Tetraethylammonium chloride	972.3	E858.3	E942.3	E950.4	E962.0	E980.4
Tetraethyl lead (antiknock compound)	984.1	E862.1	—	E950.9	E962.1	E980.9
Tetraethyl pyrophosphate	989.3	E863.1	—	E950.6	E962.1	E980.7
Tetraethylthiuram disulfide	977.3	E858.8	E947.3	E950.4	E962.0	E980.4
Tetrahydroaminoacridine	971.0	E855.3	E941.0	E950.4	E962.0	E980.4
Tetrahydrocannabinol	969.6	E854.1	E939.6	E950.3	E962.0	E980.3
Tetrahydronaphthalene	982.0	E862.4	—	E950.9	E962.1	E980.9
Tetrahydrozoline	971.2	E855.5	E941.2	E950.4	E962.0	E980.4
Tetralin	982.0	E862.4	—	E950.9	E962.1	E980.9
Tetramethylthiuram (disulfide) NEC	989.4	E863.6	—	E950.6	E962.1	E980.7
medicinal	976.2	E858.7	E946.2	E950.4	E962.0	E980.4
Tetronal	967.8	E852.8	E937.8	E950.2	E962.0	E980.2
Tetryl	983.0	E864.0	—	E950.7	E962.1	E980.6
Thalidomide	967.8	E852.8	E937.8	E950.2	E962.0	E980.2
Thallium (compounds) (dust) NEC	985.8	E866.4	—	E950.9	E962.1	E980.9
pesticide (rodenticide)	985.8	E863.7	—	E950.6	E962.1	E980.7
THC	969.6	E854.1	E939.6	E950.3	E962.0	E980.3
Thebacon	965.09	E850.2	E935.2	E950.0	E962.0	E980.0
Thebaine	965.09	E850.2	E935.2	E950.0	E962.0	E980.0
Theobromine (calcium salicylate)	974.1	E858.5	E944.1	E950.4	E962.0	E980.4
Theophylline (diuretic)	974.1	E858.5	E944.1	E950.4	E962.0	E980.4
ethylenediamine	975.7	E858.6	E945.7	E950.4	E962.0	E980.4
Thiabendazole	961.6	E857	E931.6	E950.4	E962.0	E980.4
Thialbarbital, thialbarbitone	968.3	E855.1	E938.3	E950.4	E962.0	E980.4
Thiamine	963.5	E858.1	E933.5	E950.4	E962.0	E980.4
Thiamylal (sodium)	968.3	E855.1	E938.3	E950.4	E962.0	E980.4
Thiazesim	969.0	E854.0	E939.0	E950.3	E962.0	E980.3
Thiazides (diuretics)	974.3	E858.5	E944.3	E950.4	E962.0	E980.4
Thiethylperazine	963.0	E858.1	E933.0	E950.4	E962.0	E980.4
Thimerosal (topical)	976.0	E858.7	E946.0	E950.4	E962.0	E980.4
ophthalmic preparation	976.5	E858.7	E946.5	E950.4	E962.0	E980.4
Thioacetazone	961.8	E857	E931.8	E950.4	E962.0	E980.4
Thiobarbiturates	968.3	E855.1	E938.3	E950.4	E962.0	E980.4
Thiobismol	961.2	E857	E931.2	E950.4	E962.0	E980.4
Thiocarbamide	962.8	E858.0	E932.8	E950.4	E962.0	E980.4
Thiocarbarsone	961.1	E857	E931.1	E950.4	E962.0	E980.4
Thiocarlide	961.8	E857	E931.8	E950.4	E962.0	E980.4
Thioguanine	963.1	E858.1	E933.1	E950.4	E962.0	E980.4
Thiomercaptomerin	974.0	E858.5	E944.0	E950.4	E962.0	E980.4
Thiomerin	974.0	E858.5	E944.0	E950.4	E962.0	E980.4
Thiopental, thiopentone (sodium)	968.3	E855.1	E938.3	E950.4	E962.0	E980.4
Thiopropazate	969.1	E853.0	E939.1	E950.3	E962.0	E980.3
Thioproperazine	969.1	E853.0	E939.1	E950.3	E962.0	E980.3
Thioridazine	969.1	E853.0	E939.1	E950.3	E962.0	E980.3
Thio–TEPA, thiotepa	963.1	E858.1	E933.1	E950.4	E962.0	E980.4
Thiothixene	969.3	E853.8	E939.3	E950.3	E962.0	E980.3
Thiouracil	962.8	E858.0	E932.8	E950.4	E962.0	E980.4
Thiourea	962.8	E858.0	E932.8	E950.4	E962.0	E980.4

Substance	Poisoning	Accident	Therapeutic Use	Suicide Attempt	Assault	Undetermined
		External Cause (E-Code)				
Thiphenamil	971.1	E855.4	E941.1	E950.4	E962.0	E980.4
Thiram NEC	989.4	E863.6	—	E950.6	E962.1	E980.7
medicinal	976.2	E858.7	E946.2	E950.4	E962.0	E980.4
Thonzylamine	963.0	E858.1	E933.0	E950.4	E962.0	E980.4
Thorazine	969.1	E853.0	E939.1	E950.3	E962.0	E980.3
Thornapple	988.2	E865.4	—	E950.9	E962.1	E980.9
Throat preparation (lozenges) NEC	976.6	E858.7	E946.6	E950.4	E962.0	E980.4
Thrombin	964.5	E858.2	E934.5	E950.4	E962.0	E980.4
Thrombolysin	964.4	E858.2	E934.4	E950.4	E962.0	E980.4
Thymol	983.0	E864.0	—	E950.7	E962.1	E980.6
Thymus extract	962.9	E858.0	E932.9	E950.4	E962.0	E980.4
Thyroglobulin	962.7	E858.0	E932.7	E950.4	E962.0	E980.4
Thyroid (derivatives) (extract)	962.7	E858.0	E932.7	E950.4	E962.0	E980.4
Thyrolar	962.7	E858.0	E932.7	E950.4	E962.0	E980.4
Thyrothrophin, thyrotropin	977.8	E858.8	E947.8	E950.4	E962.0	E980.4
Thyroxin(e)	962.7	E858.0	E932.7	E950.4	E962.0	E980.4
Tigan	963.0	E858.1	E933.0	E950.4	E962.0	E980.4
Tigloidine	968.0	E855.1	E938.0	E950.4	E962.0	E980.4
Tin (chloride) (dust) (oxide) NEC	985.8	E866.4	—	E950.9	E962.1	E980.9
anti–infectives	961.2	E857	E931.2	E950.4	E962.0	E980.4
Tinactin	976.0	E858.7	E946.0	E950.4	E962.0	E980.4
Tincture, iodine — *see* Iodine						
Tindal	969.1	E853.0	E939.1	E950.3	E962.0	E980.3
Titanium (compounds) (vapor)	985.8	E866.4	—	E950.9	E962.1	E980.9
ointment	976.3	E858.7	E946.3	E950.4	E962.0	E980.4
Titroid	962.7	E858.0	E932.7	E950.4	E962.0	E980.4
TMTD — *see* Tetramethylthiuram disulfide						
TNT	989.89	E866.8	—	E950.9	E962.1	E980.9
fumes	987.8	E869.8	—	E952.8	E962.2	E982.8
Toadstool	988.1	E865.5	—	E950.9	E962.1	E980.9
Tobacco NEC	989.84	E866.8	—	E950.9	E962.1	E980.9
Indian	988.2	E865.4	—	E950.9	E962.1	E980.9
smoke, second-hand	987.8	E869.4	—	—	—	—
Tocopherol	963.5	E858.1	E933.5	E950.4	E962.0	E980.4
Tocosamine	975.0	E858.6	E945.0	E950.4	E962.0	E980.4
Tofranil	969.0	E854.0	E939.0	E950.3	E962.0	E980.3
Toilet deodorizer	989.8	E866.8	—	E950.9	E962.1	E980.9
Tolazamide	962.3	E858.0	E932.3	E950.4	E962.0	E980.4
Tolazoline	971.3	E855.6	E941.3	E950.4	E962.0	E980.4
Tolbutamide	962.3	E858.0	E932.3	E950.4	E962.0	E980.4
sodium	977.8	E858.8	E947.8	E950.4	E962.0	E980.4
Tolmetin	965.69	E850.6	E935.6	E950.0	E962.0	E980.0
Tolnaftate	976.0	E858.7	E946.0	E950.4	E962.0	E980.4
Tolpropamine	976.1	E858.7	E946.1	E950.4	E962.0	E980.4
Tolserol	968.0	E855.1	E938.0	E950.4	E962.0	E980.4
Toluene (liquid) (vapor)	982.0	E862.4	—	E950.9	E962.1	E980.9
diisocyanate	983.0	E864.0	—	E950.7	E962.1	E980.6
Toluidine	983.0	E864.0	—	E950.7	E962.1	E980.6
vapor	987.8	E869.8	—	E952.8	E962.2	E982.8
Toluol (liquid) (vapor)	982.0	E862.4	—	E950.9	E962.1	E980.9
Tolylene–2,4–diisocyanate	983.0	E864.0	—	E950.7	E962.1	E980.6
Tonics, cardiac	972.1	E858.3	E942.1	E950.4	E962.0	E980.4
Toxaphene (dust) (spray)	989.2	E863.0	—	E950.6	E962.1	E980.7
Toxoids NEC	978.8	E858.8	E948.8	E950.4	E962.0	E980.4
Tractor fuel NEC	981	E862.1	—	E950.9	E962.1	E980.9
Tragacanth	973.3	E858.4	E943.3	E950.4	E962.0	E980.4
Tramazoline	971.2	E855.5	E941.2	E950.4	E962.0	E980.4
Tranquilizers	969.5	E853.9	E939.5	E950.3	E962.0	E980.3
benzodiazepine–based	969.4	E853.2	E939.4	E950.3	E962.0	E980.3
butyrophenone–based	969.2	E853.1	E939.2	E950.3	E962.0	E980.3
major NEC	969.3	E853.8	E939.3	E950.3	E962.0	E980.3

Substance	Poisoning	Accident	Therapeutic Use	Suicide Attempt	Assault	Undetermined
			External Cause (E-Code)			
phenothiazine–based	969.1	E853.0	E939.1	E950.3	E962.0	E980.3
specified NEC	969.5	E853.8	E939.5	E950.3	E962.0	E980.3
Trantoin	961.9	E857	E931.9	E950.4	E962.0	E980.4
Tranxene	969.4	E853.2	E939.4	E950.3	E962.0	E980.3
Tranylcypromine (sulfate)	969.0	E854.0	E939.0	E950.3	E962.0	E980.3
Trasentine	975.1	E858.6	E945.1	E950.4	E962.0	E980.4
Travert	974.5	E858.5	E944.5	E950.4	E962.0	E980.4
Trecator	961.8	E857	E931.8	E950.4	E962.0	E980.4
Tretinoin	976.8	E858.7	E946.8	E950.4	E962.0	E980.4
Triacetin	976.0	E858.7	E946.0	E950.4	E962.0	E980.4
Triacetyloleandomycin	960.3	E856	E930.3	E950.4	E962.0	E980.4
Triamcinolone	962.0	E858.0	E932.0	E950.4	E962.0	E980.4
ENT agent	976.6	E858.7	E946.6	E950.4	E962.0	E980.4
ophthalmic preparation	976.5	E858.7	E946.5	E950.4	E962.0	E980.4
topical NEC	976.0	E858.7	E946.0	E950.4	E962.0	E980.4
Triamterene	974.4	E858.5	E944.4	E950.4	E962.0	E980.4
Triaziquone	963.1	E858.1	E933.1	E950.4	E962.0	E980.4
Tribromacetaldehyde	967.3	E852.2	E937.3	E950.2	E962.0	E980.2
Tribromoethanol	968.2	E855.1	E938.2	E950.4	E962.0	E980.4
Tribromomethane	967.3	E852.2	E937.3	E950.2	E962.0	E980.2
Trichlorethane	982.3	E862.4	—	E950.9	E962.1	E980.9
Trichlormethiazide	974.3	E858.5	E944.3	E950.4	E962.0	E980.4
Trichloroacetic acid	983.1	E864.1	—	E950.7	E962.1	E980.6
medicinal (keratolytic)	976.4	E858.7	E946.4	E950.4	E962.0	E980.4
Trichloroethanol	967.1	E852.0	E937.1	E950.2	E962.0	E980.2
Trichloroethylene (liquid) (vapor)	982.3	E862.4	—	E950.9	E962.1	E980.9
anesthetic (gas)	968.2	E855.1	E938.2	E950.4	E962.0	E980.4
Trichloroethyl phosphate	967.1	E852.0	E937.1	E950.2	E962.0	E980.2
Trichlorofluoromethane NEC	987.4	E869.2	—	E952.8	E962.2	E982.8
Trichlorotriethylamine	963.1	E858.1	E933.1	E950.4	E962.0	E980.4
Trichomonacides NEC	961.5	E857	E931.5	E950.4	E962.0	E980.4
Trichomycin	960.1	E856	E930.1	E950.4	E962.0	E980.4
Triclofos	967.1	E852.0	E937.1	E950.2	E962.0	E980.2
Tricresyl phosphate	989.89	E866.8	—	E950.9	E962.1	E980.9
solvent	982.8	E862.4	—	E950.9	E962.1	E980.9
Tricyclamol	966.4	E855.0	E936.4	E950.4	E962.0	E980.4
Tridesilon	976.0	E858.7	E946.0	E950.4	E962.0	E980.4
Tridihexethyl	971.1	E855.4	E941.1	E950.4	E962.0	E980.4
Tridione	966.0	E855.0	E936.0	E950.4	E962.0	E980.4
Triethanolamine NEC	983.2	E864.2	—	E950.7	E962.1	E980.6
detergent	983.2	E861.0	—	E950.7	E962.1	E980.6
trinitrate	972.4	E858.3	E942.4	E950.4	E962.0	E980.4
Triethanomelamine	963.1	E858.1	E933.1	E950.4	E962.0	E980.4
Triethylene melamine	963.1	E858.1	E933.1	E950.4	E962.0	E980.4
Triethylenephosphoramide	963.1	E858.1	E933.1	E950.4	E962.0	E980.4
Triethylenethiophosphoramide	963.1	E858.1	E933.1	E950.4	E962.0	E980.4
Trifluoperazine	969.1	E853.0	E939.1	E950.3	E962.0	E980.3
Trifluperidol	969.2	E853.1	E939.2	E950.3	E962.0	E980.3
Triflupromazine	969.1	E853.0	E939.1	E950.3	E962.0	E980.3
Trihexyphenidyl	971.1	E855.4	E941.1	E950.4	E962.0	E980.4
Triiodothyronine	962.7	E858.0	E932.7	E950.4	E962.0	E980.4
Trilene	968.2	E855.1	E938.2	E950.4	E962.0	E980.4
Trimeprazine	963.0	E858.1	E933.0	E950.4	E962.0	E980.4
Trimetazidine	972.4	E858.3	E942.4	E950.4	E962.0	E980.4
Trimethadione	966.0	E855.0	E936.0	E950.4	E962.0	E980.4
Trimethaphan	972.3	E858.3	E942.3	E950.4	E962.0	E980.4
Trimethidinium	972.3	E858.3	E942.3	E950.4	E962.0	E980.4
Trimethobenzamide	963.0	E858.1	E933.0	E950.4	E962.0	E980.4
Trimethylcarbinol	980.8	E860.8	—	E950.9	E962.1	E980.9
Trimethylpsoralen	976.3	E858.7	E946.3	E950.4	E962.0	E980.4

Substance	Poisoning	Accident	Therapeutic Use	Suicide Attempt	Assault	Undetermined
			External Cause (E-Code)			
Trimeton	963.0	E858.1	E933.0	E950.4	E962.0	E980.4
Trimipramine	969.0	E854.0	E939.0	E950.3	E962.0	E980.3
Trimustine	963.1	E858.1	E933.1	E950.4	E962.0	E980.4
Trinitrin	972.4	E858.3	E942.4	E950.4	E962.0	E980.4
Trinitrophenol	983.0	E864.0	—	E950.7	E962.1	E980.6
Trinitrotoluene	989.89	E866.8	—	E950.9	E962.1	E980.9
fumes	987.8	E869.8	—	E952.8	E962.2	E982.8
Trional	967.8	E852.8	E937.8	E950.2	E962.0	E980.2
Trioxide of arsenic — *see* Arsenic						
Trioxsalen	976.3	E858.7	E946.3	E950.4	E962.0	E980.4
Tripelennamine	963.0	E858.1	E933.0	E950.4	E962.0	E980.4
Triperidol	969.2	E853.1	E939.2	E950.3	E962.0	E980.3
Triprolidine	963.0	E858.1	E933.0	E950.4	E962.0	E980.4
Trisoralen	976.3	E858.7	E946.3	E950.4	E962.0	E980.4
Troleandomycin	960.3	E856	E930.3	E950.4	E962.0	E980.4
Trolnitrate (phosphate)	972.4	E858.3	E942.4	E950.4	E962.0	E980.4
Trometamol	963.3	E858.1	E933.3	E950.4	E962.0	E980.4
Tromethamine	963.3	E858.1	E933.3	E950.4	E962.0	E980.4
Tronothane	968.5	E855.2	E938.5	E950.4	E962.0	E980.4
Tropicamide	971.1	E855.4	E941.1	E950.4	E962.0	E980.4
Troxidone	966.0	E855.0	E936.0	E950.4	E962.0	E980.4
Tryparsamide	961.1	E857	E931.1	E950.4	E962.0	E980.4
Trypsin	963.4	E858.1	E933.4	E950.4	E962.0	E980.4
Tryptizol	969.0	E854.0	E939.0	E950.3	E962.0	E980.3
Tuaminoheptane	971.2	E855.5	E941.2	E950.4	E962.0	E980.4
Tuberculin (old)	977.8	E858.8	E947.8	E950.4	E962.0	E980.4
Tubocurare	975.2	E858.6	E945.2	E950.4	E962.0	E980.4
Tubocurarine	975.2	E858.6	E945.2	E950.4	E962.0	E980.4
Turkish green	969.6	E854.1	E939.6	E950.3	E962.0	E980.3
Turpentine (spirits of) (liquid) (vapor)	982.8	E862.4	—	E950.9	E962.1	E980.9
Tybamate	969.5	E853.8	E939.5	E950.3	E962.0	E980.3
Tyloxapol	975.5	E858.6	E945.5	E950.4	E962.0	E980.4
Tymazoline	971.2	E855.5	E941.2	E950.4	E962.0	E980.4
Typhoid vaccine	978.1	E858.8	E948.1	E950.4	E962.0	E980.4
Typhus vaccine	979.2	E858.8	E949.2	E950.4	E962.0	E980.4
Tyrothricin	976.0	E858.7	E946.0	E950.4	E962.0	E980.4
ENT agent	976.6	E858.7	E946.6	E950.4	E962.0	E980.4
ophthalmic preparation	976.5	E858.7	E946.5	E950.4	E962.0	E980.4
Undecenoic acid	976.0	E858.7	E946.0	E950.4	E962.0	E980.4
Undecylenic acid	976.0	E858.7	E946.0	E950.4	E962.0	E980.4
Unna's boot	976.3	E858.7	E946.3	E950.4	E962.0	E980.4
Uracil mustard	963.1	E858.1	E933.1	E950.4	E962.0	E980.4
Uramustine	963.1	E858.1	E933.1	E950.4	E962.0	E980.4
Urari	975.2	E858.6	E945.2	E950.4	E962.0	E980.4
Urea	974.4	E858.5	E944.4	E950.4	E962.0	E980.4
topical	976.8	E858.7	E946.8	E950.4	E962.0	E980.4
Urethan(e) (antineoplastic)	963.1	E858.1	E933.1	E950.4	E962.0	E980.4
Urginea (maritima) (scilla) — *see* Squill						
Uric acid metabolism agents NEC	974.7	E858.5	E944.7	E950.4	E962.0	E980.4
Urokinase	964.4	E858.2	E934.4	E950.4	E962.0	E980.4
Urokon	977.8	E858.8	E947.8	E950.4	E962.0	E980.4
Urotropin	961.9	E857	E931.9	E950.4	E962.0	E980.4
Urtica	988.2	E865.4	—	E950.9	E962.1	E980.9
Utility gas — *see* Gas, utility						
Vaccine NEC	979.9	E858.8	E949.9	E950.4	E962.0	E980.4
bacterial NEC	978.8	E858.8	E948.8	E950.4	E962.0	E980.4
with						
other bacterial component	978.9	E858.8	E948.9	E950.4	E962.0	E980.4
pertussis component	978.6	E858.8	E948.6	E950.4	E962.0	E980.4
viral–rickettsial component	979.7	E858.8	E949.7	E950.4	E962.0	E980.4
mixed NEC	978.9	E858.8	E948.9	E950.4	E962.0	E980.4

Substance	Poisoning	Accident	Therapeutic Use	Suicide Attempt	Assault	Undetermined
			External Cause (E-Code)			
BCG	978.0	E858.8	E948.0	E950.4	E962.0	E980.4
cholera	978.2	E858.8	E948.2	E950.4	E962.0	E980.4
diphtheria	978.5	E858.8	E948.5	E950.4	E962.0	E980.4
influenza	979.6	E858.8	E949.6	E950.4	E962.0	E980.4
measles	979.4	E858.8	E949.4	E950.4	E962.0	E980.4
meningococcal	978.8	E858.8	E948.8	E950.4	E962.0	E980.4
mumps	979.6	E858.8	E949.6	E950.4	E962.0	E980.4
paratyphoid	978.1	E858.8	E948.1	E950.4	E962.0	E980.4
pertussis (with diphtheria toxoid) (with tetanus toxoid)	978.6	E858.8	E948.6	E950.4	E962.0	E980.4
plague	978.3	E858.8	E948.3	E950.4	E962.0	E980.4
poliomyelitis	979.5	E858.8	E949.5	E950.4	E962.0	E980.4
poliovirus	979.5	E858.8	E949.5	E950.4	E962.0	E980.4
rabies	979.1	E858.8	E949.1	E950.4	E962.0	E980.4
respiratory syncytial virus	979.6	E858.8	E949.6	E950.4	E962.0	E980.4
rickettsial NEC	979.6	E858.8	E949.6	E950.4	E962.0	E980.4
with						
bacterial component	979.7	E858.8	E949.7	E950.4	E962.0	E980.4
pertussis component	978.6	E858.8	E948.6	E950.4	E962.0	E980.4
viral component	979.7	E858.8	E949.7	E950.4	E962.0	E980.4
Rocky Mountain spotted fever	979.6	E858.8	E949.6	E950.4	E962.0	E980.4
rotavirus	979.6	E858.8	E949.6	E950.4	E962.0	E980.4
rubella virus	979.4	E858.8	E949.4	E950.4	E962.0	E980.4
sabin oral	979.5	E858.8	E949.5	E950.4	E962.0	E980.4
smallpox	979.0	E858.8	E949.0	E950.4	E962.0	E980.4
tetanus	978.4	E858.8	E948.4	E950.4	E962.0	E980.4
typhoid	978.1	E858.8	E948.1	E950.4	E962.0	E980.4
typhus	979.2	E858.8	E949.2	E950.4	E962.0	E980.4
viral NEC	979.6	E858.8	E949.6	E950.4	E962.0	E980.4
with						
bacterial component	979.7	E858.8	E949.7	E950.4	E962.0	E980.4
pertussis component	978.6	E858.8	E948.6	E950.4	E962.0	E980.4
rickettsial component	979.7	E858.8	E949.7	E950.4	E962.0	E980.4
yellow fever	979.3	E858.8	E949.3	E950.4	E962.0	E980.4
Vaccinia immune globulin (human)	964.6	E858.2	E934.6	E950.4	E962.0	E980.4
Vaginal contraceptives	976.8	E858.7	E946.8	E950.4	E962.0	E980.4
Valethamate	971.1	E855.4	E941.1	E950.4	E962.0	E980.4
Valisone	976.0	E858.7	E946.0	E950.4	E962.0	E980.4
Valium	969.4	E853.2	E939.4	E950.3	E962.0	E980.3
Valmid	967.8	E852.8	E937.8	E950.2	E962.0	E980.2
Vanadium	985.8	E866.4	—	E950.9	E962.1	E980.9
Vancomycin	960.8	E856	E930.8	E950.4	E962.0	E980.4
Vapor (*see also* Gas)	987.9	E869.9	—	E952.9	E962.2	E982.9
kiln (carbon monoxide)	986	E868.8	—	E952.1	E962.2	E982.1
lead — *see* Lead						
specified source NEC (*see also* specific substance)	987.8	E869.8	—	E952.8	E962.2	E982.8
Varidase	964.4	E858.2	E934.4	E950.4	E962.0	E980.4
Varnish	989.89	E861.6	—	E950.9	E962.1	E980.9
cleaner	982.8	E862.9	—	E950.9	E962.1	E980.9
Vaseline	976.3	E858.7	E946.3	E950.4	E962.0	E980.4
Vasodilan	972.5	E858.3	E942.5	E950.4	E962.0	E980.4
Vasodilators NEC	972.5	E858.3	E942.5	E950.4	E962.0	E980.0
coronary	972.4	E858.3	E942.4	E950.4	E962.0	E980.4
Vasopressin	962.5	E858.0	E932.5	E950.4	E962.0	E980.4
Vasopressor drugs	962.5	E858.0	E932.5	E950.4	E962.0	E980.4
Venom, venomous (bite) (sting)	989.5	E905.9	—	E950.9	E962.1	E980.9
arthropod NEC	989.5	E905.5	—	E950.9	E962.1	E980.9
bee	989.5	E905.3	—	E950.9	E962.1	E980.9
centipede	989.5	E905.4	—	E950.9	E962.1	E980.9

Substance	Poisoning	Accident	Therapeutic Use	Suicide Attempt	Assault	Undetermined
		External Cause (E-Code)				
hornet	989.5	E905.3	—	E950.9	E962.1	E980.9
lizard	989.5	E905.0	—	E950.9	E962.1	E980.9
marine animals or plants	989.5	E905.6	—	E950.9	E962.1	E980.9
millipede (topical)	989.5	E905.4	—	E950.9	E962.1	E980.9
plant NEC	989.5	E905.7	—	E950.9	E962.1	E980.9
marine	989.5	E905.6	—	E950.9	E962.1	E980.9
scorpion	989.5	E905.2	—	E950.9	E962.1	E980.9
snake	989.5	E905.0	—	E950.9	E962.1	E980.9
specified NEC	989.5	E905.8	—	E950.9	E962.1	E980.9
spider	989.5	E905.1	—	E950.9	E962.1	E980.9
wasp	989.5	E905.3	—	E950.9	E962.1	E980.9
Ventolin—*see* Salbutamol sulfate						
Veramon	967.0	E851	E937.0	E950.1	E962.0	E980.1
Veratrum						
album	988.2	E865.4	—	E950.9	E962.1	E980.9
alkaloids	972.6	E858.3	E942.6	E950.4	E962.0	E980.4
viride	988.2	E865.4	—	E950.9	E962.1	E980.9
Verdigris (*see also* Copper)	985.8	E866.4	—	E950.9	E962.1	E980.9
Veronal	967.0	E851	E937.0	E950.1	E962.0	E980.1
Veroxil	961.6	E857	E931.6	E950.4	E962.0	E980.4
Versidyne	965.7	E850.7	E935.7	E950.0	E962.0	E980.0
Viagra	972.5	E858.3	E942.5	E950.4	E962.0	E980.4
Vienna						
green	985.1	E866.3	—	E950.8	E962.1	E980.8
insecticide	985.1	E863.4	—	E950.6	E962.1	E980.7
red	989.89	E866.8	—	E950.9	E962.1	E980.9
pharmaceutical dye	977.4	E858.8	E947.4	E950.4	E962.0	E980.4
Vinbarbital, vinbarbitone	967.0	E851	E937.0	E950.1	E962.0	E980.1
Vinblastine	963.1	E858.1	E933.1	E950.4	E962.0	E980.4
Vincristine	963.1	E858.1	E933.1	E950.4	E962.0	E980.4
Vinesthene, vinethene	968.2	E855.1	E938.2	E950.4	E962.0	E980.4
Vinyl						
bital	967.0	E851	E937.0	E950.1	E962.0	E980.1
ether	968.2	E855.1	E938.2	E950.4	E962.0	E980.4
Vioform	961.3	E857	E931.3	E950.4	E962.0	E980.4
topical	976.0	E858.7	E946.0	E950.4	E962.0	E980.4
Viomycin	960.6	E856	E930.6	E950.4	E962.0	E980.4
Viosterol	963.5	E858.1	E933.5	E950.4	E962.0	E980.4
Viper (venom)	989.5	E905.0	—	E950.9	E962.1	E980.9
Viprynium (embonate)	961.6	E857	E931.6	E950.4	E962.0	E980.4
Virugon	961.7	E857	E931.7	E950.4	E962.0	E980.4
Visine	976.5	E858.7	E946.5	E950.4	E962.0	E980.4
Vitamins NEC	963.5	E858.1	E933.5	E950.4	E962.0	E980.4
B_{12}	964.1	E858.2	E934.1	E950.4	E962.0	E980.4
hematopoietic	964.1	E858.2	E934.1	E950.4	E962.0	E980.4
K	964.3	E858.2	E934.3	E950.4	E962.0	E980.4
Vleminckx's solution	976.4	E858.7	E946.4	E950.4	E962.0	E980.4
Voltaren—*see* Diclofenac sodium						
Warfarin (potassium) (sodium)	964.2	E858.2	E934.2	E950.4	E962.0	E980.4
rodenticide	989.4	E863.7	—	E950.6	E962.1	E980.7
Wasp (sting)	989.5	E905.3	—	E950.9	E962.1	E980.9
Water						
balance agents NEC	974.5	E858.5	E944.5	E950.4	E962.0	E980.4
gas	987.1	E868.1	—	E951.8	E962.2	E981.8
incomplete combustion of — *see* Carbon, monoxide, fuel, utility						
hemlock	988.2	E865.4	—	E950.9	E962.1	E980.9
moccasin (venom)	989.5	E905.0	—	E950.9	E962.1	E980.9
Wax (paraffin) (petroleum)	981	E862.3	—	E950.9	E962.1	E980.9
automobile	989.89	E861.2	—	E950.9	E962.1	E980.9
floor	981	E862.0	—	E950.9	E962.1	E980.9

Substance	Poisoning	Accident	Therapeutic Use	Suicide Attempt	Assault	Undetermined
		External Cause (E-Code)				
Weed killers NEC	989.4	E863.5	—	E950.6	E962.1	E980.7
Welldorm	967.1	E852.0	E937.1	E950.2	E962.0	E980.2
White						
arsenic — *see* Arsenic						
hellebore	988.2	E865.4	—	E950.9	E962.1	E980.9
lotion (keratolytic)	976.4	E858.7	E946.4	E950.4	E962.0	E980.4
spirit	981	E862.0	—	E950.9	E962.1	E980.9
Whitewashes	989.89	E861.6	—	E950.9	E962.1	E980.9
Whole blood	964.7	E858.2	E934.7	E950.4	E962.0	E980.4
Wild						
black cherry	988.2	E865.4	—	E950.9	E962.1	E980.9
poisonous plants NEC	988.2	E865.4	—	E950.9	E962.1	E980.9
Window cleaning fluid	989.89	E861.3	—	E950.9	E962.1	E980.9
Wintergreen (oil)	976.3	E858.7	E946.3	E950.4	E962.0	E980.4
Witch hazel	976.2	E858.7	E946.2	E950.4	E962.0	E980.4
Wood						
alcohol	980.1	E860.2	—	E950.9	E962.1	E980.9
spirit	980.1	E860.2	—	E950.9	E962.1	E980.9
Woorali	975.2	E858.6	E945.2	E950.4	E962.0	E980.4
Wormseed, American	961.6	E857	E931.6	E950.4	E962.0	E980.4
Xanthine diuretics	974.1	E858.5	E944.1	E950.4	E962.0	E980.4
Xanthocillin	960.0	E856	E930.0	E950.4	E962.0	E980.4
Xanthotoxin	976.3	E858.7	E946.3	E950.4	E962.0	E980.4
Xigris	964.2	E858.2	E934.2	E950.4	E962.0	E980.4
Xylene (liquid) (vapor)	982.0	E862.4	—	E950.9	E962.1	E980.9
Xylocaine (infiltration) (topical)	968.5	E855.2	E938.5	E950.4	E962.0	E980.4
nerve block (peripheral) (plexus)	968.6	E855.2	E938.6	E950.4	E962.0	E980.4
spinal	968.7	E855.2	E938.7	E950.4	E962.0	E980.4
Xylol (liquid) (vapor)	982.0	E862.4	—	E950.9	E962.1	E980.9
Xylometazoline	971.2	E855.5	E941.2	E950.4	E962.0	E980.4
Yellow						
fever vaccine	979.3	E858.8	E949.3	E950.4	E962.0	E980.4
jasmine	988.2	E865.4	—	E950.9	E962.1	E980.9
Yew	988.2	E865.4	—	E950.9	E962.1	E980.9
Zactane	965.7	E850.7	E935.7	E950.0	E962.0	E980.0
Zaroxolyn	974.3	E858.5	E944.3	E950.4	E962.0	E980.4
Zephiran (topical)	976.0	E858.7	E946.0	E950.4	E962.0	E980.4
ophthalmic preparation	976.5	E858.7	E946.5	E950.4	E962.0	E980.4
Zerone	980.1	E860.2	—	E950.9	E962.1	E980.9
Zinc (compounds) (fumes) (salts)						
(vapor) NEC	985.8	E866.4	—	E950.9	E962.1	E980.9
anti–infectives	976.0	E858.7	E946.0	E950.4	E962.0	E980.4
antivaricose	972.7	E858.3	E942.7	E950.4	E962.0	E980.4
bacitracin	976.0	E858.7	E946.0	E950.4	E962.0	E980.4
chloride	976.2	E858.7	E946.2	E950.4	E962.0	E980.4
gelatin	976.3	E858.7	E946.3	E950.4	E962.0	E980.4
oxide	976.3	E858.7	E946.3	E950.4	E962.0	E980.4
peroxide	976.0	E858.7	E946.0	E950.4	E962.0	E980.4
pesticides	985.8	E863.4	—	E950.6	E962.1	E980.7
phosphide (rodenticide)	985.8	E863.7	—	E950.6	E962.1	E980.7
stearate	976.3	E858.7	E946.3	E950.4	E962.0	E980.4
sulfate (antivaricose)	972.7	E858.3	E942.7	E950.4	E962.0	E980.4
ENT agent	976.6	E858.7	E946.6	E950.4	E962.0	E980.4
ophthalmic solution	976.5	E858.7	E946.5	E950.4	E962.0	E980.4
topical NEC	976.0	E858.7	E946.0	E950.4	E962.0	E980.4
undecylenate	976.0	E858.7	E946.0	E950.4	E962.0	E980.4
Zovant	964.2	E858.2	E934.2	E950.4	E962.0	E980.4
Zoxazolamine	968.0	E855.1	E938.0	E950.4	E962.0	E980.4
Zygadenus (venenosus)	988.2	E865.4	—	E950.9	E962.1	E980.9

SECTION 3

ALPHABETIC INDEX TO EXTERNAL CAUSES
OF INJURY AND POISONING (E CODE)

This section contains the index to the codes which classify environmental events, circumstances, and other conditions as the cause of injury and other adverse effects. Where a code from the section Supplementary Classification of External Causes of Injury and Poisoning (E800-E998) is applicable, it is intended that the E code shall be used in addition to a code from the main body of the classification, Chapters 1-17.

The alphabetic index to the E codes is organized by main terms which describe the *accident, circumstance, event,* or specific *agent* which caused the injury or other adverse effect.

> *Note—Transport accidents (E800-E848) include accidents involving:*
> *aircraft and space craft (E840-E845)*
> *watercraft (E830-E838)*
> *motor vehicle (E810-E825)*
> *railway (E800-E807)*
> *other road vehicles (E826-E829)*
>
> *For definitions and examples related to transport accidents—see Volume 1, pages 571-585.*
>
> *The fourth-digit subdivisions for use with categories E800-E848 to identify the injured person are found on pages 1447-1451.*
>
> *For identifying the place in which an accident or poisoning occurred (circumstances classifiable to categories E850-E869 and E880-E928)— see the listing in this section under "Accident, occurring."*

See the Table of Drugs and Chemicals (Section 2 of this volume) for identifying the specific agent involved in drug overdose or a wrong substance given or taken in error, and for intoxication or poisoning by a drug or other chemical substance.

The specific adverse effect, reaction, or localized toxic effect to a correct drug or substance properly administered in therapeutic or prophylactic dosage should be classified according to the nature of the adverse effect (e.g.: allergy, dermatitis, tachycardia) listed in Section 1 of this volume.

A

Abandonment
  causing exposure to weather conditions—*see*
    Exposure
  child, with intent to injure or kill E968.4
  helpless person, infant, newborn E904.0
    with intent to injure or kill E968.4
Abortion, criminal, injury to child E968.8
Abuse, (alleged) (suspected)
  adult
    by
      child E967.4
      ex-partner E967.3
      ex-spouse E967.3
      father E967.0
      grandchild E967.7
      grandparent E967.6
      mother E967.2
      non-related caregiver E967.8
      other relative E967.7
      other specified person(s) E967.1
      partner E967.3
      sibling E967.5
      spouse E967.3
      stepfather E967.0
      stepmother E967.2
      unspecified person E967.9
  child
    by
      boyfriend of parent or guardian E967.0
      child E967.4
      father E967.0
      female partner of parent or guardian
        E967.2
      girlfriend of parent or guardian E967.2
      grandchild E967.7
      grandparent E967.6
      male partner of parent or guardian E967.0
      mother E967.2
      non-related caregiver E967.8
      other relative E967.7
      other specified person(s) E967.1
      sibling E967.5
      stepfather E967.0
      stepmother E967.2
      unspecified person E967.9
Accident (to) E928.9
  aircraft (in transit) (powered) E841
    at landing, take-off E840
    due to, caused by cataclysm—*see* categories
      E908, E909
    late effect of E929.1
    unpowered (*see also* Collision, aircraft,
      unpowered) E842
    while alighting, boarding E843
  amphibious vehicle
    on
      land—*see* Accident, motor vehicle
      water—*see* Accident, watercraft
  animal, ridden NEC E828
  animal-drawn vehicle NEC E827
  balloon (*see also* Collision, aircraft,
    unpowered) E842
  caused by, due to
    abrasive wheel (metalworking) E919.3
    animal NEC E906.9
      being ridden (in sport or transport) E828
    avalanche NEC E909.2
    band saw E919.4
    bench saw E919.4

Accident—*continued*
  bore, earth-drilling or mining (land) (seabed)
    E919.1
  bulldozer E919.7
  cataclysmic
    earth surface movement or eruption E909.9
    storm E908.9
  chain
    hoist E919.2
      agricultural operations E919.0
      mining operations E919.1
    saw E920.1
  circular saw E919.4
  cold (excessive) (*see also* Cold, exposure to)
    E901.9
  combine E919.0
  conflagration—*see* Conflagration
  corrosive liquid, substance NEC E924.1
  cotton gin E919.8
  crane E919.2
    agricultural operations E919.0
    mining operations E919.1
  cutting or piercing instrument (*see also* Cut)
    E920.9
  dairy equipment E919.8
  derrick E919.2
    agricultural operations E919.0
    mining operations E919.1
  drill E920.1
    earth (land) (seabed) E919.1
    hand (powered) E920.1
      not powered E920.4
    metalworking E919.3
    woodworking E919.4
  earth(-)
    drilling machine E919.1
    moving machine E919.7
    scraping machine E919.7
  electric
    current (*see also* Electric shock) E925.9
    motor—*see also* Accident, machine, by
      type of machine
      current (of)—*see* Electric shock
  elevator (building) (grain) E919.2
    agricultural operations E919.0
    mining operations E919.1
  environmental factors NEC E928.9
  excavating machine E919.7
  explosive material (*see also* Explosion)
    E923.9
  farm machine E919.0
  fire, flames—*see also* Fire
    conflagration—*see* Conflagration
  firearm missile—*see* Shooting
  forging (metalworking) machine E919.3
  forklift (truck) E919.2
    agricultural operations E919.0
    mining operations E919.1
  gas turbine E919.5
  harvester E919.0
  hay derrick, mower, or rake E919.0
  heat (excessive) (*see also* Heat) E900.9
  hoist (*see also* Accident, caused by, due to,
    lift) E919.2
    chain—*see* Accident, caused by, due to,
      chain
    shaft E919.1

Accident—*continued*
  hot
    liquid E924.0
      caustic or corrosive E924.1
    object (not producing fire or flames)
      E924.8
    substance E924.9
      caustic or corrosive E924.1
      liquid (metal) NEC E924.0
      specified type NEC E924.8
  human bite E928.3
  ignition—*see* Ignition
  internal combustion engine E919.5
  landslide NEC E909.2
  lathe (metalworking) E919.3
    turnings E920.8
    woodworking E919.4
  lift, lifting (appliances) E919.2
    agricultural operations E919.0
    mining operations E919.1
    shaft E919.1
  lightning NEC E907
  machine, machinery—*see also* Accident,
    machine
    drilling, metal E919.3
    manufacturing, for manufacture of
      beverages E919.8
      clothing E919.8
      foodstuffs E919.8
      paper E919.8
      textiles E919.8
    milling, metal E919.3
    moulding E919.4
    power press, metal E919.3
    printing E919.8
    rolling mill, metal E919.3
    sawing, metal E919.3
    specified type NEC E919.8
    spinning E919.8
    weaving E919.8
  natural factor NEC E928.9
  overhead plane E919.4
  plane E920.4
    overhead E919.4
  powered
    hand tool NEC E920.1
    saw E919.4
      hand E920.1
  printing machine E919.8
  pulley (block) E919.2
    agricultural operations E919.0
    mining operations E919.1
    transmission E919.6
  radial saw E919.4
  radiation—*see* Radiation
  reaper E919.0
  road scraper E919.7
    when in transport under its own
      power—*see* categories E810—E825
  roller coaster E919.8
  sander E919.4
  saw E920.4
    band E919.4
    bench E919.4
    chain E920.1
    circular E919.4
    hand E920.4
      powered E920.1
    powered, except hand E919.4
    radial E919.4
  sawing machine, metal E919.3

Accident—*continued*
  shaft
    hoist E919.1
    lift E919.1
    transmission E919.6
  shears E920.4
    hand E920.4
      powered E920.1
    mechanical E919.3
  shovel E920.4
    steam E919.7
  spinning machine E919.8
  steam—*see also* Burning, steam
    engine E919.5
    shovel E919.7
  thresher E919.0
  thunderbolt NEC E907
  tractor E919.0
    when in transport under its own
      power—*see* categories E810-E825
  transmission belt, cable, chain, gear, pinion,
    pulley, shaft E919.6
  turbine (gas) (water driven) E919.5
  under-cutter E919.1
  weaving machine E919.8
  winch E919.2
    agricultural operations E919.0
    mining operations E919.1
  diving E883.0
    with insufficient air supply E913.2
  glider (hang) (*see also* Collision, aircraft,
    unpowered) E842
  hovercraft
    on
      land—*see* Accident, motor vehicle
      water—*see* Accident, watercraft
  ice yacht (*see also* Accident, vehicle NEC)
    E848
  in
    medical, surgical procedure
      as, or due to misadventure—*see*
        Misadventure
      causing an abnormal reaction or later
        complication without mention of
        misadventure—*see* Reaction, abnormal
  kite carrying a person (*see also* Collision,
    aircraft, unpowered) E842
  land yacht (*see also* Accident, vehicle NEC)
    E848
  late effect of—*see* Late effect
  launching pad E845
  machine, machinery (*see also* Accident,
    caused by, due to, by specific type of
    machine) E919.9
    agricultural including animal-powered
      E919.0
    earth-drilling E919.1
    earth moving or scraping E919.7
    excavating E919.7
    involving transport under own power on
      highway or transport vehicle—*see*
      categories E810-E825, E840-E845
    lifting (appliances) E919.2
    metalworking E919.3
    mining E919.1
    prime movers, except electric motors E919.5
      electric motors—*see* Accident, machine, by
        specific type of machine
    recreational E919.8
    specified type NEC E919.8

Blast (air)
  from nuclear explosion E996
  in
    terrorism E979.2
      from nuclear explosion E979.5
      underwater E979.0
    war operations E993
      from nuclear explosion E996
      underwater E992
  underwater E992
Blizzard E908.3
Blow E928.9
  by law-enforcing agent, police (on duty) E975
    with blunt object (baton) (nightstick) (stave)
      (truncheon) E973
Blowing up (*see also* Explosion) E923.9
Brawl (hand) (fists) (foot) E960.0
Breakage (accidental)
  cable of cable car not on rails E847
  ladder (causing fall) E881.0
  part (any) of
    animal-drawn vehicle E827
    ladder (causing fall) E881.0
    motor vehicle
      in motion (on public highway) E818
        not on public highway E825
    nonmotor road vehicle, except animal-drawn
      vehicle or pedal cycle E829
    off-road type motor vehicle (not on public
      highway) NEC E821
      on public highway E818
    pedal cycle E826
    scaffolding (causing fall) E881.1
    snow vehicle, motor-driven (not on public
      highway) E820
      on public highway E818
    vehicle NEC—*see* Accident, vehicle
Broken
  glass
    fall on E888.0
    injury by E920.8
  power line (causing electric shock) E925.1
Bumping against, into (accidentally)
  object (moving) E917.9
    caused by crowd E917.1
      with subsequent fall E917.6
    furniture E917.3
      with subsequent fall E917.7
    in
      running water E917.2
      sports E917.0
        with subsequent fall E917.5
    stationary E917.4
      with subsequent fall E917.8
  person(s) E917.9
    with fall E886.9
      in sports E886.0
    as, or caused by, a crowd E917.1
      with subsequent fall E917.6
    in sports E917.0
      with fall E886.0
Burning, burns (accidental) (by) (from) (on)
  E899
  acid (any kind) E924.1
    swallowed—*see* Table of drugs and
      chemicals
  bedclothes (*see also* Fire, specified NEC)
    E898.0
  blowlamp (*see also* Fire, specified NEC)
    E898.1

Burning, burns—*continued*
  blowtorch (*see also* Fire, specified NEC)
    E898.1
  boat, ship, watercraft—*see* categories E830,
    E831, E837
  bonfire (controlled) E897
    uncontrolled E892
  candle (*see also* Fire, specified NEC) E898.1
  caustic liquid, substance E924.1
    swallowed—*see* Table of drugs and
      chemicals
  chemical E924.1
    from swallowing caustic, corrosive
      substance—*see* Table of drugs and
      chemicals
    in
      terrorism E979.7
      war operations E997.2
  cigar(s) or cigarette(s) (*see also* Fire, specified
    NEC) E898.1
  clothes, clothing, nightdress—*see* Ignition,
    clothes
    with conflagration—*see* Conflagration
  conflagration—*see* Conflagration
  corrosive liquid, substance E924.1
    swallowed—*see* Table of drugs and
      chemicals
  electric current (*see also* Electric shock)
    E925.9
  fire, flames (*see also* Fire) E899
  flare, Verey pistol E922.8
  heat
    from appliance (electrical) E924.8
    in local application or packing during
      medical or surgical procedure E873.5
  homicide (attempt) (*see also* Assault, burning)
    E968.0
  hot
    liquid E924.0
      caustic or corrosive E924.1
    object (not producing fire or flames) E924.8
    substance E924.9
      caustic or corrosive E924.1
      liquid (metal) NEC E924.0
      specified type NEC E924.8
    tap water E924.2
  ignition—*see also* Ignition
    clothes, clothing, nightdress—*see also*
      Ignition, clothes
      with conflagration—*see* Conflagration
    highly inflammable material (benzine) (fat)
      (gasoline) (kerosine) (paraffin) (petrol)
      E894
  inflicted by other person
    stated as
      homicidal, intentional (*see also* Assault,
        burning) E968.0
      undetermined whether accidental or
        intentional (*see also* Burn, stated as
        undetermined whether accidental or
        intentional) E988.1
  internal, from swallowed caustic, corrosive
    liquid, substance—*see* Table of drugs and
    chemicals
  in
    from nuclear explosion E996
    petrol bomb E990.0
    terrorism E979.3
      from nuclear explosion E979.5
      petrol bomb E979.3

Burning, burns—*continued*
  war operations (from fire-producing device or conventional weapon) E990.9
    from nuclear explosion E996
    petrol bomb E990.0
  lamp (*see also* Fire, specified NEC) E898.1
  late effect of NEC E929.4
  lighter (cigar) (cigarette) (*see also* Fire, specified NEC) E898.1
  lightning E907
  liquid (boiling) (hot) (molten) E924.0
    caustic, corrosive (external) E924.1
      swallowed—*see* Table of drugs and chemicals
  local application of externally applied substance in medical or surgical care E873.5
  machinery—*see* Accident, machine
  matches (*see also* Fire, specified NEC) E898.1
  medicament, externally applied E873.5
  metal, molten E924.0
  object (hot) E924.8
    producing fire or flames—*see* Fire
  oven (electric) (gas) E924.8
  pipe (smoking) (*see also* Fire, specified NEC) E898.1
  radiation—*see* Radiation
  railway engine, locomotive, train (*see also* Explosion, railway engine) E803
  self-inflicted (unspecified whether accidental or intentional) E988.1
    caustic or corrosive substance NEC E988.7
    stated as intentional, purposeful E958.1
      caustic or corrosive substance NEC E958.7
    stated as undetermined whether accidental or intentional E988.1
      caustic or corrosive substance NEC E988.7
  steam E924.0
    pipe E924.8
  substance (hot) E924.9
    boiling or molten E924.0
    caustic, corrosive (external) E924.1
      swallowed—*see* Table of drugs and chemicals
  suicidal (attempt) NEC E958.1
    caustic substance E958.7
    late effect of E959
  tanning bed E926.2
  therapeutic misadventure
    overdose of radiation E873.2
  torch, welding (*see also* Fire, specified NEC) E898.1
  trash fire (*see also* Burning, bonfire) E897
  vapor E924.0
  vitriol E924.1
  x-rays E926.3
    in medical, surgical procedure—*see* Misadventure, failure, in dosage, radiation
Butted by animal E906.8

C

Cachexia, lead or saturnine E866.0
  from pesticide NEC (*see also* Table of drugs and chemicals) E863.4
Caisson disease E902.2
Capital punishment (any means) E978
Car sickness E903
Casualty (not due to war) NEC E928.9
  terrorism E979.8
  war (*see also* War operations) E995
Cat
  bite E906.3
  scratch E906.8
Cataclysmic (any injury)
  earth surface movement or eruption E909.9
    specified type NEC E909.8
  storm or flood resulting from storm E908.9
    specified type NEC E909.8
Catching fire —*see* Ignition
Caught
  between
    objects (moving) (stationary and moving) E918
      and machinery—*see* Accident, machine
  by cable car, not on rails E847
  in
    machinery (moving parts of)—*see* Accident, machine
    object E918
Cave-in (causing asphyxia, suffocation (by pressure)) (*see also* Suffocation, due to, cave-in) E913.3
Cave-in—*continued*
  with injury other than asphyxia or suffocation E916
    with asphyxia or suffocation (*see also* Suffocation, due to, cave-in) E913.3
  struck or crushed by E916
    with asphyxia or suffocation (*see also* Suffocation, due to, cave-in) E913.3
Change(s) in air pressure—*see also* Effects of, air pressure
  sudden, in aircraft (ascent) (descent) (causing aeroneurosis or aviators' disease) E902.1
Chilblains E901.0
  due to manmade conditions E901.1
Choking (on) (any object except food or vomitus) E912
  apple E911
  bone E911
  food, any type (regurgitated) E911
  mucus or phlegm E912
  seed E911
Civil insurrection —*see* War operations
Cloudburst E908.8
Cold, exposure to (accidental) (excessive) (extreme) (place) E901.9
  causing chilblains or immersion foot E901.0
  due to
    manmade conditions E901.1
    specified cause NEC E901.8
    weather (conditions) E901.0
  late effect of NEC E929.5
  self-inflicted (undetermined whether accidental or intentional) E988.3
    suicidal E958.3
  suicide E958.3
Colic, lead, painters', or saturnine —*see* category E866

Collapse
building E916
  burning (uncontrolled fire) E891.8
    in terrorism E979.3
    private E890.8
dam E909.3
due to heat—*see* Heat
machinery—*see* Accident, machine
man-made structure E909.3
postoperative NEC E878.9
structure, burning NEC E891.8
  burning (uncontrolled fire)
    in terrorism E979.3

Collision (accidental)

Note—In the case of collisions between different types of vehicles, persons and objects, priority in classification is in the following order:

> Aircraft
> Watercraft
> Motor vehicle
> Railway vehicle
> Pedal Cycle
> Animal-drawn vehicle
> Animal being ridden
> Streetcar or other nonmotor road vehicle
> Other vehicle
> Pedestrian or person using pedestrian
>   conveyance
> Object (except where falling from or set in
>   motion by vehicle etc. listed above)

In the listing below, the combinations are listed only under the vehicle etc. having priority. For definitions, *see* E code introduction.

aircraft (with object or vehicle) (fixed)
  (movable) (moving) E841
  with
    person (while landing, taking off) (without
      accident to aircraft) E844
    powered (in transit) (with unpowered
      aircraft) E841
    while landing, taking off E840
    unpowered E842
    while landing, taking off E840
animal being ridden (in sport or transport)
  E828
  and
    animal (being ridden) (herded)
      (unattended) E828
    nonmotor road vehicle, except pedal cycle
      or animal-drawn vehicle E828
    object (fallen) (fixed) (movable) (moving)
      not falling from or set in motion by
      vehicle of higher priority E828
    pedestrian (conveyance or vehicle) E828
animal-drawn vehicle E827
  and
    animal (being ridden) (herded)
      (unattended) E827
    nonmotor road vehicle, except pedal cycle
      E827
    object (fallen) (fixed) (movable) (moving)
      not falling from or set in motion by
      vehicle of higher priority E827
    pedestrian (conveyance or vehicle) E827
    streetcar E827
motor vehicle (on public highway) (traffic
  accident) E812

Collision—*continued*
after leaving, running off, public highway
  (without antecedent collision) (without
  re-entry) E816
  with antecedent collision on public
    highway—*see* categories E810-E815
  with re-entrance collision with another
    motor vehicle E811
and
  abutment (bridge) (overpass) E815
  animal (herded) (unattended) E815
    carrying person, property E813
  animal-drawn vehicle E813
  another motor vehicle (abandoned)
    (disabled) (parked) (stalled) (stopped)
    E812
    with, involving re-entrance (on same
      roadway) (across median strip) E811
  any object, person, or vehicle off the
    public highway resulting from a
    noncollision motor vehicle nontraffic
    accident E816
  avalanche, fallen or not moving E815
    falling E909
  boundary fence E815
  culvert E815
  fallen
    stone E815
    tree E815
  falling E909.2
  guard post or guard rail E815
  inter-highway divider E815
  landslide, fallen or not moving E815
    moving E909
  machinery (road) E815
  moving E909.2
  nonmotor road vehicle NEC E813
  object (any object, person, or vehicle off
    the public highway resulting from a
    noncollision motor vehicle nontraffic
    accident) E815
    off, normally not on, public highway
      resulting from a noncollision motor
      vehicle traffic accident E816
  pedal cycle E813
  pedestrian (conveyance) E814
  person (using pedestrian conveyance) E814
  post or pole (lamp) (light) (signal)
    (telephone) (utility) E815
  railway rolling stock, train, vehicle E810
  safety island E815
  street car E813
  traffic signal, sign, or marker (temporary)
    E815
  tree E815
  tricycle E813
  wall of cut made for road E815
due to cataclysm—*see* categories E908,
  E909
not on public highway, nontraffic accident
  E822
  and
    animal (carrying person, property)
      (herded) (unattended) E822
    animal-drawn vehicle E822
    another motor vehicle (moving), except
      off-road motor vehicle E822
      stationary E823
    avalanche, fallen, not moving E823
      moving E909
    landslide, fallen, not moving E823

Collision—*continued*
  vehicle
    animal-drawn—*see* Collision, animal-drawn
      vehicle
    motor—*see* Collision, motor vehicle
    nonmotor
      nonroad E848
      and
        another nonmotor, nonroad vehicle
          E848
        object (fallen) (fixed) (movable)
          (moving) not falling from or set in
          motion by aircraft, animal-drawn
          vehicle, animal being ridden, motor
          vehicle, nonmotor road vehicle,
          pedal cycle, railway train, or
          streetcar E848
      road, except animal being ridden,
        animal-drawn vehicle, or pedal cycle
        E829
      and
        animal, herded, not being ridden,
          unattended E829
        another nonmotor road vehicle, except
          animal being ridden, animal-drawn
          vehicle, or pedal cycle E829
        object (fallen) (fixed) (movable)
          (moving) not falling from or set in
          motion by, aircraft, animal-drawn
          vehicle, animal being ridden, motor
          vehicle, pedal cycle, or railway
          train E829
        pedestrian (conveyance) E829
        person (using pedestrian conveyance)
          E829
        vehicle, nonmotor, nonroad E829
  watercraft E838
    and
      person swimming or water skiing E838
    causing
      drowning, submersion E830
      injury except drowning, submersion E831
Combustion, spontaneous —*see* Ignition
Complication of medical or surgical
  procedure or treatment
  as an abnormal reaction—*see* Reaction,
    abnormal
  delayed, without mention of
    misadventure—*see* Reaction, abnormal
  due to misadventure—*see* Misadventure
Compression
  divers' squeeze E902.2
  trachea by
    food E911
    foreign body, except food E912
Conflagration
  building or structure, except private dwelling
    (barn) (church) (convalescent or residential
    home) (factory) (farm outbuilding)
    (hospital) (hotel) (institution) (educational)
    (dormitory) (residential) (school) (shop)
    (store) (theatre) E891.9
    with or causing (injury due to)
      accident or injury NEC E891.9
        specified circumstance NEC E891.8
      burns, burning E891.3
      carbon monoxide E891.2
      fumes E891.2
        polyvinylchloride (PVC) or similar
          material E891.1
      smoke E891.2

Conflagration—*continued*
  causing explosion E891.0
  in terrorism E979.3
  not in building or structure E892
  private dwelling (apartment) (boarding house)
    (camping place) (caravan) (farmhouse)
    (home (private)) (house) (lodging house)
    (private garage) (rooming house)
    (tenement) E890.9
    with or causing (injury due to)
      accident or injury NEC E890.9
        specified circumstance NEC E890.8
      burns, burning E890.3
      carbon monoxide E890.2
      fumes E890.2
        polyvinylchloride (PVC) or similar
          material E890.1
      smoke E890.2
    causing explosion E890.0
Constriction, external
  caused by
    hair E928.4
    other object E928.5
Contact with
  dry ice E901.1
  liquid air, hydrogen, nitrogen E901.1
Cramp(s)
  Heat—*see* Heat
  swimmers (*see also* category E910) E910.2
    not in recreation or sport E910.3
Cranking (car) (truck) (bus) (engine), injury
  by E917.9
Crash
  aircraft (in transit) (powered) E841
    at landing, take-off E840
    in
      terrorism E979.1
      war operations E994
    on runway NEC E840
    stated as
      homicidal E968.8
      suicidal E958.6
      undetermined whether accidental or
        intentional E988.6
    unpowered E842
  glider E842
  motor vehicle—*see also* Accident, motor
    vehicle
    homicidal E968.5
    suicidal E958.5
    undetermined whether accidental or
      intentional E988.5
Crushed (accidentally) E928.9
  between
    boat(s), ship(s), watercraft (and dock or pier)
      (without accident to watercraft) E838
      after accident to, or collision, watercraft
        E831
      objects (moving) (stationary and moving)
        E918
  by
    avalanche NEC E909.2
    boat, ship, watercraft after accident to,
      collision, watercraft E831
    cave-in E916
      with asphyxiation or suffocation (*see also*
        Suffocation, due to, cave-in) E913.3
    crowd, human stampede E917.1
    falling
      aircraft (*see also* Accident, aircraft) E841

cold—*see* Cold, exposure to
due to excessive exertion E927
heat—*see* Heat
Explosion (accidental) (in) (of) (on) E923.9
acetylene E923.2
aerosol can E921.8
aircraft (in transit) (powered) E841
  at landing, take-off E840
  in
    terrorism E979.1
    war operations E994
  unpowered E842
air tank (compressed) (in machinery) E921.1
anesthetic gas in operating theatre E923.2
automobile tire NEC E921.8
  causing transport accident—*see* categories
    E810-E825
blasting (cap) (materials) E923.1
boiler (machinery), not on transport vehicle
  E921.0
  steamship—*see* Explosion, watercraft
bomb E923.8
  in
    terrorism E979.2
    war operations E993
      after cessation of hostilities E998
      atom, hydrogen or nuclear E996
      injury by fragments from E991.9
        antipersonnel bomb E991.3
butane E923.2
caused by
  other person
    stated as
      intentional, homicidal—*see* Assault,
        explosive
      undetermined whether accidental or
        homicidal E985.5
coal gas E923.2
detonator E923.1
dynamite E923.1
explosive (material) NEC E923.9
  gas(es) E923.2
  missile E923.8
    in
    terrorism E979.2
    war operations E993
      injury by fragments from E991.9
        antipersonnel bomb E991.3
  used in blasting operations E923.1
fire-damp E923.2
fireworks E923.0
gas E923.2
  cylinder (in machinery) E921.1
  pressure tank (in machinery) E921.1
gasoline (fumes) (tank) not in moving motor
  vehicle E923.2
grain store (military) (munitions) E923.8
grenade E923.8
  in
    terrorism E979.2
    war operations E993
      injury by fragments from E991.9
homicide (attempt)—*see* Assault, explosive
hot water heater, tank (in machinery) E921.0
in mine (of explosive gases) NEC E923.2
late effect of NEC E929.8
machinery—*see also* Accident, machine
  pressure vessel—*see* Explosion, pressure
    vessel
methane E923.2

Explosion—*continued*
missile E923.8
  in
    terrorism E979.2
    war operations E993
      injury by fragments from E991.9
motor vehicle (part of)
  in motion (on public highway) E818
  not on public highway E825
munitions (dump) (factory) E923.8
  in
    terrorism E979.2
    war operations E993
of mine E923.8
  in
    terrorism
      at sea or in harbor E979.0
      land E979.2
      marine E979.0
    war operations
      after cessation of hostilities E998
      at sea or in harbor E992
      land E993
        after cessation of hostilities E998
        injury by fragments from E991.9
      marine E992
own weapons
  in
    terrorism (*see also* Suicide) E979.2
    war operations E993
      injury by fragments from E991.9
        antipersonnel bomb E991.3
pressure
  cooker E921.8
  gas tank (in machinery) E921.1
  vessel (in machinery) E921.9
    on transport vehicle—*see* categories
      E800-E848
    specified type NEC E921.8
propane E923.2
railway engine, locomotive, train (boiler) (with
  subsequent collision, derailment, fall) E803
  with
    collision (antecedent) (*see also* Collision,
      railway) E800
    derailment (antecedent) E802
    fire (without antecedent collision or
      derailment) E803
secondary fire resulting from—*see* Fire
self-inflicted (unspecified whether accidental
  or intentional) E985.5
  stated as intentional, purposeful E955.5
shell (artillery) E923.8
  in
    terrorism E979.2
    war operations E993
      injury by fragments from E991.9
stated as undetermined whether caused
  accidentally or purposely inflicted E985.5
steam or water lines (in machinery) E921.0
suicide (attempted) E955.5
terrorism—*see* Terrorism, explosion
torpedo E923.8
  in
    terrorism E979.0
    war operations E992
transport accident—*see* categories E800-E848
war operations—*see* War operations, explosion
watercraft (boiler) E837
  causing drowning, submersion (after jumping
    from watercraft) E830

Exposure (weather) (conditions) (rain) (wind)
E904.3
  with homicidal intent E968.4
  excessive E904.3
    cold (*see also* Cold, exposure to) E901.9
      self-inflicted—*see* Cold, exposure to,
        self-inflicted
      heat (*see also* Heat) E900.9
  fire—*see* Fire
  helpless person, infant, newborn due to
      abandonment or neglect E904.0
  noise E928.1
  prolonged in deep-freeze unit or refrigerator
      E901.1
  radiation—*see* Radiation
  resulting from transport accident—*see*
      categories E800-E848
  smoke from, due to
    fire—*see* Fire
    tobacco, second-hand E869.4
  vibration E928.2

F

Fall, falling (accidental) E888.9
  building E916
    burning E891.8
      private E890.8
  down
    escalator E880.0
    ladder E881.0
      in boat, ship, watercraft E833
    staircase E880.9
    stairs, steps—*see* Fall, from, stairs
  earth (with asphyxia or suffocation (by
      pressure)) (*see also* Earth, falling) E913.3
  from, off
    aircraft (at landing, take-off) (in-transit)
        (while alighting, boarding) E843
      resulting from accident to aircraft—*see*
          categories E840-E842
    animal (in sport or transport) E828
    animal-drawn vehicle E827
    balcony E882
    bed E884.4
    bicycle E826
    boat, ship, watercraft (into water) E832
      after accident to, collision, fire on E830
        and subsequently struck by (part of) boat
          E831
        and subsequently struck by (part of) boat
          E838
      burning, crushed, sinking E830
        and subsequently struck by (part of) boat
          E831
    bridge E882
    building E882
      burning (uncontrolled fire) E891.8
        in terrorism E979.3
        private E890.8
    bunk in boat, ship, watercraft E834
      due to accident to watercraft E831
    cable car (not on rails) E847
      on rails E829
    car—*see* Fall from motor vehicle
    chair E884.2
    cliff E884.1
    commode E884.6
    curb (sidewalk) E880.1

Fall, falling—*continued*
  elevation aboard ship E834
    due to accident to ship E831
  embankment E884.9
  escalator E880.0
  fire escape E882
  flagpole E882
  furniture NEC E884.5
  gangplank (into water) (*see also* Fall, from,
      boat) E832
    to deck, dock E834
  hammock on ship E834
    due to accident to watercraft E831
  haystack E884.9
  high place NEC E884.9
    stated as undetermined whether accidental
        or intentional—*see* Jumping, from, high
        place
  horse (in sport or transport) E828
  in-line skates E885.1
  ladder E881.0
    in boat, ship, watercraft E833
      due to accident to watercraft E831
  machinery—*see also* accident, machine
    not in operation E884.9
  motor vehicle (in motion) (on public
      highway) E818
    not on public highway E825
      stationary, except while alighting,
          boarding, entering, leaving E884.9
      while alighting, boarding, entering,
          leaving E824
    stationary, except while alighting, boarding,
        entering, leaving E884.9
    while alighting, boarding, entering, leaving,
        except off-road type motor vehicle
        E817
    off-road type—*see* Fall, from, off-road
        type motor vehicle
  nonmotor road vehicle (while alighting,
      boarding) NEC E829
    stationary, except while alighting, boarding,
        entering, leaving E884.9
  off road type motor vehicle (not on public
      highway) NEC E821
    on public highway E818
      while alighting, boarding, entering,
          leaving E817
    snow vehicle—*see* Fall from snow vehicle,
        motor-driven
  one
    deck to another on ship E834
      due to accident to ship E831
    level to another NEC E884.9
      boat, ship, or watercraft E834
        due to accident to watercraft E831
  pedal cycle E826
  playground equipment E884.0
  railway rolling stock, train, vehicle (while
      alighting, boarding) E804
    with
      collision (*see also* Collision, railway)
          E800
      derailment (*see also* Derailment, railway)
          E802
      explosion (*see also* Explosion, railway
          engine) E803
  rigging (aboard ship) E834
    due to accident to watercraft E831
  roller skates E885.1
  scaffolding E881.1

Fall, falling—*continued*
  scooter (nonmotorized) E885.0
  sidewalk (curb) E880.1
    moving E885.9
  skateboard E885.2
  skis E885.3
  snowboard E885.4
  snow vehicle, motor-driven (not on public
    highway) E820
    on public highway E818
      while alighting, boarding, entering,
        leaving E817
  stairs, steps E880.9
    boat, ship, watercraft E833
      due to accident to watercraft E831
    motor bus, motor vehicle—*see* Fall, from,
      motor vehicle, while alighting,
      boarding
    street car E829
  stationary vehicle NEC E884.9
  stepladder E881.0
  street car (while boarding, alighting) E829
    stationary, except while boarding or
      alighting E884.9
  structure NEC E882
    burning (uncontrolled fire) E891.8
      in terrorism E979.3
  table E884.9
  toilet E884.6
  tower E882
  tree E884.9
  turret E882
  vehicle NEC—*see also* Accident, vehicle
    NEC
    stationary E884.9
  viaduct E882
  wall E882
  wheelchair E884.3
  window E882
 in, on
  aircraft (at landing, take-off) (in-transit)
    E843
    resulting from accident to aircraft—*see*
      categories E840-E842
  boat, ship, watercraft E835
    due to accident to watercraft E831
    one level to another NEC E834
    on ladder, stairs E833
  cutting or piercing instrument or machine
    E888.0
  deck (of boat, ship, watercraft) E835
    due to accident to watercraft E831
  escalator E880.0
  gangplank E835
  glass, broken E888.0
  knife E888.0
  ladder E881.0
    in boat, ship, watercraft E833
      due to accident to watercraft E831
  object
    edged, pointed or sharp E888.0
    other E888.1
  pitchfork E888.0
  railway rolling stock, train, vehicle (while
    alighting, boarding) E804
    with
      collision (*see also* Collision, railway)
        E800
      derailment (*see also* Derailment, railway)
        E802

Fall, falling—*continued*
    explosion (*see also* Explosion, railway
      engine) E803
  scaffolding E881.1
  scissors E888.0
  staircase, stairs, steps (*see also* Fall, from,
    stairs) E880.9
  street car E829
  water transport (*see also* Fall, in, boat) E835
 into
  cavity E883.9
  dock E883.9
    from boat, ship, watercraft (*see also* Fall,
      from, boat) E832
  hold (of ship) E834
    due to accident to watercraft E831
  hole E883.9
  manhole E883.2
  moving part of machinery—*see* Accident,
    machine
  opening in surface NEC E883.9
  pit E883.9
  quarry E883.9
  shaft E883.9
  storm drain E883.2
  tank E883.9
  water (with drowning or submersion) E910.9
  well E883.1
 late effect of NEC E929.3
 object (*see also* Hit by, object, falling) E916
 other E888.8
 over
  animal E885.9
  cliff E884.1
  embankment E884.9
  small object E885.9
 overboard (*see also* Fall, from, boat) E832
 resulting in striking against object E888.1
  sharp E888.0
 rock E916
 same level NEC E888.9
  aircraft (any kind) E843
    resulting from accident to aircraft—*see*
      categories E840-E842
  boat, ship, watercraft E835
    due to accident to, collision, watercraft E831
  from
    collision, pushing, shoving, by or with
      other person(s) E886.9
      as, or caused by, a crowd E917.6
      in sports E886.0
    in-line skates E885.1
    roller skates E885.1
    scooter (nonmotorized) E885.0
    skateboard E885.2
    skis E885.3
    slipping, stumbling, tripping E885.9
    snowboard E885.4
 snowslide E916
  as avalanche E909.2
 stone E916
 through
  hatch (on ship) E834
    due to accident to watercraft E831
  roof E882
  window E882
 timber E916
 while alighting from, boarding, entering,
  leaving
  aircraft (any kind) E843

Fall, falling—*continued*
 motor bus, motor vehicle—*see* Fall, from,
  motor vehicle, while alighting, boarding
 nonmotor road vehicle NEC E829
 railway train E804
 street car E829
Fallen on by
 animal (horse) (not being ridden) E906.8
 being ridden (in sport or transport) E828
Fell or jumped from high place, so stated
 —*see* Jumping, from, high place
Felo-de-se (*see also* Suicide) E958.9
Fever
 heat—*see* Heat
 thermic—*see* Heat
Fight (hand) (fist) (foot) (*see also* Assault,
 fight) E960.0
Fire (accidental) (caused by great heat from
 appliance (electrical), hot object or hot
 substance) (secondary, resulting from
 explosion) E899
 conflagration—*see* Conflagration
 controlled, normal (in brazier, fireplace,
  furnace, or stove) (charcoal) (coal) (coke)
  (electric) (gas) (wood)
  bonfire E897
  brazier, not in building or structure E897
  in building or structure, except private
   dwelling (barn) (church) (convalescent or
   residential home) (factory) (farm
   outbuilding) (hospital) (hotel) (institution
   (educational) (dormitory) (residential))
   (private garage) (school) (shop) (store)
   (theatre) E896
  in private dwelling (apartment) (boarding
   house) (camping place) (caravan)
   (farmhouse) (home (private)) (house)
   (lodging house) (rooming house)
   (tenement) E895
  not in building or structure E897
  trash E897
 forest (uncontrolled) E892
 grass (uncontrolled) E892
 hay (uncontrolled) E892
 homicide (attempt) E968.0
 late effect of E969
 in, of, on, starting in E892
  aircraft (in transit) (powered) E841
   at landing, take-off E840
   stationary E892
   unpowered (balloon) (glider) E842
  balloon E842
  boat, ship, watercraft—*see* categories E830,
   E831, E837
  building or structure, except private dwelling
   (barn) (church) (convalescent or
   residential home) (factory) (farm
   outbuilding) (hospital) (hotel) (institution
   (educational) (dormitory) (residential))
   (school) (shop) (store) (theatre) (*see also*
   Conflagration, building or structure,
   except private dwelling) E891.9
  forest (uncontrolled) E892
  glider E842
  grass (uncontrolled) E892
  hay (uncontrolled) E892
  lumber (uncontrolled) E892
  machinery—*see* Accident, machine
  mine (uncontrolled) E892
  motor vehicle (in motion) (on public
   highway) E818

Fire —*continued*
 not on public highway E825
  stationary E892
 prairie (uncontrolled) E892
 private dwelling (apartment) (boarding
  house) (camping place) (caravan)
  (farmhouse) (home (private)) (house)
  (lodging house) (private garage) (rooming
  house) (tenement) (*see also*
  Conflagration, private dwelling) E890.9
 railway rolling stock, train, vehicle (*see also*
  Explosion, railway engine) E803
  stationary E892
 room NEC E898.1
 street car (in motion) E829
  stationary E892
 terrorism (by fire-producing device) E979.3
  fittings or furniture (burning building)
   (uncontrolled fire) E979.3
  from nuclear explosion E979.5
 transport vehicle, stationary NEC E892
 tunnel (uncontrolled) E892
 war operations (by fire-producing device or
  conventional weapon) E990.9
  from nuclear explosion E996
  petrol bomb E990.0
 late effect of NEC E929.4
 lumber (uncontrolled) E892
 mine (uncontrolled) E892
 prairie (uncontrolled) E892
 self-inflicted (unspecified whether accidental
  or intentional) E988.1
  stated as intentional, purposeful E958.1
 specified NEC E898.1
  with
   conflagration—*see* Conflagration
   ignition (of)
    clothing—*see* Ignition, clothes
    highly inflammable material (benzine)
     (fat) (gasoline) (kerosene) (paraffin)
     (petrol) E894
 started by other person
  stated as
   with intent to injure or kill E968.0
   undetermined whether or not with intent to
    injure or kill E988.1
 suicide (attempted) E958.1
  late effect of E959
 tunnel (uncontrolled) E892
Fireball effects from nuclear explosion
 in
  terrorism E979.5
  war operations E996
Fireworks (explosion) E923.0
Flash burns from explosion (*see also*
 Explosion) E923.9
Flood (any injury) (resulting from storm)
 E908.2
 caused by collapse of dam or manmade
  structure E909.3
Forced landing (aircraft) E840
Foreign body, object or material (entrance into
 (accidental))
 air passage (causing injury) E915
  with asphyxia, obstruction, suffocation E912
   food or vomitus E911
  nose (with asphyxia, obstruction, suffocation)
   E912
   causing injury without asphyxia,
    obstruction, suffocation E915

Foreign body, object or material—*continued*
  alimentary canal (causing injury) (with
      obstruction) E915
    with asphyxia, obstruction respiratory
        passage, suffocation E912
      food E911
    mouth E915
      with asphyxia, obstruction, suffocation
          E912
        food E911
    pharynx E915
      with asphyxia, obstruction, suffocation
          E912
        food E911
  aspiration (with asphyxia, obstruction
      respiratory passage, suffocation) E912
    causing injury without asphyxia, obstruction
        respiratory passage, suffocation E915
      food (regurgitated) (vomited) E911
        causing injury without asphyxia,
            obstruction respiratory passage,
            suffocation E915
    mucus (not of newborn) E912
    phlegm E912
  bladder (causing injury or obstruction) E915
  bronchus, bronchi—*see* Foreign body, air
      passages
  conjunctival sac E914
  digestive system—*see* Foreign body,
      alimentary canal
  ear (causing injury or obstruction) E915
  esophagus (causing injury or obstruction) (*see
      also* Foreign body, alimentary canal) E915
  eye (any part) E914
  eyelid E914
  hairball (stomach) (with obstruction) E915
  ingestion—*see* Foreign body, alimentary canal
  inhalation—*see* Foreign body, aspiration
  intestine (causing injury or obstruction) E915
  iris E914
  lacrimal apparatus E914
  larynx—*see* Foreign body, air passage
  late effect of NEC E929.8
  lung—*see* Foreign body, air passage
  mouth—*see* Foreign body, alimentary canal,
      mouth
  nasal passage—*see* Foreign body, air passage,
      nose
  nose—*see* Foreign body, air passage, nose
  ocular muscle E914
  operation wound (left in)—*see* Misadventure,
      foreign object
  orbit E914
  pharynx—*see* Foreign body, alimentary canal,
      pharynx
  rectum (causing injury or obstruction) E915
  stomach (hairball) (causing injury or
      obstruction) E915
  tear ducts or glands E914
  trachea—*see* Foreign body, air passage
  urethra (causing injury or obstruction) E915
  vagina (causing injury or obstruction) E915
Found dead, injured
  from exposure (to)—*see* Exposure
  on
    public highway E819
    railway right of way E807

Fracture (circumstances unknown or
    unspecified) E887
  due to specified external means—*see* manner
      of accident
  late effect of NEC E929.3
  occurring in water transport NEC E835
Freezing —*see* Cold, exposure to
Frostbite E901.0
  due to manmade conditions E901.1
Frozen —*see* Cold, exposure to

G

Garrotting, homicidal (attempted) E963
Gored E906.8
Gunshot wound (*see also* Shooting) E922.9

H

Hailstones, injury by E904.3
Hairball (stomach) (with obstruction) E915
Hanged himself (*see also* Hanging,
    self-inflicted) E983.0
Hang gliding E842
Hanging (accidental) E913.8
  caused by other person
    in accidental circumstances E913.8
    stated as
      intentional, homicidal E963
      undetermined whether accidental or
          intentional E983.0
  homicide (attempt) E963
  in bed or cradle E913.0
  legal execution E978
  self-inflicted (unspecified whether accidental
      or intentional) E983.0
    in accidental circumstances E913.8
    stated as intentional, purposeful E953.0
  stated as undetermined whether accidental or
      intentional E983.0
  suicidal (attempt) E953.0
Heat (apoplexy) (collapse) (cramps) (effects of)
    (excessive) (exhaustion) (fever) (prostration)
    (stroke) E900.9
  due to
    manmade conditions (listed in E900.1,
        except boat, ship, watercraft) E900.1
    weather (conditions) E900.0
  from
    electric heating apparatus causing burning
        E924.8
    nuclear explosion
      in
        terrorism E979.5
        war operations E996
  generated in, boiler, engine, evaporator, fire
      room of boat, ship, watercraft E838
  inappropriate in local application or packing in
      medical or surgical procedure E873.5
  late effect of NEC E989
Hemorrhage
  delayed following medical or surgical
      treatment without mention of
      misadventure—*see* Reaction, abnormal
  during medical or surgical treatment as
      misadventure—*see* Misadventure, cut

I

Ictus
caloris—*see* Heat
solaris E900.0
Ignition (accidental)
anesthetic gas in operating theatre E923.2
bedclothes
with
conflagration—*see* Conflagration
ignition (of)
clothing—*see* Ignition, clothes
highly inflammable material (benzine)
(fat) (gasoline) (kerosene) (paraffin)
(petrol) E894
benzine E894
clothes, clothing (from controlled fire) (in
building) E893.9
with conflagration—*see* Conflagration
from
bonfire E893.2
highly inflammable material E894
sources or material as listed in E893.8
trash fire E893.2
uncontrolled fire—*see* Conflagration
in
private dwelling E893.0
specified building or structure, except
private dwelling E893.1
not in building or structure E893.2
explosive material—*see* Explosion
fat E894
gasoline E894
kerosene E894
material
explosive—*see* Explosion
highly inflammable E894
with conflagration—*see* Conflagration
with explosion E923.2
nightdress—*see* Ignition, clothes
paraffin E894
petrol E894
Immersion —*see* Submersion
Implantation of quills of porcupine E906.8
Inanition (from) E904.9
hunger—*see* Lack of, food
resulting from homicidal intent E968.4
thirst—*see* Lack of, water
Inattention after, at birth E904.0
homicidal, infanticidal intent E968.4
Infanticide (*see also* Assault)
Ingestion
foreign body (causing injury) (with
obstruction)—*see* Foreign body, alimentary
canal
poisonous substance NEC—*see* Table of drugs
and chemicals
Inhalation
excessively cold substance, manmade E901.1
foreign body—*see* Foreign body, aspiration
liquid air, hydrogen, nitrogen E901.1
mucus, not of newborn (with asphyxia,
obstruction respiratory passage,
suffocation) E912
phlegm (with asphyxia, obstruction respiratory
passage, suffocation) E912
poisonous gas—*see* Table of drugs and chemicals
smoke from, due to
fire —*see* Fire
tobacco, second-hand E869.4
vomitus (with asphyxia, obstruction respiratory
passage, suffocation) E911

Injury, injured (accidental(ly)) NEC E928.9
by, caused by, from
air rifle (B-B gun) E922.4
animal (not being ridden) NEC E906.9
being ridden (in sport or transport) E828
assault (*see also* Assault) E968.9
avalanche E909.2
bayonet (*see also* Bayonet wound) E920.3
being thrown against some part of, or object
in
motor vehicle (in motion) (on public
highway) E818
not on public highway E825
nonmotor road vehicle NEC E829
off-road motor vehicle NEC E821
railway train E806
snow vehicle, motor-driven E820
street car E829
bending E927
bite, human E928.3
broken glass E920.8
bullet—*see* Shooting
cave-in (*see also* Suffocation, due to,
cave-in) E913.3
without asphyxiation or suffocation E916
cloudburst E908.8
cutting or piercing instrument (*see also* Cut)
E920.9
cyclone E908.1
earth surface movement or eruption E909.9
earthquake E909.0
electric current (*see also* Electric shock)
E925.9
explosion (*see also* Explosion) E923.9
fire—*see* Fire
flare, Very pistol E922.8
flood E908.2
foreign body—*see* Foreign body
hailstones E904.3
hurricane E908.0
landslide E909.2
law-enforcing agent, police, in course of
legal intervention—*see* Legal intervention
lightning E907
live rail or live wire—*see* Electric shock
machinery—*see also* Accident, machine
aircraft, without accident to aircraft E844
boat, ship, watercraft (deck) (engine room)
(galley) (laundry) (loading) E836
missile
explosive E923.8
firearm—*see* Shooting
in
terrorism—*see* Terrorism, missile
war operations—*see* War operations,
missile
moving part of motor vehicle (in motion)
(on public highway) E818
not on public highway, nontraffic accident
E825
while alighting, boarding, entering,
leaving—*see* Fall, from, motor vehicle,
while alighting, boarding
nail E920.8
needle (sewing) E920.4
hypodermic E920.5
noise E928.1
object
fallen on

Injury, injured—*continued*
    motor vehicle (in motion) (on public
       highway) E818
       not on public highway E825
     falling—*see* Hit by, object, falling
    paintball gun E922.5
    radiation—*see* Radiation
    railway rolling stock, train, vehicle (part of)
      E805
     door or window E806
    rotating propeller, aircraft E844
    rough landing of off-road type motor vehicle
      (after leaving ground or rough terrain)
      E821
     snow vehicle E820
    saber (*see also* Wound, saber) E920.3
    shot—*see* Shooting
    sound waves E928.1
    splinter or sliver, wood E920.8
    storm E908.9
    straining E927
    street car (door) E829
    suicide (attempt) E958.9
    sword E920.3
    terrorism—*see* Terrorism
    third rail—*see* Electric shock
    thunderbolt E907
    tidal wave E909.4
     caused by storm E908.0
    tornado E908.1
    torrential rain E908.2
    twisting E927
    vehicle NEC—*see* Accident, vehicle NEC
    vibration E928.2
    volcanic eruption E909.1
    weapon burst, in war operations E993
    weightlessness (in spacecraft, real or
      simulated) E928.0
    wood splinter or sliver E920.8
  due to
    civil insurrection—*see* War operations
     occurring after cessation of hostilities E998
    terrorism—*see* Terrorism
    war operations—*see* War operations
     occurring after cessation of hostilities E998
  homicidal (*see also* Assault) E968.9
  in, on
    civil insurrection—*see* War operations
    fight E960.0
    parachute descent (voluntary) (without
      accident to aircraft) E844
     with accident to aircraft—*see* categories
      E840-E842
    public highway E819
    railway right of way E807
    terrorism—*see* Terrorism
    war operations—*see* War operations
  inflicted (by)
    in course of arrest (attempted), suppression
      of disturbance, maintenance of order, by
      law-enforcing agents—*see* Legal
      intervention
    law-enforcing agent (on duty)—*see* Legal
      intervention
    other person
     stated as
      accidental E928.9
      homicidal, intentional—*see* Assault

Injury, injured—*continued*
    undetermined whether accidental or
      intentional—*see* Injury, stated as
      undetermined
   police (on duty)—*see* Legal intervention
  late effect of E929.9
  purposely (inflicted) by other person(s)—*see*
    Assault
  self-inflicted (unspecified whether accidental
    or intentional) E988.9
   stated as
    accidental E928.9
    intentionally, purposely E958.9
  specified cause NEC E928.8
  stated as
    undetermined whether accidentally or
      purposely inflicted (by) E988.9
    cut (any part of body) E986
    cutting or piercing instrument (classifiable
      to E920) E986
    drowning E984
    explosive(s) (missile) E985.5
    falling from high place E987.9
     manmade structure, except residential
      E987.1
     natural site E987.2
     residential premises E987.0
    hanging E983.0
    knife E986
    late effect of E989
    puncture (any part of body) E986
    shooting—*see* Shooting, stated as
      undetermined whether accidental or
      intentional
    specified means NEC E988.8
    stab (any part of body) E986
    strangulation—*see* Suffocation, stated as
      undetermined whether accidental or
      intentional
    submersion E984
    suffocation—*see* Suffocation, stated as
      undetermined whether accidental or
      intentional
  to child due to criminal abortion E968.8
Insufficient nourishment —*see also* Lack of,
  food
  homicidal intent E968.4
Insulation, effects —*see* Heat
Interruption of respiration by
  food lodged in esophagus E911
  foreign body, except food, in esophagus E912
Intervention, legal —*see* Legal intervention
Intoxication, drug or poison —*see* Table of
  drugs and chemicals
Irradiation —*see* Radiation

J

Jammed (accidentally)
  between objects (moving) (stationary and
    moving) E918
  in object E918
Jumped or fell from high place, so stated
  —*see Jumping, from, high place, stated as*
  in undetermined circumstances
Jumping
  before train, vehicle or other moving object
    (unspecified whether accidental or
    intentional) E988.0
   stated as

Jumping—*continued*
    intentional, purposeful E958.0
      suicidal (attempt) E958.0
   from
    aircraft
      by parachute (voluntarily) (without
         accident to aircraft) E844
      due to accident to aircraft—*see* categories
         E840-E842
    boat, ship, watercraft (into water)
      after accident to, fire on, watercraft E830
        and subsequently struck by (part of) boat
         E831
      burning, crushed, sinking E830
        and subsequently struck by (part of) boat
         E831
      voluntarily, without accident (to boat) with
        injury other than drowning or
        submersion E883.0
    building—*see also* Jumping, from, high
      place
    burning (uncontrolled fire) E891.8
      in terrorism E979.3
      private E890.8
    cable car (not on rails) E847
      on rails E829
    high place
      in accidental circumstances or in
        sport—*see* categories E880-E884
      stated as
        with intent to injure self E957.9
          man-made structures NEC E957.1
          natural sites E957.2
          residential premises E957.0
        in undetermined circumstances E987.9
          man-made structures NEC E987.1
          natural sites E987.2
          residential premises E987.0
        suicidal (attempt) E957.9
          man-made structures NEC E957.1
          natural sites E957.1
          residential premises E957.0
    motor vehicle (in motion) (on public
      highway)—*see* Fall, from, motor vehicle
    nonmotor road vehicle NEC E829
    street car E829
    structure—*see also* Jumping, from, high
      place
      burning NEC (uncontrolled fire) E891.8
        in terrorism E979.3
   into water
    with injury other than drowning or
      submersion E883.0
      drowning or submersion—*see* Submersion
    from, off, watercraft—*see* Jumping, from,
      boat
Justifiable homicide —*see* Assault

<h1 style="text-align:center">K</h1>

Kicked by
  animal E906.8
  person(s) (accidentally) E917.9
    with intent to injure or kill E960.0
    as, or caused by a crowd E917.1
      with subsequent fall E917.6
    in fight E960.0
    in sports E917.0
      with subsequent fall E917.5

Kicking against
  object (moving) E917.9
    in sports E917.0
      with subsequent fall E917.5
    stationary E917.4
      with subsequent fall E917.8
  person—*see* Striking against, person
Killed, killing (accidentally) NEC (*see also*
  Injury) E928.9
  in
    action—*see* War operations
    brawl, fight (hand) (fists) (foot) E960.0
      by weapon—*see also* Assault
        cutting, piercing E966
          firearm—*see* Shooting, homicide
  self
    stated as
      accident E928.9
      suicide—*see* Suicide
    unspecified whether accidental or suicidal
      E988.9
Knocked down (accidentally) (by) NEC E928.9
  animal (not being ridden) E906.8
    being ridden (in sport or transport) E828
  blast from explosion (*see also* Explosion)
    E923.9
  crowd, human stampede E917.6
  late effect of—*see* Late effect
  person (accidentally) E917.9
    in brawl, fight E960.0
    in sports E917.5
  transport vehicle—*see* vehicle involved under
    Hit by
  while boxing E917.5

<h1 style="text-align:center">L</h1>

Laceration NEC E928.9
Lack of
  air (refrigerator or closed place), suffocation
    by E913.2
  care (helpless person) (infant) (newborn)
    E904.0
    homicidal intent E968.4
  food except as result of transport accident
    E904.1
    helpless person, infant, newborn due to
      abandonment or neglect E904.0
  water except as result of transport accident
    E904.2
    helpless person, infant, newborn due to
      abandonment or neglect E904.0
Landslide E909.2
  falling on, hitting
    motor vehicle (any) (in motion) (on or off
      public highway) E909.2
    railway rolling stock, train, vehicle E909.2
Late effect of
  accident NEC (accident classifiable to E928.9)
    E929.9
    specified NEC (accident classifiable to
      E910-E928.8) E929.8
  assault E969
  fall, accidental (accident classifiable to
    E880-E888) E929.3
  fire, accident caused by (accident classifiable
    to E890-E899) E929.4
  homicide, attempt (any means) E969
  injury due to terrorism E999.1

Late effect of—*continued*
  injury undetermined whether accidentally or
    purposely inflicted (injury classifiable to
    E980-E988) E989
  legal intervention (injury classifiable to
    E970-E976) E977
  medical or surgical procedure, test or therapy
    as, or resulting in, or from
      abnormal or delayed reaction or
        complication—*see* Reaction, abnormal
      misadventure—*see* Misadventure
  motor vehicle accident (accident classifiable to
    E810-E825) E929.0
  natural or environmental factor, accident due
    to (accident classifiable to E900-E909)
    E929.5
  poisoning, accidental (accident classifiable to
    E850-E858, E860-E869) E929.2
  suicide, attempt (any means) E959
  transport accident NEC (accident classifiable
    to E800-E807, E826-E838, E840-E848)
    E929.1
  war operations, injury due to (injury
    classifiable to E990-E998) E999.0
Launching pad accident E845
Legal
  execution, any method E978
  intervention (by) (injury from) E976
    baton E973
    bayonet E974
    blow E975
    blunt object (baton) (nightstick) (stave)
      (truncheon) E973
    cutting or piercing instrument E974
    dynamite E971
    execution, any method E973
    explosive(s) (shell) E971
    firearms(s) E970
    gas (asphyxiation) (poisoning) (tear) E972
    grenade E971
    late effect of E977
    machine gun E970
    manhandling E975
    mortar bomb E971
    nightstick E973
    revolver E970
    rifle E970
    specified means NEC E975
    stabbing E974
    stave E973
    truncheon E973
Lifting, injury in E927
Lightning (shock) (stroke) (struck by) E907
Liquid (noncorrosive) in eye E914
  corrosive E924.1
Loss of control
  motor vehicle (on public highway) (without
    antecedent collision) E816
    with
      antecedent collision on public highway
        —*see* Collision, motor vehicle
        involving any object, person or vehicle
          not on public highway E816
        on public highway—*see* Collision, motor
          vehicle
      not on public highway, nontraffic accident
        E825
        with antecedent collision—*see* Collision,
          motor vehicle, not on public highway
    off-road type motor vehicle (not on public
      highway) E821

Loss of control—*continued*
    on public highway—*see* Loss of control,
      motor vehicle
  snow vehicle, motor-driven (not on public
    highway) E820
    on public highway—*see* Loss of control,
      motor vehicle
Lost at sea E832
  with accident to watercraft E830
  in war operations E995
Low
  pressure, effects—*see* Effects of, air pressure
  temperature, effects—*see* Cold, exposure to
**Lying before train, vehicle or other moving
  object** (unspecified whether accidental or
  intentional) E988.0
  stated as intentional, purposeful, suicidal
    (attempt) E958.0
Lynching (*see also* Assault) E968.9

M

**Malfunction, atomic power plant in water
  transport** E838
Mangled (accidentally) NEC E928.9
Manhandling (in brawl, fight) E960.0
  legal intervention E975
Manslaughter (nonaccidental)—*see* Assault
Marble in nose E912
Mauled by animal E906.8
Medical procedure, complication of
  delayed or as an abnormal reaction without
    mention of misadventure—*see* Reaction,
    abnormal
  due to or as a result of misadventure—*see*
    Misadventure
Melting of fittings and furniture in burning
  in terrorism E979.3
Minamata disease E865.2
Misadventure(s) to patient(s) during surgical or
  medical care E876.9
  contaminated blood, fluid, drug or biological
    substance (presence of agents and toxins
    as listed in E875) E875.9
    administered (by) NEC E875.9
      infusion E875.0
      injection E875.1
      specified means NEC E875.2
      transfusion E875.0
      vaccination E875.1
  cut, cutting, puncture, perforation or
    hemorrhage (accidental) (inadvertent)
    (inappropriate) (during) E870.9
    aspiration of fluid or tissue (by puncture or
      catheterization, except heart) E870.5
    biopsy E870.8
      needle (aspirating) E870.5
    blood sampling E870.5
    catheterization E870.5
      heart E870.6
    dialysis (kidney) E870.2
    endoscopic examination E870.4
    enema E870.7
    infusion E870.1
    injection E870.3
    lumbar puncture E870.5
    needle biopsy E870.5
    paracentesis, abdominal E870.5
    perfusion E870.2
    specified procedure NEC E870.8

Misadventure(s)—*continued*
    placement of endotracheal tube during
      anesthetic procedure E876.3
  transfusion—*see also* Misadventure, by
    specific type, transfusion
  excessive amount of blood E873.0
  mismatched blood E876.0
  wrong
    drug given in error—*see* Table of drugs and
      chemicals
    fluid in infusion E876.1
    placement of endotracheal tube during
      anesthetic procedure E876.3
Motion (effects) E903
  sickness E903
Mountain sickness E902.0
**Mucus aspiration or inhalation, not of
  newborn** (with asphyxia, obstruction
  respiratory passage, suffocation) E912
Mudslide of cataclysmic nature E909.2
Murder (attempt) (*see also* Assault) E968.9

N

Nail, injury by E920.8
Needlestick (sewing needle) E920.4
  hypodermic E920.5
Neglect —*see also* Privation
  criminal E968.4
  homicidal intent E968.4
Noise (causing injury) (pollution) E928.1

O

Object
  falling
    from, in, on, hitting
      aircraft E844
        due to accident to aircraft—*see*
          categories E840-E842
      machinery—*see also* Accident, machine
        not in operation E916
      motor vehicle (in motion) (on public
        highway) E818
        not on public highway E825
        stationary E916
      nonmotor road vehicle NEC E829
      pedal cycle E826
      person E916
      railway rolling stock, train, vehicle E806
      street car E829
      watercraft E838
        due to accident to watercraft E831
    set in motion by
      accidental explosion of pressure vessel—*see*
        category E921
      firearm—*see* category E922
      machine(ry)—*see* Accident, machine
      transport vehicle—*see* categories E800-E848
    thrown from, in, on, towards
      aircraft E844
      cable car (not on rails) E847
        on rails E829
      motor vehicle (in motion) (on public
        highway) E818
        not on public highway E825
      nonmotor road vehicle NEC E829
      pedal cycle E826
      street car E829
      vehicle NEC—*see* Accident, vehicle NEC

Obstruction
  air passages, larynx, respiratory passages
    by
      external means NEC—*see* Suffocation
      food, any type (regurgitated) (vomited)
        E911
      material or object, except food E912
      mucus E912
      phlegm E912
      vomitus E911
  digestive tract, except mouth or pharynx
    by
      food, any type E915
      foreign body (any) E915
  esophagus
    food E911
    foreign body, except food E912
    without asphyxia or obstruction of
      respiratory passage E915
  mouth or pharynx
    by
      food, any type E911
      material or object, except food E912
  respiration—*see* Obstruction, air passages
Oil in eye E914
Overdose
  anesthetic (drug)—*see* Table of drugs and
    chemicals
  drug—*see* Table of drugs and chemicals
Overexertion (lifting) (pulling) (pushing) E927
Overexposure (accidental) (to)
  cold (*see also* Cold, exposure to) E901.9
    due to manmade conditions E901.1
  heat (*see also* Heat) E900.9
  radiation—*see* Radiation
  radioactivity—*see* Radiation
  sun, except sunburn E900.0
  weather—*see* Exposure
  wind—*see* Exposure
Overheated (*see also* Heat) E900.9
Overlaid E913.0
Overturning (accidental)
  animal-drawn vehicle E827
  boat, ship, watercraft
    causing
      drowning, submersion E830
      injury except drowning, submersion E831
  machinery—*see* Accident, machine
  motor vehicle (*see also* Loss of control, motor
    vehicle) E816
    with antecedent collision on public
      highway—*see* Collision, motor vehicle
    not on public highway, nontraffic accident
      E825
      with antecedent collision—*see* Collision,
        motor vehicle, not on public highway
  nonmotor road vehicle NEC E829
  off-road type motor vehicle—*see* Loss of
    control, off-road type motor vehicle
  pedal cycle E826
  railway rolling stock, train, vehicle (*see also*
    Derailment, railway) E802
  street car E829
  vehicle NEC—*see* Accident, vehicle NEC

P

Radiation—*continued*
  isotopes, radioactive—*see* Radiation,
    radioactive isotopes
  laser(s) E926.4
    in
      terrorism E979.8
      war operations E997.0
      misadventure in medical care—*see*
        Misadventure, failure, in dosage,
        radiation
  late effect of NEC E929.8
    excessive heat from—*see* Heat
  light sources (visible) (ultraviolet) E926.2
  misadventure in medical or surgical
      procedure—*see* Misadventure, failure, in
      dosage, radiation
  overdose (in medical or surgical procedure)
    E873.2
  radar E926.0
  radioactive isotopes E926.5
    atomic power plant malfunction E926.5
      in water transport E838
    misadventure in medical or surgical
        treatment—*see* Misadventure, failure, in
        dosage, radiation
  radiobiologicals—*see* Radiation, radioactive
    isotopes
    radiofrequency E926.0
  radiopharmaceuticals—*see* Radiation,
    radioactive isotopes
  radium NEC E926.9
  sun E926.2
    excessive heat from E900.0
  tanning bed E926.2
  welding arc or torch E926.2
    excessive heat from E900.1
  x-rays (hard) (soft) E926.3
    misadventure in medical or surgical
        treatment—*see* Misadventure, failure, in
        dosage, radiation
Rape E960.1
Reaction —abnormal to or following(medical or
    surgical procedure) E879.9
  amputation (of limbs) E878.5
  anastomosis (arteriovenous) (blood vessel)
      (gastrojejunal) (skin) (tendon) (natural,
      artificial material, tissue) E878.2
    external stoma, creation of E878.3
  aspiration (of fluid) E879.4
    tissue E879.8
  biopsy E879.8
  blood
    sampling E879.7
    transfusion
      procedure E879.8
  bypass—*see* Reaction, abnormal, anastomosis
  catheterization
    cardiac E879.0
    urinary E879.6
  colostomy E878.3
  cystostomy E878.3
  dialysis (kidney) E879.1
  drugs or biologicals—*see* Table of drugs and
    chemicals
  duodenostomy E878.3
  electroshock therapy E879.3
  formation of external stoma E878.3
  gastrostomy E878.3
  graft—*see* Reaction, abnormal, anastomosis
  hypothermia E879.8

Reaction—*continued*
  implant, implantation (of)
    artificial
      internal device (cardiac pacemaker)
        (electrodes in brain) (heart valve
        prosthesis) (orthopedic) E878.1
      material or tissue (for anastomosis or
        bypass) E878.2
      with creation of external stoma E878.3
    natural tissues (for anastomosis or bypass)
      E878.2
      as transplantion—*see* Reaction, abnormal,
        transplant
      with creation of external stoma E878.3
  infusion
    procedure E879.8
  injection
    procedure E879.8
  insertion of gastric or duodenal sound E879.5
  insulin-shock therapy E879.3
  lumbar puncture E879.4
  perfusion E879.1
  procedures other than surgical operation (*see*
    also Reaction, abnormal, by specific type
    of procedure) E879.9
    specified procedure NEC E879.8
  radiological procedure or therapy E879.2
  removal of organ (partial) (total) NEC E878.6
    with
      anastomosis, bypass or graft E878.2
      formation of external stoma E878.3
      implant of artificial internal device E878.1
      transplant(ation)
        partial organ E878.4
        whole organ E878.0
  sampling
    blood E879.7
    fluid NEC E879.4
    tissue E879.8
  shock therapy E879.3
  surgical operation (*see also* Reaction,
    abnormal, by specified type of operation)
    E878.9
    restorative NEC E878.4
      with
        anastomosis, bypass or graft E878.2
        formation of external stoma E878.3
        implant(ation)—*see* Reaction, abnormal,
          implant
        transplant(ation)—*see* Reaction,
          abnormal, transplant
    specified operation NEC E878.8
  thoracentesis E879.4
  transfusion
    procedure E879.8
  transplant, transplantation (heart) (kidney)
    (liver) E878.0
    partial organ E878.4
  ureterostomy E878.3
  vaccination E879.8
Reduction in
  atmospheric pressure—*see also* Effects of, air
    pressure
    while surfacing from
      deep water diving causing caisson or
        divers' disease, palsy or paralysis
        E902.2
      underground E902.8
Residual (effect)—*see* Late effect

Submersion—*continued*
    due to accident to boat, ship, watercraft
      E830
  landslide E909.2
    overturning boat, ship, watercraft E909.2
    sinking boat, ship, watercraft E909.2
    submersion boat, ship, watercraft E909.2
    tidal wave E909.4
      caused by storm E908.0
    torrential rain E908.2
  late effect of NEC E929.8
  quenching tank E910.8
  self-inflicted (unspecified whether accidental
    or intentional) E984
  in accidental circumstances—*see* category
    E910
  stated as intentional, purposeful E954
stated as undetermined whether accidental or
  intentional E984
suicidal (attempted) E954
while
  attempting rescue of another person E910.3
  engaged in
    marine salvage E910.3
    underwater construction or repairs E910.3
  fishing, not from boat E910.2
  hunting, not from boat E910.2
  ice skating E910.2
  pearl diving E910.3
  placing fishing nets E910.3
  playing in water E910.2
  scuba diving E910.1
    nonrecreational E910.3
  skin diving E910.1
  snorkel diving E910.2
  spear fishing underwater E910.1
  surfboarding E910.2
  swimming (swimming pool) E910.2
  wading (in water) E910.2
  water skiing E910.0

Sucked
into
  jet (aircraft) E844

Suffocation (accidental) (by external means) (by
  pressure) (mechanical) E913.9
  caused by other person
    in accidental circumstances—*see* category
      E913
    stated as
      intentional, homicidal E963
      undetermined whether accidental or
        intentional E983.9
        by, in
          hanging E983.0
          plastic bag E983.1
          specified means NEC E983.3
  due to, by
    avalanche E909.2
    bedclothes E913.0
    bib E913.0
    blanket E913.0
    cave-in E913.3
      caused by cataclysmic earth surface
        movement or eruption E909.9
    conflagration—*see* Conflagration
    explosion—*see* Explosion
    falling earth, other substance E913.3
    fire—*see* Fire
    food, any type (ingestion) (inhalation)
      (regurgitated) (vomited) E911

Suffocation—*continued*
  foreign body, except food (ingestion)
    (inhalation) E912
  ignition—*see* Ignition
  landslide E909.2
  machine(ry)—*see* Accident, machine
  material, object except food entering by nose
    or mouth, ingested, inhaled E912
  mucus (aspiration) (inhalation), not of
    newborn E912
  phlegm (aspiration) (inhalation) E912
  pillow E913.0
  plastic bag—*see* Suffocation, in, plastic bag
  sheet (plastic) E913.0
  specified means NEC E913.8
  vomitus (aspiration) (inhalation) E911
homicidal (attempt) E963
in
  airtight enclosed place E913.2
  baby carriage E913.0
  bed E913.0
  closed place E913.2
  cot, cradle E913.0
  perambulator E913.0
  plastic bag (in accidental circumstances)
    E913.1
    homicidal, purposely inflicted by other
      person E963
    self-inflicted (unspecified whether
      accidental or intentional) E983.1
      in accidental circumstances E913.1
      intentional, suicidal E953.1
    stated as undetermined whether
      accidentally or purposely inflicted
      E983.1
    suicidal, purposely self-inflicted E953.1
  refrigerator E913.2
self-inflicted—*see also* Suffocation, stated as
  undetermined whether accidental or
  intentional E953.9
  in accidental circumstances—*see* category
    E913
  stated as intentional, purposeful—*see*
    Suicide, suffocation
stated as undetermined whether accidental or
  intentional E983.9
  by, in
    hanging E983.0
    plastic bag E983.1
    specified means NEC E983.8
suicidal—*see* Suicide, suffocation
Suicide, suicidal (attempted) (by) E958.9
  burning, burns E958.1
  caustic substance E958.7
    poisoning E950.7
    swallowed E950.7
  cold, extreme E958.3
  cut (any part of body) E956
  cutting or piercing instrument (classifiable to
    E920) E956
  drowning E954
  electrocution E958.4
  explosive(s) (classifiable to E923) E955.5
  fire E958.1
  firearm (classifiable to E922)—*see* Shooting,
    suicidal
  hanging E953.0
  jumping
    before moving object, train, vehicle E958.0
    from high place—*see* Jumping, from, high
      place, stated as, suicidal

War operations—*continued*
  antipersonnel E991.3
  bullet(s) (from carbine, machine gun, pistol, rifle, shotgun) E991.2
    rubber E991.0
  burn from
    chemical E997.2
    fire, conflagration (caused by fire-producing device or conventional weapon) E990.9
      from nuclear explosion E996
      petrol bomb E990.0
    gas E997.2
  burning aircraft E994
  chemical E997.2
  chlorine E997.2
  conventional warfare, specified form NEC E995
  crushing by falling aircraft E994
  depth charge E992
  destruction of aircraft E994
  disability as sequela one year or more after injury E999.0
  drowning E995
  effect (direct) (secondary) nuclear weapon E996
  explosion (artillery shell) (breech block) (cannon shell) E993
    after cessation of hostilities of bomb, mine placed in war E998
    aircraft E994
    bomb (mortar) E993
      atom E996
      hydrogen E996
      injury by fragments from E991.9
        antipersonnel E991.3
      nuclear E996
    depth charge E992
    injury by fragments from E991.9
      antipersonnel E991.3
    marine weapon E992
    mine
      at sea or in harbor E992
      land E993
        injury by fragments from E991.9
      marine E992
    munitions (accidental) (being used in war) (dump) (factory) E993
    nuclear (weapon) E996
    own weapons (accidental) E993
      injury by fragments from E991.9
        antipersonnel E991.3
    sea-based artillery shell E992
    torpedo E992
  exposure to ionizing radiation from nuclear explosion E996
  falling aircraft E994
  fire or fire-producing device E990.9
    petrol bomb E990.0
  fireball effects from nuclear explosion E996
  fragments from
    antipersonnel bomb E991.3
    artillery shell, bomb NEC, grenade, guided missile, land mine, rocket, shell, shrapnel E991.9
  fumes E997.2
  gas E997.2
  grenade (explosion) E993
    fragments, injury by E991.9
  guided missile (explosion) E993
    fragments, injury by E991.9
    nuclear E996

War operations—*continued*
  heat from nuclear explosion E996
  injury due to, but occurring after cessation of hostilities E998
  lacrimator (gas) (chemical) E997.2
  land mine (explosion) E993
    after cessation of hostilities E998
    fragments, injury by E991.9
  laser(s) E997.0
  late effect of E999.0
  lewisite E997.2
  lung irritant (chemical) (fumes) (gas) E997.2
  marine mine E992
  mine
    after cessation of hostilities E998
    at sea E992
    in harbor E992
    land (explosion) E993
      fragments, injury by E991.9
    marine E992
  missile (guided) (explosion) E993
    fragments, injury by E991.9
    marine E992
    nuclear E996
  mortar bomb (explosion) E993
    fragments, injury by E991.9
  mustard gas E997.2
  nerve gas E997.2
  phosgene E997.2
  poisoning (chemical) (fumes) (gas) E997.2
  radiation, ionizing from nuclear explosion E996
  rocket (explosion) E993
    fragments, injury by E991.9
  saber, sabre E995
  screening smoke E997.8
  shell (aircraft) (artillery) (cannon) (land based) (explosion) E993
    fragments, injury by E991.9
    sea-based E992
  shooting E991.2
    after cessation of hostilities E998
    bullet(s) E991.2
      rubber E991.0
    pellet(s) (rifle) E991.1
  shrapnel E991.9
  submersion E995
  torpedo E992
  unconventional warfare, except by nuclear weapon E997.9
    biological (warfare) E997.1
    gas, fumes, chemicals E997.2
    laser(s) E997.0
    specified type NEC E997.8
  underwater blast E992
  vesicant (chemical) (fumes) (gas) E997.2
  weapon burst E993

Washed
  away by flood—*see* Flood
  away by tidal wave—*see* Tidal wave
  off road by storm (transport vehicle) E908.9
  overboard E832

Weather exposure —*see also* Exposure
  cold E901.0
  hot E900.0

Weightlessness (causing injury) (effects of) (in spacecraft, real or simulated) E928.0

Wound (accidental) NEC (*see also* Injury) E928.9
  battle (*see also* War operation) E995
  bayonet E920.3
  in

Wound—*continued*
     legal intervention E974
     war operations E995
  gunshot—*see* Shooting
  incised—*see* Cut
  saber, sabre E920.3
   in war operations E995

RAILWAY ACCIDENTS (E800–E807)

The following fourth-digit subdivisions are for use with categories E800-E807 to identify the injured person.

.0 Railway employee

Any person who by virtue of his employment in connection with a railway, whether by the railway company or not, is at increased risk of involvement in a railway accident, such as:

catering staff on train	postal staff on train
driver	railway fireman
guard	shunter
porter	sleeping car attendant

.1 Passenger on railway

Any authorized person traveling on a train, except a railway employee

Excludes: intending passenger waiting at station (.8)
unauthorized rider on railway vehicle (.8)

.2 Pedestrian

See definition (r), Vol. 1, E code introduction

.3 Pedal cyclist

See definition (p), Vol. 1, E code introduction

.8 Other specified person

Intending passenger waiting at station

Unauthorized rider on railway vehicle

.9 Unspecified person

MOTOR VEHICLE TRAFFIC AND NONTRAFFIC ACCIDENTS
(E810–825)

The following fourth–digit subdivisions are for use with categories E810–E819 and E820–E825 to identify the injured person:

.0 Driver of motor vehicle other than motorcycle

See definition (l), Vol. 1, E code introduction

.1 Passenger in motor vehicle other than motorcycle

See definition (l), Vol. 1, E code introduction

.2 Motorcyclist

See definition (l), Vol. 1, E code introduction

.3 Passenger on motorcycle

See definition (l), Vol. 1, E code introduction

.4 Occupant of streetcar

.5 Rider of animal; occupant of animal–drawn vehicle

.6 Pedal cyclist

See definition (p), Vol. 1, E code introduction

.7 Pedestrian

See definition (r), Vol. 1, E code introduction

.8 Other specified person

Occupant of vehicle other than above

Person in railway train involved in accident

Unauthorized rider of motor vehicle

.9 Unspecified person

OTHER ROAD VEHICLE ACCIDENTS (E826–E829)

(animal–drawn vehicle, streetcar, pedal cycle, and other nonmotor road vehicle accidents)

The following fourth–digit subdivisions are for use with categories E826–E829 to identify the injured person:

.0 Pedestrian

    See definition (r), Vol. 1, E code introduction

.1 Pedal cyclist (does not apply to codes E827, E828, E829)

    See definition (p), Vol. 1, E code introduction

.2 Rider of animal (does not apply to code E829)

.3 Occupant of animal–drawn vehicle (does not apply to codes E828, E829)

.4 Occupant of streetcar

.8 Other specified person

.9 Unspecified person

WATER TRANSPORT ACCIDENTS (E830–E838)

The following fourth–digit subdivisions are for use with categories E830–E838 to identify the injured person:

.0 Occupant of small boat, unpowered

.1 Occupant of small boat, powered

See definition (t), Vol. 1, E code introduction

Excludes: water skier (.4)

.2 Occupant of other watercraft — crew

Persons:

engaged in operation of watercraft

providing passenger services [cabin attendants, ship's physician, catering personnel]

working on ship during voyage in other capacity [musician in band, operators of shops and beauty parlors]

.3 Occupant of other watercraft — other than crew

Passenger

Occupant of lifeboat, other than crew, after abandoning ship

.4 Water skier

.5 Swimmer

.6 Dockers, stevedores

Longshoreman employed on the dock in loading and unloading ships

.8 Other specified person

Immigration and custom officials on board ship

Person:
accompanying passenger or member of crew
visiting boat

Pilot (guiding ship into port)

.9 Unspecified person

AIR AND SPACE TRANSPORT ACCIDENTS (E840–E845)

The following fourth–digit subdivisions are for use with categories E840–E845 to identify the injured person:

.0 Occupant of spacecraft

.1 Occupant of military aircraft, any

Crew in military aircraft [air force] [army] [national guard] [navy]

Passenger (civilian) (military) in military aircraft [air force] [army] [national guard] [navy]

Troops in military aircraft [air force] [army] [national guard] [navy]

Excludes: occupants of aircraft operated under jurisdiction of police departments (.5)
parachutist (.7).

.2 Crew of commercial aircraft (powered) in surface to surface transport

.3 Other occupant of commercial aircraft (powered) in surface to surface transport

Flight personnel:
not part of crew
on familiarization flight

Passenger on aircraft (powered) NOS

.4 Occupant of commercial aircraft (powered) in surface to air transport

Occupant [crew] [passenger] of aircraft (powered) engaged in activities, such as:
aerial spraying (crops) (fire retardants)
air drops of emergency supplies
air drops of parachutists, except from military craft
crop dusting
lowering of construction material [bridge or telephone pole]
sky writing

.5 Occupant of other powered aircraft

Occupant [crew] [passenger] of aircraft (powered) engaged in activities, such as:
aerobatic flying
aircraft racing
rescue operation
storm surveillance
traffic surveillance

Occupant of private plane NOS

.6 Occupant of unpowered aircraft, except parachutist

Occupant of aircraft classifiable to E842

.7 Parachutist (military) (other)

Person making voluntary descent

Excludes: person making descent after accident to aircraft (.1–.6)

.8 Ground crew, airline employee

Persons employed at airfields (civil) (military) or launching pads, not occupants of aircraft

.9 Other person

052.2   **Postvaricella myelitis**
New code

053.14   **Herpes zoster myelitis**
New code

054.74   **Herpes simplex myelitis**
New code

136.3   **Pneumocystosis**
Add inclusion term

151   **Malignant neoplasm of stomach**
Add exclusion term

152   **Malignant neoplasm of small intestine, including duodenum**
Add exclusion term

171   **Malignant neoplasm of connective and other soft tissue**
Add inclusion term, revise exclusion term

174   **Malignant neoplasm of female breast**
Add "Use additional code" note

175   **Malignant neoplasm of male breast**
Add "Use additional code" note

202.0   **Nodular lymphoma**
Delete description term

211   **Benign neoplasm of other parts of digestive system**
Add exclusion term

215.5   **Abdomen**
Add inclusion term

233.1   **Cervix uteri**
Add inclusion term, revise exclusion term

235   **Neoplasm of uncertain behavior of digestive and respiratory systems**
Add exclusion term

238.1   **Connective and other soft tissue**
Add inclusion term

238.7   **Other lymphatic and hematopoietic tissues**
Delete description terms, revise exclusion terms

238.71   **Essential thrombocythemia**
New code

238.72   **Low grade myelodysplastic syndrome lesions**
New code

238.73   **High grade myelodysplastic syndrome lesions**
New code

238.74   **Myelodysplastic syndrome with 5q deletion**
New code

238.75   **Myelodysplastic syndrome, unspecified**
New code

238.76   **Myelofibrosis with myeloid metaplasia**
New code

238.79   **Other lymphatic and hematopoietic tissues**
New code

255.10   **Hyperaldosteronism, unspecified**
Revise code

277.3   **Amyloidosis**
Delete description terms

277.30   **Amyloidosis, unspecified**
New code

277.31   **Familial Mediterranean fever**
New code

277.39   **Other amyloidosis**
New code

278.0   **Overweight and obesity**
Revise "Use additional code" note

281.3   **Other specified megaloblastic anemias not elsewhere classified**
Delete exclusion term

284   **Aplastic anemia and other bone marrow failure syndromes**
Revise category

284.0   **Constitutional aplastic anemia**
Delete description terms

284.01   **Constitutional red blood cell aplasia**
New code

284.09   **Other constitutional aplastic anemia**
New code

284.1   **Pancytopenia**
New code

284.2   **Myelophthisis**
New code

284.8   **Other specified aplastic anemias**
Delete inclusion term

284.9   **Aplastic anemia, unspecified**
Revise exclusion term

285.0   **Sideroblastic anemia**
Revise exclusion term

285.2   **Anemia of chronic disease**
Revise code, add description term

285.29   **Anemia of other chronic disease**
Revise code, add description term

285.8   **Other specified anemias**
Delete inclusion term

287   **Purpura and other hemorrhagic conditions**
Revise exclusion term

288.0   **Neutropenia**
Revise subcategory

288.00   **Neutropenia, unspecified**
New code

288.01   **Congenital neutropenia**
New code

288.02   **Cyclic neutropenia**
New code

288.03   **Drug induced neutropenia**
New code

288.04   **Neutropenia due to infection**
New code

288.09   **Other neutropenia**
New code

288.4   **Hemophagocytic syndromes**
New code

288.5   **Decreased white blood cell count**
New subcategory

288.50   **Leukocytopenia, unspecified**
New code

288.51   **Lymphocytopenia**
New code

288.59   **Other decreased white blood cell count**
New code

288.6   **Elevated white blood cell count**
New subcategory

288.60   **Leukocytosis, unspecified**
New code

288.61   **Lymphocytosis (symptomatic)**
New code

288.62   **Leukemoid reaction**
New code

288.63   **Monocytosis (symptomatic)**
New code

288.64   **Plasmacytosis**
New code

288.65   **Basophilia**
New code

288.69   **Other elevated white blood cell count**
New code

288.8   **Other specified disease of white blood cells**
Delete description terms, add exclusion term

289.4   **Hypersplenism**
Revise exclusion term

289.53   **Neutropenic splenomegaly**
New code

289.83   **Myelofibrosis**
New code

289.89   **Other specified diseases of blood and blood-forming organs**
Delete description term

305.1   **Tobacco use disorder**
Add exclusion term

307.89   **Other**
Revise "Code first" note

309.81   **Posttraumatic stress disorder**
Add description term

323   **Encephalitis, myelitis, and encephalomyelitis**
Revise inclusion term, add exclusion terms

323.0   **Encephalitis, myelitis, and encephalomyelitis in viral diseases classified elsewhere**
Revise code, delete exclusion terms

323.01   **Encephalitis and encephalomyelitis in viral diseases classified elsewhere**
New code

323.02   **Myelitis in viral diseases classified elsewhere**
New code

323.1   **Encephalitis, myelitis, and encephalomyelitis in rickettsial diseases classified elsewhere**
Revise code

323.2   **Encephalitis, myelitis, and encephalomyelitis in protozoal diseases classified elsewhere**
Revise code

323.4   **Other encephalitis, myelitis, and encephalomyelitis due to infection classified elsewhere**
Revise code, delete exclusion terms

323.41   **Other encephalitis and encephalomyelitis due to infection classified elsewhere**
New code

323.42   **Other myelitis due to infection classified elsewhere**
New code

323.5   **Encephalitis, myelitis, and encephalomyelitis following immunization procedures**
Revise code, delete description terms

323.51   **Encephalitis and encephalomyelitis following immunization procedures**
New code

323.52   **Myelitis following immunization procedures**
New code

323.6   **Postinfectious encephalitis, myelitis, and encephalomyelitis**
Revise code

323.61   **Infectious acute disseminated encephalomyelitis (ADEM)**
New code

323.62   **Other postinfectious encephalitis and encephalomyelitis**
New code

323.63   **Postinfectious myelitis**
New code

323.7   **Toxic encephalitis, myelitis, and encephalomyelitis**
Revise code, new subcategory

323.71   **Toxic encephalitis and encephalomyelitis**
New code

323.72   **Toxic myelitis**
New code

323.8   **Other causes of encephalitis, myelitis, and encephalomyelitis**
Revise code, new subcategory

323.81   **Other causes of encephalitis and encephalomyelitis**
New code

323.82   **Other causes of myelitis**
New code

323.9   **Unspecified cause of encephalitis, myelitis, and encephalomyelitis**
Revise code

326   **Late effects of intracranial abscess or pyogenic infection**
Revise Note

327.5   **Organic sleep related movement disorders**
Revise exclusion term

331.83   **Mild cognitive impairment, so stated**
New code

333.6   **Genetic torsion dystonia**
Revise code

333.7   **Acquired torsion dystonia**
Revise code, new subcategory

333.71   **Athetoid cerebral palsy**
New code

333.72   **Acute dystonia due to drugs**
New code

333.79   **Other acquired torsion dystonia**
New code

333.81	**Blepharospasm** Add exclusion term
333.82	**Orofacial dyskinesia** Delete description term, add exclusion term
333.85	**Subacute dyskinesia due to drugs** New code
333.92	**Neuroleptic malignant syndrome** Add exclusion term
333.94	**Restless legs syndrome (RLS)** New code
333.99	**Other** Delete description term
336.9	**Unspecified disease of spinal cord** Revise exclusion term
337.1	**Peripheral autonomic neuropathy in disorders classified elsewhere** Revise "Code first" note
338	**Pain, not elsewhere classified** New category
338.0	**Central pain syndrome** New code
338.1	**Acute pain** New subcategory
338.11	**Acute pain due to trauma** New code
338.12	**Acute post-thoracotomy pain** New code
338.18	**Other acute postoperative pain** New code
338.19	**Other acute pain** New code
338.2	**Chronic pain** New subcategory
338.21	**Chronic pain due to trauma** New code
338.22	**Chronic post-thoracotomy pain** New code
338.28	**Other chronic postoperative pain** New code
338.29	**Other chronic pain** New code
338.3	**Neoplasm related pain (acute) (chronic)** New code
338.4	**Chronic pain syndrome** New code
341.2	**Acute (transverse) myelitis** New subcategory
341.20	**Acute (transverse) myelitis NOS** New code
341.21	**Acute (transverse) myelitis in conditions classified elsewhere** New code
341.22	**Idiopathic transverse myelitis** New code
343	**Infantile cerebral palsy** Add exclusion terms
345	**Epilepsy and recurrent seizures** Revise category
345.1	**Generalized convulsive epilepsy** Revise exclusion terms
345.4	**Localization-related (focal) (partial) epilepsy and epileptic syndromes with complex partial seizures** Revise code
345.5	**Localization-related (focal) (partial) epilepsy and epileptic syndromes with simple partial seizures** Revise code
345.8	**Other forms of epilepsy and recurrent seizures** Revise code
345.9	**Epilepsy, unspecified** Add inclusion terms and exclusion terms
348.31	**Metabolic encephalopathy** Add exclusion term
349.82	**Toxic encephalopathy** Add description term
357.4	**Polyneuropathy in other diseases classified elsewhere** Revise "Code first" note
359.6	**Symptomatic inflammatory myopathy in diseases classified elsewhere** Revise "Code first" note
360.0	**Purulent endophthalmitis** Add exclusion term
360.1	**Other endophthalmitis** Add exclusion term
377.43	**Optic nerve hypoplasia** New code
379.6	**Inflammation (infection) of postprocedural bleb** New subcategory
379.60	**Inflammation (infection) of postprocedural bleb, unspecified** New code
379.61	**Inflammation (infection) of postprocedural bleb, stage 1** New code
379.62	**Inflammation (infection) of postprocedural bleb, stage 2** New code
379.63	**Inflammation (infection) of postprocedural bleb, stage 3** New code
389.11	**Sensory hearing loss, bilateral** Revise code
389.12	**Neural hearing loss, bilateral** Revise code
389.14	**Central hearing loss, bilateral** Revise code
389.15	**Sensorineural hearing loss, unilateral** New code
389.16	**Sensorineural hearing loss, asymmetrical** New code
389.18	**Sensorineural hearing loss of combined types, bilateral** Revise code
403	**Hypertensive chronic kidney disease** Revise code, revise fifth-digit classification
404	**Hypertensive heart and chronic kidney disease** Revise code, revise fifth-digit classification

420.0 Acute pericarditis in diseases classified elsewhere
Revise "Code first" note

425.7 Nutritional and metabolic cardiomyopathy
Revise "Code first" note

429.83 Takotsubo syndrome
New code

440.24 Atherosclerosis of the extremities with gangrene
Add "Use additional code" note

445.81 Kidney
Revise "Use additional code" note

478.1 Other diseases of nasal cavity and sinuses
Delete description

478.11 Nasal mucositis (ulcerative)
New code

478.19 Other diseases of nasal cavity and sinuses
New code

496 Chronic airway obstruction, not elsewhere classified
Add exclusion term

514 Pulmonary congestion and hypostasis
Add exclusion term

517.8 Lung involvement in other diseases classified elsewhere
Revise "Code first" note

518.7 Transfusion related acute lung injury (TRALI)
New code

519.1 Other diseases of trachea and bronchus, not elsewhere classified
Delete description terms

519.11 Acute bronchospasm
New code

520.6 Disturbances in tooth eruption
Add inclusion term

521.06 Dental caries pit and fissure
Add inclusion term

521.07 Dental caries of smooth surface
Add inclusion term

521.08 Dental caries of root surface
Add inclusion term

521.8 Other specified diseases of hard tissues of teeth
Delete description terms

521.81 Cracked tooth
New code

521.89 Other specified diseases of hard tissues of teeth
New code

523.00 Acute gingivitis, plaque induced
New code

523.01 Acute gingivitis, non-plaque induced
New code

523.1 Chronic gingivitis
Delete description term

523.10 Chronic gingivitis, plaque induced
New code

523.11 Chronic gingivitis, non-plaque induced
New code

523.3 Aggressive and acute periodontitis
Revise code

523.30 Aggressive periodontitis, unspecified
New code

523.31 Aggressive periodontitis, localized
New code

523.32 Aggressive periodontitis, generalized
New code

523.33 Acute periodontitis
New code

523.4 Chronic periodontitis
Delete description term

523.40 Chronic periodontitis, unspecified
New code

523.41 Chronic periodontitis, localized
New code

523.42 Chronic periodontitis, generalized
New code

524.07 Excessive tuberosity of jaw
Add description term

524.2 Anomalies of dental arch relationship
Add description term

524.21 Malocclusion, Angle's class I
Revise code

524.22 Malocclusion, Angle's class II
Revise code

524.23 Malocclusion, Angle's class III
Revise code

524.24 Open anterior occlusal relationship
Add description term

524.25 Open posterior occlusal relationship
Add description term

524.26 Excessive horizontal overlap
Add description term

524.27 Reverse articulation
Add description term

524.29 Other anomalies of dental arch relationship
Add description term

524.33 Horizontal displacement of teeth
Add description term

524.34 Vertical displacement of teeth
Add description terms

524.35 Rotation of tooth/teeth
Revise code

524.36 Insufficient interocclusal distance of teeth (ridge)
Add description term

524.37 Excessive interocclusal distance of teeth
Add description term

524.54 Insufficient anterior guidance
Add description term

524.55 Centric occlusion maximum intercuspation discrepancy
Add description term

524.56 Non-working side interference
Add description term

525.6 Unsatisfactory restoration of tooth
New subcategory

525.60 Unspecified unsatisfactory restoration of tooth
New code

525.61 Open restoration margins
New code

525.62 **Unrepairable overhanging of dental restorative materials**
New code

525.63 **Fractured dental restorative material without loss of material**
New code

525.64 **Fractured dental restorative material with loss of material**
New code

525.65 **Contour of existing restoration of tooth biologically incompatible with oral health**
New code

525.66 **Allergy to existing dental restorative material**
New code

525.67 **Poor aesthetics of existing restoration**
New code

525.69 **Other unsatisfactory restoration of existing tooth**
New code

526.6 **Periradicular pathology associated with previous endodontic treatment**
New subcategory

526.61 **Perforation of root canal space**
New code

526.62 **Endodontic overfill**
New code

526.63 **Endodontic underfill**
New code

526.69 **Other periradicular pathology associated with previous endodontic treatment**
New code

528.0 **Stomatitis and mucositis (ulcerative)**
Revise code, add exclusion terms

528.00 **Stomatitis and mucositis, unspecified**
New code

528.01 **Mucositis (ulcerative) due to antineoplastic therapy**
New code

528.02 **Mucositis (ulcerative) due to other drugs**
New code

528.09 **Other stomatitis and mucositis (ulcerative)**
New code

528.3 **Cellulitis and abscess**
Revise exclusion term

528.71 **Minimal keratinized residual ridge mucosa**
Add description term

528.72 **Excessive keratinized residual ridge mucosa**
Add description term

528.79 **Other disturbances of oral epithelium, including tongue**
Add description term

536.8 **Dyspepsia and other specified disorders of function of stomach**
Add description term

538 **Gastrointestinal mucositis (ulcerative)**
New code

567 **Peritonitis and retroperitoneal infections**
Revise exclusion terms

567.23 **Spontaneous bacterial peritonitis**
Add exclusion term

573 **Other disorders of liver**
Revise exclusion term

581.81 **Nephrotic syndrome in diseases classified elsewhere**
Revise "Code first" note

582.81 **Chronic glomerulonephritis in diseases classified elsewhere**
Revise "Code first" note

583.81 **Nephritis and nephropathy, not specified as acute or chronic, in diseases classified elsewhere**
Revise "Code first" note

585 **Chronic kidney disease (CKD)**
Delete exclusion, add "Code first" note

585.5 **Chronic kidney disease, stage V**
Add exclusion

585.6 **End stage renal disease**
Add description term

599.6 **Urinary obstruction**
Delete exclusion term

599.69 **Urinary obstruction, not elsewhere classified**
Add coding instruction

600 **Hyperplasia of prostate**
Add inclusion term, delete "Use additional code" note

600.00 **Hypertrophy (benign) of prostate without urinary obstruction and other lower urinary tract symptoms (LUTS)**
Revise code

600.01 **Hypertrophy (benign) of prostate with urinary obstruction and other lower urinary tract symptoms (LUTS)**
Revise code, add "Use additional code" note

600.20 **Benign localized hyperplasia of prostate without urinary obstruction and other lower urinary tract symptoms (LUTS)**
Revise code

600.21 **Benign localized hyperplasia of prostate with urinary obstruction and other lower urinary tract symptoms (LUTS)**
Revise code, add "Use additional code" note

600.90 **Hyperplasia of prostate, unspecified, without urinary obstruction and other lower urinary symptoms (LUTS)**
Revise code

600.91 **Hyperplasia of prostate, unspecified, with urinary obstruction and other lower urinary symptoms (LUTS)**
Revise code, add "Use additional code" note

608.2 **Torsion of testis**
Delete description

608.20 **Torsion of testis, unspecified**
New code

608.21 **Extravaginal torsion of spermatic cord**
New code

608.22 **Intravaginal torsion of spermatic cord**
New code

608.23 **Torsion of appendix testis**
New code

608.24   **Torsion of appendix epididymis**
New code

616.8   **Other specified inflammatory diseases of cervix, vagina, and vulva**
Delete description terms

616.81   **Mucositis (ulcerative) of cervix, vagina, and vulva**
New code

616.89   **Other inflammatory disease of cervix, vagina and vulva**
New code

618.84   **Cervical stump prolapse**
New code

629.2   **Female genital mutilation status**
Add description term

629.20   **Female genital mutilation status, unspecified**
Add description term

629.21   **Female genital mutilation Type I status**
Add description term

629.22   **Female genital mutilation Type II status**
Add description term

629.23   **Female genital mutilation Type III status**
Add description term

629.29   **Other female genital mutilation status**
New code

629.81   **Habitual aborter without current pregnancy**
New code

629.89   **Other specified disorders of female genital organs**
New code

629.9   **Unspecified disorder of female genital organs**
Delete description term

641.3   **Antepartum hemorrhage associated with coagulation defects**
Add exclusion term

642.2   **Other pre-existing hypertension complicating pregnancy, childbirth, and the puerperium**
Revise description terms

646.8   **Other specified complications of pregnancy**
Delete description term

648.4   **Mental disorders**
Revise description

649   **Other conditions or status of the mother complicating pregnancy, childbirth, or the puerperium**
New category

649.0   **Tobacco use disorder complicating pregnancy, childbirth, or the puerperium**
New subcategory

649.1   **Obesity complicating pregnancy, childbirth, or the puerperium**
New subcategory

649.2   **Bariatric surgery status complicating pregnancy, childbirth, or the puerperium**
New subcategory

649.3   **Coagulation defects complicating pregnancy, childbirth, or the puerperium**
New subcategory

649.4   **Epilepsy complicating pregnancy, childbirth, or the puerperium**
New subcategory

649.5   **Spotting complicating pregnancy**
New subcategory

649.6   **Uterine size date discrepancy**
New subcategory

666.1   **Other immediate postpartum hemorrhage**
Revise description term, add exclusion term

692.3   **Due to drugs and medicines in contact with skin**
Revise exclusion term

693   **Dermatitis due to substances taken internally**
Revise exclusion term

713.7   **Other general diseases with articular involvement**
Revise "Code first" note

729.7   **Nontraumatic compartment syndrome**
New subcategory

729.71   **Nontraumatic compartment syndrome of upper extremity**
New code

729.72   **Nontraumatic compartment syndrome of lower extremity**
New code

729.73   **Nontraumatic compartment syndrome of abdomen**
New code

729.79   **Nontraumatic compartment syndrome of other sites**
New code

730.0   **Acute osteomyelitis**
Add "Use additional code" note

730.1   **Chronic osteomyelitis**
Add "Use additional code" note

730.2   **Unspecified osteomyelitis**
Add "Use additional code" note

731.3   **Major osseous defects**
New code

733.0   **Osteoporosis**
Add "Use additional code" note

733.4   **Aseptic necrosis of bone**
Add "Use additional code" note

743.8   **Other specified anomalies of eye**
Add exclusion term

768   **Intrauterine hypoxia and birth asphyxia**
Add exclusion terms

768.3   **Fetal distress first noted during labor and delivery, in liveborn infant**
Revise code

768.5   **Severe birth asphyxia**
Add exclusion term

768.6   **Mild or moderate birth asphyxia**
Add exclusion term

768.7   **Hypoxic-ischemic encephalopathy (HIE)**
New code

768.9	**Unspecified birth asphyxia in liveborn infant** Delete description term
770.8	**Other respiratory problems after birth** Add exclusion term
770.87	**Respiratory arrest of newborn** New code
770.88	**Hypoxemia of newborn** New code
775.8	**Other neonatal endocrine and metabolic disturbances** Revise code
775.81	**Other acidosis of newborn** New code
775.89	**Other neonatal endocrine and metabolic disturbances** New code
776.7	**Transient neonatal neutropenia** Revise exclusion term
779.2	**Cerebral depression, coma, and other abnormal cerebral signs** Add description term, exclusion terms
779.85	**Cardiac arrest of newborn** New code
780.31	**Febrile convulsions (simple), unspecified** Revise code
780.32	**Complex febrile convulsions** New code
780.39	**Other convulsions** Add description term
780.58	**Sleep related movement disorder, unspecified** Revise exclusion term
780.6	**Fever** Add "Code first" note
780.95	**Excessive crying of child, adolescent, or adult** Revise code
780.96	**Generalized pain** New code
780.97	**Altered mental status** New code
780.99	**Other general symptoms** Delete description term
781.2	**Abnormality of gait** Revise exclusion term
783.2	**Abnormal loss of weight and underweight** Revise "Use additional code" note
784.3	**Aphasia** Add exclusion term
784.9	**Other symptoms involving head and neck** Delete description
784.91	**Postnasal drip** New code
784.99	**Other symptoms involving head and neck** New code
785.52	**Septic shock** Delete "Code first" term
788	**Symptoms involving urinary system** Add exclusion term

788.2	**Retention of urine** Delete exclusion term, add coding note
788.3	**Urinary incontinence** Add coding note
788.4	**Frequency of urination and polyuria** Add coding note
788.6	**Other abnormality of urination** Add coding note
788.64	**Urinary hesitancy** New code
788.65	**Straining on urination** New code
790	**Nonspecific findings on examination of blood** Revise exclusion term
790.29	**Other abnormal glucose** Add description term
790.6	**Other abnormal blood chemistry** Add description term, exclusion term
793.81	**Mammographic microcalcification** Add exclusion terms
793.89	**Other abnormal findings on radiological examination of breast** Add description terms
793.9	**Other** Delete description
793.91	**Image test inconclusive due to excess body fat** New code
793.99	**Other nonspecific abnormal findings on radiological and other examinations of body structure** New code
795.04	**Papanicolaou smear of cervix with high grade squamous intraepithelial lesion (HGSIL)** Delete description term
795.06	**Papanicolaou smear of cervix with cytologic evidence of malignancy** New code
795.7	**Other nonspecific immunological findings** Add exclusion terms
795.8	**Abnormal tumor markers** New subcategory
795.81	**Elevated carcinoembryonic antigen [CEA]** New code
795.82	**Elevated cancer antigen 125 [CA 125]** New code
795.89	**Other abnormal tumor markers** New code
799.4	**Cachexia** Add "Code first" note, delete exclusion term
873.63	**Tooth (broken) (fractured) (due to trauma)** Revise code
873.73	**Tooth (broken) (fractured) (due to trauma)** Revise code
958.9	**Traumatic compartment syndrome** New subcategory
958.90	**Compartment syndrome, unspecified** New code

958.91 Traumatic compartment syndrome of upper extremity
New code

958.92 Traumatic compartment syndrome of lower extremity
New code

958.93 Traumatic compartment syndrome of abdomen
New code

958.99 Traumatic compartment syndrome of other sites
New code

995.2 Other and unspecified adverse effect of drug, medicinal and biological substance
Revise code

995.20 Unspecified adverse effect of unspecified drug, medicinal and biological substance
New code

995.21 Arthus phenomenon
New code

995.22 Unspecified adverse effect of anesthesia
New code

995.23 Unspecified adverse effect of insulin
New code

995.27 Other drug allergy
New code

995.29 Unspecified adverse effect of other drug, medicinal and biological substance
New code

995.3 Allergy, unspecified
Revise exclusion term

995.4 Shock due to anesthesia
Revise exclusion term

995.9 Systemic inflammatory response syndrome (SIRS)
Delete "Code first" note

995.91 Sepsis
Revise code

995.92 Severe sepsis
Revise code

995.93 Systemic inflammatory response syndrome due to noninfectious process without acute organ dysfunction
Revise code

995.94 Systemic inflammatory response syndrome due to noninfectious process with acute organ dysfunction
Revise code

996.45 Peri-prosthetic osteolysis
Add "Use additional code" note

996.7 Other complications of internal (biological) (synthetic) prosthetic device, implant and graft
Add "Use additional code" note

997.3 Respiratory complications
Add exclusion term

998.5 Postoperative infection
Add exclusion term

999 Complications of medical care, not elsewhere classified
Revise exclusion term

999.8 Other transfusion reaction
Add exclusion term

V07.39 Other prophylactic chemotherapy
Revise exclusion term

V18.51 Colonic polyps
New code

V18.59 Other digestive disorders
New code

V20.2 Routine infant or child health check
Add description term

V26.21 Fertility testing
Revise exclusion term

V26.3 Genetic counseling and testing
Add exclusion term

V26.31 Testing of female for genetic disease carrier status
Revise code

V26.32 Other genetic testing of female
Revise code

V26.34 Testing of male for genetic disease carrier status
New code

V26.35 Encounter for testing of male partner of habitual aborter
New code

V26.39 Other genetic testing of male
New code

V28 Encounter for antenatal screening of mother
Revise category

V45.3 Intestinal bypass or anastomosis status
Add exclusion terms

V45.77 Genital organs
Revise exclusion term

V45.86 Bariatric surgery status
New code

V54.1 Aftercare for healing traumatic fracture
Add exclusion term

V58.3 Attention to dressings and sutures
Revise code

V58.30 Encounter for change or removal of nonsurgical wound dressing
New code

V58.31 Encounter for change or removal of surgical wound dressing
New code

V58.32 Encounter for removal of sutures
New code

V58.41 Encounter for planned postoperative wound closure
Add exclusion term

V58.49 Other specified aftercare following surgery
Add description term

V65.3 Dietary surveillance and counseling
Add "Use additional code" note

V65.4 Other counseling, not elsewhere classified
Revise exclusion term

V72.11 Encounter for hearing examination following failed hearing screening
New code

V72.19 Other examination of ears and hearing
New code

V82.7   **Genetic screening**
New subcategory

V82.71   **Screening for genetic disease carrier status**
New code

V82.79   **Other genetic screening**
New code

V85   **Body Mass Index [BMI]**
Revise category

V85.5   **Body Mass Index, pediatric**
New subcategory

V85.51   **Body Mass Index, pediatric, less than 5th percentile for age**
New code

V85.52   **Body Mass Index, pediatric, 5th percentile to less than 85th percentile for age**
New code

V85.53   **Body Mass Index, pediatric, 85th percentile to less than 95th percentile for age**
New code

V85.54   **Body Mass Index, pediatric, greater than or equal to 95th percentile for age**
New code

V86   **Estrogen receptor status**
New category

V86.0   **Estrogen receptor positive status [ER+]**
New code

V86.1   **Estrogen receptor negative status [ER-]**
New code